Textbook of
Pulmonary & Critical Care Medicine

Textbook of Pulmonary & Critical Care Medicine

Volume 2

3rd Edition

Editor-in-Chief

Surinder K Jindal MD FAMS FNCCP FICS FCCP
Emeritus Professor and Ex-Head
Department of Pulmonary Medicine
Postgraduate Institute of Medical Education and Research
Chandigarh, India
(Medical Director, Jindal Clinics, Chandigarh, India)

Editors

Suhail Raoof MD Master FCCP MACP FCCM ATSF CPE
Director
Lung Institute, Northwell Health
Chief, Pulmonary, Critical Care and Sleep Medicine
Lenox Hill Hospital
New York, NY, USA

Ashutosh Nath Aggarwal MD DM FCCP
Professor and Head
Department of Pulmonary Medicine
Postgraduate Institute of Medical Education
and Research
Chandigarh, India

Ritesh Agarwal MD DM
Professor
Department of Pulmonary Medicine
Postgraduate Institute of Medical Education and Research
Chandigarh, India

Associate Editors

Aditya Jindal
Anup Singh

Forewords

JS Guleria
Atul C Mehta

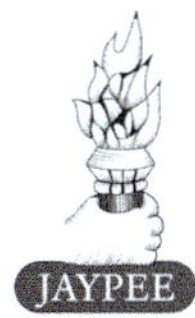

JAYPEE BROTHERS MEDICAL PUBLISHERS
The Health Sciences Publisher
New Delhi | London

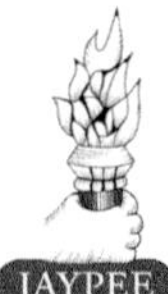

Jaypee Brothers Medical Publishers (P) Ltd

Headquarters
EMCA House, 23/23-B Ansari Road,
Daryaganj New Delhi 110 002, India
Landline: +91-11-23272143,
+91-11-23272703
+91-11-23282021, +91-11-23245672
e-mail: jaypee@jaypeebrothers.com

Corporate Office
4838/24, Ansari Road,
Daryaganj New Delhi 110 002, India
Phone: +91-11-43574357
Fax: +91-11-43574314
e-mail: jaypee@jaypeebrothers.com

Overseas Office
JP Medical Ltd.
83, Victoria Street, London
SW1H 0HW (UK)
Phone: +44-20 3170 8910
e-mail: info@jpmedpub.com

EU GPSR Authorised Representative
Logos Europe, 9 rue Nicolas Poussin
17000, La Rochelle, France
Phone: +33 (0) 6 67 93 73 78
e-mail: contact@logoseurope.eu

Website: www.jaypeebrothers.com
Website: www.jaypeedigital.com

Inquiries for bulk sales may be solicited at: jaypee@jaypeebrothers.com

Textbook of Pulmonary & Critical Care Medicine (Volume 2) / Surinder K Jindal

First Edition: 2011

Second Edition: 2017

Third Edition: 2025

Reprint: 2026

ISBN: 978-93-5696-621-5

Printed in India

Contents

Volume 1

SECTION 1: HISTORY AND DEVELOPMENT

SECTION 2: RESPIRATORY PHYSIOLOGY

SECTION 4: RESPIRATORY DIAGNOSIS

Part A: Clinical Approach

Part C: Lung Function Tests

Part D: Thoracic Endoscopy

SECTION 5: TUBERCULOSIS

SECTION 6: NONTUBERCULAR RESPIRATORY INFECTION

SECTION 7: BRONCHIAL ASTHMA

Volume 2

SECTION 8: OBSTRUCTIVE PULMONARY DISEASES

SECTION 9: ENVIRONMENTAL AND OCCUPATIONAL DISORDERS

SECTION 11: DISORDERS OF PULMONARY CIRCULATION

SECTION 13: MEDIASTINUM, CHEST WALL AND DIAPHRAGM DISORDERS

SECTION 14: SYSTEMATIC DISEASES AND PREGNANCY

SECTION 15: RESPIRATORY SLEEP DISORDERS

SECTION 16: LUNG NEOPLASMS

SECTION 17: RESPIRATORY CRITICAL CARE

SECTION 18: SURGICAL ASPECTS

SECTION 19: PERSPECTIVES OF RESPIRATORY CARE

SECTION 20: APPENDICES

SECTION

8

Obstructive Pulmonary Diseases

SECTION OUTLINE

Chronic Obstructive Pulmonary Disease: Epidemiology, Burden, and Risk Factors

CHAPTER 83

Surinder K Jindal

INTRODUCTION

From the healthcare point of view, the twenty-first century is the era of noncommunicable diseases (NCDs) besides the brief period of the pandemic of coronavirus disease 19 (COVID-19), a communicable disease. Chronic obstructive pulmonary disease (COPD) is one of the most common NCDs which constitutes a huge healthcare burden all over the world. Chronic respiratory disease, along with cardiovascular disease, diabetes, and cancers, was identified by the United Nations (UN) General Assembly as one of the four most important chronic and "lifestyle-related" diseases needing global attention.[1] It had been only the second time in the history of UN General Assembly when an international health issue was discussed and the UN called upon all its member countries to take suitable action for control of all these NCDs. Most commonly attributed to tobacco smoking, COPD was earlier considered as a disease of the Western countries. But the disease is also being recognized in increasing numbers among nonsmoker populations living in the low- and middle-income countries (LMICs) who are exposed to other harmful environmental, inhalational exposures.[2,3] The disease is largely preventable if the exposures could be avoided.

Historically, COPD has been differently described as chronic bronchitis (CB) and its subtypes, emphysema, chronic airflow limitation, obstructive bronchitis, and so on. There was always a significant overlap of clinical, pathophysiological, and diagnostic features making it difficult to distinguish one from the other. Over the decades, the term COPD has been used as all inclusive with different clinical pheno- and endotypes. The Global Initiative for Chronic Obstructive Lung Disease (GOLD) in its most recent version (GOLD 2023) defines COPD as a "heterogeneous lung condition characterized by chronic respiratory symptoms (dyspnea, cough, expectoration, and/or exacerbations) due to abnormalities of the airways (bronchitis, bronchiolitis) and/or alveoli (emphysema) that cause persistent, often progressive, airflow obstruction".[4]

As implied in the name, COPD is primarily a disease of the lungs characterized by airflow limitation. But a large number of extrapulmonary manifestations and other comorbidities are increasingly recognized as being associated with COPD. Exaggerated atherosclerosis of coronary vessels is frequently responsible for ischemic heart disease. Similarly, the involvement of cerebral vessels may cause stroke and other neurological deficits. Nutritional impairment, muscular dystrophy, and osteoporosis are partly responsible for weight loss which is a very common feature. Several neuropsychiatric disturbances such as severe anxiety and mental depression are commonly seen. Abnormalities in fluids and electrolyte balance are frequent and serious consequences of COPD which add to the disease morbidity and mortality. COPD is therefore aptly described as a systemic inflammatory disorder.

EPIDEMIOLOGY

There has been an epidemic proportion of increase in the prevalence of COPD. The increase is even more sinister than that of an infectious disease since COPD is a chronic and progressive condition which keeps on adding to the burden measured in terms of disease morbidity and mortality, reduced work productivity, and economic losses. A number of global studies including a few from India have examined the epidemiology and burden of COPD. There are wide variations in prevalence and burden indices reported in different studies. Some of these variations are attributable to factors such as the differences in the types and enormity of risk factors. The criteria used for definition and diagnosis of disease, methods of collecting data, and analysis of results are also important factors which account for variations.

Global Epidemiology and Burden

- *Prevalence*: Epidemiological data for a chronic disease like COPD are difficult and expensive to collect. Even in the developed countries, accurate epidemiologic data may not be available. COPD is a widely prevalent disease among adults all over the world. It accounts for prevalence of over 300 million cases worldwide ranging between 15 and 20% of the adult population in Europe aged over 40 years and over 6% in the United States.

The 12-site Burden of Obstructive Lung Disease (BOLD) study, based on questionnaires and spirometry, report the average prevalence of COPD as 10.1%, with wide regional variations.[5] In USA, COPD affected over 15 million adults in 2018. Similarly, in 2020–2022, about 1.17 million people in England were diagnosed with COPD, around 1.9% of the total population. The prevalence is likely to be even higher in the LMICs.

- *Burden estimates*: Disease burden implies the impact of the disease as measured by fiscal cost, mortality, morbidity, and other indicators of loss of work. It is often expressed in terms of terms of disability-adjusted life-years (DALYs) or quality-adjusted life-years. Both direct healthcare costs and loss of work result in a huge financial burden on the patients' families as well as the healthcare system.

As per the World Health Organization (WHO) fact sheet, COPD is the third most common cause of death worldwide, responsible for 3.23 million deaths in 2019 **(Table 1)**;[6] about 90% of COPD deaths in those under 70 years of age occur in LMICs.[5]

Most of the information available on COPD prevalence, morbidity, and mortality comes from high-income countries. It is known that almost 90% of COPD deaths occur in LMICs. In USA, COPD constituted the fourth leading cause of death. The Global Burden of Disease Study (GBDS) 2019 project retrieved data on the prevalence, deaths, and DALYs of COPD and its attributable risk factors for 204 countries and territories, between 1990 and 2019.[7] The counts and rates per 100,000 population, along with 95% uncertainty intervals, were presented for each estimate. The study reported 212.3 million prevalent cases of COPD globally, with COPD accounting for 3.3 million deaths and 74.4 million DALYs. In 2019, Denmark, Myanmar, and Belgium had the highest age-standardized point prevalence of COPD, while Egypt and Georgia showed the largest increases in age-standardized point prevalence across the study period.

There were differences in the mortality and DALY rates in different regions. The GBDS 2019 study revealed that the age-standardized death rates per 100,000 were the highest in Nepal (182.5) and lowest in Japan (7.4) in 2019.[7] COPD is also the seventh leading cause of poor health measured by DALY.[5] In the GBDS 2019 study, the age-standardized DALY rates per 100,000 were highest for Nepal and lowest for Barbados. The results clearly implied that COPD is a major public health problem, especially in countries with a low sociodemographic index.[7] The report also pointed that the global DALY rate in men increased up to age of 85–89 years and then decreased with advancing age, whereas for women the rate increased up to the oldest age group (≥95 years).

Factors contributing most to the DALY rates for COPD included smoking (46.0%), pollution from ambient particulate matter (20.7%), and occupational exposure to particulate matter, gases, and fumes (15.6%). Tobacco smoking accounts for over 70% of COPD cases in high-income countries. In LMICs, tobacco smoking accounts for 30–40% of COPD cases, and household air pollution (HAP) is a major risk factor.[5] The COPD burden is projected to increase in coming decades because of continued exposure to COPD risk factors and aging of the population.

Indian Epidemiology

- *Prevalence*: India, like many other LMICs, faces COPD in epidemic proportions because of the dual onslaught of risk factors of smoking and environmental pollution-related exposures. The earlier studies of 1970–1990s reported a median prevalence of 5% in male and 2.7% in female population.[8] The Indian study on Epidemiology of Asthma, Respiratory Symptoms and Chronic Bronchitis (INSEARCH) reported the prevalence of CB as 3.49% while one or the other respiratory symptom was reported in 8.5% of subjects.[9,10] Other studies from South India have reported varying prevalence of CB. An average estimated prevalence of CB between 6.5 and 7.7% was reported in one meta-analysis even though there was a great heterogeneity of different studies.[11]

In a recent meta-analysis of COPD prevalence studies from South Asian countries, 32 provided data from India; the prevalence of COPD was highest in north India (19.4%) and in men. The estimated pooled prevalence of CB was 5.0%.[12] In another meta-analysis of eight identified studies, the estimated prevalence was 7.4% and was higher among males, in the urban area, and in the northern region.[13] A similar prevalence of 7% among

TABLE 1: Global and Indian burden of COPD.

	Global	India
Cause of death	Third leading cause of death worldwide	Second most common cause of NCD-related deaths
Poor health—DALYs	Seventh leading cause of poor health worldwide	Second most leading cause of DALYs
Tobacco smoking versus nonsmoker COPD	Accounts for over 70% of COPD cases in high-income countries; LMIC tobacco smoking accounts for 30–40%	Household air pollution is a major risk factor in one-third to half of COPD

(COPD: chronic obstructive pulmonary disease; DALYs: disability-adjusted life-years)

population above 30 years was reported in another meta-analysis using six databases for studies on COPD in India between 2000 and 2020.[14]

There have been a few other small reports on COPD prevalence from different parts of India. Prevalence of 10% was reported using a pretested questionnaire and postbronchodilator spirometry in a community-based cross-sectional study in Delhi in a systematic random sample of 1,200 adults.[15] In another study from the semiurban area of Thiruvananthapuram, South India, the investigators mapped COPD cases using geographic information system (GIS) in a community-based, cross-sectional, descriptive study in 494 adults; a prevalence of 6.5% was reported which was considered comparable to national prevalence estimates.[16] The authors found GIS technology as useful to identify spatial clustering of COPD cases and its environmental risk factors.[16]

- *Burden indices*: India being a large country has great heterogeneity in the burden of COPD and asthma across different states and regions. There are also differences in epidemiological and healthcare burden across different regions. The prevalence of COPD and other major chronic respiratory diseases, deaths, and DALYs caused by them for every state of India was meticulously examined in the Global Burden of Diseases, Injuries, and Risk Factors Study (GBD) 2016 between1990 and 2016.[17] It was concluded that India had a high burden of chronic respiratory diseases such as COPD which accounted for a high rate of health loss from them, especially in the less-developed states with low epidemiological transition level (ETL)—defined as the ratio of DALYs from communicable diseases to those from NCDs and injuries combined, with a low ratio denoting high ETL and vice versa.[17]

Data from India on burden of COPD measured in terms of morbidity indices, mortality rates, and economic costs is rather sparse. COPD is reported as one of the important causes of burden from NCDs, which along with injuries, accounts for 52% of deaths in India.[18] Bronchitis and asthma were reported as the most common causes of death in both men and women in multiple surveys conducted by different agencies such as the Survey of Causes of Death, Annual Reports of Registrar General of India, Census of India I, and NFHSI I and II.[19,20]

Exacerbations of COPD multiply the disease burden by several folds in terms of both disease-related indices and economic costs. Healthcare utilization due to COPD exacerbations has been recently assessed in India with predication modeling; several discriminators have been reported to predict "prolonged hospital stay" and "prolonged intensive care".[21] A systematic review of humanistic and economic burden reported substantial economic burden and impairment of health-related quality of life (HRQoL) due to symptomatic COPD.[22] Reduced HRQoL in COPD patients in India has been also reported in an earlier study.[22]

It is also important to appreciate that the morbidity (as well as mortality) from COPD is not only due to respiratory disability from airflow limitation but also from several systemic diseases which are frequently associated with COPD due to shared risk factors and mechanisms of pathogenesis. Enhanced atherosclerosis in COPD is responsible for a higher incidence of cardio- and cerebro-vascular diseases. COPD exacerbations multiply the disease burden by several folds.

Economic burden: COPD has huge fiscal implications. Estimates of both direct costs on health expenditure and indirect economic losses are enormous. This is even more burdensome in India where most of the patients and their families have to bear out of the pocket costs in the absence of health insurance schemes, especially for outpatient, maintenance expenditures. There were significantly higher direct and indirect fiscal losses in families with one or more smokers than nonsmoker families.[23] In an earlier assessment in 2011, the direct costs on COPD were found as significantly burdensome and the estimated economic loss was about ₹350,000 million for that year.[24] It was also calculated that proper "program-based" or "guideline-based" management of COPD could significantly reduce these costs by approximately 70%.[25]

RISK FACTORS

A number of risk factors are globally recognized as important in causing COPD **(Box 1)**. Variations in the prevalence of risk factors account for the marked differences in disease prevalence in different reports. COPD is a chronic inflammatory disease of the airways secondary to long-term exposure to noxious particles and gases, particularly cigarette smoke. A recent umbrella review of risk factors suggested tobacco smoking, ambient air pollution, indoor combustion of biomass fuels, exposure to occupational dusts, low body mass index (BMI), childhood asthma, and diet as important risk factors.[26] Depending upon the presence of causative risk factors, COPD is sometimes classified into different types: (1) Genetically determined, (2) early-life event-related, (3) infection-related, (4) smoking/vaping-related, and (5) environmental exposure-related COPD.[27] Results of a systematic review and modeling study aimed to estimate global, regional, and national COPD prevalence and risk factors suggested that most COPD patients lived in LMICs, male sex, smoking, low BMI, biomass exposure, and occupational exposure to dust or smoke were important risk factors:[28]

- *Age and gender*: COPD prevalence increases with increasing age independent of smoking habit and/or other exposures.[28] The relationship is cumulative in nature; that is, the highest incidence is present in the oldest men. Globally, COPD is more commonly present in men. On the other hand, COPD in nonsmokers is more common in men in some studies while it is more

BOX 1 Some common risk factors responsible for COPD.

- *Age and gender*: Elderly and male sex*
- *Tobacco smoking*:
    - Cigarettes and pipes
    - Indian forms of smoking—*bidis, hookah, chillum*, and *chutta*
- *COPD in nonsmokers*:†
    - *Household air pollution*: Solid fuel (dried wood, animal dung, crop residue, or coal) combustion for cooking and heating
    - *Nonfuel-related indoor air pollutants*: Environmental tobacco smoke exposure, i.e., passive smoking; volatile gases, fumes, and dusts
    - *Ambient air pollution*: Vehicular and industrial exhausts—living around heavy traffic highways and in industrial areas
    - Exposures to occupational dusts and smokes created during manufacturing and finishing activities of industrial products
    - Chronic asthma—poorly controlled and severe disease
- Genetic predisposition†
- Alpha-1 antitrypsin deficiency†
- *Miscellaneous*:† Childhood respiratory infections and pulmonary tuberculosis; Childhood/early life events such as poor growth in utero, prematurity, low birth weight, low socioeconomic status, malnutrition

*Female gender is equally or more common in nonsmoker COPD.
†Compounding role in those who are smokers.

(COPD: chronic obstructive pulmonary disease)

so in women in others.[29] There are other studies which show almost equal prevalence in men and women reflecting a changing pattern of exposures to tobacco smoke, environmental tobacco smoke (ETS), indoor fuel combustion, and occupational dusts.[30] It has also been suggested that women who smoke are more susceptible to the effects of smoking than men.[31]

- *Tobacco smoking*: Smoking is the most important environmental risk factor for chronic respiratory symptoms and lung function abnormalities as has been consistently shown in numerous studies from all over the world including from India.[32-35] There is a greater annual rate of forced expiratory volume in 1 second (FEV_1) decline and a greater COPD mortality rate than nonsmokers. Smokers in various reports are found to have a three- to eight-times greater risk of developing COPD. Smoking during pregnancy is likely to adversely affect lung growth and development of fetus in utero and possibly prime the immune system for abnormal/enhanced responses in the future.[36]

    Smoking habits in India reflect large regional variations. Besides cigarettes, a large number of people use a nonconventional form of tobacco such as *hookah, chillum bidi,* and *chutta* **(Fig. 1)**. *(Hukkah and chillum consist of an earthen clay pot in which tobacco is burnt and smoked either directly, i.e., chillum, or indirectly through a pipe, i.e., hukkah; bidis contain crude, dried tobacco wrapped in a dried "tendu" leaf and smoked; chutta is like a bidi with the lighted end kept inside the mouth—reverse smoking, popular in the coastal regions of Andhra Pradesh and Orissa).*

    Bidis and other indigenous forms of tobacco smoking are shown to be at least as (or even more) harmful as cigarette smoking. Passive exposure to cigarette smoke (also known as environmental tobacco smoke or ETS) also contributes to the development of respiratory symptoms and COPD.[10]

- *COPD in nonsmokers*: It is now recognized that almost 60–70% of COPD cases belong to LMICs where nonsmoking risk factors are significantly more common. It is estimated that about 50% of global burden of COPD is therefore likely due to nonsmoking risk factors. Several harmful exposures are recognized as important risk factors for COPD in nonsmokers.
    - *Biomass fuel exhaust*: Biomass domestic fuels like crop residues, wood, and dried animal dung typically burnt in poorly functioning stoves in ill-ventilated kitchens are used for combustion for cooking and heating in over half the world households **(Figs. 2A and B)**. In majority of households, the effluent is released into the indoor living area; an indoor surrounding allows persistence of pollutants in the air and therefore exposure to those pollutants for longer periods.

        The nonspecific respiratory symptoms such as cough, phlegm, wheezing, and breathlessness are common in women using biomass fuels for cooking and heating at home. HAP exposure is shown as a cause of high prevalence of COPD, especially CB in women who do most of the cooking. Exposure to smoke exhaust from these solid fuels is the most important nonsmoking risk factor, especially in women in LMICs.[36-38] The risk of COPD in

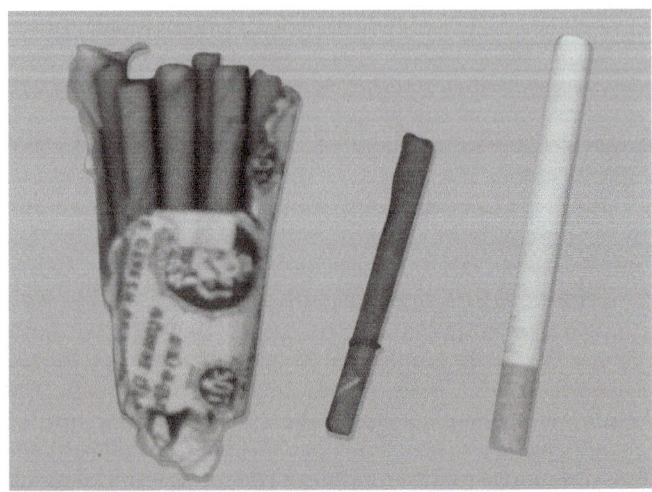

FIG. 1: Some common forms of tobacco smoked in India.

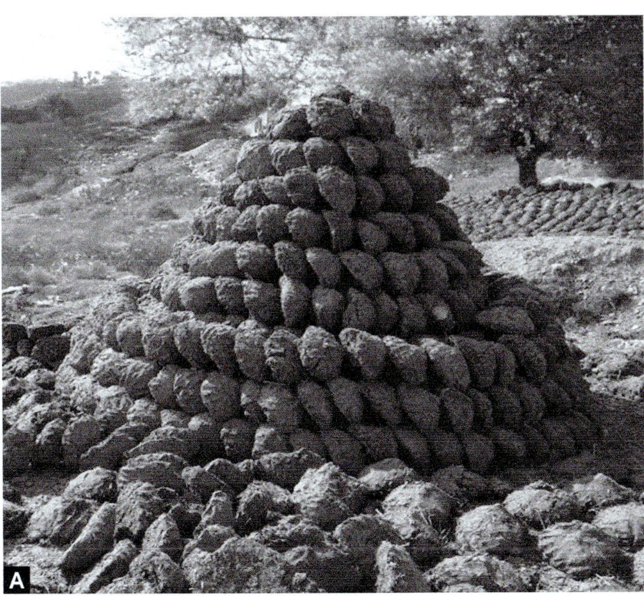

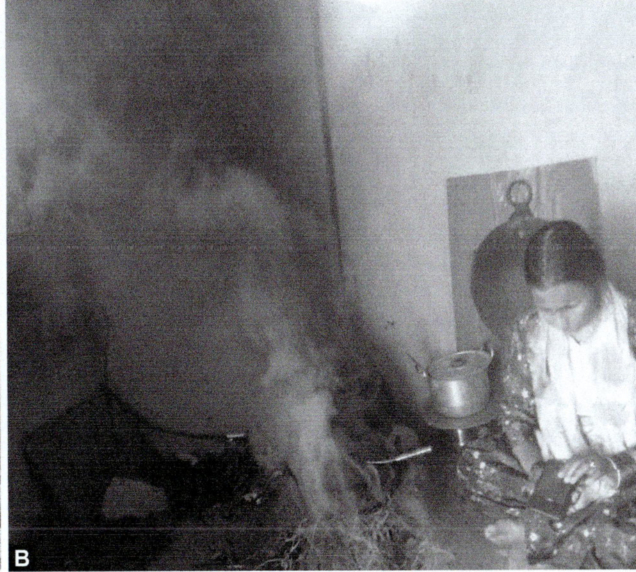

FIGS. 2A AND B: (A) Heaps of dried animal-dung cakes used for domestic combustion. (B) The house-lady exposed for long hours during periods of cooking and heating to the smoke from burning of solid fuels in the kitchen equipped with poorly designed and open three-brick stove is a common scene in the rural areas.

HAP-exposed population is about double the risk among non-HAP-exposed population **(Table 2)**.[10,39-46] COPD in nonsmoker, biomass-exposed population may in fact present with distinct phenotypic characteristics.[36]

- *Other indoor pollutants*: Indoor air pollution may also occur from other indoor pollutants such as dust, smoke, and volatile organic compounds. Exposure to ETS, i.e., side-stream smoke or passive smoking, is of particular interest as an important cause of chronic cardiorespiratory diseases including COPD and respiratory cancers in nonsmokers.[10,47] There are a few studies that show that other indoor air pollutants such as those produced during the burning of mosquito coils and incense sticks may also be associated with respiratory morbidity.[34,35] However, the evidence is limited at present.
- *Outdoor air pollution (OAP)*: Traffic and industrial exhausts and emissions constitute an important public health problem.[48,49] This is particularly important in location around heavy traffic areas such as along the highways. Ambient OAP is particularly significant in large and overcrowded metropolitan cities with high-rise buildings limiting atmospheric dispersion of pollutants. Smoke emitted through chimneys from factories and furnaces significantly contributes to OAP in industrial cities. Similarly, the smoke from open, field-burning of crop residue contributes to OAP in rural area.
- *Occupational exposures*: There is a higher risk of COPD and CB in workers occupationally exposed to gases, dusts, and fumes in different dusty occupations. Prolonged workplace exposures have been associated with COPD in several epidemiological studies, some showing exposure-response gradient relationship.[29] Burden of 14% of spirometry-defined COPD and 13% for CB was reported in occupationally exposed populations.[50] Similarly, a 6.3 times higher risk of COPD was described in a small hospital-based study in the Indian subcontinent from Bangladesh among the workers such as mechanics, cleaners, and others with self-reported exposure to vapors, gas, dust, fume, and smokes in their workplace than the nonexposed group.[51] The development of COPD is related to industrial activities such as smelting, machine maintenance, casting, and finishing
- *Chronic asthma*: Asthma is also described as a risk factor of nonsmoker COPD.[52] Airway remodeling due to chronic and persistent airway inflammation in chronic asthma is also recognized as an important cause of COPD.[53] Remodeling is characterized by thickening and fibrosis of airway walls causing irreversible airway obstruction similar to that seen in COPD. This is especially so in poorly treated patients, smoker asthmatics, or those who suffer from severe disease.
- *Miscellaneous risk factors*: Childhood respiratory tract infections and history of pulmonary tuberculosis (TB) are reported to be associated with COPD.[37,54,55] Pulmonary TB as a risk factor and/or complication of COPD is reported mostly from LMICs from TB-endemic areas and in younger adults.[56,57] It remains debatable whether TB is a true risk factor for diffuse COPD or merely a cause of impaired lung function

TABLE 2: Odds ratios of risk for COPD/chronic bronchitis in association with household pollution exposure in some of the recent studies.

Authors	Population	Odds ratio	95% Confidence intervals
Johnson et al.[39]	900 nonsmoker women	1.24	0.36–6.64
Jindal et al.[10]	169,575 adults	1.65 (coal, wood)	1.35–2.00
Sehgal et al.[40]	–	2.37	1.59–3.54
Choi et al.[41]	600 households, 547 adult women	1.54	1.00–2.37
Sana et al.[42]	5 case–control studies and 19 cross-sectional studies: • Spirometry-diagnosed COPD • Chronic bronchitis • Overall COPD	 1.20 2.11 1.38	 0.99–1.40 1.70–2.52 1.28–1.57
Chan et al.[43]	Cohort of 280,000 Chinese never-smokers • Major respiratory diseases • COPD	 1.36 1.10	 1.32–1.40 1.03–1.18
Long et al.[44]	Overall COPD: • FEV1/FVC < LLN	 1.69	 1.41–2.04
Shetty et al. [45]	Systemic review and meta-analysis: • COPD prevalence • COPD mortality	 2.08 2.13	 – –
Shi et al.[46]	12,925 adults, multimorbidity	1.81	1.67–1.98

(COPD: chronic obstructive pulmonary disease; FEV1: forced expiratory volume in 1 second; FVC: forced vital capacity; LLN: lower limit of normal)

due to postinfectious, localized parenchymal fibrosis.[58] Similarly, poor socioeconomic status, poverty, and overcrowded living conditions are described as other associations independent of known causes of COPD such as tobacco smoking. But the epidemiological evidence is not conclusive and the relationship may be partly attributable to exposure to higher concentrations of harmful exposures, higher prevalence of smoking, and malnutrition among the disadvantaged populations.

Factors which adversely influence the lung development during gestation and childhood, collectively listed as "childhood disadvantage factors", may contribute to the development of COPD later in life.[59] Low birth weight, childhood infections, ETS exposure during childhood, and malnutrition are identified as some of these factors. Genetic inheritance and alpha-1 antitrypsin deficiency are important factors but account for a small number of patients. Identification of different genetic variants likely to be associated with susceptibility to COPD is accomplished with a combined approach employing genome-wide association studies and candidate gene analysis.[60]

SUMMARY

Chronic obstructive pulmonary disease is a common and progressive disease of the lungs responsible for a huge global burden in terms of both morbidity and mortality. It is a major cause of burden on healthcare infrastructure and healthcare costs. The burden keeps on adding every year with mounting disability and numbers of new patients added to the existing load. Tobacco smoking of all kinds is the most common risk factor but nonsmoking risk factors such as household and ambient air pollution and occupational exposures are almost equally common in LMICs. Genetic factors may play a significant role in susceptible populations exposed to risk factors. Early life, childhood nutrition, and infections are also important.

REFERENCES

1. United Nations General Assembly A/66/83, 2011 (Item 119 of the Preliminary list, A/66/50). Prevention and control of non-communicable diseases-Report of the Secretary General.
2. Gnatiuc L, Caramori G. COPD in nonsmokers: the biomass hypothesis—to be or not to be? Eur Respir J. 2014;44:8-10.
3. Gordon SB, Bruce NG, Grigg J, et al. Respiratory risks from household air pollution in low and middle income countries. Lancet Respir Med. 2014;2:823-60.
4. Agustí A, Celli BR, Criner GJ, et al. Chronic Obstructive Pulmonary Disease. Global Initiative for Chronic Obstructive Lung Disease

2023 Report: GOLD Executive Summary. Eur Respir J. 2023;61(4): 2300239.

5. Buist AS, McBurnie MA, Vollmer WM, et al. BOLD Collaborative Research Group. International variation in the prevalence of COPD (the BOLD Study): a population-based prevalence study. Lancet. 2007;370(9589):741-50.
6. World Health Organization. Chronic Obstructive Pulmonary Disease. [online] Available from https://www.who.int/news-room/fact-sheets/detail/chronic-obstructive-pulmonary-disease-(copd). [Last accessed June, 2024].
7. Safiri S, Carson-Chahhoud K, Noori M, et al. Burden of chronic obstructive pulmonary disease and its attributable risk factors in 204 countries and territories, 1990-2019: results from the Global Burden of Disease Study 2019. BMJ. 2022;378:e069679.
8. Jindal SK, Aggarwal AN, Gupta D. A review of population studies from India to estimate national burden of chronic obstructive pulmonary disease and its association with smoking. Indian J Chest Dis Allied Sci. 2001;43(3):139-47.
9. Jindal SK, Aggarwal AN, Chaudhry K, et al.; Asthma Epidemiology Study Group. A multicentric study on epidemiology of chronic obstructive pulmonary disease and its relationship with tobacco smoking and environmental tobacco smoke exposure. Indian J Chest Dis Allied Sci. 2006;48(1):23-9.
10. Jindal SK, Aggarwal AN, Gupta D, et al. Indian study on epidemiology of asthma, respiratory symptoms and chronic bronchitis in adults (INSEARCH). Int J Tuberc Lung Dis. 2012;16:1270-7.
11. McKay AJ, Mahesh PA, Fordham JZ, et al. Prevalence of COPD in India: a systematic review. Prim Care Respir J. 2012;21(3):313-21.
12. Jarhyan P, Hutchinson A, Khaw D, et al. Prevalence of chronic obstructive pulmonary disease and chronic bronchitis in eight countries: a systematic review and meta-analysis. Bull World Health Organ. 2022;100(3):216-30.
13. Daniel RA, Aggarwal P, Kalaivani M, et al. Prevalence of chronic obstructive pulmonary disease in India: A systematic review and meta-analysis. Lung India. 2021;38(6):506-13.
14. Verma A, Gudi N, Yadav UN, et al. Prevalence of COPD among population above 30 years in India: A systematic review and meta-analysis. J Glob Health. 2021;11:04038.
15. India State-Level Disease Burden Initiative CRD Collaborators. The burden of chronic respiratory diseases and their heterogeneity across the states of India: the Global Burden of Disease Study 1990–2016. Lancet Glob Health. 2018;6(12):e1363-74.
16. Sinha B, Singla VR, Chowdhury R. An epidemiological profile of chronic obstructive pulmonary disease: A community-based study in Delhi. J Postgrad Med. 2017;63(1):29-35.
17. Surendran S, Mohan A, Joseph M, et al. Spatial analysis of chronic obstructive pulmonary disease and its risk factors in an urban area of Trivandrum, Kerala, India. Lung India. 2022;39(2): 110-5.
18. Narain JP, Garg R, Fric A. Non-communicable diseases in the South-East Asia region: burden, strategies and opportunities. Natl Med J India. 2011;24(5):280-7.
19. Jindal SK. COPD: The unrecognized epidemic in India. JAPI (Suppl). 2012;60:14-6.
20. Ramankumar AV, Aparjita C. Respiratory disease burden in rural India: a review from multiple data sources. Int J Epidemiol. 2005;2:2.
21. Ramaraju K, Kaza AM, Balasubramanian N, et al. Predicting Healthcare Utilization by Patients Admitted for COPD Exacerbation. J Clin Diagn Res. 2016;10(2):OC13-7.
22. Srivastava K, Thakur D, Sharma S, et al. Systematic review of humanistic and economic burden of symptomatic chronic obstructive pulmonary disease. Pharmacoeconomics. 2015;33(5):467-88.
23. Jindal SK, Sapru RP, Aggarwal AN, et al. Excess morbidity and expenditure on healthcare in families with smokers: A community study. National Med J India. 2005;18:123-6.
24. Indian Council of Medical Research Task Force Study (1993-98). Project Report, Estimation of costs of management of smoking related chronic obstructive pulmonary disease and coronary heart disease.
25. Murthy KJ, Sastry JG. Economic burden of chronic obstructive pulmonary disease. In: Rao KS (Ed). Burden of Disease in India. New Delhi: National Commission on Macroeconomics and Health; 2005.
26. Holtjer JCS, Bloemsma LD, Beijers RJHCG, et al. Identifying risk factors for COPD and adult-onset asthma: an umbrella review. Eur Respir Rev. 2023;32(168):230009.
27. Stolz D, Mkorombindo T, Schumann DM, et al. Towards the elimination of chronic obstructive pulmonary disease: a Lancet Commission. Lancet. 2022;400(10356):921-72.
28. Adeloye D, Song P, Zhu Y, et al. Global, regional, and national prevalence of, and risk factors for, chronic obstructive pulmonary disease (COPD) in 2019: a systematic review and modelling analysis. Lancet Respir Med. 2022;10(5):447-58.
29. Bang KM. Chronic obstructive pulmonary disease in non smokers by occupation and exposure: a brief review. Curr Opin Pulm Med. 2015;21:149-54.
30. Foreman MG, Zhang L, Murphy J, et al. Early-onset chronic obstructive pulmonary disease is associated with female sex, maternal factors, and African American race in the COPD Gene Study. Am J Respir Crit Care Med. 2011;184:414-20.
31. Lopez Varela MV, Montes de Oca M, et al. Sex-related differences in COPD in five Latin American cities: the PLATINO study. Eur Respir J. 2010;36:1034-41.
32. Wheaton AG, Liu Y, Croft JB, et al. Chronic Obstructive Pulmonary Disease and Smoking Status - United States, 2017. MMWR Morb Mortal Wkly Rep. 2019;68(24):533-8.
33. Perez-Padilla R, Menezes AMB. Chronic Obstructive Pulmonary Disease in Latin America. Ann Glob Health. 2019;85(1):7.
34. Jha P, Ramasundarahettige C, Landsman V, et al. 21st-century hazards of smoking and benefits of cessation in the United States. N Engl J Med. 2013;368(4):341-50.
35. Postma DS, Bush A, van den Berge M. Risk factors and early origins of chronic obstructive pulmonary disease. Lancet. 2015;385(9971):899-909.
36. Jindal SK, Jindal A. COPD in biomass exposed non smokers: a different phenotype. Exp Rev Respir Med. 2021;15(1):51-8.
37. Salvi SS, Barnes PJ. Chronic obstructive pulmonary disease in non-smokers. Lancet. 2009;374(9691):733-43.
38. Mortimer K, Gordon SB, Jindal SK, et al. Household air pollution is a major avoidable risk-factor for cardiopulmonary disease. Chest. 2012;142:1308-15.
39. Johnson P, Balakrishnan K, Ramaswamy P, et al. Prevalence of chronic obstructive pulmonary disease in rural women of Tamil Nadu: implications for refining disease burden assessments attributable to household biomass combustion. Glob Health Action. 2011;4:10.3402.
40. Sehgal M, Rizwan SA, Krishnan A. Disease burden due to biomass cooking-fuel-related household air pollution among women in India. Glob Health Action. 2014;7:25326.

41. Choi JY, Baumgartner J, Harnden S, et al. Increased risk of respiratory illness associated with kerosene fuel use among women and children in urban Bangalore, India. Occup Environ Med. 2015;72:114-22.
42. Sana A, Somda SMA, Meda N, et al. Chronic obstructive pulmonary disease associated with biomass fuel use in women: a systematic review and meta-analysis. BMJ Open Respir Res. 2018;5(1):e000246.
43. Chan KH, Kurmi OP, Bennett DA, et al. Solid Fuel Use and Risks of Respiratory Diseases. A Cohort Study of 280,000 Chinese Never-Smokers. Am J Respir Crit Care Med. 2019;199(3):352-61.
44. Long HY, Xing ZZ, Chai D, et al. Solid Fuel Exposure and Chronic Obstructive Pulmonary Disease in Never-Smokers. Front Med (Lausanne). 2021;8:757333.
45. Shetty BSP, D'Souza GA, Anand MP. Effect of Indoor Air Pollution on Chronic Obstructive Pulmonary Disease (COPD) Deaths in Southern Asia—A Systematic Review and Meta-analysis. Toxics. 2021;9(4):85.
46. Shi W, Zhang T, Li Y, et al. Association between household air pollution from solid fuel use and risk of chronic diseases and their multimorbidity among Chinese adults. Environ Int. 2022;170:107635.
47. Parasuramalu BG, Huliraj N, Prashanth Kumar SP, et al. Prevalence of chronic obstructive pulmonary disease and its association with tobacco smoking and environmental tobacco smoke exposure among rural population. Indian J Public Health. 2014;58(1):45-9.
48. Cai Y, Schikowski T, Adam M, et al. Cross-sectional associations between air pollution and chronic bronchitis: an ESCAPE meta-analysis across five cohorts. Thorax. 2014;69:1005-14.
49. Kumar R, Sharma M, Srivastava A, et al. Association of outdoor air pollution with chronic respiratory morbidity in an industrial town in Northern India. Archives Environ Health. 2004;59:471-7.
50. Blanc PD, Annesi-Maesano I, Balmes JR, et al. The Occupational Burden of Nonmalignant Respiratory Diseases: An Official American Thoracic Society and European Respiratory Society Statement. Am J Respir Crit Care Med. 2019;199:1312-34.
51. Sumit AF, Das A, Miraj IS, et al. Association between chronic obstructive pulmonary disease (COPD) and occupational exposures: A hospital based quantitative cross-sectional study among the Bangladeshi population. PLoS One. 2020;15(9): e0239602.
52. Leung C, Sin DD. Asthma-COPD Overlap: What are the Important Questions? Chest. 2022;161(2):330-44.
53. Jindal SK. Remodelling in asthma and COPD: recent concepts. Lung India. 2016;33:1-2.
54. Yang W, Li F, Li C, et al. Focus on Early COPD: Definition and Early Lung Development. Int J Chron Obstruct Pulmon Dis. 2021;16:3217-28.
55. Allwood BW, Byrne A, Meghji J, et al. Post-Tuberculosis Lung Disease: Clinical Review of an Under-Recognised Global Challenge. Respiration. 2021;100(8):751-63.
56. Ravimohan S, Kornfeld H, Weissman D, et al. Tuberculosis and lung damage: from epidemiology to pathophysiology. Eur Respir Rev. 2018;27:170077.
57. Byrne AL, Marais BJ, Mitnick CD, et al. Tuberculosis and chronic respiratory disease: a systematic review. Int J Infect Dis. 2015;32:138-46.
58. Jindal SK. Is pulmonary tuberculosis a true risk-factor for chronic obstructive pulmonary disease? Indian J Tuberc. 2022;69(2): 131-3.
59. Svanes C, Sunyer J, Plana E. Early life origins of chronic obstructive pulmonary disease. Thorax. 2010;65:14-20.
60. Marciniak SJ, Lomas DA. Genetic susceptibility. Clin Chest Med. 2014;35:29-38.

An Appraisal of Chronic Obstructive Pulmonary Disease in Low- and Middle-income Countries

CHAPTER 84

Mohammad Azizur Rahman, Pajanivel Ranganadin, Varuna Jethani

INTRODUCTION

Chronic obstructive pulmonary disease (COPD) is a disease state characterized by the presence of airflow obstruction which is generally progressive but may be partially reversible. Most patients with COPD have features of both emphysema and chronic bronchitis. Chronic bronchitis is a clinical diagnosis defined by excessive secretion of bronchial mucus (bronchorrhea) and is manifested by daily productive cough for 3 months or more in at least 2 consecutive years. On the other hand, emphysema is a pathologic diagnosis that denotes abnormal permanent enlargement of air spaces distal to the terminal bronchiole with destruction of their walls and without obvious fibrosis. Smoker's cough (pre-COPD) is defined as persistent cough in smokers as a result of the irritation and damage of the lining of lungs from smoking of cigarettes or *bidis*. In practice, smokers' cough represents a spectrum of lung disease from mild irritation to advanced COPD. Smoker's cough can be seen as the first step toward the development of COPD.

EPIDEMIOLOGY

Chronic obstructive pulmonary disease is a leading cause of morbidity and mortality worldwide with an economic and social burden that is both substantial and increasing. According to World Health Statistics, an estimated 200 million people have COPD, of which about 3.2 million die each year, making it the third leading cause of death by 2030 of which almost 90% of COPD deaths occur in low- and middle-income countries (LMICs). In South Asia, COPD was ranked fifth in causing both mortality and loss of DALYs in 2010. The estimated burden of COPD in India in 1996 was over 12 million, based on several studies sponsored by the Indian Council of Medical Research (ICMR) involving 35,295 adults of age >35 years.[1] But the epidemiological data currently available for India is still thin and underestimate the total burden of COPD.[2] The mortality data also underestimates COPD as a cause of death because the disease is more likely to be cited as contributory rather than an underlying cause of death, or may not be cited at all. Depending on severity of disease, the 5-year mortality rate for patients with COPD varies from 40 to 70%. It affects 5–19% of adults over 40 years of age, making it the fourth most common cause of hospitalization in males and seventh in females. As per the INSEARCH study, the prevalence of COPD (as measured by chronic bronchitis) is 3.49% in population above 35 years, whereas in the southern state of Kerala it is 10%.[1]

Using random effects pooled estimates, the reported prevalence of COPD in India was 7.4% (11% in urban areas and 5.6% in rural areas).[3] In addition, the commonly associated comorbidities such as cardiovascular disease, lung cancer, osteoporosis, and diabetes are reported to increase the epidemiological burden by several folds. According to a small prevalence study conducted across India, the median prevalence rate is 5.5% for males and 3.2% for females that can be contributed to associated lifestyle factors such as smoking and occupational hazard; however, recent studies suggest that nonsmoking-related COPD is higher than previously believed, particularly in the LMICs, accounting for one fourth to one third of all COPD cases. There were 60% of COPD cases in never smokers in a study in 1,200 slum dwellers in Pune, Maharashtra.[3]

RISK FACTORS OF CHRONIC OBSTRUCTIVE PULMONARY DISEASE

Tobacco smoking has been the major cause of COPD in most of the world including in India. Compared to nonsmokers, smokers have three times more risk of developing COPD; *bidi* smokers are at even higher risk than the cigarette smokers.[4] Numerous other nonmodifiable (age, gender, and genetic factors) and modifiable risk factors (indoor and outdoor air pollution, exposure to environmental tobacco smoke, and occupational dust and chemicals) have also been identified, especially among the nonsmokers. Other risk factors which are also known to play a role in the development of COPD include dietary habits, long-standing asthma, recurrent respiratory infection in early childhood, and pulmonary tuberculosis.

The major nonsmoking risk factors for COPD include the following:

- *Indoor air pollution*: The principal sources of indoor air pollutants that are related to development of COPD include smoke produced by domestic use of different cooking fuels and environmental tobacco smoke or passive smoke. Women exposed to biomass fuels and open fire have low birth weight babies and low birth weight itself associated with poor lung growth and lung function during childhood and adulthood. Indoor air pollution from solid fuel use in developing countries was estimated to account for about 1.6 million deaths annually in 2004 and about 500,000 in India in 2010, suggesting a serious impact on health. An odds ratio of 2.3 for COPD has been seen with exposure to biomass smoke in a meta-analysis of 36 global studies; further 400–550,000 premature deaths and 4–6% of the Indian national burden of disease has been attributed to annual use of biomass fuel and indoor air pollution.[5]

  Indoor exposure to domestic fuel combustion, especially from biomass fuels, has been reported as an important cause of chronic bronchitis and COPD in females in studies from India, Nepal, China, South Africa, and Turkey. It has been argued that the exposure to biomass fuel has a larger risk for COPD than tobacco smoking. Women with domestic exposure to combustion of biomass fuel develop COPD with clinical characteristics and have impaired quality of life with mortality similar in extent to those of tobacco smokers and have been developed more local scarring and pigment deposition in lung parenchyma and fibrosis in the small airway wall.

  In rural areas of developing countries, biomass fuel burning is often carried out in indoor environment with open fire using poorly functioning stoves with limited ventilation facilities, so they are exposed to fuels for 30–40 years throughout their life equivalent to 60,000 hours. The common type of cooking devices used are kerosene stoves, coal-lighted *angithi*, gas stoves operated with liquid petroleum gas (LPG), and *chullas* in which biomass fuels are used. Women and family prefer food cooked on *chullas* due to taste, which more preferable than gas-cooked food. Biomass fuel usually involves wood, crop residues, and animal dung whose burning emits a variety of toxins due to their low combustion efficiency.

  Majority of households (90% rural and 32% urban) use biomass stoves for cooking purpose. In rural India, 62% of households use firewood and 14% cook with dung cakes while 13% use straw, shrubs, grass, and agricultural crop residues to fire their stoves. In urban India, 22% use firewood, 8% use kerosene while the rest use cleaner fuels such as LPG or natural gas for cooking and heating purpose. Even the severity of pollutants varies in biomass fuels as benzene concentration in indoor kitchen using wood fuel is significantly low as compared to dung fuel used in a variety of Indian kitchen facilities.[3]

  Biomass smoke contains a large number of pollutants including ambient particulate matter of <10 μm in aerodynamic diameter (PM10), carbon monoxide, nitrogen dioxide, sulfur dioxide, formaldehyde, asbestos fibers, allergens, and polycyclic organic matter including carcinogens. The World Health Organization (WHO) standard safety standards specify that PM10 concentration is 150 μg/m^3 in 24 hours. Environment Protection Agency safety standards specify that carbon monoxide concentration should not be more than 10 ppm in 8 hours. However, burning of biomass fuel generates a mean concentration of 300–3,000 μg/m^3 PM10 in 24 hours. In homes using biomass fuel, concentration of carbon monoxide can be 2–50 ppm in 24 hours and 10–500 ppm during cooking.[6]

  In South Indian states, the concentration of respirable particulate matter ranges from 500 to 2,000 μg/m^3 during cooking with biomass fuel in household. The blood carboxyhemoglobin concentration in nonsmoking healthy females from Chandigarh and its adjoining areas in India exposed to different types of cooking fuel were two to five times significantly higher than those in nonsmoking healthy unexposed females.[7] The values of lung function were significantly lower in biofuel users compared with both kerosene and LPG users, and COPD prevalence was higher in biomass fuel users than clean fuel users.

  In a cytogenetic analysis, a higher frequency of DNA damage was found in biomass fuel users exposed for >5 years compared to LPG in Indian women. A minimum required biomass exposure index of 60 has been identified which is significantly associated with chronic bronchitis after adjusting for age, passive smoking, and occupational exposure. In the district of Mysore in the Karnataka state of India, it was observed that 1 in every 20 nonsmoking women having a biomass fuel exposure index of >110 develops chronic bronchitis. India needs to develop a policy for separate kitchen on the lines of separate toilets for hygiene, with proper ventilation, and promote use of chimneys for both cooking and heating purpose as this is also a major factor for inhalation of chemicals and carcinogens produced by fuel, so simultaneously the fuel as well as area of cooking needs to be changed to decrease the prevalence of COPD.

  There is an increased risk with the presence of exposure to two or more risk factors. In India, 56–76% of household use various types of mosquito repellents which are also responsible for some degree of indoor air pollution. Passive smoke or environmental tobacco smoke exposure among nonsmokers, especially women and children, is common in Asian countries including in India. Around 250 chemicals are known to be harmful from second-hand smoke. Parental smoking is reported to result in significant decline in forced expiratory volume in 1 second (FEV_1) among children. It is reported that patients exposed to one risk factor had a mean age of 61.32 years, two risk factors had a mean age of 52.35 years, and three risk factors had a mean age of 51.93 years implying that patients exposed to multiple risk factors develop COPD at an earlier age.[8]

- *Outdoor air pollution*: Air pollution is consistently increasing in developing countries attributable to industrialization and traffic congestion, especially in Asia. The deleterious effects of particulate pollutants are known to increase bronchial reactivity, airway oxidative stress, pulmonary and systemic inflammation, amplification of viral infection, and reduction in airway ciliary activity. India is listed as heavily polluted along with other South Asian countries in a global air pollution survey conducted by the WHO where 13 out of 20 most polluted cities were from India and there is 24.9% increase in emergency room visits for COPD due to a higher level of outdoor pollutants. A report from Mumbai after Delhi has presented with a high prevalence of COPD and health expenditure burden attributable to air pollution, because of increasing population density in cities.
- *Occupational hazards*: There is an established relationship between COPD and occupational exposure to toxic gases at workplace, grain dust in farms, and dust or fumes in factories. India is the largest producer of pesticide in Asia and is the third largest consumer in the world which overall affects the respiratory health of the population. The prevalence of COPD is higher among agricultural workers spraying cholinesterase-inhibition pesticides (18.1%) compared to control (6.9%) in Eastern India.[9] The long-term exposure of metal dust was evaluated among metal polish workers in 25 brass and steelware polishing industries at Moradabad and unexposed controls in North India where 6.7% of polishers were found to have chronic bronchitis.[10] A higher prevalence of chronic bronchitis has also been seen among railway workers (16.7%) compared to controls (8.9%) in India as peak expiratory flow rate <300 L/min was observed in 54.6% railway workers compared to only 2.2% in controls.[11]
- *Socioeconomic factor*: Socioeconomic factors which include poor dietary habits and low consumption of fresh fruits and food items having high antioxidants play an important role in the development of COPD. Poor housing conditions like mud houses with thatched/ tin house roof, no separate kitchen, and improper ventilation promote COPD development. These poor living conditions are also related to intrauterine growth retardation and childhood respiratory tract infection.
- *Other risk factors*: Male sex and increasing age are well-established nonmodifiable risk factors for COPD. On the other hand, female patients are reported to present with more dyspnea which could be due to a relatively greater degree of bronchial obstruction, more exacerbation, and higher prevalence of systemic features. Mean values of FEV1 decline in healthy men and women are around 30 mL/year and 25 mL/year, respectively. Adult smokers experience an average FEV_1 decline of 40–50 mL/year. History of pulmonary tuberculosis has been reported to be a strong predictor of COPD as this is associated with airway fibrosis and immune response to mycobacteria which can result in airway inflammation, characteristic of COPD. Chronic asthma causes lung remodeling resulting in irreversible and progressive airflow obstruction and development of COPD.

SALIENT CLINICAL FEATURES

Usually, the patient is above 40 years, male, and smoker who typically complains of chronic cough and sputum production, which is progressively increasing. There is also progressively increasing breathlessness with or without wheezing. In early COPD, physical examination is generally normal. Signs of emphysema may be seen in advanced disease: Increased anteroposterior diameter of the chest (sometimes barrel chest), reduced diaphragmatic movements during respiration, hyper-resonance on percussion, diminished breath sounds, and prolonged expiratory phase (particularly at forced expiration). In severe COPD, there may be use of accessory muscles of respiration, intercostal retractions during inspiration, "pursed-lip" breathing, and central cyanosis. Traditionally, "COPD facies" is typically described when there is bluish discoloration of lips and tip of the nose in the presence of 'pursed-lip' breathing in an advance stage of COPD. The person having "COPD facies" may or may not have "smoker's facies" (i.e., looking much older than the stated age with coarse facial features and wrinkled grayish, atrophic skin).

DIAGNOSIS AND TREATMENT OF CHRONIC OBSTRUCTIVE PULMONARY DISEASE IN LOW- AND MIDDLE-INCOME COUNTRIES

Spirometry is essentially required for COPD diagnosis; the presence of post bronchodilator FEV_1/forced vital capacity (FVC) < 0.7 defines airway obstruction. Spirometry is not available in many LMICs at the primary care level. For example, in some African countries with high COPD prevalence, the availability of spirometry is restricted to urban setup; therefore, COPD is diagnosed by clinical signs and symptoms in a rural setup.[12] The nonavailability, nonaccessibility, and operational training are significant impediments to COPD diagnosis in LMICs. Also, the screening questionnaires and prognostic tools such as indices which are widely used in high-income countries lack validation in LMICs. Consequently, more than 50%

of people with airway obstruction are not diagnosed and are deprived of the benefit from early intervention and treatment. Both healthcare workers and patients lack awareness and education on COPD leading to delayed diagnosis and consequences.[13] There are other hindering factors such as lack of appropriate training, defective and poor equipment maintenance, and lack of electricity, especially in the rural setting.

Standard treatment of stable COPD includes both pharmacological and nonpharmacological options. Most nations in high-income countries have developed their own national guidelines for COPD. However, in LMICs, there are no local guidelines customized to local and regional scenarios; only 22% of LMICs have same COPD guidelines.[14] In most LMICs, the Global Initiative for Chronic Obstructive Lung Disease (GOLD) strategy guidelines have been translated to the native language without consideration of local context and resources. Dissemination of the guidelines has been suboptimal, and many healthcare workers are not aware of the entrance of guidelines.[15] The key treatment paradox in most LMICs including India is lack of prescription of maintenance therapy and excess focus on management of symptomatic and acute episodes. Medication shortages are also common in LMICs in both the public and the private sectors. Unlike in high-income countries, most governments in LMICs do not provide social insurance coverage, resulting in significant out-of-pocket expenditure leading to nonaffordability and noncompliance.[15,16] Other significant factors which influence the treatment outcomes in LMICs are malnutrition, poverty, illiteracy, societal beliefs, and cultural taboos.

Active targeted case-finding activities which can be implemented along with the existing screening programs for tuberculosis are therefore recommended in LMICs to improve early case diagnosis. Funding support to LMICs is also recommended for policy interventions to make basic diagnostic tools like spirometry as essential medical devices. Multisectoral and intersectoral coordination is required to ensure continuity of healthcare delivery and improvement of maintenance treatment availability at an affordable cost. It is also important to improve awareness of nonpharmacological treatment options and investment in preventive strategies like biomass fuel reduction and smoking cessation support.

SUMMARY

Chronic obstructive pulmonary disease is generally progressive but partially reversible. Most patients with COPD have combined features of both emphysema and chronic bronchitis. Smoker's cough can be seen as the first step toward the development of COPD. Active targeted case-finding activities need to be implemented along with e.g., the existing screening programs for tuberculosis in LMICs to improve an early case diagnosis. Funding support to LMICs is also recommended for policy interventions. Multisectoral and intersectoral coordination is essential ensure continuity of healthcare delivery and improvement of maintenance treatment availability at an affordable cost. It is also important to improve awareness of nonpharmacological treatment options and investment in preventive strategies.

REFERENCES

1. Jindal SK, Aggarwal AN, Gupta D, et al. Indian study on epidemiology of asthma, respiratory symptoms and chronic bronchitis in adults (INSEARCH). Int J Tuberc Lung Dis. 2012;16:1270-7.
2. Lopez AD, Mathers CD, Ezzati M, et al. Global and regional burden of disease and risk factors, 2001: systematic analysis of population health data. Lancet. 2006;367:1747-57.
3. Walia GK, Vellakkal R, Gupta V. Chronic obstructive pulmonary disease and its non smoking risk factors in India. COPD. 2016;13(2):251-61.
4. Bhome AB. COPD in India. Iceberg or volcano? J Thorac Dis. 2012;4:298-309.
5. Smith KR. National burden of disease in India from indoor air pollution. Proc Natl Acad Sci USA. 2000;97:13286-93.
6. Boy E, Bruce N, Delgado H. Birth weight and exposure to kitchen wood smoke during pregnancy in rural Guatemala. Environ Health Perspect. 2002;110:109-14.
7. Behera D, Dash S, Yadav SP. Carboxyhaemoglobin in women exposed to different cooking fuels. Thorax. 1991;46:344-6.
8. Mahmood T, Singh KR, Kant S, et al. Prevalence and etiological profile of chronic obstructive pulmonary disease in non smokers. Lung India. 2017;34(2):122-6.
9. Chakrabarti B, Purkait S, Gun P, et al. Chronic exposures to cholinesterase-inhibiting pesticides adversely affect respiratory health of agricultural workers in Ind J Occup Health. 2009;51:488-97.
10. Rastogi SK, Gupta BN, Husain T, et al. Respiratory symptoms and ventilatory capacity in metal polishers. Hum Exp Toxicol. 1992;11:466-72.
11. Gupta SK, Singh SK. A study on prevalence of chronic bronchitis in workers exposed to smoke and irritant fumes in a railway workshop. Ind J Chest Dis Allied Sci. 1992;34:25-8.
12. Robertson NM, Nagourney EM, Pollard SL, et al. Urban-rural disparities in chronic obstructive pulmonary disease management and access in Uganda. COPD. 2019;6(1):17-28.
13. Pinnock H, Steed L, Jordan R. Supported self-management for COPD: making progress, but there are still challenges. Eur Res J. 2016;48(1):6-9.
14. Tabyshova A, Hurst JR, Soriano JB, et al. Gaps in COPD guidelines of low- and middle-income countries: a systematic scoping review. Chest. 2021;159(2):575-84.
15. Mills A. Health care systems in low- and middle-income countries. N Engl J Med. 2014;370(6):552-7.
16. Boland MRS, Tsiachristas A, Kruis AL, et al. The health economic impact of disease management programs for COPD: a systematic literature review and meta-analysis. BMC Pulm Med. 2013;13(1):40.

Chronic Obstructive Pulmonary Disease: Pathogenesis, Clinical Features and Diagnosis

CHAPTER 85

Aditya Jindal

INTRODUCTION

The definition of chronic obstructive pulmonary disease (COPD) continues to evolve ever since the disease was first recognized in the middle of the last century. The prototype, chronic bronchitis (CB), was essentially a symptom-based disease diagnosed by the presence of "cough with or without sputum production for at least 3 months in a year continuously for 2–3 years"; emphysema, characterized by air trapping, lung hyperinflation and bullae formation, was another distinct entity.[1] But there was a large overlap of clinical, radiological, and pathophysiological features. In due course of time, the two diagnoses were collectively termed COPD. As newer advances and observations are made, the definition of COPD had changed over time. The Global Initiative for Chronic Obstructive Lung Disease (GOLD) in its most recent version (GOLD 2023) defines COPD as a "heterogeneous lung condition characterized by chronic respiratory symptoms (dyspnea, cough, expectoration, and/or exacerbations) due to abnormalities of the airways (bronchitis, bronchiolitis) and/or alveoli (emphysema) that cause persistent, often progressive, airflow obstruction".[2]

GOLD 2023 employs several different terms to describe COPD based on either the stage or the type of presentation.[2] These terms are important to understand the development of the disease rather than the clinical types to describe COPD:

- *Early COPD*:[3] It describes the "biological" first step early in life. It is not the clinically "early" disease.
- *Mild COPD*: It is used to describe the spirometrically measured severity of airflow obstruction.
- *Young COPD*: It is seen in younger age, usually between 20 and 50 years of age. Young COPD is not synonymous with "mild" COPD.
- *Pre-COPD*:[4] It identifies individuals (of any age) with the presence of respiratory symptoms and/or other detectable structural and/or functional abnormalities without any spirometrically demonstrable airflow obstruction. These patients may (or not) develop persistent airflow obstruction in future.
- *PRISm*:[5] It describes individuals with "preserved ratio [forced expiratory volume in 1 second (FEV_1)/forced vital capacity (FVC) ≥0.7 after bronchodilation] but impaired spirometry (FEV_1 <80% of reference, after bronchodilation)". The prevalence is particularly high in current and former smokers. PRISm can progress to both normal and obstructed spirometry over time.

PATHOGENESIS AND PATHOPHYSIOLOGY

Chronic obstructive pulmonary disease is an inflammatory disorder of the airways and lung parenchyma but with a number of accompanying systemic extrapulmonary manifestations. It is characterized by sequential airflow inflammation, narrowing, and functional obstruction **(Flowchart 1)**. Inhalation of noxious particles and gases from tobacco smoking and/or other environmental pollutants such as solid-fuel exhausts results in an enhanced inflammatory response in the airways.[2,6] Concurrent airway infections add to the ongoing inflammation. The cascade of inflammatory effects of biomass fuels' smoke is likely to be similar to that of tobacco smoke wherein a number of cellular and molecular mechanisms may be involved in causing airway obstruction and COPD.[7] The airway inflammation induces intracellular damage. There are additional factors such as gastroesophageal reflux, allergic rhinitis, and sinusitis which are also associated with an increased incidence of CB and mucus hypersecretion.

In addition, there is increased oxidative stress and production of toxic radicals such as reactive oxygen species and reactive nitrogen intermediates.[8] There is increased influx of inflammatory cells (neutrophils, macrophages, and T lymphocytes) and release of a variety of cytokines in the airways and the lung parenchyma. Consequently, there are sequential pathological abnormalities as follows: Disruption of the epithelial barrier, mucous hypersecretion and ciliary dysfunction, accumulation of inflammatory mucous exudates in the small airway lumina, infiltration of inflammatory cells, and submucosal fibrosis causing thickening of the

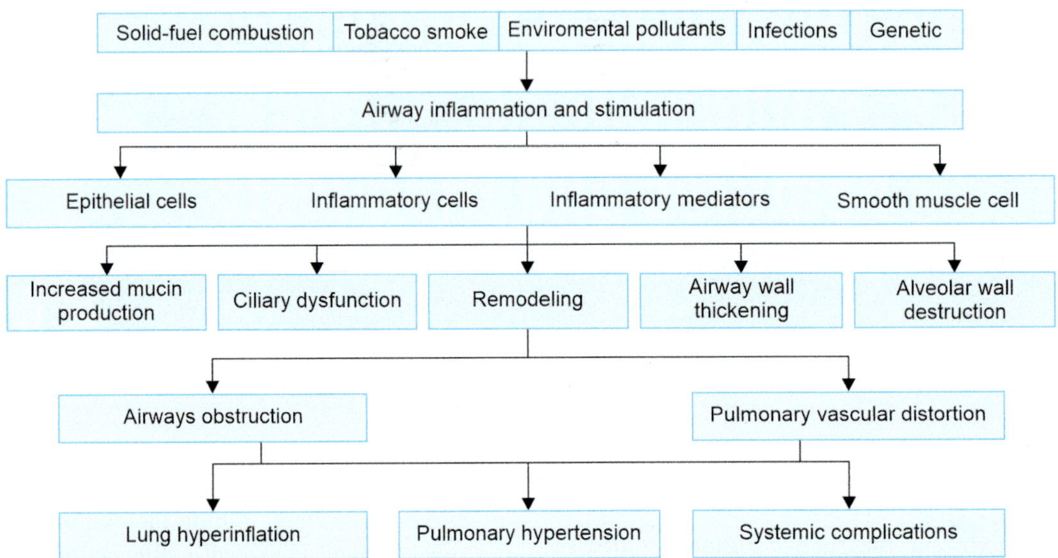

FLOWCHART 1: Simplified schema of important and sequential pathophysiological abnormalities in chronic obstructive pulmonary disease.

airway walls. The important pathological abnormalities and physiological disturbances which may occur are listed as follows:

- *Mucous hypersecretion*:[9] Chronic airway irritation by noxious particles and gases produces squamous metaplasia, bronchial submucosal gland hypertrophy, and increased numbers of goblet cells. Consequently, there is increased production of mucus which constitutes the bulk of expectoration. Normal airway mucus is a gel composed of 97% water. The solid component consists of mucins which are large glycoproteins, nonmucin proteins, cellular debris, salts, and lipids. The mucus traps inhaled toxins which are subsequently expectorated via the processes of ciliary beating and cough.
- *Ciliary dysfunction and autophagy*: Ciliary dysfunction occurs due to squamous metaplasia of epithelial cells. Mucociliary function is important to keep the airways clear and expel out inhaled particles. Impaired ciliary function results in difficulty in expectorating thick mucus plugs.[10] Autophagy (or macroautophagy) is another key process that removes damaged molecules of proteins and subcellular organelles to maintain cellular homeostasis. However, dysregulation of this process may also contributes to the pathogenesis of COPD.[11]
- *Airflow obstruction*: Submucosal gland hypertrophy and thickening result in narrowing of bronchial lumina and airflow obstruction. This is further augmented by mucus plugging in the airways, air trapping, and hyperinflation of the obstructed lung segments. Primarily, the airflow obstruction occurs in the small conducting and peripheral airways that are <2 mm in diameter.[12]
- *Airway remodeling*: Repeated injury and repair processes of chronic inflammation are responsible for structural changes of airway walls affecting airway smooth muscle, epithelium, blood vessels, and extracellular matrix.[13] Simultaneous to inflammation and narrowing, there is loss of the lung elastic recoil (due to destruction of alveolar walls) and loss of alveolar support (from alveolar attachments). Airway remodeling is generally the result of long-standing airway inflammation but can also occur in children with asthma.
- *Gas exchange abnormalities*: In advanced disease, both airways obstruction and alveolar destruction result in abnormalities of ventilation and perfusion responsible for physiological defects such as hypoventilation, shunt effect, or both and cause abnormal gas exchange.[14] Consequently, there is hypoxia with or without CO_2 retention depending upon the severity of physiological dysfunction.
- *Pulmonary hypertension*: The structural distortions of lung parenchyma and pulmonary vasculature also lead to obstruction to pulmonary blood flow and pulmonary hypertension. Pulmonary hypertension occurs later due to pulmonary arterial constriction and other contributory factors which include the presence of endothelial dysfunction and remodeling of the pulmonary arteries, i.e., smooth muscle hypertrophy and hyperplasia.[15,16] Presence of hypoxia is also likely to augment pulmonary vasoconstriction and hypertension.
  Alveolar destruction is also accompanied with destruction of the pulmonary capillary bed. Structural changes in the pulmonary arterioles result in obstruction to pulmonary blood flow and persistent pulmonary hypertension. This may lead to overloading and hypertrophy of right ventricle. Enlargement and dysfunction of right ventricle was commonly labeled as cor pulmonale in the past.[17]
- *Systemic features*: It is likely that there is significant spillover of inflammatory mediators in the systemic circulation. COPD is now recognized as a systemic

inflammatory disorder because of the frequent presence of other extrapulmonary manifestations such as weight loss, muscular wasting, osteopenia, increased risk for atherosclerotic vascular disease, depression and other metabolic disturbances.[18,19]

CLINICAL FEATURES

Chronic obstructive pulmonary disease presents with a mixture of respiratory and general systemic symptoms.[2] Presence of chronic respiratory symptoms is more characteristic, while systemic features are usually nonspecific. Variability of symptoms is common almost every week which is largely related to disease severity and acute exacerbations.[20,21]

Chronic Respiratory Symptoms

Cough with sputum production and breathlessness are the important respiratory symptoms. Cough and expectoration are usually most pronounced in the early morning on waking up. There are frequent or prolonged "winter colds", i.e., winter exacerbations. An increase in amount and purulence of expectoration may point to a COPD exacerbation. Dyspnea is mostly attributable to the presence of airway obstruction and loss of lung parenchyma due to alveolar wall destruction. This is also compounded by the associated anxiety and psychological distress as well as other physiological defects such as gas exchange abnormalities and peripheral muscle dysfunction due to deconditioning. Systemic inflammation and comorbidities such as the cardiovascular disease also add to dyspnea. Dyspnea is frequently accompanied by the presence of wheezing and chest tightness. Symptoms get aggravated during episodes of acute exacerbations often characterized by increased amount and purulence of sputum production and increased breathlessness, sometimes accompanied with signs of acute respiratory failure.

General Symptoms

Tiredness, generalized aches, anxiety, depression, and fatigue are common which are frequently accompanied with anorexia, muscle mass loss, and weight loss. Swelling over the ankles and face may occur due to multiple factors such as fluid retention, right heart failure, and hypoproteinemia. Prolonged immobility can also cause leg swelling and venous thrombosis.

There are also some differences in clinical features of COPD in nonsmoker patients exposed to solid fuel combustion than from smoker COPD **(Table 1)**.[22,23] In a recent multicenter analysis of 1,984 COPD cases, sputum production was significantly found to be more common in smokers while

TABLE 1: Common differences in clinical and diagnostic features of COPD between smokers and nonsmoker, biomass fuel-exposed patients.

Clinical features	COPD in smokers	COPD in nonsmokers (exposed to biomass fuel smoke)
Demographic features	Elderly, more common in males, usually thin	Younger, more likely in females, greater BMI
Clinical symptoms	Breathlessness more pronounced, cough	More symptoms, sputum, phlegm, dyspnea, more activity limitation, less disease control
Exacerbations	Common but lesser than in nonsmokers	More exacerbations and hospitalizations
Pulmonary function tests	• Airways obstruction on spirometry; DLCO normal or low • Normal PaO_2 and SaO_2 in early COPD, reduced in advanced disease	• Less airflow limitation; More had small AO, better FEV_1, low DLCO • Normal PaO_2 and SaO_2 in early COPD, reduced in advanced disease
Chest radiology	• May be normal • Emphysema more pronounced • Lesser bronchial wall thickening	• Normal in early COPD • Less emphysema, more bronchial wall thickening
Airway inflammation • Sputum	Neutrophilic and lymphocytic cell inflammation is more likely	More eosinophilic inflammation
• BALF	Lymphocytes and neutrophils are increased	• Less lymphocytes, increased eosinophils • Increased levels of inflammatory mediators: IL-6 and IL-8
	Lymphocytes and neutrophils	Macrophage and lymphocyte, eosinophils
General	• Lung parenchymal involvement more common in the form of emphysema • Faster decline of lung function	• Airway predominant phenotype • Chronic bronchitis phenotype • Slower rate of PF decline

(AO: airways obstruction; BALF: bronchoalveolar lavage fluid; BMI: body mass index; COPD: chronic obstructive pulmonary disease; DLCO: diffusion capacity; IL: interleukin; PaO_2: arterial oxygen partial pressure; PF: pulmonary function; SaO_2: arterial oxygen saturation)

nonsmoker COPD, which was more commonly observed in women exposed to biomass fuels, was characterized with a higher rate of exacerbations and higher healthcare resource utilization.[23] The frequency of acute symptomatic worsening, emergency visits, and hospitalization was significantly higher in nonsmoker COPD, but there were no differences in the maintenance requirement of bronchodilators, inhalational steroids, or home nebulization and intensive care unit admissions in the two groups.[23]

Physical Examination

Presence of physical signs depends upon the stage and severity of disease. Both general physical and chest examination are normal in the early stages and quiescent phases of COPD. Physical signs of airflow obstruction are seen in advanced disease when there is significant impairment of lung function. Emphysema is detected by the presence of physical signs such as hyperinflated chest which is sometimes called barrel-shaped chest, diminished chest-wall movements, hyper-resonant percussion note, and diminished breath sounds. Presence of usually bilateral and diffuse rhonchi and crepitations may be heard on auscultation, especially during an episode of exacerbation. Physical signs are more pronounced during acute exacerbations when there may be symptoms and signs of hypoxia and hypercapnia. Physical signs of pulmonary hypertension which were characteristically described in the past in patients with chronic cor pulmonale (right ventricular enlargement/failure, loud P2 heart sound) are not often demonstrable in the presence of lung hyperinflation.

DIAGNOSIS OF CHRONIC OBSTRUCTIVE PULMONARY DISEASE

Diagnosis of COPD is suspected on the basis of clinical features, while airway obstruction is confirmed on spirometry. Chest radiology and/or other investigations are required for differential diagnosis from asthma or other similar conditions.

Clinical Diagnosis

Presence of chronic respiratory symptoms as listed earlier may fairly suggest the possible diagnosis of COPD.[2,24] This is further strengthened by the detailed medical history of an exposure to risk factors, such as tobacco smoking and occupational or environmental exposures (household/outdoor). Physical examination may help either to support the diagnosis or sometimes to exclude the other possible alternative diagnoses. It is also important to look for other comorbidities for a comprehensive diagnosis. Some of the common comorbidities include the cardiovascular heart disease, osteoporosis, musculoskeletal disorders, anxiety, and depression. Lung cancer and other malignancies are also more frequent largely due to the common risk factor of tobacco use.

Lung Function Tests

Spirometry

Presence of airflow obstruction demonstrated with forced spirometry is the most reproducible and objective measurement.[2,25] Peak expiratory flow (PEF) has poor specificity and cannot be used as a substitute to spirometry for COPD diagnosis.

The following important indices on forced spirometry are assessed and interpreted for diagnosis:

- Volume of air forcibly exhaled from the point of maximal inspiration (FVC)
- Volume of air exhaled during the first second of the forced exhalation (forced expiratory volume in one second, FEV_1)
- Ratio of FEV_1/FVC

Spirometric measurements are expressed by comparison with reference values based on age, height, sex, and race.

An obstructive pattern as seen in COPD is diagnosed from the presence of a decrease in both FEV_1 and FVC. GOLD typically describes the postbronchodilator ratio of $FEV_1/FVC < 0.7$ as the spirometric criterion for airflow obstruction as simple and independent of reference values. GOLD recommends the use of the fixed FEV_1/FVC ratio over lower limit of normal (LLN) values for diagnostic simplicity and consistency. Airflow obstruction in asthma and other diseases may also show some irreversibility. But the degree of reversibility may vary over time. Repeated spirometry may be needed to assess the degree of reversibility. Repeat spirometry on a separate occasion may also be needed to assess the presence or absence of airflow obstruction when a single measurement of the postbronchodilator FEV_1/FVC ratio is between 0.60 and 0.80, which may happen as a result of biological variation. Certain differences are reported in spirometry between smoker and nonsmoker COPD; nonsmoker patients had significantly lower values of FVC and FEV_1, but there were no significant differences in percent-predicted vital capacity.

It is controversial whether screening spirometry is helpful in the general population for the diagnosis of COPD. GOLD recommends spirometry only in symptomatic patients and/or in the presence of risk factors for active case finding.

Other Lung Function Tests

Spirometry is frequently recognized to be normal in COPD; moreover, COPD symptoms, pathology, and adverse outcomes are reported in patients even in the presence of normal spirometry.[26] Imaging studies and other lung function tests such as diffusing capacity and exercise testing have been helpful in such situations.

Detailed lung function tests are required whenever there is significant discordance between the degree of airflow obstruction and the presence of symptoms.[25] Residual volume and total lung capacity can be measured with body plethysmography or by helium dilution lung volume measurement. These investigations will help to characterize the severity of COPD but are not essential to patient management. Measurement of the single breath carbon monoxide diffusing capacity of the lungs (DLCO) is helpful to evaluate the gas transfer properties of the respiratory system, especially when symptoms such as breathlessness are disproportionate to the degree of airflow obstruction.[27] There is an increased risk of death which is independent of the severity of airflow obstruction if the DLCO values are <60% predicted, and presence of low DLCO values may also suggest against surgical lung resection in patients with lung cancer. DLCO values <80% predicted are a marker of emphysema even in the absence of demonstrable airways obstruction and predict an increased risk for developing COPD over time.

Exercise tests are required to assess functional status in patients with minimal symptoms despite severe airflow obstruction.[28] Paced shuttle walk test or self-paced 6-minute walking distance is useful to evaluate exercise limitation of the patient and administer rehabilitative therapy. Walking tests are helpful to assess the effectiveness of pulmonary rehabilitation. Coexisting or alternative conditions, e.g., cardiac disease, require assessment with laboratory exercise testing using cycle or treadmill ergometry.

Simple pulse oximetry is routinely measured to evaluate arterial oxygen saturation and can be used to decide the need for supplemental oxygen therapy.[29] Arterial blood gas pressures of oxygen and carbon dioxide are measured for the presence of hypoxia and hypercapnia in suspected respiratory failure or right heart failure. Blood gas testing has potential therapeutic implications to decide about assisted mechanical ventilation.

Radiological Investigations[30,31]

Radiological examination with chest X-ray is not usually required for COPD diagnosis but helps in differential diagnosis to exclude alternate causes and/or detect complications. Chest X-ray is likely to be normal or show increased bronchovascular markings, the tram lines representing thickened bronchial walls in CB. Signs of lung hyperinflation (hyperlucency of the lungs, flattened diaphragm, widened intercostal spaces, and an increase of retrosternal air space) are present in advanced COPD with emphysema.

Computed tomography (CT) is required for assessment for concurrent lung disease and enhanced understanding of disease phenotypes, severity, treatment decisions, and outcomes. CT is also used for decision-making for lung volume reduction surgery (LVRS) or endobronchial valve placement. Computer-assisted CT analysis enables quantification of airway abnormality. CT imaging can also provide significant information about COPD comorbidities such as about coronary and pulmonary artery status, bone density, and muscle mass.

Systemic Evaluation

Evaluation of involvement of other systemic systems is done as per indication. Cardiac evaluation requires electrocardiography (ECG) and echocardiography (ECHO) in most patients. ECG and ECHO are essential to detect pulmonary hypertension and right ventricular overload in most patients. Hemodynamic studies with right heart catheterization may be required in selected patients, especially those suspected to have left ventricular and cardiovascular disease.

Hematological and biochemical investigations are required for hepatic, renal, and metabolic evaluation. Ultrasound and/or CT scanning for concerned organ systems may be indicated. Assessment for bone density is important for osteoporosis and osteopenia.

Blood eosinophil counts of ≥300 cells/μL are used to identify COPD phenotypes with greater risk of exacerbations. Screening for alpha-1 antitrypsin deficiency is indicated for younger COPD patients (<45 years age) with emphysema.[32]

Assessment for Therapy

No single treatment is ideal for all forms of COPD in view of the marked heterogeneity. Assessment to institute therapy is based on phenotypic recognition and other criteria usually related to the severity of airflow limitation, magnitude of current symptoms, previous history of moderate and severe exacerbations, and presence of other diseases (multimorbidity).[2,33,34]

- *Symptom evaluation*: Different dyspnea questionnaires and scoring methods are employed for assessment of symptoms:
    - *Dyspnea questionnaire*: Modified Medical Research Council (mMRC) dyspnea scale: This is a multidimensional health status measure which may also predict future mortality risk.
    - Multidimensional questionnaires such as the Chronic Respiratory Questionnaire (CRQ) and St. George's Respiratory Questionnaire (SGRQ) are complex for routine use. Shorter COPD Assessment Test (CAT™) is more suitable for use in the clinic.
- *Severity of airflow limitation*: It is based on the postbronchodilator value of FEV_1 (% reference).
- *Exacerbation risk (ECOPD)*, i.e., episodes of acute respiratory symptom worsening. ECOPD adversely affects the health status and lung function.

To guide initial pharmacological treatment, GOLD 2023 recommends combined assessment for classification of patients into A, B, and E (previous C and D) categories based on the level of symptoms (mMRC or CAT™) and the frequency of previous exacerbations.[2] The A and B groups constitute patients with 0 or 1 moderate exacerbation not leading to hospitalization; respectively, with symptom score = mMRC < 2, CAT < 10 (A) and mMRC ≥ 2, CAT ≥ 10 (B). Group E includes all patients with ≥2 moderate exacerbations or ≥1 leading to hospitalization. (See COPD Therapy chapter.)

SUMMARY

Chronic obstructive pulmonary disease is a chronic inflammatory disease of the airways characterized by mucus hypersecretion, bronchial wall thickening, airflow limitation, and alveolar wall destruction. Diagnosis is generally based on the history of presence of a risk factor, respiratory symptoms, and demonstration of airways obstruction on spirometry. Chest X-ray and CT scan are sometimes required to rule out an alternate diagnosis or presence of a complication. Evaluation with detailed lung function tests and other system investigations is required whenever there is a diagnostic dilemma or suspicion of comorbidities.

REFERENCES

1. A Report of the Conclusions of a CIBA Symposium. Terminology, Definitions, and Classification of Chronic Pulmonary Emphysema and Related Conditions. Thorax. 1959;14(4): 286-99.
2. Global Initiative for Chronic Obstructive Lung Disease. Global Strategy for the diagnosis, management and prevention of chronic obstructive pulmonary disease (2023 Report). [online] Available from https://goldcopd.org/2023-gold-report [Last accessed June, 2024].
3. Soriano JB, Polverino F, Cosio BG. What is early COPD and why is it important? Eur Respir J. 2018;52(6):1801448.
4. Han MK, Agusti A, Celli BR, et al. From GOLD 0 to pre-COPD. Am J Respir Crit Care Med. 2021;203(4):414-23.
5. Wan ES. The Clinical Spectrum of PRISm. Am J Respir Crit Care Med. 2022;206(5):524-5.
6. Christenson SA, Smith BM, Bafadhel M, et al. Chronic obstructive pulmonary disease. Lancet. 2022;399(10342):2227-42.
7. Barnes PJ. Inflammatory mechanisms in patients with chronic obstructive pulmonary disease. J Allergy Clin Immunol. 2016;138(1):16-27.
8. Domej W, Oettl K, Renner W. Oxidative stress and free radicals in COPD--implications and relevance for treatment. Int J Chron Obstruct Pulmon Dis. 2014;9:1207-24.
9. Fahy JV, Dickey BF. Airway mucus function and dysfunction. N Engl J Med. 2010;363(23):2233-47.
10. Perotin JM, Coraux C, Lagonotte E, et al. Alteration of primary cilia in COPD. Eur Respir J. 2018;52(1):1800122.
11. Barnes PJ, Baker J, Donnelly LE. Autophagy in asthma and chronic obstructive pulmonary disease. Clin Sci (Lond). 2022;136(10):733-46.
12. McDonough JE, Yuan R, Suzuki M, et al. Small-airway obstruction and emphysema in chronic obstructive pulmonary disease. N Engl J Med. 2011;365(17):1567-75.
13. Hirota N, Martin JG. Mechanisms of airway remodeling. Chest. 2013;144(3):1026-32.
14. Young IH, Bye PT. Gas exchange in disease: asthma, chronic obstructive pulmonary disease, cystic fibrosis, and interstitial lung disease. Compr Physiol. 2011;1(2):663-97.
15. Blanco I, Tura-Ceide O, Peinado VI, et al. Updated Perspectives on Pulmonary Hypertension in COPD. Int J Chron Obstruct Pulmon Dis. 2020;15:1315-24.
16. García AR, Piccari L Emerging phenotypes of pulmonary hypertension associated with COPD: a field guide. Curr Opin Pulm Med. 2022;28(5):343-51.
17. Shujaat A, Minkin R, Eden E. Pulmonary hypertension and chronic cor pulmonale in COPD. Int J Chron Obstruct Pulmon Dis. 2007;2(3):273-8.
18. Cavaillès A, Brinchault-Rabin G, Dixmier A, et al. Comorbidities of COPD. Eur Respir Rev. 2013;22(130):454-75.
19. Rabe KF, Hurst JR, Suissa S. Cardiovascular disease and COPD: dangerous liaisons? Eur Respir Rev. 2018;27(149):180057.
20. Miravitlles M, Izquierdo JL, Esquinas C, et al. The variability of respiratory symptoms and associated factors in COPD. Respir Med. 2017;129:165-72.
21. Espinosa de los Monteros MJ, Peña C, Hurtado EJS, et al. Variability of respiratory symptoms in severe COPD. Arch Bronconeumol. 2012;48(1):3-7.
22. Gordon S B, Bruce NG, Grigg J, et al. Respiratory risks from household air pollution in low and middle income countries. Lancet Respir Med. 2014;2:823-60.
23. Jindal SK, Aggarwal AN, Jindal A, et al. OPD exacerbation rates are higher in non-smoker patients in India. Int J Tuberc Lung Dis. 2020;24(12):1272-8.
24. Gentry S, Gentry B. Chronic Obstructive Pulmonary Disease: Diagnosis and Management. Am Fam Physician. 2017;95(7): 433-41.
25. Haynes JM, Kaminsky DA, Ruppel GL. The Role of Pulmonary Function Testing in the Diagnosis and Management of COPD. Respir Care. 2023;68(7):889-913.
26. Price D, Brusselle G. Challenges of COPD diagnosis. Expert Opin Med Diagn. 2013;7(6):543-56.
27. DeCato TW, Hegewald MJ. Diffusing Capacity, the Too Often Ignored Lung Function Test in COPD. Chest. 2021;160(2): 389-90.
28. Ward SA, Grocott MPW, Levett DZH. Exercise Testing, Supplemental Oxygen, and Hypoxia. Ann Am Thorac Soc. 2017;14(Suppl 1):S140-8.
29. Garcia-Gutierrez S, Unzurrunzaga A, Arostegui I, et al.; IRYSS-COPD group. The Use of Pulse Oximetry to Determine Hypoxemia in Acute Exacerbations of COPD. COPD. 2015;12(6):613-20.
30. Willer K, Fingerle AA, Noichl W, et al. X-ray dark-field chest imaging for detection and quantification of emphysema in patients with chronic obstructive pulmonary disease: a diagnostic accuracy study. Lancet Digit Health. 2021;3(11): e733-44.
31. Pistenmaa CL, Washko GR. Computerized Chest Imaging in the Diagnosis and Assessment of the Patient with Chronic Obstructive Pulmonary Disease. Clin Chest Med. 2020;41(3): 375-81.
32. Stockley RA. Alpha-1 Antitrypsin Deficiency: The Learning Goes On. Am J Respir Crit Care Med. 2020;202(1):6-7.
33. Vogelmeier CF, Román-Rodríguez M, Singh D, et al. Goals of COPD treatment: Focus on symptoms and exacerbations. Respir Med. 2020;166:105938.
34. Riley CM, Sciurba FC. Diagnosis and Outpatient Management of Chronic Obstructive Pulmonary Disease: A Review. JAMA. 2019;321(8):786-97.

Systemic Manifestations and Comorbidities of Chronic Obstructive Pulmonary Disease

CHAPTER 86

Agam Vora

INTRODUCTION

Decades of ongoing research in chronic obstructive pulmonary disease (COPD) have led to an improved understanding of the etiopathogenesis and clinical presentation of this disease. Comorbidities are defined as other chronic medical conditions.[1] The spectrum of comorbid diseases associated with COPD range from cardiac disease, diabetes mellitus, hypertension, osteoporosis, and obstructive sleep apnea to psychological disorders.[1] There are significant variations observed in the prevalence of these comorbid diseases across different studies. Another dilemma posed by comorbid diseases in COPD is the overlap of risk factors such as smoking, making it difficult to draw conclusions about the interrelationship between COPD and these comorbidities. Some authors now consider these comorbid disorders to be a part of the COPD sequelae.[1]

Comorbidities are associated with increased hospitalizations in patients with COPD.[2] In the Lung Health Study (*n* = 5,887 smokers), it was reported that about 12.8% of smokers were hospitalized and of these, 42% of the hospitalizations were due to cardiovascular events or pulmonary complications.[3] Comorbidities have been reported to have an impact on the duration of COPD hospitalizations.[4] Hence, it is important to address the comorbidities in COPD patients and choose the drugs used to treat COPD and comorbid conditions with care. One must be prudent about the choice of drugs since some drugs used to treat COPD may worsen the comorbid disease and vice versa. This chapter provides insights into common comorbid disorders observed in COPD patients.

CHRONIC OBSTRUCTIVE PULMONARY DISEASE AND CARDIOVASCULAR DISEASE

Vascular and heart diseases have a direct impact on survival in COPD patients. Two pathophysiological mechanisms are implicated, namely endothelial dysfunction and coagulopathy.[5] The systemic inflammation present in COPD induces a "procoagulant" state. COPD patients have abnormally high levels of tissue factor and Factor VIIa and their fibrin clots are resistant to lysis.[6,7]

Coronary heart disease and COPD share smoking as the common risk factor and both the diseases are inflammatory diseases and have clotting abnormalities The presence of symptoms of simple chronic bronchitis increases the risk of death related to a coronary event by 50%. It is estimated that with every 10% decrease in forced expiratory volume in 1 second (FEV1), all-cause mortality will increase by 14%, cardiovascular mortality will increase by 28% and the frequency of nonfatal coronary events will increase by 20%.[5]

Heart failure and COPD share pathophysiological mechanisms, such as inflammation and skeletal muscle alterations. Since the symptoms of the two diseases are similar, a delayed diagnosis of heart failure is often seen. COPD is a truly independent risk factor for death in compromised heart failure patients. Heart failure worsens the prognosis of COPD. Hyperinflation in COPD can cause a compressive effect on the heart creating a milieu for myocardial infarction.[8]

Medications

Nonselective beta-blockers may worsen lung function (decrease FEV1) in some patients with COPD, but avoiding them in COPD could result in increased cardiovascular events. Bronchodilators are associated with tachyarrhythmias. Inhaled anticholinergics can impact intraocular pressure or bladder function. Inhaled corticosteroids may increase the risk of cataracts, skin bruising, osteoporosis, diabetes, hypertension, muscle dysfunction, and adrenal insufficiency **(Table 1)**.[9]

SYSTEMIC VENOUS THROMBOEMBOLISM AND CHRONIC OBSTRUCTIVE PULMONARY DISEASE

In COPD patients, the three components of the Virchow's triad are observed (systemic venous endothelial dysfunction, coagulopathy, and venous stasis due to physical inactivity),

TABLE 1: COPD and comorbid diseases.[9]

Comorbid disease	Mechanistic pathways	Impact of comorbid disease on COPD outcomes	Impact of COPD on the comorbid disease
Cardiovascular disease	• CRP • TNF	• Affects mortality • QoL, duration and frequency of exacerbations	• Exacerbations of COPD can trigger arrhythmias • Hyperinflation in COPD has a compressive effect on the heart creating a milieu for myocardial infarction
Diabetes	• IL-6 • TNF • Adipokines	Affects mortality, QoL	Corticosteroids impair glycemic control in patients with diabetes mellitus
Osteoporosis	Metalloproteinases	Adversely affects QoL	Patients with COPD have a higher risk of developing osteoporosis, owing to the presence of risk factors such as advancing age, smoking, low physical activity, low BMI, malnutrition, declining gonadal function, and use of corticosteroids
Obstructive sleep apnea	Unclear	Affects frequency of pulmonary hypertension	Concomitant disease and overlap syndrome are reported to cause a more severe condition[10]
GERD	Aspiration	Affects the frequency of exacerbations and QoL	
Anxiety and depression	Unclear	Affects mortality, QoL	Mortality after a COPD exacerbation is greater among depressive patients

(BMI: body mass index; COPD: chronic obstructive pulmonary disease; CRP: C reactive protein; GERD: gastroesophageal reflux disease; IL: interleukin; QoL: quality-of-life; TNF: tumor necrosis factor)

which predisposes them to venous thromboembolism (VTE). VTE is reported in about 3–29% of COPD exacerbations. In the absence of specific clinical, biological, or radiological signs, VTE should be suspected in the presence of chest pain or syncope or a fall in arterial carbon dioxide tension in a patient who is usually hypercapnic during a COPD exacerbation episode **(Table 1)**.[5]

Venous thromboembolism leads to a prolongation of hospitalization by 4.4 days and an increase in 1-year mortality by 30% in exacerbations of COPD. If VTE is not diagnosed and anticoagulant therapy is not initiated, an increase in mortality rate by 25% is expected.[5]

PULMONARY HYPERTENSION AND CHRONIC OBSTRUCTIVE PULMONARY DISEASE

Pulmonary artery remodeling is observed in COPD and leads to pulmonary hypertension (PH). This remodeling is due to endothelial dysfunction and coagulopathy, lung-specific mechanisms, such as hypoxic vasoconstriction, destruction of the pulmonary capillary bed by emphysema, smoking-induced inflammatory infiltration of the vascular wall, and shear stress due to redistribution of the blood flow **(Table 1)**.[11-13]

Pulmonary hypertension is defined as mean pulmonary arterial pressure > 25 mm Hg at rest or higher than 30 mm Hg while performing exercise. The prevalence of PH in COPD is 5–40%, but moderate and severe PH only account for <5% of cases. The clinical implication of PH includes worsening gas exchange, dyspnea, and it predisposes to right ventricular (RV) dysfunction and peripheral edema. It is also associated with higher mortality. PH should be suspected in a COPD patient with dyspnea, desaturation during the 6-minute walk test, or a disproportionate reduction in the diffusing capacity of the lung for carbon monoxide in relation to the severity of the obstruction or clinical or biological (brain natriuretic peptide) signs of RV dysfunction not explained by left ventricular failure or a loud second heart sound in the pulmonic area. On echocardiography, a high maximum tricuspid regurgitation velocity (TR_{max} 3.5 m/s^{-1}) is suggestive of PH, but TR_{max} is not evaluable in one third of COPD patients owing to the low echogenicity of emphysematous lungs. Cardiac catheterization can be used to confirm the diagnosis of PH and assess its severity.[11-13]

Management

The management of COPD is not affected by the presence of PH. Long-term oxygen therapy is beneficial, which stabilizes PH in certain patients with COPD.[11,12]

PULMONARY EMBOLISM

Emerging data has indicated the presence of pulmonary embolism (PE) as a common comorbid condition of COPD. A clinical index of suspicion must be maintained since the diagnosis of PE could easily be missed due to the overlap of symptoms of PE and those of a COPD exacerbation. PE may be suspected in the patients who present with acute exacerbation of COPD with no obvious cause.[11-13]

PNEUMONIA

Pneumonia is a common comorbid disease seen in patients with COPD. Pneumonia is considered by some clinicians as a part of the spectrum of COPD. There are distinct differences in COPD patients with exacerbations presenting with or without pneumonia. In patients with pneumonia, a more abrupt onset of symptoms, more severe illness, longer stay in hospital, and higher rates of ICU admission and death were observed **(Table 1)**.[14]

Medications

Drugs used to reduce the risk of exacerbations, such as salmeterol and fluticasone, may increase the risk of pneumonia.[15] Treatment choices would have to be prudently made based on the presence of pneumonia in patients with exacerbations of COPD. Antibiotic therapy is definitely useful for the management of pneumonia but the use of antibiotics during an exacerbation of COPD offers modest benefits. Similarly, corticosteroids have a definite role in the management of exacerbations of COPD, but their role in pneumonia is not yet clear.[16,17]

LUNG CANCER

Lung cancer continues to be an important cause of death in COPD patients. The common causal link in both the disease is the overlap of risk factors such as smoking. The degree of airway obstruction is directly correlated with the development of lung cancer. Squamous cell carcinoma is strongly associated with smoking and COPD exacerbates this risk by 2.5 and 3.5 times.[18,19] Shared genetic links that predispose to both diseases have been identified (e.g., 15q25, 4q31, and 6p21).[20]

Management

Smoking cessation is the cornerstone of COPD management. Exposure to high doses of inhaled corticosteroids reduces the risk of lung cancer.[20]

MUSCULOSKELETAL DYSFUNCTION

Chronic obstructive pulmonary disease is associated with musculoskeletal dysfunction (MSD) which leads to exercise limitation and disability.[21-23] Patients with COPD have a reduced ability for repetitive muscular contractions and experience muscle fatigue. Changes in the quality of enzymes and muscle fiber atrophy have been implicated in muscular dysfunction. MSD may also be associated with osteoporosis. Other contributors to MSD in COPD patients include poor nutrition, prolonged bed rest, the use of corticosteroids, systemic inflammation, and oxidative stress.[24,25] 1–1.5% per day loss of muscle strength with prolonged bed rest has been reported.[26]

Management of Musculoskeletal Dysfunction

Current recommendations for the management of MSD include pulmonary rehabilitation and avoiding systemic corticosteroids.[27] The results of nutritional supplementation and hormonal replacement are not satisfactory.[28,29]

MALNUTRITION IN CHRONIC OBSTRUCTIVE PULMONARY DISEASE PATIENTS

Malnutrition in COPD is caused by an imbalance between energy intake and consumption. Inadequate intake is secondary to the dyspnea resulting from the effort of eating and by impaired leptin regulation, a hormone that reduces food intake. Increased energy consumption has been attributed to work of breathing, smoking, and medications such as theophylline. Increased protein catabolism is also related to systemic inflammation, hypoandrogenism and hypoxia.[5]

In COPD, patients are considered to be malnourished when their body mass index (BMI) is 20 kg/m^2. Malnutrition reduces the lean body mass (muscle). Three malnutrition profiles have been identified in COPD—underweight patients with concomitant depletion of lean body mass (60%), underweight patients with a normal lean body mass (20%), and patients with stable body weight with depletion of lean body mass.[5]

Nutritional Rehabilitation

Physical exercise as part of respiratory rehabilitation, caloric, protein, and polyunsaturated fatty acid supplementation and anabolic steroids are a part of the rehabilitation regimen.[5]

OSTEOPOROSIS IN CHRONIC OBSTRUCTIVE PULMONARY DISEASE PATIENTS

Patients with COPD have a greater risk of developing osteoporosis due to risk factors such as advancing age, smoking, low physical activity, low BMI, malnutrition, declining gonadal function, and use of corticosteroids.[30-33] The risk factors for COPD and osteoporosis are interlinked. Smoking and systemic inflammation have an impact on receptor activator of nuclear factor kappa-B ligand (RANKL) binding, and vitamin D deficiency stimulates parathormone secretion and affects osteoclast maturation through its effect on RANK/RANKL. Oral steroid therapy has an adverse impact on bone homeostasis by causing an increased expression of RANKL, decreased osteoprotegerin, and suppression of osteoclast apoptosis. Another contributing factor to osteoporosis is the presence of hypogonadism in COPD patients. The decrease in estrogen levels inhibits the action of the osteoprotegerin/RANKL complex. The lower levels of physical activity in COPD patients have a negative impact on bone metabolism.

Vertebral fractures have been reported in 29% of patients with COPD **(Table 1)**.[34]

Management

Screening of high-risk patients with a significant smoking history is recommended for early detection of osteoporosis.[5]

Dietary supplementation with calcium (recommended daily allowance 1,000–1,500 mg) and vitamin D (recommended daily allowance 400–800 IU) and lifestyle modification along with pulmonary rehabilitation are recommended.[5] The role of new treatments such as teriparatide in COPD remains to be defined, although it does have a proven benefit in glucocorticoid-induced osteoporosis.[5]

Respiratory rehabilitation with exercise retraining programs improves bone mineral density. It may also improve muscle strength and balance and reduce the risk of falling.[5]

GASTROESOPHAGEAL REFLUX

An increased prevalence of gastroesophageal reflux (GER) disease and other esophageal disorders has been reported in COPD.[35] It has been postulated that aspiration of *Helicobacter pylori* or its exotoxins may amplify the airway inflammation.[36] GER symptoms have been observed to be more common in those with an FEV1 ≤ 50%, as compared with those with an FEV1 > 50.[5]

DIABETES MELLITUS

The prevalence of diabetes in patients with COPD ranges from 1.6 to 16%. Both COPD and diabetes have smoking as a common risk factor. Current data indicate that reduced lung function is a risk factor for the development of diabetes.[37] The cytokines tumor necrosis factor alpha (TNF-α), interleukin-6 (IL-6), and C reactive protein (CRP) are elevated in both COPD and diabetes.[38,39] Corticosteroids used to treat COPD patients impair glycemic control in patients with diabetes mellitus.

Management

Metformin should be discontinued in situations where there is a risk of acute renal failure, such as intravascular contrast media (discontinued for 3 days) in radiological studies, sepsis, hepatitis or gastrointestinal disturbances involving diarrhea and vomiting, or of acute hypoxia, such as during acute cardiac or respiratory failure or perioperatively.[5]

ANXIETY AND DEPRESSION DISORDERS

First hospitalization for COPD may occur earlier in patients with presence of anxiety and/or depression. Depression affects between 20 and 60% of COPD patients. Mortality following a COPD exacerbation was greater among the depressive patients.[5]

Management

The doctor-patient relationship is essential to assess the psychological impact of the disorder. Antidepressants change the patient's perception of symptoms and improve quality of life.[5]

SLEEP DISTURBANCE

Impaired sleep quality is common in COPD. This may be attributed to distension and increased work of breathing, potentiated when lying down. Respiratory symptoms (dyspnea, cough, and expectoration) can cause arousal. One third of COPD patients are observed to have restless legs syndrome. Anxiety and reactive depression can also cause sleep disturbances. The presence of obstructive sleep apnea syndrome (OSAS) exacerbates sleep disturbances in COPD patients.[5]

Management

Noninvasive ventilation (NIV) combined with oxygen therapy slightly improves the sleep of patients with severe hypercapnic COPD compared to oxygen therapy alone.[5]

Long-acting inhaled bronchodilators do not affect sleep quality.[5] Studies of indacaterol have demonstrated that it reduces nocturnal awakenings due to dyspnea, as compared to placebo and other comparator drugs (tiotropium and salmeterol).[5]

The treatment of insomnia in COPD patients consists of restriction the time spent in bed, relaxation, and cognitive behavioral therapy. Short-term hypnotics must be avoided in patients with untreated concomitant OSAS or chronic hypercapnic respiratory failure or during exacerbations.[5]

Continuous positive airway pressure (CPAP) is recommended for OSAS. It is effective and improves prognosis.[5] CPAP therapy has been shown to improve daytime partial pressure of arterial oxygen (PaO_2) values both in OSAS and in obstructive sleep (OS).[40] NIV may be initiated immediately, depending on the severity of daytime or nocturnal hypoventilation and then a switch later to CPAP could be considered if nocturnal hypoventilation [during rapid eye movement (REM) sleep] persists during CPAP therapy. Further studies are warranted to optimize the therapeutic strategy.[5]

An emerging interesting area is the use of humidification therapy in selected patients of COPD. Studies have demonstrated that heated humidification in COPD patients could help in mucus clearance, reduce mucus viscosity, and help in expectoration. Humidification could also have an impact on long-term oxygen treatment since the inhalation of dry air could cause ciliary dysfunction, alterations in mucus properties, and impaired mucociliary clearance. In OSAS patients, humidification helps to reduce the nasal symptoms. Multicenter studies with large number of patients are warranted to identify the subsets of patients who are likely to benefit from the addition of humidification to a noninvasive therapy.[41]

SUMMARY

Comorbid disorders are a part of the COPD sequelae. Comorbidities are associated with increased hospitalizations in patients with COPD. Current research has led to emerging new insights into the complex pathophysiological relationship between COPD and some comorbid disorders. The adverse impact of the comorbidities on the outcomes of the treatment of COPD must be taken into consideration. Choosing drugs to treat COPD and its comorbidities requires a prudent approach so that neither COPD nor the comorbid disease is adversely affected.

REFERENCES

1. Chatila WM, Thomashow BM, Minai OA, et al. Comorbidities in chronic obstructive pulmonary disease. Proc Am Thorac Soc. 2008;5(4):549-55.
2. Mannino DM. COPD: epidemiology, prevalence, morbidity and mortality, and disease heterogeneity. Chest. 2002;121:121S-6S.
3. Anthonisen NR, Connett JE, Enright PL, et al.; Lung Health Study Research Group. Hospitalizations and mortality in the Lung Health Study. Am J Respir Crit Care Med. 2002;166:333-9.
4. Kinnunen T, Saynajakangas O, Tuuponen T, et al. Impact of comorbidities on the duration of COPD patients' hospital episodes. Respir Med. 2003;97:143-6.
5. Cavaillès A, Brinchault-Rabin G, Dixmier A, et al. Comorbidities of COPD. Eur Respir Rev. 2013;22(130):454-75.
6. Vaidyula VR, Criner GJ, Grabianowski C, et al. Circulating tissue factor procoagulant activity is elevated in stable moderate to severe chronic obstructive pulmonary disease. Thromb Res. 2009;124:259-61.
7. Kaczmarek P, Sladek K, Stepien E, et al. Fibrin clot properties are altered in patients with chronic obstructive pulmonary disease. Beneficial effects of simvastatin treatment. Thromb Haemost. 2009;102:1176-82.
8. Aisanov Z, Khaltaev N. Management of cardiovascular comorbidities in chronic obstructive pulmonary disease patients. J Thorac Dis. 2020;12(5):2791-802.
9. Barr RG, Celli BR, Martinez FJ, et al. Physician and patient perceptions in COPD: the COPD Resource Network Needs Assessment Survey. Am J Med. 2005;118:1415.
10. Larsson LG, Lindberg A. Concomitant obstructive sleep apnea and chronic obstructive pulmonary disease: study design—the OLIN OSAS-COPD study. Clin Respir J. 2008;2 (Suppl 1):120-2.
11. Tillie-Leblond I, Marquette CH, Perez T, et al. Pulmonary embolism in patients with unexplained exacerbation of chronic obstructive pulmonary disease: prevalence and risk factors. Ann Intern Med. 2006;144:390-6.
12. Monreal M, Munoz-Torrero JF, Naraine VS, et al.; RIETE Investigators. Pulmonary embolism in patients with chronic obstructive pulmonary disease or congestive heart failure. Am J Med. 2006;119:851-8.
13. Rutschmann OT, Cornuz J, Poletti PA, et al. Should pulmonary embolism be suspected in exacerbation of chronic obstructive pulmonary disease? Thorax. 2007;62:121-5.
14. Lieberman D, Lieberman D, Gelfer Y, et al. Pneumonic vs nonpneumonic acute exacerbations of COPD. Chest. 2002;122:1264-70.
15. Calverley PM, Anderson JA, Celli B, et al.; TORCH investigators. Salmeterol and fluticasone propionate and survival in chronic obstructive pulmonary disease. N Engl J Med. 2007;356:775-89.
16. Rabe KF, Hurd S, Anzueto A, et al. Global Initiative for Chronic Obstructive Lung Disease. Am J Respir Crit Care. 2007;176:532-55.
17. Confalonieri M, Urbino R, Potena A, et al. Hydrocortisone infusion for severe community-acquired pneumonia: a preliminary randomized study. Am J Respir Crit Care Med. 2005;171:242-8.
18. Nomura A, Stemmermann GN, Chyou PH, et al. Prospective study of pulmonary function and lung cancer. Am Rev Respir Dis. 1991;144:307-11.
19. Papi A, Casoni G, Caramori G, et al. COPD increases the risk of squamous histological subtype in smokers who develop non-small cell lung carcinoma. Thorax. 2004;59:679-81.
20. Young RP, Hopkins RJ. How the genetics of lung cancer may overlap with COPD. Respirology. 2011;16:1047-55.
21. Schols AM, Slangen J, Volovics L, et al. Weight loss is a reversible factor in the prognosis of chronic obstructive pulmonary disease. Am J Respir Crit Care Med. 1998;157:1791-7.
22. Landbo C, Prescott E, Lange P, et al. Prognostic value of nutritional status in chronic obstructive pulmonary disease. Am J Respir Crit Care Med. 1999;160:1856-61.
23. Gray-Donald K, Gibbons L, Shapiro SH, et al. Nutritional status and mortality in chronic obstructive pulmonary disease. Am J Respir Crit Care Med. 1996;153:961-6.
24. Koechlin C, Couillard A, Cristol JP, et al. Does systemic inflammation trigger local exercise-induced oxidative stress in COPD? Eur Respir J. 2004;23:538-44.
25. Oudijk EJ, Lammers JW, Koenderman L. Systemic inflammation in chronic obstructive pulmonary disease. Eur Respir J Suppl. 2003;46:5s-13s.
26. Muller EA. Influence of training and of inactivity on muscle strength. Arch Phys Med Rehabil. 1970;51:449-62.
27. Minai OA, Maurer JR, Kesten S. Comorbidities in end-stage lung disease. J Heart Lung Transplant. 1999;18:891-903.
28. Creutzberg EC, Schols AM, Weling-Scheepers CA, et al. Characterization of nonresponse to high caloric oral nutritional therapy in depleted patients with chronic obstructive pulmonary disease. Am J Respir Crit Care Med. 2000;161:745-52.
29. Wilson DO, Rogers RM, Sanders MH, et al. Nutritional intervention in malnourished patients with emphysema. Am Rev Respir Dis. 1986;134:672-7.

30. Reid IR. Osteoporosis–emerging consensus. Aust N Z J Med. 1997;27:643-7.
31. Incalzi RA, Caradonna P, Ranieri P, et al. Correlates of osteoporosis in chronic obstructive pulmonary disease. Respir Med. 2000;94:1079-84.
32. Gluck O, Colice G. Recognizing and treating glucocorticoid-induced osteoporosis in patients with pulmonary diseases. Chest. 2004;125:1859-76.
33. McEvoy CE, Ensrud KE, Bender E, et al. Association between corticosteroid use and vertebral fractures in older men with chronic obstructive pulmonary disease. Am J Respir Crit Care Med. 1998;157:704-9.
34. Jorgensen NR, Schwarz P, Holme I, et al. The prevalence of osteoporosis in patients with chronic obstructive pulmonary disease: A cross-sectional study. Respir Med. 2007;101:177-85.
35. Mokhlesi B, Morris AL, Huang CF, et al. Increased prevalence of gastroesophageal reflux symptoms in patients with COPD. Chest. 2001;119:1043-8.
36. Roussos A, Philippou N, Krietsepi V, et al. *Helicobacter pylori* seroprevalence in patients with chronic obstructive pulmonary disease. Respir Med. 2005;99:279-84.
37. Engstrom G, Janzon L. Risk of developing diabetes is inversely related to lung function: a population-based cohort study. Diabet Med. 2002;19:167-70.
38. Hu FB, Meigs JB, Li TY, et al. Inflammatory markers and risk of developing type 2 diabetes in women. Diabetes. 2004;53: 693-700.
39. Chung KF. Cytokines in chronic obstructive pulmonary disease. Eur Respir J Suppl. 2001;34:50s-9s.
40. Lacedonia D, Carpagnano GE, Aliani M, et al. Daytime PaO_2 in OSAS, COPD and the combination of the two (overlap syndrome). Respir Med. 2013;107(2):310-6.
41. Esendağlı D, Sarınç Ulaşlı S, Esquinas A. Humidification therapy; long-term effects in COPD and OSAS patients. Tuberk Toraks. 2018;66(1):57-63.

Treatment of Chronic Obstructive Pulmonary Disease

CHAPTER 87

Peter J Barnes

INTRODUCTION

Chronic obstructive pulmonary disease (COPD) is characterized in most patients by slowly progressive development of airflow limitation that is not fully reversible.[1] COPD encompasses chronic obstructive bronchiolitis with obstruction of small airways and emphysema with enlargement of airspaces and destruction of lung parenchyma, loss of lung elasticity, and closure of small airways. Chronic bronchitis, by contrast, is defined by a productive cough of more than 3 months duration for more than 2 successive years; this reflects mucous hypersecretion and is not necessarily associated with airflow limitation. Most patients with COPD have all three pathological mechanisms (chronic obstructive bronchitis, emphysema, and mucus plugging) but may differ in the proportion of emphysema and small airway disease. At present, these different phenotypes of COPD do not appear to affect the choice of therapy. However, in the future, as more specific therapies are developed, careful phenotyping and endotyping will be important in selecting optimal therapy.[2]

Chronic obstructive pulmonary disease is one of the most common chronic diseases in elderly people and one of the most frequent causes of hospital admission. Globally, COPD is now the third most common cause of death and the only one that is increasing.[3] COPD is one of the most common causes of death in India.[4] Despite the enormous advances in asthma management that have taken place over the last 10 years, there have been relatively few new developments in the management of COPD. None of the existing drug therapies significantly slows the relentless progression of airway obstruction and lung disease, so treatment is based largely on improving lung function with bronchodilators, together with changes in lifestyle. Since the airflow obstruction in COPD is largely irreversible and current therapies do not alter the course of the disease, existing drug treatments provide only limited benefit to patients. There is now an urgent search for new classes of treatment that might alter the course of disease in the future.

The management of COPD has now been formalized in guidelines produced in several countries and all propose escalating treatment, depending on the severity of airflow obstruction, symptoms, and the risk of exacerbations.[5]

PREVENTION AND RISK FACTORS

It is likely that there are important interactions between environmental factors and a genetic predisposition to develop the disease. Reducing risk factors that are known to worsen the disease is an important aspect of management.

Environmental Risk Factors

In industrialized countries, cigarette smoking accounts for most cases of COPD, but in developing countries, other environmental pollutants, such as particulates associated with cooking with biomass fuels in confined spaces, are important causes.[6] Even in developed countries, nonsmoking COPD may account for over 20% of COPD patients.[7] Much less is known about nonsmoking forms of COPD. Some cases are due to progression of asthma which loses its reversibility, but these are usually identified by early onset and a typical history of variable symptoms at least in the early history of the disease. In developing and emerging countries such as India, exposure to biomass fuels is an important cause of COPD, especially in women, and accounts for over 50% of cases.[8] Nonsmoking COPD due to biomass smoke exposure is similar in most characteristics to COPD due to cigarette smoking, with a similar pattern of airway inflammation, but small airway disease is predominant and there is less emphysema.[9]

Air pollution (particularly sulfur dioxide and particulates), exposure to certain occupational chemicals such as cadmium, and passive smoking may all be additional risk factors. Outdoor air pollution is now recognized as an increasing risk factor for COPD.[10] The role of airway hyperresponsiveness and allergy as risk factors for COPD is still uncertain and airway hyperresponsiveness may be explained by geometric factors due to fixed airway narrowing and differs from the abnormal airway responsiveness of asthma. Low birth weight is also a risk factor for COPD, probably because poor nutrition in fetal life results in small lungs, so that decline in lung function with age starts from a lower peak value. Poor nutrition may contribute to COPD and a lack of dietary antioxidants may be particularly important.

Chest infections during the first year of life are associated with COPD in later life. There is some evidence that certain latent virus infections (such as adenovirus) may predispose to the development of COPD, but this is controversial. Many patients with COPD have a history of previous tuberculosis (TB), whereas patients with COPD have an increased risk of developing TB, although the relationship between COPD and TB is not clear.[11]

The most important management strategy is to reduce exposure to environmental risk factors wherever possible to prevent disease progression. Most attention has focused on smoking cessation strategies.

Stopping Smoking

Stopping smoking is the single most beneficial management strategy and the only intervention that reduces the accelerated decline in lung function and the number of exacerbations and is important even in elderly patients. Stopping smoking also reduces the mucus hypersecretion of chronic bronchitis and markedly reduces the risks of associated cardiovascular disease.[12] Smoking cessation is more effective early in the course of disease and becomes less effective as the disease progresses to severe and very severe disease.

Nicotine is addictive and stopping smoking should be viewed as the treatment of drug addiction. Abrupt quitting is more successful than gradual reduction, but even after an intensive smoking cessation program, 75% of smokers are still smoking 1 year later. There are several ways to encourage smoking cessation. Psychological counseling, group therapy, and smoking reduction measures may be useful in some patients. Nicotine replacement therapy available as chewing gum, skin patches, nasal spray, and inhaler (including e-cigarettes) doubles long-term (6–12 months) abstinence rates. Bupropion is an atypical antidepressant that acts through stimulating noradrenergic activity and has double the quit rate of nicotine replacement therapies. Varenicline, a partial nicotinic agonist and the most effective antismoking drug, is the most effective way of quitting smoking.[13] Varenicline is usually given for 12 weeks and is well tolerated, but some patients develop nausea, insomnia, and depression.

Avoiding Biomass Fuel Exposure

It is exposure to biomass fuels (wood, charcoal, and animal dung) in unventilated houses which is a major risk factor for COPD in developing countries. This may be addressed by using alternative fuels, such as liquefied petroleum gas (LPG) or natural gas, ethanol, or biogas, although this may not be available or affordable in poor rural communities. Improving ventilation of the cooking area, reducing cooking time, or cooking outdoors may also help. Substitution of traditional open fires with locally produced improved stoves has been shown to improve respiratory health in women and to improve lung function and disease progression.[14]

Genetic Factors

Longitudinal monitoring of lung function in cigarette smokers reveals that only a minority (15–40% depending on definition) develop significant airflow obstruction due to an accelerated decline in lung function [two- to fivefold higher than the normal decline of 15–30 mL forced expiratory volume in 1 second (FEV_1)/year] compared to the normal population and the remainder of smokers who have consumed an equivalent number of cigarettes. This strongly suggests that genetic factors may determine which smokers are susceptible and develop airflow limitation. Further evidence that genetic factors are important is the familial clustering of patients with early-onset COPD and the differences in COPD prevalence between different ethnic groups. Patients with α_1-antitrypsin deficiency [proteinase inhibitor (Pi)ZZ phenotype with α_1-antitrypsin levels <10% of normal values] develop early emphysema which is exacerbated by smoking, indicating a clear genetic predisposition to COPD.[15] However, α_1-antitrypsin deficiency accounts for <1% of patients with COPD and many other genetic variants of α_1-antitrypsin that are associated with lower than normal serum levels of this proteinase inhibitor have not been clearly associated with an increased risk of COPD. This has led to a search for associations between COPD and polymorphisms of other genes that may be involved in its pathophysiology.[16]

So far, few significant associations have been detected and even those reported have not been replicated in other studies. A tenfold increased risk of COPD in individuals who have a polymorphism in the promoter region of the gene for tumor necrosis factor-alpha (TNF-α) that is associated with increased TNF-α production has been reported in a Chinese population but not confirmed in Caucasian populations. Several other genes have been implicated in COPD, but few have been replicated in different populations. Genome-wide association studies in COPD have found susceptibility related to two polymorphisms of the nicotinic receptor, which probably reflect propensity to nicotine addiction. It is unlikely that molecular genetics will identify new therapeutic targets. Even in patients with α_1-antitrypsin deficiency, replacement therapy has been poorly effective as well as very expensive. Techniques such as deoxyribonucleic acid (DNA) microarray (gene chips) to detect single nucleotide polymorphisms, proteomics to detect novel proteins, and gene expression profiling to measure which known and novel genes are expressed are now being employed in cigarette smokers who develop COPD compared with matched smokers who do not. This may identify markers of risk but may also reveal novel molecular targets for the development of treatments of the future.

BRONCHODILATORS

Bronchodilators are the mainstay of current drug therapy for COPD, although the degree of bronchodilatation is less than seen in asthma (typically about 5% improvement in FEV_1, although some patients show greater responses). Bronchodilators may improve dyspnea and exercise tolerance, despite little or no effect on spirometry, by reducing lung volumes and therefore hyperinflation (air trapping).[17] In addition, bronchodilators may reduce respiratory muscle fatigue (controversial) and improve mucociliary clearance. The choice of bronchodilator includes short and long-acting β_2-agonists (LABA), anticholinergics (muscarinic receptor antagonists), and theophylline, which will partly be determined by patient preference and cost. The preferred bronchodilators are long-acting inhaled drugs such as LABA (formoterol, salmeterol, indacaterol, vilanterol, and olodaterol) or long-acting muscarinic antagonist (LAMA: Tiotropium bromide, glycopyrrolate, umeclidinium, and aclidinium) **(Table 1)**. Long-acting inhaled bronchodilators are more effective than short-acting bronchodilators, and in general, once-daily drugs are more effective than twice-daily drugs.

TABLE 1: Bronchodilators for COPD.

Drug	Inhaler	Nebulizer	Oral	Duration (hours)
β_2-agonists				
Short acting:				
Salbutamol	MDI, DPI	Yes	Yes	4–6
Terbutaline	DPI		Yes	4–6
Fenoterol	MDI	Yes	Yes	4–6
Long acting:				
Formoterol	DPI	Yes		12
Salmeterol	MDI, DPI			12
Indacaterol	DPI			24
Olodaterol	SMI			24
Anticholinergics				
Ipratropium bromide	MDI	Yes		6–8
Oxitropium bromide	MDI			7–9
Aclidinium bromide	DPI			12
Tiotropium bromide	DPI, MDI, SMI			24
Glycopyrrolate	DPI	Yes		12–24
Umeclidinium	DPI			24
Revefenacin		Yes		24
Combinations				
SABA/SAMA:				
Salbutamol/ipratropium	MDI, SMI			6–8
Fenoterol/ipratropium	SMI			6–8
LABA/LAMA:				
Formoterol/aclidinium	DPI			12
Formoterol/glycopyrrolate	DPI			12
Indacaterol/glycopyrrolate	DPI			24
Vilanterol/umeclidinium	DPI			24
Olodaterol/tiotropium	SMI			24

Continued

Continued

Drug	Inhaler	Nebulizer	Oral	Duration (hours)
ICS/LABA:				
FP/salmeterol	MDI, DP			12
Budesonide/formoterol	DPI			12
BDP/formoterol	MDI, DPI			12
Mometasone/formoterol	DPI			12
FF/vilanterol	DPI			24
ICS/LABA/LAMA (triple):				
BDP/formoterol/glycopyrrolate	MDI, DPI			12
Budesonide/formoterol/glycopyrrolate	DPI			12
FF/vilanterol/umeclidinium	DPI			24
Theophylline				
Theophylline SR			Yes	24
Aminophylline SR			Yes	24

(BDP: beclomethasone dipropionate; COPD: chronic obstructive pulmonary disease; DPI: dry powder inhaler; FF: fluticasone furoate; FP: fluticasone propionate; ICS: inhaled corticosteroids; LABA: long-acting β_2-agonist; LAMA: long-acting muscarinic antagonist; MDI: metered dose inhaler; SAMA: short-acting β_2-agonist; SAMA: short-acting muscarinic antagonist; SMI: soft mist inhaler; SR: slow release)

Anticholinergics

Atropine is a naturally occurring compound that was introduced for the treatment of asthma, but because of side effects (particularly, drying of secretions), less soluble quaternary compounds (e.g., ipratropium bromide) were developed. Anticholinergics are probably the most effective bronchodilators in the treatment of COPD and vagal cholinergic tone appears to be the only reversible element in the airflow obstruction of COPD.

Mode of Action

Anticholinergics are specific antagonists of muscarinic receptors and inhibit cholinergic nerve-induced bronchoconstriction. A small degree of resting bronchomotor tone is present because of tonic cholinergic nerve impulses, which release acetylcholine in the vicinity of airway smooth muscle and cholinergic reflex bronchoconstriction may be initiated by irritants, cold air, and stress **(Fig. 1)**. Anticholinergics reduce air trapping by acting on small airways and thereby improve dyspnea and symptoms.

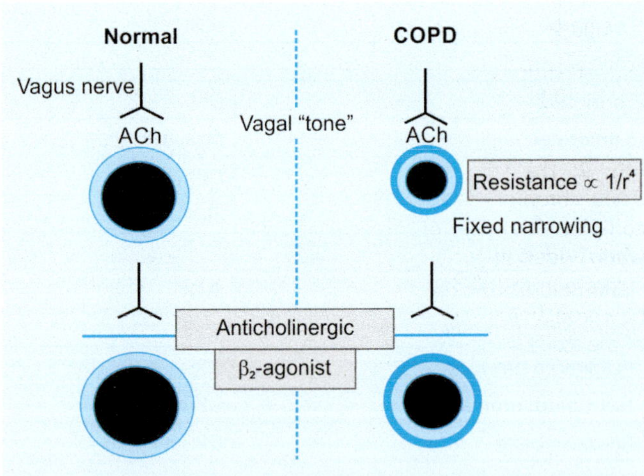

FIG. 1: Cholinergic control of airways in chronic obstructive pulmonary disease (COPD). Normally, there is a certain amount of cholinergic tone. This is exaggerated in COPD because of geometric factors related to the fixed narrowing of the airways (airway resistance R is proportional to $1/r^4$, where r is airway radius), so that airway resistance improves to a greater extent than in normal airways with an anticholinergic drug, which blocks the effect of acetylcholine (ACh) on muscarinic receptors in airway smooth muscle. Beta-agonists, which block all known bronchoconstrictor mechanisms, have a similar effect to anticholinergics, suggesting that vagal tone is the only reversible component in COPD.

Clinical Use

Ipratropium bromide and oxitropium bromide are administered three or four times daily via inhalation, whereas tiotropium bromide is given once daily by inhalation. Tiotropium is very effective in improving lung function and quality of life at all stages of disease even when added to other therapies, as shown in the large UPLIFT study[18] **(Fig. 2)**. Tiotropium also reduces severe exacerbations and hospital admissions, as well as mortality from COPD and cardiovascular disease. In addition to tiotropium, there are other LAMA now available, including glycopyrrolate, umeclidinium, olodaterol, and revefenacin, which are given once daily and aclidinium, which is administered twice daily.[19]

Anticholinergic drugs may have additive bronchodilator effects with β_2-agonists, so they may be given together in a fixed combination inhaler. For short-acting drugs, ipratropium-salbutamol inhalers are popular. Once-daily inhaled LABA-LAMA combinations are now the bronchodilators of choice in the management of COPD and have become first-line therapy.[5] LABA-LAMA combinations may be once daily (indacaterol-glycopyrrolate, vilanterol-umeclidinium, and olodaterol-tiotropium) or twice daily (formoterol-glycopyrrolate and formoterol-aclidinium) and give added bronchodilatation and greater reduction in symptoms and exacerbations.[20]

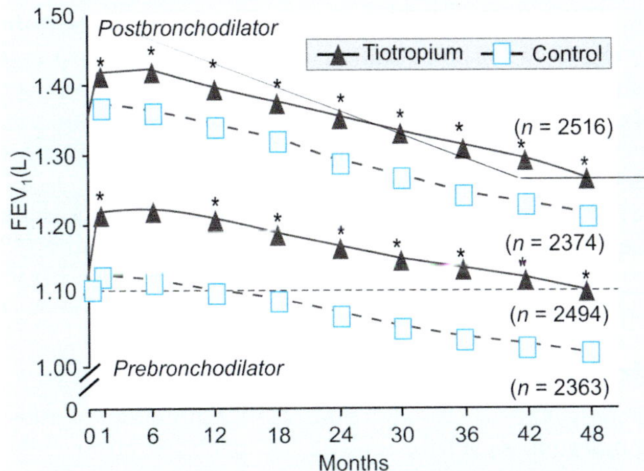

FIG. 2: The UPLIFT study. This large study of approximately 6,000 chronic obstructive pulmonary disease (COPD) patients compared tiotropium bromide (18 μg once daily) with placebo when added to current therapy. Tiotropium resulted in a greater increase in forced expiratory volume in 1 second (FEV_1) pre- and postbronchodilator, which was sustained throughout the 4 years of the study.[18]

Side Effects

Inhaled anticholinergic drugs are well tolerated and systemic side effects are uncommon because almost no systemic absorption occurs. Ipratropium bromide, even in high doses, has no detectable effect on airway secretions. Nebulized ipratropium bromide may precipitate glaucoma in elderly patients as a result of a direct effect of the nebulized drug on the eye; this is avoided by use of a mouthpiece rather than a face mask. Dry mouth occurs in about 5–10% of patients on LAMA but rarely requires discontinuation of treatment.

β_2-agonists

Short-acting β_2-agonists are used mainly as required for symptom relief but may be used four times a day on a regular basis. LABA are preferred therapy for COPD as they give better control of symptoms and are used as a maintenance therapy either once or twice a day.[21]

Mode of Action

Beta2-agonists have several beneficial effects on the airways in COPD **(Fig. 3)**. These drugs act on airway smooth muscle, causing a relaxation in large and small airways. They act as functional antagonists and reverse bronchoconstriction irrespective of the cause. Experimentally, they reduce plasma exudation and cholinergic reflexes. They also increase mucociliary clearance (when it is reduced) and have no effect on chronic inflammation. Evidence suggests that β_2-agonists may reduce adherence of bacteria to airway epithelial cells and this may reduce infective exacerbations. There is some evidence that β_2-agonists may increase the ventilatory drive to hypercapnia (but not to hypoxia).

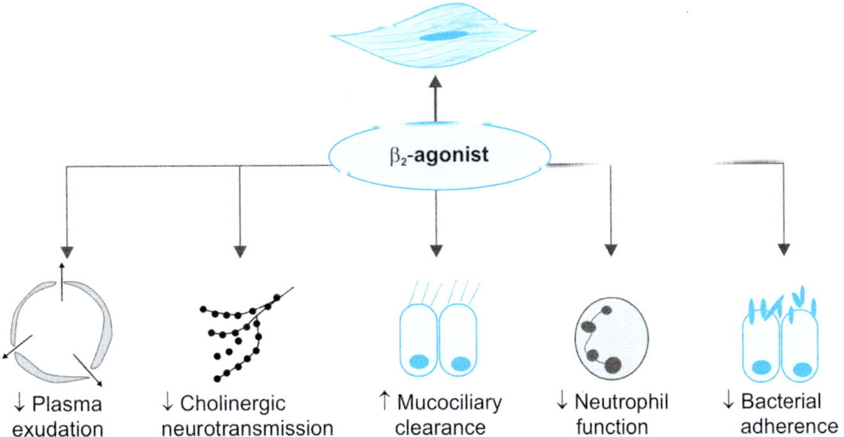

FIG. 3: Mechanism of action of β_2-agonists in chronic obstructive pulmonary disease (COPD). Although their primary action is likely to be on airway smooth muscle, there are additional effects of β_2-agonists that may be beneficial.

Side Effects

Side effects are not usually a problem; excessive use does not appear to be dangerous, even in patients with hypoxia and with cardiovascular disease.

- Muscle tremor (direct effect on skeletal muscle β_2-receptors)—more common in elderly patients
- Tachycardia (direct effect on atrial β_2-receptors, reflex effect from increased peripheral vasodilatation via β_2-receptors)
- Hypokalemia (direct effect on skeletal muscle uptake of potassium ions via β_2-receptors)—usually a small effect
- Restlessness
- Hypoxemia (increased V/Q mismatch due to pulmonary vasodilatation)

Short-acting β_2-agonists

Short-acting inhaled β_2-agonists, such as salbutamol and terbutaline, are recommended for the immediate relief of symptoms. They should not be used regularly (as tolerance to their protective effects occurs), although in patients with severe COPD regular nebulized β_2-agonists may be indicated.

Long-acting Inhaled β_2-agonists

Salmeterol and formoterol give bronchodilatation and protection against bronchoconstriction for over 12 hours. Indacaterol, vilanterol, and olodaterol are a once-daily LABA that are approved for use in COPD. There is compelling evidence that these LABAs are useful as bronchodilators in patients with COPD and that once-daily drugs are more effective than twice-daily drugs. These drugs may improve symptoms, quality of life, and exercise performance and reduce air trapping through relaxant effects on small airways. In long-term studies, they are safe and reduce exacerbations and mortality.[22,23] They have a similar efficacy to anticholinergics, but together they have additive effects as discussed earlier.

Oral β_2-agonists

Although inhaled β_2-agonists are preferred, some elderly patients have problems with using inhalers. Slow-release oral β_2-agonist preparations, such as bambuterol and slow-release salbutamol, are available. An advantage of these preparations is that they may treat peripheral airways more effectively, but the disadvantage is that side effects are more frequent than with inhaled preparations. Bambuterol is a prodrug which is slowly metabolized to terbutaline and is effective as a once-daily preparation.[24]

Theophylline

Theophylline in high doses (with plasma concentration 10–20 mg/L) is a useful additional bronchodilator in patients with severe COPD.[25] Oral administration has the advantage of treating small airways. It may have additional properties such as effects on mucociliary clearance and on respiratory muscles that are useful **(Fig. 4)**. The major limitation to the use of theophylline is its side effects when high doses are used. Lower doses of theophylline (plasma concentration 5–10 mg/L) have anti-inflammatory effects in COPD patients and specifically reduce neutrophilic inflammation.[26]

Mode of Action

Theophylline acts through nonselective inhibition of phosphodiesterases (PDE), resulting in increased intracellular concentrations of cyclic adenosine monophosphate (AMP) and cyclic guanosine monophosphate (GMP).[26] This effect is important for bronchodilator action and might also be important in reducing neutrophilic inflammation. The drug also has some adenosine receptor antagonism, which accounts for some of the side effects, but there is little evidence that this is relevant for bronchodilator effects. It is difficult to explain all of the beneficial effects of theophylline through these mechanisms alone, as many only occur at

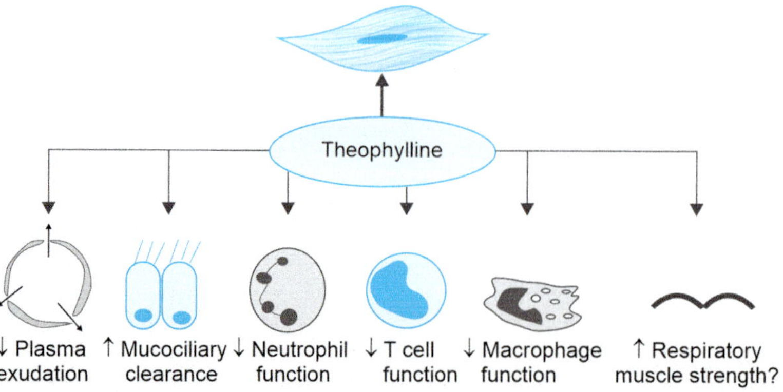

FIG. 4: Mechanism of action of theophylline in chronic obstructive pulmonary disease (COPD). There may be several mechanisms of action of this drug apart from bronchodilatation. At subbronchodilator doses, theophylline reduces neutrophilic inflammation in COPD.

concentrations higher than those used therapeutically. Low concentrations of theophylline reverse corticosteroid resistance in COPD cells in vitro through direct inhibition of oxidative stress-activated phosphoinositide-3-kinase-δ, which results in increased histone deacetylase-2 activity which restores steroid responsiveness.[27] However, two large clinical trials have failed to show any clinical benefit of low-dose theophylline in patients treated with inhaled corticosteroids (ICS).[28,29]

Recommended Use in Chronic Obstructive Pulmonary Disease

Theophylline is recommended as an additional bronchodilator in patients not controlled on regular inhaled LAMA and LABA. A slow-release preparation should be given twice daily to achieve plasma concentrations of 10–20 mg/L. The recent demonstration that theophylline has anti-inflammatory effects and reverses corticosteroid resistance in COPD may lead to the use of low doses (plasma concentration 1–5 mg/L) as a maintenance treatment combined with low doses of ICS.[26]

Side Effects

Side effects are related to plasma concentration, although some patients may be particularly susceptible to side effects. They may be reduced by slowly increasing the dose when the drug is introduced. Side effects are mainly due to PDE inhibition and include:

- Nausea and vomiting
- Headache
- Restlessness
- Gastroesophageal reflux
- Diuresis
- Cardiac arrhythmias (usually plasma concentration >20 mg/L and due to adenosine receptor antagonism)
- Epileptic seizures (usually plasma concentration >30 mg/L and due to adenosine receptor antagonism)

Clearance of Theophylline

The therapeutic effect is related to plasma concentration, which is affected by several factors that alter clearance. If in doubt, plasma concentrations should be measured.

Increased clearance (increase dose):

- Enzyme induction (rifampicin, phenobarbitone, and ethanol)
- Smoking (tobacco and marijuana)
- Childhood
- High-protein, low-carbohydrate diet
- Barbecued meat

Decreased clearance (decrease dose):

- Enzyme inhibition (cimetidine, erythromycin, ciprofloxacin, allopurinol, and ketoconazole)
- Congestive heart failure
- Liver disease
- Pneumonia
- Viral infection and vaccination
- High-carbohydrate diet

Doxofylline: It is a methylxanthine with similar bronchodilator properties to theophylline.[30] It is not an adenosine receptor antagonist, so there is reduced risk of cardiac arrhythmias or seizures. It does not significantly inhibit PDE isoenzymes which may also contribute to its better safety profile. In addition there are fewer drug interactions.

CORTICOSTEROIDS

The role of corticosteroids in the management of COPD is controversial.[31] Maintenance treatment with oral corticosteroids should be avoided as there is no evidence of benefit and a high risk of side effects, particularly muscle wasting in COPD populations. ICS are commonly prescribed in high doses on the basis that COPD is like poorly responsive asthma, but they are not beneficial in most patients with COPD. Approximately, 10% of patients with COPD have a positive response to oral corticosteroids and it is likely that these patients have coexisting asthma [asthma-COPD overlap (ACO)] and should therefore be treated as if they are asthmatic with regular ICS. These patients may be recognized by increased eosinophils in the sputum and nitric oxide in the breath.[32]

Patients with COPD have a poor response to corticosteroids in comparison to asthma with little improvement in lung function. High doses of ICS have consistently been shown a reduction (~20%) in exacerbations in patients with severe disease and this is the main clinical indication for their use. Several large studies have shown that corticosteroids fail to reduce the progression in COPD (measured by annual fall in FEV_1) and they do not significantly reduce mortality.[33,34] These results are likely to reflect the resistance of pulmonary inflammation to corticosteroids in COPD patients as a result of the reduction in histone deacetylase 2 (HDAC2).[35] However, increasing evidence suggests that blood and sputum eosinophils may predict efficacy of ICS for reducing exacerbations in COPD.[36] Thus, ICS may be added to dual bronchodilator therapy in COPD patients with two or more exacerbations or one hospital admission for exacerbation if blood eosinophil count is >300 cells/μL.[5]

Side Effects

The reduction in the frequency of exacerbations may be offset by systemic side effects of ICS, such as osteoporosis, particularly in an elderly population that may be poorly nourished with reduced mobility. There is evidence that high-dose ICS are associated with increased cataracts and that there is an increased risk of diabetes in COPD patients. Several large trials of high-dose ICS have shown an increase in pneumonia amongst COPD patients.[37]

This increased risk of pneumonia is seen mainly in patients with low blood eosinophils (<100 cells/μL) and with bacterial colonization of the lower airways. The increased risk of pneumonia may be due to suppression of antibacterial peptides by topical corticosteroids.[38] Slow withdrawal of ICS in COPD patients, even with severe disease and a history of exacerbations, is not associated with increased exacerbations, unless blood eosinophils are >300 cells/μL.[39,40]

Combination Inhalers

Inhaled corticosteroids should never be used alone in the management of COPD but always combined with a long-acting bronchodilator. ICS/LABA combinations are effective in reducing exacerbations in COPD if blood eosinophils are >300 cells/μL and are also indicated in patients with COPD who have features of asthma (ACO). However, for the majority of patients with COPD, ICS/LABA inhalers are less effective in improving lung function than LABA/LAMA combination because of the additive effects on LABA and LAMA and may be less effective at reducing exacerbations.

Several triple inhalers are now approved for use in COPD patients, including fluticasone furoate/vilanterol/umeclidinium once daily and beclomethasone/formoterol/glycopyrrolate and budesonide/formoterol/glycopyrrolate twice daily. Triple inhalers are indicated in patients on LAB/LAMA inhalers who have exacerbations if blood eosinophils >300 cells/μL.[41] There is some evidence that mortality may also be reduced compared to LABA/LAMA therapy, mainly due to a reduction in cardiovascular deaths, although more studies are needed to overcome this.[42]

PHOSPHODIESTERASE INHIBITORS

Theophylline is a weak, nonselective inhibitor of PDE, which breaks down cyclic nucleotides (cyclic AMP and cyclic GMP), resulting in bronchodilatation and anti-inflammatory effects. PDE4 inhibitors have a broad spectrum of anti-inflammatory effects in vitro and animal models of COPD show good anti-inflammatory effects.[43] Several selective PDE4 inhibits have been tested in COPD and most failed because of insufficient clinical efficacy or unacceptable side effects (most commonly nausea, vomiting, diarrhea, and headaches). Roflumilast is the only PDE4 inhibitor approved for COPD which provides only modest clinical benefit in COPD patients with severe disease and frequent exacerbations. There is a small improvement in lung function but no significant improvement in symptoms or quality of life and a small (~20%) reduction in exacerbation frequency.[44] However, many patients develop side effects and discontinue therapy. It may be indicated for patients with frequent exacerbations instead of high-dose ICS. The best responses to roflumilast are seen in COPD patients with severe disease (FEV_1 < 50% predicted), a history of chronic bronchitis with frequent exacerbations.[45]

SUPPLEMENTARY OXYGEN

Poor oxygenation is a problem in patients with severe COPD who may be considered for supplementary oxygen therapy.[46] Controlled oxygen (24%) is used acutely in the treatment of acute exacerbations in all patients who are hospitalized. Long-term oxygen therapy (LTOT, domiciliary oxygen) is indicated in selected patients with COPD. Two large multicenter trials demonstrated that long-term oxygen administration (>15 hours daily) prolongs survival (by about 30%) in patients with COPD. The goal of oxygen therapy is to increase partial pressure of arterial oxygen (PaO_2) to around 60 mm Hg or oxygen saturation of >90%; increasing PaO_2 above 60 mm Hg has little further benefit and increases the risk of CO_2 retention.[47] There is a danger of inducing respiratory failure if supplementary oxygen is used in patients with CO_2 retention, so careful assessment is required before oxygen is prescribed.

Long-term oxygen therapy may have several beneficial effects:

- Improvement in exercise capacity (increased endurance)
- Reduction in dyspnea
- Reduction in pulmonary hypertension by reducing hypoxic pulmonary vasoconstriction
- Reduction in hematocrit by reducing erythropoietin levels
- Improved quality of life and neuropsychiatric function
- Reduction in severe desaturation episodes during sleep

There are three methods of providing domiciliary oxygen therapy:

1. Long-term, low-dose oxygen for patients with chronic respiratory failure
2. Portable oxygen therapy for exercise-related hypoxia and dyspnea
3. Short-burst oxygen therapy for temporary relief of symptoms

Selection of Patients for Long-term Oxygen Therapy

In some countries, guidelines (Department of Health) have been drawn up for the provision of LTOT. LTOT should not be considered in patients who continue to smoke. All patients should be assessed by a pulmonary specialist.

Absolute indications are:

- Stable COPD with hypoxemia and edema
- FEV_1 < 1.5 L, forced vital capacity (FVC) < 2.0 L
- PaO_2 < 55 mm Hg (<7.3 kPa), partial pressure of arterial carbon dioxide ($PaCO_2$) > 45 mm Hg (>6 kPa)
- Stability demonstrated over 3 weeks on optimal therapy

Relative indications are:

- As abovementioned but without edema or $PaCO_2$ > 45 mm Hg
- Palliative (symptom relief)

Portable oxygen is indicated in patients who desaturate during exercise and its efficacy needs to be assessed during a treadmill or 6-minute walk test with patients wearing the portable oxygen cylinder. Portable oxygen may also be indicated in patients with severe exercise limitation irrespective of oxygen desaturation. Portable oxygen may also be needed in such patients during commercial airline flights (provided by airline).

ANTIBIOTICS

Infection is often the cause of progression or acute deterioration in patients with COPD; the combating of infection by the appropriate use of antibiotics is an important part of therapy.[48] In fact, the organisms causing pulmonary infections are often the same as those found normally in the upper respiratory tract. It may be difficult to know if a pathogen isolated from the sputum is responsible for the exacerbation. For most of the time, the sputum in COPD is mucoid but becomes yellow or green with exacerbations of infection and when this occurs, it is usual to begin empirical antibiotic therapy. Purulence of sputum is due to an increase in degranulating neutrophils and may not necessarily imply bacterial infection. Indeed, many exacerbations of COPD are likely to be due to upper respiratory tract virus infections, such as rhinovirus, respiratory syncytial virus, coronavirus, and parainfluenza virus.[49] This means that antibiotics are often used inappropriately, but it is difficult to tell clinically whether an infection is viral or bacterial in origin. In a meta-analysis of placebo-controlled trials of antibiotics for COPD, there was a small difference in clinical outcomes between patients treated with antibiotics and placebo, except for patients with very severe exacerbations in the intensive care unit.[50]

The common bacterial organisms responsible for exacerbations of COPD include *Haemophilus influenzae* (*H. influenzae*), *Streptococcus pneumoniae*, and *Moraxella catarrhalis* and these are the organisms that most commonly colonize the lower airways of COPD patients. The choice of antibiotic depends upon the likely organisms, the likely sensitivity of the organisms in the community, the tolerance of the patient for the drug, and the response to treatment. The treatment of choice in the community will often be either amoxycillin or cotrimoxazole (Septrin). Cotrimoxazole is not recommended as development of resistance and side effects due to the sulfonamide component are relatively common. Since many strains of *H. influenzae* are now β-lactamase producers and hence resistant to ampicillin/amoxycillin, the choice for initial therapy commonly lies between:

- Amoxycillin/clavulanic acid (augmentin)
- Erythromycin or other macrolides (clarithromycin, azithromycin)
- A cephalosporin, for example, cefaclor
- A tetracycline, for example, doxycycline

There are advantages and disadvantages of each drug and the choice may finally be based on finding out which drug works for a given patient. Cost is also a factor and there is no justification for using an expensive drug when a cheaper one works just as well. In most cases, the choice usually falls between amoxycillin, amoxycillin/clavulanic acid, or doxycycline for the typical ambulatory patient.

The antibiotic should be given in full therapeutic doses for a course lasting about 10–14 days except for clarithromycin and azithromycin which are given for shorter periods (3 days). Treatment is then stopped provided the patient has responded. If there has been a poor response, a change of antibiotic may be indicated, usually to one of the newer broad-spectrum agents such as clarithromycin if this has not already been tried. Continuous antibiotic administration is not recommended as this has not been shown to alter the course of the disease and is likely to lead to an increase in resistant organisms. Macrolide antibiotics (erythromycin and azithromycin) reduce exacerbations of COPD, but it is not certain whether this is an antibiotic or an anti-inflammatory effect of the macrolide.[51] Since long-term macrolide treatment may have adverse effects (cardiovascular risk and deafness) and increased bacterial resistance, they may be only indicated in selected patients, such as those with coexistent bronchiectasis who have persistently purulent sputum.

OTHER DRUG THERAPIES

Mucolytics

Because mucus hypersecretion is a prominent feature of chronic bronchitis, various mucolytic therapies have been used to increase the ease of mucus expectoration in the belief that this will improve lung function.[52] Chronic bronchitis is present in 30–50% of patients with COPD and is usually accompanied by a neutrophilic pattern of inflammation; neutrophil products are potent stimulants of goblet cell and mucus gland secretions in the airways.[53]

- *Stopping smoking* is the most effective way to reduce mucus hypersecretion.
- *Anticholinergics* may decrease mucus hypersecretion.
- β_2-*agonists* and *theophylline* may improve mucus clearance.
- *Steam inhalation* (with or without aromatics) may provide symptomatic relief, but there is no evidence that it improves lung function or long-term symptom control.
- Several drugs, such as *bromhexol* and *ambroxol*, reduce mucus viscosity *in vitro*, but there is little evidence from controlled trials that they improve lung function in patients with COPD and cannot be recommended as routine therapy.
- Expectorants, such as *guaifenesin* and *potassium iodide*, similarly have no proven beneficial effects.
- *Recombinant human deoxyribonuclease (DNAse)* (dornase alfa and Pulmozyme) has beneficial effects in

some patients with cystic fibrosis, but its role in COPD is not yet clear. Until there is clear evidence of benefit, it should not be used in view of its high cost.

Antioxidants

Since oxidant damage may be critical in the pathophysiology of COPD, antioxidant therapy is logical.[54] N-acetyl-cysteine (NAC) and carbocisteine were originally developed as mucolytics but have well-documented antioxidant effects. Several small studies demonstrated a beneficial effect of NAC in reducing exacerbations of COPD by approximately 25%; meta-analysis has shown little effect and no effect on the quality of life.[55] In a large prospective controlled trial, NAC failed to reduce exacerbations, improve health status, or reduce disease progression.[56] Large studies from China showed that carbocisteine and NAC significantly reduced exacerbations, especially in less severe patients.[57,58] At present, these therapies are not recommended for routine use because of relative lack of efficacy in patients already treated with inhaled bronchodilators and corticosteroids.

Vaccines

- Influenza vaccine is recommended as patients with COPD are subject to severe exacerbations with this infection and there is evidence for a reduction in acute exacerbations and hospital admissions. Influenza vaccination is cost-effective in elderly people and should be more so in patients with COPD. Influenza vaccination reduces all-cause mortality.[59] It should be given prior to the winter season.
- Coronavirus disease 2019 (COVID-19) vaccination is recommended for all patients with COPD and COPD patients may be more likely to suffer severe COVID-19 disease.
- Polyvalent pneumococcal vaccine is used in many countries to protect against the development of pneumococcal lung infections. Pneumococcal vaccination does not reduce mortality[59] and there are no convincing large trials to show a reduction in exacerbations.[60] Improved vaccines are now in development.
- OM85-BV (Broncho-Vaxom) is a mixture of bacterial products that activate macrophage function (the advantage of which is obscure!). There is some evidence that it may reduce the severity of acute exacerbations but there are no consistent clinical benefits so it cannot be recommended as a routine treatment.[61]

Treatment of Dyspnea

Breathlessness is a problem in many patients, particularly in those with severe emphysema. Several drugs, including nebulized opiates, slow-release morphine, dihydrocodeine, and benzodiazepines, may reduce the sensation of dyspnea, but the reduction in ventilatory drive is potentially dangerous and these drugs should be avoided, particularly during exacerbations.[62]

Respiratory Stimulants

There is no role for respiratory stimulants, such as doxapram or almitrine, in the long-term management of COPD, since there is no evidence that central ventilatory drive is impaired. Ventilation is limited by mechanical rather than neurophysiological factors. However, doxapram may be indicated in the management of an acute exacerbation of COPD if there is hypercapnia and hypoventilation in order to tide the patient over 24–36 hours until the underlying cause (e.g., infection) is controlled. It is likely that the use of doxapram in this situation will decline as nasal intermittent positive pressure ventilation (NIPPV) becomes more widely available.

Antitussives

Cough is often a troublesome symptom of COPD but may have a protective effect in clearing secretions. The regular use of antitussives is therefore not recommended in COPD.[63]

NONPHARMACOLOGICAL TREATMENTS

Several nonpharmacological approaches have been also used in the management of COPD and may form part of a comprehensive rehabilitation program in elderly patients.

Exercise

Exercise training to improve cardiorespiratory function is helpful; the type of exercise does not appear to be important and aerobic exercise or upper limb exercises are equally effective. Respiratory muscle training using resistive inspiratory loading may reduce breathlessness, but an analysis of several controlled studies of respiratory muscle training alone has provided no evidence of clear overall benefit.[64] Controlled breathing techniques, such as pursed lip breathing and diaphragmatic breathing, result in reduced dyspnea, particularly in patients with hyperventilation.

Nutrition

Nutrition is important in patients with COPD; many patients are malnourished and underweight, although marked cachexia is uncommon. Many COPD patients are obese because of reduced physical activity who should lose weight, particularly if there are sleep disturbances or they have metabolic syndrome or frank type 2 diabetes. Antioxidant vitamin supplements may also be used. There is no convincing evidence that improved nutrition is beneficial in COPD patients and there is no evidence that nutritional supplements with a high fat content that are marketed for use in COPD have any special value.[65] The place of androgens and anabolic steroids to build muscle bulk in COPD has not been established.[66]

Pulmonary Rehabilitation

Rehabilitation concerns prevention of deconditioning and allowing the patient to cope with his/her disease. Rehabilitation programs are successful in prospective randomized trials in terms of increased performance and quality of life and reduce exacerbations, even though they may not improve lung function.[67,68] Patients with moderate-to-severe COPD should be considered for pulmonary rehabilitation programs, which include educational advice and physiotherapy. There is evidence that pulmonary rehabilitation also increases the efficacy of bronchodilator therapy.[69]

Artificial Ventilation

Artificial ventilation devices have improved enormously. Noninvasive ventilation using NIPPV has been an important advancement in the management of acute exacerbations of COPD in hospital and more recently in the control of hypercapnic respiratory failure at home, thus reducing the need for hospitalization. There is no good evidence for the use of nocturnal NIPPV in stable COPD.[70] NIPPV corrects hypercapnia and respiratory acidosis. Good results in management of acute exacerbations have been reported, with significant reduction in mortality and time spent in hospital.[71]

Surgery

Several surgical techniques have been successfully applied to more severe emphysema. These include heart-lung transplantation, now largely replaced by single lung transplantation in carefully selected patients.[72] Lung volume reduction surgery (LVRS) by excision of badly affected emphysematous lung is effective in highly selected patients with bilateral, predominantly upper lobe emphysema and evidence of air trapping. There is sustained improvement in lung function and reduction in symptoms and exacerbations.[73] Patients with a very poor diffusing capacity had an increased mortality. More recently, bronchoscopic LVRS has been developed to avoid the surgical morbidity and mortality of LVRS. Several devices, including one-way valves, coils, sealants, airway bypass stents, and bronchoscopic thermal vapor ablation, designed to collapse and remodel hyperinflated lung, are currently being tried in clinical trials.[74]

MANAGING CHRONIC DISEASE

It is important that an accurate diagnosis is made and COPD differentiated from asthma, which is usually possible from the history. Spirometry is important to diagnose airway obstruction objectively and to stage the disease in order to determine severity and progression when measured serially. In the Global Initiative for Chronic Obstructive Lung Disease (GOLD) strategy for COPD, treatment of chronic disease follows a stepwise escalation based on disease severity, symptoms, and risk of exacerbations.[5] At all stages, smoking cessation is important, particularly in the early stages of disease and patients should routinely receive immunization against seasonal influenza and COVID-19. The choice of initial therapy is based on symptoms [COPD assessment test (CAT) score, modified Medical Research Council (mMRC) dyspnea score] and number of exacerbations in the previous year (hospitalizations and moderate exacerbations treated with antibiotics or oral corticosteroids) **(Fig. 5)**. For patients in Group A with few or no symptoms and <1 exacerbation/year, a bronchodilator to treat symptoms is recommended, whereas in Group B, patients with more symptoms (CAT ≥ 10, mMRC ≥ 2) but few if any exacerbations (most COPD patients), a LABA/LAMA combination is recommended. For Group E patients with significant exacerbations (≥2 moderate exacerbations or >1 hospitalization), a LABA/LAMA combination is recommended, unless blood eosinophils are ≥300 cells/μL when a triple inhaler should be considered. If patients require further treatment, it is important to evaluate adherence to therapy as well as inhaler technique. For patients who continue to have exacerbations, addition of roflumilast should be considered in patients with chronic bronchitis and severe disease or a macrolide such as azithromycin, especially if sputum is purulent. Pulmonary rehabilitation is also useful is some patients if it is available. In very severe patients, it is necessary to consider the use of supplementary oxygen and for very selected patients, lung volume reduction.

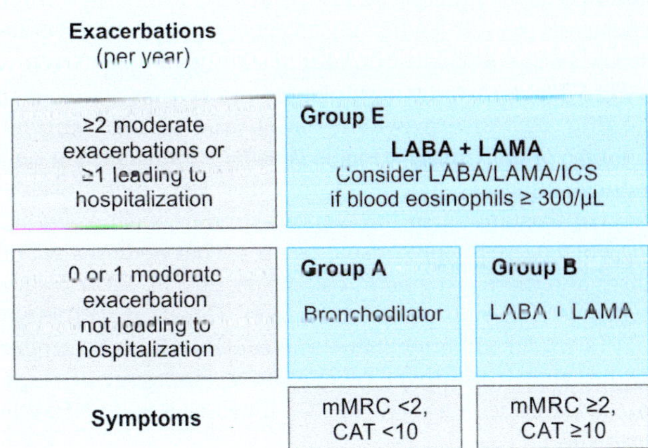

FIG. 5: Recommended initial inhaled therapy for COPD based on symptoms and exacerbation history.

(COPD: chronic obstructive pulmonary disease; ICS: inhaled corticosteroids; LABA: long-acting β_2-agonist; LAMA: long-acting muscarinic antagonist; mMRC: modified Medical Research Council Dyspnea Score; CAT: COPD assessment test)

Referral to Hospital

Referral to a respiratory physician is useful to:

- Establish the diagnosis and differentiate from asthma
- Exclude other pathology, including malignancy
- Reinforce the need to stop smoking
- Optimize therapy

Referral is indicated particularly in following conditions:

- Early onset of disease or family history of α_1-antitrypsin deficiency
- Signs of cor pulmonale
- Assessment of LTOT or nebulizer therapy
- Those with a rapid decline in lung function (>100 mL/year)
- Those with frequent infections to exclude bronchiectasis

TREATMENT OF ACUTE EXACERBATIONS

An important aim of treatment is to prevent exacerbations. Several of the treatments for chronic disease including long-acting bronchodilators (both β_2-agonists and anticholinergic), low-dose theophylline, high-dose ICS, pulmonary rehabilitation, and smoking cessation have been shown to reduce exacerbation rates and hospitalization.[5]

Chronic obstructive pulmonary disease exacerbations are one of the most common causes of emergency hospital admission. Apart from the treatment of underlying bacterial infection with antibiotics (as discussed earlier), exacerbations are treated symptomatically by increasing the dose of short-acting β_2-agonist and anticholinergic bronchodilators delivered by nebulizer. The place of antibiotics is not certain as controlled trials show little clinical benefit; this may reflect the fact that over half of the exacerbations are due to viral or noninfective causes. Oxygen (24% or 28% via Venturi mask) should be given to achieve a PaO_2 of at least 60 mm Hg without a fall in pH to <7.26 (indicating an acute change). Blood gases should be checked within 1 hour of starting oxygen therapy.

Oxygen saturation by pulse oximetry may be used to monitor response provided $PaCO_2$ and pH are normal. A course of oral corticosteroids is usually indicated but only reduces inpatient stay by about 1 day. Very high doses of oral corticosteroids, or intravenous steroids, such as hydrocortisone or methylprednisolone, are no better than low oral doses and there is a greater risk of side effects. Diuretics are indicated if there is peripheral edema. Chest physiotherapy may be useful, although there is no evidence from controlled studies that it improves recovery. Development of respiratory failure with a rising $PaCO_2$ may necessitate NPPV or intubation.

TREATMENT OF COR PULMONALE

Cor pulmonale (right heart failure) is due to the effect of chronic hypoxia on pulmonary vasculature, resulting in pulmonary hypertension and pulmonary vascular remodeling. It is usual to treat with LTOT. Diuretics are used to reduce fluid retention. Digoxin is only indicated if there is coexistent atrial fibrillation. Vasodilators may be hazardous as they lower systemic as well as pulmonary blood pressure.

FUTURE THERAPIES

There is a pressing need to develop new therapies, as existing treatments do not alter the progressive course of the disease or reduce mortality. There have been relatively few advances in the therapeutic options for the treatment of COPD, but better understanding of the molecular mechanisms involved in the pathogenesis of COPD will undoubtedly lead to improved therapies in the future. We have effective inhaled long-acting bronchodilators that reduce symptoms, improve quality of life, and reduce exacerbations. However, none of these treatments target the underlying disease mechanisms and do not reduce disease progression or mortality. There is a need to develop drugs that target the underlying disease process to reduce chronic lung inflammation.[75] Drugs that block specific mediators, such as leukotriene B_4 and TNF, have not been shown to have any benefit, which may reflect the large number of inflammatory mediators secreted in COPD. More broad-spectrum anti-inflammatory drugs, such as PDE4 inhibitors, p38 mitogen-activated protein (MAP) kinase inhibitors or Janus kinase (JAK) inhibitors. However, all these drugs have significant side effects when given orally and this limits the dose and efficacy of treatment. Attempts to overcome this by delivering drugs by inhalation have not been promising as the inhaled drugs have little efficacy.[76]

There is increasing evidence that COPD involves accelerated lung aging with the accumulation of senescent cells that release multiple inflammatory mediators. This has led to the development of drugs (senotherapies) that inhibit the development of cellular senescence by targeting the signaling pathways involved (senostatics) or drugs that selective kill off senescent cells (senolytics).[77] Several of these drugs are now in clinical development, although no studies in chronic inflammatory demyelinating polyneuropathy (CIPD) have so far been reported.

SUMMARY

The mainstay of COPD therapy is inhaled long-acting bronchodilators, which improve symptoms and reduce exacerbations. LAMA and LABA are equally effective and additive when given in combination, preferably in a fixed dose combination inhaler. ICS are indicated in patients with continued exacerbations and an increased blood eosinophil count and are most conveniently given as a fixed dose ICS/LABA/LAMA combination inhaler (triple inhaler). A macrolide antibiotic and the phosphodiesterase inhibitor roflumilast may also be added if patients continue to have exacerbations. Non-pharmacological treatments are also important, including smoking cessation, reducing household air pollution using ventilation and clean cooking stoves, and pulmonary rehabilitation. Acute exacerbations should be treated with a nebulised short-acting β_2-agonist, with the addition of a short-acting anticholinergic if necessary, a course of oral corticosteroids and antibiotics if sputum is purulent.

REFERENCES

1. Barnes PJ, Burney PGJ, Silverman EK, et al. Chronic obstructive pulmonary disease. Nat Rev Dis Primers. 2015;1:15076.
2. Barnes PJ. Endo-phenotyping of COPD patients. Expert Rev Resp Med. 2021;15(1):27-37.
3. Global Burden of Disease Collaboration. Prevalence and attributable health burden of chronic respiratory diseases, 1990-2017: a systematic analysis for the Global Burden of Disease Study 2017. Lancet Respir Med. 2020;8:585-96.
4. India State-Level Disease Burden Initiative CRD Collaborators. The burden of chronic respiratory diseases and their heterogeneity across the states of India: the Global Burden of Disease Study 1990-2016. Lancet Glob Health. 2018;6(12):e1363-74.
5. Agustí A, Celli BR, Criner GJ, et al. Global initiative for chronic obstructive lung disease 2023 Report: GOLD executive summary. Eur Respir J. 2023;61(4):2300239.
6. Salvi SS, Barnes PJ. Chronic obstructive pulmonary disease in non-smokers. Lancet. 2009;374:733-43.
7. Garcia Rodriguez LA, Wallander MA, Tolosa LB, et al. Chronic obstructive pulmonary disease in UK primary care: incidence and risk factors. COPD. 2009;6:369-79.
8. Salvi S. Tobacco smoking and environmental risk factors for chronic obstructive pulmonary disease. Clin Chest Med. 2014;35: 17-27.
9. Salvi SS, Brashier BB, Londhe J, et al. Phenotypic comparison between smoking and non-smoking chronic obstructive pulmonary disease. Respir Res. 2020;21:50.
10. Sin DD, Doiron D, Agusti A, et al. Air pollution and COPD: GOLD 2023 committee report. Eur Respir J. 2023;61(5):2202469.
11. Sarkar M, Srinivasa, Madabhavi I, et al. Tuberculosis associated chronic obstructive pulmonary disease. Clin Respir J. 2017;11: 285-95.
12. Anthonisen NR, Skeans MA, Wise RA, et al. The effects of a smoking cessation intervention on 14.5-year mortality: a randomized clinical trial. Ann Intern Med. 2005;142:233-9.
13. Cahill K, Stevens S, Lancaster T. Pharmacological treatments for smoking cessation. JAMA. 2014;311:193-4.
14. Zhou Y, Zou Y, Li X, et al. Lung function and incidence of chronic obstructive pulmonary disease after improved cooking fuels and kitchen ventilation: a 9-year prospective cohort study. PLoS Med. 2014;11:e1001621.
15. Chapman KR, Chorostowska-Wynimko J, Koczulla AR, et al. Alpha 1 antitrypsin to treat lung disease in alpha 1 antitrypsin deficiency: recent developments and clinical implications. Int J Chron Obstruct Pulmon Dis. 2018;13:419-32.
16. Silverman EK, Spira A, Paré PD. Genetics and genomics of chronic obstructive pulmonary disease. Proc Am Thorac Soc. 2009;6:539-42.
17. Cazzola M, Page CP, Calzetta L, et al. Pharmacology and therapeutics of bronchodilators. Pharmacol Rev. 2012;64:450-504.
18. Tashkin DP, Celli B, Senn S, et al. A 4-year trial of tiotropium in chronic obstructive pulmonary disease. N Engl J Med. 2008;359: 1543-54.
19. Ora J, Coppola A, Cazzola M, et al. Long-Acting Muscarinic Antagonists Under Investigational to Treat Chronic Obstructive Pulmonary Disease. J Exp Pharmacol. 2020;12:559-74.
20. Miravitlles M, Kawayama T, Dreher M. LABA/LAMA as first-line therapy for COPD: a summary of the evidence and guideline recommendations. J Clin Med. 2022;11(22):6623.
21. Burkes RM, Panos RJ. Ultra long-acting β-agonists in chronic obstructive pulmonary disease. J Exp Pharmacol. 2020;12: 589-602.
22. Calverley PM, Anderson JA, Celli B, et al. Salmeterol and fluticasone propionate and survival in chronic obstructive pulmonary disease. N Engl J Med. 2007;356:775-89.
23. Suissa S, Ernst P, Vandemheen KL, et al. Methodological issues in therapeutic trials of COPD. Eur Respir J. 2008;31:927-33.
24. Cazzola M, Calderaro F, Califano C, et al. Oral bambuterol compared to inhaled salmeterol in patients with partially reversible chronic obstructive pulmonary disease. Eur J Clin Pharmacol. 1999;54:829-33.
25. ZuWallack RL, Mahler DA, Reilly D, et al. Salmeterol plus theophylline combination therapy in the treatment of COPD. Chest. 2001;119:1661-70.
26. Barnes PJ. Theophylline. Am J Respir Crit Care Med. 2013;188: 901-6.
27. To Y, Ito K, Kizawa Y, et al. Targeting phosphoinositide-3-kinase-delta with theophylline reverses corticosteroid insensitivity in COPD. Am J Resp Crit Care Med. 2010;182:897-904.
28. Devereux G, Cotton S, Fielding S, et al. Effect of theophylline as adjunct to inhaled corticosteroids on exacerbations in patients with COPD: a randomized clinical trial. JAMA. 2018;320: 1548-59.
29. Jenkins CR, Wen FQ, Martin A, et al. The effect of low-dose corticosteroids and theophylline on the risk of acute exacerbations of COPD: the TASCS randomised controlled trial. Eur Respir J. 2021;57:2003338.
30. Cazzola M, Matera MG. The effect of doxofylline in asthma and COPD. Respir Med. 2020;164:105904.
31. Barnes PJ. Inhaled corticosteroids in COPD: a controversy. Respiration. 2010;80:89-95.
32. Brightling CE, McKenna S, Hargadon B, et al. Sputum eosinophilia and the short term response to inhaled mometasone in chronic obstructive pulmonary disease. Thorax. 2005;60:193-8.
33. Agusti A, Fabbri LM, Singh D, et al. Inhaled corticosteroids in COPD: Friend or foe? Eur Respir J. 2018;52(6):1801219.
34. Yang IA, Ferry OR, Clarke MS, et al. Inhaled corticosteroids versus placebo for stable chronic obstructive pulmonary disease. Cochrane Database Syst Rev. 2023;3(3):CD002991.
35. Barnes PJ. Role of HDAC2 in the pathophysiology of COPD. Annu Rev Physiol. 2009;71:451-64.
36. Yun JH, Lamb A, Chase R, et al. Blood eosinophil count thresholds and exacerbations in patients with chronic obstructive pulmonary disease. J Allergy Clin Immunol. 2018;141:2037-47. e2010.

37. Yang M, Du Y, Chen H, et al. Inhaled corticosteroids and risk of pneumonia in patients with chronic obstructive pulmonary disease: A meta-analysis of randomized controlled trials. Int Immunopharmacol. 2019;77:105950.
38. Singanayagam A, Glanville N, Girkin JL, et al. Corticosteroid suppression of antiviral immunity increases bacterial loads and mucus production in COPD exacerbations. Nat Comm. 2018;9(1):2229.
39. Magnussen H, Disse B, Rodriguez-Roisin R, et al. Withdrawal of Inhaled Glucocorticoids and Exacerbations of COPD. N Engl J Med. 2014;371(14):1285-94.
40. Chapman KR, Hurst JR, Frent SM, et al. Long-term triple therapy de-escalation to Indacaterol/Glycopyrronium in Patients with Chronic Obstructive Pulmonary Disease (SUNSET): a randomized, double-blind, triple-dummy clinical trial. Am J Respir Crit Care Med. 2018;198:329-39.
41. Ritondo BL, Puxeddu E, Calzetta L, et al. Efficacy and safety of triple combination therapy for treating chronic obstructive pulmonary disease: an expert review. Expert Opin Pharmacother. 2021;22(5):611-20.
42. Yang M, Li Y, Jiang Y, et al. Combination therapy with long-acting bronchodilators and the risk of major adverse cardiovascular events in patients with COPD: a systematic review and meta-analysis. Eur Respir J. 2023;61(2):2200302.
43. Hatzelmann A, Morcillo EJ, Lungarella G, et al. The preclinical pharmacology of roflumilast—a selective, oral phosphodiesterase 4 inhibitor in development for chronic obstructive pulmonary disease. Pulm Pharmacol Ther. 2010;23:235-56.
44. Wedzicha JA, Calverley PM, Rabe KF. Roflumilast: a review of its use in the treatment of COPD. Int J Chron Obstruct Pulmon Dis. 2016;11:81-90.
45. Rennard SI, Calverley PM, Goehring UM, et al. Reduction of exacerbations by the PDE4 inhibitor roflumilast--the importance of defining different subsets of patients with COPD. Respir Res. 2011;12(1):18.
46. Tarpy SP, Celli B. Long-term oxygen therapy. N Engl J Med. 1995;333:710-4.
47. Lacasse Y, Casaburi R, Sliwinski P, et al. Home oxygen for moderate hypoxaemia in chronic obstructive pulmonary disease: a systematic review and meta-analysis. Lancet Respir Med. 2022;10:1029-37.
48. Sethi S, Murphy TF. Infection in the pathogenesis and course of chronic obstructive pulmonary disease. N Engl J Med. 2008;359:2355-65.
49. Papi A, Bellettato CM, Braccioni F, et al. Infections and airway inflammation in chronic obstructive pulmonary disease severe exacerbations. Am J Respir Crit Care Med. 2006;173:1114-21.
50. Vollenweider DJ, Frei A, Steurer-Stey CA, et al. Antibiotics for exacerbations of chronic obstructive pulmonary disease. Cochrane Database Syst Rev. 2018;10:CD010257.
51. Albert RK, Connett J, Bailey WC, et al. Azithromycin for prevention of exacerbations of COPD. N Engl J Med. 2011;365(8):689-98.
52. Fahy JV, Dickey BF. Airway mucus function and dysfunction. N Engl J Med. 2010;363:2233-47.
53. Hill DB, Button B, Rubinstein M, et al. Physiology and pathophysiology of human airway mucus. Physiol Rev. 2022;102:1757-836.
54. Barnes PJ. Oxidative stress in chronic obstructive pulmonary disease. Antioxidants (Basel). 2022;11(5):965.
55. Poole P, Sathananthan K, Fortescue R. Mucolytic agents versus placebo for chronic bronchitis or chronic obstructive pulmonary disease. Cochrane Database Syst Rev. 2019;5:CD001287.
56. Decramer M, Rutten-van Molken M, Dekhuijzen PN, et al. Effects of N-acetylcysteine on outcomes in chronic obstructive pulmonary disease (Bronchitis Randomized on NAC Cost-Utility Study, BRONCUS): a randomised placebo-controlled trial. Lancet. 2005;365(9470):1552-60.
57. Zheng JP, Kang J, Huang SG, et al. Effect of carbocisteine on acute exacerbation of chronic obstructive pulmonary disease (PEACE Study): a randomised placebo-controlled study. Lancet. 2008;371(9629):2013-8.
58. Zheng JP, Wen FQ, Bai CX, et al. Twice daily N-acetylcysteine 600 mg for exacerbations of chronic obstructive pulmonary disease (PANTHEON): a randomised, double-blind placebo-controlled trial. Lancet Respir Med. 2014;2:187-94.
59. Schembri S, Morant S, Winter JH, et al. Influenza but not pneumococcal vaccination protects against all-cause mortality in patients with COPD. Thorax. 2009;64:567-72.
60. Schenkein JG, Nahm MH, Dransfield MT. Pneumococcal vaccination for patients with COPD: current practice and future directions. Chest. 2008;133:767-74.
61. Sprenkle MD, Niewoehner DE, MacDonald R, et al. Clinical efficacy of OM-85 BV in COPD and chronic bronchitis: a systematic review. COPD. 2005;2:167-75.
62. Currow DC, Abernethy AP. Pharmacological management of dyspnoea. Curr Opin Support Palliat Care. 2007;1:96-101.
63. Molassiotis A, Bryan G, Caress A, et al. Pharmacological and non-pharmacological interventions for cough in adults with respiratory and non-respiratory diseases: A systematic review of the literature. Respir Med. 2010;104:934-44.
64. Holland AE, Hill CJ, Jones AY, et al. Breathing exercises for chronic obstructive pulmonary disease. Cochrane Database Syst Rev. 2012;10:CD008250.
65. Collins PF, Elia M, Stratton RJ. Nutritional support and functional capacity in chronic obstructive pulmonary disease: a systematic review and meta-analysis. Respirology. 2013;18:616-29.
66. Liu Y, Huang C, Du J, et al. Anabolic-androgenic steroids for patients with chronic obstructive pulmonary disease: A systematic review and meta-analysis. Front Med. 2022;9:915159.
67. Casaburi R, ZuWallack R. Pulmonary rehabilitation for management of chronic obstructive pulmonary disease. N Engl J Med. 2009;360:1329-35.
68. Troosters T, Hornikx M, Demeyer H, et al. Pulmonary rehabilitation: timing, location, and duration. Clin Chest Med. 2014;35:303-11.
69. Casaburi R, Kukafka D, Cooper CB, et al. Improvement in exercise tolerance with the combination of tiotropium and pulmonary rehabilitation in patients with COPD. Chest. 2005;127:809-17.
70. Struik FM, Lacasse Y, Goldstein RS, et al. Nocturnal noninvasive positive pressure ventilation in stable COPD: a systematic review and individual patient data meta-analysis. Respir Med. 2014;108:329-37.
71. Plant PK, Owen JL, Parrott S, et al. Cost effectiveness of ward based non-invasive ventilation for acute exacerbations of chronic obstructive pulmonary disease: economic analysis of randomised controlled trial. BMJ. 2003;326(7396):956.
72. Patel N, DeCamp M, Criner GJ. Lung transplantation and lung volume reduction surgery versus transplantation in

chronic obstructive pulmonary disease. Proc Am Thorac Soc. 2008;5:447-53.

73. Criner GJ, Cordova F, Sternberg AL, et al. The National Emphysema Treatment Trial (NETT) Part II: Lessons learned about lung volume reduction surgery. Am J Respir Crit Care Med. 2011;184:881-93.
74. Lashari BH, Criner GJ. Advances in surgical and mechanical management of chronic obstructive pulmonary disease. Med Clin North Am. 2022;106:1013-25.
75. Barnes PJ. New anti-inflammatory treatments for chronic obstructive pulmonary disease. Nat Rev Drug Discov. 2013;12:543-59.
76. Singh D, Lea S, Mathioudakis AG. Inhaled phosphodiesterase inhibitors for the treatment of chronic obstructive pulmonary disease. Drugs. 2021;81:1821-30.
77. Baker J, Donnelly LE, Barnes PJ. Senotherapy: a new horizon for COPD therapy. Chest. 2020;158:562-70.

Exacerbations of Chronic Obstructive Pulmonary Disease

CHAPTER 88

Raja Dhar, Aloke Gopal Ghoshal, Tarang Kulkarni

INTRODUCTION

Exacerbation of chronic obstructive pulmonary disease (ECOPD) is a significant defining event in a patient's disease course, even if the underlying disease was mild or moderate and previously stable. These exacerbations can occur frequently and vary in severity, affecting the patient's physical and emotional health, as well as incurring significant financial costs for the patient and their family.[1] Even after recovery, these exacerbations might leave a long-term impact on pulmonary function and quality of life. ECOPD typically result in increased airway inflammation, excessive mucus production, and significant air trapping—all of which contribute to escalated breathlessness, the primary symptom of exacerbation. Additional symptoms include increased coughing and wheezing, along with a surge in sputum purulence and quantity. As exacerbations can have a notable adverse effect on a patient's health, some researchers have proposed alternative terminology, such as lung attacks[2], COPD attacks, COPD flare-ups, and COPD crises[3]. Successful treatment and future prevention of ECOPD are achievable for most patients.

DEFINITION AND SEVERITY OF CHRONIC OBSTRUCTIVE PULMONARY DISEASE EXACERBATION

According to the Global Initiative for Chronic Obstructive Lung Disease (GOLD), "An ECOPD is defined as an event characterized by increased dyspnea and/or cough and sputum that worsens in <14 days which may be accompanied by tachypnea and/or tachycardia and is often associated with increased local and systemic inflammation caused by infection, pollution, or other insult to the airways."[4] This new definition of ECOPD is different from the previous one, which relied solely on a patient's perception of increased respiratory symptoms, leading to several issues such as variability between patients, other conditions mimicking the symptoms, and a lack of measurable pathophysiological variables or a timing framework.

The GOLD 2023 guidelines classified ECOPD based on the level of healthcare management required for treatment. Exacerbations classified as "mild" are those that only require short-acting beta-agonists (SABA), while "moderate" exacerbations require SABA with antibiotics and/or oral corticosteroids. Exacerbations associated with respiratory failure, requiring mechanical ventilation, are classified as "severe."

The current definition of ECOPD is limited by its reliance on level of use of healthcare resources to determine the severity of the event. To address this limitation, the ROME Proposal for An Updated Definition and Severity Classification of ECOPD proposed a new classification system **(Table 1)** based on six objectively measured variables that

TABLE 1: Classification of severity of ECOPD.[5]

Severity	Criteria
Mild	• Dyspnea VAS score < 5 • Respiratory rate < 24 breaths/min • Heart rate < 95 beats/min • Resting SpO_2 > 92% on room air (or patient's usual oxygen requirement) and change > 3% • CRP < 10 mg/L
Moderate	• Dyspnea VAS score ≥ 5 • Respiratory rate ≥ 24 breaths/min • Heart rate ≥ 95 beats/min • Resting SpO_2 < 92% on room air (or patient's usual oxygen requirement) and change > %3 • CRP ≥ 10 mg/L • ABG: Hypoxemia (PaO_2 < 60 mm Hg) and/or hypercapnia ($PaCO_2$ > 45 mm Hg) but no acidosis (pH > 7.35)
Severe	ABG show hypercapnia and acidosis ($PaCO_2$ > 45 mm Hg and pH > 7.35)

(ABG: arterial blood gas; CRP: C-reactive protein; ECOPD: exacerbations of chronic obstructive pulmonary disease; $PaCO_2$: partial pressure of carbon dioxide; PaO_2: partial pressure of oxygen; SpO_2: oxygen saturation; VAS: visual analog scale)

serve as markers of event severity.[5] These variables include dyspnea, oxygen saturation (SpO_2), respiratory rate, heart rate, serum C-reactive protein (CRP), and in selected cases, arterial blood gases. The use of these objective measures can provide a more accurate assessment of the severity of ECOPD across different healthcare systems and practitioners, reducing subjectivity and variability in reported outcomes.

PATHOPHYSIOLOGY OF EXACERBATION OF CHRONIC OBSTRUCTIVE PULMONARY DISEASE (FLOWCHART 1)

The pathophysiology of COPD is primarily characterized by expiratory airflow limitation and the resultant dynamic hyperinflation (DHI). During an exacerbation state, there is a further increase in the airflow resistance due to the occurrence of bronchospasm, mucosal edema, and mucus plugging. This progressive airflow limitation further exacerbates the DHI, leading to an increase in the intrinsic positive end-expiratory pressure (iPEEP) and impaired gas exchange. In an attempt to compensate for these effects, patients with COPD typically adopt a rapid, shallow breathing pattern, which further worsens DHI. The impaired gas exchange resulting from an increased ratio of dead space to tidal volume (Vd/Vt) can lead to acute respiratory failure, while the increased iPEEP can lead to cardiovascular complications, such as decreased right ventricular preload and an increase in pulmonary artery pressures.

Respiratory infections have been identified as the most common triggers for exacerbations in COPD patients, with almost 70% of exacerbations being triggered by respiratory viral infections. In addition to viral and bacterial infections, atypical bacteria have also been identified as potential triggers. Various risk factors have been identified that predict an increased risk of future exacerbations, including advanced age, COPD disease duration, a history of COPD-related hospitalization, peripheral blood eosinophilia (>340/mm^3)[6], and the presence of multiple comorbidities **(Box 1)**.

In the ECLIPSE study, the history of previous exacerbations was found to be the single most important predictor of increased exacerbation risk.[7] Although forced expiratory volume in 1 second (FEV_1) levels were previously thought to be a predictor of increased exacerbation risk, recent trials have challenged this hypothesis, as FEV_1 alone may not provide a good assessment of exacerbation risk.[5] The presence of exacerbations, hospitalization, and death are more common in those with worsening airflow obstruction. This relationship is utilized in the BODE (body mass index, airflow obstruction, dyspnea, and exercise capacity) index, a tool that predicts the prognosis and evaluates the effectiveness of medications, pulmonary rehabilitation, and other therapies.[8]

BOX 1 Factors increasing chronic obstructive pulmonary disease (COPD) exacerbation risk.[6,7]

- History of previous exacerbations and hospitalization
- Advanced age
- Longer disease duration
- Increased exposure to PM2.5 and PM10 particles
- Peripheral blood eosinophilia (>340/mm^3)
- Multiple comorbidity status
- Pulmonary hypertension [pulmonary artery to aorta (PA:A) ratio > 1 on computed tomography (CT) scan]

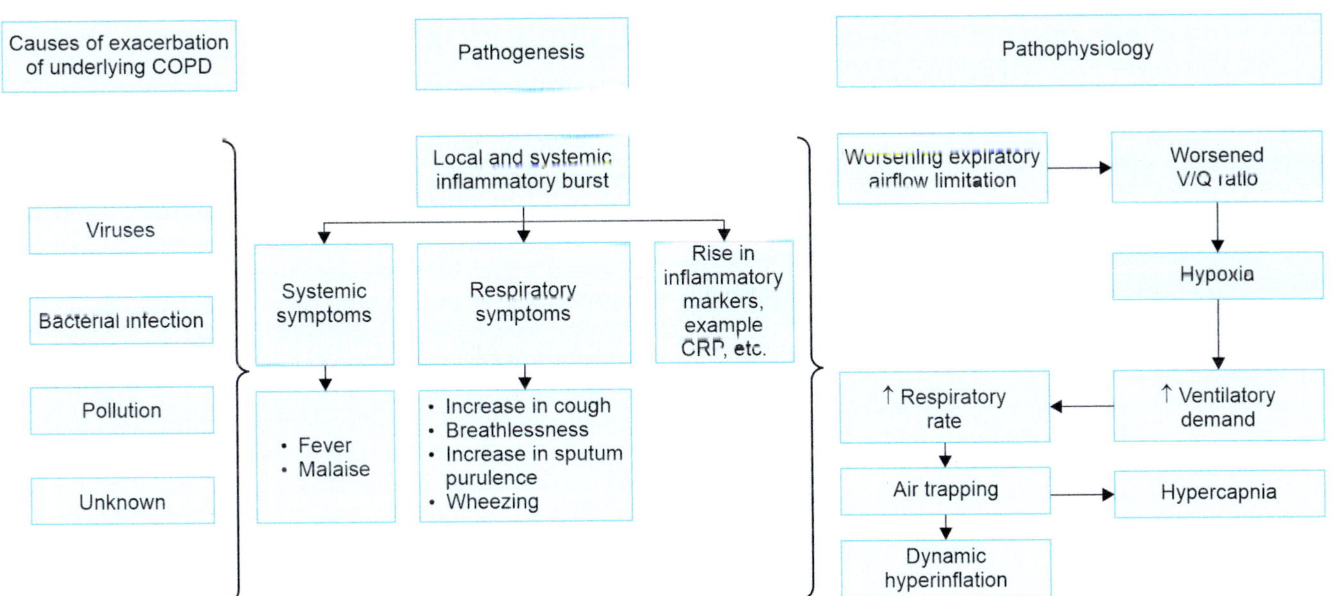

FLOWCHART 1: Pathogenesis of COPD exacerbation.
(COPD: chronic obstructive pulmonary disease; CRP: C-reactive protein; V/Q: ventilation to perfusion)

Hospitalizations due to ECOPD have been linked to exposure to poor outdoor air quality, particularly higher levels of ozone, carbon monoxide, particulate matter up to 10 microns, and nitrogen dioxide. Exposure to both PM2.5 and PM10 is linked to an increased risk of acute ECOPD (AECOPD); reducing exposure to PM2.5 and PM10 could be an effective preventive strategy against AECOPD patients.[9] Recently published CLEAN AIR study concluded that that the use of air cleaners with high efficiency particulate air (HEPA) filters and ultraviolet germicidal irradiation (UVGI) can significantly reduce indoor air pollution and exacerbation rates in patients with moderate-to-severe COPD.[10]

In addition to the aforementioned risk factors, the presence of gastroesophageal reflux disease (GERD) and pulmonary hypertension [PA:A ratio > 1 on computed tomography (CT) scans] have also been observed to be independent factors of ECOPD risk.[7] These predictors provide important information for the early identification, management, and prognostication of ECOPD patients, ultimately leading to improved patient outcomes.

In the Indian context, individuals with nonsmoking COPD have been found to have a greater incidence of exacerbations and increased utilization of healthcare resources.[11]

SYMPTOMS OF EXACERBATION OF CHRONIC OBSTRUCTIVE PULMONARY DISEASE

Patients frequently manifest one or more symptoms of acute exacerbation **(Box 2)**. Diagnostic procedures can provide valuable information to guide management decisions and to rule of differential diagnoses **(Table 2)**. Assessing the severity of underlying COPD, identifying the presence of comorbidities, and obtaining a history of prior exacerbations are all critical components of evaluating patients with exacerbations **(Box 3)**. It is important to note that some of these differentials can happen concurrently with ECOPD. Chest radiography can reveal the extent of lung involvement, while sputum and blood examination can help identify potential pathogens and rule out other potential diagnoses.

BOX 2 Symptoms of chronic obstructive pulmonary disease (COPD) exacerbation.

- Increase in cough
- Increase in breathlessness
- Increase in sputum volume and change in its color (white to green, yellow, or blood streaked)
- Fever
- Increased tiredness
- Increase in oxygen requirement (for those on long-term oxygen therapy)

TABLE 2: Differential diagnosis of AECOPD.

Condition	Investigations to exclude differentials
Pneumothorax	Chest radiograph/ultrasound
Pneumonia	• Chest radiograph • CRP/procalcitonin levels
Heart failure	• NT-proBNP levels • Echocardiography • Cardiac enzymes
Cardiac arrhythmias	Electrocardiogram
Pleural effusion	Chest radiograph/ultrasound
Pulmonary embolism	• D-dimer/compression ultrasound • CT pulmonary angiography

(AECOPD: acute exacerbations of chronic obstructive pulmonary disease; CRP: C-reactive protein; CT: computed tomography; NT-proBNP: N-terminal prohormone of brain natriuretic peptide)

BOX 3 Factors associated with a poor prognosis in chronic obstructive pulmonary disease (COPD) exacerbations.[13,14]

- Advanced age
- Lower body mass index
- Presence of comorbidities such as cardiovascular disease or lung cancer
- Prior hospitalizations for COPD exacerbations
- Clinical severity of the present exacerbation
- Need for long-term oxygen therapy

MANAGEMENT OF EXACERBATION OF CHRONIC OBSTRUCTIVE PULMONARY DISEASE (BOX 4)

The initial evaluation in a patient with suspected ECOPD requires a comprehensive strategy. Firstly, it aims to confirm the diagnosis of an exacerbation based on presenting symptoms and other pertinent clinical factors. Additionally, it seeks to assess the severity of the exacerbation, as well as to determine its underlying etiology. It is also important to identify and rule out any comorbidities that may be contributing to the severity of the exacerbation. This is essential, as it can have a profound impact on the course of treatment and overall prognosis.

The initial evaluation also aims to decide whether the patient can be safely managed on an outpatient basis or requires hospitalization. This decision is guided by several factors, including the severity of the exacerbation, the presence of comorbidities, and the patient's overall clinical status. The preference of the patient and their family should be considered when making decisions regarding treatment.

BOX 4 Essential pharmacological components of treatment of chronic obstructive pulmonary disease (COPD) exacerbation.

Bronchodilators

- Short-acting beta 2-agonist and/or ipratropium by metered dose inhaler (MDI) with spacer or handheld nebulizer as needed
- Consider adding long-acting bronchodilator, e.g., formoterol (by MDI plus spacer or nebulized route

Corticosteroids (the actual dose may vary)

- Oral prednisone 30–40 mg/day for 5 days
- Consider using an inhaled corticosteroid

Antimicrobials

May be initiated in patients with altered sputum characteristics

- Choice should be based on local bacteria resistance patterns
- Amoxicillin/ampicillin, cephalosporins
- Doxycycline
- Macrolides
- If the patient has failed prior antibiotic therapy, consider:
  - Amoxicillin/clavulanate
  - Respiratory fluoroquinolones

To consider antivirals in patients tested positive for influenza/coronavirus disease (COVID-19)

BOX 5 Indications of hospital admission and intensive care unit (ICU) with exacerbations of chronic obstructive pulmonary disease (ECOPD).

Indications of hospital admission ECOPD:

- Sudden worsening of symptoms such as dyspnea, tachypnea, worsening hypoxia, and altered mental status
- Acute respiratory failure
- Emergence of new signs such as cyanosis and worsening pedal swelling
- Presence of significant comorbidities such as heart failure, pulmonary embolism, and pneumothorax
- Insufficient home support

Indications of ICU admission with ECOPD:

- Severe shortness of breath not responding to initial management
- Altered mental status (confusion, drowsiness, etc.)
- Worsening or persistent hypoxia or respiratory acidosis despite supplemental oxygen and noninvasive ventilation
- Need of invasive ventilation
- Recent hemodynamic instability needing inotrope support

It is important to acknowledge that there can be a sudden decline in the patient's condition, leading to a change in the decision to treat them at home or in a hospital setting **(Box 5)**. The diagnosis of an exacerbation is primarily based on clinical evaluation, although investigations can be valuable in assessing the severity of the condition and planning the most effective treatment approach.

In all patients with an exacerbation referred to hospital, following should be taken:

- A chest radiograph should be obtained.
- Arterial blood gas tensions should be measured and the inspired oxygen concentration recorded.
- An electrocardiogram (ECG) should be recorded to exclude cardiac comorbidities.
- A plasma brain natriuretic peptide/N-terminal prohormone of brain natriuretic peptide (NT-proBNP) levels to exclude heart failure
- A D-dimer level could be needed if the patient has risk factors for thromboembolic disease.
- A full blood count should be performed; urea and electrolyte concentrations should be measured.
- A theophylline level should be measured in patients who are on theophylline therapy at admission.
- If sputum is purulent, a sample should be sent for microscopy and culture.
- Coronavirus disease 2019 (COVID-19)/respiratory virus panel may be needed in selected patients.
- Blood cultures should be taken if the patient has fever.

In patients with ECOPD managed at primary care, pulse oximetry may be useful to evaluate for features of severe exacerbation. Sputum specimen for culture may not be needed in this group of patients. It has been suggested that exacerbations characterized by elevated levels of sputum or blood eosinophils could exhibit greater responsiveness to systemic steroids.

PROGNOSTICATION OF CHRONIC OBSTRUCTIVE PULMONARY DISEASE EXACERBATIONS

The long-term prognosis for patients who experience a hospitalization for a ECOPD is poor, with a 5-year mortality rate of approximately 50%.[12] There are several contributing factors that are independently linked with a poorer prognosis **(Box 3)**.[13,14] Patients who exhibit a higher prevalence and severity of respiratory symptoms, diminished quality of life, impaired lung function, reduced exercise capacity, decreased lung density, and thickened bronchial walls on CT scan are also at a heightened risk of mortality after an episode of ECOPD.[15]

The primary approach to management of ECOPD involves the use of inhaled short-acting bronchodilators to reverse airflow limitation, administration of systemic glucocorticoids, addressing any underlying infection, ensuring adequate oxygenation, identifying hypercarbic acidotic respiratory failure, and minimizing the necessity for invasive mechanical ventilation. Additionally, it is crucial to prioritize smoking cessation among individuals who smoke, enhance nutritional status, emphasize of adult vaccination as per existing guidelines and address coexisting medical conditions, and implement rehabilitative interventions to prevent prolonged immobilization.

OUTPATIENT MANAGEMENT FOR EXACERBATION OF CHRONIC OBSTRUCTIVE PULMONARY DISEASE

The treatment of exacerbation has to be based on the clinical presentation of the patient. The essential components of outpatient treatment include antibiotics, bronchodilators, and other drugs **(Box 4)**.

INPATIENT MANAGEMENT OF EXACERBATION OF CHRONIC OBSTRUCTIVE PULMONARY DISEASE

As previously mentioned, the decision to admit a patient to the hospital is based on the subjective interpretation of clinical indicators, including the severity of dyspnea, assessment of respiratory failure, short-term response to emergency room treatment, presence of cor pulmonale, and the presence of complicating factors such as severe bronchitis, pneumonia, or other comorbid conditions **(Box 5)**. General consensus suggests that hospitalization is warranted for patients with severe acute hypoxemia or acute hypercarbia. Additional factors that identify patients at "high risk" include recent emergency room visits within the past 7 days, the number of doses of nebulized bronchodilators administered, home oxygen use, previous relapse rates, prior administration of aminophylline, and the use of corticosteroids and antibiotics at the time of previous emergency room discharge **(Table 3)**.[16] Pharmacologic management, in conjunction with supportive measures, remains the mainstay of managing ECOPD.

PHARMACOLOGICAL MANAGEMENT

Bronchodilators

In the treatment of AECOPD, it is recommended to use inhaled SABA as the initial bronchodilators, with or without short-acting anticholinergics [short-acting muscarinic antagonists (SAMA)].[17] There is no significant difference in lung function improvement between metered dose inhalers (MDI) and nebulizers, although nebulizers may be easier for sicker patients.[18]

If a nebulizer is chosen for bronchodilator administration, air-driven nebulizers are preferred over oxygen-driven nebulizers to avoid potential risks associated with increased partial pressure of carbon dioxide ($PaCO_2$) levels.[19] Although MDI devices have shown equal efficacy in ECOPD, nebulized therapy is often preferred due to the assumption of more reliable drug delivery to the airway.

Methylxanthines (aminophylline and theophylline) are considered second-line therapy and have not shown additional efficacy beyond inhaled bronchodilators and glucocorticoids. They also have a higher incidence of adverse effects such as nausea, vomiting, tremor, palpitations, and arrhythmias compared to placebo.[20] Recent evidence from a real world study on 2,088 patients revealed that patients on methylxanthine therapy had a better symptom control and that higher eosinophil counts were associated with a greater efficacy of methylxanthines.[21]

For severe exacerbations that do not respond promptly to short-acting bronchodilators, intravenous administration of a single dose of magnesium sulfate (2 g infused over 20 minutes) is suggested. Intravenous magnesium sulphate has bronchodilator activity by inhibiting calcium influx into airway smooth muscle cells. Evidence suggests a decrease in hospitalizations, shorter length of hospital stay, and improved dyspnea scores with intravenous magnesium compared to placebo.[22] However, caution should be exercised in patients with renal insufficiency, as well as hypermagnesemia, which can cause muscle weakness.

Systemic Corticosteroids

Use of systemic glucocorticoids has been shown to be beneficial in shortening the recovery time and improving lung function, oxygenation levels, and decreasing the risk of early relapse, treatment failure, and hospitalization. The GOLD guidelines recommend the use of prednisone 40 mg once daily for 5 days for the majority of ECOPD. It was observed

TABLE 3: Classification of exacerbations in admitted patients.[16]

	Criteria	Ideal place of admission
No respiratory failure	Respiratory rate: ≤24 breaths/min, heart rate < 95 beats/min, no use of accessory respiratory muscles; preserved mental status; maintaining SpO_2 88–92% with supplemental oxygen given via Venturi mask 24–35% FiO_2, normal $PaCO_2$	Ward
Acute respiratory failure	Respiratory rate: >24 breaths/min; using accessory respiratory muscles; preserved mental status; maintaining SpO_2 88–92% with supplmental oxygen via Venturi mask >35% FiO_2; $PaCO_2$ elevated 50–60 mm Hg	Ward/HDU
Acute respiratory failure—life-threatening	Respiratory rate: >24 breaths/min; using accessory respiratory muscles; preserved mental status; maintaining SpO_2 88–92% with supplemental oxygen via Venturi mask >40% FiO_2; $PaCO_2$ elevated 50–60 mm Hg or with presence of acidosis pH < 7.2	ICU

(FiO_2: fraction of inspired oxygen; HDU: high dependency unit; ICU: intensive care unit; $PaCO_2$: partial pressure of carbon dioxide; SpO_2: oxygen saturation)

that low-dose corticosteroids were sufficient and safe in treatment of ECOPD and the response was noninferior to higher doses of steroids.[23] Treatment with oral prednisolone was noninferior to intravenous therapy in terms of death, intensive care unit (ICU) admission, and intensification of pharmacological therapy in 90 days after exacerbation.[24] Likewise, the REDUCE trial, which evaluated a 5-day regimen of prednisone against a 14-day regimen, demonstrated that the shorter course was as effective as the longer one in terms of re-exacerbation after 6 months. Further, it resulted in decreased exposure to glucocorticoids.[25]

In cases where patients present with severe exacerbations or are unable to take oral medication, intravenous glucocorticoids are typically administered. This may be useful in conditions where there is lack of response to oral glucocorticoids at home or impaired absorption caused by decreased splanchnic perfusion. However, it is important to note that even short courses of corticosteroids may be associated with increased risks, such as pneumonia and mortality, according to one observational study.[26] Therefore, the use of these medications should be limited to patients with significant exacerbations.

Nebulized budesonide alone has shown promise as an alternative treatment for COPD exacerbations in certain patients.[27] It has been found to provide similar benefits to intravenous methylprednisolone, although the choice between these options may depend on physician's and patient's choice.

Antimicrobial Therapy

The use of antibiotics in ECOPD is a subject of debate due to various factors. There is evidence supporting the use of antibiotics when patients exhibit clinical signs of a bacterial infection, such as increased sputum purulence.[28] Observing sputum color can help guide antibiotic therapy; sputum purulence indicates a high bacterial load and a potential causative relationship. Placebo controlled studies have shown that antibiotics reduce short-term mortality, treatment failure, and sputum purulence in ECOPD.[29,30] Therefore, moderately or severely ill patients with ECOPD and increased cough and sputum purulence should be treated with antibiotics.

In addition to presence of sputum purulence, CRP testing has shown promise in reducing antibiotic prescriptions without compromising outcomes.[31] Similarly, procalcitonin-guided antibiotic treatment has shown efficacy in reducing antibiotic exposure and side effects in outpatient settings.[32,33] However, conflicting results and higher mortality rates in ICU settings call for further research before recommending procalcitonin-based protocols. Shorter antibiotic treatment durations (≤5 days) have shown comparable efficacy and may reduce the risk of antimicrobial resistance and associated complications.[34] Sputum culture testing may be necessary for patients with frequent exacerbations, severe airflow obstruction, or those requiring mechanical ventilation. Improvement in dyspnea and sputum purulence indicates clinical success.

The selection of an appropriate antibiotic should be based on the local bacterial resistance patterns. Typically, initial empirical treatment options include aminopenicillin with clavulanic acid, macrolides, tetracyclines, or in specific cases, quinolones. For patients experiencing frequent exacerbations, severe airflow obstruction, or exacerbations necessitating mechanical ventilation, escalation of antibiotics may be needed.[35] This is important because gram-negative bacteria (such as *Pseudomonas* species) or resistant pathogens that are not susceptible to the aforementioned antibiotics may be present. The choice between oral or intravenous administration depends on the patient's ability to eat and the pharmacokinetics of the antibiotic, although oral administration is generally preferred.

Antiviral therapy such as oseltamivir is typically recommended for patients whose AECOPD is triggered by the influenza virus. However, the effectiveness of antiviral treatment decreases over time. Therefore, for patients who seek medical attention 72 hours or more after the onset of illness, clinical trajectory (such as whether their condition is worsening or improving) should be considered before deciding whether to prescribe antiviral therapy. In an exacerbation due to COVID-19 infection, standard treatment including bronchodilators, systemic corticosteroids, and antibiotics should not be altered for patients. However, close monitoring is necessary to detect any deterioration in their condition. Considering their age and comorbidities, patients with COPD and COVID-19 are likely to be suitable candidates for COVID-19-specific therapy.

Oxygen Therapy

Supplemental oxygen is an essential part of acute therapy for ECOPD. The goal is to administer oxygen in a way that maintains an SpO_2 of 88–92%. This range helps minimize the risk of worsening hypercapnia, a condition where there is excessive carbon dioxide in the blood, which can occur with excessive supplemental oxygen. Titrating supplemental oxygen to SpO_2 88–92% leads to lower mortality rates compared to high-flow oxygen that is not titrated.[36]

In most cases, a high fraction of inspired oxygen (FiO_2) is not necessary to correct the hypoxemia associated with ECOPD. If hypoxemia cannot be corrected with a relatively low FiO_2, further investigation is needed to identify other potential causes of low oxygen levels, such as pulmonary emboli, acute respiratory distress syndrome, pulmonary edema, or severe pneumonia.

When delivering oxygen, Venturi masks are preferred over nasal prongs as they provide more precise and controlled oxygen delivery. Ensuring adequate oxygenation (to achieve SpO_2 between 88 and 92%), even if it results in acute hypercapnia, is crucial. Patients with chronically elevated levels of partial pressure of arterial carbon dioxide ($PaCO_2$) generally tolerate hypercapnia well. However, if hypercapnia is accompanied by symptoms such as impaired mental status, severe acidosis, or cardiac dysrhythmias, assisted ventilation may be necessary. Regular monitoring of arterial blood gases should be conducted to assess oxygenation, carbon dioxide retention, and acid-base balance. Venous blood gas analysis has shown promise in assessing bicarbonate levels and pH, but further research is needed to determine its utility in acute respiratory failure scenarios.[37]

High-flow Nasal Oxygen Therapy

High-flow nasal therapy (HFNT) utilizes specialized devices to deliver heated and humidified air-oxygen blends at varying flow rates, up to 8 L/min in infants and up to 60 L/min in adults.[38] HFNT has demonstrated several physiological benefits, including reduced respiratory rate and effort, improved gas exchange, lung volume, and compliance, as well as improved oxygenation and clinical outcomes in patients with acute hypoxemic respiratory failure.[39] It has also shown potential in improving oxygenation, ventilation, and health-related quality of life in patients with acute hypercapnia during exacerbations and stable hypercapnic COPD.[40,41] However, the interpretation of the value of HFNT for the broader COPD patient population is limited by small sample sizes, heterogeneous patient populations, and short follow-up durations. While HFNT has shown benefits in some areas, the European Respiratory Society (ERS) Clinical Practice Guidelines recommend trial with noninvasive ventilation (NIV) before considering HFNT for COPD patients with hypercapnic acute respiratory failure.[42] Hence, it is important to exercise caution when employing HFNT in hypercapnic ECOPD until additional evidence becomes available.

Assisted Ventilation (Box 6)

In severe exacerbation cases where optimal pharmacological treatment is insufficient, patients may require ventilatory support when they are unable to maintain adequate ventilation. NIV aids the patient's breathing by delivering a mixture of air and oxygen through a tightly fitted facial or nasal mask.[43]

Noninvasive positive pressure ventilation (NIPPV) is the most commonly used mode of NIV. It combines continuous positive airway pressure (CPAP) with pressure support ventilation (PSV). NIPPV improves gas exchange by enhancing alveolar ventilation without significantly altering the ventilation/perfusion mismatch or gas exchange in the lungs.

BOX 6 Indications of noninvasive ventilation (NIV).

- Respiratory acidosis [partial pressure of carbon dioxide (PCO_2) > 45 mm Hg and pH < 7.35
- Severe dyspnea with evidence of respiratory muscle fatigue such as excessive use of accessory muscles, paradoxical breathing, intercostal muscle retraction, and increased work of breathing
- Hypoxia that persists despite maximal supplemental oxygen therapy

Large, randomized controlled trials and meta-analyses consistently show that bilevel NIV is beneficial for patients with ECOPD complicated by hypercapnic acidosis.[44,45] A meta-analysis of 17 randomized trials revealed a nearly 50% reduction in mortality when NIV was combined with standard therapy compared to standard therapy alone for AECOPD patients with hypercapnia ($PaCO_2$ > 45 mm Hg).[44] The effectiveness of bilevel NIV for patients with acute nonhypercapnic respiratory failure caused by ECOPD remains uncertain when compared to patients with acute hypercapnic respiratory failure due to AECOPD. Evidence against administering NIV in this population comes from various small, randomized or prospective trials, which have reported low tolerance of bilevel NIV and no significant effect on mortality. Additionally, the impact of NIV on intubation rates in AECOPD patients without severe respiratory acidosis has also shown conflicting results.[46]

For persistent hypercapnic ventilatory failure during exacerbations despite optimal medical therapy, NIV should be the preferred treatment. NIPPV should be offered to patients experiencing respiratory acidosis (pH < 7.36) and/or excessive breathlessness despite optimal medical therapy and oxygenation. Arterial blood gases should be measured for all patients being considered for mechanical ventilation.

- If the pH is <7.30, NIPPV should be administered in controlled environments such as intermediate ICUs and/or high-dependency units.
- If the pH is <7.25, NIPPV should be given in the ICU with intubation readily available.
- It is crucial to ensure that NIV is administered by a dedicated team with the necessary training and expertise, well versed in its application and limitations.
- The combination of CPAP (e.g., 4–8 cmH_2O) and PSV (e.g., 10–15 cmH_2O) is the most effective mode of NIPPV.
- NIV should also be considered for patients who have difficulty weaning off the ventilator.
- In the first few hours, the level of assistance and monitoring for NIPPV is the same as for mechanical ventilation.
- When initiating NIV, there should be a well-defined plan for each patient regarding the course of action in the event of deterioration, as well as clear indicators for when further intervention is required.

Invasive Mechanical Ventilation (Box 7)

The main objectives of using invasive mechanical ventilation in patients with ECOPD are as follows: Correcting abnormalities in oxygenation and ventilation, reducing the workload of breathing, and preventing DHI.[47]

Preventing DHI is particularly crucial in this patient population due to its potential complications, such as barotrauma, which can prolong the duration of mechanical

BOX 7 Indications of invasive mechanical ventilation.

- Altered mental status (drowsiness, confusion, agitation, etc.)
- Postcardiac or respiratory arrest
- Inability to tolerate noninvasive ventilation (NIV)
- Failure of NIV trial
- Arrhythmias or severe ventricular dysfunction
- Severe hypoxemia in patients not able to tolerate NIV

ventilation and even lead to cardiovascular collapse or death. When mechanical ventilation is required for COPD-related acute respiratory failure, volume-targeted ventilation modes are recommended over pressure support or pressure-limited modes. Among volume-targeted modes, preference is given to volume-controlled modes (e.g., volume control continuous mandatory ventilation) or synchronized intermittent mandatory ventilation with PSV (SIMV/PSV) if volume-controlled modes result in excessive ventilation. It is not uncommon for mode adjustments to be made during the course of the patient's illness, particularly when complications arise.

The optimal ventilator settings for acute respiratory failure in COPD patients are those that align with the goals of mechanical ventilation. The initial settings will depend on the cause of respiratory failure and the selected mode of ventilation. Subsequent adjustments should be based on the patient's clinical condition, comfort, gas exchange, and propensity for DHI. iPEEP, also known as auto-PEEP, is common in mechanically ventilated COPD patients due to a high prevalence of spontaneous or ventilator-induced DHI. Auto-PEEP can lead to issues such as patient–ventilator dyssynchrony, increased breathing effort, barotrauma, cardiovascular collapse, and even death. Preventing and treating DHI involve reducing respiratory rate and/or tidal volume, increasing inspiratory flow rate, applying external PEEP, and addressing underlying airflow obstruction with bronchodilators and glucocorticoids if present.[48,49]

The mortality rate for COPD patients requiring mechanical ventilation for acute respiratory failure is high (37–64%).[50] Poor prognostic indicators in this population include a lack of response to NIV, multiorgan failure, active malignancy, high acute physiologic and chronic health evaluation (APACHE) score, and isolation of virulent pathogens such as *Pseudomonas* and *Aspergillus* species from airway secretions.[51,52]

The extracorporeal carbon dioxide (CO_2) removal (ECCO_2R) device is capable of eliminating a portion of CO_2 from the blood through extracorporeal circulation. However, due to its low-flow system, it does not contribute to oxygenating the blood.[53] Recent technological advancements and improved understanding of the technique have expanded its application to patients with ECOPD with hypercapnic respiratory failure.[54] When used in combination with NIV, ECCO_2R has the potential to enhance the effectiveness of CO_2 removal, leading to a reduction in respiratory rate.[55] This can subsequently mitigate DHI and iPEEP. As a result, the workload of breathing can be diminished.[6] Importantly, the absence of sedation allows patients to actively engage in physiotherapy, which helps prevent muscle deconditioning.

DISCHARGE PLANNING

The criteria for patient discharge in cases of COPD generally rely on observing significant improvement in COPD symptoms, stability of the patient's condition, and the absence of frequent nebulizer treatments. If the patient has returned to a state similar to their prehospital baseline, discharge to home is usually appropriate. However, certain patients may no longer require hospital-level care but are unable to manage independently at home due to frailty or severe exercise intolerance. In such cases, a period of inpatient rehabilitation may be more suitable.

When determining whether a patient can be discharged to home, their ability to perform activities of daily living (ADLs) at home should be assessed, along with the need for assistive devices such as walkers, elevated toilet seats, bedside commodes, or shower chairs. Patients who receive a new prescription for long-term oxygen therapy typically require additional instructions on using oxygen delivery systems (e.g., tanks, concentrators, and portable systems) and following safe practices to avoid tripping hazards associated with oxygen tubing and exposure to open flames. These patients should be reassessed 2–3 months after discharge to evaluate the ongoing need for supplemental oxygen and determine the appropriate dosage.

The disease course of COPD varies widely, ranging from a gradual decline in exercise tolerance and oxygenation to an unexpected and sudden end-of-life situation. Given the challenges in predicting the clinical course, an exacerbation requiring hospitalization, especially one necessitating intensive care, provides an opportunity to initiate discussions about a palliative care consultation. Palliative care encompasses various essential aspects, including addressing the patient's comprehension of their illness and prognosis, evaluating and effectively managing symptoms, engaging in discussions regarding care goals and advance care planning, coordinating and assisting in the planning of end-of-life care, including the determination and appropriate timing of institutional care.

PREVENTION OF EXACERBATION OF CHRONIC OBSTRUCTIVE PULMONARY DISEASE (TABLE 4)

Various pharmacological interventions have demonstrated efficacy in reducing the frequency of ECOPD, including long-acting muscarinic antagonists, long-acting beta-agonists, inhaled glucocorticoids, and roflumilast. The choice among these medications depends on the severity of symptoms and the patient's risk of exacerbations.

TABLE 4: Interventions reducing risk of exacerbation of COPD.

Interventions	Modalities	Summary of evidence
General measures	Smoking cessation	Data from observational studies report reduction in ECOPD[57]
	Pulmonary rehabilitation	• Significant reduction in hospital admission and improvement in exercise tolerance and quality of life • Optimal timing for initiation post exacerbation not clear[58]
	Vitamin D supplementation[83]	Metanalysis showed reduction of exacerbation in patients with vitamin D level < 10 ng/mL[59]
	Lung volume reduction therapies	Postoperative improvement in lung function leads to reduction in exacerbations[60,61]
	Personal protective measures (e.g., wearing masks, hand washing, etc.)	Decline of exacerbations during COVID-19 pandemic was attributed to personal protective measures
	Air purification systems	Exposure to both PM2.5 and PM10 is linked to an increased risk of ECOPD. Recent study suggests that reducing exposure to PM2.5 and PM10 could be an effective preventive strategy against ECOPD[9]
	Vaccinations	Updated GOLD guidelines recommend influenza vaccination, PCV20, and dTAP vaccines for patients with COPD[4]
Bronchodilators	LABA	Associated with reduction of exacerbation irrespective of previous exacerbation history[62]
	LAMA	Improvement in symptoms, including cough and sputum; rate of exacerbations and effectiveness of pulmonary rehabilitation
	LABA + LAMA	Multiple RCTs confirm that combination LABA + LAMA is more effective at reducing exacerbation than monotherapy
Corticosteroid-containing regimen	LABA + ICS LABA + LAMA + ICS	ICS-containing regimen used in patients with history of recurrent/hospitalization exacerbation, eosinophil level > 300 cells/μL, history of concomitant asthma
Mucoregulatory agents	N-acetyl cysteine Carbocysteine	Reduction in risk of exacerbations seen with N-acetyl cysteine therapy in patients with chronic bronchitis phenotype[63,64]
Anti-inflammatory agents	Roflumilast	Reduction in moderate–severe exacerbations in chronic bronchitis and severe/very severe COPD with recurrent exacerbations[65]
	Macrolides	Azithromycin (250 mg/day or 500 mg three times per week) or erythromycin (250 mg two times per day) over a 1-year period resulted in a decreased risk of exacerbations.[66,67] Reduced benefit seen in individuals who are active smokers

(COPD: chronic obstructive pulmonary disease; COVID-19: coronavirus disease 2019; dTAP: diphtheria, tetanus, and acellular pertussis; ECOPD: exacerbations of COPD; GOLD: Global Initiative for Chronic Obstructive Lung Disease; ICS: inhaled corticosteroid; LABA: long-acting β2-agonist; LAMA: long-acting muscarinic antagonist; PCV20: pneumococcal conjugate vaccine; RCT: randomized controlled trial)

Observational studies conducted in multiple countries have revealed a substantial decrease in hospital admissions related to ECOPD during the COVID-19 pandemic.[56] This decline has been attributed to the implementation of preventive measures such as wearing masks, practicing social distancing, and maintaining good hand hygiene.

For patients experiencing recurrent exacerbations despite optimal therapy with long-acting bronchodilators and glucocorticoid inhalers, prophylactic use of azithromycin may be considered to reduce the frequency of exacerbations. NIV has shown benefits for hypercapnic patients requiring ventilation during hospitalization for a ECOPD and implementing nocturnal NIV at home can significantly reduce the risk of rehospitalization. Various measures which have been used for prevention of acute exacerbations include both pharmacological and nonpharmacological interventions[57-67].

SUMMARY

It is important to identify risk factors and implement pharmacological and nonpharmacological interventions to reduce exacerbation frequency and improve patient outcomes. Individualized treatment plans and comprehensive discharge planning are highlighted as key elements in reducing readmissions and optimizing long-term management. More data is required to address these gaps in order to enhance prevention and management strategies for ECOPD.

REFERENCES

1. Koul PA, Nowshehri AA, Khan UH, et al. Cost of Severe Chronic Obstructive Pulmonary Disease Exacerbations in a High Burden Region in North India. Ann Glob Health. 2019;85(1):13.
2. Holverda S, Rutgers MR, Kerstjens HAM. Time to rename COPD exacerbations: implementing the term lung attack. Lancet Respir Med. 2020;8(4):e25.
3. Bafadhel M, Criner G, Dransfield MT, et al. Exacerbations of chronic obstructive pulmonary disease: time to rename. Lancet Respir Med. 2020;8(2):133-5.
4. Global Initiative for Chronic Obstructive Lung Disease (GOLD). (2023). 2023 GOLD Report. [online] Available from https://goldcopd.org/2023-gold-report-2/ [Last accessed June, 2024].
5. Celli BR, Fabbri LM, Aaron SD, et al. An Updated Definition and Severity Classification of Chronic Obstructive Pulmonary Disease Exacerbations: The Rome Proposal. Am J Respir Crit Care Med. 2021;204(11):1251-8.
6. Vedel-Krogh S, Nielsen SF, Lange P, et al. Blood Eosinophils and Exacerbations in Chronic Obstructive Pulmonary Disease. The Copenhagen General Population Study. Am J Respir Crit Care Med. 2016;193(9):965-74.
7. Hurst JR, Vestbo J, Anzueto A, et al. Susceptibility to exacerbation in chronic obstructive pulmonary disease. N Engl J Med. 2010;363(12):1128-38.
8. Marin JM, Carrizo SJ, Casanova C, et al. Prediction of risk of COPD exacerbations by the BODE index. Respir Med. 2009;103(3):373-8.
9. Li N, Ma J, Ji K, et al. Association of PM2.5 and PM10 with Acute Exacerbation of Chronic Obstructive Pulmonary Disease at lag0 to lag7: A Systematic Review and Meta-Analysis. COPD. 2022;19(1):243-54.
10. Hansel NN, Putcha N, Woo H, et al. Randomized Clinical Trial of Air Cleaners to Improve Indoor Air Quality and Chronic Obstructive Pulmonary Disease Health: Results of the CLEAN AIR Study. Am J Respir Crit Care Med. 2022;205(4):421-30.
11. Salvi SS, Barnes PJ. Chronic obstructive pulmonary disease in non-smokers. Lancet. 2009;374(9691):733-43.
12. Hoogendoorn M, Hoogenveen RT, Mölken MPR van, et al. Case fatality of COPD exacerbations: a meta-analysis and statistical modelling approach. Eur Respir J. 2011;37(3):508-15.
13. Piquet J, Chavaillon JM, David P, et al. High-risk patients following hospitalisation for an acute exacerbation of COPD. Eur Respir J. 2013;42(4):946-55.
14. Singanayagam A, Schembri S, Chalmers JD. Predictors of Mortality in Hospitalized Adults with Acute Exacerbation of Chronic Obstructive Pulmonary Disease. A Systematic Review and Meta-analysis. Ann Am Thorac Soc. 2013;10(2):81-9.
15. Garcia-Aymerich J, Pons IS, Mannino DM, et al. Lung function impairment, COPD hospitalisations and subsequent mortality. Thorax. 2011;66(7):585-90.
16. Celli BR, Barnes PJ. Exacerbations of chronic obstructive pulmonary disease. Eur Respir J. 2007;29(6):1224-38.
17. NICE. (2018). Chronic obstructive pulmonary disease in over 16s: diagnosis and management. [online] Available from https://www.nice.org.uk/guidance/ng115 [Last accessed June, 2024].
18. van Geffen WH, Douma WR, Slebos D, et al. (2016). Bronchodilators delivered by nebuliser versus inhalers for lung attacks of chronic obstructive pulmonary disease. [online] Available from https://www.cochrane.org/CD011826/AIRWAYS_bronchodilators-delivered-nebuliser-versus-inhalers-lung-attacks-chronic-obstructive-pulmonary [Last accessed June, 2024].
19. Bardsley G, Pilcher J, McKinstry S, et al. Oxygen versus air-driven nebulisers for exacerbations of chronic obstructive pulmonary disease: a randomised controlled trial. BMC Pulm Med. 2018;18(1):157.
20. Duffy N, Walker P, Diamantea F, et al. Intravenous aminophylline in patients admitted to hospital with non-acidotic exacerbations of chronic obstructive pulmonary disease: a prospective randomised controlled trial. Thorax. 2005;60(9):713-7.
21. Zhan Z, Ma Y, Huang K, et al. Methylxanthine Treatment in Patients Hospitalized for Acute Exacerbation of Chronic Obstructive Pulmonary Disease in China: A Real-World Study Using Propensity Score Matching Analysis. Front Pharmacol. 2022;13:802123.
22. Ni H, Aye SZ, Naing C. Magnesium sulfate for acute exacerbations of chronic obstructive pulmonary disease. Cochrane Database Syst Rev. 2022;5(5):CD013506.
23. Pu X, Liu L, Feng B, et al. Efficacy and Safety of Different Doses of Systemic Corticosteroids in COPD Exacerbation. Respir Care. 2021;66(2):316-26.
24. de Jong YP, Uil SM, Grotjohan HP, et al. Oral or IV prednisolone in the treatment of COPD exacerbations: a randomized, controlled, double-blind study. Chest. 2007;132(6):1741-7.
25. Leuppi JD, Schuetz P, Bingisser R, et al. Short-term vs Conventional Glucocorticoid Therapy in Acute Exacerbations of Chronic Obstructive Pulmonary Disease: The REDUCE Randomized Clinical Trial. JAMA. 2013;309(21):2223-31.
26. Sivapalan P, Ingebrigtsen T, Rasmussen D, et al. COPD exacerbations: The impact of long versus short courses of oral corticosteroids on mortality and pneumonia: Nationwide data on 67 000 patients with COPD followed for 12 months. BMJ Open Respir Res. 2019;6:407.
27. Gunen H, Hacievliyagil SS, Yetkin O, et al. The role of nebulised budesonide in the treatment of exacerbations of COPD. Eur Respir J. 2007;29(4):660-7.
28. Miravitlles M, Kruesmann F, Haverstock D, et al. Sputum colour and bacteria in chronic bronchitis exacerbations: a pooled analysis. Eur Respir J. 2012;39(6):1354-60.
29. Quon BS, Gan WQ, Sin DD. Contemporary management of acute exacerbations of COPD: a systematic review and metaanalysis. Chest. 2008;133(3):756-66.
30. Ram FSF, Rodriguez-Roisin R, Granados-Navarrete A, et al. Antibiotics for exacerbations of chronic obstructive pulmonary disease. Cochrane Database Syst Rev. 2006;(2):CD004403.
31. Butler CC, Gillespie D, White P, et al. C-Reactive Protein Testing to Guide Antibiotic Prescribing for COPD Exacerbations. N Engl J Med. 2019;381(2):111-20.
32. Daubin C, Valette X, Thiollière F, et al. Procalcitonin algorithm to guide initial antibiotic therapy in acute exacerbations of COPD admitted to the ICU: a randomized multicenter study. Intensive Care Med. 2018;44(4):428-37.
33. Schuetz P, Wirz Y, Sager R, et al. Procalcitonin to initiate or discontinue antibiotics in acute respiratory tract infections. Cochrane Database Syst Rev. 2017;10(10):CD007498.
34. Falagas ME, Avgeri SG, Matthaiou DK, et al. Short- versus long-duration antimicrobial treatment for exacerbations of chronic bronchitis: a meta-analysis. J Antimicrob Chemother. 2008;62(3):442-50.
35. Adams SG, Melo J, Luther M, et al. Antibiotics Are Associated With Lower Relapse Rates in Outpatients With Acute Exacerbations of COPD. Chest. 2000;117(5):1345-52.

36. Austin MA, Wills KE, Blizzard L, et al. Effect of high flow oxygen on mortality in chronic obstructive pulmonary disease patients in prehospital setting: randomised controlled trial. BMJ. 2010;341:c5462.
37. McKeever TM, Hearson G, Housley G, et al. Using venous blood gas analysis in the assessment of COPD exacerbations: a prospective cohort study. Thorax. 2016;71(3):210-5.
38. Roca O, Hernández G, Díaz-Lobato S, et al. Current evidence for the effectiveness of heated and humidified high flow nasal cannula supportive therapy in adult patients with respiratory failure. Crit Care. 2016;20:109.
39. Lin SM, Liu KX, Lin ZH, et al. Does high-flow nasal cannula oxygen improve outcome in acute hypoxemic respiratory failure? A systematic review and meta-analysis. Respir Med. 2017;131: 58-64.
40. Nagata K, Horie T, Chohnabayashi N, et al. Home High-Flow Nasal Cannula Oxygen Therapy for Stable Hypercapnic COPD: A Randomized Clinical Trial. Am J Respir Crit Care Med. 2022;206(11):1326-35.
41. Bonnevie T, Elkins M, Paumier C, et al. Nasal High Flow for Stable Patients with Chronic Obstructive Pulmonary Disease: A Systematic Review and Meta-Analysis. COPD. 2019;16(5-6): 368-77.
42. Oczkowski S, Ergan B, Bos L, et al. ERS Clinical Practice Guidelines: high-flow nasal cannula in acute respiratory failure. Eur Respir J. 2022;59(4):2101574.
43. Rochwerg B, Brochard L, Elliott MW, et al. Official ERS/ATS clinical practice guidelines: noninvasive ventilation for acute respiratory failure. Eur Respir J. 2017;50(2):1602426.
44. Osadnik CR, Tee VS, Carson-Chahhoud KV, et al. Non-invasive ventilation for the management of acute hypercapnic respiratory failure due to exacerbation of chronic obstructive pulmonary disease. Cochrane Database Syst Rev. 2017;7(7):CD004104.
45. Lindenauer PK, Stefan MS, Shieh MS, et al. Outcomes associated with invasive and noninvasive ventilation among patients hospitalized with exacerbations of chronic obstructive pulmonary disease. JAMA Intern Med. 2014;174(12):1982-93.
46. Keenan SP, Powers CE, McCormack DG. Noninvasive positive-pressure ventilation in patients with milder chronic obstructive pulmonary disease exacerbations: a randomized controlled trial. Respir Care. 2005;50(5):610-6.
47. Davidson AC, Banham S, Elliott M, et al. BTS/ICS guideline for the ventilatory management of acute hypercapnic respiratory failure in adults. Thorax. 2016;71 Suppl 2:ii1-35.
48. Thorevska NY, Manthous CA. Determinants of dynamic hyperinflation in a bench model. Respir Care. 2004;49(11): 1326-34.
49. de Chazal I, Hubmayr RD. Novel aspects of pulmonary mechanics in intensive care. Br J Anaesth. 2003;91(1):81-91.
50. Makris D, Desrousseaux B, Zakynthinos E, et al. The impact of COPD on ICU mortality in patients with ventilator-associated pneumonia. Respir Med. 2011;105(7):1022-9.
51. Gadre SK, Duggal A, Mireles-Cabodevila E, et al. Acute respiratory failure requiring mechanical ventilation in severe chronic obstructive pulmonary disease (COPD). Medicine (Baltimore). 2018;97(17):e0487.
52. Domenech A, Puig C, Martí S, et al. Infectious etiology of acute exacerbations in severe COPD patients. J Infect. 2013;67(6): 516-23.
53. Morelli A, Del Sorbo L, Pesenti A, et al. Extracorporeal carbon dioxide removal (ECCO2R) in patients with acute respiratory failure. Intensive Care Med. 2017;43(4):519-30.
54. Combes A, Auzinger G, Capellier G, et al. $ECCO_2R$ therapy in the ICU: consensus of a European round table meeting. Crit Care. 2020;24(1):490.
55. Azzi M, Aboab J, Alviset S, et al. Extracorporeal CO_2 removal in acute exacerbation of COPD unresponsive to non-invasive ventilation. BMJ Open Respir Res. 2021;8(1):e001089.
56. Alsallakh MA, Sivakumaran S, Kennedy S, et al. Impact of COVID-19 lockdown on the incidence and mortality of acute exacerbations of chronic obstructive pulmonary disease: national interrupted time series analyses for Scotland and Wales. BMC Med. 2021;19(1):124.
57. Au DH, Bryson CL, Chien JW, et al. The Effects of Smoking Cessation on the Risk of Chronic Obstructive Pulmonary Disease Exacerbations. J Gen Intern Med. 2009;24(4):457-63.
58. Puhan MA, Gimeno-Santos E, Cates CJ, et al. Pulmonary rehabilitation following exacerbations of chronic obstructive pulmonary disease. Cochrane Database Syst Rev. 2016;12(12): CD005305.
59. Jolliffe DA, Greenberg L, Hooper RL, et al. Vitamin D to prevent exacerbations of COPD: systematic review and meta-analysis of individual participant data from randomised controlled trials. Thorax. 2019;74(4):337-45.
60. Washko GR, Fan VS, Ramsey SD, et al. The Effect of Lung Volume Reduction Surgery on Chronic Obstructive Pulmonary Disease Exacerbations. Am J Respir Crit Care Med. 2008;177(2):164-9.
61. Abia-Trujillo D, Yu Lee-Mateus A, Garcia-Saucedo JC, et al. Prevention of acute exacerbation of chronic obstructive pulmonary disease after bronchoscopic lung volume reduction with endobronchial valves. Clin Respir J. 2022;16(1):43-8.
62. Wedzicha JA, Buhl R, Lawrence D, et al. Monotherapy with indacaterol once daily reduces the rate of exacerbations in patients with moderate-to-severe COPD: Post-hoc pooled analysis of 6 months data from three large phase III trials. Respir Med. 2015;109(1):105-11.
63. Poole P, Sathananthan K, Fortescue R. Mucolytic agents versus placebo for chronic bronchitis or chronic obstructive pulmonary disease. Cochrane Database Syst Rev. 2019;2019(5):CD001287.
64. Cazzola M, Calzetta L, Page C, et al. Influence of N-acetylcysteine on chronic bronchitis or COPD exacerbations: a meta-analysis. Eur Respir Rev. 2015;24(137):451-61.
65. Calverley PMA, Rabe KF, Goehring UM, et al. Roflumilast in symptomatic chronic obstructive pulmonary disease: two randomised clinical trials. Lancet. 2009;374(9691):685-94.
66. Ni W, Shao X, Cai X, et al. Prophylactic use of macrolide antibiotics for the prevention of chronic obstructive pulmonary disease exacerbation: a meta-analysis. PloS One. 2015;10(3):e0121257.
67. Albert RK, Connett J, Bailey WC, et al. Azithromycin for prevention of exacerbations of COPD. N Engl J Med. 2011;365(8):689-98.

Palliative Care and End-of-life Communication in Advanced Chronic Obstructive Pulmonary Disease

CHAPTER 89

Sujeet Rajan, Rohit Joshi

INTRODUCTION

Palliative care and end-of-life communication is by far the most challenging part of managing advanced chronic obstructive pulmonary disease (COPD) for respiratory physicians. Physicians managing COPD must be both confident and competent in caring for their patients in the final phase of their illness. Both the patient and his family must be assisted to face inevitable death. It is not surprising that in a study of 100 patients with COPD, 58% preferred a plan of comfort care over a plan to extend life and 78% did not want ventilation in intensive care.[1] Decisions to limit support in terminal illness have become routine in Europe and in the United States. In India, however, these decisions are far more difficult due to the lack of palliative care orientation, unawareness of ethical issues, culture of "fighting till the end," and legal and administrative prejudices.[2]

DEFINITIONS

At the end of life, potentially important decisions are needed. The correct definition of each possible intervention is extremely important. The definitions below are from the International Consensus Conference on end-of-life care in the intensive care unit (ICU) published in 2004.[3,4]

Withholding: A planned decision not to introduce therapies that are otherwise warranted (i.e., intubation, renal replacement therapy, increased doses of vasopressor infusions, surgery, transfusion, nutrition, and hydration).

Withdrawal: Discontinuation of treatments that have been started (i.e., decreasing inspiratory oxygen fraction to 21%, extubating, turning off the ventilator, and suspending the vasopressors)

Terminal sedation: Pain and symptom treatment with the possible side effect of shortening life

Euthanasia: From the Greek words *eu* and *thanatos* meaning "good death." It means that a doctor is intentionally killing a person who is suffering unbearably and hopelessly at the latter's voluntary, explicit, repeated, well-considered, informed request.

Physician-assisted suicide: Means that a doctor is intentionally helping/assisting/cooperating in the suicide of a person who is suffering unbearably and hopelessly at the latter's voluntary, explicit, repeated, well-considered, informed request. These acts do not include withholding or withdrawing treatments although these may occur prior to physician-assisted suicide.

Cardiopulmonary resuscitation (CPR) failure: Defined as death despite the use of a ventilator or cardiac massage

Brain death: Documented cessation of cerebral function and meeting the criteria for brain death

Palliative care: Any interventions aimed to prevent and relieve suffering by controlling symptoms and providing other support to patients and families in order to maintain and improve their quality of living during all stages of chronic life-threatening (or terminal) illness.

End-of-life care: It is the care (comfort, supportive or symptom care) provided to a person in their final stages of life.

PALLIATIVE CARE BEFORE END-OF LIFE

Palliative care need not be a separate stage at the end of life when all disease-modifying options have been exhausted.[5] Any chronic life-threatening illness needs parallel palliative care with disease-specific therapy before being declared as terminal. Palliative care needs to start at a much earlier stage and be an integral part of standard care, based on needs rather than just prognosis.

For patients with chronic lung disease, this information will often not often be as simple to classify as whether the patient is in "active treatment" or "palliative only." Instead, it should indicate that the patient has advanced disease and that standard treatments have often resulted in recovery and are also the best way of relieving symptoms, but should the patient fail to respond, it would be appropriate to switch the focus to the relief of symptoms and to ensure that a peaceful, dignified, and natural death is achieved. For this disease trajectory, it is imperative that specific disease-modifying treatments and palliative care must run parallelly.

ADVANCED TERMINAL CHRONIC OBSTRUCTIVE PULMONARY DISEASE

Advanced terminal COPD comes under the spectrum of "end-stage lung disease" which basically implies that the patient now has very severe airflow obstruction, often with a forced expiratory volume in 1 second (FEV_1) of 0.5 L. There is chronic hypoxemia with or without hypercapnia. The terminal phase of COPD is difficult to define; it can vary from one patient to another based on the actual lung function, presence of pulmonary hypertension, personality, and attitude toward illness, and of course, the social status of the patient. At one spectrum, one could get a patient with an FEV_1 of 45% of predicted, from a lower socioeconomic stratum who has almost permanently confined himself to his home, to another from a higher socioeconomic stratum with an FEV_1 of 34% who is raring to play golf.

A good way to define terminal disease is when survival is expected to be <2 years. This allows the primary care physician with help from the specialist to guide the patient and the family on how the future is likely to evolve. Though 2 years sound a realistic end point before which to start communicating, it is not so easy in COPD, which reflects certain death at an uncertain time. In fact, most patients with COPD do not die of progressive respiratory failure but of cardiac disease or cancers. This was clearly evident from the review of the mortality data from the TORCH (TOwards a Revolution in COPD Health) study.[6] Therefore, a reasonably healthy COPD patient may actually and very often die suddenly of myocardial infarction. This may not be easily predictable. However, that needs to be a factored point when discussing end-of-life issues with the patient.[7]

Prognosis of Advanced Chronic Obstructive Pulmonary Disease

Equally important is to realize the prognosis of patients with COPD. **Table 1** lists a good guide in deciding when to bring up the topic for discussion with patients discharged after an acute exacerbation of chronic bronchitis (AECB).

A Canadian study suggested that after 6 months of discharge from a hospital following AECB, only 25% of patients were well and with a good quality of life; 44% of them had been readmitted by then.[8] This illustrates how important it is to bring up this issue at the stage of hospital discharge from an AECB. The author will discuss other situations to define advanced terminal COPD, but equally important is the presence of pulmonary hypertension and right ventricle (RV) dysfunction, the presence of which itself is indicative of a 4-year mortality of 73%.[9] The timing of death, however, remains almost impossible to predict. As mentioned in the example earlier of myocardial infarction as a cause of death, the timing of death is poorly estimated even within a week of death.[10]

TABLE 1: Postdischarge mortality in two studies.

Ai Ping et al.[7]	Breen et al.[8]
6 months: 39%	6 months: 41%
1 year: 43%	1 year: 49%
3 years: 61%	2 years: 58%
5 years: 76%	3 years: 64%

Perceived and Implicit Bias in Chronic Obstructive Pulmonary Disease

Despite having a comparable symptom burden, patients with COPD and interstitial lung disease (ILD) receive fewer indicators of palliative care on average than those with metastatic cancer.[11]

It is ethically unacceptable that patients with COPD who experience symptom burdens as high as or higher than those patients with other diseases do not receive similar levels of care. Patients with similar palliative care needs merit similar treatment, regardless of their primary diagnosis.[12]

Palliative care may be withheld or reduced in patients with COPD and other smoking-related lung diseases, especially when patients are unable to quit smoking.[13] The bias against smoking-related diseases can be often unintentional and still perceived by the patient,[14,15] making patients often feel they deserve the disease.

Differing expectations between the physician and patient often introduce some bias.[12] Some physicians may question the benefit of palliative care in a patient who continues to smoke, failing to realize that socioeconomic status could be playing a significant role in the tobacco addiction. COPD patients are often from lower socioeconomic status, further worsening the chances of smoking cessation or receiving desirable support.

Physicians must be aware of this implicit bias and understand that COPD patients' may experience discrimination based on their addiction to tobacco, both in the hospital setting and at their homes.

Issues Involved in Treating Advanced Terminal Chronic Obstructive Pulmonary Disease

When the disease gets worse and as the pharmacological options become limited, the care gets harder and more challenging. Some of the questions to handle at this stage are as follows:

- Handling the fear of a dying patient—the fear of suffocation or choking to death is real; watching someone going through this stage can be equally devastating for the family.
- When the next exacerbation occurs, should the patient be *actively* treated to prolong life or treated so as to allow smooth transition from life to death?

- How *much* active treatment is appropriate? Should the next exacerbation be treated at home (especially in a financially drained patient) or at a hospital?
- If treated at home, should noninvasive ventilation (NIV) be used (machines can now be rented or bought by patients)?
- If treated in the hospital, should the patient be treated in the room/ward or ICU (distanced from relatives and loved ones)?
- If a decision has been taken that patient is not to be transferred to ICU, what is the maximum time for the patient to remain in the ward/room setting?
- If a decision to transfer to ICU is taken, is the patient agreeable to be *invasively* ventilated?
- If it is *no* to the above question, what will be the maximum care offered to the patient in the ICU, which cannot be given in a room/ward?
- If the patient has said no to any of the above "active treatment" options, has an "advance directive" been obtained from the patient?
- Are the relatives taking most of the decisions for the patient (common in Indian scenario, where shielding the patient from an adverse diagnosis or prognosis is common)? Is the patient educated enough to take a better decision himself? If so, is the "relatives" opinion/decision final?
- If the patient is unconscious (with no advance directives), how does the discussion with family ensue?

GOOD DEATH IN CHRONIC OBSTRUCTIVE PULMONARY DISEASE: IMPLICATIONS

An excellent study identified five issues that a patient may wish to see addressed before he dies.[16] As a physician, it is important to be very sensitive to the following issues:

1. Adequate relief of symptoms, especially pain and dyspnea
2. No inappropriate prolongation of life
3. Sense of control of their own person
4. Relief of the burden to their family
5. Strengthening of family relationships

Patients with COPD are not always able to die quietly, peacefully, or in their own homes. The patient and the families' descriptions of breathlessness challenge the definitions of a "good death." Patients often die in the ICU or hospital and it could be argued that dying in an environment away from the home setting has meant that we have lost our ability to communicate with the dying patient.[17]

It is also understood that it is difficult to provide the same level of security, symptom relief, and support that can be provided in a hospital[5] as compared to home. Caregivers with inadequate training or awareness leads to further anxiety and insecurity in the family setting.

For the COPD patient, this is a constant dilemma. By suffering at home all the time, he has already experienced a "social" death for years. He is often "dying and living" at the same time. At the end, when brought to a hospital, he is additionally subjected to the regular procedures of a "hospital management," which could range from simple intravenous lines to endotracheal intubation and invasive ventilation. Having undergone a prolonged period of reduced physical and social functioning, they are actually hardly "living" in the true sense much before they die. The COPD patient, therefore, challenges the concept of a "good death." This remains one of the most difficult situations in dealing with patients with any kind of advanced lung disease.[18]

APPROPRIATE TIME TO BEGIN DISCUSSIONS ON END-OF-LIFE ISSUES WITH CHRONIC OBSTRUCTIVE PULMONARY DISEASE PATIENTS

As mentioned earlier, when survival is expected to be below 2 years, the time has come to start a discussion with the patient. Studies have shown that patients appreciate physicians who discuss these issues with them, in contrast to many physicians believing that patients may not be ready for the same.[19] Patients appreciated physicians who are honest and straightforward, willing to talk about dying, good at listening, give bad news in a sensitive way, and most importantly, are sensitive to the timing of such discussions. By avoiding the topic, patients are less satisfied. Introduction of the topic actually allows patients to engage in a good discussion and maintain a sense of hope with less depression, even when the prognosis is poor.

Patients perceive their physicians based on *what* (the content) they communicate and *how* (the process) they do it largely. Unfortunately, most of these discussions take place outside the ICU and often when the patient himself is unable to take a decision on his own. This delay in communication must be avoided and every attempt should be made at the outpatient level to start such discussions where appropriate and of course after a full review of diagnostic tests and ongoing treatments. Sometimes, even a second opinion helps before deciding that the patient and the family needs such a discussion. End-of-life discussions in COPD can be started in the presence of different disease criteria (**Box 1**).

Despite these criteria, <15% of ICU patients retain decision-making capacity, so it is impossible to discuss

BOX 1 **Different criteria in COPD when end-of-life discussion can happen.**

- FEV_1 < 30% (during the stable period)
- Oxygen dependence
- One or more hospitalizations in the past 1 year with AECB
- Left heart failure
- Weight loss/cachexia and increasing dependence on others
- Age > 70 years

(AECB: acute exacerbations of chronic bronchitis; COPD: chronic obstructive pulmonary disease; FEV_1: forced expiratory volume in 1 second)

the decision with them in ICU.[20] Also, though the patient's family is often involved in decision-making in India (largely shielding the patient); studies have shown that relatives rate the communication with hospital staff as poor.

Additionally, many of these discussions occur outside an ICU and during an exacerbation,[21] hardly the appropriate place to start of such discussions, but sadly this is where most such discussions occur.

Identifying the High-risk Patient

More recently, a decision tree [Classification and Regression Tree (CART)] has been proposed and validated. It can identify patients at a high risk of mortality in the next 5 years and takes into account five easily available parameters in clinical practice:[22]

1. Age
2. FEV_1
3. Dyspnea
4. Physical activity
5. Number of hospital admissions in the previous 2 years

It would be worth using such decision trees in prognosticating severe COPD in clinical practice.

PRINCIPLES OF END-OF-LIFE COMMUNICATION IN CHRONIC OBSTRUCTIVE PULMONARY DISEASE

- *Ethical principles*: The basic ethical principles consist of beneficence, nonmaleficence, autonomy, and justice, i.e., fairness in the physician's approach. Physician should not provide investigation or treatment that will harm or serve no purpose. Avoid imposing futile treatments on the patient. Treatment aimed at a specific symptom may have adverse effects that may shorten life, e.g., morphine. When the benefits of alleviating the patient's suffering outweigh the risks, then such therapy is acceptable and is not considered euthanasia.
- *Cultural principles*: Surprisingly, there is very little information on how the influence of culture affects the patient and family. Culture encompasses the patient's beliefs, life's experiences, values, attitudes, and assumptions. This is not necessarily related to the ethnicity of the patient. Culture can affect the entire way in which a patient approaches his life, disease, and death. This culture needs to be respected by the physician. Eye contact with the patient, physical touch, and privacy often varies between cultures. The entire communication process of "breaking bad news" can vary between cultures and understandably, this can have profound effects on management planning. Respect given to the patient's cultural preferences has a tremendous positive impact on the patient and the family. Trust is immensely improved and strengthened when this aspect of the patient's whole is also respected.
- *Incompetent patient*: Depression can often affect the decision-making process of COPD patients. This must be carefully looked for before labeling the patient as poorly responsive to suggestions or incompetent in making a decision. For the actual incompetent patient, one has to often ask the family for end-of-life directives. Ideally, this should be the spouse or children. It is important here to understand if the patient had ever expressed any desires about the way he should be managed toward the end of his life. Often, the patient has expressed such views to the family, such as not being ventilated or brought to ICU at all. Our culture often shields the patient from bad news, despite the patient realizing, long before the family, that he is headed in a downward trajectory.

Sadly, even in competent patients, the family often incorrectly states a patient's wishes.[23] When life and death decisions are at play, the family must be told that the decision is not their responsibility, but that they are simply guiding the physicians in their decisions.

Place Where End-of-life Communication Should be Done

Communication is most often done outside an ICU cubicle! This should be avoided as far as possible. A large quiet room with privacy and confidentiality is the best. Emotional outbursts are not uncommon by family members. In some cultures, the patient is asked as to whom he would like to have present in the room. In others, the patient is often left out of the discussion, leaving this to responsible family members whom he entrusts with all decisions pertaining to his life and death. It is important to counsel these members extensively.

When such discussions occur, ensure that everyone's opinion in the room is heard out and try to end it on a final collective decision that everyone agrees to.

How and What Needs to be Done[24]

- After listening well to the patient and the family, you will be able to understand their expectations and come to a consensus on what needs to be done. The levels at which things for advanced COPD can be planned are outlined further:
  - *Level 4*: All conditions investigated and treated, including CPR
  - *Level 3*: Above, except CPR (the patient can still be intubated and ventilated)
  - *Level 2*: Potentially reversible conditions are investigated and treated (can be done at home or hospital)
  - *Level 1*: Main focus is on palliative care—symptom relief is the focus of all treatment [intravenous feeds and Ryle's tube (RT) feeds are avoided].
- As mentioned earlier, when planning the foreseeable level of care, always use words such as "if" rather than "when." "When" seems to be a prediction of doom, but

"if" is more often seen as uncertainty and allows patients to balance hope and acceptance.

- Discuss the implications and consequences of treatments, in the light of the disease prognosis. It is imperative that patients and their families understand the "misery of doing everything." Often, patients with unlimited financial resources believe that "everything" must be done for a dying patient. "Everything" includes more drugs with adverse effects, mechanical ventilation, more procedures on an ill patient, and not to forget the ongoing mental stress to the patient and the family members, many of whom have not been actively involved in this decision to do "everything."
- *Do not forget about depression and COPD*: Depression often affects decision-making by the COPD patient and this should not preclude the introduction of an intervention when it can actually help to improve the patient's quality of life.
- *Manage symptoms as possible in the following ways*:
    - *Dyspnea*: Over 50% patients suffer from dyspnea and 90% by the end of their life. Dyspnea is often aggravated by anxiety, low-dose anxiolytics such as alprazolam can often help, especially if backup NIV is available. Pharmacologic therapy is often limited after nebulized bronchodilators and systemic steroid have been used. Though oxygen and NIV help, morphine may need to be used when dyspnea worsens. The only drugs with a proven effect on dyspnea are opioids. An excellent recent randomized, placebo-controlled trial was performed on patients with refractory dyspnea, the large majority having COPD.[25] Not only did the dyspnea scores improve significantly with morphine, but the patients reported much better sleep too. The only concern was distressing constipation despite laxatives. Though the Global initiative for chronic Obstructive Lung Disease (GOLD) guidelines state that opioids are contraindicated in COPD management, physicians should refer to the American Thoracic Society (ATS) Clinical Policy Statement on Palliative Care where the principle holds that relief of suffering is adequate justification of the use of opioids to control dyspnea or pain.[26] Sadly, in many countries, "morphine phobia" among clinicians and the general population leads to inappropriate management of terminal pain and dyspnea.

The benefits are largely related to reduced ventilation and the sensation of dyspnea. Unlike pain management, the long-term effects are not so beneficial and side effects are common. Relaxation breathing, upright posture, and sometimes, music therapy can also help in palliative care. Slow-paced music is usually preferred over fast pace. Music therapy is shown to be superior to progressive muscle relaxation in acute exacerbations.[27]

- *Cough*: Often, suppressive therapy works for cough. Sometimes, systemic steroids are needed. Inhaled local anesthetics can help at times. Physiotherapy may help to control secretions, but adequate hydration goes a long way in ensuring that thick secretions do not impair the ability of the patient to protect his airway.
- *Insomnia*: Not uncommon in advanced COPD, usually due to orthopnea. Anxiety, depression and theophylline can also contribute. Oxygen to relieve nocturnal desaturation often helps. Nonbenzodiazepine sedatives such as zolpidem and amitriptyline may help. Benzodiazepines should be avoided as far as possible.
- *Fatigue*: Lack of exercise, low body mass index, and insomnia—all contribute to fatigue. Never miss out treatable causes such as anemia (iron or B_{12} deficiency) or thyroid disease. Sleep disturbance is often a cause of fatigue and must be addressed.
- *Delirium*: Confusion occurs in a large number of patients as they approach death. Medications, especially opioids and metabolic disturbances can contribute. After correction of hypoxia and hyponatremia, haloperidol can be tried as a good first-line choice for this symptom. As the need for haloperidol increases, more aggressive sedation may be required and the family should be informed about this requirement.
- *Cachexia and weight loss*: A poor prognostic sign, this catabolic state often is a result of increased minute ventilation. Mouth breathing and aerophagy aggravate anorexia. High-calorie supplements can help. Sometimes, prokinetics help by improving gastric emptying. Foods liked by patient should be provided, including alcohol. Though weight loss can be explained to families as a body's way of shutting down, it is often followed by desperate attempts to feed (and often overfeed) the patient. This must be avoided as metabolism will increase further, putting further load on the respiratory system.
- *Judicious use of NIV*: NIV has significantly helped many COPD patients die a more comfortable death. Just the ability to speak and eat a bit too makes NIV so much less intrusive than an endotracheal tube or a tracheostomy. NIV at home has also reduced the number of terminally ill COPD patients reaching the hospital for the inevitable. Though the machines are expensive to purchase, rentals on a daily or monthly basis are now available in several cities.

In the era before NIV, COPD patients admitted to an ICU for an acute exacerbation aged > 65 years had a mortality rate of 30%, which doubled after 1 year to 60%. A more recent retrospective study aimed at looking at long-term survival of patients treated with NIV for the first time. Survival here was 72%, 52%, and 26% at 1, 2, and 5 years, respectively.[28] The survival rate was also influenced by the need for readmission. Those who needed readmission had a 20% survival chance at 5 years.

Though we are aware that numerous studies have shown improved survival with invasive ventilation and NIV, these patients require physiotherapy and intensive nursing for weeks after recovery. In the rare situations where even tracheostomies have been done and the patient is sent home, the quality of life can really take a huge dip, despite improved "survival." Many of these patients live the last phase of their lives in a hospital or protected environment, with reduced privacy and restricted policies to meet their relatives.[29]

In the final analysis, NIV has improved survival, but the quality of life of COPD patients on long-term NIV needs to be seriously examined in the Indian setting. It is always helpful to proceed according to the decision-tree to appropriate the management of COPD.[30]

SUMMARY

End-of-life communication and palliative care are cardinal in the overall management of severe, advanced COPD. As the disease gets more and more severe, less and less specific therapies are likely to benefit the patient and more supportive and palliative care becomes the order of the day. It is imperative that not just respiratory physicians but also primary care physicians better understand the process of dying in these patients. It will help them deal with death much better.

REFERENCES

1. Claessens MT, Lynn J, Zhong Z, et al. Dying with lung cancer or chronic obstructive pulmonary disease: Insights from SUPPORT. Study to Understand Prognoses and Preferences for Outcomes and Risks of Treatments. J Am Geriatr Soc. 2000;48(5 Suppl):S146-53.
2. Mani RK. End-of-life care in India. Intensive Care Med. 2006;32(7):1066-8.
3. Lambertus JC, Thijs G, Antonelli M, et al. Challenges in end-of-life care in the ICU. Statement of the 5th International Consensus Conference. Intensive Care Med. 2004;30:770-84.
4. Carlucci A, Guerrieri A, Stefano N. Eur Respir Rev. 2012; 12(126):347-54.
5. Bourke S, Peel E. Palliative care of chronic progressive lung disease. Clin Med. 2014;14(3):325.
6. Calverley PM, Anderson JA, Celli B, et al. Salmeterol and fluticasone propionate and survival in chronic obstructive pulmonary disease. N Engl J Med. 2007;356(8):775-89.
7. Ai-Ping C, Lee KH, Lim TK. In-hospital and 5-year mortality of patients treated in the ICU for acute exacerbation of COPD: a retrospective study. Chest. 2005;128(2):518-24.
8. Connors AF Jr, Dawson NV, Thomas C, et al. Outcomes following acute exacerbation of severe chronic obstructive lung disease. The SUPPORT investigators (Study to Understand Prognoses and Preferences for Outcomes and Risks of Treatments). Am J Respir Crit Care Med. 1996;154(4 Pt 1):959-67.
9. Breen D, Churches T, Hawker F, et al. Acute respiratory failure secondary to chronic obstructive pulmonary disease treated in the intensive care unit: a long term follow up study. Thorax. 2002;57(1):29-33.
10. Budev MM, Arroliga AC, Wiedemann HP, et al. Cor pulmonale: an overview. Semin Respir Crit Care Med. 2003;24(3):233-44.
11. Brown CE, Engelberg RA, Nielsen EL, et al. Palliative care for patients dying in the ICU with chronic lung disease compared to metastatic cancer. Ann Am Thorac Soc. 2016;13(5):684-9.
12. Brown CE, Jecker NS, Curtis JR. Inadequate palliative care in chronic lung disease. An issue of health care inequality. Ann Am Thorac Soc. 2016;13(3):311-6.
13. Johnson JL, Campbell AC, Bowers M, et al. Understanding the social consequences of chronic obstructive pulmonary disease: the effects of stigma and gender. Proc Am Thorac Soc. 2007;4:680-2.
14. Banaji MR, Greenwald AG. Blindspot: hidden biases of good people. New York: Delacorte Press; 2013.
15. FitzGerald C. A neglected aspect of conscience: awareness of implicit attitudes. Bioethics. 2014;28:24-32.
16. Singer PA, Martin DK, Kelner M. Quality end-of-life care: patients' perspectives. JAMA. 1999;281(2):163-8.
17. Costello J. Dying well: nurses' experiences of 'good and bad' deaths in hospital. J Adv Nurs. 2006;54(5):594-601.
18. Russel SJ, Russel RE. Challenges in end-of-life communication in COPD. Breathe. 2007;4(2):133-9.
19. Wenrich MD, Curtis JR, Shannon SE, et al. Communicating with dying patients within the spectrum of medical care from terminal diagnosis to death. Arch Intern Med. 2001;161(6):868-74.
20. Curtis JR, Engelberg RA, Nielsen EL, et al. Patient–physician communication about end-of-life care for patients with severe COPD. Eur Respir J. 2004;24:200-5.
21. Singh VP, Rao V, Prem V, et al. Comparison of the effectiveness of music and progressive muscle relaxation for anxiety in COPD—A randomized controlled pilot study. Chron Respir Dis. 2009;6(4):209-16.
22. GOV.UK. (2008). End-of-life care strategy: promoting high quality care for all adults at the end of life. [online] Available from https://www.gov.uk/government/publications/end-of-life-care-strategy-promoting-high-quality-care-for-adults-at-the-end-of-their-life [Last accessed June, 2024].
23. Layde PM, Beam CA, Broste SK, et al. Surrogates' predictions of seriously ill patients' resuscitation preferences. Arch Farm Med. 1995;4(6):518-23.
24. Bourbeau J, Nault D, Borycki E. The Final Illness: Palliative Care in Terminal COPD. In: Warren P, Barnett B, Cathcart A, et al. (Eds). Comprehensive Management of Chronic Obstructive Pulmonary Disease, 1st edition. Hamilton, Ontario: BC Decker; 2002. pp. 319-38.
25. Abernethy AP, Currow DC, Frith P, et al. Randomised double-blind, placebo-controlled crossover trial of sustained-release morphine for the management of refractory dyspnoea. BMJ. 2003;327:523-28.
26. Lanken PN, Terry PB, Delisser HM, et al. An official American Thoracic Society clinical policy statement: palliative care for patients with respiratory diseases and critical illnesses. Am J Respir Crit Care Med. 2008;177:912-27.
27. Senef MG, Wagner DP, Wagner RP, et al. Hospital and 1-year survival of patients admitted to intensive care units with acute exacerbation of chronic obstructive pulmonary disease. JAMA. 1995;274:1852-7.
28. Chung LP, Winship P, Phung S, et al. Five year outcome in COPD patients after their first episode of acute exacerbation treated with non-invasive ventilation. Respirology. 2010;15:1084-91.
29. Soler-Cataluna JJ, Martinez Garcia MA, Roman Sanchez P, et al. Severe acute exacerbations and mortality in patients with chronic obstructive pulmonary disease. Thorax. 2005;60:925-31.
30. Esteban C, Arostegui I, Moraza J, et al. Development of a decision tree to assess the severity and progress of stable COPD. Eur Respir J. 2011;38:1294-300.

CHAPTER 90

Pulmonary Rehabilitation

Deepak Talwar, Mir Shad Ali, Dhruv Talwar

INTRODUCTION

Pulmonary rehabilitation (PR) is an integral and essential component of clinical management and health maintenance of patients with chronic respiratory disease who remain symptomatic or continue to have decreased function despite standard medical treatment. PR is a complex multidisciplinary intervention of proven benefits in chronic obstructive pulmonary disease (COPD). PR includes multiple components which may vary as per needs and requirements of an individual patient. Defined initially by the American Collage of Chest Physicians in 1974, the American Thoracic Society (ATS) published the first official statement on PR in 1981. 6-minute walk test (6MWT) and respiratory-related quality of life (QOL) questionnaires led to clinical trials demonstrating effectiveness in patients, particularly in COPD. Role of PR is better discussed in the context of COPD which constitutes the most important indication as of today.

DISABILITY ASSOCIATED WITH CHRONIC OBSTRUCTIVE PULMONARY DISEASE

Exercise intolerance and functional impairment are common consequences of COPD.[1] The distinctive characteristics of exercise intolerance in this population include dyspnea, muscle fatigue, hypoxia, bronchospasm, fear, and anxiety-surrounding activity.[2] To avoid these symptoms, patients with COPD spend significantly less time walking and standing and more time sitting and lying in daily life, causing substantial disability. The spiral of inactivity is also affected by symptoms of anxiety and depression experienced by many patients with COPD. The sensation of dyspnea generates feelings of anxiety, but anxiety itself can manifest as dyspnea. Low mood is frequently reported by patients with COPD related to their disability and loss of function but may also be due to a preexisting phenomenon predisposing to smoking. The effects of low mood on motivation and self-esteem may further impact on the inactivity **(Fig. 1)**.

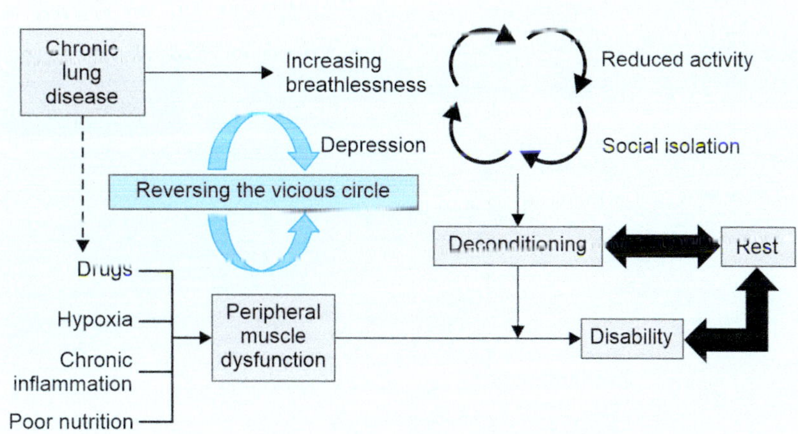

FIG. 1: The relationship between chronic lung disease, muscle deconditioning, and disability spiral of inactivity.

SYSTEMIC CONSEQUENCES OF CHRONIC OBSTRUCTIVE PULMONARY DISEASE

Muscles dysfunction, nutrition, bone density, gonadal hormones, hemoglobin, and mood[3-5] influence exercise tolerance and health-related QOL (HRQL). Muscles of locomotion are altered on multiple levels **(Fig. 2)**. Morphologically, there is a reduction in muscle mass and strength of the quadriceps compared to age-matched healthy controls.[5] The muscle fiber types are altered with an increase in proportion of the type IIX, fast twitch, glycolytic fibers (more fatigable) compared to the type I, slow twitch, oxidative fibres.[6,7] Muscle metabolism is altered with a reduction in oxidative enzymes and a reduction in mitochondrial density. During exercise, energy metabolism is altered with a more rapid loss of phosphocreatine at lower workloads than age-matched healthy controls and a failure of adenosine triphosphate (ATP) replenishment to meet the demand.[8]

Skeletal muscle dysfunction contributes to reduced exercise tolerance by promoting an earlier rise in the level of lactic acid, which when buffered, increases carbon dioxide (CO_2) production which in turn increases the ventilatory load applied to a system which already has an impaired ventilatory capacity. Whether the skeletal muscle dysfunction relates to deconditioning or whether it relates to an underlying inflammatory myopathy remains an area of interest. Patients with COPD enter a vicious cycle of inactivity which also influences the function of their leg muscles. Moreover, reduced ambulatory muscle function can be reversed with exercise training. In favor of an underlying systemic inflammatory process are the increased levels of systemic markers of inflammation as well as oxidative stress and nutritional depletion. Hypoxia and medications such as corticosteroids also contribute toward the skeletal muscle alteration.

ROLE OF PULMONARY REHABILITATION

Pulmonary rehabilitation is a complex multidisciplinary intervention with variable composition as per needs and requirements of an individual respiratory patient.[8] Components of PR, for example, breathing exercises, walking exercises, muscle training, bronchial hygiene, disease-related education, psychological support, and respiratory medications including oxygen have been included for many centuries as a part of good medical care **(Fig. 3)**. Demonstration of dose-dependent effect of exercise training on physiological benefit in COPD was shown to improve exertional dyspnea.[8,9] It was recommended in management of COPD in the Global Initiative for Chronic Obstructive Lung Disease (GOLD) 2–4 stages as an element of nonpharmacological treatment in 2001 on the

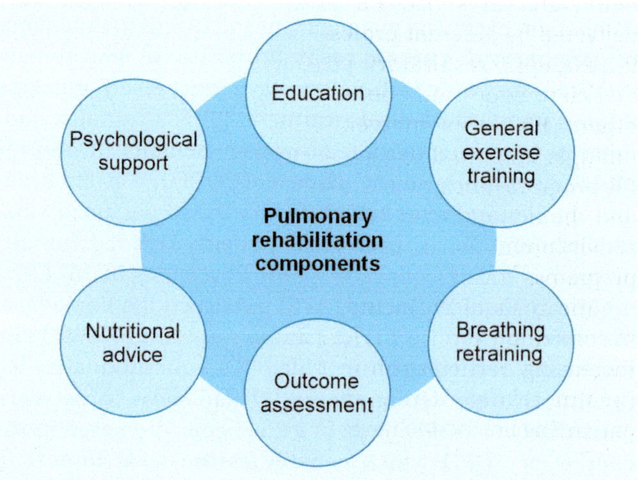

FIG. 3: Components of pulmonary rehabilitation.

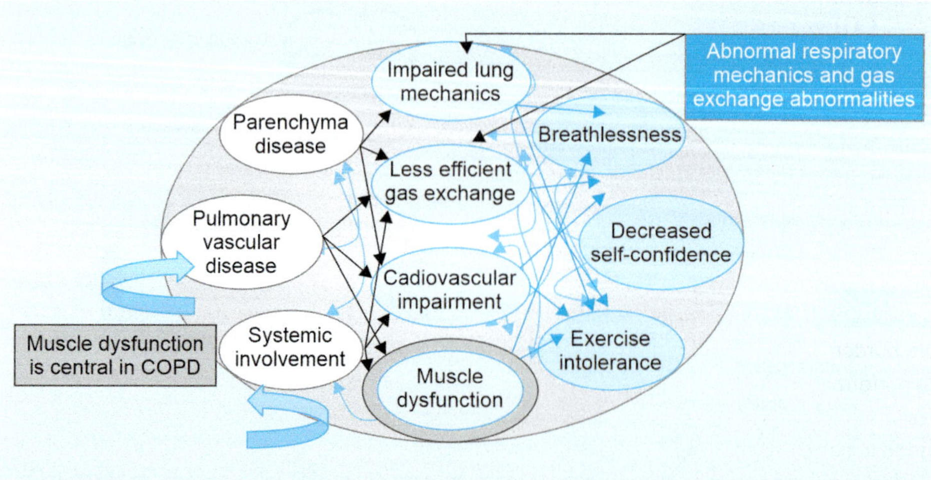

FIG. 2: Breathlessness in chronic obstructive pulmonary disease (COPD) is multifactorial and muscle dysfunction is a key player which remains unaddressed in pharmacotherapy and is targeted in pulmonary rehabilitation.

basis of unequivocal impact of PR in COPD not only on exercise capacity and QOL but also on subsequent need for healthcare. Also, as physical inactivity is related to shortened survival and recurrent hospitalizations, PR targets in improving activity with collateral benefit.[10]

DEFINITION AND GOALS OF PULMONARY REHABILITATION

The ATS/European Respiratory Society (ERS) statement provides a workable definition of PR as a comprehensive intervention based on a thorough patient assessment followed by patient-tailored therapies, which include, but are not limited to, exercise training, education, and behavioral change designed to improve physical and emotional condition of persons with chronic respiratory disease and to promote the long-term adherence to health-enhancing behaviors. In short, PR combines different therapies delivered by different professionals with relevant expertise, for example, respiratory physician, respiratory therapist, dietician, education counselor, exercise physiologist, and others. PR as an intervention is given to the patient at multiple times in disease trajectory of chronic lung disease. PR programs include several evidence-based components and should not be mistaken for more general programs of activity promotion, convalescence, or pure self-management programs.[11]

The goals of PR include minimizing symptom burden, maximizing exercise performance, promoting autonomy, increasing participation in everyday activities, enhancing (health related) QOL, and effecting long-term health-enhancing behavior change **(Box 1)**.

INDICATIONS FOR PULMONARY REHABILITATION—WHO TO REFER?

Traditionally, COPD patients constitute the target population for PR and therefore, COPD remained the subject of the original studies. PR provided to individuals with chronic respiratory diseases other than COPD (such as interstitial lung disease, bronchiectasis, cystic fibrosis, asthma, pulmonary hypertension, lung cancer, lung volume reduction surgery, and lung transplantation) has also demonstrated improvements in symptoms, exercise tolerance, and QOL.

BOX 1 Goals of pulmonary rehabilitation.

- Minimize symptom burden
- Maximize exercise performance
- Promote autonomy
- Increase participation in day-to-day activities
- Improve health-related quality of life
- Effectuate long-term health-enhancing behavior change

The spiral of inactivity, which also applies to other chronic respiratory diseases, provides a rationale for rehabilitation which has been reported to be beneficial in other conditions **(Fig. 1)**. Exertional dyspnea that interferes with function as assessed by the Medical Research Council (MRC) Dyspnea Scale is the predominant clinical criterion for referral for PR.[12,13] This is a simple, self-assessed scale and can easily be used to screen those who may benefit from rehabilitation.

International guidelines suggest referral for PR for Grades III–V, but there is evidence to suggest that patients with milder levels of breathlessness may also benefit.[14] The World Health Organization (GOLD) recommends rehabilitation for any symptomatic patients with GOLD stage 2 and above [forced expiratory volume in 1 second (FEV_1) < 80% predicted]. Both the primary respiratory disease and existing comorbid conditions should be optimally managed prior to enrolment. Patients with obstructive disease should receive optimal airway care. Any preexisting depression should be addressed as it is known to be associated with poor compliance and response to rehabilitation. Diagnostic assessment and optimizing management should occur prior to commencing PR. Patients need to be able to participate in endurance exercises and those with a predominantly orthopedic, neurological, or peripheral vascular limitation to exercise are commonly excluded. Safety criteria should be adhered to, for example, a myocardial infarction sustained within 3 months, unstable angina, moderate-to-severe aortic stenosis or uncontrolled blood pressure will all exclude patients from being enrolled **(Table 1)**. Patients with unstable cardiovascular disease must be assessed and treated appropriately prior to inclusion to a program. Nonclinical factors may be pivotal. These include a reasonable level of comprehension, realistic expectations of the program, motivation to improve, an ability to follow instructions, acceptable health literacy, and a supportive home and family.

ASSESSMENT FOR PULMONARY REHABILITATION PROGRAM

Before starting a training program, the assessment should systematically address the inclusion and exclusion criteria and further inform the patients about the process of PR. An assessment of dyspnea, exercise performance, and health status is standard and can inform both individual progress and program quality.[15] An exercise assessment is needed to individualize the exercise prescription, evaluate the potential need for supplemental oxygen, help rule out some cardiovascular comorbidities, and help ensure the safety of the intervention. Patients with resting hypoxia should exercise with supplemental oxygen. The criterion for ambulatory oxygen varies from place to place. Those who desaturate markedly on exercise <85% are often offered supplementary oxygen during training. In many countries, the expense of oxygen makes it prohibitive except in patients with profound hypoxemia.

TABLE 1: Indications and contraindications of patients for pulmonary rehabilitation.

Indications	Contraindications
• Persistent respiratory symptoms, especially dyspnea • Limitation of functional status despite optimal medication • Impaired health-related quality of life • Decreased occupational performance • Psychosocial problems attendant on the underlying respiratory illness • Difficulty with medical regimen • Difficulty performing day-to-day activities • Nutritional depletion • Increased use of medical resources • Gas exchange abnormalities	• Conditions that substantially increase risk during rehabilitation, e.g., unstable angina • Conditions that substantially interfere with rehabilitative process • Uncontrolled diabetes • Psychiatric illness, e.g., dementia • Severe exercise-induced hypoxemia, not correctable with oxygen supplementation • Inability to exercise due to orthopedic or other reasons

COMMON OUTCOME MEASURES

Outcome assessment requires a minimum of two time points—one before PR (baseline) and one immediately after completing rehabilitation. The most common outcome measures in PR consist of evaluating an individual's ability to exercise, symptoms, and HRQL.

Exercise Capacity

Measures of exercise capacity range from simple field tests to cardiopulmonary exercise (CPX) tests (CPET). The most commonly used field tests of exercise capacity are the 6MWT and the incremental shuttle walk test (ISWT) or endurance shuttle walk test (ESWT).

Cardiopulmonary Exercise Tests

The gold standard measurement of exercise capacity is maximal oxygen consumption (VO_{2max}). A maximal, incremental, symptom-limited cardiopulmonary test with expiratory gas analysis can provide this as well as comprehensive information about the precise limitation to exercise. However, it involves expensive equipment and expertise. CPET are performed on a cycle ergometer, but a treadmill can also be used particularly if cycling is not familiar. Endurance tests can be performed using the same equipment set at an intensity relative to the peak performance. Although the variability of endurance testing is greater than for maximal testing, endurance tests are often a more sensitive outcome measure for PR.

6-minute Walk Test

The most commonly used field test is the 6MWT.[16] This test is clinically favored because it is functional and does not require extensive or expensive equipment. The test is completed over a 30-meter flat course. It is self-paced and standardized instructions are given. The 6MWT can be influenced by encouragement, which is therefore standardized. Patient is asked to walk as far as he can at his own pace for 6 minutes and the result is usually presented as the distance walked, although the speed can be calculated. The test is reproducible after two practice tests and is responsive. Unlike other field tests, normal reference values are available. It is likely closer to peak exercise capacity, although the distance walked is referred to as a measure of functional capacity. The 6MWT distance is highly correlated with other outcomes of COPD such as mortality and is featured in the multidimensional severity index, the BODE [body mass index (BMI), airflow obstruction, dyspnea, and exercise] index.[17] It may be useful information for formulating an initial exercise prescription (usually as a percentage of the overall speed), but the intensity will vary between individuals. It is reliable, valid, and interpretable, all important qualities for its use in clinical research.[16]

Shuttle Walk Distance Tests

There are two types of shuttle walk distance tests—the incremental and the endurance.

Incremental Shuttle Walk Test

The ISWT is a symptom-limited, externally paced test that utilizes an audible pacing timer to incrementally increase pacing frequency conducted along a 10-meter (33 feet) course and reflects maximal exercise capacity.[18] The walking speed increases every minute until the patient is too breathless or fatigued to continue or can cannot keep pace with the external pacing signal. The result is presented as the total distance achieved. It is reproducible after a single practice test. In contrast to the 6MWT, the ISWT has a graded physiological response. However, normal reference values are not currently available. The test is also reliable, valid, and interpretable,[18,19] making it an excellent evaluative test just like the 6MWT.

Endurance Shuttle Walk Test

The ESWT can be used to test submaximal exercise capacity. This test is a standardized, externally controlled, constant-paced walking test for the assessment of endurance capacity.

It is similarly symptom limited and uses the same 10-meter course as the ISWT.[20] After a 2-minute warm-up, the patients walk at the set speed until they can no longer maintain the required speed or are too breathless or fatigued to continue. The result is presented as the time walked after the warm-up and is reproducible after a familiarization test. The ISWT and ESWT can be used to develop individualized exercise prescriptions for PR. The ISWT is initially performed to determine exercise capacity and then a paced walk speed corresponding to 85% of capacity is used to determine the walking speed for the ESWT. The duration of the walk can then be progressed throughout the program. Both the ISWT and ESWT are responsive outcome measures.

Health Status

Health-related QOL has become an important outcome for assessing chronic disease interventions. Most disease-specific questionnaires have components that assess dyspnea and activity limitation. The two most commonly used and therefore the best understood are the Chronic Respiratory Questionnaire (CRQ)[21] and St George's Respiratory Questionnaire (SGRQ).[22] They are both reproducible and evaluative, but the SGRQ has the advantage of also being discriminative. Generic questionnaires such as the Medical Outcomes Short Form-36 Questionnaire (SF-36) can also be used. This has the advantage of being able to compare across different disease populations and has normative values, but it is more discriminative than evaluative and may not identify small disease-specific changes. The recently developed COPD assessment test (CAT) is short, easy to administer, and provides an overview of a patient's health status.[23] It has been shown to be sensitive to PR.[24]

Dyspnea

The MRC scale is often used as an outcome measure for dyspnea. It is a valid, reproducible instrument but not designed to be an evaluative tool.[25] It is however a valuable guide for staging the severity of COPD. The Baseline Dyspnea Index and the Transition Dyspnea Index (BDI/TDI) are disease specific, valid, reproducible, and interpretable. Together with the SGRQ and the CRQ, the BDI–TDI is among the most frequently employed measures of outcome in PR.[26]

Clinically Important Difference

For many of the outcome measures described, a "clinically meaningful" change has been evaluated. This adds to clinical interpretation of results from an intervention. A minimum clinically important difference exists for the 6MWT, ISWT, ESWT, CRQ, SGRQ, and the BDI/TDI. If achieved, it provides a rationale for introducing or withdrawing a management intervention.

CORE COMPONENTS OF A PULMONARY REHABILITATION PROGRAM

The core components of a program are summarized in **Box 2**.

General Exercise Training

Exercise training is an essential component to PR and has the largest supporting evidence base of all the other components. For exercise training to be effective the total training load must reflect the individual's specific requirements, it must exceed loads encountered during daily life to improve aerobic capacity and muscle strength (i.e., the training threshold) and must progress as improvement occurs. PR is based on following principles in exercise training:

- *Intensity*: Higher intensity produces greater results (e.g., >60% of VO_{2max} or at 60–80% W_{max}).
- *Specificity*: Only muscles trained produce the desired effect.
- *Reversibility*: Stopping regular exercise training decreases the effect.

Exercise regimen is designed to improve endurance, strength, or both.

Lower Limb Endurance Training

Lower limb endurance training is mandatory for individuals who wish to improve exercise tolerance and reduce dyspnea on exertion. It is individually prescribed, based on an assessment exercise test and progressed throughout the program. High-intensity training is recommended in the healthy population for achieving cardiorespiratory fitness. Similar principles apply to patients with COPD and high-intensity training produces greater physiologic benefits than lower-intensity training.[27] However, many are so constrained by dyspnea that they are often unable to achieve the ideal training intensity, but the highest intensity feasible should be the aim. The framework recommended by the American College of Sports Medicine [ACSM's Guidelines for Exercise Testing and Prescription on Frequency, Intensity, Time, and Type (FITT)] can be applied in PR.[28] Intensity can be prescribed from the CPET performed on

BOX 2 Core components of a pulmonary rehabilitation program.

- *General exercise training*:
  - Lower limb endurance training (continues and interval training)
  - Lower and upper limb resistance training
- Multidisciplinary education
- Psychological support
- Nutritional support
- Self-management

a treadmill or a cycle ergometer or from the various field tests. The training speed or load can be calculated from the measured (CPX) or predicted (field tests) percentage of peak oxygen consumption (typically, 60–80% for high intensity) or from peak heart rate (similarly, 60–80% predicted for high intensity). A Borg dyspnea or fatigue score of 4–6 [moderate to (very) severe] or rating of perceived exertion of 12–14 (somewhat hard) is often considered a target training intensity.[29] Walking and cycling are both effective training modalities.

Interval Training

Interval training is a modification of endurance training in which high-intensity exercise is regularly interspersed with periods of rest or lower-intensity exercise. Interval training has a good rationale for allowing the muscles to recover during the lower-intensity periods; studies have not identified interval training as being more effective than constant load training for those with COPD.[30]

Resistance (Strength) Training

Resistance (strength) training has received much attention over the last two decades and is recommended by international guidelines. Although muscle strength is improved compared to endurance training alone, this has not translated to additional improvements in exercise tolerance or health status. The effect of strength training on daily physical activity is yet to be thoroughly investigated. The ACSM recommends that to enhance muscle strength in adults, 1–3 sets of 8–12 repetitions should be undertaken on 2–3 days each week.[31] Initial loads equivalent to either 60–70% of the one repetition maximum and progressed through the program. The studies advocating resistance training were performed on gym equipment. Lower limb exercise often consists of sit to stand, step ups, and leg raises, which can be progressed throughout the program, but these exercises have not been thoroughly evaluated **(Figs. 4A to D)**. Ankle weights can also be employed to add resistance. Upper limb resistance training is commonly performed using free weights and currently, unsupported endurance exercises are recommended in the guidelines There are theoretical reasons why improving upper limb strength may help dyspnea and activities of daily living, but the results of small studies so far

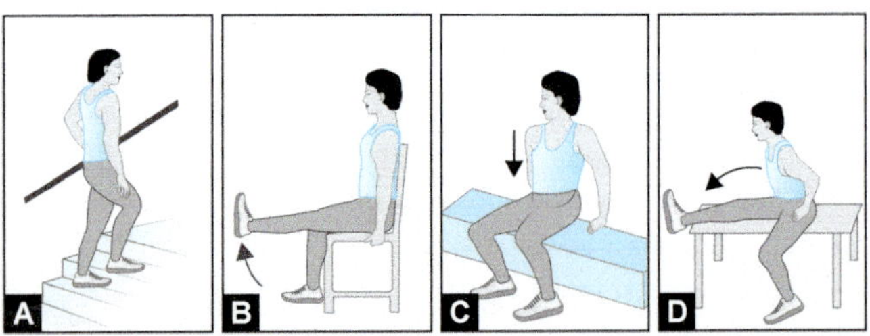

FIGS. 4A TO D: Exercises for lower extremity in sitting and standing position.

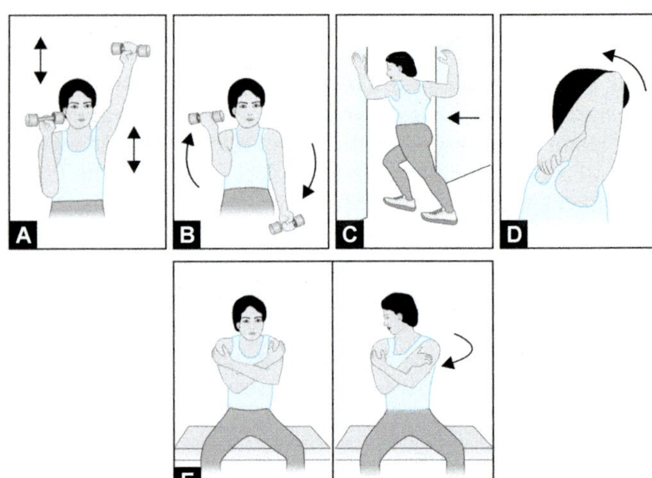

FIGS. 5A TO E: Exercises for upper extremity in sitting and standing position.

are varied.[32] Nevertheless, most PR programs include upper limb exercise **(Figs. 5A to E)**.

Multidisciplinary Education

It is widely accepted that education is a logical and necessary component of PR, but less is known about which topics are essential. Education is commonly delivered in a group setting but should be supplemented with individual support and other ongoing educational materials such as computer-based, online learning modules.

Psychological Support in Pulmonary Rehabilitation

Psychological support is a core component of PR as many patients experience symptoms of anxiety or depression. Prevalence of anxiety and depression in COPD is 36% and 40%, respectively, and depression is known to increase the risk of acute exacerbation and hospitalizations in COPD. Patient may be provided with vocational counseling, education strategies to cope stress, and involvement of family members to resolve conflicts. However, patients with severe psychological problems need formal evaluation by psychiatrist. Psychological status should be first assessed using a standardized measuring tool such as the Hospital Anxiety and Depression Scale (HADS).[33] The process of PR has been shown to improve low mood and reduce anxiety.[34]

Nutritional Support in Pulmonary Rehabilitation

Weight as well as fat-free mass (FFM) estimates of the patient needs consideration in PR. Caloric supplementation is provided to meet the extra demands for energy from PR

BOX 3 Examples of topics for the education component.

- Disease education
- Breathing strategies
- Secretion clearance techniques
- Nutritional advice
- Relaxation
- Effective use of respiratory devices and oxygen therapy
- Benefits advice
- Energy conservation during activities of daily living
- Travel
- Sexual intercourse advice
- Early recognition and treatment of exacerbation
- Pharmacology
- Proper inhaler technique

and if any deficit preexisting (BMI < 21 kg/m^2). It is recommended to monitor BMI periodically to see the effect of nutritional support as it has also been shown to improve QOL.

Education: Self-management

Self-management trains individuals in gaining personal care and health behavior skills and promote confidence (self-efficacy) in applying these skills on an everyday basis. It increases patients' involvement and control of their disease and improves their sense of well-being. It has been shown to reduce resources' utilization, especially those attributable to unscheduled visits to the hospital.[35] Patients learn to cope and react to their disease. With new skills of decision-making, early symptom recognition, and action plans patients can recognize and respond to respiratory exacerbations and avoid hospital admissions. Exercise, nutritional management, and the correct administration of medications are all assisted by self-management education **(Box 3)**.

DURATION AND FREQUENCY OF A PULMONARY REHABILITATION PROGRAM

Ideally, rehabilitation should continue as long as gains are being made. There is no consensus on optimal duration of PR, but it is ideally set by continued progress toward goals and optimization of benefit. In reality, it is also influenced by financial resources and traveling burden. Generally, longer programs (>12 weeks) may help sustain benefits and considered to produce greater gains and maintenance of benefits achieved on short term.[36-38] But a minimum of 8 weeks is recommended to gain substantial benefit.[38-40] Our study showed that as short as 3 weeks after discharge from hospital for COPD adverse event (AE) is effective considering difficulties in sustaining long-term programs.[41] Also, length of PR is also dependent on the setting, i.e., hospital based, community based, or home based and if one can be followed by the other as per convince and teams decisions. 2–3 days/week are recommended in outpatient programs and inpatient programs are usually planned for 5 days/week.[11]

LONG TERM/MAINTENANCE

Benefits appear to diminish over 6–12 months after discontinuation of PR most commonly due to the following reasons:

- Decrease in treatment adherence, especially to long-term regular exercise
- Progression of underlying disease
- Development of comorbidities
- Acute exacerbations[42]

Benefits can be maintained by establishing ongoing communication of the patient with PR team through weekly telephone calls and monthly reinforcement visits or weekly supervised outpatient-based exercise plus unsupervised home exercise. Other strategies include continuous rehabilitation, maintenance programs, and repeated courses. It is not clear what form of maintenance therapy should take or how it should be applied; more research in this area is needed. Repeating a course of rehabilitation does seem to have the ability to reproduce the short-term gain but without long-term advantage.[43] In many healthcare systems, cost is an obstacle. Reduction of adherence is difficult, but it is likely that those who benefited little from the program will not subsequently maintain their exercise habits. Rolling programs have the advantage over fixed entry programs in which patients may enter or reenter at any time.

OXYGEN

Supplemental oxygen and increased flow rates may be needed to maintain adequate oxygenation during exercise may be required in patients already on long-term oxygen therapy. Oxygen supplementation increases exercise tolerance and reduces breathlessness in individuals with COPD in the laboratory setting,[44] even in those with mild hypoxemia or exercise oxygen desaturation.[45] However, the effects of training with supplemental oxygen have been variable.[40,47] Carrying the weight of the cylinder may negate any additional benefits. Although liquid oxygen is lighter to carry, it is expensive and not widely available.

MOBILITY AIDS

The use of a rollator to assist with ambulation have been shown to increase functional exercise capacity and reduce dyspnea on exertion in some individuals with COPD. Rollators provide more stable support, improve balance, and enable the user to sit comfortably on the seat provided.

Rollators have been shown to improve walking distance, especially among the more limited patients-unassisted 6MWD < 375 m.[48] These benefits are sustained if the patients continue to use the rollator at home.[49] Rollators also have the advantage of being able to carry oxygen or other small items such as groceries.

PULMONARY REHABILITATION TEAM

Pulmonary rehabilitation is implemented by a dedicated, interdisciplinary team, which includes generally following specialists depending upon availability and resource utilization:

- Respiratory physicians
- Exercise physiologists
- Respiratory therapists
- Physiotherapists
- Psychologists/behavioral specialist
- Nutritionists
- Occupational therapists
- Social workers
- Patient educator
- Nurse practitioner

However, resources and availability of healthcare professionals limit most of PR programs and hence, some of the teammates play dual or more roles to fill in for nonavailable staff members.[11]

QUALITY ASSURANCE AND AUDIT

Programs should set up a regular audit to ensure that the results are in keeping with acceptable standards. Group aggregate data on walking distance and health status are frequently used. Feedback from patients can be collected by anonymous satisfaction questionnaire and data on compliance and dropout rates should also be recorded.

LOCATION AND SETTINGS OF PULMONARY REHABILITATION

Although programs have been conventionally developed where patient visits PR center in the hospital or clinic two or three times a week, PR has been shown to be effective inpatient settings too. Recently, successful PR programs have demonstrated to be delivered in other settings, for example, primary care (physiotherapists' clinic), home or secondary care (community or nursing homes), and systemic review has confirmed beneficial effects of home-based PR, but such programs are to be considered for most severely disabled, provided supervision by experts is available which is rare.[50,51]

EXACERBATIONS

Exacerbations represent one of the most common reasons for hospital admission and result in a substantial proportion of COPD-related healthcare costs and are called the real enemy of PR as all the components that improve with PR—dyspnea, exercise tolerance, muscle strength, and HRQL—are reduced following an acute exacerbation.[42,52,53] Many patients do not reach their pre-exacerbation level of functioning and clinical practice is of repeat referral for a shorter (booster) program. There is evidence that undergoing PR immediately postexacerbation is beneficial and not associated with adverse effects.[54] PR immediately postexacerbation has a strong rationale, but there are significant challenges in engaging patients immediately postexacerbation[55] and whether morbidity can be improved in long-term needs to be investigated. Although evidence supports early mobilization strategies within the intensive care setting, a recently published randomized controlled trial showed no benefit of a similar strategy during hospitalization for an exacerbation of COPD.[56] Managing patients postexacerbation remains an area for further research.

TRAINING ADJUNCTS OR STRATEGIES

Ventilatory limitation is a major barrier to exercise training. The use of proportional assist ventilation (noninvasive ventilation), by means of a tight-fitting mask, has shown improvement in endurance under laboratory conditions.[57] The use of a helium-hyperoxic mixture improves endurance time and enables a faster progression of training intensity, resulting in greater improvements in HRQL.[58] As helium is less dense, turbulence is reduced, and laminar flow is improved, thereby reducing the work of breathing.

An approach that reduces the ventilatory load by limiting the muscle mass being exercised has generated considerable interest.[59] The reduced muscle mass reduces the amount of lactic acid. As the latter is buffered to release CO_2, this reduction enables a lower ventilatory drive and therefore increases endurance. A training study has demonstrated that this is one of the few approaches to exercise training in COPD that will improve the peak oxygen consumption.[60]

HOME-BASED PULMONARY REHABILITATION

Home-based PR is an alternative model that could improve uptake and access. Initial reports suggested that home-based PR is safe and may improve clinical outcomes; however, these studies had limitations due to trial methods and protocols. As a result, there has been little uptake in clinical practice, with home-based PR offered in <5% of centers worldwide. Present pandemic has affected future research and also need for more home-based programs. A recent home-based PR program using minimal resources and little direct supervision has been shown to deliver short-term improvements in functional exercise capacity and HRQL that are at least equivalent to conventional center-based PR in COPD patients.[61] QOL outcomes were also equivalent at

12 months following program completion. More work to be done to evaluate essential components as well as duration of such programs and appears to be a definite way forward in providing PR.

VIRTUAL PULMONARY REHABILITATION

Considering limitations in providing PR to large number of needy patients and looking at vast geography of our country, the need for novel alternative models of PR are required to improve both equity of access and patient-related outcomes. Present covid times made tele- and video consultations acceptable and patient friendly and work is going on for providing virtual PR services which can reach majority of needy patients, eliminating the need for visit to hospitals and rehabilitation centers. Preliminary data suggests that tele PR is effective and needs more large-scale studies to implement it on wide scale. But it would require support of sufficient trained staff to provide such guidance without compromising safety of the patients. However, it would be premature to conclude that virtually supervised home-based PR program may be the future of PR.

SUMMARY

Pulmonary rehabilitation addresses the systemic effects of chronic respiratory disease, which are complex and involve peripheral muscle dysfunction. Although the role of PR in COPD has been established beyond doubt and has been shown to be far superior to any other therapy at patient oriented multiple outcome areas, its role in other chronic respiratory diseases is still evolving. Role of PR has been extended from stable patients to patients in hospitals and immediately after discharge while being treated for exacerbation. PR has also been recommended early in critical illness with neuromuscular stimulation started in mechanically ventilated patients. PR is also recommended in mild and early COPD due to the presence of physical inactivity in these patients also. Home-based and community-based programs are being developed to circumvent the difficulties of traveling to PR centers. Furthermore, the Internet and telemonitoring has advanced the scope of PR where it can be assisted remotely. PR is an exciting field whose growth and acceptance as mainstream management opens the way for further innovations.

REFERENCES

1. American Association of Cardiovascular and Pulmonary Rehabilitation. In: Bolton CE, Bevan-Smith EF, Blakey JD, et al. (Eds). Guidelines for Pulmonary Rehabilitation Programs, 3rd edition. Champaign, IL: Human Kinetics; 2004.
2. Pauwels RA, Buist AS, Calverley PM, et al. Global strategy for the diagnosis, management, and prevention of chronic obstructive pulmonary disease. NHLBI/WHO Global Initiative for Chronic Obstructive Lung Disease (GOLD) Workshop summary. Am J Respir Crit Care Med. 2001;163(5):1256-76.
3. Agusti A, Soriano JB. COPD as a systemic disease. COPD. 2008;5(2):133-8.
4. Agusti AG, Noguera A, Sauleda J, et al. Systemic effects of chronic obstructive pulmonary disease. Eur Respir J. 2003;21(2): 347-60.
5. Similowski T, Agusti A, MacNee W, et al. The potential impact of anaemia of chronic disease in COPD. Eur Respir J. 2006;27(2): 390-6.
6. Maltais F, Sullivan MJ, LeBlanc P, et al. Altered expression of myosin heavy chain in the vastus lateralis muscle in patients with COPD. Eur Respir J. 1999;13(4):850-4.
7. Steiner MC, Evans R, Deacon SJ, et al. Adenine nucleotide loss in the skeletal muscles during exercise in chronic obstructive pulmonary disease. Thorax. 2005;60(11):932-6.
8. Casaburi RA. Brief history of pulmonary rehabilitation. Respir Care. 2008;53:1185-9.
9. ZuWallack RA. History of pulmonary rehabilitation back to future. Pneumonol Alergol Pol. 2009;77:298-301.
10. Griffiths TL, Burr ML, Campbell IA, et al. Results at 1 year of outpatient multidisciplinary pulmonary rehabilitation: a randomised controlled trial. Lancet. 2000;355(9201):362-8.
11. Spruit MA, Singh SJ, Garvey C, et al. An official American Thoracic Society/European Respiratory Society statement: key concepts and advances in pulmonary rehabilitation. Am J Respir Crit Care Med. 2013;188(8):e13-64.
12. Nishimura K, Izumi T, Tsukino M, et al. Dyspnea is a better predictor of 5-year survival than airway obstruction in patients with COPD. Chest. 2002;121(5):1434-40.
13. Crisafulli E, Clini EM. Measures of dyspnea in pulmonary rehabilitation. Multidiscip Respir Med. 2010;5(3):202-10.
14. Evans RA, Singh SJ, Collier R, et al. Pulmonary rehabilitation is successful for COPD irrespective of MRC dyspnoea grade. Respir Med. 2009;103(7):1070-5.
15. Brooks D, Sottana R, Bell B, et al. Characterization of pulmonary rehabilitation programs in Canada in 2005. Can Respir J. 2007;14(2):87-92.
16. ATS Committee on Proficiency Standards for Clinical Pulmonary Function Laboratories. ATS statement: guidelines for the six-minute walk test. Am J Respir Crit Care Med. 2002;166(1): 111-7.
17. Celli BR, Cote CG, Marin JM, et al. The body-mass index, airflow obstruction, dyspnea, and exercise capacity index in chronic obstructive pulmonary disease. N Engl J Med. 2004;350(10):1005-12.
18. Singh SJ, Morgan MD, Hardman AE, et al. Comparison of oxygen uptake during a conventional treadmill test and the shuttle walking test in chronic airflow limitation. Eur Respir J. 1994;7(11):2016-20.
19. Singh SJ, Morgan MD, Scott S, et al. Development of a shuttle walking test of disability in patients with chronic airways obstruction. Thorax. 1992;47(12):1019-24.
20. Revill SM, Morgan MD, Singh SJ, et al. The endurance shuttle walk: a new field test for the assessment of endurance capacity in chronic obstructive pulmonary disease. Thorax. 1999;54(3):213-22.

21. Schunemann HJ, Goldstein R, Mador MJ, et al. A randomised trial to evaluate the self-administered standardised chronic respiratory questionnaire. Eur Respir J. 2005;25(1):31-40.
22. Jones PW, Quirk FH, Baveystock CM, et al. A self-complete measure of health status for chronic airflow limitation. The St. George's Respiratory Questionnaire. Am Rev Respir Dis. 1992;145(6):1321-7.
23. Jones PW, Harding G, Berry P, et al. Development and first validation of the COPD Assessment Test. Eur Respir J. 2009;34(3):648-54.
24. Dodd JW, Hogg L, Nolan J, et al. The COPD assessment test (CAT): response to pulmonary rehabilitation. A multicentre, prospective study. Thorax. 2011;66(5):425-9.
25. Bestall JC, Paul EA, Garrod R, et al. Usefulness of the Medical Research Council (MRC) dyspnoea scale as a measure of disability in patients with chronic obstructive pulmonary disease. Thorax. 1999;54(7):581-6.
26. Mahler DA, Waterman LA, Ward J, et al. Validity and responsiveness of the self-administered computerized versions of the baseline and transition dyspnea indexes. Chest. 2007;132(4):1283-90.
27. Vallet G, Ahmaidi S, Serres I, et al. Comparison of two training programmes in chronic airway limitation patients: standardized versus individualized protocols. Eur Respir J. 1997;10(1):114-22.
28. Garber CE, Blissmer B, Deschenes MR, et al.; American College of Sports Medicine. American College of Sports Medicine position stand: quantity and quality of exercise for developing and maintaining cardiorespiratory, musculoskeletal, and neuromotor fitness in apparently healthy adults: guidance for prescribing exercise. Med Sci Sports Exerc. 2011;43:1334-59.
29. Horowitz MB, Littenberg B, Mahler DA. Dyspnea ratings for prescribing exercise intensity in patients with COPD. Chest. 1996;109:1169-75.
30. Beauchamp MK, Nonoyama M, Goldstein RS, et al. Interval versus continuous training in individuals with chronic obstructive pulmonary disease—a systematic review. Thorax. 2010;65(2):157-64.
31. American College of Sports Medicine. American College of Sports Medicine position stand: progression models in resistance training for healthy adults. Med Sci Sports Exerc. 2009;41:687-708.
32. Janaudis-Ferreira T, Hill K, Goldstein R, et al. Arm exercise training in patients with chronic obstructive pulmonary disease: a systematic review. J Cardiopulm Rehabil Prev. 2009;29(5): 277-83.
33. Bjelland I, Dahl AA, Haug TT, et al. The validity of the Hospital Anxiety and Depression Scale. An updated literature review. J Psychosom Res. 2002;52(2):69-77.
34. Paz-Diaz H, Montes de Oca M, López JM, et al. Pulmonary rehabilitation improves depression, anxiety, dyspnea and health status in patients with COPD. Am J Phys Med Rehabil. 2007;86(1):30-6.
35. Bourbeau J, Julien M, Maltais F, et al. Reduction of hospital utilization in patients with chronic obstructive pulmonary disease: a disease-specific self-management intervention. Arch Intern Med. 2003;163(5):585-91.
36. Ries AL, Bauldoff GS, Carlin BW, et al. Pulmonary rehabilitation: Joint ACCP/AACVPR evidence-based clinical practice guidelines. Chest. 2007;131(5 Suppl):4S-42S.
37. Pitta F, Troosters T, Probst VS, et al. Are patients with COPD more active after pulmonary rehabilitation? Chest. 2008;134: 273-80.
38. Rossi G, Florini F, Romagnoli M, et al. Length and clinical effectiveness of pulmonary rehabilitation in outpatients with chronic airway obstruction. Chest. 2005;127:105-9.
39. Beauchamp MK, Janaudis-Ferreira T, Goldstein RS, et al. Optimal duration of pulmonary rehabilitation for individuals with chronic obstructive pulmonary disease—a systematic review. Chron Respir Dis. 2011;8:129-40.
40. Troosters T, Casaburi R, Gosselink R, et al. Pulmonary rehabilitation in chronic obstructive pulmonary disease. Am J Respir Crit Care Med. 2005;172:19-38.
41. Ali MS, Talwar D, Jain SK. The Effect of a Short-term Pulmonary Rehabilitation on Exercise Capacity and Quality of Life in Patients Hospitalised with Acute Exacerbation of Chronic Obstructive Pulmonary Disease. Indian J Chest Dis Allied Sci. 2014;56:13-9.
42. Cote CG, Dordelly LJ, Celli BR. Impact of COPD exacerbations on patient-centered outcomes. Chest. 2007;131(3):696-704.
43. Foglio K, Bianchi L, Ambrosino N. Is it really useful to repeat outpatient pulmonary rehabilitation programs in patients with chronic airway obstruction? A 2-year controlled study. Chest. 2001;119(6):1696-704.
44. Emtner M, Porszasz J, Burns M, et al. Benefits of supplemental oxygen in exercise training in nonhypoxemic chronic obstructive pulmonary disease patients. Am J Respir Crit Care Med. 2003;168:1034-42.
45. Somfay A, Porszasz J, Lee SM, et al. Dose–response effect of oxygen on hyperinflation and exercise endurance in nonhypoxaemic COPD patients. Eur Respir J. 2001;18:77-84.
46. Garrod R, Paul EA, Wedzicha JA. Supplemental oxygen during pulmonary rehabilitation in patients with COPD with exercise hypoxaemia. Thorax. 2000;55(7):539-43.
47. Nonoyama ML, Brooks D, Lacasse Y, et al. Oxygen therapy during exercise training in chronic obstructive pulmonary disease. Cochrane Database Syst Rev. 2007;(2):CD005372.
48. Probst VS, Troosters T, Coosemans I, et al. Mechanisms of improvement in exercise capacity using a rollator in patients with COPD. Chest. 2004;126(4):1102-7.
49. Gupta R, Goldstein R, Brooks D. The acute effects of a rollator in individuals with COPD. J Cardiopulm Rehabil. 2006;26(2): 107-11.
50. Van Wetering CR, Hoogendoorn M, Mol SJ, et al. Short- and long-term efficacy of a community-based COPD management programme in less advanced COPD: a randomised controlled trial. Thorax. 2010;65(1):7-13.
51. Maltais F, Bourbeau J, Shapiro S, et al. Effects of home-based pulmonary rehabilitation in patients with chronic obstructive pulmonary disease: a randomized trial. Ann Intern Med. 2008;149(12):869-78.
52. Spruit MA, Gosselink R, Troosters T, et al. Muscle force during an acute exacerbation in hospitalised patients with COPD and its relationship with CXCL8 and IGF-I. Thorax. 2003;58(9):752-6.
53. Pitta F, Troosters T, Probst VS, et al. Physical activity and hospitalization for exacerbation of COPD. Chest. 2006;129(3): 536-44.
54. Puhan M, Scharplatz M, Troosters T, et al. Pulmonary rehabilitation following exacerbations of chronic obstructive pulmonary disease. Cochrane Database Syst Rev. 2009;(1): CD005305.

55. Jones SE, Green SA, Clark AL, et al. Pulmonary rehabilitation following hospitalisation for acute exacerbation of COPD: referrals, uptake and adherence. Thorax. 2014;69(2):181-2.
56. Greening NJ, Williams JE, Hussain SF, et al. An early rehabilitation intervention to enhance recovery during hospital admission for an exacerbation of chronic respiratory disease: randomised controlled trial. BMJ. 2014;349:g4315.
57. Hawkins P, Johnson LC, Nikoletou D, et al. Proportional assist ventilation as an aid to exercise training in severe chronic obstructive pulmonary disease. Thorax. 2002;57(10):853-9.
58. Eves ND, Sandmeyer LC, Wong EY, et al. Helium-hyperoxia: a novel intervention to improve the benefits of pulmonary rehabilitation for patients with COPD. Chest. 2009;135(3):609-18.
59. Dolmage TE, Goldstein RS. Response to one-legged cycling in patients with COPD. Chest. 2006;129(2):325-32.
60. Dolmage TE, Goldstein RS. Effects of one-legged exercise training of patients with COPD. Chest. 2008;133(2):370-6.
61. Holland AE, Cox NS, Houchen-Wolloff L, et al. Defining Modern Pulmonary Rehabilitation—An Official American Thoracic Society Workshop Report. Ann Am Thorac Soc. 2021;18:e12-29.

Bullous Lung Diseases

CHAPTER 91

Aditya Jindal, Gyanendra Agrawal

INTRODUCTION

Bullous lung diseases are characterized by the presence of bullae, i.e., air-containing pockets or emphysematous space that have a diameter of >1 cm in the distended state within the lungs. A bulla will cause a local protrusion from the surface of the resected lung. The specific terminology "bullous lung disease" is reserved for an entity characterized by the presence of bullae in one or both lung fields, with normal intervening lung.[1] This entity is different in etiology and pathogenesis from "bullous emphysema," a condition in which bullae occur due to alveolar septal destruction and hyperinflation in conjunction with the emphysematous changes in the nonbullous lung.[2-4] "Giant bullous lung disease" is said to be present if the bullae occupy at least one-third of the hemithorax and compress the surrounding lung parenchyma.[2] It is a rare form of bullous lung disease which may frequently need differential diagnosis from pneumothorax.[4]

It is important to differentiate between the terms bulla, bleb, and cyst. "Bleb" is an accumulation of air between the two layers of visceral pleura and lined by the elastic lamina whereas "bulla" is present deep to the internal elastic layer of the visceral pleura and is confined by connective tissue septa of the lung. In contrast, "cyst" is lined by epithelium and can be present in the lung parenchyma or mediastinum. Progressive cystic lung disease can lead to formation of lung bullae.[5] Pathologically, three types of bullae are recognized which differ in location, size of neck, and amount of contained residual lung tissue, the clinical significance of which is unclear.

PATHOGENESIS

The pathogenesis of bullae formation is complex and poorly understood. Bulla arises from destruction, dilatation, and confluence of airspaces distal to terminal bronchioles, the walls of which are composed of attenuated and compressed parenchyma. Of all the hypotheses, that of an underlying paraseptal emphysema is the most popular. The structural weakness of the interalveolar septa caused by elastolysis, which itself may be secondary either to a constitutional disorder or to enhanced proteolysis, is the predominant mechanism for the development of paraseptal emphysema. Airspaces in paraseptal emphysema may become confluent and develop into bullae, which may be large. Airway obstruction caused either by loss of airway support or by inflammatory changes in the walls of small airways also contribute to progressive enlargement of these airspaces, ultimately resulting in the formation of bullous emphysema.

In patients of "bullous lung disease" with normal intervening lung, a mechanism different from that of bullae occurring in conjunction with emphysema is more likely. Several hypotheses have been proposed over the years, but none has been proved. Two hypotheses which have attracted most of the attention are "paper bag hypothesis" and a "ball valve mechanism" for bulla formation. Chronic inflammation of the airways, especially terminal bronchioles, causes airway obstruction, which acts as ball valve allowing air to enter during inspiration, leading to progressive air trapping and tension airspaces. However, this theory of bulla formation by positive pressure within the airspace has been refuted by the studies of dynamic computerized tomography and intrabulla pressure measurements. Moreover, in studies performed in subjects with bullae who were taken to altitudes of 18,500 feet (at an ascent rate of 1,000 ft/min), a little increase in bulla volume was noted, probably reflecting good communication between bullae and airways and adequate pressure equalization.

The pressure in bullae is normally negative and the same as that of pleural pressure.[6] The lung surrounding the bulla is less compliant than the bulla itself. Therefore, the pressure required to inflate the surrounding lung is greater than that necessary to inflate the bulla. During inspiration, when bullae and the adjacent lung parenchyma are subjected to the same negative pleural pressure, bulla fills preferentially than the surrounding lung like a "paper bag." This "paper bag compliance" is seen up to a critical lung volume, after which they become stiff and much less compliant than lung.[7] Bullae communicate with the rest of the bronchial tree, but air enters or leaves the bullae quite slowly. Bullae generally

BOX 1 Causes of bullae in the lungs.

- *Extraneous/environmental*:
  - Tobacco smoking
  - Cannabis and marijuana smoking
  - HIV infection
  - Post-tubercular fibrosis
  - Electronic cigarette smoking (vaping)
- *Rare familial disorders*:
  - Alpha-1 antitrypsin deficiency
  - Fabry's disease
  - Cutis laxa
  - Ehlers–Danlos syndrome
  - Marfan's syndrome
  - Neurofibromatosis
- *Miscellaneous*:
  - Ankylosing spondylitis
  - Sarcoidosis
  - Langerhans cell histiocytosis
  - Idiopathic pulmonary fibrosis
- Idiopathic bullous disease

do not act as clinically important dead space. During tidal breathing, PO_2 in bullae is higher than arterial PO_2.

ETIOLOGY

Bullae may originate in a variety of clinical and pathogenetic settings **(Box 1)**. Smoking and alpha 1-antitrypsin deficiency are the two most important risk factors for bullous emphysema.[8-10] Chronic cannabis and marijuana smoking is also believed to cause bullae formation through microscopic injury to the airways or other unknown mechanisms.[11,12] Vaping, i.e., use of electronic cigarettes, is also associated with the rapid development of bullous lung disease.[13] Marijuana smoking has been implicated as the cause of large upper zone bullae in some individuals. Concomitant use of marijuana and tobacco frequently makes it difficult to isolate the damaging effects of marijuana on lung microstructure and function.[14]

A hereditary predisposition to bullous emphysema is also suggested in view of its association with a variety of rare familial disorders, including Fabry's disease, cutis laxa, Ehlers–Danlos syndrome, and Marfan syndrome.[15-19] In a cohort of 166 patients of Marfan syndrome, 16 (9.6%) had apical blebs or bullae.[19] Upper zone "fibrobullous disease" is also reported in ankylosing spondylitis, usually seen in patients of long-standing disease of 15–20 years' duration with marked spinal involvement.[20] It is possible that some patients labeled as having giant bullous disease harbor an unusual condition like pulmonary sarcoidosis, Langerhans cell histiocytosis, idiopathic pulmonary fibrosis, or progressive massive fibrosis.[21-23] Post-tubercular fibrosis may sometimes present as bullous disease.[24] Bullae are occasionally described in association with other rare conditions such as neurofibromatosis, Proteus syndrome, and absent unilateral pulmonary artery.[25-27]

The cause cannot be ascertained in a subset of patients with bullous disease, which is then labeled as idiopathic bullous disease. Pleural blebs or bullae were seen in 6% of 250 young healthy adults on thoracoscopic examination performed for thoracic sympathectomy for essential hyperhidrosis.[28] Transport and retail trade industrial workers exposed to exhaust gas had a significant increased risk for bullae on chest radiographs performed on 27,361 men in their 50s in Japan.[29]

CLINICAL PRESENTATION

As a rule, small bullae usually produce no symptoms, signs, or discernible alterations in pulmonary function and are detected during routine chest radiography. Rupture of one or more bullae may lead to spontaneous pneumothorax.[30] Most of the causes of bullae formation are therefore responsible for recurrent pneumothraces.[19,20,30]

The most common presenting symptom in bullous lung disease is of gradually progressive exertional dyspnea. Occasionally, the patients may develop sudden severe increase in breathlessness due to either pneumothorax or overdistension due to air-trapping. Chest pain may occur in a patient with bullous lung disease.[4] This is also due to overdistension of the large bullae or development of pneumothorax. Overdistension causes a diffuse dull aching type of chest pain, usually located retrosternally. Hemoptysis is an uncommon presentation and usually indicates hemorrhage inside the bullae. Increase in cough and sputum production, in patients with known bullous disease, usually heralds the presence of infection in a bulla.

The findings on physical examination are usually dominated by the presence of associated disease. Occasionally, giant bullae may cause localized hyper-resonant note and decreased breath sounds. Giant bullae may commonly present with vanishing lung syndrome.[3,31]

RADIOLOGIC FEATURES

Small bullae rarely become visible on the chest radiograph, but they are easily visible by computed tomography. Apical bullae may sometimes be misinterpreted as cavitation on plain radiographs. They can be differentiated if it is remembered that cavities are centered within areas of consolidation and they do not merely overlap them.

High-resolution computed tomography is an important tool as it can locate the bullae with considerable accuracy, even when their presence is not suspected on the basis of clinical and radiographic data.[3] It also helps in assessing the extent and localization of bullae and associated diffuse nonbullous emphysema. It also allows assessment of associated diseases such as bronchiectasis, infected cysts, pleural disease, and pulmonary hypertension.[1] Computed

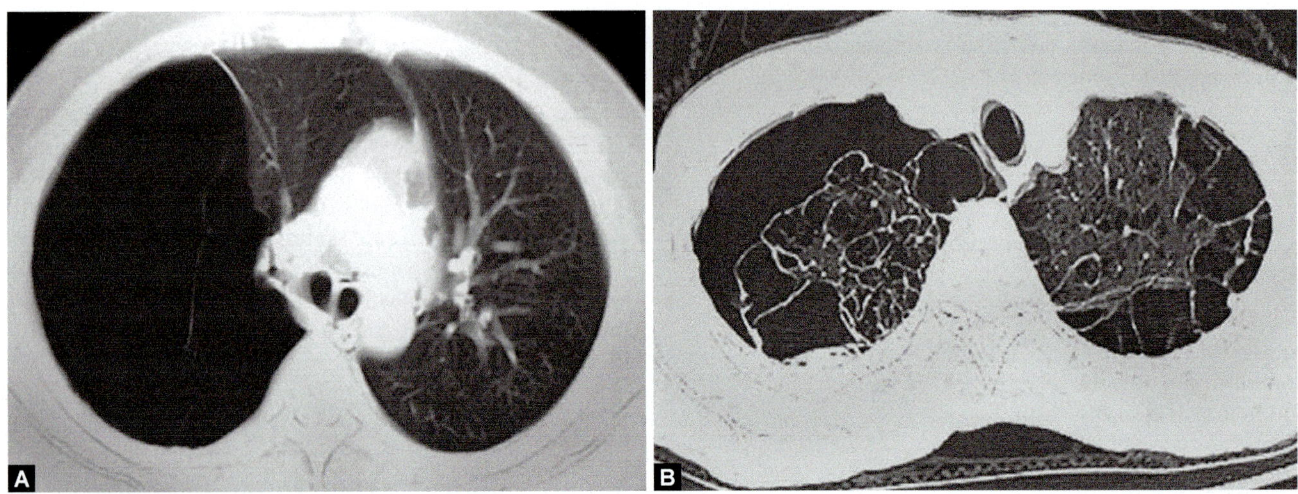

FIGS. 1A AND B: High-resolution CT scan in (A) bullous lung disease and (B) bullous emphysema.

tomography scans can help in differentiating bullous lung disease from bullous emphysema. The intervening lung parenchyma is normal in bullous lung disease as opposed to changes of emphysema seem in emphysematous bullae **(Figs. 1A and B)**.

A bulla is seen as an avascular transradiant area separated from the rest of lung parenchyma by a thin curvilinear wall. The wall is usually of hairline thickness. They are of variable sizes ranging from 1 cm to almost half of the hemithorax. Bullae are more common in the upper zones, especially those associated with paraseptal emphysema. The difficult distinction between bullous disease and pneumothorax can be made with CT through the "double-wall sign" (i.e., air visible on either side of the wall of bulla). CT has also been used to create 3D reconstructions of bullae, which can then be used to calculate bullae volumes.

PULMONARY FUNCTION TESTS

Detailed pulmonary function tests (PFTs) have an important place in the assessment of these conditions and to differentiate bullous disease from bullous emphysema.[1,32] This distinction is important since patients with bullous emphysema are poor surgical candidates as compared to patients with bullous lung disease. PFTs can also help to make an objective assessment of the severity of underlying disease, quantifying the size of bulla, and monitor the response to treatment.

Spirometry in patients with bullous lung disease usually shows restrictive defect, presumably as a result of the bulla compressing intervening normal lung, whereas a predominant obstructive defect is seen in patients having bullous emphysema. The diffusing capacity is reduced to a greater extent in bullous emphysema as compared to bullous lung disease; this test correlates better with morphologic estimates of emphysema than do most other tests. The diffusing capacity fails to increase normally during exercise. With exercise, the arterial oxygenation, ratio of dead space to tidal volume, and alveolar-arterial difference in PaO_2 tend to remain normal or near-normal in patients with a few circumscribed bullae and otherwise normal lungs, as compared to patients with bullous emphysema where they uniformly decrease, indicating progressive alveolar hypoventilation.

In patients with bullous lung disease, the lung volumes should be assessed by both the helium dilution technique and body plethysmography. A known volume of gas and a trace amount of helium (an inert gas, very little of which absorbs into the pulmonary circulation) are breathed in and out of a reservoir in the helium dilution technique. The helium is diluted by the gas that was previously present in the lung. With the knowledge of the gas in the reservoir and the initial and final helium concentrations, the functional residual capacity and the total lung capacity (TLC) can be calculated. However, because of inadequate time to equilibrate with slowly communicating and non-communicating air spaces such as bullae, this technique may underestimate the TLC. So, lung volumes should also be measured with body plethysmography, which measures the total volume of the thorax. The difference in TLC measured by body plethysmography and that by the helium dilution technique approximates the volume of the bullae.[1]

Bullae volume = TLC by body plethysmography - TLC by helium dilution

In some patients with bullous emphysema, respiratory muscle strength improves after bullectomy, as assessed by the measurements of maximal inspiratory and transdiaphragmatic pressures.[33] In patients with bullous emphysema, due to reduction in the pulmonary vascular bed, the resting pulmonary artery pressures are increased which further exaggerate during exercise. However, isolated bullae act like amputated segments of the lung and resting pulmonary arterial pressure and blood flow are within normal limits.

NATURAL HISTORY

Systematic long-term studies on the natural history of bullous lung disease are lacking. Patients with bullous disease should be monitored by chest radiography at regular intervals to ensure that the disease is stable. Bullae usually enlarge over months and years at a variable rate; the period of stability may be followed by a sudden expansion. In some patients, often young men, there may be the inexorable progression of idiopathic giant bullous disease. The alternative name given for the devastating nature of this condition is "vanishing lung syndrome." In some patients, bulla may disappear either spontaneously or following infection and hemorrhage, or with medical therapy alone.[34,35]

COMPLICATIONS

The main complications of bullae are pneumothorax, infection, or hemorrhage. When infected, bullae usually contain fluid and develop an air-fluid level. Air-fluid levels within the bullae **(Figs. 2A and B)** are relatively uncommon.[36] Fluid may be frequently resorbed and cause complete resolution of the bulla. The hairline wall often becomes thickened, and indeed this may be the only sign of infection. An infected bulla differs from an abscess in that the patient is less ill, the wall of the ring shadow is thinner and has a sharp margin, and there is less adjacent pneumonitis. Sometimes, a fungus colonizes a bulla and may form a mycetoma or fungal ball. Hemorrhage inside the bulla is a less common complication and it manifests as hemoptysis or a decrease in the hemoglobin level.[35] As with infection, bulla may disappear after bleeding occurs. Pneumothorax may occur due to the rupture of the bulla in pleural cavity or as a complication of paraseptal emphysema. Patients tend to have a prolonged air leak in such cases.[37]

Isolated cases of carcinomas arising in bullous lung diseases have been reported during the past 40 years. The majority of lung cancers associated with bullous disease are non-small-cell tumors. The frequency of lung cancer in subjects with bullous disease is approximately 32 times higher than in those without these abnormalities.[38] High-resolution computed tomography signs which could suggest the presence of carcinoma include mural nodule, mural thickening, fluid within bulla, and change in bulla diameter. The possible carcinogenic mechanism of bullous disease remains uncertain. The proposed mechanisms are: (1) carcinogens may inhibit antielastase enzymes, resulting in interalveolar-septal destruction with subsequent bulla formation; (2) constitutional or congenital factors may cause bullous disease and simultaneously may also predispose to lung cancer; and (3) impaired ventilation of bullae may facilitate the deposition of carcinogens.

TREATMENT

An asymptomatic patient diagnosed to have bullous lung disease should be reassured and educated about the disease. All attempts should be made to quit smoking. The patients should be asked to avoid activities that promote rupture of bulla like "scuba-diving." Appropriate treatment for the associated disease like asthma or chronic obstructive pulmonary disease (COPD) should be given. There are case reports of spontaneous resolution of progressively enlarging giant bullous emphysema after medical therapy for COPD was instituted.[34] Appropriate antibiotics and chest physiotherapy should be started as soon as the diagnosis of infected bullae is established.

Because of the impairment of respiratory function, and the higher incidence of coexisting infection and cancer, the giant bulla should be resected in all patients, even if they are asymptomatic. Enlarging bullae causing incapacitating

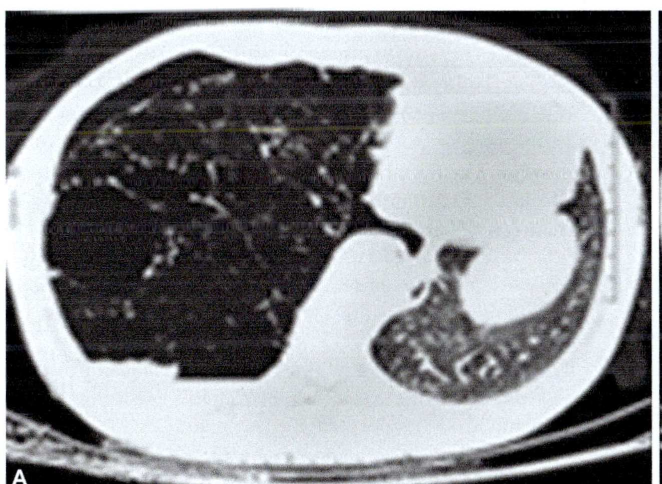

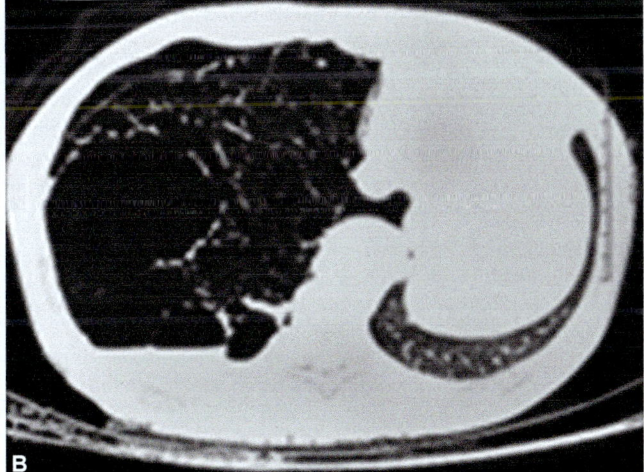

FIGS. 2A AND B: Giant bullae with fluid levels.

BOX 2 Indications of bullectomy.

- Giant bullae
- *Symptomatic bullous lung disease*:
  - Incapacitating dyspnea
  - Chest pain
- *Complications*:
  - Infection
  - Recurrent pneumothorax
  - Cancer

dyspnea or chest pain or impending respiratory insufficiency also need to be resected. Any lung mass associated with bullae should be considered as an indication for surgery. Other indications of bullectomy include infected bullae and that causing recurrent pneumothorax **(Box 2)**.

Even in bullectomy cases without the evidence of parenchymal lesions, the surgical resection should be as complete as possible. Pathological examination of the resected specimen should be performed because of the suspected existing occult or small-sized lung cancer. Bullectomy can be done via either video thoracoscopy (using a stapling device) or conventional thoracotomy. Giant bullae in vanishing lung syndrome have also been removed by video-assisted thoracoscopic surgery.[39] Thoracoscopic bullaplasty performed in fully awake patients is reported to be well tolerated and effective.[40] Autologous pleural reinforcement of staple line in surgery is another safe and cost-effective measure.[41] Mortality and complication rates are usually lower with thoracoscopy than with other surgical approaches.

Lung volume reduction surgery (LVRS) is the surgical removal of 20–30% of nonbullous emphysematous lung from each side. The greatest benefit from surgery is seen in a patient with a large bulla (occupying 50% or more of hemithorax), a moderate reduction in forced expiratory volume in 1 second (FEV_1), a rapid onset of dyspnea, and no evidence of generalized emphysema.[42,43] The physiologic basis of functional improvement after bullectomy is similar to that following LVRS.[44] Other treatment approaches for giant bullae include reduction pneumoplasty and Brompton's procedure (endocavitary aspiration with sclerosis and pleurodesis).[45]

SUMMARY

Bullous lung diseases include a wide spectrum of illnesses characterized with presence of air spaces of larger than 1 cm in diameter. Giant bullae may sometimes be responsible for vanishing lung syndrome. Bullae are common in smokers but also occur in association with cannabis and marijuana smoking and several other hereditary diseases. Distinction should be made between widespread obstructive airways disease with concomitant bullae and bullous lung disease, since surgical lung resection in generalized emphysema offers a less certain therapeutic response than does resection of giant bullae in the absence of widespread obstructive lung disease. As a rule, surgical intervention is avoided in bullae associated with either obstructive or fibrotic lung disease, unless there is a life-threatening complication.

REFERENCES

1. Agarwal R, Aggarwal AN. Bullous lung disease or bullous emphysema? Respir Care. 2006;51(5):532-4.
2. Stern EJ, Webb WR, Weinacker A, et al. Idiopathic giant bullous emphysema (vanishing lung syndrome): imaging findings in nine patients. AJR Am J Roentgenol. 1994;162(2):279-82.
3. Sharma N, Justaniah AM, Kanne JP, et al. Vanishing lung syndrome (giant bullous emphysema): CT findings in 7 patients and a literature review. J Thorac Imaging. 2009;24(3):227-30.
4. Ghattas C, Barreiro TJ, Gemmel DJ. Giant bullae emphysema. Lung. 2013;191:573-4.
5. Anwar A, Kokosi M, Aldik G. Progressive cystic lung disease with bullous destruction. Clin Med (Lond). 2022;22(5):478-81.
6. Morgan MD, Edwards CW, Morris J, et al. Origin and behaviour of emphysematous bullae. Thorax. 1989;44(7):533-8.
7. Ting EY, Klopstock R, Lyons HA. Mechanical properties of pulmonary cysts and bullae. Am Rev Respir Dis. 1963;87:538-44.
8. Paulose-Ram R, Tilert T, Dillon CF, et al. Cigarette smoking and lung obstruction among adults aged 40-79: United States, 2007-2012. NCHS Data Brief 2015;(181):1-8.
9. Doney B, Hnizdo E, Syamlal G, et al. Prevalence of chronic obstructive pulmonary disease among US working adults aged 40-70 years. National Health Interview Survey Data 2004-2011. J Occup Environ Med. 2014;56:1088-93.
10. Stockley RA. Apha1-antitrypsin review. Clin Chest Med. 2014;35:39-50.
11. Tashkin DP. Marijuana and Lung Disease. Chest. 2018;154(3):653-63.
12. Gracie K, Hancox RJ. Cannabis use disorder and the lungs. Addiction. 2021;116(1):182-90.
13. Kalra SS, Pais F, Harman E, et al. Rapid development of bullous lung disease: a complication of electronic cigarette use. Thorax. 2020;75(4):359.
14. Howden ML, Naughton MT. Pulmonary effects of marijuana inhalation. Expert Rev Respir Med. 2011;5:87-92.
15. Brown LK, Miller A, Bhuptani A, et al. Pulmonary involvement in Fabry disease. Am J Respir Crit Care Med. 1997;155:1004-10.
16. Franzen D, Krayenbuehl PA, Lidove O, et al. Pulmonary involvement in Fabry disease: overview and perspectives. Eur J Intern Med. 2013;24:707-13.
17. Ayres JG, Pope FM, Reidy JF, et al. Abnormalities of the lungs and thoracic cage in the Ehlers-Danlos syndrome. Thorax. 1985;40(4):300-5.
18. Dyhdalo K, Farver C. Pulmonary histologic changes in Marfan syndrome: a case series and literature review. Am J Clin Pathol. 2011;136:857-63.

19. Karpman C, Aughenbaugh GL, Ryu JH. Pneumothorax and bullae in Marfan syndrome. Respiration. 2011;82:219-24.
20. Alfaiate CDS, Durão VMR, Patrício JS, et al. Apical fibrobullous lung disease in ankylosing spondylitis: case report and literature review. Eur Clin Respir J. 2022;9(1):2086359.
21. Jeebun V, Forrest IA. Sarcoidosis: an underrecognized cause for bullous lung disease? Eur Respir J. 2009;34:999-1001.
22. Vassallo R, Harari S, Tazi A. Current understanding and management of pulmonary Langerhans cell histiocytosis. Thorax. 2017; 72:937-45.
23. Ryu JH, Tian X, Baqir M, et al. Diffuse cystic lung diseases. Front Med. 2013;7:316-27.
24. Yen YT, Wu MH, Cheng L, et al. Image characteristics as predictors for thoracoscopic anatomic lung resection in patients with pulmonary tuberculosis. Ann Thorac Surg. 2011;92(1): 290-5.
25. Nardecchia E, Perfetti L, Castiglioni M, et al. Bullous lung disease and neurofibromatosis type-1. Monaldi Arch Chest Dis. 2012;77(2):105-7.
26. Lim GY, Kim OH, Kim HW, et al. Pulmonary manifestations in Proteus syndrome: pulmonary varicosities and bullous lung disease. Am J Med Genet A. 2011;155A(4):865-9.
27. Betigeri VM, Betigery AV, Saichandran BV, et al. Bullous lung disease and bronchiectasis in unilateral absent right pulmonary artery. Gen Thorac Cardiovasc Surg. 2013;61:100-3.
28. Amjadi K, Alvarez GG, Vanderhelst E, et al. The prevalence of blebs or bullae among young healthy adults: a thoracoscopic investigation. Chest. 2007;132:1140-5.
29. Mitsumune T, Senoh E, Kayashima E. Occupations associated with bullae on chest radiographs in Japanese middle-aged men. Int Arch Occup Environ Health. 2005;78:185-8.
30. Van Berkel V, Kuo E, Meyers BF. Pneumothorax, bullous disease and emphysema. Surg Clin North Am. 2010;90:935-53.
31. Mani D, Guinee DG Jr, Aboulafia DM. Vanishing lung syndrome and HIV infection: an uncommon yet potentially fatal sequel of cigarette smoking. J Int Assoc Physicians AIDS Care (Chic). 2012;11(4):230-3.
32. Lor KL, Liu CP, Chang YC, et al. Predictive Modelling of Lung Function using Emphysematous Density Distribution. Sci Rep. 2019;9:19763.
33. Travaline JM, Addonizio VP, Criner GJ. Effect of bullectomy on diaphragm strength. Am J Respir Crit Care Med. 1995;152 (5 Pt 1):1697-701.
34. Chang WH. Complete spontaneous resolution of a giant bulla without rupture or infection: a case report and literature review. J Thorac Dis. 2017;9(6):E551-5.
35. Withey S, Tamimi A. Spontaneous pulmonary haemorrhage into an existing emphysematous bulla. BMJ Case Rep. 2016;2016:bcr2015213144.
36. Henao-Martinez AF, Fernandez JF, Adams SG, et al. Lung bullae with air-fluid levels: what is the appropriate therapeutic approach? Respir Care. 2012;57(4):642-5.
37. Smit HJ, Wienk MA, Schreurs AJ, et al. Do bullae indicate a predisposition to recurrent pneumothorax? Br J Radiol. 2000; 73(868):356-9.
38. Ema T. Large cell carcinoma on the bullous wall detected in a specimen from a patient with spontaneous pneumothorax: report of a case. J Thoracic Dis. 2014;6:E234-6.
39. Van Bael K, La Meir M, Vanoverbeke H. Video-assisted thoracoscopic resection of a giant bulla in vanishing lung syndrome: case report and a short literature review. J Cardiothorac Surg. 2014;9:4.
40. Pompeo E, Tacconi F, Frasca L, et al. Awake thoracoscopic bullaplasty. Eur J Cardiothorac Surg. 2011;39(6):1012-7.
41. Baysungur V, Tezel C, Ergene G, et al. The autologous pleural buttressing of staple lines in surgery for bullous lung disease. Eur J Cardiothorac Surg. 2010;38(6):679-82.
42. Sardenberg RA, Younes RN, Deheizelin D. Lung volume reduction surgery: an overview. Rev Assoc Med Bras. 2010;56(6): 719-23.
43. De Giacomo T, Rendina EA, Venuta F, et al. Bullectomy is comparable to lung volume reduction in patients with end-stage emphysema. Eur J Cardiothorac Surg. 2002;22(3):357-62.
44. Kösek V, Thiel B, Nikolova K, et al. Lung volume reduction surgery: from National Emphysema Treatment Trial to non-intubated awake video-assisted thoracoscopic surgery. Ann Transl Med. 2020;8(21):1468.
45. Giller DB, Scherbakova GV, Giller BD, et al. Surgical treatment of bilateral vanishing lung syndrome: a case report. J Cardiothorac Surg. 2020;15:201.

Upper and Central Airway Obstruction

CHAPTER 92

VR Pattabhi Raman, Arun Raja

INTRODUCTION

Upper airway obstruction (UAO) is defined as the obstruction of the airways at or proximal to carina, including the nose, mouth, pharynx, and larynx.[1] The problems relevant to these areas are usually dealt with by the otorhinolaryngologists; therefore, readers interested in details are advised to refer to otorhinolaryngology textbooks. Chronic UAO poses a diagnostic dilemma and is frequently misdiagnosed and managed as bronchial asthma. On the other hand, acute UAO poses a therapeutic challenge and is best managed in a well-equipped setting that has physicians trained in difficult airway management. Also, obstructive sleep apnea (OSA), an important disorder causing UAO, is dealt with separately in this textbook. This chapter essentially focuses on disorders that cause obstruction between the vocal cords and the carina.

TYPES OF UPPER AIRWAYS OBSTRUCTION

Upper airway obstruction can be classified as acute and chronic. Tracheal obstruction at the level of thoracic inlet, including in the vocal cords and the cervical portion of trachea, is called extrathoracic UAO, whereas obstruction in the thoracic portion of trachea till the carina is called intrathoracic UAO. This distinction is helpful as the changes in the airway dynamics that happen during a respiratory cycle are different in the two segments. The intrathoracic segment of trachea increases in dimension during inspiration and decreases during expiration, whereas it is the opposite in the extrathoracic trachea and the airways above. The pressure that affects the caliber of upper airways in the extrathoracic region is atmospheric pressure **(Fig. 1)** and the intrathoracic pressure is the pleural pressure.[2] It is therefore easy to imagine how narrowed (extrathoracic) upper airways cause snoring, which is typically associated with inspiratory collapse of the airways.

The nature of obstruction, whether it is stiff or pliable, determines whether there will be changes in severity in

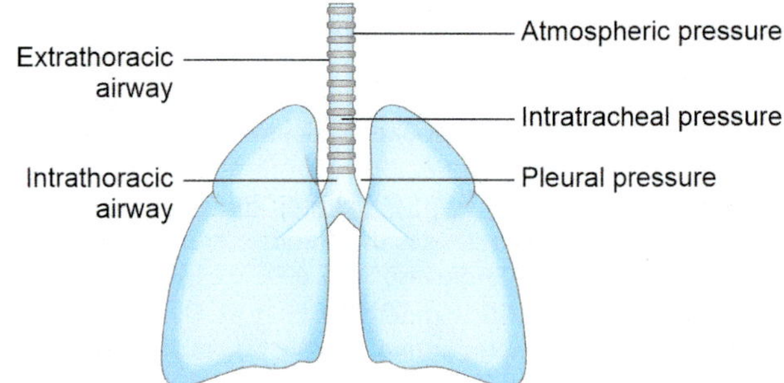

FIG. 1: Pressure affecting upper airways.
Source: Modified from Acres and Kryger (1981).[2]

relation to changes in the transmural pressure. A stiff lesion as in some cases of postintubation tracheal stenosis (PITS) does not allow dynamic differences in the diameter of the stenosis and in the airflow between inspiration and expiration.[2] This is called fixed airway obstruction. In cases of bilateral abductor palsy of vocal cords, there are differences in the caliber and the airflow during the respiratory cycle. Because of the extrathoracic nature of the obstruction, inspiration worsens and expiration lessens the obstruction. This is an example of variable airway obstruction. Based on these parameters, UAO can be divided into fixed obstruction, variable extrathoracic obstruction, and variable intrathoracic obstruction.

ANATOMIC DIFFERENCES OF THE AIRWAY IN INFANTS/CHILDREN AND ITS CONSEQUENCES

Airways in children are much smaller than those of an adult. Tongue is larger compared with that of an adult. Cephalad position of larynx in infants and toddlers. In infants and toddlers, epiglottis is short and narrow angled. It is away from the long axis of trachea. Vocal cords have a lower attachment anteriorly. Larynx is funnel shaped in children < 10 years of age, and the narrowest portion of the airway is below the vocal cords at the level of cricoid cartilage.

In teenagers and adults, larynx is cylinder shaped and the narrowest portion is at the glottic inlet.[3] The narrowest point of larynx in a neonate is the cricoid ring area. It is characterized by the following features.

- Mucus membrane is loosely attached to the underlying non-fibrous structure thus making it prone to edema.
- Cartilaginous support is soft making is susceptible to collapse during inspiration.

Even minor edema/obstruction can significantly reduce the airway diameter and increase resistance to airflow. Posterior displacement of the tongue may cause severe airway obstruction. Controlling the position of the tongue with the laryngoscope blade may be difficult during tracheal intubation. High position of the larynx makes the angle between the base of the tongue and glottic opening more acute.[3] Therefore, straight blades are more useful in creating direct visual plane from mouth to glottis. Controlling the epiglottis with laryngoscope blade may be more difficult. A blindly placed endotracheal tube may get caught at the anterior commissure of the cord. The size of the endotracheal tube must be selected based on the size of the cricoid ring rather than glottic opening. Obstruction of glottic and subglottic areas results in turbulent and high-velocity airflow resulting in stridor which is low pitched and extends into exhalation.[3]

CLINICAL FEATURES

Acute airway obstruction usually presents as severe breathlessness and agitation. Stridor is the usual diagnostic sign. Stridor is frequently audible unaided and a stethoscope is seldom required. The patient may also present very late in the course of the disease. The presence of stridor in UAO means a fairly severe narrowing. Tracheal lumen of <8 mm produces symptoms after exercise[4] and of <5 mm produces stridor.[5] A high index of suspicion is usually required in chronic UAO. Chronic obstruction is frequently misdiagnosed and managed as asthma/chronic obstructive pulmonary disease (COPD) for a variable period of time before the recognition of upper airway problem. Diligent history-taking including history of intubation and of thyroid surgery could serve as a clue. Many cases of chronic UAO have periods of worsening, which get better with antibiotics and steroids, further delaying the diagnosis. Certain features, such as hemoptysis, and refractoriness to asthma treatment, should alert the physicians about the possibility of UAO and the need for further investigations.

DIAGNOSIS

Radiology

Plain X-ray is seldom useful. It may show obvious mediastinal lymphadenopathy or sometimes a tracheal tumor with extramural extension. At times, the penetrated film may show the site of obstruction. Computed tomography (CT) is very valuable for diagnosing airway obstruction, particularly the reconstructed images **(Fig. 2)** which provide details about the site, the extent, and the nature of obstruction. The diameter at the narrowest portion and the length of the stenosis are critical details that are required to plan treatment. The present-generation multiplanar CT provides this information in a very short time. Some patients with very severe stenosis may not be able to lie down flat and hold their breath for the study. Magnetic resonance imaging (MRI) is not very commonly sought. It may give valuable information by its superior contrast resolution.

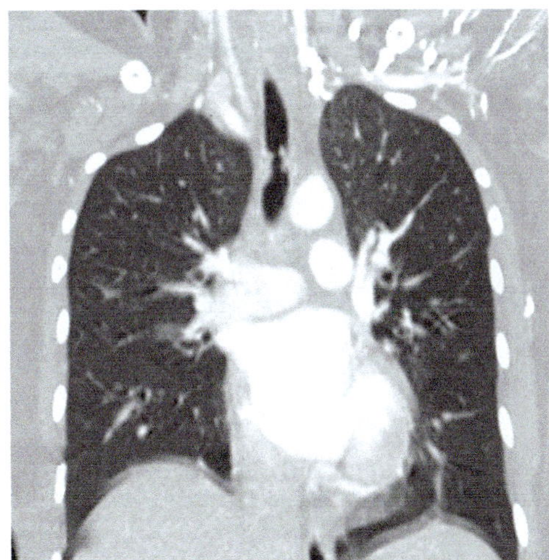

FIG. 2: Reconstructed CT image of a patient with tracheal stenosis.

Spirometry

In normal subjects, during a forced expiration from total lung capacity (TLC), the maximum airflow is achieved during the first 25% of the vital capacity (VC), which is dependent directly on effort and inversely on resistance. In the remaining 75%, the flow is limited in such a way that an increase in effort (and the associated increase of pleural pressure) does not result in increased flows.[4] With UAO, flow at higher lung volume may be limited by obstruction. UAO causes more pronounced decrease in peak expiratory flow (PEF) than in forced expiratory volume in 1 second (FEV_1).[6] Therefore, an increased ratio of FEV_1 (mL) divided by PEF (L/mL) can alert the clinician to the need for an inspiratory and expiratory flow-volume loop.[7] This ratio is called Empey's Index; a value of >8 suggests the presence of central airway obstruction (CAO) or UAO.[8] Poor initial effort by the patient can also increase the index. Hence, it is very important that the patient's inspiratory and expiratory efforts are maximal and the technician should confirm this in the quality pattern of repeatable plateau of forced inspiratory flow, with a preserved expiratory flow loop indicating variable extrathoracic UAO **(Fig. 3A)**, the pattern of cut off of forced expiratory flow

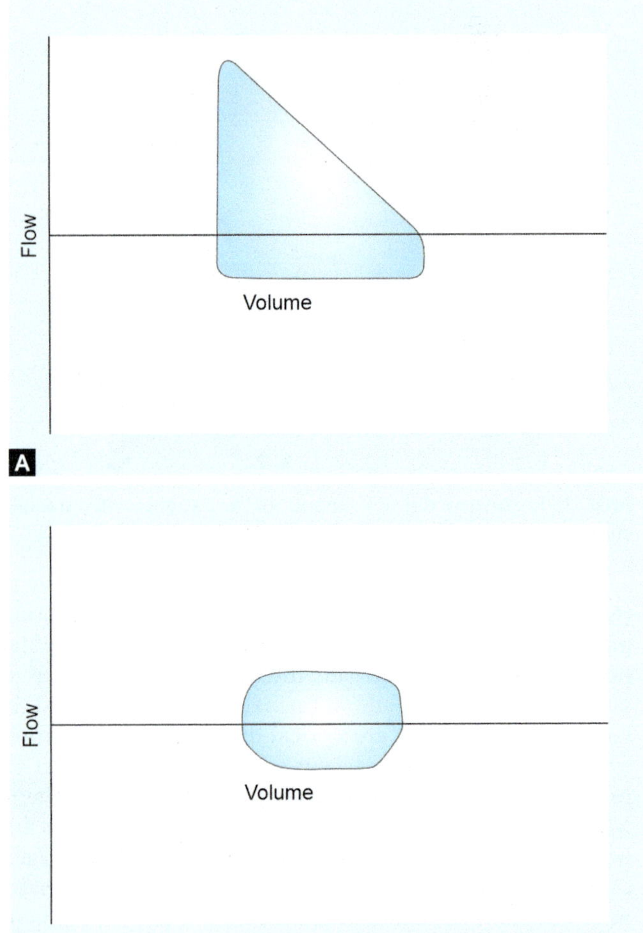

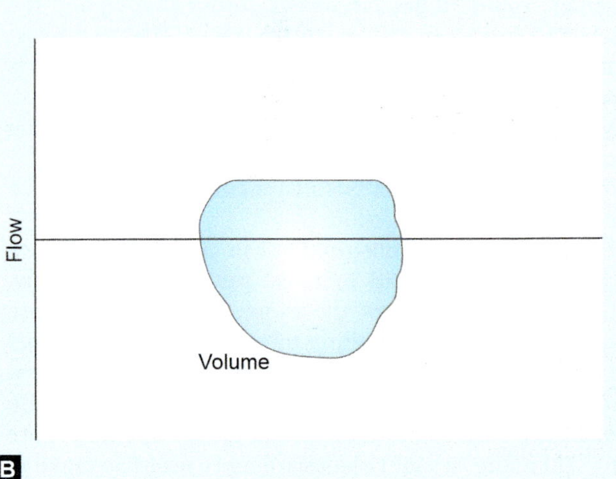

FIGS. 3A TO C: Flow–volume loop in UAO. (A) Variable extrathoracic obstruction; (B) Variable intrathoracic obstruction; (C) Fixed airway obstruction.

Source: Adapted from Miller RD, Hyatt RE. Obstructing lesions of the larynx and trachea: clinical and physiologic characteristics. Mayo Clin Proc. 1969;44:145-61.

with a preserved inspiratory flow loop is consistent with variable intrathoracic obstruction.[8] **(Fig. 3B)**. A combined inspiratory and expiratory plateauing of the flow volume loops which is repeatable is consistent with a fixed UAO **(Fig. 3C)**. When a patient's effort is good, the absence of classic patterns does not rule out UAO. The presence of specific UAO patterns would also warrant confirmation of the presence of UAO; hence, bronchoscopy is required as the next important step.

Bronchoscopy

Bronchoscopy is considered the procedure of choice as it provides the most useful information in UAO. It is ideal to have an idea about the lesion with a CT done before bronchoscopy so that planning could be better. The cause of the anatomical obstruction can be diagnosed in the case of an intramural pathology like a tumor. Care however has to be taken while passing a flexible bronchoscope through a very narrow lumen, since even a minor hemorrhage can become catastrophic by causing critical airway narrowing. It is wise to employ rigid bronchoscopy in such a case of severe obstruction. During rigid bronchoscopy, ventilation can be done during the procedure and therefore oxygenation is easy. Moreover, the larger bore of the rigid barrel allows the passage of instruments simultaneously, and procedures like biopsy can be safely done. Also, the barrel of the bronchoscope could be used to tamponade bleeding points and to mechanically dilate the stenosis. Another significant advantage of rigid bronchoscopy is the deployment of stents, making it the investigation of choice in severe UAO.

In cases of extrinsic compression, bronchoscopy could be valuable in assessing the mucosa, to evaluate for transmural invasion. It also helps in assessing the extent of involvement to guide a definitive therapy. In cases of functional obstruction, such as in tracheomalacia (TM), bronchoscopy is mandatory. Here, flexible bronchoscopy scores over rigid bronchoscopy in identifying abnormal airway dynamics during respiration as it requires a conscious and cooperative patient, which is not possible in an anesthetized patient undergoing rigid bronchoscopy.

ACUTE UPPER AIRWAY OBSTRUCTION

Acute UAO due to different causes, as discussed in the following text, may often present as a life-threatening emergency requiring urgent attention.[9]

Foreign Body

Typically seen in children aged between 2 and 4 years, aspiration of foreign bodies can be also seen in older children and elderly individuals. In the elderly patients, it commonly occurs in the presence of comorbidities with depressed consciousness and poor swallowing reflex.[10] In pediatric population, choking is the most common symptom followed by a protracted cough.[11] There is a male preponderance and more often when there is an elderly sibling. No predilection between right and left bronchial trees is seen; at that age, the bronchial division makes a similar angle on both the sides. History may not be forthcoming in all cases, and a high index of suspicion is required. Radiography is useful only in the case of radiopaque foreign bodies or when there is expiratory hyperinflation.[11] Normal chest X-ray does not exclude foreign body aspiration. Early intervention is important, especially when vegetable matter like groundnut or bean is aspirated since granulation happens rather rapidly and at times so profusely that it may not be visible in bronchoscopy.[12,13] Also, delayed removal may not result in complete healing of the granulation tissue. Groundnut is probably the most common foreign body among children in India.[13]

Though rigid bronchoscopy is considered the gold standard for the retrieval of an aspirated foreign body, there is a definite role for flexible pediatric bronchoscopes for both diagnosis and retrieval of pediatric foreign bodies.[14,15] In a retrospective study analyzing emergency calls for UAO among age group under 5 years – aspiration of liquid (formula feeds/juice) was common under 1 year age and solid aspiration was typically seen in children over 1 year of age. Symptoms resolved in 59% of patients even before arrival of paramedic and intervention was required only in 2% of them.[10] In infants < 1 year of age and unresponsive, five backslaps and chest thrusts should be given by holding the baby in a head-down position; in children > 1 year of age and unresponsive, Heimlich maneuver should be given for immediate dislodgement of the foreign body.

Acute Laryngeal Edema

Acute laryngeal edema may happen following anaphylactic reactions causing life-threatening angioedema, the prototype being the penicillin allergy or nonsteroidal anti-inflammatory drugs (NSAID) allergy in aspirin-sensitive asthma. The deterioration is rapid and early intervention is crucial. Parenteral administration of adrenaline can be life-saving. This has to be distinguished from a rare autosomal-dominant condition called hereditary angioedema which occurs due to deficiency of C1 inhibitor enzyme due to mutations of its gene.[17] Localized swelling that is self-limiting can happen at any site of the body including the skin, genitalia, and gastrointestinal tract. Angioedema is characterized variable age of onset and absence of urticaria. It is a life-threatening when it happens in the larynx, especially if untreated. The attacks are not precipitated by allergy but by trauma and stress.[18] Prophylaxis is useful if started early (with tranexamic acid) or attenuated with androgens like danazol.[19] In patients refractory to prophylaxis of danazol, pasteurized plasma-derived C1 inhibitor (pC1-INH) concentrate has been found to be useful in reducing the recurrence.[20] In acute attacks, pC1-INH concentrate (intravenous dose of 20 U/kg) and newer drugs like icatibant and bradykinin receptor-2 antagonist (30 mg subcutaneous injection) have been shown to provide rapid relief.[21]

Another important cause of nonallergic laryngeal edema is the administration of angiotensin-converting enzyme inhibitors (ACEIs) which, like hereditary angioedema, is not associated with itching or urticaria. Prompt recognition and stopping the drug will stop the recurrence. Increased incidence of angioedema in renal transplant recipients receiving a combination of ACEIs and mammalian target of rapamycin (mTOR) inhibitors has been also described.[22]

Infection

Infection as a cause of acute UAO typically occurs in children.[9] The usual infections which may present with UAO are croup, epiglottitis, tracheitis, retropharyngeal abscess, and peritonsillar abscess. Acute epiglottitis is caused by either *Haemophilus influenzae* or beta-hemolytic streptococci and Ludwig's angina is characterized by a rapidly progressing cellulitis involving submandibular space. The treatment involves rapid airway stabilization, antibiotics, and surgical drainage of the pus. Viral croup, often caused by parainfluenza virus, is managed by nebulized adrenaline and parenteral corticosteroids. Bacterial tracheitis is usually caused by *Staphylococcus aureus* infection. Bronchoscopic appearance shows the presence of erythema, edema, thick secretions, and at times plaques in the trachea.

CHRONIC UPPER AIRWAY OBSTRUCTION

Vocal Cord Dysfunction

Vocal cord dysfunction is a syndrome in which the vocal cords adduct during inspiration producing UAO-like features. Patients are usually females in the age group of 20–40 years.[23,24] It masquerades the diagnosis of refractory asthma with multiple attacks and is usually managed similar to asthma. In an Indian study that evaluated difficult-to-control asthma, vocal cord dysfunction was seen in about 23.5% and was also frequently found to coexist with asthma.[25] Usual triggers include exercise, psychological stress, irritants, rhinosinusitis, and gastroesophageal reflux disease (GERD).[26]

The "wheeze" typically appears at lower lung volumes since the obstruction happens during the inspiration and for the same reason, the chest X-ray does not show hyperinflation. Spirometry done during the episode may show the classical loop of extrathoracic UAO. Flexible laryngoscopy is considered the gold standard for diagnosis, especially when done during the episode. The classical description during inspiration consists of adduction of the vocal cords, with a small diamond-shaped chink in the posterior region of the vocal cords. Reassurance and breathing exercises may reduce the intensity during the acute episode; rapid shallow breathing (like panting), speech therapy, psychological counseling, and avoidance of triggers would help in long-term management.[23,27]

Tracheobronchomalacia

Tracheomalacia refers to the weakness of tracheal walls, frequently due to reduction and/or atrophy of the longitudinal elastic fibers of the pars membrane, or cartilage integrity, such that the airway is softer and more susceptible to collapse.[28] TM may be localized or diffuse and usually affects the intrathoracic portion of trachea. If main bronchi are also involved, it is called tracheobronchomalacia (TBM).

Pediatric TM: TM is the most common congenital abnormality of trachea. There is a strong association with prematurity, mucopolysaccharidosis, tracheoesophageal fistula, and some congenital heart diseases.[28,29] There is a male preponderance. Acquired causes include long-standing tracheostomy and pressure from vascular slings. Congenital TM is usually self-limiting and the children outgrow the disease by the age of 2–3 years. Severe cases are managed by the use of continuous positive airway pressure (CPAP) or by surgical procedures like aortopexy.[30,31] Aortopexy which is a procedure where the aortic arch is stitched to the sternum and thus relieves the pressure on the trachea is gaining popularity in surgical approach to pediatric TM, especially if it becomes life threatening. Some authors report the success of thoracoscopic aortopexy with its advantages including shorter hospital stay and no additional complications.

Adult TM and TBM: There is an increased awareness in recognizing and implicating TM as an important cause for pulmonary symptoms. This can be attributed to the advances in CT technology and virtual bronchoscopy, increasing availability of bronchoscopes, and better therapeutic options. TM in adults is predominantly seen in the middle-aged male individuals who are also smokers. Adult cases most commonly happen following the trauma, including after intubation, tracheostomy, external chest trauma, and lung transplantation. Emphysema, chronic bronchitis, chronic inflammation like relapsing polychondritis (RP), and chronic extrinsic compression of the trachea are the other important reasons.

Acquired TM is commonly seen in association with long-term intubation and tracheostomy. It is usually a short-segment stenosis. A comprehensive in-depth review on TM describes that the length of malacic segment secondary to postintubation in usually < 3 cm.[28] More than 50% decrease in airway caliber occurring during expiration is diagnostic of TM. Three types are described:[28]

1. Saber-sheath type (Ω)—lateral wall narrowing
2. Scabbard type (⌓)—AP narrowing-crescentic type
3. Circumferential type (O)—all round narrowing

The TM secondary to COPD is usually diffuse and also difficult to treat. The patient presents with symptoms such as cough, dyspnea, and wheeze. Dynamic CT, which is noninvasive, is useful for diagnosis. The multidetector CT technology shows very good promise.[32]

Symptomatic cases need to be treated depending on the etiology. Focal TM in postintubation or post-traumatic cases should be resected, if possible. Alternatively, it can be managed with tracheostomy, if the segment can be bypassed. The advantage of tracheostomy in such a situation is that the tube acts like a stent. Long flange tracheostomy tubes are available for the purpose. The tracheostomy can also be an interface for CPAP application. However, tracheostomy can also predispose to TM of a different segment of trachea. In TM secondary to COPD, the optimization of medications for COPD can help reduce symptoms. Severe cases can be managed with silicone stents. However, it is not effective in all patients and there is a high chance of migration of these stents. Metallic stents should be avoided because of the difficulty of removal and replacement.

Based on a retrospective study which included 58 patients who had silicone stent placement for severe TBM, majority (57%) of them had COPD followed by OSA (28%), GERD (28%), and asthma (22%).[33] A comparison of baseline stent placement in patients with and without PD showed that in those with COPD, it was associated with an improvement in quality of life as assessed by St George's respiratory questionnaire (SGRQ), American Thoracic Society (ATS) dyspnea index, and Karnofsky performance status (KPS) whereas in patients without COPD it was associated with only in significant improvement in dyspnea index.[33] The most common complication was mucous plugging seen in 21 patients followed by infection in 14 and stent migration in 10.[33] Another retrospective study which included 103 patients with TBM and COPD received stent followed by tracheobronchoplasty (TBP), stent alone, and TBP alone and were followed up after 1 month. Stenting was performed in 91%, stenting followed by TBP in 25%, and TBP alone in 1%. Compared to baseline stenting was associated with significant improvement in mean transitional dyspnea index (TDI) and significant improvement in SGRQ score.[34] Different surgical techniques have been tried. Strengthening the posterior membranous portion using various prostheses like crystalline polypropylene mesh has been tried with variable success.[35]

Polychondritis

Relapsing polychondritis (RP) is a rare disease. It is a multisystem disorder with unknown etiology, characterized by recurrent progressive inflammation and degeneration of the cartilage and the connective tissue.[36,37] RP affects people between 2 and 80 years of age and has equal gender distribution. The airway complications in about 50% of the cases are seen more often in females than in males and carry a poorer prognosis.

Diagnostic Criteria

Presence of three or more of the following six McAdam criteria[38] is employed for diagnosis:

1. Chondritis of larynx, trachea, or bronchitis
2. Chondritis of nasal cartilages
3. Chondritis of both auricles
4. Audiovestibular damage (sensorineural hearing loss, tinnitus, and vertigo)
5. Ocular inflammation (conjunctivitis, keratitis, episcleritis, uveitis)
6. Nonerosive seronegative inflammatory polyarthritis

These initial criteria were modified to include histological features and therapeutic responses. The modified criteria by Damiani and Levine[39] include the presence of any one of the following combinations to make a diagnosis:

- Three or more of initial McAdam's criteria (no tissue confirmation needed)
- One or more of the initial McAdam's criteria with positive histological confirmation by biopsy of the cartilage
- At least two McAdam's criteria with response to steroids and/or dapsone

Clinical Features

Clinical features depend on the cartilage that is involved. It is important to understand that apart from cartilaginous structure of the external ear, nose, peripheral joints, larynx, and tracheobronchial tree, other proteoglycan-rich structures can become involved, including the heart, blood vessels, and inner ear.[40]

Airway Complications

The prevalence of symptomatic airway involvement was reported in 21% with female preponderance in about 70% patients.[37] The usual symptoms were progressive dyspnea, cough, stridor, hoarseness, chest discomfort, and features of respiratory failure. The presence of airway symptoms was the first manifestation of RP in about 50% of patients with airway manifestation. Airway obstruction in RP can occur due to any of the following:

- Acute airway inflammatory swelling and airway narrowing
- TBM due to progressive destruction of the cartilage
- Formation of fibrous tissue and cicatricial contraction at a later stage

Investigations

Pulmonary function tests show a mixed pattern.[37] Dynamic CT scan and bronchoscopy **(Fig. 4)** provide the vital details in RP regarding the extent and severity of the airway problem. Typical CT findings include the presence of diffuse tracheobronchial stenosis (better seen with reconstructed CT images), dynamic expiratory collapse, or anterior bronchial wall thickening with posterior sparing. PET-CT is also used to diagnose and identify site for transbronchial needle aspiration (TBNA).[41] Typical bronchoscopic findings include supraglottic and false vocal cord edema, subglottic stenosis, or TM.[37]

Treatment

Many medications, such as steroids, mycophenolate mofetil, methotrexate, and dapsone, have been tried, but the response to treatment is variable. Newer biological agents like rituximab, etanercept, and abatacept show some promise. Bronchoscopic techniques, such as balloon dilatation, and tracheobronchial stenting used alone or in combination might give some respite from symptoms for patients with airway complications.[42] Interventional procedures provide a good short-term relief. However, long-term outcome is quite variable.

Tracheopathia Osteochondroplastica

Tracheopathia osteochondroplastica is a rare, slowly progressive disorder of unknown etiology. Endoluminal projections of bony and cartilaginous nodules that arise from the submucosa of the trachea usually affect lower two-third of trachea. There appears to be a male predominance and usually presents in the sixth or seventh decade of life.[43,44] The nodules characteristically spare the posterior

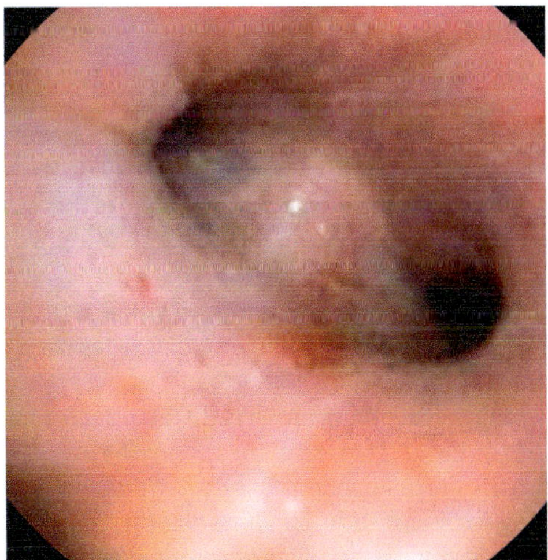

FIG. 4: Relapsing polychondritis. 55-year-old lady: Biopsy-proven relapsing polychondritis. Note the absence of cartilage prominence at the level of distal trachea.

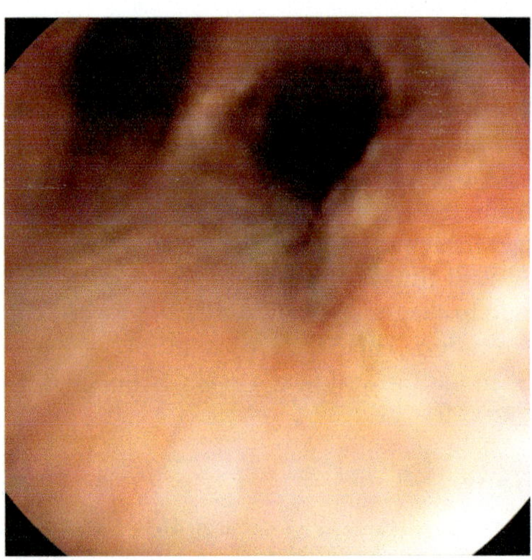

FIG. 5: Case of Tracheopathia osteochondroplastica. Note the nodules seen only on the cartilaginous portion of trachea and sparing of membranous portion.

membrane **(Fig. 5)** but may be present in the proximal, main bronchi also. The presentation is usually with chronic cough, dyspnea in advanced cases, and minimal hemoptysis due to the ulceration of the overlying mucosa.[45] Diagnosis is based on typical bronchoscopic appearances; biopsy is not generally needed. There is no definitive treatment. Severe obstruction may warrant therapeutic interventions.

Tracheobronchial Amyloidosis

Tracheobronchial amyloidosis is very rare, characterized by endoluminal accumulation of abnormal proteins in the form of fibrils, which cause obstructive symptoms. TBA is due to localized deposition of immunoglobulin light chain (AL) secreted by clonal plasma cell residing deep to the airway.[46] The age of disease onset ranges from childhood to old age. Women tend to present at a younger age than men. Females are more commonly affected than men.[47] In a retrospective review of 17 biopsy-proven TBA cases over a 26-year period, Capizzi and colleagues from the Mayo Clinic described dyspnea, cough, hemoptysis and hoarseness as presenting symptoms.[48] Distribution of TBA typically following these patterns.

- Proximal airway involvement from subglottis to carina.
- Mid airway involvement from distal trachea to main bronchi.
- Distal airway involving airways distal to secondary carina.

Endobronchial TBA can be focal or diffuse and has characteristic appearance of yellow deposits with raised hard edges with capillary prominence on an erythematous base.[47] The diagnosis is challenging; often, patients are misdiagnosed and treated as refractory asthma. The median delay in diagnosis of TBA was 11 months.[47] Diagnosis is made by bronchoscopy and biopsy with specific Congo red staining. Response to medications like steroids and melphalan is suboptimal; severe obstruction warrants debulking.

Tuberculosis

Endobronchial tuberculosis (TB) is defined as TB disease which affects the tracheobronchial tree. It occurs because of spread of organism by infected sputum or direct extension to the bronchus from adjacent active parenchymal foci. Endobronchial diseases are mostly seen in patients with extensive cavitatory pulmonary diseases.[49] The true incidence in patients with sputum-positive pulmonary TB is difficult to estimate because bronchoscopy is usually avoided. Endobronchial TB is seen more commonly in females, perhaps because they tend to retain the infected secretions in the bronchial tree and avoid expectoration. It is also more common in the left than right-side bronchi, probably because the left main bronchus is narrow and lengthy and hence the infected sputum may remain in contact with the bronchi for a longer time. Since the infected sputum cannot remain in the trachea, endotracheal TB **(Fig. 6)** is very rare. Symptoms include productive cough, hemoptysis, and shortness of breath, and a characteristic barking cough was described in some.

On CT imaging, endobronchial spread can manifest as centrilobular nodules with a tree-in-bud appearance, segmental bronchi narrowing, concentric bronchial thickening, and bronchiectasis.[49] In a retrospective study of 38 patients with endobronchial TB, a characteristic sign of localized wheezing was seen only in 6% of the patients, TB lesions were predominantly seen in the main bronchi and upper bronchi, and only 5% had lower tracheal involvement.[50]

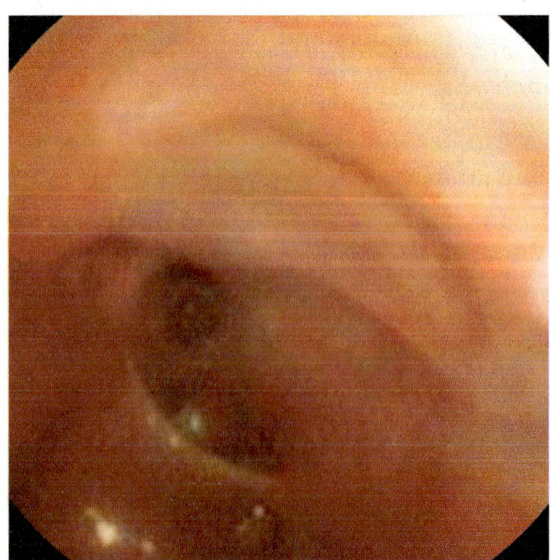

FIG. 6: A 21-year-old lady, a known case of sputum-positive pulmonary tuberculosis, developed severe respiratory distress despite therapy. She had endotracheal fibrostenosis in distal trachea, which was dilated.

The disease is quite refractory to chemotherapy alone. Different appearances may be seen on bronchoscopy: Active caseating, edematous-hyperemic, fibrostenotic, tumorous, granular, ulcerative, and nonspecific bronchitis. Once the lesion becomes fibrostenotic, which is a final path for all the types,[51] it becomes resistant to therapy. Hence, early identification by bronchoscopy is encouraged in a suspected patient. Suspicion arises if a patient with TB develops wheeze or breathlessness. Surgery is ideal if the involved segment is small. If the disease is extensive, balloon dilatation or thermal deobstruction followed by silicone stenting can be tried.[52] Traditionally, steroids have been used to prevent the development of stenosis and for treatment of endobronchial TB, but recent evidences have shown not much benefit with steroids.[53]

Sarcoidosis

Endobronchial involvement is usually seen in the elderly age groups, smokers during advanced stages of parenchymal involvement, and with thickening of bronchovascular bundles on high-resolution CT. It carries a relatively poorer prognosis.[54] Flow limitation is seen in about 9% of patients with sarcoidosis. Sarcoidosis can affect every part of upper airway. Sarcoid involvement of the supraglottic airways, larynx, and central and peripheral airways is also described.[55] OSA syndrome is seen more often in patients with sarcoidosis, especially lupus pernio.[56]

Tracheal obstruction secondary to sarcoidosis is very rare. The classic endobronchial sarcoidosis is characterized by mucosal islands of waxy yellow mucosal nodules, measuring 2–4 mm in diameter. The nodules are sparse in the trachea but abundant in the main, lobar, and segmental bronchi. Other changes are mucosal erythema, granular mucosa, cobblestone mucosa, mucosal plaques, bronchial stenosis, airway distortion due to cicatricial changes in parenchyma, bronchiectasis, extrinsic compression due to mediastinal lymphadenopathy, or airway hyperresponsiveness.[55]

Tracheal Stenosis

Tracheal stenosis is an important cause of UAO. It usually occurs secondary to trauma following prolonged intubation, i.e., PITS, and after tracheostomy, i.e., post-tracheostomy tracheal stenosis (PTTS). Idiopathic stenosis is rare. Mechanical ventilation has made a great difference in the outcome of many sick patients with respiratory failure, but the use of endotracheal tube has resulted in a group of diseases that have become more common than before. Despite the use of low-pressure cuffs, which have reduced the incidence of tracheal stenosis significantly, the incidence of PITS and PTTS is high, i.e., 0.6–21%.[57-59] It is seen predominantly in females, presumably because of smaller tracheal lumen and hence is prone to injury.

Classification

Brichet et al.[60] classified the postintubation tracheal stenosis based on bronchoscopic appearance into three types:

1. *Web-like membranous stenosis*: A short segment (<1 cm) concentric stenosis with no cartilage damage **(Fig. 7A)**.
2. *Pseudoglottic stenosis*: "A"-shaped stenosis secondary to lateral impacted fracture of cartilage in patients following tracheostomy. Since the stenosis resembles a vocal cord, it is called pseudoglottic stenosis **(Fig. 7B)**.
3. *Complex stenosis*: It includes all other varieties, including extensive (>1 cm), circumferential hour-glass-like contraction scarring, or malacia. Basically, there is a cartilage damage along with the narrow lumen **(Figs. 7C and D)**. The membranous and complex types are most common.

Pathogenesis

Usage of high-pressure cuff in an intubated patient predisposes to mucosal ischemia, which also worsens in the presence of hypotension when the capillary pressure is lower. Pressure necrosis and chondritis result, which lead either to the development of cicatricial tissue and membranous type of stenosis or to the cartilage damage causing a complex stenosis.[58]

Stenosis usually develops at the site of the cuff, through the distal end of the tube, because of repetitive injury. Management of tracheal stenosis depends on the type of stenosis, presence of comorbidities, functional status of the patient, and length of the stenosis. Tracheal sleeve resection is a permanent solution considered the gold standard; it carries 3% mortality in trained hands. A multidisciplinary approach incorporating both surgical and bronchoscopic techniques is preferably employed.[60]

Bronchoscopic Management

Bronchoscopic management is sufficient in a majority of cases of membranous stenosis and can be very useful as either a standalone therapy or a bridge to surgery in very sick patients. Bronchoscopy is used for both achieving and maintaining an effective lumen. Some of the procedures to tackle membranous stenosis can be done with a flexible bronchoscope, but it is important that the bronchoscopist is trained in rigid bronchoscopy as well. Better ventilation, better control of secretions and of bleeding during the procedure, and, more importantly, the option of deploying silicone stents make rigid bronchoscopy the procedure of choice.

The general recommendation by the Food and Drug Administration (FDA) is to avoid metallic stents for such benign causes of tracheal obstruction. Since the stent placement for benign lesions (PITS being the prototype) is usually temporary, it is customary to remove the stent and assess after 12–18 months of deployment to see the tracheal function effectively without the stent. Deploying metal stents is easy, can be done through flexible scope, and can be

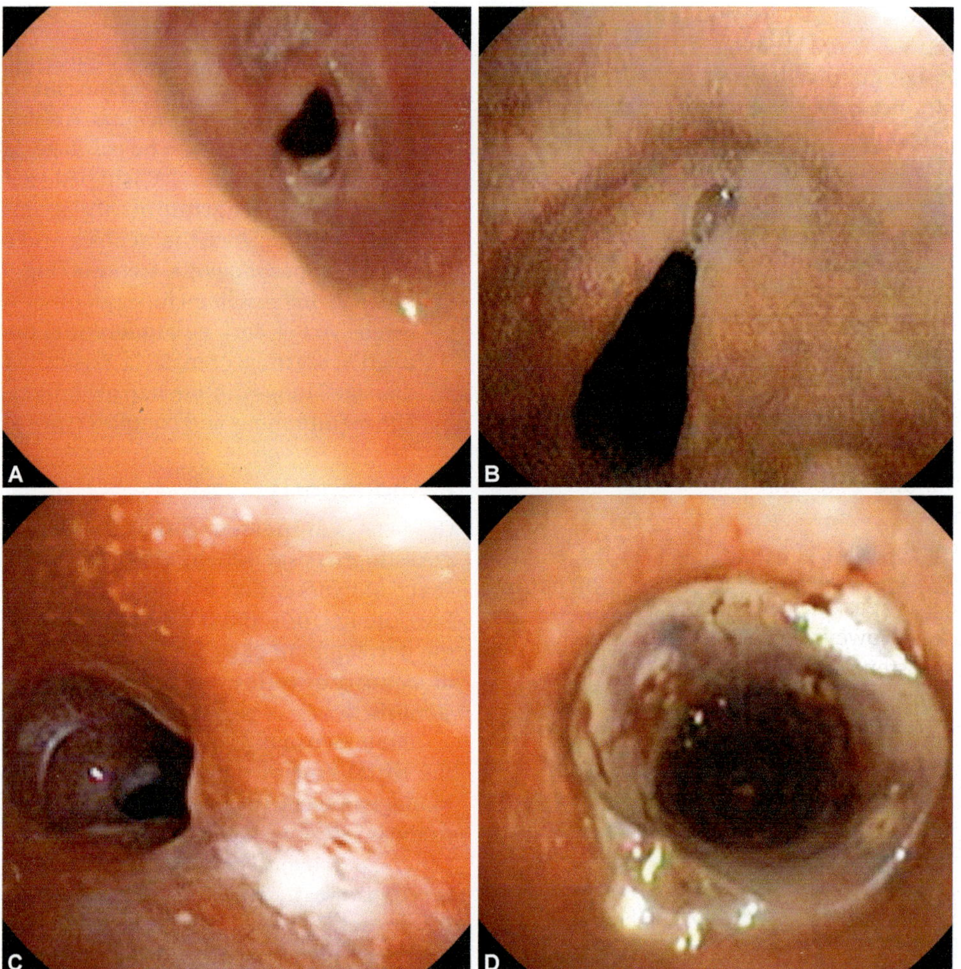

FIGS. 7A TO D: (A) A 24-year-old lady, postintubation. (B) Example of pseudoglottis stenosis. There is membranous stenosis with a remarkable resemblance to vocal cords. (C and D) Complex stenosis. A complex stenosis involving more than one cartilage, managed. These patients are typically managed by dilatation followed by silicone stenting.
Courtesy: Dr Ravindra Mehta, Bengaluru, Karnataka, India.

done with little training; hence, it is very popular. However, removal of stent after it is deployed is a messy affair. It cannot be removed in toto and needs a trained physician with rigid bronchoscopy skills. Hence, a silicone stent is the standard choice for supporting stenosis secondary to cartilage weakness. In membranous stenosis, a stent is not required after dilatation since the cartilage is not involved, and the stability of airway is not affected. In complex stenosis, however, the underlying cartilage is damaged and collapsible. Therefore, despite achieving a good lumen by bronchoscopic means, it has to be followed by leaving a stent at the end of the procedure.

Managing patients with tracheal stenosis is all about two important components: (1) to achieve an effective lumen and (2) to maintain the lumen:

1. *Achieving effective lumen*: Many techniques are described, which are broadly classified as mechanical or thermal. Dilatation using rigid bronchoscope-barrels of increasing diameters, dilators, balloon dilatation, and making nicks in the membrane using rigid scissors are some of the techniques. Laser and electrocautery can be used to cut the membranes with Mercedes Benz incisions, which are mucosa sparing. They prove to be curative in about 65% cases when repeated up to three times.[61]
2. *Maintaining the lumen*: For membranous stenosis, achieving an effective lumen would suffice. However, in complex stenosis, because of cartilaginous weakness, achieving effective lumen shall usually be followed by silicone stenting.

It is important to realize the importance of being gentle with the airways since the best approach to tracheal stenosis is to prevent its occurrence. Using appropriate cuff pressures and noninvasive ventilation when indicated are important considerations. Newer endotracheal tubes that do not have cuffs and have the ability to mold to the shape of the intratracheal airways have been tested in animals and show good promise in reducing tracheal injury.[62]

Idiopathic Tracheal Stenosis

Idiopathic tracheal stenosis is a rare condition. It is seen almost exclusively in females and involves the upper trachea, predominantly the immediate subglottic portion.[63] Many causes have been proposed; it may represent some form of fibromatosis.[63] Immunohistochemical staining for estrogen receptors is usually positive. GERD is seen in about a third of cases. Usual treatment consists of dilatation, tracheostomy, or, if feasible, resection of the involved cartilage.

Extrinsic Compression

Extrinsic compression of trachea occurs from the enlargement of surrounding structures such as the malignant lymph nodes, thyroid enlargement (both benign and malignant), esophageal tumors, and occasionally vascular problems. Vascular problems may more often cause TM secondary to a long-standing pressure effect than anatomical obstruction. In a patient with esophageal malignancy for whom surgery is not done due to any reason, stenting the esophagus is a popular intervention. However, in the presence of partial tracheal obstruction, stenting the esophagus may precipitate severe airway obstruction. In such a situation, the trachea is stented first, followed by esophageal stenting **(Fig. 8)**.

Both benign and malignant disorders of thyroid can cause UAO. Airway obstruction is an indication for surgery in both benign and malignant thyroid problems. Mechanisms of airway obstruction include extrinsic tracheal compression (e.g., benign intrathoracic or substernal goiter), tracheal invasion by a growth, vocal cord paralysis (e.g., recurrent nerve paralysis after thyroidectomy), or a combination of the above **(Fig. 9)**.[64] The incidence of airway obstruction secondary to thyroid enlargement varies widely in the literature, ranging from 16 to 60% based on the population studied.[65] Surgical resection with reconstruction is the treatment of choice, but many patients are inoperable due to extensive spread of tumor into adjacent structures. Tracheostomy can be technically difficult in the case of a large bulky thyroid mass, is ineffective, and may be extremely risky to attempt in patients with intrathoracic tumor involvement of the trachea and entails risk of airway loss. Therapeutic rigid bronchoscopy is an alternative and efficacious treatment modality for management of malignant CAO. In a series of 30 patients with thyroid disorders causing UAO who were also not candidates for surgery due to various reasons, there is a great utility of rigid bronchoscopy and laser application in providing both immediate and long-term benefits.

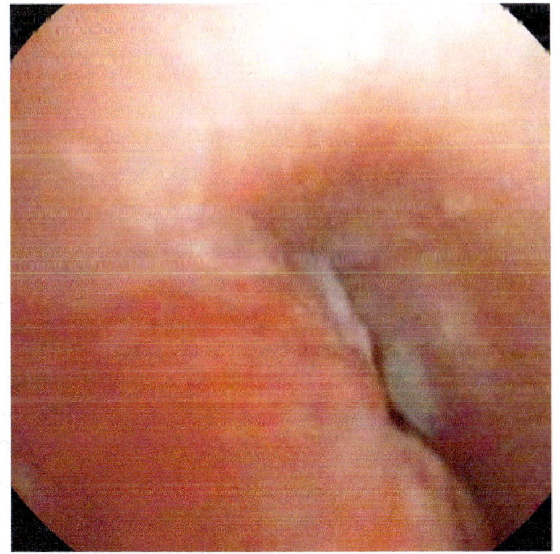

FIG. 8: A 60-year-old lady with esophageal malignancy causing near-total occlusion at the subglottic region.

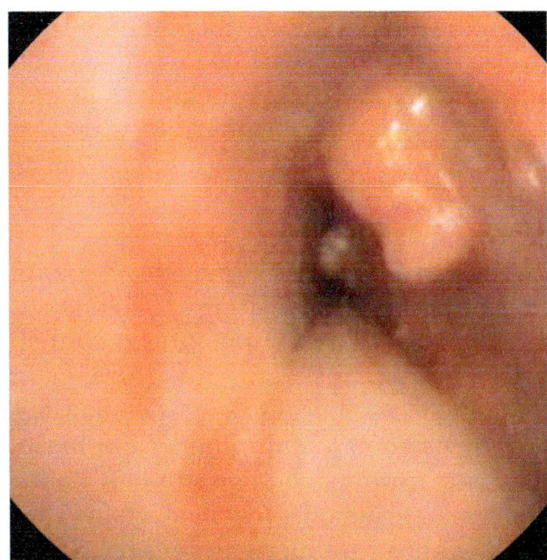

FIG. 9: An elderly lady with thyroid malignancy causing both extrinsic compression and tumor infiltration of upper trachea.

Granulomatosis with Polyangiitis

Upper airways are commonly involved in granulomatosis with polyangiitis (GPA) most of the times. Nasal and oral ulcerations, epistaxis, sinusitis and otitis, cough, nasal cartilage destruction causing septal perforation, saddle nose deformity, and stridor are common upper airway manifestations.[66] Usual features are ulceration of larynx and trachea. However, a rare but a significant airway problem is subglottis stenosis. This has been reported to develop during treatment with steroid and cyclophosphamide.[67] It is typically dealt with by interventional techniques like laser application or dilatation.[68] Intralesional long-acting corticosteroids have been also found to be effective.[69]

Tumors

Primary tracheal tumors are very rare, seen in about 0.2 per 100,000 persons of whom about 80% are malignant.[70] Primary tracheal tumors can arise from the respiratory epithelium, salivary glands, and mesenchymal structures of the trachea.[71] Squamous and adenoid cystic carcinoma account for about two-thirds of tumors from trachea. The other malignant tumors are mucoepidermoid carcinoma, arising from the submucosal glands. Neuroendocrine neoplasms are seen more in bronchi than in trachea and include typical and atypical carcinoids, large-cell neuroendocrine tumors, and small-cell carcinoma. The difference between the primary tracheal tumors and the bronchogenic malignancies is that the tracheal tumors have a better long-term prognosis and need a more aggressive approach in providing good palliation or a cure.[72] Benign tumors of the trachea include tumors from surface epithelium like papilloma, papillomatosis, tumors from glands (like pleomorphic adenoma, mucous gland adenoma, myoepithelioma, and oncocytoma), and tumors from mesenchymal structures [like fibroma, benign fibrous histiocytoma, hemangioma, paraganglioma (chemodectoma), hemangiopericytoma, glomus tumor, chondroma, lipoma, and leiomyoma granular cell tumors]. Endotracheal metastases are much less common than endobronchial metastasis. Endobronchial metastasis commonly arises from renal, colon, or bronchogenic malignancy, melanoma, and osteosarcoma. Presentation of metastases as UAO is very rare.[71]

Other Causes

Bilateral vocal cord palsy can happen secondary to thyroid malignancy or thyroid surgery. Others include the neurological diseases or idiopathic causes. Cases of bilateral vocal cord palsy have been reported following nasogastric tube, systemic lupus erythematosus (SLE), and esophageal surgeries.[73-75] Other rare and diverse causes of UAO have been described as anecdotal case reports.

THERAPEUTIC CONSIDERATIONS

As is true with many other conditions in medicine, treating the primary cause of the UAO is important. However, it is also important to manage the obstruction. Obstruction can be secondary to intrinsic pathology like in the case of tumors/tracheal stenosis or extrinsic compression like due to mediastinal node/thyroid/esophageal pathology. Functional obstruction without significant anatomic narrowing can happen secondary to TM. In cases where surgery is feasible, especially in short segment complex stenosis or tracheal tumors, it should be offered. Several other interventional approaches provide a good quality of life in most of the conditions.

In the cases of intramural pathology, achieving a patent lumen is accomplished by techniques like rigid bronchoscopy, laser, electrocautery, and argon plasma coagulation, while airway stenting is necessary for extramural compression or TM where maintaining lumen is the key issue.[76-79] Silicone stents are preferred over metallic stents because the latter are difficult to remove after deployment. Most of the cases of UAO secondary to tracheal stenosis could be managed using flexible bronchoscopy, for balloon dilatation, laser application, stent placement, and brachytherapy.[78] But rigid bronchoscopy is generally preferred because of a better control of airway, ventilation, and for deployment of silicone stents.

SUMMARY

Upper airway obstruction can present with an acute life-threatening emergency; obstruction can also occur due to intrinsic pathology or extrinsic compression. Tracheal stenosis frequently follows tracheostomy done for prolonged assisted ventilation in an intensive care unit. Functional obstruction can occur in conditions such as trachea bronchomalacia. The most important issue in management consists of achieving a patent lumen which is accomplished by different techniques depending upon the cause. For malignant obstruction, one may require rigid bronchoscopy, laser, electrocautery, and argon plasma coagulation, while airway stenting is necessary.

REFERENCES

1. Rotman HH, Liss HP, Weg JG. Diagnosis of upper airway obstruction by pulmonary function testing. Chest. 1975;68(6):796-9.
2. Acres JC, Kryger MH. Clinical significance of pulmonary function tests: upper airway obstruction. Chest. 1981;80(2):207-11.
3. Lahiri K. Upper airway obstruction. Indian J Pediatr. 1996;63(5):665-71.
4. Al-Bazzaz F, Grillo H, Kazemi H. Response to exercise in upper airway obstruction. Am Rev Respir Dis. 1975;111(5):631-40.
5. Geffin B, Grillo HC, Cooper JD, et al. Stenosis following tracheostomy for respiratory care. JAMA. 1971;216(12):1984-8.
6. Pellegrino R, Viegi G, Brusasco V, et al. Interpretative strategies for lung function tests. Eur Respir J. 2005;26(5):948-68.
7. Empey DW. Assessment of upper airways obstruction. Br Med J. 1972;3(5825):503-5.
8. Miller RD, Hyatt RE. Obstructing lesions of the larynx and trachea: clinical and physiologic characteristics. Mayo Clin Proc. 1969;44:145-61.
9. Eskander A, de Almeida JR, Irish JC. Acute Upper Airway Obstruction. N Engl J Med. 2019;381(20):1940-9.
10. Boyd M, Chatterjee A, Chiles C, et al. Tracheobronchial foreign body aspiration in adults. South Med J. 2009;102(2):171-4.
11. Swanson KL, Edell ES. Tracheobronchial foreign bodies. Chest Surg Clin N Am. 2001;11(4):861-72.
12. Moura e Sá J, Oliveira A, Caiado A, et al. Tracheobronchial foreign bodies in adults--experience of the Bronchology Unit of Centro Hospitalar de Vila Nova de Gaia. Rev Port Pneumol. 2006;12(1):31-43.
13. Gulati SP, Kumar A, Sachdeva A, et al. Groundnut as the commonest foreign body of tracheobronchial tree in winter in

Northern India. An analysis of fourteen cases. Indian J Med Sci. 2003;57(6):244-8.
14. Tang LF, Xu YC, Wang YS, et al. Airway foreign body removal by flexible bronchoscopy: experience with 1027 children during 2000-2008. World J Pediatr WJP. 2009;5(3):191-5.
15. Swanson KL, Prakash UBS, Midthun DE, et al. Flexible bronchoscopic management of airway foreign bodies in children. Chest. 2002;121(5):1695-700.
16. Vilke GM, Smith AM, Ray LU, et al. Airway obstruction in children aged less than 5 years: the prehospital experience. Prehosp Emerg Care. 2004;8(2):196-9.
17. Papadopoulou-Alataki E. Upper airway considerations in hereditary angioedema. Curr Opin Allergy Clin Immunol. 2010; 10(1):20-5.
18. Weis M. Clinical review of hereditary angioedema: diagnosis and management. Postgrad Med. 2009;121(6):113-20.
19. Gompels MM, Lock RJ, Abinun M, et al. C1 inhibitor deficiency: consensus document. Clin Exp Immunol. 2005;139(3):379-94.
20. Kreuz W, Martinez-Saguer I, Aygören-Pürsün E, et al. C1-inhibitor concentrate for individual replacement therapy in patients with severe hereditary angioedema refractory to danazol prophylaxis. Transfusion (Paris). 2009;49(9):1987-95.
21. Craig TJ, Levy RJ, Wasserman RL, et al. Efficacy of human C1 esterase inhibitor concentrate compared with placebo in acute hereditary angioedema attacks. J Allergy Clin Immunol. 2009;124(4):801-8.
22. Duerr M, Glander P, Diekmann F, et al. Increased incidence of angioedema with ACE inhibitors in combination with mTOR inhibitors in kidney transplant recipients. Clin J Am Soc Nephrol CJASN. 2010;5(4):703-8.
23. Malaty J, Wu V. Vocal Cord Dysfunction: Rapid Evidence Review. Am Fam Physician. 2021;104(5):471-5.
24. Morris MJ, Deal LE, Bean DR, et al. Vocal cord dysfunction in patients with exertional dyspnea. Chest. 1999;116(6):1676-82.
25. Hira HS, Singh A. Significance of upper airway influence among patients of vocal cord dysfunction for its diagnosis: Role of impulse oscillometry. Lung India Off Organ Indian Chest Soc. 2009;26(1):5-8.
26. Deckert J, Deckert L. Vocal cord dysfunction. Am Fam Physician. 2010;81(2):156-9.
27. Mahoney J, Hew M, Vertigan A, et al. Treatment effectiveness for Vocal Cord Dysfunction in adults and adolescents: A systematic review. Clin Exp Allergy J Br Soc Allergy Clin Immunol. 2022;52(3):387-404.
28. Carden KA, Boiselle PM, Waltz DA, et al. Tracheomalacia and tracheobronchomalacia in children and adults: an in-depth review. Chest. 2005;127(3):984-1005.
29. Jacobs IN, Wetmore RF, Tom LW, et al. Tracheobronchomalacia in children. Arch Otolaryngol Head Neck Surg. 1994;120(2): 154-8.
30. Kamran A, Jennings RW. Tracheomalacia and Tracheobronchomalacia in Pediatrics: An Overview of Evaluation, Medical Management, and Surgical Treatment. Front Pediatr. 2019;7:512.
31. Kamran A, Baird CW, Jennings RW. Tracheobronchomalacia, Tracheobronchial Compression, and Tracheobronchial Malformations: Diagnostic and Treatment Strategies. Semin Thorac Cardiovasc Surg Pediatr Card Surg Annu. 2020;23:53-61.
32. Wagnetz U, Roberts HC, Chung T, et al. Dynamic airway evaluation with volume CT: initial experience. Can Assoc Radiol J. 2010;61(2):90-7.
33. Ernst A, Majid A, Feller-Kopman D, et al. Airway stabilization with silicone stents for treating adult tracheobronchomalacia: a prospective observational study. Chest. 2007;132(2):609-16.
34. Ernst A, Odell DD, Michaud G, et al. Central airway stabilization for tracheobronchomalacia improves quality of life in patients with COPD. Chest. 2011;140(5):1162-8.
35. Hanawa T, Ikeda S, Funatsu T, et al. Development of a new surgical procedure for repairing tracheobronchomalacia. J Thorac Cardiovasc Surg. 1990;100(4):587-94.
36. Shimizu J, Murayama MA, Mizukami Y, et al. Innate immune responses in Behçet disease and relapsing polychondritis. Front Med. 2023;10:1055753.
37. Ernst A, Rafeq S, Boiselle P, et al. Relapsing polychondritis and airway involvement. Chest. 2009;135(4):1024-30.
38. McAdam LP, O'Hanlan MA, Bluestone R, et al. Relapsing polychondritis: prospective study of 23 patients and a review of the literature. Medicine (Baltimore). 1976;55(3):193-215.
39. Damiani JM, Levine HL. Relapsing polychondritis—report of ten cases. Laryngoscope. 1979;89(6 Pt 1):929-46.
40. Trentham DE, Le CH. Relapsing polychondritis. Ann Intern Med. 1998;129(2):114-22.
41. Lei W, Zeng DX, Chen T, et al. FDG PET-CT combined with TBNA for the diagnosis of atypical relapsing polychondritis: report of 2 cases and a literature review. J Thorac Dis. 2014;6(9):1285-92.
42. Sarodia BD, Dasgupta A, Mehta AC. Management of airway manifestations of relapsing polychondritis: case reports and review of literature. Chest. 1999;116(6):1669-75.
43. Lundgren R, Stjernberg NL. Tracheobronchopathia osteochondroplastica. A clinical bronchoscopic and spirometric study. Chest. 1981;80(6):706-9.
44. Jindal S, Nath A, Neyaz Z, et al. Tracheobronchopathia osteochondroplastica—a rare or an overlooked entity? J Radiol Case Rep. 2013;7(3):16-25.
45. Decalmer S, Woodcock A, Greaves M, et al. Airway abnormalities at flexible bronchoscopy in patients with chronic cough. Eur Respir J. 2007;30(6):1138-42.
46. Berk JL, O'Regan A, Skinner M. Pulmonary and tracheobronchial amyloidosis. Semin Respir Crit Care Med. 2002;23(2):155-65.
47. O'Regan A, Fenlon HM, Beamis JF, et al. Tracheobronchial amyloidosis. The Boston University experience from 1984 to 1999. Medicine (Baltimore). 2000;79(2):69-79.
48. Capizzi SA, Betancourt E, Prakash UB. Tracheobronchial amyloidosis. Mayo Clin Proc. 2000;75(11):1148-52.
49. Shahzad T, Irfan M. Endobronchial tuberculosis-a review. J Thorac Dis. 2016;8(12):3797-802.
50. Hoheisel G, Chan BK, Chan CH, et al. Endobronchial tuberculosis: diagnostic features and therapeutic outcome. Respir Med. 1994;88(8):593-7.
51. Chung HS, Lee JH. Bronchoscopic assessment of the evolution of endobronchial tuberculosis. Chest. 2000;117(2):385-92.
52. Low SY, Hsu A, Eng P. Interventional bronchoscopy for tuberculous tracheobronchial stenosis. Eur Respir J. 2004;24(3):345-7.
53. Mishra NR, Panigrahi MK, Bhatt GC, et al. Corticosteroid as an Adjunct in the Treatment of Endobronchial Tuberculosis: A Systematic Review & Meta-analysis. Curr Pediatr Rev. 2020; 16(1):53-60.
54. Handa T, Nagai S, Fushimi Y, et al. Clinical and radiographic indices associated with airflow limitation in patients with sarcoidosis. Chest. 2006;130(6):1851-6.

55. Polychronopoulos VS, Prakash UBS. Airway involvement in sarcoidosis. Chest. 2009;136(5):1371-80.
56. Turner GA, Lower EE, Corser BC, et al. Sleep apnea in sarcoidosis. Sarcoidosis Vasc Diffuse Lung Dis Off J WASOG. 1997;14(1): 61-4.
57. Rumbak MJ, Graves AE, Scott MP, et al. Tracheostomy tube occlusion protocol predicts significant tracheal obstruction to air flow in patients requiring prolonged mechanical ventilation. Crit Care Med. 1997;25(3):413-7.
58. Raghuraman G, Rajan S, Marzouk JK, et al. Is tracheal stenosis caused by percutaneous tracheostomy different from that by surgical tracheostomy? Chest. 2005;127(3):879-85.
59. James P, Parmar S, Hussain K, et al. Tracheal Stenosis after Tracheostomy. Br J Oral Maxillofac Surg. 2021;59(1):82-5.
60. Brichet A, Verkindre C, Dupont J, et al. Multidisciplinary approach to management of postintubation tracheal stenoses. Eur Respir J. 1999;13(4):888-93.
61. Mehta AC, Lee FY, Cordasco EM, et al. Concentric tracheal and subglottic stenosis. Management using the Nd-YAG laser for mucosal sparing followed by gentle dilatation. Chest. 1993;104(3):673-7.
62. Gordin A, Chadha NK, Campisi P, et al. Effect of a novel anatomically shaped endotracheal tube on intubation-related injury. Arch Otolaryngol Head Neck Surg. 2010;136(1):54-9.
63. Mark EJ, Meng F, Kradin RL, et al. Idiopathic tracheal stenosis: a clinicopathologic study of 63 cases and comparison of the pathology with chondromalacia. Am J Surg Pathol. 2008;32(8): 1138-43.
64. Noppen M, Poppe K, D'Haese J, et al. Interventional bronchoscopy for treatment of tracheal obstruction secondary to benign or malignant thyroid disease. Chest. 2004;125(2):723-30.
65. Madan K, Shrestha P, Garg R, et al. Bronchoscopic management of critical central airway obstruction by thyroid cancer: Combination airway stenting using tracheal and inverted-Y carinal self-expanding metallic stents. Lung India. 2017;34(2): 202-5.
66. Alam DS, Seth R, Sindwani R, et al. Upper airway manifestations of granulomatosis with polyangiitis. Cleve Clin J Med. 2012;79 (Suppl 3):S16-21.
67. Strange C, Halstead L, Baumann M, et al. Subglottic stenosis in Wegener's granulomatosis: development during cyclophosphamide treatment with response to carbon dioxide laser therapy. Thorax. 1990;45(4):300-1.
68. Schokkenbroek AA, Franssen CFM, Dikkers FG. Dilatation tracheoscopy for laryngeal and tracheal stenosis in patients with Wegener's granulomatosis. Eur Arch Otorhinolaryngol. 2008;265(5):549-55.
69. Solans-Laqué R, Bosch-Gil J, Canela M, et al. Clinical features and therapeutic management of subglottic stenosis in patients with Wegener's granulomatosis. Lupus. 2008;17(9):832-6.
70. Pearson FG, Cardoso P, Keshavjee S. Primary tumours of the upper airway. In: Pearson FG, Deslauriers J, Ginsberg RJ, et al. (Eds). Thoracic Surgery, 1st edition. New York: Churchill Livingstone; 1995. pp. 285-99.
71. Macchiarini P. Primary tracheal tumours. Lancet Oncol. 2006;7(1):83-91.
72. Maziak DE, Todd TR, Keshavjee SH, et al. Adenoid cystic carcinoma of the airway: thirty-two-year experience. J Thorac Cardiovasc Surg. 1996;112(6):1522-31; discussion 1531-2.
73. Brousseau VJ, Kost KM. A rare but serious entity: nasogastric tube syndrome. Otolaryngol Head Neck Surg. 2006;135(5):677-9.
74. Jayachandran NV, Agrawal S, Rajasekhar L, et al. Bilateral vocal cord palsy as a manifestation of systemic lupus erythematosus. Lupus. 2010;19(1):109-10.
75. Hamer PW, Thompson SK, Rees GL, et al. Bilateral recurrent laryngeal nerve palsy after Ivor Lewis oesophagectomy. ANZ J Surg. 2009;79(12):959-60.
76. Senitko M, Oberg CL, Abraham GE, et al. Microwave Ablation for Malignant Central Airway Obstruction: A Pilot Study. Respir Int Rev Thorac Dis. 2022;101(7):666-74.
77. Guedes F, Branquinho MV, Sousa AC, et al. Central airway obstruction: is it time to move forward? BMC Pulm Med. 2022;22(1):68.
78. Rahman NA, Fruchter O, Shitrit D, et al. Flexible bronchoscopic management of benign tracheal stenosis: long term follow-up of 115 patients. J Cardiothorac Surg. 2010;5:2.
79. Sabath BF, Casal RF. Airway stenting for central airway obstruction: a review. Mediastinum Hong Kong China. 2023;7:18.

Chronic Respiratory Failure

Jennifer Trevor, Lanier O'Hare

CHAPTER 93

INTRODUCTION

The primary function of the respiratory system is to facilitate the uptake of oxygen into the blood and the elimination of carbon dioxide (CO_2). The term *respiratory failure* is used when the lungs are unable to effectively perform this function. Respiratory failure can be further subdivided into hypoxemic (type I), i.e., PaO_2 of < 55 mm Hg with a low or normal PCO_2, or hypercapnic (type II), defined as a PCO_2 of >50 mm Hg with a normal or low PaO_2. These two categories can be further divided into acute or chronic variants. Chronic hypercapnic respiratory failure is differentiated from acute failure based on a normal pH due to compensated serum bicarbonate levels. Chronic hypoxemic respiratory failure differs from acute hypoxemic respiratory failure in the time to onset of the disorder and change from baseline.[1,2] Hypoxemic and hypercapnic respiratory failures differ in their etiologies and management. In addition to treating the underlying cause, hypoxemic failure is managed with supplementary oxygen, while hypercapnic failure is managed with interventions that improve ventilation.

CHRONIC HYPOXEMIC RESPIRATORY FAILURE

Physiology

The process of ventilation and gas exchange is regulated by the central nervous system (CNS), chest wall, diaphragm, and elastic properties of the lung. Dysfunction of any of these systems can interrupt the process of oxygenation.[3] Once oxygen is in the alveolar space, its entry into the blood is determined by the diffusion gradient of oxygen across the alveolar-capillary membrane, the properties of the membrane itself, and the rate at which blood flows through the capillary bed. The diffusion gradient is determined by the difference in the partial pressure of oxygen between the alveoli and the capillary blood. In a healthy lung, oxygen diffuses rapidly across this barrier, making oxygenation of the blood dependent on the rate at which the capillaries are perfused.

Once an oxygen molecule reaches the circulation, it binds to hemoglobin or dissolves within the plasma. The concentration of oxygen in the blood, or the arterial oxygen content (CaO_2), can be described as follows:

$$CaO_2 = (1.34 \times Hgb \times SaO_2) + (0.003 \times PaO_2)$$

(SaO_2 = Oxygen saturation of hemoglobin, Hgb, and PaO_2 = dissolved oxygen in plasma)

SaO_2 is measured with pulse oximetry or by arterial blood gas (ABG) assessment, and PaO_2 is measured by ABG. As described in the above equation, the arterial oxygen concentration is largely driven by the concentration of Hgb.

Pathophysiology

There are five commonly cited etiologies for hypoxemic respiratory failure: Low inspired oxygen fraction, alveolar hypoventilation, diffusion impairment, ventilation/perfusion (V/Q) mismatch, and right-to-left shunt **(Table 1)**.

TABLE 1: Chronic hypoxemic (type I) respiratory failure.

Categories of hypoxemic respiratory failure	Etiology of chronic hypoxemic respiratory failure
Low inspired FiO_2	Altitude (typically not chronic)
Alveolar hypoventilation	COPD, obstructive sleep apnea, obesity hypoventilation syndrome, causes of type II respiratory failure
Diffusion impairment	Interstitial lung disease
V/Q mismatch	• *Shunt*: Atelectasis, mucus plug • *Dead space*: Emphysema, pulmonary embolism
Right-to-left shunt	Hepatopulmonary syndrome, intracardiac shunts

(COPD: chronic obstructive pulmonary disease; V/Q: ventilation/perfusion)

Low Inspired Oxygen Fraction

Low inspired oxygen fraction (FiO_2) may occur in situations of low barometric pressure, where the percentage of oxygen may be normal, but less oxygen is available due to low pressure, such as at high altitudes. This concept is illustrated by the alveolar gas equation:

$$PAO_2 = (Patm - PH_2O) \times FiO_2 - (PaCO_2/RQ)$$

where PAO_2 is alveolar oxygen concentration, Patm is atmospheric pressure (760 mm Hg at sea level), PH_2O is the partial pressure of water assumed (45 mm Hg), FiO_2 is the fraction of inspired oxygen (0.21), $PaCO_2$ is the partial pressure of CO_2 in alveoli (typically 40–45 under normal physiologic conditions), and RQ is the respiratory quotient, which is typically assumed to be 0.82. This equation describes why increases in altitude can reduce alveolar oxygen concentration through reduction in atmospheric pressure.

Alveolar Hypoventilation

Alveolar hypoventilation, as an etiology of chronic hypoxemic respiratory failure, encompasses disorders that are caused by chronically decreased ventilation. These causes overlap with those that cause chronic hypercapnic respiratory failure. Applying the alveolar gas equation, we can infer that conditions which chronically increase the alveolar carbon dioxide content ($PACO_2$) will cause a concurrent decrease in the alveolar oxygen content (PAO_2). This will in turn decrease the amount of available oxygen in the alveoli which can diffuse into the capillaries, thereby decreasing the arterial oxygen content. Therefore, conditions resulting in a severe increase in $PACO_2$ can cause combined hypoxemic and hypercapnic respiratory failure. These conditions include chronic obstructive pulmonary disease (COPD), obstructive sleep apnea (OSA), obesity, and hypoventilation syndrome, among others. We can also derive from the above equation that increasing the total amount of inspired oxygen (FiO_2) will overcome the hypoxemic portion of the respiratory failure.

Diffusion Impairment

Diffusion impairment refers to conditions that affect the ability of oxygen to cross from the alveoli into the capillaries. While CO_2 diffuses rapidly across this barrier, oxygen transport can be profoundly interrupted in pathologic states. In the healthy lung, oxygen in the alveoli diffuses across the thin cell membrane of a type I pneumocyte, through the interstitium, and then through the endothelium of the capillaries into bloodstream.[4] Any disease which involves these membranes may increase the diffusion time and lead to hypoxemia. Common chronic etiologies of diffusion impairment include interstitial lung diseases (ILDs), which damage the interstitium of the lung through inflammatory cell infiltration and fibrin deposition, eventually resulting in fibrosis. Scarring of the interstitial space decreases the ability of oxygen to diffuse across it.[5-7] These processes can be overcome by increasing the fraction of oxygen in the alveoli through use of supplemental oxygen, which will increase the diffusion gradient, and thereby increasing the available oxygen for diffusion into the bloodstream.

Ventilation/Perfusion Mismatch

Ventilation/perfusion defects occur when there is inadequate interaction between the air in the alveoli and blood supplied by the capillary bed. Within this category, two etiologies exist: When a portion of the lung is perfused but not ventilated, this is referred to as a "shunt"; conversely, when a ventilated portion of the lung is not perfused, this is referred to as "dead space". There also exists overlap between these two groups. The most common example of V/Q mismatch is COPD, a mix of two separate disease processes—emphysema and chronic bronchitis.[8] Both the breakdown of alveolar architecture seen in emphysema and the presence of inflammation and secretions in the airways in chronic bronchitis contribute to hypoxemia.[9] Other examples of V/Q mismatch causing hypoxemia include acute pulmonary embolism, wherein a well-ventilated portion of the lung becomes abruptly unperfused resulting in dead space,[10,11] and atelectasis causing hypoxemia through shunt development.

Right-to-left Shunt

A right-to-left shunt is a more extreme version of a V/Q mismatch. In this condition, blood passes through the lung without being exposed to oxygen or bypasses the pulmonary circulation completely. Blood that does not undergo gas exchange has the same gas content as systemic venous blood and alters the gas properties of oxygenated blood when they mix. The effect on the total arterial oxygen content when the unoxygenated fraction mixes with the oxygenated fraction can be calculated by the shunt fraction equation as follows:

$$Qs/Qt = (CcO_2 - CaO_2)/(CcO_2 - CvO_2)$$

In the above equation, Qs is the blood flow through the shunt per minute, while Qt is the total cardiac output per minute. Qs/Qt is the shunt fraction, which represents the portion of the total cardiac output that is composed of shunted blood. CcO_2 is the pulmonary end-capillary O_2 content, which under normal conditions is approximately equal to the alveolar O_2 content (PaO_2). CaO_2 is the arterial O_2 content and CvO_2 is the mixed venous O_2 content. Several different methods for measuring shunt fraction exist. One common, minimally invasive, technique is the 100% oxygen method, where the shunt fraction is calculated from the arterial and venous blood gas following administration of 100% O_2.

Common causes of a right-to-left shunt include intracardiac shunts, pulmonary arteriovenous malformations, and hepatopulmonary syndrome. In these conditions, blood from the right side of the heart bypasses the pulmonary circulation and the lung and is therefore nonresponsive to supplemental oxygen, unlike other causes of chronic hypoxemic respiratory failure.[12]

CHRONIC HYPERCAPNIC RESPIRATORY FAILURE

Physiology

Carbon dioxide is a waste product of aerobic metabolism which diffuses into the alveoli and is eliminated by respiration. It reaches equilibrium across the alveoli almost instantly, so disease processes that affect alveolar gas exchange do not alter the removal of CO_2 by the body. As such, removal of CO_2 is more dependent on the mechanical process of ventilation and patency of the airway than on the process of diffusion. Ventilation can be defined as follows:

$$\text{Minute ventilation} = \text{Respiratory rate} \times \text{Tidal volume}$$

wherein respiratory rate is defined as the number of breaths per minute and tidal volume is the volume of each exhaled breath. Decreasing the respiratory rate or the tidal volume will decrease the minute ventilation, which will lead to increased retention of CO_2. In a healthy state, the medullary respiratory center of the brain interacts with the muscles of respiration to alter the minute ventilation to maintain CO_2 homeostasis.

Pathophysiology

Adequate ventilation requires effective interaction of the CNS, peripheral nervous system, chest wall, chest wall and abdominal muscles, diaphragm, and airway **(Table 2)**. Dysfunction of any of these systems can lead to inadequate ventilation, which leads to CO_2 retention. $PaCO_2$ of >50 mm Hg is considered hypercapnic respiratory failure which can happen in several disease processes as follows:[13]

- *Central nervous system*: The brain and the spinal cord provide the respiratory drive to achieve the minute ventilation required to maintain a normal physiologic pCO_2 and pH. This is mediated through chemoreceptors located in the aortic and carotid bodies that detect changes in pCO_2 and pH in the blood. These chemoreceptors communicate with the pons in the brainstem to either increase the tidal volume (apneustic center) or decrease tidal volume (pneumotaxic center). The pons then communicates with the medulla, also located within the brainstem, to make fine adjustments in tidal volume and respiratory rate needed to maintain a normal physiologic pH. Problems that affect the ability of the CNS to interpret the physiologic environment of the body, or to communicate with the body to stimulate the muscles involved in the ventilatory process, can lead to chronic hypercapnic respiratory failure, such as seen in the presence of physical damage to CNS tissue due to trauma or mass effect by tumors or degenerative processes like neuromuscular diseases such as amyotrophic lateral sclerosis (ALS).
- *Chest wall*: The primary muscles of inspiration include the external intercostal muscles and the diaphragm. During inspiration, the chest wall expands to inflate the lungs through contraction of these muscles which elevate the ribs and sternum, creating negative pressure to allow for the inflow of air. Expiration is largely a passive phenomenon where relaxation allows for the outflow of air; however, other sets of intercostal muscles and abdominal muscles can provide additional force to propel air from the lung. Common diseases of the chest wall that can lead to chronic hypercapnic respiratory failure include spinal malformations, morbid obesity, and trauma. Obesity is an important cause of chronic respiratory failure, which impairs the ability of the chest cavity to expand and reduces diaphragmatic excursion, resulting in decreased tidal volumes and increased dead-space ventilation leading to CO_2 retention.[14]
- *Neuromuscular*: Neuromuscular diseases result in chronic hypercapnic respiratory failure through degeneration of the peripheral nervous system, with or without CNS involvement. In addition, myopathies lead to degradation of muscle fibers that can affect the muscles of the chest wall. The loss of coordinated movement of the muscles of respiration leads to respiratory failure as seen in myasthenia gravis and poliomyelitis (which affect the peripheral nerve fibers innervating muscle tissue) and in inflammatory myopathies, polymyositis and muscular dystrophy (which result in degeneration of the muscle fibers).[15,16]
- *Pulmonary*: COPD is the best example of hypercapnic respiratory failure due to lung parenchymal disease. There are multiple mechanisms of airways obstruction, alveolar hypoventilation, and hypercapnia in COPD. The early collapse of small airways also results in air trapping and impaired elimination of CO_2.[8] In addition, hyperinflation of the lungs from emphysematous destruction of alveoli reduces diaphragmatic excursion which also contributes to the development of chronic hypercapnic respiratory failure.

TABLE 2: Chronic hypercapnic (type II) respiratory failure.

Affected system	Example of observed pathology
Central nervous system (CNS)	CNS trauma, central sleep apnea, amyotrophic lateral sclerosis
Chest wall	Chest wall trauma, kyphoscoliosis/spinal deformities, obesity
Neuromuscular	Poliomyelitis, myasthenia gravis, polymyositis, muscular dystrophy
Pulmonary	Chronic obstructive pulmonary disease

MANAGEMENT OF CHRONIC RESPIRATORY FAILURE

Supplemental oxygenation to reverse hypoxemia, positive-pressure ventilation (PPV) to correct hypercapnia, and management of the underlying cause of chronic respiratory failure constitute the mainstay of therapy. Additional therapies are focused on respiratory rehabilitation, nutrition, exercise, and other supports which can greatly improve the quality of life.

Management of Chronic Hypoxemic Respiratory Failure

Long-term oxygen therapy (LTOT) is the standard of care for chronic hypoxemia which may likely improve survival for most patients **(Table 3)**.[17,18] LTOT may also improve quality of life[19] and reduce hospital admissions.[20] Most current guidelines recommend LTOT for COPD patients with severe hypoxemia despite optimal medical management. Hypoxemia is best determined by ABG assessment, ideally with two separate determinations obtained while breathing room air for 20–30 minutes. Indications for LTOT include a PaO_2 of 55 mm Hg or $SpO_2 < 88\%$.[21] Further qualified indications include PaO_2 of 55–59 mm Hg in the presence of cor pulmonale or polycythemia (hematocrit > 55%), as these are end-organ sequelae of chronic hypoxia.[22]

The goal of chronic oxygen supplementation is to maintain $SpO_2 > 90\%$, including during periods of sleep and with exertion.[21] Supplemental oxygen use for a minimum of 15 h/day is considered necessary to be effective.[23]

Management of Chronic Hypercapnic Respiratory Failure

Positive-pressure ventilation **(Table 4)** provides respiratory support without the use of endotracheal intubation and can be administered via a facial interface such as a mouth or nasal piece, nasal mask, or full-face mask.

Continuous Positive Airway Pressure

Continuous positive airway pressure (CPAP) utilizes a constant level of positive pressure throughout the respiratory cycle. This pressure prevents the periodic collapse of airways in patients with sleep-disordered breathing such as OSA and obesity hypoventilation syndrome (OHS) characterized by recurrent episodes of hypoxemia, hypercapnia, and sleep fragmentation caused by nocturnal apneic or hypopneic events.[24] CPAP is the first line of therapy in treating even mild symptomatic OSA and OHS. Most patients with OHS have concomitant OSA, and CPAP similarly prevents nocturnal airway occlusions in OHS patients.[24] Patients who continue to have episodes of hypoventilation while on CPAP are often placed on noninvasive positive-pressure ventilation (NIPPV).

TABLE 3: Home supplemental oxygen therapy.

Supplemental oxygen modality	Typical maximum flow rates
Concentrator	10 L/min
Portable metal cylinders	15 L/min
Portable concentrator	6 L/min
Liquid oxygen	6 L/min

TABLE 4: Noninvasive ventilation modalities.

NIV modalities	Pressure delivery
Continuous positive airway pressure (not considered NIV/NIPPV)	Constant level of pressure is applied throughout the respiratory cycle
Bilevel positive airway pressure	Continuous positive pressure plus additional inspiratory support pressure during inspiration
Average volume assured pressure support	Continuous positive airway pressure plus variable inspiratory support pressures to achieve a target volume

(NIPPV: noninvasive positive-pressure ventilation; NIV: noninvasive ventilation)

Noninvasive Positive-pressure Ventilation

- Similar to CPAP, bilevel positive pressure ventilation (BiPAP) delivers targeted pressures throughout the respiratory cycle. Unlike CPAP, it delivers a higher inspiratory pressure and a lower expiratory pressure to create a gradient that drives ventilation. In this mode, pressure is the independent variable, while the tidal volume is the dependent variable based largely on lung and chest wall compliance. Use of BiPAP can be most helpful in patients with advanced COPD and severe OSA/OHS, where neuromuscular function and respiratory drive are largely intact, but additional ventilatory support may be required due to chest wall and pulmonary limitation.[25]
- An alternative mode of NIPPV is average volume-assured pressure support (AVAPS). AVAPS functions like BiPAP, except instead of targeting a pressure, it targets a volume by adjusting pressure to achieve the desired target. Here, the volume serves as the independent variable and the pressure is the dependent variable. It can also provide automatic expiratory positive airway pressure (EPAP) adjustments to maintain airway patency while minding comfort. This mode can be especially useful in patients with progressive neuromuscular dysfunction to assist in maintaining adequate minute ventilation as their disease advances.[26]

Though the delivery of inspiratory pressure is often triggered by the patient's inspiratory effort, some NIPPV devices can be programmed with a backup rate to ensure that the patient receives a mandatory minimal respiratory rate or minute ventilation. This is particularly important for those with chronic progressive neuromuscular conditions or those with central processes that affect respiratory drive, such as central sleep apnea.

Long-term/Domiciliary Invasive Positive-pressure Ventilation

Invasive mechanical ventilation may be necessary for patients requiring prolonged respiratory support and for patients for whom NIV is either ineffective or contraindicated.[27] Long-term invasive ventilation generally necessitates tracheostomy placement which has the advantages of fewer oral ulcerations, improved airway security, better patient comfort, facilitation of pulmonary toilet, and possibly less pneumonia.[28]

Indications for long-term invasive ventilation include neuromuscular disease, CNS disorders or damage, anatomical defects of the thoracic wall or airways, COPD, restrictive parenchymal lung disease, and sequelae of pneumonia.[27] Long-term ventilation is sometimes required after acute respiratory failure, following failure to wean from the ventilator and failed attempts at extubation.

Ventilators can apply positive pressure in multiple ways. Ventilators augment the patient's intrinsic respiratory effort. This is usually achieved by providing a target volume or pressure of insufflated air in coordination with the patient's inspiration or as a separate mandatory breath. Positive end expiratory pressure is often provided as well. A wide degree of variability is present in ventilator features, including ability to utilize pressure and/or volume modes, ramping up or down the rate of airflow, maximum oxygen delivery rate, and variable mechanical breath triggers.[29]

Patients with sufficiently mild and stable disease may be candidates for home invasive ventilation. Though more cost effective than prolonged inpatient care, home invasive ventilation requires an adequate home setting, effective caregiver support and training, and continued close healthcare support.[30]

All home ventilator devices should be equipped with backup batteries, alarms, and safety systems, and they should maximize patient mobility. The degree of ventilator sophistication should be targeted to the patient's needs to maximize cost-effectiveness and ease of use.[29] Initiation and maintenance of long-term invasive ventilation generally portend a grim prognosis.[31,32] As there may be significant discordance between the likely outcomes and patient/physician expectations, a realistic assessment of the risks and benefits should be undertaken prior to tracheostomy.[32,33]

Adjunctive Management of Chronic Respiratory Failure

Nutrition

Low body mass index (BMI) is associated with increased short-term mortality in COPD and ILD and is associated with progressive respiratory failure. Nutritional deficiencies and low BMI in chronic respiratory failure contribute to worsening hypoxia through reduced respiratory muscle capacity and low physical activity resulting in deconditioning. Hypoxia increases circulating levels of leptin resulting in attenuation of appetite, further compounding the problem. To augment nutritional status, a nutritional assessment at regular intervals should be performed and include weight measurement. Multimodal nutritional rehabilitation inclusive of nutritional education and supplements may improve clinical outcomes in chronic respiratory failure.[34]

Pulmonary Rehabilitation

Chronic lung disease resulting in respiratory failure is associated with both poor functional capacity and exercise tolerance due to impaired ventilatory and gas exchange, peripheral muscle dysfunction, and/or cardiac dysfunction. Exercise intolerance is one of the primary limiting factors to participation in activities of daily living. COPD guidelines recommend pulmonary rehabilitation citing strong evidence that it reduces anxiety and depression as well as improves exercise tolerance and health status. Pulmonary rehabilitation improves functional status, particularly for those individuals with moderate to severe COPD.[35] It also improves quality of life and dyspnea for individuals with COPD and (ILD).[36]

Palliative Care

Chronic respiratory failure often results in significant symptomatic and psychosocial burden for patients. Symptoms commonly include unrelenting cough, dyspnea, and fatigue, all of which may have a profound impact on the quality of life. Additionally, depression and anxiety are commonly experienced. Such morbidity can result in increased acute exacerbations, readmissions, healthcare utilization, and mortality. Palliative care serves, in part, to reduce or relieve symptom burden to improve quality of life in patients with end-stage illness. In addition to evaluating symptoms, palliative care serves to assist in clinical decision-making, assesses the efficacy of interventions, and monitors health status. Palliative care has been recommended for individuals with symptomatic or life-threatening respiratory disease at any point in the disease trajectory.

SUMMARY

It is important for physicians to recognize risk factors and other common pulmonary diseases responsible for the development of chronic respiratory failure. New technologies and nonpharmacologic interventions now allow these patients to live longer and have better lives. However, use of these technologies and interventions should be applied judiciously with patients' personal goals and preferences being paramount.

ACKNOWLEDGMENTS

We extend our special thanks to Nicholas Raush, MD, and John Willoughby, MD, for their previous contributions to this chapter.

REFERENCES

1. British Thoracic Society Standards of Care C. Non-invasive ventilation in acute respiratory failure. Thorax. 2002;57(3): 192-211.
2. Roussos C, Koutsoukou A. Respiratory failure. Eur Resp J. 2003;47:3s-14s.
3. Pellegrino R, Viegi G, Brusasco V, et al. Interpretative strategies for lung function tests. Eur Resp J. 2005;26(5):948-68.
4. Borland CD, Cox Y. Effect of varying alveolar oxygen partial pressure on diffusing capacity for nitric oxide and carbon monoxide, membrane diffusing capacity and lung capillary blood volume. Clin Sci. 1991;81(6):759-65.
5. Ware LB, Matthay MA. The acute respiratory distress syndrome. New Engl J Med. 2000;342(18):1334-49.
6. Gross TJ, Hunninghake GW. Idiopathic pulmonary fibrosis. New Engl J Med. 2001;345(7):517-25.
7. Kozu R, Shingai K, Hanada M, et al. Respiratory Impairment, Limited Activity, and Pulmonary Rehabilitation in Patients with Interstitial Lung Disease. Phys Ther Res. 2021;24(1):9-16.
8. Balkissoon R, Lommatzsch S, Carolan B, et al. Chronic obstructive pulmonary disease: a concise review. Med Clin North Am. 2011;95(6):1125-41.
9. Rodriguez-Roisin R, Drakulovic M, Rodriguez DA, et al. Ventilation-perfusion imbalance and chronic obstructive pulmonary disease staging severity. J Appl Physiol. 2009;106(6): 1902-8.
10. Lapner ST, Kearon C. Diagnosis and management of pulmonary embolism. BMJ. 2013;346:f757.
11. Burrowes KS, Clark AR, Tawhai MH. Blood flow redistribution and ventilation-perfusion mismatch during embolic pulmonary arterial occlusion. Pulm Circ. 2011;1(3):365-76.
12. Sommer RJ, Hijazi ZM, Rhodes JF. Pathophysiology of congenital heart disease in the adult: part III: Complex congenital heart disease. Circulation. 2008;117(10):1340-50.
13. Shneerson J. Hypercapnic respiratory failure: from the past to the future. Thorax. 2007;62(12):1024-6.
14. Piper AJ, Grunstein RR. Obesity hypoventilation syndrome: mechanisms and management. Am J Resp Crit Care Med. 2011;183(3):292-8.
15. Drachman DB. Myasthenia gravis. New Engl J Med. 1994; 330(25):1797-810.
16. Latronico N, Bolton CF. Critical illness polyneuropathy and myopathy: a major cause of muscle weakness and paralysis. Lancet Neurol. 2011;10(10):931-41.
17. Continuous or nocturnal oxygen therapy in hypoxemic chronic obstructive lung disease: a clinical trial. Nocturnal Oxygen Therapy Trial Group. Ann Intern Med. 1980;93(3):391-8.
18. Long term domiciliary oxygen therapy in chronic hypoxic cor pulmonale complicating chronic bronchitis and emphysema. Report of the Medical Research Council Working Party. Lancet. 1981;1(8222):681-6.
19. Eaton T, Lewis C, Young P, et al. Long-term oxygen therapy improves health-related quality of life. Respir Med. 2004;98(4): 285-93.
20. Ringbaek TJ, Viskum K, Lange P. Does long-term oxygen therapy reduce hospitalisation in hypoxaemic chronic obstructive pulmonary disease? Eur Respir J. 2002;20(1):38-42.
21. Celli BR, MacNee W, Force AET. Standards for the diagnosis and treatment of patients with COPD: a summary of the ATS/ERS position paper. Eur Respir J. 2004;23(6):932-46.
22. Petty TL. Long-term outpatient oxygen therapy in advanced chronic obstructive pulmonary disease. Chest. 1980;77(2 Suppl):304.
23 Katsenos S, Constantopoulos SH. Long-Term Oxygen Therapy in COPD: Factors Affecting and Ways of Improving Patient Compliance. Pulm Med. 2011;2011:325362.
24. Chanda A, Kwon JS, Wolff AJ, et al. Positive pressure for obesity hypoventilation syndrome. Pulm Med. 2012;2012:568690.
25. Barutçu HS, Altinay E, Ogus H, et al., Comparison of AVAPS and BIPAP modes in patients with postoperative hypercapnic respiratory failure after open heart surgery. ERJ Open Res. 2020;6(suppl 4):29.
26. Maheshwari A, Khatri J, Soni G, et al. Role of Average Volume Assured Pressure Support Mode (AVAPS) in the Management of Acute Exacerbation of Chronic Obstructive Pulmonary Disease With Type 2 Respiratory Failure. Cureus. 2022;14(12):e32200.
27. King AC. Long-term home mechanical ventilation in the United States. Resp Care. 2012;57(6):921-30; discussion 30-2.
28. Combes A, Luyt CE, Nieszkowska A, et al. Is tracheostomy associated with better outcomes for patients requiring long-term mechanical ventilation? Crit Care Med. 2007;35(3):802-7.
29. Gregoretti CPN, Ghannadian S, Carlucci A, et al. Choosing a ventilator for home mechanical ventilation. Breath ERJ. 2013;9(5):394-409.
30. McKim DA, Road J, Avendano M, et al. Home mechanical ventilation: a Canadian Thoracic Society clinical practice guideline. Can Respir J. 2011;18(4):197-215.
31. Bigatello LM, Stelfox HT, Berra L, et al. Outcome of patients undergoing prolonged mechanical ventilation after critical illness. Crit Care Med. 2007;35(11):2491-7.
32. Cox CE, Martinu T, Sathy SJ, et al. Expectations and outcomes of prolonged mechanical ventilation. Crit Care Med. 2009;37(11):2888-94; quiz 904.
33. Carson SS, Kahn JM, Hough CL, et al. A multicenter mortality prediction model for patients receiving prolonged mechanical ventilation. Crit Care Med. 2012;40(4):1171-6.
34. Baldemir R, Alagoz A. The Relationship Between Mortality, Nutritional Status, and Laboratory Parameters in Geriatric Chronic Obstructive Pulmonary Disease Patients. Cureus. 2021;13(12):e20526.
35. Corhay JL, Dang DN, Van Cauwenberge H, et al. Pulmonary rehabilitation and COPD: providing patients a good environment for optimizing therapy. Int J Chron Obstruct Pulm Dis. 2014;9:27-39.
36. Dowman L, Hill CJ, May A, et al. Pulmonary rehabilitation for interstitial lung disease. Cochrane Database Syst Rev. 2021;2(2): CD006322.

SECTION

9

Environmental and Occupational Disorders

SECTION OUTLINE

CHAPTER 94

Lung Disease in Coal Workers

Harakh V Dedhia, Daniel E Banks†*

INTRODUCTION

Coal is not a pure mineral. It is formed by the accumulation of vegetable matter covered by sedimentary rock (thereby sealing it from air) and subjected to pressure and temperature over the ages. This causes the physical and chemical properties of the matter to change. The matter dries, becomes warmer, and loses oxygen content, all the while increasing the relative carbon content.[1]

The first step in this conversion of vegetable matter to coal is the formation of peat, a moist spongy material. This transformation of an organic deposit can occur in a stagnant waterbed relatively quickly (at a rate of ~1 foot per 100 years). An approximately 100-foot accumulation of peat compresses to form a 1-foot-wide coal seam. In the simplest terms, coal is comprised of moisture (which lessens with time), pure coal (carbon), and mineral and other matter.[2]

The process of conversion (coalification) from organic matter follows a transformation of wood with other organic matter to peat to lignite to bituminous coal to anthracite coal **(Table 1)**.[3] Rank describes the extent of change from vegetation to mineral-free coal and the terms "brown coal" and "black coal" refer to coal of low and high rank, respectively. The composition of coal mine dust varies with the coal seam. Most of the dust is composed of carbon, although in some seams it may only approximate 60% of the dust, with >50 different elements and their oxides.[4] These "contaminants" are organic materials present when the process leading to coal formation begins. Dusts of high rank typically contain more silica than the dusts of lesser rank, and anthracite seams often have roofs and floors of quartz, which contaminate the coal during mining. Exposures to these dusts can be generated on the surface, by initially removing the overburden of soil and then drilling and blasting the underlying coal in relatively small sites (known as "strip mining"), or on a much larger scale associated with earth moving and digging great pits (described as "open cast mining"), or by underground mining—mining associated with substantial infrastructure where miners directly drill into the coal seam and move coal from below ground to the surface. Although in general underground miners may have the greatest risk for developing lung disease, miners engaged in each of these manners of coal mining are at risk.

TABLE 1: Coal characteristics.

Coal rank	% Volatile matter	% Carbon	% Ash	% Moisture	BTU*/pound
Peat (dried)	70	25	5	10	8,000–12,000
Lignite	41	36	9	14	5,500–7,000
Bituminous	32	55	10	3	12,000–14,000
Anthracite	5	87	5	3	>13,000

*1 BTU (British thermal unit) is equivalent to the amount of heat necessary to raise the temperature of 1 pound of water from approximately 4–5°F.

Source: Adapted from Haught (1955).[3]

The world is in transition regarding the use of coal as an energy source. The paths that the US and India have taken regarding coal utilization are very different.

Although one may consider the "underground" and "strip" mines of the state of West Virginia as yielding the greatest coal production in the US, the most productive state for coal production, Wyoming, produces three times as much coal using the "open cast mining" method. Yet, coal production continues its dramatic decline. Peak coal production in the US was approximately 1.17 billion tons in 2008. In 2021, the most recent year when data is available, the yield was 577 million tons.[5] This approximates the lowest yearly level of coal production since 1965. This decline in coal production is largely the result of less demand for US coal internationally and dramatically less demand for coal in the domestic electric power sector, also reflected in the continuing retirement of coal-fired power plants. There

**Dr Harakh Dedhia is deceased.*

†The authors are employees of the US government. This work was prepared as part of their official duties. The views expressed herein are their own and do not reflect the official policy or position of the US Government.

is a strong political effort to stay this course as carbon and carbon dioxide are released when coal is consumed. These greenhouse gases are recognized as major sources of concern with respect to changes in the global climate. In addition, low-carbon energy-generation technologies, e.g., wind and solar, have gained momentum as costs have declined and there is strong political support for this approach.

In India, the picture is different. Coal is described by the Ministry of Coal as the "Indian energy choice."[6] India is now the world's second largest coal producer after China. As the need for energy has increased, coal consumption has increased 700% over the past 40 years and in the face of a rising population and expanding economy, the government appears committed to this path. Growth in coal production will continue. With a relatively limited amount of petroleum and natural gas, restrictions placed on the development of hydroelectric projects, and political disagreements associated with nuclear power, coal will remain in the forefront of India's energy structure. Total coal production has increased from 556 million tons in 2012 to 745 million tons in 2021 with approximately 90% of production from open cast mines. The Coal Ministry has announced a production target of 1.31 billion tons for 2024–2025 and 1.5 billion tons the following year.[7] India's proven coal reserves are estimated to be 92 billion tons (with three or four more times this amount likely). These deposits are dispersed over 27 major coalfields, mainly in the eastern and south-central parts of the country. Lignite, or soft coal, reserves approximate 36 billion tons, the great majority located in the southern state of Tamil Nadu.

EPIDEMIOLOGIC FEATURES OF COAL-INDUCED LUNG DISEASE

Through serial coal mine dust measurements and measuring objective features attributable to dust inhalation on the chest radiograph of the miner, we can understand exposures associated with the development of lung disease and identify the adequacy of the permissible dust exposures that are in place.

Our system of classifying the radiological severity of pneumoconiosis began with the work of Davies and Mann, and Oldham.[8,9] These investigators postulated that the number of small opacities visualized on the chest radiograph reflects the severity of pneumoconiosis and introduced the concept of the "major" categories of simple pneumoconiosis (based on the profusion and extent of opacities). Liddell is later credited as the first to divide each major category into three subcategories.[10] These notions were incorporated into the initial International Labor Organization (ILO) 1958 Classification of the Radiographs of Pneumoconiosis, in which a continuum of the profusion of opacities is separated into four distinct categories—from 0 to 3.[11] The next steps validated this work by relating these standardized abnormalities on the chest radiograph to spirometry and demographic data.

The Union for International Cancer Control (UICC) Working Group on Asbestos and Cancer in 1964 recognized the need to improve comparability and build on this classification.[12] Further changes of this scheme form what is basically the current ILO system, initially introduced as the 1970 UICC/Cincinnati classification.[13] Changes included the division of pleural changes into "calcified" and "noncalcified", as well as changes in the manner that small opacities were described. A 12-point scale reflecting a series of "shades of gray" within the four major categories was added. In addition, the lung was separated into three zones for more descriptive imaging, rather than characterized as a single entity, and small opacities separated into "rounded" and "irregular" shapes, and these opacities further separated into different sizes ("p", "q", "r"' and "s", "t", "u"). Copies of "standardized" radiographs were made available from several investigators. The 1968 ILO classification system was modified to incorporate asbestos-related diseases based in part on the UICC/Cincinnati classification system.

The 1980 ILO classification system made several more refinements.[14] These included a set of 22 standard chest radiographs (available to all interested parties), which were examples of the size and shape of opacities by profusion categories. An estimate of film quality became a part of the protocol, and the description of pleural changes was more detailed.

In 2000, the ILO gave the scheme a "face lift." Standard films illustrating "u" shape shadows and pleural abnormalities were changed. Film quality was now judged on a scale from unimpeachable ("+") to unusable ("u"). If not "+", then written comments are needed. Obliteration of the costophrenic angle was necessary for "diffuse pleural thickening." New symbols for chest radiological findings were also included.[15,16] An ILO reference detailing the revision in 2011 has five chapters which are identical to the information in the 2000 revision, and a sixth chapter which addresses viewing, interpretating, and storing digital radiographic images.[17] The most recent revision, in 2022, presented the ILO classification of guidelines for interpretation with accompanying standardized digitally acquired images.[18]

Although the chest radiograph is the foundation for the diagnosis of coal workers' pneumoconiosis (CWP), it is insensitive at low profusion of macules and nodules.[19,20] In this setting, high-resolution computed tomography (HRCT) scanning was considered more informative. At an international expert meeting, the development of a standardized HRCT reporting system was proposed.[21] The International Classification of HRCT for Occupational and Environmental Respiratory Diseases (ICOERD) was developed. Not surprisingly, compared with the ILO system for radiograph interpretation, HRCT was superior in detecting pneumoconiosis in the early stage and, overall, there was good correlation between the profusion of opacities by ILO radiograph category and the grade of the HRCT scan. However, there was an important divergence. Using the ILO classification for radiographs, there was a consistent stepwise negative correlation between ILO category and an individual's forced expiratory volume in 1 second (FEV_1) and forced vital capacity (FVC) percent predicted values, whereas this relationship did not exist using the HRCT grading scheme. In conclusion, when this disparity and the cost, radiation exposure, and accessibility were considered, the authors determined that there was insufficient evidence to support the routine use of an HRCT approach.[22]

CLINICAL FEATURES OF COAL DUST EXPOSURE

The inhalation of coal dust over time and its persistent presence in the lung affect the rate of lung function decline in miners. For example, when aging from 40 to 60 years, a healthy 5′6″ (167 cm) Chinese man will lose approximately 25 mL/year in FVC and 27.5 mL/year in FEV_1.[23] In a population from western India, the loss in lung function for a man of the same height over the same time was determined to be 21.5 and 16 mL/year, respectively.[24] In mining populations from the US, England, and France, independent of the presence or absence of pneumoconiosis or dust-induced bronchitis in participating miners, the mean FEV_1 and mean FVC decline approximated 45 mL/year. Cigarette smoking increased the rate of decline approximately 20 mL/year for each parameter.[25-28]

However, in some mining populations, the poor quality of air dramatically affected the rate of decline and the development of disease. For example, in a group of Hong Kong granite quarry workers, those with pneumoconiosis and radiographic progression had a mean decline in FEV_1 and FVC of 97 and 95 mL/year, respectively.[29] In 138 West Virginia coal miners with advanced lung disease due to dust inhalation [progressive massive fibrosis (PMF)], lung function declined sharply averaging 87 mL/year for FEV_1 and 74 mL/year for FVC over a 12.2-year period.[30] In 73 Romanian gold miners with pneumoconiosis, the mean decline in FEV_1 was 187 mL/year when measured over a 3-year period.[31] In five populations of Chinese miners with lung function measured over 2 years, the mean decline of the group as a whole was 277 mL (138 mL/year) for FEV_1 and 406 mL (203 mL/year) for FVC.[32] In all of these examples, the lung function declines far exceeded the predicted rate of change in a "general healthy population." Engineering controls and dust monitoring of workplace exposures must be in place to protect the miner.[33]

Coal workers' pneumoconiosis (in nearly all cases associated with silica exposure) with advanced presentations of this disease attributed to dust exposure described as "progressive massive fibrosis" and coal mine dust-induced chronic bronchitis have been recognized for generations as the outcomes of coal dust exposure in the lung. In addition, emphysema, caused by the distortion of the lung associated with these dust exposures and the development of opacities, is recognized.[34] In one report of autopsies performed on coal miners, based on the extent of opacities, the amount of emphysema was reported to be to the degree as seen in smokers.[35] Yet, our understanding has changed over the past several years as investigators have put forward insights into the changes in the lung with coal dust exposure, and a new, broad generic term of "coal mine dust lung disease" (CMDLD) has been introduced.[36] The discussion regarding pulmonary illnesses attributable to coal dust inhalation now includes the above-mentioned illnesses, plus a relatively newly recognized entity described as "dust-fibrosis," detailed below and recognized as coal mine dust-induced, but inconsistent with long-held concepts familiar to many. Determinants of the pulmonary presentation following exposure to coal dust are primarily attributed to the extent and duration of exposure, as well as particle size, but other more unpredictable features may come into play.

Industrial Bronchitis

Industrial bronchitis is a common diagnosis among workers exposed to dusts, including coal dust.[37] It manifests as a productive cough, which persists for at least 3 months per year for at least 2 years (chronic bronchitis) associated with workplace dust exposure. In a defining autopsy study, coal dust exposure resulted in an increase in the maximal gland: wall ratio (independent of smoking), but no relationship between mucous gland size and the amount of lung dust or presence or absence of pneumoconiosis was found.[38] These data suggest that mucous gland enlargement is related to the inhalation of larger (nonrespirable) dust particles that are trapped in the airway which behave as irritants and present a chronic burden to the mucociliary escalator, whereas CWP is the result of the deposition of respirable-size dust particles in the alveolar space and ultimately their progression into the lung interstitium.

Older reports showed that the prevalence of bronchitis in coal miners varied by smoking history, age, and job.[39] In all reports, smoking miners had bronchitis more frequently than nonsmokers and the prevalence of bronchitis increased with a miner's age (a surrogate for years of dust exposure). Marine identified 543 lifetime nonsmokers among 14,888 British coal miners (3.6%) studied between 1953 and 1967 who were <65 years of age, worked at the coal face in most instances, did not have PMF, and had participated in three surveys regarding miners' health including spirometry over 10 years.[40] Of these, 17% had bronchitis at the third survey. In a second report addressing the respiratory status of American coal miners, 16% had bronchitis.[41] A recent report of >12,000 Australian miners assessed at least once by respiratory questionnaire and spirometry from 2001 to 2012 showed that even though dust exposure levels had declined, cough (15.1%), wheeze

(13.3%), phlegm (11.3%), and breathlessness (9.8%) continued to develop. Intriguingly, even though exposures are less, the prevalence of disease is like that identified in older studies. Those who reported phlegm (bronchitis) had greater dust exposures than those without phlegm. Exposure to greater amounts of dust of a respirable size showed a negative association with lung function parameters (FEV_1, FVC, and FEV_1/FVC ratio), although of a relatively small amount. Cigarette smokers showed considerably greater respiratory symptoms and greater lung function decline.[42]

Coal Workers' Pneumoconiosis with Progressive Massive Fibrosis

Coal workers' pneumoconiosis results from the inhalation and deposition of coal mine dust, and the lung's reaction to its presence. Three criteria are necessary for this diagnosis.[43] They include:

1. A chest radiograph consistent with the features of CWP
2. A work history (typically underground coal mining) sufficient in exposure and latency to result in pneumoconiosis
3. The absence of other illnesses which may mimic CWP

It is the third parameter which allows us to make the diagnosis of CWP with confidence and without histologic confirmation. Clinical features, such as dyspnea, cough, and sputum production, are important in addressing the degree of a miner's impairment but are not a part of the diagnostic criteria. The radiographic appearance of CWP cannot be differentiated from silicosis, and coal miners often develop disease associated with exposure to both dusts. CWP is dose related. Among underground miners **(Fig. 1)**, those working at the face with exposure to higher concentrations of coal mine dust have a higher prevalence of CWP than surface workers **(Fig. 2)** or those whose jobs caused them to enter the face area intermittently.[44]

Coal workers' pneumoconiosis is categorized as simple pneumoconiosis or PMF. The traditional understanding of CWP includes a recognition of rounded nodules which predominate and tend to appear first in the upper zones and then in the mid and lower zones as the number of opacities increase. The typical radiograph in simple rounded pneumoconiosis shows small opacities, ranging in size from pinhead to 1 cm in diameter. With prolonged excessive exposure, these small opacities may coalesce and form larger opacities, typically in the upper zone, recognized as a PMF lesion > 2 cm in diameter. These opacities exert tension and are associated with distortion of lung architecture typically leading to deviation of the trachea and major airways to the side of the most prominent area of coalescence, loss of upper zone lung volume, elevation of the hila, and basilar emphysema (typically of a panacinar type). Importantly, CWP can progress after the cessation of coal mine dust exposure.[45] When the radiographic changes of PMF occur in an asymmetric manner, that is, when the appearance of the conglomerate lesion on one side of the chest appears quite different from the other, then the reader should consider a differential diagnosis of carcinoma, tuberculosis, or abnormalities caused by bacterial infections.[46]

In a population comparing miners without CWP to those with CWP, respiratory symptoms and physical signs were no more prevalent in those with simple CWP.[47] The frequent presence of a chronic cough and sputum production, even in the presence of CWP, is reasonably attributable to "industrial bronchitis." Alternatively, these

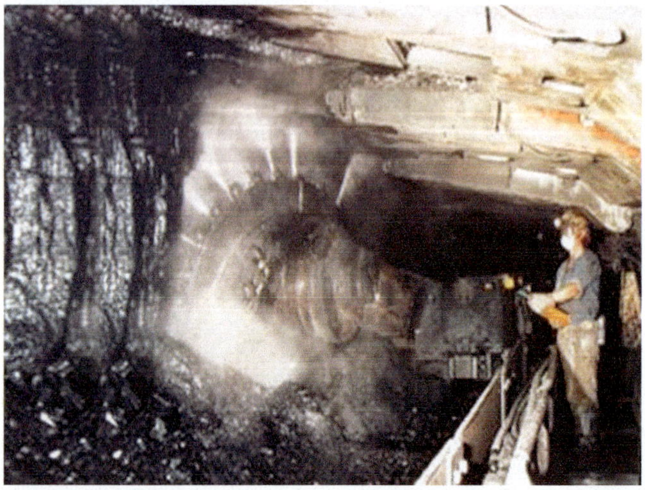

FIG. 1: Aggressive aspect of underground mining and how productive this process is. The cutting head is cooled and generated dust limited by the spray. The miner is protected by roof cave-ins by standing under the overhead supports.

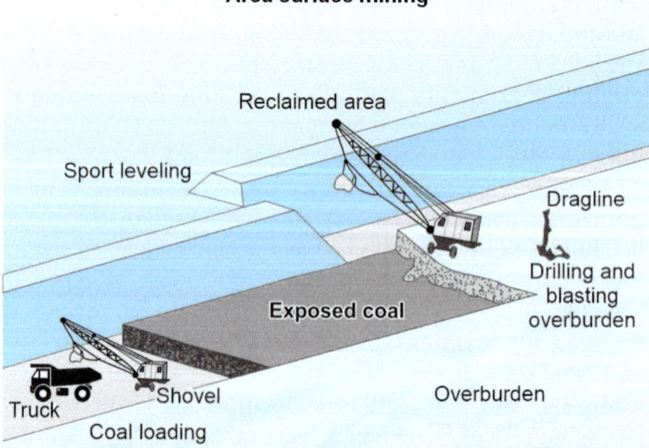

FIG. 2: Surface mining removes coal located near the surface. This process requires removing the overburden (earth and rock covering the coal seam) with heavy earth-moving equipment, such as draglines, power shovels, excavators, and loaders. Once exposed, miners drill, place explosive charges, and fracture the coal. This allows for the systematic removal of coal using trucks or conveyors and the transport to a coal preparation plant.

same clinical features in a smoking miner may be partially attributable to bronchitis caused by the inflammatory stimulus of cigarette smoke. Finger clubbing is not a feature of CWP and, if recognized, should prompt further investigations. Yet, when PMF is recognized on the chest radiograph, the worker frequently describes dyspnea, cough, and sputum production, although it is recognized that the degree of impairment and presence or absence of symptoms do not correlate well with the extent of chest radiographic abnormalities. A comprehensive description of PMF has recently been published.[48]

The effect of CWP on the heart has been described by several investigators. Lapp performed cardiac catheterization during rest and exercise in miners with CWP, some with airways obstruction.[49] Those with an underlying obstructive lung disease or PMF had increased pulmonary artery pressures. In those without these two illnesses, increased pressures occurred in the presence of pinpoint ("p") opacities on their radiograph. This type of opacity is associated with diminished diffusion and a decreased vascular bed.[50] A later autopsy study of British coal miners addressed the relationship between coal dust exposure and right ventricular hypertrophy (RVH) comparing those with simple CWP or no pneumoconiosis to those with PMF. The prevalence of RVH was the same in those with simple CWP as in those without pneumoconiosis (~15%) and was related to the extent of airways obstruction. In this population, right ventricle enlargement did not occur unless the miner was a smoker with associated severe airflow obstruction or PMF.[51]

Typically, CWP is a slowly progressive illness, with radiographic features progressing over a period of many years. The development of these conglomerate changes occur on a background of small opacities in nearly all instances, and the risk for PMF increases as the profusion of opacities becomes greater.[52] Development of PMF is associated with an accelerated decline in lung function (compared to those without disease or those with simple pneumoconiosis), as well as an increased rate of morbidity and mortality.[53] Risk factors which may explain why miners with simple pneumoconiosis progress to PMF include the following:

1. Inhalation of significant amounts of silica dust as a component of coal mine dust. This appears to be the most common pathway for a miner to develop PMF, with this conclusion buttressed by the recent reports of the presence of large amounts of silica in these conglomerate lesions and the apparent inability to identify other explanations in nearly all instances.[54,55] When there is mixed dust exposure—silica and coal—silica dust appears to be the driving force in the development and progression of this disease.
2. Infection with a mycobacterial organism (the appearance of a cavity in a PMF lesion or an aggressive rate of radiographic progression should prompt the examination of the sputum for mycobacterial infection)

Yet, none of these explanations appear to satisfactorily explain the development of PMF in all cases. As an example, PMF has been reported in carbon electrode workers. This suggests that silica exposure is not necessary for PMF to occur.[56] Of interest, empiric treatment of miners with simple CWP in Wales with antituberculous drugs did not prevent PMF.[57]

Finally, earlier studies suggested that autoantibodies reactive to lung tissue antigens were present in the sera of miners, suggesting a role in the tissue response and PMF development.[58] Several studies have addressed the prevalence of rheumatoid factor in mining populations. Soutar reported the antinuclear autoantibody (ANA) prevalence in British miners to be 17% with nearly half showing a dilution of 1:40 or greater and the rheumatoid factor prevalence to be 11%. The incidence increased as the severity of disease increased and was most frequently noted in those with PMF. This was confirmed by American studies.[59] The implication was that an immunologic process is a part of the development of PMF. However, this was shown not to be the case in a large population of coal miners collected from healthy blood donors.[60] In this report, there was a similar distribution of antinuclear factors between miners and nonminers. Yet, in this population, rheumatoid factor was more common in miners than nonminers and present in 5.3% of coalminers, particularly in the few miners with PMF. The combined prevalence of both factors increased with age at all disease levels but showed an association with pneumoconiosis category in men older than the age of 60 years. Overall, the immunologic contribution to the development of PMF is now less certain.

Dust-related Diffuse Fibrosis

Dust-related diffuse fibrosis (DDF), a form of interstitial disease, is caused by inhalation of coal dust and can be mistaken for idiopathic pulmonary fibrosis (IPF) if an exposure history is not taken.[37] Workers with exposures to coal mine dust, silica, and mixed dusts are at risk.[61] This pulmonary presentation of coal dust exposure features irregular opacities bilaterally in the bases. The recognition of this as a separate entity in miners has been bolstered by recognizing that nearly 40% coal miners employed for >25 years show irregular opacities (not the typical rounded nodular opacities of CWP) consistent with DDF and that those opacities were more frequent in the lower compared to the upper lung zone.[62] These findings have been validated in French miners[63] and, most recently, in a population of coal miners from New Mexico, US.[64] Compared to our understanding of CWP, relatively little systematic research has been performed on this presentation of coal dust in the lung.[53]

Coal Dust Exposure and Cancer

Evidence for carcinogenicity for coal dust is conflicting. To begin, coal mine dust often contains silica, an agent recognized as carcinogenic by the International Agency for Research on Cancer (IARC).[65] In a large study of US underground coal miners with a 26-year follow-up, there was no excess or relationship in the rate of lung cancer with increasing dust exposure. The authors note that silica dust levels were not measured.[66]

Li et al. recently reported a meta-analysis on the association of coal mine dust and mortality risk of lung cancer.[67] This group identified 22 reports which recognized the standardized mortality ratio with 95% confidence limits in coal miner and comparison populations. Although there was an increased risk of mortality from lung cancer for coal miners [1.16; 95% confidence interval (CI) 1.03, 1.30], there was great heterogeneity among the results of the studies. Of the 22, 5 studies showed no increase in mortality among coal miners without statistical significance, another 5 showed no increase in mortality among coal miners with statistical significance, 7 showed an increase in mortality among coal miners with statistical significance, and, finally, 5 showed an increase in mortality among the coal miners without statistical significance. Of particular interest are the Chinese studies. They showed the strongest risk for lung cancer in miners and had a predominant effect on the results of the meta-analysis. No Indian studies were included in this review.

Immunologic Considerations

There is an increased association with immunologically mediated disease in individuals with silica exposure. In mining, silica is present in coal mine dust, and the reports consistently suggest that this agent, rather than coal dust, is the offending agent. A random phone survey in selected counties in Appalachia, the heart of underground mining in America, revealed that about one third of cases of rheumatoid arthritis could be attributed to mining.[68] Similarly, in a group of silica-exposed individuals in Sweden, the risk for rheumatoid arthritis was two-fold compared to silica nonexposed.[69] In a group of 60 consecutive cases of scleroderma, Rodnan described 26 cases with a history of employment as a coal miner or employment in an occupation where silica exposure was encountered.[70] Although the course of scleroderma did not vary in the two groups, it appears that chronic fibrogenic dust exposure may also be a risk factor for the development of scleroderma.

A special case of nodular lung reaction—development of "crops" of small, rounded opacities in miners who either have rheumatoid arthritis or are recognized to develop rheumatoid arthritis within the subsequent 5–10 years—is described as Caplan Syndrome.[71] Opacities vary in diameter from 0.5 to 5 cm and are usually multiple, occur in both lungs, and are situated peripherally. Grossly, the lesions resemble a larger silicotic nodule. Microscopically, the amount of dust in the lesion is small, there is a necrotic area in the center, and there is a surrounding cellular zone infiltrated with lymphocytes and plasma cells. In many nodules, there is a peripheral zone of active inflammation with neutrophils and a few macrophages. This observation has been further enhanced when similar radiographic appearances were seen in miners without arthritis, but in whom the circulating rheumatoid factor was demonstrated.[72]

The clinician may be presented with the diagnostic dilemma of attempting to distinguish a primary or metastatic neoplasm from an unusual presentation of PMF. When large opacities of PMF occur bilaterally on a background of simple CWP, one can be reasonably confident that the lesions are less likely to represent neoplastic disease. When there is a sparse background of simple CWP or none, when there are crops of nodules (as in Caplan syndrome), or when the presence of PMF develops in an asymmetric manner, differentiation from neoplasm may indeed be difficult.[73]

PATHOLOGY OF COAL WORKERS' PNEUMOCONIOSIS

As the normal dust clearance mechanisms of the lung are overwhelmed, dust deposition increases in the alveolar spaces. With the initiation and progression of fibrosis, the lung lesions increase in size and number. A focal collection of coal dust in pigment-laden macrophages around dilated respiratory bronchioles, which taper off toward the alveolar duct, is initially apparent.[74] This is the coal macule, the characteristic lesion of CWP **(Figs. 3 and 4)**.[75] A fine network of reticulin within this collection of cells may be visible early on. Focal emphysema is a specific entity that is an integral part of the simple lesion of simple CWP **(Fig. 5)**. It is characterized by the enlargement of the air spaces immediately adjacent to the dust macule.[76] It is common to identify silicotic nodules, as well as an opacity with features of the coal macule and the silicotic nodule, when mixed

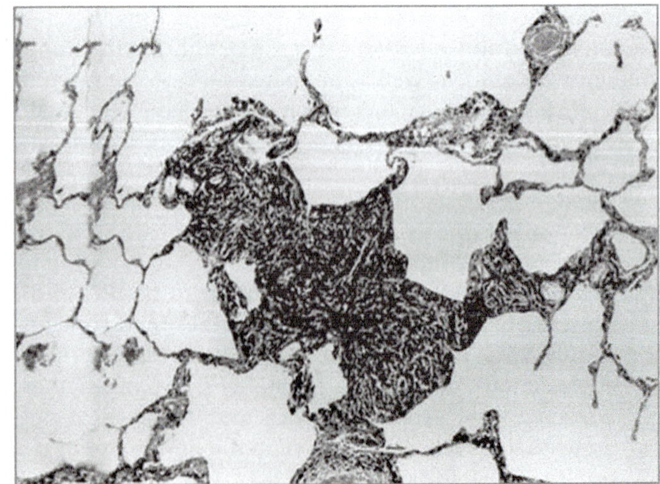

FIG 3: Photomicrograph of a coal macule. There is coal dust, reticulin fibers, and coal dust-laden macrophages, with minimal fibrosis. The periphery of the nodule shows air space enlargement.

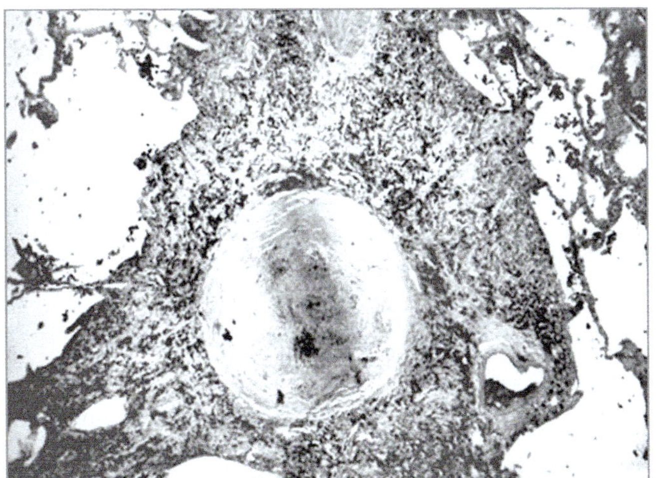

FIG. 4: Photomicrograph of a lung biopsy from a roof bolter with the histologic evidence of both a coal macule and a silicotic nodule. This reflects the accumulation of exposure to coal and silica dusts, which have occurred over his working lifetime. On the periphery, there is coal dust with coal-laden macrophages. Centrally, there are the whorls of fibrosis characteristic of a silicotic nodule. The cellularity is most prominent in the periphery of the lesion.

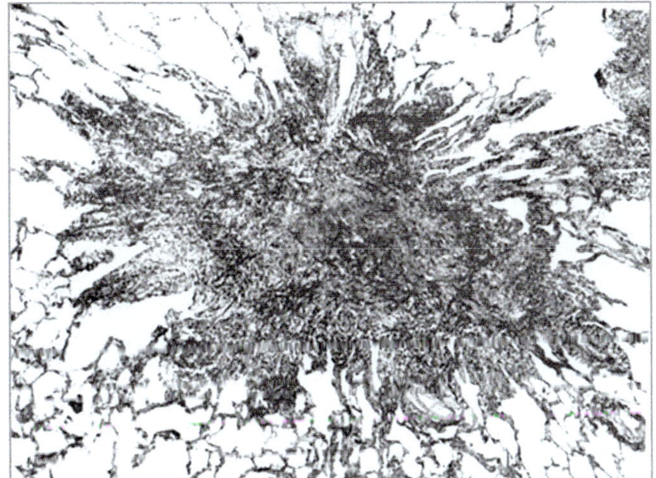

FIG. 5: Coal nodule surrounding a respiratory bronchiole. As the macule enlarges, smooth muscle atrophies and the bronchiole enlarges. Of interest in this photomicrograph are the enlarged air spaces surrounding the macule, a feature described as focal emphysema.

dust exposures occur. On gross examination of the lung, larger collections of dust are described as coal nodules, classified as micronodular, if they are 7 mm in diameter or less, and macronodular, if they are larger than this. These are palpable, whereas coal macules are not.

What impact these histologic abnormalities have on lung function has been the subject of considerable discussion.

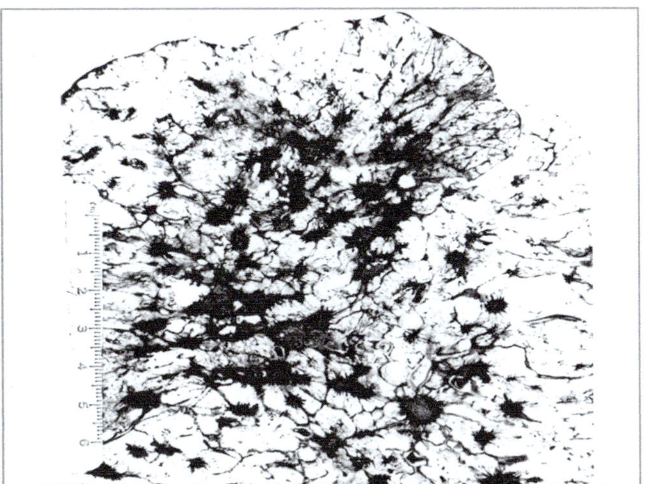

FIG. 6: Gough section of the lung. Simple coal workers' pneumoconiosis (category 1) is percent on a background of diffuse emphysema. The black deposits are the coal macules. The degree of emphysema is widespread.

In nonsmoking, nonobstructed miners without CWP, Morgan[77] showed an increase in the residual volume (RV); the RV was 105% of a group of nonminers. This increased to 108% and 114% of controls in miners with category 1 or categories 2 and 3 simple CWP. Morgan considered this to be attributable to focal emphysema. He also considered this hyperinflation to be the result of coal macules narrowing the airways with the alteration of the peripheral flow rates by increasing resistance and resulting in air trapping.

Histologically, PMF is diagnosed when one or more nodules attain a size of 2 cm or greater in diameter, typically on a background of simple CWP[78] **(Fig. 6)**. The 2-cm diameter is an arbitrary choice of a minimal diameter that has allowed better correlation with clinical and radiographic measurements. Gross examination of the lung in PMF reveals a solid, heavily pigmented lung, which is rubbery to hard in texture. These features are most common in the posterior portions of the upper lobes or the superior segments of the lower lobes. These lesions tend to occur asymmetrically, occasionally showing first in one lung and then the other, leading to a suspicion of malignancy. When these lesions are ashed: incinerated in order to identify and quantify mineral deposited in lung tissue, they appear to be composed of varying amounts of coal, silica, calcium, and other substances. About one fourth of the proteinaceous material in the center of these fibrotic lesions is collagen.[79] These large pneumoconiotic lesions may also cavitate and the worker may expectorate an ink-like fluid (a clinical sign described as melanoptysis), or when these cavitary lesions are cut, they may drain ink-like fluid. Airways and vessels adjacent to the lesions are distorted and destroyed within the lesions. Excessive silica exposures in surface coal mine drillers can also result in PMF lesions and result in "cor pulmonale" and respiratory failure **(Figs. 7 to 9)**.

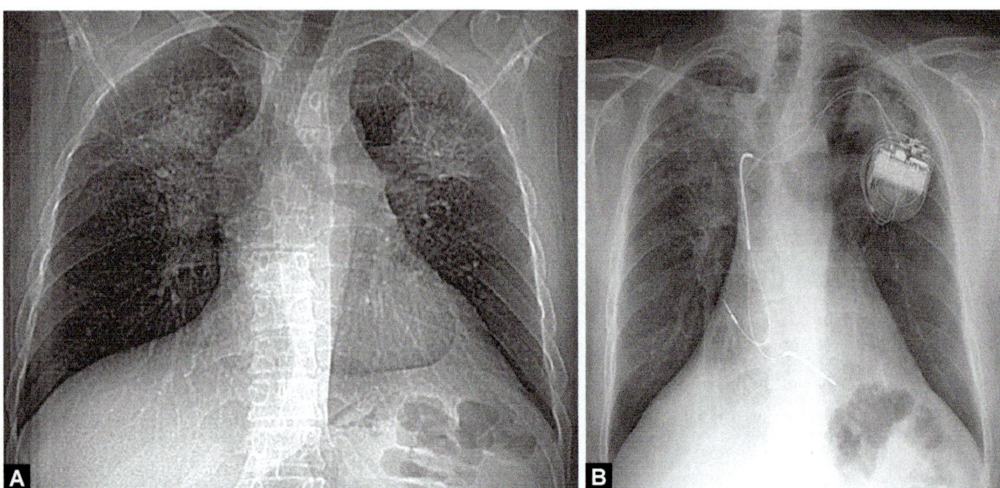

FIGS. 7A AND B: (A) Multiple, small-rounded densities bilaterally, predominantly located in the upper lung zones. Mass-like densities are also present in the upper zones, and the overall appearance is typical for progressive massive fibrosis (PMF). (B) The picture is taken 6 years later. It shows progression of PMF over time. In the time between figures (A) and (B), a pacemaker-defibrillator with intracardiac two leads had been inserted.

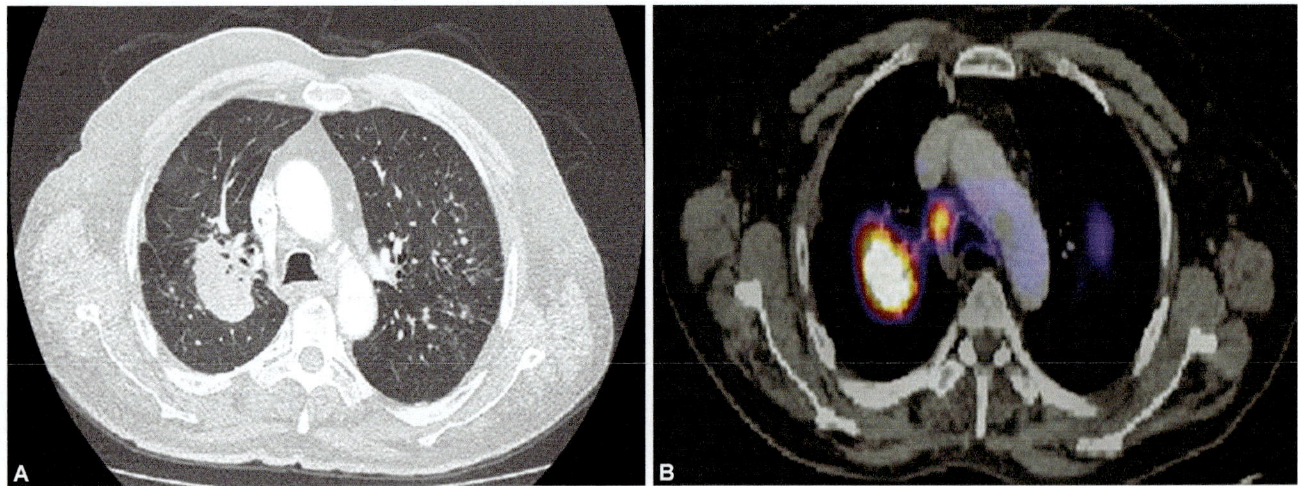

FIGS. 8A AND B: (A) Chest CT (computed tomography) scan in a surface coal mine driller, which shows bilateral upper lobe fibrosis, more prominent on the right compared to the left, and a right upper lobe (RUL) mass. (B) A PET (positron emission tomography) scan taken near the time of figure 8A shows asymmetric progressive massive fibrosis (PMF) lesions (right more than left) as well as right peritracheal adenopathy.

How Coal Mine Lung Dust Disease Develops: Cellular and Immunologic Factors

Coal mine dust lung disease is the result of coal dust-induced cell damage with the activation of the fibrotic process. Development of bronchoalveolar lavage (BAL) as a means for sampling lung cells and fluid has provided an opportunity to study the lung's response to the inhalation of various dusts as well as the mechanisms of inflammation and fibrosis. Lapp provided a well-outlined approach to addressing how coal dust causes lung damage.[80]

The potential mechanisms include:

- Direct cytotoxicity of coal dust
- The release of oxidants, enzymes, and cell membrane constituents from alveolar macrophages (AMs) in association with cell death due to coal dust exposure
- Stimulation of cytokine release from AMs to recruit effector cells (other macrophages or neutrophils) and stimulate fibroblast proliferation and collagen synthesis around coal dust deposition

Coal dust is much less fibrogenic than silica.[81] As an example, a mixture of 10% silica and 90% coal is far more cytotoxic to AMs than pure coal dust. However, both

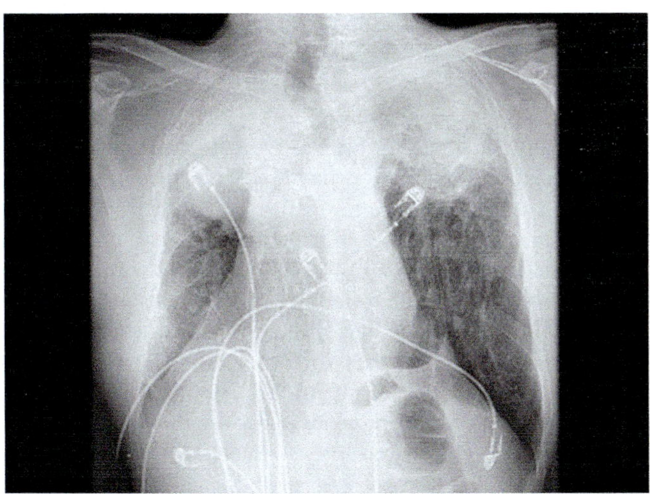

FIG. 9: A radiograph shows large opacities in both upper zones with associated calcification and fibrosis consistent with the diagnosis of progressive massive fibrosis (PMF).

dusts, when cleaved, show surface radicals by electron spin resonance spectroscopy. The free radicals generated by crushing anthracite coal are more numerous than those generated from crushing bituminous coal leading to speculation regarding free radical release from different coal ranks and the suggestion that exposure to anthracite coal increases the risk for the development and progression of disease.[82]

Long-term coal dust exposure increases the number of alveolar cells recovered by BAL.[83] In addition, an elevation in the number of blood monocytes and an increased rate of mitosis have been recognized in cells from animals undergoing chronic coal dust inhalation.[84] This suggests that there was recruitment of cells into the lung from the alveolar capillaries and the interstitium of the lung. Recruited "young" AMs appear to be more active in phagocytosis than older AMs. This may imply a more effective clearance of particles.[85]

Exposure of AMs to particles can result in the release of proteolytic enzymes, reactive oxygen species [i.e., hydrogen peroxide (H_2O_2), hydroxyl radical (OH), and superoxide anion (O_2^-)], and leukotrienes via breakdown of arachidonic acid in the cell membrane. Again, silica is a much stronger stimulus to the release of these agents than coal dust.[86] Excessive release of these reactive oxygen species has the potential to overwhelm the naturally protective antioxidant system within the lung and begin and perpetuate the process of inflammation and fibrosis.

Alveolar macrophages secrete a wide variety of mediators, which can attract neutrophils into the affected area and then stimulate them to release reactive oxygen species and enzymes. Similarly, the macrophage-derived inflammatory factors can act as chemotactic agents for neutrophils (e.g., tumor necrosis factor, interleukin 8, and leukotrienes) and increase neutrophil adherence and reactive enzyme release (platelet-derived growth factor and platelet-activating factor).[87] The presence of these factors escalates the inflammatory process. Finally, secretions of many of the above factors by AMs are likely to enhance fibroblast growth and/or stimulate the production of collagen.

Genetic differences may help to explain the variation in response to inhaled coal mine dust, especially the attack rates and progression of CWP. Data showed no difference in the histocompatibility antigens in coal miners to explain the development or progression of CWP.[88]

MANAGEMENT OF COAL MINE DUST-INDUCED LUNG DISEASE

There is no proven therapy for pneumoconiosis. Primary prevention of lung disease in miners must include continuing efforts at reducing coal mine dust exposure. This is managed by engineering controls. Engineering controls typically include diluting the generated dust through ventilation at the coal face, designing the saw on the cutting machine at the coal face ("the shearer drum") in a way which may alter the flow of dust away from the workers, and using water and wetting agents to suppress dust. The major challenge to the physician once lung disease has developed is the recognition and management of airflow obstruction, respiratory infection, hypoxemia, respiratory failure, cor pulmonale, arrhythmias, and pneumothorax.

A thorough initial database for each worker allows accurate assessment of the worker's respiratory health and serves as a starting point for potentially observing the response to therapy or progression of disease. Workers presenting with respiratory symptoms should have careful evaluation. The initial history and examination should be supplemented by chest radiograph, spirometry with bronchodilator inhalation, measurement of diffusing capacity, an electrocardiogram, and, in some instances, resting arterial blood gas.

Smoking cessation is important regardless of symptoms of respiratory disease, chest radiograph abnormalities, or pulmonary function status. Physician's encouragement to stop smoking should be supplemented by support from smoking cessation groups, use of nicotine substitutes or other medications that may assist in stopping smoking, and behavior modification techniques.

Symptomatic reversible airflow obstruction should be treated with inhaled bronchodilator and/or long-acting muscarinic antagonist therapy as indicated. Hypoxemia can be a serious complication in those with advanced dust disease. It is typically present first during exercise but can develop to occur with rest and during sleep. Chronic hypoxemia can lead to complications of polycythemia, pulmonary hypertension, cor pulmonale, and cerebral dysfunction. Therapy with low-flow oxygen is indicated when the arterial oxygen tension is <55 mm Hg or when clinical evidence of cor pulmonale is present.

Miners should receive appropriate immunization with influenza, pneumococcal, and COVID-19 vaccines. Bacterial and viral episodes of bronchitis or pneumonia should be promptly recognized and appropriately treated. Similarly, miners with concomitant exposure to silica dust (most often roof bolters, drillers, and motormen) deserve special attention regarding mycobacterial infection. A large clinical trial to prevent tuberculosis in miners with isoniazid therapy was unsuccessful.[89] Symptoms of weight loss, fever, sweat, change in sputum production, or malaise should be promptly investigated with a chest radiograph and examination of the sputum through stain and culture for acid-fast bacillus (AFB). Active mycobacterial infection in this population can be successfully treated with the usual drug regimens.[90,91] However, these trials were performed prior to the widespread development and recognition of drug-resistant organisms. In coal miners with a significant history of concurrent silica exposure, the treatment for tuberculosis may need to be more aggressive, and long-term follow-up is indicated in view of the reports of recurrent pulmonary tuberculosis in patients with PMF after the completion of apparently adequate therapy.[92] Treatment needs to be individualized in each case. Pneumothorax can be particularly troublesome in miners with pneumoconiosis. Those with bullous disease in the presence of advanced complicated pneumoconiosis are at the greatest risk. Typically, once the lung collapses, it is difficult to expand, a feature attributable to the decreased compliance associated with interstitial lung disease. Therapy with one or several chest tubes may be therapeutic; however, in those with a pneumothorax that cannot be expanded, an open procedure and pleurodesis may be indicated.

Respiratory failure may complicate advanced PMF as it does in other chronic respiratory diseases. Ventilatory support measures are indicated when the failure is precipitated by a treatable complication. The application of ventilatory support measures should be discussed with the patient before the need arises. In general, miners with advanced pneumoconiosis are poor candidates for long-term mechanical ventilatory therapy.

Overall, improved mining methods and lower dust levels, as well as medical surveillance programs, have the potential to reduce exposures, yet new cases of both simple and complicated pneumoconiosis continue to be recognized.[53] If the worker with CMDLD is unable or declines to leave the workplace, then he/she should be encouraged to transfer from jobs with high-dust exposure to jobs with low-dust exposure. It is our opinion that any worker with simple CWP should be encouraged to leave dust exposure. Those with category 2 or great pneumoconiosis are at clear risk for progression even in the absence of additional coal dust exposure, even after ceasing exposure.[52,93]

Are there interventions which may alter the natural history of pneumoconiosis? There are no long-term proven therapies; however, a report reviewing serial lung function of Chinese miners receiving whole lung lavage showed that the rate of decline in lung function slowed over a 2-year period.[32] Although we recognize that numerous mechanisms associated with pneumoconiosis may be affected by biologic agents,[94] we are unaware of the therapeutic trials of these agents in affected miners. One may understand hesitation among clinicians in prescribing these medications because of a lack of evidence of clinical effectiveness as well as concerns about immunosuppression and potential adverse effects. Finally, with the relatively recent understanding of coal dust-induced lung fibrosis and its resemblance to IPF, trials to treat non-IPF progressive fibrotic diseases (excluding miners with coal mine dust disease) have shown that pirfenidone treatment may be of benefit, can be safely used, and is well tolerated.[95,96]

SUMMARY

Coal workers' pneumoconiosis is a disease distinct and separate from silicosis. Although the coal particle is not nearly as fibrogenic as the silica particle, excessive exposures over a period overwhelm effective clearance mechanisms and initiate chronic interstitial lung disease. Simple CWP is clearly related to the amount of dust deposited within the lungs. In nearly all cases, PMF occurs on a background of simple CWP and is the result of dust deposition, in particular the amount of silica in coal mine dust, plus other inadequately defined host factors. Immunological and local cellular factors may contribute to the development of this form of the disease.

Progressive massive fibrosis is clearly associated with alterations in the ventilatory, mechanical and vascular function of the lungs. These abnormalities in PMF contribute to the premature morbidity and mortality of this disease.

A better understanding of a newly recognized entity, coal-related diffuse fibrosis, may help us understand the full implication of coal dust exposure. A systematic study is needed for clinicians to understand how this contributes to respiratory impairment.

Prevention remains the cornerstone of eliminating this occupational lung disease. Unfortunately, in those with this illness, a better understanding of how to alter the well-recognized natural history of those with advanced disease is needed. Although there is no proven therapy for coal mine dust disease, perhaps the relatively untested perspectives presented in this report may show promise. The education of workers and employers regarding the hazards of coal dust exposure and the measurement and effective control of dust exposure remain the sole means of eliminating this disease.

ACKNOWLEDGMENTS

The authors appreciate the comprehensive review of this manuscript by Drs John Parker and Jessica Deslauriers.

REFERENCES

1. Stahl R. Coal and derivatives. In: Encyclopedia of Occupational Health and Safety, 3rd (revised) edition. Geneva: International Labour Organization; 1989.
2. Thomas L. Handbook of Practical Coal Geology. Chichester: John Wiley & Sons; 1992. pp. 1-322.
3. Haught OL. Coal and Coal Mining in West Virginia. Morgantown, WV: Geological and Economic Survey; 1955. pp. 1-32.
4. NIOSH. Criteria for a recommended standard: occupational exposure to respirable coal mine dust. Cincinnati, OH: US Department of Health and Human Services. Public Health Service. DHHS (NIOSH); 1995. pp. 95-106.
5. U.S. Energy Information Administration. Independent Statistics and Analysis Coal. [online] Available from tableES1.pdf (eia.gov). [Last accessed June, 2024].
6. Indian Ministry of Coal. [online] Available from https://www.coal.nic.in/ [Last accessed June, 2024].
7. India Express Newspaper. (2023). Centre says domestic coal production to touch 1.31 billion tonnes by FY25. [online] Available from https://indianexpress.com/article/business/economy/india-coal-production-2023-2024-8464233/ [Last accessed June, 2024].
8. Davies I, Mann KJ. Proc 9th Int. Congress Industrial Med. Bristol: John Wrights; 1948. pp. 769-72.
9. Oldham PD. Numerical scoring of radiological simple pneumoconiosis. Inhaled Part. 1970;2:621-32.
10. Liddell FD. An experiment in film reading. Br J Ind Med. 1963; 20:300-12.
11. International Labour Office. Meeting of experts on the international classification of radiographs of the pneumoconiosis. Occup Safety Health. 1959;9:2.
12. International Union Against Cancer (UICC): report and recommendations of the working group on asbestos and cancer. Br J Ind Med. 1965;22:165-71.
13. UICC–Cincinnati classification of the radiographic appearances of pneumoconiosis. A cooperative study by the UICC committee. Chest. 1970;58(1):57-67.
14. International Labour Office. Guidelines for the use of ILO international classification of radiographs of pneumoconiosis, revised edition. Geneva: International Labour Office; 1980.
15. Henry DA. International Labor Office Classification System in the age of imaging: relevant or redundant. J Thorax Imaging. 2002;17(3):179-88.
16. Hering KG, Jacobsen M, Bosch-Galethe E, et al. Further development of the International Pneumoconiosis classification–from ILO 1980 to ILO 2000/German Federal Republic version. Pneumologie. 2003;57(10):576-84.
17. Guidelines for the use of the ILO International Classification of Radiographs of Pneumoconioses 2011 revision. [online] Available from 11060331guide E.indd (ilo.org) [Last accessed June, 2024].
18. Guidelines for the use of the ILO International Classification of Radiographs of Pneumoconioses 2011 revision. [online] Available from wcms_867859.pdf (ilo.org) [Last accessed June, 2024].
19. Wagner GR, Attfield MD, Parker JE. Chest radiography in dust-exposed miners: promise and problems, potential and imperfections. Occup Med. 1993;8(1):127-41.
20. Vallyathan V, Brower PS, Green FH, et al. Radiographic and pathologic correlation of coal worker's pneumoconiosis. Am J Respir Crit Care Med. 1996;154(3):741-8.
21. Tossavainen A. International expert meeting on new advances in the radiology and screening of asbestos-related diseases. Scand J Work Environ Health. 2000;26:449–54.
22. Sener MU, Simsek C, Ozkara S, et al. Comparison of the International Classification of High-Resolution Computed Tomography for occupational and environmental respiratory diseases with the International Labor Organization International Classification of Radiographs of Pneumoconiosis. Ind Health. 2019;57:495-502.
23. Jian W, Gao Y, Hao C, et al. Reference values for spirometry in Chinese aged 4–80 years. J Thorac Dis. 2017;9(11):4538-49.
24. Agarwal D, Parker RA, Pinnock H, et al. Normal spirometry predictive values for the Western Indian adult population. Eur Respir J. 2020;56:1902129.
25. Attfield MD. Longitudinal decline in FEV1 in United States coalminers. Thorax. 1985;40:132-7.
26. Love RG, Miller BG. Longitudinal study of lung function in coal-miners. Thorax. 1982;37:193-7.
27. Goodwin S, Attfield M. Temporal trends in coal workers' pneumoconiosis prevalence. Validating the National Coal Study results. J Occup Environ Med. 1998;40:1065-71.
28. Dimlich-Ward H, Bates DV. Reanalysis of a longitudinal study of pulmonary function in coal miners in Lorraine, France. Am J Ind Med. 1994;25:613-23.
29. Ng TP, Chan SL, Lam KP. Radiological progression and lung function in silicosis: a ten year follow up study. BMJ. 1987;295:164-8.
30. Wade AW, Petsonk EL, Young B, et al. Severe occupational pneumoconiosis among West Virginian coal miners. One hundred thirty-eight cases of Progressive Massive Fibrosis compensated between 2000 and 2009. Chest. 2011;139:1458-62.
31. Cocarla A, Kozlov I, Oarga M, et al. Longitudinal study of the FEV1, cumulative exposure to dusts and silicosis in gold miners. Rom J Intern Med. 2003;41(2):179-88.
32. Zeng Y, Jiang Y, Banks DE. The Effectiveness of Whole Lung Lavage in Pneumoconiosis: A Systematic Review and Meta-Analysis. J Occup Environ Med. 2022;64:e492-9.
33. Banks DE, Bauer MA, Castellan RM, et al. Silicosis in surface coal mine drillers. Thorax. 1983;38:275-8.
34. Coggon D, Newman-Taylor A. Coal mining and chronic obstructive lung disease: a review of the evidence. Thorax. 1998;53:398-407.
35. Kuempell ED, Wheeler MW, Smith RJ, et al. Contributions of dust exposure and cigarette smoking to emphysema severity in coal miners in the United States. Am J Resp Crit Care Med. 2009;180:257-64.
36. Petsonk EL, Rose C, Cohen R. Coal mine dust lung disease. New lessons from old exposure. Am J Respir Crit Care Med. 2013;187:1178-85.
37. Morgan WK. Industrial bronchitis. Brit J Ind Med. 1978;35(4):285-91.
38. Douglas AN, Lamb D, Ruckley VA. Bronchial gland dimensions in coalminers: influence of smoking and dust exposure. Thorax. 1982;37(10):760-4.

39. Kibelstis JA, Morgan EJ, Reger R, et al. Prevalence of bronchitis and airway obstruction in American bituminous coal miners. Am Rev Respir Dis. 1973;108(4):886-93.
40. Marine WM, Gurr D, Jacobsen M. Clinically important respiratory effects of dust exposure and smoking in British coal miners. Am Rev Respir Dis. 1988;137(1):106-12.
41. Seixas NS, Robins TG, Attfield MD, et al. Exposure response relationships for coal mine dust and obstructive lung disease following enactment of the Federal Coal Mine Health and Safety Act of 1969. Am J Ind Med. 1992;21(5):715-34.
42. Rumchev K, Van Hoang D, Lee AH. Exposure to dust and respiratory health among Australian miners. Intern Arch Occup Environ Health. 2023;96:355-63.
43. Balaan MR, Weber SL, Banks DE. Clinical aspects of coal workers' pneumoconiosis and silicosis. Occup Med. 1993;8(1):19-34.
44. Jacobsen M, Rae S, Walton WH, et al. The relation between pneumoconiosis and dust-exposure in British coal mines. In: Walton WH (Ed). Inhaled Particles III. Surrey: Unwin Brothers; 1971. pp. 903-17.
45. Donnan PT, Miller BG, Scarisbrick DA. Progression of simple pneumoconiosis in ex-coal miners after cessation of exposure to coal mine dust. Edinburgh: Institute of Occupational Medicine (Edinburgh) Technical Memorandum Series; 1997.
46. Castranova, V, Vallyathan V. Silicosis and coal workers' pneumoconiosis. Environ Health Perspect. 2000;108(Suppl 4): 675-84.
47. Rom WN, Kanner RE, Renzetti, AD. Respiratory disease in Utah coal miners. Am Rev Respir Dis. 1981;123(4 pt 1):372-7.
48. Weissman DN. Progressive massive fibrosis: An overview of the recent literature. Pharmacol Ther. 2022;240:108232.
49. Lapp NL, Seaton A, Kaplan KC, et al. Pulmonary haemodynamics in coal workers' pneumoconiosis. In: Walton WH (Ed). Inhaled Particles III. Surrey: Unwin Brothers; 1971. pp. 645-57.
50. Lyons JP, Clarke WG, Hall AM, et al. Transfer factor (diffusing capacity) for the lung in simple pneumoconiosis of coal workers. Brit Med J. 1967;4(5582):772-4.
51. Fernie JM, Douglas AN, Lamb D, et al. Right ventricular hypertrophy in a group of coal workers. Thorax. 1983;38(6):436-42.
52. Almberg KS, Friedman LS, Rose CS, et al. Progression of coal workers' pneumoconiosis absent further exposure. Occup Environ Med. 2020;77(11):748-51.
53. Attfield M, Castranova V, Hale JM, et al. Coal mine dust exposures and associated health outcomes; a review of information published since 1995. 2022. DHHS (NIOSH) Publication No. 2011–172. Available from https://www.cdc.gov/niosh/docs/2011-172/pdfs/2011-172.pdf
54. Cohen RA, Petsonk EL, Rose C, et al. Lung pathology in US coal workers with rapidly progressive pneumoconiosis implicates silica and silicates. Amer J Resp Crit Care Med. 2016;193(6): 673-80.
55. Cohen RA, Rose CS, Go LHT, et al. Pathology and mineralogy demonstrate respirable crystalline silica is a major cause of severe pneumoconiosis in US coal miners. Ann Am Thorac Soc. 2022;19(9):1469-78.
56. Collis EL, Gilchrist JC. Effects of dust upon coal trimmers. J Ind Hyg Toxicol. 1928;10:101-9.
57. Watson AJ, Black J, Doig AT, et al. Pneumoconiosis in carbon electrode workers. Br J Ind Med. 1959;16:274-85.
58. Soutar CA, Turner-Warwick M, Parkes WR. Circulating antinuclear antibody and rheumatoid factor in coal pneumoconiosis. Br Med J. 1974;3:145-7.
59. Pearson DJ, Mentnech MS, Elliott JA, et al. Serologic changes in pneumoconiosis and Progressive Massive Fibrosis of coal workers. Am Rev Respir Dis. 1981;124:696-9.
60. Boyd JE, Robertson MD, Davis JD. Autoantibodies in coalminers; their relationship to the development of progressive massive fibrosis. Am J Ind Med. 1982;3:201-8.
61. Go LHT, Cohen RA. Coal Workers' Pneumoconiosis and Other Mining-Related Lung Disease New Manifestations of Illness in an Age-Old Occupation. Clin Chest Med. 2020;41:687-96.
62. Laney AS, Petsonk EL. Small pneumoconiotic opacities on U.S. coal worker surveillance chest radiographs are not predominately in the upper lung zones. Am J Ind Med. 2012;55: 793-8.
63. Brichet A, Tonnel AB, Brambilla E, et al. Chronic interstitial pneumonia with honeycombing in coal workers. Sarcoidosis Vasc Diffuse Lung Dis. 2002;19:211-9.
64. Rehman M, Sood A, Pollard C, et al. Characterizing patterns of small pneumoconiotic opacities on chest radiographs of New Mexico coal miners. Arch Environ Occup Health. 2022;77(4): 263-7.
65. IARC (International Agency for Research on Cancer) Monographs on the Evaluation of Carcinogenic Risks to Humans, Vol 68. Silica, some silicates, Coal Dust and Para-aramid fibrils. Lyon: IARC; 1997. Available from https://monographs.iarc.who.int/wp-content/uploads/2018/08/14-002.pdf
66. Attfield MD, Kuempel ED. Mortality among U.S. underground coal miners: A 23-year follow-up. Am J Ind Med. 2008;51: 231-45.
67. Li L, Jiang M, Li X, et al. Association between Coal mine Dust and Mortality Risk of Lung Cancer: A Meta-Analysis. BioMed Res Int. 2021:6624799.
68. Schmajuk G, Truopin L, Yelin E, et al. Prevalence of arthritis and Rheumatoid Arthritis in coal mining counties of the U.S. Arthritis Care Res (Hoboken). 2019;71(9):1209-15.
69. Stolt P, Kallberg H, Lundberg I, et al. Silica exposure is associated with increased risk of developing rheumatoid arthritis: results from the Swedish EIRA study. Ann Rheum Dis. 2005;64:582-6.
70. Rodnan GP, Benedek TG, Medsger TA, et al. The association of progressive systemic sclerosis (scleroderma) with coal miners pneumoconiosis and other forms of silicosis. Ann Intern Med. 1967;66(2):323-34.
71. Caplan A. Certain unusual radiological appearances in the chest of coal-miners suffering from rheumatoid arthritis. Thorax. 1953;8(1):29-37.
72. Caplan A, Payne RB, Withey JL. A broader concept of Caplan's syndrome related to rheumatoid factors. Thorax. 1962;17: 205-12.
73. Hodous TK, Attfield MD. Progressive massive fibrosis developing on a background of minimal simple coal worker's pneumoconiosis. Proceedings of the VII International Pneumoconiosis Conference. U.S. Department of Health and Human Services, Public Health Service, Center for Disease Control, National Institute for Occupational Safety and Health. DHHS (NIOSH). 1990;90:122-6.
74. Hepplestone AG. The pathogenesis of simple pneumoconiosis in coal workers. J Pathol Bacteriol. 1954;67(1):51-63.
75. Hepplestone AG. The essential lesion of pneumoconiosis in Welsh coal workers. J Pathol Bacteriol. 1947;59:453-60.
76. Kleinerman J, Green F, Harley-RA, et al. Pathology standards for coal workers' pneumoconiosis. Arch Pathol Lab Med. 1979;103:374-432.

77. Morgan WK, Burgess DB, Lapp NL, et al. Hyperinflation of the lungs in coal miners. Thorax. 1971;26(5):585-90.
78. Shennan DH, Washington JS, Thomas DJ, et al. Factors predisposing to the development of progressive massive fibrosis in coal miners. Br J Ind Med. 1981;38(4):321-6.
79. Wagner JC. Etiologic factors in complicated coal workers' pneumoconiosis. Ann NY Acad Sci. 1972;200:401-4.
80. Lapp NL, Castranova V. How silicosis and coal workers' pneumoconiosis develops - a cellular assessment. In: Occupational Medicine: State of the Art Reviews. Philadelphia: Hanley and Belfus, Inc; 1993. pp. 35-65.
81. Adamis Z, Timlár T. Studies on the effect of quartz, bentonite, and coal dust mixtures on macrophages *in vitro*. Br J Exp Pathol. 1978;59:411-9.
82. Dalal NS, Suryan MM, Vallayathan V, et al. Detection of reactive free radicals in fresh coal mine dusts and their implication for pulmonary injury. Ann Occup Hyg. 1989;33(1):79-84.
83. Lapp NL, Lewis D, Schwegler-Berry D. Bronchoalveolar lavage in asymptomatic underground coal miners. In: Ramani RV (Ed). Proceedings of Respiratory Dusts in the Mineral Industry. Englewood: Society of Mining Engineering; 1991. pp. 159-69.
84. Adamson IY, Bowden DH. Adaptive responses of the pulmonary macrophagic system to carbon: II. Morphologic studies. Lab Invest. 1978;38(4):430-8.
85. Castranova V, Bowman L, Reasor MV, et al. The response of rat alveolar macrophages to chronic inhalation of coal dust and/or diesel inhalation. Environ Res. 1985;36(2):405-19.
86. Vallyathan V, Schwegler D, Reasor M. Comparative in vivo cytotoxicity and relative pathogenicity of mineral dusts. In: Dodgson J, McCallum RI, Bailey MR, et al (Eds). Inhaled Particles VI. Oxford: Pergamon; 1989. pp. 279-89.
87. Lee JS, Shin JH, Lee JO, et al. Serum levels of interleukin-8 and tumor necrosis factor-alpha in coal workers' pneumoconiosis: one-year follow-up study. Safety Health Work. 2010;1:69-79.
88. Heise ER, Mentnech MS, Olenchock SA, et al. HLA-A1 and coal workers' pneumoconiosis. Am Rev Respir Dis. 1979;119(6): 903-8.
89. Churchyard GJ, Fielding KL, Lewis JJ. A trial of mass isoniazid preventive therapy for tuberculosis control. N Engl J Med. 2014;370(4):301-10.
90. Ball JD, Berry G, Clarke WG, et al. A controlled rial of anti-tuberculosis chemotherapy in the early complicated pneumoconiosis of coal workers. Thorax. 1969;24(4):399-406.
91. Dubois P, Gyselen A, Prignot J. Rifampicin-combined chemotherapy in coal workers pneumoconio-tuberculosis. Am Rev Respir Dis. 1977;115(2):221-8.
92. Morgan EJ. Silicosis and tuberculosis. Chest. 1979;75(2): 202-3.
93. Hughes JM, Jones RN, Gilson JC, et al. Determinants of progression in sandblasters' silicosis. Ann Occup Hyg. 1982;26: 701-12.
94. Jalloul A, Banks DE. Can We Translate Our Understanding of the Pathogenic Mechanisms of Silicosis into a Therapeutic Plan? Clin Pulm Med. 2010;17(6):266-75.
95. Maher TM, Corte TJ, Fischer A, et al. Pirfenidone in patients with unclassifiable progressive fibrosing interstitial lung disease: a double-blind, randomised, placebo-controlled, phase 2 trial. Lancet Respir Med. 2020;8(2):147-57.
96. Behr J, Prasse A, Kreuter M, et al. Pirfenidone in patients with progressive fibrotic interstitial lung diseases other than idiopathic pulmonary fibrosis (RELIEF): a double-blind, randomised, placebo-controlled, phase 2b trial. Lancet Respir Med. 2021;9(5):476-86.

CHAPTER 95

Silicosis

Surinder K Jindal, PS Shankar

INTRODUCTION

Silicosis is a type of pneumoconiosis which comprises a group of lung diseases caused by chronic inhalation of inorganic dusts. Silicosis commonly results from workplace exposure to crystalline silica dust which induces marked degree of inflammation and fibrotic scarring in the form of nodular lesions. Even though the respiratory problems due to dusts date back to the ancient Greek and Roman civilizations, the term *silicosis* (from the Latin *silex* or flint) was first used in the 19th century. Silicosis remains among the most serious potentially fatal occupational diseases.[1-4] The total number of deaths however was down from 50,000 in 1990 to 43,000 in 2013 in the Global Burden of Disease Study.[2]

SILICA AND SILICOSIS

Silica, also known as silicon dioxide (SiO_2), is a chemical compound which is widely distributed in nature and contributes to about 28% of the earth's crust. Silicon is highly reactive and does not remain in a state of an element. It combines either with oxygen to form free silica (SiO_2) or with oxygen and other cations such as magnesium, aluminum, or iron to form silicates. Examples of silicates include mica, soapstone, talc, tremolite, and cement. Silica and silicates form the bulk of most kinds of rocks, clays, and sands. Silica exists in two distinct forms as crystalline and amorphous: "Crystalline" refers to silicon and oxygen atoms oriented and related to each other in a fixed pattern. In amorphous form, silicon and oxygen atoms are distributed in a random fashion.

The term silicosis is applied for the lung disorders caused by inhalation of the free silica. The inhaled SiO_2 is usually in crystalline form, most often as quartz. Crystalline silica produces different polymorphs at different temperatures and pressure. Alpha quartz (simply referred to as quartz) is stable over most temperatures and pressures found on the earth's surface. It forms the most common polymorph found in the earth's crust. Cristobalite and tridymite are other crystalline forms of silica; they are stable at high temperatures and low pressures. Beta quartz is stable at high temperatures. Free silica refers to quartz, cristobalite, and tridymite.

Because of the colorless and nonirritant properties, exposure to silica in large amounts goes unrecognized. It does not produce any immediate effect in most instances. Chronic exposure leads to a progressive fibrosing disease which may also predispose to tuberculosis. In high-pressure environment at different temperatures as found in different industrial processes (such as ceramic manufacturing and foundry process), quartz may be heated to high temperatures at high pressures. The examples of amorphous forms of silica include opal, diatomaceous earth, silica-rich fiberglass, mineral wools, and silica glass. Generally, they are harmless to humans except the fiberglass.

Silicosis is encountered in mining and quarrying of hard rock, anthracite coal, and metals. The sandstone industry, sand blasting, stone quarrying and dressing, granite industry, grinding of metals, iron and steel foundries, brick yards, silica milling, flint crushing, glass making, ceramic manufacturing, and manufacture of abrasive soaps are some of the occupations related to silica exposure. There is exposure to silica particles of respirable size with an aerodynamic diameter of 0.5–5 μm.

PROBLEM OF SILICOSIS IN INDIA

Silica sand is an inexpensive and useful component of a variety of manufacturing processes. Rock cutting and rock carving to build temples, sculpturing stone containing granite, mining, and metallurgy have been in existence in India since a very long period of time. The condition originally described in miners at Kolar Gold Mines was benign since the free silica dust did not possess fibrogenic property.[5] Several reports on occurrence of silicosis in mining and industrial workers became available thereafter, such as in slate pencil and agate-grinding industry.[6,7] Workers who are at high potential risk of silica exposure include those employed in occupations such as mining and quarrying gold, mica, and coal mines, those employed in ceramic and pottery industry, agate and slate pencil industry, brick workers and stone cutters, and workers engaged in manufacture of nonmetallic products such as refractory products, structural clay, glass mica, and manufacture of basic metals and alloys such as iron and steel, copper, ferroalloys, aluminum, and others.[8-16] The development and progression of silicosis frequently occurs after exposure to silica has stopped.

The epidemiologic studies carried out in India have shown marked variation in the prevalence of silicosis. The prevalence rate has varied from 3.5% in ordnance factories to 54.6% in slate pencil industry. The variation is due to the fact of variability of concentration of silica in work environment of different occupations, duration of exposure, and the physical properties of the silica.

The Indian National Institute of Occupational Health (NIOH) has undertaken environmental and medical surveys in several industries and found the prevalence of silicosis to be very high in most instances. The prevalence of silicosis was attributed to a high concentration of total and respirable dust and the great percentage of free silica in the dust; the free silica levels between 55 and 60% of total dust were reported at some of the industrial sites; up to half of the workers were reported to suffer from silicosis. The average duration of exposure before the development of silicosis, in most of these surveys, was approximately 10–12 years or less. The human cost was great, with approximately 55% of slate pencil industry workers having silicosis nearly 18% developing progressive massive fibrosis (PMF) and 22% dying within 16 months of diagnosis.

Environmental Pneumoconiosis

An interesting form of nonoccupational pneumoconiosis is reported in some parts of India, mostly from the high-altitude villages in Central Ladakh and Kaza in the Himalayas. Silicosis was common in the older inhabitants of villages exposed to frequent dust storms containing free silica.[17,18] Silica exposure was unrelated to any specific occupation. This condition appears to be similar to that described due to dust storms in the desert areas.[19]

PROBLEM OF SILICOSIS IN OTHER ASIAN COUNTRIES

There are occasional published reports of silicosis from other Asian countries, where the environmental and working conditions in factories are similar to those in India.[20-30] The problem of silicosis in China and Hong Kong, which accounts for an important health concern, has been extensively investigated. The problem has been described from Japan among workers involved in occupations such as ceramic industry, tunnel construction, and whetstone cutting, as well as more frequently in industrial work force in Southeastern countries such as Thailand, Singapore, and Vietnam.[20-30] The prevalence of silicosis was 10% in Vietnam among refractory brick workers.[27] This was almost linearly related to the duration of work.[28] A survey among workers in 33 factories in Thailand revealed radiologic silicosis in 61 (9%) workers; 13 (1.9%) had pulmonary tuberculosis.[29] 31 of the 33 factories had measurements of either total dust or respirable dust exceeding threshold limit values.

PATHOGENESIS[31-33]

Crystalline silica particles are inhaled while the respirable-sized particles are deposited in the distal airways and alveoli. Alveolar macrophages ingest the silica particles, migrate into the interstitium, enter the lymphatics, and are transported to the regional lymph nodes.

The interaction of silica and the pulmonary alveolar macrophages is a crucial event in the development of silicosis. Macrophage injury or death will release intercellular proteolytic enzymes that are likely to take part in the lung injury. There is also the release of cytokines which attract other inflammatory cells such as neutrophils and T-lymphocytes. The injured macrophages and the other inflammatory cells release superoxide anions and hydroxyl radicals and they cause injury to the lung tissue. Silica-activated macrophages and lymphocytes also release many inflammatory mediators, such as interleukin-1 and tumor necrosis-alpha factor that contribute to the production of fibrosis. Silica has great fibrogenic potential and the dying macrophages liberate a fibroblast-stimulating factor which causes excessive production and release of collagen by fibroblasts.

TYPES OF SILICOSIS

Silicosis has a long latency period; three different patterns of silicosis have been recognized, i.e., chronic, accelerated, or acute forms primarily based on the degree and duration of exposure and onset of symptoms. The presentations of the disease reflect the variable intensity of exposure and rate of silica deposition in the lungs, retention of total amount of crystalline silica, latency periods, and natural histories.

Chronic (or Classic) Silicosis

The physiology of chronic silicosis involves chronic inflammation due to accumulation of a variety of inflammatory mediators and fibrogenic elements. The rate of progression of the disease depends upon the rate and amount of silica deposition and retention in the lungs. The condition can be simple or complicated.

The simple chronic silicosis develops following exposure to low-to-moderate concentration of free silica for 20 years or more. Initially, there is collection of silica-laden macrophages in the loose reticulin fibers in the peribronchial, perivascular, paraseptal, and subpleural areas. Later, there is formation of silicotic nodules in which the central area gets organized with a concentric whorl-like arrangement of collagen. The lesions may have variable degrees of calcification. The nodules are seen in the pulmonary parenchyma, typically in the upper lobes, and the hilar and peribronchial lymph nodes. A few birefringent silica particles may be demonstrated in the center of silicotic nodules under polarized light. They represent inhaled silicate particles mixed with SiO_2. The inflammation continues in the periphery of the nodule, which gets enlarged by including adjacent pulmonary structures. Such a stage is referred to as PMF.

These nodules are referred to as "histologic tornadoes" with a "quiet" center of hyaline and collagen fibers concentrically arranged around the centre.[34] In the periphery, there is collection of inflammatory cells such as macrophages and lymphocytes. Later, it becomes the seat of a fibrotic reaction.

In complicated silicosis, the nodules coalesce to form large masses of hyalinized tissue. The masses may have a variable diameter of 2 cm or more. The blood vessels and bronchioles are obliterated. The amount of silica or inflammatory cells is negligible. They are found in the apices of the lung and tend to be bilaterally symmetrical in distribution. There can be central necrosis and cavitation. These patients exhibit an increased susceptibility to infection with *Mycobacterium tuberculosis (M.tb)* as a result of which the lesion may get cavitated.

Accelerated Silicosis

The condition is encountered in persons who are exposed to heavy amounts of silica, often with duration of 5–10 years. Accelerated silicosis occurs over a relatively shorter time course when compared with chronic silicosis. The rate of progression is more rapid. The condition progresses even after removal of the person from the continued silica exposure. Pathologically, there is filling of alveolar spaces with eosinophilic granular material. The collagen vascular diseases such as systemic sclerosis, systemic lupus erythematosus, and rheumatoid arthritis are sometimes associated with this type of silicosis.

Acute Silicosis

Acute silicosis is rare but often fatal. It is likely to occur in workers as a consequence of intense exposure to very high concentrations of silica over a period varying from several months up to about 5 years. Cases have been encountered in sandblasters, in silica flour manufacturing, and rock drilling. The mechanism of injury is different from that seen in chronic silicosis. There is a stronger inflammatory response due to the presence of freshly fractured silica exhibiting abundant cleaved particle surfaces. Lungs exhibit consolidation without silicotic nodules. The lungs involved by acute silicosis show presence of hypertrophic type II pneumonocytes lining the alveoli. They are responsible for the production of an excess amount of proteinaceous material and surfactant protein. The alveolar spaces are filled with eosinophilic proteinaceous material. This is referred to as silicoproteinosis. There is diffuse alveolar damage and desquamative pneumonitis.

CLINICAL FEATURES

The most common presentation of silicosis is in the form of uncomplicated chronic silicosis. Chronic silicosis develops only after decades of repeated exposures to high concentrations of silica dust. Generally, it is asymptomatic even when the radiographic appearance suggests fairly advanced silicosis. Dyspnea on exertion is considered to be the most frequent and directly related symptom of silicosis. There can be cough and sputum production from nonspecific bronchitis or from cigarette smoking. Chest pain and hemoptysis indicate the likely complication of tuberculosis. Acute silicosis presents with dyspnea, fatigue, weight loss, fever, and pleuritic pain. Pneumothorax, rarely bilateral, is also reported.[35]

In addition to the development of pneumoconiosis in silica-exposed workers, there are several reports on increased respiratory symptoms and impaired lung function in industrial workers, miners, stone cutters, and others in the absence of a definitive radiological diagnosis of silicosis.[36,37] This nonspecific symptomatology is attributed to chronic dust exposure. Stunting of lung growth is reported on long-term exposure to respirable dust in childhood and early adult life.[38]

DIAGNOSIS

Clinical and radiological features that distinguish silicosis from other fibrotic disease including the following:

- Occupational exposure to a substantial amount of silica
- Silicotic nodule
- Involvement of hilar lymph nodes

There is a close resemblance radiologically between silicosis and miliary tuberculosis. However, the size of nodules seen in tuberculosis are less than those seen in silicosis. The radiographs of patients with silicosis usually exhibit an increased translucency as against general loss of translucency in tuberculosis.

The symptoms in a patient with simple nodular silicosis are markedly less compared to patients with miliary tuberculosis. Further, the incidence of miliary tuberculosis in adults is less common and exhibits toxic manifestations. The distinction between PMF and postprimary tuberculosis may pose difficulties sometimes. The conglomerate shadows of PMF do not show cavitation. The PMF often exhibits large fibrotic masses with an upward displacement of the mediastinal and hilar structures from volume loss. The lower lung zones may be hyperinflated and emphysematous. The onset of cavitation should prompt a search for active mycobacterial disease. Associated features such as pleural effusion, localized increase in size of opacities, and distortion of intrathoracic structures due to fibrosis are noted in tuberculosis.

Acute silicosis produces a homogeneous ground glass appearance on chest radiograph. It has to be distinguished from pulmonary edema, alveolar hemorrhage, pulmonary alveolar proteinosis, pneumonia, and bronchoalveolar cell carcinoma.

RADIOGRAPHIC PATTERNS

The diagnosis of silicosis is established by a history of occupational exposure and chest radiograph with typical nodules. Exclusion of other diseases and very rarely, histologic examination of lung tissue may be necessary.

Chest radiography is vital for the diagnosis of silicosis. There is a clear relationship between total dust exposure and severity of radiographic changes. In the initial stages, there is reticulation of the lung fields due to thickening of the perivascular and intercommunicating lymphatics. The diagnosis of silicosis is possible only after the appearance of nodules.

The classic radiographic features of simple silicosis are rounded opacities ranging in size from 1 to 10 mm and occurring predominantly in the upper lung zones. They can be categorized using the International Labour Organization's (ILO) International Classification of Radiographs of Pneumoconiosis by size, shape, and profusion category.[39] The small, rounded opacities are grouped into three diameter ranges designated as "*p*" (up to 1.5 mm), "*q*" (1.5–3.0 mm), and "*y*" (1.0–10 mm). As the disease progresses, the opacities are also seen in the mid- and lower-lung zones. The nodules are of homogeneous density and are usually bilaterally symmetrical.

In addition to the size and shape of the nodules, the abundance (profusion of nodules within the parenchyma of the lung are also important. By comparison with standard films provided by the ILO, the profusion of nodules in the patient's films can be categorized in order of increasing severity as category 1, 2, or 3.

Hilar lymphadenopathy is also seen sometimes in advanced nodular parenchymal shadows **(Fig. 1)**. There can be "eggshell" calcification of the lymph nodes and it is strongly suggestive of silicosis. However, the eggshell calcification is not specific and it may be seen with sarcoidosis, radiation-treated Hodgkin disease, blastomycosis, scleroderma, amyloidosis, or histoplasmosis.[40]

On continued dust exposure, the nodule increase in size and number ultimately covering most parts of the lungs. They may unite and form conglomerate shadows, which are described as PMF. The ILO classifies these large opacities as A, B, and C based on size or on total cross-sectional area relative to the size of right upper zone (or on both). With coalescence of the nodules, the upper lobes become fibrotic and contract, making the conglomerate nodules appear to migrate toward the hilar areas. The hilar structures are pulled upward, leaving areas of compensatory emphysema at their margins and in the lung bases. With these alterations, the small, rounded opacities that were evident previously on the radiograph become less visible or at times disappear. Pleural abnormalities are not commonly encountered, but they may be seen sometimes in lesions.

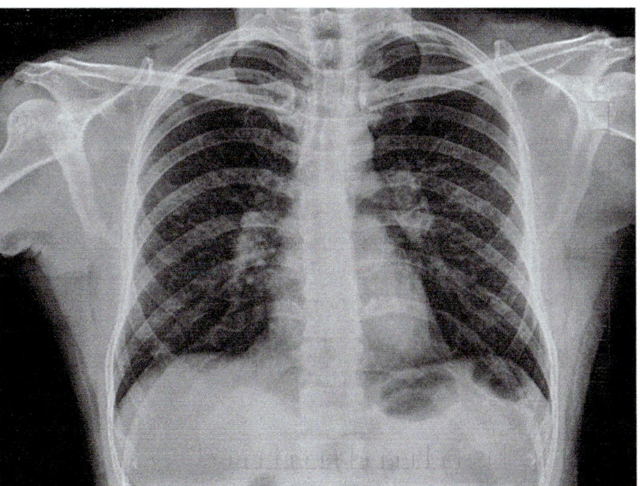

FIG. 1: Chest radiograph of a patient of silicosis demonstrating hilar lymphadenopathy and small nodular infiltrates.

Acute silicosis may present with radiographic alveolar filling pattern, leading to a ground glass appearance and association with conglomerate silicotic nodules is rarely seen. Pulmonary tuberculosis in the patient with silicosis may be associated with pleural effusion, localized increase in size of opacities, and cavitation.

PULMONARY FUNCTIONS

Pulmonary function tests help in the evaluation of persons with suspected silicosis. There are no specific patterns of ventilatory impairment in silicosis. There can be significant airflow limitation. Both peak expiratory flow (PEF) and forced vital capacity (FVC) are reported to reduce in chronically exposed individuals.[36-38] Tobacco smoking in the presence of other dust exposure further aggravates the presence of airway obstruction. In patients with PMF, restrictive ventilatory impairment is seen in association with arterial hypoxemia. The pulmonary function changes occur earlier and are more marked in acute and accelerated silicosis. They make a rapid progress compared to chronic form of the disease.

OTHER INVESTIGATIONS

Bronchoalveolar lavage (BAL) study is rarely indicated. It may be undertaken when exposure history and clinical presentations are atypical. The BAL fluid of workers exposed to quartz dust will demonstrate an increased number of cells, protein, and quartz in the macrophages. The amount of mineral dust in BAL fluid cells is related to the intensity of exposure and duration of employment.

Lung biopsy (open or thoracoscopic) is rarely needed to establish the diagnosis. It may be indicated in some clinical settings when complications are present. This is particularly important when lung malignancy is suspected as a complication.

The demonstration of tubercle bacilli in the sputum of patients suffering from silicotuberculosis is difficult in many instances. The walling in of the tubercle foci by the silicotic fibrosis prevents the elimination of tubercle bacilli in the sputum.

COMPLICATIONS (BOX 1)

There is an increased susceptibility to pulmonary tuberculosis rarely to fungal infection.[41-44] In presence of worsening of respiratory symptoms and rapidly changing or progressive lesions on chest radiographs, mycobacterial infection (*M.tb* or atypical mycobacteria) should be suspected and investigated. Tuberculosis can either complicate silicosis or pose a problem in the differential diagnosis. It is thought that macrophage dysfunction caused by the presence of silica appears to be the cause of increased susceptibility to tuberculosis and other infections.

Patients with PMF are prone to mycobacterial infections and spontaneous pneumothorax. The prevalence of tuberculosis has varied from 1.9 to 3.6% in brick makers, metal workers, and coal miners with silicosis. According to NIOH reports, tuberculosis was present in 4.8% of coal miners and 48% of stone cutters.[41] Silicotuberculosis has been identified as an important comorbidity in several other Asian populations.[42,43]

Reports appearing in the past few decades continue to identify a clinically important rate of tuberculosis in silicotics. Tuberculosis exhibits some specific characteristics in persons with silicosis **(Box 2)**.

Free silica impairs macrophage function, thereby increasing the chances of mycobacterial infection.[45] Important predisposing factors relate to social circumstances and to living and working conditions. Tobacco smoking is an important predisposition. Most of these workers live in crowded and unsanitary conditions, while their jobs are in dusty environments and silica exposures are not controlled. The chances of spread of infection are higher in such surroundings. Many reports of silicotuberculosis cited earlier do not necessarily attribute the presence of tuberculosis to underlying silicosis. However, when the conditions are present together, there is increased morbidity and mortality, with clear evidence of rapid silicosis progression. Studies from Singapore have reported the occurrence of tuberculosis as a significant factor associated with the development of PMF and a strong predictor of mortality in patients with silicosis. Occasionally, silicosis is complicated by fungal invasion **(Fig. 2)**. Aspergillosis complicating a cavitary silicotic nodule is also reported.[46]

There is an increased incidence of autoimmunity and diseases such as rheumatoid arthritis in patients with silicosis. These patients exhibit positive latex fixation tests, antinuclear antibodies, and increased levels of immunoglobulins. Necrotizing rheumatoid nodule in silicosis is a characteristic clinical picture known as Caplan syndrome. Chronic silicosis gradually leads to development of pulmonary hypertension, chronic cor pulmonale, and chronic

BOX 1 Important complications seen in patients of silicosis.

- Pulmonary hypertension and chronic cor pulmonale
- Chronic respiratory failure
- Respiratory infections
- Silicotuberculosis
- Silicomycosis
- Autoimmune disorders
- Necrotizing nodules—Caplan syndrome
- Scar carcinoma
- Acute/accelerated silicosis—alveolar proteinosis
- Massive pulmonary fibrosis

BOX 2 Characteristics of tuberculosis in silicotics.

- Frequent occurrence
- Increased risk
- Severe and persistence respiratory symptoms
- Rapid progression to fibrosis
- Poor response to antituberculosis therapy
- Necessity of longer duration of therapy

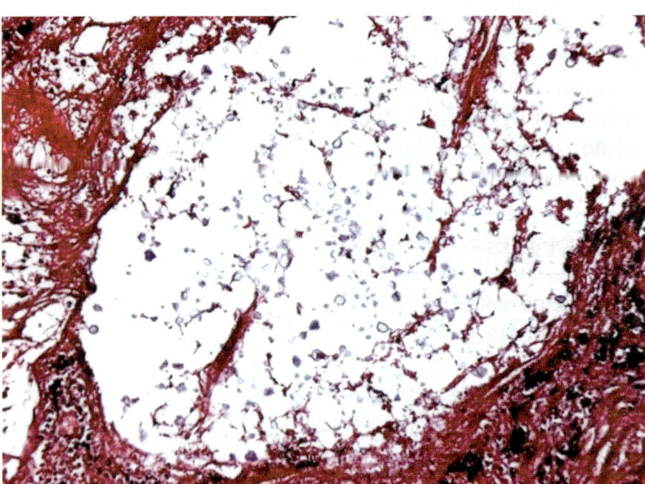

FIG. 2: Postmortem lung histology—photomicrograph showing silicomycosis. Clusters of *Cryptococci* and fibrocollagenous material with extensive blackish pigment, which revealed needle-shaped silica particles under polarized light examination.
Courtesy: Dr Ashim Das, Department of Pathology, PGIMER, Chandigarh.

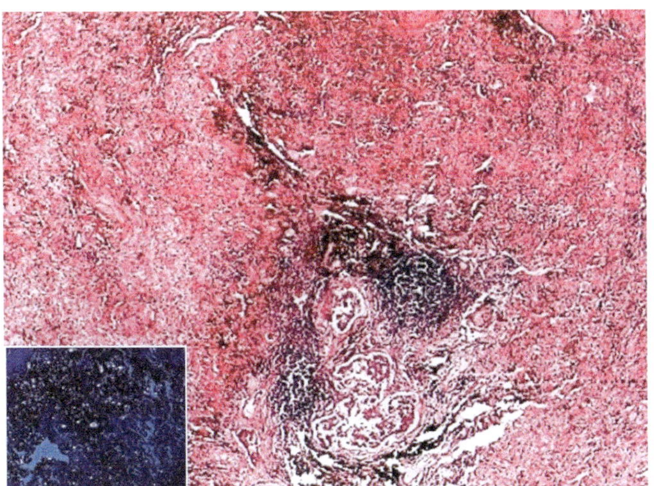

FIG. 3: Postmortem lung histology—photomicrograph showing pigment deposition, fibrotic nodular formation, and adenocarcinoma.

Courtesy: Dr Ashim Das, Department of Pathology, PGIMER, Chandigarh.

respiratory failure. The onset of these complications is rapid in case of massive fibrosis.

There is an increased relationship between quartz exposure, silicosis, and development of bronchogenic carcinoma and there is an increased mortality from lung cancer among workers exposed to silica dust.[47-49] This is mostly an adenocarcinoma which commonly occurs over a silicotic scar in the lung **(Fig. 3)**. Tobacco smoking is an added risk for carcinogenesis.

PROGNOSIS

Patients with conglomerate fibrosis progress to cor pulmonale and respiratory failure. The clinical course of patients with acute silicosis is inexorably downward with pulmonary fibrosis, restrictive lung disease, and ultimately respiratory failure resulting in death. Silicosis especially when "acute" may be complicated by secondary alveolar proteinosis with marked respiratory distress and failure.

TREATMENT

There is no specific treatment for silicosis and the therapy is directed largely at the complications of the disease. Corticosteroids have been used with varying success and have limited efficacy in the treatment of silicosis.[34,50] The polymers such as polyvinyl pyridine N-oxide (PVPNO) and polybetaine though showed protective effects in experimental animals, found not suitable for human disease. Tetrandrine, though found to diminish fibrosis and collagen synthesis in silica-exposed animals has not found to be effective in humans and has shown to be teratogenic.

Following the diagnosis of silicosis, it is advisable to avoid further exposure to silica-containing dusts. The individual should be promptly removed from such surroundings. In advanced disease or if it has developed following a short exposure, further dust exposure has to be avoided. The comorbid conditions such as chronic obstructive pulmonary disease should be identified and managed.[51] Severe airflow obstruction and cor pulmonale are treated with bronchodilators, diuretics, and oxygen. Tobacco smoking, if present, must be stopped.

Treatment of tuberculosis in these workers poses tremendous problems. Results of standard chemotherapeutic protocols for tuberculosis in the presence of silicosis are less effective than therapy for tuberculosis alone.[44] A partial explanation for the poor response has been attributed to impaired macrophage function and poor penetration of the drugs into fibrotic nodules. It is generally recommended that patients with tuberculosis should receive at least four antimycobacterial drugs such as isoniazid, rifampicin, and pyrazinamide for 2 months followed by two antituberculosis drugs (isoniazid and rifampicin) for a total of 9 months or longer. The exact duration of therapy remains debatable.

Acute silicosis with respiratory failure needs aggressive treatment that includes whole-lung lavage in an attempt to improve gas exchange and to remove alveolar debris. However, the benefit is not established.[52] Though a short-term controlled trial of systemic corticosteroids improved lung function in patients with silicosis, majority of studies have not shown any benefit.

PREVENTION

Prevention remains the main goal of silicosis. Several countries and international agencies have recommended and adopted different preventive measures in this direction.[53-57] The strategy generally consists of medical screening and surveillance and dust control measures.

Medical Surveillance

Workers exposed to silica dust should undergo periodic medical examination to screen for adverse health effects and dust measurements in work environment. The medical examination consists of pre-employment and periodic examinations, including chest radiographs, sputum examination for tubercle bacilli, and spirometry. The pre-employment medical examination provides the baseline data for each individual. The periodic medical examination helps in early detection of silicosis and silicotuberculosis. Health education is important to get active cooperation of the workers at risk.

Dust Control Measures

Silicosis does not develop without exposure to dust. The dust levels in the workplace correlate well with the incidence and severity of the disease. Hence, elimination or suppression of dust at the workplace forms the essence in the control of silicosis. The work process should be isolated and enclosed. Adequate ventilation should be provided. Personal protection is important.

Exposure to dust can be reduced by use of improved ventilation and local exhaust, use of substitution innocuous substances that are less hazardous than silica, isolation and enclosure of the sources of dust, use of wet abrasive techniques, humidification of work environment, and personal protection. Masks are advocated only when other dust control measures have failed. The dust masks are of little value when the dust concentrations are high as the dust particles will clog the pores in the filter. Further, masks are less suited for hot and humid climate. In its efforts to control and prevent silicosis, India has also implemented several of these measures including the workmen compensation for disability.[58-60]

SUMMARY

Silicosis is an old disease which remains a major occupational health hazard in India, responsible for high morbidity and mortality in industrial workers. Workers exposed to high concentrations of free crystalline silica in unprotected settings are at great risk for developing pulmonary fibrosis. The disease is progressive and irreversible. All measures should be undertaken to avoid and control dust exposure. The lack of therapy emphasizes the importance of primary prevention in our approach to the problem.

REFERENCES

1. Gupta A. Silicosis - An uncommonly diagnosed common occupational disease. ICMR Bull. 1999;29:95-100.
2. GBD 2013 Mortality and Causes of Death, Collaborators. Global, regional, and national age-sex specific all-cause and cause-specific mortality for 240 causes of death, 1990–2013: a systematic analysis for the Global Burden of Disease Study 2013. Lancet. 2014;385(9963):117-71.
3. Blanc PD, Seaton A. Pneumoconiosis Redux. Coal Workers' Pneumoconiosis and Silicosis Are Still a Problem. Am J Respir Crit Care Med. 2016;183:603-5.
4. Yi X, He Y, Zhang Y, et al. Current status, trends, and predictions in the burden of silicosis in 204 countries and territories from 1990 to 2019. Front Public Health. 2023;11:1216924.
5. Gowda AMS. Pneumoconiosis in the Kolar Gold Fields. Proceedings of sixth International Conference of Pneumoconiosis. 1983;2:1219.
6. Saiyed HN, Parikh DJ, Ghodasara NB, et al. Silicosis in slate pencil workers. An environmental/medical study. Am J Industr Med. 1985;8:127.
7. Sadhu SG, Parikh DJ, Sharma YK, et al. A follow up study of health status of small scale agate industry workers. Ind J Industr Med. 1995;41:401.
8. Govindagoudar MB, Singh PK, Chaudhry D, et al. Burden of Silicosis among stone crushing workers in India. Occup Med (Lond). 2022;72(6):366-71.
9. Dave SK. Classical silicosis: Epidemiology, clinical manifestations, diagnosis and treatment. Industr Safe Chron. 2000;3:50-7.
10. Jindal SK. Silicosis in India: Past and Present. Curr Opin Pulm Med. 2013;19:163-8.
11. Gangopadhyay PK, Bhattacharya SK, Mazumdar PK, et al. Occupational health problems of mica processing male workers. Indian J Industr Med. 1994;40:8.
12. Srivastava AK, Gupta BN, Chandra H, et al. Pulmonary disease due to multimetal exposure in glass bangle workers. Ind J Industr Med. 1988;34:20.
13. Malik SK, Behera D, Awasthi GK, et al. Pulmonary silicosis in emery polish workers. Ind J Chest Dis Allied Sci. 1985;27:116-21.
14. Saiyed HN, Ghodasara NB, Sathwara NG, et al. Dustiness, silicosis and tuberculosis in small scale pottery workers. Indian J Med Res. 1995;102:138.
15. Saini RK, Yousif M, Allaqaband GR, et al. Silicosis in stone cutters in Kashmir. J Indian Med Assn. 1984;82:118.
16. Tiwari RR, Sharma YK. Respiratory health of female stone grinders with free silica dust exposure in Gujarat, India. Int J Occup Environ Health. 2008;14:280-2.
17. Norboo T, Angchuk PT, Yahya M, et al. Silicosis in a Himalayan village population: role of environmental dust. Thorax. 1991;46:341-3.
18. Franco G, Massola A. Non-occupational pneumoconiosis at high altitude villages in central Ladakh. Br J Industr Med. 1992;49:452-3.
19. Goudie AS. Desert dust and human health disorders. Environ Int. 2014;63:101-13.
20. Wang XR, Christiani DC. Occupational lung disease in China. Int J Occup Environ Health. 2002;9:320-5.
21. Law YW, Leung MC, Leung CC, et al. Characteristics of workers attending the pneumoconiosis clinic for silicosis assessment in Hong Kong: retrospective study. Hong Kong Med J. 2001;7:343-9.
22. Jiang CQ, Xiao LW, Lam TH, et al. Accelerated silicosis in workers exposed to agate dust in Guangzhou, China. Am J Industr Med. 2001;40:87-91.
23. Huang J, Shibata E, Takeuchi Y, et al. Comprehensive health evaluation of workers in the ceramic industry. Br J Industr Med. 1993;50:112-6.
24. Lee HS, Phoon WH, Ng TP. Radiological progression and its predictive risk factors in silicosis. Occup Environ Med. 2001;58:467-71.
25. Kalampakorn S. Occupational health nursing in Thailand. Insight into international occupational health. AAOHN J. 2003;51:79-83.
26. Yingratanasuk T, Seixas N, Barnhart S, et al. Respiratory health and silica exposure of stone carvers in Thailand. Int J Occup Environ Health. 2002;8:301-8.
27. Lan TN, Son PH, Trung le V, et al. Distribution of silica-exposed workers by province and industry in Vietnam. Int J Occup Environ Health. 2002;9:128-33.
28. Chien VC, Chai SK, Hai DN, et al. Pneumoconiosis among workers in a Vietnamese refractory brick facility. Am J Ind Med. 2002;42:397-402.

29. Aungkasuvapala N, Juengprasert W, Obhasi N. Silicosis and pulmonary tuberculosis in stone-grinding factories in Saraburi, Thailand. J Med Assoc Thai. 1995;78:662-9.
30. Graham WG. Silicosis. Clin Chest Med. 1992;13:253-67.
31. Grossman BT, Churg A. Mechanisms in the pathogenesis of asbestosis and silicosis. Am J Respire Crit Care Med. 1998; 157:1666-80.
32. Vallyathan V, Shi X, Dalal NS, et al. Generation of free radicals from freshly fractured silica dust. Am Rev Respir Dis. 1988;138:1213-9.
33. Fuzimura N. Pathology and pathophysiology of pneumoconiosis. Curr Opin Pulm Med. 2000;6:140-4.
34. Sharma SK, Pande JN, Verma K. Effect of prednisolone treatment in chronic silicosis. Am Rev Respir Dis. 1991;143:814-21.
35. Gupta KB, Manchanda M, Kaur P. Bilateral spontaneous pneumothorax in silicosis. Ind J Chest Dis Allied Sci. 2006;48: 201-3.
36. Singh SK, Chowdhary GR, Chhangani VD, et al. Quantification of reduction in forced vital capacity of sand stone quarry workers. Int J Environ Res Public Health. 2007;4:296-300.
37. Tiwari RR, Narain R, Patel BD, et al. Spirometric measurements among quartz stone ex-workers of Gujarat, India. J Occup Health. 2003;45:88-93.
38. Green DA, McAlpine G, Semple S, et al. Mineral dust exposure in young Indian adults: an effect on lung growth? Occup Environ Med. 2008;65:306-10.
39. International Labour Office. Guidelines of the use of ILO International Classification of Radiographs of Pneumoconiosis of coal miners. Br Jr Industr Med. 1956;13:85.
40. Gross BH, Schneider HJ, Proto AV. Eggshell calcification of lymph nodes: an update. AJR Am J Roentgenol. 1980;135: 1265-8.
41. Kashyap SK. Occupational pneumoconiosis and tuberculosis. Ind J Tuberculosis. 1994;41:73-6.
42. Taguchi O, Saitoh Y, Saitoh K, et al. Mixed dust fibrosis and tuberculosis in comparison with silicosis and macular pneumoconiosis. Am J Ind Med. 2000;37:260-4.
43. Chang KC, Leung CC, Tam CM. Tuberculosis risk factors in a silicotic cohort in Hong Kong. Int J Tuberc Lung Dis. 2001;5: 177-84.
44. Barboza CE, Winter DH, Seiscento M, et al. Tuberculosis and silicosis: epidemiology, diagnosis and chemoprophylaxis. J Bras Pneumol. 2008;34:959-66.
45. Morgan EJ. Silicosis and tuberculosis. Chest. 1979;75:202-3.
46. Parakh UK, Sinha R, Bhatnagar AK, et al. Chronic necrotizing pulmonary aspergillosis: a rare complication in a case of silicosis. Ind J Chest Dis Allied Sci. 2005;47:199-203.
47. Tsuda T, Mino Y, Babazono A, et al. A case-control study of lung cancer in relation to silica exposure and silicosis in a rural area in Japan. Ann Epidemiol. 2002;12:288-94.
48. Cocco P, Rice CH, Chen JQ, et al. Lung cancer risk, silica exposure and silicosis in Chinese mines and pottery factories: the modifying role of other workplace lung carcinogens. Am J Ind Med. 2001;40:674-82.
49. Cocco P, Rice CH, Chen JQ, et al. Non-malignant respiratory diseases and lung cancer among Chinese workers exposed to silica. J Occup Environ Med. 2000;42:639-44.
50. Banks DE, Chang YH, Weber SL, et al. Strategies for the treatment of pneumoconiosis. Occup Med. 1993;8:204-32.
51. Rushton L. Chronic obstructive pulmonary disease and occupational exposure to silica. Rev Environ Health. 2007;22: 255-72.
52. Wilt H, Banks DE, Weissman DN, et al. Reduction of lung dust burden in pneumoconiosis by whole lung lavage. J Occup Environ Med. 1996;38:619-24.
53. World Health Organization. Report on Council of Pneumoconiosis (Prevention, early diagnosis and treatment) WHO-OCH 90.1. Geneva: WHO; 1990.
54. Krefft S, Wolff J, Rose C. Silicosis: An Update and Guide for Clinicians. Clin Chest Med. 2020;41(4):709-22.
55. Aguado-Agudo M, Rodríguez-Sanz J, Martín-Biel L, et al. Complicated silicosis. Med Clin (Barc). 2023;161(4):183.
56. Edwards GM. Silicosis-lessons from Australia's Dust Diseases Taskforce (2019-21). Occup Med (Lond). 2022;72(6):354-56.
57. Hoy RF, Jeebhay MF, Cavalin C, et al. Current global perspectives on silicosis-Convergence of old and newly emergent hazards. Respirology. 2022;27(6):387-98.
58. Rupani MP. Challenges and opportunities for silicosis prevention and control: need for a national health program on silicosis in India. J Occup Med Toxicol. 2023;18:11.
59. Sishodiya PK. Silicosis–An Ancient Disease: Providing Succour to Silicosis Victims, Lessons from Rajasthan Model. Indian J Occup Environ Med. 2022;26(2):57-61.
60. India Environment Portal. (2019). Order of the Supreme Court of India regarding the issue of fixing compensation to victims of silicosis, 05/03/2019. [online] Available from http://www.indiaenvironmentportal.org.in/category/2536/thesaurus/silicosis/ [Last accessed June, 2024].

Metal-induced Lung Diseases

CHAPTER 96

Nikhil C Sarangdhar, Dilip V Maydeo

INTRODUCTION

Several million workers are employed worldwide in industries or occupations associated with exposure to different metals and metallic compounds. Exposure to metals, whether environmental, occupational, or otherwise, affects the respiratory system in several ways; the nature and extent of such effects is not always uniform but is largely dependent on the physicochemical properties of the metal, the degree, extent and duration of exposure, the presence of ambient air pollution at the workplace, and susceptibility factors in the host.[1] Several metals and their compounds have been associated with respiratory symptoms, impairment of pulmonary function, and development of different types of lung diseases.[2-4] There is a varied clinical spectrum of metal-induced lung diseases which includes metal fume fever, allergic sensitization, asthma, chronic obstructive pulmonary disease (COPD), tracheobronchitis, bronchiolitis, interstitial lung diseases (ILD) including fibrosing ILD, hypersensitivity pneumonitis, pneumoconioses, pleural effusions, pulmonary edema, and others.[5-12]

Apart from occupational exposure to metals, environmental factors such as pollution and host factors such as genetic susceptibility, smoking, and the presence of underlying respiratory illness and other risk factors also influence the development and progression of metal-induced lung disease.[13,14] Environmental pollution augments the lung damage caused by metals, as several environmental pollutants have sensitizing properties, whereas others act as irritants to the respiratory tract. Early identification of disease, cessation of exposure to metals, and prompt treatment and rehabilitation of patients are all key components of disease management, as chronicity and severity of metal-induced lung disease are associated with progression to respiratory failure, in which treatment options are largely limited.

CLINICAL CLASSIFICATION OF METAL-INDUCED LUNG DISEASES

Airway diseases such as asthma occur in response to the inhalation of antigenic metals such as cobalt (Co), chromium, or nickel. Metal fume fever is an acute, short-term response mediated by the release of specific cytokines, typically in response to zinc oxides. Parenchymal fibrosis and granulomatous lung disease are other consequences of metal inhalation. Hard metal is a polycrystalline compound material produced by compacting powdered Co and tungsten carbide (WC) through a process called sintering, hence, the term "sintered carbides" (or cemented carbides). The term "hard metal lung disease" (HMLD) is used to denote a broad spectrum of lung diseases caused by exposure to hard metals and include obstructive pathologies such as asthma, bronchitis, and obliterative bronchiolitis, as well as fibrotic pathologies such as interstitial fibrosis, pneumoconiosis, and others. Chronic beryllium disease (CBD) is a granulomatous lung disorder caused by beryllium exposure in the workplace and is characterized by the accumulation of beryllium-specific $CD4^+$ T cells in bronchoalveolar lavage (BAL) fluid.[9]

The long list of metal-induced lung diseases by no means completely links several types or bizarre manifestations of pulmonary diseases with exposure(s) to different metal(s) **(Table 1)**. This has also led to the recognition of not only a wide range of pulmonary pathologies but also a growing list of metals that are implicated in the pathogenesis of metal-induced lung diseases.

EPIDEMIOLOGY AND RISK FACTORS

The development of metal-induced lung disease is dependent on several factors, including the nature of the offending metal, its physicochemical properties, the dose, extent and duration of exposure, the presence of ambient pollution or exhaust ventilation at the workplace, and host factors.[2,3] Hard metal-induced asthma has been described in several industries involved with metal processing and production. Cobalt (Co) asthma is well recognized in automobile industry and even low levels of Co exposure are associated with airway inflammation and lung function impairment in both smoking and nonsmoking industry workers. Inhalation of zinc oxide from activities such as welding and cutting of zinc-covered metal pieces is commonly implicated in metal fume fever. The prevalence of disease and levels of exposure that lead

TABLE 1: Clinical classification of metal-induced lung diseases.

Type of lung disease	Clinical presentation	Metal or alloys implicated
Fever	Metal fume fever	Zinc, tin, beryllium, copper, cadmium, silver, and magnesium
Allergy	Allergic sensitization	Beryllium, nickel, chromium, zinc, tin, tungsten, manganese, platinum, gold, silver, copper, aluminum, molybdenum, vanadium, zirconium, indium, iridium, iron, lead, mercury, titanium, and palladium
Upper respiratory tract inflammation	Rhinitis	Aluminum, chromium, cobalt, manganese, nickel, palladium, platinum, rhodium, titanium, and steel
	Tracheitis	Cadmium, manganese, mercury, nickel, zinc, and vanadium
	Laryngitis	Nickel, gold, and steel
Obstructive airway disease	Tracheobronchitis	Beryllium, cadmium, manganese, mercury, nickel, zinc, and vanadium
	Bronchiolitis	Beryllium, cadmium, manganese, mercury, nickel, zinc, and vanadium
	Asthma	Cobalt, tungsten, hard metal, nickel, chromium, aluminum, iron, manganese, mercury, platinum, platinum, palladium, vanadium, rhodium, zinc, zirconium, and steel
	Emphysema and chronic obstructive pulmonary disease (COPD)	Cadmium, copper, and selenium
Fibrosing parenchymal or interstitial lung disease	Chronic beryllium disease (CBD)	Beryllium
	Hard metal lung disease (HMLD)	Hard metal (tungsten carbide and cobalt alloy) Cobalt
	Diffuse fibrosing interstitial lung disease	Aluminum, cobalt, silica, titanium, copper, molybdenum, beryllium, hard metal, and rare earths
	Hypersensitivity pneumonitis	Beryllium, cobalt, hard metal, gold, iron, titanium, tantalum, nickel, chromium, zinc, zirconium, and metal working fluids (MWF)
	Sarcoidosis	Beryllium, silica, aluminum, and zirconium
	Pneumoconiosis	Iron, silica, asbestos, aluminum, beryllium, and hard metal
Acute lung injury	Chemical pneumonitis	Beryllium, cadmium, manganese, mercury, nickel, zinc, and vanadium
	Pulmonary edema and acute respiratory failure	Beryllium, cadmium, manganese, mercury, nickel, zinc, and vanadium
Disorders of alveolar surfactant	Pulmonary alveolar proteinosis (secondary)	Silica, aluminum, titanium, indium, nickel, copper, and zirconium
Mediastinal involvement	Mediastinal lymphadenopathy	Beryllium, silica, aluminum, zirconium (and all metals causing lung cancer)
Pleural disease	Pneumothorax	Beryllium, hard metal, silica, aluminum, and zirconium
	Pleural effusions and/or thickening	Asbestos, aluminum, chromium, iron, zinc, copper, and molybdenum
Pulmonary malignancy	Lung cancer	Nickel, cadmium, copper, chromium, zinc, lead, iron, steel, mercury, uranium, arsenic, and radon

to granulomatous lung disease have been most extensively studied for beryllium and hard metal.[2,3] But for isolated case reports or small series, there is relative paucity of literature regarding lung diseases in workers exposed to other metals. Several factors which contribute to the lower rates, include lower exposure to respirable and ultrafine particles, selective particle deposition, and clearance in the upper airways that protects the lower airways from exposure. Workplace factors such as ambient air pollution and levels of respirable fraction of metallic particles are also linked to the development of lung disease in a dose-response manner. The nature, extent, and duration of occupational or environmental exposure to metals is particularly important. Genetic susceptibility in the host also plays a contributory role. Dietary intake of metals such as iron, zinc, copper, molybdenum, and others in trace amounts affects immune functions, homeostatic balance, and the lung microbiome, therefore implicated in the development of different pulmonary as well as extrapulmonary diseases.[15]

Finally, a history of smoking or vaping and the presence of underlying lung disease such as asthma in workers are all associated with increased symptoms and significant decline in lung function.[1] Occupational exposures to welding fumes, metal working fluids (MWF), titanium dioxide nano particles, and newer metals such as indium are also implicated as causes of different types of metal-induced lung diseases.[2,10,14]

PATHOGENESIS

The pathogenesis of metal fume fever appears to involve an increase in proinflammatory cytokine release in the lung, with elevated levels of tumor necrosis factor-alpha (TNF-α) and interleukins 6 and 8 (IL-6 and 8). Metal-induced asthma and bronchitis are usually the result of allergen-induced sensitization and airway hyperreactivity, analogous to the immunoglobulin E (IgE)-mediated atopic reaction, though nonallergenic mechanisms may at times also be responsible. Pulmonary inflammation and damage in COPD, particularly in emphysema is believed to be the end result of several mechanisms, particularly protease/antiprotease imbalance and oxidative stress.[7] Copper is an important cofactor for some intercellular and intracellular enzymes, including the antioxidant enzyme superoxide dismutase (SOD) and selenium is a cofactor of glutathione peroxidase; these enzymes protect organs and tissues from damage mediated by free radicals.

Metals are also implicated in the pathogenesis of pleural disease. Estimates of metal levels in pleural fluids revealed that (1) metals such as zinc and copper were found elevated in exudates as compared to transudates; (2) benign exudates contained significantly higher levels of zinc than malignant exudates and transudates; and (3) iron and copper levels were significantly elevated in malignant effusions.[11] Exposure to air pollution, especially gaseous pollutants was associated with change in the pleural fluid levels of metals such as zinc and molybdenum in patients with parapneumonic effusions.[13] These two studies suggest that metals play an important role in pleural fluid transport and dynamics, with the capacity to affect immune and inflammatory responses in pleural effusions of varying etiology.[11,13]

Several metals that cause parenchymal or ILD do so by inducing granulomatous immune responses in the lung; these can be broadly classified into the following types:

- *Antigen-specific cell-mediated immunity*: Beryllium, titanium, zirconium, aluminum, Co, and gold
- *Giant cell granuloma*: Hard metal (WC and Co), Co, and titanium
- *Foreign body-type reaction*: Copper and barium

Other metals can also trigger specific immune responses. Aluminum, Co, gold, and zirconium stimulate a delayed-type hypersensitivity response to intradermal injection, analogous to the purified protein derivative used in tuberculin skin testing, in certain susceptible individuals. Aluminum, Co, gold, and titanium can also trigger in vitro lymphocyte proliferation. The immune response to beryllium serves as a prototype for immunologically driven granulomatous lung disease.[16] Histopathological features often seen in lung tissue samples obtained from patients with CBD include poorly formed noncaseating epithelioid granulomas, often indistinguishable from those observed in sarcoidosis, with lymphocytic and mononuclear cell infiltrate imposed on the background of diffuse interstitial inflammation and fibrosis.[3]

The pathology of HMLD is characterized by the presence of large "cannibalistic" multinucleated histiocytes (giant cells) in the alveolar airspaces and BAL fluid, in the background of mild alveolitis with or without other changes such as focal peribronchiolar inflammation, diffuse or centrilobular interstitial fibrosis, and honeycombing, termed as giant cell interstitial pneumonia (GCIP or GIP) **(Figs. 1A and B)**.[17] The multinucleate giant cells are considered to originate from the fusion of monocyte-macrophage lineage cells as part of the response to acute lung injury or inflammation and their formation is believed to augment the inherent defensive capacity of alveolar macrophages.[18] GIP is often described as a desquamative interstitial pneumonia-like reaction with

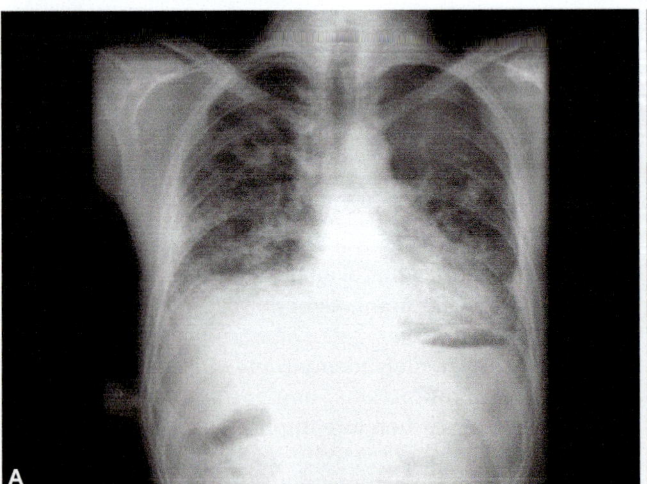

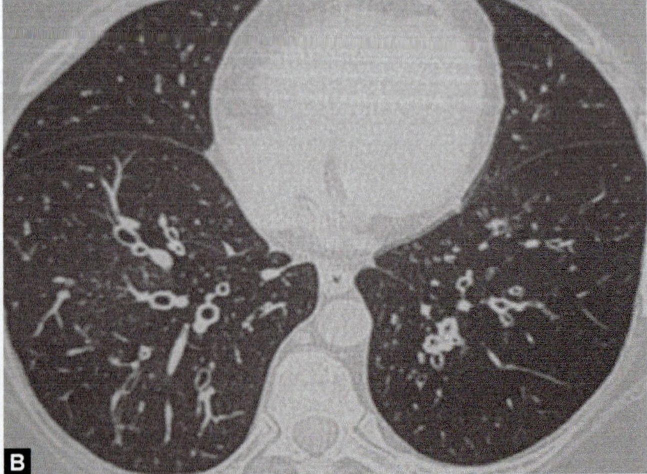

FIGS. 1A AND B: (A) Chest radiography and (B) computed tomography (CT) appearance of patients with hard-metal lung disease (HMLD).

numerous large, multinucleated histiocytes (cannibalistic giant cells) that ingest other inflammatory cells in the alveolar spaces.[19]

Carcinogenesis has been linked to excessive exposure to some metals and to a deficiency of others. Metals serve as cofactors for nearly half the proteins in the body and greatly influence the formation and structure of many crucial proteins apart from the catalytic activity of several enzymes necessary in homeostasis.[20] Metals implicated in the pathogenesis of lung cancer originate from several direct sources including mining, smelting, oil refineries, petrol and diesel industry, chemicals, pesticides, paints, tanning, MWF, pulp and paper industry, and sewage and indirect sources such as metal piping and traffic and combustion by-products from thermal power plants.[3,20,21] In addition to these sources, they exist in trace amounts in the environment in air, water, soil, and in cigarette and e-cigarette smoke as well. Several mechanisms are implicated in carcinogenesis due to metals, including chronic inflammation, oxidant injury due to free radicals, activation of oncogenic-signaling pathways, and vascular angiogenesis.[20,21]

CLINICAL AND RADIOLOGICAL FEATURES, LUNG FUNCTION IMPAIRMENT AND ASSESSMENT

The typical course of metal fume fever is heralded by the development of a sweet metallic taste and dry throat along with an influenza-like illness (ILI) with symptoms such as fever, chills, myalgias, and respiratory complaints such as chest tightness, nonproductive cough, and dyspnea; these occur within 4–8 hours following exposure and spontaneously resolve within 48 hours. Chest radiography and pulmonary function tests are usually normal. Recurrence of symptoms on return to work after a short period of absence akin to the Monday morning fever has also been noted. A few cases may present with more severe manifestations such as acute pneumonitis, acute respiratory distress syndrome, pericarditis, and aseptic meningitis. It is important to distinguish metal fume fever from acute metal fume toxicity which develops following acute high-intensity exposure to metal fumes but instead of being self-limiting progresses to fulminant respiratory distress and respiratory failure.

The diagnosis of metal-induced asthma and bronchitis rests on documentation of respiratory symptoms (wheeze and chest tightness) and correlation with patch tests, peak flow rates, and/or bronchoprovocation tests. In patients with normal spirometry at presentation, bronchoprovocation tests, either nonspecific with methacholine or histamine [with a provocative concentration (PC_{20}) of 8–16 mg/mL] or with specific irritants may be necessary to support diagnosis. Metal-induced occupational asthma must be differentiated from bronchitis by the onset of symptoms as well as the nature of airway hyperresponsiveness **(Table 2)**.

TABLE 2: Differentiation of metal-induced occupational asthma and bronchitis.

Metal-induced occupational asthma	Metal-induced bronchitis
• Acute symptoms, more severe • Persistent AHR • IgE mediated • Amplification of airway response on repeated exposure • Eosinophilic BAL	• Chronic symptoms, less severe • Variable AHR • Can be IgE or non-IgE mediated • Attenuation of airway response over time • Neutrophilic BAL

(AHR: airway hyperresponsiveness; BAL: bronchoalveolar lavage; IgE: immunoglobulin E)

An acute pneumonitis-like picture is seen in response to high-dose exposure (e.g., copper sulfate solution and beryllium). Disease symptoms typically begin with the subtle onset of dyspnea on exertion, nonproductive cough, fatigue, weight loss, and low-grade fever. Chest examination may reveal fine crackles. Chest imaging demonstrates different patterns of irregular or reticulonodular infiltrates in response to different metals **(Table 3)**. Tuberculosis is an important differential diagnosis, especially in the developing high-burden countries.

About a third of patients with CBD demonstrate mediastinal and hilar lymphadenopathy that is easily confused with sarcoidosis. Patients with suspected disease should undergo pulmonary function tests. They typically show airflow obstruction early in the disease process, with subsequent mixed patterns of obstruction and restriction, and pure restriction in advanced or end-stage disease. Blood gas exchange abnormalities during exercise are notable in patients with CBD, and hypoxemia can occur with advanced fibrosis in parenchymal disease associated with beryllium, copper, and rare earth (lanthanide) metals. Pulmonary function tests and blood gases may also be normal, as reported in the few cases of zirconium-associated lung disease.

The presentation of HMLD closely resembles hypersensitivity pneumonitis, with some patients having episodes of work-related subacute disease and some patients evolving, more or less rapidly, to lung fibrosis.[22-25] Occasionally, HMLD is found in conjunction with other connective tissue disorders such as rheumatoid arthritis or with complications such as pneumothorax. One important aspect of HMLD is that the disease may occur after a short duration of exposure, thus suggesting that individual susceptibility, rather than cumulative exposure, plays a major role.

Thoracic imaging plays an important role, with the disease being frequently noticed on a routine chest radiograph **(Fig. 1A)**. Computed tomography (CT) or high-resolution CT (HRCT) of the chest reveals the extent of involvement **(Fig. 1B)**. Radiology is also helpful for

TABLE 3: Radiographic and physiological abnormalities of lung diseases associated with exposure to metals.

Metal and industries	Chest radiograph or HRCT findings	Pulmonary physiology
Aluminum: Aircraft, welding, grinding, polishing	• Upper lobe predilection • Bilateral reticular shadows or infiltrates • Small modules resembling silicosis • Subpleural or diffuse honeycombing resembling IPF	Restrictive, hypoxemia
Barium: Oil well drilling, electronics, superconductors, rodenticides, radiocontrast dyes	• Sharply circumscribed small radiopaque nodules may be rounded or reticular • Acute pneumonitis with pulmonary edema if ingested	• Not well established • Hypoxemia with decreased DLCO if chemical aspiration
Beryllium: Ceramics, electronics, semiconductors, aerospace, nuclear weapons, defense	• Diffuse involvement or with upper lobe predilection • Shadows range from small nodular opacities with perilymphatic distribution to larger conglomerate masses • Smooth or nodular interlobular septal thickening • Ground-glass opacities, airway wall thickening • Mediastinal or hilar adenopathy	• *Early stage*: Obstruction • *Advanced stage*: Mixed pattern of obstruction and restriction • *End-stage disease*: Restriction with decreased DLCO • Hypoxemia
Cobalt: Diamond-cutting tools, paints and dyes, dentistry, batteries, radiotherapy	• Irregular or rounded opacities, centrilobular nodules, multifocal bilateral fibrotic consolidation • Traction bronchiectasis • May resemble NSIP, UIP, HP or sarcoidosis	• Obstruction if airway disease • Restriction with decreased DLCO if fibrosis
Copper: Plating, vineyard spraying, electronics, power cables, motors, heating elements	• Micronodular or fine miliary pattern • Small nodular opacities at lung bases • Fibrosis in upper lung fields or diffusely distributed • UIP or NSIP pattern, respiratory bronchiolitis, emphysema	• Obstruction if airway disease • Restriction with hypoxemia if pulmonary fibrosis hypoxemia
Gold: Jewelry, dentistry, medical, electronics, bullion	• Alveolar opacities along the bronchovascular bundles • Interstitial fibrosis • Bronchiolitis obliterans with organizing pneumonia	• Obstruction if airway disease • Restriction with hypoxemia if pulmonary fibrosis
Hard metal: Construction, shipbuilding, machines, saw and drill bits	• UIP or NSIP pattern • Bibasilar and subpleural distribution • Septal thickening and reticular fibrosis • Traction bronchiectasis and bronchiolectasis • Subpleural cysts and honeycombing	• Obstruction, restriction or mixed pattern • Decreased DLCO with hypoxemia if interstitial fibrosis
Iron: Iron ore mining, smelting, steel industry, welding	Widespread ill-defined centrilobular nodules or patchy areas of ground-glass attenuation without zonal predominance	• Restrictive, with or without hypoxemia and with normal or reduced DLCO
Lanthanides (rare earths): Wind turbines, electric vehicles, laser crystals, radar systems, movie or film projection	• Small reticulonodular infiltrates • Diffuse interstitial lung fibrosis • Emphysema	• Obstruction, restriction or mixed pattern • Hypoxemia with decreased DLCO if advanced
Titanium: Nanotechnology, jet engines, fan blades, missiles	• Reticulonodular infiltrates • Ground-glass opacities with peribronchial distribution • NSIP pattern	• Restriction • Hypoxemia with decreased DLCO
Zirconium: Anticorrosives, ceramics, die casting and mold coating, refractory paints, aerospace	• Bilateral irregular or ground-glass opacities • Pulmonary edema • Interstitial pneumonia with mild fibrosis • NSIP or HP pattern	• May be normal • Restriction with hypoxemia and reduced DLCO if fibrosis

(DLCO: diffusing capacity of the lungs for carbon monoxide; HP: hypersensitivity pneumonitis; HRCT: high-resolution computed tomography; IPF: idiopathic pulmonary fibrosis; NSIP: nonspecific interstitial pneumonia; UIP: usual interstitial pneumonia)

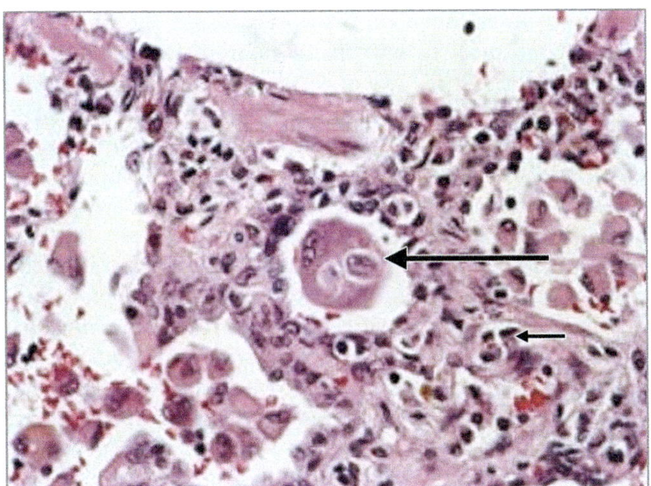

FIG. 2: Histopathologic appearance of giant cell interstitial pneumonia, showing giant cells (thick arrow) filling airspaces, with thickening of the interstitium and infiltration of the alveolar walls by mononuclear cells (thin arrow).

correlation with histological findings as well as follow up assessment.[22,26,27]

Definitive diagnosis of granulomatous lung disease is made on lung biopsy, for which endoscopic or surgical samples may be obtained. Typical histological findings include poorly formed noncaseating granulomas resembling those found in sarcoidosis in CBD or multinucleate giant cells in HMLD **(Fig. 2)**. Other histologic features include interstitial mononuclear cell infiltration **(Fig. 2)** with T-lymphocytic and/or histiocytic predominance, along with varying degrees of fibrosis.[22,26-28] In HMLD, sometimes, as was observed in tungsten workers in Japan, a usual interstitial pneumonia (UIP) pattern with predilection for upper lobe involvement on CT might be encountered; however, the remarkably classic histological pattern of GIP helps to differentiate it from UIP.[24]

DIAGNOSTIC APPROACH

A careful occupational and environmental history may implicate the etiologic metal involved. The history should include a listing of jobs that entailed metal dust or fume exposures, metals used, and conditions of exposure (use of respiratory protection and availability of exhaust ventilation). Knowledge of several unusual or unique occupational lung diseases should prompt questioning about a patient's occupational history, which may sometimes uncover an occupational rather than an idiopathic ILD.

The challenge lies in establishing a "cause-effect" relationship between metal exposure and lung disease.[4] This can be achieved by demonstration of metallic particles or content in lavage fluid or in biopsy specimens by particle analysis or spectrometry.[4,19,29,30] A diagnosis of metal-induced lung disease is consistent with suggestive histopathologic features which include patterns of desquamative interstitial pneumonia or hypersensitivity pneumonitis with acute or chronic inflammatory cell infiltrates centered predominantly around the bronchioles and varying degrees and extent of interstitial fibrosis in general, and the presence of giant cell interstitial pneumonia or sarcoid-like epithelioid granulomas in HMLD and CBD in particular. Alternatively, demonstration of specific immune reactions to the metal by patch testing for aluminum, beryllium, Co, gold, or zirconium exposure or in vitro lymphocyte proliferation tests for aluminum, beryllium, Co, gold, and titanium also serve to establish specific immune response. Interestingly, Co alone, instead of hard metal may be detected in approximately 10% of lung samples from patients with HMLD as shown in two studies and can be also be measured quantitatively in lavage due to its high solubility in body fluids.[19,26,31] Assessment of respiratory function by spirometry, lung volumes, and diffusion capacity is important in workers with a high occupational risk of exposure to metal particles and lung function tests play an important role in early detection, establishing respiratory dysfunction, classifying the extent and severity of disease, as well as follow-up and treatment monitoring.

Careful clinicoradiologic-histopathologic correlation is required before the diagnosis of metal-induced lung disease can be confidently made and is achieved by the following:[22,32]

- Established history of exposure (occupational, environmental, or otherwise) to metal dust or fluids
- Cough and dyspnea on exertion over a prolonged period
- Radiologic features suggestive of ILD or pneumoconiosis
- Histopathologic findings of ILD or a giant cell interstitial pneumonia pattern
- Demonstration of metallic particles in lung tissue or lavage fluid samples by electron microscopy and energy-dispersive X-ray fluorescence spectrometry techniques or by a combination of both, such as electron probe microanalysis wavelength-dispersive spectrometry (EPMA-WDS)

A relevant occupational or exposure, combined with lung function assessment and suggestive findings on chest HRCT and BAL are, in most cases, amply sufficient to establish the diagnosis. It is necessary to differentiate metal-induced lung disease from others with similar clinical and radiological manifestations; in this regard, tuberculosis and lung cancer are two important mimics with considerable clinical and radiological overlap which need to be kept in mind, particularly in the developing countries. A comprehensive history and diligent physical examination coupled with efforts directed toward establishing diagnosis of metal-induced lung disease through specific histopathological findings or other investigations should help considerably in resolving any diagnostic dilemma.

TREATMENT

There exists limited data to prove that reducing future exposure to metals positively affects the course of illness; nevertheless, doing so is considered medically prudent, as a few isolated case reports have shown symptomatic improvement and near-complete resolution of parenchymal abnormalities on HRCT within periods as short as 2 months and 2 years after the cessation of exposure, respectively, even in the absence of any concurrent therapy.[22] Medical treatment is indicated in symptomatic patients and is largely aimed at reducing lung inflammation and palliating the secondary consequences of hypoxemia, pulmonary hypertension, and right heart failure. Therapy is mainly directed at controlling the disease.

Treatment of metal fume fever is usually supportive with analgesics and antipyretics as most cases are self-limiting. Symptomatic patients of metal-induced ling disease can be treated with oral glucocorticosteroids (prednisolone or prednisone) starting with 0.5–1 mg/kg/day or every other day for 3–6 months, which is then tapered down to the lowest alternate-day dose needed to maintain symptomatic and physiologic improvement.[22] Inhaled corticosteroids (ICS) or oral corticosteroids and bronchodilators may be effective for disease associated with relatively mild symptoms and airway obstruction or inflammation and ICS may also be tried as maintenance therapy following a course of oral corticosteroids.[33,34] There are reports of successful treatment and considerable improvement with ICS alone.[33] Methotrexate may be tried in those who do not respond to prednisone or respond only at a dose associated with intolerable side effects, but it must be remembered that it itself may cause lung damage.[35] It can be started at the initial oral dose of 2.5–5 mg/week and subsequently increased up to 10–15 mg/week. Corticosteroids may then be tapered to the lowest dose that maintains improvement. Azathioprine has been tried in patients with disease progression despite corticosteroid therapy. Anti-TNF-α receptor blocker etanercept has the potential to inactivate mediators that participate in the development of fibrosis.[36]

Supplemental oxygen, limited use of diuretics, and angiotensin-converting enzyme inhibitors may be used to manage pulmonary hypertension and right-sided heart failure. Lung transplantation may be attempted as a last resort in symptomatic patients with severe progressive fibrotic lung disease in spite of optimal medical treatment and after cessation to exposure. Whole-lung lavage may be a viable treatment option in patients who develop alveolar proteinosis. Stressing the importance of and encouraging smoking and vaping cessation is of paramount importance in workers who smoke or vape. Pulmonary rehabilitation helps affected patients function with their impairment.

PREVENTION

Primary prevention (exposure reduction) and secondary prevention (relocation) form the mainstay of preventive strategies in metal-induced lung diseases. Primary prevention is the best treatment given our limited ability to halt or reverse the progression of disease once the patient has progressed to persistent inflammation and end-stage pulmonary fibrosis. Metal exposure must be eliminated or if this is not possible for any reason, at least it should be reduced on a priority basis. The best hope for prevention is to substitute safer working materials, encourage or enforce use of respirators or masks, limit the number of exposed workers, and implement industrial hygiene and environmental controls. All workers exposed to respirable metallic particles should be screened at the time of employment and regularly followed up for symptoms, along with physiological assessment by pulmonary function testing.[37] Reporting of occupational lung disease in metal workers should be made mandatory by legislative measures. Education about the hazards from exposure to metallic dust must be freely available to workers and employers, as well as healthcare providers. Screening and follow-up of metal workers should include a complete evaluation of respiratory complaints, smoking history, along with documentation and spirometric and radiographic data and the level of dust exposure.[38,39] Medical surveillance should also include information about the cumulative burden of disease which should be monitored over a period of time. Physicians who recognize metal-induced lung disease should also attempt to determine whether ongoing workplace exposure presents a continuing health risk to affected workers. Personal protective equipment and wet processes have been found effective in reducing deleterious effects of lung injury due to inhaled metallic particles and their salts.[39] Airborne levels of respirable dusts can be minimized by exhaust ventilation. In exposed workers who smoke or vape, emphasis on smoking and vaping cessation is of paramount importance.

SUMMARY

A myriad basket of risk factors are implicated in the pathogenesis of metal-induced lung disease. The clinical manifestations of metal-induced lung disease are diverse and may range from metal fume fever to occupational asthma to end-stage diffuse parenchymal fibrosing lung disease, all of which if left undetected or untreated, have the potential to lead to respiratory failure. Presence of a history of exposure to metals or their compounds, symptoms or clinical findings of lung disease, coupled with radiographic features and lung function impairment are sufficient to establish a working diagnosis of metal-induced lung disease. Treatment options include exposure and smoking cessation, corticosteroids, immunomodulators, and lung transplantation. Health standards should be established to protect workers employed in industries or occupations that pose a high risk of exposure to metals or their compounds. Engineering and administrative controls should focus toward enforcing best practices, such as periodic screening and assessment of workers at risk, monitoring and reducing exposure levels to safe limits, encouraging use of personal protective equipment such as masks and prompt treatment, as well as rehabilitation of those affected. Of key importance are strategies that promote understanding, early detection, and prevention of exposure to reduce their socioeconomic impact and health burden.

REFERENCES

1. Wyman AE, Hines SE. Update on metal-induced occupational lung disease. Curr Opin Allergy Clin Immunol. 2018;18(2):73-9.
2. Mayer A, Hamzeh N. Beryllium and other metal-induced lung disease. Curr Opin Pulm Med. 2015;21(2):178-84.
3. Nemery B. Metal toxicity and the respiratory tract. Eur Respir J. 1990;3(2):202-19.
4. Ruediger HW. Hard Metal Particles and Lung Disease: Coincidence or Causality? Respiration. 2000;67:137-8.
5. Roach K, Roberts J. A comprehensive summary of disease variants implicated in metal allergy. J Toxicol Environ Health B Crit Rev. 2022;25(6):279-341.
6. Walters GI, Robertson AS, Moore VC, et al. Cobalt asthma in metal-workers from an automotive engine valve manufacturer. Occup Med (Lond). 2014;64(5):358-64.
7. Fei Q, Weng X, Liu K, et al. The Relationship between Metal Exposure and Chronic Obstructive Pulmonary Disease in the General US Population: NHANES 2015-2016. Int J Environ Res Public Health. 2022;19(4):2085.
8. Kelleher P, Pacheco K, Newman L. Inorganic dust pneumonias: The metal-related parenchymal disorders. Environ Health Perspect. 2000,108:685-96.
9. Fontenot AP, Amicosante M. Metal induced diffuse lung disease. Semin Respir Crit Care Med. 2008;29(6):662-9.
10. Gupta A, Rosenman KD. Hypersensitivity pneumonitis due to metal working fluids: Sporadic or under reported? Am J Ind Med. 2006;49(6):423-33.
11. Fitzgerald DB, Popowicz ND, Joseph J, et al. Trace element levels in pleural effusions. Health Sci Rep. 2021;4(2):e262.
12. Nakano T, Ito T, Kanazawa M, et al. Pulmonary edema caused by inhalation of vapors from water-soluble paint. Acute Med Surg. 2018;5(4):337-41.
13. Bai KJ, Chuang KJ, Chen JK, et al. Alterations by Air Pollution in Inflammation and Metals in Pleural Effusion of Pneumonia Patients. Int J Environ Res Public Health. 2019;16(5):705.
14. Riccelli MG, Goldoni M, Poli D, et al. Welding Fumes, a Risk Factor for Lung Diseases. Int J Environ Res Public Health. 2020;17(7):2552.
15. Healy C, Munoz-Wolf N, Strydom J, et al. Nutritional immunity: the impact of metals on lung immune cells and the airway microbiome during chronic respiratory disease. Respir Res. 2021;22(1):133.
16. Newman LS, Lloyd J, Daniloff E. The natural history of beryllium sensitization and chronic beryllium disease. Environ Health Perspect. 1996;104:937-43.
17. Moriyama H, Kobayashi M, Takada T, et al. Two dimensional analysis of elements and mononuclear cells in hard metal lung disease. Am J Respir Crit Care Med. 2007;176:70-7.
18. Kumarguru BN, Natarajan M, Biligi DS, et al. Giant Cell Lesions of Lungs: A Histopathological and Morphometric Study of Seven Autopsy Cases. J Clin Diagn Res. 2015;9(11):EC12-6.
19. Naqvi AH, Hunt A, Burnett BR, et al. Pathologic spectrum and lung dust burden in giant cell interstitial pneumonia (hard metal disease/cobalt pneumonitis) review of 100 cases. Arch Environ Occup Health. 2008;63(2):51-70.
20. Callejón-Leblic B, Arias-Borrego A, Pereira-Vega A, et al. The Metallome of Lung Cancer and its Potential Use as Biomarker. Int J Mol Sci. 2019;20(3):778.
21. Huang HH, Huang JY, Lung CC, et al. Cell-type specificity of lung cancer associated with low-dose soil heavy metal contamination in Taiwan: an ecological study. BMC Public Health. 2013;13:330.
22. Sergio P, Ceruti M, Manotti L, et al. Hard metal lung disease: Unexpected CT findings. Indian J Radiol Imaging. 2017;27(2):256-9.
23. Khoor A, Roden AC, Colby TV, et al. Giant cell interstitial pneumonia in patients without hard metal exposure: analysis of 3 cases and review of the literature. Hum Pathol. 2016;50:176-82.
24. Tanaka J, Moriyama H, Terada M, et al. An observational study of giant cell interstitial pneumonia and lung fibrosis in hard metal lung disease. BMJ Open. 2014;4(3):e004407.
25. Zheng M, Marron RM, Sehgal S. Hard Metal Lung Disease: Update in Diagnosis and Management. Curr Pulmonol Rep. 2009;9:37-46.
26. Nemery B, Abraham JL. Hard metal lung disease: still hard to understand. Am J Respir Crit Care Med. 2007;176(1):2-3.
27. Dunlop P, Muller NL, Wilson J, et al. Hard metal lung disease: high resolution CT and histologic correlation of the initial findings and demonstration of interval improvement. J Thorac Imaging. 2005;20(4):301-4.
28. Choi JW, Lee KS, Chung MP, et al. Giant cell interstitial pneumonia: high-resolution CT and pathologic findings in four adult patients. Am J Radiol. 2005;184:268-72.
29. Broding HC, Michalke B, Goen T, et al. Comparison between exhaled breath condensate analysis as a marker for cobalt and tungsten exposure and biomonitoring in workers of a hard metal alloy processing plant. Int Arch Occup Environ Health. 2009;82(5):565-73.
30. Takada T, Moriyama H, Suzuki E. Elemental analysis of occupational and environmental lung diseases by electron probe microanalyzer with wavelength dispersive spectrometer. Respir Investig. 2014;52(1):5-13.
31. Abraham JL, Burnett BR, Hunt A. Development and use of a pneumoconiosis database of human pulmonary inorganic particulate burden in over 400 lungs. Scanning Microsc. 1991;5(1):95-104; 105-8.
32. Chong S, Lee KS, Chung MJ, et al. Pneumoconiosis: Comparison of Imaging and Pathologic Findings. Radiographics. 2006;26:59-77.
33. Nureki S, Miyazxaki E, Nishio S, et al. Hard metal lung disease successfully treated with inhaled corticosteroids. Intern Med. 2013;52(17):1957-61.
34. Sundaram P, Agrawal K, Mandke JV, et al. Giant cell pneumonitis induced by cobalt. Indian J Chest Dis Allied Sci. 2001;43(1):47-9.
35. Dawson JK, Quah E, Earnshaw B, et al. Does methotrexate cause progressive fibrotic interstitial lung disease? A systematic review. Rheumatol Int. 2021;41(6):1055-64.
36. Raghu G, Brown KK, Costabel U, et al. Treatment of idiopathic pulmonary fibrosis with etanercept: an exploratory, placebo-controlled trial. Am J Respir Crit Care Med. 2008;178(9):948-55.
37. Verougstraete V, Mallants A, Buchet JP, et al. Lung function changes in workers exposed to cobalt compounds: A 13 year follow-up. Am J Respir Crit Care Med. 2004;170(2):162-6.
38. Martyny JW, Hoover MD, Mroz MM, et al. Aerosols generated during beryllium machining. J Occup Environ Med. 2000;42(1):8-18.
39. Briffa J, Sinagra E, Blundell R. Heavy metal pollution in the environment and their toxicological effects on humans. Heliyon. 2020;6(9):e04691.

CHAPTER 97

Berylliosis

Clayton T Cowl

INTRODUCTION

Situated in the periodic table of elements as the lightest of the alkaline earth metals, beryllium has an atomic number of 4 and is considered the lightest of these metals. Although discovered in 1798 initially by Nicolas-Louis Vauquelin as a compound in an oxide form associated with beryl (an extremely hard compound of beryllium aluminum silicate from which gemstones such as emerald and aquamarine are included), the metal itself was identified by Friedrich Wöhler and Antoine Bussy in 1828 when they discovered that potassium could be utilized to reduce chloride from the compound and create the pure metal state.[1]

Beryllium has been used in a variety of industrial settings due to its light weight with just two-thirds the density of aluminum and its tensile strength at six times the stiffness of steel, and it is nonmagnetic. The United States is the largest producer of beryllium ore with additional sources coming from China, Mozambique, and Brazil. Other physical properties prompting its use included a high melting point as well as thermal and electrical conductivity.[2]

Often used as an alloy in military munitions with copper compounds, beryllium use escalated in the early 20th century including the lead-up to World War II. When it was shown to have a high neutron multiplication reaction at low neutron absorption rates, it became widely used as part of civilian nuclear reactors. The metal was also used for fluorescent lamp production using the compound beryllium oxide.[3]

Acute berylliosis, now considered rare and reported only from very concentrated exposures to beryllium compounds particularly within confined spaces or with industrial catastrophes, has been largely mitigated with the development of increased regulations and environmental hygiene standards. It was first noted in the early 1930s in Europe and in the United States by the 1940s as industrial uses expanded and wartime manufacturing was burgeoning. The acute form of the disease arose as a caustic irritant inhalation mostly affecting the upper respiratory tract but with prolonged or highly concentrated inhaled exposures could result in a diffuse parenchymal pneumonitis with bronchiolitis obliterans injury to the proximal and distal airways.[4]

Rather than acute beryllium-induced respiratory disease, more common are three major categories into which patients may be characterized: Specifically, those exposed to beryllium without sensitization, those with blood lymphocytes considered beryllium-sensitized without apparent pulmonary disease, and an entity referred to as chronic beryllium disease (CBD) that involves a cell-mediated hypersensitivity reaction to components of beryllium metal resulting in a chronic granulomatous inflammatory response, appearing very similar to sarcoidosis. It is hypothesized that clinically there is a spectrum of disease that begins with sensitization and progresses to more advanced disease.[5]

CLINICAL AND RADIOLOGICAL FEATURES

Early stages of CBD are often asymptomatic. Latency from initial exposure to actual symptom development has been reported to be as long as two decades.[6] Although lymph node, skin, and hepatic involvement have been reported, the respiratory system is the primary organ affected and is responsible for the vast majority of the morbidity and mortality of the condition. When symptoms do present, common nonspecific complaints are often the first clinical manifestation of this uncommon nonpneumoconiotic form of interstitial lung disease. Chronic cough, burning substernal discomfort, and dyspnea are most frequent in association with generalized fatigue, night sweats, unexplained weight loss, and joint and myofascial pain as the disease progresses.[7,8] As with all occupational or environmental lung diseases, the clinician must consider exposure history and obtain a detailed description of specific maneuvers of the individual's occupation, the amount of exposure, whether any form of personal protective equipment was worn, and if there were coworkers affected by similar symptoms.[9] When the history suggests the potential for beryllium exposure, obtaining a blood beryllium lymphocyte proliferation test can detect hypersensitivity to the metal and may be the first sign of CBD.[10] Physical examination may reveal advanced disease, particularly when consideration of CBD has been delayed due to the failure of considering workplace exposures. For example, Velcro crackles, digital clubbing, cyanosis, or even evidence for pulmonary artery hypertension and cor pulmonale may be detected as the disease progresses into more advanced stages and at that point can be associated with peripheral edema, hepatomegaly, and distention of neck veins from venous backflow.[11] Fever has been reported in some individuals with CBD.[12] Hyperuricemia, hypercalcemia, and nephrocalcinosis have also been noted.[13] Mild elevation in hepatic transaminases may occur in association with hepatic granulomas. Dermatologic manifestations may present as acute contact dermatitis from soluble beryllium salts, or in the case of some machinists and ceramic workers who have been reported to have sustained implantation of beryllium metal alloys or salts, a nodular scar or ulcer of the skin may result. Dermatopathology of these nodules reveals granulomatous change with sensitivity on lymphocyte proliferation testing. Mantoux and Kveim testing were negative in patients who were studied previously with these lesions. Local excision of the skin nodules appeared to be curative in cases reported.[14] Nodules, when present, may be noted on the hands, arms, and chest.

Wide variation in spirometric findings has been noted in cohorts of workers screened for the condition including normal, obstructive, restrictive, or mixed patterns, and either normal or reduced diffusing capacity for carbon monoxide (DLCO).[15,16] A widening alveolar-arterial (A–a) oxygen gradient with exercise, unexplained hypoxemia with exertion, or other ventilatory limitations may be the very earliest signs of abnormality in individuals developing CBD.[16]

Patients confirmed to have sensitivity to beryllium via the lymphocyte stimulation test should undergo flexible bronchoscopy to ascertain whether the individual has only sensitivity to the metal or actual CBD. Much like sarcoidosis, bronchoalveolar lavage (BAL) in individuals with CBD typically reveals significant CD4+ lymphocytosis and cells cultured with beryllium in the BAL lymphocyte proliferation test reveal an increased response.[7] Transbronchial lung biopsies are associated with granulomatous inflammation and when combined with sensitivity to beryllium on a blood or BAL lymphocyte proliferation test, a diagnosis of CBD can be confirmed.

Radiographically, the abnormalities of CBD are essentially identical to those of sarcoidosis and are often misdiagnosed when an occupational history is not obtained.[17] Common findings include round and/or reticular lesions spread diffusely in the pulmonary parenchyma, but in some cases are confined to the apical lung regions. Half of CBD cases demonstrate hilar adenopathy, but bulky lymphadenopathy is not typically noted. As the disease progresses, parenchymal retraction and fibrotic scarring may be observed on chest radiography or CT imaging. In more severe cases, mass-like conglomerations of granulomatous inflammation along with bullous emphysematous changes may be noted. Over time, severe fibrosis and pleural thickening may also be evident. Unlike sarcoidosis, spontaneous resolution of radiographic abnormalities seen in CBD have not been reported.[10] **Box 1** outlines general similarities and differences between sarcoidosis and CBD.

BOX 1 General patterns between sarcoidosis and chronic beryllium disease.

***Sarcoidosis*:**

- Precise exposure or environmental factors unclear
- Hilar and mediastinal adenopathy common
- Noncaseating granulomatous inflammation within lymph nodes and pulmonary parenchymal nodules
- Lymphocytic alveolitis with T-lymphocyte CD4/CD8 > 3.5 in more than half of cases
- Erythema nodosum
- Hypercalcemia
- Cardiac involvement
- Central nervous system dysfunction
- Hypercalcemia
- Bone abnormalities in chronic disease
- Parotid involvement
- Spontaneous radiographic resolution may occur
- Hepatic involvement
- Responsive to corticosteroids during active disease

***Chronic beryllium disease*:**

- Associated with occupational or environmental history of beryllium exposure
- Hilar adenopathy somewhat uncommon
- Diffuse round and reticular abnormalities appearing radiographically identical to sarcoidosis without massive lymphadenopathy occasionally seen in sarcoidosis
- Granulomatous inflammation present in biopsy specimens
- Long latency period between exposure and disease development
- Prevalence is low even in exposed populations (1–5%)
- Proliferative response to beryllium lymphocyte stimulation testing
- Responsive to corticosteroids during active disease

DIAGNOSIS

It is important to note that CBD cases have only been reported in individuals who have been documented to have had direct industrial exposures to the metal such as grinding, heating, abrading, or directly handling beryllium alloys, metals, salts, or oxides. Other individuals working in close proximity to beryllium compounds within an industrial environment or family members exposed to contaminated work clothes of individuals working in these environments have also been documented to have developed CBD. There have not been reported cases of CBD in people with nonindustrial exposure. In addition, the latency between initial beryllium exposure and development of disease averages 10 years in duration.[19] Because it remains unclear whether total cumulative exposure to beryllium or peak exposure concentration to the metal results in more significant disease, determining a safe and effective regulatory threshold for beryllium exposure continues to be debatable. The US Occupational Safety and Health Administration has mandated to employers a legal level of exposure to no more than 0.2 ug/m^3 of beryllium over an 8-hour time-weighted average or a short-term exposure limit of 2 μg/m^3 over a sampling time frame of 15 minutes.[20]

Interestingly, the prevalence of exposed workers who actually develop CBD is quite low, reported at 1–5%.[21] Since it is believed that only a small subset of exposed populations actually develop CBD, a genetic component to development has been hypothesized.[22] Additionally, it is believed that an immunologic reaction to beryllium is what instigates development of CBD based on studies that looked at skin patch testing after which a delayed-type hypersensitivity phenomenon was noted in patients with documented CBD, that there exists a granulomatous response in individuals with CBD, and that sensitization can be reliably reproduced in animal models and the sensitivity can be transferred to animals without prior beryllium exposure.[23]

Confirmatory diagnosis of CBD involves both demonstration of granulomatous involvement in the pulmonary parenchyma or other tissues and measurement of beryllium sensitivity measured by a beryllium lymphocyte proliferation test. Use of cells from BAL fluid is preferred, but blood proliferation testing levels may also be utilized. Of note, availability of laboratories offering the beryllium lymphocyte proliferation test is scarce.

TREATMENT

In most cases, given the detection of CBD in its earlier stages, use of corticosteroids for affected individuals with subpar pulmonary function or progressive respiratory deterioration has been effective in controlling disease symptoms and radiographic abnormalities tend to resolve over weeks to months.[24] Due to known untoward side effects of corticosteroids, it is recommended that dosing of steroids be tapered to the lowest effective level with close clinical monitoring of radiographic imaging, spirometry, and clinical symptoms. In cases of progressive, corticosteroid-resistant cases of CBD, use of steroid-sparing immunosuppressive agents such as methotrexate and azathioprine may be considered. Lung transplantation for individuals with end-stage pulmonary disease may be considered if other contraindications are not present. Patients with CBD require lifelong surveillance testing and clinical follow-up.

BERYLLIUM EXPOSURE AND LUNG CANCER RISK

There remains controversy as to whether occupational exposure to beryllium results in development of lung cancer in humans, noting that beryllium has been described as a human carcinogen based upon animal models and some epidemiologic studies.

Lung cancer incidence was noted to be greater among cohorts of individuals with either acute or chronic beryllium disease within a registry model. A cohort mortality study involving 689 patients in a registry with confirmed beryllium disease that included females and more than a decade of follow-up showed a standardized mortality ratio (SMR) of 2.00 (95% confidence interval = 1.33–2.89) based on 28 observed lung cancer deaths that remained unchanged after adjusting for prior tobacco abuse/dependence. Lung cancer excess was consistent for both sexes and did not appear to increase with duration of exposure to beryllium or with time elapsed since the first exposure to this element. However, the number of individuals noted to have acute beryllium disease was higher compared to CBD (SMR = 2.32 vs. 1.57).[25]

A separate historical cohort study of more than 16,000 workers employed between 1925 and 2008 at 15 different facilities focused on whether mortality among workers was more significant with insoluble versus soluble beryllium compounds. Interestingly, employment in plants with soluble beryllium compound exposures was associated with increased mortality only among workers hired prior to 1955 and there was no trend with duration of employment. Retrospectively, mortality from CBD increased among individuals hired prior to that time within beryllium facilities handling soluble and mixed beryllium. There was no increase in lung cancer mortality when the entire cohort was taken into consideration and lung cancer motility was not increased within the cohort of workers hired in 1955 or later within facilities handling soluble beryllium or at any time within facilities handling insoluble beryllium.[26]

After adjustment for confounding variables, a slight increase in lung cancer mortality across various exposure categories was noted within two different lower exposure beryllium plants for individuals employed at the facilities between 1940 and 2005.[27] It has been hypothesized that excess mortality has been present primarily among workers employed within the early phase of the beryllium manufacturing industry that included the time frame from the 1920s through the mid-1950s, noting that there had been no relationship between duration of employment and cumulative exposure, but both average and maximum exposures to the metal were associated with a higher cancer risk.[28] Increased incidence of lung cancer may be elevated even at the current exposure limits of 2.0 μg/m^3 8-hour weighted average as mandated by the US Occupational Safety and Health Administration, but a direct causal effect has not been proven for those levels in humans.[29]

PREVENTION

Avoidance is the primary strategy for minimizing health effects of beryllium or its compounds. Increased regulation and aggressive screening programs have been effective in attenuating the prevalence of significant respiratory impairment. Comprehensive preventive programs have been introduced by several large producers of beryllium and beryllium-related products that include an emphasis on respiratory and dermal protection, use of engineering controls including improved ventilatory processes, dust mitigation through filtration and improved air flows, and educating workers and their supervisors within high-risk areas of production facilities.[30]

SUMMARY

Acute beryllium disease is rarely if ever seen today but CBD continues to be diagnosed in certain workers with prior industrial exposures. Latency for beryllium-related disease development is typically more than one decade, and the clinical findings mimic sarcoidosis radiographically. Use of the beryllium lymphocyte stimulation test is useful as part of the diagnostic assessment. If diagnosed relatively early after clinical manifestations arise, injured individuals often respond to protracted courses of oral corticosteroids. Although risk for lung cancer has been pointed out in animal models and some epidemiological studies involving current or prior beryllium exposure as being increased, a direct causal relationship between CBD and lung cancer continues to be debated. Prevention strategies have been highly successful in reducing prevalence of the disease, including implementation of engineering controls and personal protective equipment in at risk workers.

REFERENCES

1. Kolanz ME. Introduction to beryllium: uses, regulatory history, and disease. Appl Occup Environ Hyg. 2001;16(5):559-67.
2. Armiento G, Bellatreccia F, Cremisini C, et al. Beryllium natural background concentration and mobility: a reappraisal examining the case of high Be-bearing pyroclastic rocks. Environ Monit Assess. 2013;185(1):559-72.
3. National Center for Biotechnology Information. PubChem Element Summary for Atomic Number 4, Beryllium. https://pubchem.ncbi.nlm.nih.gov/element/Beryllium. [Last accessed July 2, 2024].
4. Mayer A, Hamzeh N. Beryllium and other metal-induced lung disease. Curr Opin Pulm Med. 2015;21(2):178-84.
5. Newman LS, Mroz MM, Balkissoon R, et al. Beryllium sensitization progresses to chronic beryllium disease: a longitudinal study of disease risk. Am J Respir Crit Care Med. 2005;171(1):54-60.
6. Williams WJ. Beryllium disease. Postgrad Med J. 1988;64:511-6.
7. Maier LA. Clinical Approach to Chronic Beryllium Disease and Other Nonpneumoconiotic Interstitial Lung Diseases. J Thorac Imaging. 2002;17(4):273-84.
8. Tepper LB, Hardy H, Chamberlin RI. Toxicity of beryllium compounds. In: Browning E (Ed). Elsevier Monographs on Toxic Agents. Amsterdam: Elsevier; 1961. pp. 1-190.
9. Middleton DC. Chronic beryllium disease: uncommon disease, less common diagnosis. Environ Health Perspect. 1998;106(12): 765-7.
10. Newman LS. Significance of the blood beryllium lymphocyte proliferation test. Environ Health Perspect. 1996;104(Suppl 5): 953-6.
11. Freiman DG, Hardy HL. Beryllium disease. The relation of pulmonary pathology to clinical course and prognosis based on a study of 130 cases from the U.S. beryllium case registry. Hum Pathol. 1970;1(1):25-44.
12. Rossman MD. Chronic beryllium disease: diagnosis and management. Environ Health Perspect. 1996;104(Suppl 5): 945-7.
13. Kelley WN, Goldfinger SE, Hardy HL. Hyperuricemia in chronic beryllium disease. Ann Intern Med. 1969;70(5):977-83.
14. Cummings KJ, Deubner DC, Day GA, et al. Enhanced preventive programme at a beryllium oxide ceramics facility reduces beryllium sensitisation among new workers. Occup Environ Med. 2007;64(2):134-40.
15. Andrews JL, Kazemi K, Hardy HL. Patterns of lung dysfunction in chronic beryllium disease. Am Rev Respir Dis. 1969;100(6): 791-800.
16. Pappas GP, Newman LS. Early pulmonary physiologic abnormalities in beryllium disease. Am Rev Respir Dis. 1993;148(3): 661-6.
17. Fireman E, Haimsky E, Noiderfer M, et al. Misdiagnosis of sarcoidosis in patients with chronic beryllium disease. Sarcoidosis Vasc Diffuse Lung Dis. 2003;20(2):144-8.
18. Sharma N, Patel J, Mohammed TL. Chronic beryllium disease: computed tomographic findings. J Comput Assist Tomogr. 2010;34(6):945-8.
19. Eisenbud M, Lisson J. Epidemiological aspects of beryllium-induced nonmalignant lung disease: a 30-year update. J Occup Med. 1983;25(3):196-202.
20. Occupational Safety & Health Administration (OSHA). Code of Federal Regulations, Part 1910.1024. Beryllium. [online] Available from https://www.osha.gov/laws-regs/regulations/standardnumber/1910/1910.1024AppA [Last accessed June, 2024].
21. Balmes JR, Abraham JL, Dweik RA, et al. An official American Thoracic Society statement: diagnosis and management of beryllium sensitivity and chronic beryllium disease. Am J Respir Crit Care Med. 2014;190(10):e34-59.
22. Richeldi L, Sorrentino R, Saltini C. HLA-DPB1 glutamate 69: a genetic marker of beryllium disease. Science. 1993;262(5131): 242-4.
23. Alekseeva OG. Study of the ability of beryllium compounds to produce delayed type allergy. Gig Tr Prof Zabol. 1965;9(11):20-5.

SECTION 9: ENVIRONMENTAL AND OCCUPATIONAL DISORDERS

24. Sood A. Current treatment of chronic beryllium disease. J Occup Environ Hyg. 2009;6(12):762-5.
25. Steenland K, Ward E. Lung cancer incidence among patients with beryllium disease: a cohort mortality study. J Natl Cancer Inst. 1991;83(19):1380-5.
26. Boffetta P, Fordyce TA, Mandel JS. A mortality study of beryllium workers. Cancer Med. 2016;5(12):3596-605.
27. Schubauer-Berigan MK, Couch JR, Deddens JA. Is beryllium-induced lung cancer caused only by soluble forms and high exposure levels? Occup Environ Med. 2017;74(8):601-3.
28. Boffetta P, Fryzek JP, Mandel JS. Occupational exposure to beryllium and cancer risk: a review of the epidemiologic evidence. Crit Rev Toxicol. 2012;42(2):107-18.
29. Schubauer-Berigan MK, Deddens JA, Couch JR, et al. Risk of lung cancer associated with quantitative beryllium exposure metrics within an occupational cohort. Occup Environ Med. 2011;68(5):354-60.
30. Thomas CA, Deubner DC, Stanton ML, et al. Long-term efficacy of a program to prevent beryllium disease. Am J Ind Med. 2013;56(7):733-41.

The Health Risks of Asbestos Fiber Inhalation

CHAPTER 98

Jessica R Deslauriers, Harakh V Dedhia, Daniel E Banks†*

INTRODUCTION

The term "asbestos" describes six different occurring fibrous crystals (crocidolite, amosite, chrysotile, anthophyllite, tremolite, and actinolite) with a great number of industrial uses. An association between environmental or occupational exposure to asbestos and the occurrence of chest diseases is well established and reported **(Box 1)**.

The relationship of workplace asbestos exposure to alterations in the pleura and to the development of mesothelioma, lung cancer, and asbestosis has been clarified in the past decades. Although the case in nearly all instances, direct occupational exposure is not necessary for disease. Unrecognized asbestos exposure may be indirect, occurring in the construction industry, the shipyards, or asbestos workers' homes. Of particular importance is the latency period between exposure and clinically detectable disease, usually exceeding 20 years. When these illnesses are under consideration, a detailed occupational, environmental, and family history is necessary to recognize the role of asbestos exposure in disease.

During the second half of the last century, diseases associated with asbestos fiber inhalation, such as asbestosis, lung cancer, and mesothelioma, dramatically declined in populations at risk. This decline in the rate of diagnosis of asbestosis has occurred despite an increase in life expectancy. For example, in 1950, 40-year-old white men in the United States were projected to live 31.2 more years. In 2011, this same population had a projected survival of 38.6 years. Non-white men in this age group had a projected survival of 27.3 and 35.5 years at these points in time, respectively.[1] With this increase in life expectancy comes the associated increase in the latency period. It is reasonable to expect that workers with asbestos exposure would have a longer time to first develop disease and second progress to more severe disease. Workers at risk for mesothelioma would also have a longer time to develop this illness, and one would reasonably expect that this illness would likely occur more frequently. Similarly, those with asbestos exposure with the greatest risk for lung cancer, cigarette smokers, would have a prolonged time to develop lung cancer, even after they stopped smoking. With these insights, if asbestos exposures had remained the same, these additional years of survival measured in this population would have resulted in more frequent and more severe dust-induced chest illnesses.

What caused this dramatic lessening in the number of cases of asbestosis? Regulatory agencies have become sensitized to the adverse respiratory effects of asbestos exposure and responded by lessening permissible exposure limits (PELs) and enforcing these standards. This has resulted in a substantial decrease (typically of several orders of magnitude) in respirable exposures. These lesser exposures are reflected in longer survival. Although there are no reports which clearly identify the prevalence of asbestos-related illnesses which are truly "representative" of a generation of workers, we have taken the liberty to cite several studies which may be considered "representative" of the decade(s) that the workers were employed, the year of publication, and the risk for asbestosis as reflected in the exposures of the time. These reports show the dramatic decline in asbestosis **(Fig. 1)**.

Decisions made by governmental agencies regarding standard setting have been driven by epidemiologic studies as well as asbestos importation/production policies. These studies have used years of employment and dust measurements as dependent variables and the development

BOX 1 Asbestos-related pulmonary effects.

- Asbestosis (asbestos pneumoconiosis)
- Pleural plaques
- Pleural effusion (benign)
- Diffuse pleural thickening
- Pleural mesothelioma
- Lung cancer

*Deceased.

†The authors are employees of the US government. This work was prepared as part of their official duties. The views expressed herein are their own and do not reflect the official policy or position of the US Government.

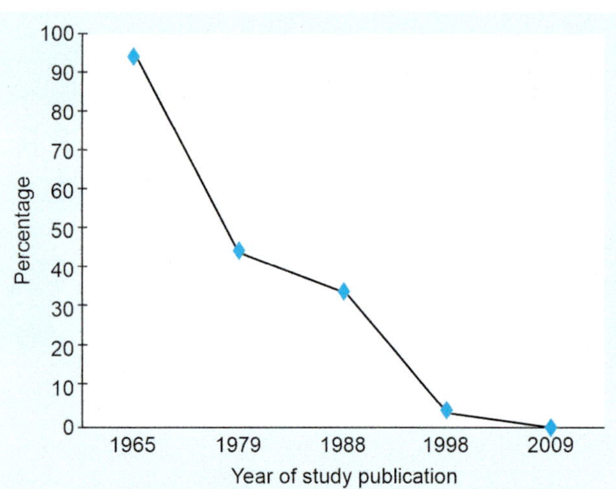

FIG. 1: Percent prevalence of asbestosis in selected cross-sectional studies by decade. The following cross-sectional studies were cited to plot the change in the prevalence of asbestosis in specific working populations by decade.

Note:

- *1965*: In a population of 121 asbestos workers with a 40-year latency of asbestos exposure, 94.2% had a radiologic diagnosis of asbestosis. (Selikoff IJ, Churg J, Hammond EC. The occurrence among insulation workers in the United States. Ann NY Acad Sci. 1965;132:139-55.)
- *1979*: In 359 present and retired shipyard workers with ≥10 years of exposure, 44% had parenchymal interstitial disease. (Polakoff PL, Horn BR, Scherer OR. Prevalence of radiographic abnormalities among northern California shipyard workers. Ann N Y Acad Sci. 1979;330:333-9.)
- *1988*: In 1,016 workers in the sheet metal industry employed > 35 years, parenchymal interstitial fibrosis (consistent with asbestosis) was diagnoses in 33.1%. (Selikoff IJ, Lilis R. Radiological abnormalities among sheet metal workers in the construction industry in the United States and Canada: relationship to asbestos exposure. Arch Environ Health. 1991;46:30-6.)
- *1998*: In electricians with >20 years of union membership, the prevalence of small opacities was 2.1%. (Hessel PA, Melenka LS, Michaelchuk D, et al. Lung health among electricians in Edmonton, Alberta, Canada. J Occup Environ Med. 1998;40:1007-12.)
- *2009*: In a follow-up from the 1988 study cited above, 2181 sheet-metal workers with a negative chest radiograph for pneumoconiosis in the initial study were retested from 1986 to 2004. 5.3% had radiographic changes consistent with asbestosis. Of those with a positive radiograph, 91.3% worked ≥29 years. No worker who began employment after 1970 had parenchymal interstitial fibrosis (consistent with asbestosis). The data point of zero prevalence is plotted above. (Welch LS, Halle E. Asbestos-related disease among sheet-metal workers 1986-2004: radiographic changes over time. Am J Ind Med. 2009;52:519-22.)

of disease {as manifest by decrements in lung function tests [typically, forced expiratory volume in 1 second (FEV_1) and forced vital capacity (FVC)] and chest radiographic abnormalities [as interpreted by the International Labour Organization (ILO) classification]} as outcomes. The understanding that these variables determine outcomes in a relatively predictable manner (i.e., dose-dependent) is a key to protecting the worker. Using these data, workers have been protected (as shown by the relatively recent decline in mortality). Yet, these same summaries by governmental agencies reflect the long-term continuing adverse effects of dust exposure on the American worker **(Fig. 2)**.

Asbestos has not been mined in the United States since 2002. The United States is dependent on imports to meet manufacturing needs. In 2022, US asbestos consumption was estimated to be 260 tons, a 75% decrease during the past decade. Most of this is used in the chlor-alkali industry to manufacture semipermeable diaphragms.[2] Asbestos mining in India has also stopped over the past decade, with no working mines reported in 2020.[3] Asbestos consumption in India has also decreased, reported as 350,000 metric tons in 2017.[4] A great percentage of asbestos used in India is mixed with cement to form roofing sheets. Though asbestos is a known carcinogen, India remains the second highest asbestos consumer globally.

Our challenge is to know about illnesses so we may detect them early. We need to be able to educate potentially exposed workers and their families about the health risks of asbestos. Prevention of these illnesses is best accomplished by eliminating asbestos from the workplace. If this cannot be accomplished, we must limit asbestos exposure through appropriate engineering controls.

ASBESTOS FIBERS

Asbestos is classified as serpentine or amphibole, based on structural and chemical properties. Chrysotile is a serpentine asbestos which accounts for 95% of world production. The fibers are long, silky, pliable, and heat resistant but poorly resistant to sea water and chemical digestion. Because of its flexibility, it is commonly woven into textiles. The larger deposits are in Russia's Ural Mountains and in Quebec, although some deposits are found in Vermont, USA. The category of amphibole asbestos fibers, in contrast to serpentine, is straight and rod-like and resistant to acids, heat, and alkali. Crocidolite, amosite, and anthophyllite are the common commercial varieties of amphiboles. Crocidolite and amosite have been mined in South Africa, and anthophyllite is found in Finland. In Quebec, the asbestos deposit contains 99% chrysotile and 1% tremolite, making this deposit unique. Chrysotile, crocidolite, and amosite are the most used fibers. Among the three amphiboles, anthophyllite is used least due to its short and brittle nature.[5]

A summary of the uses of asbestos throughout time is of interest.[6] Asbestos was first used in industrial applications around 1870. Since then, world annual asbestos production increased until it approximated 5 million tons in 1975, the year of peak production. Since then, the health effects have been better understood and production has declined by approximately 60%. Estimated worldwide utilization of asbestos fibers decreased from approximately 2 million tons in 2010 to roughly 1.2 million tons annually over the past several years.[7] Asbestos mining is typically an open pit operation where mechanical shovels and bulldozers mine and then load trucks or train cars with the mined product for transport to a processing mill. The raw material is further processed by fracturing, sorting, and screening to separate the asbestos from undesired ores. Milling further concentrates

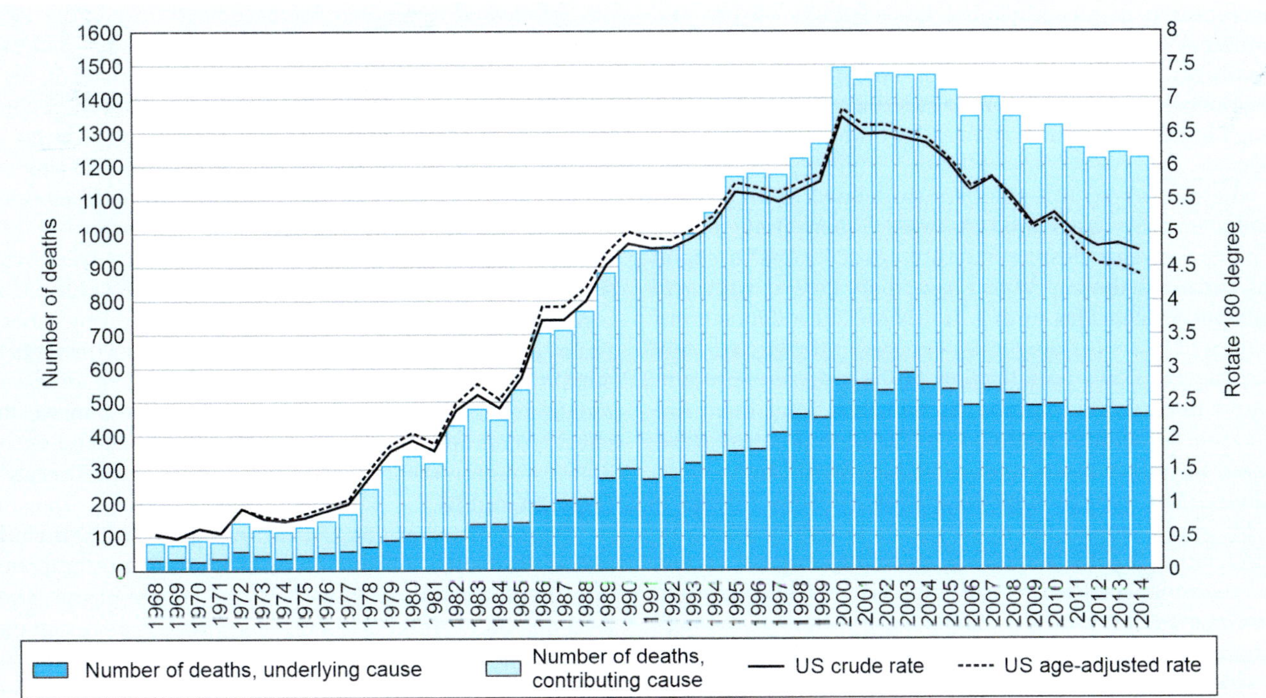

FIG. 2: Data from the US National Institute for Occupational Safety and Health (NIOSH) show a continuing adverse effect of asbestos dust exposures on the health of the American worker. Although the attributable mortality rates have declined over time, asbestos exposure continues to adversely affect worker productivity and lifespan.

Source: NIOSH Work-Related Lung Disease (WoRLD) surveillance system. (2017). Asbestosis: Number of deaths, crude and age-adjusted death rates, U.S. residents aged 15 and over, 1968–2014. [online] Available from https://wwwn.cdc.gov/eWorld/Data/Asbestosis_Number_of_deaths_crude_and_age-adjusted_death_rates_US_residents_age_15_and_over_19682010/915 [Last accessed June, 2024].

the fibers by eliminating contaminants and allows for sorting fibers by types and quality.

Although many manufactured products are composed of multiple fiber types, the longest asbestos fibers are used mainly for textiles and insulation, the intermediate length fibers are used in asbestos cement production and friction and filter production, and the shortest fibers are used in the vinyl asbestos tiles and as an admixture to industrial paints. Mill tailings from the mining process have been used in road construction. In the past decades, the major end users have been the construction, shipbuilding, and automobile and railroad equipment industry. Today, much of the insulation and friction materials are made of nonasbestos replacement fiber materials.

Potential work exposures occur during mining, milling, handling, and manufacturing processes. Asbestos is virtually indestructible and remains in the environment indefinitely. Once the fibers are incorporated into a manufactured item, there is little health risk unless the item is disrupted. Additional work exposures can occur during the destruction of previously manufactured material associated with building renovation or demolition (asbestos abatement).

Parenchymal Penetration by Fibers

Asbestos fibers which are not cleared by airway cilia penetrate deep into the lung parenchyma. Fiber deposition in the lung is largely ruled by fiber diameter, with fiber length being less important. Crocidolite, the thinnest, penetrates deepest, anthophyllite, the widest in diameter, penetrates least; amosite is intermediate in size and penetration. While the chrysotile fiber is long, despite the similarity in diameter to crocidolite, penetration is less due to its curly, serpentine shape. Typically, fibers with diameters >5 μm do not penetrate in the lower lung but those less than this may penetrate deeply and enter cell membranes to be carried within macrophages into the interstitium and pleural space. The length of the fiber is also important. Fibers 200–300 μm long can be found in the lung as their diameter is <5 μm. Fibers <3 μm in length can be phagocytosed and carried to the lymphatic vessels to be drained, whereas those longer than 5 μm are incompletely phagocytosed and remain in the tissue, sustaining the cellular and molecular events leading to disease.

Long fibers are cleared less rapidly than short fibers.[8] For example, fibers that are most carcinogenic for the development of mesothelioma have lengths >8 μm and diameters <0.25 μm.[9] Crocidolite is about 10 times more carcinogenic than chrysotile for mesothelial cells and crocidolite fibers are more prone to induce pleural fibrosis.[10] Lung fibrosis, however, is affected by both types of asbestos fibers.

The lung's response to fibers embedded in lung tissue results in asbestos-related disease. Fibers may remain in place for years despite macrophage attempts to engulf and surround them.[11] With time, fibers coated with acid mucopolysaccharides form a matrix for "iron deposition." Coating of fibers is thought to decrease fibrogenicity. Light microscopy allows visualization of these ferritin-protein-coated fibers which appear as relatively long bead-like structure. Sometimes referred to as "asbestos bodies," these coated fibers are more appropriately termed "ferruginous bodies." The typical fiber length of asbestos bodies is 20–50 μm, although fibers <5 μm in length can also be found. Other inhaled fibers (e.g., talc, fibrous glass, cotton, and diatomaceous earth) are handled in a like manner. Thus, coated fibers are not diagnostic of asbestos, although ferruginous bodies have most commonly been found to have an asbestos core.[12]

Although ferruginous bodies can be found in the lung tissue of virtually all of us, identifying these fibers in digested tissue, sputum, and cells garnered by lung lavage may provide a fundamental index of asbestos exposure.[13,14] In the sputum of asbestos workers, the quantity of ferruginous bodies present has been correlated with the duration of asbestos exposure.[15] Ninety-six percent of urban dwellers over the age of 40 years had ferruginous bodies present in their lungs. The number of ferruginous bodies has been shown to be greater in the lungs of blue-collar workers and, in particular, steel workers.[16]

Asbestos fibers induce fibrosis of the lung and cancers of the lung and pleura.[17,18]

Fibrosis begins as an inflammatory reaction which evokes a repair process, resulting in persistent scarring. Cancers begin as a multistep process in which the target cell deoxyribonucleic acid (DNA) suffers increasing amounts of damage (genetic mutations) through a variety of molecular injuries.[19] Experimental animal studies and in vitro studies of cell cultures have shown that all types of asbestos fibers can cause cell damage which, if sufficiently severe, results in cell death, gene mutation, chromosomal aberration, aneuploidies, and malignant cell transformation.[20]

ASBESTOSIS

In the US, although the prevalence of asbestos-related diseases has become less over time, health issues continue to be recognized, particularly in the older or retired worker. In a report from the 1990s, mortality from asbestosis peaked 40–45 years after the workers' initial occupational exposure to asbestos.[21] As noted above, asbestos consumption increased substantially during and after World War II, with a peak in 1975, followed by a steep decrease beginning in the 1980s, yet asbestosis-related mortality has persisted.[22] Asbestos-containing materials that continue to be used in some workplaces and material already in place which becomes disturbed represent risks for the current generation. All personal exposure limit (PEL) determinations and exposure regulations are directed toward preventing the development of asbestosis and not other manifestations of exposure.

The term "asbestosis" refers only to parenchymal fibrosis associated with asbestos exposure. The chronic and progressive inflammation and injury produced by asbestos fibers continues from the time of exposure, through the subclinical phase, to the time when clinical disease is identifiable by the classic methods of lung function testing, chest radiography, and more sophisticated imaging such as high-resolution computerized tomography (HRCT) scan[23,24] **(Figs. 3A and B)**.

Signs and symptoms of asbestosis are those of the other diffuse interstitial fibrotic diseases but may not be present or only minimally noted early in the course of the illness. Dyspnea on exertion is the usual symptom of presentation, which worsens as the disease progresses and lung function declines. Nonproductive cough and chest pain are present in some cases but occur late in the disease. When the cough is productive, it is likely attributable to bronchitis. Chest tightness and chest discomfort can be attributed to muscle pain appearing only when the cough and the dyspnea become severe. Hemoptysis is not expected and should be fully investigated as it suggests lung carcinoma. These symptoms may occur during the working years or even begin after exposure has ceased, becoming clinically apparent only after retirement.[25]

Persistent crackles are the most important physical finding. They are a clinical indication that disease is present and their appearance coincides with detectable changes in lung function and chest radiograph abnormalities, in most cases. They are typically first heard in the lower posterior and lateral lung fields in the late-inspiratory phase and, as the disease progresses, increase in amount to become audible in the mid and late phases of inspiration. Other adventitious sounds are usually absent. Finger clubbing may be present but does not necessarily relate to asbestosis severity. Cyanosis and reduced chest expansion are late manifestations of the disease.

The diagnosis of asbestosis has three requirements:

1. A duration of exposure and latency period sufficient to explain these features
2. Chest radiographic features consistent with asbestosis
3. The absence of other illnesses which might explain the radiologic features[26,27]

Neither the presence of respiratory symptoms nor abnormalities in physiologic testing are necessary to make the diagnosis of asbestosis, although there is little question that the addition of this clinical evidence increases the strength of the argument that asbestosis is present. Only in

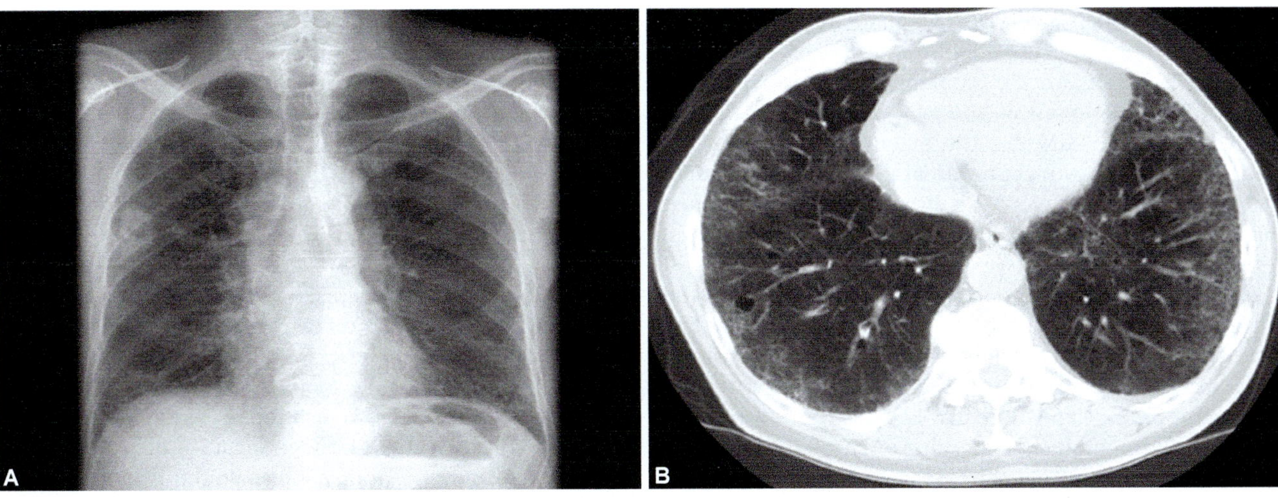

FIGS. 3A AND B: Chest X-ray and CT scan of a 71-year-old man with a lung nodule. (A) The chest radiograph shows increased interstitial lung markings at both bases. Mild honeycombing was noted. A cavitary mass is noted in the right upper zone. (B) Slices from the CT scan show fibrotic changes consistent with asbestosis

BOX 2 Clinical manifestations seen in some patients with asbestosis.

- Subjective respiratory complaints
- Restrictive pulmonary function tests (FVC <80% predicted)
- Finger clubbing
- Basilar crepitations
- Chest radiograph with increased basilar lung markings
- Known asbestos exposure

(FVC: forced vital capacity)

the rarest of occasions is an open lung biopsy with assessment of the mineral content of the lung necessary for the diagnosis. Disability determination is made on a clinical basis in the absence of tissue diagnosis. It is not an indication for biopsy (**Box 2**).

The meaning of the term "sufficient exposure and latency period" has changed over the past 75 years, beginning when epidemiologic studies on populations of asbestos workers were first reported. The driving determinant of change has been the recognition that exposures need to be monitored and the initiation and enforcement of a protective PEL established by federal agencies throughout the world. In the US, this has decreased over time and the allowable exposures have become less. Yet, based on changes in exposure limits, absolute values describing a "sufficient exposure and latency period" cannot be presented, but the decline in asbestosis in populations where exposure has been recognized suggests that the regulations have been effective, and the evaluating physician may need to consider greater years of exposures and longer latency periods than previously. As a practical consideration, in 1997, the Helsinki Criteria stated that the latency period must be at least 10 years.[28] In the absence of recognized persistent excessive exposures, the development of disease may require a working lifetime of exposure in a workplace where asbestos exposure has been recognized to explain the illness. Yet, cases may even develop after "a working lifetime." Follow-up evaluations may need to go for additional years as a worker who had no radiographic evidence of asbestosis after 30 years of work, may retire, and then be recognized to have this disease several years later.[29]

The chest radiograph classically shows irregular basilar opacities which, in time, may progress to honeycombing. The radiographic specificity for asbestosis, which may be identical to other diffuse fibrotic processes, is enhanced when bilateral pleural thickening and, in particular, pleural calcification accompany basal parenchymal fibrosis. In the United States, examinations are used to test physician proficiency in interpreting chest radiographs of individuals with suspected lung disease due to dust inhalation.[30]

High-resolution computed tomography scan has not been shown to be justified as a screening tool in the evaluation of the presence or absence of interstitial disease in asbestos-exposed workers, but it has a place in the clinical investigation of these individuals. For example, it can better define pleural-based abnormalities and interstitial changes compared to the chest radiograph or routine chest tomography. When lung cancer or mesothelioma is considered, the HRCT scan better defines the anatomic extension of disease. Compared to the conventional CT scan, HRCT scan has improved our assessment of the interstitium and allows us to better appreciate interstitial and emphysematous changes.[31]

A decline in diffusing capacity is the most sensitive measurement of asbestos effect. Decrement in FEV_1, peak flow rate, and pO_2 are less sensitive and may show little change over time.[32] Yet, when asbestosis becomes clinically important, it is classically associated with restriction of lung volumes [total lung capacity (TLC) <80% predicted]. These other physiologic parameters, as well as the rate of FVC decline, become more pronounced as the disease progresses. Although a decrease in small airway flow rates due to peribronchial accumulation of asbestos fibers with associated fibrosis may occur, smoking plays an independent role in the development of airway obstruction in heavily exposed workers.[33] Grossly, the extent of fibrosis in the asbestotic lung varies from minimal amounts at the bases (in a subpleural distribution) to a diffusely fibrotic, shrunken lung. Progressive massive fibrosis occurs rarely and, if present, suggests mixed dust exposure.

Microscopically, asbestosis is fibrosis associated with asbestos bodies (visualized by light microscopy) or uncoated asbestos fibers (identified by transmission electron microscopy). Both fibers and fibrosis must be present. Dust accumulation and fibrosis occur at the level of the respiratory bronchiole and may have features thought to sometimes be consistent with respiratory bronchiolitis. The alveolar septae become thickened and infiltrated with mononuclear cells, neutrophils, and macrophages. With progression, diffuse alveolar wall thickening occurs with replacement of parenchyma by connective tissue. The extent and prominence of fibrosis correlates with other parameters of disease severity, such as the progressive radiographic changes and worsening lung function tests.[34]

The most likely respiratory illness which can be mistaken for asbestosis is idiopathic pulmonary fibrosis (IPF). In addressing this, the occupational and environmental exposure history is of great importance. In addition, there are several histologic differences aside from the absence of asbestos fibers in IPF. First, the interstitial fibrosis of asbestosis is accompanied by very little inflammation; second, the fibroblastic foci identified in IPF, a disease typically more rapidly progressive than asbestosis, are absent in asbestosis; and third, asbestosis is very often accompanied by fibrosis of the visceral pleura, a feature that is not a part of IPF.[35]

MEDICAL REMOVAL PROTECTION/ EXPOSURE PREVENTION

Does removing the worker with asbestosis from the work environment affect progression? Once recognized, asbestosis can be a chronic and progressive disease. Yet, the evolution of asbestosis has changed significantly since the original report in 1907 by Murray who reported 10 workers with asbestosis who died before the age of 30 years.[36] In 1965, asbestos exposure in a population of Corsican miners and millers ceased. At that time, only 14% showed radiographic changes of category 1/1 profusion or greater parenchymal fibrosis, and 6% had bilateral pleural lesions; in 1979, these percentages in these retired workers reached 40% and 27%, respectively.[37] Epidemiological studies of asbestos-exposed individuals beginning in the 1970s have repeatedly documented a higher incidence of asbestosis and lung cancer among workers with greater cumulative dose.[38] Yet, more recently studied populations have shown different outcomes. In 1988, 33.1% of sheet metal workers employed for more than 35 years had radiographic evidence of parenchymal interstitial fibrosis (consistent with asbestosis).[39] A follow-up study of the same workplace was reported in 2009. Of those, 5.3% currently employed had chest radiographic changes consistent with asbestosis. Of these cases, 91.3% had worked ≥29 years. No worker beginning after 1970 showed disease.[40] Currently, with attention to PELs, effective engineering controls, and early disease recognition, the number of cases and the number of cases which progress to asbestosis is dramatically less. Most cases are recognized in workers after the age of 50 years and fewer than 20% of recognized cases progress.

Is there an effective therapy? The medical management of the patient with asbestosis is supportive. Steroids are not helpful. As cited above, there is evidence to support that ceasing exposure reduces the rate of progression.[41] Once diagnosed, the worker must avoid further exposure to asbestos dust.

ASBESTOS FIBERS AND THE PLEURAL SPACE

Asbestos fibers have a natural, unexplained predilection for transport to the pleura. The result is an unusual array of benign and malignant manifestations of exposure—these changes are not typically identified in any other lung disease, although there have been rare cases of silica exposure associated with pleural changes.[42,43] Exposure to no other fibrogenic dust is associated with these outcomes on such a regular basis. In addition to mesothelioma, asbestos-induced pleural disease includes the nonmalignant entities of benign asbestos pleurisy, diffuse pleural thickening, pleural plaques, and rounded atelectasis. These nonmalignant disorders are important because they are relatively common in those exposed and in some instances, result in abnormal lung function and symptoms. Intriguingly, these benign pleural changes may occur in the absence of a radiologically or pathologically visible parenchymal response. Despite some insights into how fibers enter the pleural space, an explanation for the very different responses has been elusive. Whether the pleural pathology known to be associated with asbestos exposure occurs (or fails to occur) and whether the changes of diffuse pleural thickening following an exudative pleural effusion or whether the development of pleural plaques or even rounded atelectasis occurs in a worker with recognized clinically significant exposure are unable to be predicted.

It is not known how asbestos fibers are transported to the pleural space. Investigators have presented numerous theories.[44,45] Parkes considered that the most likely means of transport is via the lymphatics with probable additional contributions of gravity and respiratory motion.[46] Taskinen et al. considered three potential mechanisms of how dust may be handled in the lung: (1) Penetration through the lung, the visceral pleura, and the pleural cavity with uptake into the parietal pleura, (2) propagation through the blood vessels, and (3) transport via lymphatic vessels. In a worker exposed to coal and siliceous dust, they showed autopsy evidence of linear pigmentation along the intercostal vessels, the location of the lymphatic vessels, just anterior to the parietal pleura. These authors proposed that particles from the lung were first carried in macrophages or transported free in the lymphatic vessels into the lymph nodes of the lung. When the nodes were full, this contaminated lymph flowed retrograde into the intercostal lymphatic vessels anterior to the parietal pleura. They dismissed penetration of particles through the pleura as the outline of the lymphatic vessels was "clear-cut" and dismissed penetration of particles through the blood vessels because the particles were not visible in the blood vessel wall. Coal and silica particles were also identified in the lymphatic vessels, strengthening their argument.[47]

In 2008, Miserocchi et al. explained how fibers are translocated from the airway into the interstitium and from there into the pleural space using principles of fluid dynamics.[48] First, fibers in the alveolar lining fluid reach the interstitium through phagocytosis by type I alveolar lining cells which allow a "pass-through" into the interstitium by combined osmotic (through active sodium absorption) and hydraulic (the interstitial pressure is less than the airway pressure) gradients. Alveolar epithelial cell injury also damages fibroblasts and myofibroblasts and results in an inflammatory response with the laying down of increased amounts of extracellular matrix; the start of the pathologic process of asbestosis. Second, asbestos fibers can exit the lung through lymphatic vessels. Very fine fibers can be cleared in 24 hours.[49] The lymphatic circulation inevitably drains into the blood, and, in that way, fibers may be dispersed to all organs.[50] Fibers in lymphatic vessels and in the blood can enter the pleural space dragged by water flux gradients. Third, movement of fibers from the lung parenchyma into the pleural space can occur directly. If there is an inflammatory response in the lung (such as asbestos-induced alveolitis), the interstitial pressure is raised, and this can drive fibers in the lung parenchyma through minute pores in the visceral pleura into the pleural space.

Although fibers are transported into the pleural space (be it via the lymphatic vessels, the systemic circulation, or through direct pleural penetration), the differing pleural responses are unexplained. Yet, diffuse pleural thickening and pleural plaques frequently co-exist. For example, the intense inflammatory features of an exudative pleural effusion which resolves and scars to form diffuse pleural thickening are very different from the insidiously progressive essentially acellular and avascular pleural fibrosis.[51] Furthermore, it appears that diffuse pleural thickening is considerably more frequent than plaques in workers with crocidolite exposure, suggesting the role of amphibole fibers in its etiology.[52]

Pleural Effusions

Effusions attributable to asbestos exposure may be clinically manifest as being without symptoms with radiologic features of a blunted costophrenic angle as the sole manifestation of the inflammatory process to a "full-blown" bout of pleurisy with chest pain on inspiration, fever, dyspnea, and a substantial collection of hemorrhagic fluid in the affected pleural space. The effusions are exudative in nature and attribution to asbestos exposure is typically a "diagnosis of exclusion." These may occur in individuals who have a history of asbestos exposure and a latency period most often of approximately 10–15 years, although sometimes less (such effusions as recognized to be the earliest presentations of an asbestos-induced chest effect).[53] These may be attributed to asbestos after chemical and cellular assessment of the fluid in the pleural space, as well as a sample of the pleural tissue provides no clear diagnosis. This may require serial chest radiographs over an observation period of 2 or 3 years as these effusions typically resolve slowly and spontaneously over a period of months.[54,55] Finally, it should be noted that the "cause and effect" relationship of an exudative pleural effusion with clinical features of acute pleurisy leading to diffuse pleural thickening is often presumptive, with the effusion never recognized but thought to have occurred on a subclinical basis.[56,57]

Not surprisingly, these exudative effusions leave a "scarred" pleural space as they resolve. This is manifest by the radiographic appearance of obliteration of the costophrenic angle and described as diffuse pleural thickening. Asbestos-related pleural effusions do not predict the development of lung cancer, pleural plaques, or mesothelioma, although exudative effusions often accompany lung cancer as well as mesothelioma.[58,59]

Diffuse Pleural Thickening: Fibrosis of the Visceral Pleura

Diffuse pleural thickening is a disease of the visceral pleura. It is not specific for asbestos exposure and is often associated with fibrosis due to an inflammatory reaction caused by tuberculosis, surgery, hemorrhagic chest trauma, or drug reaction. In addition, the radiologic features of pleural thickening were more than three times more likely in obese [body mass index (BMI) > 30 kg/m^2) asbestos workers.[60]

In association with asbestos exposure, the mechanism(s) which cause diffuse pleural thickening are unknown but appear to be the result of exudative benign pleurisy in most cases. In other cases, where there is no history of a previous episode of benign pleurisy, perhaps the confluence of pleural plaques or the extension of subpleural parenchymal fibrosis into the visceral pleura has caused diffuse thickening. In the most aggressive cases, diffuse pleural thickening can extend into the interlobular spaces of the lung and affect the fissures, leading to restriction of lung expansion, even in the absence of interstitial lung fibrosis.[61] Although it had been originally thought that those who develop diffuse pleural thickening had greater exposure to asbestos than those who developed pleural plaques, no difference in asbestos burden in those with plaques versus those with diffuse pleural thickening was shown by addressing exposures and duration of exposure in shipyards **(Figs. 4A to C)**.[62]

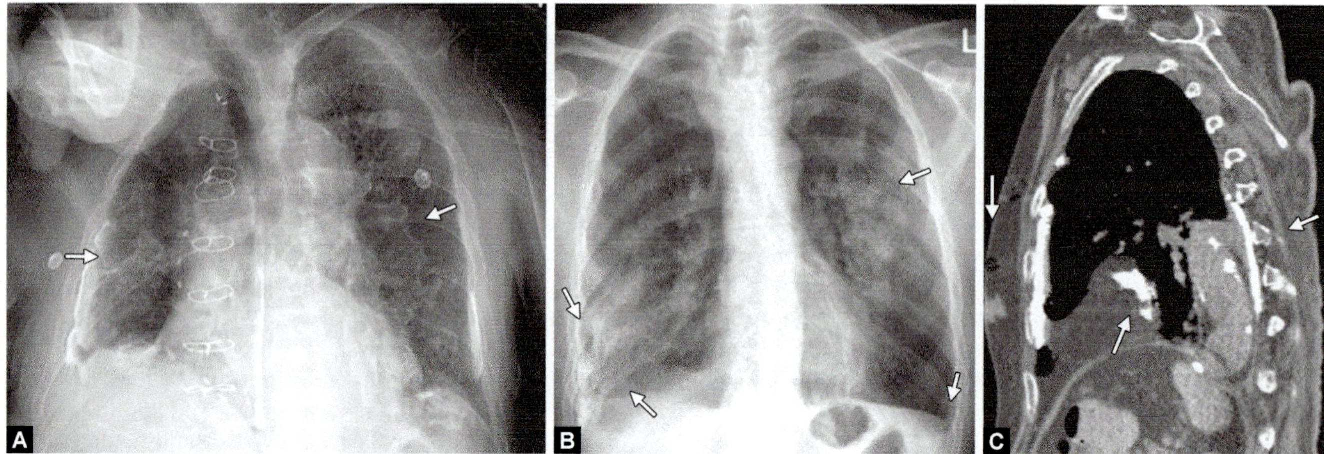

FIGS. 4A TO C: These three chest images show features emphasizing diffuse pleural thickening. The first radiograph shows extensive pleural changes in an asbestos-exposed worker who has had previous coronary artery bypass surgery. Specifically, there is calcified pleural thickening in both right and left pleural bases and lower pleural margins. In addition, there are calcified *en face* pleural plaques most notable on the left chest and a discrete calcified pleural plaque along the left chest wall. The second radiograph shows extensive pleural calcifications with obliteration of both costophrenic angles. Particularly noticeable is a calcified discrete pleural plaque on the right chest wall. The final figure is a chest CT scan (sagittal cuts) showing heavily calcified pleural plaques on the left side (along the anterior chest wall, the posterior and outlining the basal lobule). Calcifications of the descending aorta are also noted.

Diffuse pleural thickening may be responsible for dyspnea on exertion and perhaps a dry cough. Decreased respiratory excursion may be noted if the lung is "trapped" and moves little on the affected side. Diffuse pleural thickening may restrict lung function modestly if limited, but if extensive and bilateral, this may cause a significant restriction of lung function due to a "trapped lung" and result in respiratory insufficiency and failure in the most severe instances. Although the radiographic features of diffuse pleural thickening often appear to show a more extensive pleural effect compared to the radiographic features of benign pleural plaques, data show no difference in mean exposures between workers with these two types of radiographic features. A wide distribution of exposures was recognized in both groups.

On the radiograph, diffuse pleural thickening appears as a continuous, smooth pleural opacity extending more than one-fourth of the pleural surface with blunting of the costophrenic angle. If diffuse pleural thickening is bilateral, the foremost concern is asbestos exposure. The relationship between these radiographic changes and asbestos exposure is a clinical perception and does not require histologic confirmation unless malignant pleural disease is considered. Because this primarily affects the visceral pleura in the posterior and posterolateral lower zones, the CT scan provides a better visualization than the chest radiograph. Diffuse pleural thickening can be complicated by extension of fibrosis in the interlobar and interlobular fissures to form "crow's feet" (a focal abnormality of the visceral pleura which appear as small, pleural and parenchymal fibrous strands which appear to extend into the lung). Rounded atelectasis (the folded lung) is also known as Blesovsky syndrome. This is thought to be the result of visceral pleural fibrosis which has been "drawn back" into the lung.[63]

Pleural Plaques: Fibrosis of the Parietal Pleura

One of the radiographic hallmarks of asbestos exposure is pleural plaques. These are located on the parietal pleura, are not associated with pleural adhesions, and cause no pulmonary function impairment. Workers with pleural plaques are without symptoms or signs of chest disease. How pleural plaques develop is poorly understood. First, the relationship between exposure and the development of plaques is not clear. Using chest radiographs, work from British shipyard population surveys showed that the prevalence of plaques increased with increasing doses of asbestos inhaled.[64] In direct opposition to this conclusion, using CT scanning of the chest, there was no relationship between the plaque surface area and cumulative amount of asbestos exposure, smoking history, or time since the first asbestos exposure.[65] Asbestos bodies are not typically found in the pleural abnormality, yet short and thin fibers may be recognized in the pleural space soon after inhalation exposure. Unlike diffuse pleural thickening, plaques appear to be more likely related to chrysotile compared to amphibole exposures.[66] Even though pleural plaques are strongly associated with past asbestos exposure, they may occur in subjects with low-level or even sporadic asbestos exposure (based on fiber counts collected by bronchoalveolar lavage) using HRCT scans to identify the extent of fiber involvement.[67] Thompson has suggested that inhaled fibers gradually penetrate toward the base and periphery of the lung in a migration propelled by the continual movement of the lung.[68] He hypothesized that the common basal and posterior pleural plaques are a result of these areas being dependent when the subject is upright and during sleep. The tendinous part of the diaphragm, the ribs, and the vertebral bodies block fiber penetration, and thus pleural plaques are typically located over these structures. Perhaps the thin and pointed nature of the fibers in the pleural space facilitate tissue penetration, scratching of the pleural tissue, and initiation of an inflammatory reaction, followed by organization, all leading to the pleural plaque.

Grossly, plaques are firm, raised areas with a nearly white, glistening surface. Microscopically, collagen fibers are oriented in a parallel fashion in the submesothelial layers of the parietal pleura at the level of the costal margins, the diaphragms, and the paraspinal areas. They are covered by the typical mesothelial lining which does not contribute to the development of the plaque. They can be found in the pericardium and, less often, in other mediastinal pleura. Visceral pleural plaques occur much less frequently but can extend in the interlobar fissures. Therefore, the plaque is extrapleural.[69] This plus the slow, nonexudative growth of the plaque may explain the lack of adhesions. Pleural calcification occurs in areas of collagen degeneration and implies that the plaque has been present for 20 or more years.[70] Generally, neither asbestos bodies nor asbestos fibers are found in the plaques.

The earliest finding on the chest radiograph of a pleural plaque is frequently a thin line of soft-tissue density at the lateral margin of the seventh or eighth rib. This early change may be difficult to distinguish from normal "companion" shadows. The routine chest radiograph is thought to define only 8–15% of all pleural plaques.[71] Oblique views may assist in their recognition. The conventional CT scan recognizes plaques much earlier and at a less well-defined stage than the chest radiograph. Diaphragmatic plaques which were not always well appreciated with the conventional CT scan may be better evaluated with the HRCT scan. Computed tomography scans can clearly differentiate plaques from extrapleural fat pads, a sometimes-difficult distinction on the plain chest radiograph, particularly in those overweight or obese. Furthermore, in the presence of extensive and calcified pleural plaques, the CT scan permits a clearer appreciation of the lung parenchyma than the plain radiograph **(Figs. 5A to C)**.

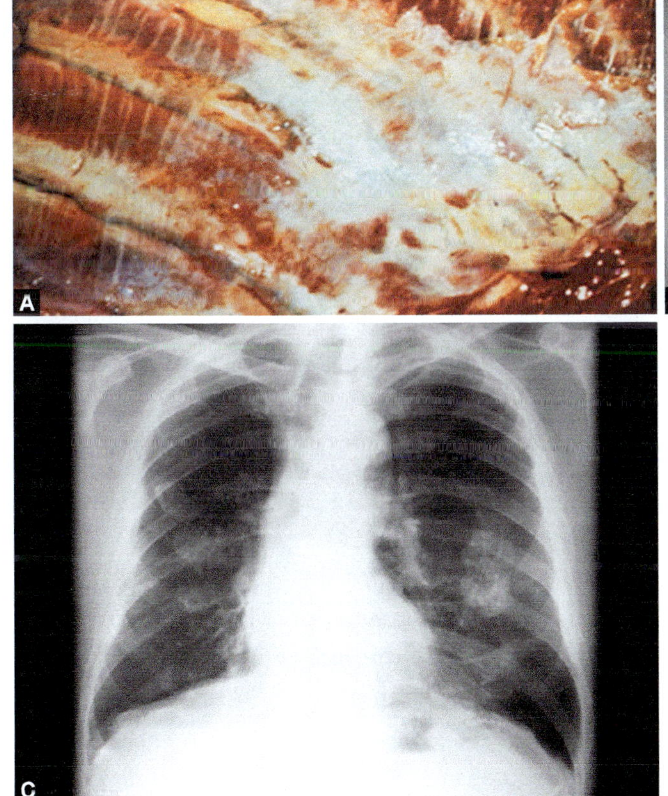

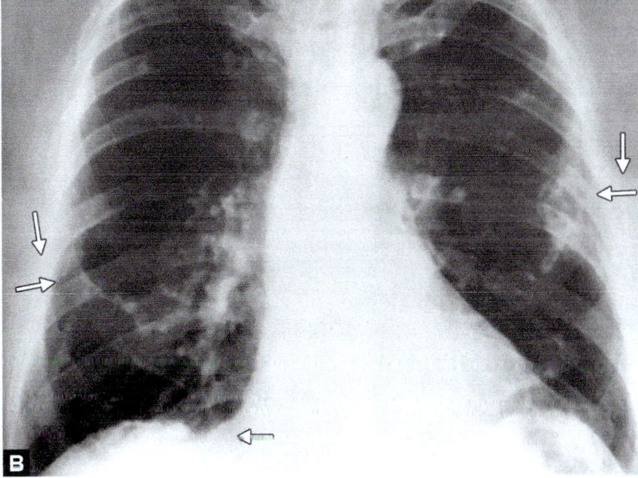

FIGS. 5A TO C: (A) Parietal plaque on the thoracic wall with an irregular thick plaque. (B) Pleural thickening along both lateral chest walls which shows a calcified pleural plaque of the right hemidiaphragm. (C) Several calcified *en face* discrete pleural plaques located on the chest wall, bilateral calcified pleural thickening along the lateral chest wall, and bilateral diaphragm thickening.

(A) *Courtesy*: Asbestos Related Disease: Clinical, Epidemiologic, Pathologic, and Radiologic Characteristics and Manifestations. Virginia: American College of Radiology; 1982.

MALIGNANT MESOTHELIOMA

Mesothelioma, on the other hand, is recognized as the most sensitive and specific marker of adverse health effects attributed to asbestos.[72] It is estimated that asbestos exposure causes the vast majority (80%) of cases of malignant mesothelioma.[73] Latency period from initial asbestos exposure, rather than dose, is the driving factor in the development of mesothelioma. The typical latency period for malignant mesothelioma approximates 30 years from the initial exposure. LaVecchi et al. addressed 3,343 asbestos workers with exposures active from 1950 or hired from 1950 to 1986 and followed from 1986 to 2003. There were 135 deaths from mesothelioma. In this report, there was no difference in mesothelioma rates between those who had retired less than 3 years before the end of the study compared to those who had retired more than 30 years ago, supporting the argument that the risk associated with the latency period since the initial exposure was more important than the overall dose.[74] Similarly, in a population of British tradesmen, the duration of exposure in the distant past (at a younger age), had the most impact on the development of mesothelioma. There was no difference in the mesothelioma risk for carpenters starting at a young age and working <10 years versus those who worked for ≥10 years starting after the age of 30 years. Exposure at a younger age and even for a short time (<10 years) appears to have profound implications for the development of mesothelioma.[75]

Pleural mesothelioma arises from the mesothelial cells of the pleura. Tumors may be solitary or diffuse. Solitary mesotheliomas are benign, well circumscribed, variable in size, and usually fibrous in histologic type, although epithelial elements may be present. They are unrelated to asbestos exposure and curable by surgical excision. It is a rare tumor but with increasing incidence and a poor prognosis.[76]

Diffuse malignant mesothelioma has a gross appearance which is more diagnostic than its variable histologic appearance.[77] In its early stages, it appears as multiple gray or white nodules on the pleural surface **(Figs. 6 and 7)**. It spreads along the pleural surface, encasing the lung with a resulting loss of volume. Distant metastases beyond the regional lymph nodes are rare, unless advanced disease is present. The tumor has a predilection for growth along incision or biopsy sites. This malignancy spreads by direct extension into adjacent structures of the chest wall, interlobar fissures, lung parenchyma, mediastinum, pericardium, diaphragm, esophagus, large vessels of the mediastinum, contralateral pleura, and peritoneal cavity **(Fig. 8)**. Death is usually caused by restriction of one or more of these vital structures.

Malignant mesothelioma may also be of peritoneal origin—this occurs in <25% cases. In the abdomen, the gross appearance of the tumor is quite similar to direct invasion of the abdominal structures. Microscopically, malignant mesothelioma may have one of three histologic patterns: Epithelial, sarcomatous, or mixed. Usually, one pattern predominates, but elements of the other two may be present.[78]

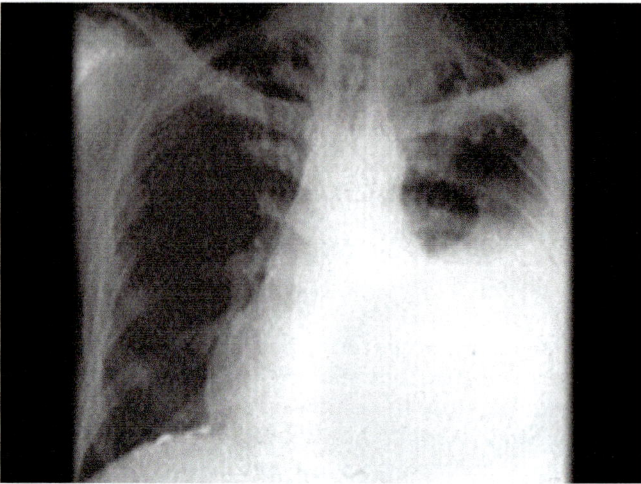

FIG. 6: This radiograph shows a large left-sided pleural effusion. Following thoracentesis, the left lateral chest wall showed a "bumpy" nodular appearance. Histologic staining of the mass showed malignant mesothelioma. Note displacement of the heart to the right and calcifications on the right hemidiaphragm.

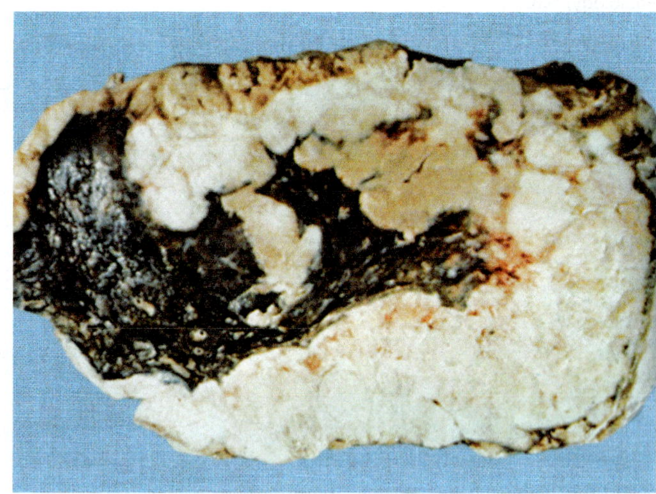

FIG. 7: This lung was removed at autopsy from an insulator with a 35-year history of asbestos exposure. The lung is encased by the gray-colored mesothelioma.

Courtesy: Asbestos Related Disease: Clinical, Epidemiologic, Pathologic, and Radiologic Characteristics and Manifestations. Virginia: American College of Radiology; 1982.

Although inhalation of asbestos fibers is a major risk factor for the development of mesothelioma, not all mesotheliomas are associated with asbestos fiber inhalation. Exposure to amphibole fibers is much more likely to induce mesothelioma than exposure to chrysotile fibers, yet all commercially available fibers have been recognized to cause mesothelioma.[79,80] The relationship between mesothelioma and asbestos exposure was first well documented in 1960.[81] A study of 17,800 asbestos insulators uncovered 66 mesotheliomas.[82] Most occurred 30 or more years from

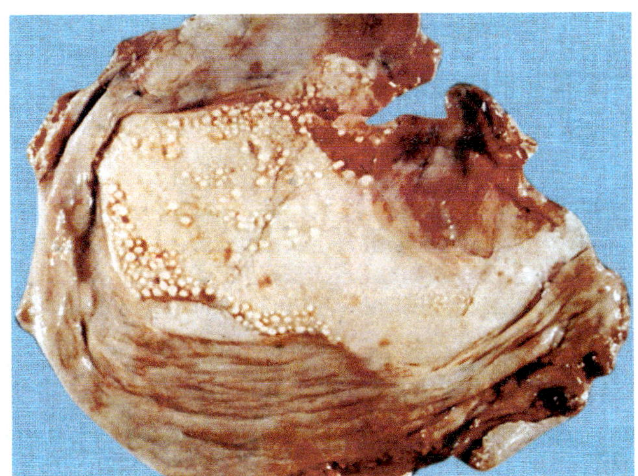

FIG. 8: This photograph shows the peritoneal surface of the diaphragm of a pipefitter with a 30-year asbestos exposure history. The main tumor mass was within the peritoneal cavity and involved the small intestine and pelvis. The discrete white nodules reflect seeding of the mesothelioma along the inferior aspect of the diaphragm.

Courtesy: Asbestos Related Disease: Clinical, Epidemiologic, Pathologic, and Radiologic Characteristics and Manifestations. Virginia: American College of Radiology; 1982.

the onset of exposure. It was soon recognized that persons having household contacts with asbestos workers are also at an increased risk for the development of mesothelioma.[83] Residents of communities where asbestos is mined/processed may also be at an increased risk **(Fig. 9)**. Overall, in the absence of asbestos exposure, malignant mesothelioma is a rare disease with an incidence of one to two cases per year per million people in the general population of North America. In the asbestos-exposed populations, the rates can be 5- to 20-fold higher, with a gradient of 10–1 for crocidolite to chrysotile exposures.[84,85]

Clinical clues suggesting mesothelioma include symptoms which develop insidiously and include progressive dyspnea and weight loss. Most patients with mesothelioma cite chest pain, often only partially relieved by analgesics, as the reason that they consult a physician. The presenting sign is usually a unilateral pleural effusion that progressively increases in size. As the disease progresses, affected supraclavicular nodes may become palpable and ribs may become tender as a result of local tumor invasion. Both superior and inferior vena cava obstruction can occur with resultant congestion, edema, and ascites. Digital clubbing may be present.

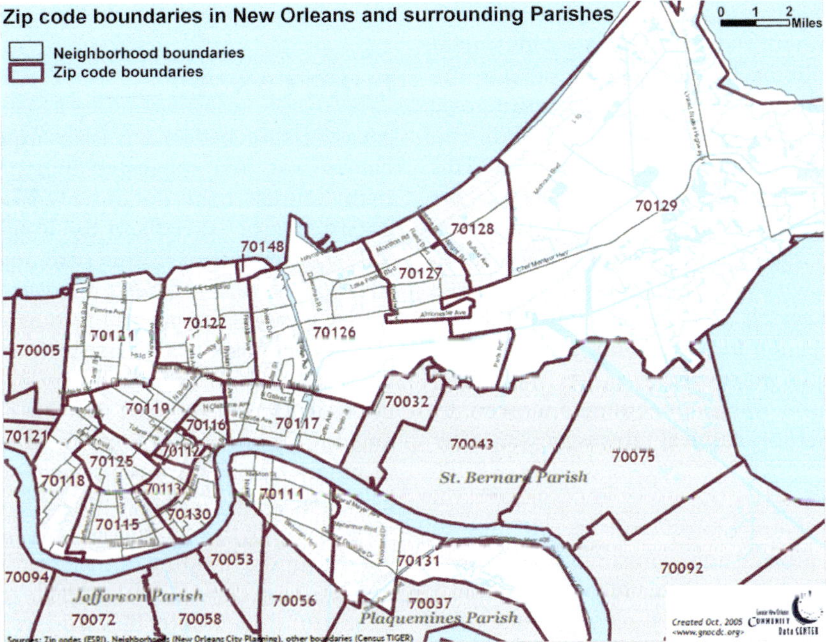

FIG. 9: A 28-year-old accountant presented with dull chest pain for several months. Evaluation showed a large pleural effusion and diagnostic workup showed malignant mesothelioma. Lung tissue assessed for asbestos fibers showed two different types in the lung. Importantly, when asked, she reported that she had recently finished her CPA (Certified Public Accountant) accreditation and had no known exposure to asbestos. The story was a puzzle until the MDs realized that her two places of residence in her life were several blocks from an asbestos cement manufacturing plant that had ceased operation in New Orleans several years earlier. Using the Louisiana state registry, we showed that there was a cluster of mesothelioma cases in women (but not men) residing in this 70116 zip code in the previous decade, with a decrease in the number of cases as one went further away from this address. This led us to conclude, based on epidemiologic data, that the risk for developing mesothelioma may well have been associated with the presence of the asbestos cement plant in the residential area.

Source: Zip codes (ESRI), Neighborhoods (New Orleans City Planning), other boundaries (Census TIGER).

Malignant mesothelioma should be considered in the differential diagnosis of all cases of unexplained exudative pleural effusion, particularly if asbestos exposure is documented. Clinical clues suggesting mesothelioma include contralateral pleural plaques and pleural calcification. In fact, among workers with asbestosis and/or asbestos-related pleural disease, there has been a significant increase in the risk for mesothelioma.[86-88] The issue under discussion, at least in some of these reports, is the adequacy of accurately identifying plaques by chest radiograph.[89,90] Commonly, mesothelioma is seen in the absence of basilar interstitial fibrosis, the classic radiologic finding of asbestosis.[91]

During thoracentesis, it may be difficult to enter the pleural space due to thickened pleura. The effusion is exudative, viscous, and very cellular, with normal, malignant and inflammatory cells. Cytologic examination of the fluid is often of limited diagnostic value because it is frequently difficult to differentiate benign from malignant mesothelial cells. Hyaluronic acid may be greatly elevated in effusions associated with malignant mesotheliomas.[92] Repeated thoracentesis or placement of an indwelling catheter in the pleural space may be necessary to palliate dyspnea in the presence of rapid fluid reaccumulation.

There are several innovations regarding biomarkers for the diagnosis of malignant mesothelioma.[93] For example, serum osteopontin levels can distinguish individuals with exposure to asbestos without cancer from those with similar exposure and mesothelioma.[94] Nevertheless, despite the interest in understanding the serologic and immunologic changes associated with mesothelioma, there remains no method for the early recognition of mesothelioma. This illness is most often diagnosed at advanced stages when the tumor has become unresectable and spread on the pleural surfaces with malignant cells in the pleural fluid. The natural history is one of direct extension of malignant growth into the mediastinum and great vessels, chest wall, and pericardium and heart. Surgical resection for cure is not possible. In a series of selected patients diagnosed at earlier stages and treated with extrapleural pneumonectomy followed by radiation and chemotherapy, survival rates were 38% after 2 years and 15% after 5 years.[95] In a combined series of 3,400 patients, the median survival period was 6–12 months.[96]

Although an open thoracotomy with pleural biopsy may well be needed to provide adequate amounts of tissue to establish a certain diagnosis, recent recommendations suggest that an earlier and equally reliable diagnosis may be gained through the use of thoracoscopy (except in cases of preoperative contraindication).[97] In addition, because standard staining procedures are insufficient in approximately 10% of cases, these consultants propose using specific immunohistochemistry markers on pleural biopsies. The patient's performance status and histological subtype are important prognostic factors of clinical importance in the management of pleural mesothelioma. Other potential parameters should be recorded at baseline and reported in clinical trials. Mesothelioma exhibits a high resistance to chemotherapy and only a few patients are candidates for radical surgery. To date, surgery, radiotherapy, chemotherapy, and immunotherapy or cytokine therapy, or a combination of the above, have been equally unsuccessful in curing this disease although may improve prognosis for a period. Gene therapy has not yet reached clinical practice.[98] Patients who are considered candidates for a multimodal approach to therapy should be enrolled in a prospective trial at a specialized center.

It has been very difficult to estimate the predicted number of mesothelioma cases and when these cases may reach their peak. In the US, mesothelioma cases were previously projected to peak in 2005. However, malignant mesothelioma deaths have increased over the past couple of decades, with 2,597 deaths reported in 2015. Cases have increased in persons over the age of 85 years old, apparently reflecting a long latency period associated with prior exposures. Unexpectedly, cases continue to develop in younger adult populations, suggesting that clinically important asbestos exposure occurred perhaps 30 years prior, a time when asbestos use was less regulated.[99] In India, it is not possible to predict when mesothelioma cases might peak, given the lack of reliable reporting of mesothelioma and the continuing use of asbestos.[100] Yet, it is reasonable to assume that this disease will persist. Preventing asbestos exposure is the main way to decrease malignant mesothelioma rates.

LUNG CANCER

An association between asbestos exposure and bronchogenic cancer was first suggested in 1935, and since that time many studies have documented this relationship.[101] The persistence of asbestos in the lung parenchyma results in a lifelong exposure to this carcinogen. Of note, although the worker with asbestos exposure is at an elevated risk for lung cancer, progression to asbestosis is an important risk for lung cancer.[102] Thus, despite removal of the worker from a contaminated environment, the worker's lungs are continually exposed and the risk for cancer increased. In an early report, 60% of English workers with asbestosis died of lung cancer.[103] An extensive discussion of lung cancer, asbestosis, and asbestos exposure, including screening for lung cancer in this population, has been published.[104]

Our understanding of the specific process that asbestos induces lung cancer is incomplete. Some consider asbestos to be a tumor promoter based on its weak activity in standard tests which address a carcinogen's potential (i.e., its ability to produce chromosomal abnormalities). Based on this perspective, the fibers increase the susceptibility of the lung to other carcinogens (such as cigarette smoke). Others consider asbestos to be a tumor initiator, and note the excess number of lung cancers in animals not exposed to other carcinogens as well as the excess of pulmonary malignancies even in lifetime nonsmokers. A separate and quite contentious issue reflects whether asbestosis is necessary for the genesis of lung carcinoma. This is supported by epidemiological studies which have shown an excess number of lung cancers in a great majority of reports addressing the outcomes of the most heavily exposed workers with the highest prevalence of radiographic opacities consistent with asbestosis.[105] However, alternative views contend that lung cancers occur in the absence of radiologic or histologic evidence of asbestosis and that the extent of asbestos exposure, the risk for developing asbestosis, the effects of cigarette smoking, and the ensuing risk for lung cancer all run parallel and increase with time, making the measurable risk for asbestosis alone, as it applies to lung cancer, difficult to separate from these other parameters.[106-109] Likewise, decreasing or ceasing exposure to tobacco smoke or asbestos decreases the risk of lung cancer development.[110]

Our understanding of asbestos-related lung cancers in the absence of clinically recognizable asbestosis is further complicated by the multiplicative risk of smoking. In one report where asbestos exposure was high, the risk of lung cancer in cigarette smoking asbestos workers was compared to a group without asbestos exposure.[111] Asbestos workers who smoked one pack of cigarettes per day over many years had an 87-fold increase in the risk of developing lung cancer compared to nonsmoking, nonasbestos-exposed controls. In nonsmoking asbestos workers, this risk was only five-fold. This has led to the postulate that the exposure to smoking and to asbestos causes a multiplicative risk for lung cancer. More recently, data from different asbestos-exposed populations and the risks for lung cancer were measured. Although the fiber dose required to develop lung cancer was similar among different populations of asbestos insulators, it was very different among populations of workers exposed to asbestos in the manufacture of textiles and in workers employed in the manufacture of asbestos cement. The disparities are not clear and have led many to challenge the hypothesis that there is not a "multiplicative risk," but rather a synergistic effect of asbestos exposure and cigarette smoking altered by other interacting elements in the causation of lung cancer. Suggestions regarding smoking history; fiber type; underlying obstructive lung disease; exposure to contaminant metals, ionizing radiation, and chemicals such as benzopyrene and polycyclic aromatic hydrocarbons; the presence or absence of asbestosis; and the question of individual susceptibility have been considered as possible explanations for these differences.[112]

Asbestos-related cancers are not distinct in type, nature, or their location within the lung from those solely associated with cigarette smoking. The histologic distribution of asbestos-related cancers approximates 35% epidermoid, 25% small-cell, 30% adenocarcinoma, and 10% large-cell carcinoma, a distribution like the cell types of cancer in those who smoke without asbestos exposure.[113]

Asbestos-related lung tumors present in the same manner as lung tumors caused by other carcinogens, except when the symptoms of asbestosis are present. In the presence of asbestosis, it is accepted that lung cancers should be compensated. In the absence of asbestosis, compensation has been debated, some refusing compensation for all cases whereas others favoring compensation for cases of long exposure (>20 years).

OTHERS ASBESTOS-RELATED CANCERS

Numerous reports have found an association between asbestos exposure and nonrespiratory cancers. In 2006, the Institute of Medicine completed a meta-analysis to comprehensively evaluate whether a causal association exists between asbestos and five other, nonrespiratory cancers (colorectal, stomach, esophageal, laryngeal, and pharyngeal cancers).[114] Of particular interest are the differing perspectives regarding the relationship between laryngeal cancer and asbestos exposure. Through a systematic review of case–control and cohort studies, the members of the Institute of Medicine concluded that there is sufficient evidence to support a causal association between asbestos exposure and laryngeal cancer. Yet, others have published reports which disagree.[115-117] Causality could not be established for the other types of nonrespiratory cancer.

AN ASSESSMENT OF THE EXTENT OF ASBESTOS-RELATED DISEASE IN INDIA

A great percentage of asbestos used in India is mixed with cement to form roofing sheets. Although the epidemic of asbestos-related disease in the US appears to be waning due to lesser amounts of importation of asbestos, the pattern of asbestos usage in India suggests that the Indian epidemic is closer to its beginning.

In the absence of banning the use of asbestos, control of asbestos dust exposure in the workplace is the most effective way to prevent disease. In the past, although peak asbestos fiber counts in the workplace air sometimes exceeded 100 fibers/cc of air, more typical exposures ranged from 5 to 20 fibers/cc. The current allowable US limit to airborne exposures is 0.1 fiber/cc of air expressed as an 8-hour time-weighted average with a maximum exposure of limitation of 1.0 fiber/cc of air as averaged over a sampling period of 30 minutes for all fiber types.[118] In India, asbestos exposure is regulated under the Factories Act (1948), in which asbestosis is listed as a notifiable disease in the schedule 3 of the Act.[119] Under this act, the limit of exposure is 1 fiber/cc. Asbestos is also regulated under the Environment Protection Act (1986) which sets a limit of 4 fibers/cc for environmental emissions.[120]

Reviews provide considerable insight into the prevalence of asbestosis in India, although in other reports, authors are increasingly vigorous in maintaining that asbestosis occurs much more commonly than it is reported.[121-123] In one report, approximately 100,000 workers have been exposed to asbestos and less than 30 workers have been compensated. This same report recognized 41 workers with asbestosis in one asbestos-processing plant where asbestos brought into the workplace in bags is processed and made into finished products such as asbestos textiles and brake and clutch linings.[124]

A 1996 epidemiologic study reported lung impairment and radiologic abnormalities in 54.8% of asbestos millers and 19.5% of asbestos miners.[125] In some workplaces, exposures are reported to be excessive. In a study of asbestos cement factory workers, exposures were two to three times higher than the threshold limit value (TLV) among asbestos pipe cutters but below the TLV in other areas. In this group, the FVC was less in the group employed for 16–20 years, but in workers employed for more than 20 years, the mean values of all pulmonary function parameters studied were reduced, implying a "mixed" defect in lung function. When smokers were compared to nonsmokers, there was no measurable effect.[126] In another report of asbestos miners, exposures were below the PEL in the mine, but the ambient exposures in the mill were 200–400 fibers/cc.[127] These exposures were lessened to 15–20 fibers/cc with appropriate engineering controls.[128] Others have reported grossly increased exposures in asbestos milling.[129] With such exposure data, it is not surprising that a 1989–1990 report by the Indian National Institute of Occupational Health (NIOH) showed an asbestosis prevalence of 4% among miners and 21% among millers.[130]

The prevalence of asbestosis in asbestos cement factories and the asbestos textile industry workers is variably described from 3 to 9%.[131,132] Perhaps this is not surprising when relatively recent questionnaire information gained from workers at several small asbestos manufacturing plants showed that less than half knew that asbestos was present in the workplace, that less than three fourth knew asbestos was harmful, and that only 10% had received safety training.[133]

SCREENING THE ASBESTOS-EXPOSED WORKER FOR LUNG CANCER

Based on the Surveillance, Epidemiology and End Results (SEER) program data in the US, the 5-year survival of lung cancer from 2013 to 2019 was 25.4% when all stages and histological cell types are included.[134] In one report, asbestos exposure is thought to contribute to up to 15% of all lung cancers[135] and is the leading occupational cause of lung cancer mortality.[136] Approximately 3% and 8% of the lung cancer cases occurring during the years 2001–2005 can be attributed to asbestos exposure.[137]

Low-dose chest CT (LDCT) allows a low-resolution image of the entire thorax in a single breath-hold with low radiation exposure, effectively identifying nodules as small as 2–3 mm in diameter. It has been widely recommended as the preferred method for lung cancer screening in high-risk populations, which includes exposure to occupational lung carcinogens.[138] Compared to the chest radiograph, LDCT identifies many more nodules and the number of nodules that turn out to be malignant (typically in an early and therefore resectable stage) overwhelmingly exceed nodules that are benign. Indeed, this has been the experience in asbestos-exposed populations.[139-141] Often, using a three-dimensional reconstruction of images, the physician can gain insight into nodules that are more likely to be malignant.

The National Lung Screening Trial screened more than 50,000 current and ex-smokers between the ages of 55 years and 74 years with at least 30 pack-years of smoking. Results supported LDCT as the superior, more sensitive method for earlier detection of lung cancer in high-risk populations. Overall, LDCT reduced the risk of dying from lung cancer in heavy smokers by approximately 20%.[142] Although the trial did not address the risk of cancer attributable to asbestos and the usefulness of such an approach in the care of asbestos-exposed workers, more recent studies and workgroups have supported the inclusion of LDCT in screening for asbestos-exposed workers. A review published in 2022 recommended LDCT screening in asbestos-exposed populations for workers ≥50 years who had ≥5 years of asbestos exposure and other lung cancer risk factors (such as tobacco exposure or lung disease).[143]

SUMMARY

An accurate and detailed work history remains the gold standard for assessing prior asbestos fiber inhalation.[144] If the exposure history is not clear, the presence of pleural abnormalities of diffuse pleural thickening or pleural plaques can serve as a surrogate for past asbestos exposure. Although a great number of articles have addressed the adverse respiratory health effects associated with asbestos exposure, numerous questions regarding the determinants of pleural disease (specifically, mesothelioma and pleural plaques) and how fibers interact with the pleural space remain. Specifically, why some workers with similar workplace exposures have very different radiographic manifestations is not understood. Some develop pleural plaques, while others may have an exudative pleural effusion which may end up with diffuse pleural thickening. How do pleural plaques develop when there is only minimal evidence of inflammation in the pleural space? How does the persistence of fibers in the lung of one worker result in mesothelioma while in another there is no visible effect?

Next, it is reasonable to state that there is sufficient data to justify the current exposure regulations which protect the worker from the development of asbestosis. Yet, there is no exposure evidence available which addresses the maximal allowable levels of asbestos exposure which will protect the worker from the development of pleural changes, mesothelioma, or the risk of lung cancer. Asbestos exposure regulations are not based on these outcomes of exposure.

Third, it remains unclear how asbestosis apparently transforms into lung malignancy. Yet, even more unclear is how fibers which may cause inflammation, but no discernable lung disease, increase the risk of malignancy.[145] Overall, this appears to be increasingly consequential. In the past, the weight of evidence about the relationship between asbestos exposure and lung cancer appeared to favor the conclusion that asbestosis was necessary to attribute lung cancer to asbestos exposure. At present, this conclusion has been increasingly challenged as research continues.

Finally, these illnesses are the result of decisions to incorporate asbestos in the environment. Although asbestos remains in buildings and will continue to pose a threat to those employed in the demolition of buildings, banning the importation and utilization of this material would dramatically lessen the number of illnesses attributable to asbestos exposure and provide a lasting impact on the occurrence of these diseases in future generations.

REFERENCES

1. Infoplease. (2023). Life Expectancy by Age, 1850–2011. [online] Available from http://www.infoplease.com/ipa/A0005140.html [Last accessed June, 2024].
2. US Geological Survey (USGS). (2023). Asbestos Mineral Commodity Summaries. Reston, VA: USGS. [online] Available from https://pubs.usgs.gov/periodicals/mcs2023/mcs2023-asbestos.pdf. [Last accessed June, 2024].
3. Indian Bureau of Mines. Indian Minerals Yearbook 2020, 59th Edition, Asbestos. (ibm.gov.in) [Last accessed July 2024].
4. Centre for Environmental Health. Asbestos in India. [online] Available from ceh.org.in [Last accessed June, 2024].
5. Constantinidis K. Asbestos exposure—its related disorders. Br J Clin Pract. 1977;31(7-8):89-101.
6. Alleman J, Mossman BT. "Asbestos revisited." Scientific American. 1997;54-7-13. [online] Available from https://www.scientificamerican.com/article/asbestos-revisited/ [Last accessed June, 2024].
7. USGS. (2022). Asbestos. Mineral Commodity Summaries 2022. [online] Available from https://data.usgs.gov/datacatalog/data/USGS:61ead2e5d34e8b818ad9f38d [Last accessed June, 2024].
8. Morgan A, Holmes A. Solubility of asbestos and man-made mineral fibers in vitro and in vivo: its significance in lung disease. Environ Res. 1986;39(2):475-84.
9. Roggli VL. Rare pneumoconioses: metalloconiosis. In: Saldana MS (Ed). Pathology of Pulmonary Diseases. Philadelphia: J B Lippincott; 1994. pp. 411-22.
10. Dufresne A, Begin R, Churg A, et al. Mineral fibre content of lungs in mesothelioma cases seeking compensation in Québec. Lung Cancer. 1996;15(2):270-1.
11. Brian JD, Valberg PA. Models of lung retention based on ICRP task group report. Arch Environ Health. 1974;28(1):1-11.
12. Churg A, Warnock ML, Green N. Analysis of the cores of ferruginous (asbestos) bodies from the general population. II. True asbestos bodies and pseudoasbestos bodies. Lab Invest. 1979;40(1):31-8.
13. Churg A, Green FHY. Pathology of Occupational Lung Disease, 1st edition. New York: Igaku-Shoin Ltd; 1989.
14. Bignon J, Sébastien P, Gaudichet A. Measurement of asbestos retention in human respiratory system related to health effects. In: Proceedings of the Workshop on Asbestos. National Bureau of Standards, Washington, DC. Special publication #506, 1979; pp. 95-119.
15. Farlev ML, Greenberg SD, Shuford EH, et al. Ferruginous bodies in sputa of former asbestos workers. Acta Cytol. 1977;21(5):693-700.
16. Churg A, Warnock ML. Correlation of quantitative asbestos body counts and occupation in urban patients. Arch Pathol Lab Med. 1977;101(12):629-34.
17. Rom WN, Travis WD, Brody AR. Cellular and molecular basis of the asbestos-related diseases. Am Rev Respir Dis. 1991;143(2):408-22.
18. Bégin R, Ostiguy R, Fillion R, et al. Recent advances in the early diagnosis of asbestosis. Semin Roentgenol. 1992;27:121.
19. Bégin R, Cantin A, Berthiaume Y, et al. Clinical features to stage alveolitis in asbestos workers. Am J Ind Med. 1985;8(6):521-36.
20. Banks DE, Morris M, Jindal SK. Oxidative stress and asbestosis. In: Ganguly NK, Jindal SK, Biswa S, et al. (Eds). Oxidative Stress in Applied Basic Research and Clinical Practice - Studies on Respiratory Disorders, Vol. 27. New York: Springer Nature; 2014. pp. 203-24.
21. Centers for Disease Control and Prevention (CDC). Changing pattern of pneumoconiosis mortality-United States. 1968-2000. MMWR. 2004;53(28):627-32.
22. Selikoff IJ, Hammond EC, Seidman H. Latency of asbestos disease among insulation workers in the United States and Canada. Cancer. 1980;46(12):2736-40.
23. Staples CA, Gamsu G, Ray CS, et al. High-resolution computed tomography and lung function in asbestos-exposed workers with normal chest radiographs. Am Rev Respir Dis. 1989;139(6):1502-8.
24. Bégin R, Ostiguy G, Filion R, et al. Computed tomography in the early detection of asbestosis. Br J Ind Med. 1993;50(8):689-98.
25. Becklake MR, Liddell FD, Manfreda J, et al. Radiological changes after withdrawal from asbestos exposure. Br J Ind Med. 1979;36(1):23-8.
26. American Thoracic Society. Medical section of the American Lung Association: The diagnosis of nonmalignant diseases related to asbestos. Am Rev Respir Dis. 1986;134(2):363-8.
27. Harber P, Smitherman J. Asbestosis: diagnostic dilution. J Occup Med. 1991;33(7):786-93.
28. Asbestos, asbestosis, and cancer: the Helsinki criteria for diagnosis and attribution. Scand J Work Environ Health. 1997;23:311-6.
29. Banks DE. Unanswered questions regarding asbestos exposure: Concerns for the next generation. In: Huang YC, Ghio A, Maier L (Eds). A Clinical Guide to Occupational and Environmental Lung Diseases. Totowa, NJ: Springer. pp. 153-69. [online] Available from https://doi.org/10.1007/978-1-62703-149-3_8 [Last accessed June, 2024].
30. NIOSH and CDC. Chest radiography: B Reader Information for Medical Professionals. [online] Available from https://www.cdc.gov/niosh/chestradiography/php/about/index.html [Last accessed June, 2024].
31. Huuskonen O, Kivisaari L, Zitting A, et al. High-resolution computed tomography classification of lung fibrosis for

SECTION 9: ENVIRONMENTAL AND OCCUPATIONAL DISORDERS

patients with asbestos-related disease. Scand J Work Environ Health. 2001;27(2):106-12.
32. Britton MG, Hughes DT, Wever AM. Serial pulmonary function tests in patients with asbestosis. Thorax. 1977;32(1):45-52.
33. Abejie BA, Wang X, Kales SN, et al. Patterns of pulmonary dysfunction in asbestos workers: a cross-sectional study. J Occup Med Toxicol. 2010;5:12.
34. Craighead JE, Abraham JL, Churg A, et al. The pathology of asbestos - associated diseases of the lung and pleural cavities: diagnostic criteria and proposed grading scheme. Arch Path Lab Invest. 1982;106:544.
35. Roggli VI, Gibbs AR, Attanoos R, et al. Pathology of asbestosis–An update of the diagnostic criteria: Report of the asbestosis committee of the College of American Pathologists and Pulmonary Pathology Society. Arch Path Lab Med. 2010;134(3):462-80.
36. Murray H. Report of the Commission on compensation of industrial disease. London: Her Majesty's Stationary Office; 1907. 3496: 127.
37. Viallat JR, Boutin C, Pietri JF, et al. Late progression of radiographic changes in Canari chrysotile mine and mill ex-workers. Arch Environ Health. 1983;38(1):54-8.
38. Gregor A, Parkes RW, du Bois R, et al. Radiographic progression of asbestosis: preliminary report. Ann N Y Acad Sci. 1979;330: 147-56.
39. Selikoff IJ, Lilis R. Radiological abnormalities among sheet metal workers in the construction industry in the United States and Canada: relationship to asbestos exposure. Arch Environ Health. 1991;46:30-6.
40. Welch LS, Halle E. Asbestos-related disease among sheet-metal workers 1986-2004: radiographic changes over time. Am J Ind Med. 2009;52:519-22.
41. Sébastien P, Dufresne A, Massé S, et al. Asbestos fibres lung retention and the outcome of asbestosis with or without exposure cessation. Ann Occup Hygiene. 1994;18(Suppl 1):672.
42. Arakawa H, Honma K, Saito Y, et al. Pleural Disease in Silicosis: Pleural thickening, effusion, and invagination. Radiology. 2005;235(2):685-93.
43. Xeren EH, Colby TV, Roggli VL. Silica-induced pleural disease: An unusual case mimicking malignant mesothelioma. Chest. 1997;112:436-8.
44. Lawson JP. Pleural calcification as a sign of asbestosis. Clin Radiol. 1963;14:414-7.
45. Asbestos Working Group, a special committee of the ACR task force on pneumoconiosis. Asbestos-related diseases: clinical, epidemiologic and radiologic characteristics and manifestations. Chicago: American College of Radiology; 1982. p. 25.
46. Parkes WR. Asbestos-related disorders. Br J Dis Chest. 1973;67(4):261-300.
47. Taskinen E, Ahlman K, Wiikeri M. A current hypothesis of the lymphatic transport of inspired dust to the parietal pleura. Chest. 1973;64:193-6.
48. Miserochi G, Sancini S, Mantegazza F, et al. Translocation pathways for inhaled asbestos fibers. Environ Health. 2008;7:4.
49. Oberdorster G, Morrow PE, Spurny K. Size dependent lymphatic short term clearance of amosite fibers in the lung. Ann Occup Hyg. 1988;32 (inhaled particles VI):149-56.
50. Dodson RF, O'Sullivan MF, Huang J, et al. Asbestos in extrapulmonary sites: omentum and mesentery. Chest. 2000;117:486-93.
51. Begin R. Asbestos-related lung disease. In: Banks DE, Parker JE (Eds). Occupational Lung Disease: An International Perspective. London: Chapman and Hall; 1999. pp. 219-38.
52. deKlerk NH, Musk AW, Cookson WOC, et al. Natural history of pleural thickening after exposure to crocidolite. BJIM. 1989;46:461-7.
53. Epler GR, McLoud TC, Gaensler EA. Prevalence and incidence of benign asbestos pleural effusion in a working population. JAMA. 1982;247(5):617-22.
54. Cugell DW, Kemp DW. Asbestos and the pleura: a review. Chest. 2004;125:1103-17.
55. Cohen M, Sahn SA. Resolution of pleural effusions. Chest. 2001;119(5):1547-62.
56. Rudd RM. New developments in asbestos-related pleural disease. Thorax. 1996;51:210-6.
57. Miles SE, Sandrini A, Johnson AR, et al. Clinical consequences of asbestos-related diffuse pleural thickening: A review. J Occup Med. 2008;3:20.
58. Robinson BW, Musk AW. Benign asbestos pleural effusion: diagnosis and course. Thorax. 1981;36(12):896-900.
59. Gaensler EA, Kaplan AI. Asbestos pleural effusion. Ann Intern Med. 1971;74(2):178-91.
60. Lee YC, Runnion CK, Pang SC, et al. Increased body mass index is related to apparent circumscribed pleural thickening on plain chest radiographs. Am J Ind Med. 2001;39(1):112-6.
61. Hillerdal G. The pathogenesis of pleural plaques and pulmonary asbestosis: Possibilities and impossibilities. Eur J Respir Dis. 1980;61(3):129-38.
62. Smith KA, Sykes LJ, McGavin CR. Diffuse pleural fibrosis—an unreliable indicator of heavy asbestos exposure? Scand J Work Environ Health. 2003;29(1):60-3.
63. Genevois PA, de Maertenlaer V, Madani A, et al. Asbestosis, pleural plaques and diffuse pleural thickening: three distinct benign responses to asbestos exposure. Eur Respir J. 1998;11(5):1021-7.
64. Harries PG. Mackenzie FA, Sheers G, et al. Radiological survey of men exposed to asbestos in naval dockyards. BJIM. 1972;29:274-9.
65. Van Cleemput J, De Raeve H, Verschakelen JA, et al. Surface of localized pleural plaques quantitated by computed tomography scanning: no relation with cumulative asbestos exposure and no effect on lung function. Am J Respir Crit Care Med. 2001;163:705-10.
66. Sebastien P, Janson X, Gaudichet A. Asbestos retention in human respiratory tissues: comparative measures in lung parenchyma and parietal pleura. In: Wagner JC, Davis W (Eds). Biologic Effects of Mineral Fibres, Vol 1. Lyons: IARC Scientific Publication No. 30. 1980. pp. 237-46.
67. Orlowski E, Pairon JC, Ameille J, et al. Pleural plaques, asbestos exposure, and asbestos bodies in bronchoalveolar lavage fluid. Am J Ind Med. 1994;26(3):349-58.
68. Thompson JG. The pathology of pleural plaques. Proceedings of the International Conference, Johannesburg 1969. Johannesburg: Cape Town University Press; 1970. pp. 138-41.
69. Becklake MR. Asbestos-related diseases of the lung and other organs: their epidemiology and implications for clinical practice. Am Rev Resp Dis. 1976;114(1):187-227.
70. Fletcher DE, Edge JR. The early radiological changes in pulmonary and pleural asbestosis. Clin Radiol. 1970;21(4):355-65.
71. Hourihane DO, Lessof L, Richardson PC. Hyaline and calcified pleural plaques as an index of exposure to asbestos. Br Med J. 1966;1(5496):1069-74.

72. Weill H, Hughes JM, Churg AM. Changing trends in U.S. mesothelioma incidence. Occup Environ Med. 2004;61:438-41.
73. Hajj GNM, Cavarson CH, Pinto CAL, et al. Malignant pleural mesothelioma: an update. J Bras Pneumol. 2021;47(6): e20210129.
74. LaVecchia C, Boffetta P. Role of stopping exposure and recent exposure to asbestos in the risk of mesothelioma. Eur J Cancer Prevent. 2012;21:227-30.
75. Rake C, Gilham C, Hatch J, et al. Occupational, domestic, and environmental mesothelioma risks in the British population: a case-control study. Br J Cancer. 2009;100:1175-83.
76. Demicco EG, Park MS, Araujo DM, et al. Solitary fibrous tumor: a clinicopathological study of 110 cases and proposed risk assessment model. Modern Pathol. 2012;25:1298-306.
77. Saccone A, Goblenz A. Endothelioma of the pleura with a report of two cases. Am J Clin Pathol. 1943;13:186.
78. Churg J, Rosen SH, Moolten S. Histological characteristics of mesothelioma associated with asbestos. Ann N Y Acad Sci. 1965;32(1):614-22.
79. McDonald JC, McDonald AD. The epidemiology of mesothelioma in historical context. Eur J Respir. 1996;9(9):1932-42.
80. Dufresne A, Begin R, Churg A, et al. Mineral fiber content of lungs in patients with mesothelioma seeking compensation in Quebec. Am J Resp Crit Care Med. 1996;153(2):711-8.
81. Wagner JC, Sleggs CA, Marchand P. Diffuse pleural mesothelioma and asbestos exposure in the North Western Cape Province. Br J Ind Med. 1960;17:260-71.
82. Selikoff IJ, Hammond EC. Asbestos-associated disease in United States shipyards. CA Cancer J Clin. 1978;28(2):87-99.
83. Anderson HA, Lilis R, Daum SM, et al. Asbestosis among household contacts of asbestos factory workers. Ann N Y Acad Sci. 1979;330:387-99.
84. Bégin R, Gauthier JJ, Desmeules M, et al. Work-related mesothelioma in Québec, 1967-1990. Am J Ind Med. 1992;22(4): 531-42.
85. Selikoff IJ, Churg J, Hammond EC. Relation between exposure to asbestos and mesothelioma. N Engl J Med. 1965;272:560-5.
86. Cvitanovic S, Znaor L, Konsa T, et al. Malignant and nonmalignant asbestos-related pleural and lung disease: 10-year follow-up study. Croat Med J. 2003;44(5):618-25.
87. Edge JR. Asbestos related disease in Barrow-in-Furness. Environ Res. 1976,11(2):244 7.
88. Hillerdal G. Pleural plaques and risk for bronchial carcinoma and mesothelioma. A prospective study. Chest. 1994;105(1):144-50.
89. Smith DD. Plaques, cancer and confusion. Chest. 1994;105(1):8-9
90. Banks DE, Shi R, McLarty J, et al. American College of Chest Physicians consensus statement on the respiratory health effects of asbestos: Results of a Delphi study. Chest. 2009; 135(6):1619-27.
91. Legha SS, Muggia FM. Pleural mesothelioma: Clinical features and therapeutic implications. Ann Intern Med. 1977;87(5):613.
92. Rasmussen KN, Farber V. Hyaluronic acid in 247 pleural fluids. Scand J Respir Dis. 1967;48:366.
93. Oksa P, Wolff H, Vehmas T. Asbestos, asbestosis, and cancer – Helsinki Criteria for diagnosis and attribution 2014: recommendations. Scand J Work Environ Health. 2015;41(1):5-15.
94. Pass HI, Lott D, Lonardo F, et al. Asbestos Exposure, Pleural Mesothelioma, and Serum Osteopontin Levels. N Engl J Med. 2005;353:1564-73.
95. Sugarbaker DJ, Flores RM, Jaklitsch MT, et al. Resection margins, extrapleural nodal status, and cell type determine postoperative long-term survival in trimodality therapy of malignant pleural mesothelioma: results in 183 patients. J Thorac Cardiovasc Surg. 1999;117:54-63.
96. Churg A, Cagle PT, Roggli VL. Tumors of the serosal membranes. In: AFIP Atlas of Tumor Pathology, Series IV, Fascicle 3. Washington, DC: American Registry of Pathology; 2006.
97. Scherpereel A, Astoul P, Baas P, et al. Guidelines of the European Respiratory Society and the European Society of Thoracic Surgeons for the management of malignant pleural mesothelioma. Eur Respir J. 2010;35(3):479-95.
98. Vachani A, Moon E, Wakeam E. Gene therapy for mesothelioma and lung cancer. Am J Respir Cell Mol Biol. 2010;42(4):385-93.
99. Mazurek JM, Syamlal G, Wood JM, et al. Malignant Mesothelioma Mortality — United States, 1999–2015. MMWR. 2017;66:214-8.
100. Joshi TK, Bhuva UB, Katoch P. Asbestos ban in India: challenges ahead. Ann N Y Acad Sci. 2006;1076:292-308.
101. Lynch KM, Smith WA. Pulmonary asbestosis III: Carcinoma of lung in asbestos-silicosis. Am J Cancer. 1935;24:56.
102. Oksa P, Klockars M, Karjalainen A, et al. Progression of asbestosis predicts lung cancer. Chest. 1998;113(6):1517-21.
103. Wagner JC. Proceedings: Asbestos carcinogenesis. Br J Cancer. 1975;32(2):258-9.
104. Wolff H, Vehmas T, Oksa P, et al. Asbestos, asbestosis, and cancer, the Helsinki criteria for diagnosis and attribution 2014: recommendations. Scand J Work Environ Health 2015;41(1): 5-15.
105. Weiss W. Asbestosis: A marker for the increased risk of lung cancer among workers exposed to asbestos. Chest. 1999;115(2):536-49.
106. Banks DE, Wang ML, Parker JE. Asbestos exposure, asbestosis, and lung cancer. Chest. 1999;115(2):320-2.
107. Tossavainen A. Consensus report. Asbestos, asbestosis, and cancer: the Helsinki criteria for diagnosis and attribution. Scand J Work Environ Health. 1997;23:311-6.
108. Reid A, de Klerk N, Ambrosini GL. The effect of asbestosis on lung cancer risk beyond the dose related effect of asbestos alone. Occup Environ Med. 2005;62(12):885-9.
109. Finkelstein MM. Radiographic asbestosis is not a prerequisite for asbestos-associated lung cancer in Ontario asbestos-cement workers. Am J Ind Med. 1997;32(4):341-8.
110. Klebe S, Leigh J, Henderson DW, et al. Asbestos, Smoking and Lung Cancer: An Update. Int J Environ Res Public Health. 2019;17(1):258.
111. Hammond EC, Selikoff IJ, Seidman H. Asbestos exposure, cigarette smoking and death rates. Ann N Y Acad Sci. 1979;330:473-90.
112. Henderson DW, Rodelsperger K, Woitowitz HJ, et al. After Helsinki: a multidisciplinary review of the relationship between asbestos exposure and lung cancer, with emphasis on studies published during 1997–2004. Pathology. 2004;36(6):517-50.
113. Churg A. Lung Cancer Cell Type and Asbestos Exposure. JAMA. 1985;253:2984-5.
114. Institute of Medicine (US) Committee on Asbestos: Selected Health Effects. Asbestos: Selected Cancers. Washington, DC: National Academies Press (US); 2006.
115. Browne K, Gee JB. Asbestos exposure and laryngeal cancer. Ann Occup Hyg. 2000;44(4):239-50.

116. Ferster APO, Schubart J, Kim Y, et al. Association between laryngeal cancer and asbestos exposure: A Systematic Review. JAMA Otolaryngol Head Neck Surg. 2017;143(4):409-16.
117. Peng WJ, Mi J, Jiang YH. Asbestos exposure and laryngeal cancer mortality. Laryngoscope. 2016;126(5):1169-74.
118. US Occupational Safety and Health (OSHA). Toxic and Hazardous Substances [online] Available from https://www.osha.gov/pls/oshaweb/owadisp.show_document?p_table=STANDARDS&p_id=9995 [Last accessed June, 2024].
119. Ministry of Labour, Government of India. The Factories Act [Act 63 of 1948]. [online] Available from https://labour.gov.in/sites/default/files/The-Factories-Act-1948.pdf [Last accessed June, 2024].
120. Government of India. Environmental Protection Act, 1986. [online] Available from https://www.indiacode.nic.in/bitstream/123456789/4316/1/ep_act_1986.pdf [Last accessed June, 2024].
121. Jindal SK, Aggarwal AN, Gupta D. Dust-induced interstitial lung disease in the tropics. Curr Opin Pulm Med. 2001;7(5):272-7.
122. Dave SK, Beckett WS. Occupational asbestos exposure and predictable asbestos-related disease in India. Am J Ind Med. 2005;48(2):137-43.
123. Murlidhar V. Occupational health physicians: unwilling or unable to practice ethically. Ind J Med Ethics. 2002;10:26-7.
124. Murlidhar V, Kanhere V. Asbestosis in an asbestos composite mill in Mumbai: A prevalence study. Environ Health. 2005;4:24.
125. Dave SK, Bjaia LJ, Mazumdar PK, et al. The correlation of chest radiograph and pulmonary function tests in asbestos miners and millers. Ind J Chest Dis Allied Sci. 1996;38(2):81-9.
126. Dave SK, Ghodasara NB, Mohandrao N, et al. The relation of exposure to asbestos and smoking habit with pulmonary function tests and chest radiograph. Indian J Public Health. 1997;41(1):16-24.
127. Bhagia LJ, Dave SK, Shah SH, et al. Environmental sampling and control of asbestos fibers in India. A review. In: Proc IVth Annual Conf. IASTA Bull. 1992; II (4):82.
128. Bhagia LJ, Dave SK, Shah SH, et al. Size distribution of airborne asbestos fibers in milling. Indian Aerosol Sci Tech Assoc (IASTA). 1994;7:1.
129. Mukherjee AK, Rajmohan HR, Dave SK, et al. An environmental survey in chrysotile asbestos milling processes in India. Am J Ind Med. 1992;22(4):543-51.
130. National Institute of Occupational Health, Ahmedabad. Annual Report: Prevalence of asbestosis in asbestos miners, 1989–1990. pp. 9-18.
131. Dave SK. Epidemiology, clinical manifestations, diagnosis and treatment. Indian J Clin Pract. 1993;3:40-9.
132. Udwadia FE, Kharas D. Occupational and environmental diseases in India. (Part 1). J Environ Med. 2000;2:122-37.
133. Tiwar RR, Saha A. Awareness and handling practices of asbestos in asbestos workers. J Environ Occup Sci. 2014;3(4):186-9.
134. National Cancer Institute: Surveillance, Epidemiology and End Results program. Cancer Stat Fact: lung and bronchus cancer. [online] Available from http://seer.cancer.gov/statfacts/html/lungb.html [Last accessed June, 2024].
135. Alberg AJ, Samet JM. Epidemiology of Lung Cancer. Chest. 2003;123:21-49.
136. GBD 2015 Risk Factors Collaborators. Global, regional, and national comparative risk assessment of 79 behavioural, environmental and occupational, and metabolic risks or clusters of risks, 1990–2015: A systematic analysis for the Global Burden of Disease Study 2015. Lancet. 2016;388: 1659-724.
137. McCormack V, Peto J, Byrnes G, et al. Estimating the asbestos-related lung cancer burden from mesothelioma mortality. Br J Cancer. 2012;106:575-84.
138. Delva F, Margery J, Laurent F, et al. Cancer Prof Working Group. Medical follow-up of workers exposed to lung carcinogens: French evidence-based and pragmatic recommendations. BMC Public Health. 2017;17:191.
139. Fasola G, Belveder O, Aita M, et al. Low-dose computed tomography screening for lung cancer and pleural mesothelioma in an asbestos-exposed population: Baseline results of a prospective, nonrandomized feasibility trial – An Alpe-Adtia Thoracic Multidisciplinary group study (ATOM 002). The Oncologist. 2007;12:1215-24.
140. Mastrangelo G, Ballarin MN, Bellini E, et al. Feasibility of a screening programme for lung cancer in former asbestos workers. Occup Med. 2008;58:175-80.
141. Clin B, Morlas F, Guittet L, et al. Performance of chest radiograph and CT scan for lung cancer screening in asbestos-exposed workers. Occup Environ Med. 2009;66:529-34.
142. National Lung Screening Trial Research Team. Reduced Lung-Cancer Mortality with Low-Dose Computed Tomographic Screening. N Engl J Med. 2011;365:395-409.
143. Markowitz SB. Lung Cancer Screening in Asbestos-Exposed Populations. Int J Environ Res Public Health. 2022;19(5):2688.
144. Bégin R, Christman JW. Detailed occupational history: the cornerstone in diagnosis of asbestos-related lung disease. Am J Resp Crit Care Med. 2001;163(3 Pt 1):598-9.
145. Lehtimäki L, Oksa P, Järvenpää R, et al. Pulmonary inflammation in asbestos-exposed subjects with borderline parenchymal changes on HRCT. Resp Med. 2010;104(7):1042-9.

Bronchial Anthracofibrosis

CHAPTER 99

Ashok Shah, Chandramani Panjabi, Vikas Pilaniya

INTRODUCTION

The term "anthracosis," coined in 1813, refers to the bluish-black discoloration of the bronchial mucosa or lung parenchyma caused by inhalation of soot.[1] Predominantly seen among coal workers, smokers, and city dwellers, it is often an incidental finding on bronchoscopy and occurs due to deposition of carbon as well as other mineral elements such as iron, lead, and cadmium on the bronchial mucosa. Endobronchial pigmentation with airway narrowing was first described in eight female patients with perforated tuberculous lymph nodes; six had anthracotic pigmentation in the right middle lobe (RML).[2] This appears to be the first ever description of a clinical entity that is now termed "bronchial anthracofibrosis (BAF)".

The term BAF was later introduced on bronchoscopic, visualization of anthracotic pigmentation associated with narrowing or obliteration of the bronchi in 28 nonsmoking elderly subjects, 20 of whom were females with long-standing exposure time to wood smoke.[3] Active tuberculosis (TB) was confirmed in 17/20 patients leading to the hypothesis that TB was responsible for the occurrence of BAF. Current evidence, however, incriminates long-standing exposure to the smoke generated by incomplete combustion of biomass fuel in poorly ventilated kitchens as the causative factor. BAF was first documented in India in 2008 in a 65-year-old lady with a history of prolonged exposure to wood fuel smoke who presented with a middle lobe syndrome (MLS).[4]

BRONCHIAL ANTHRACOFIBROSIS AND BIOMASS FUEL SMOKE EXPOSURE

It is estimated that more than half the world's population is dependent on biomass fuel for cooking and heating. Incomplete combustion of biomass fuel in traditional Indian stoves "chullas" generates smoke which when combined with poor ventilation creates an unhealthy atmosphere for ladies who cook on an average around 6 hours/day making a cumulative lifetime exposure of about 60,000 hours.[5] These women, as they age, are prone to various health hazards such as chronic obstructive pulmonary disease (COPD), asthma, TB, and lung cancer.[6] Respiratory symptoms like dyspnea and postnasal drip were significantly higher in north Indian women exposed to biomass fuel smoke.[5] Prolonged exposure to this smoke has now been incriminated as the primary causative agent for the occurrence of BAF.

Pathogenesis

The exact pathogenesis of anthracofibrosis is still unknown. Initially, it was thought that TB infection was the causative agent which explains the high coexistence of TB in anthracotic patients.[7,8] Silica containing pigmentation causes alteration in the immune mechanisms of the lungs, thereby increasing the chances of *Mycobacterium tuberculosis (M.tb)* infection.[9] Long-term exposure to air pollutants, cigarette smoke, and biomass fuel smoke causes carbon and silica accumulation in lymph nodes.[10] Whenever these lymph nodes, infected with *M. tuberculosis*, rupture into the adjacent tracheobronchial tree, it causes black pigmentation and leads to inflammation and fibrosis of bronchial tree.[2,11,12] The very fact that some BAF patients receiving TB treatment clinically improved favors this hypothesis.[3]

Prolonged exposure to biomass fuel smoke has emerged as the key etiological factor in the occurrence of BAF. Carbonaceous particles are deposited in lung by two ways: (1) these microparticles are directly engulfed by macrophages that are responsible for removing inhaled particles, and remain in the submucosa,[13] and (2) due to deficient mucociliary clearance and abnormal macrophage activity, inhaled particles may remain in the bronchial tree where they are then directly taken up by bronchial epithelial cells.[14] The inhaled particles mostly accumulate at the branching portion of the bronchus, where there is a relatively lower clearance rate.[15] These deposited carbonaceous particles cause fibrosis of the bronchial wall and surrounding interstitium, resulting in hypertrophy of the bronchial wall and narrowing of the bronchus.[16]

Demographic Features

The epidemiological data on BAF are limited. A female preponderance has been reported in most series.[3,6,17] The median age of patients varied between 60 and 75 years in different studies.[3,6,17,18] It has been suggested that BAF is more likely to develop in subjects from the Indian subcontinent than in those from other Asian countries.[19]

Clinical Features

Most patients of BAF present with dyspnea and cough.[6] Some studies have reported cough to be more common than dyspnea.[3,16,20] Hemoptysis and expectoration (both black and watery), are also common.[20] Nonspecific chest pain and fatigue are other symptoms which have been observed less frequently. However, symptoms can vary as BAF is known to be associated with several diseases.[6] The frequency of symptoms may vary between studies.[11,20-23] New onset of fever and weight loss, associated subsequently with complications such as broncholithiasis and vocal cord palsy, has been observed in few patients.[12,24,25] Pulmonary hypertension has also been reported in a Japanese coalmine worker with silicosis and BAF.[26] The most common auscultation finding in patients with BAF is wheezing.[3] Rales or decreased intensity of breath sounds may also be noted. One possible explanation for this variation in clinical features and examination findings may be the association of BAF with different diseases.[6]

Natural Course

Anthracofibrosis is a chronic disorder which is commonly misdiagnosed as chronic bronchitis. Most patients with bronchial anthracotic lesions have a stationary and inactive course that might be interrupted by acute attacks.[18] When a known case of anthracofibrosis is not responding to conventional therapy or is having an unexpectedly poor clinical course, additional clinical evaluation is performed using bronchoscopy or chest CT scans.[27] Pulmonary infections, including TB and pneumonia, and exacerbation of COPD are the most common associated diseases presenting with persistent localized wheezing or abnormal chest X-ray findings with or without respiratory symptoms. It has been suggested that pneumonia or acute exacerbation of COPD may occur repeatedly during the clinical course of BAF.[16,27]

Pulmonary Function Test

Majority of patients with BAF have abnormal pulmonary function tests (PFTs), and biomass fuel smoke-induced BAF usually appears clinically as an obstructive airway disease.[27] Nonetheless, a restrictive ventilatory defect may also be seen.[28] This was reflected in the spirometric findings in one study from India where the most common ventilatory defect was a nonobstructive pattern (suggestive of restriction/mixed defect). Biomass fuel smoke exposure probably leads to activation of pulmonary fibroblasts and an increased production of fibronectin.[29] This could possibly explain the restrictive or mixed pattern on spirometry, because of increased fibrosis. In addition, a normal spirometric finding can also be seen in patients with biomass fuel smoke exposure. No defect on spirometry was the most common finding in an Indian study in patients with BAF as well as anthracosis.[28]

Radiological Features (Table 1)

Although BAF is diagnosed by bronchoscopy, radiological features often provide the initial diagnostic clue. Radiological manifestations of BAF, which are diverse and characteristic, can be divided as primary and secondary.[17,28,30] The primary imaging features are due to BAF per se. These include multifocal bronchial narrowing and peribronchial cuffing and are considered to be radiological hallmarks.[3,4,6,28] The secondary findings are due to the presence of associated diseases, namely pulmonary TB, COPD, pneumonia, and malignancy. These clinical conditions contribute to the radiological picture in the form of collapse, consolidation, and mass lesions.[6,28,30] A pictorial essay from India highlights the spectrum of radiological appearances of BAF.[31]

Airway Lesions

Multifocal bronchial narrowing, the radiological hallmark of BAF, usually involves the segmental or lobar branches of the right upper and middle lobes **(Fig. 1)**. Sparing of trachea and the mainstem bronchi is observed. Pigmentary deposits are commonly found at the branching points within the tracheobronchial tree, and this subsequently leads to an inflammatory response along with bronchial stenosis.[30,32] Multifocal bronchial stenosis, most commonly in the RML bronchus, was reported in 23/58 (39.7%) patients

TABLE 1: Radiological features of BAF.[6,32,44,45]

Chest skiagram	CT scan	FDG-PET
Atelectasis	Multifocal bronchial narrowing	Increased uptake in lymph node
Consolidation	Atelectasis	Increased uptake in mass lesion
Linear shadows	Peribronchial cuffing	To rule out malignant conditions
Reticulono-dular pattern	Mediastinal lymphadenopathy	
Mass lesion	Pulmonary fibrosis and interstitial nodules	

(BAF: bronchial anthracofibrosis; FDG-PET: fludeoxyglucose positron emission tomography)

with BAF.[30] In a prospective study from India that enrolled 80 patients with a longstanding history of exposure to biomass fuel smoke, 24/60 (40%) patients, who consented for fiberoptic bronchoscopy (FOB), were diagnosed with BAF.[28]

Peribronchial soft-tissue thickening or cuffing on high-resolution computed tomography (HRCT) can also be an initial clue to the diagnosis of BAF.[30] However, this "picturesque" radiological finding is also observed in many patients with pulmonary sarcoidosis.[33] On HRCT, bronchiectasis has also been observed in some patients with BAF. Three of the 24 patients from India with BAF had bronchiectasis on HRCT.[28]

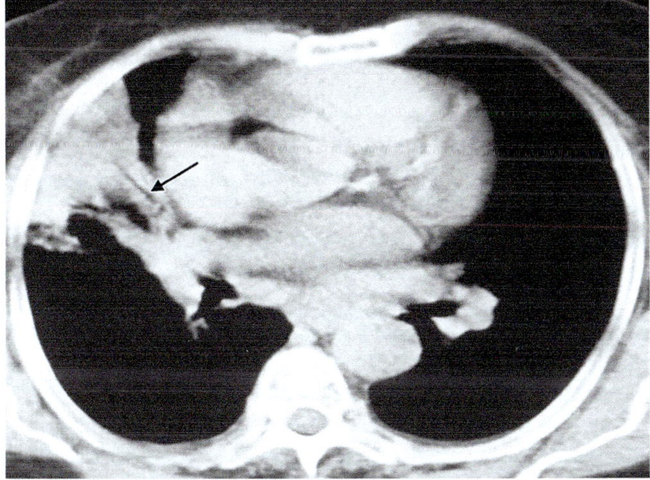

FIG. 1: Contrast-enhanced CT of the thorax showing multifocal bronchial stenosis (arrow) along with segmental collapse of the right middle lobe (RML) in a 67-year-old female with bronchial anthracofibrosis (BAF).

Parenchymal lesions

Among the secondary radiological features of BAF, lobar or segmental collapse is a common finding. Collapse is caused by bronchostenosis/bronchial obstruction or extrinsic compression of the affected bronchi. The RML is most commonly involved and these patients often present with MLS **(Figs. 2A and B)**. The classical radiological feature of MLS was the initial presentation of the first case of BAF from India.[4] The Golden S sign, classically described in patients with bronchial malignancies, can also occur in patients with BAF, either due to bronchial stenosis and complete obstruction or due to extrinsic compression by enlarged lymph nodes.[34] Pulmonary TB and malignancies should be excluded in patients having signs of lung collapse on imaging.[35]

Consolidation is another common finding. In nearly a fourth of the patients, the consolidation is usually due to associated pneumonia.[6] Bronchial narrowing is found majorly in the bronchi of the lobes having consolidation. These consolidations can easily be misdiagnosed as pneumonias or even tuberculous pneumonias. All efforts should be made to distinguish these clinical conditions from consolidations due to BAF.

The occurrence of a mass lesion is uncommon. When seen, malignancy should be ruled out, either by a CT-guided transthoracic biopsy or by bronchoscopic means. The appearance of irregular margins, spiculations, and cavitation in the mass lesion should raise the suspicion for malignancy.[31] Parenchymal fibrotic bands are also found in patients with BAF. On HRCT, such lesions were seen in approximately half of patients.[28,30] These linear opacities are about 1–3 mm in thickness and invariably extend up to the visceral pleura.

Nodular or reticulonodular interstitial opacities are also seen in patients with BAF.[36-39] Both usual interstitial

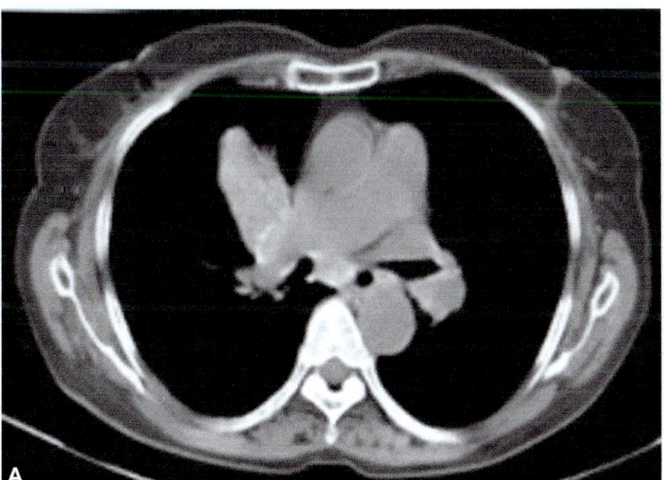

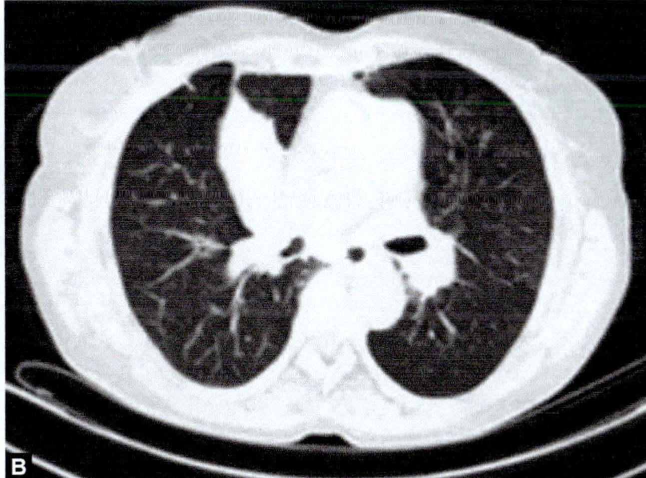

FIGS. 2A AND B: CT thorax showing collapse consolidation of the lateral segment of the right middle lobe, suggestive of middle lobe syndrome (MLS), in a 62-year-old female diagnosed with bronchial anthracofibrosis (BAF).

pneumonia (UIP) and nonspecific interstitial pneumonia (NSIP) patterns have been reported.[31,36] The presence of cavitating nodules in such patients are sometimes the first clue to the diagnosis of malignancy. Other interstitial patterns include ground glassing, mosaic pattern, and centrilobular micro- and macronodules.[31] These interstitial shadows are usually a manifestation of inflammation, small airways involvement, and air trapping.

Mediastinal Lymphadenopathy

Enlargement of mediastinal lymph nodes is not uncommon in BAF.[16,17,30] Sometimes, these nodes may develop calcification as well.[40] A clinicoradiological prediction model has shown that in addition to female gender, advanced age, and active TB, calcified lymphadenopathy is also a predisposing factor for BAF. When necrosis is observed, underlying TB must be excluded. The advent of endobronchial ultrasound (EBUS) guided lymph node evaluation has helped in confirming the diagnosis. Extrinsic bronchial compression from enlarged nodes can lead to lobar or segmental collapse. Bronchostenosis occurs when the nodes erode into a bronchus.

Pleural Involvement

Pleural effusion or thickening is encountered in patients with BAF having associated TB or malignancy[30] having pleural effusion. In the Indian context, there should be a high index of suspicion for pulmonary TB in BAF patients having pleural effusion.

Radiological Findings in Bronchial Anthracofibrosis Associated with Tuberculosis

A distinct radiological pattern is seen in BAF with TB.[35] The various CT findings include consolidations (either single or multiple), cavities, "tree-in-bud" nodules, mediastinal lymphadenopathy, and pleural involvement.[40] The lymph nodes, on contrast CT, invariably show enhancement suggestive of necrosis.[41] A retrospective analysis of the CT findings in 49 patients with BAF and 35 patients with endobronchial TB revealed that bronchostenosis and multiple lobar involvement were significantly more involved in BAF, but the main bronchus was invariably preserved.[42]

Fludeoxyglucose Positron Emission Tomography

On PET scans, increased fludeoxyglucose (FDG) uptake has been seen in hilar and mediastinal lymph nodes as well as in anthracotic pulmonary nodules in patients with BAF.[43,44] The reported SUV_{max} value within the lymph nodes was 4.76 (1–16.8) and was indistinguishable from malignant or granulomatous conditions in 201 lymph nodes from 106 patients with a mean duration of exposure to biomass of 35.5 years.[43]

Positron emission tomography (PET) scans may also be helpful to diagnose any malignancy associated with BAF. However, the specificity of PET to distinguish malignancy from a benign condition is very low. For any intense uptake observed in hilar and mediastinal lymph nodes on PET scans, benign and malignant conditions should be ruled out by histopathological examination.[44]

Bronchoscopic Features

Bronchoscopic visualization is the only confirmatory modality for the diagnosis. Bluish-black mucosal pigmentation in bronchial mucosa having normal shape and opening of the bronchi without any evidence of narrowing or distortion is suggestive of bronchial anthracosis, while multiple pigmented anthracotic lesions that appear more dense and associated bronchial distortion/stenosis **(Fig. 3)** are the pathognomonic features of BAF on FOB **(Table 2)**.[20,31] Anthracotic pigmentation is frequently observed involving the mucosa around the bronchial branching points, chiefly in both upper lobes[16] and the RML.[37] The frequency of involvement of RML and right upper lobe (RUL) varied in different studies. In some studies, the RML bronchus was the most commonly affected, while in others, RUL was most commonly involved.[17,19,37] Bronchial narrowing predominantly occurred at the level of the lobar and segmental bronchi, particularly in the RUL and RML.[7,16,17,37] Multifocal narrowing was observed in more than two-thirds of the patients.[16] There is a significant tendency to bleed after bronchial biopsy.

In one of the earliest large studies,[20] bilateral bronchial involvement on bronchoscopy was observed in 62.5% of the patients. Lobar bronchi were affected in 83.2%, main bronchus in 37%, and segmental bronchi in 35% of patients. Bronchial narrowing and/or obstruction were observed in 37.4% of the total patients.[20]

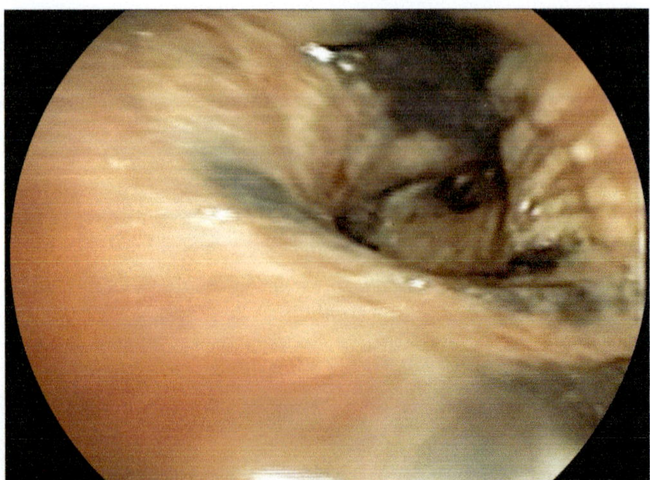

FIG. 3: Fiberoptic bronchoscopic image showing bluish-black anthracosis with narrowing and distortion of the middle lobe bronchus suggestive of bronchial anthracofibrosis (BAF).

Diagnostic Criteria

A set of diagnostic criteria has evolved that include (1) long-standing history of biomass fuel smoke exposure, (2) multifocal bronchial stenosis on HRCT when present, and (3) confirmed on bronchoscopy by visualization of (i) bluish-black mucosal anthracotic pigmentation along with (ii) narrowing/distortion of the affected bronchus **(Flowchart 1)**.

TABLE 2: Differences between anthracosis and bronchial anthracofibrosis.[6,31]

	Anthracosis	Bronchial anthracofibrosis
Clinical profile	History of smoking, biomass fuel smoke exposure, coal mine workers	Elderly subjects with significant biomass fuel smoke exposure, rural households
Severity of disease	Mild	Severe
Radiology	• Can be normal • Parenchymal fibrotic bands	• Multifocal bronchial narrowing • Segmental collapse/consolidation • Peribronchial cuffing • Middle lobe syndrome • Mediastinal lymphadenopathy
Functional status	Usually preserved	Significantly affected adversely
Visual findings on bronchoscopy	Bluish-black pigmentation of bronchial mucosa	• Bluish-black pigmentation of bronchial mucosa with stenosis • Narrowing/distortion of the affected bronchus

Source: Adapted from reference 31.

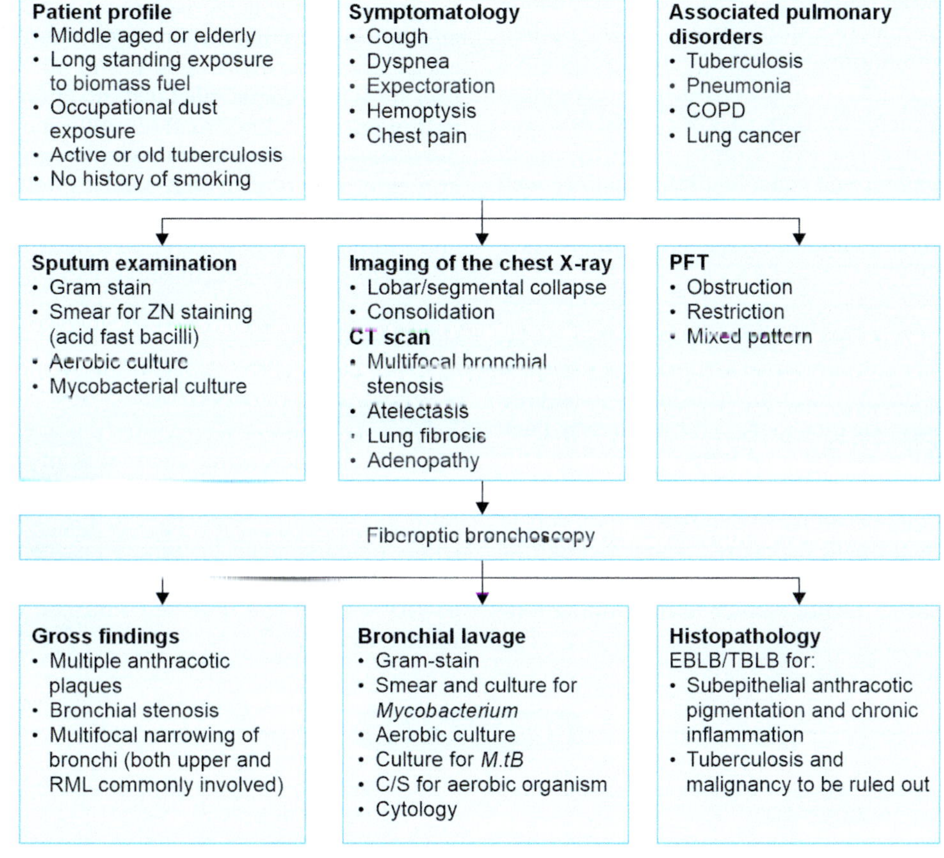

FLOWCHART 1: Proposed diagnostic algorithm of BAF.

(BAF: bronchial anthracofibrosis; COPD: chronic obstructive pulmonary disease; *M.tb: Mycobacterium tuberculosis*; PFT: pulmonary function test; ZN: Ziehl–Neelsen)

Source: Adapted from reference 6.

BRONCHIAL ANTHRACOFIBROSIS AND TUBERCULOSIS

A strong association has been documented between BAF and TB.[3,25,45] Although there is no clear and defined reason for this increased association, factors, namely alterations of the pulmonary immune defense mechanisms due to toxic substances in wood smoke,[46] higher prevalence of TB with increasing age,[47] and increased sensitivity to *M. tuberculosis* due to silica-containing pigmentation,[9] have been proposed. In addition, an increased risk of TB with repeated exposure to biomass fuel smoke also strengthens the association.[48] Recently, endobronchial TB was incriminated as the cause of BAF in an adolescent boy with no history of exposure to any source of carbon.[49]

BRONCHIAL ANTHRACOFIBROSIS AND OTHER RESPIRATORY CONDITIONS

Bronchial anthracofibrosis has also been associated with COPD and pneumonia. In four different studies, 596 patients with BAF were evaluated for underlying COPD and pneumonia.[16,36,50,51] Features of airflow obstruction were found in a quarter of these patients, while pneumonia was seen in approximately a third. It was thence opined that COPD and pneumonia were frequently associated with nontuberculous BAF.[51] Since exposure to biomass fuel smoke is a risk factor for both COPD[22,23] and BAF, the association between these two entities is pretty much obvious. Because pneumonic consolidation is mainly seen in lobes with bronchial narrowing,[50] the structural bronchial abnormalities in BAF are implicated as a major predilection for pneumonia.

A few studies[36,52] have also depicted an association between BAF and bronchial asthma. In an Indian study, a significantly higher prevalence of asthma was observed among elderly subjects from households using biomass fuels than from those using cleaner fuels.[52] It has already been demonstrated that biomass fuel smoke exposure reduced the peak expiratory flow rates in asthmatics and worsened their symptoms.[53] Since there is an increased risk of lung cancer following biomass fuel smoke exposure,[54,55] it is but natural that patients with BAF, by virtue of long-term exposure to biomass smoke, have a higher chance of developing lung cancer.[16,56]

Studies from India

In a study on the occurrence of BAF in respiratory symptomatics with biomass fuel smoke exposure, 24 of 60 had BAF on bronchoscopy, 17 had bronchial anthracosis, and 19 had normal appearance.[28] On HRCT, segmental collapse and consolidation were significantly higher in patients with BAF with the RML being the most affected (15/24; 62.5%). Multifocal bronchial narrowing was specific to BAF. Furthermore, these 24 patients had significantly poorer functional status.

In a review of 31 patients with BAF,[35] four had an associated diagnosis of TB. The study highlighted that once a diagnosis of TB is established in a patient with longstanding exposure to biomass fuel smoke, the invasive procedure required for the diagnosis of BAF may not be considered and the diagnosis could possibly remain confined to pulmonary TB.

Prevention and Treatment

Globally, there is great dependency on biomass fuels such as coal, wood, dung, and crop residues[57] for household activities for cooking and heating in poorly ventilated areas. Since BAF has also been suggested to be an occupational lung disorder,[58-60] prevention of dust and fumes exposure at the workplace must also be emphasized.

There is no specific treatment for BAF. Drugs such as antibiotics for concomitant respiratory infections, bronchodilators, mucolytic agents, and inhaled corticosteroids provide symptomatic relief with no effect on the underlying pathogenesis.[44] Empirical antitubercular treatment has been suggested for patients who live in areas where TB is endemic, in whom it may lead to definite improvement of chest radiograph findings.[59] Mechanical dilation or endobronchial stents could also be used in patients with endobronchial anthracofibrosis.[60] Two cases with severe symptomatic bronchial stenosis responded to endobronchial stent placement.

SUMMARY

There is an increasing awareness of the distinct clinic-radiological and bronchoscopic features of BAF as a specific pulmonary entity, especially in the developing countries where biomass fuel is in common usage.[61] When present on HRCT, MLS along with multifocal narrowing is suggestive of BAF while it can only be confirmed on visualization by bronchoscopy.[17,32]

REFERENCES

1. Klotz O. Pulmonary anthracosis - a community disease. Am J Public Health (NY). 1914;4:887-916.
2. Cohen AG. Atelectasis of the right middle lobe resulting from perforation of tuberculous lymph nodes into bronchi in adults. Ann Intern Med. 1951;35:820-35.
3. Chung MP, Lee KS, Han J, et al. Bronchial stenosis due to anthracofibrosis. Chest. 1998;113:344-50.
4. Kala J, Sahay S, Shah A. Bronchial anthracofibrosis and tuberculosis presenting as a middle lobe syndrome. Prim Care Respir J. 2008;17:51-5.

5. Behera D, Jindal S K. Respiratory symptoms in Indian women using domestic cooking fuels. Chest. 1991;100:385-8.
6. Gupta A, Shah A. Bronchial anthracofibrosis: an emerging pulmonary disease due to biomass fuel exposure. Int J Tuberc Lung Dis. 2011;15:602-12.
7. Long R, Wong E, Barrie J. Bronchial anthracofibrosis and tuberculosis: CT features before and after treatment. AJR Am J Roentgenol. 2005;184(suppl):S33-6.
8. Gómez-Seco J, Pérez-Boal I, Guerrero-González J, et al. Anthracofibrosis or anthracostenosis. Arch Bronconeumol. 2012;48:133-6.
9. Allison AC, Hart PD. Potentiation by silica of the growth of *Mycobacterium tuberculosis* in macrophage cultures. Br J Exp Pathol. 1968;49:465-76.
10. Wynn GJ, Turkington PM, O'Driscoll BR. Anthracofibrosis, bronchial stenosis with overlying anthracotic mucosa: possibly a new occupational lung disorder: a series of seven cases from one UK hospital. Chest. 2008;134:1069-73.
11. Singh V, Meena H, Bairwa R. Clinico-radiological profile and risk factors in patients with anthracosis. Lung India. 2015;32: 102-6.
12. Mirsadraee M, Katebi M. Loose body in the main bronchus due to broncholithiasis. Tanaffos. 2010;9:63-6.
13. Kradin RL, Spirn PW, Mark EJ. Intrapulmonary lymph nodes. Clinical, radiologic, and pathologic features. Chest. 1985; 87:662-7.
14. Churg A. The uptake of mineral particles by pulmonary epithelial cells. Am J Respir Crit Care Med. 1996;154:1124-40.
15. Gore DJ, Patrick G. A quantitative study of the penetration of insoluble particles into the tissue of the conducting airways. Ann Occup Hyg. 1982;26:149-61.
16. Kim YJ, Jung CY, Shin HW, et al. Biomass smoke induced bronchial anthracofibrosis: presenting features and clinical course. Respir Med. 2009;103:757-65.
17. Kim HY, Im JG, Goo JM. Bronchial anthracofibrosis (inflammatory bronchial stenosis with anthracotic pigmentation): CT findings. AJR Am J Roentgenol. 2000;174:523-27.
18. Amoli K. Anthracotic airway disease: Report of 102 cases. Tanaffos. 2009;8:14-22.
19. Hwang J, Puttagunta L, Green F, Shimanovsky A, Barrie J, Long R. Bronchial anthracofibrosis and tuberculosis in immigrants to Canada from the Indian subcontinent. Int J Tuberc Lung Dis. 2010;14:231-7.
20. Sigari N, Mohammadi S. Anthracosis and anthracofibrosis. Saudi Med J. 2009;30:1063-6.
21. Mirsadraee M. Anthracosis of the lungs: etiology, clinical manifestations and diagnosis: a review. Tanaffos. 2014;13:1 13.
22. Dennis R J, Maldonado D, Norman S, et al. Wood smoke exposure and risk for obstructive airways disease among women. Chest. 1996;109:115-9.
23. Orozco-Levi M, Garcia-Aymerich J, Villar J, et al. Wood smoke exposure and risk of chronic obstructive pulmonary disease. Eur Respir J. 2006;27:542-6.
24. Touhidi M, Keshmiri M, Ataran D, et al. Tuberculous bronchostenosis presenting as anthracofibrosis. Med J Mashhad Univ Med Sci. 2002;45:73-6.
25. Bircan HA, Bircan S, Oztürk O, et al. Mediastinal tuberculous lymphadenitis with anthracosis as a cause of vocal cord paralysis. Tuberk Toraks. 2007;55:409-13.
26. Yazaki K, Yoshida K, Hyodo K, et al. Pulmonary hypertension due to silicosis and right upper pulmonary artery occlusion with bronchial anthracofibrosis. Respir Med Case Rep. 2021;34: 101522.
27. Mirsadraee M, Asnaashari A, Attaran D. Pattern of pulmonary function test abnormalities in anthracofibrosis of the lungs. Tanaffos. 2012;11:34-7.
28. Pilaniya V, Kunal S, Shah A. Occurrence of bronchial anthracofibrosis in respiratory symptomatics with exposure to biomass fuel smoke. Adv Respir Med. 2017;85:12735.
29. Krimmer D, Ichimaru Y, Burgess J, et al. Exposure to biomass smoke extract enhances fibronectin release from fibroblasts. PLoS One. 2013;8:e83938.
30. Kahkouee S, Pourghorban R, Bitarafan M, et al. Imaging findings of isolated bronchial anthracofibrosis: A computed tomography analysis of patients with bronchoscopic and histologic confirmation. Arch Bronconeumol. 2015;51:3227.
31. Shah A, Kunal S, Gothi R. Bronchial anthracofibrosis: the spectrum of radiological appearances. Indian J Radiol Imaging. 2018;28:333-41.
32. Kim HJ, Kim SD, Shin DW, et al. Relationship between bronchial anthracofibrosis and endobronchial tuberculosis. Korean J Intern Med. 2013;28:330-8.
33. Criado E, Sánchez M, Ramírez J, et al. Pulmonary sarcoidosis: typical and atypical manifestations at high-resolution CT with pathologic correlation. Radiographics. 2010;30:156786.
34. Gupta P. The Golden S sign. Radiology. 2004;233:7901.
35. Kunal S, Shah A. The concomitant occurrence of pulmonary tuberculosis with bronchial anthracofibrosis. Indian J Tuberc. 2017;64:59.
36. Lee HS, Maeng JH, Park PG, et al. Clinical features of simple bronchial anthracofibrosis which is not associated with tuberculosis. Tuberc Respir Dis. 2002;53:510-8.
37. Torun T, Gungor G, Ozmen I, et al. Bronchial anthracostenosis in patients exposed to biomass smoke. Turkish Respir J. 2007;8: 48-51.
38. Kunal S, Pilaniya V, Shah A. Bronchial anthracofibrosis with interstitial lung disease: an association yet to be highlighted. BMJ Case Rep. 2016;pii:bcr2015213940.
39. Kunal S, Pilaniya V, Shah A. The co-occurrence of bronchial anthracofibrosis and interstitial lung disease. Arch Bronconeumol. 2017;53:2189.
40. Choe HS, Lee IJ, Lee Y. The CT findings of bronchial anthracofibrosis: Comparison of cases with or without active tuberculosis. J Korean Radiol Soc. 2004;50:10914.
41. Dhamija A, Basu A, Sharma V, et al. Mediastinal adenopathy in India: through the eyes of endobronchial ultrasound. J Assoc Physicians India. 2015;63:158.
42. Park HJ, Park SH, Im SA, et al. CT differentiation of anthracofibrosis from endobronchial tuberculosis. AJR Am J Roentgenol. 2008;191:247-51.
43. Yilmaz Demirci N, Alici IO, Yilmaz A, et al. Risk factors and maximum standardized uptake values within lymph nodes of anthracosis diagnosed by endobronchial ultrasound-guided transbronchial needle aspiration. Turk J Med Sci. 2015;45: 984-90.
44. Jamaati H, Sharifi A, Mirenayat MS, et al. What do we know about anthracofibrosis? A literature review. Tanaffos. 2017;16: 175-89.

45. Hemmati SH, Shahriar M, Molaei NA. What causes anthracofibrosis? Either tuberculosis or smoke. Pak J Med Sci. 2008;24:395-8.
46. Zelikoff JT, Chen LC, Cohen MD, et al. The toxicology of the inhaled woodsmoke. J Toxicol Environ Health. 2002;5:269-82.
47. Rajagopalan S. Tuberculosis and aging: A global health problem. Clin Infect Dis. 2001;33:1034-9.
48. Mishra VK, Retherford RD, Smith KR. Biomass cooking fuels and prevalence of tuberculosis in India. Int J Infect Dis. 1999;3:119-29.
49. Greimel T, Strenger V, Egger M, et al. Bronchial anthracofibrosis in an adolescent with tuberculosis without environmental carbon exposure. Pediatr Pulmonol. 2023;58:2408-10.
50. No TM, Kim IS, Kim SW, et al. The clinical investigation for determining the etiology of bronchial anthracofibrosis. Korean J Med. 2003;65:665-74.
51. Jang SJ, Lee SY, Kim SC, et al. Clinical and radiological characteristics of non-tuberculous bronchial anthracofibrosis. Tuberc Respir Dis. 2007;63:139-44.
52. Mishra V. Effect of indoor air pollution from biomass combustion on prevalence of asthma in the elderly. Environ Health Perspect. 2003;111:71-7.
53. Behera D, Chakrabarti T, Khanduja KL. Effect of exposure to domestic cooking fuels on bronchial asthma. Indian J Chest Dis Allied Sci. 2001;43:27-31.
54. Kleinerman RA, Wang Z, Wang L, et al. Lung cancer and indoor exposure to coal and biomass in rural China. J Occup Environ Med. 2002;44:338-44.
55. Ramanakumar AV, Parent ME, Siemiatycki J. Risk of lung cancer from residential heating and cooking fuels in Montreal, Canada. Am J Epidemiol. 2007;165:634-42.
56. Kunal S, Jain S, Shah A. Middle lobe syndrome: An exceptional presentation of concomitant lepidic adenocarcinoma and bronchial anthracofibrosis. Monaldi Arch Chest Dis. 2017;87:864.
57. Moran-Mendoza O, Pérez-Padilla JR, Salazar-Flores M, et al. Wood smoke-associated lung disease: a clinical, functional, radiological and pathological description. Int J Tuberc Lung Dis. 2008;12:10928.
58. Kim MH, Lee HY, Nam KH, et al. The clinical significance of bronchial anthracofibrosis associated with coal workers' pneumoconiosis. Tuberc Respir Dis. 2010;68:67-73.
59. Tutluer S, Tanriover MD, Emri S. Systemic glucocorticoid and anti-tuberculosis therapy in a patient with coexisting tuberculosis and anthracosis. Sarcoidosis Vasc Diffuse Lung Dis. 2013;30:308-11.
60. El Raouf BA, Kramer MR, Fruchter O. Bronchial anthracofibrosis: treatment using airway stents. Int J Tuberc Lung Dis. 2013;17:1118-20.
61. Shah A. Bronchial anthracofibrosis: A perilous consequence of exposure to biomass fuel smoke [Editorial]. Indian J Chest Dis Allied Sci. 2015;57:1513.

Respiratory Disability

CHAPTER 100

Mahesh PA, Greeshma MV

INTRODUCTION

Respiratory disability or impairment, characterized by alterations in lung structure and/or function, can profoundly impact an individual's quality of life. It often manifests through the distressing symptom of dyspnea upon exertion along with other symptoms such as cough, expectoration, or tiredness, leaving those affected struggling to perform routine activities. For cases associated with occupational disability, it may necessitate a formal evaluation for impairment and disability.

The underlying causes of pulmonary disability are diverse, spanning a spectrum of respiratory diseases, including airway conditions such as asthma and chronic obstructive pulmonary disease (COPD), parenchymal diseases, interstitial lung diseases, and pleural diseases. A pulmonary physician may be called upon to assess and determine the degree of impairment, for finalizing benefits or compensation programs. Moreover, physicians may also be asked to provide critical insights into an individual's capacity to engage in gainful employment.

IMPAIRMENT AND DISABILITY

Occupational health and safety considerations are critical, as they not only help prevent the onset of pulmonary disability but also ensure that individuals with preexisting conditions receive the necessary safeguards and accommodations to continue working without compromising their health. Impairment is primarily situated at the level of organs or organ systems, while whole-person impairment pertains to the extent of functional loss relative to the overall body's functioning. Conversely, disability concerns the individual's limitations in performing typical, everyday activities.[1-3]

Impairment, a cornerstone concept in the evaluation of pulmonary disability, is intricately tied to the degree of loss in the normal use or function of a particular body part or organ. The World Health Organization (WHO) provides a comprehensive definition of impairment as "any loss or abnormality of psychological, physiologic, or anatomic structure or function".[4] This definition underscores the encompassing nature of impairment, highlighting that it spans not only the physical but also the mental and physiological aspects of an individual's health. The American Medical Association (AMA) further elucidates this concept, defining impairment as "a loss, loss of use, or derangement of any body part, organ system, or organ function".[5] In essence, impairment encapsulates a wide spectrum of deviations from the ideal state of health and functioning.

Disability, a central concept within the realm of pulmonary impairment evaluation, holds paramount significance in assessing an individual's overall functional capacity. It encompasses the manifold ways in which a respiratory condition can profoundly affect an individual's life and their ability to engage in everyday activities. This profound impact extends beyond the mere presence of a medical diagnosis; it is rooted in how that diagnosis translates into tangible limitations in the person's life.[6,7] The WHO offers a comprehensive definition of disability as "any restriction or lack of ability to perform any activity within the range considered normal for a human being".[4] This definition underscores the pivotal concept that disability is not merely confined to the realm of medical parameters but extends to the real-world abilities and limitations that individuals experience. It encapsulates the notion that disability is not solely about what one cannot do, but how their condition influences what they can do in comparison to the typical capabilities of a human being.

The rising tide of patients seeking evaluation for pulmonary impairment and disability can be attributed to several interwoven factors such as the increasing prevalence of COPD and heightened awareness of the industrial and environmental hazards. As our understanding of respiratory health deepens and more individuals are exposed to potentially harmful agents in their work and living environments, the need for comprehensive assessment and support for those affected becomes increasingly apparent. **(Flowchart 1)**.[8-10]

Legislative changes and societal shifts have fostered a more accepting environment for individuals with pulmonary impairment to obtain compensation. Healthcare professionals, especially those in pulmonary rehabilitation,

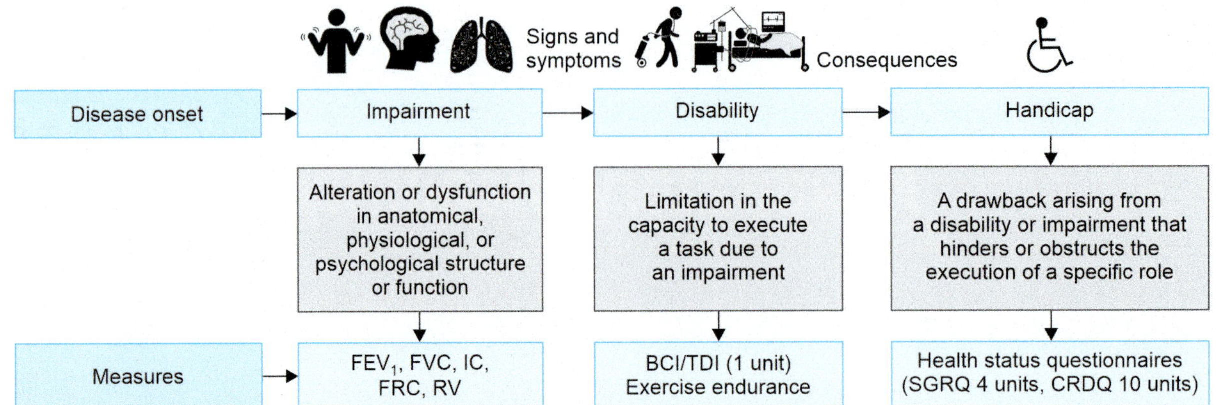

FLOWCHART 1: Relationship between workplace impairment and disability and assessment of impairment, disability, and handicap.
(BDI: baseline dyspnea index; CRDQ: chronic respiratory disease questionnaire; FEV1: forced expiratory volume in 1 second; FRC: functional residual capacity; FVC: forced vital capacity; IC: inspiratory capacity; 6-MWD: 6-minute walking distance; RV: residual volume; SGRQ: St George's Respiratory Questionnaire; TDI: transition dyspnea index)

increasingly fulfil dual roles as both caregivers and evaluators of respiratory impairment. Pulmonologists are now commonly expected to assess and quantify pulmonary disability, a task demanding a synthesis of medical knowledge, legal understanding, and ethical practice.[11] This multifaceted role requires a delicate balance of medical expertise, legal acumen, and ethical considerations. Prior to a determination that a medical condition has led to permanent impairment or disability, the exhaustion of reasonable options or the optimization of medical treatment is mandatory and this is referred to as "maximum medical improvement" (MMI). At this stage, the medical condition has reached a point where further significant improvements in its treatment or management are unlikely, and it serves as the baseline from which to assess the degree of impairment or disability.[6]

CLINICAL APPROACH TO RESPIRATORY DISABILITY EVALUATION

It is useful to maintain a standard approach for each subject though it needs to be individualized based on the exposed occupation or environment of the subject being assessed for disability. Developing a comprehensive algorithm for evaluating pulmonary disability due to occupational exposures requires a multidisciplinary approach involving pulmonologists, occupational medicine specialists, and experts in occupational health.[12-14] The algorithm should consider various factors, including medical history, clinical assessments, pulmonary function tests (PFTs), imaging studies, and exposure history **(Box 1)**. A comprehensive occupational history must chronologically detail job durations, activities, and potential inhalational hazards such as dust, fumes, gases, or smoke, quantifying exposure levels and frequency. Ventilation quality and respiratory protection usage, alongside any immediate work-related symptoms, warrant investigation. Document chemical exposures meticulously, especially those with significant health implications, using Safety Data Sheets for insight into chemical hazards. Additionally, examine the patient's home environment for heating, cooling, and humidification systems, pet-related allergens, hot tub usage, and hobby-associated exposures.[15,16]

HISTORY, SYMPTOMS, FUNCTIONAL LIMITATIONS, AND PHYSICAL EXAMINATION

The key symptoms—chronic dyspnea, cough, and wheezing—are crucial indicators of potential work-related respiratory impairment. Dyspnea, a subjective experience of uncomfortable breathing, is a sensitive but nonspecific symptom of respiratory dysfunction.[17-19] The Medical Research Council (MRC) dyspnea scale assists in quantifying its impact on daily activities. Chronic cough and sputum production, persisting over 4 weeks, reflect airway irritation or damage and inform impairment severity. Wheezing, particularly when associated with workdays, suggests occupational lung diseases such as work-related asthma. A temporal pattern of symptom relief during nonwork periods can pinpoint occupational etiology, aiding in disability assessments.[20-22]

The correlation of these symptoms with job activities, regular symptom monitoring, and standardized evaluations is important in occupational health protocols to safeguard workers and facilitate appropriate compensation and rehabilitation.[23] Difficulties arise when the subject is exposed to nonoccupational detrimental stimuli such as smoking and biomass fuels for cooking or heating at home or when subjects have preexisting disease conditions such as asthma or bronchiectasis before they have joined for work. Some of the hazardous occupations include construction, manufacturing, agriculture, mining, welding and metal

BOX 1 Steps of an algorithm for evaluating pulmonary disability due to occupational and environmental exposures.

Step 1: Initial assessment

- *Patient history*:
  - Obtain a detailed medical and occupational history
  - Document specific job tasks, duration of exposure, and types of exposures (e.g., dust, chemicals, fumes)
  - Occupational exposure history: Consult with an occupational medicine specialist to determine the extent of exposure and its relation to the patient's condition
  - Identify any preexisting lung conditions or comorbidities
- *Symptoms and functional limitations*:
  - Assess the patient's respiratory symptoms (e.g., cough, dyspnea, wheezing)
  - Evaluate how these symptoms affect the patient's daily activities and quality of life

Step 2: Physical examination

- *Respiratory examination*:
  - Conduct a thorough respiratory examination, including inspection, palpation, percussion, and auscultation
  - Look for signs of respiratory distress, chest deformities, or clubbing
- *General examination*:
  - Assess the general health and nutritional status of the patient
  - Assess for extrapulmonary conditions contributing to the general impairment

Step 3: Pulmonary function tests (PFTs)

- *Spirometry*: Perform spirometry to assess lung function, including FEV1 (forced expiratory volume in 1 second) and FVC (forced vital capacity)
- *DLCO (diffusing capacity of the lungs for carbon monoxide)*: Measure DLCO to assess gas exchange in the lungs
- *Lung volume measurements*: Consider additional lung volume measurements, such as total lung capacity (TLC) and residual volume (RV), if needed
- *Cardiopulmonary exercise test*: Exercise testing plays a crucial role in assessing and diagnosing certain medical conditions, especially when there is a significant mismatch between a patient's symptoms and resting physiology. This discrepancy often indicates that the patient's symptoms are triggered or exacerbated by physical exertion, and exercise testing can help provide a more precise measurement of work capacity, identify the underlying issues, and guide treatment decisions

Step 4: Imaging studies

- *Chest X-ray*: Perform a chest X-ray to evaluate the presence of parenchymal abnormalities, occupational lung diseases, or other lung conditions
- *High-resolution CT (HRCT) scan*: Consider HRCT for a more detailed assessment of lung parenchyma, especially if chest X-ray findings are inconclusive

Step 5: Additional testing

- *Laboratory tests*: Conduct blood tests, including arterial blood gases (if necessary) and specific biomarkers (e.g., serum markers for pneumoconiosis)
- *Bronchoscopy*: Consider bronchoscopy if there is a suspicion of airway involvement or the need to obtain bronchoalveolar lavage (BAL) or biopsy samples

Step 6: Disease-specific impairment assessment

- Asthma, chronic obstructive pulmonary disease (COPD), bronchiectasis, lung cancer, hypersensitivity pneumonitis

Step 7: Pulmonary disability evaluation

- *Functional impairment assessment*: Determine the extent of pulmonary disability by evaluating the impact of lung function impairment on the patient's ability to work and perform daily activities and divide them into five classes

Step 8: Apportionment and workplace protection

- *Apportionment*: Develop a personalized apportionment plan, based on previous noxious exposures, for example, tobacco smoking, and previous diseases, for example, asthma
- *Workplace protection*: Follow the NIOSH model for careful evaluation of workplace exposure to hazardous chemicals and use of respirators

work, chemical industry, and office work with poor indoor air quality and health workers.[24]

- *Construction workers*: Evaluation of the risks necessitates detailed inquiries into their specific trade—be it carpentry, masonry, or electrical work—and any contact with respiratory hazards such as dust, asbestos, or chemicals. Assessing their personal protective equipment usage, such as respirators, is crucial for determining risk mitigation practices. The length of their career in construction, including involvement in renovations or demolitions, is essential to understanding the cumulative exposure. Additionally, it is critical to determine if they have been diagnosed with occupational lung diseases such as pneumoconiosis, which includes conditions such as asbestosis and silicosis, as these could be compounded by their occupational activities.[25,26]
- *Manufacturing employees*: Key inquiries should include their specific sector, such as metalworking or electronics, and exposures to solvents, dust, or fumes. Assessing their work in confined spaces, chemical handling, and occupational health training is crucial for evaluating respiratory risks.[25,27]
- *Agricultural workers*: They are susceptible to respiratory hazards present in farming environments. It is important to understand their primary agricultural tasks, whether they engage in crop farming or animal husbandry. Inquiring about exposures to agricultural dust, pesticides, or mold is vital as these factors can significantly impact respiratory health. Furthermore, understanding their use of respiratory protection while working with livestock or in dusty environments provides insights into their safety practices. Asking whether they have experienced symptoms such as coughing, wheezing, or shortness of breath after working on the farm helps identify potential respiratory issues related to their occupation.[28,29]
- *Miners*: They work in underground or excavation settings, often encountering respiratory hazards. It is essential to inquire about the type of mining they engage in, whether it is coal, metal, or stone mining. Understanding whether they have been exposed to underground dust, gases, or diesel exhaust helps assess their respiratory exposure. Inquiring about their regular screening for occupational lung diseases is essential for monitoring their health. Additionally, asking whether they use respiratory protection devices and practice safe mining techniques provides insights into their safety practices.[30,31]
- *Welders and metalworkers*: In welding or metalwork, exposure to fumes, dust, or gases is common. It is important to assess their protective equipment use, ventilation, and any respiratory symptoms or conditions like metal fume fever.[32]
- *Chemical industry workers:* Chemical workers handle substances that may pose respiratory risks. Evaluating their knowledge of these hazards, adherence to safety protocols, and any respiratory issues is key for occupational health assessment.[33-35]
- *Office workers with indoor air quality concerns*: Indoor air quality issues can affect office workers' respiratory health. Assessing symptoms related to workplace air, such as mold or poor ventilation, and any improvement outside work is necessary, along with history of allergies or asthma.[36,37]
- *Healthcare professionals*: Facing potential exposure to airborne pathogens and chemicals, healthcare workers' safety measures, and experiences of respiratory symptoms, especially after medical procedures, must be evaluated for occupational health risks, including latex allergy.[34,38]

DISABILITY ASSESSMENT

A patient's respiratory condition is examined in terms of its impact on daily life, particularly on activities of daily living (ADLs). This comprehensive evaluation illuminates the disease's disability and how it hinders functional independence.[39] *Basic self-care*: Assessing the ability to perform basic self-care tasks, like bathing and personal grooming, is critical for gauging self-sufficiency and the effects of pulmonary conditions on these essential activities.

- *Mobility*: Mobility assessment includes evaluating ease of walking, capacity for brisk walking, and resilience in uphill movements, all of which reflect the patient's functional status compared to peers. Determining their capability to climb stairs also offers insight into their respiratory system's functional capacity.[40]
- *Home maintenance*: The capacity to manage indoor and outdoor household tasks is scrutinized to understand the patient's ability to maintain their living environment, providing a lens into their functional limitations.[41]
- *Hobbies and activities*: Beyond the realm of necessities, life is enriched by customary hobbies, exercise routines, and job-related tasks. The impact of respiratory conditions on engagement in hobbies, exercises, and occupational tasks is also vital, offering a broader view of the patient's functional limitations.[42,43]

  In the assessment of ADLs, standardized methods are available, with some tailored to specific diseases. The AMA Guides present a detailed list of ADLs for disability evaluation, and dyspnea scales help quantify symptom severity. Yet, the disparity between subjective dyspnea and objective PFTs underscores the necessity for a nuanced assessment that combines both.[44,45] A comprehensive physical examination including height and weight measurements is important to provide information on respiratory health. Signs of right heart failure, such as jugular venous distention, a palpable left parasternal heave, liver engorgement, and peripheral edema, are documented as evidence of advanced respiratory impairment in severe cases.[46,47]
- *Pulmonary function test (spirometry, DLCO, cardiopulmonary exercise testing)*: The evaluation of respiratory impairment in lung disease focuses on lung function, as

TABLE 1: Classification of respiratory impairment and disability (ATS).

Classification of respiratory impairment (ATS)		
Normal	≥80% predicted FVC ≥80% predicted FEV1 >75% FEV1/FVC ≥80% predicted DLCO	Work ability—normal
Mildly impaired	≥80% predicted FVC ≥80% predicted FEV1 >75% FEV1/FVC ≥80% predicted DLCO	Work ability—usually able to perform most jobs
Moderately impaired	51–59% predicted FVC 41–59% predicted FEV1 41–59% FEV1/FVC 41–59% predicted DLCO	Work ability—diminished ability to perform many jobs
Severely impaired	<50% predicted FVC <40% predicted FEV1 <40% FEV1/FVC <40% predicted DLCO	Work ability—unable to meet physical demands of most jobs including travel to work

(ATS: American Thoracic Society; DLCO: diffusing capacity of the lungs for carbon monoxide; FEV1: forced expiratory volume in 1 second; FVC: forced vital capacity)

a metric to rate impairment, without assigning a specific whole-person impairment percentage often used in disability compensation.[48] The American Thoracic Society (ATS) framework **(Table 1)** categorizes impairment into four levels based on PFT outcomes, describing the individual's capacity for work-related functions, aiding in determining occupational limitations and necessary accommodations.[48-50]

Unlike the ATS classification, the AMA classification of respiratory impairment **(Table 2)** serves as a structured framework for evaluating the impact of respiratory conditions on an individual's overall health and impairment. This classification system categorizes individuals into four distinct classes based on specific criteria related to pulmonary function and exercise capacity.[5]

- *Chest Imaging*: Standard posteroanterior and lateral chest radiographs serve as initial investigative modalities for the detection of parenchymal abnormalities, pleural changes, and other structural anomalies potentially indicative of occupational lung diseases, such as pneumoconiosis, asbestosis, or silicosis. However, the intrinsic limitation of two-dimensional X-rays in delineating complex interstitial lung diseases often necessitates the deployment of high-resolution computed tomography (HRCT), which offers cross-sectional imaging with axial, coronal, and sagittal planes. HRCT excels in characterizing the morphology and distribution of lung parenchymal alterations, which contribute significantly to the International Labour Office (ILO) classification of radiographs of pneumoconiosis. Furthermore, HRCT's sensitivity in detecting early interstitial lung disease can influence prognostication and compensation decisions in occupational health adjudication. When quantifying impairment, radiologists must integrate the radiological

TABLE 2: Classification of respiratory impairment and disability (according to American Medical Association).

Class 0	Severity grade—nil ≥80% predicted FVC ≥80% predicted FEV1 >LLN/ >75% predicted FEV1/FVC >75% predicted DLCO	No current signs of the disease, no symptoms, intermittent dyspnea does not require treatment
Class 1: 2–10% impairment	Severity grade (A—2%, B—4%, C—6%, D—8%, E—10%) 70–79% predicted FVC 65–79% predicted FEV1 65–74% predicted DLCO	• Controlled dyspnea with intermittent or continuous treatment • Physical finding not present/intermittent mild
Class 2: 11–23% impairment	Severity grade (A—11%, B—14%, C—17%, D—20%, E—23%) 70–79% predicted FVC 65–79% predicted FEV1 65–74% predicted DLCO	• Constant mild/ intermittent moderate dyspnea with continuous treatment • Constant mild/ intermittent moderate physical findings with constant treatment
Class 3: 24–40% impairment	Severity grade (A—24%, B—28%, C—32%, D—36%, E—40%) 50–59% predicted FVC 45–54% predicted FEV1 45–54% predicted DLCO	• Constant moderate/ intermittent severe dyspnea with continuous treatment • Constant moderate/ intermittent severe physical findings with continuous treatment
Class 4: 45–65% impairment	Severity grade (A—45%, B—50%, C—55%, D—60%, E—65%) <50% predicted FVC <45% predicted FEV1 <45% predicted DLCO	• Constant severe/ intermittent extreme dyspnea with continuous treatment • Constant severe/ intermittent extreme physical findings with continuous treatment

(DLCO: diffusing capacity of the lungs for carbon monoxide; FEV1: forced expiratory volume in 1 second; FVC: forced vital capacity; LLN: lower limit of normal)

Source: Adapted from Evaluation of impairment/disability secondary to respiratory disorders. AMA Guides® to the Evaluation of Impairment, 6th edition. Chicago, IL: American Medical Association; 2008.

findings with PFT results, as well as the patient's clinical presentation and exposure history, to provide a comprehensive appraisal of functional impairment attributable to workplace-inhaled toxins, ensuring that such evaluations are grounded in evidence-based criteria and are consistent with current best practices in thoracic imaging and occupational health standards.[51,52]

The ILO radiological classification system is a globally recognized method for standardizing the radiographic assessment of pneumoconiosis, a group of lung diseases caused by the inhalation of different dusts. The system was developed to provide a consistent and reproducible means of recording and communicating the radiographic abnormalities found in the chest radiographs of workers exposed to dust.[53,54]

Standard radiographs: The ILO classification is based on a set of standard radiographs that serve as reference images representing different types and severities of abnormalities. Radiologists compare the individual's chest X-ray with these standards to determine the presence and extent of disease.

Technical quality of radiograph: Before classifying the radiographic findings, the technical quality of the radiograph is assessed (e.g., inspiration, rotation, penetration), as this can significantly affect the interpretation.

Parenchymal abnormalities: These are classified according to size (classified as p, q, r, s, t, u), shape, and profusion (concentration) of small opacities **(Box 2)**. Profusion is based on the number of abnormalities seen in the affected zones of the lung fields and is graded on a scale from 0/0 (normal) to 3/3 (most severe).

BOX 2 ILO categorization of parenchymal lung abnormalities.

- *Small opacities*:
  - p-type: Rounded opacities with diameters of up to 1.5 mm
  - q-type: Rounded opacities with diameters of 1.5–3 mm
  - r-type: Rounded opacities with diameters of 3–10 mm
  - s-type: Irregular opacities with widths of up to 1.5 mm
  - t-type: Irregular opacities with widths of 1.5–3 mm
  - u-type: Irregular opacities with widths of 3–10 mm
- *Large opacities*: Classified as A, B, or C depending on their size:
  - Category A: Any opacity with an area equivalent to the size of a chest X-ray film segment (subsegmental)
  - Category B: Opacities with an area greater than category A but less than the equivalent of the upper right lung zone
  - Category C: Any opacity with an area greater than the upper right lung zone
- *Pleural abnormalities*: The ILO system also includes the classification of pleural abnormalities, including pleural thickening and calcification. The thickening is assessed in terms of extent (localized or diffuse), width at the chest wall, and obliteration of the costophrenic angle

(ILO: International Labour Organization)

Symbols: The ILO system uses specific symbols to note other radiographic findings that are not classified within the standard categories but may be significant in the evaluation of pneumoconiosis, such as bullae (B) or evidence of tuberculosis (tb).

Completeness and comparability: A section of the ILO form addresses the issue of whether the radiograph is acceptable for classification and whether previous radiographs are available for comparison, which is important for determining disease progression.

The ILO classification is used in occupational health to assess eligibility for compensation, monitor disease progression, and implement preventive measures in workplace settings. The goal is to have an internationally uniform approach that allows for comparison between different populations and time periods. It is a vital tool for epidemiological studies, health surveillance programs, and research on the health effects of inhalational exposures in the workplace.[55]

- *Other investigations*:
  - *Blood investigations*: In occupational lung disease evaluation, blood tests including a complete blood count (CBC) and comprehensive metabolic panel (CMP) are foundational, while arterial blood gas (ABG) analysis is vital for assessing respiratory function, potentially guiding oxygen or ventilator therapy.[56,57] For pneumoconiosis, specific biomarkers such as Clara cell protein (CC16), C-reactive protein (CRP), serum amyloid A (SAA), and cytokines like interleukin 1 (IL-1) and tumor necrosis factor alpha (TNF-alpha) are indicative of inflammation and disease severity. Surfactant proteins A and D (SP-A and SP-D), secreted by alveolar cells, are markers for pulmonary fibrosis, signaling epithelial damage. Research into molecular markers offers prospects for understanding disease pathways and therapeutic interventions.[58,59]
  - *Bronchoscopy*: This is a diagnostic cornerstone when other methods fall short, enabling visualization and tissue sampling to distinguish between benign and malignant conditions.[60] Bronchoalveolar lavage (BAL) reveals cellular details that can indicate alveolitis and the presence of macrophages laden with dust or birefringent particles, suggestive of mineral dust exposure. Differential cell counts, cytology, and culture of the BAL fluid can also aid in the diagnosis of infections or neoplastic conditions. BAL fluid analysis for oxidative stress and fibrosis biomarkers assists in evaluating disease progression. Despite risks, transbronchial biopsy is a decisive tool, providing histopathological evidence crucial for diagnosing and managing interstitial lung diseases.[61,62]
  - *Bronchoprovocation testing*: This plays a critical role in the assessment of occupational pulmonary impairment, particularly in cases where work-related

asthma (WRA) or other forms of occupation-related airway hyper-reactivity are suspected. This form of testing is designed to assess the responsiveness of the airways to specific or nonspecific stimuli that could mimic exposure in the workplace environment.[63]

- *Specific inhalation challenge (SIC)*: In the context of occupational exposures, SIC is considered the gold standard for diagnosing occupational asthma **(Box 3)**. This test involves controlled exposure to the suspected occupational agent in a laboratory setting while closely monitoring lung function and symptoms. A positive test, characterized by a significant decline in forced expiratory volume in 1 second (FEV1) following exposure, confirms the diagnosis of occupational asthma.[64-66]

For each specific bronchoprovocation test, the concentration of the agent and the duration of exposure are carefully controlled to minimize the risk to the individual being tested. The patient's respiratory function is closely monitored during and after exposure, using spirometry to detect any changes indicative of an asthma reaction. Positive reactions are characterized by a decrease in forced expiratory volume in 1 second (FEV1) and can be accompanied by symptoms such as coughing, wheezing, chest tightness, and shortness of breath. Due to the potential risks associated with specific bronchoprovocation testing, it is usually carried out in specialized centers with appropriate facilities and expertise, where immediate medical intervention is available if necessary.[63]

- *Nonspecific bronchoprovocation testing*: These tests involve the inhalation of nonspecific agents such as methacholine, histamine, or mannitol that can trigger bronchoconstriction. If hyper-responsiveness is demonstrated by a significant decrease in FEV1, it may suggest a diagnosis of asthma but does not necessarily confirm the occupational origin. However, when combined with a thorough occupational history and improvement of symptoms away from work, it supports the diagnosis of WRA.[67]

- *Clinical implications*:[68]
  - *Diagnosis of occupational asthma*: Bronchoprovocation testing is essential for diagnosing occupational asthma, distinguishing it from nonoccupational asthma, and identifying specific workplace triggers.
  - *Assessment of airway hyper-responsiveness*: It aids in the assessment of airway hyper-responsiveness, which can be a feature of occupational asthma or other work-related airway disorders.
  - *Quantifying impairment*: The degree of bronchial responsiveness can also help quantify the level of impairment and may be useful in making decisions regarding fitness for work, work modifications, or disability assessment.
  - *Monitoring and surveillance*: Regular bronchoprovocation testing can be part of surveillance programs for workers at risk of developing occupational asthma, allowing for early detection and intervention.
- *Limitations and considerations*:
  - *Interpretation*: Interpretation of bronchoprovocation tests must be performed with caution and in the context of the patient's occupational, clinical, and exposure history.
  - *Safety*: The tests should be conducted in a controlled environment due to the risk of inducing significant bronchospasm, and resuscitative equipment should be available.
  - *False positives/negatives*: Both false-positive and false-negative results can occur, which may require correlation with other diagnostic modalities such as peak flow variability testing or immunologic assays.

BOX 3 Specific challenges for occupational exposures.

- *Isocyanates*: Common in the automotive and painting industries for products like spray-on foams, paints, and coatings
- *Wood dusts*: Particularly in carpentry, sawmilling, and furniture-making occupations
- *Flour and grain dust*: Commonly tested in bakers, millers, and agricultural workers
- *Animal proteins and enzymes*: Laboratory animal workers, veterinary staff, or those working in animal processing plants may be tested for sensitivity to animal dander or proteins
- *Latex*: Healthcare workers are commonly tested for latex allergy due to the use of latex gloves and medical devices containing latex
- *Acids and anhydrides*: Employed in the chemical and plastics industries, causing respiratory sensitivity in some workers
- *Colophony*: Used in soldering fumes and may cause asthma in electronics industry workers
- *Ammonia*: Commonly encountered in agricultural, food processing, and industrial cleaning environments
- *Persulfate salts*: Used in hair bleaching products and can affect hairdressers
- *Formaldehyde*: Found in numerous manufacturing processes, particularly where resin products are used
- *Metals*: Such as platinum salts and nickel sulfate, which are used in refining and electroplating industries

DISEASE-SPECIFIC IMPAIRMENT EVALUATIONS

Asthma

One of the best studied diseases for occupational impairment assessments is workplace asthma. In the specialized context of pulmonary disability assessment for asthma, the ATS guidelines and AMA Guides provide a structured approach for quantifying impairment due to asthma. Recognizing the episodic and variable nature of airflow limitation and bronchial hyper-responsiveness inherent to asthma, the ATS established an evaluation paradigm that considers both the severity of airway obstruction and the level of medication required to achieve control.[5,69]

The subject is discussed in length in the chapter on "Occupational Asthma".

For a definitive and comprehensive evaluation, the individual must have reached MMI and should be at an optimal therapeutic baseline, which implies the least amount of medication necessary to maintain controlled asthma has been determined, and sufficient time has been allowed for the medication to exhibit its full effect. The postbronchodilator FEV1, the degree of reversibility indicated by percentage change with bronchodilator, and methacholine challenge results (i.e., PC20) and the medicine needed for maximum improvement to be sustained are pivotal metrics. The requirement for minimum medication use needs to be documented by the treating physician in the records, when the patient has exacerbations on stopping or reducing the dosage. The composite score, derived from these individual metrics, delineates the class of impairment ranging from Class 0 (no impairment) to Class V (asthma uncontrolled despite maximal therapy). The AMA Guides elaborate on this by assigning a corresponding range of whole-person impairment percentages for each class, facilitating a uniform assessment.[5]

The ATS has put forth a structured system for evaluating the impairment associated with asthma, detailed in their impairment rating guidelines. This evaluation method is designed to consider various aspects of asthma severity and control and is broken down into several sections.[69]

Summary of impairment rating classes: The total score from Sections A, B, and C determines the impairment class.

A total score of 0 indicates no impairment (class 0).

A score ranging from 1 to 3 corresponds to class I impairment.

Class II impairment is defined by scores from 4 to 6.

Class III corresponds to scores between 7 and 9.

Scores from 10 to 11 are categorized as class IV impairment.

Finally, class V signifies severe impairment, where asthma is not controlled despite maximal treatment, exemplified by FEV1 remaining less than 50% even with the use of 20 mg or more of prednisone daily. This comprehensive scoring system allows clinicians to assign an impairment rating that reflects the functional limitations and therapeutic requirements of individuals with asthma, especially when evaluating for occupational health and disability.

Chronic Obstructive Pulmonary Disease

Several occupations are associated with an increased risk of developing COPD. Individuals engaged in mining, operating blast furnaces, steelworks, and rolling and finishing mills confront considerably higher risks, in additional to employees in grocery distribution, those working in automotive repair shops, maids, farmworkers, those specialized in vehicle or mobile equipment maintenance, operators of material-moving machinery, and laborers outside the construction sphere. Such risks are often correlated with specific environmental exposures; workers face asbestos in the furnace and metalworking industries, aerosol paints in vehicle repair, pesticides in agricultural settings, and pervasive dust and ash among operators and laborers handling materials. These associations signal a need for targeted preventive measures and health surveillance in these high-risk sectors and roles.[70,71]

One of the primary methods of assessing COPD is through pulmonary function testing. The most important PFT in COPD is spirometry, particularly the FEV1 and the FEV1/FVC (forced vital capacity) ratio. The FEV1 value, expressed as a percentage of the predicted value for a person's age, gender, height, and ethnicity, is used to categorize the severity of COPD. Beyond spirometry, other tests like diffusion capacity [diffusing capacity of the lungs for carbon monoxide (DLCO)], ABGs, and HRCT scans may be used to further elucidate the extent of pulmonary impairment and gas exchange abnormalities.[72]

AMA Guides for pulmonary impairment ***(Box 1)***: The AMA's "Guides to the Evaluation of Permanent Impairment" provides a structured approach for rating pulmonary impairment. COPD impairment is often categorized by the individual's FEV1 score postbronchodilator use: Mild impairment may be indicated by an FEV1 of 60–80% of predicted. Moderate impairment is often assigned to individuals with FEV1 values of 50–59% of predicted. Severe impairment might be considered when FEV1 falls below 50% of the predicted value.[5]

ATS recommendations ***(Table 1)***: The ATS also provides guidance, suggesting that other factors should be considered in addition to spirometric values, such as patient symptoms (e.g., dyspnea scale), impact on daily living activities, frequency and severity of exacerbations, need for supplemental oxygen, hospitalizations related to respiratory illness, presence of secondary pulmonary hypertension, and/or cor pulmonale (right-sided heart failure due to lung disease).[69]

Bronchiectasis

The evaluation and rating of pulmonary disability in bronchiectasis present unique challenges due to the episodic nature of the condition. Traditional PFTs may not fully capture the extent of impairment in bronchiectasis because patients often experience recurrent bouts of infection and inflammation that lead to intermittent respiratory symptoms and dysfunction. These exacerbations can significantly impair ADLs despite periods of seemingly normal lung function.[73]

The AMA Guides to the Evaluation of Permanent Impairment, Fifth Edition, recognize the limitations of standard PFTs in bronchiectasis. As such, these guidelines concede that typical pulmonary testing is only relevant in a restricted number of cases when assessing bronchiectasis. Instead, the AMA Guides permit the evaluating physician to determine impairment based on the frequency, intensity, and severity of infectious and inflammatory episodes, as well as their impact on a patient's ADLs. This assessment must be backed by objective evidence that could include, but is not limited to, imaging studies, sputum production, and the presence of systemic symptoms.[74]

In practice, when evaluating bronchiectasis, a physician should carefully document the pattern and severity of the patient's symptoms, the frequency and outcome of exacerbations, the extent of any hospitalizations, the response to treatment, and the overall effect on the patient's quality of life and ability to perform ADLs. This comprehensive approach allows for a more nuanced and accurate determination of disability in patients with bronchiectasis, ultimately leading to a fairer representation of their impairment and needs for assistance or compensation.

Lung Cancer

There are two distinct approaches to rating permanent impairment resulting from lung cancer, acknowledging the grave nature of the diagnosis. From the onset of diagnosis, individuals with lung cancer are deemed to be severely impaired. This initial classification reflects the significant impact that lung cancer typically has on an individual's respiratory function, overall health status, and ability to perform ADLs.

After 1 year from the diagnosis, the impairment assessment is revisited. If there is ongoing evidence of the primary tumor or if there has been a recurrence of the disease, the individual continues to be categorized as severely impaired. This sustained classification as severely impaired indicates that the cancer remains active or progressive and is likely to be continuing to significantly affect the patient's respiratory capacity and functional status.

On the other hand, if after 1 year there is no evidence of residual tumor or recurrence, the impairment rating is then determined using the standard respiratory disease methodology outlined in the AMA Guides. This methodology involves a detailed evaluation of the individual's respiratory function through PFTs, which measure parameters such as FVC and FEV1. The results of these tests are used to classify impairment within a defined grading system.[6,75]

The ATS has also issued guidelines for the assessment of impairment due to respiratory diseases, which can be applied to cases of lung cancer. The ATS guidelines emphasize the need for comprehensive evaluations that may include PFTs, exercise tolerance tests, assessments of gas exchange, and the consideration of clinical symptoms and signs. In addition to objective measurements, both the AMA and ATS acknowledge the importance of considering the patient's subjective experience of their condition, including symptoms such as dyspnea, pain, and the impact on their ability to perform daily activities and to work. When evaluating lung cancer in the context of occupational exposure, it is also important to consider the individual's exposure history and the potential causative role of workplace carcinogens. This is particularly relevant for cases where lung cancer may be attributed to occupational hazards, and it can have implications for workers' compensation or disability benefits.[76]

Hypersensitivity Pneumonitis

Occupational hypersensitivity pneumonitis (OHP), also known as extrinsic allergic alveolitis, is a complex respiratory syndrome caused by inhaling various environmental antigens related to specific workplaces. This condition represents an immunologically mediated inflammatory disease affecting the lung parenchyma and small airways. It is triggered by repeated exposure to organic dusts, chemical agents, or proteins that are inhaled in the occupational environment. The causative agents of OHP are diverse and are often associated with specific jobs. For example, workers in agriculture may develop farmer's lung after inhaling moldy hay dust containing thermophilic actinomycetes. Bird fancier's lung, another form of OHP, is triggered by exposure to avian proteins found in droppings or feathers. Industrial settings, such as plastics manufacturing and electronics, can expose workers to chemicals (acid anhydrides, persulfates, metal salts) that may also trigger hypersensitivity responses.[77,78]

Respiratory disability in OHP is primarily determined by the degree of lung function impairment and the presence of fibrosis. Over time, chronic inflammatory response may lead to lung scarring, significantly reducing lung volumes and gas exchange capabilities. Consequently, patients may suffer from a reduction in exercise tolerance, progressive dyspnea, and chronic hypoxemia, leading to a profound impact on their quality of life and ability to perform ADLs or maintain employment.[9,79]

The assessment of impairment in individuals with OHP is challenging due to the episodic nature of the disease and the variability in clinical presentation. The approach to impairment assessment typically includes a combination of patient history, symptom evaluation, PFTs, and sometimes HRCT scans. PFTs can reveal restrictive patterns, reduced diffusing capacity, or mixed obstructive–restrictive deficits. Serial PFTs may be necessary to assess the progression of the disease. In addition to objective testing, the patient's subjective experience of symptoms and the impact on their ADLs are considered. For example, an individual's ability to perform tasks that require physical exertion, such as lifting, walking, or climbing stairs, can be compromised. The AMA Guides provide a structured approach for assigning a percentage of impairment, which can be used for determining eligibility for disability benefits or workers' compensation. Preventive strategies, including the identification and control of exposure to the offending antigens, are crucial in managing OHP. Early diagnosis and intervention can prevent the progression of the disease and reduce the degree of impairment. Workplace monitoring and the use of protective equipment are important measures to prevent the onset of OHP in susceptible individuals.[5,76,80]

APPORTIONMENT

In the complex domain of respiratory impairment evaluations, particularly in the context of occupational health, clinicians are frequently required to dissect and quantify the impact of individual disease processes on the overall impairment. This intricate process of apportionment arises predominantly in workers' compensation cases, aiming to precisely attribute a portion of the total impairment to the work-related factors, thereby affecting the monetary compensation, while generally not altering the scope of medical or wage compensation benefits. The challenge within this process lies in the inherent lack of a concrete scientific framework to guide the exact apportionment. Despite being a systematic requirement, the process can often be characterized as speculative due to the absence of definitive evidence to support precise calculations.

The influence of nonoccupational factors, particularly cigarette smoking, emerges as a predominant consideration in this equation. Smoking-related or biomass smoke exposure conditions need to be frequently dissected from work-related contributions, with studies highlighting significant differences in the manifestation of symptoms and physical limitations between smokers and nonsmokers within the same occupational groups. For instance, literature indicates notable contrasts in how smoking workers experience their condition compared to their nonsmoking counterparts. Furthermore, the primary limitation in physical activity among certain populations may be rooted in cardiovascular, obesity, or poor physical conditioning rather than respiratory deficiencies. While methodologies for such specific apportionment have been suggested in the literature, they lack validation through rigorous scientific scrutiny and thus remain without consensus in the medical community. If preexisting evidence of respiratory impairment exists, such as baseline diagnostic test results acquired before the occupational exposure or the onset of a work-related disease, that would be very useful for deciding apportionment. This involves a comparison of the individual's prior baseline to their current level of function, thereby enabling a more substantiated allocation of impairment. However, this process is invariably complex and must be approached with meticulous consideration of all contributing factors to ensure fairness and accuracy within the bounds of the current understanding and legal frameworks.[6,81]

WORKPLACE PROTECTION

In India, the National Institute for Occupational Safety and Health (NIOSH) plays a pivotal role in developing guidelines to protect workers' respiratory health. Their recommendations are meticulously designed to prevent occupational respiratory diseases and ensure a safe breathing environment for workers across various industries. An in-depth look at the NIOSH guidelines for respiratory protection in the workplace is as follows:

Respiratory protection standard: NIOSH has established a respiratory protection standard, which emphasizes the importance of a comprehensive respiratory protection program. This program must include a detailed evaluation of respiratory hazards in the workplace, selection of appropriate respirators, fit testing, regular training for workers, proper respirator use, maintenance, and storage procedures.

Hazard identification and exposure assessment: The first step in the NIOSH guidelines is to identify and assess respiratory hazards that workers may encounter. This involves monitoring air quality and determining the types and concentrations of harmful airborne contaminants present in the workplace.

Engineering controls: NIOSH strongly advocates for the use of engineering controls as the primary means to control airborne contaminants. These controls include local exhaust ventilation systems, process enclosure, and substitution of less toxic materials.

Work practice controls: In conjunction with engineering controls, NIOSH recommends the implementation of work practice controls. These involve modifying work practices and schedules to reduce the duration and level of exposure, along with administrative controls like training and safe work procedures.

Respiratory protection devices: When engineering and work practice controls are not feasible or do not reduce exposure to acceptable levels, the use of certified respiratory protection devices is recommended. NIOSH certifies respirators and provides guidance on the selection of devices based on the hazard type, exposure levels, and specific needs of the workforce.

Fit testing and user seal checks: To ensure the effectiveness of respirators, NIOSH mandates fit testing for all users of tight-fitting facepiece respirators. This ensures a proper seal and optimal protection. Additionally, users must perform seal checks each time a respirator is donned.

Training and education: Education and training are key components of the NIOSH guidelines. Workers must be educated about the respiratory hazards they face, the importance of using respiratory protection, and the correct use and maintenance of respirators.

Program evaluation: To maintain the efficacy of the respiratory protection program, NIOSH suggests regular evaluations. This includes assessing the ongoing appropriateness of selected respirators, the continued effectiveness of fit testing, and the adequacy of worker training.

Medical evaluation: Before an employee uses a respirator, a medical evaluation is necessary to determine the worker's ability to use a respirator safely. This evaluation must be conducted by a qualified healthcare professional.

Record-keeping: Maintaining records is vital for the success of the respiratory protection program. NIOSH guidelines recommend keeping detailed records of hazard assessments, respirator fit testing, training, medical evaluations, and maintenance.

SUMMARY

The landscape of disease-related and occupational pulmonary disability is continuously evolving. The traditional reliance on clinical pulmonary function testing for assessing respiratory disability is becoming inadequate due to several emerging factors. Traditional methods focus too narrowly on quantifying functional loss and fail to consider the broader societal and individual impacts of impairments. There is a need for updated studies and more nuanced methodologies to accurately address the complexities of contemporary occupational activities and provide personalized assessments. Moreover, the dynamic nature of today's workplaces—with their diverse and changing respiratory demands—requires updated studies to ensure that assessments remain relevant and applicable. Additionally, current assessment methods confront specific challenges when applied to conditions such as asthma, where the interplay between environmental triggers and impaired lung function complicates the assessment of work-related capabilities. Recent advances in our understanding of respiratory impairment emphasize the profound societal and individual consequences of these conditions. It is becoming clear that a broader perspective is essential—one that goes beyond the mere quantification of functional loss to encompass the multifaceted ways in which impairments can culminate in disability. There is a compelling need to develop more nuanced and precise methodologies that can cater to the complexities of contemporary occupational activities both at home and in the workplace.

REFERENCES

1. Sharma S, Hashmi MF, Badireddy M. Dyspnea on Exertion. In: StatPearls. Treasure Island, FL: StatPearls Publishing; 2023. [online] Available from http://www.ncbi.nlm.nih.gov/books/NBK499847/ [Last accessed June, 2024].
2. Harber P. Respiratory disability: what is it, how can we measure it, what causes it and is it important? Thorax. [online] Available from https://thorax.bmj.com/content/64/4/280 [Last accessed June, 2024].
3. Harber P. Respiratory disability and impairment: what is new? Curr Opin Pulm Med. 2015;21(2):201-7.
4. World Health Organization. International Classification of Functioning, Disability and Health (ICF). [online] Available from https://www.who.int/standards/classifications/international-classification-of-functioning-disability-and-health [Last accessed June, 2024].
5. AMA Guides. (2008). AMA Guides to the Evaluation of Permanent Impairment, 6th Edition. [online] Available from https://ama-guides.ama-assn.org/books/book/3/AMA-Guides-to-the-Evaluation-of-Permanent [Last accessed June, 2024].
6. Soud A. Performing a Lung Disability Evaluation: How, When, and Why? J Occup Environ Med. 2014;56(0 10):S23-9.
7. Chen JJ. Functional Capacity Evaluation and Disability. Iowa Orthop J. 2007;27:121-7.
8. World Health Organization. (2023). Chronic obstructive pulmonary disease (COPD). [online] Available from https://www.who.int/news-room/fact-sheets/detail/chronic-obstructive-pulmonary-disease-(copd) [Last accessed June, 2024].
9. Devine JF. Chronic Obstructive Pulmonary Disease: An Overview. Am Health Drug Benefits. 2008;1(7):34-42.
10. Verma A, Gudi N, Yadav UN, et al. Prevalence of COPD among population above 30 years in India: A systematic review and meta-analysis. J Glob Health. 11:04038.
11. Katz PP, Gregorich S, Eisner M, et al. Disability in valued life activities among individuals with COPD and other respiratory conditions. J Cardiopulm Rehabil Prev. 2010;30(2):126-36.
12. Gupta D, Agarwal R, Aggarwal AN, et al. Guidelines for diagnosis and management of chronic obstructive pulmonary disease: joint recommendations of Indian Chest Society and National College of Chest Physicians (India). Indian J Chest Dis Allied Sci. 2014;56 Spec No:5-54.
13. Gupta D, Agarwal R, Aggarwal AN, et al. Guidelines for diagnosis and management of chronic obstructive pulmonary disease: Joint ICS/NCCP (I) recommendations. Lung India. 2013;30(3):228-67.
14. Agarwal R, Dhooria S, Aggarwal AN, et al. Guidelines for Diagnosis and Management of Bronchial Asthma: Joint Recommendations of National College of Chest Physicians (India) and Indian Chest Society. Indian J Chest Dis Allied Sci. 2015;57 Spec No:5-52.
15. NIOSH and CDC. (2023). Occupational and environmental exposure history. [online] Available from https://www.cdc.gov/niosh/learning/b-reader/clinical/diagnostic/6.html [Last accessed June, 2024].
16. Ponce MC, Sankari A, Sharma S. Pulmonary Function Tests. In: StatPearls. Treasure Island, FL: StatPearls Publishing; 2023. [online] Available from http://www.ncbi.nlm.nih.gov/books/NBK482339/ [Last accessed June, 2024].
17. Tarlo SM. Occupational Lung Disease. Goldman's Cecil Medicine. 2012;567-74.
18. Dyspnea. Am J Respir Crit Care Med. 1999;159(1):321-40.
19. Burkhardt R, Pankow W. The Diagnosis of Chronic Obstructive Pulmonary Disease. Dtsch Arztebl Int. 2014;111(49):834-46.

20. Medical Research Council (MRC) Dyspnoea Scale. Physiopedia. [online] Available from https://www.physio-pedia.com/Medical_Research_Council_(MRC)_Dyspnoea_Scale [Last accessed June, 2024].
21. Bestall J, Paul E, Garrod R, et al. Usefulness of the Medical Research Council (MRC) dyspnoea scale as a measure of disability in patients with chronic obstructive pulmonary disease. Thorax. 1999;54(7):581-6.
22. Kim S, Oh J, Kim YI, et al. Differences in classification of COPD group using COPD assessment test (CAT) or modified Medical Research Council (mMRC) dyspnea scores: a cross-sectional analyses. BMC Pulm Med. 2013;13(1):35.
23. Vlahovich KP, Sood A. A 2019 Update on Occupational Lung Diseases: A Narrative Review. Pulm Ther. 2020;7(1):75-87.
24. Johns Hopkins Medicine. Occupational Lung Diseases. [online] Available from https://www.hopkinsmedicine.org/health/conditions-and-diseases/occupational-lung-diseases [Last accessed June, 2024].
25. Boadu EF, Okeke SR, Boadi C, et al. Work-related respiratory health conditions among construction workers: a systematic narrative review. BMJ Open Respir Res. 2023;10(1):e001736.
26. McCormick B. (2023). Construction Workers at Increased Risk of Respiratory Hazards, Diseases. AJMC. [online] Available from https://www.ajmc.com/view/construction-workers-at-increased-risk-of-respiratory-hazards-diseases [Last accessed June, 2024].
27. Abdalla S, Apramian SS, Cantley LF, et al. Occupation and Risk for Injuries. In: Mock CN, Nugent R, Kobusingye O, Smith KR (Eds). Injury Prevention and Environmental Health, 3rd edition. The International Bank for Reconstruction and Development/The World Bank; 2017. [online] Available from http://www.ncbi.nlm.nih.gov/books/NBK525209/ [Last accessed June, 2024].
28. Rumchev K, Gilbey S, Mead-Hunter R, et al. Agricultural Dust Exposures and Health and Safety Practices among Western Australian Wheatbelt Farmers during Harvest. Int J Environ Res Public Health. 2019;16(24):5009.
29. International Labour Office. Safety and Health in Agriculture. [online] Available from https://www.ilo.org/wcmsp5/groups/public/@ed_protect/@protrav/@safework/documents/publication/wcms_110193.pdf [Last accessed June, 2024].
30. CDC and NIOSH. (2022). Mining Topic - Respiratory Diseases. [online] Available from https://www.cdc.gov/niosh/mining/topics/RespiratoryDiseases.html [Last accessed June, 2024].
31. Laney AS, Weissman DN. Respiratory Diseases Caused by Coal Mine Dust. J Occup Environ Med. 2014;56(0 10):S18-22.
32. Health and Safety Executive (HSE). [online] Available from Welding: Health risks from welding - HSE. https://www.hse.gov.uk/welding/health-risks-welding.htm [Last accessed June, 2024].
33. Papadopoli R, Nobile CGA, Trovato A, et al. Chemical risk and safety awareness, perception, and practices among research laboratories workers in Italy. J Occup Med Toxicol. 2020;15(1):17.
34. Occupational Safety and Health Administration. Chemical hazards and toxic substances - overview. [online] Available from https://www.osha.gov/chemical-hazards [Last accessed June, 2024].
35. Tupper C, Swift CJ. OSHA Chemical Hazards and Communication. In: StatPearls. Treasure Island, FL: StatPearls Publishing; 2023. [online] Available from http://www.ncbi.nlm.nih.gov/books/NBK580552/ [Last accessed June, 2024].
36. Tanir F, Mete B, Tanir F, et al. Impacts of the indoor air quality on the health of the employee and protection against these impacts. In: Air Quality and Health. IntechOpen; 2022. [online] Available from doi:10.5772/intechopen.102708 [Last accessed June, 2024].
37. Carrer P, Wolkoff P. Assessment of Indoor Air Quality Problems in Office-Like Environments: Role of Occupational Health Services. Int J Environ Res Public Health. 2018;15(4):741.
38. Mohanty A, Kabi A, Mohanty AP. Health problems in healthcare workers: A review. J Family Med Prim Care. 2019;8(8):2568-72.
39. Bevacqua BK. Pre-operative pulmonary evaluation in the patient with suspected respiratory disease. Indian J Anaesth. 2015;59(9):542-9.
40. Elsevier. (2020). Care plan: Self-Care Deficit, Adult. [online] Available from https://elsevier.health/en-US/preview/self-care-deficit-cpg [Last accessed June, 2024].
41. K-State. Essential living skills – essential home maintenance. [online] Available from https://bookstore.ksre.ksu.edu/pubs/s134c.pdf Available from https://elsevier.health/en-US/preview/self-care-deficit-cpg [Last accessed June, 2024].
42. Kohl HW III, Cook HD. Environment C on PA and PE in the S, Board F and N, Medicine I of Physical Activity and Physical Education: Relationship to Growth, Development, and Health. In: Educating the Student Body: Taking Physical Activity and Physical Education to School. Washington, DC: National Academies Press (US); 2013. [online] Available from https://www.ncbi.nlm.nih.gov/books/NBK201497/ [Last accessed June, 2024].
43. Spruit MA, Burtin C, De Boever P, et al. COPD and exercise: does it make a difference? Breathe (Sheff). 2016;12(2):e38-e49.
44. Edemekong PF, Bomgaars DL, Sukumaran S, Schoo C. Activities of Daily Living. In: StatPearls. Treasure Island, FL: StatPearls Publishing; 2023. [online] Available from http://www.ncbi.nlm.nih.gov/books/NBK470404/ [Last accessed June, 2024].
45. Pizarro-Pennarolli C, Sánchez-Rojas C, Torres-Castro R, et al. Assessment of activities of daily living in patients post COVID-19: a systematic review. PeerJ. 2021;9:e11026.
46. Tuteur PG. Chest examination. In: Walker HK, Hall WD, Hurst JW (Eds). Clinical Methods: The History, Physical, and Laboratory Examinations, 3rd edition. Boston: Butterworths; 1990.
47. MSD Manual Professional Edition. (2023). Evaluation of the pulmonary patient - pulmonary disorders. [online] Available from https://www.msdmanuals.com/professional/pulmonary-disorders/approach-to-the-pulmonary-patient/evaluation-of-the-pulmonary-patient [Last accessed June, 2024].
48. ATS/ACCP Statement on Cardiopulmonary Exercise Testing. Am J Respir Crit Care Med. 2003;167(2):211-77.
49. Ranu H, Wilde M, Madden B. Pulmonary Function Tests. Ulster Med J. 2011;80(2):84-90.
50. Ranavaya MI. The Challenge of Evaluating Asthma Impairment and Disability. Guides Newsletter. 1997;2(3):1-4.
51. Wielpütz MO, Heußel CP, Herth FJF, et al. Radiological Diagnosis in Lung Disease. Dtsch Arztebl Int. 2014;111(11):181-7.
52. Hovinga M, Sprengers R, Kauczor HU, et al. CT imaging of interstitial lung diseases. In: Schoef UJ, Meinel FG (Eds). Multidetector-Row CT of the Thorax. pp. 105-30.
53. International Labour Organization. (2022). Guidelines for the use of the ILO International Classification of Radiographs of Pneumoconioses. [online] Available from https://www.ilo.org/wcmsp5/groups/public/---ed_dialogue/---lab_admin/documents/publication/wcms_867859.pdf [Last accessed June, 2024].

54. NIOSH and CDC. (2023). Chest Radiography: ILO Classification. [online] Available from https://www.cdc.gov/niosh/topics/chestradiography/ilo.html [Last accessed June, 2024].
55. International Labour Organization. (1980). Guidelines for the use of ILO international classification of radiographs of pneumoconioses. [online] Available fromhttps://www.ilo.org/wcmsp5/groups/public/@ed_protect/@protrav/@safework/documents/genericdocument/wcms_861208.pdf [Last accessed June, 2024].
56. Meyer KC. Diagnosis and management of interstitial lung disease. Transl Respir Med. 2014;2:4.
57. Deyrup AT, D'Ambrosio D, Muir J, et al. Essential laboratory tests for medical education. Acad Pathol. 2022;9(1):100046.
58. Tzouvelekis A, Kouliatsis G, Anevlavis S, et al. Serum biomarkers in interstitial lung diseases. Respir Res. 2005;6(1):78.
59. Cheng CW, Chien MH, Su SC, et al. New markers in pneumonia. Clin Chim Acta. 2013;419:19-25.
60. Kebbe J, Abdo T. Interstitial lung disease: the diagnostic role of bronchoscopy. J Thorac Dis. 2017;9(Suppl 10):S996-S1010.
61. MedlinePlus Medical Test. Bronchoscopy and bronchoalveolar lavage (BAL): [online] Available from https://medlineplus.gov/lab-tests/bronchoscopy-and-bronchoalveolar-lavage-bal/ [Last accessed June, 2024].
62. Davidson KR, Ha DM, Schwarz MI, et al. Bronchoalveolar lavage as a diagnostic procedure: a review of known cellular and molecular findings in various lung diseases. J Thorac Dis. 2020;12(9):4991-5019.
63. Braman SS, Corrao WM. Bronchoprovocation testing. Clin Chest Med. 1989;10(2):165-76.
64. Vandenplas O, Suojalehto H, Aasen TB, et al. Specific inhalation challenge in the diagnosis of occupational asthma: consensus statement. Eur Respir J. 2014;43(6):1573-87.
65. Preisser AM, Koschel D, Merget R, et al. Workplace-related inhalation test – Specific inhalation challenge: S2k Guideline of the German Society for Occupational and Environmental Medicine e.V. (DGAUM), the German Society for Pneumology and Respiratory Medicine e.V. (DGP) and the German Society for Allergology and Clinical Immunology e.V. (DGAKI). Allergologie Select. 2021;5:315.
66. World Allergy Organization. Diagnosis of occupational asthma. https://www.worldallergy.org/education-and-programs [Last accessed 15 June, 2024].
67. Lee MK, Yoon HK, Kim SW, et al. Nonspecific Bronchoprovocation Test. Tuberc Respir Dis (Seoul). 2017;80(4):344-50.
68. MSD Manual Professional Edition. (2023). Work-related asthma - pulmonary disorders. [online] Available from https://www.msdmanuals.com/en-in/professional/pulmonary-disorders/environmental-and-occupational-pulmonary-diseases/work-related-asthma [Last accessed June, 2024].
69. Nici L, Donner C, Wouters E, et al. American Thoracic Society/European Respiratory Society Statement on Pulmonary Rehabilitation. Am J Respir Crit Care Med. 2006;173(12):1390-413.
70. Silver SR, Alarcon WA, Li J. Incident chronic obstructive pulmonary disease associated with occupation, industry, and workplace exposures in the Health and Retirement Study. Am J Ind Med. 2021;64(1):26-38.
71. Rushton L. Occupational causes of chronic obstructive pulmonary disease. Rev Environ Health. 2007;22(3):195-212.
72. Kakavas S, Kotsiou OS, Perlikos F, et al. Pulmonary function testing in COPD: looking beyond the curtain of FEV1. npj Prim Care Respir Med. 2021;31.
73. Emmons EE. Bronchiectasis: Practice Essentials, Background, Pathophysiology. [online] Available from https://emedicine.medscape.com/article/296961-overview?form=fpf [Last accessed June, 2024].
74. AMA Guides. AMA Guides® to the Evaluation of Permanent Impairment: an overview. [online] Available from https://www.ama-assn.org/delivering-care/ama-guides/ama-guides-evaluation-permanent-impairment-overview [Last accessed June, 2024].
75. AMA Guides Sixth 2023: Current medicine for permanent impairment ratings. [online] Available from https://www.ama-assn.org/delivering-care/ama-guides/ama-guides-sixth-2023-current-medicine-permanent-impairment-ratings [Last accessed June, 2024].
76. American Thoracic Society Documents. American Thoracic Society/European Respiratory Society Statement on Pulmonary Rehabilitation. [online] Available from https://www.thoracic.org/statements/resources/respiratory-disease-adults/atserspr0606.pdf [Last accessed June, 2024].
77. Science.gov. Occupational hypersensitivity pneumonitis. [online] Available from https://www.science.gov/topicpages/o/occupational+hypersensitivity+pneumonitis [Last accessed June, 2024].
78. Quirce S, Vandenplas O, Campo P, et al. Occupational hypersensitivity pneumonitis: an EAACI position paper. Allergy. 2016;71(6):765-79.
79. Agarwal AK, Raja A, Brown BD. Chronic Obstructive Pulmonary Disease. In: StatPearls. Treasure Island, FL: StatPearls Publishing; 2023. [online] Available from http://www.ncbi.nlm.nih.gov/books/NBK559281/ [Last accessed June, 2024].
80. Cocchiarella L. Andersson GBJ. AMA Guides to the Evaluation of Permanent Impairment, Fifth Edition. Philadelphia: American Medical Association; 2001.
81. Hamid A, Saleem W, Yaqub G, et al. Comparative assessment of respiratory and other occupational health effects among elementary workers. 2019;25(3):394-401.

CHAPTER 101

Occupational Asthma

Lt Col (Dr) Rahul Tyagi, Saurabh Mittal

INTRODUCTION

Asthma is a common heterogeneous disorder characterized by chronic inflammation of the airways.[1] Diagnosis of work-related asthma (WRA) is considered when the patient has signs and symptoms compatible with asthma diagnosis related to workplace exposure. WRA is not a single disorder, but rather a heterogeneous condition that encompasses asthma symptoms developing de novo due to exposure to sensitizers or high-level irritant and nonspecific exposures causing exacerbation of underlying asthma.[2] Around 16% of asthma diagnosed in adults is attributed to occupational exposures.[3] More than 400 agents causing WRA have been identified but yet new agents are being reported constantly adding to the list.[2] Early identification and removal of exposures are essential to improve the prognosis in cases of WRA. Hence, physicians dealing with adult asthma must keep a close watch for WRA in adults presenting with signs and symptoms of asthma. WRA includes two entities called occupational asthma (OA) and work-aggravated asthma (WAA).[4]

Work-related asthma: Asthma developing de novo due to exposures occurring at the workplace or pre-existing asthma made worse by workplace exposure constitutes WRA.

Occupational asthma: Airborne exposures in the working environment causing employees to develop signs and symptoms of asthma is known as occupational asthma.[4] OA encompasses allergic/sensitizer-induced OA and irritant-induced OA.[4]

Work-aggravated asthma: A patient having pre-existing asthma or developing adult-onset asthma and reporting symptomatic worsening due to nonspecific factors at the workplace is known as WAA.[4]

ECONOMIC BURDEN

Occupational asthma has significant financial implications both for the employee and the employer. For the employee, it is a financial burden as he may have to change to a less-paying job or risk worsening of asthma, and for the employer, it is a loss due to the nonavailability of a skilled worker.[5] In one estimate, OA cost to the economy in the United Kingdom including both healthcare and societal cost were around 1.1 billion pounds per decade.[5] It has also been noted that patients with OA have prolonged impairment of work-related quality of life and a higher prevalence of psychiatric disorders, thus further increasing the societal and health care costs.[6] A significant proportion of OA patients have severe asthma and a large study found around 16% of OA patients to have severe asthma. Persistent work exposure, longer disease duration, low education level, childhood asthma, and sputum production are associated with severe OA.[7]

A population-based survey from India has also shown an increased risk of asthma among men in various occupations such as plant and machine operators, mining, construction, manufacturing, and transport.[8] Surprisingly, the study found no increased risk for women in the same occupation. This shows that despite OA being relatively under diagnosed and under recognized in India, a significant proportion of our workforce is at risk for occupational asthma which is likely to result in enormous healthcare-related and societal costs.

OCCUPATIONAL ASTHMA: AGENTS AND CAUSATION

Occupational asthma due to allergic sensitization requires a period of repeated exposure. "Latent period" is used to describe the duration between initial exposure and onset of symptoms. The highest risk of OA development is seen within the first year of exposure, although latent periods ranging from a few weeks to many years have been reported.[9] Individual susceptibility does play a role in the development of OA but these individual factors have still not been consistently identified. Presently, the main determinant considered for the development of OA is the level of allergen exposure in the workplace.[4]

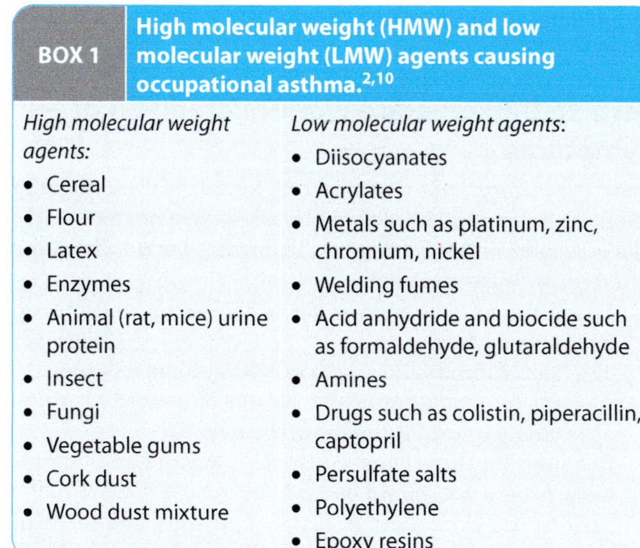

BOX 1 **High molecular weight (HMW) and low molecular weight (LMW) agents causing occupational asthma.[2,10]**

High molecular weight agents:	*Low molecular weight agents:*
• Cereal	• Diisocyanates
• Flour	• Acrylates
• Latex	• Metals such as platinum, zinc, chromium, nickel
• Enzymes	• Welding fumes
• Animal (rat, mice) urine protein	• Acid anhydride and biocide such as formaldehyde, glutaraldehyde
• Insect	• Amines
• Fungi	• Drugs such as colistin, piperacillin, captopril
• Vegetable gums	• Persulfate salts
• Cork dust	• Polyethylene
• Wood dust mixture	• Epoxy resins

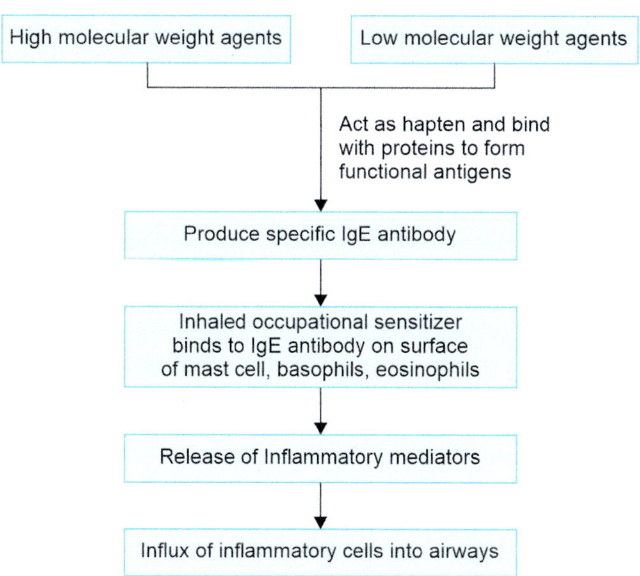

FLOWCHART 1: Mechanism of development of sensitizer-induced occupational asthma-immunologic IgE mediated.[12]

More than 400 agents causing OA have been identified. Agents causing OA may be divided into high molecular weight (HMW) and low molecular weight (LMW) agents **(Box 1)**.[10] While HMW agents have a longer latency, more occulonasal symptoms, and a predominantly eosinophil-driven pathology, LMW agents have shorter latency, less occulonasal symptoms, and accompanying dermatitis more commonly. More than 70% of the cases of OA are caused by isocyanates, flour, acrylates, quaternary ammonium compounds, persulfates, metal, wood, and latex.[11]

Occupational asthma with sensitizers can be IgE-mediated or non-IgE-mediated. Most HMW agents and a few LMW agents (in combination with respiratory proteins) induce the production of specific IgE antibodies directed against the antigen and follow a cascade of different steps **(Flowchart 1)**. These IgE antibodies bind to the surface of mast cells, basophils, and eosinophils. Subsequent exposure to the antigen causes cross-linking of IgE resulting in the release of chemical mediators (histamine, prostaglandin, and cysteinyl-leukotrienes).[12]

Antigen presentation by dendritic cells results in antigen-activated CD4 cells differentiating into Th2 cells which produce interleukin (IL)-4, -5, and -13, activate B cells, promote IgE-synthesis, recruitment of mast cells, and eosinophilia. Some LMW agents also cause OA by non-IgE mediated immunological mechanisms, which may be driven by Th1 inflammation, IL 1/IL 15.[2]

Clinical, functional, and inflammatory characteristics in patients who had been diagnosed as OA using specific inhalation challenge (SIC) were compared in a multicenter, retrospective study to determine if OA caused by HMW and LMW agents had distinct phenotypes.[11] A total of 1,180 patients with OA (LMW agents n = 635; HMW agent n = 544) were included. HMW agents showed significant association with work-related rhinitis, conjunctivitis, atopy, early asthmatic reaction, higher risk of airflow limitation, and higher baseline blood eosinophilia. LMW agents were associated with increased chest tightness at work, daily sputum, late asthmatic reactions, and a higher risk of severe exacerbations.[11]

DIAGNOSIS

A high index of suspicion is necessary for the diagnosis of OA. Despite studies showing that a significant proportion of adult-onset asthma can be attributed to occupational exposures, diagnostic delays remain significant. Patients with OA experienced a mean delay of 4 years for assessment in secondary care after initial presentation to primary care.[13] In an assessment of the quality of diagnosis of OA, the median time from onset of symptoms to diagnosis of OA in Finland was 3.2 years.[14] In a similar study from Canada, the mean time to diagnosis was 4.9 years.[15] Reported causes for increased delay in diagnosis include lack of inquiry at primary care about the relation of symptoms to work, fear of work time loss, lower household income, and educational level.[15]

No single test can be considered diagnostic of OA and the approach to diagnosis will vary depending on patient circumstances, healthcare echelon available, experience of the physician, and availability of testing facilities.

A detailed history is necessary for the diagnosis of OA. In all patients presenting with adult-onset asthma, having a resurgence of asthma symptoms or having unexplained worsening of asthma symptoms should be asked in detail regarding their occupational history. Patients must be asked about the following in detail:

- Nature of their work
- Exposures at workplace

- Onset, duration, and progression of symptoms; any latency between suspected exposure and first symptom onset
- Relation of symptoms to workplace and similar symptoms in coworkers
- Any history of asthma before entering the present work
- Nasal/eye symptoms
- Control measures being taken at the workplace (masks, filters, exhausts)

Investigations for diagnosis of OA need to be three-pronged, i.e., they should provide a physiological confirmation of asthma, demonstrate a work relatedness of symptoms, and demonstrate respiratory sensitization to workplace exposures.[16] Questionnaires have also been used for the identification of OA. Questionnaires that identify symptoms such as wheezing and breathlessness which improve on days away from work have been found to have high sensitivity but low specificity for OA.[17]

Diagnostic Tests for Occupational Asthma

Ideally, diagnostic tests for OA should be carried out before the commencement of treatment as these tests become less sensitive if exposure is terminated or treatment is started.[18]

Tests for Confirmation of Asthma

Spirometry

All patients with suspected OA should undergo spirometry (both pre- and postbronchodilator) for physiological confirmation of asthma diagnosis. Forced expiratory volume in 1st second (FEV1), forced vital capacity (FVC), and peak expiratory flow (PEF) must be measured and interpreted according to internationally recommended guidelines.[19] Spirometry may show airflow obstruction with reversibility but may also be normal in a significant number of patients.[4] However, it is useful, even if normal, as it serves as a baseline for future comparison.

Bronchoprovocation Testing

In subjects with suspicion of OA who are not having any airflow limitation on spirometry, demonstration of nonspecific bronchial hyperreactivity (NSBHR) using a bronchoprovocation test is necessary.[2] Direct (methacholine, or histamine) and indirect [exercise, adenosine monophosphate (AMP), mannitol, hypertonic saline] tests have been described for bronchial hyperreactivity (BHR) testing. Histamine and methacholine challenge with a 20% fall in FEV1 are reliable and well-standardized.[20] Compared to SIC the sensitivity, specificity, and positive and negative predictive values of the methacholine challenge test done at least once at work are 98.1%, 39.1%, 44%, and 97.7%. In settings with the nonavailability of SIC, appropriate clinical settings with spirometry, serial PEF monitoring, and bronchoprovocation testing can be used to make a diagnosis of OA.[21]

Tests to Demonstrate Work-relatedness of Symptoms

Peak expiratory flow monitoring: Serial PEF monitoring offers a cheap and simple way to assess response to workplace-related inhaled antigens. Following need to be done when recording serial PEF:

- Teach the patient how to use a PEF meter and how to log the recordings.
- The best of three values each time should be recorded.
- At least four readings daily should be recorded which are equally spaced throughout the day.
- Readings for three consecutive days at work and periods away from work should be available.
- Also record work timings, tasks, exposures, and medications used.

Work relationship of PEF can be measured by calculating mean values of PEF at work and comparing them with mean PEF values away from work. Also, the diurnal variation in PEF can be used to ascertain the work-relatedness of airflow changes.[22]

Various patterns of PEF variability compatible with OA are:

- *Early decrease in PEF*: Within 1 hour of exposure
- *Late decrease in PEF*: May occur after leaving work also
- Progressive worsening of PEF over the week with each passing day at work
- Nonprogressive but similar daily worsening of PEF on days at work
- Significant fall in PEF on first weekday of work and lesser falls on subsequent days

In a systematic review, the pooled sensitivity and specificity of serial PEF monitoring for diagnosis of OA was found to be 82% and 88% respectively.[22]

Tests for Demonstration of Respiratory Sensitization to Workplace Exposures

Skin prick test or specific IgE: A positive skin prick test/raised specific IgE antibodies to a workplace allergen confirm sensitization but cannot be considered diagnostic of OA and cannot predict future risk of OA also.

Specific inhalational challenge testing: SIC is considered the reference standard for diagnosis of OA as it mimics workplace exposure in a controlled setting.[23] Other than confirming the diagnosis of OA, when other methods have failed to provide definite results, SIC can also be used for the identification of the cause of OA, identifying a new agent as the cause of OA, and for research purposes.[23]

Specific inhalational challenge should only be carried out at specialized centers with the availability of the facility for managing adverse reactions such as acute severe asthma and anaphylaxis. SIC should be conducted under close supervision by a trained physician and the patient should be fully covered to avoid exposure through the skin. The agent should be delivered in the same physical form (gas, fume, aerosol, or liquid) and chemical form as encountered in the workplace. Increase the duration of exposure or concentration of the agent but the concentration should not exceed the occupational exposure limit (OEL) to avoid irritant response. A SIC is considered positive when there is a sustained fall in FEV1 of more than 15% from a prechallenge value. A "control" substance exposure should be done for around 30 minutes on a day prior to the active challenge. On both control and challenge days, the patient should be monitored in the hospital for 6–8 hours after the test.[23]

Management

- *Avoidance of exposure*: Avoidance of exposure is an essential step in the management of occupational asthma. A systematic review comparing the effects of total avoidance versus reduction in exposure showed that mere reduction in exposure is associated with a lower likelihood of improvement and recovery of symptoms and a higher risk of symptom worsening and NSBHR.[24] However, considering the socioeconomic impact, total avoidance may not be always feasible. In these cases, a reduction in exposure should be ensured. The various methods to achieve this include:
  - *Use of personal protective equipment (PPE)*: Use of masks, hoods, and suits with hoods having a fresh air system can be used.
  - *Structural changes*: Structural changes such as enclosing the equipment/processes that produce fumes, vapors, or aerosols can reduce the operator's exposure. Improving ventilation and increasing the frequency of air exchange can reduce the concentration of airborne agents.
  - Use of an alternative agent, if available
  - *Change of location*: A change of job location of the affected individual, to a site where he is not likely to get exposed to the offending agent, may be required to ensure avoidance.
- *Medical management:* Medical management of OA is similar to asthma not related to work and should follow standard treatment guidelines.[4] Allergen immuno therapy and anti-IgE antibody have also been used in the management of OA, but only limited evidence is available at present.[4]

The prognosis in OA mainly depends on the level and duration of exposure. Hence, early identification and avoidance/reduction of exposure are the main determinants of the outcomes in patients with OA.

TABLE 1: Clinical phenotypes of irritant-induced asthma (IIA).[2]

Phenotype	Duration of exposure	Level of exposure	The onset of asthma symptoms
Definite IIA	Single exposure	High level	Few hours
Probable IIA	Multiple	High level	Days to weeks
Possible IIA	Chronic	Moderate level	Delayed

IRRITANT-INDUCED ASTHMA

Irritant-induced asthma (IIA) denotes asthma related to irritant exposure at work. Based on the level of exposure and onset of symptoms, it has been divided into three clinical phenotypes (**Table 1**).

Acute-onset IIA is also known as reactive airway dysfunction syndrome (RADS) and is seen after a single high-level exposure in patients without pre-existing asthma. Patients develop asthma-like symptoms within 24 hours of exposure.[25] The symptoms should persist for a few weeks for a diagnosis of acute-onset IIA. Various exposures described to cause acute IIA include chromate,[26] closed space smoke inhalation,[27] airborne particulates after a disaster,[28] and various other exposures such as sodium hypochlorite, chlorine, aqua regia, polyethylene glycol esters, and others.[29]

Patients with IAA can continue in occupation with measures to avoid further high-level exposures. During the acute symptom phase bronchodilators, steroids and oxygen should be given. If these patients develop persistent asthma-like symptoms, complete removal from the workplace may be warranted.

CONCLUSION

Occupational asthma is a common disorder and should always be considered in patients with adult onset asthma. The first step in the management of OA is a correct diagnosis which will require a detailed history and spirometry, serial PEFR monitoring, bronchoprovocation testing, or specific inhalation challenge testing based on local expertise and availability. Treatment requires avoidance of exposure as the most important factor while pharmacotherapy follows standard asthma management guidelines.

REFERENCES

1. Global Initiative for Asthma. (2023). Global Strategy for Asthma Management and Prevention, 2023. [online] Available from www.ginasthma.org. [Last accessed July, 2024].
2. Tiotiu AI, Novakova S, Labor M, et al. Progress in Occupational Asthma. Int J Environ Health Pub Health. 2020;17(12):4553.
3. Blanc PD, Annesi-Maesano I, Balmes JR, et al. The occupational burden of nonmalignant respiratory diseases. An official American thoracic Society and European respiratory Society statement. Am J Respir Crit Care Med. 2019;199:1312-34.
4. Barber CM, Cullinan P, Feary J, et al. British Thoracic Society Clinical Statement on occupational asthma. Thorax. 2022;77: 433-42.
5. Ayres JG, Boyd R, Cowie H, et al. Costs of occupational asthma in the UK. Thorax. 2011;66(2):128-33.
6. Moullec G, Lavoie KL, Malo JL, et al. Long-term socioprofessional and psychological status in workers investigated for occupational asthma in quebec. J Occup Environ Med. 2013;55(9): 1052-64.
7. Vandenplas O, Godet J, Hurdubaea L, et al; European network for the PHenotyping of OCcupational ASthma (E-PHOCAS) investigators. Severe occupational asthma: Insights from a multicenter european cohort. J Allergy Clin Immunol Pract. 2019;7(7):2309-18.e4.
8. Agrawal S, Pearce N, Millett C, et al. Occupations with an increased prevalence of self-reported asthma in Indian adults. J Asthma. 2014;51(8):814-24.
9. Nicholson PJ, Cullinan P, Burge PS. Occupational asthma: Prevention, identification & management: Systematic review & recommendations. British Occupational. London: Health Research Foundation; 2010.
10. Maestrelli P, Henneberger PK, Tarlo S, et al. Causes and Phenotypes of Work-related Asthma. Int J Environ Res Public Health. 2020;17(13):4713.
11. Vandenplas O, Godet J, Hurdubaea L, et al; European network for the PHenotyping of OCcupational ASthma (E-PHOCAS) investigators. Are high- and low-molecular-weight sensitizing agents associated with different clinical phenotypes of occupational asthma? Allergy. 2019;74(2):261-72.
12. Zacharisen MC. Occupational asthma. Med Clin North Am. 2002;86(5):951-71.
13. Fishwick D, Bradshaw L, Davies J, et al. Are we failing workers with symptoms suggestive of occupational asthma? Prim Care Respir J. 2007;16(5):304-10.
14. Sauni R, Kauppi P, Helaskoski E, et al. Audit of quality of diagnostic procedures for occupational asthma. Occup Med (Lond). 2009;59(4):230-6.
15. Poonai N, van Diepen S, Bharatha A, et al. Barriers to diagnosis of occupational asthma in Ontario. Can J Public Health. 2005;96(3):230-3.
16. Kongsupon N, Walters GI, Adab P, et al. Screening tools for work-related asthma and their diagnostic accuracy: a systematic review protocol. BMJ Open. 2022;12(9):e058054.
17. Baur X, Sigsgaard T, Aasen TB, et al; ERS Task Force on the Management of Work-related Asthma. Guidelines for the management of work-related asthma. Eur Respir J. 2012;39(3):529-45.
18. Cullinan P, Vandenplas O, Bernstein D. Assessment and management of occupational asthma. J Allergy Clin Immunol Pract. 2020;8:3264-75.
19. Graham BL, Steenbruggen I, Miller MR, et al. Standardization of spirometry 2019 update. An official American thoracic Society and European respiratory Society technical statement. Am J Respir Crit Care Med. 2019;200:e70-88.
20. Quirce S, Campo P, Domínguez-Ortega J, et al. New developments in work-related asthma. Expert Rev Clin Immunol. 2017;13:271-81.
21. Trivedi V, Apala DR, Iyer VN. Occupational asthma. Curr Opin Pulm Med. 2005;11(4).
22. Moore VC, Jaakkola M, Burge P. A systematic review of serial peak expiratory flow measurements in the diagnosis of occupational asthma. Ann Respir Med. 2010;1:31-44.
23. Vandenplas O, Suojalehto H, Aasen TB, et al.; ERS Task Force on Specific Inhalation Challenges with Occupational Agents. Specific inhalation challenge in the diagnosis of occupational asthma: consensus statement. Eur Respir J. 2014;43(6):1573-87.
24. Vandenplas O, Dressel H, Wilken D, et al. Management of occupational asthma: cessation or reduction of exposure? A systematic review of available evidence. Eur Respir J. 2011;38(4): 804-11.
25. Vandenplas O, Wiszniewska M, Raulf M, et al; European Academy of Allergy and Clinical Immunology. EAACI position paper: irritant-induced asthma. Allergy. 2014;69(9):1141-53.
26. Nagasaka Y, Nakano N, Tohda Y, et al. Persistent reactive airway dysfunction syndrome after exposure to chromate. Nihon Kyobu Shikkan Gakkai Zasshi. 1995;33(7):759-64. [Japanese].
27. Tyagi R, Mohanty CS, Hande V. Reactive airway dysfunction syndrome: Are we missing these patients? Med J Armed Forces India. 2020;76(3):342-44.
28. Banauch GI, Alleyne D, Sanchez R, et al. Persistent hyperreactivity and reactive airway dysfunction in firefighters at the World Trade Center. Am J Respir Crit Care Med. 2003;168(1):54-62.
29. Walters GI, Huntley CC. Updated review of reported cases of reactive airways dysfunction syndrome. Occup Med (Lond). 2020;70(7):490-5.

High-altitude-related Illness

CHAPTER 102

Air Cmde Ajay Handa, Col Vikas Marwah, Lt Col Robin Choudhary

INTRODUCTION

Ascent to high altitude poses various challenges on the human body which includes extreme cold temperatures, low atmospheric pressures, and hypoxia which can cause specific altitude-related illnesses such as acute mountain sickness (AMS), high-altitude pulmonary edema (HAPE), and high-altitude cerebral edema (HACE). These illnesses can be sometimes severe and if unrecognized can even cause fatal outcome. There is an immense interest in collaborative networks and scientific production of data aimed at studying the mechanisms of adaptation to altitude and AMS.[1]

Individuals with preexisting lung diseases are at a higher risk of these high-altitude-related illnesses due to limited physiological reserve. There is scarcity of data regarding the risk of developing altitude-related illnesses and the effect of high altitude on the underlying lung disease. In the present era of changing lifestyles and desire for adventure, many people with lung diseases are traveling to high-altitude areas (HAA) for leisure and are likely to develop catastrophic problems unless they undergo proper evaluation before travel and follow advice regarding adequate acclimatization.[2] A recent review summarizes the information on different aspects including pathophysiology, clinical features, and recommendation for management and prevention of altitude-related illnesses.[3] The relevance of high-altitude related illnesses for practicing physicians and internists is ever increasing with ease of travel to these destinations.

PHYSICAL CHANGES WITH ALTITUDE

The increasing altitude most commonly leads to decrease in barometric pressure and lower inspired oxygen and fall in alveolar oxygen partial pressure (P_AO_2) and arterial oxygen tension (P_aO_2) values. Also, there is a reduction in density of air and ambient temperature with altitude gain, leading to greater water losses through the respiratory tract. There are less dust mite allergens in the HAA due to cold temperatures and reduced humidity.[4] Both altitude and cold weather are risks factors associated with various cardiovascular problems.[5]

PHYSIOLOGICAL ADAPTATION TO HIGH ALTITUDE

Acclimatization constitutes of various adaptive changes that occur in the respiratory, cardiovascular, and hematological systems to enable humans to survive in HAA. It includes a compensatory increase in ventilation due to the decreased P_aO_2 called hypoxic ventilatory response (HVR). The exercise capacity at high altitude is limited due to an increased work of breathing and respiratory muscle oxygen consumption.[2]

The low P_AO_2 (reduced alveolar–capillary gradient) combined with lower mixed venous oxygen levels adversely affects the exchange in the alveolar capillaries which delays alveolar–capillary equilibration.[6] Exercise leads to aggravation of these problems by increased cardiac output, shortened capillary transit time, and greater venous oxygen desaturation causing further arterial desaturation.[7]

The delivery of oxygen to tissues is maintained despite the decrease in blood oxygen content, by the increased cardiac output and increased red cell mass (hypoxia-induced erythropoietin production by kidneys). A hemoglobin-oxygen dissociation curve is shifted to right. High levels of 2,3-diphosphoglycerate in red blood cells, which counteract the effect of hyperventilation-induced respiratory alkalosis at altitude.[2]

Pulmonary vasoconstriction is triggered by alveolar hypoxia in order to maintain ventilation–perfusion ratio leading to a rise in pulmonary arterial pressure. This response maybe dysregulated in some patients leading to HAPE and altitude-related pulmonary hypertension.[8-11]

There are changes in lung volumes in HAA due to low atmospheric pressure. Most studies have shown a reduction in vital capacity and increases in total lung capacity (TLC) and residual volume. The responsible mechanisms include pulmonary vascular congestion, interstitial edema, abdominal distension, and reduced respiratory muscle strength. The peak expiratory flow rate (PEFR) is increased and airways resistance is reduced due to the decreased air density at high altitude.[12,13] The data regarding changes in forced expiratory volume in 1 second (FEV1) are conflicting.

ALTITUDE-RELATED SPECIFIC ILLNESSES

Acute Mountain Sickness

Acute mountain sickness affects 22–53% of travelers to altitudes between 1,850 and 4,240 m.[14] AMS consists of nonspecific symptoms occurring at altitudes of ≥2,500 m in unacclimatized individuals. The onset of AMS is after usually 4–12 hours of arrival at the new altitude. The symptoms are usually most pronounced on the first night and resolve spontaneously when appropriate measures are taken.[15] There is a risk of development of one of three forms of acute altitude illness over 2,500 m:[16] (1) AMS, (2) HACE, and (3) HAPE.

The diagnosis of AMS is clinical and is based on the presence of headache with any of the following: Fatigue, anorexia, nausea, vomiting, giddiness, and insomnia, the risk factors being altitude exposure and the rate of ascent. Other risk factors for AMS include reduction in SaO_2, body mass index (BMI) > 24 kg/m^2, and smoking.[17,18] There are no specific physical examination findings or laboratory studies. The development of moderate-to-severe AMS was predicted to be related to lower end-exercise SpO_2 and no previous exposure to altitude of above 5,000 m.[19]

Acute mountain sickness can be prevented by adequate acclimatization, undertaking a slow ascent to HAA. For those persons with risk factors, acetazolamide and dexamethasone are proven to be effective prophylactic agents. Treatment of severe AMS requires immediate descent by at least 300 m, oxygen inhalation, non-narcotic analgesics, and oral acetazolamide in doses of 250 mg twice a day. Both oral dexamethasone at a dose of 4 mg twice a day as well as inhaled corticosteroids such as budesonide at a dose of 200 μg twice a day were found to be useful for prevention of severe AMS compared to placebo.[20] The effect of dexamethasone is related to the altitude and dosage.[21] A recent Cochrane review recommends acetazolamide for the prevention of AMS in dosage of 250–750 mg/day.[22]

High-altitude Cerebral Edema

High-altitude cerebral edema is a life-threatening illness characterized by the presence of ataxia, altered mental status, or both in a patient with preceding symptoms of either AMS or HAPE. It is usually seen at altitudes above 4,000 m. The main risk factor is a rapid ascent to high altitude. The clinical hallmarks of HACE are truncal ataxia and decreased level of consciousness, which can rapidly progress to coma without treatment.[16] Preventive measures are the same as for AMS. Management primarily includes an immediate descent to a lower altitude. Emergency treatment and recompression in a portable hyperbaric chamber along with supplemental oxygen can be lifesaving. Affected patients should also be treated with dexamethasone (dose of 8 mg followed by 4 mg q 6 hourly intravenously).[23] If HACE is not recognized and treated immediately, there can be progressive cerebral edema with herniation and death.

High-altitude Pulmonary Edema

High-altitude pulmonary edema is a noncardiogenic pulmonary edema that affects 0.2–15% of high-altitude travelers.[24,25] It mostly occurs at altitudes above 3,000 m. It is seen after 2–5 days of ascent and can either develop following symptoms of AMS or HACE or de novo. Cases of HAPE are often seen in unacclimatized persons who ascend to altitude for pilgrimage to the Amarnath shrine in Kashmir located at an altitude of 3,882 m.[26,27] The risk factors include altitude, overexertion, rate of ascent, and cold-air exposure at altitude. Individuals susceptible to HAPE demonstrate exaggerated pulmonary vascular responses to hypoxia and exercise at HAA.[8,9]

The early symptoms are dry cough and decreased exercise performance. As HAPE worsens, patients develop dyspnea on minimal activity and productive cough with characteristic pink frothy sputum. Physical examination reveals low-grade fever, resting tachycardia, tachypnea, cyanosis, and bilateral crackles. Prevention of HAPE is pivotal and involves undertaking a slow ascent to HAA in a staged manner and avoiding overexertion. Patients giving a history of underlying respiratory diseases or pulmonary hypertension are ideal candidates for prophylaxis with nifedipine SR 20 mg twice daily and/or use of inhaler Salmeterol 125 μg twice daily.[28,29] Management of this fatal disorder is descent to lower altitude if possible or immediate recompression in a portable hyperbaric chamber with supplemental oxygen and nifedipine 10 mg stat followed by nifedipine SR 30 mg twice daily. In few cases, continuous positive airway pressure (CPAP) and noninvasive ventilation (NIV) with oxygen have been used as an adjunctive therapy.[30] Severe cases of HAPE may require invasive ventilatory support to correct refractory hypoxemia and prevent mortality.

Subacute Mountain Sickness

Subacute mountain sickness (SAMS) is an entity described in Indian soldiers posted to altitudes between 5,800 and 6,700 meters for an average of 10 weeks.[31] Anand et al. reported 21 cases of right heart failure who presented with dyspnea, cough, and exercise-induced angina and had clinical evidence of pedal edema, polycythemia, cardiomegaly, pericardial effusion, and ascites. The postulated mechanism was an exaggerated hypoxic pulmonary vasoconstriction response leading to heart failure.[32] Treatment involved transfer to lower altitudes causing rapid resolution of the disorder.

Chronic Mountain Sickness

Chronic mountain sickness (CMS) affects long-term residents staying over 1 year at HAA. The mean prevalence of CMS at altitudes between 2,350 and 4,150 meters in Himachal Pradesh has been reported as 6.17%; this increases to 13.73% above 3,000 m.[33] CMS is of two types: Seroche Monge's disease and pulmonary hypertension without polycythemia. Monge's disease is described as a syndrome marked by the triad of polycythemia, hypoxemia, and impaired mental status (headache, fatigue, impaired concentration, irritability), and clinical examination includes clubbing and cyanosis.[34] There occurs vascular remodeling due to prolonged hypoxic pulmonary vasoconstriction; the oxygen content of the blood is high along with increased diffusion capacity.[35] Right ventricular failure is uncommon. Treatment includes descent and stay at lower altitudes, periodic phlebotomy, diuretics, and respiratory stimulants. The other form of CMS has pulmonary hypertension and right heart failure without polycythemia.[36] Treatment includes descent and stay at lower altitudes. These persons are advised to avoid HAA as the disease is known to recur on high-altitude exposure.

EFFECTS OF HIGH ALTITUDE ON EXISTING LUNG DISEASES

Chronic Obstructive Pulmonary Disease

There are many physiological derangements in patients with COPD; most of them have impaired gas exchange. In severe COPD, there could be sarcopenia, reduced muscle strength, and mild-moderate pulmonary hypertension. These patients are likely to have hypoxemia and worsening pulmonary hypertension at high-altitude exposure. There is data to support that long term residence at high altitude was associated with increased mortality and higher incidence of cor pulmonale in COPD patients; therefore, patients with moderate-to-severe COPD must be advised to avoid long-term stay or permanent residence in HAA.[37]

As per the guidelines of the American Thoracic Society, P_aO_2 should be maintained above 50 mm Hg during commercial flight.[30] Guidelines by Aerospace Medical Association set this threshold at 55 mm Hg.[39] This value is reasonable as P_aO_2 values in this range ensure arterial oxygen saturation above 85% and lies above the steep portion of the hemoglobin-oxygen dissociation curve. Using the above data for travel to HAA, patients with COPD with PaO_2 levels < 50–55 mm Hg are advised to use their inhaled medications and use supplemental oxygen during stay at HAA.[40] Most of these studies have included moderate-to-severe COPD without CO_2 retention, and therefore results cannot be extrapolated to severe COPD with hypercapnia. The duration of exposure in these studies was shorter than what an individual would experience during stay at high altitude. Another important issue in the COPD patient with severe bullous disease is predisposition to bulla expansion and pneumothorax due to decrease in ambient pressure at high altitude. These concerns maybe theoretical since the bullae probably communicate with the airways to a greater extent than expected, allowing for pressure equalization to occur.

COPD patients with baseline FEV1 < 1.5 L should be assessed prior to travel to a HAA to determine the need for supplemental oxygen. Prediction of the P_aO_2 at high altitude should be based on the following regression equation provided by Dillard et al.:[38]

$$P_aO_2 \text{ altitude} = (0.5196 \times P_aO_2SL) + (11.856 \times FEV1) - 1.76$$

Those with predicted P_aO_2 < 50–55 mm Hg should undergo optimization of treatment and hypoxic challenge test before travel to high-altitude destinations. If unavoidable, high-altitude travel is to be done with supplemental oxygen. Patients should increase the flow rate of oxygen by 2 L/min when engaging in physical activity. COPD patients with preexisting moderate-to-severe pulmonary hypertension should be counseled against traveling to high altitude due to the high risk of developing HAPE or acute right heart failure. If the travel cannot be avoided, patients should travel with supplemental oxygen and should be started on oral nifedipine SR 20 mg twice daily for duration of stay at altitude. Extreme caution should be advised to COPD patients intending to travel to altitudes > 3,048 m, as there is no data available to guide recommendations above this elevation.[2]

Bronchial Asthma

There is a reduced allergen load at high altitude due to lower ambient temperature and humidity and asthma exacerbations are inversely related to altitude.[1] On the other hand, factors such as hypoxia, hypocapnia, and cold air can aggravate bronchial hyper-responsiveness (BHR) and worsen asthma control. Protection of the nose and mouth in cold winds by using appropriate head gear helps to warm inspired air and must be advised to all asthmatic subjects visiting HAA. The reduced air density at altitude should be beneficial for airflow limitation akin to effects of Heliox in asthma exacerbations, but these effects have not been studied systematically. The available data from field trials of mild asthmatic subjects suggests that asthmatics can travel up to the altitudes of 5,000 m without any adverse effects in duration of short-term trips. Those with severe asthma will need optimization of therapy and bronchoprovocation testing and hypoxic challenge test before travel in high-altitude destinations.[41] Severe asthmatics should be advised against travel to HAA as they are likely to deteriorate and there is lack of medical facilities at most places. Patients are to continue baseline medications and carry ample supply of inhalers and oral prednisolone for asthma exacerbations. Peak expiratory flow must be measured by patients and must be monitored twice daily to guide self-management plans as prescribed before travel.

Disorders with Pulmonary Hypertension

The main pathogenetic mechanism for HAPE is exaggerated pulmonary vasoconstriction in response to hypoxia. Several reports reflect a risk for HAPE in patients with preexisting pulmonary arterial hypertension (PAH) including those with altitude-related PAH.[2] The severity of PAH in these reports has been varied and to ascertain a threshold level for the risk is not feasible. The patients with PAH may develop sudden rise in pulmonary artery pressure causing acute right heart failure or progression to SAMS on exposure to HAA. Patients with PAH are to avoid traveling to HAA. Those patients who cannot avoid travel are advised prophylaxis with nifedipine SR 20 mg BD and to use supplemental oxygen for duration of stay. Phosphodiesterase inhibitor (sildenafil) and dexamethasone have also been used for prevention of HAPE.[42,43]

Pulmonary Thromboembolic Disorders

A patient with a history of venous thromboembolism is at an increased risk for recurrence at HAA. In a large retrospective study of over 20,000 patients, there were 46 cases of vascular thrombosis (44 venous and 2 arterial) from HAA versus 17 cases from low-altitude areas. The calculated odds ratio of thromboembolic events at high altitude was 30.5.[44] The mean duration of stay at HAA in those who developed thromboembolic events was 10 months. There are case reports of preexisting thrombophilic states with thromboembolic events at altitude in some patients. These include presence of factor V Leiden mutation, protein C deficiency, hyperhomocysteinemia, and use of oral contraceptive pills. Thus, persons with preexisting thrombophilias need to be explained the increased risk for thromboembolism at altitude exposure.[2]

Patients with a history of venous thromboembolism who travel to high altitude should continue anticoagulant drugs and monitor coagulogram before and after return from altitude. Females using oral contraceptives should be advised to discontinue the medications during their high-altitude exposure. These patients should be advised to maintain good hydration and regular ambulation. An alternative strategy is to start low-dose aspirin during the stay at HAA.[2]

Interstitial Lung Disease

Among all the respiratory diseases, least data is available on the effects of high altitude in patients with interstitial lung disease. There are reports of worsening dyspnea, resting hypoxemia, and exercise-induced desaturation in patients with ILD.[45] In addition, severe ILD patients have pulmonary hypertension and are at an increased risk of HAPE.

Patients with ILD require assessment for need of supplemental oxygen based on the regression equation proposed by Christensen et al.:[46]

$$P_aO_2 \text{ altitude} = 50.74 + (0.396 \times P_aO_2SL) + (0.0336 \times TLC)$$

Patients with P_aO_2 levels < 50–55 mm Hg should undergo thorough assessment with hypoxia challenge test and receive supplemental oxygen during stay at altitude. Those with ILD-associated pulmonary hypertension should be advised to avoid travel and if unavoidable they are required to be started on nifedipine prophylaxis for HAPE.[2]

Pneumothorax

Patients who underwent thoracic surgery and those with pneumothorax are advised to wait for 2 weeks for radiographic resolution of pneumothorax before traveling to HAA. Patients with residual pneumothorax or bronchopleural fistula should undergo chest tube drainage before travel to HAA. Screening of patients who are at high risk for secondary spontaneous pneumothorax by CT chest prior to high-altitude travel is advisable.[2]

Ventilatory Disorders

Obesity is a risk factor for altitude-induced pulmonary hypertension. Further, those with obesity hypoventilation syndrome (OHS) and obstructive sleep apnea (OSA) are at an increased risk for developing right heart failure, AMS, and HAPE. These patients are advised to avoid traveling to HAA. If the travel cannot be avoided, administer supplemental oxygen and start acetazolamide 125–250 mg BD. Patients with pulmonary hypertension should also start nifedipine SR 20 mg BD for prophylaxis against HAPE. Those patients using domiciliary bilevel or CPAP therapy are advised to use their device regularly during sleep at HAA.[2]

Obstructive Sleep Apnea Syndrome

For a patient with OSA traveling to HAA, carrying along a CPAP device can be quite inconvenient. Practical issues such as lack of electricity may lead to patients with OSAS unable to continue CPAP.[47] Exposure to HAA worsens the sleep-related events due to increased central apnea-hypopnea events without changing the rate of obstructive events. Thus, acclimatization does not affect the rate of obstructive apneic events in patients with OSAS. Sleep quality gets impaired and daytime psychomotor skills are decreased.[47] Alternative treatment options for OSAS at altitude include tab Acetazolamide at a dose of 250 mg twice daily, causing significant improvement in nocturnal oxygenation, reducing central sleep events, and improving sleep quality and sleep efficiency when compared to no treatment at all. Acetazolamide also prevented excessive blood pressure rise and weight gain at altitude. There was no effect on obstructive sleep events, and no significant effects on daytime performance were noted.[48] Therefore, for patients with OSA who refuse to use CPAP device, acetazolamide can be beneficial for OSAS patients during stay at high attitudes.

The combination therapy that provided a better nocturnal oxygenation and a better control of sleep apnea at altitude is of value in OSAS patients traveling to altitude destinations.[49] The current literature suggests that CPAP treatment should preferably be continued in an autoadjusting mode with addition of acetazolamide as an adjunctive to achieve a better sleep efficiency and higher arterial oxygen saturation. CPAP devices are thus capable of adjusting to the lower barometric pressure of altitude.

SUMMARY

The pathophysiology of high-altitude-related illnesses has been well studied in healthy individuals, but the risks of high-altitude exposure in patients with preexisting lung disease have not been systematically studied. The deranged physiologic functions in a patient with lung disease can be aggravated at high altitude and cause worsening of hypoxemia and respiratory failure and predispose to occurrence of HAPE. The presence of lung disease does not always preclude travel to high altitude provided thorough assessment is done beforehand and disease is well controlled with medications. Initiation of appropriate prophylactic medications to prevent altitude-related illnesses before travel and continued use till return to lower altitude is recommended. Most importantly, adequate attention must be paid to acclimatization taking rest days at various stages, carry out limited physical activity for 24–48 hours, and be aware of early recognition symptoms to seek medical attention.

REFERENCES

1. Zila-Velasque JP, Grados Espinoza P, Morán-Mariños C, et al. Adaptation and altitude sickness: A 40-year bibliometric analysis and collaborative networks. Front Public Health. 2023; 11:1069212.
2. Luks AM, Swenson ER. Travel to high altitude with pre-existing lung disease. Eur Respir J. 2007;29:770-92.
3. Netzer N, Strohl K, Faulhaber M, et al. Hypoxia-related altitude illnesses. J Travel Med. 2013;20(4):247-55.
4. West JB, Lahiri S, Maret KH, et al. Barometric pressures at extreme altitudes on Mt. Everest: physiological significance. J Appl Physiol. 1983;54:1188-94.
5. Whayne TF Jr. Altitude and cold weather: are they vascular risks? Curr Opin Cardiol. 2014;29(4):396-402.
6. West JB, Hackett PH, Maret KH, et al. Pulmonary gas exchange on the summit of Mount Everest. J Appl Physiol. 1983;55: 678-87.
7. Torre-Bueno JR, Wagner PD, Saltzman HA, et al. Diffusion limitation in normal humans during exercise at sea level and simulated altitude. J Appl Physiol. 1985;58:989-95.
8. Maggiorini M, Melot C, Pierre S, et al. High-altitude pulmonary edema is initially caused by an increase in capillary pressure. Circulation. 2001;103:2078-83.
9. Berger MM, Hesse C, Dehnert C, et al. Hypoxia impairs systemic endothelial function in individuals prone to high-altitude pulmonary edema. Am J Respir Crit Care Med. 2005;172:763-7.
10. Dehnert C, Grunig E, Mereles D, et al. Identification of individuals susceptible to high-altitude pulmonary oedema at low altitude. Eur Respir J. 2005;25:545-51.
11. Dunham-Snary KJ, Wu D, Sykes EA, et al. Hypoxic pulmonary vasoconstriction: From molecular mechanisms to medicine. Chest. 2017;151:181-92.
12. Mason NP, Barry PW, Pollard AJ, et al. Serial changes in spirometry during an ascent to 5300 m in the Nepalese Himalayas. High Alt Med Biol. 2000;1:185-95.
13. Pollard AJ, Mason NP, Barry PW, et al. Effect of altitude on spirometric parameters and the performance of peak flow meters. Thorax. 1996;51:175-8.
14. Hackett PH, Roach RC. High-altitude illness. N Engl J Med. 2001;345:107-14.
15. Estrada N, Franco M, Medina D, et al. Interventions for preventing high altitude illness: Part 1. Commonly-used classes of drugs. Cochrane Database Syst Rev. 2017;6.
16. Luks AM, Swenson ER, Bärtsch P. Acute high-altitude sickness. Eur Respir Rev. 2017;26(143):160096.
17. Hsu TY, Weng YM, Chiu YH, et al. Rate of ascent and acute mountain sickness at high altitude. Clin J Sport Med. 2014; 25(2):95-104.
18. Vinnikov D, Brimkulov N, Krasotski V, et al. Risk factors for occupational acute mountain sickness. Occup Med (Lond). 2014;64(7):483-9.
19. Cobb AB, Levett DZH, Mitchell K, et al. Physiological responses during ascent to high altitude and the incidence of acute mountain sickness. Physiol Rep. 2021;9(7):e14809.
20. Zheng CR, Chen GZ, Yu J, et al. Inhaled budesonide and oral dexamethasone prevent acute mountain sickness: a double-blind randomized controlled trial. Am J Med. 2014;127(10): 1001-9.e2.
21. Tang E, Chen Y, Luo Y. Dexamethasone for the prevention of acute mountain sickness: systematic review and meta analysis. Int J Cardiol. 2014;173(2):133-8.
22. Swenson ER. Pharmacology of acute mountain sickness: old drugs and newer thinking. J Appl Physiol (1985). 2016;120(2): 204-15.
23. Singh I, Kapila CC, Khanna PK, et al. High-altitude pulmonary oedema. Lancet. 1965;1:229-34.
24. Hultgren HN, Grover RF, Hartley LH. Abnormal circulatory responses to high altitude in subjects with a previous history of high-altitude pulmonary edema. Circulation. 1971;44: 759-70.
25. Bhagi S, Srivastava S, Singh SB. High altitude pulmonary edema: Review. J Occup Health. 2014;56(4):235-43.
26. Koul PA, Khan UH, Hussain T, et al. High altitude pulmonary edema among "Amarnath Yatris". Lung India. 2013;30(3):193-8.
27. Oelz O, Maggiorini M, Ritter M, et al. Nifedipine for high altitude pulmonary oedema. Lancet. 1989;2:1241-4.
28. Sartori C, Allemann Y, Duplain H, et al. Salmeterol for the prevention of high-altitude pulmonary edema. N Engl J Med. 2002;346:1631-6.

29. Walmsley M. Continuous positive airway pressure as adjunct treatment of acute altitude illness. High Alt Med Biol. 2013; 14(4):405-7.
30. Anand IS, Malhotra RM, Chandrashekhar Y, et al. Adult subacute mountain sickness-a syndrome of congestive heart failure in man at very high altitude. Lancet. 1990;335:561-5.
31. Maggiorini M, Leon-Velarde F. High-altitude pulmonary hypertension: a pathophysiological entity to different diseases. Eur Respir J. 2003;22:1019-25.
32. Sahota IS, Panwar NS. Prevalence of chronic mountain sickness in high altitude districts of Himachal Pradesh. Indian J Occup Environ Med. 2013;17(3):94-100.
33. Monge CC, Whittembury J. Chronic mountain sickness. Johns Hopkins Med J. 1976;139(Suppl.):87-9.
34. Naeije R, Vanderpool R. Pulmonary hypertension and chronic mountain sickness. High Alt Med Biol. 2013;14(2):117-25.
35. Aldashev AA, Sarybaev AS, Sydykov AS, et al. Characterization of high-altitude pulmonary hypertension in the Kyrgyz: association with angiotensin-converting enzyme genotype. Am J Respir Crit Care Med. 2002;166:1396-402.
36. Cote TR, Stroup DF, Dwyer DM, et al. Chronic obstructive pulmonary disease mortality. A role for altitude. Chest. 1993;103: 1194-7.
37. Standards for the diagnosis and care of patients with chronic obstructive pulmonary disease. American Thoracic Society. Am J Respir Crit Care Med. 1995;152:S112-3.
38. Medical guidelines for air travel. Aerospace Medical Association, Air Transport Medicine Committee, Alexandria, VA. Aviat Space Environ Med. 1996;67(Suppl. 10):B1-16.
39. Dillard TA, Rosenberg AP, Berg BW. Hypoxemia during altitude exposure. A meta-analysis of chronic obstructive pulmonary disease. Chest. 1993;103:422-5.
40. Golan Y, Onn A, Villa Y, et al. Asthma in adventure travelers: a prospective study evaluating the occurrence and risk factors for acute exacerbations. Arch Intern Med. 2002;162:2421-6.
41. Sydykov A, Mamazhakypov A, Maripov A, et al. Pulmonary Hypertension in Acute and Chronic High Altitude Maladaptation Disorders. Int J Environ Res Public Health. 2021;18(4): 1692.
42. Maggiorini M, Brunner-La Rocca H, Peth S, et al. Both tadalafil and dexamethasone may reduce the incidence of high altitude pulmonary edema: a randomized trial. Ann Intern Med. 2006; 145:497-506.
43. Anand AC, Jha SK, Saha A, et al. Thrombosis as a complication of extended stay at high altitude. Natl Med J India. 2001;14: 197-201.
44. Seccombe LM, Kelly PT, Wong CK, et al. Effect of simulated commercial flight on oxygenation in patients with interstitial lung disease and chronic obstructive pulmonary disease. Thorax. 2004;59:966-70.
45. Christensen CC, Ryg MS, Refvem OK, et al. Effect of hypobaric hypoxia on blood gases in patients with restrictive lung disease. Eur Respir J. 2002;20:300-5.
46. Nussbaumer-Ochsner Y, Schuepfer N, Ulrich S, et al. Exacerbation of sleep apnoea by frequent central events in patients with the obstructive sleep apnoea syndrome at altitude: a randomised trial. Thorax. 2010;65:429-35.
47. Nussbaumer-Ochsner Y, Latshang TD, Ulrich S, et al. Patients with obstructive sleep apnea syndrome benefit from acetazolamide during an altitude sojourn: a randomized, placebo-controlled, double-blind trial. Chest. 2012;141:131-8.
48. Latshang TD, Nussbaumer-Ochsner Y, Henn RM, et al. Effect of acetazolamide and autoCPAP therapy on breathing disturbances among patients with obstructive sleep apnea syndrome who travel to altitude: a randomized controlled trial. JAMA. 2012;308:2390-8.
49. Patz DS, Swihart B, White DP. CPAP pressure requirements for obstructive sleep apnea patients at varying altitudes. Sleep. 2010;33:715-8.

Aviation and Space Travel

Air Cmde Ajay Handa, Lt Col (Dr) Rahul Tyagi

CHAPTER 103

AIR TRAVEL

INTRODUCTION

Air travel has become a common mode of transportation in the present-day society. About 2.2 billion people travelled by air during 2021, despite the corona virus disease pandemic.[1] It is estimated that approximately 24–130 inflight medical emergencies (IMEs) occur per million air travelers, around 10% of which are due to respiratory disorders.[2] Among respiratory diseases, chronic obstructive pulmonary disease (COPD) is the main disease resulting in IME and requiring preflight medical screening.[3] Due to an aging population, the prevalence of respiratory diseases is increasing worldwide and most such patients would prefer to travel by air to minimize discomfort. It is imperative that health care providers identify high-risk individuals and screen them to minimize the risk of air travel in patients who have reduced physiological reserves.[4]

RESPIRATORY PHYSIOLOGY WITH ALTITUDE

Commercial aircraft fly at 10,000–13,000 m above sea level (ASL), but the relative cabin altitude is kept at 8,000 feet (2,438 m ASL) since significant hypoxemia can occur above this altitude.[5] Most travelers will maintain a partial pressure of arterial oxygen (PaO_2) of 60–65 mm Hg and oxygen saturation (SpO_2) of 89–94%. This mild hypoxemia is usually well tolerated in healthy subjects; it may however compromise an underlying pulmonary or cardiovascular disease.[5] Such patients need thorough preflight evaluation and recommendation on requirement of supplemental in-flight oxygen.

Ascent to high altitude also results in expansion of gases due to decrease in ambient pressure (Boyle's law). The expansion of gas trapped in close cavities such as the middle ear and intestine can cause discomfort. The gas within a lung bulla will expand by 30% at 2,450 m ASL and may cause rupture and complications such as pneumothorax, pneumomediastinum, and air embolism.[6] Patients of COPD with emphysematous bullae are at an increased risk for pneumothorax and respiratory failure during air travel and are therefore advised to avoid air travel.

Patient with COPD have a higher risk of developing significant hypoxemia during air travel.[7] Yet, the awareness and standard approach to assessment of these patients prior to flying are lacking. In a questionnaire-based study, only 30% pulmonologists were found to have informed COPD patients about air travel risk. Preflight assessment (PFA) was done by around 60% pulmonologists, and there was no standard approach used for the same.[7] This suggests a lack of standardized approach to evaluation of patients with respiratory illness prior to flying. This not only jeopardizes patient safety but may also lead to significant financial losses if a flight is diverted due to medical emergency.

PREFLIGHT ASSESSMENT

The aim of PFA is to identify those likely to develop significant hypoxemia onboard the flight. Patients on long-term oxygen therapy (LTOT) and those with cardiorespiratory illnesses constitute important categories. Patients with severe COPD, bronchial asthma, restrictive lung diseases, past venous thromboembolism, recent pneumothorax, and pulmonary tuberculosis are also at high risk of deterioration during air travel.[8] COPD is the most common cause of referral for PFA.[9] Preflight evaluation must be done for patients with the following conditions:[4]

- Preexisting requirement of oxygen/noninvasive ventilator (NIV) support
- Bullous lung disease
- Forced expiratory volume in 1 second (FEV_1) < 1.5 L or FEV_1 < 30% predicted
- Comorbidities such as cardiac disease and pulmonary hypertension
- Any significant symptoms during previous air travel

In other respiratory diseases, common indications for referral for PFA are:[10]

- Restrictive disorders with a forced vital capacity <1 L
- Recent pneumothorax

- Significant respiratory illness within last 6 weeks
- Previous history of deep venous thrombosis/pulmonary thromboembolism

Preflight assessment should include the detailed history of general health, presence of symptoms, any recent worsening of symptoms suggestive of exacerbation, and treatment being taken followed by thorough general and systemic examination.[4] It is worth noting that no resting measures of lung function [such as SpO_2 at sea level (SpO_2 SL) and FEV1] can reliably predict inflight hypoxemia.[10]

It is important to discuss the various challenges which may arise during air travel, in a patient with a significant cardiorespiratory illness. The patient needs to be informed clearly regarding the following aspects:[10]

- Prior arrangements for inflight oxygen with the airlines and at destination if the patient is on LTOT/NIV
- Patient should carry their emergency medicines in handbag
- Patients should be advised to hydrate well, avoid alcohol, and keep moving every 1–2 hours, specially on long haul flights.

Resting SpO_2 at sea level on room air needs to be recorded; SpO_2 less than 95% on room air will need further evaluation.[4,10] These patients should undergo an arterial blood gas analysis. A value of PaO_2 of >70 mm Hg was earlier considered safe for flying without oxygen.[11] However, studies in COPD have shown that sea level PaO_2 may not be appropriate to predict desaturation in flying.[12,13] Other tests used for preflight evaluation include pulmonary function testing, use of predictive equations, walk tests, and hypoxic challenge test.

Airline medical authorities traditionally use the 50 m walk test for screening passengers—those who are able to walk 50 m are considered "fit to fly". The test is a crude assessment of cardiorespiratory status and needs to be supervised. Failure to complete the distance or developing moderate-to-severe respiratory distress should alert the physician for referral for assessment for inflight oxygen by a respiratory physician.

Nomograms and equations for predicting PaO_2 at altitude using blood gas parameters and spirometry at ground level have been developed for COPD patients exposed to hypoxia **(Box 1)**.[14] In clinical practice, such equations are most frequently applied to predict fitness and requirement of on-board oxygen. Predicted PaO_2 values < 50 mm Hg are indication of supplemental inflight oxygen.

There are no guidelines as to which of the equations is to be used. Some authors use regression equation for calculating predicted PaO_2 at altitude. If the calculated value is 50 ± 3 mm Hg, a hypoxic challenge test is advised for definitive recommendations.

BOX 1 Equations for calculating predicted PaO_2 at 2,450 m.

- PaO_2 altitude = 0.84 + 0.68 (PaO_2 ground)
- PaO_2 altitude = 0.295 (PaO_2 sea level) + 0.086 (FEV_1% predicted) + 23.211
- PaO_2 altitude = 0.245 (PaO_2 sea level) + 0.171 (FEV_1/FVC% predicted) + 21.028

Hypoxia Altitude Stimulation Test/ Hypoxic Challenge Test

Patient with respiratory disorders who have identifiable risk factors (hypercapnia, FEV1 < 50% of predicted, restrictive pulmonary disorders, cardiac or cerebrovascular diseases which may worsen with hypoxia, recent admission for an exacerbation of chronic pulmonary or cardiac disease) and having a ground SpO_2 of 92–95% will require this test to determine the need for supplemental inflight oxygen **(Table 1)**.[15,16]

The test was first described by Henry Gong Jr in 1984.[14] The hypoxia altitude stimulation test (HAST) or hypoxic challenge test remains the gold standard for PFA regarding oxygen supplementation. The subject is exposed to 15% oxygen (in nitrogen) using nonrebreathing facemask or body plethysmograph. Continuous monitoring with pulse oximetry and electrocardiography is done to prevent severe desaturation and to detect cardiac arrhythmias. The subjects are asked to breathe the gas mixture for 20 minutes or until equilibration and arterial blood gas analysis is done before and after exposure. If the PaO_2 during the test is >55 mm Hg, no supplemental oxygen is required. If the PaO_2 falls to below 50 mm Hg, the patient is given oxygen (usually at 2 L/min). The test is repeated with oxygen to ensure adequate hypoxia correction. Values of PaO_2 between 50 and 55 mm Hg are considered borderline needing 6—minute walk test (6MWT) and clinical judgment by physician.[15]

Patients who are subjected to hypoxic challenge are categorized based on the measured PaO_2 after 20 minutes at FiO_2 15% and advised accordingly based on PaO_2 **(Table 2)**. Despite being considered the gold standard test for assessment for need for inflight oxygen supplementation, the hypoxic challenge test did not predict the development of problems in air travel. There was no difference in PaO_2 levels during hypoxic challenge test at 2,438 m between those with COPD who subsequently developed respiratory symptoms in flight during air travel and those who did not.[17]

Another simple algorithm based on SpO_2 SL and SpO_2 after 6MWT (SpO_2 6MWT) has been found to have

TABLE 1: British Thoracic Society (BTS) recommendations for initial screening.

Pulse oximetry	Recommendation
SpO_2 > 95%	Oxygen not required
SpO_2 92–95% without risk factors	Oxygen not required
SpO_2 92–95% with risk factors	Hypoxic simulation altitude test
SpO_2 < 92%	Inflight oxygen

TABLE 2: British Thoracic Society (BTS) recommendations after hypoxia altitude stimulation test (HAST).

Blood gas report	Recommendation
PaO_2 > 55 mm Hg	Oxygen not required
PaO_2 50–55 mm Hg	Borderline, advised 6-minute walk test, and clinical judgment to advise inflight oxygen supplementation
PaO_2 < 50 mm Hg	Inflight oxygen @ 2 L/min to be used

sensitivity of 100% and specificity of 80% in predicting the need for inflight oxygen in moderate-to-severe COPD patients.[18] Patients with SpO_2 SL >95% combined with SpO_2 6MWT >84% could be allowed to travel by air without further assessment. Inflight supplemental oxygen was recommended if SpO_2 SL was 92–95% combined with SpO_2 6MWT <84% or if SpO_2 SL <92%.

PRESCRIBING INFLIGHT OXYGEN

Any patient with PaO_2 of <70 mm Hg at sea level at rest will require supplemental oxygen during air travel.[19] Most commercial airlines will provide oxygen inflight based on advance request and physician's prescription. The expenses are required to be borne by the travelers. The oxygen supply is usually provided from cylinders so the rate of flow and duration must be specified so that an adequate amount of oxygen is available during the journey. The rate of oxygen of 2 L/min is suitable for most passengers. Those on LTOT are advised to increase the flow rate of 2 L/min above the usual flow rate.[20]

Most airlines provide oxygen through simple face mask, and passengers are advised to carry their nasal prongs to prevent rebreathing. The oxygen and cabin air inside the aircraft are devoid of moisture and can lead to drying of tracheobronchial mucosa and precipitation of bronchospasm. The airlines must be informed for humidified oxygen for patients with asthma and COPD. In addition, such patients must be advised to carry their medications in their hand baggage for use in emergency situations.[21]

Airlines do not provide oxygen during waiting period and stopovers. Some airports restrict oxygen use in the airport because of the risk of explosion. Oxygen-dependent patients must make additional arrangements for use during the waiting periods at the airports. Patients cannot use their own cylinders or concentrators but may be able to take these items with them as baggage for use at their destination. It is also important for these patients to carry their medical documents and extra drug supplies during travel **(Box 2)**.

COVID-19 AND AIR TRAVEL

COVID-19 transmission during flight is well documented.[23,24] International Civil Aviation Organization (ICAO) had released guidelines for safe travel during the pandemic.[25] The suggestions for passengers to avoid getting infected include using well-fitting face masks with face shields throughout the flight, regular hand cleaning with alcohol-based disinfectant, and avoid touching of eyes, face, and nose.

BOX 2 Guidelines for oxygen dependent patients prior to air travel.[22]

- Obtain medical certificate of fitness to fly
- Carry prescription of inflight oxygen requirement
- Inform the airlines while booking tickets and 48–72 hours before the date of journey
- Inform airlines the need for oxygen before boarding and during stopovers
- Preferably take nonstop flight to destination
- Carry extra tubing and personal nasal cannula
- Carry extra copies of prescriptions and medical certificate
- Carry emergency supply of medications in hand baggage

SUMMARY

Air travel is safe and comfortable mode of travel for the vast majority of people. Patients who have cardiorespiratory diseases are at a risk of significant hypoxemia during air travel. Most of these individuals would be able to complete the journey uneventfully with supplemental oxygen. All the present recommendations are based on results of effects of simulated hypoxia on patients with lung diseases.

SPACE TRAVEL

INTRODUCTION

Space travel is at present undergoing a revolution with both government and commercial agencies preparing for long-distance air travel as well as space tourism.[26] Current evidence regarding human health in space travel is very limited. The condition of zero gravity or weightlessness (microgravity) for assessing its effects on the human body can be achieved by two methods, i.e., parabolic flight in aircraft and space flight. The parabolic flights in commercial jet aircraft are associated with small periods of microgravity with periods of hypergravity (increased gravitational forces) during these maneuvers. Parabolic flights are more easily available and less expensive compared to space flights. They have the disadvantage of creating motion sickness in the passengers during this "roller coaster" flight. The US, Russia, and European Union countries have regular parabolic flights for their research work.

The flights in spacecraft are infrequent and extremely expensive. The advantage is that space flights have sustained periods of microgravity from 1 week to up to a year. Most research work has been done onboard Russian space station Mir and International Space Station (ISS) led by the USA. These space stations offer a convenient environment for studying the effects of space on human physiology. The number of subjects is limited to a maximum of four as the crew serve as subjects and operators or both. The evaluation includes preflight and postflight testing of various parameters and comparison with data under microgravity.[27]

MICROGRAVITY AND WEIGHTLESSNESS

There are some ground-based experiments which mimic weightlessness, such as 6° head-down tilt (HDT) and thermoneutral water immersion (TWI). These have been useful to study the cardiovascular and musculoskeletal responses. But the significant effect of gravity on the lungs and pulmonary vasculature cannot be eliminated. Further HDT and TWI cause larger reductions in resting lung volumes than microgravity, which cannot be ignored.[28]

To understand the effect of microgravity and weightlessness in space on the respiratory system, we can take a cue from the common knowledge that even though there are no structural differences between the upper and lower parts of the human lungs, gravitational forces lead to marked functional differences between these areas. The alveoli at the top of the lung are more expanded compared with the bottom of the lung because of the weight of the lungs on the lower parts. On the other hand, alveolar ventilation is higher at the bottom of the lung as compared to the apex. Gravity also influences the intrapleural pressure, parenchymal stress, and pulmonary blood flow which result in regional differences in lung function.[29,30] There is greater disparity in the pulmonary blood flow between the top and bottom of the lung with greater flows near the bases than the apices. This is due to the effect of hydrostatic forces on the low-pressure pulmonary circulation. As a result of the profound effects of gravity on alveolar ventilation and pulmonary perfusion, ventilation-perfusion ratio ($\dot{V}/\dot{Q}$) is higher at the apices than the lung bases and there are regional differences in gas exchange in the lungs.[31]

The influence of gravity on the lung on earth and increasing the gravitational effect has been studied. Most of the changes in lung function are attributable to gravity. The conclusions of these studies cannot be extrapolated to zero gravity conditions. Many studies on respiratory and cardiac functions in the absence of gravity have been performed in the last decade and a half. The results of some of these studies are summarized in the succeeding paragraphs **(Table 3)**.

TABLE 3: Summary of results of studies on effects on pulmonary and cardiac functions during space travel.

Effects	Initial findings	Prolonged duration exposure
Lung volumes and flows		
VC	Reduced	Normalized
FRC	Reduced	Normalized
RV	Unchanged	
PEFR	Unchanged	
FEF 25–75%	Unchanged	
Pulmonary diffusion		
DLCO	Increased	Increased
Gas exchange		
Tidal volume	Reduced	
Respiratory rate	Increased	
Minute ventilation	Marginal decrease	
Physiological dead space	Reduced	
Oxygen consumption	Unchanged	
CO_2 production	Unchanged	
Cardiac function		
Cardiac output	Increased	–
Heart rate	Increased	–
Stroke volume	Unchanged	–
Response to exercise		
Cardiac	Reduced	–
Ventilatory	Unchanged	–
Ventilatory control		
Hypoxic drive	Reduced	–
CO_2 drive	Unchanged	–
Sleep		
Sleep efficiency	Poor	Poor
Sleep apneas syndrome	Reduction in events and snoring	

(DLCO: diffusing capacity of the lungs for carbon monoxide; FEF: forced expiratory flow; FRC: functional residual capacity; PEFR: peak expiratory flow rate; RV: residual volume; VC: vital capacity)

Effects on Lung Volume and Spirometry

The first study of space on lung volumes was done in the 1970s and showed that vital capacity (VC) reduced by 5–10%.[32] The subsequent studies have shown that VC reduces by 5–6% for the first 2 days and normalizes by day 4. This was explained by the early inflight increased intrathoracic blood volume which subsequently reduces to normal as plasma volume reduces in sustained space flight.[33] As the effect of gravity was removed, the functional residual capacity (FRC) reduced by 5–10%, due to cranial shift of diaphragm and outward movement of ribcage.[34] Residual volume (RV) remains unchanged with microgravity.[35]

Peak expiratory flow (PEF) was found to be unaffected in most studies. During initial space flight, there is reduction in the PEF due to lack of a firm platform to push against during the forced expiration. Subsequent recovery is noticed due to better performance after adaptation to microgravity. There is change in forced expiratory flow (FEF) in effort independent portion at lower volumes (FEF 25–75%), which suggests that behavior of central and peripheral airways and respiratory muscles is unaffected in space.[36]

Effects on Diffusion Capacity and Pulmonary Perfusion

There is a substantial increase in diffusion capacity by 28% over the baseline and it remains elevated over the course of flight due to an increase in pulmonary capillary blood volume and membrane diffusing capacity.[37] These phenomena are attributed to transition of the lung from its zone 1, 2, 3 $\dot{V}/\dot{Q}$ configurations on ground level to predominant zone 2 or zone 3 in space causing more uniform capillary filling.[37]

Effects on Gas Exchange and Ventilation–Perfusion Relationship

The tidal volume is reduced and breathing frequency is increased; thus, the minute ventilation is only marginally reduced. Moreover, the physiological dead space is reduced; thus, the effective alveolar ventilation remains the same. In spite of these ventilatory changes, oxygen consumption and carbon dioxide production are unchanged in space.[38] The peak oxygen consumption however reduces by 22% on return to ground and gradually recovers over the next 6–9 days to preflight levels, postulated to be due to circulatory blood volume changes.

Effect on Cardiac Output and Exercise

Cardiac output increases after 2 weeks in space as a result of increased heart rate with constant stroke volume.[39] The ventilatory response to exercise remain unchanged in microgravity, but the cardiac response to exercise is less in short-duration space flights when compared to ground-level changes. No data is available for long-duration space flights.[40]

Ventilatory Control and Sleep in Space

There is substantial reduction in the ventilatory response to hypoxia with halving of hypoxic drive, whereas the response to carbon dioxide remains unchanged. This change in the hypoxic response is possibly due to an increase in blood pressure at the level of the carotid bodies due to zero gravity. The systemic blood pressure remains unchanged, but the blood pressure at the carotid bodies is higher due to abolition of hydrostatic pressure difference normally present on ground.[41] There is poor sleep efficiency during space flights due to poor ventilatory control and altered circadian rhythm. The subjects with obstructive sleep apneas syndrome have improvement in sleep quality with reduction in events and snoring. The cause of sleep deficiency in space is not related to respiratory system changes.[42]

ASSESSMENT PRIOR TO SPACE TRAVEL

Requirements for PFA before space travel will depend on the duration of space travel. While suborbital flights have only brief microgravity exposures of 3–5 minutes, orbital flights can have microgravity exposures up to 30 days.[26] The aim of preflight screening is to identify conditions which may cause sudden incapacitation requiring either disqualifying or appropriate treatment. The following screening is recommended prior to space travel:[26]

- Detailed history and physical examination
- Metabolic screening
- Assessment of aerobic capacity (VO_2 max)
- Assessment of muscle strength and pulmonary functions
- Health screening test as per age recommendations (mammography, prostate specific antigen, colonoscopy)

SUMMARY

The comprehensive data on changes in respiratory physiology in space have found that the effects are generally benign and unlikely to limit the activities of astronauts in space. The experience in this field is limited at present. More challenges are likely to be recognized in the coming years as the humans enter the era of interplanetary travel.

REFERENCES

1. Statista. Global air travel statistics. [online] Available from https://www.statista.com/statistics/564717/airline-industry-passenger-traffic-globally/ [Last accessed June, 2024].
2. Martin-Gill C, Doyle TJ, Yealy DM. In-Flight Medical Emergencies: A Review. JAMA. 2018;320(24):2580-90.
3. Khan IA, Pierucci P, Ambrosino N. COPD patients' pre-flight check: A narrative review. Monaldi Arch Chest Dis. 2022; 92(4).
4. Ergan B, Akgun M, Pacilli AMG, et al. Should I stay or should I go? COPD and air travel. Eur Respir Rev. 2018;27(148):180030.
5. Powell-Dunford N, Adams JR, Grace C. Medical Advice for Commercial Air Travel. Am Fam Physician. 2021;104(4):403-10.
6. Dillard TA, Rosenberg AP, Berg BW. Hypoxaemia during altitude exposure. A meta-analysis of chronic obstructive pulmonary disease. Chest. 1993;103:422-5.
7. Ergan B, Arıkan H, Akgün M. Are pulmonologists well aware of planning safe air travel for patients with COPD? The SAFCOP study. Int J Chron Obstruct Pulmon Dis. 2019;14:1895-900.
8. Dillard TA, Berg BW, Rajagopal KR, et al. Hypoxaemia during air travel in patients with COPD. Ann Intern Med. 1989;111:362-7.

9. Coker RK, Shiner RJ, Partridge MR. Is air travel safe for those with lung disease? Eur Respir J. 2007;30:1057-63.
10. Josephs LK, Coker RK, Thomas M; BTS Air Travel Working Group; British Thoracic Society. Managing patients with stable respiratory disease planning air travel: a primary care summary of the British Thoracic Society recommendations. Prim Care Respir J. 2013;22(2):234-8.
11. Aerospace Medical Association. Medical Guidelines for Air Travel, 2nd edition. Aviat Space Environ Med. 2003;74(Suppl):A1-19.
12. Akero A, Christensen CC, Edvardsen A, et al. Hypoxaemia in chronic obstructive pulmonary disease patients during a commercial flight. Eur Respir J. 2005;25:725-30.
13. Christensen CC, Ryg M, Refvem OK, et al. Development of severe hypoxaemia in chronic obstructive pulmonary disease patients at 2,438 m (8,000 ft) altitude. Eur Respir J. 2000;15:635-9.
14. Gong H, Tashkin DP, Lee EY, et al. Hypoxia-altitude simulation test. Am Rev Respir Dis. 1984;130:980-6.
15. Dine CJ, Kreider ME. Hypoxia altitude simulation test. Chest. 2008;133(4):1002-5.
16. British Thoracic Society Standards of Care Committee. Managing passengers with respiratory disease planning air travel: British Thoracic Society recommendations. Thorax. 2002;57:289-304.
17. Edvardsen A, Ryg M, Akerø A, et al. COPD and air travel: does hypoxia-altitude simulation testing predict in-flight respiratory symptoms? Eur Respir J. 2013;42:1216-23.
18. Edvardsen A, Akerø A, Christensen CC, et al. Air travel and chronic obstructive pulmonary disease: a new algorithm for pre-flight evaluation. Thorax. 2012;67:964-9.
19. Cramer D, Ward S, Geddes D. Assessment of oxygen supplementation during air travel. Thorax. 1996;51:202-3.
20. Vohra KP, Klocke RA. Detection and correction of hypoxemia associated with air travel. Am Rev Respir Dis. 1993;148:1215-9.
21. Khilnani GC, Bhatta N. Air travel and supplemental oxygen in patients with cardiopulmonary diseases. J Assoc Physicians India. 2002;50:811-5.
22. Handa A. Oxygen therapy during air travel. In: Jindal SK, Agarwal R (Eds). Oxygen Therapy. New Delhi: Jaypee Brothers Medical Publishers; 2009. pp. 221-6.
23. Chen J, He H, Cheng W, et al. Potential transmission of SARS-CoV-2 on a flight from Singapore to Hangzhou, China: an epidemiological investigation. Travel Med Infect Dis. 2020;36:101816.
24. Hoehl S, Karaca O, Kohmer N. et al. Assessment of SARS-CoV-2 transmission on an international flight and among a tourist group. JAMA Netw Open. 2020;3(8):e2018044.
25. Harries AD, Martinez L, Chakaya JM. SARS-CoV-2: how safe is it to fly and what can be done to enhance protection? Trans R Soc Trop Med Hyg. 2021;115(1):117-9.
26. Krittanawong C, Singh NK, Scheuring RA, et al. Human Health during Space Travel: State-of-the-Art Review. Cells. 2022;12(1):40.
27. Prisk GK. The lung in space. Clin Chest Med. 2005;26:415-38.
28. Derion T, Guy HJB, Tsukimoto K, et al. Ventilation perfusion relationships in the lung during head-out water immersion. J Appl Physiol. 1992;72:64-72.
29. West JB, Matthews FL. Stresses, strains, surface pressures in the lung caused by its weight. J Appl Physiol. 1972;31:332-45.
30. West JB, Dollery CT. Distribution of blood flow and ventilation-perfusion ratio in the lung, measured with radioactive CO_2. J Appl Physiol. 1960;15:405-10.
31. West JB. Regional differences in gas exchange in the lung of erect man. J Appl Physiol. 1962;17:893-8.
32. Sawin CF, Nicogossian AE, Rummel JA, et al. Pulmonary function evaluation during the Skylab and Apollo-Soyuz Missions. Aviat Space Environ Med. 1976;47:168-72.
33. Buckey JC, Gaffney FA, Lane LD, et al. Central venous pressure in space. N Engl J Med. 1993;328:1853-4.
34. Elliott AR, Prisk GK, Guy HJB, et al. Lung volumes during sustained microgravity on Spacelab SLS-1. J Appl Physiol. 1994;77:2005-14.
35. Bettinelli D, Kays C, Bailliart O, et al. Effect of gravity and posture on lung mechanics. J Appl Physiol. 2002;93:2044-52.
36. Guy HJB, Prisk GK, Elliott AR, et al. Maximum expiratory flow-volume curves during short periods of microgravity. J Appl Physiol. 1991;70:2587-96.
37. Prisk GK, Guy HJB, Elliott AR, et al. Pulmonary diffusing capacity, capillary blood volume and cardiac output during sustained microgravity. J Appl Physiol. 1993;75:15-26.
38. Prisk GK, Elliott AR, Guy HJB, et al. Pulmonary gas exchange and its determinants during sustained microgravity on Spacelabs SLS-1 and SLS-2. J Appl Physiol. 1995;79:1290-8.
39. Prisk GK, Fine JM, Elliott AR, et al. Effect of 6° head down tilt on cardiopulmonary function: comparison with microgravity. Aviat Space Environ Med. 2002;73:8-16.
40. Shykoff BE, Farhi LE, Olszowka AJ, et al. Cardiovascular response to submaximal exercise in sustained microgravity. J Appl Physiol. 1996;81:26-32.
41. Fritsch-Yelle JM, Charles JB, Jones MM, et al. Microgravity decreases heart rate and arterial pressure in humans. J Appl Physiol. 1996;80:910-4.
42. Elliott AR, Shea SA, Dijk D-J, et al. Microgravity reduces sleep-disordered breathing in normal humans. Am J Respir Crit Care Med. 2001;164:478-85.

SECTION

10

Diffuse Parenchymal Interstitial Lung Diseases

SECTION OUTLINE

Diagnosis and Classification of Interstitial Lung Diseases

CHAPTER 104

Alok Nath, Zafar Neyaz

INTRODUCTION

Interstitial lung diseases (ILDs) are a heterogeneous and complex group of more than 200 conditions that cause scarring/fibrosis of the lung parenchyma. With time, it has been realized that this disease does not confine itself merely to the interstitium but may involve other parenchymal components such as endothelium, terminal airways, and alveoli; hence, the term *diffuse parenchymal lung disease* (DPLD) is used interchangeably. Our understanding of the grouping of these disorders has historically been based on histopathological findings or the underlying etiology and has undergone modification repeatedly in the wake of better understanding of the disease process. Yet, we lag in understanding the exact pathophysiologic mechanisms leading to the development of fibrosis and label a considerable number of cases as idiopathic. A comprehensive diagnostic approach is needed to confirm the condition. It is imperative to assess the patient in detail, make an accurate and timely diagnosis, and provide management as may deem fit on a case-to-case basis.

HISTORICAL ASPECT

The earliest description of ILDs dates back to the 1800s when a German physician Von Buhl reported *chronic interstitial pneumonia*.[1] Later, the disease was labeled as the parenchymal fibrous scarring *cirrhosis of the lung*.[2] Till then, the evidence was confined to case reports. Thereafter, Louis Hamman and Arnold Rich described in detail the clinical, radiological, and pathological features of the fulminant progressive ILD that was later named after them as the "Hamman-Rich syndrome".[3] Around that era, ILDs with even a protracted course were reported as chronic "Hamman-Rich syndrome".

The first landmark classification of ILDs was given by *Liebow and Carrington* in 1969 based on histopathology.[4] The most common pattern encountered was called the usual interstitial pneumonia (UIP), and others depending on the predominant finding were classified as bronchiolitis obliterans with interstitial pneumonia (BIP), lymphocytic interstitial pneumonia (LIP), desquamative interstitial pneumonia (DIP), and giant cell interstitial pneumonia (GIP). While the most common pattern was UIP, the ILD associated with it was called chronic fibrosing alveolitis (CFA). Decades later, this classification was modified to include a new group of nonspecific interstitial pneumonia (NSIP); otherwise, the classification was more or less similar **(Table 1)**. NSIP was kept as a provisional category and was essentially a diagnosis of exclusion.[5,6]

TABLE 1: Initial classifications of interstitial lung diseases (ILDs).

Liebow and Carrington (1969)	Katzenstein (1997)	Müller and Colby (1997)
Usual interstitial pneumonia	Usual interstitial pneumonia	Usual interstitial pneumonia
Desquamative interstitial pneumonia (DIP)	DIP/respiratory bronchiolitis interstitial lung disease	DIP
Bronchiolitis obliterans interstitial pneumonia and diffuse alveolar damage (DAD)	Acute interstitial pneumonia	Bronchiolitis obliterans with organizing pneumonia (BOOP)
Lymphoid interstitial pneumonia	Nonspecific interstitial pneumonia	Acute interstitial pneumonia
Giant cell interstitial pneumonia		Nonspecific interstitial pneumonia

CLASSIFICATIONS

In the year 2002, the American Thoracic Society (ATS) and European Respiratory Society (ERS) provided a joint statement and standardized the ILD classification for the first time. The four major classes were categorized as ILD of known causes, idiopathic interstitial pneumonias (IIPs), granulomatous DPLD and other forms. IIPs were further subclassified into idiopathic pulmonary fibrosis (IPF) and IIP other than IPF **(Fig. 1)**. The clinical, radiological, and pathological features of each category were defined clearly. The diagnosis of IIPs was determined by histopathology and the pattern with respective diagnosis was clearly defined. In the algorithm of diagnosis, following the high-resolution tomography of the chest, bronchoalveolar lavage or a transbronchial lung biopsy (TBLB) was recommended which, if inconclusive, warranted surgical lung biopsy (SLB).[7]

Later, in 2013, an update of the IIP classification was published in which IIPs were classified into three major categories: Major IIPs, rare IIPs, and unclassifiable IIPs. The major IIPs were further subgrouped into chronic fibrosing, smoking related, and acute or subacute types. It was here that NSIP was designated as a definitive diagnosis for the first time. In the situation of inadequate or discordant clinic-radiological or pathological data, the category of unclassifiable IIPs was defined. The rare histologic subtypes such as idiopathic lymphoid interstitial pneumonia (LIP), acute fibrinous organizing pneumonia, idiopathic pleuroparenchymal fibroelastosis, and interstitial pneumonia with bronchiolocentric distribution were also described.[8] This classification is followed till date **(Box 1)**.

More recently, it has been proposed that classification be based on the disease course and probable outcome. Thus, those ILDs that are characterized by radiological or histopathological features of fibrosis are proposed to be labeled as fibrosing ILDs and include IPF, idiopathic NSIP, connective tissue ILDs such as rheumatoid arthritis and systemic sclerosis-associated ILD, interstitial pneumonia with autoimmune features, hypersensitivity pneumonitis (HSP), sarcoidosis, occupational and unclassifiable ILDs, etc.[9] Given the high probability of progression, these ILDs have been lately christened as progressive fibrosing ILDs (PF-ILD) or progressive pulmonary fibrosis (PPF) and criteria for diagnosis have been recently updated in an official ATS/ERS/JRS/ALAT clinical practice guideline **(Table 2)**.[10] The objective behind this classification is identifying patients who may be a candidate for available antifibrotic therapies because data from a couple of studies have demonstrated benefit of antifibrotic drugs like pirfenidone and nintedanib in these patients.[11,12]

There has been a paradigm shift in the approach to the diagnosis of ILDs and nowadays the emphasis has shifted from etiology to clinical behavior of the disease which has underscored its importance in the treatment and prognosis of a group of ILDs rather than an individual clinical entity. Given the heterogeneity of the presentation, clinical behavior of ILDs, and significant interobserver differences in interpretation of radiological and histological features, it is quite difficult to make a confident diagnosis based on individual finding on clinical, serological, radiological,

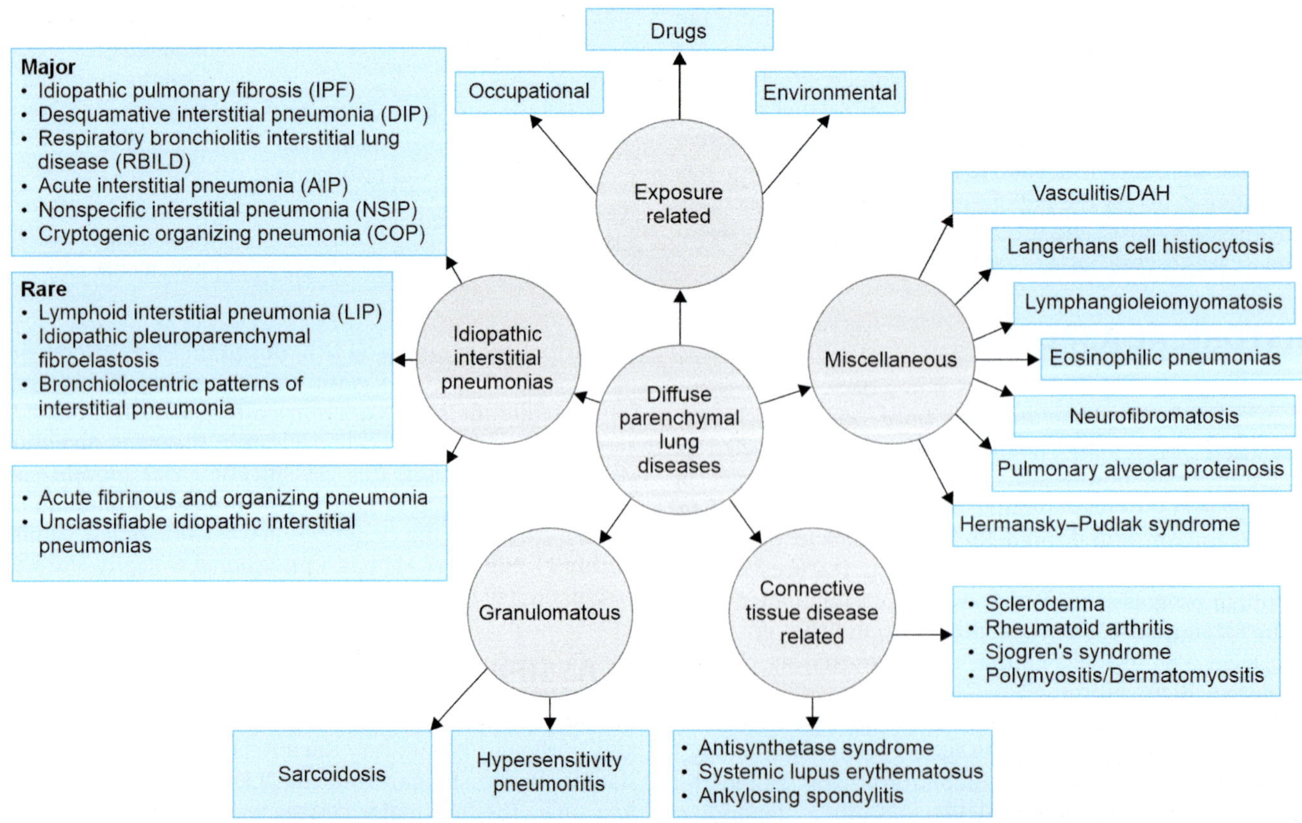

FIG. 1: The American Thoracic Society (ATS)/European Respiratory Society (ERS) 2002 classification of diffuse parenchymal lung diseases (DPLDs) into the four main categories of those with known causes, idiopathic, granulomatous, and other forms.

BOX 1 Current American Thoracic Society/European Respiratory Society (ATS/ERS) classification of interstitial lung disease (ILDs).

- *Major idiopathic interstitial pneumonias*:
  - Idiopathic pulmonary fibrosis
  - Idiopathic nonspecific interstitial pneumonia
  - Respiratory bronchiolitis–interstitial lung disease
  - Desquamative interstitial pneumonia
  - Cryptogenic organizing pneumonia
  - Acute interstitial pneumonia
- *Rare idiopathic interstitial pneumonias*:
  - Idiopathic lymphoid interstitial pneumonia
  - Idiopathic pleuroparenchymal fibroelastosis
- Unclassifiable idiopathic interstitial pneumonias
- Acute fibrinous and organizing pneumonia
- Bronchiolocentric patterns of interstitial pneumonia

TABLE 2: Definition and diagnostic criteria of progressive pulmonary fibrosis (PPF).

Definition	In a patient with ILD of known or unknown etiology other than IPF who has radiological evidence of pulmonary fibrosis, PPF is defined as at least two of the following three criteria occurring within the past year with no alternative explanation
Diagnostic criteria	• Worsening respiratory symptoms • Physiological evidence of disease progression (either of the following): ○ Absolute decline in FVC ≥5% predicted within 1 year of follow-up ○ Absolute decline in DLCO (corrected for Hb) ≥10% predicted within 1 year of follow-up • Radiological evidence of disease progression (one or more of the following): ○ Increased extent or severity of traction bronchiectasis and bronchiolectasis ○ New ground-glass opacity with traction bronchiectasis ○ New fine reticulation ○ Increased extent or increased coarseness of reticular abnormality ○ New or increased honeycombing ○ Increased lobar volume loss

(DLCO: carbon monoxide diffusion capacity; FVC: forced vital capacity; ILD: interstitial lung disease)

and histopathological examination, and this has led to more and more emphasis on multidisciplinary discussion (MDD) among all the stakeholders like pulmonologist, rheumatologist, radiologist, and histopathologist involved in the management in which all the available information is combined and discussed to achieve a diagnosis with "highest confidence".

DIAGNOSIS

The diagnostic approach to ILDs has an initial broad spectrum that subsequently gets narrowed to the suggestive category. In this chapter, the basic approach as well as the distinguishing features of the major ILDs as have been established over the years of research are described.

Clinical History

Personal History

A careful and detailed medical history is an indispensable component of clinical evaluation and accurate diagnosis of ILDs. The majority of ILDs have a protracted course, but the duration of illness can be helpful in identifying ILDs because several of them may have acute and subacute presentation also.

The basic details provide a clue in that IPF is more common in elderly males while connective tissue related ILDs (CTD ILDs) are more common in females.[13] Similarly occupational lung diseases are more commonly described in males.[14,15] The presentation may vary from being symptomatic to incidental finding on radiological investigation. The most common presenting symptom is dry cough or at rest followed in frequency by dyspnea. Other symptoms are not so common and may occur in specific ILDs. Substernal dull chest pain may be felt in sarcoidosis, and wheezing can be present in ILDs involving the airways such as HSP, sarcoidosis, or eosinophilic pneumonias.[15] Diffuse alveolar hemorrhage or vasculitis can present with hemoptysis, and pleuritic chest pain may occur in CTD-associated serositis. Likewise, pneumothorax may be the presenting symptom in cystic ILDs.[15] The duration, progression, and severity should be inquired into as individual ILDs have their own disease course (**Box 2**).

History suggestive of autoimmune disorders is often present in CTD-associated ILDs. Scleroderma patients may give history of gastric reflux, skin tightness and thickening, telangiectasias, Raynaud's phenomenon, or digital pitting; bilateral symmetrical inflammatory deforming polyarthritis may be present in rheumatoid arthritis, malar skin rash may be present in lupus, while rash on extensor aspect (erythema nodosum) may be seen in sarcoidosis. Patients with Sjogren syndrome can provide history of sicca symptoms. An overlap of symptoms may be seen; on the other hand, symptoms like fatigue, malaise, and weakness may be common to all. Detailed inquiry regarding skin rash and other skin symptoms and presence of heliotrope rash, Gottron's papules, or "mechanic's hands" may reveal the diagnosis of dermatomyositis as these features are almost pathognomonic of this disease. Papular eruptions, lupus pernio, and erythema nodosum are sometimes seen in sarcoidosis.[16]

Occupational and Environmental History

A history of exposure to organic or inorganic dust is extremely important, especially in HSP. HSP is one of the

BOX 2 Classification of interstitial lung diseases (ILDs) based on the duration of illness.

- *Acute (days)*:
  - Acute interstitial pneumonia
  - Cryptogenic organizing pneumonia
  - Drug induced ILDs
  - Diffuse alveolar hemorrhage syndromes
  - Eosinophilic lung diseases
  - Acute hypersensitivity pneumonitis
- *Subacute (weeks to months)*:
  - Connective tissue disease-related ILDs
  - Cryptogenic organizing pneumonia
  - Drug induced ILDs
  - Hypersensitivity pneumonitis
- *Chronic (months to years)*:
  - Hypersensitivity pneumonitis
  - Connective tissue disease-related ILDs
  - Idiopathic pulmonary fibrosis
  - Nonspecific interstitial pneumonia
  - Occupation-related lung disease (e.g., silicosis, asbestosis)

potentially treatable forms of ILD which is underdiagnosed because of absence of elicitation of history of appropriate exposure. History of exposure is not available in almost 70% of cases of HSP. Therefore, a detailed history of the patient with special reference to place of residence (urban or rural), occupation, participation in agricultural activities, presence of any industrial establishment in close vicinity, cattle rearing (sheep rearing, poultry farming, exposure to pigeon droppings and feathers), living conditions (dampness in house), etc., should be taken. The official ATS/JRS/ALAT clinical practice guideline for the diagnosis and management of HSP recommends development and validation of questionnaires for evaluation of exposure among these patients according to geographical locale.

Similarly, past and present occupational history is important to assess organic and inorganic exposures if any. Comprehensive details about the kind of exposure at workplace should be elicited like history of construction work, plumbing, and electrical work. Inorganic dust like coal, asbestos, silica, and beryllium and metal exposure are important causes of ILD and should be inquired specifically. Overall, a detailed occupational history and employment in industrial establishments should be taken for the presence of any offending exposure at the workplace. Some of the common occupations and related ILDs are depicted in **Table 3**.

Drugs and Family History

Several pharmacological agents have been described to cause ILDs which can range from acute pneumonitis to chronic fibrosing disease; therefore, a meticulous history of recent and past intake of drugs or radiation therapy should be taken.[17,18] Besides various and chemotherapeutic agents and radiation therapy used in the management of malignancies, nonsteroidal anti-inflammatory drugs (NSAIDs), nitrofurantoin, sulfasalazine, and amiodarone are among the common agents which can cause ILD. The list of drugs causing ILD is exhaustive, but the common drugs associated are listed in **Table 4**.

The majority of ILDs are not familial in origin but approximately 2–20% of IIPs are estimated to be familial in origin. A careful family history may sometimes be positive in patients with IIPs. Certain other ILDs like lymphangioleiomyomatosis (LAM), neurofibromatosis, and Hermansky–Pudlak syndrome are also genetically linked.[19]

Physical Examination

General examination may reveal features of underlying collagen vascular disease such as rash, joint swelling, and/or deformity. Patients with scleroderma may have skin tightening, sclerodactyly, digital pitting/scars and telangiectasia and oral ulcers. Gottron's papules and mechanic's hands indicate polymyositis or dermatomyositis. The presence of neurofibromas, café-au-lait spots, and Lisch nodules along with neurocognitive impairment is a classical finding in neurofibromatosis. Similarly, a combination of albinism and nystagmus may clinch the diagnosis of Hermansky–Pudlak syndrome, and facial angiofibromas, periungual fibromas, and Shagreen patch are typical in tuberous sclerosis.

Respiratory system examination may be at times normal in nonfibrosing ILDs; however, it may reveal fine-end inspiratory crackles usually heard in the basal areas in fibrosing ILDs. The presence of rhonchi or inspiratory squeaks indicate an underlying ILD with bronchiolar involvement like HSP and sarcoidosis. Clubbing is a common finding in IPF. Signs of pulmonary hypertension and right heart failure should be looked for including elevated jugular venous pressure, pedal edema, right ventricular heave, and loud P2.[14,15]

Imaging

Chest Radiograph

Chest X-ray may be the first abnormal investigation that points toward ILD. It has a sensitivity specificity of nearly 80% in detection of ILDs, but CXR can provide a confident diagnosis in only ~23% of cases.[20] It provides a gross approximation of the lung volume status and predominant zone involvement. Most ILDs cause volume loss; however, those associated with concomitant airway involvement or coexistent emphysema, or cystic lung diseases may have preserved lung volumes. ILDs like IPF, chronic HSP, and asbestosis are lower lobe predominant while sarcoidosis, silicosis, acute to subacute HSP, coal

TABLE 3: Common occupations and related interstitial lung diseases.

Occupation	Related ILDs	Offending exposure
• Electrician • Plumber • Pipe fitter • Construction worker • Ship builder	Asbestosis	Asbestos
• Stone cutters • Miners • Sand blasters	Silicosis	Crystalline silica dust
Metal grinder	• Giant cell interstitial pneumonia • Hard metal lung disease	Hard metals, cobalt, tungsten carbide
Metal worker	Berylliosis	Beryllium
Factory workers	• Stannosis • Hard metal lung disease • Antimoniosis • Siderosis • Alveolar proteinosis • Aluminosis • Metal fume fever • Metalworking fluid lung	• Tin oxide • Cobalt • Antimony • Iron oxide • Aluminum • Copper • Aerosolized metalworking fluid (*Mycobacteroides immunogenum, Pseudomonas* species)
Coal worker	Coal worker's pneumoconiosis	Coal dust
• Paint sprayer • Plastic worker	Chemical worker's lung	Isocyanates
• Farm worker • Mushroom farmer	• Farmer's lung • Mushroom worker's lung	• Moldy hay, silage, grain (*Thermophilic actinomycetes*) • Mushroom compost (*Thermoactinomyces sacchari*)
Office worker	Humidifier lung	Contaminated forced air systems (*Vulgaris, T. sacchari, Thermoactinomyces candidus*)
Lifeguards	Hot tub lung	Contaminated hot tubs (*Mycobacterium avian* complex species)
Trumpet players	Wind instrument lung	Contaminated trombone, bagpipe, saxophone (*Fusarium* species, *Penicillium* species, *Mycobacteroides chelonae, Candida* species, *Cryptococcus* species)
Woodworkers	Woodworker's lung	Moldy oak, cedar, mahogany (*Alternaria* species wood dusts)
Aviculturists	Pigeon breeder's lung	Pigeon droppings
	Bird fancier's lung	Avian droppings, feathers, serum parakeets, budgerigars, love birds, cockatiels, chickens

worker's pneumoconiosis, and pulmonary Langerhans cell histiocytosis (LCH) are upper lobe predominant. Likewise peripheral involvement is characteristic of IPF and chronic eosinophilic pneumonitis. Sequential chest radiographs may provide evidence of migratory opacities as may be seen in cryptogenic organizing pneumonia (COP) or HSP **(Table 5)**. Mediastinal or hilar enlargement can be seen in sarcoidosis, silicosis, or berylliosis.

Radiological findings may vary from linear reticulations to reticulonodular shadows. Sometimes, cystic shadows forming a honeycomb pattern may be apparent.[21]

Computed Tomography

High-resolution tomography of the chest plays a pivotal role in establishing the diagnosis of ILDs even allowing clinicoradiological diagnosis in select situations. Based on computed tomography (CT), ILDs can be broadly categorized as fibrotic and nonfibrotic types. The classic findings of fibrosis include traction bronchiectasis, honeycombing, and reticulations. The specific spatial distribution of these findings leads to recognizable patterns such as UIP or NSIP. Important patterns are described as in the following text.

TABLE 4: Therapeutic agents causing interstitial lung disease.

Group	Drug
Chemotherapeutic agents	• Azathioprine • Bleomycin • Busulfan • Chlorambucil • Melphalan • Mitomycin C • Nitrosoureas • Procarbazine • Vinblastine • Methotrexate • Procarbazine
Immunomodulatory drugs	• Pembrolizumab • Nivolumab, Ipilimumab
Monoclonal antibodies and TKIs	• Bevacizumab • Cetuximab • Trastuzumab • Rituximab • Gefitinib, erlotinib, imatinib, ceritinib
Antibiotics	• Nitrofurantoin • Minocycline, cephalosporins • Isoniazid
Antiarrhythmics	• Amiodarone • Angiotensin-converting enzyme inhibitors • β-blockers • Dipyridamole • Flecainide, tocainide
NSAIDs	• Salicylates • Sulfasalazine • Dextropropoxyphene
Recreational agents	• Heroin • Methadone • Methylphenidate • Cocaine
Miscellaneous	• Aspirated oil • Oxygen • Anorexigens • Dantrolene • Methysergide • Radiation • Tocolytic agents • Tricyclic antidepressants • L-tryptophan

(NSAIDs: nonsteroidal anti-inflammatory drugs)

TABLE 5: Diagnostic considerations based on a chest radiograph.

Low lung volumes	IPF; CTD-related ILD; chronic HP; asbestosis; chronic drug-induced fibrosis; chronic COP, CEP, or DIP
Preserved lung volumes	RB-ILD, CPFE, LCH, LAM, sarcoidosis, tuberous sclerosis, neurofibromatosis, bronchiolitis
Upper zone predominance	Sarcoidosis, silicosis, CWP, HP, LCH, berylliosis, CEP, Caplan syndrome, RA
Lower zone predominance	IPF, CTD-associated ILD, asbestosis, DIP, chronic HP
Peripheral predominance	IPF, COP, CEP
Mediastinal/hilar adenopathy	Sarcoidosis, malignancy, silicosis, berylliosis, CTD-associated ILD

(CEP: chronic eosinophilic pneumonia; COP: cryptogenic organizing pneumonia; CPFE: combined pulmonary fibrosis and emphysema; CTD: connective tissue disease; CWP: coal worker's pneumoconiosis; DIP: desquamative interstitial pneumonia; HP: hypersensitivity pneumonitis; IPF: idiopathic pulmonary fibrosis; LAM: lymphangioleiomyomatosis; LCH: Langerhans' cell histiocytosis; RA: rheumatoid arthritis; RBILD: respiratory bronchiolitis ILD)

Usual Interstitial Pneumonia

The UIP pattern is characterized by heterogeneous parenchymal involvement in basal subpleural predominance of honeycombing and reticulations along with traction bronchiectasis/bronchiolectasis **(Figs. 2 and 3)**. It was previously subclassified as UIP, possible UIP, probable UIP, and non-UIP in this order based on the deviation from the usual pattern.[19] It was later modified as UIP **(Figs. 4A and B)**, probable UIP, and indeterminate for UIP and alternative diagnosis **(Table 6)**.[10,22] The UIP pattern is seen in IPF, rheumatoid arthritis (RA)-ILD, and advanced HSP although the distribution of the findings may vary.

Nonspecific Interstitial Pneumonia

Predominant ground glassing with basal peripheral predominance with reticulations is seen in NSIP **(Figs. 5A and B)**. The classic finding of subpleural sparing is seen only in about 20–30%. The fibrotic variant of NSIP can demonstrate honeycombing and traction bronchiectasis although not as extensive as UIP and often associated with ground-glass opacities (GGOs) **(Figs. 6A and B)**.[23]

Respiratory Bronchiolitis–ILD/Desquamative Interstitial Pneumonia

Main high-resolution CT (HRCT) features of respiratory bronchiolitis–ILD (RBILD) **(Fig. 7)** are GGOs, poorly defined centrilobular nodules aka centrilobular ground-glass nodules, diffuse lung distribution, centrilobular emphysema, and/or bronchial wall thickening. Although both RBILD and DIP are exclusively described as smoking-associated ILDs, they may not necessarily represent a

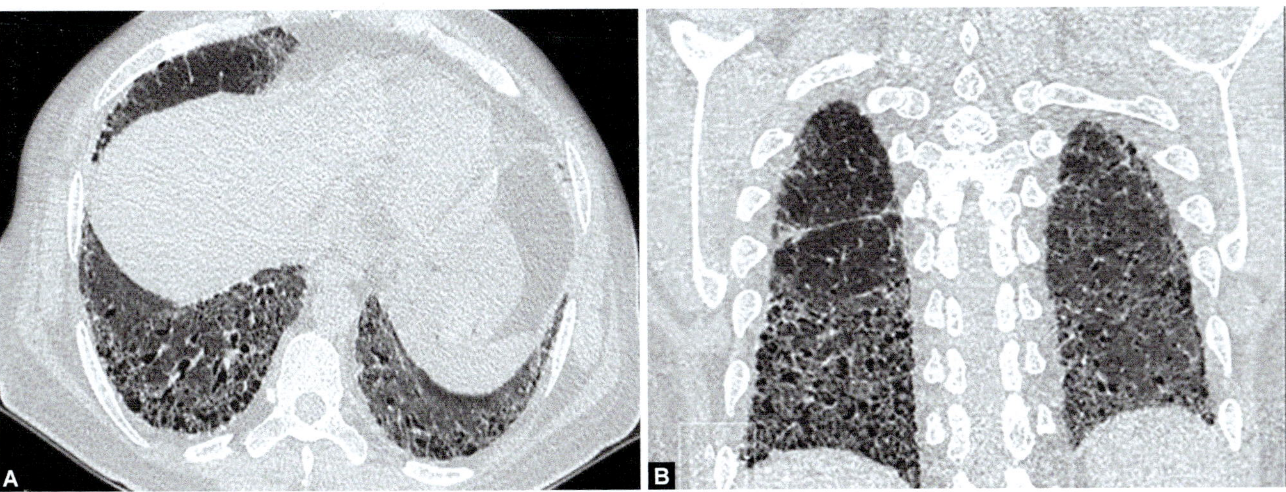

FIGS. 2A AND B: Usual interstitial pneumonia. (A) Axial high-resolution computed tomography (HRCT) image showing reticular thickening and tractional bronchiectasis with honeycombing; (B) Coronal reconstruction showing a marked apicobasal gradient.

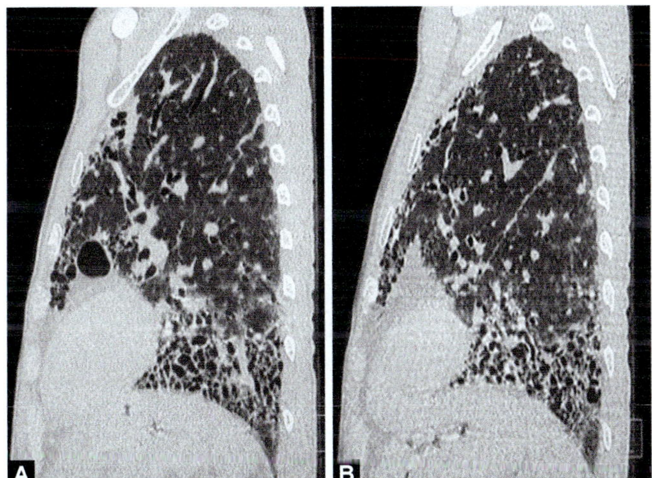

FIGS. 3A AND B: Usual interstitial pneumonia. Propeller blade distribution of abnormality involving anterior portion of upper lobes and posterior portion of lower lobes.

spectrum of the same disease. DIP is characterized by more extensive involvement with some pathognomonic features like diffuse GGOs, thickening of alveolar septa: bilateral and symmetric (86%), basal and peripheral (60%), patchy (20%) and diffuse (20%), irregular linear opacities and microcysts (50% of patients) **(Figs. 8A and B)**.[7,8]

Cryptogenic Organizing Pneumonia

Cryptogenic organizing pneumonia is one of the ILDs with a good prognosis and excellent response to glucocorticoids. HRCT may show peripheral or peribronchial patchy consolidations (sometimes with subpleural area spread), lower lobe preponderance, with air bronchograms and mild cylindrical bronchial dilatation.[7,8] GGOs with a tendency to migration and rarely a mass or nodule with central hypodensity, typically described as an "atoll sign", are some of characteristic lesions on HRCT **(Fig. 9)**.

Acute Interstitial Pneumonia

Acute interstitial pneumonia occurs in all age groups with a mean age of approximately 50 years, and there is no sex predominance nor is it associated with smoking. HRCT shows diffuse GGO with a mosaic pattern which is usually bibasilar but can be diffuse and can involve upper lobes also **(Fig. 10)**. Presence of consolidation with lung architectural distortion, traction bronchiectasis, and cysts has also been described.[7,8] Survivors show areas of hypoattenuation, lung cysts, reticular abnormality, and architectural distortion on follow-up HRCT.

Lymphoid Interstitial Pneumonia

Mostly described in association with diseases such as Sjögren syndrome, AIDS (particularly children), immunodeficiency syndromes, and autoimmune thyroid disease, LIP is characterized by uniform or patchy areas of bilateral GGO are typically characterized by uniform or patchy areas of bilateral GGO (>80%) however, a few, perivascular, thin-walled cysts are also seen on HRCT thorax **(Fig. 11)**. These cysts measure 1–30 mm and are seen predominantly in the mid-lung zones, adjacent to blood vessels. Centrilobular and subpleural nodules with thickening of the interlobular septa are also typical.[7,8] Perivascular honeycombing in areas of previous airspace abnormality and reticular pattern (>50%) is seen.

Other Rare Radiological Patterns

Pleuropulmonary elastosis is one of the rare radiological patterns in which there is pleural thickening in the upper zones, which is sometimes also associated with signs of fibrosis, such as traction bronchiectasis. Subpleural consolidations and/or reticulations in upper and middle

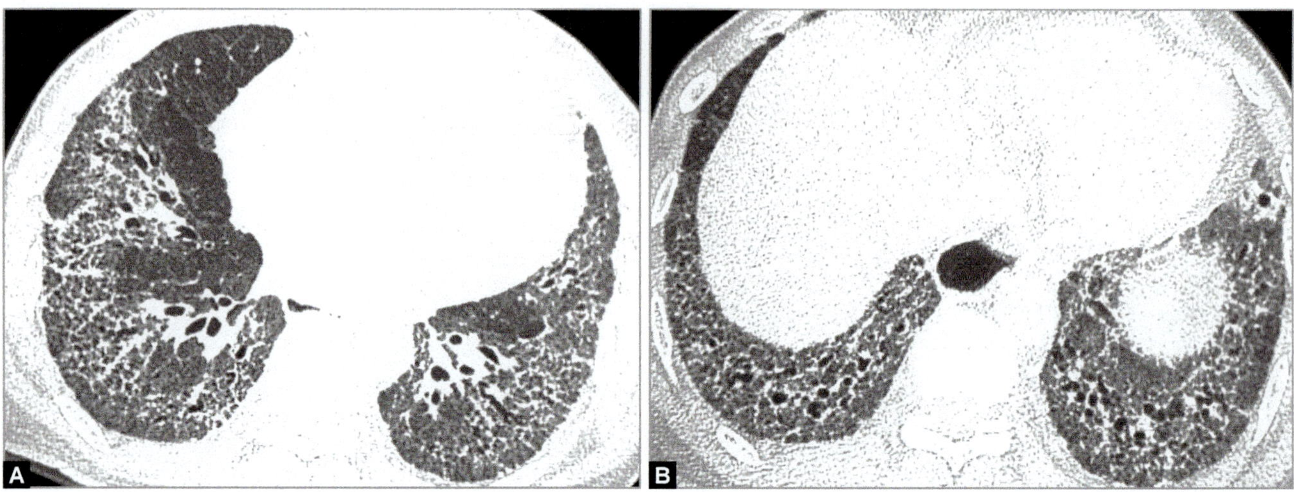

FIGS. 4A AND B: Probable usual interstitial pneumonia. Reticular thickening involving both lungs more in the subpleural region. No honeycombing could be appreciated.

TABLE 6: Radiologic patterns on high resolution computerized tomography.

UIP	Probable UIP	Indeterminate for UIP	Alternative diagnosis
• Subpleural and basal predominant; distribution is often heterogeneous • Honeycombing with or without peripheral traction bronchiectasis or bronchiolectasis	• Subpleural and basal predominant; distribution is often heterogeneous • Reticular pattern with peripheral traction bronchiectasis or bronchiolectasis • May have mild GGO	• Subpleural and basal predominant • Subtle reticulation; may have mild GGO or distortion (early UIP pattern) • CT features and/or distribution of lung fibrosis that do not suggest any specific etiology (truly indeterminate)	Findings suggestive of another diagnosis, including: *CT features*: • Cysts • Marked mosaic attenuation • Predominant GGO • Profuse micronodules • Centrilobular nodules • Nodules • Consolidation *Predominant distribution*: • Peribronchovascular • Perilymphatic • Upper or mid-lung *Others*: • Pleural effusion • Dilated esophagus • Distal clavicular erosions • Extensive lymphadenopathy • Pleural effusions, pleural thickening (consider CTD/drugs)

(CTD: connective tissue disorder; GGO: ground-glass opacity; UIP: usual interstitial pneumonia)

zones can also be seen. Pleural irregularities could extend to the interlobar fissures leading to chronic fibrosis and further leading to volume loss. Acute fibrinous and organizing pneumonia is another uncommon pattern which has been described in the last ATS/ERS classification of ILDs. The principal HRCT findings are bilateral basal opacities and areas of consolidation closely mimicking AIP, but typical hyaline membranes are absent on histology and the dominant histologic pattern is intra-alveolar fibrin deposition and associated organizing pneumonia. It may be idiopathic or associated with cardiovascular disease (CVD), HSP, or drug reaction. As this pattern can be seen in eosinophilic pneumonia, this diagnosis should be excluded by absence of tissue and peripheral eosinophilia.[8]

It becomes imperative to follow this "pattern-based approach" in clinical practice because this is the steering

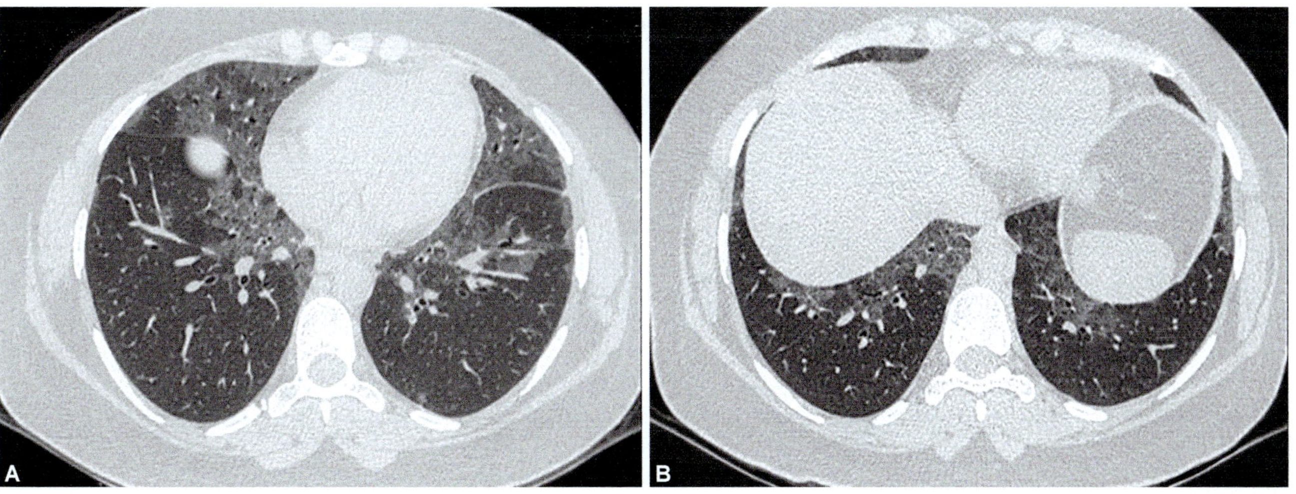

FIGS. 5A AND B: Cellular nonspecific interstitial pneumonia. (A) Ground-glass opacity involving subpleural region more in lower lobes; (B) Similar findings at a lower level.

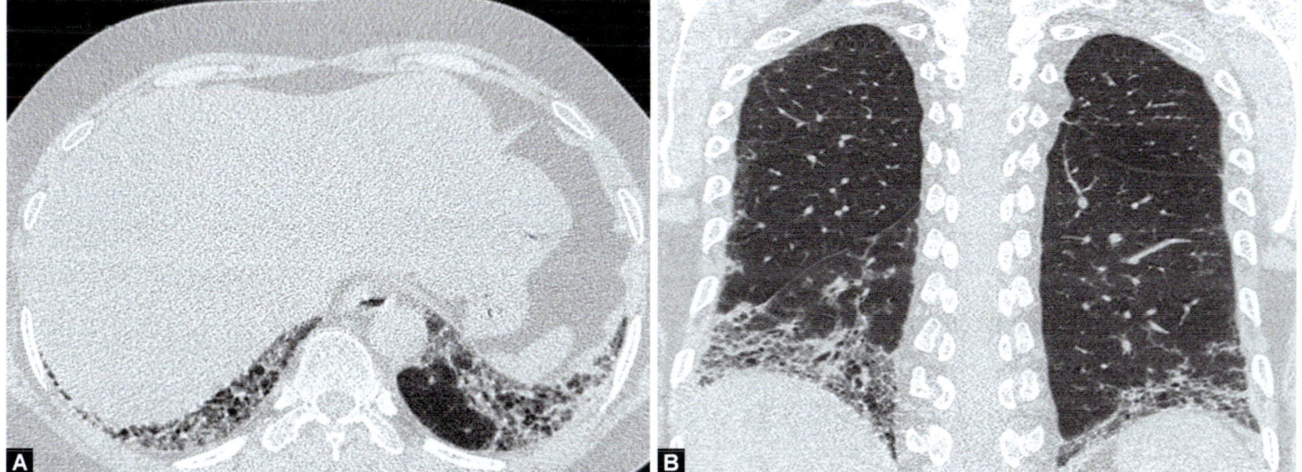

FIGS. 6A AND B: Fibrotic nonspecific interstitial pneumonia. (A) Reticular thickening with tractional bronchiectasis involving both lungs. Subpleural sparing is also appreciated. (B) Similar findings at a lower level with dilated esophagus.

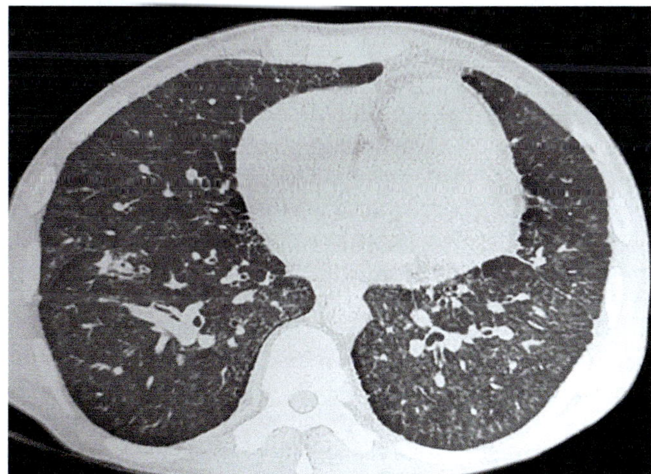

FIG. 7: Respiratory bronchiolitis-associated ILD. Ill-defined centrilobular, nodules with diffuse lung distribution, centrilobular emphysema, and/or bronchial wall thickening.

step in clinical evaluation of ILD. Once the clinician has made a confirmed diagnosis or reasonably excluded UIP pattern, the next step is to distinguish these imaging patterns from other described patterns and that helps in substantially narrowing the differential diagnosis and helps in planning further serological or sometimes histopathological examination to make the final diagnosis and also in differentiating between other causes of a UIP pattern (e.g., CTD-ILD, fibrotic HSP). Some radiological appearances have been linked to specific etiologies like the "three-density sign" previously described as "headcheese sign"; that is, juxtaposition of lobular regions of low, normal, and high attenuation indicative of a mixed infiltrative and obstructive process suggests HSP **(Figs. 12A and B)**.[24]

Recently, some important radiological signs have been described which suggest an underlying CTD as a potential etiology such as a dilated fluid- or air-filled esophagus, presence of exuberant honeycombing **(Fig. 13)**, i.e., honey-

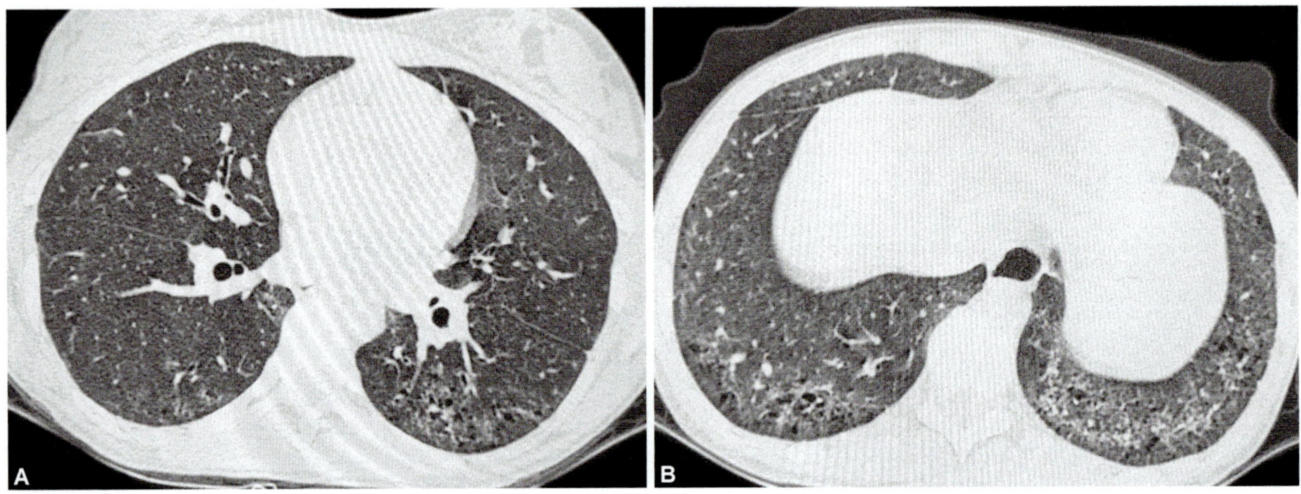

FIGS. 8A AND B: Desquamating interstitial pneumonia. Subtle reticular thickening with small cysts. Also see dilated esophagus; the patient has mixed connective tissue disorder.

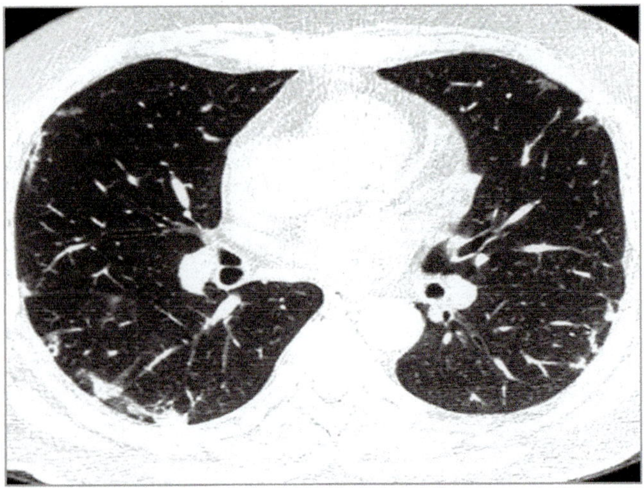

FIG. 9: Organizing pneumonia. Multiple peripheral small areas of consolidation.

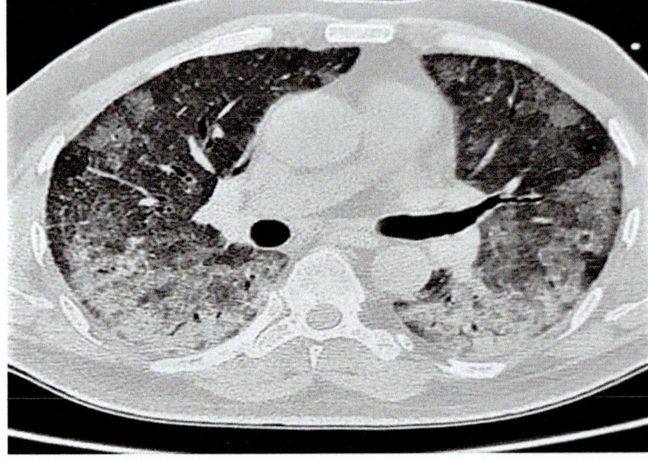

FIG. 10: Diffuse ground-glass opacities with a mosaic pattern and patchy consolidation without any lobar predilection. Architectural distortion, traction bronchiectasis, and cysts may also be seen.

combing that is disproportionately severe compared with other features of fibrosis, fibrosis in the anterior upper lobes of the lung "anterior upper lobe sign", and isolation of fibrosis in the lung bases with a sharp demarcation of normal and abnormal lung parenchyma or the "straight-edge sign".[25] "Atoll sign" or "reverse halo sign" characterized by central GGO surrounded by denser consolidation in the shape of a crescent or ring suggests COP, and "galaxy sign" which is the presence of a mass-like lesion composed of coalescing granulomatous nodules more concentrated in the center than at the periphery is a feature of sarcoidosis.

Laboratory Investigations

A battery of investigations is needed to evaluate any patient with ILD and like any other disease, blood counts along with baseline liver and renal function tests and electrolyte studies are warranted in ILDs as well and may give an information about an underlying disease or comorbidity; for example, an elevated eosinophil count may point toward eosinophilic lung disease, elevated gamma globulin fraction of serum protein might give a clue toward underlying autoimmune illness, and elevated serum or urine calcium is a marker for underlying sarcoidosis or other granulomatous pathologies. A complete urine analysis should be obtained in all cases, while specific investigation such as albumin-to-creatinine ratio or 24-hour urinary protein measurement is required when indicated.[26-29]

Once a pattern is identified on HRCT and a definite UIP pattern is excluded, a detailed serological workup is needed in almost all patients with ILD **(Table 7)**. Although there are no guidelines for serological screening for patients with ILD, most of pulmonologists now recognize that all patients of undiagnosed ILD should be subjected to a panel of serological parameters as listed in **Table 7**. It is suggested that the advanced panel that includes myositis-specific and myositis-associated antibodies, etc., should be sent if basic extractable nuclear antigen (ENA) screen is negative or there is a clinical or radiological clue and the clinical suspicion is high. Presence of clinical features suggestive of underlying CTD may not be present at the time of diagnosis of ILD, and it now almost an established fact that ILD may be a presenting feature in various CTDs and as a result of this ambiguity in diagnosis and evaluation of ILD, the ERS/ATS task force suggested the nomenclature of interstitial pneumonia with autoimmune features (IPAF) for patients with undifferentiated forms of CTD-associated ILD in 2015. These patients do not completely fulfil the criteria for a particular CTD but can have clinical, radiological, serological, or histopathological features to suggest an underlying CTD. The criteria for classification and diagnosis of IPAF are listed in **Table 8**.

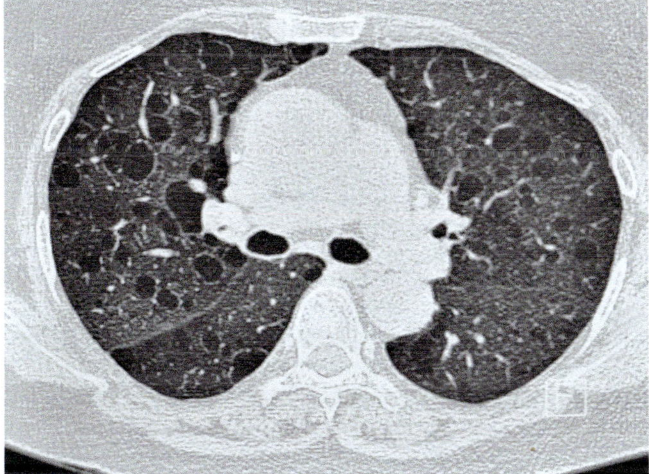

FIG. 11: Lymphoid interstitial pneumonia. Images at the level of the midthorax show multiple scattered cysts of variable sizes throughout the lungs with surrounding ground-glass opacities and interstitial thickening.

Pulmonary Function Tests

The assessment of lung function is done via spirometry that usually demonstrates a restrictive pattern but may show mixed patterns in airway-centric ILDs like sarcoidosis and HSP. Some patients may also demonstrate an obstructive pattern if they have a concomitant obstructive airway disease. Lung volumes are typically decreased but they may be preserved in patients with Langerhans cell histiocytosis, LAM, combined pulmonary fibrosis with emphysema (CPFE), or coexistent COPD.

The diffusion capacity [diffusing capacity of the lungs for carbon monoxide (DLCO)] is reduced and impaired even before the restriction is evident on spirometry. A scoring system called the "GAP index" has been devised and is used for monitoring patients with IPF which estimates mortality in years, based on patient gender, age, and degree of physiologic impairment using forced vital capacity (FVC) and DLCO.[30]

Sequential spirometry assessment is useful in assessing the functional course of the disease. Oximetry and arterial blood gas analysis is important to assess hypoxemia. Exercise capacity assessment tools such as 6-minute walk test (6MWT) or shuttle walk test (SWT) are useful tools in monitoring response to therapy in patients with ILD and should be done in all the patients periodically along with spirometry and DLCO.[31-34]

Bronchoalveolar Lavage

Bronchoalveolar lavage studies have a limited role in the diagnosis of ILDs and are useful only in corroboration with

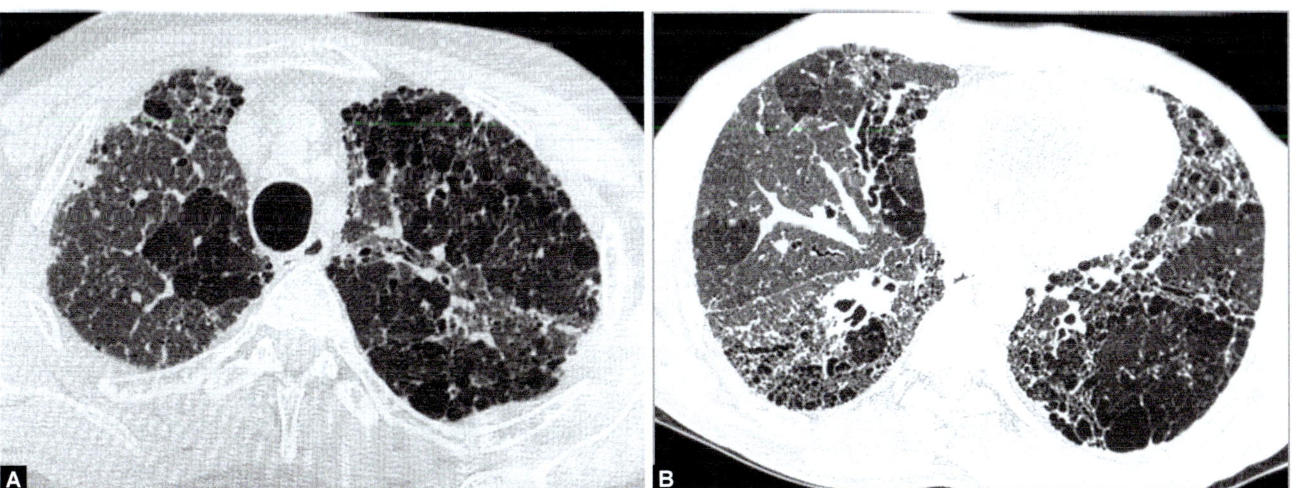

FIGS. 12A AND B: Chronic hypersensitivity pneumonitis. Reticular thickening and tractional bronchiectasis with honeycombing in both lungs. Multiple areas of mosaic attenuation with normal, low, and high attenuation area—"the three-density sign".

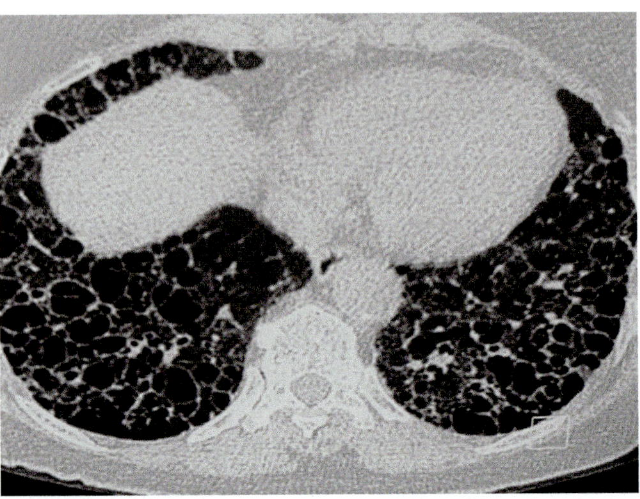

FIG. 13: Exuberant honeycombing. Diffuse honeycomb cysts constitute nearly all of the fibrotic regions of the lungs on this cross-section.

TABLE 7: Autoantibodies in evaluation of interstitial lung disease (ILD).

Autoantibody	Associated disease
Antinuclear antibody (ANA)	Systemic lupus erythematosus (SLE), scleroderma, mixed connective tissue disease (MCTD)
SSA/Anti-Ro/Anti-La	Sjögren syndrome, inflammatory myopathies
• Scl-70 • Anticentromere antibody	Scleroderma
• PM/Scl 75 (polymyositis, scleroderma) • PM/Scl 100	Myositis and scleroderma overlap
• RF (rheumatoid factor) • Anti-CCP (anti-cyclic citrullinated peptide)	Rheumatoid arthritis
• RNP (ribonucleoprotein) • Antihistone antibody	MCTD
• Antineutrophilic cytoplasmic antibodies (p-ANCA, c-ANCA) • Myeloperoxidase antibody (MPO) • Proteinase 3 antibody (PR-3)	ANCA-associated vasculitis
• *Myositis-specific antibodies*: Jo-1, PL-7, PL-12, EJ, OJ, KS, MDA-5 • *Myositis-associated antibodies*: PM-Scl, Ro-52, Ku	• Inflammatory myopathies: Polymyositis • Dermatomyositis • Antisynthetase syndrome

other findings although in some conditions like diffuse alveolar hemorrhage, asbestos, or silica-related lung disease and pulmonary alveolar proteinosis, it may be diagnostic also. Differential cytology on BAL may be useful in narrowing the differential diagnosis of certain ILDs like eosinophilic pneumonias (eosinophil count > 25%), HSP, and sarcoidosis. A lymphocytic predominant BAL (lymphocyte > 25%) may also be an indication for a favorable response to glucocorticoid therapy in a given clinical setting. A predominant lymphocytic BAL may also suggest granulomatous diseases, NSIP, drug-induced ILD, LIP, or lymphoma. BAL is typically neutrophilic in IPF, diffuse alveolar damage, and AIP. In a lymphocyte-predominant BAL, flow cytometry may be used to study lymphocyte subsets and a CD4:CD8 ratio of >3.5 may increase confidence for the diagnosis of sarcoidosis. It may also be employed in ruling out infections in patients with ILD if there is suspicion of active infection prior to starting immunosuppression or evaluating for infective causes of ILD like viral pneumonias and pneumocystis pneumonia (PCP).[35-38]

Tissue Diagnosis

Lung biopsy is the final diagnostic modality for accurate diagnosis of ILD. TBLB may be obtained in airway-centric diseases like HSP and sarcoidosis, but the diagnostic yield of TBLB is quite low in characterization of ILD; therefore, SLB is the preferred modality for most of the IIPs.[39] The most commonly employed technique is video-assisted thoracoscopic surgery (VATS). The common postprocedure complications after SLB include pain at the local site, persistent air leak, bleeding, and infection. The risk–benefit ratio should be assessed prior to subjecting a patient to lung biopsy, especially in an elderly patient and in comorbid conditions; its significance lies in guiding management and in prognostication. The mortality rates and exacerbation of disease after SLB are quite high and moreover many patients are not fit for a surgical biopsy under general anesthesia.

Transbronchial cryobiopsy (TBLC) is a reasonably good approach for diagnosis of ILD because it can provide larger and better-preserved tissue samples compared with those obtained using traditional biopsy forceps. TBLC is a bronchoscopic biopsy technique in which a flexible catheter with blunt metal is advanced into the lung in the same manner as TBLB and a compressed gas, like carbon dioxide or nitrous oxide, is released at high flow at the tip of the probe causing rapid gas expansion and cooling of the tip of the probe to −79°C when using carbon dioxide or −89°C when using nitrous oxide which leads the surrounding tissue to freeze adhere to the probe which is extracted by quickly pulling back the probe. It can be done by flexible bronchoscopy with bronchial blocker or by rigid bronchoscopy under sedation. Cryobiopsy appears to have a lower rate of mortality and acute exacerbation compared with SLB but

TABLE 8: Criteria for classification of interstitial pneumonia with autoimmune features.

Diagnostic criteria: • Presence of an interstitial pneumonia (by HRCT or surgical lung biopsy) + • Exclusion of alternative etiologies + • Not satisfying criteria of a defined connective tissue disease + • At least one feature from at least two of following domains:		

Clinical domain:
• Distal digital fissuring (i.e., "mechanic hands")
• Distal digital tip ulceration
• Inflammatory arthritis or polyarticular morning joint stiffness ≥ 60 minutes
• Palmar telangiectasia
• Raynaud's phenomenon
• Unexplained digital edema
• Unexplained fixed rash on the digital extensor surfaces (Gottron's sign)
	Serologic domain:
	• ANA ≥ 1:320 titer, diffuse, speckled, homogeneous patterns or
	  ○ ANA nucleolar pattern (any titer) *or*
	  ○ ANA centromere pattern (any titer)
	• Rheumatoid factor ≥ 2× upper limit of normal
	• Anti-CCP
	• Anti-dsDNA
	• Anti-Ro (SS-A)
	• Anti-La (SS-B)
	• Anti-ribonucleoprotein
	• Anti-Smith
	• Anti-topoisomerase (Scl-70)
	• Anti-tRNA synthetase (e.g., Jo-1, PL-7, PL-12; EJ, OJ, KS, Zo)
	• Anti-PM-Scl 12, anti-MDA-5
		Morphologic domain:
		• Suggestive radiology patterns on HRCT:
		  ○ NSIP
		  ○ OP
		  ○ NSIP with OP overlap
		  ○ LIP
		• Histopathology patterns or features by surgical lung biopsy:
		  ○ NSIP
		  ○ OP
		  ○ NSIP with OP overlap
		  ○ LIP
		  ○ Interstitial lymphoid aggregates with germinal centers
		  ○ Diffuse lymphoplasmacytic infiltration (with or without lymphoid follicles)
		• Multicompartment involvement (in addition to interstitial pneumonia):
		  ○ Unexplained pleural effusion or thickening
		  ○ Unexplained pericardial effusion or thickening
		  ○ Unexplained intrinsic airways disease
		  ○ Unexplained pulmonary vasculopathy

(ANA: antinuclear antibody; HRCT: high-resolution computed tomography; NSIP: nonspecific interstitial pneumonia; OP: organizing pneumonia)

has a substantially high risk of pneumothorax.[40] It is associated with lesser complications and therefore shorter duration of hospital stay as compared to the SLB.

Multidisciplinary Discussion

Due to diverse clinical presentation and radiologic and histopathologic appearance, it is often not possible to characterize the type of ILD one is dealing with. Therefore, a MDD has become an integral part of evaluation of ILD.[11] MDD is nothing but to put together all the evidence and a detailed discussion among the pulmonologist, rheumatologist, radiologist, and histopathologist. The process of making the diagnosis of ILD is dynamic requiring close communication between the stakeholders. It does not imply that histologic diagnosis will lose its importance in this approach, but it implies on what occasions a biopsy is needed and when associated complications can be avoided.[35,36] This approach has now become the gold standard for the evaluation of ILDs. At primary or secondary healthcare settings wherein a diagnostic ambiguity is encountered and MDD is not feasible, a timely referral to a tertiary care center should be considered because it gives an opportunity for optimal diagnostic evaluation and access to standard treatment options including enrollment in lung transplant programs. Telehealth programs can play a very important role in providing MDD at remote places where all the facilities are not available.

FUTURE DIRECTIONS

The classification of ILD is ever evolving because of fast development in its etiology, morphology, and disease behavior. There is tremendous magnitude of research going on to identify biomarkers for diagnosis and prediction of disease behavior of various ILD subtypes. Insights into molecular biology based on genomic, epigenomic, and proteomic data may provide better understanding about the mechanisms involved in the disease process and also identify potential therapeutic targets.

SUMMARY

The approach to an ILD patient begins with a detailed clinical history and thorough physical examination. The radiological studies help to distinguish fibrosing from nonfibrosing ILDs and the pattern on the HRCT thorax may even be diagnostic. Laboratory studies provide supplementary clues while the autoimmune serological workup may again be diagnostic. If the etiology is still unclear, lung biopsy may be done if feasible. A MDD among experts is warranted to reach the final diagnosis.

REFERENCES

1. Buhl L. Lungenentzündung, Tuberkulose und Schwindsucht: zwölf Briefe an einen Freund. Oldenbourg; 1873.
2. Wolters PJ, Blackwell TS, Eickelberg O, et al. Time for a change: is idiopathic pulmonary fibrosis still idiopathic and only fibrotic? Lancet Respir Med. 2018;6(2):154-60.
3. Hamman L, Rich AR. Fulminating diffuse interstitial fibrosis of the lungs. Trans Am Clin Climatol Assoc. 1935;51:154.
4. Liebow AA. Definition and classification of interstitial pneumonias in human pathology. Prog Respir Res. 1975;8:1-31.
5. Müller NL, Coiby TV. Idiopathic interstitial pneumonias: high-resolution CT and histologic findings. Radiographics. 1997; 17(4):1016-22.
6. Katzenstein AL, Myers JL. Idiopathic pulmonary fibrosis: clinical relevance of pathologic classification. Am J Resp Crit Care Med. 1998;157(4):1301-15.
7. Travis WD, King TE, Bateman ED, et al. American Thoracic Society/European Respiratory Society international multidisciplinary consensus classification of the idiopathic interstitial pneumonias. Am J Respir Crit Care Med. 2002;165(2):277-304.
8. Travis WD, Costabel U, Hansell DM, et al. An official American Thoracic Society/European Respiratory Society statement: update of the international multidisciplinary classification of the idiopathic interstitial pneumonias. Am J Respir Crit Care Med. 2013;188(6):733-48.
9. Cottin V, Hirani NA, Hotchkin DL, et al. Presentation, diagnosis and clinical course of the spectrum of progressive-fibrosing interstitial lung diseases. Eur Respir Rev. 2018;27(150):180076.
10. Raghu G, Remy-Jardin M, Richeldi L, et al. Idiopathic Pulmonary Fibrosis (an Update) and Progressive Pulmonary Fibrosis in Adults: An Official ATS/ERS/JRS/ALAT Clinical Practice Guideline. Am J Respir Crit Care Med. 2022;205(9):e18-e47.
11. Flaherty KR, Well AU, Cottin V, et al. Nintedanib in progressive fibrosing interstitial lung diseases. N Engl J Med. 2019;381: 1718-27.
12. Behr J, Prasse A, Kreuter M, et al. Pirfenidone in patients with progressive fibrotic interstitial lung diseases other than idiopathic pulmonary fibrosis (RELIEF): a double-blind, randomised, placebo-controlled, phase 2b trial. Lancet Respir Med. 2021;9:476-86.
13. Han MK, Murray S, Fell CD, et al. Sex differences in physiological progression of idiopathic pulmonary fibrosis. Eur Respir J. 2008;31(6):1183-8.
14. Han MK, Arteaga-Solis E, Blenis J, et al. Female sex and gender in lung/sleep health and disease. Increased understanding of basic biological, pathophysiological, and behavioral mechanisms leading to better health for female patients with lung disease. Am J Respir Crit Care Med. 2018;198(7):850-8.
15. Schwarz MI. Approach to the evaluation and diagnosis of interstitial lung disease. In: Schwarz MI, King TE (Eds). Interstitial Lung Disease, 4th edition. London: BC Decker Inc; 2003. pp. 1-30.
16. Omote N, Taniguchi H, Kondoh Y, et al. Lung-dominant connective tissue disease: clinical, radiologic, and histologic features. Chest. 2015;148(6):1438-46.
17. Rake C, Gilham C, Hatch J, et al. Occupational, domestic and environmental mesothelioma risks in the British population: a case-control study. Br J Cancer. 2009;100(7):1175-83.
18. Camus P, Kudoh S, Ebina M. Interstitial lung disease associated with drug therapy. Br J Cancer. 2004;91(Suppl 2):S18-S23.
19. Devine MS, Garcia CK. Genetic interstitial lung disease. Clin Chest Med. 2012;33(1):95-110.
20. Afzal F, Raza S, Shafique M. Diagnostic accuracy of X-ray chest in interstitial lung disease as confirmed by high resolution computed tomography (HRCT) chest. Pak Armed Forces Med J. 2017;67:593-8.
21. Walsh SL, Devaraj A, Enghelmayer JI, et al. Role of imaging in progressive-fibrosing interstitial lung diseases. Eur Respir Rev. 2018;27(150):180073.
22. Raghu G, Collard HR, Egan JJ, et al. An official ATS/ERS/JRS/ALAT statement: idiopathic pulmonary fibrosis: evidence-based guidelines for diagnosis and management. Am J Respir Crit Care Med. 2011;183(6):788-824.
23. Silva CI, Müller NL, Hansell DM, et al. Nonspecific interstitial pneumonia and idiopathic pulmonary fibrosis: changes in pattern and distribution of disease over time. Radiology. 2008;247(1):251-9.
24. Magee AL, Montner SM, Husain A, et al. Imaging of hypersensitivity pneumonitis. Radiol Clin North Am. 2016;54(6): 1033-46.
25. Chung JH, Cox CW, Montner SM, et al. CT features of the usual interstitial pneumonia pattern: differentiating connective tissue disease–associated interstitial lung disease from idiopathic pulmonary fibrosis. Am J Roentgenol. 2018;210(2):307-13.
26. Adegunsoye A, Ryerson CJ. Diagnostic Classification of Interstitial Lung Difrome in Clinical Practice. Clin Chest Med. 2021;42(2):251-61.
27. Seaman DM, Meyer CA, Gilman MD, et al. Diffuse cystic lung disease at high-resolution CT. Am J Roentgenol. 2011;196(6): 1305-11.
28. Criado E, Sánchez M, Ramírez J, et al. Pulmonary sarcoidosis: typical and atypical manifestations at high-resolution CT with pathologic correlation. Radiographics. 2010;30(6):1567-86.
29. Behr J. Approach to the diagnosis of interstitial lung disease. Clin Chest Med. 2012;33(1):1-10
30. Ley B, Ryerson CJ, Vittinghoff E, et al. A multidimensional index and staging system for idiopathic pulmonary fibrosis. Ann Intern Med. 2012;156(10):684-91.
31. Martinez FJ, Flaherty K. Pulmonary function testing in idiopathic interstitial pneumonias. Proc Am Thorac Soc. 2006;3(4):315-21.
32. Hegewald MJ. Diffusing capacity. Clin Rev Allergy Immunol. 2009;37(3):159-66.

33. Lama VN, Flaherty KR, Toews GB, et al. Prognostic value of desaturation during a 6-minute walk test in idiopathic interstitial pneumonia. Am J Respir Crit Care Med. 2003;168(9):1084-90.
34. Villalba WO, Sampaio-Barros PD, Pereira MC, et al. Six-minute walk test for the evaluation of pulmonary disease severity in scleroderma patients. Chest. 2007;131(1):217-22.
35. Caminati A, Harari S. IPF: New insight in diagnosis and prognosis. Respir Med. 2010;104(Suppl 1):S2-S10.
36. Meyer KC. Bronchoalveolar lavage as a diagnostic tool. Semin Respir Crit Care Med. 2007;28(5):546-60.
37. Kantrow SP, Meyer KC, Kidd P, et al. The CD4/CD8 ratio in BAL fluid is highly variable in sarcoidosis. Eur Respir J. 1997;10(12):2716-21.
38. Meyer KC, Raghu G. Bronchoalveolar lavage for the evaluation of interstitial lung disease: is it clinically useful? Eur Respir J. 2011;38(4):761-9.
39. Raj R, Raparia K, Lynch DA, et al. Surgical lung biopsy for interstitial lung diseases. Chest. 2017;151(5):1131-40.
40. Ravaglia C, Bonifazi M, Wells AU, et al. Safety and diagnostic yield of transbronchial lung cryobiopsy in diffuse parenchymal lung diseases: a comparative study versus video-assisted thoracoscopic lung biopsy and a systematic review of the literature. Respiration. 2016;91:215-27.
41. Valenzi E, Kass DJ. Diagnosis from Afar: is remote multidisciplinary discussion appropriate for interstitial lung disease care? Ann Am Thorac Soc. 2019;16(4):434-6.

Idiopathic Pulmonary Fibrosis

CHAPTER 105

Zein Kattih, Joseph Parambil, Stephen Machnicki, Suhail Raoof

INTRODUCTION

Idiopathic pulmonary fibrosis (IPF) is a progressive, fibrosing interstitial pneumonia with unknown cause. IPF is associated with specific clinical manifestations, radiologic findings, and histopathologic findings that distinguish it from other forms of interstitial lung disease. Certain genetic mutations may be responsible for the development of IPF in a subset of patients. Fibrosis associated with IPF is irreversible and ultimately leads to death or requires transplantation.

PATHOGENESIS OF IDIOPATHIC PULMONARY FIBROSIS

The pathogenesis of IPF is a combination of genetic, environmental, and behavioral factors that ultimately lead to fibrosis. This fibrosis is characterized by the presence of extracellular matrix deposition, parenchymal scar formation, and parenchymal remodeling which leads to architectural distortion.[1] In over 95% of cases, IPF is a sporadic disease. In the remaining small subset of patients with familial IPF, genetic factors have been identified to be associated with the development of IPF.[1] These factors include the human telomerase reverse transcriptase (TERT) or human telomerase RNA (TERC) components of the telomerase complex that lead to telomere shortening and the MUC5B promoter polymorphism.[2] The MUC5B promoter polymorphism is commonly see in IPF while the genetic abnormalities of telomere mutations are uncommon and have not been consistently shown to be present in sporadic IPF.

IDIOPATHIC PULMONARY FIBROSIS IN INDIA

There are significant variations in IPF prevalence estimate countrywise **(Table 1)**.[3] Retrospective studies of single centers in India have suggested a prevalence of IPF in India which is higher than the prevalence in western countries **(Table 1)**.[4] In a retrospective cohort study of patients identified to have ILD, 17% of patients were diagnosed with IPF.[4] This same study conducted in the Tricity region comprising three districts around Chandigarh estimated a crude annual incidence for IPF of 2.1–4.3 per 100,000 and an estimated prevalence of 5.8–11.6 per 100,000.[5] A prospective registry of patients with ILD in India was created encompassing 27 centers across 19 cities in India.[5] In this cohort, the incidence of IPF was reported as 1.7%.[5] Overall, there is heterogeneity in reported incidence and prevalence of IPF, and the diagnosis is likely underrecognized and underreported in India.

TABLE 1: Idiopathic pulmonary fibrosis (IPF) prevalence estimate by country.[3]

Country	Source	Mean unadjusted prevalence	Mean adjusted prevalence
USA	Raghu et al.[8]	0.67 (per 10,000)	2.4 (per 10,000)
UK	Strongman et al.	1.16 (per 10,000)	0.78 (per 10,000)
South Korea	Kim et al.[23]	3.52 (per 10,000)	4.51 (per 10,000)
Japan	Kondoh et al.[17]	0.59 (per 10,000)	0.89 (per 10,000)
India (single center)	Kaul et al.[3]	19.62 (per 100,000)	20.29 (per 10,000)
India (Tricity)	Dhooria et al.[5]	NA	5.8–11.6 (per 100,000)

CLINICAL MANIFESTATIONS

The initial presenting symptoms of IPF include shortness of breath and cough. These symptoms are usually mild and nonspecific, which leads to delayed diagnosis.[6] Physical examination may present with fine, inspiratory crackles, particularly at the bases, especially throughout inspiration.[7]

Clubbing may be present in the digits. Pulmonary function tests commonly reveal a restrictive pattern with reduction in forced vital capacity (FVC), forced end expiratory volume in 1 second (FEV1), and a reduced diffuse capacity for carbon monoxide (DLCO).[6]

IMAGING FINDINGS (TABLE 2)

Idiopathic pulmonary fibrosis is associated with radiologic findings of usual interstitial pneumonia (UIP) pattern on high resolution CT imaging of the chest **(Figs. 1 to 4)**. Volumetric acquisition and noncontrast thin-section CT images (≤1.5-mm slices) are suggested to characterize these abnormalities.[8] This pattern is characterized by the presence of reticulation along with honeycombing and traction bronchiectasis and associated architectural distortion in a craniocaudal gradient and with a subpleural predominance.[8] Importantly, there is a lack of predominance of other features such as cysts, ground-glass changes, micronodules, or consolidation, which should prompt consideration of alternative diagnosis. These features would make the diagnosis of IPF less likely and suggest the possibility of other interstitial lung disease (ILD).

The imaging findings are defined radiographically in the 2018 revised Fleischner criteria as UIP pattern, probable UIP pattern, or indeterminate pattern, and alternative diagnosis to UIP described as under:[9] UIP pattern on CT has a basilar distribution and subpleural predominance which is often heterogeneous. Computed tomography (CT) features of honeycombing, reticular pattern, traction

TABLE 2: Radiologic and histopathologic categories of UIP.

	UIP/IPF (usual interstitial pneumonia/idiopathic pulmonary fibrosis)	Probable UIP/IPF	Indeterminate for UIP/IPF	Features most consistent with an alternative diagnosis
Findings on chest computed tomography	• Subpleural and basilar predominant • Heterogeneous distribution • Honeycombing, reticulation, traction bronchiectasis/ bronchiolectasis present • No features of non-UIP	Similar to UIP/IPF but no honeycombing	• Variable distribution • Some features of non-UIP pattern with fibrosis	• May not have reticulation • Other nontypical features may include: ○ Greater involvement of the upper lobes ○ Sparing of subpleural spaces ○ Air trapping or mosaic attenuation
Histopathologic findings	Presence of: • Dense fibrosis causing architecture remodeling with honeycombing • Patchy fibrosis • Subpleural and/or paraseptal • Fibroblast foci at the edge of dense scars	Similar features as UIP/IPF Or Honeycomb fibrosis	Fibrosing process and non-UIP pattern	Non-UIP pattern or UIP pattern with miscellaneous features

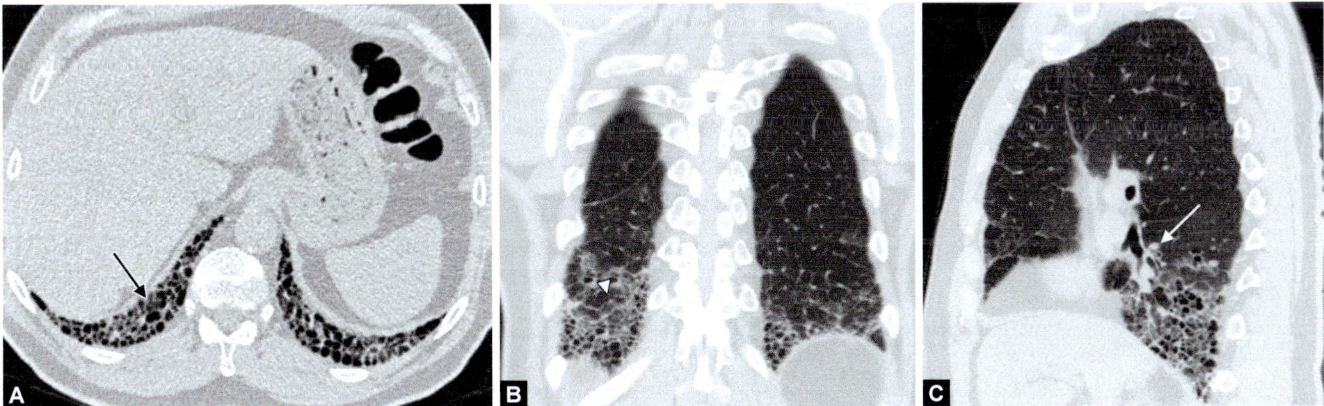

FIGS. 1A TO C: (A) Axial, (B) coronal, and (C) sagittal CT images of the lungs demonstrate subpleural and basilar predominant honeycombing (black arrow), traction bronchiectasis (white arrow), and irregular reticulation (arrowhead), consistent with a usual interstitial pneumonia (UIP) pattern.

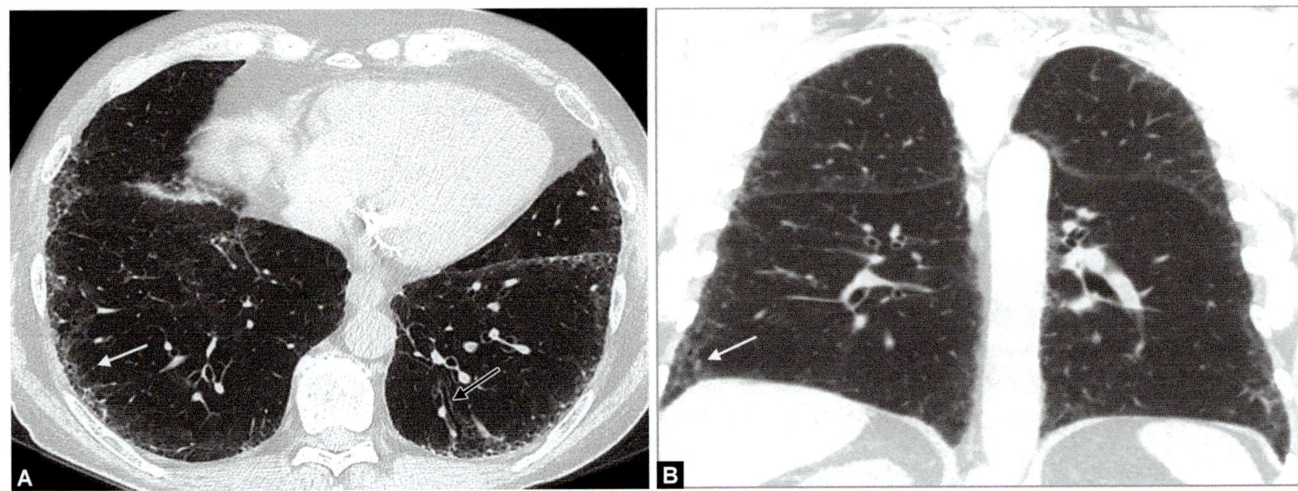

FIGS. 2A AND B: (A) Axial and (B) coronal CT images with lung windows showing loss of smooth interfaces with subpleural and basilar predominant reticulation (white arrows) and traction bronchiectasis (black arrow), without honeycombing consistent with a probably usual interstitial pneumonia (UIP) pattern.

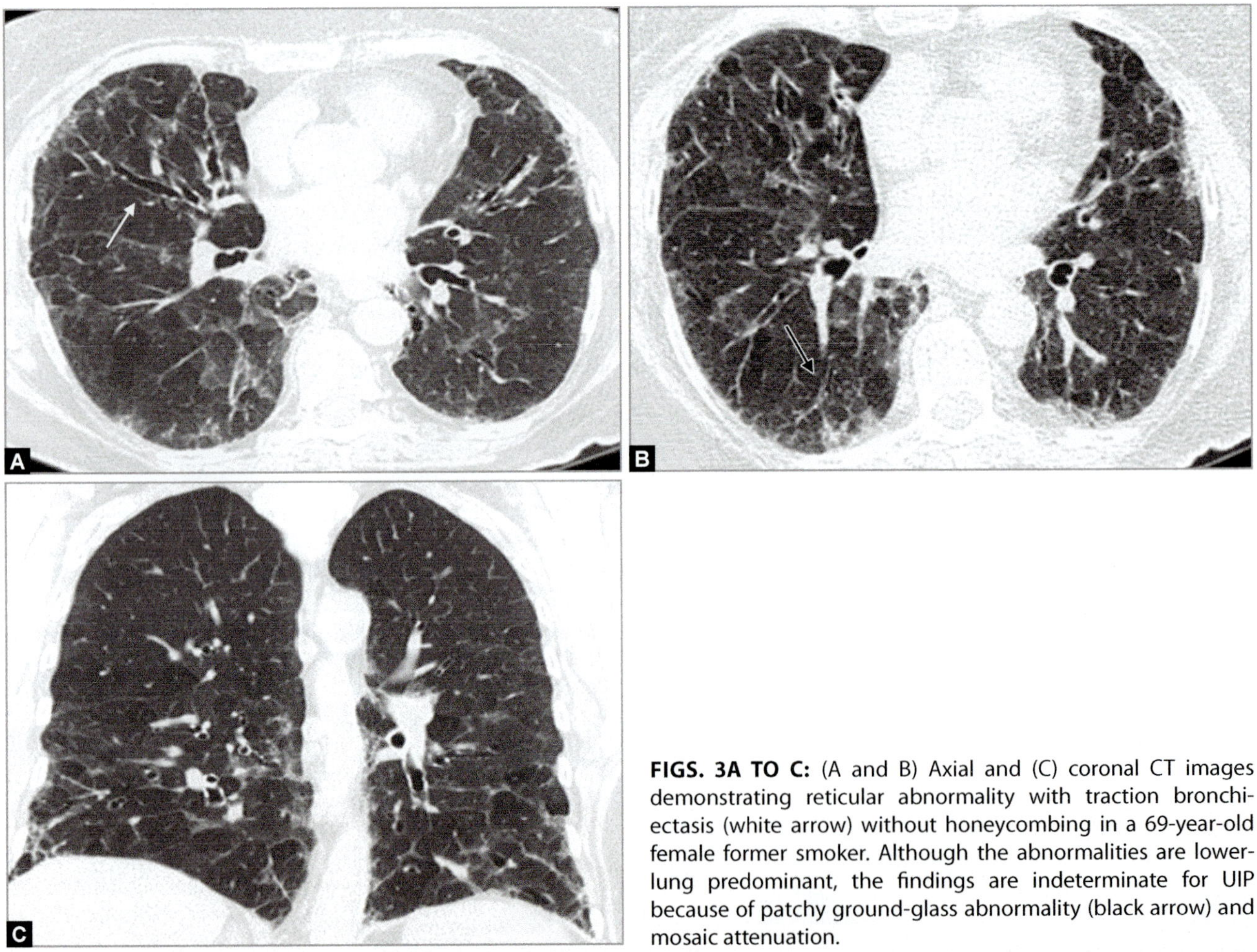

FIGS. 3A TO C: (A and B) Axial and (C) coronal CT images demonstrating reticular abnormality with traction bronchiectasis (white arrow) without honeycombing in a 69-year-old female former smoker. Although the abnormalities are lower-lung predominant, the findings are indeterminate for UIP because of patchy ground-glass abnormality (black arrow) and mosaic attenuation.

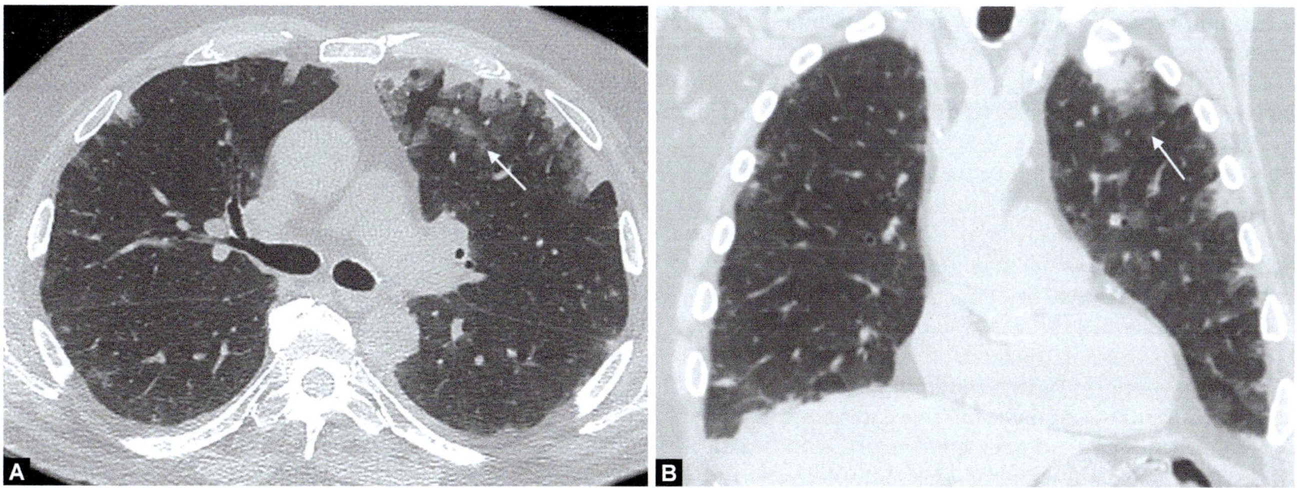

FIGS. 4A AND B: (A) Axial and (B) coronal CT images of the lungs demonstrating alternative diagnosis to usual interstitial pneumonia (UIP) due to presence of peripheral consolidation (white arrows) in patient with chronic eosinophilic pneumonia.

bronchiectasis/bronchiolectasis and absence of non-UIP features are present. Honeycombs are defined as clustered cystic air spaces which are typically 3–10 mm in diameter with well-defined walls and in the subpleural area. Probable UIP pattern demonstrates the same basal and subpleural predominant distribution with features of reticular pattern and traction bronchiectasis/bronchiolectasis but without honeycombing. Mini-IPS format on CT imaging can demonstrate dilated airways which beading and extension to the outer area of the lung, and this mode of CT imaging can evaluate for mimics of honeycombing such as subpleural cysts. Indeterminate UIP pattern has variable or diffuse involvement with fibrosis and may have some inconspicuous features suggestive of a non-UIP pattern (such as ground glass opacities or air trapping). Ground glass opacity in this case which is associated with the reticular pattern is usually fibrotic.

Finally, CT pattern consisting of an alternative diagnosis for UIP may have peribronchovascular involvement, cysts, nodules, air trapping or mosaic attenuation, ground-glass opacities, consolidations, and an absence of a craniocaudal gradient. UIP pattern and many cases of probable UIP pattern have high probability of identifying a UIP pattern on histopathological assessments if the clinical context of IPF is fulfilled. If the clinical context occurs in men who are smokers and greater than 60 years of age, a confident clinical diagnosis of IPF can be made based on clinical-radiographic features alone. In the indeterminate pattern, since this association with pathologic UIP is less robust, sampling of the pulmonary parenchyma with biopsy might become necessary to make the eventual diagnosis of IPF.

HISTOLOGIC FEATURES (TABLE 2)

Histologic features of IPF are a patchwork appearance with areas of fibrosis alternating with areas of normal lung parenchyma. There are characteristic fibroblast foci at the leading edge of the fibrosing process and finally microscopic honeycombing is noted as dilated airspaces lined by bronchiolar epithelium.[7] Features that would suggest an alternative diagnosis include lack of a patchwork pattern of fibrosis or evidence of histology which is consistent with an alternative diagnosis.[8]

MULTIDISCIPLINARY DISCUSSION

The diagnosis of IPF is more frequently suspected in males in their seventh decade at age above 60 years with a history of current or past cigarette smoking.[7] Patients can present at younger ages, around 40 years of age, when IPF is associated with familiar pulmonary fibrosis or when there are clinical clues to suggest a genetic predisposition.[2] Workup should include evaluation for evidence of other causes of interstitial lung disease (see separate chapter entitled "ILD other than IPF").

Patients with IPF or suspected of having IPF should undergo further diagnostic testing. Baseline characteristics including oxygen saturation at rest and with ambulation during a 6-minute walk test (6MWT), assessment of dyspnea score, full pulmonary function testing, high-resolution CT chest imaging to evaluate the imaging pattern and evaluations for concurrent pulmonary hypertension are all indicated.[10]

Lung Biopsy

In patients who are suspected of having IPF based on clinical features with radiological findings which are probable or indeterminate for UIP, biopsy is often indicated. A surgical lung biopsy is recommended in patients who are at low surgical risk,[11] though recent years have seen an increase utility of transbronchial biopsy, transbronchial cryobiopsy, and genomic classifier use.[11] Surgical lung biopsy may be associated with a mortality of 6% at 3 months in patients with fibrotic lung disease.[12] This is more likely if the lung involvement is more severe. For example, the mortality due to surgical lung biopsy is 11% if DLCO < 50%. In addition, there is significant morbidity from prolonged air leak in 3.3% cases,[13] increased costs due to prolonged length of stay in the hospital of 6.1 days.[12] Thus, 90% patients who require tissue diagnosis may not get referred for this procedure.[14]

Genomic classifiers such as the Envisia® genomic classifier utilize total RNA extracted from transbronchial biopsy samples and perform next-generation RNA sequencing to evaluate for fibrotic sequences.[15] These genomic classifiers have been utilized to detect gene expression signature which is concordant with the UIP pathology pattern.[15] However, this genomic classifier is not specific for IPF, merely the UIP histologic pattern, which limits its utility. The most recent updates to guidelines suggest that transbronchial cryobiopsy be considered an acceptable alternative for diagnosis in centers with experience performing and interpreting these.[11] Though national guidelines do not make a recommendation regarding genomic classifier testing, institutional recommendations exist but vary.[11] Some institutions have developed a suggested algorithmic approach to genetic testing in which recommends Envisia® genomic classifier via transbronchial biopsy in patients with a CT demonstrating indeterminate UIP pattern and in whom surgical or cryobiopsy is not performed **(Flowchart 1)**.

Step	
Step 1	• Rule out secondary causes • CVD/Sarcoid • Drug-induced • Occupational • Recurrent aspiration
Step 2	• Possible hypersensitivity pneumonitis? • History • Specific antigen panel • Consider BAL with cell count (lymph >20–30%) • Surgical biopsy only if necessary
Step 3	• Is CT suggestive of UIP or probable UIP pattern? • If so, biopsy probably not necessary if clinical context is fulfilled
Step 4	• Indeterminate UIP pattern (UIP 50% likely) • Surgical biopsy or cryobiopsy feasible? • If no, consider Envisia (R) genomic classifier via TBBx • Alternative to UIP pattern (UIP 25% likely) • Tissue sampling with bronch with TBBx and BAL or cryobiopsy or surgical biopsy • Present case to multidisciplinary meeting

FLOWCHART 1: Recommended 4-step algorithm in diagnosing fibrotic lung disease.

(BAL: bronchoalveolar disease; CVD: cardiovascular disease; UIP: usual interstitial pneumonia)

Source: Reproduced with permission from the Lung Institute, Northwell Health.

Genetic and Telomere Testing

In familial IPF, genetic factors have been identified to be associated with the disease. These factors include rare variants in the human telomerase reverse transcriptase (TERT) or human telomerase RNA (TERC) components of the telomerase complex, and common variants in the MUC5B promoter polymorphism.[2] Individuals with shortened telomeres or telomere-related mutations have more rapid disease progression and decreased transplant-free survival.[2] The presence of telomere-related mutation has implications in consideration for lung transplantation and requires consideration of post-transplantation immunosuppressive medications.[2]

MONITORING OF CLINICAL PROGRESSION

Idiopathic pulmonary fibrosis is a progressive disease, which is ultimately fatal. The natural history of IPF can present with either rapid progression, slow progression, or a stuttering course that is marred with episodes of acute exacerbation or worsening.[10] The majority of patients exhibit a stuttering course or a course of slow progression.[9] Lung function reliably declines in these patients by about 150–200 mL per year.[10] Monitoring of 6MWT and degree of dyspnea are useful markers of clinical progression. FVC decrease by >10%, DLCO decrease by >15%, and increase in honeycombing and fibrosis on CT scan over a 1-year period are suggestive of disease progression.[10]

TREATMENT AND MANAGEMENT

Treatment modalities for IPF are limited to recent antifibrotic medications as well as nonmedication management strategies. Several trials have evaluated the efficacy of therapies which have proven ineffective. These include the combination of N-acetylcysteine, prednisone, and azathioprine which was evaluated in the PANTHER-IPF trial.[16] Immunosuppressive medications such as cyclophosphamide and mycophenolate have also shown no benefit.[17] Oral steroids have been demonstrated to show some utility as antitussives and in improving subjective reports of quality of life. In some individuals with short telomere lengths, oral steroids may result in more rapid decline of PFTs and more frequent exacerbations.[2]

Antifibrotic Medications

Nintedanib and pirfenidone are antifibrotic agents which are approved for use in IPF. In INPULSIS-1 and INPULSIS-2, nintedanib was shown to reduce the decline in FVC over a 52-week period.[18] Patients in the INPULSIS-1 study treated with nintedanib had an annual decline of 114.7 mL in FVC compared with 239.9 mL in the placebo group with a 125.3 mL annual difference.[18] In the INPULSIS-2 study, there was a 93.7 mL per year difference in FVC decline between those treated with nintedanib and those who received placebo.[18] Similarly, in the RELIEF trial, pirfenidone was shown to reduce decline in FVC at 48 weeks compared with placebo with a difference of 1.69 FVC % predicted.[19] There was also a higher proportion of patients treated with pirfenidone demonstrating <5% relative annual FVC decline compared with those receiving placebo.[19] In the phase 3 ASCEND study, pirfenidone reduced disease progression, and increased exercise tolerance and progression-free survival.[20]

Therapies currently under investigation include recombinant human pentraxin-2, a medication which acts as an anti-fibrotic and inhaled treprostinil.[6]

Supplemental Oxygen

Guidelines currently strongly recommend supplemental O_2 use for patients with IPF who have hypoxemia at rest.[21]

Comorbid Conditions and Referral for Lung Transplantation

Echocardiogram does not accurately evaluate the presence of pulmonary hypertension in patients with fibrosis (citation). Right heart catheterization is required for diagnosis of comorbid pulmonary hypertension that may be contributing to patient symptoms.[11] In patients treated for PH, there is a strong recommendation against the use of ambrisentan due to potential for harm.[11] Recently, inhaled treprostinil was approved to treat pulmonary hypertension in IPF based on the favorable results of the INCREASE trial. The International Society of Heart and Lung Transplantation (ISHLT) suggests consideration of referral to lung transplantation in patients with rapid decline in FVC or DLCO, oxygen desaturation, or decrease in 6MWT distance **(Box 1)**.[22] Unilateral or bilateral lung transplantation can be performed.

BOX 1 Indications for lung transplantation in interstitial lung disease.

Timing of referral:

- Referral should be made at time of diagnosis
- Any form of pulmonary fibrosis with forced vital capacity (FVC) < 80% predicted or diffusing capacity of the lungs for carbon monoxide (DLCO) < 40% predicted
- Any form of pulmonary fibrosis with one of the following in the past 2 years:
    - Relative decline of FVC ≥ 10%
    - Relative decline of DLCO ≥ 15%
    - Relative decline in FVC ≥ 5% in combination with worsening of respiratory symptoms or radiologic progression
    - Supplemental oxygen requirement either at rest or on exertion
    - For inflammatory idiopathic pulmonary fibroses (IPF), progression of disease (either on imaging or pulmonary function) despite treatment
    - For patient with connective tissue disease or familial pulmonary fibrosis, early referral is recommended

Timing of listing:

- Any form of pulmonary fibrosis with one of the following in the past 6 months, despite appropriate treatment
- Absolute decline of FVC ≥ 10%
- Absolute decline of DLCO ≥ 15%
- Absolute decline in FVC ≥ 5% with radiologic progression
- Desaturation to <88% on 6MWT or >50 m decline in 6MWT distance in the past 6 months
- Pulmonary hypertension on right heart catheterization or on 2-dimentional echocardiography (in the absence of diastolic dysfunction)
- Hospitalization because of respiratory decline, pneumothorax, or acute exacerbation

Source: Adapted from the International Society for Heart and Lung Transplantation (ISHLT) 2021 Consensus document.[22]

ACUTE EXACERBATIONS OF IDIOPATHIC PULMONARY FIBROSIS

About 5–10% of patients with IPF will have an acute exacerbation, a clinically significant respiratory deterioration characterized by new, diffuse ground-glass abnormalities superimposed on the chronic fibrotic changes on imaging **(Figs. 5A to C)**.[1] This reported incidence varies widely in the literature and has been suggested to be between 1% and 50%.[23] Acute exacerbations are defined as an acute change in the respiratory status that typically occur in days to weeks and no less than 1 month.[1] These symptoms must not be attributable to heart failure or fluid overload.[1] Acute exacerbations are associated with significant respiratory failure, hospitalization, and death, and up to 46% of deaths due to IPF are preceded by acute exacerbation.[1] Exacerbations may be triggered by multiple causes including viral or bacterial infections, postoperatively, due to drug toxicity, or aspiration.[1] Chronic factors, such as underlying epithelial cell dysfunction, fibroblast accumulation, and fibroblast activation and acute factors, such as stress injuries and acute lung injuries, contribute to acute exacerbations of IPF.[1] Risk factors for acute exacerbation include poor lung function, advanced disease, prior history of acute exacerbation, existing pulmonary hypertension, coexisting coronary artery disease, and smoking history.[23]

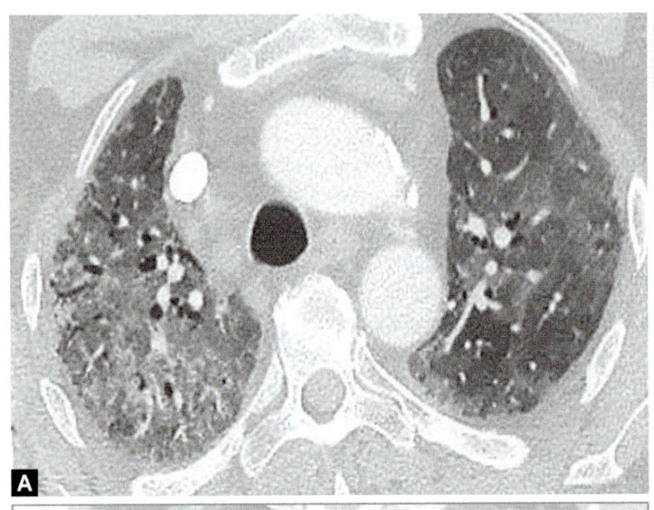

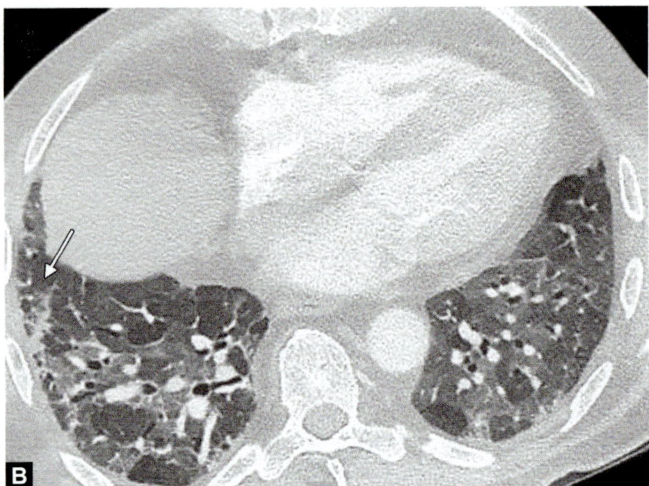

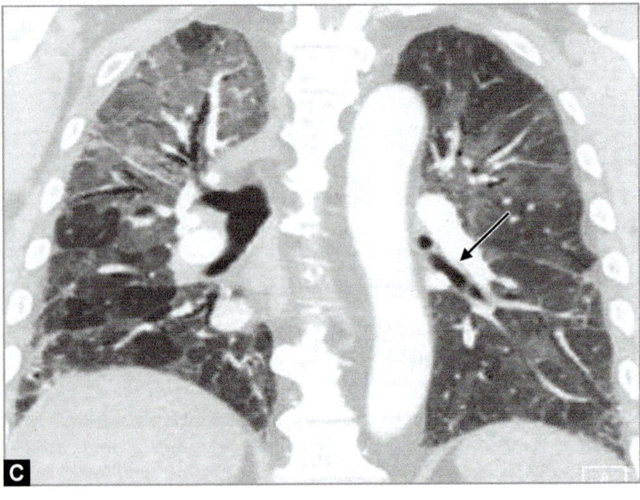

FIGS. 5A TO C: Axial CT images through the left upper (A) and right upper (B) lung zones and coronal (C) image demonstrating diffuse, bilateral ground-glass opacification on a background of a subpleural and basilar predominant reticular pattern with traction bronchiectasis (black arrow). This was a 79-year-old male with history of IPF who presented with acute respiratory failure. There was no evidence pulmonary edema or infection.

Pathologic findings in acute IPF reveals underlying UIP with acute lung injury patterns of either diffuse alveolar damage or organizing pneumonia.[24] Median survival in patients with acute exacerbation of IPF is estimated to be around 3–4 months.[1] The role of biopsy in these patients is limited due to small tissue sample obtained from transbronchial biopsy and significant risk of deterioration, morbidity and mortality with surgical lung biopsy during acute exacerbation.[1]

Currently, there are no effective therapies for acute exacerbations of IPF. Supportive care remains at the forefront of management. Supplemental oxygen delivery and palliation of symptoms is crucial.[1] Use of mechanical ventilation in patients with IPF is controversial, since upward of 90% of patients will die.[21] Shared decision-making and the assistance of palliative care is necessary. Most patients who present with acute exacerbation receive steroids,[21] though this weak recommendation is primarily due to anecdotal or case report evidence of utility. Use of antifibrotic agents may reduce the incidence of acute exacerbation but are not indicated during the acute exacerbation.

SUMMARY

Idiopathic pulmonary fibrosis is a progressive disease of the lungs which is characterized by fibrosis that demonstrates specific imaging findings of UIP, nonspecific clinical symptoms, and evidence on workup of deterioration in pulmonary functions. The emergence of antifibrotic therapy for this disease has allowed the slowing of progression of disease. However, there remains no mechanism for disease reversal. Symptomatic management, monitoring of symptoms and pulmonary functions, repeat imaging, and management of acute exacerbations are the hallmarks of management of this disease process.

REFERENCES

1. Collard HR, Ryerson CJ, Corte TJ, et al. Acute exacerbation of Idiopathic Pulmonary Fibrosis. An International Working Group Report. AJRCCM. 2016;194:11.
2. Courtwright AM, El-Chemaly S. Telomeres in Interstitial Lung Disease: The Short and the Long of It. Ann Am Thorac Soc. 2019;16(2):175-81.
3. Kaul B, Cottin V, Collard HR, et al. Variability in global prevalence of interstitial lung disease. Front Med (Lausanne). 2021;8:751181.
4. Singh S, Collins BF, Sharma BB, et al. Interstitial lung disease in India. Results of a prospective registry. Am J Respir Crit Care Med. 2017;195(6):801-13.
5. Dhooria S, Sehgal IS, Agarwal R, et al. Incidence, prevalence, and national burden of interstitial lung diseases in India: Estimates from two studies of 3089 subjects. PLoS One. 2022; 17(7):e0271665.
6. Glass DS, Grossfeld D, Fenna HA, et al. Idiopathic pulmonary fibrosis: Current and future treatment. Clin Respir J. 2022;16(2): 84-96.
7. Cottin V, Cordier JF. Velcro crackles: the key for early diagnosis of idiopathic pulmonary fibrosis? Eur Respir J. 2012;40(3): 519-21.
8. Raghu G, Remy-Jardin M, Myers JL, et al. Diagnosis of Idiopathic Pulmonary Fibrosis. An Official ATS/ERS/JRS/ALAT Clinical Practice Guideline. Am J Respir Crit Care Med. 2018;198(5): e44-68.
9. Lynch DA, Sverzellati N, Travis WD, et al. Diagnostic criteria for idiopathic pulmonary fibrosis: A Fleischner Society White Paper. Lancet Respir Med. 2018;6(2):138-53.
10. Raghu G. Idiopathic pulmonary fibrosis: lessons from clinical trials over the past 25 years. Eur Respir J. 2017;50.
11. Raghu G, Remy-Jardin M, Richeldi L, et al. Idiopathic Pulmonary Fibrosis (an Update) and Progressive Pulmonary Fibrosis in Adults: An Official ATS/ERS/JRS/ALAT Clinical Practice Guideline. Am J Respir Crit Care Med. 2022;205(9):e18-47.
12. Kreider ME, Hansen-Flaschen J, Ahmad NN, et al. Complications of video-assisted thoracoscopic lung biopsy in patients with interstitial lung disease. Ann Thorac Surg. 2007;83:1140-4.
13. Ravaglia C, Bonifazi M, Wells AU, et al. Safety and diagnostic yield of transbronchial lung cryobiopsy in diffuse parenchymal lung diseases: A comparative study versus video-assisted thoracoscopic lung biopsy and a systematic review of the literature. Respiration. 2016;91(3):215-27.
14. Margaritopoulos GA, Wells AU. The role of transbronchial biopsy in the diagnosis of diffuse parenchymal lung diseases: con. Rev Port Pneumol. 2012;18(2):61-3.
15. Choi Y, Lu J, Hu Z, et al. Analytical performance of Envisia: a genomic classifier for usual interstitial pneumonia. BMC Pulm Med. 2017;17(1):141.
16. Raghu G, Anstrom KJ, King TE Jr, et al. Prednisone, azathioprine, and N-acetylcysteine for pulmonary fibrosis. N Engl J Med. 2012;366(21):1968-77.
17. Kondoh Y, Taniguchi H, Yokoi T, et al. Cyclophosphamide and low-dose prednisolone in idiopathic pulmonary fibrosis and fibrosing nonspecific interstitial pneumonia. Eur Respir J. 2005;25(3):528-33.
18. Richeldi L, du Bois RM, Raghu G, et al. Efficacy and safety of nintedanib in idiopathic pulmonary fibrosis. N Engl J Med. 2014;370(22):2071-82.
19. Behr J, Prasse A, Kreuter M, et al. Pirfenidone in patients with progressive fibrotic interstitial lung diseases other than idiopathic pulmonary fibrosis (RELIEF): a double-blind, randomised, placebo-controlled, phase 2b trial. Lancet Respir Med. 2021;9(5):476-86.
20. King TE Jr, Bradford WZ, Castro-Bernardini S, et al. A phase 3 trial of pirfenidone in patients with idiopathic pulmonary fibrosis. N Engl J Med. 2014;370(22):2083-92.
21. Raghu G, Rochwerg B, Zhang Y, et al. An official ATS/ERS/JRS/ALAT clinical practice guideline: Treatment of idiopathic pulmonary fibrosis. An update of the 2011 clinical practice guideline. Am J Respir Crit Care Med. 2015;192:16.
22. Leard LE, Holm AM, Valapour M, et al. Consensus document for the selection of lung transplant candidates: An update from the International Society for Heart and Lung Transplantation. J Heart Lung Transplant. 2021;40(11):1349-79.
23. Kim DS. Acute exacerbation of idiopathic pulmonary fibrosis. Encyclopedia of Respiratory Medicine, 2nd edition. London: Academic Press Inc. Ltd; 2021. pp. 199-217.
24. Churg A, Muller NL, Silva CI, et al. Acute exacerbation (acute lung injury of unknown cause) in UIP and other forms of fibrotic interstitial pneumonias. Am J Surg Pathol. 2007;31(2):277-84.

Interstitial Lung Disease other than Idiopathic Pulmonary Fibrosis

CHAPTER 106

Zein Kattih, Joseph Parambil, Arunabh Talwar, Stephen Machnicki, Suhail Raoof

INTRODUCTION

Interstitial lung diseases (ILD) are a group of heterogenous diseases of the lung that are characterized by overlapping clinical, pathological, and radiological features. These diseases are often associated with nonspecific symptoms, radiological findings, and pathological features that make it difficult to distinguish the various subtypes. Treatment of ILD includes use of antifibrotic agents and addressing the underlying mechanism of disease.

PATHOGENESIS OF INTERSTITIAL LUNG DISEASE

Inflammation due to underlying immune diseases is the most common cause of the inflammatory processes found in ILD. Ultimately, the persistent release of cytokines or autoantibodies in the case of autoimmune diseases leads to fibrosis of the lung parenchyma.[1] Other manifestations of inflammatory processes include inflammation due to environmental exposures, such as in hypersensitivity pneumonitis (HP), and granuloma formations, such as in sarcoidosis.[1] Granulomas are formed by tightly aggregated macrophages that congregate into multinucleate cells. The epithelial damage in susceptible individuals in combination with factors such as genetics, age, and environmental factors lead to an abnormal wound healing response, epithelial injury, and, ultimately, scarring and fibrosis.[1]

CLASSIFICATION OF INTERSTITIAL LUNG DISEASE

Interstitial lung disease includes diseases such as idiopathic pulmonary fibrosis (IPF) (see Chapter 105), nonspecific interstitial pneumonia (NSIP), cryptogenic organizing pneumonia (OP), acute interstitial pneumonia, respiratory bronchiolitis-associated ILD, connective tissue disease-related interstitial lung disease (CTD-ILD), desquamative interstitial pneumonia, and lymphoid interstitial pneumonia, among others.[2] These diseases can be idiopathic, autoimmune-related, exposure-related, ILDs with cysts, or secondary to sarcoidosis **(Flowchart 1)**.[1]

Connective tissue disease-related ILDs are reviewed separately (see Chapters 108 and 109). Occupational ILD requires reduction in the exposure to the agent.[3] The most well-recognized agents that can lead to ILD include asbestos and silica.[3] These exposures include metals and inorganic fibrous and nonfibrous dust, including silicosis, asbestosis, and chronic beryllium disease.[3] Other diseases such as shrinking lung syndrome, polymyositis and dermatomyositis,

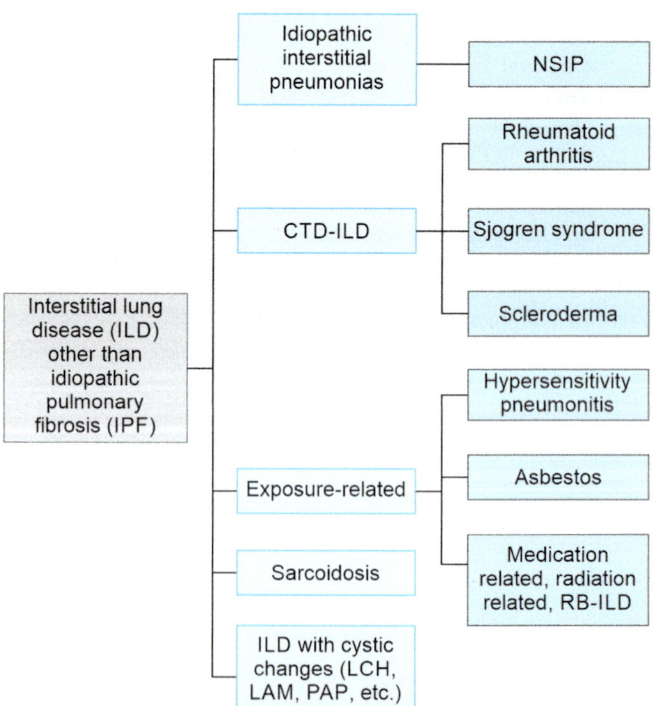

FLOWCHART 1: Subtypes of most common interstitial lung diseases. Subtypes which are underlying are more prevalent.

(CTD-ILD: connective tissue disease-related ILD; ILD: interstitial lung disease; IPF: idiopathic pulmonary fibrosis; LAM: lymphangioleiomyomatosis; LCH: Langerhans' cell histiocytosis; NSIP: nonspecific interstitial pneumonia; PAP: pulmonary alveolar proteinosis; RB-ILD: respiratory bronchiolitis-ILD)

Sjogren syndrome, and mixed CTD confer increased risk for developing ILD.[4] More rare diseases include ILD associated with lysosomal storage diseases such as acid sphingomyelinase deficiency which is associated with ILD,[5] though the most common pulmonary association in these diseases is chronic obstructive pulmonary disease (COPD)-like symptoms.[5]

Diagnosis and classification depend on radiologic findings, clinical findings, and exposure history. Pathology is frequently required for diagnosis. Multidisciplinary discussion is imperative for many of these patients.

EPIDEMIOLOGY

There is a wide range of reported incidence of ILD across various populations depending on ethnicity and geographic location.[1] The existing epidemiologic data is inconsistent. The prevalence of IPF reported in the literature varies between 7 and 1,650 patients per 100,000 patients.[6] Furthermore, even when reporting the subtype of ILD, there is a wide range reported. For instance, systemic sclerosis-associated ILD (SSc ILD) prevalence has been reported between 26.1% and 88.1%, and silicosis prevalence ranges from 5.6% to 37%.[6] Overall, there is a lack of uniformity in estimates of incidence and prevalence in ILD, which is especially evident given the heterogeneity of the group of diseases.

Epidemiology in India

A prospective registry of patients with ILD in India was created encompassing 27 centers across 19 cities.[7] In this cohort, there was an incidence of 47.3% HP, 13.9% CTD-ILD, 13.7% IPF, 8.5% idiopathic NSIP, 7.8% sarcoid, 3% pneumoconiosis, and 5.7% other ILDs.[7] Most of these patients presented with dyspnea (90%) and cough (82.2%).[7] ILD in India is likely underdiagnosed and underreported. HP was significantly more frequent in this cohort study in India when compared with population studies in countries such as Belgium, France, and the United States.[7,8] Of interest, many of the patients who presented with HP in this study had exposure to air coolers which are known to grow mold and spores that can trigger immune responses in predisposed patients.[7]

In a more recent retrospective cohort study, sarcoidosis was identified as the most common ILD subtype (37.3%) in India followed by CTD-ILD (19.3%), IPF (17%), and HP (14.4%).[8] The estimated crude annual incidence of ILD is 10.1–20.2 per 100,000 population.[8] In a retrospective cohort study of patients identified to have ILD, 17% of patients were diagnosed with IPF.[8] This same study of the Tricity region comprising three districts (Chandigarh, Panchkula, and Sahibzada Ajit Singh Najar) estimated a crude annual incidence of ILD to be 4.03 per 100,000 averaged over the 5 years' duration of the study.[8] Specifically, the crude annual incidence and prevalence per 100,000 people were estimated as follows: Sarcoidosis (incidence: 3.9–7.8; prevalence: 24.2–48.3), CTD-ILD (1.7–3.5; 8.5–17.0), HP (1.4–2.9; 6.2–12.3), IPF (2.1–4.3; 5.8–11.6), and other ILDs (0.9–1.7; 4.4–8.9).[8]

CLINICAL MANIFESTATIONS

As with IPF, ILD presents with nonspecific symptoms which can be progressive dyspnea and cough, and symptoms may occur up to years before diagnosis.[1] A hallmark on examination includes fine crackles on auscultation, particularly at the bases. This finding has been reported in up to 60–79% of patients with ILD.[1] Extrapulmonary manifestations such as joint pain or dysphagia should prompt consideration of underlying autoimmune diseases.[1] A thorough history regarding symptoms and exposure history is required. Pulmonary function tests (PFTs), review of medications, and chest imaging with high-resolution computed tomography (HRCT) are crucial. Guidelines do not exist for screening for ILD. In patients suspected of or confirmed to have ILD, initial evaluation with autoantibody testing is recommended. In sarcoid, angiotensin-converting enzyme (ACE) levels and anti-interleukin 2 receptor levels can be evaluated.[9] If HP is suspected, levels of serum IgG antibodies for a specified antigen should be measured, usually via a HP panel.[9]

On pulmonary function testing, diffusion capacity of carbon monoxide (DLCO) will be reduced. Patients may have evidence of hypoxemia with ambulation on a 6-minute walk test (6MWT) or at rest.

Fibrotic Hypersensitivity Pneumonitis (see Chapter 113)

Hypersensitivity pneumonitis is characterized by inflammation or fibrosis of the lung parenchyma and small airways due to an exaggerated immune response to an inhaled antigen in a susceptible individual.[10] Common antigens that lead to HP include thermophilic *Actinomyces* species, bird proteins, bacteria such as *Mycobacterium*, and fungi such as *Aspergillus*.[11] HP is less common in smokers.[11]

Hypersensitivity pneumonitis is classified based on HRCT chest findings and pathologic findings. Typical features of nonfibrotic HP include profuse, poorly defined centrilobular ground-glass opacities that affect all lung zones, or inspiratory mosaic attenuation with three density sign, or inspiratory mosaic attenuation and air-trapping associated with centrilobular nodules *and* lack of features suggesting an alternative diagnosis.[12] Features typical of fibrotic HP include signs of fibrosis with either profuse poorly defined centrilobular, ground-glass nodules affecting all lung zones or inspiratory mosaic attenuation with three-density sign *and* lack of features suggesting an alternative diagnosis.[12] Other imaging findings can be compatible with fibrotic HP or indeterminate for fibrotic HP.[12] HRCT chest images in deep inspiration and in expiration are the preferred imaging modality to diagnose HP radiologically.[10]

Hypersensitivity pneumonitis is diagnosed based on the characteristic CT chest findings and a definite history of exposure to an antigen.[8] Bronchoalveolar lavage (BAL) with lymphocyte predominance confers confidence of the diagnosis. However, atypical findings or an unclear history require multidisciplinary discussion and frequently require transbronchial biopsy, transbronchial lung cryobiopsy or surgical lung biopsy.[8,10]

A histopathology review of HP will demonstrate fibrotic changes and architectural distortion superimposed on acute or subacute changes, and these findings can mimic other diseases such as usual interstitial pneumonia (UIP) or NSIP.[11] Distinguishing features include bronchiolocentric accentuation of inflammation, peribronchial fibrosis, bronchiolar epithelial hyperplasia, and the presence of granulomas or multinucleated giant cells.[11] The presence of plasma cells predominating over lymphocytes, extensive lymphoid hyperplasia, extensive well-formed sarcoid or necrotizing granulomas, and aspirated particles suggests an alternative diagnosis to HP.[10]

Advanced Sarcoidosis (see Chapter 116)

Sarcoidosis is the most common ILD subtype in India across population studies.[8] The average age of this patient population is 44.4 years (±11.4 years), and only 7.9% are smokers.[8] The pathogenesis of the disease is suspected to be due to inflammatory response characterized by large numbers of macrophages and helper T cells in the setting of genetic and environmental factors (Singh 20). Some bacterial or viral exposures including *Mycoplasma or Borrelia*, as well as organic and inorganic agents, have been suggested to be involved in sarcoidosis.[13] Clinical presentation of sarcoidosis varies widely and can be nonspecific or asymptomatic.[13] Most patients have normal spirometry, but restrictive and obstructive patterns can be seen.[8] HRCT chest usually demonstrates upper lung predominant perilymphatic distribution of nodules with or without mediastinal or hilar lymphadenopathy.[7] Features that favor sarcoidosis as a diagnosis include perilymphatic lesion location, lesions around the bronchovascular bundles and fibrous septa, and lesions near the visceral pleura.[13]

In general, patients require biopsy for diagnosis. Combined endobronchial biopsy, transbronchial lung biopsy, and transbronchial needle aspiration maximize the yield for sarcoidosis.[7] Histology demonstrates features typical for sarcoid granulomas including well-formed, concentrically arranged layers of immune cells with a central core of macrophage aggregates and multinucleated giant cells.[13]

IMAGING FINDINGS

Various patterns can be identified on high-resolution CT chest in patients with ILD. Imaging findings suggestive of UIP are more likely to suggest IPF **(Figs. 1A to C)**. The presence of other features such as ground-glass opacities, consolidations, micronodules, or pleural changes suggests a diagnosis alternative to UIP **(Figs. 2A and B)**. In rheumatoid arthritis, the UIP pattern can be present. Fibrotic HP **(Figs. 3A and B)** can be distinguished because of the presence of reticulation in combination with ground-glass opacities and centrilobular nodules with associated architectural distortion.[11] Reticulation can be predominantly subpleural or peribronchovascular.[11] Stage IV sarcoidosis can present with varying imaging findings on CT chest, including fibrosis, hilar retraction, honeycombing, nodules, pleural thickening, and air trapping **(Figs. 4A and B)**.

In NSIP, radiology is often sufficient for diagnosis of definite or probable NSIP **(Figs. 5A and B)**. NSIP has predominant lower lobe involvement in a craniocaudal distribution, either in a diffuse or predominantly peripheral distribution, most commonly associated with reticular changes, traction bronchiectasis, and volume loss.[14] Ground-glass attenuation is present in 44% of patients.[14] Features that would favor the diagnosis of NSIP include

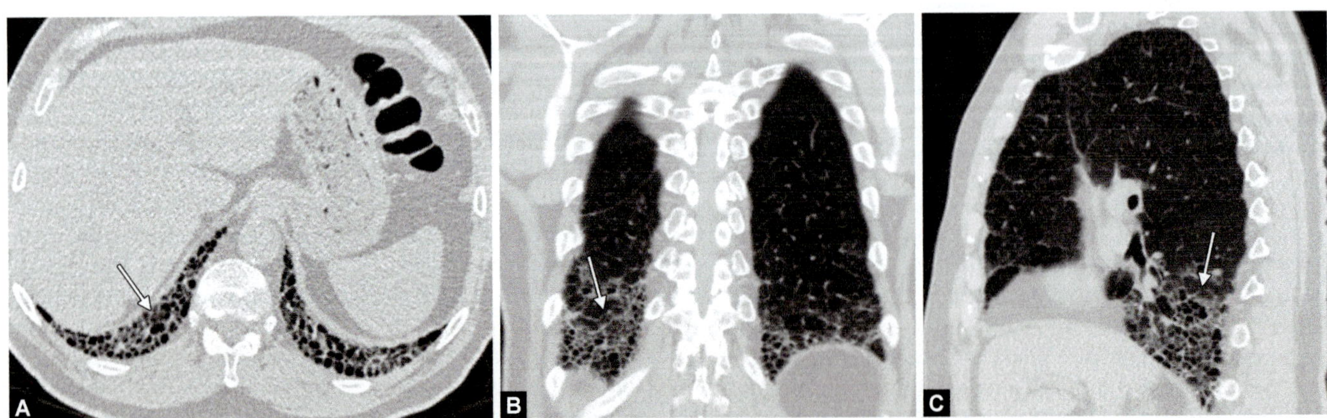

FIGS. 1A TO C: (A) Axial, (B) coronal, and (C) sagittal CT images of the lungs demonstrate subpleural and basilar predominant honeycombing, traction bronchiectasis, and irregular reticulation (white arrows), consistent with a usual interstitial pneumonia (UIP) pattern.

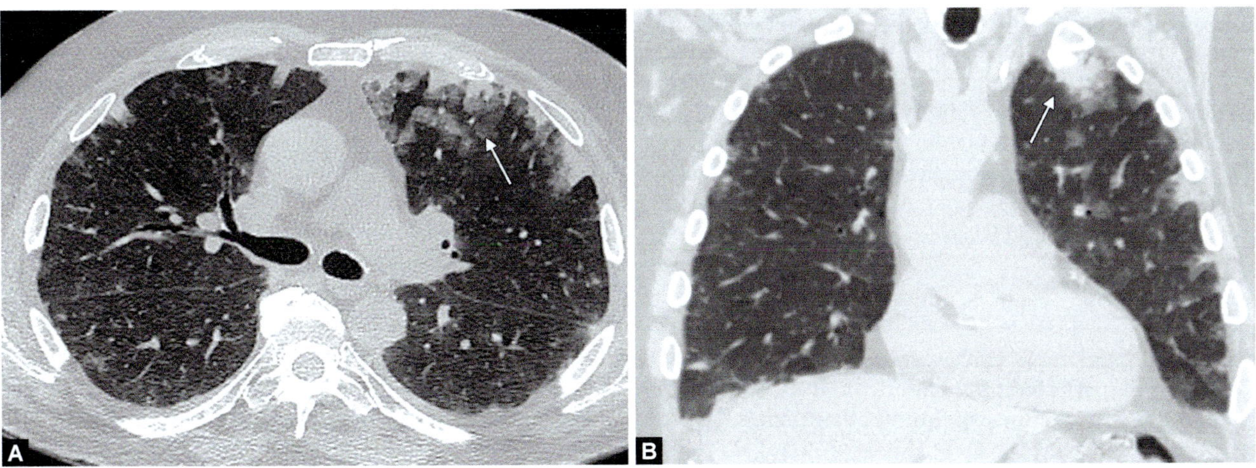

FIGS. 2A AND B: (A) Axial and (B) coronal CT images of the lungs demonstrate alternative diagnosis to usual interstitial pneumonia (UIP) due to presence of consolidations (white arrows). In this patient, peripheral consolidations were due to chronic eosinophilic pneumonia.

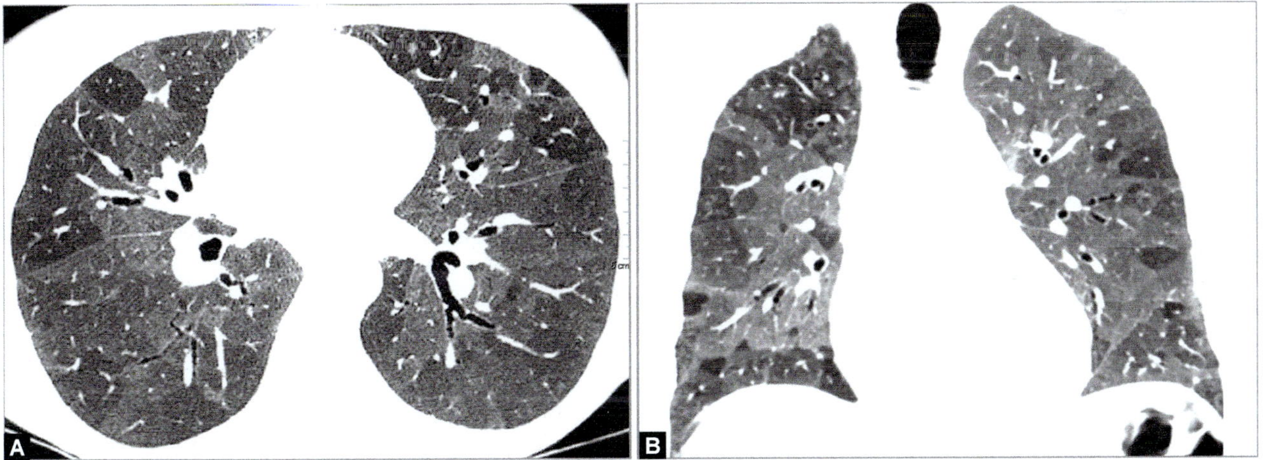

FIGS. 3A AND B: CT images in the lung in (A) axial and (B) coronal planes that demonstrate inspiratory mosaic attenuation with three-density sign with ground-glass opacities and traction bronchiectasis.

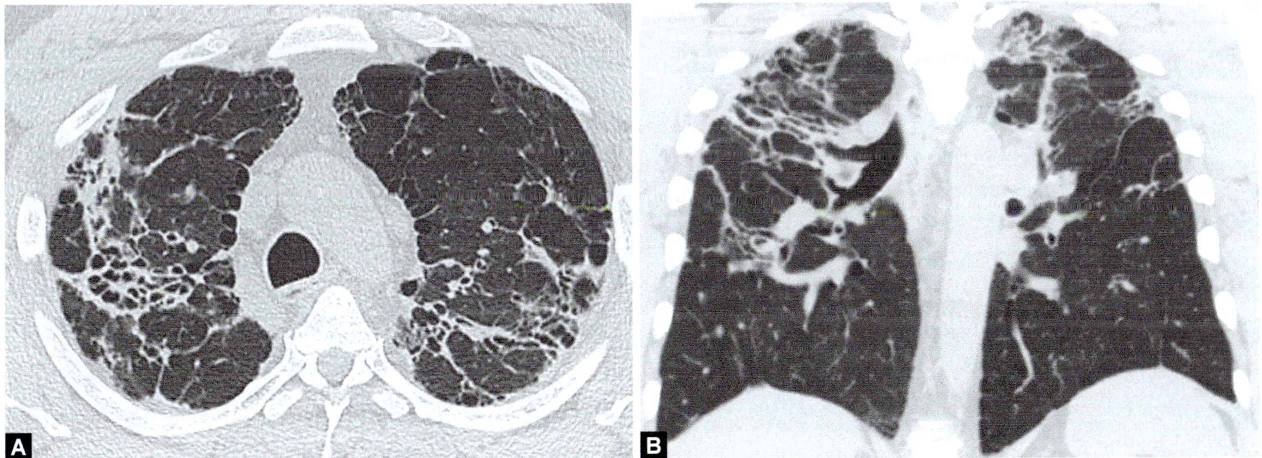

FIGS. 4A AND B: (A) Axial and (B) coronal images from noncontrast chest CT demonstrate upper lobe predominant bronchiectasis and architectural distortion with air trapping. There is upward and outward retraction of the right hilum. Mild paraseptal emphysema is also present.

subpleural sparing and ground-glass opacities, while the presence of honeycombing would favor the diagnosis of UIP.[14] The key defining feature of NSIP is uniformity of interstitial involvement that ranges from a nonfibrotic to a fibrosing process.[14] In SSc-ILD, findings include peripheral predominant ground-glass opacities with subpleural sparing and traction bronchiectasis that may be consistent with fibrotic NSIP **(Figs. 6A and B)**.

DIAGNOSIS

Various additional tools exist to aid in the diagnosis of ILD when it is suspected. The American Thoracic Society official practice guidelines recommend utilizing BAL to evaluate cell patterns and evaluate for infectious processes.[15] When the predominant macrophages include smoking-related inclusions, desquamative interstitial pneumonia or respiratory bronchiolitis-ILD (RB-ILD) would be suspected.[15] Predominance of lymphocytes suggests consideration of granulomatous disease, NSIP, drug reaction, lymphoid interstitial pneumonia, OP, or lymphoma.[15] An extremely elevated lymphocyte count is suggestive of HP.[11] Eosinophil predominance suggests eosinophilic pneumonia. Pathological examination of NSIP shows interstitial thickening by uniform fibrosis with preserved alveolar architecture and varying degrees of cellular inflammation consisting of lymphocytes and plasma cells.[14] Most patients demonstrate a fibrosing pattern of NSIP (84%).[14] In patients with fibrotic NSIP, histology demonstrates areas of interstitial fibrosis with enlarged airspaces which are indistinguishable from honeycombing.[14]

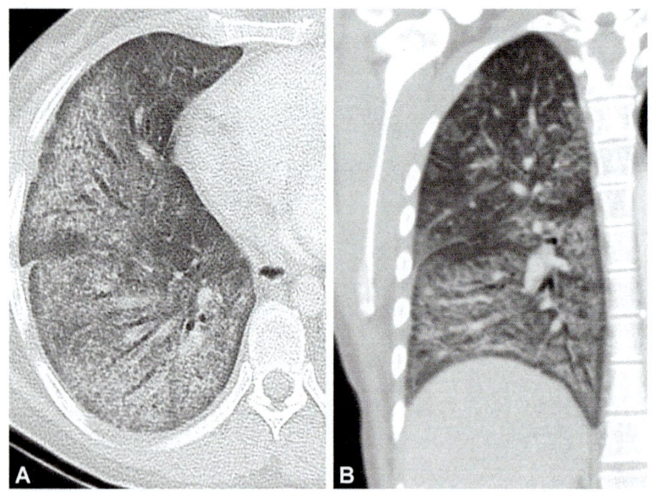

FIGS. 5A AND B: CT images of the lung in (A) axial and (B) coronal planes that demonstrate abnormal reticulation and traction bronchiectasis. There is conspicuous ground-glass opacity and subpleural sparing consistent with nonspecific interstitial pneumonia (NSIP).

Transbronchial lung biopsy procures small samples of tissue but is the initial procedure of choice in patients in whom small samples may be diagnostic, particularly bronchocentric diseases.[9] Transbronchial biopsy is not recommended in patients suspected of having IPF due to low diagnostic yield. Endobronchial biopsy in addition to transbronchial biopsy increases diagnostic yield in sarcoidosis.[9] Surgical lung biopsy may be performed when the diagnosis is uncertain in low-risk patients.[9] Consideration can be made for obtaining transbronchial cryobiopsy as an alternative to surgical lung biopsy. Referral to pulmonary rehabilitation is recommended by most societies.[16] Multidisciplinary discussion adds consensus to clinical diagnosis.[16]

Genetic Testing

Genetic testing in ILD is most frequently performed in the diagnosis of IPF or when there is clinical suspicion for a genetic disease such as Hermansky–Pudlak disease.[2] Immunological inflammation appears to be a more prominent pathogenesis in SSc-ILD, for instance, compared with IPF.[2] Genetic

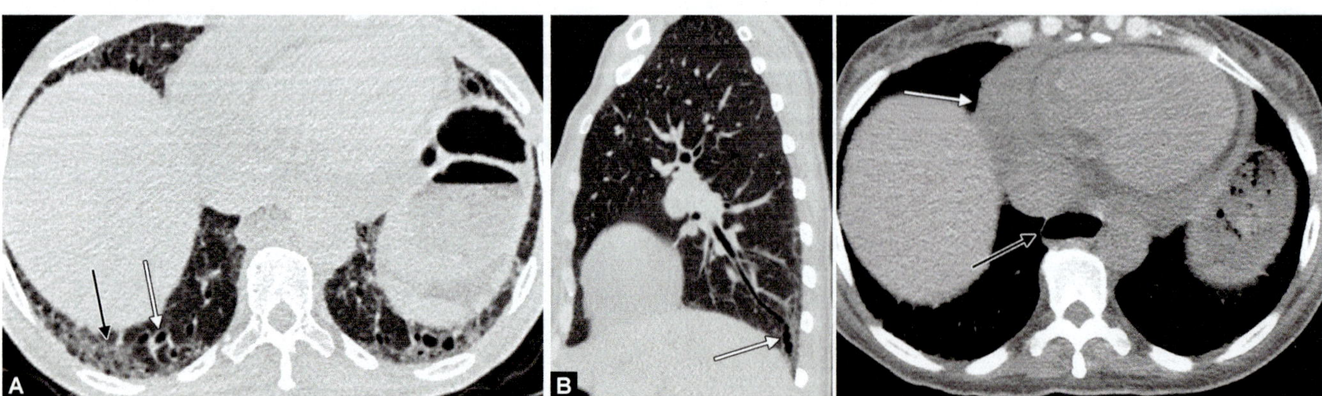

FIGS. 6A AND B: (A) Axial and (B) sagittal images from chest CT demonstrate subpleural and peripheral predominant ground-glass opacity (black arrow) with associated traction bronchiectasis (white arrows), consistent with fibrotic nonspecific interstitial pneumonia (NSIP). (Right) Axial CT image with soft-tissue windowing from the same patient with scleroderma demonstrates a dilated esophagus (black arrow) and a pericardial effusion (white arrow).

pathways that are affected in ILD include polymorphisms related to telomere length, surfactant biogenesis, cellular mitogenesis, and host defenses.[1] Telomere-related mutations are associated with IPF, including shortened telomeres or telomere-related mutations.[17] This association has not been established with other types of ILD. Telomere-related mutations have been found in 12% of rheumatoid arthritis-related ILD and are more common in pleuroparenchymal fibroelastosis.[17] In patients being considered for lung transplantation, genetic testing to evaluate for the presence of telomere-related mutations may confer prognostic value during post-transplantation and help guide immunosuppressive management.[17]

TREATMENT AND MANAGEMENT

Predominantly inflammatory ILDs compared with predominant fibrosing features require different management approaches, and ultimately, treatment is directed at the underlying pathophysiology. The principles of treatment include targeting active disease with medications and targeting symptomatic improvement. This can be achieved by utilizing supplemental oxygen or nighttime noninvasive ventilation, pulmonary rehabilitation, optimizing co-morbidities, and consideration for referral for lung transplantation **(Flowchart 2)**. Treatment of fibrotic HP includes prolonged corticosteroid therapy.[11]

Recent advances include the development of antifibrotic agents which were initially directed at treating IPF, namely nintedanib and pirfenidone.[18,19] **Table 1** lists commonly utilized medications for ILD, mechanisms of action of these medications, and several side effects.

Anti-inflammatory Medications

Several immunomodulatory therapies have been studied for the treatment of varying types of ILD.[18] Small, randomized trials have suggested that steroids lead to more rapid

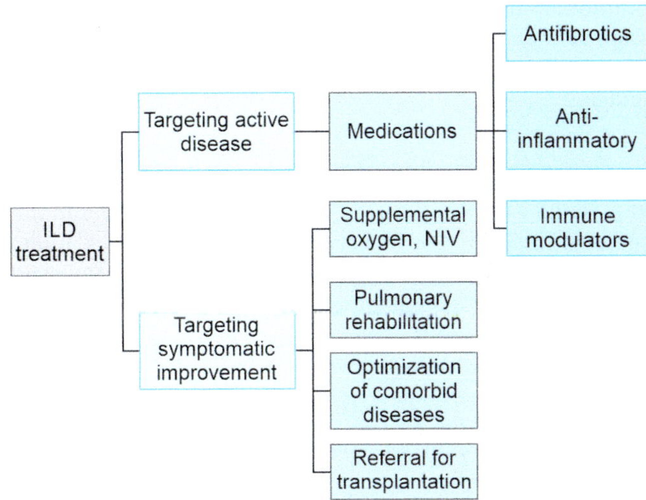

FLOWCHART 2: Suggested considerations for treatment of ILD.
(ILD: interstitial lung disease; NIV: noninvasive ventilation)

TABLE 1: Common medications utilized for the treatment of ILD with mechanism and common side effects.

Medication	Mechanism of action	Common side effects
Mycophenolate mofetil	*Immunosuppressive*: Inhibits inosine monophosphate dehydrogenase and exerts a cytostatic effect on lymphocytes	Nausea, vomiting, diarrhea, other gastrointestinal symptoms, pancytopenias
Cyclophosphamide	*Immunosuppressive*: Alkylating agent preventing cell division and decreasing DNA synthesis	Nausea, vomiting, diarrhea, bladder carcinoma, bone marrow suppression
Azathioprine	*Immunosuppressive*: Blocks pathway for purine synthesis and stops DNA replication	Nausea, vomiting, diarrhea, pancytopenias, rash, chronic immunosuppression
Rituximab	*Immunosuppressive*: Monoclonal antibody directed against CD20 antigen on B lymphocytes	Infusion-related reactions, progressive multifocal leukoencephalopathy, immune suppression, hepatitis B reactivation
Tacrolimus	*Immunosuppressive*: Inhibits T lymphocyte activation and suppresses cell immunity, preventing calcineurin phosphatase activity	Increased risk of infections and malignancy, nephrotoxicity, neurotoxicity, drug-induced thrombotic microangiopathy
Prednisone (or other corticosteroids)	*Anti-inflammatory*: Suppresses migration of polymorphonuclear leukocytes and reduces capillary permeability	Hyperglycemia, adrenal suppression, Cushing syndrome, GI side effects, increased risk of infections
Nintedanib	*Antifibrotic*: Tyrosine kinase inhibitor that blocks intracellular signaling of fibroblasts	Abdominal pain, nausea, vomiting, hepatotoxicity, pruritis, and skin rash
Pirfenidone	*Antifibrotic*: Decreases fibroblast proliferation and decreases production of fibrosis-associated proteins and cytokines	Abdominal pain, nausea, vomiting, hepatotoxicity, agranulocytosis, skin rash

improvement in FVC in patients with acute HP compared with placebo.[18] Other data is lacking for steroid use, though it remains the most common first-line treatment for many ILDs in clinical practice.[18] Cryptogenic OP should be treated with prolonged steroids weaned over 6–12 months.[9] ILD with polymyositis or dermatitis warrants early treatment with steroids and cyclophosphamide or other immunosuppressive to prevent disease progression.[9] Sarcoidosis, if mild, does not require treatment. Severe disease due to sarcoidosis requires steroids and immunosuppressives.[9] Comorbid pulmonary hypertension should be considered if there is a disproportionate abnormality on PFTs compared with the degree of pulmonary parenchymal abnormality seen on imaging.[9]

Antifibrotic Medications

The evidence for antifibrotics nintedanib and pirfenidone remains largely in IPF. However, their role and clinical utility has been increasingly recognized in fibrosing phenotypes of ILD, particularly inflammatory ILD which has progressed to a fibrotic phenotype.[18]

Nonpharmacological Management

Treatment of comorbid conditions including pulmonary hypertension, sleep-disordered breathing, and symptomatic management of dyspnea and cough are indicated.[4] Supplemental oxygen therapy is offered to patients with severe resting hypoxemia or exertional dyspnea associated with hypoxemia.[18] Other management strategies include referral for pulmonary rehabilitation, which is associated with short-term improvement in exercise endurance and quality of life.[18] Preventative medicine, including vaccination, is crucial. Multidisciplinary support including involvement of palliative care and referral to lung transplantation may be indicated.[18] Patients who meet selection criteria, usually including age younger than 65 years, should be referred to lung transplantation if the total lung capacity is lower than 40% of predicted or if there is progressive decline in FVC more than 10% or in FVC more than 15% at 6 months follow-up.[9]

Treatment of respiratory failure in ILD **(Flowchart 3)** is focused on supplemental oxygen via portable or home concentrators or rolling tanks or high-flow nasal cannula. Nighttime noninvasive positive-pressure ventilation can be used in patients who have obstructive sleep apnea or sleep-disordered breathing or in those with hypercapnia. Pulmonary rehabilitation and endurance and resistance training can increase 6MWT distance and improve quality of life.[20]

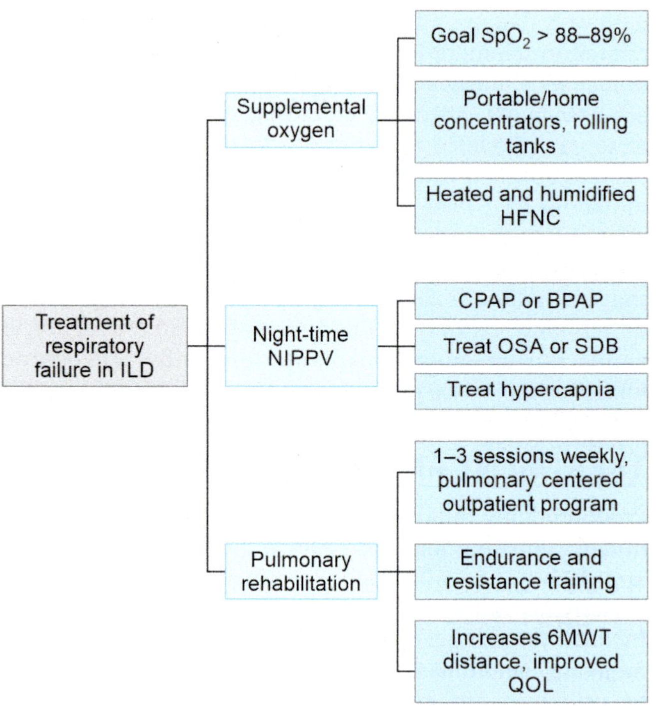

FLOWCHART 3: Treatment of respiratory failure in ILD.
(6MWT: 6-minute walk test; BPAP: bilevel positive airway pressure; CPAP: continuous positive airway pressure; HFNC: high-flow nasal cannula; ILD: interstitial lung disease; NIPPV: noninvasive positive-pressure ventilation; OSA: obstructive sleep apnea; QOL: quality of life; SDB: sleep-disordered breathing)

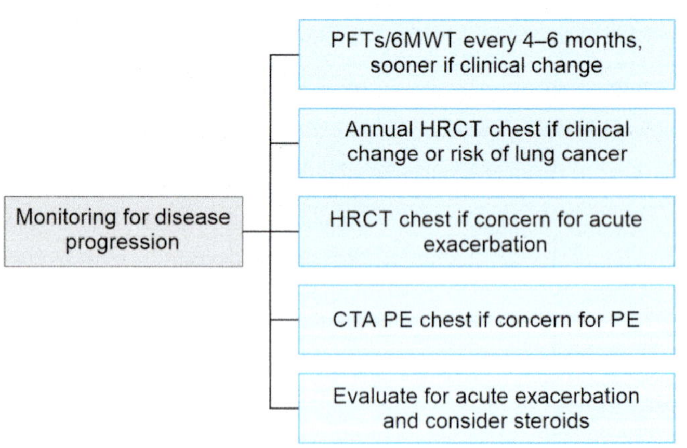

FLOWCHART 4: Suggested monitoring for ILD progression.
(6MWT: 6-minute walk test; CT PE: computed tomography pulmonary embolism protocol; HRCT: high-resolution CT chest; ILD: interstitial lung disease; PFT: pulmonary function test)

PROGNOSIS

The prognosis of ILD depends on the underlying phenotype of disease. Disease monitoring **(Flowchart 4)** is aimed at following pulmonary function and evaluating lung parenchyma via high-resolution imaging. PFTs and 6MWT can be repeated every 4–6 months or sooner if there is clinical change. Annual HRCT chest is indicated for surveillance or repeated sooner if there is clinical change concerning for acute exacerbation.[20] CT angiography (CTA) pulmonary embolism (PE) can be performed if there is concern for PE.[20] Correlation between the presence of COVID-19 and ILD demonstrated that patients with ILD who were hospitalized with COVID-19 were more likely to die compared to those without ILD.[19] Some forms of ILD such as exposure-related nonfibrotic HP may be reversible with exposure avoidance. Other forms of ILD are progressive and irreversible and associated with decline in lung function and ultimately death.[1] One study suggested that 52.4% of patients with UIP have a decline of 10% in FVC or more at 52 weeks, while 43.2% of patients with NSIP showed this decline. Risk factors for poor outcomes include lower baseline lung function, age above 60 years, need for oxygen supplementation, continued exposure to causative agent, underlying telomere shortening or dysfunction, loss of > 10% FVC in the prior year, and poor response to attempted therapy.[1]

ACUTE EXACERBATIONS OF INTERSTITIAL LUNG DISEASES

Acute exacerbation of ILD is adapted from the definition of acute exacerbation of IPF, which is defined as an acute, clinically significant deterioration without an identified cause **(Flowchart 5)**.[21] Acute exacerbations of ILD can be triggered by environmental exposures, viral or bacterial infections, PE, or inflammatory processes.[19] Management of acute exacerbations of ILD remains uncertain. Prospective trials and evidence are lacking to guide treatment.[19] Steroids remain the mainstay of treatment, though evidence is lacking for their efficacy.[19] Other medications like immunosuppressives, including medications such as tocilizumab, an anti-IL-6 receptor antibody, have limited evidence based on case reports and case series.[19] Acute exacerbations are more common in IPF and in ILD are associated with up to 50% 90-day mortality.[1] In acute exacerbations, clinicians must be careful to identify progressive pulmonary fibrosis as a phenotype of presentation of acute ILD exacerbations (see Chapters 110 and 111).

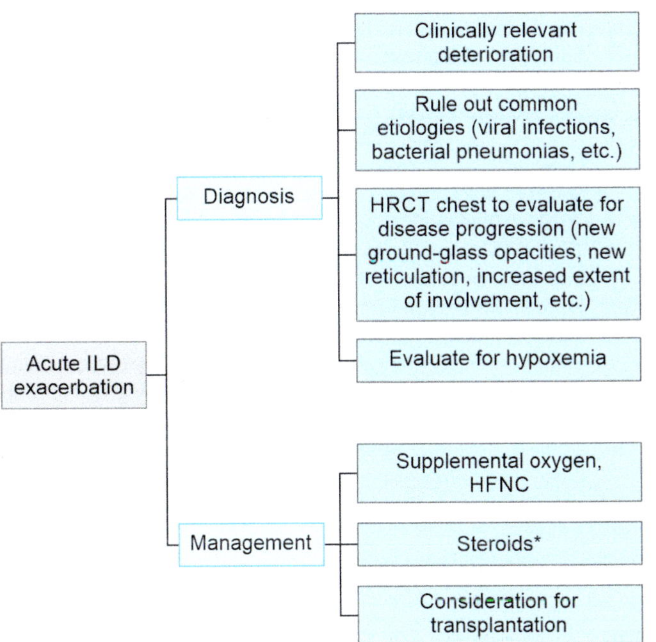

*Limited evidence for use of steroids in acute exacerbations of ILD, though this is the mainstay of treatment.

FLOWCHART 5: Suggested approach to acute ILD exacerbation.

(HFNC: high-flow nasal cannula; HRCT: high-resolution CT; ILD: interstitial lung disease)

SUMMARY

Interstitial lung diseases are a group of heterogenous diseases characterized by progressive clinical symptoms, decline in pulmonary function, and abnormalities on CT imaging. Obtaining a thorough exposure history is essential. Evaluation for underlying associated autoimmune disorders and consideration for genetic factors are important. Treatment of ILD is aimed at treating the underlying mechanism of disease and can include steroids, immunosuppressive therapy, or antifibrotics. Multidisciplinary discussions are essential for clinical consensus.

REFERENCES

1. Wijsenbeek M, Suzuki A, Maher TM. Interstitial lung diseases. Lancet. 2022;400(10354):769-86.
2. Grutters JC, du Bois RM. Genetics of fibrosing lung diseases. Eur Respir J. 2005;25(5):915-27.
3. Glazer CS, Newman LS. Occupational interstitial lung disease. Clin Chest Med. 2004;25(3):467-78, vi.
4. Mathai SC, Danoff SK. Management of interstitial lung disease associated with connective tissue disease. BMJ. 2016;352: h6819.
5. Borie R, Crestani B, Guyard A, et al. Interstitial lung disease in lysosomal storage disorders. Eur Respir Rev. 2021;30(160): 200363.
6. Shah Gupta R, Koteci A, Morgan A, et al. Incidence and prevalence of interstitial lung diseases worldwide: a systematic literature review. BMJ Open Respir Res. 2023;10(1):e001291.
7. Singh S, Collins BF, Sharma BB, et al. Interstitial Lung Disease in India. Results of a Prospective Registry. Am J Respir Crit Care Med. 2017;195(6):801-13.
8. Dhooria S, Sehgal IS, Agarwal R, et al. Incidence, prevalence, and national burden of interstitial lung diseases in India: Estimates from two studies of 3089 subjects. PLoS One. 2022;17(7):e0271665.
9. Wells AU, Denton CP. Interstitial lung disease in connective tissue disease—mechanisms and management. Nat Rev Rheumatol. 2014;10(12):728-39.
10. Koster MA, Thomson CC, Collins BF, et al. Diagnosis of Hypersensitivity Pneumonitis in Adults, 2020 Clinical Practice Guideline: Summary for Clinicians. Ann Am Thorac Soc. 2021;18(4):559-66.
11. Selman M, Pardo A, King TE Jr. Hypersensitivity pneumonitis: insights in diagnosis and pathobiology. Am J Respir Crit Care Med. 2012;186(4):314-24.

12. Fernández Pérez ER, Travis WD, Lynch DA, et al. Executive Summary: Diagnosis and Evaluation of Hypersensitivity Pneumonitis: CHEST Guideline and Expert Panel Report. Chest. 2021;160(2):595-615.
13. Crouser ED, Maier LA, Wilson KC, et al. Diagnosis and Detection of Sarcoidosis. An Official American Thoracic Society Clinical Practice Guideline. Am J Respir Crit Care Med. 2020;201(8):e26-e51.
14. Travis WD, Hunninghake G, King TE Jr, et al. Idiopathic nonspecific interstitial pneumonia: report of an American Thoracic Society project. Am J Respir Crit Care Med. 2008;177(12):1338-47.
15. Meyer KC, Raghu G, Baughman RP, et al. An official American Thoracic Society clinical practice guideline: the clinical utility of bronchoalveolar lavage cellular analysis in interstitial lung disease. Am J Respir Crit Care Med. 2012;185(9):1004-14.
16. Dodia N, Amariei D, Kenaa B, et al. A comprehensive assessment of environmental exposures and the medical history guides multidisciplinary discussion in interstitial lung disease. Respir Med. 2021;179:106333.
17. Courtwright AM, El-Chemaly S. Telomeres in Interstitial Lung Disease: The Short and the Long of It. Ann Am Thorac Soc. 2019;16(2):175-81.
18. Johannson KA, Chaudhuri N, Adegunsoye A, et al. Treatment of fibrotic interstitial lung disease: current approaches and future directions. Lancet. 2021;398(10309):1450-60.
19. Podolanczuk AJ, Wong AW, Saito S, et al. Update in Interstitial Lung Disease 2020. Am J Respir Crit Care Med. 2021;203(11):1343-52.
20. Raghu G, Remy-Jardin M, Ryerson CJ, et al. Diagnosis of Hypersensitivity Pneumonitis in Adults. An Official ATS/JRS/ALAT Clinical Practice Guideline. Am J Respir Crit Care Med. 2020;202(3):e36-e69.
21. Collard HR, Ryerson CJ, Corte TJ, et al. Acute exacerbation of Idiopathic Pulmonary Fibrosis: An international Working Group Report. Am J Respir Crit Care Med. 2016;194(3):265-75.

Interstitial Lung Abnormalities

CHAPTER 107

Zein Kattih, Hiroto Hatabu, Stephen Machnicki, Kevin K Brown, Suhail Raoof

INTRODUCTION

Interstitial lung abnormalities (ILA) are a collection of subtle parenchymal abnormalities seen on noncontrast computed tomography (CT) of the chest. These findings can be incidentally noted and used to be considered of unclear clinical significance. They may not have been observed or reported by the radiologist. Recent studies suggest that these abnormalities have clinical significance and are associated with health implications and adverse outcomes.[1-3] Thus, ILA is an important entity to define, and identification of ILA confers prognostic value.

DEFINITION AND CLASSIFICATION OF INTERSTITIAL LUNG ABNORMALITIES

Interstitial lung abnormality is a radiologic finding on CT chest imaging consisting of nondependent changes in >5% of any lung zone.[2] Lung zones are defined as upper, middle, and lower zones, and these zones are demarcated by the level of the inferior aortic arch and the right inferior pulmonary vein **(Fig. 1)**.[3] These radiologic abnormalities include ground-glass opacities, reticular abnormalities, traction bronchiectasis, nonemphysematous cysts, and honeycombing.[2] These findings are equivocal when they are focal and unilateral which would not define them as ILA.[2] Moreover, persistence on prone imaging is a requirement for diagnosis.[2] Nonemphysematous cysts are lucencies with irregular, well-defined walls, characteristics which distinguish them from both emphysema and honeycombing.[2]

Interstitial lung abnormalities as a diagnosis can only be applied to patients who do not have a history that is suggestive of an increased risk for interstitial lung disease (ILD). These risk factors include occupational exposures, history or symptoms of connective tissue disease (CTD), and history of familial interstitial diseases or abnormalities.[3] Patients who are identified to have these abnormalities on CT chest are then categorized clinically.[3] In patients who are symptomatic, a diagnosis of ILA cannot be made. These patients will be diagnosed with preclinical or subclinical ILD. In patients at high risk of ILD who are asymptomatic, the diagnosis of ILA cannot be made, and these patients will be diagnosed with early ILD.[2] Patients who are asymptomatic and who are not at high risk of ILD based on clinical history are diagnosed with ILA.

Interstitial lung abnormality has been classified into nonsubpleural nonfibrotic, subpleural nonfibrotic, and subpleural fibrotic subtypes.[2] Subpleural fibrotic ILA is characterized by a predominance of subpleural reticular abnormalities that may or may not be associated with architectural distortion. These abnormalities are associated with fibrotic changes such as honeycombing, traction bronchiectasis, or bronchiectasis.[2] ILA with a nonsubpleural pattern does not usually progress.[2] Subpleural fibrotic ILA is more frequently associated with worsened morbidity and mortality.[2]

Pathologic correlation with CT imaging findings of ILA remains rarely described in the literature. When evaluated, histopathology may reveal areas of fibrotic changes or findings consistent with usual interstitial pneumonia.[2]

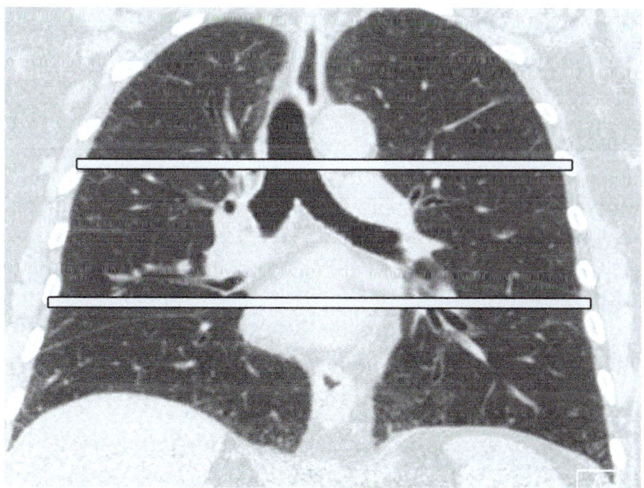

FIG. 1: Upper, middle, and lower lung zones. These lung zones are demarcated by the level of the inferior aortic arch and the right inferior pulmonary vein (white lines). Reticulations are present in the lower lung zone and comprise <5% of the lung zone, consistent with interstitial lung abnormalities (ILA).

INCIDENCE AND RISK FACTORS

Overall, general population cohort studies suggest a 10% incidence of ILA with a mean age of 70 years.[4] The incidence of ILA correlates with age.[5] There is a 4% incidence of ILA in patients younger than 60 years of age, and that incidence increases to 47% in patients older than 70 years of age.[5] Smoking is a risk factor for ILA, and the incidence of ILA in smokers is 4–9% overall and 17% in smokers over the age of 60 years.[5] The incidence of ILA in patients with stage IV lung cancer was reported to be about 3.9% in one study.[6] Various risk factors have been described for ILA that confer an increased likelihood of clinical progression.[3] A history of smoking, history of occupational exposures, and progressive decline of pulmonary lung function are all risk factors for clinical progression of ILA.[5] Other risk factors have been described in cohort and population studies. One study in a population of asymptomatic patients over 60 years of age and enrolled in a lung aging program demonstrated a correlation between increased serum concentrations of the minor allele frequency of the MUC5B promoter polymorphism and ILA.[4] There was also a significant association between resisting levels and ILA.[4] Other serum markers including matrix metalloproteinase-7 (MMP-7), interleukin 6, galectin-3, and common promoter polymorphism in MUC5B have all been associated with a risk of developing ILA.[7]

Longitudinal studies suggest that up to 40% of ILA will progress when evaluated over the ensuing 5-year period.[8]

IMAGING

Imaging Modalities

High-resolution computed tomography (HRCT) is the modality of choice to identify ILA.[2] However, ILA can also be incidentally identified on low-dose computed tomography (LDCT) performed for screening for lung cancer. Densitometry has been utilized to assess the proportion of high attenuation areas between -660 and -250 Hounsfield units.[3] Normal lung attenuation is around −750 Hounsfield units, and those with −250 Hounsfield units may signify lung consolidation.[3] Computer-aided detection and quantification techniques have also been attempted to quantify ILA. Greater computer-aided detection percentage fibrosis extent in patients with lung cancer predicted worse disease-free survival.[9] Prone imaging is especially relevant to this diagnosis to distinguish ILA from dependent atelectasis.[2]

Imaging Findings

Typical findings of ILA include ground-glass opacities, reticulations, traction bronchiectasis or architectural distortion, honeycombing, and nonemphysematous cysts. These abnormalities must take up more than 5% of the CT chest to be considered significant.[2] It is important to identify mimics of ILA that may suggest an alternative diagnosis. These include diffuse centrilobular nodularity, dependent lung abnormalities that resolve when prone imaging is obtained, osteophyte-related paraspinal fibrosis, interlobular septal thickening, focal unilateral abnormalities, and pleural parenchymal fibroelastosis.[2] Identification of these abnormalities should prompt evaluation for a process that is not ILA.

Interstitial lung abnormalities have been classified into nonsubpleural nonfibrotic **(Fig. 2)**, subpleural nonfibrotic **(Fig. 3)**, and subpleural fibrotic **(Fig. 4)**.[2] Nonsubpleural nonfibrotic ILA is that without subpleural localization and with the typical findings of ILA and progresses slowly

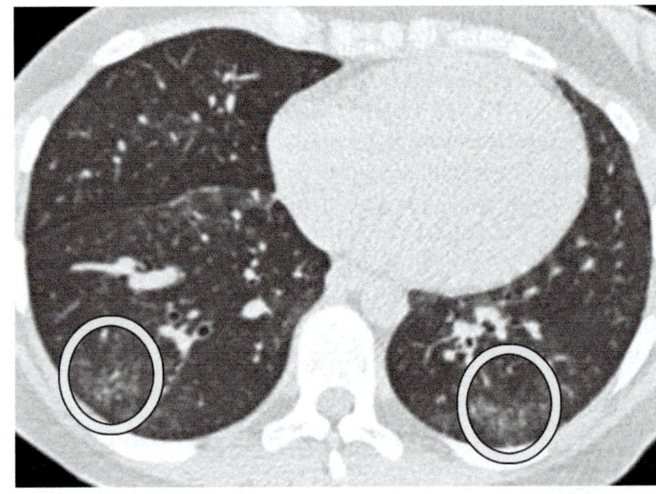

FIG. 2: Axial CT image from a 62-year-old female smoker demonstrates areas of ground-glass opacity centrally in both lungs (white circle) consistent with nonsubpleural nonfibrotic interstitial lung abnormalities (ILA).

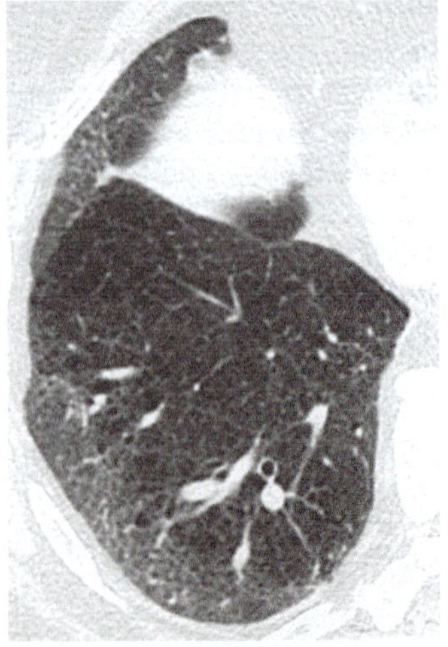

FIG. 3: Axial CT image through the right lung base demonstrates peripheral ground-glass opacity consistent with subpleural fibrotic interstitial lung abnormalities (ILA).

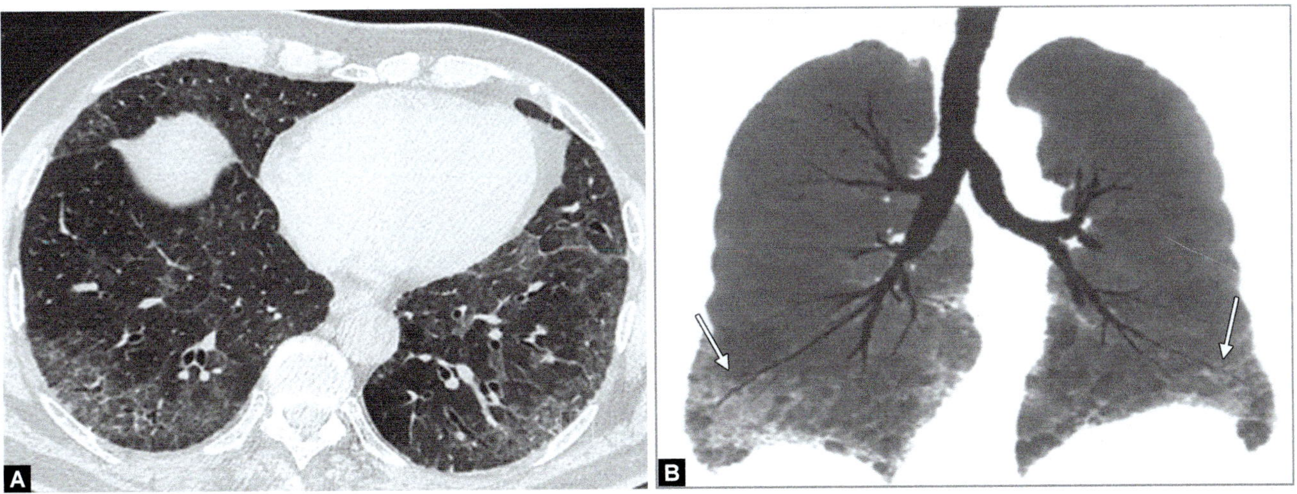

FIGS. 4A AND B: Images from dedicated follow-up chest CT of a 78-year-old male who had undergone a CT scan of the abdomen and pelvis for complaint of abdominal pain and had abnormalities noted at the lung bases. (A) Axial image through lung bases demonstrates subpleural and basilar predominant ground-glass opacity, reticulation, and traction bronchiectasis. These findings portend a worse prognosis compared with ground-glass changes. (B) Coronal minimum intensity projection (MinIP) image demonstrates the traction bronchiectasis (arrows).

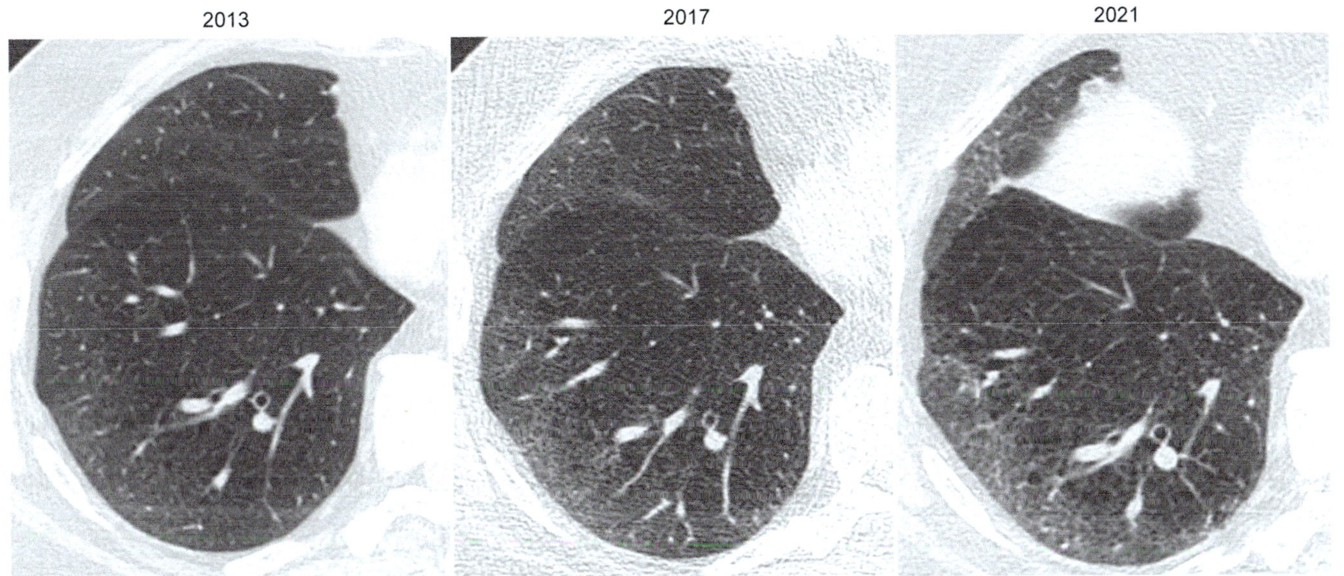

FIG. 5: Subpleural ground-glass opacity demonstrated on axial CT chest progressing slowly over 8 years.

(Fig. 5).[3] Subpleural fibrotic ILA is characterized by predominance of subpleural reticular abnormalities that are associated with architectural distortion and fibrotic changes such as honeycombing or traction bronchiectasis.[2] Extensive honeycombing/reticulation with clinical symptoms is not consistent with ILA and is instead consistent with ILD **(Figs. 6A and B)**. These classifications provide insight into the risk of progression of ILA.

CLINICAL OUTCOMES

Interstitial Lung Abnormality Progression

Several cohort studies have attempted to correlate ILA radiologic progression with physiologic progression. The definition of progression has been poorly defined. Current

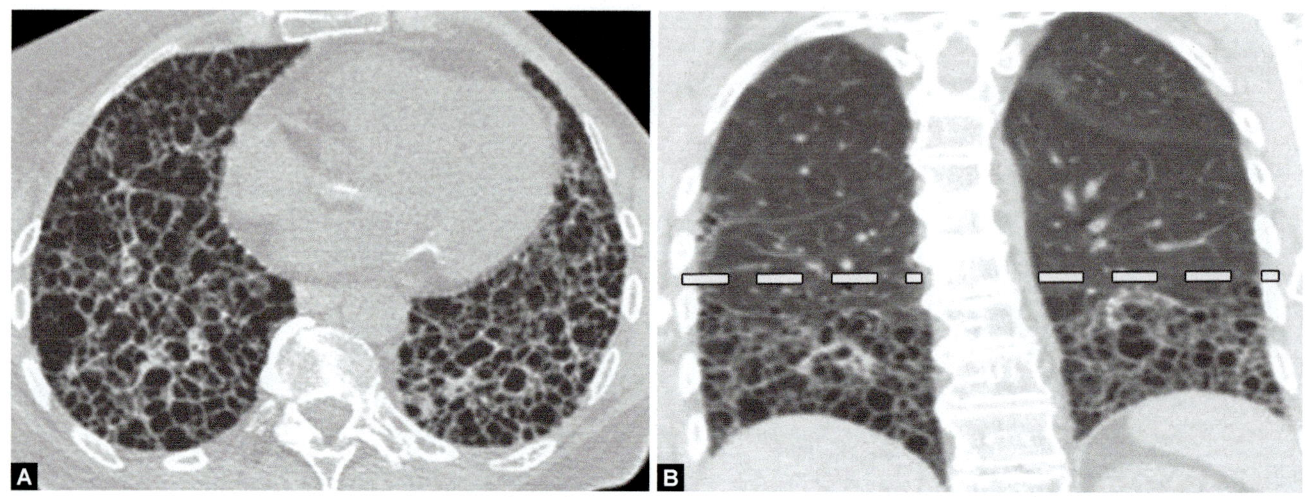

FIGS. 6A AND B: (A) Axial and (B) coronal CT images from a 74-year-old female demonstrate exuberant honeycombing at the lung bases bilaterally. There is a straight upper edge of the honeycombing on the coronal image (dashed lines). These findings are suggestive of CTD-associated ILD and not consistent with ILA. The patient was found to have rheumatoid arthritis.

standards suggest that progression is present when patients meet two of three criteria. These criteria are decline of pulmonary function tests [either > 10% decline in forced vital capacity (FVC), >15% decline in diffusing capacity for carbon monoxide (DLCO), or a 50-m decline in 6-minute walk distance (6MWD)], an initiation or worsening of respiratory symptoms, and an increase of >30% of lesions compared to a previous HRCT or the appearance of new lesions.[4] When two of these three criteria were present, patients were categorized as having ILA progression.

In the Framingham study, ILA radiologic progression correlated with accelerated decline of FVC compared to patients without ILA.[8] Compared with the normal physiologic decline of 30 mL/yr of FVC expected in normal populations with age, patients with ILA and evidence of radiologic progression had a 60 mL/yr FVC decline.[8] Overall, FVC was 9% lower in ILA patients and DLCO was 12% lower in ILA patients when compared to a cohort of similar patients without ILA.[8] In contrast, patients with IPF have an annual decline of about 200 mL/yr.[8]

The reported rate of progression of ILA varies widely between 20 and 48%.[3] A study of the National Lung Screening Trial (NLST) cohort found a progression rate of 20% over 2 years,[10] and the AGES-Reykjavik study found a progression rate of 48% over 5 years.[3] In patients with COPD and ILA, there was over a two times increased risk of exacerbation compared to patients without ILA.[11] In this cohort of COPD patients, the decline in forced expiratory volume in 1 second (FEV1) was significantly sharper in patients with ILA compared with those without ILA.[11] ILA occurred with COPD in 40.5% of patients.[11] Patients with ILA and COPD had lower baseline FEV1, FVC, DLCO, and 6MWD compared to those without ILA.[11]

Mortality

The presence of ILA on imaging is associated with a higher rate of all-cause mortality.[12] These mortality rates remain lower than those mortality rates in clinically significant pulmonary fibrosis like in diseases such as idiopathic pulmonary fibrosis (IPF). In smokers, particularly, the presence of ILA is associated with increased all-cause mortality with a hazard ratio (HR) of 2.0.[5] This increase in all-cause mortality persisted even in patients without lung cancer with a HR of 1.6.[5] This association remained regardless of the ILA subclassification, and this increase was only partly attributable to an increased risk of lung cancer and nonpulmonary malignancies.[5] Several other cohort studies have attempted to evaluate the correlation of ILA with mortality.[8,12,5,13] In the general population, the Framingham Heart Study found a HR of 2.7 [95% confidence interval (CI) 1.1-6.5] for all-cause mortality in patients with ILA compared with those without ILA.[8] Similarly in the AGES-Reykjavik study, there was 1.3 (95% CI 1.2–1.4) HR for all-cause mortality in patients with ILA compared to those without ILA after use of adjusted Cox proportional hazard model to adjust for confounders such as age, sex, body mass index, pack-years of smoking, and current or former smoking status.[12] In populations of smokers being screened through lung cancer screening programs too, this association between ILA and all-cause mortality is present. In the COPDGene study, HR is 1.8 (95% CI 1.1–2.8) for all-cause mortality in patients with ILA,[5] and in the ECLIPSE study, HR is 1.4 (95% CI 1.1–2.0).[12] In these patients with COPD, there is an associated between ILA and more frequent exacerbations of COPD as well as more rapid decline in FEV1 and FVC.[11] ILA is also associated with increased mortality in patients with severe aortic stenosis who undergo transcatheter aortic valve replacement.[14] A recent meta-analysis suggested a pooled mortality risk higher in patients with ILA compared to those without with an odds ratio of 3.56 over a medial follow-up of 5 years.[15] The prevalence in this meta-analysis was 7% in lung cancer screening studies and an overall pooled prevalence of 10%.[15]

Association with Lung Cancer

The presence of ILA on imaging has been associated with an increased incidence of lung cancer. The AGES-Reykjavik study found a HR of 2.77 (95% CI 1.76–4.36) in ILA patients compared with patients with ILA for the development of lung cancer.[12] A cohort study from the NLST found an incidence rate ratio of 1.33 (95% CI 1.07–1.65) in patients with ILA compared to those without.[16] This study of over 53,000 patients from 33 medical centers in the United States noted a 20.2% incidence of ILA on baseline LDCT imaging.[16] There were 2% lung cancer cases in the ILA group compared with 1.5% cases in the non-ILA group before adjusting for the presence of radiologic emphysema.[16] Lung cancer deaths were higher in the ILA group compared with the non-ILA group, 1.3% versus 0.8%, respectively, with a HR of 1.82 (CI 1.37–2.42).[16] The overall survival in patients with stage IV non-small-cell lung cancer (NSCLC) and with ILA is shorter compared to those without ILA.[6] Patients with lung cancer and ILA have an increased risk of chemotherapy-associated drug toxicity, extensive radiation pneumonitis, and acute lung injury post surgery.[17-19] In treatment-naive patients with advanced-stage NSCLC too, the overall survival is decreased in patients with ILA compared to those without ILA.[18]

In patients with subclinical ILD, defined as ILD which is untreated and oxygen-free, who were treated with stereotactic body radiation therapy (SBRT) for NSCLC or metastatic lung tumors, one study found no significant correlation between subclinical ILD and grade 2 through grade 5 radiation pneumonitis.[17] However, in these patients, the rate of extension of radiation pneumonitis was higher in patients with subclinical ILD compared to those without.[17] Moreover, preexisting radiologic ILA was associated with an increased risk of grade 2 or higher radiation pneumonitis at 1 year in patients with small cell lung cancer receiving thoracic radiation therapy.[19] In early-stage NSCLC, the presence of ILA on CT chest was a predictor of postoperative pulmonary complications in otherwise healthy, elderly patients.[20] Moreover, the incidence of immunotherapy-associated ILD, specifically anti-PD-1 antibodies such as nivolumab or pembrolizumab, was higher in patients with ILA compared to those without ILA.[21] Those at higher risk were those with ground-glass opacities which suggest a lymphocytic infiltration in these patients, and these medications cause lymphocyte proliferation.[21] In general, patients with preexisting ILA given radiation therapy are at a higher risk of progression and IPF.

DISEASE MONITORING

Current guidelines do not outline specific interval follow-up for patients identified to have ILA. Published algorithmic approaches suggest all ILA patients receive risk factor reduction counseling and guidance.[3] All patients should be screened for potential correlations by history including any smoking, inhalational exposures, drug toxicities, occult systemic diseases, recurrent aspirations, acid reflux symptoms, or other similar symptoms. Patients should also be screened with CTD labwork in those with relevant history. When ILAs are identified, patients can be classified into those at high risk of progression when fibrotic changes are present and those at low risk when those changes are not present.[2] Moreover, patients should be reassessed for clinical symptoms and radiologic progression at regular intervals.[2] Consideration for a first clinical follow-up at 3–12 months after initial identification is suggested.[2] Repeat CT chest imaging can be performed at 12–24 months after initial identification of ILA or sooner if there is concern for or evidence of clinical progression.[3] In patients with ILA who are undergoing surgery or immunotherapy, clinicians should be aware of the increased risk of acute exacerbation of acceleration in these patients.[2]

SUMMARY

Interstitial lung abnormality describes radiologic abnormalities on CT imaging that are diagnosed incidentally who are not at high risk for ILD. They are correlated with age and smoking status, and about 40% of these patients will show progression of ILA within 5 years of identification. The presence of ILA is associated with increased morbidity and mortality. Identification and monitoring of ILA is clinically relevant, particularly subpleural fibrotic ILA which is associated with progression and worsened morbidity and mortality.

REFERENCES

1. Hatabu H, Hunninghake GM, Lynch DA. Interstitial Lung Abnormality: Recognition and Perspectives. Radiology. 2019; 291(1):1-3.
2. Hatabu H, Hunninghake GM, Richeldi L, et al. Interstitial lung abnormalities detected incidentally on CT: a position paper from the Fleischner Society. Lancet Respir Med. 2020;8(7):726-37.
3. Hata A, Schiebler ML, Lynch DA, et al. Interstitial Lung Abnormalities: State of the Art. Radiology. 2021;301(1):19-34.
4. Buendía-Roldán I, Fernandez R, Mejía M, et al. Risk factors associated with the development of interstitial lung abnormalities. Eur Respir J. 2021;58(2):2003005.

5. Hoyer N, Wille MMW, Thomsen LH, et al. Interstitial lung abnormalities are associated with increased mortality in smokers. Respir Med. 2018;136:77-82.
6. Araki T, Dahlberg SE, Hida T, et al. Interstitial lung abnormality in stage IV non-small cell lung cancer: A validation study for the association with poor clinical outcome. Eur J Radiol Open. 2019;6:128-31.
7. Hunninghake GM, Hatabu H, Okajima Y, et al. MUC5B promoter polymorphism and interstitial lung abnormalities. N Engl J Med. 2013;368:2192-200.
8. Araki T, Putman RK, Hatabu H, et al. Development and Progression of Interstitial Lung Abnormalities in the Framingham Heart Study. Am J Respir Crit Care Med. 2016;194(12):1514-22.
9. Iwasawa T, Okudela K, Takemura T, et al. Computer-aided Quantification of Pulmonary Fibrosis in Patients with Lung Cancer: Relationship to Disease-free Survival. Radiology. 2019; 292(2):489-98.
10. Jin GY, Lynch D, Chawla A, et al. Interstitial lung abnormalities in a CT lung cancer screening population: prevalence and progression rate. Radiology. 2013;268(2):563-71.
11. Lee TS, Jin KN, Lee HW, et al. Interstitial Lung Abnormalities and the Clinical Course in Patients with COPD. Chest. 2021;159(1): 128-37.
12. Putman RK, Hatabu H, Araki T, et al. Evaluation of COPD Longitudinally to Identify Predictive Surrogate Endpoints (ECLIPSE) Investigators; COPDGene Investigators. Association between Interstitial Lung Abnormalities and All-cause Mortality. JAMA. 2016;315(7):672-81.
13. Gudmundsson G, Putman RK, Araki T, et al. Interstitial lung abnormalities in the AGES-Reykjavik study. Eur Resp J. 2016;48 (Suppl 60):PA798.
14. Kadoch M, Kitich A, Alqalyoobi S, et al. Interstitial lung abnormality is prevalent and associated with worse outcome in patients undergoing transcatheter aortic valve replacement. Respir Med. 2018;137:55-60.
15. Grant-Orser A, Min B, Elmrayed S, et al. Prevalence, Risk Factors, and Outcomes of Adult Interstitial Lung Abnormalities: A Systematic Review and Meta-analysis. Am J Respir Crit Care Med. 2023;208(6):695-708.
16. Whittaker Brown SA, Padilla M, Mhango G, et al. Interstitial Lung Abnormalities and Lung Cancer Risk in the National Lung Screening Trial. Chest. 2019;156(6):1195-203.
17. Yamaguchi S, Ohguri T, Ide S, et al. Stereotactic body radiotherapy for lung tumors in patients with subclinical interstitial lung disease: the potential risk of extensive radiation pneumonitis. Lung Cancer. 2013;82(2):260-5.
18. Nishino M, Cardarella S, Dahlberg SE, et al. Interstitial lung abnormalities in treatment-naïve advanced non-small-cell lung cancer patients are associated with shorter survival. Eur J Radiol. 2015;84(5):998-1004.
19. Li F, Zhou Z, Wu A, et al. Preexisting radiological interstitial lung abnormalities are a risk factor for severe radiation pneumonitis in patients with small-cell lung cancer after thoracic radiation therapy. Radiat Oncol. 2018;13(1):82.
20. Im Y, Park HY, Shin S, et al. Prevalence of and risk factors for pulmonary complications after curative resection in otherwise healthy elderly patients with early stage lung cancer. Respir Res. 2019;20(1):136.
21. Nakanishi Y, Masuda T, Yamaguchi K, et al. Pre-existing interstitial lung abnormalities are risk factors for immune checkpoint inhibitor-induced interstitial lung disease in non-small cell lung cancer. Respir Investig. 2019;57:451-9.

Connective Tissue Disease-Interstitial Lung Disease

CHAPTER 108

Simon Meredith, Joseph Parambil, Kevin K Brown, Dominick Guerrero, Stephen Machnicki, Suhail Raoof

INTRODUCTION

The interstitial lung diseases (ILD) are a large group of pulmonary disorders, pathologically characterized by varying degrees of chronic inflammation and fibrosis. Within the large number of causes and associations, the autoimmune-mediated connective tissue diseases (CTD) are among the most common.[1-3] Among the CTD, those that commonly affect the lungs are systemic sclerosis (SSc), rheumatoid arthritis (RA), dermatomyositis (DM), polymyositis (PM), Sjögren syndrome (SS), systemic lupus erythematosus (SLE), and mixed connective tissue disease (MCTD).[4]

While the histologic and chest imaging pattern of lung involvement is often distinct from idiopathic pulmonary fibrosis (IPF), there can be significant overlap.[5] The most common patterns are nonspecific interstitial pneumonia (NSIP) and usual interstitial pneumonia (UIP). Given the ability of CTD-ILD to mimic IPF, and as the overall prognosis of CTD-ILD is significantly better, current guidelines recommend that all patients with a fibrosing ILD be screened for an underlying CTD.[6] In this chapter, we will review the underlying CTDs most commonly seen in ILD patients, their respective high resolution computed tomography (HRCT) and pathological findings, and general approach to treatment.

PATHOGENESIS

The mechanism of lung injury in CTD-ILD is unknown. However, it is recognized that the underlying disordered immune system can lead to an inflammatory injury with subsequent aberrant repair. This appears to differ from the noninflammatory fibrosis that characterizes IPF. As mentioned in previous chapters, this fibrosis appears to begin with injury to the alveolar epithelial cell membrane causing release of profibrotic cytokines and infiltration by fibroblasts and myofibroblasts.[7-9] The combination of these processes results in deposition of extracellular matrix.

Genetic mutations that lead to telomere shortening and the overexpression of the MUC5B protein may play a role in the development and progression of certain forms of CTD-ILD.[10-13] These mutations have been most commonly identified in RA-associated ILD and less commonly in SSc-associated ILD.[14]

Autoantibodies appear to play a significant role in CTD-ILD specifically in RA, SSc, and myositis related-ILDs.[15] The autoantibodies are found to be in association with infiltrating lymphocytes and plasma cells in the lung tissue that cause tissue injury. The resultant injury stimulates fibroblasts' accumulation and prime further the fibrotic cascade.[16-18]

RHEUMATOID ARTHRITIS

Rheumatoid arthritis is a systemic CTD with typical articular manifestations and pathologically characterized by cellular infiltration of the joint. It is associated with both genetic ["shared epitopes" in class II major histocompatibility complex (MHC) region or human leukocyte antigen (HLA)-DRB1 alleles] and environmental risk factors such as exposure to tobacco smoke. Autoantibodies are a common, but not a universal feature of the disease, and include rheumatoid factor and antibodies against post-translationally modified proteins like citrullination [anti-citrullinated protein antibody (ACPA)].

Pulmonary involvement is a common systemic feature and can include pleural, airway, pulmonary vasculature, and parenchymal involvement.[19] This section will focus on lung parenchymal involvement in ILD seen in different kinds of CTDs. Both SSc and inflammatory myopathies exhibit parenchymal and vascular involvement more commonly. Pleural and airway involvement is more commonly seen in RA and to some extent in MCTD.[20]

The diagnosis of RA-ILD requires a multidisciplinary approach involving radiologists, pathologists, rheumatologists, and pulmonologists. As clinically significant ILD can complicate RA both years after and years before the diagnosis, both patients with known RA and those who present with an apparent idiopathic interstitial pneumonia are at risk. The workup begins with chest imaging and pulmonary physiology. Physiology typically demonstrates a restrictive defect with a reduction in forced vital capacity (FVC) and a reduction in diffusion capacity of the lung for carbon monoxide (DLCO). On chest imaging, four major patterns can be seen on HRCT of the chest. These include UIP (37%) **(Fig. 1)**, NSIP (30%) **(Fig. 2)**, obliterative bronchiolitis (17%) **(Figs. 3A and B)**, and organizing pneumonia (OP) **(Fig. 4)** (8%).[21-24] The UIP pattern is the most common in RA-ILD and is characterized by subpleural basilar predominant reticulation with traction bronchiectasis and focal honeycombing.[24,25] The NSIP pattern is also seen and is characterized by basilar predominant ground glass with or without associated reticulations, usually with subpleural sparing and lack of honeycombing.[25,26] Since tobacco smoking history is common, emphysema is often seen on HRCT with combined pulmonary fibrosis and emphysema in nearly 50% of the RA-ILD patients **(Fig. 1)**.[26]

After obtaining chest imaging and determining the pattern present, the next step is determining the need for lung biopsy. When the HRCT of the chest pattern is determined to be UIP, it is well documented that surgical lung biopsy (SLB) is not needed, as the radiologic pattern is highly correlated with its histopathologic counterpart.[27,28] In cases of chest imaging patterns other than UIP, the risk and benefits of lung biopsy must be weighed. In cases where the clinical and serological diagnosis strongly points toward RA-ILD, lung biopsy is not necessary to determine the diagnosis. However, in cases where the lung injury precedes the articular or other clinical features of the underlying CTD (10–20% of patients), lung biopsy may be useful.[29-32] This is predicated on patient preference and the associated risks of the procedure chosen. Lung biopsy, either surgical or via transbronchial cryobiopsy, may show typical histopathological features and/or features.

SYSTEMIC SCLEROSIS

Systemic sclerosis is a systemic autoimmune disease that affects many organ systems including the skin, gastrointestinal tract, kidneys, heart, as well as the lungs with fibrosis and vascular changes.[30-33] Autoantibodies are common and include antinuclear antibodies accompanied with anti-topoisomerase I (anti-Scl-70), anti-Th/To, anti-U3 ribonucleoprotein (RNP), anti-U11/U12 RNP, or occasionally anticentromere antibodies.[34-36] The most common pulmonary presentations of SSc are fibrotic lung disease and/or pulmonary arterial hypertension. These two complications account for 60% of SSc-associated deaths.

The workup of a patient suspected of having SSc-ILD includes pulmonary function testing (PFT), HRCT imaging of the chest, and possible lung biopsy. The most common HRCT pattern in SSc-ILD patients is fibrotic NSIP **(Fig. 5)**. While NSIP is the most common pattern, in up to one third of SSc-ILD patients, a UIP pattern may be seen. PFT is also important in monitoring progression. PFTs typically demonstrate a reduction in FVC with reduction in DLCO.

Determination of the need for lung biopsy is based on combining the clinical context with HRCT and PFT. If the underlying diagnosis of CTD is unclear or other important diagnostic possibilities are in the differential, then lung biopsy may be needed for histologic pattern confirmation and treatment planning.

IDIOPATHIC INFLAMMATORY MYOPATHIES

Polymyositis and DM are inflammatory myopathies that present with a constellation of muscular pain and weakness, with skin involvement in the form of a distinctive rash. Autoantibodies occur in 50% of cases and are classified as myositis-specific antibodies (MSAs) or myositis-associated antibodies (MAAs). Nearly 93% of patients with myositis-related ILD will have MSA antibodies present.[37-39] The MSAs that are most commonly associated with pulmonary involvement are the antisynthetase antibodies, with the most common being anti Jo-1 and occasionally anti-PL-7 and anti-PL-12. Autoantibodies against RNA helicase encoded by melanoma differentiation-associated gene 5 (anti-MDA-5) needs to be recognized as these patients often present with rapidly progressing ILD.[26,40-43] AntiMDA-5 positive patients often present with amyopathic DM and typically have skin findings of a heliotrope rash and/or Gottron's papules and can have ischemic skin necrosis. These patients also have worse outcomes due to the rapid progression of their lung disease. Antibodies associated with a poor prognosis are given in **Table 1**. ILD is common with 20–40% of patients presenting with ILD, with pulmonary manifestations preceding musculoskeletal manifestations in a significant number of patients.

The diagnosis of myositis-associated ILD is made by combining the clinical features with HRCT findings, PFTs, and lung biopsy findings (if needed). Typical HRCT patterns **(Fig. 6)** in these patients are NSIP **(Fig. 2)** and OP **(Fig. 3)** or a mixture of the two—NSIP + OP. A UIP pattern can be seen in these patients but is less common.[44] Physiologic findings are similar to the other CTD, with a restrictive ventilatory defect and a reduction in gas transfer.

SJÖGREN SYNDROME AND MIXED CONNECTIVE TISSUE DISEASE

Two final diseases that can manifest with ILD are SS and MCTD.[45,46] SS usually demonstrates the presence of anti-SSA/Ro and anti-SSB/La antibodies,[45] while MCTD is defined serologically by the presence of anti-U1 antibodies.[45] Pulmonary involvement occurs in 75% of MCTD patients and similar to SSc, ILD and pulmonary hypertension are the most common manifestations.

The HRCT findings for both diseases are similar with the most common chest imaging pattern reported being NSIP;

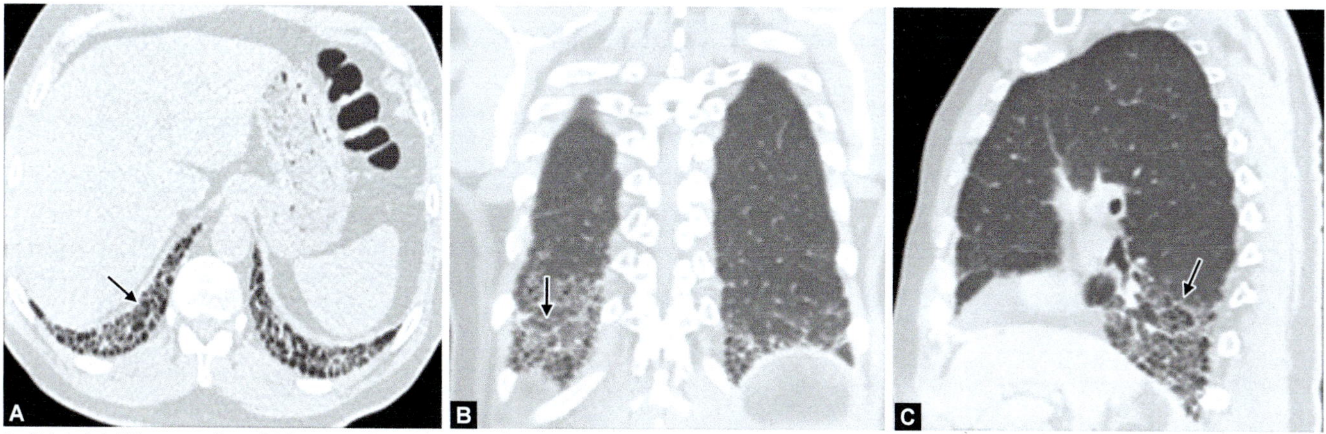

I. (A) Axial, (B) coronal, and (C) sagittal CT images of the lungs demonstrate subpleural and basilar predominant honeycombing, traction bronchiectasis, and irregular reticulation (arrows), consistent with a UIP pattern.

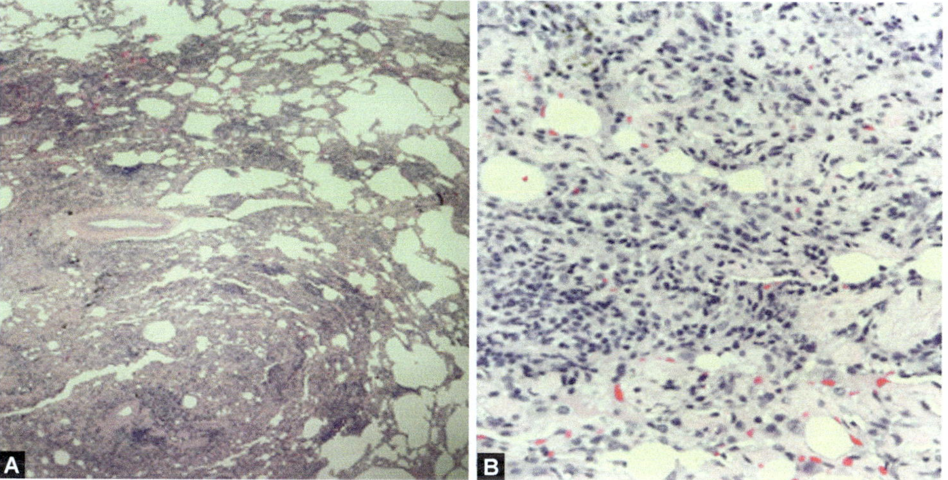

II. Histologic findings of patchy interstitial infiltrate (A, 20×) consisting of lymphocytes, histiocytes, and plasma cells (B, 200×). In this case, the interstitial infiltrate showed some bronchiolocentricity; however, the patient was confirmed to have rheumatoid arthritis and other etiologies were ruled out.

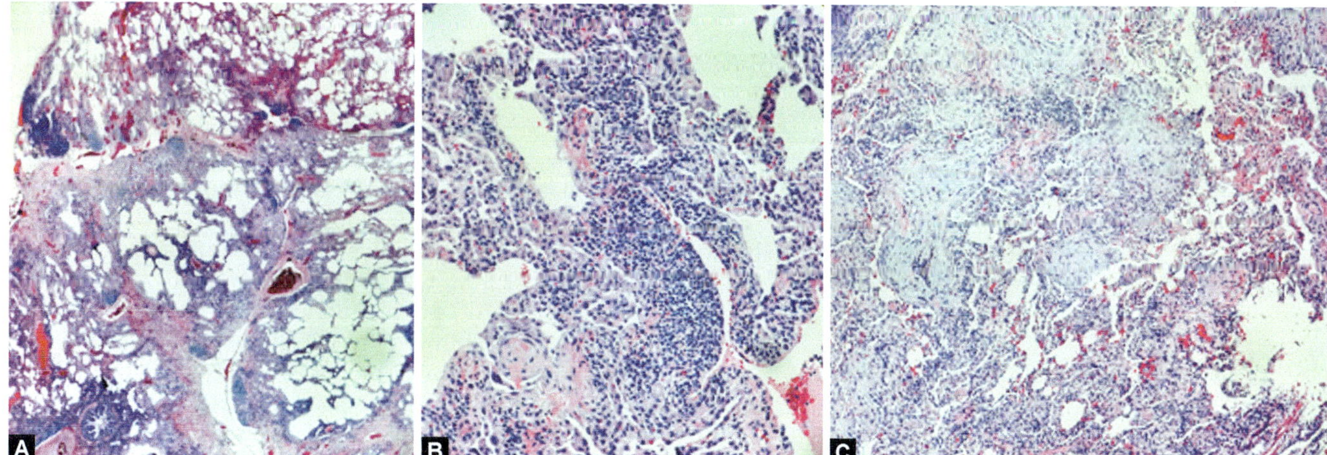

III. Histologic findings of fibrosis and cellular interstitial pneumonia with UIP features, areas of honeycombing and patches of uninvolved lung (A, 20×). Areas of lymphocytic cellular interstitial infiltrate were readily identifiable (B, 200×). Interstitial fibroblastic foci were also seen (C, 200×). The patient carried a diagnosis of rheumatoid arthritis.

FIGS. 1I TO III: Example of UIP pattern which is typical in RA-related interstitial lung disease but can also be present in other CTD-ILDs. Also displayed are two lung biopsies from separate patients: The first displaying a pattern in a confirmed RA-ILD case and the second displaying the typical UIP pattern seen in a second case of RA-ILD.

(CTD: connective tissue disease; ILD: interstitial lung disease; RA: rheumatoid arthritis; UIP: usual interstitial pneumonia)

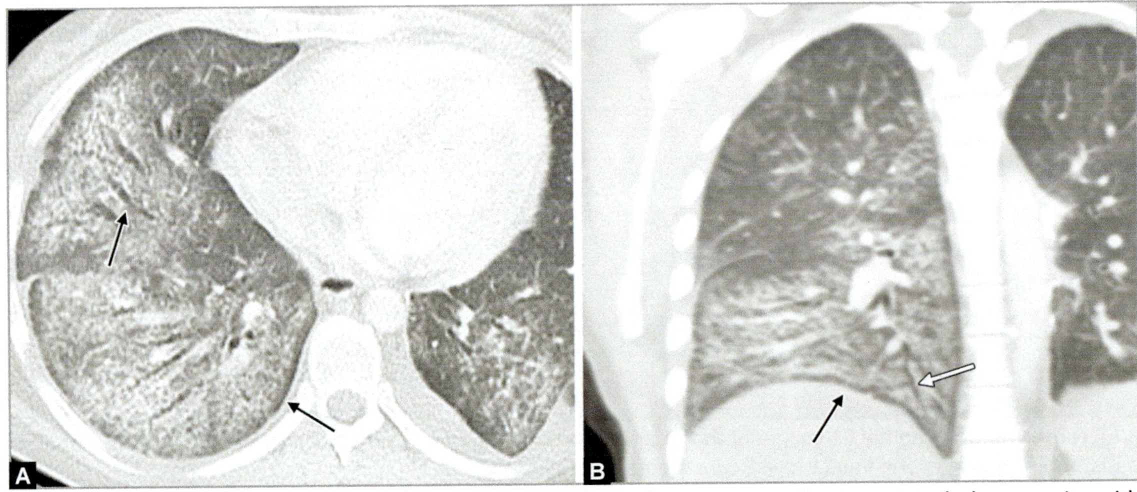

I. (A) Axial and (B) coronal CT images focusing on right lung demonstrate extensive ground-glass opacity with subpleural sparing (black arrows) and traction bronchiectasis (white arrows), consistent with fibrotic NSIP.

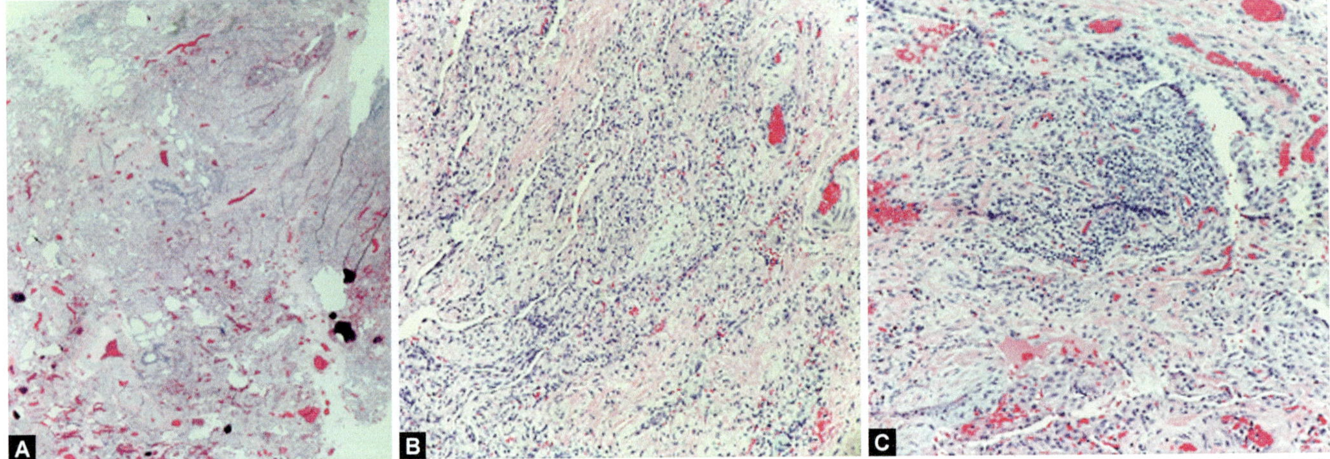

II. Histologic findings of diffuse fibrosing pneumonitis with microscopic honeycombing (A, 20×), myxoid fibroblastic foci (B, 200×), and cellular chronic interstitial inflammation (C, 200×), from a right upper lobe wedge biopsy. The interstitial pneumonitis in this case is relatively progressed with prominent fibrosis.

FIGS. 2I AND II: Fibrotic NSIP pattern which can be seen in a large number of diseases as well as its respective pathology from a sperate patient who underwent lung biopsy.
(NSIP: nonspecific interstitial pneumonia)

UIP is seen less commonly. Sjögren's disease can present with a primary airways disease, follicular bronchiolitis, in 15% of cases.[42-44] On chest imaging, follicular bronchiolitis will show scattered nodules with perivascular cysts.[44]

TREATMENT

Treatment for patients with CTD-ILD is based on the pathologic presence of varying degrees of cellular inflammation and fibrosis. For the inflammatory component immunosuppressive therapy, while corticosteroid therapy is often the initial approach, steroid-sparing agents such as mycophenolate, azathioprine, or occasionally cyclophosphamide are generally added quite early in the therapeutic course.[30] However, it is important to keep in mind that in SSc patients, corticosteroids are known to be associated with the development of renal crisis,[47-50] and those with anti-RNA polymerase III antibodies are at an increased risk.

In the RA-ILD population with UIP pattern, treatment with steroids followed by cyclophosphamide or mycophenolate may show a modest improvement in FVC and DLCO and stabilization of disease on HRCT.[51-56] However, cyclophosphamide carries risks of infection, malignancies, bone marrow suppression, and hemorrhagic cystitis. The added risks from cyclophosphamide make mycophenolate a more attractive steroid-sparing agent.[51-56] Methotrexate is the most common first-line agent used to treat RA articular disease. In patients in whom steroids and first-line RA disease-modifying agents have failed, second-line

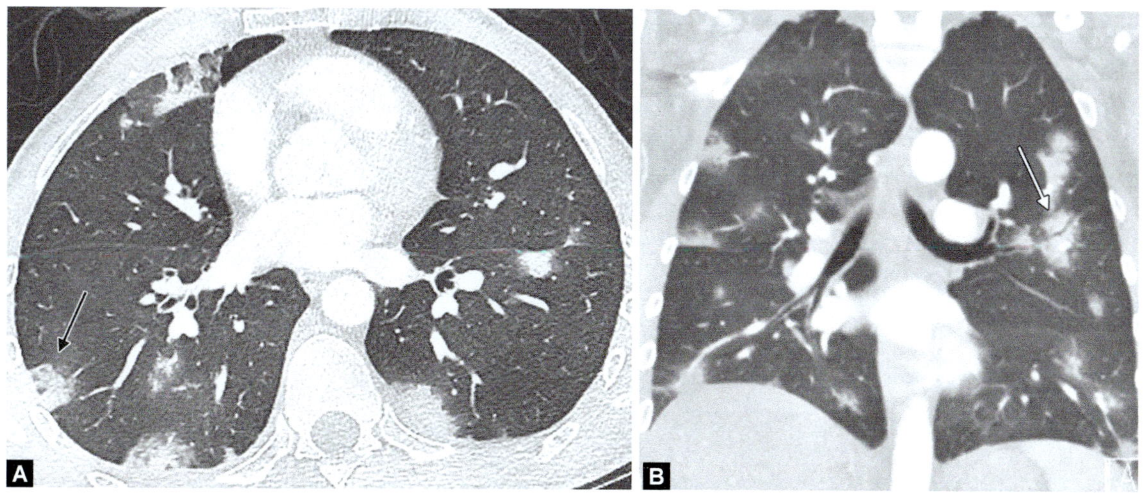

FIGS. 3A AND B: HRCT finding of organizing pneumonia that is seen in some rheumatoid arthritis patients as well as other connective tissue diseases. (A) Axial and (B) coronal images of the lungs demonstrate multiple nodular and mass-like areas of consolidation bilaterally. Most of the areas of consolidation have either a peribronchovascular (white arrow) or subpleural (black arrow) distribution. This pattern is suggestive of organizing pneumonia.

(HRCT: high-resolution computed tomography)

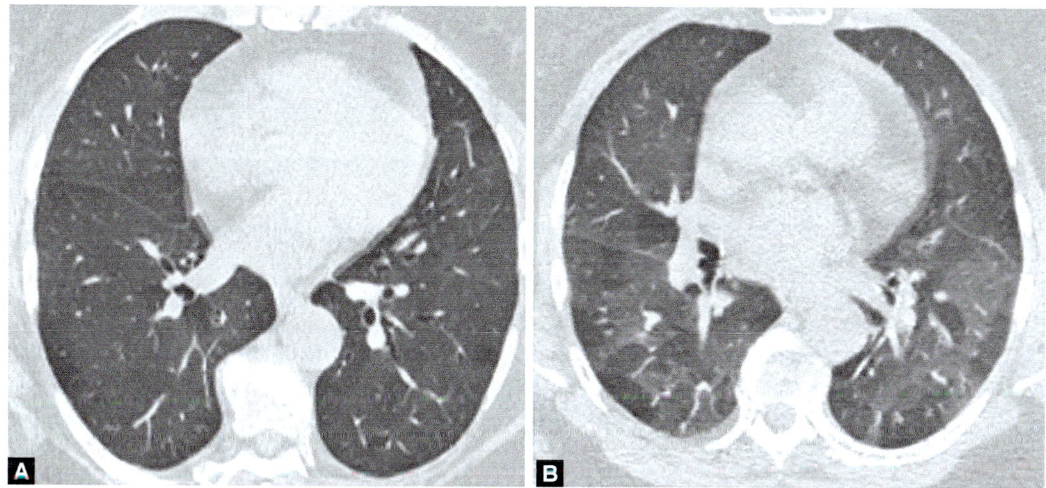

FIGS. 4A AND B: HRCT finding of obliterative bronchiolitis that is seen in some rheumatoid arthritis patients. Axial CT images obtained at (A) end-inspiration and (B) end-expiration. The lungs appear normal at end-inspiration, but there is a mosaic attenuation pattern consistent with air-trapping on the expiration images. Patient was found to have obliterative bronchiolitis.

(HRCT: high-resolution computed tomography)

therapy is often initiated. The RECITAL trial compared rituximab to cyclophosphamide in progressive CTD-ILD patients and found both to be equally effective. This trial demonstrated that when patients with progression of CTD-ILD are given either cyclophosphamide or rituximab, FVC is increased and respiratory symptoms decreased. The rituximab arm showed fewer side effects and a similar level of treatment response.[57] Rituximab is being used with increased frequency in treating CTD-ILD due to this more favorable safety profile.[57] In contrast to patients with a UIP pattern, those with an NSIP or OP pattern may demonstrate regression of radiographic changes in response to immunosuppressive therapy.

In patients whose disease progression is due to an increase in lung fibrosis, antifibrotic therapy with pirfenidone and nintedanib can be considered. The INBUILD study looked at fibrotic ILD patients who showed progression of their disease despite appropriate standard therapy. 25% of the study population were made up of CTD-ILDs.[17,58] While the patients in the placebo arm

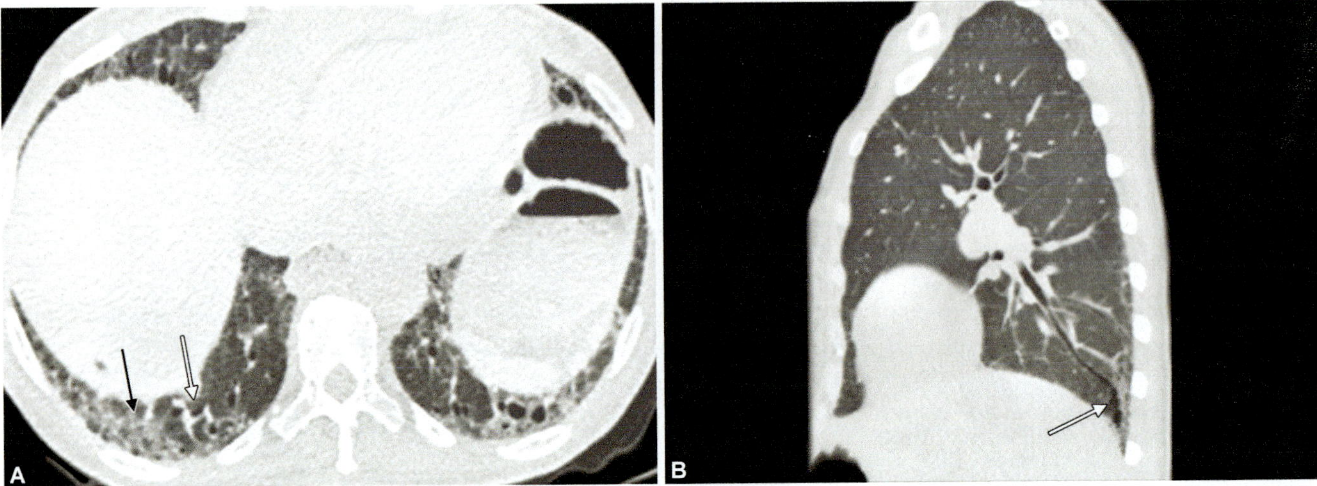

I. (A) Axial and (B) sagittal images from chest CT demonstrate subpleural and peripheral predominant ground-glass opacity (black arrow) with associated traction bronchiectasis (white arrows), consistent with fibrotic NSIP.

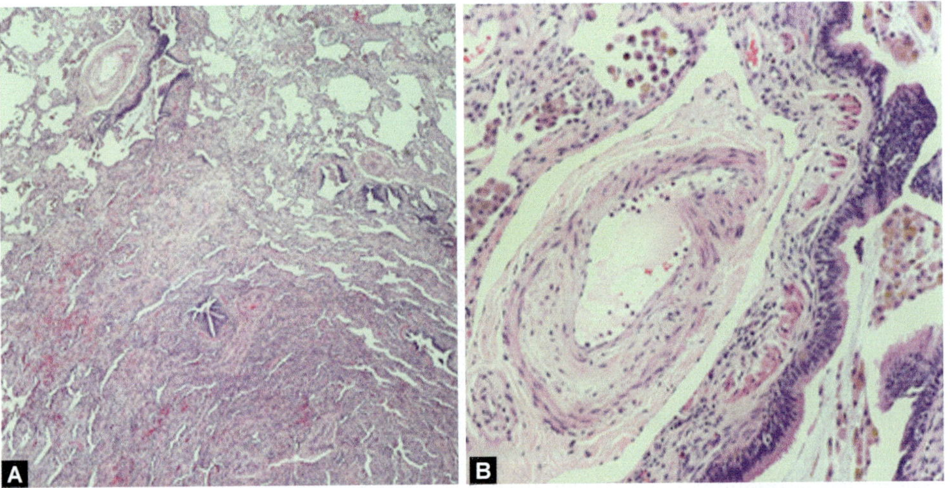

II. (A) Histologic findings show lung tissue with diffuse, pan-lobular moderate interstitial fibrosis, without inflammation. Significant arthropathy is identified with intimal proliferation (B, 200×).

FIGS. 5I AND II: A fibrotic NSIP pattern which is typical for systemic sclerosis ILD but can be seen in a multitude of CTD-ILDs as highlighted in Table 3. Figure 5II A and B display is also the lung biopsy of a scleroderma patient with these HRCT findings.

showed a rate of decline in FVC similar to the rate of decline seen in IPF patients, those in the nintedanib arm showed a significant reduction in the rate of FVC decline at 52 weeks.[17] Similar findings were seen in the SENCSIS study of nintedanib treatment in patients with scleroderma.[59]

Connective tissue disease-ILD can be difficult to treat, especially in patients with SSc, RA-ILD, and anti-MDA5 myositis. Rapid progression of disease often warrants additional immunosuppression. In scleroderma patients, the addition of rituximab to standard therapy may slow progressive lung function decline when compared to cyclophosphamide alone.[60-62] Anti-MDA5-associated ILD is another form that may progress rapidly. In these patients, upfront triple therapy in the form of corticosteroids, cyclophosphamide, and calcineurin inhibitors shows a difference in overall survival of 40–50%.[63-66] Given the rapid progression of anti-MDA5 myositis, further treatment development is on the horizon with studies showing that tofacitinib has potential in refractory cases.[67]

IDIOPATHIC INTERSTITIAL PNEUMONIA WITH AUTOIMMUNE FEATURES

Many patients with an ILD may clinically present with signs and/or symptoms suggestive of a CTD but do not meet diagnostic criteria for a specific autoimmune disorder. This phenomenon has led to the ongoing concept of idiopathic interstitial pneumonia with autoimmune features (IPAF).[1] For the diagnosis of IPAF, a patient must have an interstitial pneumonia on HRCT of the chest, alternative explanations for the presence of the ILD must have been excluded, and

TABLE 1: Autoantibodies associated with CTD-ILD. These autoantibodies for the respective CTDs have been associated with rapid progression of ILD and are markers of worse outcomes.[21,22,26,49,54,74]

Rheumatoid arthritis	Systemic sclerosis	Inflammatory myopathies	Sjögren's disease	Mixed connective tissue disease
Rheumatoid factor	Anti-Scl-70	*MSA antibodies*	Anti-SSA/Ro	Anti-U1 RNP
Anti-CCP	Anti-Th/To	Anti-Jo-1	Anti-SSB/La	
	Anti-U3 RNP	Anti-PL-7		
	Anti-U11/U12 RNP	Anti-PL-12		
	Anticentromere	Anti-Ku		
		Anti-MDA-5		
		MAA antibodies		
		Anti-U1-RNP		
		Anti-Ro52/60		

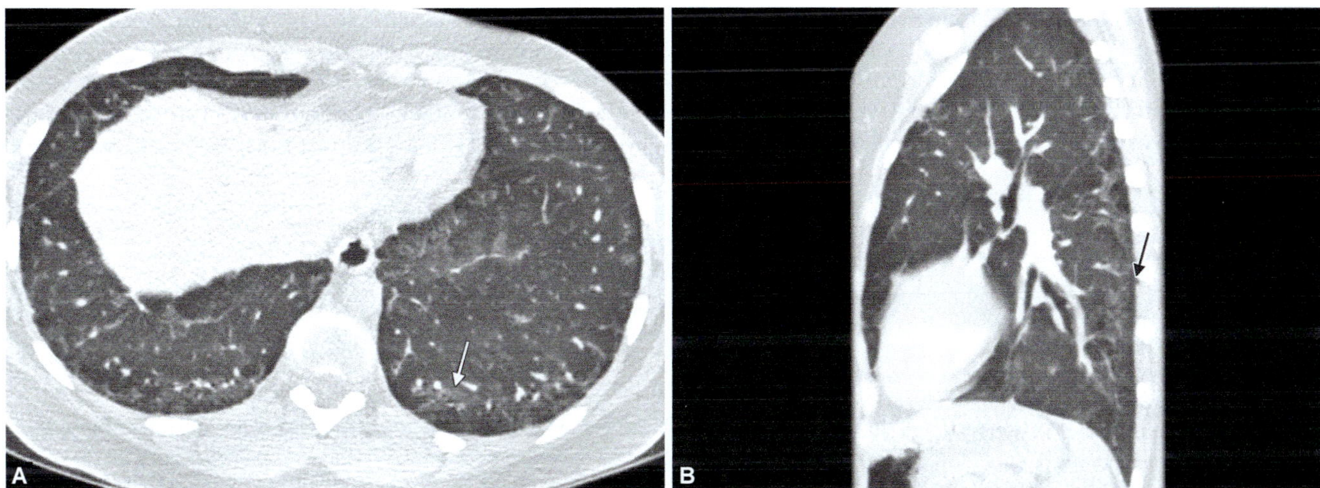

I. (A) Axial and (B) sagittal chest CT images demonstrate predominantly peripheral ground-glass opacity and traction bronchiolectasis (white arrow) in each lower lobe. Subpleural sparing nicely demonstrated on sagittal image (black arrow).

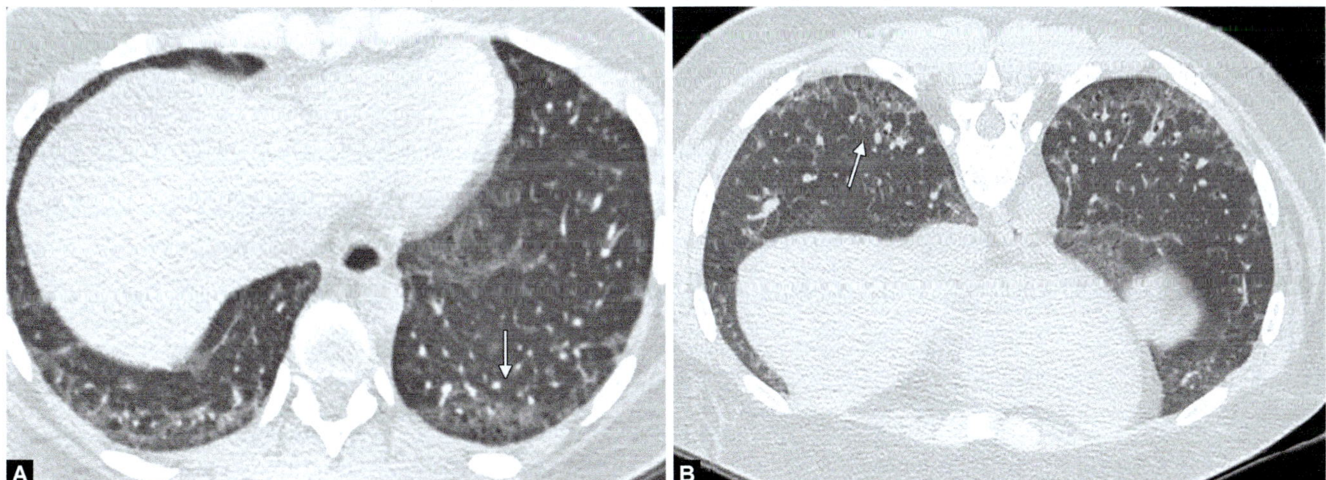

II. These axial images of the chest from the same patient obtained with the patient (A) supine and (B) prone demonstrate that the ground-glass opacity (white arrows) in the dependent portion of the lower lobes on the supine image is persistent on the prone image, proving that it is a true abnormality and not related to dependent atelectasis.

FIGS. 6I AND II: Typical finding of dermatomyositis ILD as demonstrated by the respective arrows displaying subpleural ground-glass, reticulations, and areas of subpleural sparring.

the necessary criteria for a specific CTD are not met. In this setting, one feature from two of the three (clinical, serologic, and morphologic) domains will make the IPAF diagnosis.[68]

The clinical domain focuses on physical examination findings. These include distal digital fissuring (mechanics hands), inflammatory arthritis or polyarticular morning stiffness lasting > 60 minutes, Raynaud's phenomenon, and unexplained fixed rash on the digital extensor surfaces (Gottron's sign).[53,68] The serological domain requires autoantibodies known to be associated with CTD **(Table 1)**. Antinuclear antibodies can fulfil this criteria; however, the titer must be ≥1:320. The final domain is the morphologic which consists of three sections. (1) Interstitial pneumonia patterns suggested by HRCT imaging. (2) Histopathologic features identified by SLB. (3) Evidence of additional thoracic compartment involvement by imaging, right heart catheterization, PFT, or histopathology.[53,68] UIP patterns are not included as having a UIP pattern does not increase the likelihood of CTD.[53,68] The criteria for the diagnosis of IPAF require at least one feature from two of the three domains, i.e., clinical, serological, and morphological.[68]

The diagnosis of IPAF is an area of ongoing clinical research as it is unclear if these patients carry a prognosis more similar to those with IPF or CTD-ILD. Case series and large retrospective studies have included IPAF patients who were treated with immunosuppressive therapy in the form of prednisone, mycophenolate, and/or rituximab. These patients showed maintenance or improvement in their pulmonary function. However, the INBUILD trial included IPAF patients and found that these patients, when they had progressed despite standard treatment, showed a significant reduction in the rate of FVC decline, indicating that the best approach to treatment for these patients remains an ongoing area of clinical investigation.

SUMMARY

Connective tissue disease-ILD encompasses a variety of autoimmune diseases and requires the clinician to combine the pattern on PFTs, HRCT, and potentially pathology to achieve the final diagnosis. These diseases may present with pulmonary manifestations prior to their autoimmune manifestations and some can have rapid disease progression. These require prompt multidisciplinary diagnosis and treatment with immunosuppressive and potentially antifibrotic medications.

REFERENCES

1. Lederer DJ, Martinez FJ. Idiopathic Pulmonary Fibrosis. N Engl J Med. 2018;378(19):1811-23.
2. Jeganathan N, Sathananthan M. Connective Tissue Disease-Related Interstitial Lung Disease: Prevalence, Patterns, Predictors, Prognosis, and Treatment. Lung. 2020;198(5):735-59.
3. Ng KH, Chen DY, Lin CH, et al. Risk of interstitial lung disease in patients with newly diagnosed systemic autoimmune rheumatic disease: A nationwide, population-based cohort study. Semin Arthritis Rheum. 2020;50(5):840-5.
4. Kim EA, Lee KS, Johkoh T, et al. Interstitial lung diseases associated with collagen vascular diseases: radiologic and histopathologic findings. Radiographics. 2002;22 Spec No:S151-65.
5. American Thoracic Society; European Respiratory Society. American Thoracic Society/European Respiratory Society International Multidisciplinary Consensus Classification of the Idiopathic Interstitial Pneumonias. Am J Respir Crit Care Med. 2002;165(2):277-304.
6. Katzenstein AL, Myers JL. Idiopathic pulmonary fibrosis: clinical relevance of pathologic classification. Am J Respir Crit Care Med. 1998;157(4 Pt 1):1301-15.
7. Korfei M, Ruppert C, Mahavadi P, et al. Epithelial endoplasmic reticulum stress and apoptosis in sporadic idiopathic pulmonary fibrosis. Am J Respir Crit Care Med. 2008;178(8):838-46.
8. Kaunisto J, Salomaa ER, Hodgson U, et al. Demographics and survival of patients with idiopathic pulmonary fibrosis in the FinnishIPF registry. ERJ Open Res. 2019;5(3):00170-2018.
9. Snetselaar R, van Batenburg AA, van Oosterhout MFM, et al. Short telomere length in IPF lung associates with fibrotic lesions and predicts survival. PLoS One. 2017;12(12):e0189467.
10. Juge PA, Lee JS, Ebstein E, et al. MUC5B Promoter Variant and Rheumatoid Arthritis with Interstitial Lung Disease. N Engl J Med. 2018;379(23):2209-19.
11. Stuart BD, Lee JS, Kozlitina J, et al. Effect of telomere length on survival in patients with idiopathic pulmonary fibrosis: an observational cohort study with independent validation. Lancet Respir Med. 2014;2(7):557-65.
12. Juge PA, Borie R, Kannengiesser C, et al.; FREX consortium. Shared genetic predisposition in rheumatoid arthritis-interstitial lung disease and familial pulmonary fibrosis. Eur Respir J. 2017;49(5):1602314.
13. Ruiz V, Ordóñez RM, Berumen J, et al. Unbalanced collagenases/TIMP-1 expression and epithelial apoptosis in experimental lung fibrosis. Am J Physiol Lung Cell Mol Physiol. 2003;285(5):L1026-36.
14. Evans CM, Fingerlin TE, Schwarz MI, et al. Idiopathic Pulmonary Fibrosis: A Genetic Disease That Involves Mucociliary Dysfunction of the Peripheral Airways. Physiol Rev. 2016;96(4):1567-91.
15. Lafyatis R, O'Hara C, Feghali-Bostwick CA, et al. B cell infiltration in systemic sclerosis-associated interstitial lung disease. Arthritis Rheum. 2007;56(9):3167-8.
16. Cotton CV, Spencer LG, New RP, et al. The utility of comprehensive autoantibody testing to differentiate connective tissue disease associated and idiopathic interstitial lung disease subgroup cases. Rheumatology (Oxford). 2017;56(8):1264-71.
17. Flaherty KR, Wells AU, Cottin V, et al.; INBUILD Trial Investigators. Nintedanib in Progressive Fibrosing Interstitial Lung Diseases. N Engl J Med. 2019;381(18):1718-27.
18. Norton S, Koduri G, Nikiphorou E, et al. A study of baseline prevalence and cumulative incidence of comorbidity and extra-articular manifestations in RA and their impact on outcome. Rheumatology (Oxford). 2013;52(1):99-110.
19. McInnes IB, Schett G. The pathogenesis of rheumatoid arthritis. N Engl J Med. 2011;365(23):2205-19.

20. Kelly CA, Saravanan V, Nisar M, et al.; British Rheumatoid Interstitial Lung (BRILL) Network. Rheumatoid arthritis-related interstitial lung disease: associations, prognostic factors and physiological and radiological characteristics—a large multicentre UK study. Rheumatology (Oxford). 2014;53(9):1676-82.
21. Koduri G, Norton S, Young A, et al.; ERAS (Early Rheumatoid Arthritis Study). Interstitial lung disease has a poor prognosis in rheumatoid arthritis: results from an inception cohort. Rheumatology (Oxford). 2010;49(8):1483-9.
22. Bendstrup E, Møller J, Kronborg-White S, et al. Interstitial Lung Disease in Rheumatoid Arthritis Remains a Challenge for Clinicians. J Clin Med. 2019;8(12):2038.
23. Fischer A, du Bois R. Interstitial lung disease in connective tissue disorders. Lancet. 2012;380(9842):689-98.
24. Raghu G, Remy-Jardin M, Richeldi L, et al. Idiopathic Pulmonary Fibrosis (an Update) and Progressive Pulmonary Fibrosis in Adults: An Official ATS/ERS/JRS/ALAT Clinical Practice Guideline. Am J Respir Crit Care Med. 2022;205(9):e18-e47.
25. Travis WD, Costabel U, Hansell DM, et al.; ATS/ERS Committee on Idiopathic Interstitial Pneumonias. An official American Thoracic Society/European Respiratory Society statement: Update of the international multidisciplinary classification of the idiopathic interstitial pneumonias. Am J Respir Crit Care Med. 2013;188(6):733-48.
26. Gutsche M, Rosen GD, Swigris JJ. Connective Tissue Disease-associated Interstitial Lung Disease: A review. Curr Respir Care Rep. 2012;1:224-32.
27. Antoniou KM, Walsh SL, Hansell DM, et al. Smoking-related emphysema is associated with idiopathic pulmonary fibrosis and rheumatoid lung. Respirology. 2013;18(8):1191-6.
28. Flaherty KR, Thwaite EL, Kazerooni EA, et al. Radiological versus histological diagnosis in UIP and NSIP: survival implications. Thorax. 2003;58(2):143-8.
29. Shaw M, Collins BF, Ho LA, et al. Rheumatoid arthritis-associated lung disease. Eur Respir Rev. 2015;24(135):1-16.
30. Nakamura Y, Suda T, Kaida Y, et al. Rheumatoid lung disease: prognostic analysis of 54 biopsy-proven cases. Respir Med. 2012;106(8):1164-9.
31. Turesson C, Matteson EL, Colby TV, et al. Increased CD4+ T cell infiltrates in rheumatoid arthritis-associated interstitial pneumonitis compared with idiopathic interstitial pneumonitis. Arthritis Rheum. 2005;52(1):73-9.
32. Tyndall AJ, Bannert B, Vonk M, et al. Causes and risk factors for death in systemic sclerosis: a study from the EULAR Scleroderma Trials and Research (EUSTAR) database. Ann Rheum Dis. 2010;69(10):1809-15.
33. Khanna D, Tashkin DP, Denton CP, et al. Ongoing clinical trials and treatment options for patients with systemic sclerosis-associated interstitial lung disease. Rheumatology (Oxford). 2019;58(4):567-79.
34. Goldin JG, Lynch DA, Strollo DC, et al.; Scleroderma Lung Study Research Group. High-resolution CT scan findings in patients with symptomatic scleroderma-related interstitial lung disease. Chest. 2008;134(2):358-67.
35. Park MS. Recent Advances in Predicting Mortality and Progression of Systemic Sclerosis-Associated Interstitial Lung Disease. Tuberc Respir Dis (Seoul). 2020;83(4):326-8.
36. Hamaguchi Y. Autoantibody profiles in systemic sclerosis: predictive value for clinical evaluation and prognosis. J Dermatol. 2010;37(1):42-53.
37. Chen IJ, Jan Wu YJ, Lin CW, et al. Interstitial lung disease in polymyositis and dermatomyositis. Clin Rheumatol. 2009;28(6):639-46.
38. Marie I, Josse S, Hatron PY, et al. Interstitial lung disease in anti-Jo-1 patients with antisynthetase syndrome. Arthritis Care Res (Hoboken). 2013;65(5):800-8.
39. Chua F, Higton AM, Colebatch AN, et al. Idiopathic inflammatory myositis-associated interstitial lung disease: ethnicity differences and lung function trends in a British cohort. Rheumatology (Oxford). 2012;51(10):1870-6.
40. Lega JC, Fabien N, Reynaud Q, et al. The clinical phenotype associated with myositis-specific and associated autoantibodies: a meta-analysis revisiting the so-called antisynthetase syndrome. Autoimmun Rev. 2014;13(9):883-91.
41. Koenig M, Fritzler MJ, Targoff IN, et al. Heterogeneity of autoantibodies in 100 patients with autoimmune myositis: insights into clinical features and outcomes. Arthritis Res Ther. 2007;9(4):R78.
42. Cao H, Pan M, Kang Y, et al. Clinical manifestations of dermatomyositis and clinically amyopathic dermatomyositis patients with positive expression of anti-melanoma differentiation-associated gene 5 antibody. Arthritis Care Res (Hoboken). 2012;64(10):1602-10.
43. Papiris SA, Manali ED, Kolilekas L, et al. Investigation of Lung Involvement in Connective Tissue Disorders. Respiration. 2015;90(1):2-24.
44. Ramos-Casals M, Brito-Zerón P, Seror R, et al.; EULAR Sjögren Syndrome Task Force. Characterization of systemic disease in primary Sjögren's syndrome: EULAR-SS Task Force recommendations for articular, cutaneous, pulmonary and renal involvements. Rheumatology (Oxford). 2015;54(12):2230-8.
45. Shiboski SC, Shiboski CH, Criswell L, et al.; Sjögren's International Collaborative Clinical Alliance (SICCA) Research Groups. American College of Rheumatology classification criteria for Sjögren's syndrome: a data-driven, expert consensus approach in the Sjögren's International Collaborative Clinical Alliance cohort. Arthritis Care Res (Hoboken). 2012;64(4):475-87.
46. Alves MR, Isenberg DA. "Mixed connective tissue disease": a condition in search of an identity. Clin Exp Med. 2020;20(2):159-66.
47. Nguyen B, Assassi S, Arnett FC, et al. Association of RNA polymerase III antibodies with scleroderma renal crisis. J Rheumatol. 2010;37(5):1068; author reply 1069.
48. Mehta P, Machado PM, Gupta L. Understanding and managing anti-MDA 5 dermatomyositis, including potential COVID-19 mimicry. Rheumatol Int. 2021;41(6):1021-36.
49. O'Dwyer DN, Armstrong ME, Cooke G, et al. Rheumatoid Arthritis (RA) associated interstitial lung disease (ILD). Eur J Intern Med. 2013;24(7):597-603.
50. Marigliano B, Soriano A, Margiotta D, et al. Lung involvement in connective tissue diseases: a comprehensive review and a focus on rheumatoid arthritis. Autoimmun Rev. 2013;12(11):1076-84.
51. Hallowell RW, Horton MR. Interstitial lung disease in patients with rheumatoid arthritis: spontaneous and drug induced. Drugs. 2014;74(4):443-50.
52. Kelly CA, Nisar M, Arthanari S, et al. Rheumatoid arthritis related interstitial lung disease-improving outcomes over 25 years: a large multicentre UK study. Rheumatology (Oxford). 2021;60(4):1882-90.

53. Fischer A, Brown KK, Du Bois RM, et al. Mycophenolate mofetil improves lung function in connective tissue disease-associated interstitial lung disease. J Rheumatol. 2013;40(5):640-6.
54. Cassone G, Sebastiani M, Vacchi C, et al. Efficacy and safety of mycophenolate mofetil in the treatment of rheumatic disease-related interstitial lung disease: a narrative review. Drugs Context. 2021;10:2020-8-8.
55. Conway R, Low C, Coughlan RJ, et al. Methotrexate and lung disease in rheumatoid arthritis: a meta-analysis of randomized controlled trials. Arthritis Rheumatol. 2014;66(4):803-12.
56. Kremer JM. Methotrexate Pulmonary Toxicity: Deep Inspiration. Arthritis Rheumatol. 2020;72(12):1959-62.
57. Maher TM, Tudor VA, Saunders P, et al.; RECITAL Investigators. Rituximab versus intravenous cyclophosphamide in patients with connective tissue disease-associated interstitial lung disease in the UK (RECITAL): a double-blind, double-dummy, randomised, controlled, phase 2b trial. Lancet Respir Med. 2023;11(1):45-54.
58. Cottin V, Richeldi L, Rosas I, et al.; INBUILD Trial Investigators. Nintedanib and immunomodulatory therapies in progressive fibrosing interstitial lung diseases. Respir Res. 2021;22(1):84.
59. Distler O, Highland KB, Gahlemann M, et al.; SENSCIS Trial Investigators. Nintedanib for Systemic Sclerosis-Associated Interstitial Lung Disease. N Engl J Med. 2019;380(26):2518-28.
60. Tashkin DP, Roth MD, Clements PJ, et al.; Scleroderma Lung Study II Investigators. Mycophenolate mofetil versus oral cyclophosphamide in scleroderma-related interstitial lung disease (SLS II): a randomised controlled, double-blind, parallel group trial. Lancet Respir Med. 2016;4(9):708-19.
61. Iqbal K, Kelly C. Treatment of rheumatoid arthritis-associated interstitial lung disease: a perspective review. Ther Adv Musculoskelet Dis. 2015;7(6):247-67.
62. Mankikian J, Caille A, Reynaud-Gaubert M, et al.; EVER-ILD investigators and the OrphaLung network. Rituximab and mycophenolate mofetil combination in patients with interstitial lung disease (EVER-ILD): a double-blind, randomised, placebo-controlled trial. Eur Respir J. 2023;61(6):2202071.
63. Fischer A, Antoniou KM, Brown KK, et al.; "ERS/ATS Task Force on Undifferentiated Forms of CTD-ILD". An official European Respiratory Society/American Thoracic Society research statement: interstitial pneumonia with autoimmune features. Eur Respir J. 2015;46(4):976-87.
64. Cottin V, Crestani B, Cadranel J, et al. French practical guidelines for the diagnosis and management of idiopathic pulmonary fibrosis - 2017 update. Full-length version. Rev Mal Respir. 2017;34(8):900-68.
65. Maher TM, Corte TJ, Fischer A, et al. Pirfenidone in patients with unclassifiable progressive fibrosing interstitial lung disease: design of a double-blind, randomised, placebo-controlled phase II trial. BMJ Open Respir Res. 2018;5(1):e000289.
66. Hallowell RW, Danoff SK. Diagnosis and Management of Myositis-Associated Lung Disease. Chest. 2023;163(6):1476-91.
67. Ida T, Furuta S, Takayama A, et al. Efficacy and safety of dose escalation of tofacitinib in refractory anti-MDA5 antibody-positive dermatomyositis. RMD Open. 2023;9(1):e002795.
68. Lee CT, Oldham JM. Interstitial Pneumonia with Autoimmune Features: Overview of proposed criteria and recent cohort characterization. Clin Pulm Med. 2017;24(5):191-6.

Connective Tissue Disease–Associated Interstitial Lung Diseases: An Indian Perspective

CHAPTER

109

Vijay Hadda, Sujay Halkur Shankar

INTRODUCTION

Connective tissue diseases (CTDs) are a variety of systemic autoimmune disorders leading to immune-mediated destruction of organs via circulating autoantibodies. The lung can be involved in all CTDs, and interstitial lung disease (ILD) is one among many manifestations that can occur in CTDs.[1] CTD-associated ILD is the second most common diagnosis in tertiary ILD referral centers. Due to its prevalence, most data on CTD ILD comes from systemic sclerosis (SSc) associated ILD which includes management-related clinical trials. These data are extrapolated to ILD due to other CTDs based on corroborative findings from observational or cohort studies.

EPIDEMIOLOGY

Interstitial lung disease frequently complicates the course of patients with autoimmune myopathy, SSc, Sjögren's syndrome (SS), rheumatoid arthritis (RA), and systemic lupus erythematosus (SLE) with estimated prevalence of 40%, 30–40%, 40%, 10%, and 8–12%, respectively.[2] Data suggest that among ILDs, the relative frequency of CTD-associated ILD shows great global variability with prevalence ranging from 7.5% of cases in Belgium to 33% of cases in Canada and 34.8% cases in Saudi Arabia.[3]

Indian data is available from two large studies which report that CTD-associated ILD comprises between 14 and 19% of the cohort among all patients with ILD attending pulmonary medicine clinics.[4,5] The age at diagnosis ranges between 45 and 55 years with a diagnosis of ILD being made after a mean duration of about 4.5 years since symptom onset. CTD-associated ILD is more common women, with males comprising only about 19–25% of the population. The two most common CTDs associated with ILD are SSc and RA, respectively.[4,5]

PATHOGENESIS

The pathogenesis of CTD-associated ILD involves a cascade of events following a trigger which ultimately leads to inflammation of the pulmonary parenchyma and fibrosis. External triggers/innate autoimmunity along with genetic predisposition leads to the initiation, amplification, and persistence of inflammation in the lung. Established external triggers include infection, smoking, toxic fume exposure, and gastroesophageal reflux disease (GERD) (microaspiration) among others. **Figure 1** depicts the pathogenesis of ILD in patients with CTD.

Genetic Predisposition

Certain genetic variants that were initially studied in idiopathic pulmonary fibrosis (IPF) have also been associated with CTD-associated ILD. Shorter telomere length (regardless of the presence of mutations) has been associated with the presence of ILD in patients with CTD when compared to healthy controls. In patients with interstitial pneumonia with autoimmune features (IPAF), shorter telomere length has been associated with faster lung function decline and poorer transplant-free survival.[6,7]

MUC5B is a gene associated with mucus production and maintenance of immune homeostasis in the lung. Mutations in this gene are associated with impaired mucociliary clearance and disruption of repair mechanisms. Mutations in the *MUC5B* gene have been observed in patients of IPAF and RA ILD with a stronger association with usual interstitial pneumonia (UIP) pattern on imaging.[8,9]

Inflammation

Triggers described earlier lead to alveolar epithelial damage which is pivotal for the establishment of inflammation in the lung parenchyma. The severity of epithelial injury as evidenced by elevated levels of KL-6 in studies has been associated with severity of lung injury and progression of ILD. Epithelial injury leads to the release of proinflammatory cytokines and chemokines [including interleukin 8 (IL-8), tumor necrosis factor alpha (TNF-α), and others] causing influx of activated macrophages and lymphocytes inciting worsening lung injury.[10]

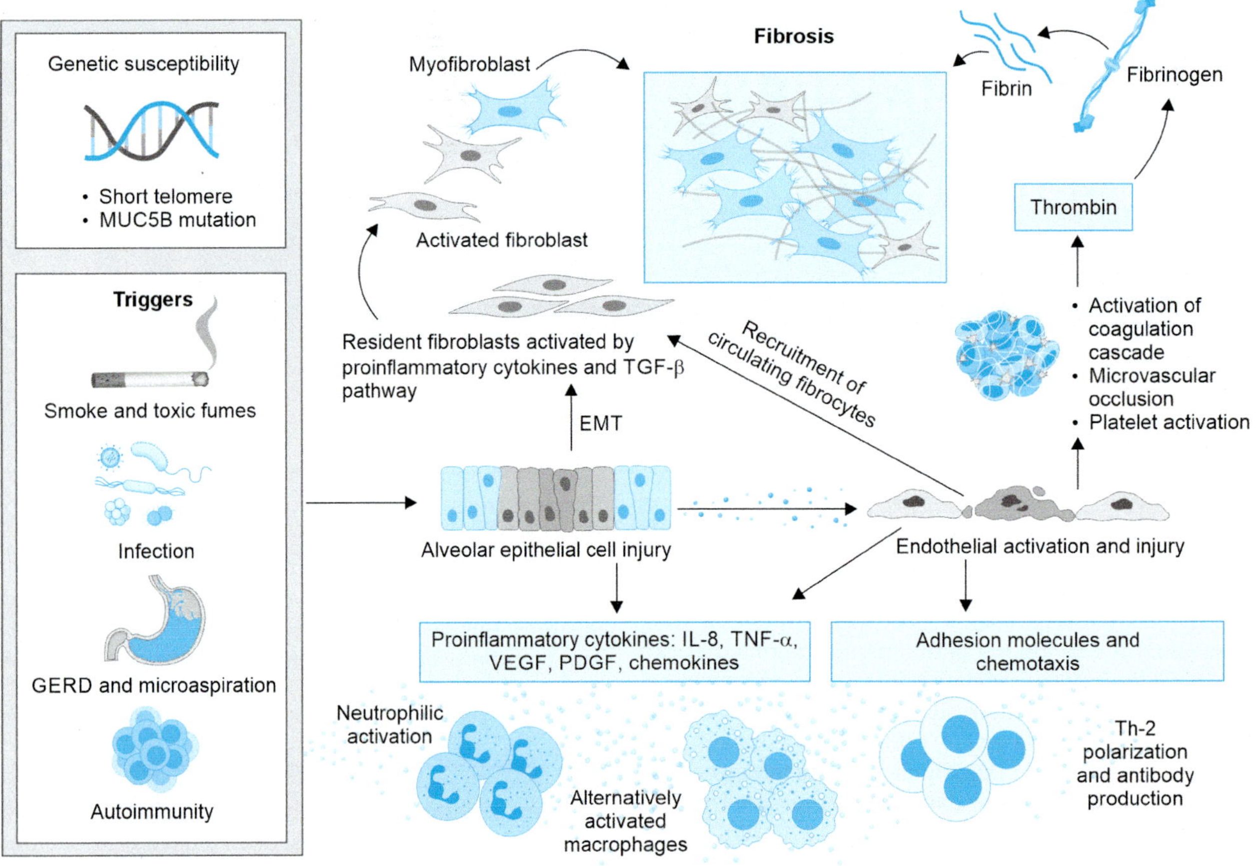

FIG. 1: Pathogenesis of CTD-associated ILD. In patients with CTD who are genetically susceptible, a trigger leads to initial damage of the alveolar epithelium with subsequent damage and activation of capillary endothelial cells. These damaged cells lead to the release of proinflammatory cytokines and chemokines that lead to homing of inflammatory cells and establishment of pulmonary inflammation. The inflammatory milieu and the damaged epithelium lead to activation of resident fibroblasts along with recruitment of additional fibroblasts (through EMT and homing of circulating fibrocytes). The activated fibroblasts transform into myofibroblasts which in tandem with fibrin deposition from the coagulation cascade leads to pulmonary fibrosis.

(CTD: connective tissue disease; EMT: epithelium-mesenchymal transformation; ILD: interstitial lung disease; PDGF: platelet-derived growth factor; TNF-α: tumor necrosis factor alpha; VEGF: vascular endothelial growth factor; TGF-β: transforming growth factor beta)

Courtesy: BioRender.com.

Fibrosis

Inflammation and epithelial damage also initiate profibrotic pathways driven by transforming growth factor beta (TGF-β). This leads to the activation of resident fibroblasts transforming them into myofibroblasts. There is also recruitment of circulating fibrocytes from blood, epithelium-mesenchymal transformation (conversion of alveolar epithelial cells to fibroblasts), and recruitment and transformation of bone marrow stem cells. Fibroblasts and myofibroblasts lead to the deposition of collagen in the extracellular matrix in tandem with fibrin deposition by the activated coagulation cascade. The result is fibrosis of the pulmonary parenchyma. Attenuation of repair mechanisms by alveolar type II pneumocytes and abnormal persistence of myofibroblasts after resolution of inflammation lead to the persistence of fibrosis.[10,11]

NATURAL HISTORY AND PROGNOSIS

The natural history of CTD-associated ILD is more complex than the progressive course of IPF. Even among patients with the same CTD, the disease course can be variable. Presentation may be subclinical following a slow and progressive course, or with acute manifestations and clinically significant rapid progression leading to severe deterioration of lung function and respiratory failure. The prognostic factors associated with development and progression of ILD and worse outcome include pattern and extent of ILD on HRCT, baseline lung function, rate of pulmonary function deterioration, and clinical features related to the primary CTDs such as age, gender, and clinical phenotype.

A study on SSc-associated ILD demonstrated that only a small proportion of patients follow a rapidly progressive course unresponsive to therapy, while most patients have a heterogenous course with periods of stability interspersed between periods of progression. Only about 30% patients had a progressive course over 1 year and about 67% of patients had a progressive course over a period of 5 years.[12]

The overall prognosis of CTD-associated ILD is favorable with 1- and 3-year survival in India of about 95 and 85%, respectively. This is significantly better than ILD due to other diagnoses.[13] Thus, close monitoring of lung function of these patients is important to identify and treat patients with progression early.

APPROACH TO DIAGNOSIS OF CTD-ASSOCIATED ILD

In most cases of CTD-associated ILD, the diagnosis of underlying CTD is already established at the time of ILD diagnosis. However, ILD can be the presenting (*forme fruste*) or the only feature of undiagnosed CTD. In the former scenario, one needs to decide when to treat, what to treat with, and how to monitor. In the latter scenario, it can be a diagnostic challenge, and correct classification of the underlying CTD is vital for therapeutic decisions and prognosis.

Hence, the diagnosis of CTD-associated ILD requires intelligent clinical and radiological evaluation. Many times, a multidisciplinary team approach is required for diagnosis, as applicable to other ILDs, with pulmonologists/physicians, radiologists, pathologists, and rheumatologists on board.

Clinical Features

CTD-associated ILD occurs more commonly in women and in nonsmokers when compared to idiopathic interstitial pneumonia (IIP). The diagnosis of CTD-associated ILD is made when a patient satisfies the classification criteria of the suspected CTD *plus* a high-resolution computed tomographic (HRCT) scan of the thorax shows evidence of ILD **(Table 1)**.[14] The clinical signs of the underlying CTD may be subtle, and thus careful history taking and examination must be conducted. The ILD per se manifests with symptoms of persistent and/or progressive shortness of breath and dry cough. However, it is important to ask for extrapulmonary manifestations like musculoskeletal pain, weakness, fever/fatigue, arthritis/arthralgia, photosensitivity, Raynaud's phenomenon, and sicca symptoms.

The examination of the eyes, hands, joints, and skin is very informative for the diagnosis of CTD. On examination, it is important to look for Raynaud's phenomenon, mechanic's hands, sclerodactyly, digital tip ulcerations, palmar and facial telangiectasia, Gottron's papules, proximal muscle weakness, and small and large joint arthritis. Some patients will show findings that are gross **(Figs. 2A to G)**; however, many a times, the finding can be very subtle that may require examination by a rheumatologist. Of note, ILD may be the first presentation of CTD in a small proportion of cases.

Depending on the clinical suspicion, ancillary testing such as nail fold capillaroscopy, Schirmer's test, minor salivary gland biopsy, skin biopsy, muscle biopsy, and electromyography can aid in the diagnosis of different CTDs.[14]

Radiology

High-resolution CT with thin slice (1–1.5 mm) is the radiologic modality of choice for the delineation of CTD-associated ILD. For optimal evaluation of parenchymal details, a volumetric scan that includes sequences obtained during full inspiration and expiration, and prone position

TABLE 1: Clinical and radiological characteristics of connective tissue diseases.

Disease	ILD prevalence	Clinical features	ILD pattern
Systemic sclerosis	Detectable in up to 75%; clinically evident. 25–45%	Raynaud's phenomenon, sclerodactyly, digital ulcers/pits, telangiectasia, skin thickening, GERD	Most common: NSIP Others: UIP, OP
Rheumatoid arthritis	Detectable in 30–60%; clinically evident: 10–30%	Symmetric polyarthritis with early morning stiffness, subcutaneous nodules	Most common: UIP Others: NSIP, OP
Idiopathic inflammatory myositis	Seen in 30–50%	Proximal muscle weakness, shawl sign, Gottron's papules, heliotrope rash, mechanic's hands	Most common: NSIP Others: OP, UIP, AIP/DAD
Systemic lupus erythematosus	Detectable in up to 30%; clinically evident: 3–11%	Malar rash, photosensitivity, alopecia, cytopenias, oral ulcers, serositis	Most common: NSIP Other: LIP, OP, UIP, AIP/DAD
Mixed connective tissue disease	Seen in 20–85%	Puffy fingers, synovitis, acrosclerosis, myositis, Raynaud's phenomenon	Most common: NSIP Other: UIP, OP
Sjögren's syndrome	Seen in 10–30%	Dry eyes, dry mouth, arthralgia/arthritis, salivary gland enlargement	Most common: NSIP Other: LIP, OP, UIP

(AIP: acute interstitial pneumonia; DAD: diffuse alveolar damage; ILD: interstitial lung disease; NSIP: nonspecific interstitial pneumonia; OP: organizing pneumonia; UIP: usual interstitial pneumonia)

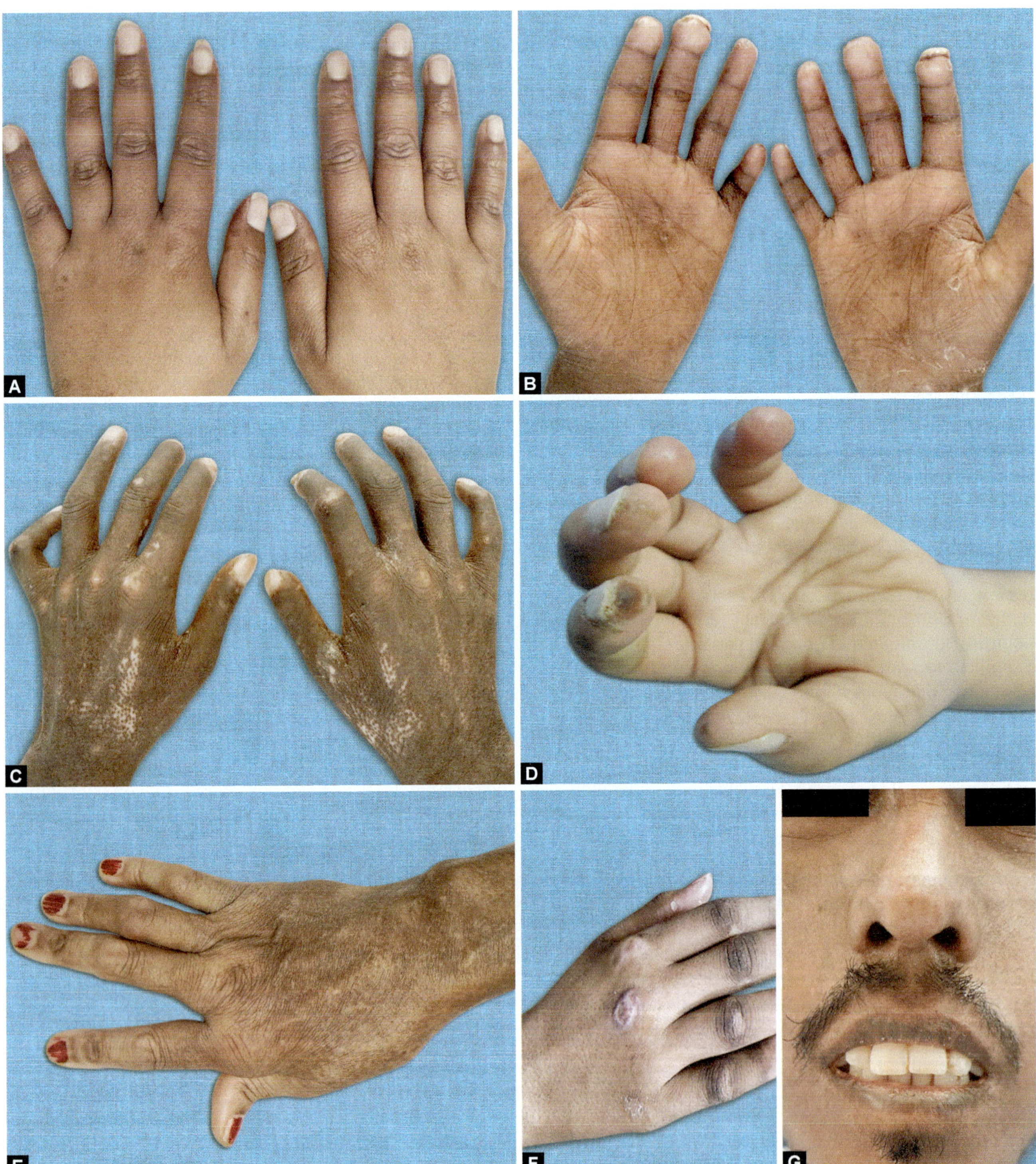

FIGS. 2A TO G: Extrapulmonary clinical examination findings that aid in the identification of CTD-associated ILD. (A) Healed Gottron's papules in a patient of dermatomyositis; (B) Sclerodactyly and resorption of digits in systemic sclerosis; (C) Sclerodactyly with skin tightening giving claw-like appearance of hand along with salt and pepper pigmentation of skin in systemic sclerosis; (D) Digital pits and ulceration; (E) Ulnar deviation of hand with Boutonniere deformity of third and fourth digits in rheumatoid arthritis; (F) Cutaneous ulceration in anti-MDA5 antibody disease; (G) Thinning of lips with microstomia and prominence of anterior teeth giving a fish-mouth appearance in systemic sclerosis.

(CTD: connective tissue disease; ILD: interstitial lung disease)

are required. While any radiologic pattern of ILD may be observed in CTD-associated ILD, nonspecific interstitial pneumonia (NSIP) pattern followed by OP pattern are the most common. An exception is in RA-ILD where UIP is the most common pattern.[15]

Certain patterns on HRCT may indicate CTD as the underlying cause of ILD. Four radiologic patterns of UIP, which include straight edge sign, exuberant honeycombing sign, anterior upper lobe sign, and the four corners sign, may differentiate CTD-associated ILD from IPF.[16] Also, extrapulmonary findings on HRCT, such as the presence of pleural effusion (RA/SLE), esophageal dilatation (SSc), and dilated pulmonary artery (SSc), can give clues to the underlying undiagnosed CTD.

Autoantibodies

Most guidelines suggest testing for autoantibodies even in the absence of overt clinical features of CTD to differentiate CTD-associated ILD from IIPs. ANA, anticyclic citrullinated peptide (anti-CCP), rheumatoid factor, and myositis panel are recommended in all patients. Extractable nuclear antigens and additional selected myositis antibody panels may be performed in selected patients. Repeat testing, if the initial panel is negative, is also recommended as seroconversion rate may be as high as 25%.[17-19] The results of autoantibody testing must always be interpreted in the clinical context and the mere presence of autoantibody must not be taken at face value. Discussion with the rheumatologist/immunologist may be fruitful for a better interpretation of the presence of autoantibodies. **Table 2** details the different autoantibodies and their associated CTDs.

TABLE 2: Autoantibody profile and their association with connective tissue diseases.

Autoantibody	ANA IIF staining pattern	Associated CTDs
• t-RNA synthetase antibodies • Myositis-specific antibodies • Anti-Jo-1, PL-7, PL-12, MDA-5	Cytoplasmic, speckled	Idiopathic inflammatory myopathy, antisynthetase syndrome
Anti PM/Scl-75/100	Nucleolar	Systemic sclerosis/ polymyositis
Anti-Ro/SSA and Anti-La/SSB	Nuclear, speckled	Sjögren's syndrome
• Anti-topoisomerase/ SCL-70 • Anti-RNA polymerase III	Nucleolar	Diffuse cutaneous systemic sclerosis
Anticentromere	Centromeric	Systemic sclerosis CREST syndrome
• Anti-ds-DNA • Anti-Sm	Nuclear, homogeneous Nuclear, speckled	SLE
Anti-U1 RNP	Nuclear, speckled	MCTD
RF and anti-CCP	–	Rheumatoid arthritis

(ANA: antinuclear antibody; CREST: calcinosis, Raynaud's phenomenon, esophageal dysmotility, sclerodactyly, and telangiectasia; CTD: connective tissue disease; MCTD: mixed connective tissue disease; IIF: indirect immunofluorescence; SLE: systemic lupus erythematosus)

Other Investigations

Bronchoalveolar lavage (BAL) is not routinely required for the diagnosis of CTD-associated ILD. BAL may only be useful to rule out infections or if diffuse alveolar hemorrhage is suspected. Similarly, lung biopsy (transbronchial or surgical) is not advised in patients with established CTD. The pattern of involvement on histopathology may alter prognosis; however, it seldom changes management strategies unlike in patients with IIPs. This makes lung biopsy in this setting redundant and a risky procedure.[11] Lung biopsy, however, may be required to rule out other pathologies such as infiltrates of nonimmune etiology (like drug toxicity) or concurrent malignancy when suspected. At our center, we do not advise lung biopsy for established CTD-associated ILD.

CONNECTIVE TISSUE DISEASE CHARACTERISTICS

Systemic sclerosis (SSc): ILD along with pulmonary hypertension are the most common pulmonary manifestations of SSc. ILD usually develops within the first 5 years of development of the first non-Raynaud's symptom and rarely beyond 15 years of diagnosis.[20] The risk factors for the development and progression of ILD in SSc are male gender, older age, African ethnicity, diffuse cutaneous SSc, and the presence of antitopoisomerase antibodies. The presence of anticentromere antibodies may be protective for the development of ILD.[9,21,22] ILD is associated with increased mortality in patients with SSc with a 10-year mortality of 40%.[20]

Rheumatoid arthritis: Though RA is more common in women, men more commonly develop ILD. Other risk factors include smoking, older age, active joint disease, and high titers of rheumatoid factor and anti-CCP.[23,24] The presence of ILD is a risk factor for mortality (three times higher risk) in patients with RA.[25] The annual mortality due to ILD in patients with RA and ILD may be as high as 35%.[26] RA-ILD with UIP pattern have lower 5-year survival rates (36%) than those with NSIP pattern (94%).[24]

Idiopathic inflammatory myositis (IIM): ILD usually develops within the first 2 years of presentation of myositis and can be the presenting feature of the disease in about

8–37% of patients.[27] Risk factors for the development of ILD include mechanic's hands and the presence of anti-Jo1, anti-MDA5, and anti-Ro52 antibodies.[28] Dermatomyositis-related ILD has a more rapid and severe course than polymyositis-associated ILD.[29] The prevalence of ILD in patients with anti-MDA5 antibodies can be 80% or higher. Patients with anti-MDA-5 antibodies develop rapidly progressive ILD that may be resistant to conventional treatment. This disease has a mortality of about 50% despite appropriate therapy.[30]

Mixed connective tissue disease (MCTD): ILD is the most frequent pulmonary manifestation of MCTD. The risk factors for developing ILD include Raynaud's phenomenon, dysphagia, anti-Ro52 antibodies, anti-Sm antibodies, and elevated C-reactive protein (CRP). Almost 25% of these patients develop a progressive fibrosing phenotype over a period of 4 years from diagnosis.[31,32]

Sjögren's syndrome: Lung involvement is usually more severe and frequent in secondary SS. The risk factors for the development of ILD include male sex, smoking, older age, and ANA positivity. The presence of ILD is associated with four times higher mortality in patients with primary SS. The 5-year mortality of these patients is about 20%.[33-37]

Interstitial pneumonia with autoimmune features (IPAF): In many patients with ILD, there are features suggestive of background autoimmunity (antibody positivity or clinical symptoms), but the established classification criteria for a specific CTD are not met. Such patients are classified as having IPAF which lies on the spectrum between IIP and CTD-associated ILD. The classification criteria for the same have now been established by the American Thoracic Society/European Respiratory Society (ATS/ERS) task force.[38,39]

Nearly one-third of previously deemed IIP or ILD due to undifferentiated CTD could be reclassified based on the IPAF classification criteria. The recognition of this entity becomes important as they have better prognosis than IIPs.[40,41]

MANAGEMENT

The optimal treatment strategy for individual CTD-associated ILD is currently unknown. Recently, the Thoracic Society of Australia and New Zealand published its position statement on the diagnosis and management of CTD-associated ILD.[42] However, graded evidence-based recommendations are still lacking. Broadly, the management components of CTD-associated ILD are as follows.

Staging and Progression

The treatment decisions in CTD-associated ILD are based on disease staging and detection of progression. CTD-associated ILD can be divided into limited or extensive disease based on forced vital capacity (FVC) and parenchymal involvement on HRCT, with extensive disease having higher mortality rates. Patients with <20% involvement of lung parenchyma on HRCT *and* an FVC of >70% are classified as having limited disease. Those with >20% of lung parenchyma involvement on HRCT *or* an FVC <70% are classified as having extensive disease.[43]

Short-term spirometry trends have also been associated with mortality and have been used to define disease progression. For CTD-associated ILD, progression is defined as a relative decline from baseline of FVC by ≥10% *or* an FVC decline of 5–9% with diffusing capacity for carbon monoxide (DLCO) decline of ≥15% over a period of 12 months.[44,45]

Decision to Treat

Patients with extensive disease or those with limited disease with documented progression as described above will usually require treatment. The decision to treat patients with stable limited disease or subclinical disease is still not well defined. These patients are usually closely monitored, and treatment is directed at the underlying CTD. ILD-specific treatment is initiated at the time of progression.[42] Some physicians may also decide to treat such patients if they have risk factors for progression. These risk factors vary with different CTDs. However, common risk factors for progression include male sex, UIP pattern on HRCT, smoking, older age, and an underlying CTD diagnosis of SSc.[46]

There is a need for the development of biomarkers to help identify patients who are likely to progress and thus benefit from early initiation of treatment. Biomarkers such as KL-6, SP-D, CCL-18, and CRP have been studied in SSc-ILD for the identification of this patient population. Among these, KL-6 (a glycoprotein expressed by injured and regenerating type II pneumocytes) is the most widely studied in both SSc and RA-associated ILD. Higher levels are associated with both extensive disease and progression with prognostic implications.[47-49]

Monitoring

The Indian consensus statement for the management of ILD suggests monitoring with PFT and DLCO every 6 months till stabilization of disease followed by 12 monthly follow-up in non-IPF ILD. They also suggest that 6-minute walk distance may not be reliable in CTD-associated ILD due to confounding factors. HRCT chest is recommended on a clinical basis when there is clinical worsening or PFT decline.[19]

Treatment

Nearly all controlled trials in the management of CTD-associated ILD come from SSc-associated ILD. These results are extrapolated to the management of other

CTD-associated ILDs as well. Treatment options include pharmacologic therapy and supportive care.

Pharmacotherapy

- *Glucocorticoids (GC):* They are the first line of immunosuppression used due to their rapid onset of action. The usual dosage in CTD-associated ILD is a starting dose of 0.5 mg/kg/day of prednisolone to taper down to a maintenance of about 10 mg/day.[42] Special considerations are to be noted in SSc and IIM-associated ILD. Steroid doses of >15 mg/day of prednisolone in SSc are avoided due to the possibility of the development of scleroderma renal crisis.[50] Higher doses of up to 1 mg/kg/day of prednisolone are usually initiated in patients with IIM-associated ILD due to the severity of disease and rapidity of progression.[51]
- *Cyclophosphamide (CYC):* It is an alkylating agent that can be administered either orally in doses up to 2 mg/kg/day or intravenously as monthly injections of 600 mg/m^2. Therapy is usually not extended beyond 6–9 months due to cumulative dose-related toxicity. The SLS I compared oral CYC against placebo over a period of 12 months. This was studied in patients with SSc within 7 years of symptom onset with evidence of alveolitis (on HRCT or BAL fluid). CYC led to an improvement in FVC from baseline of 2.53% against placebo ($p < 0.05$). There were significantly higher proportions of leucopenia and neutropenia in the CYC group.[52,53] Therefore, CYC is the drug of choice for SSc-ILD. The duration of immunosuppression in these studies was 12 months; the effect of longer duration of immunosuppression is not known.
- *Mycophenolate mofetil (MMF):* This is an oral immunosuppressant that inhibits inosine monophosphate dehydrogenase and has a cytostatic action on lymphocytes. This drug is dosed at 2–3 g/day in divided doses. In patients who do not tolerate MMF, enteric-coated mycophenolate sodium can be used (500 mg MMF = 360 mg mycophenolate sodium).[42,54]

  The SLS II trial studied subjects with SSc (<7 years since the onset of disease) with evidence of ILD on HRCT. The %FVC change from baseline was similar between the two groups, but CYC was associated with more leucopenia and thrombocytopenia.[55]

  The added advantage of MMF over CYC is the ability to give prolonged immunosuppression without the risk of cumulative dose related toxicity. Following the SLS II trial, MMF became the standard of care in SSc-ILD.
- *Rituximab (RTX):* RTX is an anti-CD20 monoclonal antibody that is administered intravenously with an induction of 1 g given 2 weeks apart followed by 1 g given every 6 months.[42] RTX (RECITAL trial) was studied in CTD-associated ILD including patients with SSc, IIM, and MCTD with severe or progressive ILD. There were numerically higher adverse events in the CYC group with higher number of administration-related adverse events and gastrointestinal disorders.[56] This study showed that RTX was comparable to CYC with fewer adverse effects in CTD-associated ILD.
- *Tocilizumab (TCZ):* TCZ is an anti-IL6 monoclonal antibody that is administered subcutaneously in a dose of 162 mg weekly. TCZ (focuSSced trial) was studied in patients with SSc (with or without ILD) where it was compared against placebo for a duration of 48 weeks. Based on this trial, TCZ is now approved for the management of SSc-ILD.
- *Azathioprine (AZA)*: AZA is a purine synthesis inhibitor that is administered orally in doses up to 2–2.5 mg/kg/day in divided doses [if thiopurine S-methyltransferase (TPMT) levels are normal].[42,54] The evidence for AZA comes mainly from retrospective cohorts. It has been shown to lead to stabilization of lung function in about 66% patients. It is also shown to be similar in efficacy to MMF. The major drawback of this drug is the toxicity leading to drug discontinuation which can be as high as 28%.[57,58]
- *Calcineurin inhibitors (CNI):* Tacrolimus (TAC) is a CNI which is administered orally in doses of 1 mg twice a day and is titrated to maintain a serum trough level of 5–8 ng/mL.[42] The evidence for TAC is mainly in IIM-related ILD from retrospective studies.[59]
- *Antifibrotics:* These include nintedanib (administered orally as 150 mg twice a day) and pirfenidone (administered orally up to a maximum dose of 801 mg thrice a day) that were originally described in the management of IPF.

  Nintedanib (SENCIS trial) has been studied in patients with SSc-ILD with at least 10% fibrosis on HRCT for a duration of 52 weeks. Half of these patients were receiving background MMF. The annual decline in FVC (mL) was about 41 mL lower when compared to placebo (statistically significant). Diarrhea was more commonly seen in the nintedanib group.[60]

  Pirfenidone (TRAIL1 trial) was studied in patients of RA-ILD with 10% fibrosis on HRCT over 52 weeks. In patients with UIP pattern on HRCT, pirfenidone led to a significant slowing in the FVC decline which was not observed in non-UIP pattern on HRCT. Pirfenidone was also studied against placebo in patients with SSc-ILD (with or without fibrosis on HRCT) taking MMF. It did not lead to a significant difference in the change in %FVC at 18 months compared to placebo.[61]

  The results of these studies suggest that adding antifibrotics in patients with CTD-ILD and fibrosis on HRCT may help slow the decline of lung function. There is also evidence for the addition of antifibrotics in progressive pulmonary fibrosis phenotype of CTD-ILD.[62,63]

Special Considerations in Treatment

- *SSc*: Apart from the above-mentioned medications, autologous stem cell transplant has been studied in patients with progressive diffuse cutaneous SSc.

In comparison to CYC, it led to an improvement in FVC and extent of ILD on HRCT but not in DLCO.[64]

- *Rheumatoid arthritis:* There was an initial consideration that MTX (due to its pulmonary toxicity) may worsen RA-ILD. However, retrospective studies have shown a protective role of MTX on lung function with a mortality benefit.[65,66] Abatacept (a CTLA-4 inhibitor) has been studied in RA-ILD and has showed disease stability or improvement in nearly 89% patients.[67]
- *IIM-related ILD:* These ILDs can present in a fulminant form with patients failing on two or even three immunosuppressants. Such patients may be given a trial of IV immunoglobulin therapy or plasma exchange as a rescue therapy.[68,69]

Supportive Care

Nonpharmacologic therapy is as important as pharmacotherapy for the management of ILD. Important measures in this bracket include smoking cessation, oxygen therapy (in patients with resting hypoxia), vaccination (including COVID-19, pneumococcal, and influenza), pulmonary rehabilitation, management of GERD, and identification and treatment of pulmonary hypertension. Furthermore, patient-centered care such as management of depression/anxiety, symptom relief, and end-of-life discussions are essential.[42,70]

Lung Transplant

The presence of CTD-associated ILD is neither a relative nor an absolute contraindication for lung transplant. Evidence exists to show that outcomes of lung transplant in CTD-associated ILD at 1 and 5 years are similar to other ILDs. The extrathoracic manifestations such as renal disease, active myositis, and severe GERD may hinder the selection of patients for transplant. These extrathoracic contraindications need to be identified and evaluated as per existing guidelines.[71] The recurrence of CTD after transplant is limited to case reports and more data is required to assess the incidence.[72]

SUMMARY

Connective tissue disease-associated ILD includes a spectrum of diseases with a heterogenous natural history but overall good prognosis. The clinical course may vary from a stable and nonprogressive disease to a rapidly progressive fulminant condition. Accurate diagnosis and timely treatment are crucial for the best outcome. Early suspicion and diagnosis are imperative to treatment. Though the optimal immunosuppression strategy is not known, a multitude of drugs exist for the management of CTD-associated ILD. Supportive care and evaluation for lung transplant are complementary to pharmacologic management of these patients.

REFERENCES

1. Cottin V, Hirani NA, Hotchkin DL, et al. Presentation, diagnosis and clinical course of the spectrum of progressive-fibrosing interstitial lung diseases. Eur Respir Rev. 2018;27(150):180076.
2. Fischer A, Strek ME, Cottin V, et al. Proceedings of the American College of Rheumatology/Association of Physicians of Great Britain and Ireland Connective Tissue Disease-Associated Interstitial Lung Disease Summit: A Multidisciplinary Approach to Address Challenges and Opportunities. Arthritis Rheumatol. 2019;71(2):182-95.
3. Kaul B, Cottin V, Collard HR, et al. Variability in Global Prevalence of Interstitial Lung Disease. Front Med. 2021;8:751181.
4. Singh S, Collins BF, Sharma BB, et al. Interstitial Lung Disease in India. Results of a Prospective Registry. Am J Respir Crit Care Med. 2017;195(6):801-13.
5. Dhooria S, Sehgal IS, Agarwal R, et al. Incidence, prevalence, and national burden of interstitial lung diseases in India: Estimates from two studies of 3089 subjects. PLoS One. 2022; 17(7):e0271665.
6. Snetselaar R, van Moorsel CHM, Kazemier KM, et al. Telomere length in interstitial lung diseases. Chest. 2015;148(4):1011-8.
7. Newton CA, Oldham JM, Ley B, et al. Telomere length and genetic variant associations with interstitial lung disease progression and survival. Eur Respir J. 2019;53(4):1801641.
8. Juge PA, Lee JS, Ebstein E, et al. MUC5B Promoter Variant and Rheumatoid Arthritis with Interstitial Lung Disease. N Engl J Med. 2018;379(23):2209-19.
9. Distler O, Assassi S, Cottin V, et al. Predictors of progression in systemic sclerosis patients with interstitial lung disease. Eur Respir J. 2020;55(5):1902026.
10. Wells AU, Denton CP. Interstitial lung disease in connective tissue disease--mechanisms and management. Nat Rev Rheumatol. 2014;10(12):728-39.
11. Cerro Chiang G, Parimon T. Understanding Interstitial Lung Diseases Associated with Connective Tissue Disease (CTD-ILD): Genetics, Cellular Pathophysiology, and Biologic Drivers. Int J Mol Sci. 2023;24(3):2405.
12. Hoffmann-Vold AM, Allanore Y, Alves M, et al. Progressive interstitial lung disease in patients with systemic sclerosis-associated interstitial lung disease in the EUSTAR database. Ann Rheum Dis. 2021;80(2):219-27.
13. Singh S, Bairwa M, Collins BF, et al. Survival predictors of interstitial lung disease in India: Follow-up of Interstitial Lung Disease India registry. Lung India. 2021;38(1):5-11.
14. Fischer A, Lee JS, Cottin V. Interstitial Lung Disease Evaluation: Detecting Connective Tissue Disease. Respiration. 2015;90(3): 177-84.
15. Yoo H, Hino T, Hwang J, et al. Connective tissue disease-related interstitial lung disease (CTD-ILD) and interstitial lung abnormality (ILA): Evolving concept of CT findings, pathology and management. Eur J Radiol Open. 2022 7;9:100419.
16. Chung JH, Cox CW, Montner SM, et al. CT Features of the Usual Interstitial Pneumonia Pattern: Differentiating Connective

Tissue Disease–Associated Interstitial Lung Disease From Idiopathic Pulmonary Fibrosis. Am J Roentgenol. 2018;210(2):307-13.

17. Raghu G, Remy-Jardin M, Myers JL, et al. Diagnosis of Idiopathic Pulmonary Fibrosis. An Official ATS/ERS/JRS/ALAT Clinical Practice Guideline. Am J Respir Crit Care Med. 2018;198(5):e44-68.
18. Hu Y, Wang LS, Wei YR, et al. Clinical Characteristics of Connective Tissue Disease-Associated Interstitial Lung Disease in 1,044 Chinese Patients. Chest. 2016;149(1):201-8.
19. Singh S, Sharma BB, Bairwa M, et al. Management of Interstitial Lung Diseases: A consensus statement of the Indian Chest Society (ICS) and National College of Chest Physicians (NCCP). Lung India. 2020;37(4):359-78.
20. Benan M, Hande I, Gul O. The natural course of progressive systemic sclerosis patients with interstitial lung involvement. Clin Rheumatol. 2007;26(3):349-54.
21. Qiu M, Nian X, Pang L, et al. Prevalence and risk factors of systemic sclerosis-associated interstitial lung disease in East Asia: A systematic review and meta-analysis. Int J Rheum Dis. 2021;24(12):1449-59.
22. Mayes MD, Lacey JV, Beebe-Dimmer J, et al. Prevalence, incidence, survival, and disease characteristics of systemic sclerosis in a large US population. Arthritis Rheum. 2003;48(8):2246-55.
23. Kadura S, Raghu G. Rheumatoid arthritis-interstitial lung disease: manifestations and current concepts in pathogenesis and management. Eur Respir Rev. 202130(160):210011.
24. Atzeni F, Gerardi MC, Barilaro G, et al. Interstitial lung disease in systemic autoimmune rheumatic diseases: a comprehensive review. Expert Rev Clin Immunol. 2018;14(1):69-82.
25. Bongartz T, Nannini C, Medina-Velasquez YF, et al. Incidence and mortality of interstitial lung disease in rheumatoid arthritis: A population-based study. Arthritis Rheum. 2010;62(6):1583-91.
26. Olson AL, Swigris JJ, Sprunger DB, et al. Rheumatoid Arthritis–Interstitial Lung Disease–associated Mortality. Am J Respir Crit Care Med. 2011;183(3):372-8.
27. Hallowell RW, Paik JJ. Myositis-associated interstitial lung disease: a comprehensive approach to diagnosis and management. Clin Exp Rheumatol. 2022;40(2):373-83.
28. Cocconcelli E, Zanatta E, Bellani S, et al. Predictors of Interstitial Lung Disease (ILD) in patients with Idiopathic Inflammatory Myopathy-associated (IIM). Eur Respir J. 2022;60(suppl 66):24E6306.
29. Saketkoo LA, Ascherman DP, Cottin V, et al. Interstitial Lung Disease in Idiopathic Inflammatory Myopathy. Curr Rheumatol Rev. 2010;6(2):108-19.
30. Nombel A, Fabien N, Coutant F. Dermatomyositis With Anti-MDA5 Antibodies: Bioclinical Features, Pathogenesis and Emerging Therapies. Front Immunol. 2021;12:773352.
31. Santacruz JC, Mantilla MJ, Rodriguez-Salas G, et al. Interstitial Lung Disease in Mixed Connective Tissue Disease: An Advanced Search. Cureus. 2023;15(3):e36204.
32. Végh J, Szilasi M, Soós G, et al. [Interstitial lung disease in mixed connective tissue disease]. Orv Hetil. 2005;146(48):2435-43.
33. Ramos-Casals M, Brito-Zerón P, Seror R, et al. Characterization of systemic disease in primary Sjögren's syndrome: EULAR-SS Task Force recommendations for articular, cutaneous, pulmonary and renal involvements. Rheumatol Oxf Engl. 2015;54(12):2230-8.
34. Vitali C, Tavoni A, Viegi G, et al. Lung involvement in Sjögren's syndrome: a comparison between patients with primary and with secondary syndrome. Ann Rheum Dis. 1985;44(7):455-61.
35. Kim YJ, Choe J, Kim HJ, et al. Long-term clinical course and outcome in patients with primary Sjögren syndrome-associated interstitial lung disease. Sci Rep. 2021;11(1):12827.
36. Yazisiz V, Göçer M, Erbasan F, et al. Survival analysis of patients with Sjögren's syndrome in Turkey: a tertiary hospital-based study. Clin Rheumatol. 2020;39(1):233-41.
37. Flament T, Bigot A, Chaigne B, et al. Pulmonary manifestations of Sjögren's syndrome. Eur Respir Rev. 2016;25(140):110-23.
38. Fischer A, Antoniou KM, Brown KK, et al. An official European Respiratory Society/American Thoracic Society research statement: interstitial pneumonia with autoimmune features. Eur Respir J. 2015;46(4):976-87.
39. Mackintosh JA, Wells AU, Cottin V, et al. Interstitial pneumonia with autoimmune features: challenges and controversies. Eur Respir Rev. 2021;30(162):210177.
40. Oldham JM, Adegunsoye A, Valenzi E, et al. Characterisation of patients with interstitial pneumonia with autoimmune features. Eur Respir J. 2016;47(6):1767-75.
41. Graney BA, Fischer A. Interstitial Pneumonia with Autoimmune Features. Ann Am Thorac Soc. 2019;16(5):525-33.
42. Jee AS, Sheehy R, Hopkins P, et al. Diagnosis and management of connective tissue disease-associated interstitial lung disease in Australia and New Zealand: A position statement from the Thoracic Society of Australia and New Zealand. Respirology. 2021;26(1):23-51.
43. Goh NSL, Desai SR, Veeraraghavan S, et al. Interstitial lung disease in systemic sclerosis: a simple staging system. Am J Respir Crit Care Med. 2008;177(11):1248-54.
44. Goh NS, Hoyles RK, Denton CP, et al. Short-Term Pulmonary Function Trends Are Predictive of Mortality in Interstitial Lung Disease Associated With Systemic Sclerosis. Arthritis Rheumatol Hoboken NJ. 2017;69(8):1670-8.
45. Khanna D, Mittoo S, Aggarwal R, et al. Connective Tissue Disease-associated Interstitial Lung Diseases–Report from OMERACT CTD-ILD Working Group. J Rheumatol. 2015;42(11):2168-71.
46. Chan C, Ryerson CJ, Dunne JV, et al. Demographic and clinical predictors of progression and mortality in connective tissue disease-associated interstitial lung disease: a retrospective cohort study. BMC Pulm Med. 2019;19(1):192.
47. Bonhomme O, André B, Gester F, et al. Biomarkers in systemic sclerosis associated interstitial lung disease: review of the literature. Rheumatol Oxf Engl. 2019;58(9):1534-46.
48. Stock C, Hoyles R, D'Accord C, et al. Serum KL-6 as a marker of disease progression in SSc-ILD. ERS International Congress 2018 abstracts; 2018.
49. Kim HC, Choi KH, Jacob J, et l. Prognostic role of blood KL-6 in rheumatoid arthritis–associated interstitial lung disease. PLoS One. 2020;15(3):e0229997.
50. Cappelli S, Randone SB, Camiciottoli G, et al. Interstitial lung disease in systemic sclerosis: where do we stand? Eur Respir Rev. 2015;24(137):411-9.
51. Hallowell RW, Danoff SK. Diagnosis and Management of Myositis-Associated Lung Disease. Chest. 2023;163(6):1476-91.
52. Tashkin DP, Goldin J, Arriola E, et al. Cyclophosphamide versus Placebo in Scleroderma Lung Disease. N Engl J Med. 2006;354(25):2655-66.

53. Tashkin DP, Elashoff R, Clements PJ, et al. Effects of 1-Year Treatment with Cyclophosphamide on Outcomes at 2 Years in Scleroderma Lung Disease. Am J Respir Crit Care Med. 2007;176(10):1026-34.
54. van den Bosch L, Luppi F, Ferrara G, et al. Immunomodulatory treatment of interstitial lung disease. Ther Adv Respir Dis. 2022;16:17534666221117002.
55. Tashkin DP, Roth MD, Clements PJ, et al. Mycophenolate mofetil versus oral cyclophosphamide in scleroderma-related interstitial lung disease (SLS II): a randomised controlled, double-blind, parallel group trial. Lancet Respir Med. 2016;4(9):708-19.
56. Maher TM, Tudor VA, Saunders P, et al. Rituximab versus intravenous cyclophosphamide in patients with connective tissue disease-associated interstitial lung disease in the UK (RECITAL): a double-blind, double-dummy, randomised, controlled, phase 2b trial. Lancet Respir Med. 2023;11(1):45-54.
57. Boerner EB, Cuyas M, Theegarten D, et al. Azathioprine for Connective Tissue Disease-Associated Interstitial Lung Disease. Respiration. 2020;99(8):628-36.
58. Huapaya JA, Silhan L, Pinal-Fernandez I, et al. Long-Term Treatment With Azathioprine and Mycophenolate Mofetil for Myositis-Related Interstitial Lung Disease. Chest. 2019;156(5):896-906.
59. Sharma N, Putman MS, Vij R, et al. Myositis-associated Interstitial Lung Disease: Predictors of Failure of Conventional Treatment and Response to Tacrolimus in a US Cohort. J Rheumatol. 2017;44(11):1612-8.
60. Distler O, Highland KB, Gahlemann M, et al. Nintedanib for Systemic Sclerosis–Associated Interstitial Lung Disease. N Engl J Med. 2019;380(26):2518-28.
61. Solomon JJ, Danoff SK, Woodhead FA, et al. Safety, tolerability, and efficacy of pirfenidone in patients with rheumatoid arthritis-associated interstitial lung disease: a randomised, double-blind, placebo-controlled, phase 2 study. Lancet Respir Med. 2023;11(1):87-96.
62. Flaherty KR, Wells AU, Cottin V, et al. Nintedanib in Progressive Fibrosing Interstitial Lung Diseases. N Engl J Med. 2019;381(18):1718-27.
63. Behr J, Prasse A, Kreuter M, et al. Pirfenidone in patients with progressive fibrotic interstitial lung diseases other than idiopathic pulmonary fibrosis (RELIEF): a double-blind, randomised, placebo-controlled, phase 2b trial. Lancet Respir Med. 2021;9(5):476-86.
64. Spierings J, Chiu YH, Voortman M, et al. Autologous stem-cell transplantation in systemic sclerosis-associated interstitial lung disease: early action in selected patients rather than escalation therapy for all. Ther Adv Musculoskelet Dis. 2021; 13:1759720X211035196.
65. Juge PA, Lee JS, Lau J, et al. Methotrexate and rheumatoid arthritis associated interstitial lung disease. Eur Respir J. 2021; 57(2):2000337.
66. Kur-Zalewska J, Kisiel B, Kania-Pudło M, et al. A dose-dependent beneficial effect of methotrexate on the risk of interstitial lung disease in rheumatoid arthritis patients. PLoS One. 2021; 16(4):e0250339.
67. Tardella M, Di Carlo M, Carotti M, et al. Abatacept in rheumatoid arthritis-associated interstitial lung disease: short-term outcomes and predictors of progression. Clin Rheumatol. 2021; 40(12):4861-7.
68. Huapaya JA, Hallowell R, Silhan L, et al. Long-term treatment with human immunoglobulin for antisynthetase syndrome-associated interstitial lung disease. Respir Med. 2019;154: 6-11.
69. Komai T, Iwasaki Y, Tsuchida Y, et al. Efficacy and safety of plasma exchange in interstitial lung diseases with anti-melanoma differentiation-associated 5 gene antibody positive clinically amyopathic dermatomyositis. Scand J Rheumatol. 2023;52(1):77-83.
70. Wijsenbeek MS, Holland AE, Swigris JJ, et al. Comprehensive Supportive Care for Patients with Fibrosing Interstitial Lung Disease. Am J Respir Crit Care Med. 2019;200(2):152-9.
71. Crespo MM, Lease ED, Sole A, et al. ISHLT consensus document on lung transplantation in patients with connective tissue disease: Part I: Epidemiology, assessment of extrapulmonary conditions, candidate evaluation, selection criteria, and pathology statements. J Heart Lung Transplant. 2021;40(11): 1251-66.
72. Rama Esendagli D, Ntiamoah P, Kupeli E, et al. Recurrence of primary disease following lung transplantation. ERJ Open Res. 2022;8(2):00038-2022.

Progressive Pulmonary Fibrosis

CHAPTER 110

Simon Meredith, Joseph Parambil, Suhail Raoof

INTRODUCTION

Interstitial lung disease (ILD) is a broad group of lung diseases that is characterized by inflammatory and/or fibrotic infiltration of the lung parenchyma. Of these, a fibrotic disease tends to carry worse prognosis than an inflammatory nonfibrotic disease. Fibrotic ILD is often detected on high-resolution CT (HRCT) scan in the form of reticulation, traction bronchiectasis, traction bronchiolectasis, honeycombing, and architectural distortion. Fibrotic changes of various types can be defined on pathological specimens following lung biopsy.[1,2] For the determination of a fibrotic interstitial process, it is extremely important to combine the HRCT findings, pathology results, and clinical picture, usually in a multidisciplinary discussion (MDD) format. Of the various diagnoses, idiopathic pulmonary fibrosis (IPF) is the most common fibrosing lung disease but there are other forms of pulmonary fibrosis.[1,2] IPF carries the worst prognosis among these and is characterized by inexorable progression. The non-IPF fibrotic lung diseases might progress as well at varying paces, and the progression of these non-IPF fibrotic ILDs is defined as progressive pulmonary fibrosis (PPF).[1] A correct assessment of this progression is paramount as PPF patients carry a worse outcome than those with a non-progressive fibrosing ILD that is not IPF.[1,2]

In this chapter, we discuss the pathophysiology as well as the physiological and radiographic signs that define this entity. We also discuss the approach to its management, especially with regards to the use of antifibrotic medications as well as the prognosis of PPF.

DEFINITION

Progressive pulmonary fibrosis is defined as progression of lung fibrosis in non-IPF ILD patients. The ATS/ERS/JRS/ALAT (American Thoracic Society/European Respiratory Society/Japanese Respiratory Society/Asociación Latino-americana de Tórax) guidelines define three major criteria for establishing the diagnosis of PPF:[1]

1. Worsening respiratory symptoms
2. Decline in physiologic function
3. CT chest with evidence of progressive fibrotic changes with no other explanation for the clinicophysiologic decline

The identification of a PPF phenotype confers a worse prognosis to these patients.[1,3] Among the various non-IPF fibrotic ILDs, approximately one-fourth will develop a progressive fibrotic phenotype leading to an irreversible decline in lung function. The various fibrotic ILDs that have demonstrated a progressive fibrotic phenotype include fibrotic hypersensitivity pneumonitis (HP), connective tissue disease (CTD)-related fibrotic ILD, fibrosing idiopathic pneumonia with autoimmune features, pleuroparenchymal fibroelastosis, and idiopathic fibrotic nonspecific interstitial pneumonia (NSIP).[1,3]

PHYSIOLOGICAL PROGRESSION

Physiological progression of pulmonary fibrosis is assessed through pulmonary function testing (PFT). Two physiologic parameters are central in monitoring patients with a fibrosing ILD: Forced vital capacity (FVC) and diffusion capacity for carbon monoxide (DLCO).[1,5]

Progressive fibrosis was defined by two of the following three criteria in a 12-month period:

1. Worsening respiratory symptoms
2. Physiologic evidence of disease progression via either:
    - Absolute decline in FVC of 5% predicted or more within 1 year
    - Absolute decline in DLCO of 10% predicted or more within 1 year
3. An increased extent of fibrosis on HRCT

RADIOLOGICAL PROGRESSION

High-resolution CT scan of the chest is one of the three pillars in determination of PPF. The progressive fibrosis pattern has been seen in patients with both a UIP pattern of fibrosis and an alternative pattern. The UIP pattern will show changes such as reticulation, traction bronchiectasis, traction bronchiolectasis, and honeycombing, usually

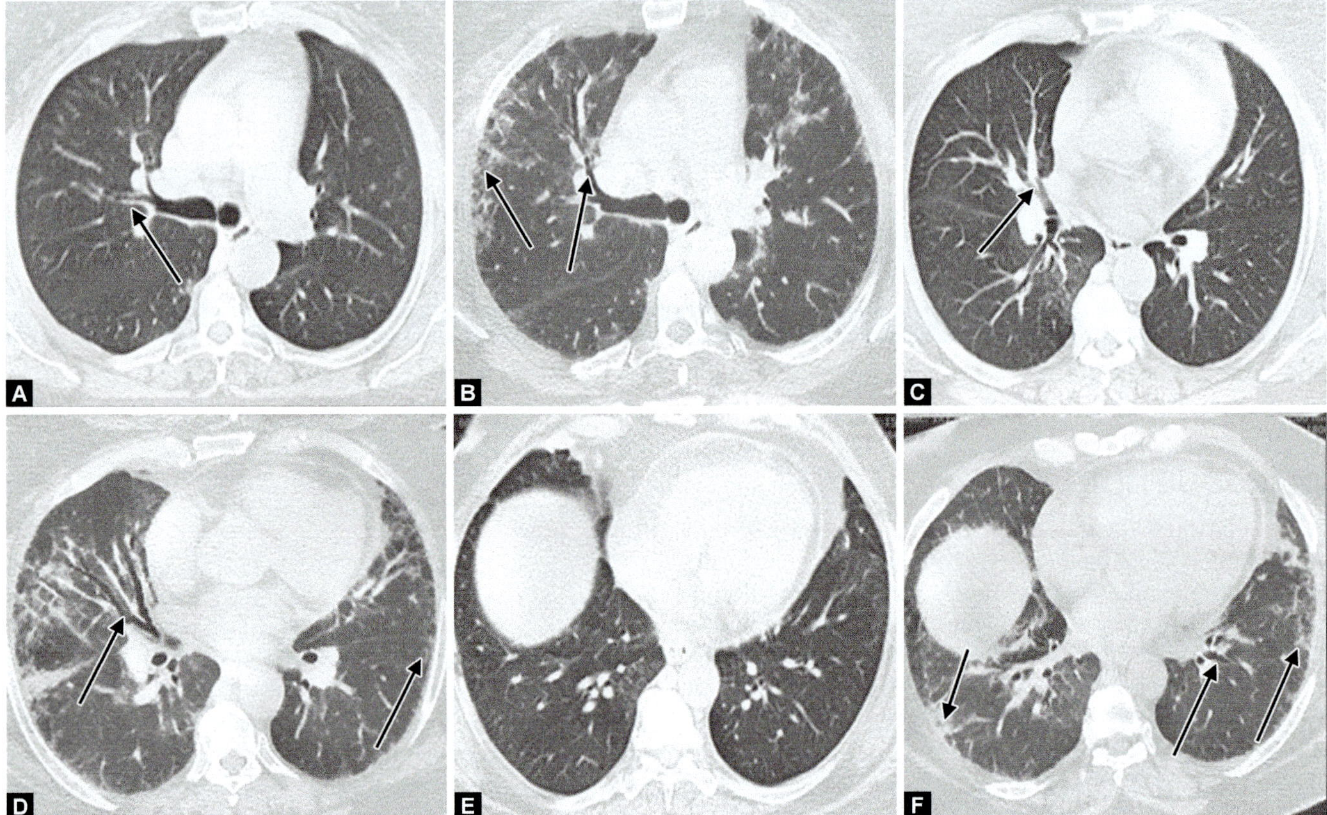

FIGS. 1A TO F: Example of progressive pulmonary fibrosis. Images A, C, and E demonstrate the presenting CT images in the upper, middle, and lower lung zones. The arrows delineate areas of traction bronchiectasis on presentation. The patient rapidly progressed leading to the images B, D, and F a few months later. These images show progression in the upper, middle, and lower lung zones with arrows delineating worsening traction bronchiectasis, reticulation, and consolidation.

in a basal and peripheral predominance **(Fig. 1)**.[6,7] The alternative patterns of fibrosis usually include fibrotic HP pattern, fibrotic NSIP pattern, and an unclassifiable pattern of fibrosis. **Figures 1 and 2** illustrate two examples of radiologic progression in HP pattern and an unclassifiable pattern of fibrosis. Progressive fibrosis on CT is usually defined as an increase in the fibrotic changes involving at least 10% of the lung parenchyma or more. Both **Figures 1 and 2** display small and large amounts of pulmonary progression.[8]

CLINICAL APPROACH

The initial step in any fibrotic ILD is to make an accurate diagnosis through a MDD including clinical symptoms, physiological symptoms, radiographic findings, and pathological features, if necessary.[9,10] **Flowchart 1** illustrates the overall algorithmic approach to managing these patients. After determining that the patient has a fibrotic lung disease, identification of the cause is also imperative as this will drive options of treatment. The causes of the fibrosing ILD can vary from CTD, inflammatory myositis, HP to IPF, to name a few.[9,10] Determination of the causative disease will help to guide the clinician in determining the next step in treatment.[9,10]

Following diagnosis of fibrosing ILD, the clinician should plan to monitor the patient closely to determine if progression is occurring. Determination of progression requires monitoring of pulmonary function, radiologic imaging, and clinical status. Current ATS/ERJ guidelines recommend monitoring of pulmonary function every 3–4 months.[1,11] Reduction in FVC by 5% with either symptom or radiographic progression has been associated with signs of worsening mortality in IPF patients. Similarly, the progressive decline of FVC in the placebo arm of the INBUILD trial was on par with FVC progressive decline of the IPF patients in the INPULSIS cohort.[12-15] All these studies point to the importance for the clinician to monitor the FVC as well as DLCO on the PFT.

Radiological monitoring is the second part of clinical monitoring for progression. Current guidelines and practices recommend at least annual chest CT monitoring.[1,11] Earlier repeat of chest CT is important if the patient begins to show further clinical signs of progression. Tests such as serum NT-proBNP (N-terminal prohormone of brain natri-

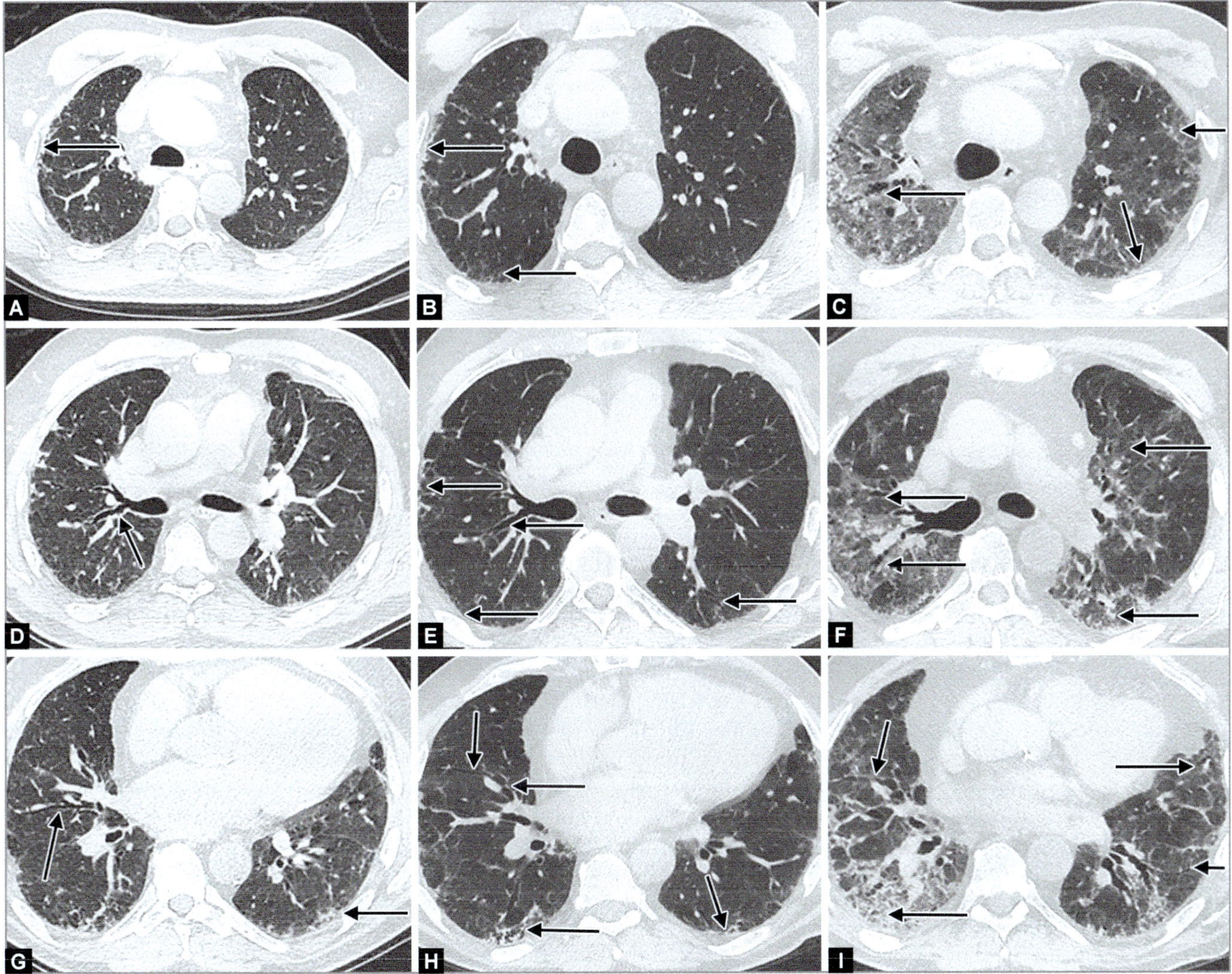

FIGS. 2A TO I: Example of progressive pulmonary fibrosis in a patient with hypersensitivity pneumonitis. Images A, D, and G represent the patient at presentation in the upper, middle, and lower lobes. The second series of images B, E, and H are performed 6 months later showing progression of disease with worsening reticulation and traction bronchiectasis as delineated via the arrows. Images C, F, and I show further progression that occurred over the course of a month with now diffuse reticulation in upper, middle, and lower lung zones as well as much more traction bronchiectasis.

uretic peptide), 6-minute walk test (6MWT), and echo cardiogram can be useful additions in clinical monitoring for progression.

PROGNOSIS

Non-IPF fibrosing ILDs that show progression have similar prognosis to IPF patients with 18–32% developing PPF within 61–80 months as demonstrated by three previous studies.[16-18] The PROGRESS study looked at the median overall survival in non-IPF patients with progressive pulmonary fibrosis. These patients had a survival rate of 76%, 57.7%, 44.5%, and 33.7% at 1, 3, 5, and 8 years, respectively.[18-23] Patients from the PROGRESS trial showed an estimated median overall survival of 4.1 years with traditional IPF patients having a median overall survival of 4.5 years.[21-23] Patients with organizing pneumonia, NSIP, and myositis-associated ILD, as well as those of younger age and with previous response to therapy, are more responsive to treatment; on the other hand, those of older age, underlying usual interstitial pneumonia, history of infections, and absence of initial response to therapy are more likely to progress despite the treatment.[24]

TREATMENT

The approach to treatment for progressive fibrotic ILD originates from the data in IPF. As mentioned earlier,

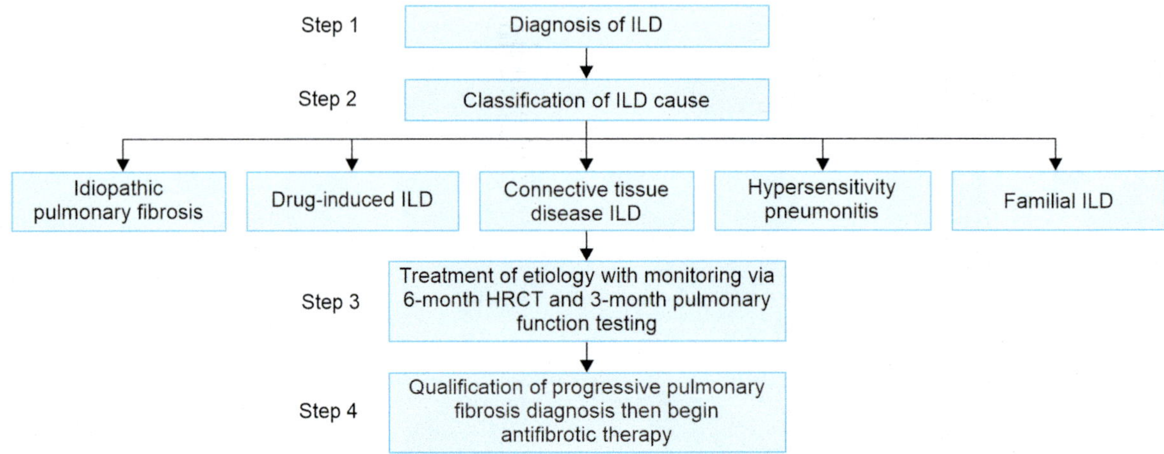

FLOWCHART 1: Algorithmic approach illustrating the diagnosis, monitoring, and management of progressive pulmonary fibrosis.

regardless of the underlying ILD pattern patients who show signs of progression have a median overall survival equal to IPF patients at 4–5 years.[21-23] The current standard of care for treatment of IPF patients is antifibrotic therapy, nintedanib or pirfenidone. Nintedanib binds to tyrosine kinase receptors as well as intracellular adenosine triphosphate site for growth factor receptors.[24] Binding of these sites prevents fibroblast proliferation and migration which leads to less extracellular matrix deposition and slows the progression of fibrotic ILD and IPF.[24] Pirfenidone is designed to interfere with transforming growth factor beta (TGF-β) and other growth factors to effectively reduce TGF-β activity on type II alveolar cells, leading to less collagen and extracellular matrix deposition and thus reducing the progression of pulmonary fibrosis.[25-27]

While determining the approach to treatment, the current first line therapy in treating patients with no-IPF fibrotic ILD, including those with progression, is antifibrotic therapy. However, it is important to note that antifibrotic therapy should not be considered first line outside of IPF, systemic sclerosis (SSc)-ILD, and rheumatoid arthritis (RA)-associated ILD.[28] The data supporting the use of antifibrotic therapy comes from the INBUILD and SENSCIS trials. INBUILD looked at non-IPF patients with progressive fibrotic lung disease and the effects of nintedanib on their progression.[18,23] SENSCIS scleroderma ILD patients, who were on immunosuppressive therapy with steroids and mycophenolate mofetil, were treated with additive nintedanib versus placebo over 52 weeks. Patients treated with nintedanib showed a reduction in decline in FVC compared to placebo by 50 mL versus 90 mL per year, respectively.[18-23] As mentioned previously in this chapter, FVC absolute reduction of 10% carries the worst prognosis for a patient on par with IPF patients' overall survival.[20-23] Nintedanib showed a reduction in the progression of the FVC. Based on these findings, the current guidelines make a recommendation for the use of nintedanib in progressive fibrotic ILD of the non-IPF origin.[1]

Pirfenidone has been recommended for use in IPF patients; however, in non-IPF fibrotic ILD patients who progress, the answer is not clear. Two studies have evaluated its use—the RELIEF trial and another looking at unclassifiable ILD patients.[29,30] The RELIEF trial enrolled chronic HP, CTD ILD, NSIP, and asbestosis-induced lung fibrosis patients.[29] Unfortunately, it was stopped early due to slow recruitment and was unable to show more than a trend toward reduction in FVC by pirfenidone, but statistical significance was not reached.[29] The unclassifiable ILD study was also unable to show statistically significant reduction in progression-free survival at 24 weeks.[29,30] Given the lack of supportive evidence, the current guidelines recommend further research into the topic and favor nintedanib over pirfenidone.[1]

Given the large multitude of diseases, it is imperative that the clinician uses a step-wise approach to the treatment of these patients. The first step is determination of the underlying etiology of ILD. As mentioned earlier in this chapter, these causes can range from IPF to non-IPF causes such as HP, OP, CTD, or myositis.[9,10] In the non-IPF causes, immunosuppressive therapy is the beginning step to treatment. Typically, this begins with corticosteroid therapy with the addition of steroid-sparing therapy in CTD and myositis.[18-23] Some caveats do exist, however, with anti-MDA-5, scleroderma ILD, and RA-ILD. These diseases typically have a higher rate of rapid progression and warrant more aggressive upfront immunosuppression.[31-33]

Connective tissue diseases such as RA-ILD and scleroderma ILD have been shown to benefit from dual suppressive therapy upfront with mycophenolate mofetil and corticosteroid therapy with the addition of rituximab if the disease is not controlled.[31,32] In the case of anti-MDA-5, upfront triple therapy in the form of corticosteroids, cyclophosphamide, and calcineurin inhibitors shows a difference of 40–50% in overall survival.[33] Even with these aggressive immunosuppressive approaches, the patient may still show further fibrotic change that would then warrant additive antifibrotics to the immunosuppressives.[34]

The evidence as to how long to treat these patients with combined immunosuppressive and antifibrotic therapy with PPF is unclear.[34] The underlying etiology of the PPF dictates the likelihood of response and indicates the patient's overall prognosis.[34] Younger age patients and those showing previous response to therapy or flareup of symptoms on stoppage of therapy and patients with diseases such as OP, NSIP, and myositis-ILD are less likely to progress with treatment. On the other hand, older-age patients, those with history of infection or showing lack of initial improvement with treatment, or those with underlying UIP are more likely to progress despite treatment.[34] Tofacitinib, a Janus kinase (JAK) inhibitor, may be a future therapy for those who have refractory anti-MDA5 myositis ILD.[35]

SUMMARY

Progressive pulmonary fibrosis is defined by symptomatic, physiological, and radiographic progression of the fibrotic ILD despite appropriate treatment. It is imperative that the treating clinician monitors these patients closely as PPF carries a median overall survival rate of 4–5 years similar to IPF patients. Monitoring entails 3–6-month follow-up with open-ended questioning to determine symptomatic progression with serial 6MWT and PFT looking for physiologic progression. When these signs are present, then HRCT imagining is imperative. Once PPF is identified, treatment with antifibrotic agents is recommended with a paucity of data lacking but the guidelines are in favor of nintedanib as the initial therapy of choice.

REFERENCES

1. Raghu G, Remy-Jardin M, Richeldi L, et al. Idiopathic Pulmonary Fibrosis (an Update) and Progressive Pulmonary Fibrosis in Adults: An Official ATS/ERS/JRS/ALAT Clinical Practice Guideline. Am J Respir Crit Care Med. 2022;205(9):e18-e47.
2. Mikolasch TA, Garthwaite HS, Porter JC. Update in diagnosis and management of interstitial lung disease. Clin Med (Lond). 2017;17(2):146-53.
3. Karimi-Shah BA, Chowdhury BA. Forced vital capacity in idiopathic pulmonary fibrosis—FDA review of pirfenidone and nintedanib. N Engl J Med. 2015;372(13):1189-91.
4. Quanjer PH, Tammeling GJ, Cotes JE, et al. Lung volumes and forced ventilatory flows. Eur Respir J. 1993;6(Suppl 16):5-40.
5. Modi P, Cascella M. Diffusing Capacity of the Lungs for Carbon Monoxide. [Updated 2023 Mar 13]. In: StatPearls [Internet]. Treasure Island (FL): StatPearls Publishing; 2023 Jan-. [online] Available from https://www.ncbi.nlm.nih.gov/books/NBK556149/ [Last accessed June, 2024].
6. Plantier L, Cazes A, Dinh-Xuan AT, et al. Physiology of the lung in idiopathic pulmonary fibrosis. Eur Respir Rev. 2018;27(147):170062.
7. Yamauchi H, Bando M, Baba T, et al. Clinical Course and Changes in High-resolution Computed Tomography Findings in Patients with Idiopathic Pulmonary Fibrosis without Honeycombing. PLoS One. 2016;11(11):e0166168.
8. Silva CI, Müller NL, Hansell DM, et al. Nonspecific interstitial pneumonia and idiopathic pulmonary fibrosis: changes in pattern and distribution of disease over time. Radiology. 2008;247(1):251-9.
9. Carnevale A, Silva M, Maietti E, et al. Longitudinal change during follow-up of systemic sclerosis: correlation between high-resolution computed tomography and pulmonary function tests. Clin Rheumatol. 2021;40(1):213-9.
10. Glenn LM, Troy LK, Corte TJ. Diagnosing interstitial lung disease by multidisciplinary discussion: A review. Front Med (Lausanne). 2022;9:1017501.
11. Takizawa A, Kamita M, Kondoh Y, et al. Current monitoring and treatment of progressive fibrosing interstitial lung disease: a survey of physicians in Japan, the United States, and the European Union. Curr Med Res Opin. 2021;37(2):327-39.
12. Zappala CJ, Latsi PI, Nicholson AG, et al. Marginal decline in forced vital capacity is associated with a poor outcome in idiopathic pulmonary fibrosis. Eur Respir J. 2010;35(4):830-6.
13. Reichmann WM, Yu YF, Macaulay D, et al. Change in forced vital capacity and associated subsequent outcomes in patients with newly diagnosed idiopathic pulmonary fibrosis. BMC Pulm Med. 2015;15:167.
14. Richeldi L, du Bois RM, Raghu G, et al.; INPULSIS Trial Investigators. Efficacy and safety of nintedanib in idiopathic pulmonary fibrosis. N Engl J Med. 2014;370(22):2071-82.
15. Guler SA, Winstone TA, Murphy D, et al. Does Systemic Sclerosis-associated Interstitial Lung Disease Burn Out? Specific Phenotypes of Disease Progression. Ann Am Thorac Soc. 2018;15(12):1427-33.
16. Reiseter S, Gunnarsson R, Mogens Aaløkken T, et al. Progression and mortality of interstitial lung disease in mixed connective tissue disease: a long-term observational nationwide cohort study. Rheumatology (Oxford). 2018;57(2):255-62.
17. Zamora-Legoff JA, Krause ML, Crowson CS, et al. Progressive Decline of Lung Function in Rheumatoid Arthritis-Associated Interstitial Lung Disease. Arthritis Rheumatol. 2017;69(3):542-9.
18. Distler O, Highland KB, Gahlemann M, et al.; SENSCIS Trial Investigators. Nintedanib for Systemic Sclerosis-associated Interstitial Lung Disease. N Engl J Med. 2019;380(26):2518-28.
19. Raghu G, Collard HR, Egan JJ, et al.; ATS/ERS/JRS/ALAT Committee on Idiopathic Pulmonary Fibrosis. An official ATS/ERS/JRS/ALAT statement: idiopathic pulmonary fibrosis: evidence-based guidelines for diagnosis and management. Am J Respir Crit Care Med. 2011;183(6):788-824.
20. Swigris JJ, Brown KK, Abdulqawi R, et al. Patients' perceptions and patient-reported outcomes in progressive-fibrosing interstitial lung diseases. Eur Respir Rev. 2018;27(150):180075.
21. Moor CC, Heukels P, Kool M, et al. Integrating Patient Perspectives into Personalized Medicine in Idiopathic Pulmonary Fibrosis. Front Med (Lausanne). 2017;4:226.
22. Lammi MR, Baughman RP, Birring SS, et al. Outcome Measures for Clinical Trials in Interstitial Lung Diseases. Curr Respir Med Rev. 2015;11(2):163-74.

23. Nasser M, Larrieu S, Boussel L, et al. Estimates of epidemiology, mortality and disease burden associated with progressive fibrosing interstitial lung disease in France (the PROGRESS study). Respir Res. 2021;22(1):162.
24. Maher TM, Brown KK, Kreuter M, et al. INBUILD trial investigators. Effects of nintedanib by inclusion criteria for progression of interstitial lung disease. Eur Respir J. 2022;59(2):2004587.
25. Prasse A, Pechkovsky DV, Toews GB, et al. A vicious circle of alveolar macrophages and fibroblasts perpetuates pulmonary fibrosis via CCL18. Am J Respir Crit Care Med. 2006;173(7):781-92.
26. Agostini C, Gurrieri C. Chemokine/cytokine cocktail in idiopathic pulmonary fibrosis. Proc Am Thorac Soc. 2006;3(4):357-63.
27. Miyazaki Y, Araki K, Vesin C, et al. Expression of a tumor necrosis factor-alpha transgene in murine lung causes lymphocytic and fibrosing alveolitis. A mouse model of progressive pulmonary fibrosis. J Clin Invest. 1995;96(1):250-9.
28. Khalil N, Xu YD, O'Connor R, et al. Proliferation of pulmonary interstitial fibroblasts is mediated by transforming growth factor-beta1-induced release of extracellular fibroblast growth factor-2 and phosphorylation of p38 MAPK and JNK. J Biol Chem. 2005;280(52):43000-9.
29. Behr J, Prasse A, Kreuter M, et al.; RELIEF investigators. Pirfenidone in patients with progressive fibrotic interstitial lung diseases other than idiopathic pulmonary fibrosis (RELIEF): a double-blind, randomised, placebo-controlled, phase 2b trial. Lancet Respir Med. 2021;9(5):476-86.
30. Maher TM, Corte TJ, Fischer A, et al. Pirfenidone in patients with unclassifiable progressive fibrosing interstitial lung disease: a double-blind, randomised, placebo-controlled, phase 2 trial. Lancet Respir Med. 2020;8(2):147-57.
31. Tashkin DP, Roth MD, Clements PJ, et al; Scleroderma Lung Study II Investigators. Mycophenolate mofetil versus oral cyclophosphamide in scleroderma-related interstitial lung disease (SLS II): a randomised controlled, double-blind, parallel group trial. Lancet Respir Med. 2016;4(9):708-19.
32. Iqbal K, Kelly C. Treatment of rheumatoid arthritis-associated interstitial lung disease: a perspective review. Ther Adv Musculoskelet Dis. 2015;7(6):247-67.
33. Mehta P, Machado PM, Gupta L. Understanding and managing anti-MDA 5 dermatomyositis, including potential COVID-19 mimicry. Rheumatol Int. 2021;41(6):1021-36.
34. Rajan SK, Cottin V, Dhar R, et al. Progressive pulmonary fibrosis: an expert group consensus statement. Eur Respir J. 2023;61(3):2103187.
35. Ida T, Furuta S, Takayama A, et al. Efficacy and safety of dose escalation of tofacitinib in refractory anti-MDA5 antibody-positive dermatomyositis. RMD Open. 2023;9(1):e002795.

Progressive Pulmonary Fibrosis: An Indian Perspective

CHAPTER 111

Sujeet Rajan, Rohit Joshi

INTRODUCTION

In a patient with interstitial lung disease (ILD) of known or unknown etiology other than idiopathic pulmonary fibrosis (IPF) who has radiological evidence of pulmonary fibrosis, the condition would be called a fibrosing ILD other than IPF. Significant interest has emerged in this group of patients as a significant number (between 18% and 32%)[1-5] of them are thought to progress, and some quite rapidly. When fibrosis progresses in a patient with a fibrosing ILD, the condition is termed progressive pulmonary fibrosis (PPF).

DEFINITION

The most simplistic definition for PPF would be what the recent American Thoracic Society (ATS) guidelines have recommended—basically at least two of the following three criteria occurring within the past 1 year with no alternative explanation:

1. Worsening respiratory symptoms
2. Physiological evidence of disease progression [forced vital capacity (FVC), diffusing capacity for carbon monoxide (DLCO)]
3. Radiological evidence of disease progression—one or more of six criteria[1,6]

The deficiency in the above approach would be that a duration of 1 year would be too less, and that progression of fibrosis, whether it occurs in 3 months or 2 years, and is currently irreversible, whatever pharmacotherapy you may offer the patient.

Following a good history, the minimal diagnostic investigations for a patient suspected to have a fibrosing ILD should be a pulmonary function test and high-resolution computed tomography (HRCT) of the lungs. These serve as very important baseline investigations following which symptoms, serial measurements of lung function, and repeat CT scans (if appropriately indicated) can help to determine whether the patient has a PPF or not.

CRITERIA FOR PROGRESSIVE PULMONARY FIBROSIS

Pulmonary Function Criteria for Progressive Pulmonary Fibrosis

Forced vital capacity is the physiological parameter most often used to follow patients with IPF because it is associated with prognosis.[7] A decline in FVC >10% predicted is a predictor of mortality. Smaller declines in FVC (5–10%) have also been associated with a worse prognosis. Although some trials have used a relative change in FVC to assess progression of pulmonary fibrosis, the ATS guideline committee preferred to use absolute change because it forecasts poorer outcomes and is regarded as an important predictor of mortality in IPF.[8] FVC has been used to define disease progression in recent trials on patients with PPF, including the INBUILD (Efficacy and Safety of Nintedanib in Patients with Progressive Fibrosing Interstitial Lung Disease) trial,[9] the RELIEF (Exploring Efficacy and Safety of Oral Pirfenidone for Progressive, Non-IPF Lung Fibrosis) trial,[10] and a trial of patients with unclassifiable ILD (uILD).[11] Integrated with DLCO trends, clinical and radiological criteria, FVC is a clear predictor of future progression.[6]

Though guidelines define an absolute decline in DLCO >10% as clinically meaningful, DLCO has not been the most useful endpoint in pulmonary fibrosis clinical trials, likely because of measurement variability, techniques across laboratories, and lack of specificity for progression. Despite these limitations, DLCO changes can be a strong predictor of mortality in patients with fibrosing ILDs.

Though 6-minute walk test desaturation correlates to some extent with DLCO levels, it should not be viewed as a surrogate marker for DLCO with existing levels of evidence, and poor reproducibility of the test again.

The INBUILD trial criteria (below) seem to be the most practical to use to assess progression and are currently the most frequently used criteria in most randomized clinical trials in IPF and non-IPF progressive ILDs.

INBUILD criteria:

- Relative decline in FVC ≥ 10% predicted
- Relative decline in FVC ≥5 to <10% predicted *and* worsened respiratory symptoms
- Relative decline in FVC ≥5 to <10% predicted *and* increased extent of fibrosis on HRCT
- Worsened respiratory symptoms *and* increased extent of fibrosis on HRCT

In general, PFTs are recommended at least every 3–4 months in the first year, and then less frequently if values and symptoms remain stable.

Radiological Criteria for Progressive Pulmonary Fibrosis

A good-quality CT is critical to diagnose and understand the progression of a fibrosing ILD. Progression of fibrosis is assessed on transverse, coronal, and sagittal contiguous HRCT sections of CT examinations compared side by side, after adjustment for lung volume changes in the best way possible. Progression of fibrosis can be noted by visualizing increased traction bronchiectasis and bronchiolectasis, new ground-glass opacities with traction bronchiectasis, new fine reticulation, increased coarseness of the reticularity, new or increased honeycombing, and increased lobar volume loss.[6]

A greater extent of fibrotic changes is known to be predictive of mortality in IPF, rheumatoid arthritis–related ILD, systemic sclerosis–related ILD, fibrotic hypersensitivity pneumonitis (fHP), pulmonary sarcoidosis, and uILD.[12] An important future research goal would be to validate a formal radiologically derived scoring system based on HRCT, to predict the progression of ILD, both at baseline and in patients with PPF.

High-resolution CT scans need to be done as frequently as PFTs—frequency of scans can vary from case to case and is usually guided by symptoms and PFT decline.

If progression of symptoms cannot be explained on pulmonary workup, other investigations may need to be performed, including possibly echocardiography and N-terminal prohormone of brain natriuretic peptide (NT-proBNP) levels, to assess for pulmonary hypertension and/or left ventricular dysfunction.

Recent studies seem to suggest that the extent of fibrosis on the HRCT (>20%), irrespective of the underlying pattern, predicts progression of almost 50% of the patients within 1 year. This increases to 52% if you add a usual interstitial pneumonia (UIP) pattern to this. This extent of fibrosis on HRCT could be used as a singular marker of progressive disease in the future, with the predictive power of progression similar to a diagnosis of IPF.[13,14]

Bronchoalveolar Lavage Criteria for Progression

Though there is little data in this space, a recent study revealed that bronchoalveolar lavage (BAL) lymphocytosis patients with non-UIP pattern and/or limited extent of fibrosis on HRCT had the lowest rates of progression.[13] There are however limitations to this study as the results may not be universally applicable to all ILD populations, and especially those in whom BAL is contraindicated.

Also, there is limited data on whether BAL lymphocytosis is only an indicator of low risk of progression (without and with therapy) or whether anti-inflammatory therapy contributes or is even necessary to achieve the nonprogression outcome. More randomized, placebo-controlled clinical treatment trials will be necessary to understand this better.

TREATING PROGRESSIVE PULMONARY FIBROSIS

Pharmacotherapy

As we are aware, pharmacotherapy does not reverse fibrosis but can only slow progression. Two antifibrotics are currently available for use in PPF—pirfenidone and nintedanib.

Based on current evidence, nintedanib seems to have been studied slightly more, especially with the INBUILD trial.[9] The results with pirfenidone from the uILD trial are also promising, but not as robust.[11]

It is important to emphasize here that *progression of fibrosis despite adequate management of the underlying ILD* is true PPF. This should also not be confused with acute exacerbations of the underlying ILD, which would need a completely different approach to investigation and treatment.

There is no standardized management for progressive fibrosing ILDs, especially when you have diseases that can progress as disparate as scleroderma and asbestosis. fHP provides an excellent example here, being the most common ILD in the Indian context. Choosing initial treatment can depend on various factors which include the ability to achieve antigen avoidance or eviction, the amount of inflammation on the CT at presentation, disease severity and the presence of a UIP pattern at presentation, age and comorbidities in a particular patient, adverse effects of traditional management, and of course patient preferences.

True progression of fibrosis (assessed after careful evaluation of the above factors) would imply that antifibrotic prescription is justified. The choice of drug could then depend on various factors which are well illustrated in **Table 1**.

Upfront antifibrotic and immunosuppressive therapy is not currently recommended, and we would currently

TABLE 1: Comparison of antifibrotic agents.

	Pirfenidone	Nintedanib
Number of tablets	3–12*	2
Side effects	Nausea, anorexia, weight loss, photosensitivity, rash, elevated liver enzymes	Diarrhea, weight loss, elevated liver enzymes
Outdoor occupation/hobby		+
Anticoagulation therapy	+	
Ischemic heart disease	+	
Cost†		
Newly planned/major surgery	+	
Impact on quality of life	+	+
Prevention of acute exacerbation and/ or respiratory-related hospitalizations	+	+

Note: A "+" possibly denotes the preferred drug of choice.

*Pill burden will vary, depending on the strengths available in different countries.

†It is important to understand that the cost of these drugs varies across countries, insurance providers, and healthcare providers (public vs. private).

recommend that if there is a treatable component of the disease; then consider appropriate management specific to that disease, exhaust such management options fully before considering sequential addition of antifibrotic drugs, after being reasonably confident of fibrosis progression.

The patients who are more likely to benefit with prolonged immunosuppression would include:

- Those who have organizing pneumonia (OP) and nonspecific interstitial pneumonia (NSIP) patterns on CT imaging
- Those who have myositis ILD
- Possibly younger patients, but carefully evaluated as they would then be exposed for more years to immunosuppression
- Those who have nonpulmonary symptoms that flare up on stoppage of steroids
- Those having a previous objective response to corticosteroids or immunosuppression

The patients less likely to benefit with prolonged immunosuppression would be:

- Those with a UIP pattern
- Older patients—here the risk of adverse effects, especially infection, would also be higher
- Those with recurrent infections
- Those who do not demonstrate any clinical or physiological improvement and therefore are at risk of more adverse effects[1]

On occasion, low-dose corticosteroids may need to be given where nonpulmonary symptoms (like joint pains) could flare up on their cessation or where pulmonary function in sarcoid clearly declines on their withdrawal—a steroid-dependent lung situation.

Assessment and Treatment of Acid Reflux

Chronic microaspiration can also aggravate symptoms and often disease in a fibrosing ILD. Antifibrotics themselves can cause significant acid-peptic symptoms. It is important to evaluate acid-peptic disease in patients with fibrosing ILDs well. This can often be a cause and/or aggravating factor of cough in these patients. Upper GI endoscopic evaluation can often be of immense help, not just to assess the upper GI mucosa, but also to evaluate for hiatal hernia, and *Helicobacter pylori* disease, the latter being eminently treatable.

Supplemental Oxygen

The main reason to prescribe supplemental oxygen is for symptomatic relief. Lack of good randomized controlled trials (RCTs) of long-term oxygen therapy (LTOT) in ILD has been an issue, and so the guidelines for LTOT in chronic obstructive pulmonary disease (COPD) are usually followed by clinicians. Ambulatory oxygen (albeit at high flow rates very often) has been shown to improve quality of life in exercise-induced hypoxia, and ATS guidelines have given a conditional recommendation for ambulatory oxygen in patients with ILD having severe exertional hypoxemia.

Vaccinations

Conjugate pneumococcal vaccination and polysaccharide pneumococcal vaccination are recommended for all patient with progressive fibrosing ILDs. The polysaccharide vaccine needs to be given in two doses, at least 5 years apart. The gap between the conjugate and polysaccharide vaccine needs to be anywhere between 2 months and 1 year.

All patients should also receive vaccination against herpes zoster. Vaccination guidelines should be strictly adhered to in these patients and especially those patients on long-term immunosuppressants.

Pulmonary Rehabilitation

There is no generic prescription for pulmonary rehabilitation. Each patient with PPF is different in that sense. The severity of the underlying disease, patient preferences and needs, comorbidities, and availability of rehabilitation services locally will all determine how the patient ultimately receives pulmonary rehabilitation, whether at home or at a healthcare facility. Pulmonary rehabilitation largely aims to improve quality of life and enable activities of daily living.

Palliative and Supportive Care

Holistic care from a palliative or supportive care consultant can go a long way in improving the quality of lives of patients with PPF. Simply assessing the patient with a different set of eyes can bring out issues that were never investigated or looked into before. Asking questions about what they have given up in life to avoid breathlessness is one such example and a recent consensus statement gives suggestions on many more such questions.

Nonpharmacological interventions such as patient positioning, acupressure, hand-held battery-operated portable fans, and low-dose opioids are some of the remarkable interventions that can help in alleviating chronic breathlessness.

Palliative care focusses around goals of care. These should always be discussed with the patient and the caregivers—this significantly improves clarity on treatment strategies when the patient is declining progressively at home or in a hospital setting.

Lung Transplantation

Over the past few years, lung transplantation has gradually come of age in India. Though an expensive option, and fraught with its own set of issues, it remains a significant option for patients willing to consider it, and who have caregivers that can support them through the process. PPF patients are largely evaluated for transplant by the same criteria that apply to IPF. However, this group of patients is often significantly younger than IPF patients, and therefore the average age of referral is lower.

FUTURE DIRECTIONS

Research needs in PPF include determining the reasons that a subset of patients with ILD of different etiologies develop a progressive and irreversible fibrotic phenotype in a relatively short time despite initial treatment, including triggers, genetic predisposition, and the role of vascular remodeling.[15,16] More research in serum biomarkers is also required to identify those at risk of PPF.[17,18] Large HRCT datasets from different geographies will be useful for disease pattern recognition, prognostication, and identifying progression[19-23] and for the characterization of incidentally detected interstitial lung abnormalities (ILAs).[24] ILAs are being increasingly recognized as a possible precursor of a fibrosing ILD, though it is important to realize that this is still a radiological finding, rather than a disease. There is need to prioritize research related to the use of antifibrotics and immunosuppressants in combination, and whether upfront, or sequentially.

SUMMARY

Antifibrotics, oxygen therapy, pulmonary rehabilitation, vaccination and finally lung transplantation are management options for progressive pulmonary fibrosis. It is imperative for respiratory physicians to understand definition of PPF for timely management of these patients.

REFERENCES

1. Rajan SK, Cottin V, Dhar R, et al. Progressive pulmonary fibrosis: an expert group consensus statement. Eur Respir J. 2023;61: 2103187.
2. Faverio P, Piluso M, De Giacomi F, et al. Progressive fibrosing interstitial lung diseases: prevalence and characterization in two Italian referral centers. Respiration. 2020;99:838-45.
3. Guler SA, Winstone TA, Murphy D, et al. Does systemic sclerosis-associated interstitial lung disease burn out? Specific phenotypes of disease progression. Ann Am Thorac Soc. 2018; 15:1427-33.
4. Nasser M, Larrieu S, Si-Mohamed S, et al. Progressive fibrosing interstitial lung disease: a clinical cohort (the PROGRESS study). Eur Respir J. 2021;57:2002718.
5. Reiseter S, Gunnarsson R, Mogens Aalokken T, et al. Progression and mortality of interstitial lung disease in mixed connective tissue disease: a long-term observational nationwide cohort study. Rheumatology. 2018;57:255-62.
6. Raghu G, Remy-Jardin M, Richeldi L, et al. Idiopathic Pulmonary Fibrosis (an Update) and Progressive Pulmonary Fibrosis in Adults: An Official ATS/ERS/JRS/ALAT Clinical Practice Guideline. Am J Respir Crit Care Med. 2022;205(9):e18-e47.
7. Karimi-Shah BA, Chowdhury BA. Forced vital capacity in idiopathic pulmonary fibrosis–FDA review of pirfenidone and nintedanib. N Engl J Med. 2015;372:1189-91.
8. du Bois RM, Weycker D, Albera C, et al. Forced vital capacity in patients with idiopathic pulmonary fibrosis: test properties and minimal clinically important difference. Am J Respir Crit Care Med. 2011;184:1382-9.
9. Flaherty KR, Wells AU, Cottin V, et al.; INBUILD Trial Investigators. Nintedanib in progressive fibrosing interstitial lung diseases. N Engl J Med. 2019;381:1718-27.
10. Behr J, Prasse A, Kreuter M, et al. RELIEF Investigators. Pirfenidone in patients with progressive fibrotic interstitial lung diseases other than idiopathic pulmonary fibrosis (RELIEF): a double-blind, randomised, placebo-controlled, phase 2b trial. Lancet Respir Med. 2021;9:476-86.
11. Maher TM, Corte TJ, Fischer A, et al. Pirfenidone in patients with unclassifiable progressive fibrosing interstitial lung disease:

a double-blind, randomised, placebo-controlled, phase 2 trial. Lancet Respir Med. 2020;8:147-57.

12. Kolb M, Vasakova M. The natural history of progressive fibrosing interstitial lung diseases. Respir Res. 2019;20:57.
13. Barnett JL, Maher TM, Quint JK, et al. Combination of BAL and computed Tomography Differentiates Progressive and Non-Progressive Fibrotic Lung Diseases. Am J Respir Crit Care Med. 2023;208(9):975-82.
14. Behr J. To Progress or Not to Progress, That is the Question! Progression in Fibrotic ILD. Am J Respir Crit Care Med. 2023; 208(9):949-51.
15. Waxman A, Restrepo-Jaramillo R, Thenappan T, et al. Inhaled treprostinil in pulmonary hypertension due to interstitial lung disease. N Engl J Med. 2021;384:325-34.
16. Wijsenbeek M, Cottin V. Spectrum of fibrotic lung diseases. N Engl J Med. 2020;383:958-68.
17. Moodley YP, Corte TJ, Oliver BG, et al. Analysis by proteomics reveals unique circulatory proteins in idiopathic pulmonary fibrosis. Respirology. 2019;24:1111-4.
18. Todd JL, Neely ML, Overton R, et al.; IPF-PRO Registry investigators. Peripheral blood proteomic profiling of idiopathic pulmonary fibrosis biomarkers in the multicentre IPF-PRO Registry. Respir Res. 2019;20:227.
19. Humphries SM, Swigris JJ, Brown KK, et al. Quantitative high-resolution computed tomography fibrosis score: performance characteristics in idiopathic pulmonary fibrosis. Eur Respir J. 2018;52:1801384.
20. Gao M, Bagci U, Lu L, et al. Holistic classification of CT attenuation patterns for interstitial lung diseases via deep convolutional neural networks. Comput Methods Biomech Biomed Eng Imaging Vis. 2018;6:1-6.
21. Walsh SLF, Calandriello L, Silva M, et al. Deep learning for classifying fibrotic lung disease on high-resolution computed tomography: a case-cohort study. Lancet Respir Med. 2018;6: 837-45.
22. Walsh SLF, Humphries SM, Wells AU, et al. Imaging research in fibrotic lung disease; applying deep learning to unsolved problems. Lancet Respir Med. 2020;8:1144-53.
23. Wang C, Moriya T, Hayashi Y, et al. Weakly supervised deep learning of interstitial lung disease types on CT images. In: Mori K, Hahn HK (Eds). Medical Imaging 2019: Computer Aided Diagnosis. Bellingham, WA: International Society for Optics and Photonics; 2019. p. 109501H.
24. Bermejo-Pelaez D, Ash SY, Washko GR, et al. Classification of interstitial lung abnormality patterns with an ensemble of deep convolutional neural networks. Sci Rep. 2020;10:338.

CHAPTER 112

Organizing Pneumonia

Brenda D Garcia, Diane Stover, Stephen Machnicki, Suhail Raoof

INTRODUCTION

Organizing pneumonia (OP) is an enigmatic and rare diagnosis of which there are two major types, cryptogenic OP (COP) and secondary OP (SOP).[1] It often manifests clinically with vague symptoms and radiographic patterns that are not specific; thus, the diagnosis is often delayed or misdiagnosed as other more common pulmonary diseases such as infection.

Making the diagnosis of OP relies on the entire clinical presentation with associated imaging and often requires the use of other supplementary data which may include histopathological findings. In general, OP is classified on the continuum of interstitial lung disease and interstitial pneumonias. It can be COP, formally known as bronchiolitis obliterans organizing pneumonia (BOOP), which has no specific etiology, or secondary OP (SOP), which can be associated with a variety of causes. When treated appropriately, it has an overall very good prognosis.[2,3]

EPIDEMIOLOGY

Presentation can occur at any age; however, it is more commonly seen later in life within the fifth and sixth decades.[4,5] No differences have been found between genders. Interestingly, contrary to usual pulmonary diseases, cigarette or tobacco smoking has been found to be a protective factor against the development of OP and disease is seen about twice as often in nonsmokers or former smokers.[6]

CAUSES

Cryptogenic OP as mentioned refers to an idiopathic or unknown inciting cause of signs and symptoms, while SOP is due to a known or associated cause. At times, it may be difficult to illicit an inciting factor. Causes of SOP are most often attributed to an inflammatory reaction to infection but also can be found with various connective tissue diseases, medications or drugs, or radiation toxicity **(Fig. 1)**. Despite the treatment of preceding infection or removal of offending agent, findings of OP can persist and it becomes a separate diagnosis. Additional associations of SOP include organ transplant, malignancies, and aspiration.[2,6,7] **Table 1** shows a list of common causes for SOP.

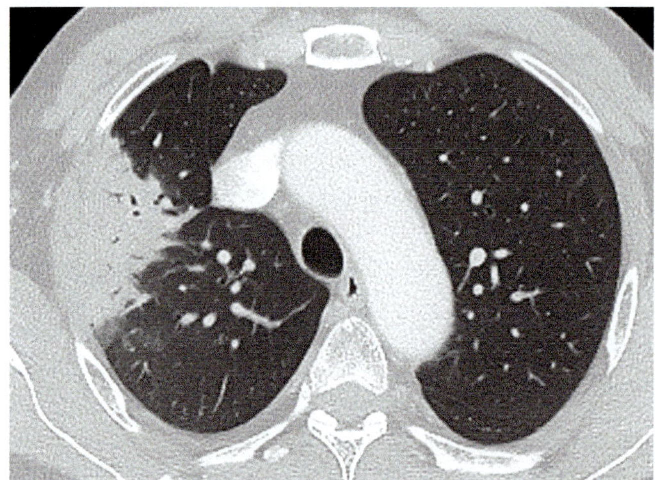

FIG. 1: A 54-year-old male with a past medical history of high-grade B-cell non-Hodgkin lymphoma treated with chemotherapy and radiation presented with fever. Axial contrast-enhanced CT image with lung windows shows peripherally located consolidation in the right upper lobe. He was found to have organizing pneumonia on biopsy.

CLINICAL FEATURES

Symptoms of OP can be vague and nonspecific. Patients may present with subacute flu-like symptoms such as generalized malaise, cough, night sweats, low-grade fever, chills, and poor appetite. Dyspnea on exertion may also be present depending on acuity of presentation or amount of parenchymal involvement; however, only rarely is significant hypoxemia present that necessitates mechanical ventilation.[1,2,7-9] In some instances, patients may be asymptomatic with pulmonary findings discovered incidentally on chest radiograph. Clinically, no significant difference has been found between the symptoms and signs of COP versus SOP.[5,8]

TABLE 1: Causes of secondary organizing pneumonia.

Types of organizing pneumonia	Cryptogenic organizing pneumonia	Secondary organizing pneumonia
Causes (list is not comprehensive)	Idiopathic; no inciting or secondary causes can be found	*Infections*: • Bacterial • Viral • Fungal • Parasitic
		Autoimmune connective tissue diseases: • Rheumatoid arthritis • Granulomatosis with polyangiitis • Systemic lupus erythematosus • Sjögren syndrome • Systemic sclerosis • Dermatomyositis/polymyositis • Inflammatory bowel disease • Sarcoidosis • Sweet syndrome
		Drug induced:* • Amiodarone • Bleomycin • Beta blockers • Nitrofurantoin • Methotrexate • Carbamazepine
		Inhalant exposure: • Cocaine • Textile fumes and dye • Sulfur dioxide • Vaping
		Association with other lung pathologies: • Aspiration • Lung cancer • Lung abscess • Metastatic disease • Hypersensitivity pneumonitis • Usual interstitial pneumonia • Nonspecific interstitial pneumonia • Chronic eosinophilic pneumonia • Diffuse alveolar damage
		Hematologic malignancy: • Diffuse large B-cell lymphoma • Non-Hodgkin lymphoma • Leukemia
		Immunodeficiency: • Common variable immunodeficiency disease • Human immunodeficiency virus
		Transplantation: • Lung • Liver • Allogeneic bone marrow
		Thoracic radiation therapy

*See full list at pneumotox.com.

ALGORITHMIC APPROACH TO DIAGNOSIS

Given the generalized symptoms, diagnosis can be difficult and often delayed due to the broad differential diagnosis that is initially considered. Additionally, the generalized symptoms and imaging findings can overlap with underlying causes of SOP, for instance, the presence of infection or resolving infection, various connective tissue diseases, and malignancy.

In general, high clinical suspicion must be maintained to make the diagnosis of OP. Important considerations include the presence of symptoms of "untreated" or refractory pulmonary infection or chest imaging consistent with infection despite adequate treatment **(Figs. 2A to C)**. Chest imaging findings include ongoing migrating, patchy parenchymal consolidations, or new focal opacities on follow-up scans **(Figs. 3A to C)**. Lastly, attention must be given to the presence of any typical known secondary cause of OP or recent inciting incident that can be attributed to the clinical syndrome.

As with most inflammatory diseases, and similarly in OP, the presence of leukocytosis, elevated C-reactive protein, and elevated erythrocyte sedimentation rate can be present. Pertinent negatives include presence of significantly elevated leukocytosis or eosinophilia. More often, other laboratory data do not play a large role in diagnosis; however, monitoring inflammatory markers, especially CRP, during treatment is often helpful to assess treatment response or disease relapse.[6,9] Pulmonary function testing is usually abnormal and may show a restrictive ventilatory defect and reduction in diffusing capacity of the lung for carbon monoxide (DLCO); however, it may also be normal or show a mixed pattern, especially if other underlying pulmonary disorders are present.[5]

Once consideration to the above is made, further imaging is required in the form of high-resolution chest computed tomography (CT) to characterize the parenchymal

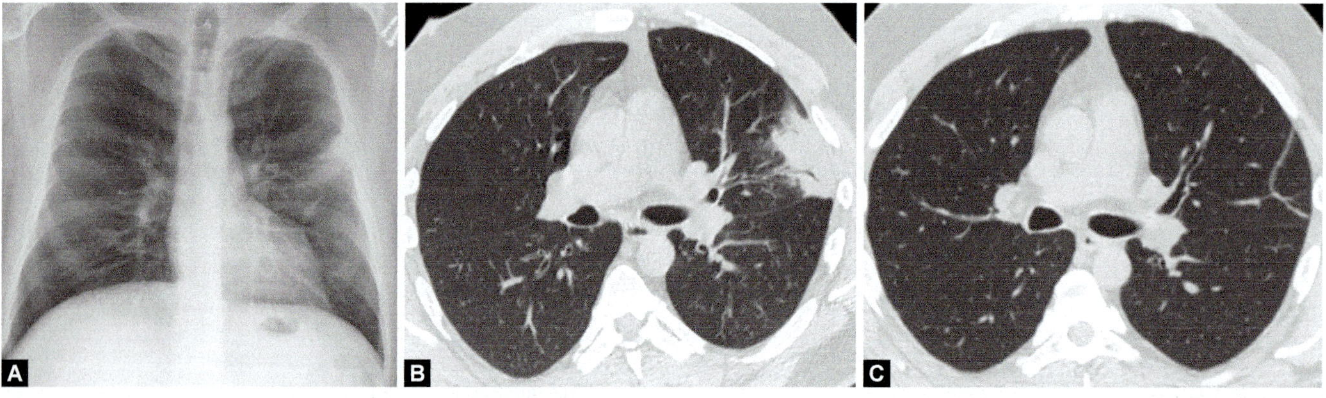

FIGS. 2A TO C: A 40-year-old male with daily marijuana use presented with cough, shortness of breath, and leukocytosis. (A) Posteroanterior chest radiograph at presentation shows peripheral consolidation in the left upper lobe, presumed to be pneumonia. (B) Axial image with lung windows from unenhanced chest CT performed 2 weeks later after no improvement in symptoms following a course of antibiotics demonstrates persistent peripheral consolidation with air bronchogram in the left upper lobe. Biopsy results consistent with organizing pneumonia. (C) Axial CT image after treatment with steroids and resolution of symptoms showing resolution of consolidation, with a curvilinear band remaining.

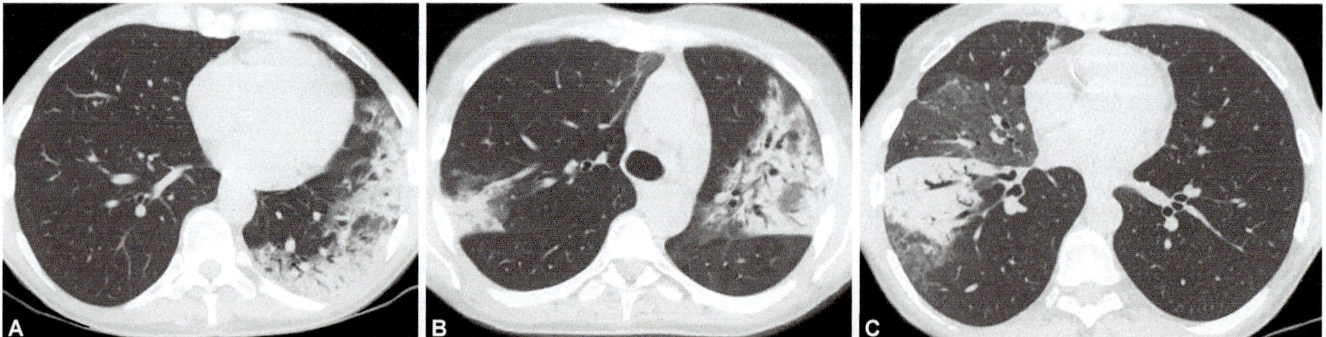

FIGS. 3A TO C: A 62-year-old male presented with cough and dyspnea. Axial images with lung windows from unenhanced CT scans obtained in (A) November 2019, (B) December 2019, and (C) October 2020 demonstrating the migratory consolidative opacities and the presence of air bronchograms that are typical of organizing pneumonia.

pattern of pulmonary involvement. There are variably described and recognized patterns within the literature regarding high-resolution chest CT indicators of OP which are classified by typical findings of predominant lesions. Just as with the symptoms of COP and SOP, there are no radiographic features unique for either. Here, we will describe three predominant radiographic patterns of OP used by Cherian et al.[2] These are consolidation predominant, nodular predominant, and linear or reticular predominant patterns of OP on chest CT.

1. Consolidation predominant presents with peripheral **(Figs. 1 to 3)** and peribronchovascular parenchymal opacities which obscure the margins of vessels and airway walls **(Figs. 4A and B)**, often with air bronchograms, or rarely can feature ground-glass opacities or a crazy paving pattern **(Figs. 5 to 7)**. The consolidation is often migrating or waxing and waning **(Figs. 3A to C)**.
2. A nodular predominant pattern involves presence of solitary **(Fig. 8)** or multiple micro- or macronodules **(Figs. 9 to 11)** or masses. These nodules can rarely present with ground-glass or tree-in-bud appearances.
3. A linear or reticular predominant pattern typically involves traction bronchiectasis, band-like arcade or arch-like pattern **(Figs. 12 and 13)**, or subpleural lines. Rarely, an atoll (reverse halo) sign **(Figs. 6, 14, and 15)** or perilobular lines exist.

Using the above information, a diagnosis is sometimes made, and treatment initiated. However, if there is a concern for alternative diagnoses or if a diagnosis of OP cannot be confidently made, a multidisciplinary discussion may be

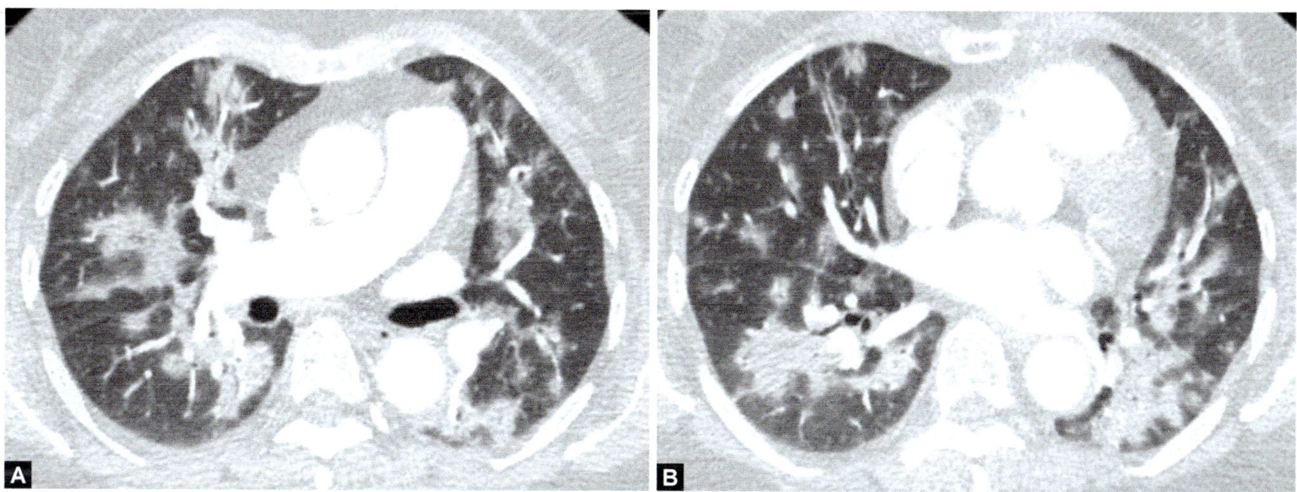

FIGS. 4A AND B: Axial images from a contrast-enhanced CT scan performed on a 44-year-old woman who presented with chest pain and shortness of breath demonstrate multiple foci of peribronchovascular consolidation in both lungs. Biopsy is consistent with organizing pneumonia.

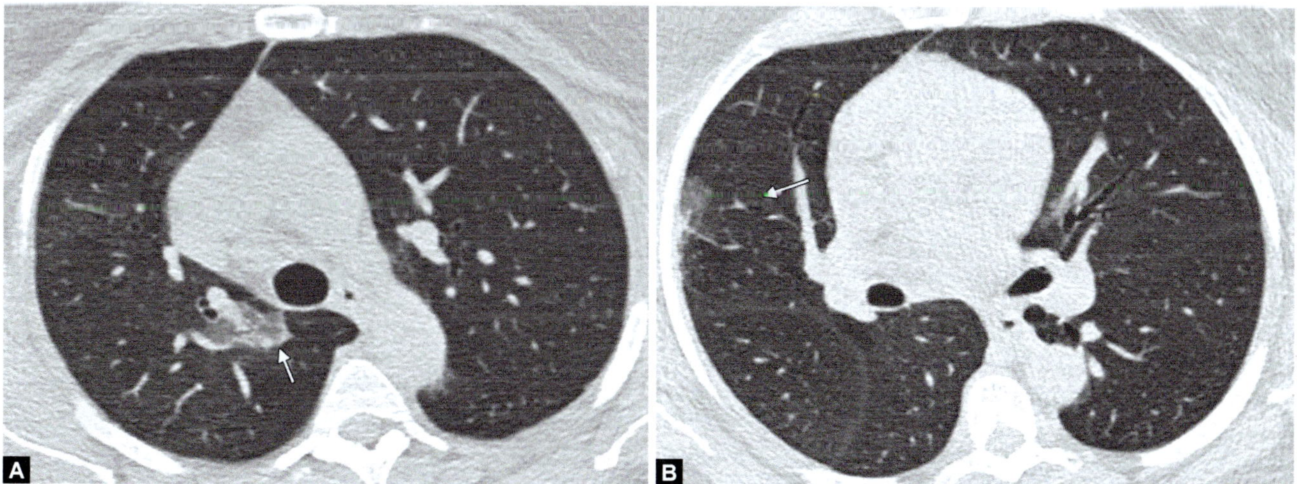

FIGS. 5A AND B: A 57-year-old female with dyspnea. Axial images from unenhanced chest CT demonstrate (A) peribronchovascular and (B) peripheral ground-glass opacities. Biopsy results are consistent with organizing pneumonia.

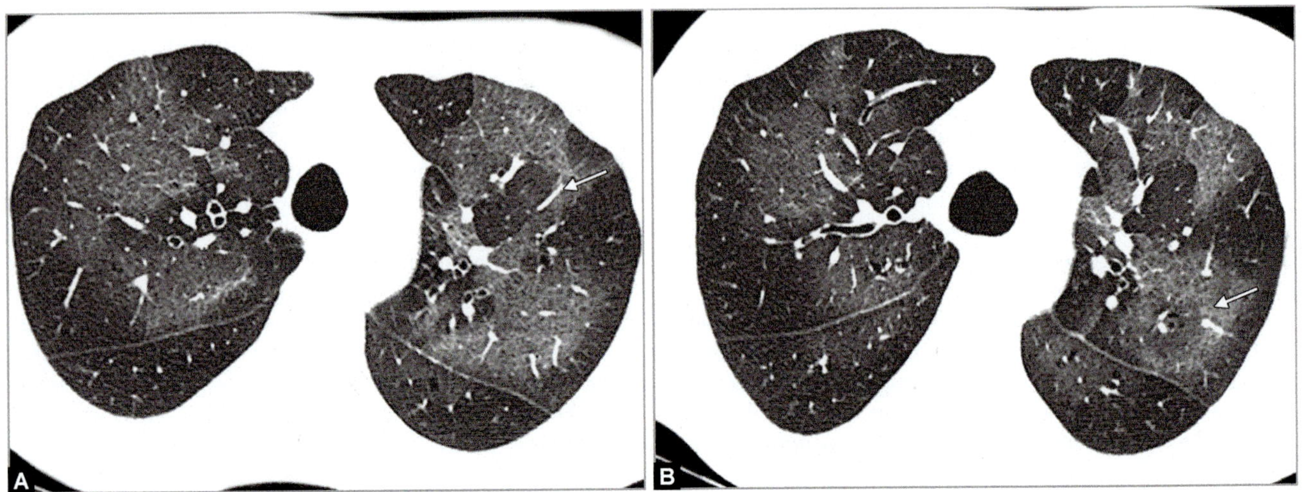

FIGS. 6A AND B: A 41-year-old female with persistent cough despite treatment. Axial images from unenhanced CT scan demonstrates large ground-glass opacity bilaterally. There is also thickening of the intralobular and interlobular septa, producing a crazy-paving pattern. Central areas of less dense opacification in the left upper lobe produce a reverse halo sign or atoll sign (arrows). Transbronchial biopsy consistent with organizing pneumonia.

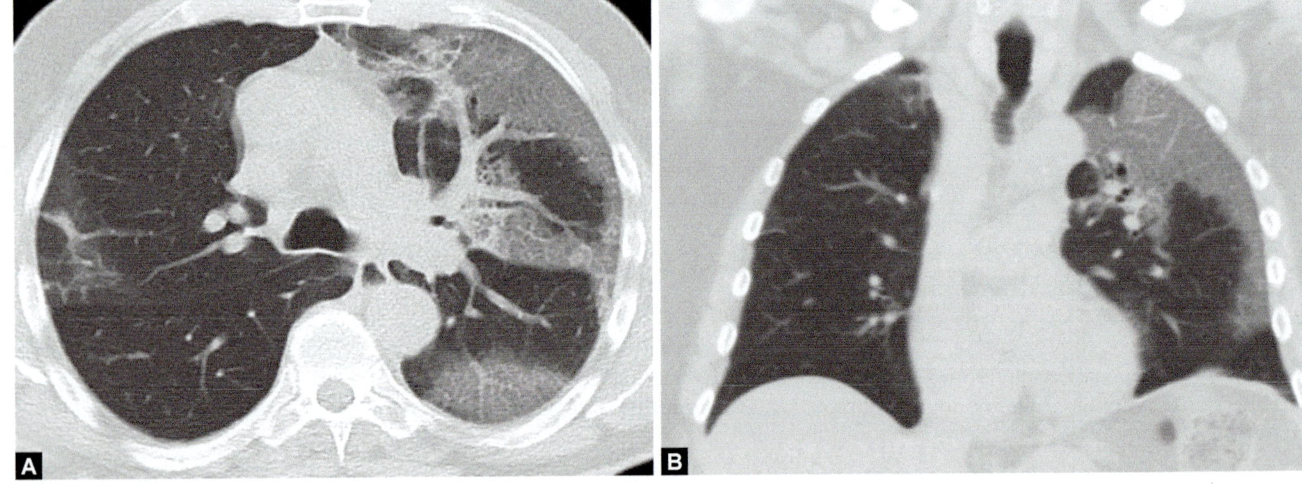

FIGS. 7A AND B: A 76-year-old male with dyspnea on exertion and history of amiodarone use. (A) Axial and (B) coronal images with lung windows from unenhanced chest CT demonstrate peripherally located ground-glass opacity with thickening of the interlobular septa and intralobular lines in the left lung, producing a crazy paving pattern. The opacities resolved on follow-up scan after drug stopped and treatment with steroids.

useful in determining next steps in the diagnostic evaluation. An algorithmic approach **(Flowchart 1)** may be helpful in diagnosing OP.

Potentially, further diagnostic workup can include bronchoscopy with bronchoalveolar lavage, with or without transbronchial or cryobiopsies to further assist with diagnosis or rule out other possible etiologies of disease.[10] Bronchoalveolar lavage findings in OP typically include a mixed cellular pattern with lymphocytic predominance (approximately 25% or greater) with decreased CD4/CD8 ratio, mildly elevated neutrophils (approximately 10%), and some eosinophils (approximately 5%).[5,6,9-11]

Alternatively, tissue biopsy alone via CT guidance or surgical lung biopsy can be pursued if the diagnosis is still unclear, if there has been clinical worsening despite treatment, or if an alternative diagnosis is strongly suspected. A multidisciplinary approach can and should be taken if a diagnosis of OP is suspected or is unclear and the diagnosis pursued with discussion of risks and benefits with the patient.

DIFFERENTIAL DIAGNOSIS

Relying solely on the above imaging categories, the differential diagnosis can vary; thus, the above algorithmic approach to diagnosis can be considered. Alternatively, OP can mimic other diagnoses given symptoms and radiographic features that are similar to malignancy

(Figs. 8 to 11), infection, inhalational exposures, radiation or drug toxicity, sarcoidosis, chronic connective tissue diseases, eosinophilic pneumonias, other interstitial lung diseases, and many others.[2,6,12] As seen in **Figures 10A and B**, COP and SOP can be fluorodeoxyglucose (FDG)-avid on positron emission tomography–computed tomography (PET/CT) mimicking malignancy.[13,14]

HISTOLOGY

As most symptomatic patients are subjected to long-term treatment with immune suppression for weeks, months, or even years and given the possibility of alternative diagnoses, a definitive pathological diagnosis may be beneficial.

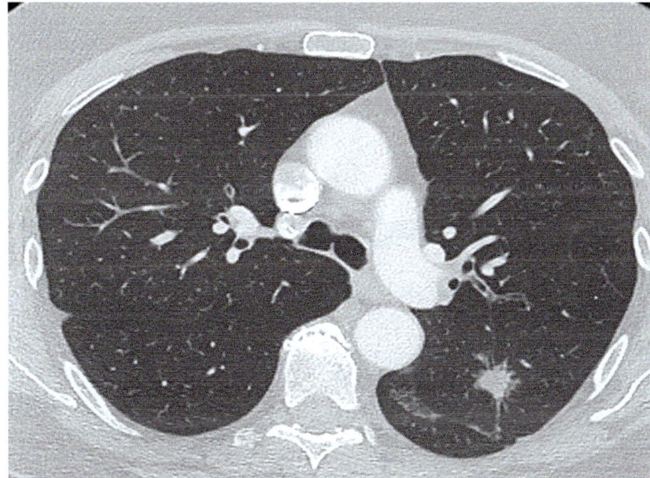

FIG. 8: A 68-year-old female underwent a contrast-enhanced chest CT for the evaluation of chest pain. Axial image from that CT scan showing a 13-mm spiculated solid nodule in the left upper lobe, suspicious for lung cancer. Transbronchial biopsy consistent with organizing pneumonia.

Typical findings of OP pattern include polypoid plugs of loose connective tissue within the airway lumens that extend into distal airways. Spaces within the alveolar ducts and alveoli are most affected and may contain alveolar exudates. Bronchiolar involvement, type II pneumocyte hyperplasia, or interstitial fibrosis is not typically seen. Most of the connective tissue is of the same age with overall preservation of the architecture of the lung parenchyma. Large specimens may show multicentric foci of OP patterns; however, in less involved or focal areas of involvement, the pattern can be focal or a single nodule of the above pattern.[2,15] Histologically, there is a spectrum of disease findings that have been described in addition to the typical OP pattern and can be found in other disease entities such as in collagen vascular disease and hypersensitivity pneumonitis or in overlap syndromes, for instance acute fibrinous organizing pneumonia (AFOP) and granulomatous organizing pneumonia (GOP) **(Figs. 5A and B)**.[12,15,16]

TREATMENT

The first-line treatment for patients with symptomatic OP from idiopathic or secondary causes includes initiation of corticosteroids. There is no consensus regarding the duration of treatment; however, a prolonged course of treatment is often pursued.[3,7,17] Generally, the treatment period can extend over 6 months to 1 year using an initial high dose of 0.5–1.5 mg/kg and progressively tapered at the discretion of the treating physician based on clinical, radiographical, and inflammatory marker trends.[2,6,7,17,18] Macrolides as monotherapy can be an alternative treatment option in nonsevere, mild cases or as a bridge after corticosteroids.[1,7,19]

Treatment of OP with corticosteroids yields successful resolution in most cases. It is rare that other immuno-

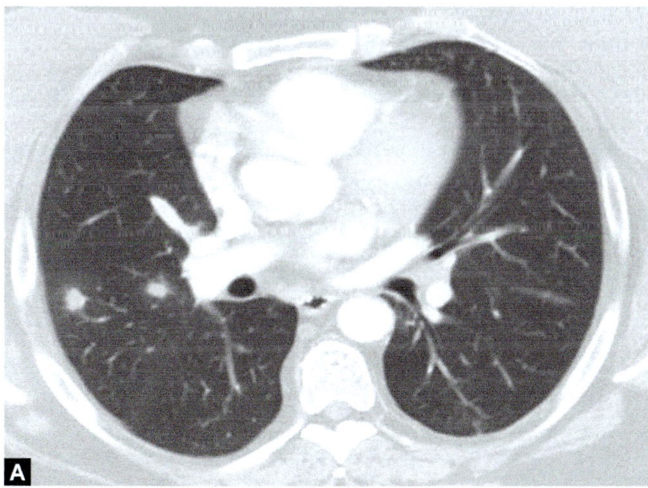

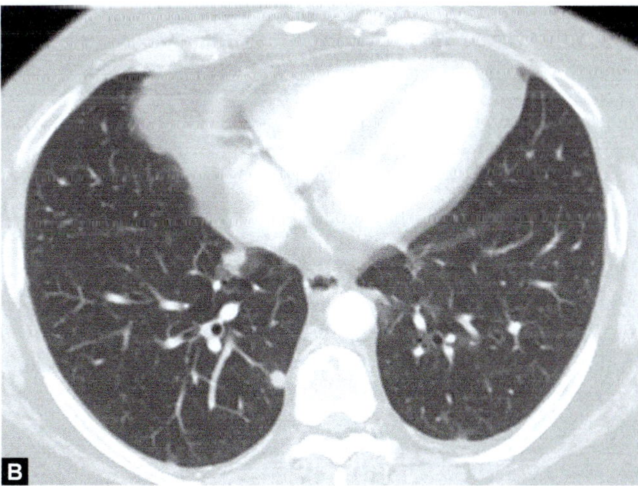

FIGS. 9A AND B: Axial images with lung windows from a contrast-enhanced chest CT performed on a 52-year-old female with history of breast cancer treated with chemotherapy who presented with worsening shortness of breath. Multiple solid nodules were detected in the right lower lobe, suspicious for metastases. Biopsy results are consistent with organizing pneumonia.

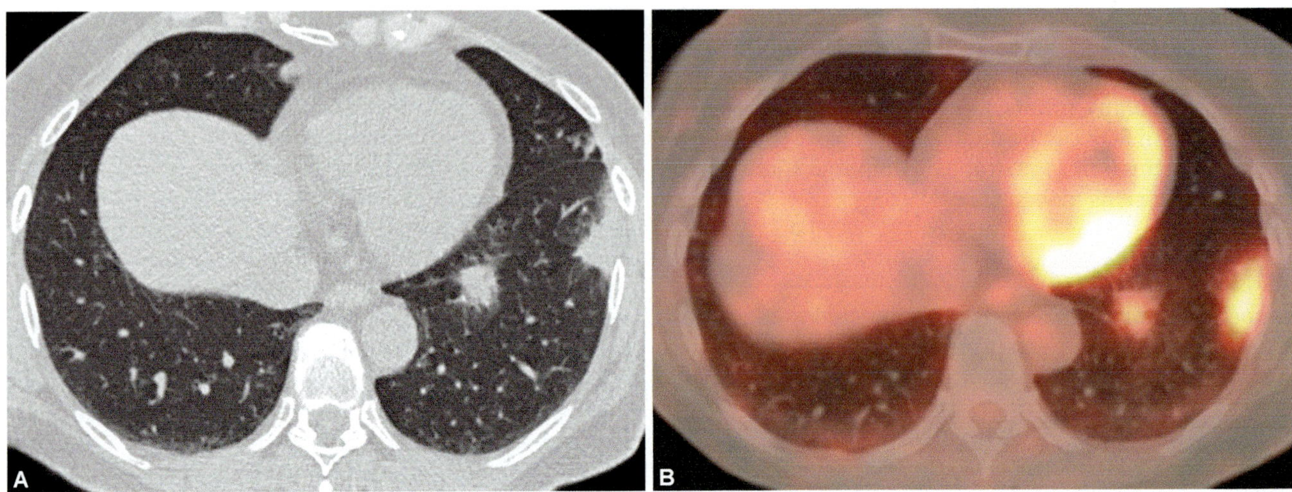

FIGS. 10A AND B: A 70-year-old female with history of breast cancer presented with cough and dyspnea. (A) Axial image with lung windows from unenhanced chest CT demonstrates a peripheral mass and a central nodule in the left lower lobe. (B) Fused PET/CT image from flourodeoxyglucose-18 PET/CT scan demonstrates the mass and nodule to be hypermetabolic, suspicious for metastatic disease. Biopsy of the mass is consistent with organizing pneumonia.

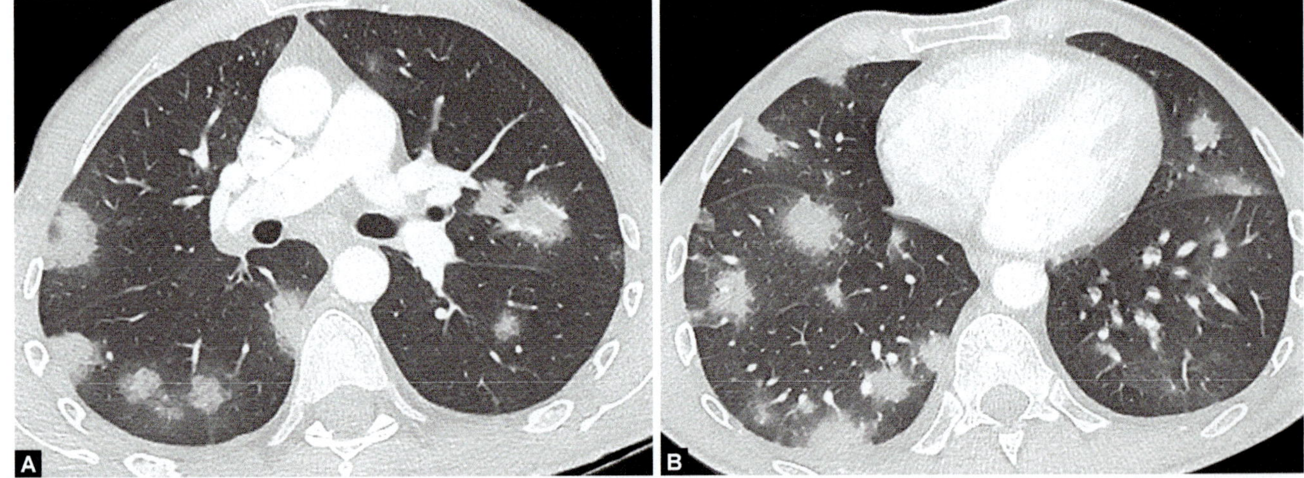

FIGS. 11A AND B: Axial CT scan images obtained on a 32-year-old male with chronic persistent cough and dyspnea on exertion for 1 year and 20-pound weight loss. Multiple solid nodules and masses bilaterally are seen. Biopsy is consistent with organizing pneumonia.

suppressive treatments such as rituximab, cyclophosphamide, azathioprine, or mycophenolate are utilized for refractory cases. Although the general response to treatment is excellent, there is a high rate of relapse, especially when a change in steroid dose is made too abruptly or treatment has been stopped or completed **(Fig. 13B)**. Despite the high rate of relapse, which occurs in up to 50% of cases, outcomes are still favorable and not affected.[6,8,17] Relapse has also been attributed to delayed diagnosis.[17]

MONITORING/PROGNOSIS

Given the known frequent rate of relapsed OP, physicians must be astute to consider an alternative diagnosis, especially if there is no response to treatment, if there is no change in clinical course, or if no histopathological diagnosis has been confirmed. Monitoring clinical symptoms, imaging, and inflammatory markers is useful while treatment is ongoing, recently changed, or completed.

Overall, the survival outcomes of patients with COP or SOP are the same between groups. However, there may be a trend for lower survival rate in those with OP compared with the general population, particularly those with secondary OP, due to underlying predisposing conditions.[4,5,7,8]

SUMMARY

Organizing pneumonia is an important clinical condition classified in the broad category of interstitial lung disease. It is either cryptogenic in origin or secondary to a large

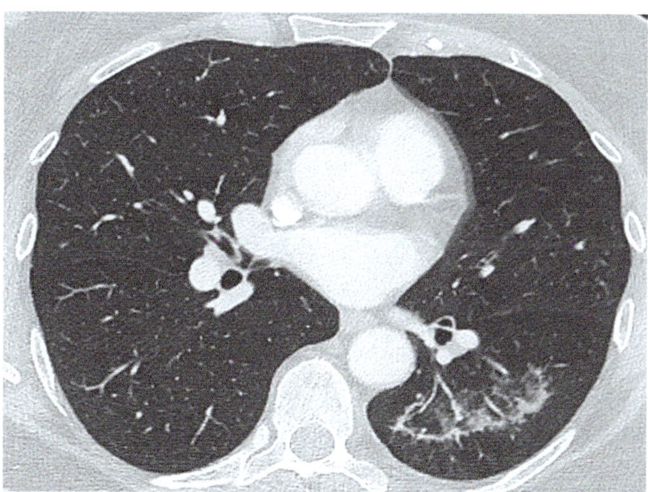

FIG. 12: A 64-year-old female complaining of chest pain. Axial image from contrast-enhanced CT scan demonstrates an incomplete peripheral solid band with patchy central ground-glass opacity. Transbronchial biopsy is consistent with organizing pneumonia.

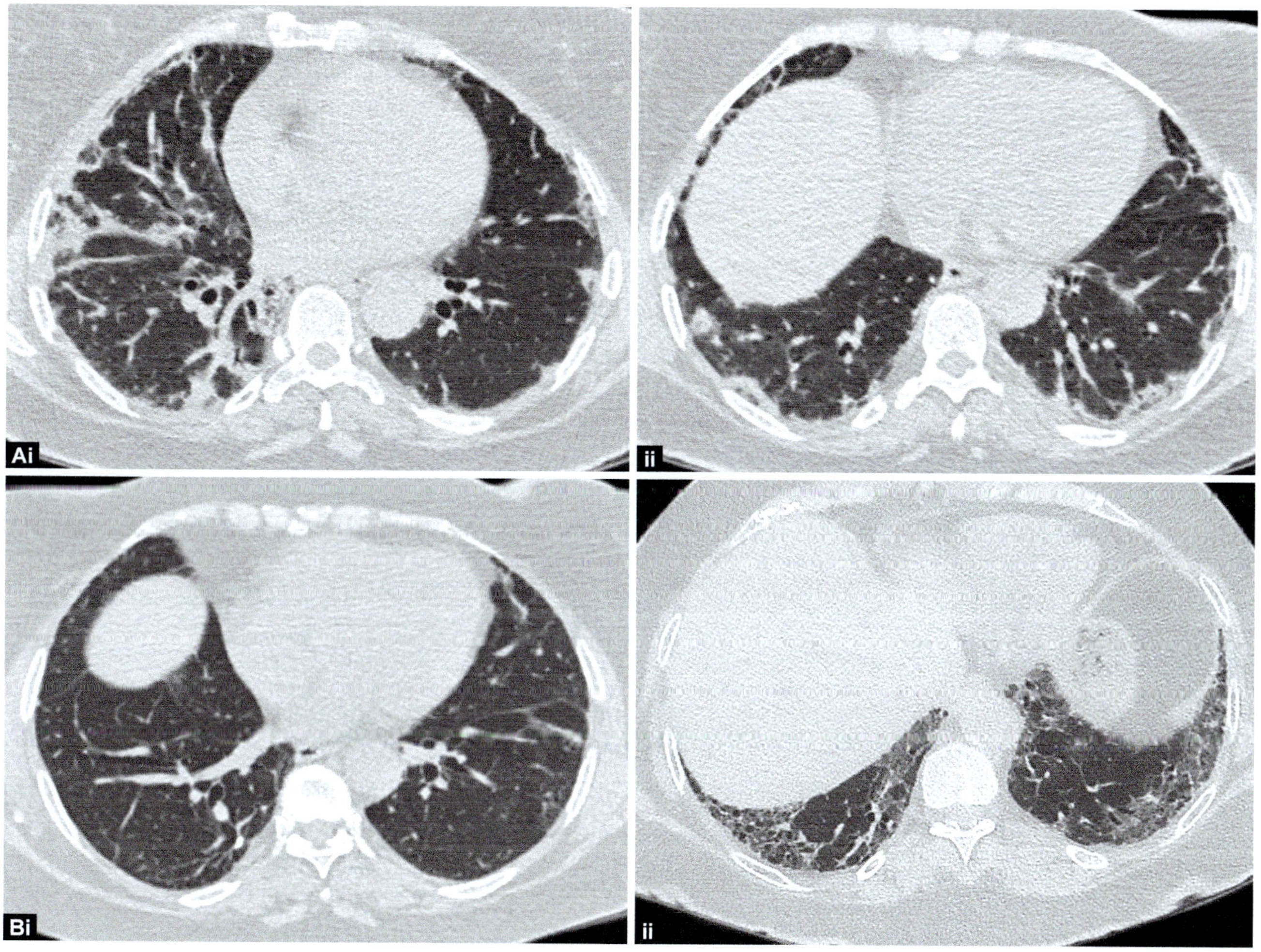

FIGS. 13A AND B: (A) A 61-year-old female with acute shortness of breath and cough. Axial images from unenhanced chest CT demonstrate peripheral predominant perilobular opacities in the lower lung zones bilaterally, producing an "arcade" pattern. Surgical lung biopsy is consistent with organizing pneumonia. The patient had a history of occupational exposure in the textile industry. (B) Same patient as (A) (i) Axial unenhanced image 9 months after treatment with steroids shows resolution of the peripheral opacities. (ii) Axial image following cessation of steroids and clinical relapse demonstrates development of peripheral ground-glass opacity, traction bronchiectasis, and honeycombing, consistent with fibrosis.

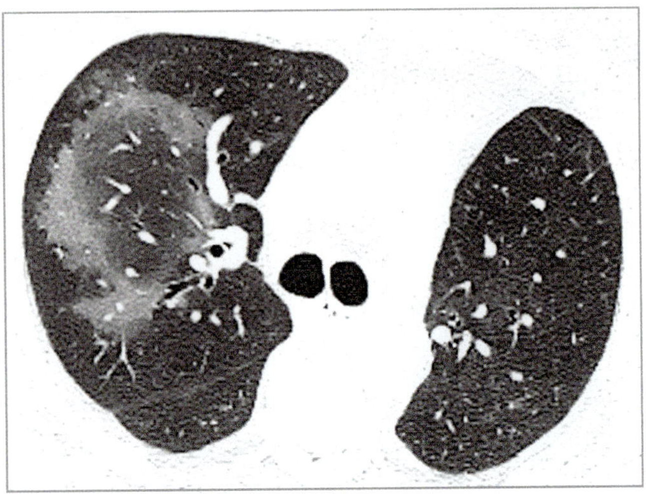

FIG. 14: A 61-year-old male with history of left lower lobectomy for lung adenocarcinoma presented with cough. Axial image with lung windows from unenhanced CT scan demonstrates a large ground-glass opacity with a lucent center in the right upper lobe, producing a reverse halo sign or atoll sign.

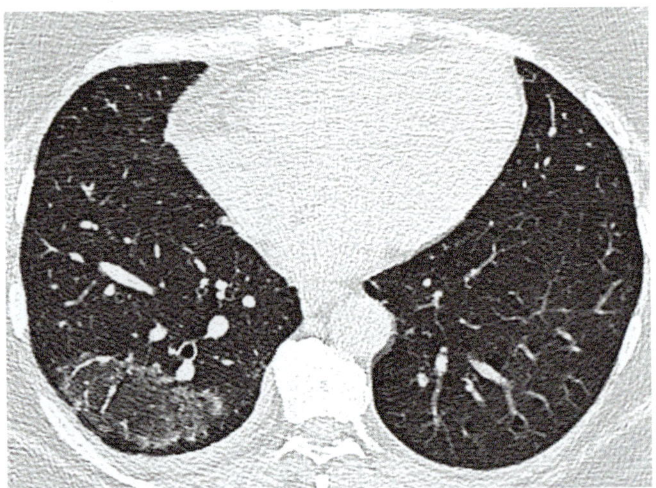

FIG. 15: A 49-year-old female previously treated with right upper lobectomy and radiation therapy for carcinoid tumor. She was asymptomatic at the time of this surveillance scan. Axial unenhanced CT image with lung windows demonstrates a reverse halo sign or atoll sign, with a mass-like opacity with a peripheral dense rim and ground-glass centrally. The finding resolved without treatment on a follow-up scan in 3 months.

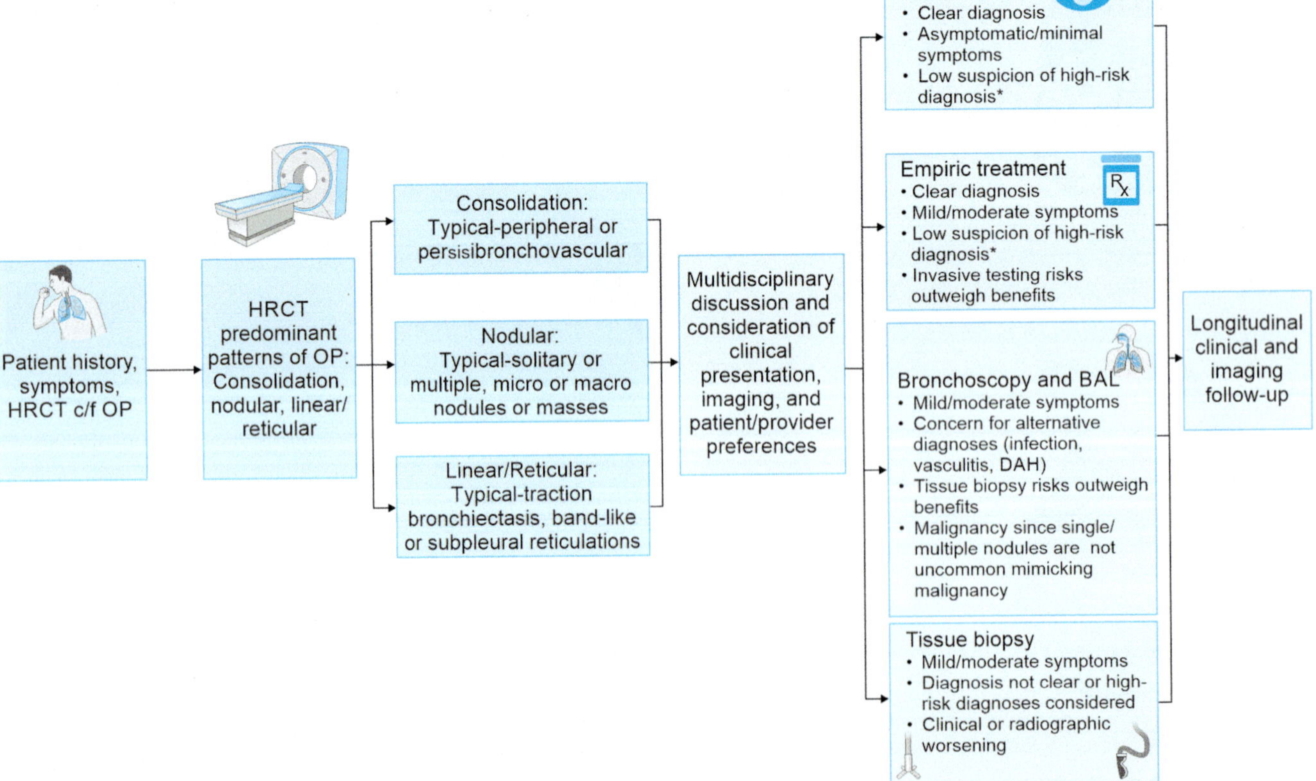

FLOWCHART 1: Approach to diagnosis of organizing pneumonia.

(DAH: diffuse alveolar hemorrhage; OP: organizing pneumonia; HRCT: high-resolution computed tomography)

Source: Adapted from reference 2.

number of other etiologies including infections, drugs, and different systemic diseases. It often presents with nonspecific symptoms and radiographic patterns, therefore delaying the diagnosis. Initial response to treatment with corticosteroids and/or other immunosuppressive drugs, besides treatment of the underlying disease, is often good.

REFERENCES

1. Epler GR, Colby TV, McLoud TC, et al. Bronchiolitis obliterans organizing pneumonia. N Engl J Med. 1985;312(3):152-8.
2. Cherian SV, Patel D, Machnicki S, et al. Algorithmic Approach to the Diagnosis of Organizing Pneumonia: A Correlation of Clinical, Radiologic, and Pathologic Features. Chest. 2022;162(1):156-78.
3. King TE Jr, Lee JS. Cryptogenic Organizing Pneumonia. N Engl J Med. 2022;386(11):1058-69.
4. Gudmundsson G, Sveinsson O, Isaksson HJ, et al. Epidemiology of organising pneumonia in Iceland. Thorax. 2006;61(9):805-8.
5. Drakopanagiotakis F, Paschalaki K, Abu-Hijleh M, et al. Cryptogenic and secondary organizing pneumonia: clinical presentation, radiographic findings, treatment response, and prognosis. Chest. 2011;139(4):893-900.
6. Cordier JF. Cryptogenic organising pneumonia. Eur Respir J. 2006;28(2):422-46.
7. Alasaly K, Muller N, Ostrow DN. Cryptogenic organizing pneumonia. A report of 25 cases and a review of the literature. Medicine (Baltimore). 1995;74(4):201-11.
8. Lohr RH, Boland BJ, Douglas WW, et al. Organizing pneumonia. Features and prognosis of cryptogenic, secondary, and focal variants. Arch Intern Med. 1997;157(12):1323-9.
9. Cordier JF, Loire R, Brune J, Idiopathic bronchiolitis obliterans organizing pneumonia. Definition of characteristic clinical profiles in a series of 16 patients. Chest. 1989;96(5):999-1004.
10. Poletti V, Cazzato S, Minicuci N, et al. The diagnostic value of bronchoalveolar lavage and transbronchial lung biopsy in cryptogenic organizing pneumonia. Eur Respir J. 1996;9(12):2513-6.
11. Jara-Palomares L, Gomez-Izquierdo L, Gonzalez-Vergara D, et al. Utility of high-resolution computed tomography and BAL in cryptogenic organizing pneumonia. Respir Med. 2010; 104(11):1706-11.
12. Enomoto N, Sumikawa H, Sugiura H, et al. Clinical, radiological, and pathological evaluation of "NSIP with OP overlap" pattern compared with NSIP in patients with idiopathic interstitial pneumonias. Respir Med. 2020;174:106201.
13. Shin L, Katz DS, Yung E. Hypermetabolism on F-18 FDG PET of multiple pulmonary nodules resulting from bronchiolitis obliterans organizing pneumonia. Clin Nucl Med. 2004;29(10):654-6.
14. Erdogan Y, Özyürek BA, Özmen O, et al. The Evaluation of FDG PET/CT Scan Findings in Patients with Organizing Pneumonia Mimicking Lung Cancer. Mol Imaging Radionucl Ther. 2015;24(2):60-5.
15. Travis WD, Costabel U, Hansell DM, et al. An official American Thoracic Society/European Respiratory Society statement: Update of the international multidisciplinary classification of the idiopathic interstitial pneumonias. Am J Respir Crit Care Med. 2013;188(6):733-48.
16. Feinstein MB, DeSouza SA, Moreira AL, et al. A comparison of the pathological, clinical and radiographical, features of cryptogenic organising pneumonia, acute fibrinous and organising pneumonia and granulomatous organising pneumonia. J Clin Pathol. 2015;68(6):441-7.
17. Lazor R, Vandevenne A, Pelletier A, et al. Cryptogenic organizing pneumonia. Characteristics of relapses in a series of 48 patients. The Groupe d'Etudes et de Recherche sur les Maladles "Orphelines" Pulmonaires (GERM"O"P). Am J Respir Crit Care Med. 2000;162(2 Pt 1):571-7.
18. Bradley B, Branley HM, Egan JJ, et al. Interstitial lung disease guideline: the British Thoracic Society in collaboration with the Thoracic Society of Australia and New Zealand and the Irish Thoracic Society. Thorax. 2008;63(Suppl 5):v1-58.
19. Stover DE, Mangino D. Macrolides: a treatment alternative for bronchiolitis obliterans organizing pneumonia? Chest. 2005; 128(5):3611-7.

CHAPTER

113

Hypersensitivity Pneumonitis

Ambika Sharma, Sheetu Singh, Kevin K Brown

INTRODUCTION

Hypersensitivity pneumonitis (HP), also called extrinsic allergic alveolitis, is an interstitial lung disease (ILD), characterized by inflammation and/or fibrosis affecting the lung parenchyma and smaller airways, as the result of exposure to specific inhaled antigens in susceptible individuals. It is believed to be mediated by both cellular and humoral immune responses.[1,2] Multiple specific antigens have been implicated in the etiology of HP, but in about half of cases, the type and source of the specific exposure are not identified.[3]

It is hypothesized that certain individuals, based on their underlying genetics, are susceptible to developing an excessive immune response within the lung when exposed to specific inhaled antigens. There are certain factors, such as air pollution, viral infections, and pesticide exposure that may facilitate the development of this reaction. Exposure to these may lead to airway inflammation, allowing other inhaled antigens to be retained in the smaller airways and alveoli, thus, predisposing to HP.[4]

Hypersensitivity pneumonitis can have varied clinical presentations ranging from self-limited to an intermittent relapsing, to a progressive fibrotic disease similar to idiopathic pulmonary fibrosis (IPF).[1] The recent guidelines have been proposed in an attempt to harmonize the definition of HP, diagnostic criteria, and strategies for evaluation of the disease.[2,5] Yet, many uncertainties persist. In this chapter, we will highlight the latest update on the epidemiology, pathogenesis, classification, diagnostic approach and treatment of HP.

EPIDEMIOLOGY

The prevalence of HP is variable and depends upon the geographic location, environmental factors, occupational history, gender, and genetic susceptibility. The overall incidence of HP is 0.3–0.9 per 100,000 population.[1] In a high-risk group such as bird breeders, the incidence can be as high as 56.4 per 100,000.[5] When calculated as a proportion of all ILD patients, it varies from 2 to 47% in various studies and registries. Studies from India and USA have reported female predominance.[6-8] A recent study from India estimated the crude annual incidence rate to be 1.4–2.9 per 100,000 population, while the estimated prevalence was 6.2–12.3 per 100,000 population.[9]

Common exposures found to be responsible for HP in the ILD India registry were birds, air-cooling devices, molds, and rural residence. A regional variation was noted most likely due to differing cultural practices, geographies, climate, and environmental exposures.

ETIOPATHOGENESIS

Hypersensitivity pneumonitis is a disease associated with exaggerated immune response following exposure to inhaled antigens in susceptible individuals. Several possible inciting agents and their sources have been reported. These agents are usually proteins derived from microorganisms, fungi or animals.[3] **Table 1** elaborates on the possible antigens and common sources. The location of exposure can be occupational, within a household or associated with recreational or vocational activities. There is no clear correlation between the extent of exposure (duration, frequency, particle size, and solubility) and the onset and severity of the disease. Tobacco smoking can also modify both the presentation and course of the disease.[10] Individual susceptibility plays an important role. After exposure, there is both a cellular [T- helper cell type 1 (Th-1)] and humoral (antigen-specific IgG antibody) immune response that leads to lymphocytic and granulomatous inflammation.[3] In some patients, abnormal fibroblast activity can contribute to the development of a fibrosing component. This varied response may be explained by variants in genes involved in the innate and adaptive immune response. Polymorphism in MHC class II has been associated with susceptibility, and other associations include shorter telomere length, abnormal proteasomes, and transport proteins, as well as tissue inhibitors of matrix and metalloproteinases (TIMP). Co-occurrence of respiratory viral infection and exposure to pesticides have been described to increase the risk of disease development. A MUC5B (Mucin 5B)

TABLE 1: Common sources of antigens known to cause hypersensitivity pneumonitis (HP).

Antigen source	Possible antigen	HP disease
Moldy hay	Thermophilic actinomycetes	Farmer's lung
Moldy pressed sugarcane (Bagasse)	Thermophilic actinomycetes	Bagassosis
Moldy compost and mushrooms	• Thermophilic actinomycetes • *Aspergillus* species • Mushroom spores	Mushroom workers disease
Contaminated barley	*Aspergillus clavatus*	Malt worker's lung
Compost	*Aspergillus* species	Compost lung
Mold on tobacco	*Aspergillus* species	Tobacco workers disease
Domestic birds	Bird proteins	Bird Fancier's lung
Pigeon droppings	Serum, feathers, droppings	Pigeon breeder's disease
Parakeets	Serum, feathers, droppings	Budgerigar Fancier's lung
Grains	Grain weevil	Grain lung
Chicken feather protein	Chicken feathers	Chicken breeder's lung
Duvet and pillow	Goose proteins	Duvet lung
Silkworm larvae	Silkworm larvae proteins	Sericulturist's lung
Wood cutting	Plant protein	Woodman's disease
Mold on grapes	*Botrytis cinerea*	Wine grower's lung
Isocyanates	Altered proteins	Hypersensitivity pneumonitis
Detergent enzymes	*Bacillus subtilis*	Detergent worker's disease (Washing powder lung)
Contaminated basement	*Cladosporium* species, *Penicillium* species	Basement lung
Contaminated hot tub water	*Mycobacterium avium* complex	Hot-tub lung
House dust	*Trichosporon asahii*	• Japanese summer house • Hypersensitivity pneumonitis
Contaminated humidifiers, air-conditioners, heating systems	• Thermophilic actinomycetes • *Penicillium*, *Cephalosporium*, *Amoebae*, *Klebsiella* species, *Candida* species.	Ventilator lung

promoter polymorphism is more prevalent in patients with fibrosis.[11,12]

CLINICAL FEATURES

The clinical presentation of HP is divided into nonfibrotic and fibrotic. Nonfibrotic HP is essentially the acute or subacute onset of symptoms after a relevant exposure. High-resolution computed tomography (HRCT) reveals ground-glass haziness, centrilobular nodules, air trapping and little or no reticulations. Fibrotic HP on the other hand is generally recognized as the result of long-term exposure. HRCT demonstrates reticulation, traction bronchiectasis, and honeycombing often overlaid upon the imaging features of nonfibrotic HP.[5,13,14] This new classification suggested by the American Thoracic Society (ATS)/European Respiratory Society (ERS) guidelines is in contrast to the traditional classification of acute, subacute, and chronic HP. This change was suggested since the onset and duration of symptoms do not have prognostic or therapeutic implications. With a growing role of antifibrotics in progressive fibrosing ILD, presence or absence of pathologic fibrosis may have important treatment implications.[5]

Common symptoms are cough, dyspnea, flu-like symptoms (low grade fever, malaise), chest tightness, and wheezing. On physical examination, mid-inspiratory squeaks (chirping rales or squeaks), crackles, and wheeze are noted. Fibrotic HP may have a more subtle onset with some combination of progressive dyspnea, inspiratory crackles on examination, digital clubbing, and hypoxemia.[3] In many patients, the presentation can be mixed and may not follow the above pattern.[13,14]

DIAGNOSTIC EVALUATION

There is no specific diagnostic test for HP and the histopathologic pattern seen on surgical lung biopsy is no longer considered the gold standard. **Flowchart 1** includes an algorithm for the stepwise evaluation and diagnosis of HP. A careful history is always necessary and required to establish a potential link between an inhaled exposure and episodes of respiratory symptoms. There is no validated questionnaire which can be recommended currently to identify the exposure.[15] Multidisciplinary discussion (MDD) with careful review of the clinical, radiological, and pathological findings plays an important role in evaluation of patients with ILD suspected to have HP **(Table 2)**. MDD helps reduce the number of ILD patients with an unclassifiable disease, increases diagnostic confidence, and may change proposed management.[16]

Specific serum antigen testing can be performed to look for immune sensitization but the predictive value of a specific IgG antibodies is poor and the test cannot differentiate between disease and sensitization.[17] A positive IgG in the right clinical context, however, can be suggestive and can help focus the search for a particular exposure. Skin tests for immediate hypersensitivity to avian, animal, and fungal antigens are not helpful, as they test for IgE-mediated, rather than IgG-mediated hypersensitivity. An exposure challenge test can be done at expert centers, which may be highly specific and sensitive for HP. However, utmost care needs to be taken as the patient may develop an acute exacerbation.[18]

Pulmonary Function Test

Pulmonary function tests (PFTs) are useful in assessing the severity of physiologic impairment, however, has no diagnostic importance. It also does not help differentiate

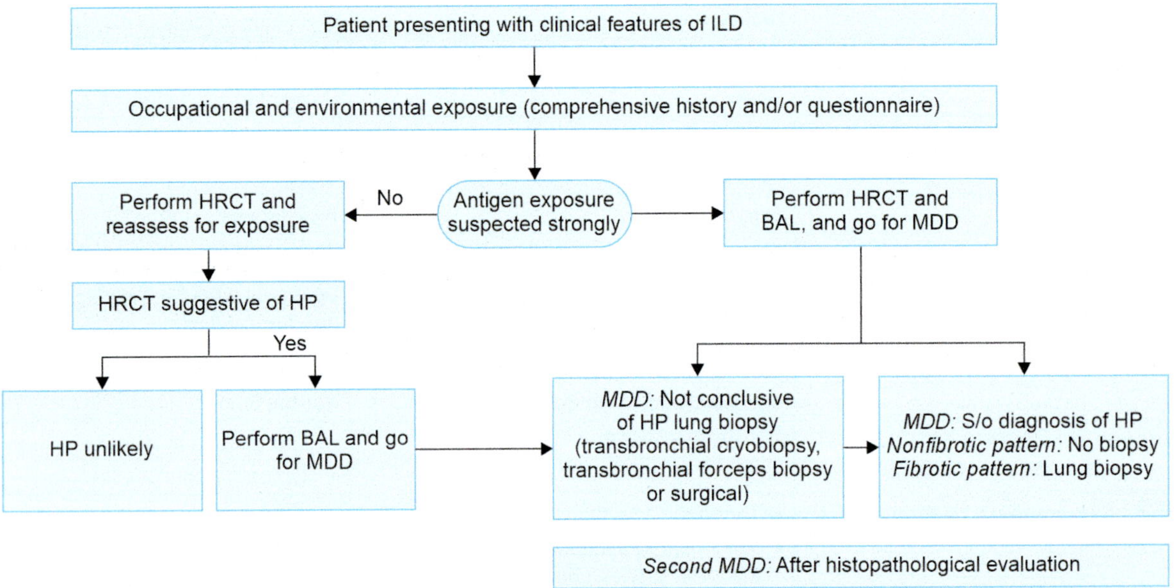

FLOWCHART 1: Approach to diagnosis of hypersensitivity pneumonitis.
(BAL: bronchioalveolar lavage; HRCT: high-resolution computed tomography; ILD: interstitial lung disease; MDD: multidisciplinary discussion)

TABLE 2: Radiological findings evident on high-resolution computed tomography of the chest in hypersensitivity pneumonitis (HP).

Nonfibrotic HP	Fibrotic HP
Features of lung infiltration (ground glass opacities, mosaic attenuation)	Irregular fine or coarse reticulation with architectural lung distortion
Abnormalities suggestive of small airway disease: Ill-defined small < 5 mm centrilobular nodules on inspiratory image plus air trapping on expiratory image	Septal thickening
Ground-glass opacity is due to extensive interstitial inflammation	Traction bronchiectasis in area of ground-glass opacities
Mosaic pattern typically reflects coexistent lobules affected by pneumonitis (increased attenuation) interspersed with lobule of normal or slightly decreased attenuation (due to bronchial obstruction)	Honeycombing
Air trapping	Three density patterns (previously called as the Head cheese sign) comprising normal lung, ground glassed lung and air trapped more black lung

nonfibrotic from fibrotic disease. Serial PFT can help monitor disease activity. Spirometry usually reveals a restrictive defect, but an obstructive pattern or mixed obstructive and restrictive ventilatory abnormalities can be seen. The diffusing capacity of carbon monoxide (DLCO) is invariably reduced.

High-resolution Computed Tomography

High-resolution CT plays an important role in diagnosis of HP and evaluation of ILD.[19] Imaging technique is important and interpretation is based on volumetric scanning of chest with special emphasis on creating motion-free images and optimal image quality at reduced radiation dose. Images are obtained in the supine position. One series at deep inspiration and the other series after prolonged expiration are recommended. Comparing the images obtained from both inspiratory and expiratory maneuvers is important in identifying the air trapping commonly seen in HP.

Not surprisingly, the histological pattern of disease at the time of diagnosis has an impact on the imaging characteristics.[20] With bronchiocentric inflammation, the typical HRCT pattern demonstrates small ill-defined ground-glass nodules distributed across all lung zones **(Fig. 1)**. There may be lobular air trapping evident on expiratory imaging. The CT pattern with the greatest specificity for HP is the "three-density pattern" (also called Head Cheese sign) **(Fig. 2)**. This combination of variable densities is due to patchy distribution of normal appearing lung, high attenuation areas of ground-glass opacity (GGO) and lucent areas (lobules of decreased attenuation and vascular sections).The three-density pattern may be seen in fibrotic disease **(Fig. 3)**. Other signs of underlying fibrosis include reticular abnormalities and/or ground glass with associated traction bronchiectasis, loss of lung volume, and honeycombing.[21,22]

Ground-glass opacity is due to extensive interstitial inflammation. In HP, this is typically patchy in distribution

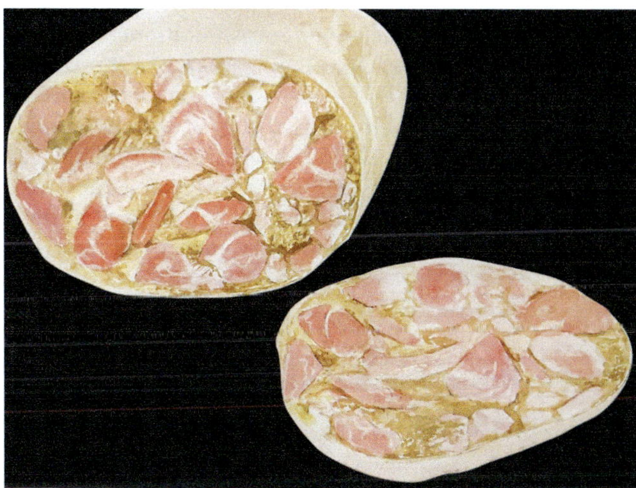

FIG. 2: Head cheese sign or three-density pattern (pictographic representation). The head cheese sign (more recently termed the three-density pattern) refers to a juxtaposition of regions with three (or sometimes more) different densities/regions of different attenuation within the lungs.

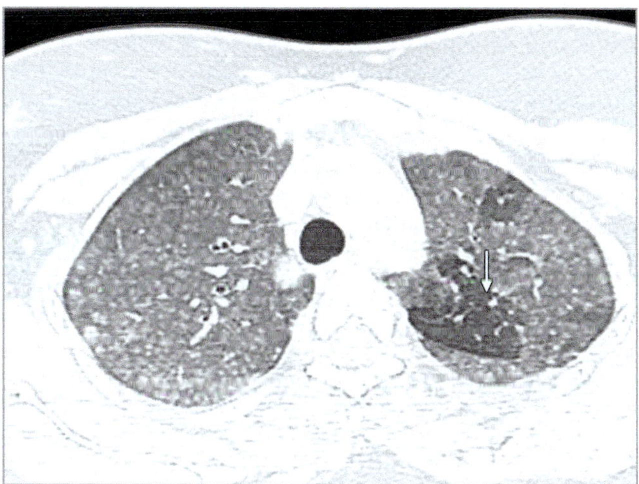

FIG. 1: High-resolution computed tomography image seen in nonfibrotic hypersensitivity pneumonitis. Axial section high-resolution computed tomography image of a 40-year-old lady with history of pigeon exposure depicts centrilobular nodules and air-trapping (arrow) predominantly in bilateral upper lobes.

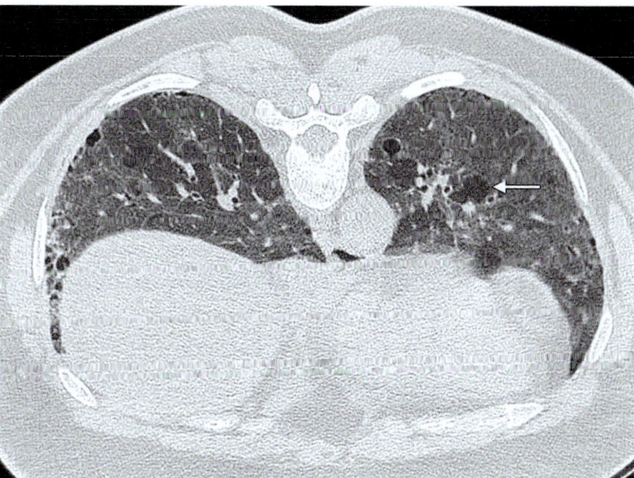

FIG. 3: High-resolution computed tomography image seen in fibrotic hypersensitivity pneumonitis. A 52-year-old lady with history of working in farms with hay exposure of >30 years presented with exertional dyspnea. High-resolution computed tomography showed ground-glass haziness, air trapping (arrow), septal thickening and honeycombing. The classical three-density sign can be seen suggestive of fibrotic hypersensitivity pneumonitis.

in combination with normal lung and air-trapping, referred as mosaic attenuation. In nonfibrotic HP, this pattern reflects coexistent lobules affected by cellular infiltration (increased attenuation) interspersed with lobules having a normal or slightly decreased attenuation (due to small airway obstruction). They are bilateral, symmetrical and diffuse.[21,22]

Bronchoalveolar Lavage Analysis

When carefully performed and processed, bronchoalveolar lavage (BAL) has diagnostic implications. In the correct clinical context, a BAL lymphocyte count of >30% increases the diagnostic probability of HP. This is seen commonly in cellular, nonfibrotic HP.[23] However, such findings can be seen in other forms of ILD, such as sarcoidosis and non-specific interstitial pneumonia (NSIP).[24] BAL lymphocytosis is also a predictor of response to corticosteroids. The performance of BAL as part of the diagnostic evaluation is included in both the ATS/JRS/ALAT and CHEST guidelines.[2,5]

Lung Biopsy and Histopathological Examination

Lung biopsy is an invasive procedure and is recommended in patients with suspected HP where there is no clear diagnosis after combining the clinical context and chest imaging and MDD review.[5] The decision to perform a lung biopsy should be individualized with a careful assessment of the risks versus benefits. The following options for tissue sampling are available: transbronchial forceps biopsy, transbronchial cryobiopsy, or surgical lung biopsy. The traditional transbronchial forceps biopsy is associated with a low tissue yield, relatively small pieces of lung, and the expected complications such as bleeding and pneumothorax. Surgical biopsy, though the gold standard, is limited by patient reluctance, lack of surgical expertise, and higher risk of severe complication including risk of exacerbations, persistent air leak, and prolonged ventilation. Cryobiopsy uses freezing techniques to obtain larger pieces of lung with minimal crush artifacts. Its yield has been reported to approach that of surgical lung biopsies in obtaining a diagnosis of ILD, though complications are not rare.[25]

Biopsies should be examined by pathologist experienced in ILD, while combining the clinical context and chest imaging findings. Typical nonfibrotic HP exhibits four key features: (1) Small airway involvement, (2) uniform cellular interstitial inflammation, (3) predominantly lymphocytic with atleast a single granuloma, and/or (4) multinucleated giant cell **(Fig. 4)**. The histological pattern of fibrotic HP may be very similar to UIP as seen in IPF. Typical fibrotic HP has three key features: (1) Airway centric fibrosis with or without widespread peribronchial metaplasia, (2) fibrosing interstitial pneumonia, and (3) poorly formed granuloma **(Figs. 5A and B)**.[26]

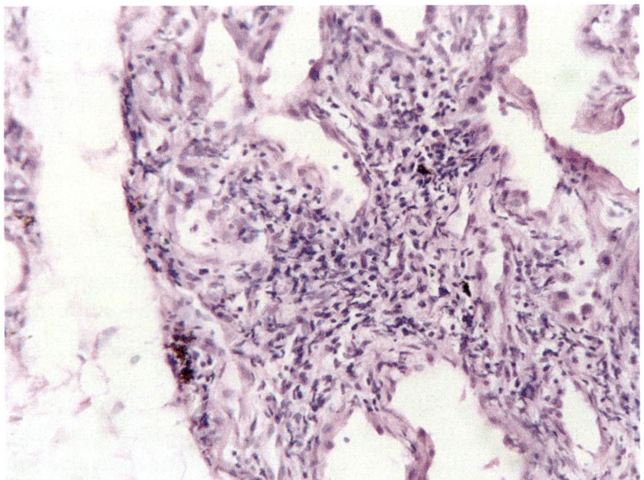

FIG. 4: Histopathological findings in nonfibrotic hypersensitivity pneumonitis. Cryobiopsy of the lung from a 42-year-old female teacher with significant exposure to pigeons and symptoms of cough and dyspnea since last 3 months. The high-power resolution (40×) demonstrates poorly formed granuloma with interstitial lymphocytic infiltrates suggestive of nonfibrotic hypersensitivity pneumonitis.

Courtesy: Dr Arundhati Agarwal.

DISEASE PROGRESSION AND OUTCOMES

The clinical course in HP is frequently variable, with many variables contributing to the pattern and outcome. In some patients with sensitization to known antigen exposure, who can eliminate the antigen, the disease can fully resolve while in others, periods of clinical and functional stability can occur.[27] Patients without a known exposure may develop a chronic, progressive disease, often associated with poor prognosis. In patients with fibrotic HP, the course is characterized by worsening symptoms, an increasing extent of fibrotic abnormalities on HRCT, deteriorating PFT and early mortality.[8,28] The follow-up data of the ILD India registry showed an average 1-year, 2-year, 3-year and 4-year survival of 83.3% (78.6–88.1), 76.1% (70.6–81.6), 66.9% (60.1–73.7) and 51.6% (40.3–63.0), respectively. Older age is associated with a worse outcome, irrespective of baseline disease severity. In addition, women have better prognosis than men. Other factors such as duration of antigen exposure, history of smoking, low forced vital capacity (FVC) at disease presentation, lower BAL lymphocytosis, presence of fibrosis on HRCT, UIP or fibrosing NSIP pattern on HRCT are all associated with unfavorable outcomes. HRCT features associated with longer survival include air trapping and mosaic attenuation.[29] Regular clinical, physiologic, and chest imaging monitoring are required to understand disease activity. Spirometry, diffusion studies, 6-minute walk tests (at 3–6 monthly

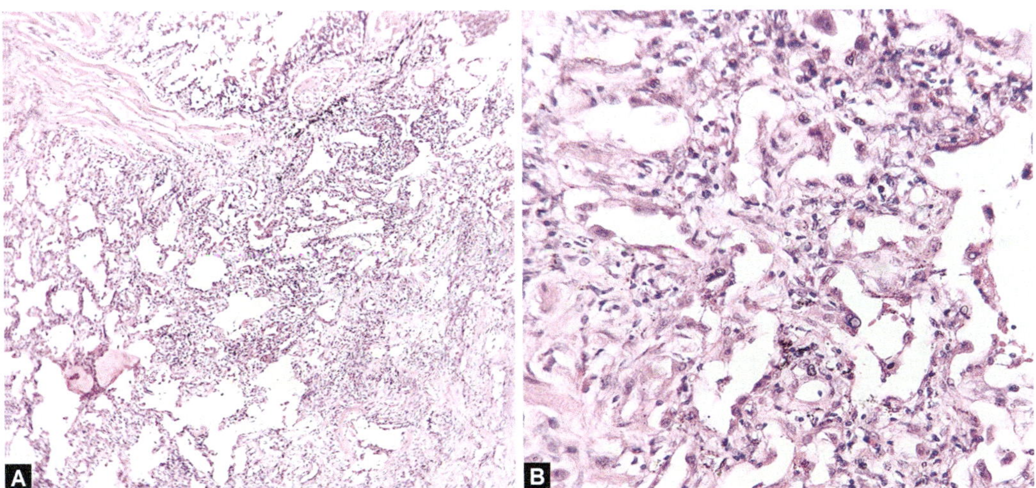

FIGS. 5A AND B: Histopathological findings in fibrotic hypersensitivity pneumonitis. Cryo lung biopsy specimen from a 50-year-old female with significant exposure to grain dust. (A) Low-power (10×) view and (B) high-power (40×) view. The biopsy reveals diffuse fibrosis and interstitial lymphocytic infiltrate, with peribronchiolar dominant distribution suggestive of fibrotic hypersensitivity pneumonitis.

Courtesy: Dr Arundhati Agarwal.

intervals) and repeated HRCT scans (yearly or early in case of deterioration) are all useful.[30]

There are various outcome prediction scores. ILD-GAP index (gender, age, and physiology) is used to predict mortality. Physiology scoring is done as per predicted FVC and DLCO. A modified ILD-GAP index was developed for application across all ILD subtypes to provide disease-specific survival estimates using a single-risk prediction model.[31] DLCO is not readily available in all ambulatory settings, especially in India and is also associated with significant technical challenges. Kobayashi et al., have described a "modified GAP score" (M-GAP) including FVC, age, and gender, but excluding DLCO to predict acute exacerbations and survival in patients with lung cancer and ILD.[32] The M-GAP score has been used to predict survival in the Indian ILD registry and there was good correlation for 1-year survival prediction.[33] Similar to other forms of fibrosing ILD, a decline in FVC by 10% or greater over period of 6–12 months, is associated with an increased risk of all-cause mortality (median survival: 53 months vs. 139 months).[34]

MANAGEMENT OF HYPERSENSITIVITY PNEUMONITIS

Nonpharmacological Measures and Supportive Care

Antigen identification and its avoidance is the cornerstone in treatment of HP. Though often difficult to achieve in clinical practice, it is the only way to achieve complete disease resolution and even in the absence of cure, it helps to improve the clinical condition and prolong survival.[27] When the exposure is not obvious, an occupational or environmental hygienist, if available, might be consulted to perform an assessment of indoor spaces or workplace and provide advice on how to eliminate or reduce the exposures. When, despite the active investigation, the antigen is not identified and the patient is worsening, a change in environment should be considered, if feasible. Additional supportive management, when appropriate, include: Domiciliary or ambulatory oxygen therapy, pulmonary rehabilitation, age-appropriate vaccinations, participation in patients' groups and counseling. Appropriate training for oxygen usage will help to ensure safety and adherence. Common comorbidities such as gastroesophageal reflux disease, pulmonary hypertension and obstructive sleep apnea should be identified and managed appropriately. Emphasis should be made on improving the quality of life and functional status.

Pharmacological Measures

In patients with mild disease without evidence of clinical progression, no treatment may be needed beyond antigen identification and abatement. Patients presenting with moderate-to-severe symptoms (often with resting or exertional hypoxemia) with features of predominant inflammatory (nonfibrotic) disease (GGO on HRCT, BAL lymphocytosis), will generally respond to corticosteroids with an improvement in symptoms, physiology/gas exchange, and chest imaging. Oral prednisolone (0.5–1.0 mg/kg/day) can be given for 4–6 weeks with gradual tapering over next 3 months. No prospective studies have evaluated the efficacy of corticosteroids in treating fibrotic HP. While short-term improvement may be seen, prolonged use (particularly high dose) of corticosteroids does not provide long-term benefit or durable slowing of disease progression. In fact, observational cohorts have suggested that fibrotic HP patients treated with corticosteroids may have shorter survival compared to those who were not treated.[35] Corticosteroids are known to have multiple significant adverse effects and, hence, are recommended only when there are signs of active inflammation and/or severe lung function impairment.[36]

Steroid-sparing immunosuppressants such as azathioprine (AZA) and mycophenolate mofetil (MMF) have been used to treat fibrotic HP. This helps in reducing the dose of corticosteroids and preservation of lung function.[37] In a retrospective study of 70 patients with chronic HP managed with AZA or MMF, there was increase in DLCO at 1 year of follow-up and reduction in dose of prednisolone but there was no improvement in FVC,[38] while others have suggested that while no physiologic benefit should be anticipated when compared to corticosteroids alone, significantly fewer treatment-related adverse effects can be expected.[39] Rituximab has also been used with anecdotal benefit.

In patients with fibrotic HP, agents that inhibit fibrogenesis pathways may be of use. However, there is no consensus on if and/or when to initiate antifibrotic therapy. Nintedanib is an intracellular inhibitor of tyrosine kinase. It has been licensed in many countries for the treatment of fibrosing ILD associated with progressive phenotype. INBUILD trial has looked into the role of nintedanib in progressive fibrosing ILD. It enrolled 663 patients with fibrosing ILD other than IPF and also included 173 patients with HP (26%). Results showed significant slowing in the rate of decline in FVC, reduced acute exacerbation of ILD, or death.[40] Pirfenidone is another FDA-approved drug for treatment of IPF. There is no RCT evaluating its role in HP; however, there are few retrospective and cohort studies. As per data of prematurely terminated RELIEF study done in patients with progressive pulmonary fibrosis due to CTD, fibrotic NSIP, and HP, slowing of the rate of FVC decline was suggested in group who received Pirfenidone.[41]

Over all, there is not enough evidence-based data to suggest a straightforward treatment algorithm for HP. However, in clinical practice, treatment options can be chosen based on the presence of either nonfibrotic or fibrotic disease presentation. **Flowchart 2** depicts an algorithm for stepwise management of HP.

Lung transplantation remains a final modality for patients with progressive fibrotic ILD which can improve survival. Among 31 patients with HP, who underwent lung transplantation at a single center in United States between 2000 to 2013, the 1-, 3-, and 5-year survival rates were 96%, 89%, and 89%, respectively. The outcomes for transplant in HP patients are better than those patients with idiopathic pulmonary fibrosis (IPF). The recurrence of HP in the transplanted lung has been demonstrated.[42]

PREVENTION OF HYPERSENSITIVITY PNEUMONITIS

The incidence of HP can be reduced by interventions that minimize exposure to antigens known to be associated with the development of disease in susceptible individuals. Examples include avoidance of contact with birds or their

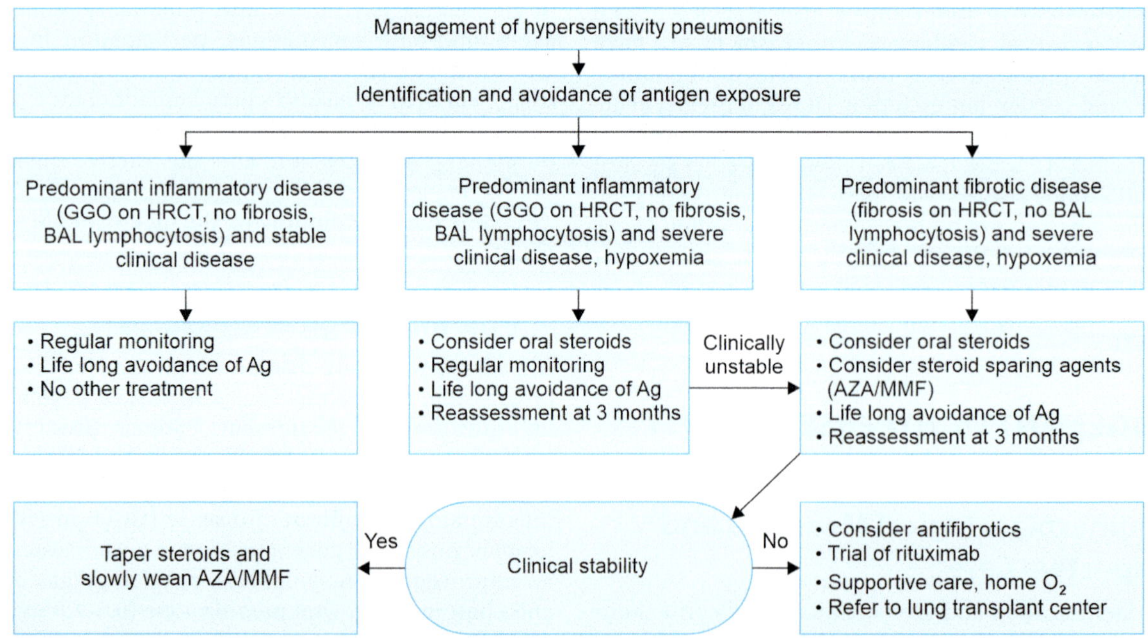

FLOWCHART 2: Management of hypersensitivity pneumonitis.

(AZA: azathioprine; BAL: bronchioalveolar lavage; GGO: glass-ground opacities; HRCT: high-resolution computed tomography; MMF: mycophenolate mofetil)

droppings, reducing microbial contamination of the work or home environment, and using protective equipment. For patients with HP, these interventions can help mitigate further exposure. Occupational exposures can be reduced by using technologies that help in reduction of generation and containment of aerosols. Alteration in the handling and storage of potential sources of microbial antigens can diminish the occurrence of HP. Humidity and temperature play an important role in the growth of many fungi, the antigenic source for many HP patients. Ensuring humidity <60% and good ventilation will lead to reduction in growth of these fungi on organic products and surfaces. Avoiding recirculation of water can reduce growth of microorganism in humidifiers and air conditioning systems.

SUMMARY

Hypersensitivity pneumonitis (HP) is a complex lung condition caused by an immune response to a specific inhaled antigen. Detecting HP requires a high level of suspicion and a diagnosis can be made when there is exposure to the triggering substance along with patterns seen on high-resolution computed tomography scans that are typical of HP. Non-fibrotic HP typically improves when the triggering substance is removed, although in some cases, systemic corticosteroids may be necessary. Conversely, fibrotic HP often does not resolve completely, and fibrosis progression may continue even after the triggering substance is removed.

REFERENCES

1. Hamblin M, Prosch H, Vašáková M. Diagnosis, course and management of hypersensitivity pneumonitis. Eur Respir Rev. 2022;31(163):210169.
2. Fernández Pérez ER, Travis WD, Lynch DA, et al. Executive summary: Diagnosis and evaluation of hypersensitivity pneumonitis: CHEST Guideline and Expert Panel Report. Chest. 2021;160(2):e97-e156.
3. Selman M, Pardo A, King TE Jr. Hypersensitivity pneumonitis: insights in diagnosis and pathobiology. Am J Respir Crit Care Med. 2012;186(4):314-24.
4. Singh S, Collins BF, Bairwa M, et al. Hypersensitivity pneumonitis and its correlation with ambient air pollution in urban India. Eur Respir J. 2019;53(2):1801563.
5. Raghu G, Remy-Jardin M, Ryerson CJ, et al. Diagnosis of Hypersensitivity Pneumonitis in Adults. An Official ATS/JRS/ALAT Clinical Practice Guideline. Am J Respir Crit Care Med. 2020;202(3):e36-69.
6. Singh S, Collins BF, Sharma BB, et al. Interstitial Lung Disease in India. Results of a Prospective Registry. Am J Respir Crit Care Med. 2017;195(6):801-13.
7. Dhooria S, Agarwal R, Sehgal IS, et al. Spectrum of interstitial lung diseases at a tertiary center in a developing country: A study of 803 subjects. PLoS One. 2018;13(2):e0191938.
8. Fernández Pérez ER, Kong AM, Raimundo K, et al. Epidemiology of Hypersensitivity Pneumonitis among an Insured Population in the United States: A Claims-based Cohort Analysis. Ann Am Thorac Soc. 2018;15(4):460-9.
9. Dhooria S, Sehgal IS, Agarwal R, et al. Incidence, prevalence, and national burden of interstitial lung diseases in India: Estimates from two studies of 3089 subjects. PLoS One. 2022;17(7):e0271665.
10. Dangman KH, Storey E, Schenck P, et al. Effects of cigarette smoking on diagnostic tests for work-related hypersensitivity pneumonitis: data from an outbreak of lung disease in metalworkers. Am J Ind Med. 2004;45:455.
11. Girard M, Israël-Assayag E, Cormier Y. Impaired function of regulatory T-cells in hypersensitivity pneumonitis. Eur Respir J. 2011;37:632.
12. Ley B, Torgerson DG, Oldham JM, et al. Raryre protein-altering telomere-related gene variants in patients with chronic hypersensitivity pneumonitis. Am J Respir Crit Care Med. 2019;200:1154-63.
13. Salisbury ML, Myers JL, Belloli EA, et al. Diagnosis and treatment of fibrotic hypersensitivity pneumonia: where we stand and where we need to go. Am J Respir Crit Care Med. 2017;196: 690-9.
14. Vasakova M, Morell F, Walsh S, et al. Hypersensitivity pneumonitis: perspectives in diagnosis and management. Am J Respir Crit Care Med. 2017;196:680-9.
15. Petnak T, Moua T. Exposure assessment in hypersensitivity pneumonitis: a comprehensive review and proposed screening questionnaire. ERJ Open Res. 2020;6.
16. Walsh SL, Wells AU, Desai SR, et al. Multicentre evaluation of multidisciplinary team meeting agreement on diagnosis in diffuse parenchymal lung disease: a case-cohort study. Lancet Respir Med. 2016;4(7):557-65.
17. Fenoglio CM, Reboux G, Sudre B, et al. Diagnostic value of serum precipitins to mould antigens in active hypersensitivity pneumonitis. Eur Respir J. 2007;29:706.
18. Muñoz X, Sánchez-Ortiz M, Torres F, et al. Diagnostic yield of specific inhalation challenge in hypersensitivity pneumonitis. Eur Respir J. 2014;44:1658.
19. Raghu G, Remy-Jardin M, Myers JL, et al.; American Thoracic Society, European Respiratory Society, Japanese Respiratory Society; Latin American Thoracic Society. Diagnosis of idiopathic pulmonary fibrosis: An official ATS/ERS/ JRS/ALAT clinical practice guideline. Am J Respir Crit Care Med. 2018;198:e44-68.
20. Silva CI, Churg A, Müller NL. Hypersensitivity pneumonitis: spectrum of high-resolution CT and pathologic findings. AJR Am J Roentgenol. 2007;188:334.
21. Sahin H, Brown KK, Curran-Everett D, et al. Chronic hypersensitivity pneumonitis: CT features comparison with pathologic evidence of fibrosis and survival. Radiology. 2007;244:591.
22. Hanak V, Golbin JM, Hartman TE, et al. High-resolution CT findings of parenchymal fibrosis correlate with prognosis in hypersensitivity pneumonitis. Chest. 2008;134:133.
23. Adams TN, Newton CA, Batra K, et al. Utility of bronchoalveolar lavage and transbronchial biopsy in patients with hypersensitivity pneumonitis. Lung. 2018;196:617.
24. Meyer KC, Raghu G, Baughman RP, et al. American Thoracic Society Committee on BAL in Interstitial Lung Disease. An official American Thoracic Society clinical practice guideline: the clinical utility of bronchoalveolar lavage cellular analysis in interstitial lung disease. Am J Respir Crit Care Med. 2012;185(9): 1004-14.

25. Lentz RJ, Argento AC, Colby TV, et al. Transbronchial cryobiopsy for diffuse parenchymal lung disease: A state-of-the-art review of procedural techniques, current evidence, and future challenges. J Thorac Dis. 2017;9:2186.
26. Castonguay MC, Ryu JH, Yi ES, et al. Granulomas and giant cells in hypersensitivity pneumonitis. Hum Pathol. 2015;46:607.
27. Fernández Pérez ER, Swigris JJ, Forssén AV, et al. Identifying an inciting antigen is associated with improved survival in patients with chronic hypersensitivity pneumonitis. Chest. 2013;144(5):1644-51.
28. Salisbury ML, Gu T, Murray S, et al. Hypersensitivity pneumonitis: radiologic phenotypes are associated with distinct survival time and pulmonary function trajectory. Chest. 2019;155:699-711.
29. Chung JH, Zhan X, Cao M, et al. Presence of air trapping and mosaic attenuation on chest computed tomography predicts survival in chronic hypersensitivity pneumonitis. Ann Am Thorac Soc. 2017;14:1533-8.
30. Singh S, Sharma BB, Bairwa M, et al. Management of interstitial lung diseases: A consensus statement of the Indian Chest Society (ICS) and National College of Chest Physicians (NCCP). Lung India. 2020;37(4):359-78.
31. Ryerson CJ, Vittinghoff E, Ley B, et al. Predicting survival across chronic interstitial lung disease: the ILD-GAP model. Chest. 2014;145(4):723-8.
32. Kobayashi H, Naito T, Omae K, et al. ILD-NSCLC-GAP index scoring and staging system for patients with non-small cell lung cancer and interstitial lung disease. Lung Cancer. 2018;121:48-53.
33. Singh S, Bairwa M, Collins BF, et al. Survival predictors of interstitial lung disease in India: Follow-up of Interstitial Lung Disease India registry. Lung India. 2021;38(1):5-11.
34. Gimenez A, Storrer K, Kuranishi L, et al. Change in FVC and survival in chronic fibrotic hypersensitivity pneumonitis. Thorax. 2018;73(4):391-2.
35. De Sadeleer LJ, Hermans F, De Dycker E, et al. Effects of corticosteroid treatment and antigen avoidance in a large hypersensitivity pneumonitis cohort: a single-centre cohort study. J Clin Med. 2018;8:14.
36. De Sadeleer LJ, Hermans F, De Dycker E, et al. Impact of BAL lymphocytosis and presence of honeycombing on corticosteroid treatment effect in fibrotic hypersensitivity pneumonitis: a retrospective cohort study. Eur Respir J. 2020;55:1901983.
37. Terras Alexandre A, Martins N, Raimundo S, et al. Impact of azathioprine use in chronic hypersensitivity pneumonitis patients. Pulm Pharmacol Ther. 2020;60:101878.
38. Morisset J, Johannson KA, Vittinghoff E, et al. Use of mycophenolate mofetil or azathioprine for the management of chronic hypersensitivity pneumonitis. Chest. 2017;151(3):619-25.
39. Adegunsoye A, Oldham JM, Fernández Pérez ER, et al. Outcomes of immunosuppressive therapy in chronic hypersensitivity pneumonitis. ERJ Open Res. 2017;3:00016-2017.
40. Wells AU, Flaherty KR, Brown KK, et al. INBUILD trial investigators. Nintedanib in patients with progressive fibrosing interstitial lung diseases-subgroup analyses by interstitial lung disease diagnosis in the INBUILD trial: a randomised, double-blind, placebo-controlled, parallel-group trial. Lancet Respir Med. 2020;8(5):453-60.
41. Behr J, Prasse A, Kreuter M, et al. Pirfenidone in patients with progressive fibrotic interstitial lung diseases other than idiopathic pulmonary fibrosis (RELIEF): a double-blind, randomised, placebo-controlled, phase 2b trial. Lancet Respir Med. 2021;9:476-86.
42. Leard LE, Holm AM, Valapour M, et al. A consensus document for the selection of lung transplant candidates: an update from the International Society for Heart and Lung Transplantation. J Heart Lung Transplant. 2021;40:1349-79.

Radiation Pneumonitis: Radiation-induced Lung Injury

CHAPTER 114

Brenda D Garcia, Stephen C Machnicki, AGabriella Wernicke

INTRODUCTION

Patients with primary lung cancer or metastatic cancer to the lungs often get radiation as a type of curative, also known as definitive, or palliative treatment. Radiation therapy can be used either alone or as a supplemental treatment with systemic therapy or prior to or after surgery. Typically, patients undergoing radiation therapy for various malignancies are inoperable candidates and have locally advanced disease or oligometastatic disease.

As with any treatment or procedure, there are potential side effects and toxicities of receiving radiation therapy. It is important to realize when radiation produces radiation-induced lung toxicity or pneumonitis, terms used interchangeably, it is via a temporal subacute and dose-dependent effect. Over time, radiation-induced pneumonitis may lead to radiation-induced pulmonary fibrosis as a later stage result of the prior subacute toxicity. The pathophysiology of radiation pneumonitis is complex and multifactorial. Advances in radiation oncology, understanding of delivery techniques, and personalized treatment plans have led to improved survival and less toxicity.[1-3]

TYPE OF RADIATION

Several types of radiation therapy exist, which have different indications and uses. There are three general categories of radiation which are external radiation, internal radiation, and systemic radiation. Modalities which are directed toward the lungs are largely in the category of external beam radiation. External beam radiation types include intensity-modulated radiation therapy and stereotactic body radiation therapy, also known as stereotactic ablative radiotherapy. Stereotactic body radiation is a modality that is now widely used for early stages of lung cancer in nonsurgical candidates as well as in oligometastatic malignancies in the lungs from any type of solid tumor.[4]

EPIDEMIOLOGY

The range of patients that are affected by radiation-induced pneumonitis is approximately 10–30%; however, the reported incidence varies across the literature due to definitions of clinically significant radiation-induced pneumonitis and the underlying malignancy.[1,5,6] Often, the clinical presentation of radiation-induced pneumonitis may be difficult to distinguish from other pulmonary conditions due to other concurrent pulmonary processes and may be underrecognized.

MECHANISM OF LUNG INJURY

The mechanisms involved in the occurrence of radiation pneumonitis are complex and multifactorial. Radiation-induced lung injury begins with broken chemical bonds of proteins, DNA, and lipids leading to cytotoxicity and release of reactive oxygen species and free radicals soon after exposure to radiation. A cascade of chemokines of resident pulmonary cells recruit inflammatory cells which in turn produces inflammation and cytokine release, vascular permeability, exudates, and ultimately fibrosis.[7-9]

RISK FACTORS

The development of radiation pneumonitis is associated with many risk factors. It is known that radiation-induced lung injury is dose dependent; however, there are also patient-related risk factors and existing lung disease that are associated with its development such as increased age and comorbidities may be associated with increased risk, but literature has not been able to recommend an optimal age for receiving radiation therapy.[10] Existing lung diseases, such as chronic obstructive lung disease and interstitial lung disease, have been noted to have a significantly increased incidence of radiation pneumonitis.[11,12] Interestingly, ongoing smoking may possibly be a protective factor from the development of radiation-induced lung injury.[10,13]

Location of the thoracic tumor, either central or peripheral tumors, and dosage technique such as single fraction or multifaction doses also impact the incidence of radiation pneumonitis. Central tumors treated with radiation commonly receive lower dose regimens due to mediastinal structures such as the heart compared with tumors located more in the periphery. Thus, centrally positioned tumors are noted to have radiation toxicity. Single fractions given at higher dosage, especially ≥ 30 Gray, rather than multiple fractions over time at lower doses are also related to increased occurrence of radiation toxicity.[14,15]

Radiation is often used in combination with other therapies, including immune checkpoint inhibitors (ICIs). Pneumonitis is a complication of ICI therapy with an incidence of 3–19%.[16] Recent studies have suggested an expanded role of ICI therapy in patients with non-small-cell lung cancer (NSCLC), including early stage.[17] Given the increased use of ICI in conjunction with radiation in the treatment of lung cancer, the concern of increased risk of pneumonitis is raised. In a meta-analysis of 20 clinical trials involving 2,027 patients, combination therapy of ICI and radiation therapy was associated with improved overall survival but with an increased risk of mild pneumonitis.[18] In a large retrospective cohort study of 18,780 patients, there was no increased risk of pneumonitis with combination treatment of ICI and radiation therapy compared with each therapy alone.[19]

Advancements in cancer genetics have allowed the identification of mutations and rearrangements that allow for the development of targeted therapies, including tyrosine kinase inhibitors (TKIs). Compared with ICI therapy, pneumonitis is rare among patients treated with TKIs. Among patients with anaplastic lymphoma kinase (ALK) rearranged NSCLC treated with TKIs, pneumonitis was reported in approximately 0.4–2.9% of patients, with lethal pneumonitis being reported in 0.09%.[20] Similarly, among patients with *EGFR* mutations treated with TKIs, pneumonitis was reported in approximately 1% of patients.[21] In a meta-analysis of 28 studies involving 1,640 patients, combination therapy with TKI and radiation therapy was not associated with an increased risk of grade > 3 pneumonitis.[22]

Prior radiation treatment is also associated with radiation-induced lung injury as recall radiation pneumonitis may occur. Recall radiation pneumonitis is a rare inflammatory reaction that may occur in patients who have had radiation therapy, and an inciting medication such as systemic cancer therapy or other biologics has been initiated. Often, recall radiation pneumonitis may require temporary or permanent cessation of the inciting medication.[23-25]

SIGNS AND SYMPTOMS

Most patients will not have any symptoms after receiving radiation therapy. However, if there are clinically significant symptoms of radiation toxicity, usually symptoms will occur approximately 6–8 weeks after radiation treatment. Symptoms are nonspecific and typical of other pulmonary diseases such as dry cough, shortness of breath at rest or dyspnea on exertion, low-grade fever, pleuritic pain, or, in more severe cases, hypoxemia.[9] The clinical significance of symptoms may not correlate with imaging findings; thus, grading systems have been implemented to establish severity and will be discussed in the following text.

DIAGNOSIS

Emphasis regarding the importance of recognition of typical symptoms, timing of symptoms, and exclusion of other causes is crucial in the diagnosis of radiation-induced lung injury. There are currently no laboratory tests to establish the diagnosis of radiation pneumonitis; however, laboratory tests are useful in diagnosing alternative causes of symptoms.[26] Timing of imaging and imaging findings on high-resolution chest computerized tomography in the field of radiation will be the cornerstone of diagnosis. Some of the characteristic cases of radiation pneumonitis on imaging are shown in **Figures 1 to 9**. Chest radiographs may not be helpful as they will only show nonspecific airspace opacities. Bronchoscopy with bronchoalveolar lavage and lung biopsies are not

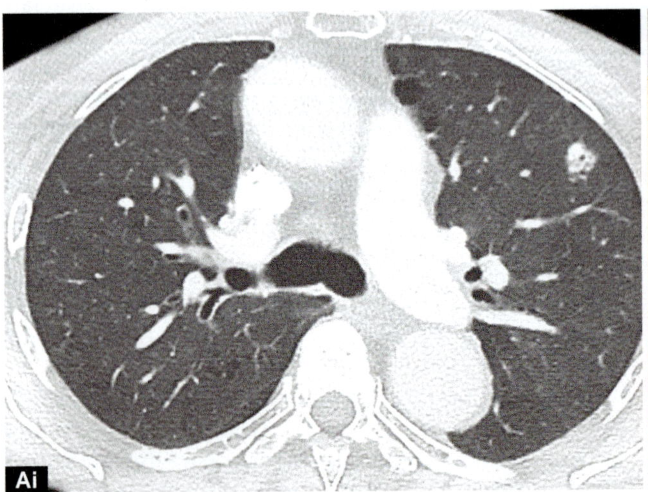

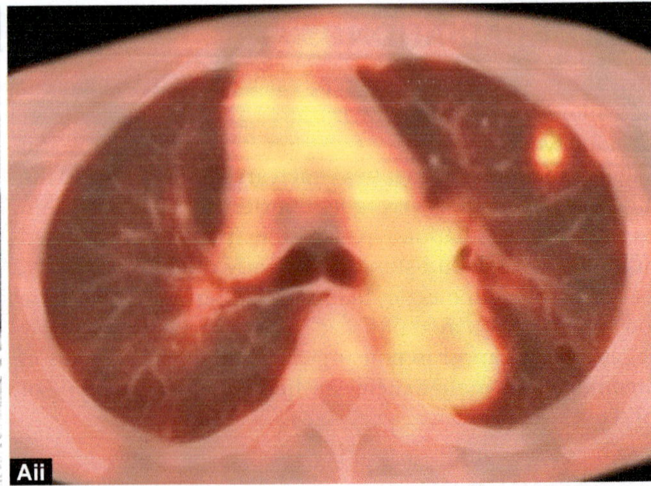

FIGS. 1A AND B: *Continued*

Continued

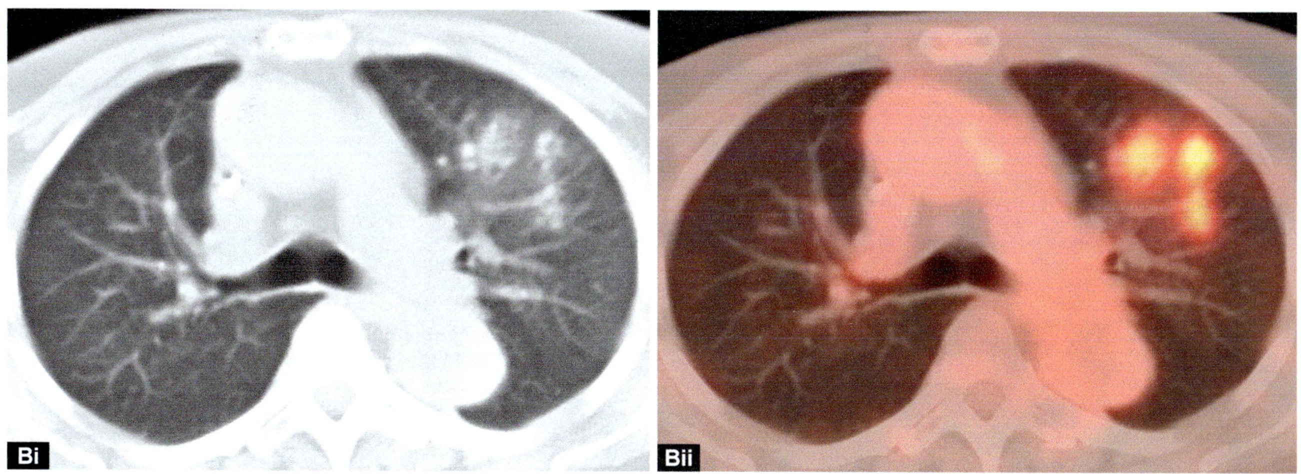

FIGS. 1A AND B: A 76-year-old female with a history of both primary lung adenocarcinoma and vaginal cancer. (A) Studies performed prior to treatment of her cancers. Axial contrast-enhanced CT scan image with lung windows (i) and fused PET-CT image (ii) from ^{18}F-FDG-PET scan showing an 11-mm solid nodule with central air bronchogram in the left upper lobe to be mildly FDG-avid, with SUV max of 1.8 g/mL. (B) Images from ^{18}F-FDG-PET-CT performed 3 months following SBRT 50 Gy to the left upper lobe. Axial CT scan image (i) and fused PET-CT image (ii) show new nodular ground-glass opacities adjacent to the tumor in the left upper lobe. The areas of GGO are FDG-avid, with SUV max of 3.6 g/mL. The treated tumor had not significantly changed. The findings are consistent with radiation pneumonitis.

(CT: computed tomography; ^{18}F-FDG: ^{18}F-fluorodeoxyglucose; GGO: ground glass opacity; PET: positron emission tomography; SBRT: stereotactic body radiation therapy; SUV: standardized uptake value)

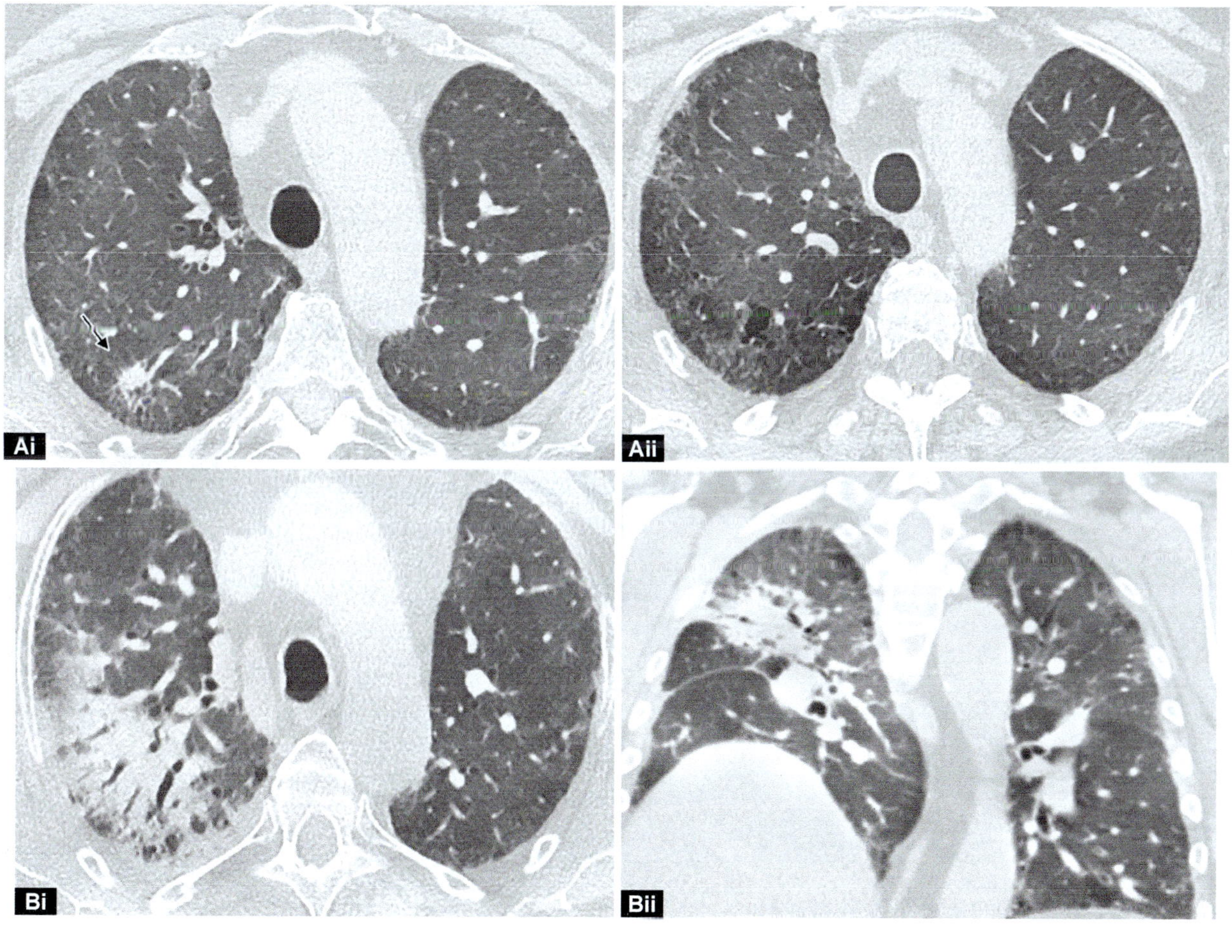

FIGS. 2A TO C: *Continued*

Continued

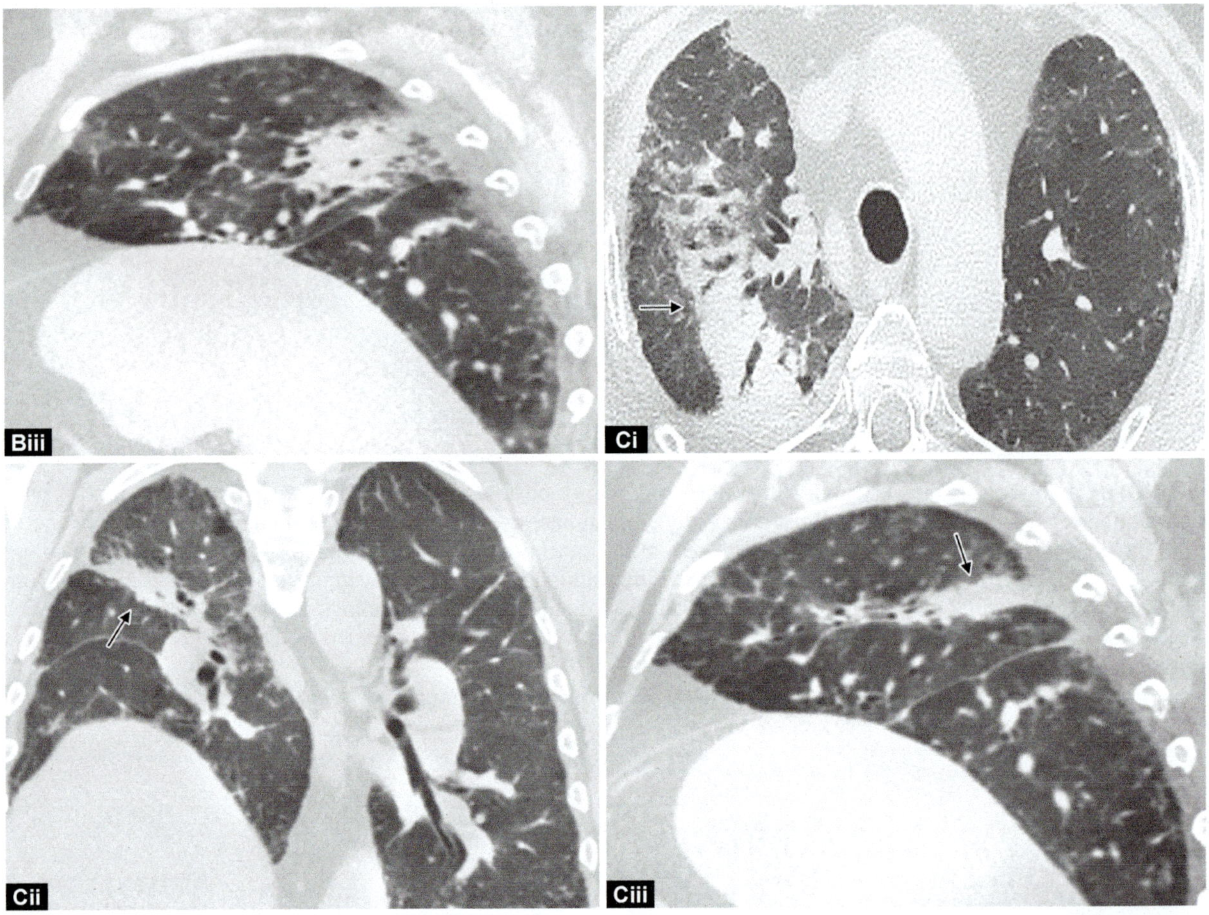

FIGS. 2A TO C: An 81-year-old male with squamous cell carcinoma of the right upper lobe. (A) Axial unenhanced CT images prior to treatment demonstrate a 13-mm solid nodule in the right upper lobe. Centrilobular emphysema is evident, as well as reticular changes and ground-glass opacity, consistent with interstitial lung abnormality. (B) Following completion of SBRT with dose of 48 Gy. Axial, coronal, and sagittal chest CT scan images performed 3 months. Airspace consolidation with traction bronchiectasis and volume loss conforming to irradiated field at 3 months. (C) Following completion of SBRT 8 months, progresses to chronic consolidation with greater volume loss, traction bronchiectasis, and development of nonanatomic, linear borders (black arrows) consistent with radiation-induced pulmonary fibrosis.

(CT: computed tomography; SBRT: stereotactic body radiation therapy)

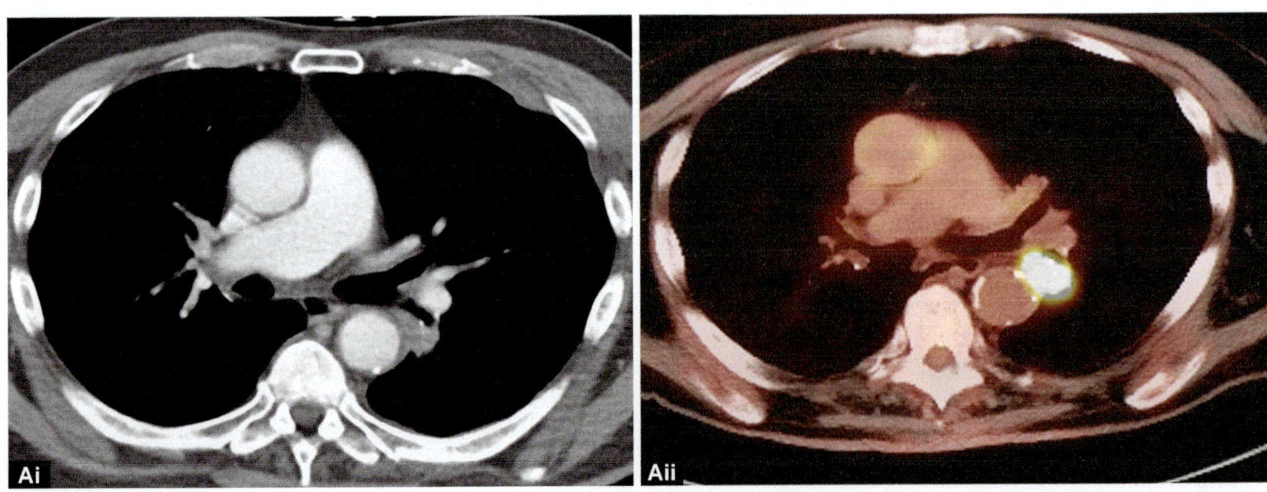

FIGS. 3A TO C: *Continued*

Continued

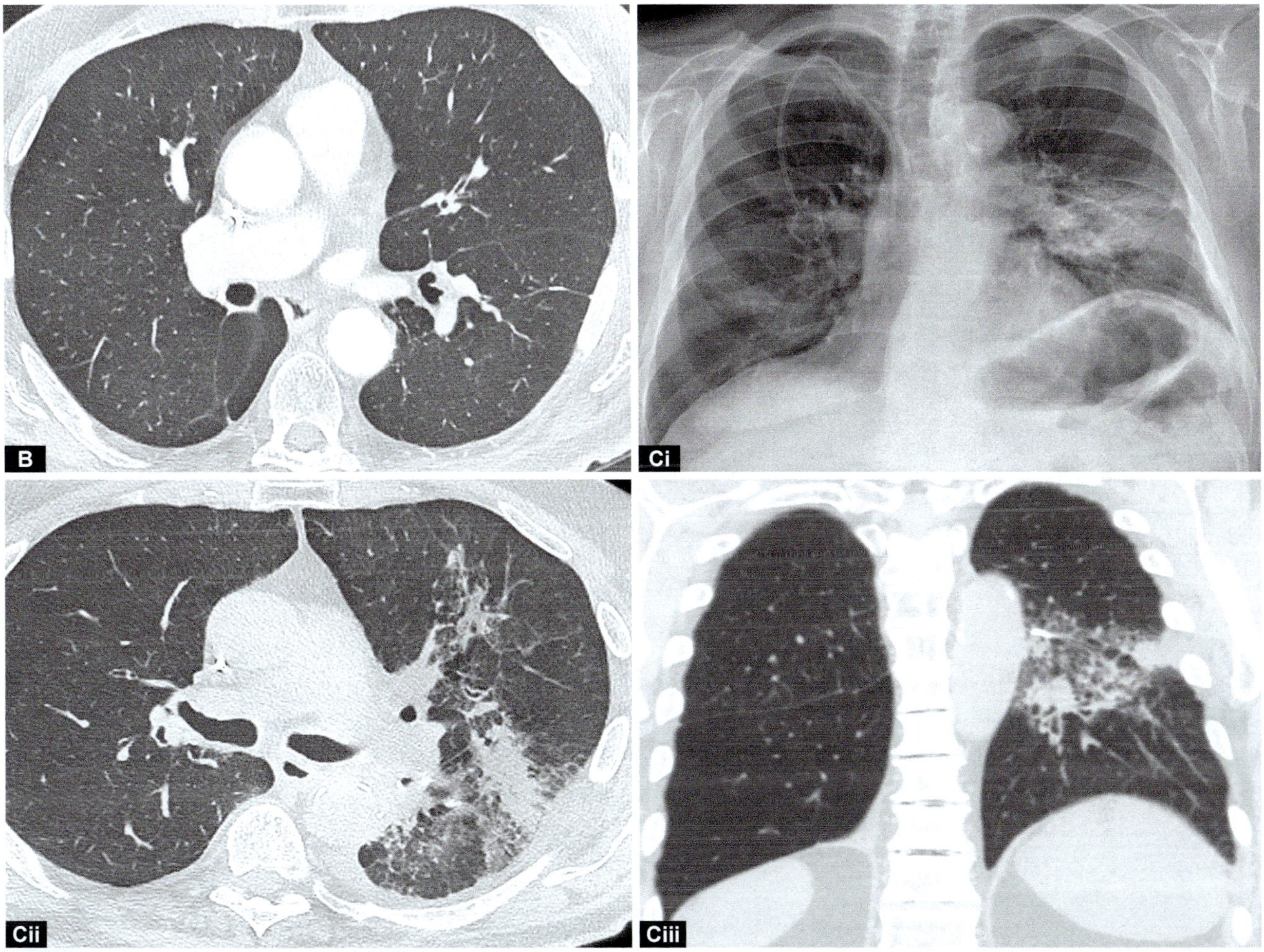

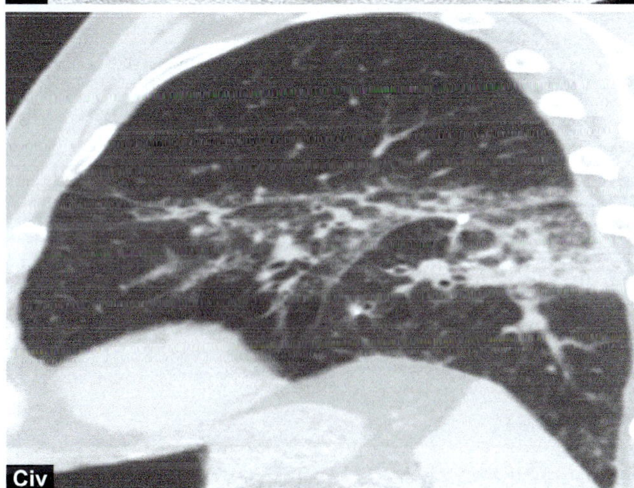

FIGS. 3A TO C: An 85-year-old male with a history of left lower lobe sublobar resection for lung adenocarcinoma developed left hilar lymph node recurrence on surveillance imaging. (A) Axial images from contrast-enhanced chest CT with mediastinal windows (i) and fused ^{18}F-FDG-PET-CT scan demonstrate a hypermetabolic lymph node in the left hilum. Endobronchial ultrasound biopsy confirmed recurrent lung adenocarcinoma. (B) Axial CT image with lung windows 3 months following completion of chemotherapy and radiotherapy showed resolution of the left hilar adenopathy. The left lung is clear. (C) The patient developed cough, wheezing, and shortness of breath 2 months after consolidation durvalumab. No improvement with antibiotics for presumed pneumonia. Posteroanterior chest radiograph and axial, coronal, and sagittal CT images demonstrate ground-glass opacity, reticulation, and airspace consolidation with linear borders in the left lung. Consistent with radiation recall pneumonitis.

(CT: computed tomography; ^{18}F-FDG: ^{18}F-fluorodeoxyglucose; PET: positron emission tomography)

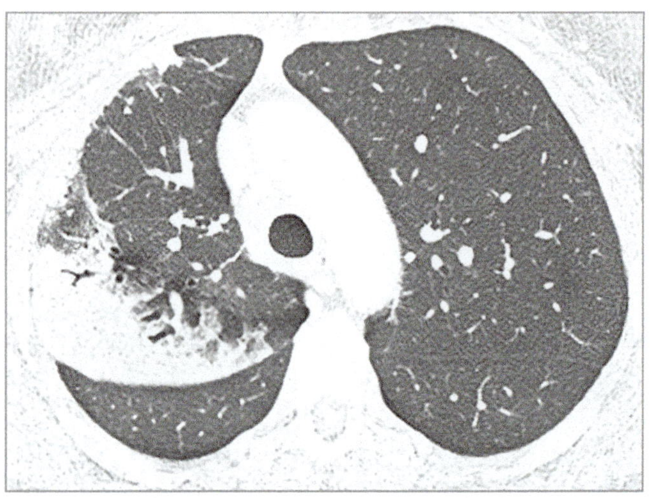

FIG. 4: Radiation-induced organizing pneumonia: Axial unenhanced computed tomography (CT) image. There is peripheral consolidation in the right upper lobe in a woman previously treated with radiation for breast cancer, biopsy-proven organizing pneumonia.

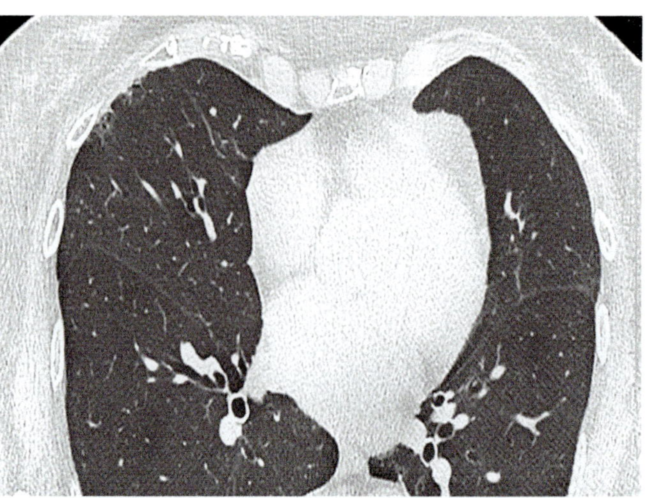

FIG. 6: A 79-year-old female who received radiation to right breast as part of treatment for breast cancer. Axial unenhanced chest computed tomography (CT) image demonstrates subpleural reticulation, ground-glass opacity, and traction bronchiectasis in the right middle lobe adjacent to the chest wall, a common appearance of radiation-induced fibrotic changes in a patient treated for breast cancer.

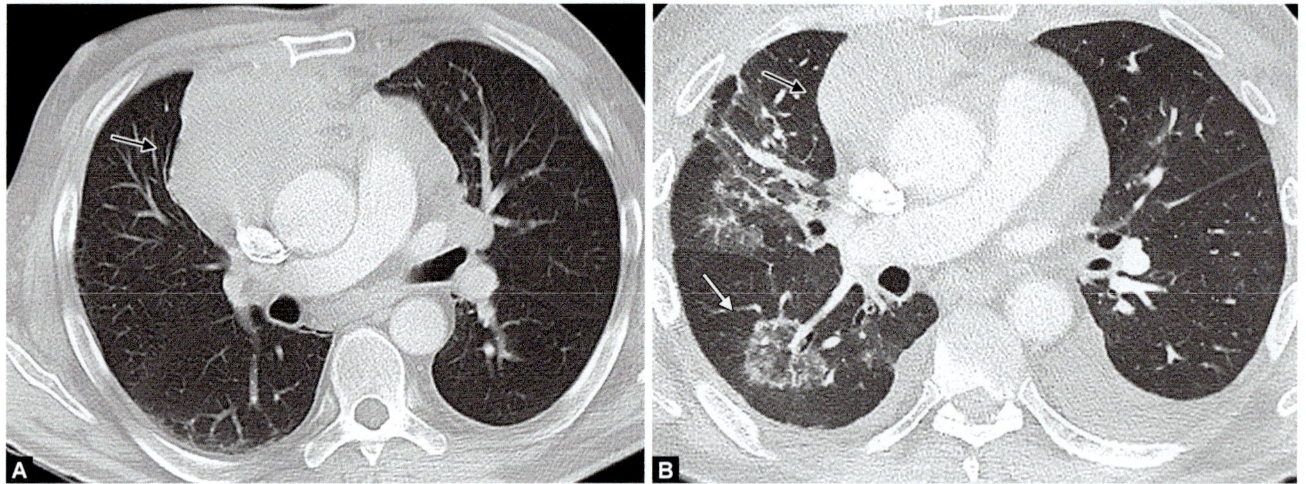

FIGS. 5A AND B: A 67-year-old male with stage IV squamous cell carcinoma of lung completed 45 Gy of radiation again to mediastinal mass. Axial contrast-enhanced computed tomography (CT) scan images of lungs prior to (A) and 3 months after completion of radiation therapy (B). The mediastinal mass decreases in size after treatment (black arrows). There are new ground-glass opacities in the right lung on post-treatment scan, with a reversed halo sign in the right lower lobe (white arrow). These findings are consistent with radiation pneumonitis.

necessary for the diagnosis of radiation pneumonitis unless there is a high suspicion for an alternative diagnosis such as infection, progression of malignancy, or organizing pneumonia, etc. Bronchoalveolar lavage has been shown in studies to show lymphocytic predominance and with predominance of T lymphocytes with CD4 predominant subset with normal ranges of CD4/CD8 ratios.[27,28]

STAGING

High-resolution chest computerized tomography findings vary depending on early-stage or late-stage radiation-induced lung injury. In early or acute initial stage, radiological findings on chest computerized tomography will be ground-glass opacities, and/or associated diffuse or patchy airspace

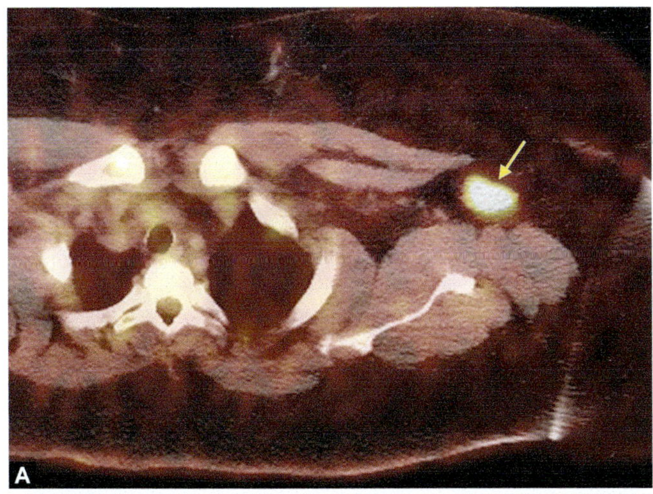

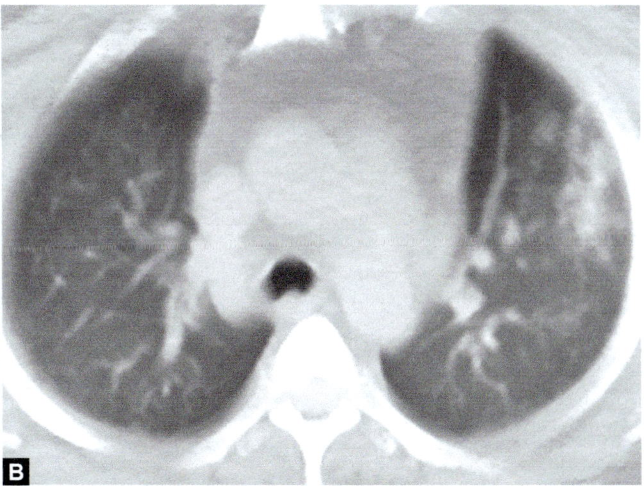

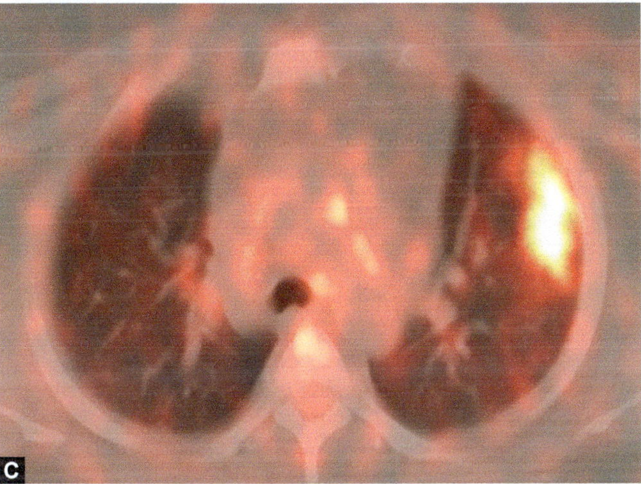

FIGS. 7A TO C: A 42-year-old female with nodular lymphocyte predominant Hodgkin's lymphoma in a left axillary lymph node. Treated with radiation therapy consisting of 30 Gy in 15 fractions. Fused axial image from ^{18}F-FDG-PET-CT scan (A) demonstrates a hypermetabolic lymph node in the left axilla (arrow), consistent with lymphoma. Axial chest CT image with lung windows (B) and fused axial image from ^{18}F-FDG-PET-CT scan (C) performed 3 months after completion of radiation therapy demonstrate new ground-glass opacity with a linear border and increased FDG activity in the left upper lobe, consistent with radiation pneumonitis. The patient was asymptomatic at the time of this surveillance scan.

(CT: computed tomography; ^{18}F-FDG: ^{18}F-fluorodeoxyglucose; PET: positron emission tomography)

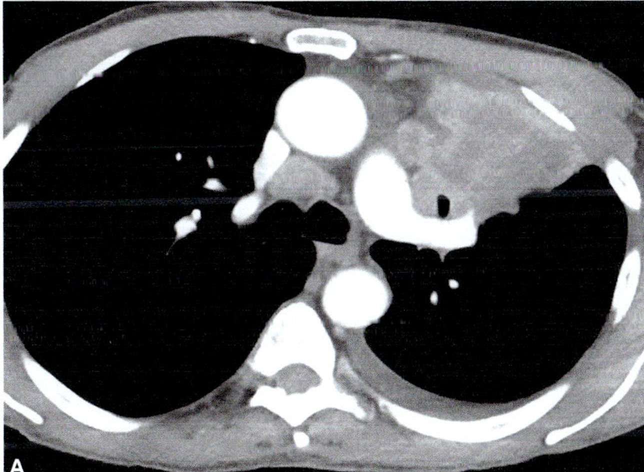

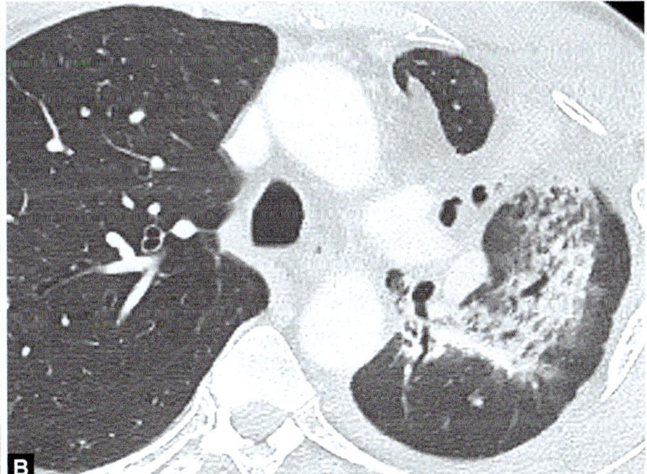

FIGS. 8A AND B: A 57-year-old male with stage IV NSCLC with brain metastases. Completed 45 Gy in 15 fractions to left lung. Axial CT scan images with mediastinal windows prior to treatment (A) and with lung windows (B) 3 months following completion of radiation therapy. Large left upper lobe mass, metastatic mediastinal lymph node, and malignant left pleural effusion present on pretreatment image. The left upper lobe mass has decreased in size after treatment and there is new airspace consolidation with traction bronchiectasis and a linear lateral border in the left lung, consistent with radiation-induced pulmonary fibrosis.

(CT: computed tomography; NSCLC: non-small cell lung cancer)

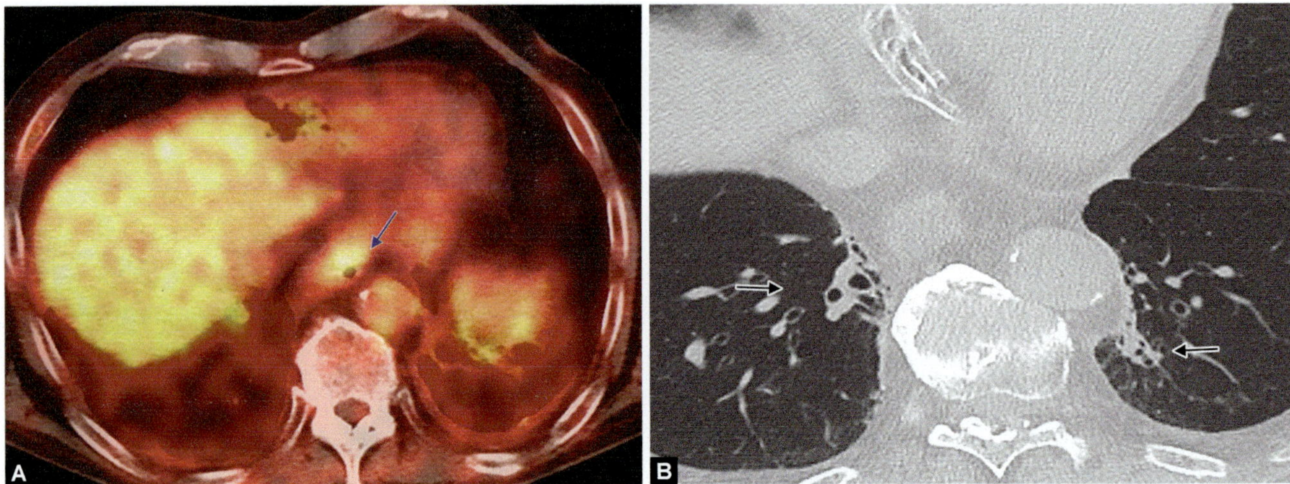

FIGS. 9A AND B: A 79-year-old male with esophageal adenocarcinoma treated with definitive chemoradiation to 50.4 Gy. Pretreatment fused axial image from ^{18}F-FDG-PET-CT (A) showing a hypermetabolic mass in the distal esophagus (blue arrow). Axial image with lung windows from CT scan performed 5 years after treatment shows paramediastinal traction bronchiectasis, volume loss, and reticular changes in each lower lobe, consistent with radiation-induced pulmonary fibrosis (black arrows).
(CT: computed tomography; ^{18}F-FDG: ^{18}F-fluorodeoxyglucose; PET: positron emission tomography)

TABLE 1: Radiation pneumonitis severity grading scale.

Radiation pneumonitis grading scale	Grade 1	Grade 2	Grade 3	Grade 4	Grade 5
Patient symptoms	Asymptomatic/ mild symptoms	Moderate • Cough, low-grade fever • Physical activities are somewhat limited	Severe • Physical activities completely limited • Supplemental oxygen required	Severe respiratory compromise requiring continuous oxygen supplementation or mechanical ventilation	Death
Radiographic findings	Minimal radiographic changes	Patchy radiographic changes	Diffuse/Dense radiographic changes	Diffuse/Dense radiographic changes	Diffuse/Dense radiographic changes

Source: Adapted from the Radiation Therapy Oncology Group and the National Institutes of Health/National Cancer Institute Common Terminology Criteria for Adverse Events.

consolidations or nodules, and/or atelectasis in the field of irradiation. There may or may not be an associated pleural effusion. In later stage or fibrotic stages, there will be radiographic changes of volume loss, septal wall thickening, linear or mass-like fibrosis, bronchiectasis, persistent pleural effusion, or pleural thickening in the same affected areas.[4,9,29-31]

These acute or late stages can be separated usually by chronicity by radiographic changes and appearance within the first 6 months or after 6 months or later after radiation treatment, respectively.

GRADING BY IMAGING

As mentioned above, grading systems of clinical severity and radiographic findings of radiation pneumonitis have been established. The most used grading systems are from the Radiation Therapy Oncology Group and from the United States National Institutes of Health/National Cancer Institute using the Common Terminology Criteria for Adverse Events.[32,33] An adapted version of the grading systems by the Radiation Therapy Oncology Group and Common Terminology Criteria for Adverse Events is given in **Table 1**.[32,33]

TREATMENT

The indication for treatment of acute radiation pneumonitis is determined by clinical presentation of the patient's symptoms. Once the diagnosis of radiation pneumonitis has been made, patients with grade 1 asymptomatic or only mild symptoms may be monitored clinically with supportive care. Corticosteroids and other supportive treatment are necessary in patients with increased symptoms. Inhaled corticosteroids have been used for treatment; however, systemic corticosteroids are the mainstay of treatment in patients with moderate or severe symptoms with or without the use of other supportive treatments such as supplemental oxygen.[4,34] Dosing of systemic corticosteroids is usually high doses of oral or intravenous steroids depending on clinical severity. The starting doses of oral corticosteroids are typically 1 mg/kg for 2–4 weeks and then tapered over up to 6–12 weeks and if severity requires the use of intravenous steroids, the dose is typically 2–4 mg/kg initially and then again slowly tapered over several weeks.[4]

Once the late stage or fibrotic changes have occurred, there are currently no guidelines for treatment to reverse or prevent changes and patients are managed using supportive care including supplemental oxygen if needed.[4]

PREVENTION/PROPHYLAXIS/PREDICTION

As can be expected, the more extensive or diffuse parenchymal involvement or if acute interstitial pneumonitis or acute respiratory distress syndrome patterns are seen on chest computerized tomography, there is increased association with high-grade radiation pneumonitis or death from radiation pneumonitis, especially if the previously mentioned risk factors are present.[35] Few studies have shown benefit in using amifostine and pentoxifylline to prevent radiation pneumonitis; however, these are not commonly used due to limited patient tolerability and limited evidence at this time.[36,37] More recently, evidence regarding the use of antifibrotics in radiation-induced fibrosis is emerging.[4,38,39] Awareness of risk factors, using predictive models, and overall advancements in radiation oncology using individualized radiation delivery and dosage methods may predict and reduce the occurrence of radiation pneumonitis.[2,5,11,13-15,40,41]

REFERENCES

1. Ling DC, Hess CB, Chen AM, et al. Comparison of Toxicity Between Intensity-Modulated Radiotherapy and 3-Dimensional Conformal Radiotherapy for Locally Advanced Non-small-cell Lung Cancer. Clin Lung Cancer. 2016;17(1):18-23.
2. Finazzi T, Haasbeek CJA, Spoelstra FOB, et al. Clinical Outcomes of Stereotactic MR-Guided Adaptive Radiation Therapy for High-Risk Lung Tumors. Int J Radiat Oncol Biol Phys. 2020;107(2): 270-8.
3. Kurz C, Buizza G, Landry G, et al. Medical physics challenges in clinical MR-guided radiotherapy. Radiat Oncol. 2020;15(1):93.
4. Hanania AN, Mainwaring W, Ghebre YT, et al. Radiation-Induced Lung Injury: Assessment and Management. Chest. 2019;156(1):150-62.
5. Wijsman R, Dankers F, Troost EGC, et al. Comparison of toxicity and outcome in advanced stage non-small cell lung cancer patients treated with intensity-modulated (chemo-)radiotherapy using IMRT or VMAT. Radiother Oncol. 2017;122(2):295-99.
6. Nishioka A, Ogawa Y, Hamada N, et al. Analysis of radiation pneumonitis and radiation-induced lung fibrosis in breast cancer patients after breast conservation treatment. Oncol Rep. 1999;6(3):513-7.
7. Arroyo-Hernandez M, Maldonado F, Lozano-Ruiz F, et al. Radiation-induced lung injury: current evidence. BMC Pulm Med. 2021;21(1).9.
8. Roy S, Salerno KE, Citrin DE. Biology of Radiation-Induced Lung Injury. Semin Radiat Oncol. 2021;31(2):155-61.
9. Kasmann L, Dietrich A, Staab-Weijnitz CA, et al. Radiation-induced lung toxicity – cellular and molecular mechanisms of pathogenesis, management, and literature review. Radiat Oncol. 2020;15(1):214.
10. Vogelius IR, Bentzen SM. A literature-based meta-analysis of clinical risk factors for development of radiation induced pneumonitis. Acta Oncol. 2012;51(8):975-83.
11. Rancati T, Ceresoli GL, Gagliardi G, et al. Factors predicting radiation pneumonitis in lung cancer patients: a retrospective study. Radiother Oncol. 2003;67(3):275-83.
12. Ueki N, Matsuo Y, Togashy Y, et al. Impact of pretreatment interstitial lung disease on radiation pneumonitis and survival after stereotactic body radiation therapy for lung cancer. J Thorac Oncol,. 2015;10(1):116-25.
13. Tucker SL, Liu HH, Liao Z, et al. Analysis of radiation pneumonitis risk using a generalized Lyman model. Int J Radiat Oncol Biol Phys. 2008;72(2):568-74.
14. Guckenberger M, Baier K, Polat B, et al. Dose-response relationship for radiation-induced pneumonitis after pulmonary stereotactic body radiotherapy. Radiother Oncol. 2010;97(1): 65-70.
15. de Jong EEC, Guckenberger M, Andratschke N, et al. Variation in current prescription practice of stereotactic body radiotherapy for peripherally located early stage non-small cell lung cancer: Recommendations for prescribing and recording according to the ACROP guideline and ICRU report 91. Radiother Oncol. 2020;142:217-23.
16. Suresh K, Voong KR, Shankar B, et al. Pneumonitis in Non-Small Cell Lung Cancer Patients Receiving Immune Checkpoint Immunotherapy: Incidence and Risk Factors. J Thorac Oncol. 2018;13(12):1930-9.
17. Wakelee H, Liberman M, Kato T, et al. Perioperative Pembrolizumab for Early-Stage Non-Small-Cell Lung Cancer. N Engl J Med. 2023;389:491-503.
18. Geng Y, Zhang Q, Feng S, et al. Safety and Efficacy of PD-1/PD-L1 inhibitors combined with radiotherapy in patients with non-small-cell lung cancer: a systematic review and meta-analysis. Cancer Med. 2021;10(4):1222-39.
19. Neibart SS, Malhotra J, Roy JA, et al. Pneumonitis in advanced non-small cell lung cancer: no interaction between immune checkpoint inhibition and radiation therapy. J Thorac Dis. 2023;15(5):2458-68.
20. Qie W, Zhao Q, Yang L, et al. Incidence of pneumonitis following the use of different anaplastic lymphoma kinase tyrosine kinase inhibitor regimens: An updated systematic review and meta-analysis. Cancer Med. 2023;12(13):13873-84.

21. Suh CH, Park HS, Kim KW, et al. Pneumonitis in advanced non-small-cell lung cancer patients treated with EGFR tyrosine kinase inhibitor: Meta-analysis of 153 cohorts with 15,713 patients: Meta-analysis of incidence and risk factors of EGFR-TKI pneumonitis in NSCLC. Lung Cancer. 2018;123:60-9.
22. Li X, Wang F, Jia H, et al. Efficacy and safety of EGFR inhibitors and radiotherapy in locally advanced non-small-cell lung cancer: a meta-analysis. Future Oncol. 2022;18(27):3055-65.
23. Lu X, Wang J, Zhang T, et al. Comprehensive Pneumonitis Profile of Thoracic Radiotherapy Followed by Immune Checkpoint Inhibitor and Risk Factors for Radiation Recall Pneumonitis in Lung Cancer. Front Immunol. 2022;13:918787.
24. Ding X, Ji W, Li J, et al. Radiation recall pneumonitis induced by chemotherapy after thoracic radiotherapy for lung cancer. Radiat Oncol. 2011;6:24.
25. McGovern K, Ghaly M, Esposito M, et al. Radiation recall pneumonitis in the setting of immunotherapy and radiation: a focused review. Future Sci OA. 2019;5(5):FSO378.
26. Wang Z, Huo B, Wu Q, et al. The role of procalcitonin in differential diagnosis between acute radiation pneumonitis and bacterial pneumonia in lung cancer patients receiving thoracic radiotherapy. Sci Rep. 2020;10(1):2941.
27. Toma CL, Serbescu A, Alexe M, et al. The bronchoalveolar lavage pattern in radiation pneumonitis secondary to radiotherapy for breast cancer. Maedica (Bucur). 2010;5(4):250-7.
28. Nakayama Y, Makino S, Fukuda Y, et al. Activation of lavage lymphocytes in lung injuries caused by radiotherapy for lung cancer. Int J Radiat Oncol Biol Phys. 1996;34(2):459-67.
29. Benveniste MF, Gomez D, Carter BW, et al. Recognizing Radiation Therapy-related Complications in the Chest. Radiographics. 2019;39(2):344-66.
30. Ikezoe J, Takashima S, Morimoto S, et al. CT appearance of acute radiation-induced injury in the lung. AJR Am J Roentgenol. 1988;150(4):765-70.
31. Dahele M, Palma D, Lagerwaard F, et al. Radiological changes after stereotactic radiotherapy for stage I lung cancer. J Thorac Oncol. 2011;6(7):1221-8.
32. Cox JD, Stetz J, Pajak TF. Toxicity criteria of the Radiation Therapy Oncology Group (RTOG) and the European Organization for Research and Treatment of Cancer (EORTC). Int J Radiat Oncol Biol Phys. 1995;31(5):1341-6.
33. Common Terminology Criteria for Adverse Events. Version 5.0. Published November 27, 2017. [online] Available from https://ctep.cancer.gov/protocoldevelopment/electronic_applications/docs/ctcae_v5_quick_reference_5x7.pdf [Last accessed August, 2024].
34. Henkenberens C, Janssen S, Lavae-Mokhtari M, et al. Inhalative steroids as an individual treatment in symptomatic lung cancer patients with radiation pneumonitis grade II after radiotherapy - a single-centre experience. Radiat Oncol. 2016;11:12.
35. Thomas R, Chen YH, Hatabu H, et al. Radiographic patterns of symptomatic radiation pneumonitis in lung cancer patients: Imaging predictors for clinical severity and outcome. Lung Cancer. 2020;145:132-9.
36. Antonadou D, Coliarakis N, Synodinou M, et al. Randomized phase III trial of radiation treatment +/- amifostine in patients with advanced-stage lung cancer. Int J Radiat Oncol Biol Phys. 2001;51(4):915-22.
37. Ozturk B, Egehan I, Atavci S, et al. Pentoxifylline in prevention of radiation-induced lung toxicity in patients with breast and lung cancer: a double-blind randomized trial. Int J Radiat Oncol Biol Phys. 2004;58(1):213-9.
38. Chen C, Zeng B, Xue D, et al. Pirfenidone for the prevention of radiation-induced lung injury in patients with locally advanced oesophageal squamous cell carcinoma: a protocol for a randomised controlled trial. BMJ Open. 2022;12(10):e060619.
39. Simone NL, Soule BP, Gerber L, et al. Oral pirfenidone in patients with chronic fibrosis resulting from radiotherapy: a pilot study. Radiat Oncol. 2007;2:19.
40. Bradley JD, Hope A, El Naqa I, et al. A nomogram to predict radiation pneumonitis, derived from a combined analysis of RTOG 9311 and institutional data. Int J Radiat Oncol Biol Phys. 2007;69(4):985-92.
41. Zhang XJ, Sun JG, Sun J, et al. Prediction of radiation pneumonitis in lung cancer patients: a systematic review. J Cancer Res Clin Oncol. 2012;138(12):2103-16.

Drug-induced Respiratory Diseases

CHAPTER 115

Kavitha Venkatnarayan, Uma Maheswari Krishnaswamy

INTRODUCTION

The ever-expanding repertoire of pharmaceutical agents has made the diagnosis of drug-induced respiratory diseases (D-IRD) increasingly challenging. Drug toxicity can involve any part of the respiratory system including airways, parenchyma, interstitium, pleura, pulmonary vasculature, and respiratory muscles. A comprehensive knowledge of the common offending drugs and typical manifestations of their toxicities is desirable for every clinician.

Diligent history taking and a high index of suspicion are important since practically any drug has the potential to cause pulmonary toxicity. It is important to note that toxicity due to a single drug may have variable clinical, radiological, and temporal features. D-IRD is a diagnosis of exclusion as patients often present with nonspecific constitutional and pulmonary symptoms. Periodic surveillance for symptoms, functional impairment, and radiological changes may help in early diagnosis.

DRUG-INDUCED RESPIRATORY DISEASE

Common agents associated with D-IRD include chemo therapeutic drugs, anti-inflammatory agents, cardiovascular drugs, antibiotics, and other miscellaneous drugs. Several risk factors like male sex, increasing age, smoking, and underlying lung disease increase the probability of developing pulmonary toxicity. Diagnosing D-IRD may be challenging due to variability in the timing and dose of drug exposure, nonspecific clinical, radiological and pathological findings, presence of an underlying disease which itself can have pulmonary manifestations, and reluctance of patients to reveal the history of use of alternative medicines and recreational drugs.

Pulmonary function tests (PFTs) are routinely performed for pre- and post-treatment evaluation of pulmonary toxicity. But the results are neither sensitive nor specific for D-IRD and may show restrictive defect in those with pulmonary parenchymal involvement. Diffusion capacity for carbon monoxide (DLCO), though nonspecific, may serve as one of the earliest markers of pulmonary toxicity. Hence, the diagnosis is predominantly based on the temporal association between drug initiation and development of lung disease, symptomatic and radiological improvement on drug withdrawal and essentially exclusion of alternative etiologies. Although not always feasible, in some instances, rechallenge with the drug may be possible with the attendant risk of recurrence of pulmonary toxicity.

Since varied toxicities and radiological findings have been reported for each drug in literature, we focus only on the common D-IRDs encountered in clinical practice for the purpose of this chapter. A web-based repository, Pneumotox v2.2 (www.pneumotox.com) provides a comprehensive update on the pulmonary toxicities of various drugs.

Cancer Chemotherapy and Pulmonary Toxicity

The past decade has witnessed new paradigms in cancer chemotherapy with the emergence of several drugs for targeted therapy and immunotherapy, which have paved the way for personalized therapy in almost all malignancies. Although the emergence of these drugs has changed the outlook for cancer patients, they are also the harbingers of potential novel toxicities. These toxicities may not always be evident during clinical trials, and every clinician needs to be vigilant about the development of unknown side effects of these drugs. Diagnosing D-IRD secondary to chemotherapeutic agents may be more complex due to several reasons: use of multidrug regimens, multimodality treatment including radiotherapy and immunosuppression predisposing to opportunistic infections which mimic D-IRD. Apart from the novel therapeutic agents, conventional cytotoxic drugs are also associated with pulmonary toxicity. Pulmonary toxicity of some commonly used chemotherapeutic agents will be discussed in the subsequent paragraphs.

Common terminology criteria for adverse events (CTCAE version 5.0) **(Table 1)** help classify the severity of adverse events in patients receiving cancer therapy uniformly and also aid in decisions regarding future management prospects.[1]

TABLE 1: Common terminology criteria for adverse events (CTCAE version 5.0).

Adverse event	Grade 1	Grade 2	Grade 3	Grade 4	Grade 5
Pneumonitis	Asymptomatic; intervention not indicated	Symptomatic; limiting instrumental ADL; medical intervention indicated	Severe symptoms; limiting self-care ADL; oxygen indicated	Life-threatening respiratory compromise; urgent intervention indicated (e.g., ventilatory support)	Death
Pulmonary fibrosis	Radiologic pulmonary fibrosis <25% of lung volume associated with hypoxia	Evidence of pulmonary hypertension; radiographic pulmonary fibrosis 25–50% associated with hypoxia	Severe hypoxia; evidence of right-sided heart failure; radiographic pulmonary fibrosis >50–75%	Life-threatening consequences; intubation with ventilatory support indicated; radiographic pulmonary fibrosis >75% with severe honeycombing	Death
Pulmonary hypertension	Minimal dyspnea; findings on physical examination or other evaluation	Moderate dyspnea, cough; requiring evaluation by cardiac catheterization and medical intervention	Severe symptoms, associated with hypoxia, right heart failure; oxygen indicated	Life-threatening airway consequences; urgent intervention indicated (e.g., tracheotomy or intubation)	Death
Pleural effusion	Asymptomatic; intervention not indicated	Symptomatic; intervention (diuretics/ thoracentesis) indicated	Symptomatic with hypoxia; chest tube insertion and/or pleurodesis indicated	Life-threatening respiratory or hemodynamic compromise; urgent intervention indicated (e.g., ventilatory support)	Death

Pulmonary Toxicity of Agents Used in Lung Cancer Chemotherapy

Taxanes

They promote cell death by inhibiting microtubule disassembly essential for mitosis. Taxanes in combination with platinum-based compounds are an integral part of lung cancer chemotherapy, especially non-small cell lung cancer (NSCLC), where they form a part of adjuvant as well as neoadjuvant regimens.

Pulmonary toxicity due to taxanes can be in the form of an acute type I hypersensitivity reaction manifesting within few minutes to hours of therapy with bronchospasm, dyspnea, and hypotension. These reactions have been reported to be due to the diluents used in the compound and are lesser with docetaxel and newer compounds like nab-paclitaxel (nano-particle albumin-bound paclitaxel). Type IV delayed hypersensitivity reactions may also occur and mainly manifest as interstitial lung diseases (ILDs). The typical time frame of presentation is within 3 weeks of therapy with smoking, underlying emphysema, or pre-existing ILD and concurrent radiotherapy increasing the risk of toxicity. Combination of taxanes with gemcitabine has been reported to increase the risk significantly and has to be avoided.[2]

Radiological findings include ground-glass opacities, nonspecific interstitial pneumonia (NSIP), or organizing pneumonia (OP) pattern. Diagnosis is established based on the temporality of events and exclusion of alternative etiology including infections. Lung biopsy is usually not indicated but has been reported to show interstitial inflammation with mononuclear and lymphohistiocytic infiltration and poorly formed granulomas. Management includes discontinuation of taxane therapy and steroids along with appropriate ventilatory and supportive treatment based on the severity of involvement.

Tyrosine Kinase Inhibitors (TKIs)

TKIs are commonly used for advanced NSCLC with positive epidermal growth factor receptor (EGFR) or anaplastic lymphoma kinase (ALK) mutations. D-ILD is a rare adverse effect of TKIs with a reported incidence of 1% for EGFR-TKI and <1% with ALK-TKIs. Various mechanisms have been postulated including direct cytotoxicity to the alveolar epithelium and alveolar capillary endothelium. Risk factors and clinical presentation are similar to other D-ILDs. Radiological findings range from nonspecific ground-glass opacities to OP pattern and acute interstitial pneumonitis.[3] Typically, patients present with suggestive symptoms within 4 weeks of initiation of therapy. Management includes cessation of TKI therapy and institution of corticosteroids after excluding infections. Rechallenge with the drug is usually avoided unless the initial involvement was minimal and asymptomatic. Presence of AIP-like pattern and poor performance status predict higher mortality and poorer prognosis.[2]

Tyrosine kinase inhibitors targeting Bcr-Abl oncoprotein have revolutionized the management of myeloproliferative disorders like chronic myelogenous leukemia. Although pulmonary complications are more common with dasatinib, they have been reported with all generations of these drugs including imatinib, bosutinib, nilotinib, and ponatinib. Pleural effusions and chylothorax are the most frequent complications usually associated with dasatinib and bosutinib. Drug-induced pulmonary hypertension (PH) is commonly seen with dasatinib and rarely with bosutinib and ponatinib.[4] D-ILDs are rare with these TKIs and are typically seen with imatinib. Clinical presentation and radiological findings are nonspecific and similar to other D-ILDs with ground-glass opacities and OP pattern with or without evidence of fibrosis. Discontinuation of the drug with initiation of corticosteroids leads to complete resolution in a quarter of the patients, while 15% may have persistent fibrosis.[5]

Immune Checkpoint Inhibitors

Immunotherapy, which enhances antitumor immunity of the body, has improved the outlook for various malignancies in the recent years including lung malignancies. Immune checkpoint inhibitors (ICI) increase the ability to fight cancer cells by blocking intrinsic downregulators such as programmed cell death 1 (PD-1) or its ligand, programmed cell death ligand 1 (PD-L1) and cytotoxic T-lymphocyte antigen 4 (CTLA 4). However, the resulting alteration in the immunologic homeostasis can have various adverse reactions. Immune-related adverse events most commonly involve gastrointestinal, dermatological, hepatic, and endocrine systems.[6]

Pulmonary toxicity is reported to be between 1% and 7% in most of the clinical trials involving these agents. Pulmonary involvement is more likely with anti-PD-1 inhibitors than with anti-CTLA-4 antibodies. The spectrum of pulmonary involvement ranges from subacute presentations with features of OP, NSIP, hypersensitivity pneumonitis, and sarcoid-like reactions to acute presentations like acute interstitial pneumonia and acute respiratory distress syndromes. Pneumonitis is more common in those receiving ICI as first-line therapy or those with a history of previous radiotherapy, NSCLC, and any pre-existing lung diseases.[7]

Management of immune-related adverse events **(Flowchart 1)** includes discontinuation of the implicated drug. Corticosteroids may be warranted in those not responding to drug withdrawal or with ≥grade 2 toxicity. In steroid refractory cases, infliximab, cyclophosphamide, or mycophenolate mofetil has been recommended with the attendant risk of superadded infections. Rechallenge with the offending drug depends on the severity of the initial immune-related adverse event. In patients with high-grade pulmonary toxicity, permanent discontinuation of the drug is advisable.[8]

Other Chemotherapeutic Agents

- *Bleomycin*: It is an antitumor antibiotic used in the management of various malignancies including lymphomas, germ cell tumors, and head and neck malignancies. Bleomycin-induced lung injury has been classically used as an animal model for the study of pulmonary fibrosis. Lung tissue is particularly susceptible to injury owing to low levels of the enzyme bleomycin hydrolase to metabolize the drug. Bleomycin induces generation of reactive oxygen radicals by combining with Fe^{3+} ions. Endothelial injury secondary to oxidative stress, perivascular edema, and inflammation; activation of cytokines including tumor necrosis factor α (TNF-α), transforming growth factor β (TGF-β), and interleukin 6 (IL-6); and eventual activation of fibroblasts leading to fibrosis have been postulated as the possible underlying pathogenetic mechanisms.[9]

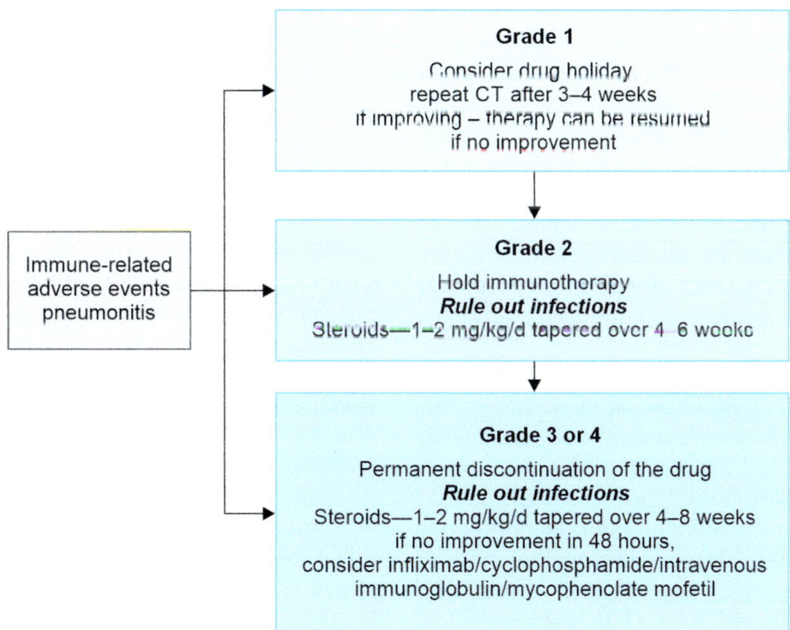

FLOWCHART 1: Algorithm for management of immunotherapy-related pneumonitis.

Use of bleomycin as a part of a combination chemotherapy regimen, higher cumulative dose > 400 units, concurrent or sequential radiotherapy within a month ("radiation recall"), and exposure to high concentrations of supplemental oxygen and smoking are some of the well-documented risk factors which can increase the propensity to develop pulmonary toxicity.

Lung involvement may be in the form of an acute hypersensitivity reaction with eosinophilic infiltrates and peripheral eosinophilia, an acute chest pain syndrome which lasts during the drug infusion and subsides with the completion of the infusion or the more common bleomycin-induced pneumonitis. Clinical and radiological findings are nonspecific and similar to other drug-induced ILDs (D-ILD). Similar to other D-ILDs, cessation of therapy may be sufficient for the milder spectrum with systemic steroids warranted in the more severe spectrum where rechallenge with the drug is not advisable.[10]

Although PFTs are routinely performed for pretreatment screening in many centers, their role in predicting toxicity remains controversial. Baseline PFTs are still advisable as they can be used as a reference in future in case of toxicity. They may also aid in the diagnosis of toxicity with DLCO showing the most significant correlation. In patients aged more than 40 years, a baseline CT is recommended as they have a higher risk of developing pneumonitis. Patients receiving a cumulative dose of >300 units should be evaluated with a post-treatment CT scan.[11]

- *Methotrexate*: This is an antimetabolite agent used as a chemotherapeutic and an immune modulatory drug. Methotrexate-related pulmonary toxicity has been most commonly described in patients with rheumatoid arthritis (RA), which is an inflammatory disorder with predominant joint symptoms. Pulmonary involvement is the most common extra-articular manifestation of RA and can affect any part of the respiratory system with ILD being the most prevalent manifestation. Paradoxically, ILD in these patients has also been linked to the use of methotrexate, an important disease-modifying agent used in RA. Age more than 60 years, hypoalbuminemia, underlying pleuropulmonary disease secondary to RA, and diabetes mellitus are some of the factors purported to increase the risk for methotrexate-induced pulmonary toxicity.

Methotrexate pneumonitis has an acute to subacute course with clinical manifestations seen within the first year of therapy. Patients present with nonspecific symptoms of cough and progressive dyspnea with or without fever. Mild peripheral blood eosinophilia may be seen with a restrictive defect on pulmonary function testing. Common patterns on radiology include NSIP or OP pattern, unlike the usual interstitial pneumonia (UIP) pattern seen commonly with RA-ILD. Bronchiole-centric pattern leading to tree-in-bud appearance may also be seen less frequently. Bronchoalveolar lavage (BAL) may show lymphocytosis with lung biopsies revealing interstitial lymphohistiocytic and eosinophilic infiltrates with or without noncaseating granulomas.[12] Diagnostic criteria proposed by Kremer and colleagues may help approach patients with suspected methotrexate-induced pulmonary toxicity, although they are not validated in prospective studies **(Box 1)**.[13]

BOX 1 Diagnostic criteria for methotrexate pneumonitis.[13]

Major criteria:

- Hypersensitivity pneumonitis by histopathologic examination (no infectious etiology noted)
- Radiologic evidence of pulmonary interstitial or alveolar infiltrates
- Blood and sputum cultures negative for pathogenic organisms

Minor criteria:

- Dyspnea of acute onset <8 weeks' duration
- Nonproductive cough
- White blood cell counts ≤15,000/mm^3 with or without eosinophilia
- Oxygen saturation ≤90% on room air
- DLCO ≤ 70% predicted

Notes:
Definite diagnosis: Major criteria 1 or major 2 *and* 3 and at least 3 minor criteria.
Probable diagnosis: Major 2 and 3 *and* 2 minor criteria.

Other Drugs Causing Pulmonary Toxicity

Amiodarone

Amiodarone is a commonly used antiarrhythmic agent to treat supraventricular and ventricular arrhythmias. This iodine-containing drug and its metabolite *N*-desethylamiodarone are highly lipid soluble and accumulate in various organs including the liver, lung, adipose tissue, and spleen. With increasing awareness and use of lower doses, the incidence of amiodarone-induced pulmonary toxicity has decreased from 5–15% to <2%. However, being aware of potential pulmonary toxicity is of utmost importance as the latter can occur at any dose. Amiodarone impairs normal phospholipid metabolism and leads to accumulation of phospholipids inside the cells which appear as lamellar inclusion bodies. This may lead to direct cellular injury or injury mediated by the production of reactive oxygen species.[14]

Male gender, advanced age, presence of an underlying lung disease, and a higher cumulative dose of the drug (>400 mg/day for >2 months) are some risk factors associated with an increased risk of toxicity. Requirement for supplemental oxygen therapy and mechanical ventilation is also reported to potentiate toxicity. Pulmonary parenchymal involvement has been widely documented with amiodarone and may manifest as OP, interstitial pneumonitis, or mass-like lesions. Pleural involvement may also be seen in the form of exudative effusions. Clinical presentation may vary from nonspecific symptoms like progressive dyspnea and cough with constitutional symptoms to a presentation as acute respiratory failure. Radiology plays a pivotal role in diagnosis, with computed tomographic imaging showing high attenuation parenchymal lesions due to the accumulation of the iodinated compound which has a prolonged half-life in the lung **(Fig. 1)**. High attenuation can also be seen in the liver and spleen; this is indicative of drug exposure and does not essentially imply toxicity. Pleural effusions and pleural thickening may also be seen.[15]

Bronchoalveolar lavage findings are nonspecific and may reveal lymphocytosis with predominance of CD8+ T cells. Histopathological findings may include features of interstitial pneumonitis characterized by type II pneumocyte hyperplasia with alveolar septal inflammation and interstitial fibrosis. Alveolar spaces filled with foamy macrophages with membrane-bound lamellar bodies on ultrastructural examination is another characteristic feature. However, these inclusions can also be seen in patients merely exposed to amiodarone without any other evidence of toxicity. Less frequent findings include bronchiolitis obliterans, diffuse alveolar damage, and alveolar hemorrhage.

Diagnosis is usually based on the temporal relation between drug use and development of symptoms coupled with characteristic radiology. BAL may show polymorphonuclear leukocytes with CD8+ T cells and foamy macrophages. Biopsy is rarely required for diagnosis and should be avoided as any form of thoracic surgery may worsen the disease. Discontinuation of therapy and switching to alternative agents where feasible generally lead to resolution. Some patients may warrant corticosteroids therapy in tapering doses for 4–12 months. Prognosis is generally favorable if diagnosed early. Hence, patients beginning amiodarone therapy should be informed about the possible toxicity and

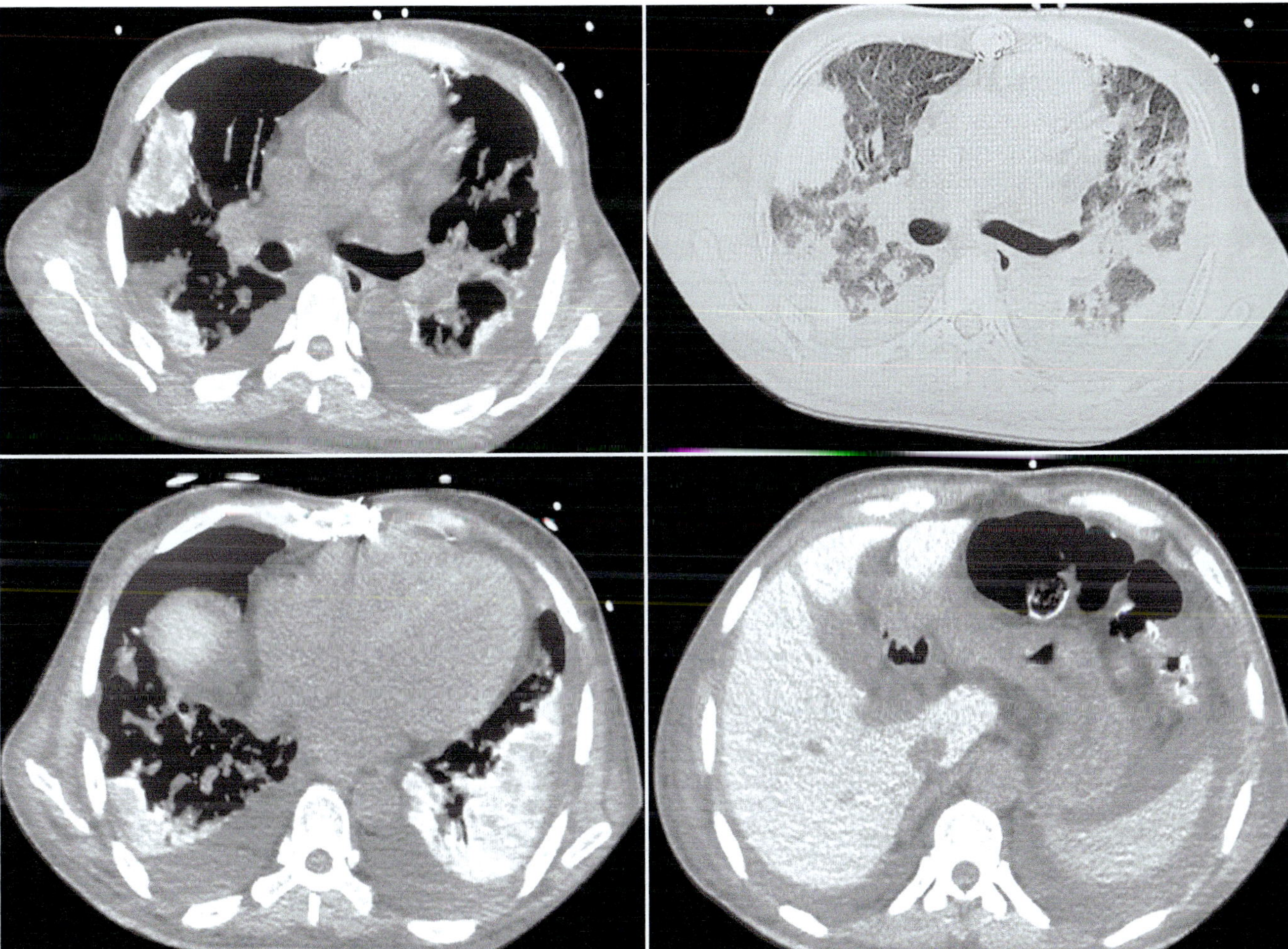

FIG. 1: Computed tomography of a patient on amiodarone showing characteristic high attenuation consolidation in right upper and bilateral lower lobes with septal thickening and fibrosis. Also noted is diffuse high attenuation in the liver and bilateral pleural effusion.

the symptoms of the same. Annual screening radiography and regular monitoring for symptoms are recommended to facilitate early diagnosis.[16]

Nitrofurantoin

Nitrofurantoin is commonly used to treat urinary tract infections (UTIs) and as prophylaxis to prevent recurrent UTI. Pulmonary toxicity with nitrofurantoin can present with acute, subacute, and chronic forms and is usually reported in elderly females. Acute and subacute forms are secondary to hypersensitivity reactions and are dose independent. They typically present within a week to a month of therapy with fever, dyspnea, cough, and peripheral and BAL eosinophilia.[17] Chronic nitrofurantoin-induced lung disease presents with progressive dyspnea and dry cough. The postulated mechanisms include oxidative injury and immune-complex-mediated reactions. Radiological manifestations include bilateral ground-glass opacities, septal thickening, honeycombing, traction bronchiectasis, and OP. BAL usually reveals lymphocytosis. Treatment includes discontinuation of the drug and steroids in symptomatic and severe cases may hasten the recovery.[18]

Miscellaneous Agents

There are several other forms of drug-induced pulmonary toxicities such as pulmonary vasculitis and hemorrhage, bronchospasm, autoimmune diseases, eosinophilia, granulomatous inflammation, and other manifestations which are frequently attributed to the use of one or the other drug **(Table 2)**.

TABLE 2: Other common drug-induced pulmonary toxicities.

Other manifestations	Associated drugs
Drug-induced systemic lupus erythematosus	• β-blockers • Amiodarone • Angiotensin-converting enzyme inhibitors • Hydralazine • Procainamide • Isoniazid • Methyldopa • Minocycline and tetracycline
Pulmonary–renal syndromes	• Phenytoin • Hydralazine • Propylthiouracil • D-penicillamine • Cocaine
Bronchospasm	• β-blockers • Aspirin • Adenosine • Nonsteroidal anti-inflammatory drugs
Eosinophilic pneumonia	• Sulfasalazine, mesalamine • Angiotensin-converting enzyme inhibitors • Amiodarone • Nitrofurantoin • Methotrexate
ANCA-associated vasculitis	D-penicillamine
Pulmonary hemorrhage	Bevacizumab
Tracheoesophageal fistula	Bevacizumab
Granulomatous inflammation	Interferon-γ
Alveolar hypoventilation	• Opioids • Sedative hypnotics

(ANCA: antineutrophil cytoplasmic antibody)

Drug-induced Pulmonary Hypertension

A number of drugs and toxins are associated with the development of PH **(Box 2)**. This is typically precapillary hypertension defined by mean pulmonary artery pressure > 20 mm Hg, pulmonary artery wedge pressure ≤ 15 mm Hg, and pulmonary vascular resistance > 2 Wood units.[19] Drug-induced pulmonary arterial hypertension (D-PAH) accounts for approximately 10% of PAH cases. Anorexigens were amongst the first class of drugs identified to cause D-PAH. Other well-reported association was with toxic rapeseed oil with methamphetamines, TKIs and interferons being more common in today's era.

Drug-induced pulmonary arterial hypertension should be suspected in patients presenting with unexplained dyspnea and other features of PH. A diagnosis of D-PAH is made in the presence of relevant exposure and after careful exclusion of alternative etiologies. In patients with mild PH, discontinuation of the offending drug and follow up after 3–4 months for any worsening pulmonary hemodynamics and symptoms are required to decide on the need to initiate therapy. Those with more severe forms of PH and intermediate- and high-risk PH should be initiated on PH-specific therapy. Discontinuation of such therapy may be feasible on follow-up if the hemodynamics improve **(Flowchart 2)**. The choice of therapy is similar to other group 1 PH cases and has been discussed elsewhere.

Drug-induced Pleural Disease

Drug-induced pleural diseases are infrequent compared to parenchymal involvement. They can manifest as pleural effusion, pleural thickening, or acute pleurisy. The underlying pathophysiology is not well understood. However, possible mechanisms reported include oxidative injury to the mesothelial cells, suppression of antioxidant defenses, acute hypersensitivity reaction, and chemical-induced pleural inflammation.[20]

Drug-induced pleural effusion **(Box 1)** is commonly lymphocyte predominant and exudative in nature. Presence of pleural fluid eosinophilia (>10% eosinophils) may point toward a drug-induced etiology, but is neither a consistent nor a specific finding. Some drugs are specifically associated with eosinophilic effusions **(Table 3)**.[21]

Of the TKIs, dasatinib is strongly implicated in the development of pleural effusion with a reported prevalence of 28% over a 5-year period of drug administration.[22] The volume

BOX 2 Association of drugs with pulmonary hypertension.[19]

Drugs with definite association:

- Aminorex
- Benfluorex
- Dasatinib
- Dexfenfluramine
- Fenfluramine
- Methamphetamines
- Toxic rapeseed oil
- Selective serotonin reuptake inhibitors#

Drugs with possible association:

- Alkylating agents (cyclophosphamide, mitomycin c)*
- Amphetamines
- Bosutinib
- Cocaine
- Interferon-α and -β
- L-Tryptophan
- Leflunomide
- Solvents (trichloroethylene)*
- St. John's wort

#Associated with increased risk of 'persistent pulmonary hypertension of newborn' in mothers exposed during pregnancy.
*Associated with pulmonary veno-occlusive disease.

TABLE 3: Drugs associated with pleural effusions.[21]

Class of drugs	Drugs
Cardiovascular drugs	• β-blockers • Amiodarone • Minoxidil
Ergot alkaloids	• Bromocriptine • Methysergide
Chemotherapeutic agents	• Bleomycin • Mitomycin • Methotrexate • Dasatinib • Procarbazine • Cyclophosphamide • Docetaxel
Eosinophilic effusions	• Valproic acid • Dantrolene • Isotretinoin • Nitrofurantoin • Propylthiouracil • Gliclazide

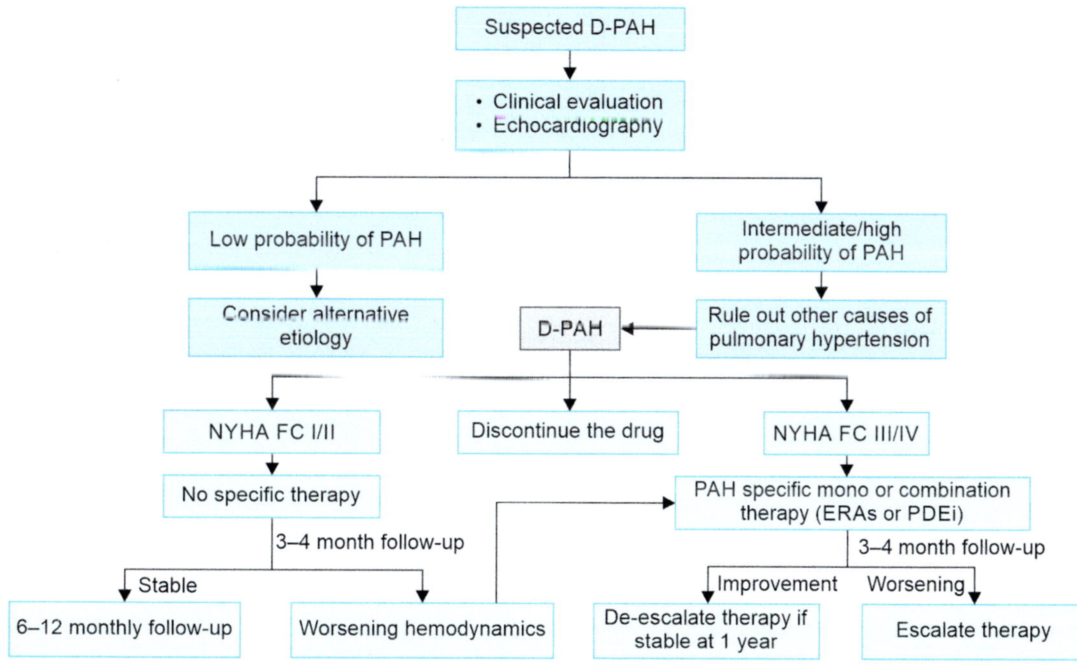

FLOWCHART 2: Management algorithm for drug-induced pulmonary hypertension.

(D-PAH: drug-induced pulmonary hypertension; ERAs: endothelin receptor antagonists; NYHA: New York Heart Association; PDEi: phosphodiesterase inhibitors)

of fluid may vary from minimal to massive effusions, and pleural fluid analysis generally reveals exudative, lymphocyte-predominant effusions. Chylothorax has also been reported with dasatinib. However, chylothorax may be underdiagnosed given the absence of a classic milky appearance of fluid in these cases and lack of routine triglyceride analysis.[4]

As there may be multiple causes leading to an effusion, pleural fluid analysis should be done in all effusions amenable to thoracentesis. Characterization of the fluid as transudate or exudate, predominant cellularity, and microbiological investigations to rule out infections should be performed. Patients with minimal effusion can be followed up with continuation of the drug. Those with symptomatic effusions may need dose reduction, discontinuation, or change of therapy along with steroid therapy.

SUMMARY

The list of drugs used for different respiratory or other systemic indications may cause undesirable pulmonary manifestations referred to as drug-induced respiratory diseases. Such toxicity can involve any part of the respiratory system including the airways, lung parenchyma, pleura, pulmonary vasculature, and respiratory muscles. It is important to have a comprehensive knowledge of the common offending drugs and typical manifestations of their toxicities for early recognition and appropriate management.

REFERENCES

1. Common Terminology Criteria for Adverse Events (CTCAE). (2017). [online] Available from https://ctep.cancer.gov/protocoldevelopment/electronic_applications/docs/CTCAE_v5_Quick_Reference_8.5x11.pdf [Last accessed July, 2024].
2. Long K, Suresh K. Pulmonary toxicity of systemic lung cancer therapy. Respirology. 2020;25(S2):72-9.
3. He Y, Zhou C. Tyrosine kinase inhibitors interstitial pneumonitis: diagnosis and management. Transl Lung Cancer Res. 2019;8(S3): S318-20.
4. Weatherald J, Bondeelle L, Chaumais MC, et al. Pulmonary complications of Bcr-Abl tyrosine kinase inhibitors. Eur Respir J. 2020;56(4):2000279.
5. Zhang P, Huang J, Jin F, et al. Imatinib-induced irreversible interstitial lung disease. Medicine (Baltimore). 2019;98(8):e14402.
6. Postow MA, Sidlow R, Hellmann MD. Immune-related Adverse Events Associated with Immune Checkpoint Blockade. N Engl J Med. 2018;378(2):158-68.
7. Martins F, Sofiya L, Sykiotis GP, et al. Adverse effects of immune-checkpoint inhibitors: epidemiology, management and surveillance. Nat Rev Clin Oncol. 2019;16(9):563-80.
8. Thompson JA, Schneider BJ, Brahmer J, et al. Management of Immunotherapy-related Toxicities, Version 1.2019. J Natl Compr Cancer Netw JNCCN. 2019;17(3):255-89.
9. Reinert T, da Rocha Baldotto CS, Nunes FAP, et al. Bleomycin-Induced Lung Injury. J Cancer Res. 2013;2013:1-9.
10. Sleijfer S. Bleomycin-induced pneumonitis. Chest. 2001;120(2): 617-24.
11. Watson RA, De La Peña H, Tsakok MT, et al. Development of a best-practice clinical guideline for the use of bleomycin in the treatment of germ cell tumours in the UK. Br J Cancer. 2018;119(9):1044-51.
12. Fragoulis GE, Conway R, Nikiphorou E. Methotrexate and interstitial lung disease: controversies and questions. A narrative review of the literature. Rheumatology. 2019;58(11):1900-6.
13. Kremer JM, Alarcón GS, Weinblatt ME, et al. Clinical, laboratory, radiographic, and histopathologic features of methotrexate-associated lung injury in patients with rheumatoid arthritis: a multicenter study with literature review. Arthritis Rheum. 1997;40(10):1829-37.
14. Feduska ET, Thoma BN, Torjman MC, et al. Acute Amiodarone Pulmonary Toxicity. J Cardiothorac Vasc Anesth. 2021;35(5):1485-94.
15. Wolkove N, Baltzan M. Amiodarone pulmonary toxicity. Can Respir J. 2009;16(2):43-8.
16. Goldschlager N, Epstein AE, Naccarelli GV, et al. A practical guide for clinicians who treat patients with amiodarone: 2007. Heart Rhythm. 2007;4(9):1250-9.
17. Milazzo E, Orellana G, Briceño-Bierwirth A, et al. Acute lung toxicity by nitrofurantoin. BMJ Case Rep. 2021;14(4):e237571.
18. Batzlaff C, Koroscil M. Nitrofurantoin-Induced Pulmonary Toxicity: Always Review the Medication List. Cureus. 2020;12(8): e9807.
19. Humbert M, Kovacs G, Hoeper MM, et al. 2022 ESC/ERS Guidelines for the diagnosis and treatment of pulmonary hypertension. Eur Respir J. 2023;61(1):2200879.
20. Lin CM, Rhiannon JJ, Chan ED. Drug-induced pleural disease. Adverse Drug Reaction Bull. 2013;281(1):1083-6.
21. Huggins JT, Sahn SA. Drug-induced pleural disease. Clin Chest Med. 2004;25(1):141-53.
22. Cortes JE, Saglio G, Kantarjian HM, et al. Final 5-Year Study Results of DASISION: The Dasatinib versus Imatinib Study in Treatment-Naïve Chronic Myeloid Leukemia Patients Trial. J Clin Oncol. 2016;34(20):2333-40.

Sarcoidosis

CHAPTER 116

Sahajal Dhooria

INTRODUCTION

Sarcoidosis is a multisystem granulomatous disorder of an unknown cause. The disease occurs worldwide and affects young and middle-aged adults of both sexes. The thoracic lymph nodes and lungs are the most frequently involved organs, but sarcoidosis can involve the eyes, skin, bones, joints, heart, liver, kidneys, and the nervous system. The inciting agent for the granulomatous response in sarcoidosis remains unknown. The most accepted hypothesis favors an environmental antigen or a microbial agent in a genetically susceptible host. In the past, sarcoidosis was considered rare in India and other developing countries. However, due to increasing awareness and the availability of better diagnostic modalities, sarcoidosis is now more readily diagnosed. Still the differentiation from tuberculosis (TB), which is far more prevalent in developing countries and is a close clinical mimic of sarcoidosis, remains a challenge.

HISTORY

In 1877, Jonathon Hutchinson, a general practitioner in London, first described sarcoidosis in a patient with chronic multiple, raised, purplish cutaneous patches over the hands and feet.[1] However, the term "sarcoidosis" was first used by Caesar Boeck. He described the histological findings of epithelioid cells and giant cells in a skin biopsy specimen and termed it "multiple benign sarkoid of the skin". The term implied that the histology resembled "sarcoma" but was benign.[2] The major landmarks in the description and understanding of the disease are summarized in **Table 1**.[3-5]

TABLE 1: Some important historical landmarks in sarcoidosis.

Year(s)	Landmark
1869	Hutchinson describes skin lesions
1889	Besnier describes "lupus pernio"
1904	Kreibich describes sarcoid bone cysts
1909	Heerfordt describes uveo-parotid fever
1916–17	Schaumann recognizes multiple organ involvement and separates sarcoidosis from lymphoma
1939	Association of hypercalcemia or hypercalciuria with sarcoidosis is described
1941	Kveim describes a test to help diagnose sarcoidosis, Siltzbach later refines and popularizes the test, James christens the test as Kveim–Siltzbach test
1946	Löfgren links erythema nodosum, bilateral hilar lymphadenopathy, fever, and polyarthritis
1951	Glucocorticoids are first used to treat sarcoidosis
1958	Wurm and colleagues propose radiographic staging, the First International Conference held in London, UK
1975	Serum angiotensin-converting enzyme (ACE) is first recognized as a possible biochemical marker by Lieberman
1987	Rizzato and James form the World Association of Sarcoidosis and other Granulomatous Disorders (WASOG)

EPIDEMIOLOGY

The incidence and prevalence of sarcoidosis vary across the world possibly because of differences in genetics, environmental exposures, diagnostic facilities available, and diagnostic pathways followed. Sarcoidosis occurs in 1–15 individuals per 100,000 population every year (annual incidence) depending on the geographical location.[6] The prevalence is between 50 and 160 per 100,000 population.[7] Northern European countries have the highest incidence followed by North America and Australia. The East Asian countries have a lower incidence. In India, the prevalence of sarcoidosis appears to be higher in the northern regions than in the northeastern and southern parts, possibly due to genetic and environmental differences. We recently described the spectrum and estimated the incidence, prevalence, and national burden of sarcoidosis and other diffuse parenchymal lung diseases (DPLD) in India based on data from our center, a tertiary care institute in northern India.[8,9] Sarcoidosis was the most common DPLD in our region followed by connective tissue disease-related interstitial lung disease (CTD-ILD), idiopathic pulmonary fibrosis (IPF), hypersensitivity pneumonitis (HP), and other ILDs. The annual incidence of sarcoidosis was estimated to be about 4–8 per 100,000 population; the prevalence estimates were 25–50 per 100,000 population. The national burden was estimated at 1.25–2.5 lakh patients.[9]

RISK FACTORS

The risk factors for sarcoidosis include (1) nonmodifiable elements such as demographic aspects (age, sex, race) and genetic variation and (2) modifiable factors such as environmental exposures to microbial or nonmicrobial antigens.[10]

Demographic Factors

Sarcoidosis is diagnosed typically in individuals in the 35–50 years age group. Some studies show a bimodal age distribution with peaks at 25–29 and 65–69 years. The overall female-to-male ratio for the occurrence of sarcoidosis is 1:1. However, in the 20–45 years age group, more males than females are diagnosed, whereas the converse is true for the 50–65-year age interval. In the United States, Black Americans have the highest incidence of sarcoidosis followed by White, Hispanic, and Asian Americans. The landmark ACCESS study, conducted across 10 centers in the United States, found that women tended to have more ocular and neurological involvement, whereas men had a higher risk of hypercalcemia.[11] African-Americans were more likely to have uveitis, skin, and liver disease.

Genetic Predisposition

Associations between sarcoidosis and several loci of the human leukocyte antigen (*HLA*) gene have been established for long. Like several T-cell-mediated diseases, sarcoidosis is associated with the major histocompatibility complex (MHC), encoded by the genes on chromosome 6. Strong associations have been described with HLA-DRB1*11:01 in diverse ethnicities, while race-specific associations exist with 12:01, 15:03, 15:01, and 04:01. The DRB1*03:01 is an interesting variant that demonstrates association with not only increased risk of the disease but also disease resolution. Genome-wide association studies (GWAS) have found novel associations in the last two decades.[12,13] Several variants in the *ANXA11* gene have been reported to be linked with sarcoidosis in different populations. Single nucleotide polymorphisms (SNPs) in the genes of the IL23/T-helper (Th)17-signaling pathway have been found to increase the risk. Another associated SNP has been described in the butyrophilin-like 2 (*BTNL2*) gene that suppresses T-cell activation. Several of the above variants differ by ancestry, suggesting that there may be more than one pathway to disease. For example, variants in the *NOTCH4* gene and the X-linked inhibitor of apoptosis (XIAP) associated factor 1 (*XAF1*) gene have been found to increase the risk in African-Americans.

Certain HLA subtypes may increase the risk for organ-specific manifestations. HLA-DRB1*04:01 is linked with uveitis, HLA-DRB1*03:01 with Löfgren syndrome, and HLA-DQB1*06:01 with cardiac sarcoidosis. Variants in the nucleotide-binding oligomerization domain-containing protein 2 (NOD2) pathway, transforming growth factor-β (TGF-β), and activated mitogen-activated protein (MAP) kinase are linked to skin and musculoskeletal involvement, while a SNP in *ZNF592*, a zinc finger gene, may be associated with neurosarcoidosis.

Sarcoidosis is a disease that exemplifies the role of gene–environment interaction. The estimated heritability of sarcoidosis is 66%.[14] Some studies indicate that certain genetic variation might make individuals susceptible to developing a granulomatous response to particular environmental exposures. HLA DRB1*1101 and insecticide exposure may be associated with cardiac sarcoidosis and hypercalcemia, while the same HLA type is associated with pulmonary sarcoidosis when exposure to molds and musty odors is present.

Clustering of sarcoidosis occurs in families. Nearly 6% of patients in the United Kingdom have an affected relative.[15] In the United States, the relative risk (RR) of sarcoidosis for family members is 4.7 with siblings having the highest (RR 5.8) risk.[16] Familial clustering is higher for White than Black families. The majority of familial "clusters" involve only parent–child pairs or sibling pairs; more complex pedigrees are rare. This suggests a summation of more than one minor genetic influence rather than a single causative gene mutation.

Blau syndrome, an autosomal-dominant chronic granulomatous disease clinically identical to sporadic infantile-onset sarcoidosis, had its gene locus mapped to 16p12-q21, and subsequently both diseases were found to be associated with mutations in the *CARD15* gene.[17] However, no association with these variants has been found in adult sarcoidosis.[18] Recently, many of class II MHC alleles have been implicated in different aspects of sarcoidosis. HLA-DR5, HLA-DR6, HLA-DR8, and HLA-DR9 seem to confer risk of sarcoidosis in Japanese patients, although HLA-DR9 is protective in the Scandinavian population. In German patients, HLA-DR5 is associated with chronic disease and HLA-DR3 with acute forms. Likewise, in Scandinavians, HLA-DR14 and HLA-DR15 are associated with chronic forms and HLA-DR17 with self-limiting ones.[19] The ACCESS study identified a significant association between HLA-DRB1 alleles (specifically HLA-DRB1*1101) and the development of the disease, in both Blacks and Caucasians.[20] The HLA-DRB1*1501 allele is associated with a reduced risk of sarcoidosis in Blacks but an increased risk in Whites. This indicates that, in general, alleles similar to class II HLA may be associated with sarcoidosis in both the populations. Similarly, other studies have identified specific alleles of

HLA-DQB1 as determining susceptibility to sarcoidosis in the African-American population.[21-23] In a study from India, the presence of DRB1*11 and DRB1*14 and absence of DRB1*07 and DQB1*0201 alleles were found to be independent predictors of sarcoidosis.[24]

Environmental and Occupational Risk Factors

Several environmental exposures have been implicated in the etiopathogenesis of sarcoidosis.[25] A recent systematic review found associations of 81 airborne occupational exposures with pulmonary sarcoidosis in the available literature.[26] Occupational silica, pesticide, and mold or mildew exposures had significant associations. Metal dusts such as that of aluminum and nickel have also been suspected, but significant association is lacking. World Trade Center demolition dust amongst exposed firefighters has been proposed to have increased the incidence of sarcoidosis amongst this population.[27,28] This has been seriously questioned based on the possibility of the observer effect (observing a phenomenon changes it, for example, more incidental sarcoidosis cases will be identified, if one is looking for them) and lack of direct causal evidence.[29] Barnard et al., based on data from the ACCESS study, observed a greater risk among workers with industrial exposure to organic powders, particularly in those who worked for suppliers of building materials, hardware, and gardening material.[30] A negative association with current smoking has also been reported, but is not consistent across studies.[31-33] All the above are weak associations with odds ratios generally < 2, and causality is questionable. Only with beryllium exposure, which causes an illness similar to sarcoidosis, the cause-effect relationship is convincing.[34] The data on seasonality in sarcoidosis occurrence is also conflicting.[35,36] Seasonal clustering of sarcoidosis was found during summer months in a study from northern India.[37]

Infectious Agents as Risk Factors

Several microbes have been associated with sarcoidosis implicated due to histochemical evidence or presence of their genetic material in the granuloma. These include *Leptospira* species, *Mycoplasma* species, herpes virus, retrovirus, *Chlamydia pneumoniae*, *Borrelia burgdorferi*, *Rickettsia helvetica*, and *Pneumocystis jiroveci*.[38,39] The strongest associations are with the genera *Mycobacterium* and *Propionibacterium*.[40-42]

A meta-analysis suggested a 30% (range, 0–50%) prevalence of mycobacterial DNA in sarcoid samples.[43] A study from our center found mycobacterial DNA with polymerase chain reaction (PCR) for the 65 kDa protein gene in 48% of samples [bronchoalveolar lavage (BAL) or biopsy] from newly diagnosed patients of sarcoidosis.[44] Aspects that favor mycobacteria being triggers for sarcoidosis include the presence of granulomatous inflammation, mycobacterial disease reported to occur before, during, or after sarcoidosis, and the finding of mycobacteria in occasional sarcoid granulomas.[45-50] Passage experiments have also suggested that mycobacteria with characteristics of *Mycobacterium tuberculosis* (*M.tb*) may be the incriminating agents.[51-54] Recent studies on humoral immunity to mycobacterial antigens from sarcoidosis patients have renewed interest in a potential role of mycobacteria in sarcoidosis.[55] It has been shown that mycobacterial ESAT-6 and katG are recognized by sarcoidosis CD4+ T cells when presented by the sarcoidosis susceptibility allele, DRB1*1101.[56] Interestingly, a study from our center also found similar frequency of circulating antibodies to the RD1 antigens used in interferon gamma release assays [IGRAs; early secreted antigenic target (ESAT-6) and culture filtrate protein (CFP-10)] in patients with pulmonary TB and sarcoidosis, indicating a possible pathogenetic role of mycobacterial antigens in sarcoidosis.[57] However, the antibody response to a combination of epitopes from the RD1 and RD2 antigens is significantly different between TB and sarcoidosis.[58]

It is possible that the presence of mycobacterial infection or Bacillus Calmette–Guérin (BCG) vaccination in a genetically predisposed host may be involved in the development of autoimmunity.[59] It has also been suggested that the organism might exist in a cell wall-deficient L-form and may be difficult to isolate.[60] Nevertheless, the jury is still out on the issue whether the TB bacillus causes sarcoidosis.

PATHOGENESIS AND IMMUNOLOGY

Granulomatous inflammation is the central feature of sarcoidosis pathogenesis. The granulomatous reaction is a protective response to an inciting agent. It limits inflammation and protects tissues. Though the exact antigen inciting this response in sarcoidosis is yet unclear, it may, in fact, be different in different patients and different geographic regions. Essentially, there are four stages involved in pathogenesis (**Flowchart 1**). First, the inciting antigen encounters antigen-processing cells (APCs), mostly alveolar macrophages. The second stage is the interaction between APCs and CD4+ T lymphocytes to initiate the formation of a simple granuloma. The third stage includes further recruitment of CD4+ T lymphocytes and elicitation of type 1 helper T (Th1) cells and type 2 helper (Th2) responses, which lead to the final stage of formation and maintenance of complex granulomas. Macrophages differentiate to form epithelioid cells under the influence of several cytokines. These epithelioid cells fuse to form multinucleated giant cells and gain secretary properties. Granulomas secrete many chemicals including calcitriol and angiotensin-converting enzyme. These events, however, are shaped by genetic susceptibility, possibly due to various functional polymorphisms.[61,62]

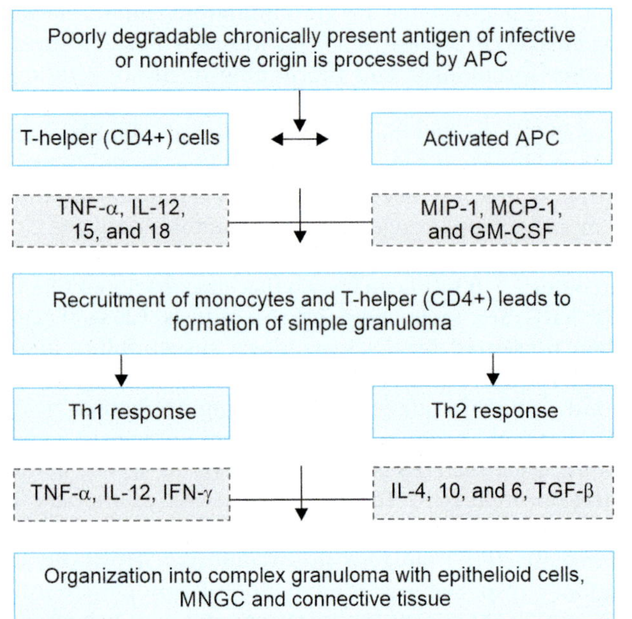

FLOWCHART 1: Hypothesis of development of granulomatous inflammation in sarcoidosis.

(APC: antigen-processing cell; GM-CSF: granulocyte-macrophage colony-stimulating factor; IFN-γ: interferon-γ; MCP-1: monocyte chemotactic protein-1; MIP-1: macrophage inflammatory protein 1; MNGC: multinucleated giant cell; TGF-β: transforming growth factor-β; TNF-α: tumor necrosis factor-α)

What controls the course of granulomas?

The granulomatous inflammation in sarcoidosis is characterized by an altered balance of Th1/Th2 responses with a dominant expression of Th1 cytokines [interferon γ (IFN-γ) and interleukin 2 (IL-2)] with low levels of expression of Th2 cytokines (IL-4 and IL-5).[63,64] First, CD4+ helper T cells accumulate and release IL-2 in the alveoli and interstitium.[63,65,66] A progressive and selective oligoclonal expansion of αβ T cells follows.[67-69] The alveolar macrophages secrete several cytokines [IL-1, IL-6, IL-8, IL-15, tumor necrosis factor α (TNF-α), IFN-γ, granulocyte-macrophage colony-stimulating factor (GM-CSF)] and chemokines [RANTES (regulated on activation, normal T cell expressed and secreted), macrophage inflammatory protein (MIP-1α), IL-16], most of which favor granuloma formation and lung damage.[70-73] IL-12 contributes to proliferation of activated T cells in early disease. Elevated levels of IL-6 and IL-8 have been reported in the BAL fluid of active sarcoidosis, and these may modify the disease process. IL-15 may aid in the proliferation of T and B cells.[74] IL-12 and IL-18 are also increased in the lungs of sarcoidosis and stimulate IFN-γ production.[63,75] The chemoattractant cytokines like IL-8, IL-15, IL-16, and RANTES recruit CD4+ T cells from peripheral blood to the site of inflammation, while IL-2 induces in situ T-cell proliferation.[76,77]

The progression and maintenance of granulomatous reaction are also helped by accumulation of monocyte macrophages that have an antigen-presenting capacity and express increased levels of activation markers (HLA-DR, HLA-DQ, CD71) and adhesion molecules (CD49a, CD54, CD102). The mechanism(s) that result in spontaneous resolution or progression to chronic disease and fibrosis are unclear but may be linked to host susceptibility and genetic factors. TGF-β is an inhibitor of IL-12 and IFN-γ production. Its production is increased in those patients who recover, suggesting a key role for TGF-β in the downregulation of granulomatous inflammation of sarcoidosis.[78] Oxidative stress may also have a role to play in the pathogenesis of sarcoidosis.[79]

Sarcoidosis is thus a delayed-type hypersensitivity response to an unknown antigen. It is unlike the classic autoimmune diseases that are characterized by an inflammatory response to an autoantigen and are usually associated with circulating autoantibodies. However, several clinical and immunological observations, such as the association of sarcoidosis to autoimmune diseases or the presence of autoantibodies in the serum of patients with sarcoidosis, suggest that humoral-mediated immune response might also play a role in the pathogenesis of sarcoidosis.[80] Therefore, the role of autoimmune or autoinflammatory phenomenon has recently been emphasized.[80-83] Further research is needed in this area.

Another clinically important phenomenon in sarcoidosis is the depression of delayed-type hypersensitivity in the skin. Commonly utilized as a diagnostic tool, this is often impaired in active sarcoidosis and not seen when sarcoidosis resolves. A subgroup of CD4+ T cells may account for this cutaneous anergy by abolishing IL-2 production and inhibiting T-cell proliferation.[84,85] It is also suggested that the anergic state may be related to diminished dendritic cell function.[86]

PATHOLOGY

In sarcoidosis-affected lungs, the common site of involvement is along the bronchovascular bundles (lymphangitic pattern), which makes transbronchial biopsy a preferred method for obtaining histological diagnosis. Pulmonary vascular involvement also occurs frequently.[87] Sarcoidosis can involve any extrapulmonary organ, but especially the lymph nodes, skin, eye, liver, spleen, joints, and heart. The histological features are similar across the body tissues affected.[88-90]

The hallmark of sarcoidosis is the presence of non-necrotic, compact, 'naked' granulomas. On histology, a sarcoid granuloma is comprised of lymphocytes, macrophages, well-differentiated epithelioid cells, multinucleated giant cells, fibroblasts, and mast cells. Sarcoid granulomas have CD4+ T cells in the center and CD8+ T cells and B lymphocytes in the periphery.[89,91-93] Histologic findings differ based on disease stage. Initially, the sarcoid granuloma is a compact structure consisting of radially arranged pale, pink epithelioid cells seen most often in the center. Lymphocytes and fibroblasts form a peripheral rim but a prominent lymphocyte cuffing of the granuloma periphery is absent (the so called 'naked' granulomas). Multinucleated Langhans' type giant cells, usually only a few, are often seen in the granuloma. Usually, there is no necrosis. Occasionally, focal coagulative or fibrinoid necrosis is seen.[92,94,95] The so-called caseous necrosis that manifests as soft and pale-to-pink (on hematoxylin and eosin stain), proteinaceous mass with debris and lysed cells is typically observed in TB and other infections and is not seen with sarcoidosis. Nonspecific cytoplasmic inclusions can be seen in sarcoidosis, such as asteroid bodies, Schaumann's bodies, Hamazaki-Wesenberg bodies, and calcium oxalate crystals. Granulomatous inflammation may resolve completely with or without therapy. If it persists, granulomas get hyalinized. Fibrosis and scarring occur in chronic sarcoidosis, especially with long-standing and untreated disease.[92,94]

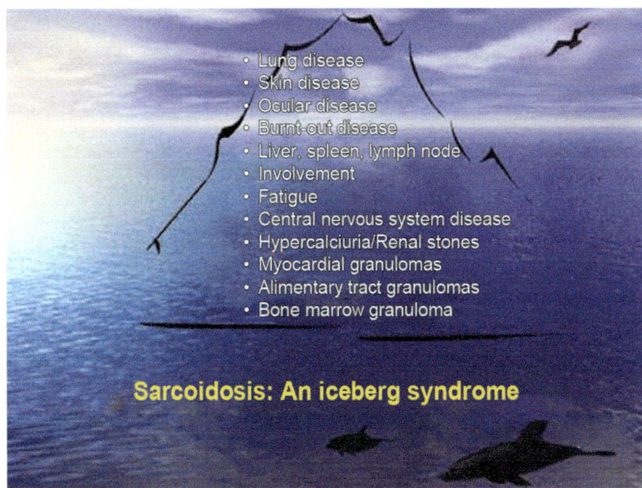

FIG. 1: Sarcoidosis is an "iceberg syndrome". The pathological involvement of various organs may not be clinically apparent.

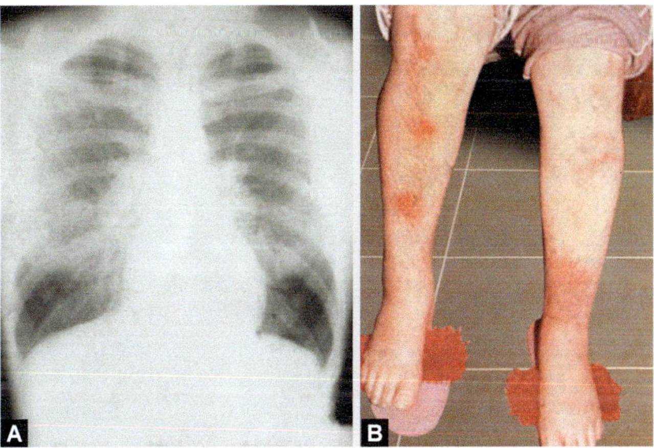

FIGS. 2A AND B: Löfgren syndrome: Bilateral hilar adenopathy with erythema nodosum.

CLINICAL FEATURES

Sarcoidosis is a multisystem disorder. The lungs and lymph nodes are the most common sites affected by granulomatous inflammation. When intrathoracic (mediastinal and hilar) lymph nodes are involved with or without the lungs, the disease gets categorized as pulmonary sarcoidosis. Involvement of other organs represents extrapulmonary sarcoidosis. The eyes, skin, and joints are the commonly affected extrapulmonary sites **(Table 2)**. The liver, kidneys, peripheral nervous system, heart, and central nervous system (CNS) are affected in a minority. The symptoms of sarcoidosis depend on the extent and severity of organ involvement. About 20–50% of sarcoidosis patients may be asymptomatic. They might be identified incidentally by way of lymph node enlargement observed on chest imaging performed for screening or other indications. Pathological involvement of organs may remain clinically silent, making sarcoidosis an iceberg syndrome **(Fig. 1)**.

Pulmonary Involvement

Clinical

Pulmonary sarcoidosis commonly presents in a TB-like or an ILD-like manner, or as part of well-defined constellations of symptoms such as the Löfgren syndrome. A TB-like presentation includes subacute onset of fever, fatigue, weight loss, and cough. It usually manifests with enlarged lymph nodes with or without lung abnormalities. Alternatively, an insidious presentation with cough and dyspnea resembles ILDs. Radiologically, it shows lung abnormalities with or without lymph node enlargement. Löfgren syndrome is a triad of fever, erythema nodosum (EN), and bilateral hilar lymphadenopathy in the chest **(Figs. 2A and B)**. Arthritis, especially involving the ankles, completes the tetrad of Löfgren.

TABLE 2: Organ involvement in sarcoidosis.

Organ involved	Proportion of patients
Lungs and lymph nodes	90%
Eyes, skin, joints	10–30% each
Liver, kidney, heart, salivary glands, nervous system	5–10% each
Hypercalcemia/hypercalciuria	5–10%
Bone marrow	<5%

Chest pain is a common complaint in sarcoidosis and may be multifactorial. It is mostly unrelated to exertion and may be pleuritic. Pleural inflammation, pneumothorax, and pulmonary embolism need to be excluded before considering the chest pain nonspecific. Wheezing as a complaint is rare and might be due to bronchial involvement; comorbid asthma should also be considered as a diagnostic possibility in patients with prominent and especially episodic wheezing. Sarcoidosis is not associated with hemoptysis, unless it is complicated by infection of damaged lung parenchyma (bronchiectasis, fibrocystic/fibrocavitary abnormalities) with bacteria or fungi. Hemoptysis should also alert the physician toward the possibility of pulmonary TB, a close differential of sarcoidosis.

Radiologic Findings

Over 90% of patients with sarcoidosis may have an abnormal chest radiograph. Over half of the patients demonstrate bilateral hilar enlargement. Symmetric bihilar and mediastinal lymphadenopathy is characteristic of sarcoidosis. Generally, the lymph nodes are big with distinct, smooth margins, with a clear line of translucency between the mediastinal shadow and the nodes historically referred to as "potato nodes". Unilateral hilar adenopathy is rare, and alternate diagnoses such as TB in endemic regions must be considered. Lung infiltrates may be encountered in about a quarter to half of the patients. Typically, the infiltrates are bilateral and symmetric and are most common in the upper and mid lung fields.[96,97] A simple chest radiographic staging system suggested decades ago by Scadding is still commonly used **(Table 3 and Figs. 3A to D)**.[98]

Overall, higher radiographic stages have been associated with poorer outcomes. [99,100] Hilar adenopathy alone com-

TABLE 3: Chest radiographic staging of sarcoidosis.

Stage	Features
0	No features of sarcoidosis on chest radiograph
1	Bilateral hilar adenopathy, often with right paratracheal adenopathy
2	Hilar and mediastinal adenopathy with lung infiltrates
3	Lung infiltrates without adenopathy as described in stage 1
4	Advanced parenchymal lung disease, including fibrosis, honeycomb lung, traction bronchiectasis, cysts, bullae, and emphysema, with or without adenopathy

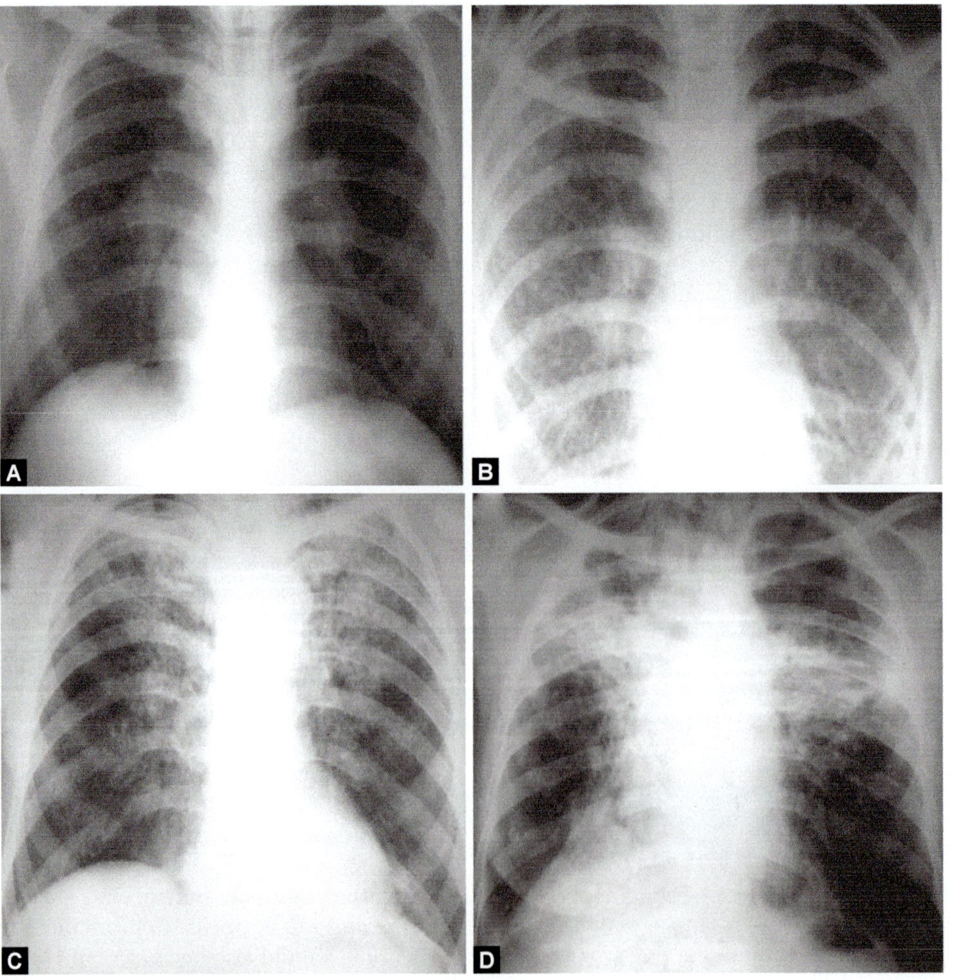

FIGS. 3A TO D: Typical chest radiographs in sarcoidosis. (A) Stage I, showing bilateral hilar and paratracheal lymphadenopathy; (B) Stage II, hilar and paratracheal lymphadenopathy with pulmonary infiltrates; (C) Stage III, pulmonary infiltrates with no lymphadenopathy; (D) Stage IV, pulmonary fibrosis with architectural distortion.

monly regresses spontaneously, while stage IV or fibrotic sarcoidosis leads to permanent sequelae and is prone to complications such as progressive pulmonary fibrosis (PPF), pulmonary hypertension (PH), aspergilloma, or chronic pulmonary aspergillosis (CPA). The stages are not useful for predicting an individual patient's prognosis as several other factors such as the extent of involvement, lung function, and treatment might also affect outcomes.[101]

Chest computed tomography (CT) offers better disease evaluation than a chest radiograph. Mostly, a thin-section (≤1.5 mm) CT along with a contrast-enhanced CT should be ordered. The previous noncontiguous high-resolution CT (HRCT) technique has been replaced by volumetric scanning with thin-section reconstruction in most good centers. For sarcoidosis, the volumetric technique is preferred, but the older technique of HRCT is still acceptable. As chest CT is more sensitive than radiography, the combination of lymph node and lung involvement observed on CT may not mirror chest radiography and thus may not correspond to the respective Scadding stages.

Chest CT reveals various patterns in sarcoidosis. There may be intrathoracic adenopathy that is mostly symmetric, multistation, bulky, and devoid of hypodense areas that suggest necrosis **(Figs. 4A to D)**. The system used to classify lymph node stations for lung cancer is often used to refer to the respective lymph nodes in sarcoidosis too.[96,102] Upper-mid predominant peribronchovascular septal thickening with a perilymphatic distribution of nodules (peribronchovascular, perifissural, and subpleural nodules) is the typical lung finding.[102,103] Predominant centrilobular nodules are uncommon in sarcoidosis and should invoke a suspicion of TB. Coalescing nodules may result in consolidation or mass-like lesions with or without air bronchograms. Patchy areas of consolidation are especially common in the lower lobes. When these conglomerate nodules are surrounded by small nodules, it appears like a galaxy of stars and therefore it is called the "sarcoid galaxy sign" **(Figs. 4A to D)**.[104] Cavitation, in general, must alert the physician toward the possibility of an alternate diagnosis such as an infection (TB, mycosis) or others. Rarely, primary areas of granulomatous inflammation undergo breakdown resulting in primary cavitary sarcoidosis, in the absence of any fibrosis or infection.[105] Fibrotic disease typically has an upper lobe predominance with lung volume loss, architectural distortion, reticulation, traction bronchiectasis, and airway-centered fibrosis. Fibrocystic change may result

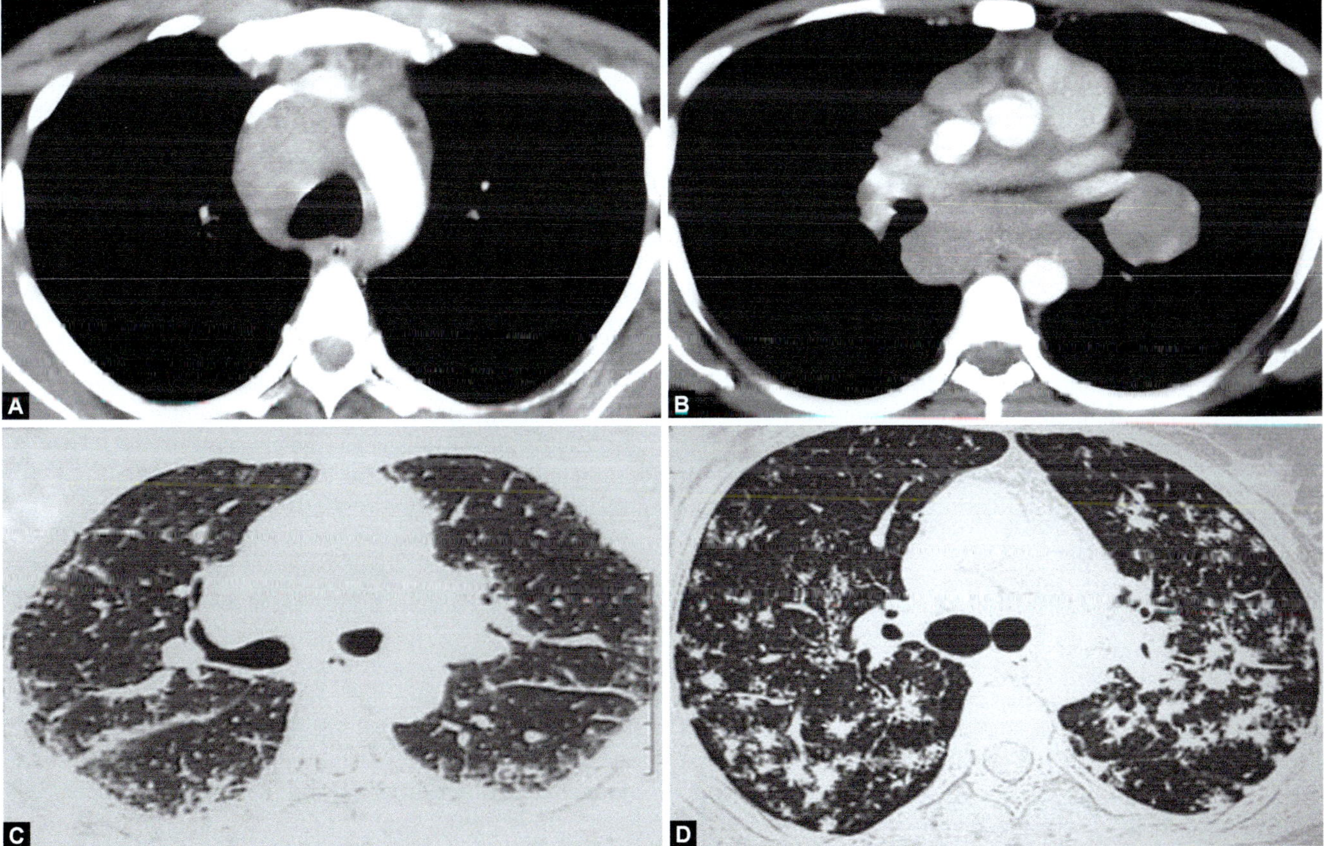

FIGS. 4A TO D: Some representative CT pictures in sarcoidosis. (A) Paratracheal lymphadenopathy. (B) Hilar/interlobar and subcarinal lymphadenopathy. Lymph nodes are typically homogenous with no central necrosis. (C) Pulmonary nodular infiltrates with typical lymphangitic distribution. (D) "Sarcoid galaxy" sign: Large conglomerate nodules surrounded by small nodules.

BOX 1	Major radiologic phenotypes of sarcoidosis on chest computed tomography.

- Multiple peribronchovascular, perifissural, or subpleural micronodules
- Multiple larger peribronchovascular nodules
- Scattered larger nodules
- Consolidation as the predominant or sole abnormality
- Bronchocentric reticulation with or without dense parenchymal opacification, without cavitation
- Bronchocentric reticulation and dense parenchymal opacification, with cavitation
- Large bronchocentric masses (i.e., PMF lookalike)

(PMF: progressive massive fibrosis)

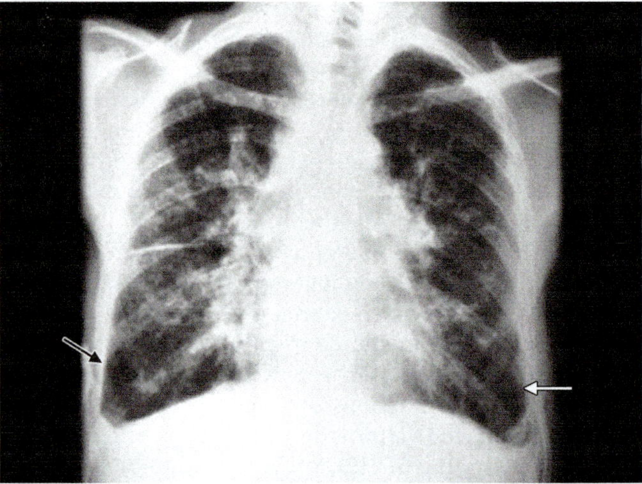

FIG. 5: Bilateral pleural thickening in sarcoidosis.

in cavity-like areas that may get colonized by fungi causing fungal balls.

Upper lobe predominant peribronchovascular septal thickening and lower lobe predominant consolidation are often encountered as distinct, mutually exclusive phenotypes. The "reverse halo" or "atoll" sign has also been described with sarcoidosis apart from the more common differentials such as organizing pneumonia and mucormycosis.[106] Ground-glass opacities may be present occasionally and generally represent granulomatous inflammation or sarcoidosis-unrelated causes such as infection or pulmonary edema.[107] Mosaic attenuation/perfusion suggests small airway disease or PH. Few areas of interlobular septal thickening, especially in the lower lobes, are not uncommon in sarcoidosis. Recently, a Delphi consensus statement of international experts have suggested seven distinct radiological phenotypes of pulmonary sarcoidosis on the chest CT **(Box 1)**.[108] Some of these phenotypes are associated with particular physiological defects or prognosis. For example, a predominant reticular pattern is associated with restrictive physiology, while a bronchocentric pattern of fibrosis is associated with an obstructive defect on spirometry. Lobar volume loss may be a marker of poor outcomes. Bronchocentric reticulation with or without dense parenchymal opacification may predict a poor response to treatment.

Functional Abnormalities

Pulmonary function abnormalities can be seen in more than half of the patients with sarcoidosis.[109] Spirometry is a simple and repeatable test that can be used to assess disease severity at baseline. About 40–50% of patients have normal spirometry.[110] A restrictive ventilatory defect is the most commonly encountered abnormality. Airflow obstruction may be seen in about 10–20% of individuals. It might occur due to endobronchial granulomatous inflammation, due to large hilar nodes leading to the distortion and narrowing of larger bronchi, or due to the architectural distortion caused by lung fibrosis.[111,112] Lung function deficits correlate with the radiologic and histologic disease burden.[113-115] Diffusion capacity of the lungs for carbon monoxide (DLCO) should also be assessed in all patients, at least at the baseline. Lung volume assessment may be required to identify a mixed obstructive and restrictive defect in specific situations. Exercise capacity assessment is a desirable parameter to be assessed in patients. A complete cardiopulmonary exercise testing is usually not required. A 6-minute walk test is mostly sufficient to assess the exercise capacity and exertional desaturation.

Presence of breathlessness in the wake of normal spirometry or symptom severity disproportionate to the extent of lung function abnormalities must trigger evaluation for myocardial sarcoidosis and PH. PH in sarcoidosis may occur due to primary granulomatous involvement of the pulmonary vessels or secondary to advanced lung disease.[116] PH and its severity are an important prognostic markers.[116,117]

Pleural effusion is observed in about 5% of patients.[118,119] These effusions are mostly small, more often right-sided, and have relatively few cells (mostly lymphocytes). They are characteristically exudative by the Light's protein criterion and transudative by the LDH criteria.[118] Chylothorax, hemothorax, and pneumothorax occur rarely.[120-122] Pleural thickening of unclear significance on chest CT may be seen in up to one-third of the patients **(Fig. 5)**.[123]

Complications

Hemoptysis, at times serious, can occur due to various reasons such as fungal ball formation in a preexisting cyst or cavity, bronchiectasis (most often due to traction caused by parenchymal fibrosis), and necrotizing sarcoid angiitis.[124,125] Rare consequences of mediastinal lymphadenopathy include the superior vena cava syndrome,[126] mediastinal lymph node calcification, and mediastinal fibrosis.[127] Rarely, giant bullae resulting from sarcoidosis may result in the "vanishing lung syndrome."[128,129]

Extrapulmonary Involvement

Apart from lungs and thoracic lymph nodes, the skin, eye, joints, liver, spleen, kidney, heart, and nervous system may be involved. Also, both pulmonary and extrapulmonary organ involvement can be associated with fever, night sweats, weight loss, fatigue, myalgia, and arthralgia.[130]

Skin

Skin is affected in 25–30% of patients with systemic sarcoidosis, making it the second most involved organ. The specific findings of cutaneous sarcoidosis include lesions with granulomas on histological examination. Other skin abnormalities are devoid of granulomas and are considered nonspecific.[131] Papules and papulonodules are the most common specific cutaneous manifestations and are typically present on the face, but also on the trunk and extremities. They are numerous, small (<1 cm), firm, nonscaly, flesh-colored, brown, or hypopigmented. Plaques are oval or annular, well demarcated, firm, sometimes scaly brown lesions mostly present on the trunk, buttocks, shoulders, and arms. Lupus pernio is a characteristic lesion seen in sarcoidosis. It appears as smooth, shiny plaques on the central face, specifically the nose, cheeks, lips, forehead, and ears. The plaques may get scaly and can disfigure the face as they erode the underlying cartilage and bone. Lupus pernio is often associated with a chronic and refractory course and often requires aggressive systemic therapy. Skin sarcoidosis may also manifest as firm, mobile, round to oval, erythematous, flesh-colored, violaceous, or hyperpigmented nodules, especially on the extremities and the trunk. Uncommonly, granulomatous lesions may appear as ichthyosiform, atrophic, or ulcerative lesions. The mucosa, nails, or hair (scarring or nonscarring alopecia) may be affected; rarely erythroderma may occur. EN is the most common nonspecific skin lesion of sarcoidosis. It presents with tender nodules on the extremities.

Eye

About 10–30% of patients with sarcoidosis develop eye abnormalities; in some series, the proportion is as high as 60%.[132] The eye may be an isolated affected site or might be a part of multiorgan involvement. Sarcoidosis can affect any part of the eye and its adnexa.[132] Uveitis is the most common finding. Lacrimal gland enlargement and conjunctivitis are also frequent. Uveitis is bilateral in 75–90% cases. Anterior uveitis is the most frequent followed by posterior, intermediate, and panuveitis. Other possibilities with similar ocular involvement include TB, syphilis, viral infections, multiple sclerosis, birdshot retinochoroidopathy, Vogt–Koyanagi–Harada syndrome, and others. Subtle and specific differences in ocular findings and the systemic features of these diseases can help differentiate between disorders. Some of the common findings of ocular sarcoidosis include "mutton-fat" keratic precipitates, iris (Koeppe's) nodules, trabecular meshwork nodules, peripheral anterior synechia, "string of pearls" vitreous opacities, chorioretinal peripheral lesions, "candle-wax drippings" on the retina, optic disc nodules, and optic neuritis.[132] Heerfordt syndrome refers to a triad of uveitis, parotitis, and fever (uveoparotid fever), sometimes accompanied by facial nerve palsy.

Cardiac

Heart involvement occurs in 5–10% of patients; in some series, up to 40% of patients were affected.[133] Manifestations can range from asymptomatic disease (detected only at autopsy) to life-threatening conditions with left ventricular (LV) systolic failure, ventricular arrhythmias, or atrioventricular conduction abnormalities. Electrocardiography and echocardiography are useful in identifying heart blocks, arrhythmias, ventricular wall motion abnormalities, regional wall thickening, valvular dysfunction, LV ejection fraction (LVEF), and increased ventricular wall thickness.[134] Cardiac magnetic resonance is the modality of choice for diagnosing cardiac sarcoidosis, as it has high sensitivity and specificity in the right setting. It helps visualize inflamed and scarred myocardium, which typically occurs in a patchy distribution. Delayed or late gadolinium enhancement characteristically appears in the basal interventricular septum. Radionuclide scanning using technetium-99m (Tc-99m) agents or gallium-67 (Ga-67) citrate can detect active mycocardial inflammation. 18F-fluorodeoxyglucose (FDG) positron emission tomography (PET), especially combined with CT, detects active inflammation but may miss 1 in 10 cases, while may be falsely positive in a quarter of the cases.

Neurosarcoidosis

The CNS is affected in up to 10% of patients.[135] Neurosarcoidosis can mimic diverse neurological conditions. Diagnosis is based on confirmation of sarcoidosis from other organs or organ systems since pathologic confirmation is rarely possible from the CNS. CNS infection and malignancy should be reasonably excluded.[136] Sarcoidosis may affect any part of the nervous system causing a cranial nerve palsy, mononeuropathy or polyneuropathy, aseptic meningitis, seizures, mass lesions in the brain or spinal cord, and encephalopathy.[137,138] Rarely, it may also mimic multiple sclerosis.[139] Seventh cranial nerve palsy is the most common manifestation of neurosarcoidosis and may antedate other disease manifestations by months. Small fiber neuropathy is a nongranulomatous manifestation of systemic disease that presents with nonlength-dependent pain and paresthesia. It can occur in up to 40% of patients.

Abnormalities of Calcium Metabolism

Hypercalcemia has been reported to occur in about 15% (range, 2–63%) of patients; hypercalciuria occurs in about 40%.[140] Serum and urine calcium levels should be measured at diagnosis and periodically during follow-up, especially if immunosuppression is not administered. Hypercalcemia in sarcoidosis is due to excess extrarenal calcitriol production.[141] Alveolar macrophages present within granulomas contain the enzyme 1-α hydroxylase which converts precursor vitamin D to active calcitriol.[142] Normally, high levels of calcitriol cause feedback inhibition of 1α-hydroxylase; calcitriol also causes upregulation of the 24-hydroxylase, the enzyme which converts 25-hydroxyvitamin D to 24, 25-hydroxyvitamin D, the metabolically inactive form of vitamin D. Both the feedback mechanisms are lost in alveolar macrophages which lead to continuous production of calcitriol.[143] An excess production of parathyroid-hormone-related peptide (PTHrp), which like parathyroid hormone causes upregulation of 1α hydroxylase, might also be responsible.[144] But, unlike the parathyroid hormone, PTHrp is not regulated by calcium but by IL-2 and TNF-α, both of which are increased in sarcoidosis.[145] It is possible that these cytokines released by the alveolar macrophages act in a paracrine fashion to upregulate PTHrp production by macrophages.[143] Hypercalciuria or hypercalcemia can lead to nephrolithiasis and renal failure. Rarely, hypercalcemia may cause acute pancreatitis.[146]

Other Extrapulmonary Organ Involvement

Sarcoidosis causes clinically apparent peripheral lymphadenopathy in more than 10% of patients.[147] Sarcoidosis may also affect the upper airways, and the gastrointestinal, hematological, musculoskeletal, endocrine, and genitourinary systems.[148] In the upper respiratory tract, sarcoidosis may involve the nasopharynx, hypopharynx, larynx, or sinuses. Rarely, vocal cord palsy may occur.[149,150] Histological involvement of the liver may be seen in 50–65% patients. Liver function abnormalities are seen in less than 35%, the most common being an elevated serum alkaline phosphatase or gamma-glutamyl transferase **(Figs. 6A and B)**.[151-155] Similarly, spleen may also be involved with minimal or no symptoms. Significant splenomegaly with hypersplenism is seen more commonly in Afro-Americans **(Fig. 7)**.[156-159] Peritoneal involvement occurs rarely in sarcoidosis **(Figs. 8A and B)**.

Bone sarcoidosis occurs in about 4% of patients and manifests as small cysts or cortical defects in the small bones of the hands or feet. It is possibly more frequent in females and in patients with lupus pernio.[160] Joint involvement in Löfgren syndrome carries a good prognosis.[161] Chronic sarcoid arthritis is uncommon and typically affects knees, ankles, wrists, hands, and/or feet.[162,163] Rarely, joint destruction or Jaccoud deformity occurs due to persistent inflammation.

DIAGNOSIS

The diagnosis of sarcoidosis rests on a triad of clinical, radiologic, and histologic criteria. Although sarcoidosis can be diagnosed in up to 80% of patients using clinical data and CT imaging, histological confirmation adds confidence to the diagnosis. Tissue samples also permit microbiological tests to exclude differentials such as TB. The 2020 American Thoracic Society (ATS) guidelines exclude the need for tissue diagnosis in typical presentations such as Löfgren syndrome.[164] But we opine that histologic and microbiologic examinations are crucial in high TB burden areas, as TB is a great masquerader. For example, Poncet's arthritis due to TB can be mistaken for Löfgren syndrome in some cases. The diagnostic possibilities in patients with intrathoracic lymphadenopathy are enumerated in **Box 2**.

Histological Diagnosis

In general, the least invasive method of obtaining a histological diagnosis should be selected.[165] Skin and peripheral lymph nodes, if involved, are the easiest to access. In most other patients, the appropriate method is to sample the mediastinal lymph nodes, the airway mucosa,

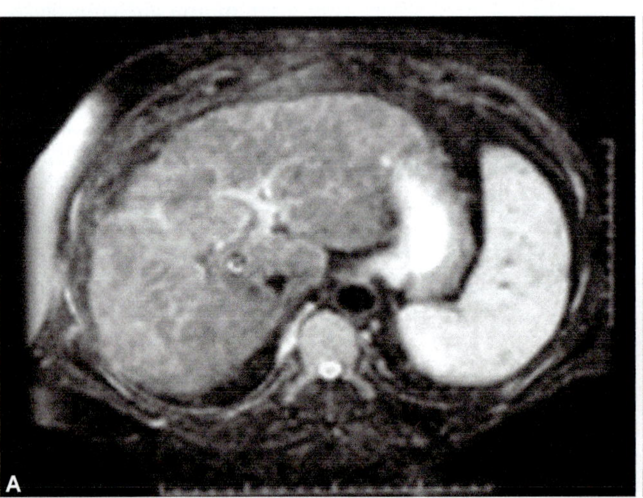

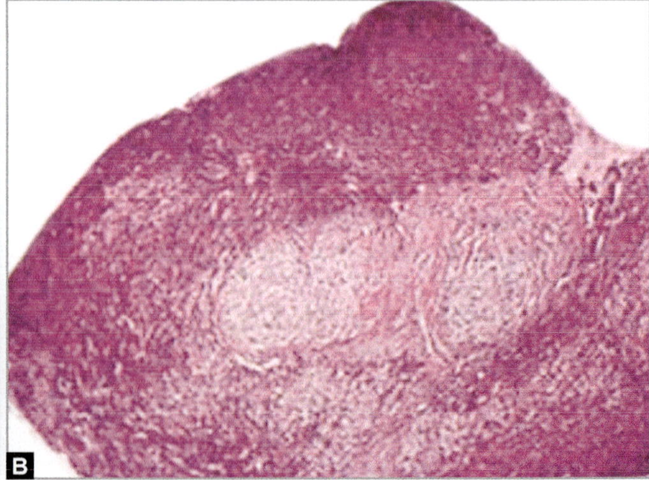

FIGS. 6A AND B: Hepatic sarcoidosis.

and/or the lung parenchyma. Transbronchial lung biopsy (TBLB) using the standard bronchoscopic forceps during flexible bronchoscopy has traditionally been the most used procedure for diagnosing pulmonary sarcoidosis.[166-168] Its yield varies from 40 to 80% depending on operator experience, patient population, forceps types, and other factors.[169-174] Granulomatous inflammation may be encountered in lung biopsies from radiologically normal lungs. Combining endobronchial biopsy (EBB) with TBLB improves the diagnostic yield by about 10%.[171,175] Endobronchial abnormalities are more commonly seen in patients with respiratory symptoms.[175] Narrow-band imaging may help to better visualize the endobronchial abnormalities in sarcoidosis.[176,177] The transbronchial lung cryobiopsy (TBLC), also known as bronchoscopic lung cryobiopsy (BLC), is a relatively novel technique that yields much larger lung tissue than the standard forceps

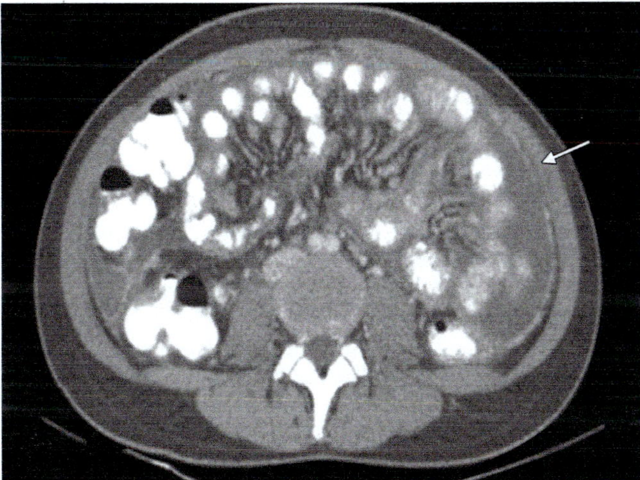

FIG. 7: A patient with sarcoidosis and massive splenomegaly. Enlarged spleen and hypersplenism are common in African-American patients.

BOX 2 Common pathological differential diagnosis of sarcoidosis.

- *Bacterial*:
  - Mycoplasma
  - Brucella
- *Mycobacterial*:*
  - TB
  - Atypical mycobacteria
- *Fungal infections*:*
  - Cryptococcosis
  - Aspergillosis
  - Histoplasmosis
  - Coccidioidomycosis
  - Blastomycosis
  - Pneumocystis
- Hypersensitivity pneumonias
- Drug reactions*
- *Pneumoconiosis*:
  - Beryllium (chronic beryllium disease)*
  - Titanium
  - Aluminum
- *Malignancy*:
  - Lymphoma*
  - Lung cancer
  - Metastatic malignancy
- *Others*:
  - Wegener's granulomatosis (sarcoid-type granulomas are rare)
  - Chronic interstitial pneumonia (UIP, LIP)
  - Necrotizing sarcoid granulomatosis (NSG)
  - Granulomatous lesions of unknown significance (GLUS syndrome)

Note: Conditions marked with (*) can also present with hilar and mediastinal lymphadenopathy.

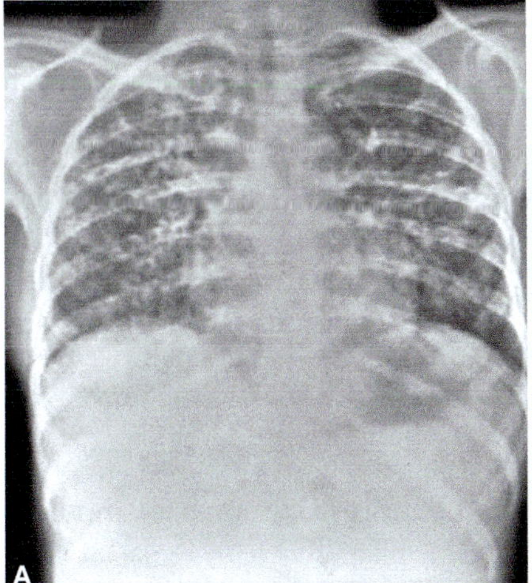

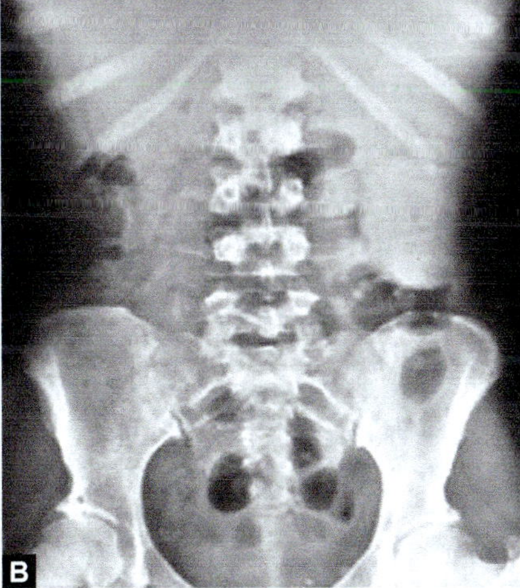

FIGS. 8A AND B: Peritoneal sarcoidosis is rare and it resembles tuberculous peritonitis.

TBLB.[178-182] It has become a preferred method to perform lung biopsy in ILDs.[183] It has a high sensitivity (>90%) in sarcoidosis but is not routinely required.[184]

In stage I and II disease, in which mediastinal lymph nodes are involved, transbronchial needle aspiration (TBNA) during flexible bronchoscopy is useful.[185-187] TBNA performed without ultrasound image guidance, often called "blind" or conventional TBNA, has an average yield of around 60% (varies from 6 to 90% in different studies).[188] Adding TBLB to TBNA increases the yield by 20%.[188] Currently, endobronchial ultrasound (EBUS) is the preferred bronchoscopic modality to perform TBNA. EBUS-guided TBNA (EBUS-TBNA) has a yield ranging from 50 to 90% averaging at around 80% in diagnosing sarcoidosis. A recent large trial reported a significantly higher yield of EBUS-TBNA as compared to a combination of EBB and TBLB.[189] However, a later study has reaffirmed the utility of conventional bronchoscopic techniques (TBNA plus TBLB plus EBB) by demonstrating their equivalence to a combination of EBUS-TBNA and TBLB.[172,190] Certain technical aspects of the procedure may influence the yield of EBUS-TBNA as well.[191-194]

Tuberculin Skin Test

Skin sensitivity to the mycobacterial purified protein derivative is depressed in sarcoidosis even in the background of high prevalence of TB. Thus, almost 90% of sarcoidosis patients do not react to a 5 tuberculin units skin test. A positive (induration ≥ 10 mm) tuberculin skin test (TST) should make the clinician strive to identify any other diagnostic clues to active TB. The IGRA may be positive and represent latent TB infection (LTBI) even in active sarcoidosis. It is thus not useful in differentiating active TB from sarcoidosis.[195]

Miscellaneous Investigations

Serum Angiotensin-converting Enzyme

Angiotensin-converting enzyme is produced by the epithelioid cells of sarcoid granulomas. [196] A rise in serum angiotensin converting enzyme (SACE) activity in active sarcoidosis has been found in a few reports from this country as well.[197,198] However, the test is neither sensitive nor specific to be useful as a diagnostic tool.[199,200] It may be normal in patients with sarcoidosis. Other disorders such as diabetes mellitus, cirrhosis, acute hepatitis, chronic renal disease, silicosis, Gaucher's disease, leprosy, asbestosis, and berylliosis may demonstrate elevated SACE levels. Overall, the sensitivity and specificity of elevated SACE levels are 55% and 90%, respectively.[201] Also, there is no apparent association between SACE level and radiographic staging.[199] Despite the low specificity, SACE can be an ancillary test to monitor disease activity. The presence of inhibitors may interfere with SACE assessment unless sensitive radioimmunoassay techniques are used.[202] Some studies have suggested that SACE levels may vary with genetic factors, and the use of genotype-corrected SACE levels may make it a more useful diagnostic tool.[203-205]

Soluble Interleukin 2 Receptor

Soluble IL-2 receptor (sIL-2R) is a cytokine released in blood by activated T lymphocytes.[206] High levels of sIL-2R suggest a diagnosis of sarcoidosis, although a broad overlap exists with HP and IPF. Serum levels might also serve as a prognostic biomarker for chronicity. A recent meta-analysis reported 85% sensitivity and 88% specificity for this test in diagnosing sarcoidosis.[207]

Bronchoalveolar Lavage

Bronchoalveolar lavage has a high positive predictive value for the diagnosis of sarcoidosis with an elevated ratio of CD4/CD8 in BAL fluid. However, the samples require >15% lymphocytes on cell count to be useful.[208] A CD4:CD8 ratio >3.5 shows a high specificity of over 90% for sarcoidosis, but the sensitivity is low (50–60%).[189,209] Considering the poor availability, it is not a cost-effective modality today in India.

Kveim Test

The Kveim–Siltzbach test is a historical test for diagnosing sarcoidosis. It used to be performed by intradermal injections of human sarcoid tissue. Four weeks later, the papule that forms at the site of the injection was biopsied. The mechanism of the Kveim test vis à vis sarcoidosis is still not clearly understood.[210-212] Limitations include unavailability of a validated good-quality antigen, duration of disease affecting test results, and the long period required to obtain the test results.[213]

Gallium Scanning

Gallium scanning demonstrates inflammation throughout the body and is associated with specific findings in sarcoidosis. Uptake in the hilar lymph nodes and right paratracheal nodes results in the "lambda sign," whereas lacrimal and salivary gland uptake results in the "panda sign."[214] Its use has largely fallen out of favor due to the advances in bronchoscopic techniques and availability of a better radionuclide study, PET.

Positron Emission Tomography Scanning

18-FDG PET may be used as an adjunct to routine investigations to identify occult sites for biopsy, to assess disease activity especially in extrapulmonary sites, and to monitor treatment response.[215,216] It is especially useful in cardiac sarcoidosis, where it can help in identifying a potentially life-threatening disease in an asymptomatic patient.[217] However, it is not useful for differentiating sarcoidosis from other inflammatory diseases, especially TB.[218] F-methyltyrosine-PET (FMT-PET) uses an amino acid that is preferentially taken up and expressed on the surface of tumor cells and is negative in patients with sarcoidosis.[219]

Assessment of Activity

Assessing disease activity and severity is critical and sometimes challenging as no single variable in isolation is accurate.[220] 18-FDG PET imaging, serum biomarkers [e.g., SACE, soluble IL-2-receptor, lysozyme, neopterin, soluble intracellular adhesion molecule (ICAM)-1, IFN-γ] or BAL fluid molecules (e.g., high lymphocytes, activation marker expression on T-cells, CD4/C8 ratio, macrophage TNF-α release, collagenase, procollagen-III-peptide, vitronectin, fibronectin, hyaluronan) have been studied for this purpose.[221-223] sIL-2R and SACE have some clinical utility, while PET is emerging as a useful tool.[224,225] The magnitude of the initial SACE levels has no prognostic significance. However, an initially elevated SACE level will usually come down within a few weeks of starting glucocorticoid (GC) treatment and thus help gauge the disease activity. Studies suggest that 18-FDG PET might help in assessing the total burden of disease activity in systemic sarcoidosis and can prove particularly useful in cardiac and fibrotic pulmonary sarcoidosis.[225] Yet, as of now, the best way to assess the activity of sarcoidosis is through multidimensional assessment of symptoms, organ function, and imaging.[114]

Sarcoidosis–tuberculosis Enigma

The relationship between sarcoidosis and TB remains a riddle. The remarkable similarity of sarcoidosis to TB in both the clinical and the histological features has perplexed investigators for decades, and a possible link between the two conditions has been debated.[226-230] The possible relationship has implications on pathogenesis, diagnosis, and treatment.[231] Certain features can help in distinguishing between the two. In a study, we found that compared to TB, patients with sarcoidosis were older, had a higher body mass index, resided in urban areas, were better educated, had higher per capita income, and had a higher socioeconomic status.[232] All these differences were also significant when sarcoidosis patients were compared to healthy controls albeit to a lesser degree. Tobacco smoking, environmental tobacco smoke exposure, and biomass fuel use were more commonly seen in TB patients.

Both TB and sarcoidosis can present with similar constitutional symptoms (fever, easy fatigability, anorexia, and weight loss) and respiratory symptoms (cough and breathlessness), although expectoration and hemoptysis are distinctly more frequent in fibrocavitary TB. In general, patients with untreated TB have more signs and symptoms compared to sarcoidosis. But the severity and magnitude may not always help in the differential diagnosis.

Hilar lymphadenopathy, the most common clinical presentation of sarcoidosis, is also a manifestation of TB.[233] However, the nodes in sarcoidosis only rarely show a central hypodensity on CT scan, which is a frequently observed finding in TB.[102] In sarcoidosis, bilateral hila are involved. Unilateral hilar enlargement or asymmetric distribution and widely variable sizes of lymph nodes favor TB. In such cases, lymphoma is also a diagnostic consideration. The characteristics of mediastinal lymph nodes on EBUS can help in differentiating sarcoidosis from TB.[234] The presence of heterogeneous echotexture or coagulation necrosis sign in lymph nodes on EBUS imaging has good specificity and positive predictive value for the diagnosis of TB.[234,235] Fibrosis, especially in apical regions, can occur in both conditions although cavitation is rarer in sarcoidosis.[236] Similarly, miliary distribution of lesions, characteristically described in TB, can also occur in sarcoidosis **(Figs. 9A to D)**.[237-239] A simple "rule of thumb" is that patients with miliary TB are usually "sick" due to the disseminated infection, while those with miliary sarcoidosis are relatively well preserved.

The tuberculin sensitivity of the skin is depressed in sarcoidosis even in the background of high prevalence of TB and a <10 mm reaction to 5 TU tuberculin test has about 90% sensitivity for sarcoidosis.[195] A negative TST excludes TB except in seriously sick or otherwise immunosuppressed individuals. Diagnosis of TB in TST-negative individuals is required to be supported by strong bacteriological evidence.[240] A positive tuberculin test in sarcoidosis should also be looked with high suspicion as discussed above. In India, TST is positive in about 30–50% of general population and in 64–85% in the 25–45 year age group.[241-243]

Interferon gamma release assays have higher sensitivity and specificity for detecting *M.tb* infection than the conventional TST, as they utilize antigens specific for *M.tb* complex.[244] Clinicians in high prevalence countries erroneously diagnosing active TB based on a positive IGRA test. We have observed that IGRA being a more sensitive test than TST continues to remain positive in many patients with sarcoidosis, and in high prevalence countries it should not be a deterrent for making a diagnosis of sarcoidosis, since it merely represents an underlying TB infection.[245,246]

Although non-necrotizing granulomas are the usual finding in sarcoidosis, necrosis can occur. Prior to the widespread use of transbronchial biopsy, necrosis was reported in up to 30% of large biopsy specimens from the lung and lymph nodes in sarcoidosis. The incidence of necrosis is far lower in smaller specimens such as TBLB because of the small number of granulomas usually sampled. Compared with the "caseous" necrosis seen in TB granulomas, the necrosis in the granulomas of sarcoidosis is most often focal, involving small areas and very few granulomas, and is not discernable on gross examination of the specimen.[247] The foci of necrosis are acidophilic with a fibrinoid, granular appearance and usually located within the centers of granulomas.

Several features such as the site and type of organ involvement may help in distinguishing TB from sarcoidosis. For example, lacrimal glands, parotid glands, and myocardium are rarely involved in TB. Thus, labial biopsy may have a high discriminatory value.[248] Subtle differences which may help in differential diagnosis from TB are summarized in **Table 4**. Rarely, the two diseases

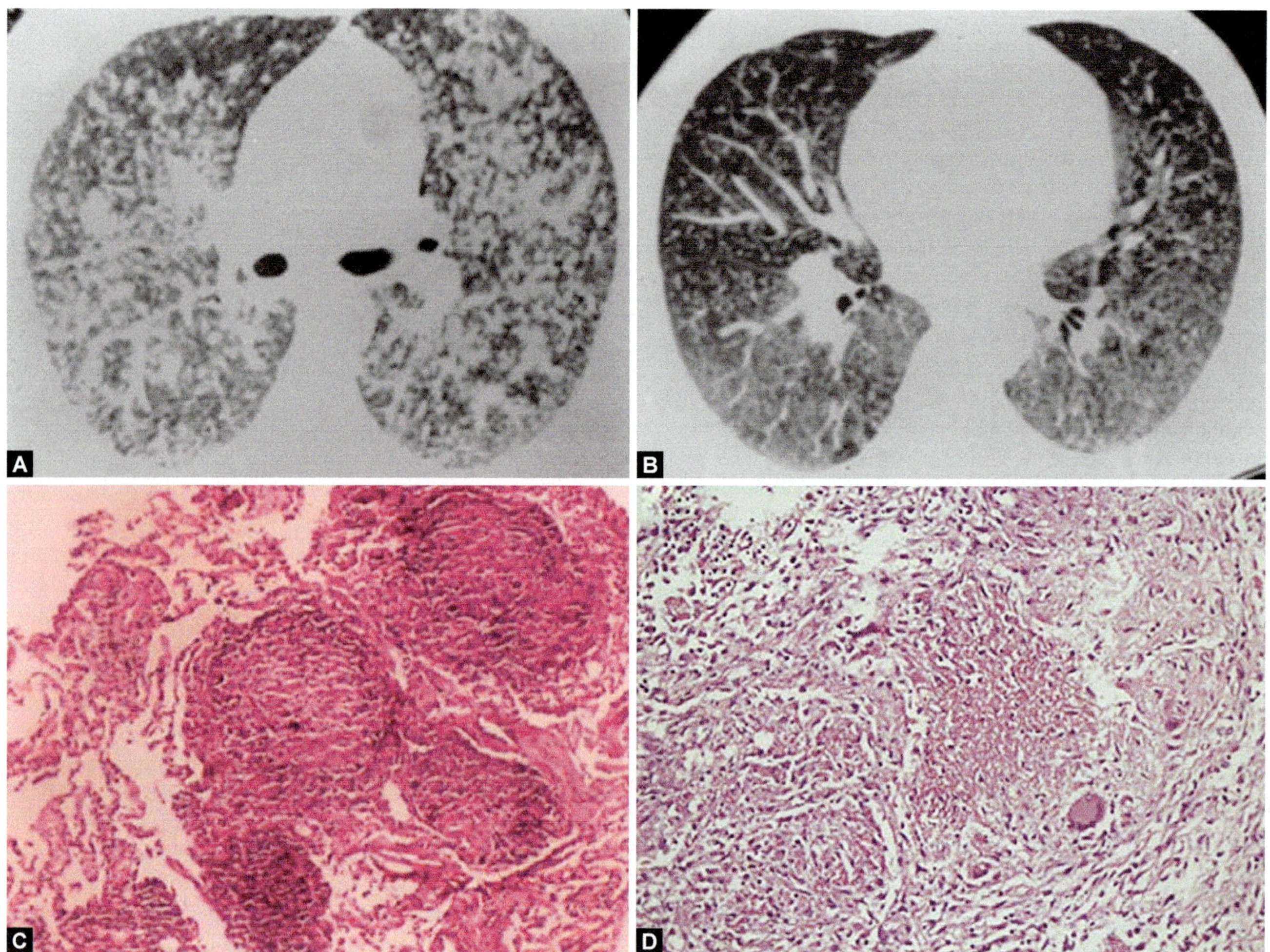

FIGS. 9A TO D: (A and C) Miliary sarcoidosis versus (B and D) miliary TB. On CT, the nodules in sarcoidosis are larger than TB with typical lymphangitic distribution. On histopathology the granulomas in sarcoidosis are typically compact, with no necrosis and minimal lymphocytic cuffing (C) compared to large areas of necrosis and intense lymphomononuclear cell infiltrates in TB (D).

TABLE 4: Useful features to differentiate sarcoidosis from TB.

Indicator	Sarcoidosis	TB
Demographic		
Age	Generally older (third to fourth decade)	Younger
Body mass index	Higher	Lower
Socioeconomic status	Higher	Lower
Clinical		
History of close contact with patient having TB infection	Not present	May be present
Constitutional symptoms	Asymptomatic or with mild fever, anorexia, and loss of weight	More prominent fever, anorexia, and weight loss
Cough	Mainly dry, hemoptysis is rare	Usually productive, hemoptysis is common

Continued

Continued

Indicator	Sarcoidosis	TB
Peripheral lymph node involvement	Seen in about 10% patients only	Cervical and axillary lymph node involvement is common
Lacrimal, parotid, and myocardial involvement	May be seen	Rare
Pleural, peritoneal, meningeal, and adrenal involvement	Rare	May be seen
Radiology		
Intrathoracic lymph node involvement	Typically symmetric bihilar and paratracheal; smooth, discrete, and solid-looking nodes	Asymmetric, large, may be conglomerate, usually with central areas of hypodensity
Radiology: Necrotizing pneumonia, cavitation and pleural involvement with effusion	Rare	Common
Chest CT	Micro- and macro- nodules which have characteristic distribution in peribronchovascular region, subpleural interstitium and interlobular septa	Micronodules, randomly distributed with tree-in-bud appearance
Clinicoradiologic correlation	• Clinicoradiologic dissociation, i.e., patient relatively asymptomatic despite extensive pulmonary involvement • Even with advanced radiologic abnormalities, usually the "patients walk-in"	Good correlation. Patients with extensive involvement; usually the patients are "brought in"
Other investigations		
Tuberculin skin test	Nearly always negative	Nearly always positive
Increased SACE level	More common	Less common
Increased serum calcium or hypercalciuria	May be seen	Not seen
Sputum: Positive for *M.tb* on smear or culture	False-positive acid-fast bacilli or rarely coexisting TB with sarcoidosis. Patient should never receive glucocorticoids alone	Confirmatory for TB
PCR of biopsy tissues is positive for *M.tb* DNA	Qualitative tests can be positive in up to half of the patients in high TB prevalence countries; quantitative tests show low copy numbers	Positive with high copy numbers if quantitative tests are done
Biopsy of involved site **(Figs. 9A to D)**	Non-necrotic, compact granulomas, sparse lymphocytic cuffing around granuloma ("naked") with inclusion bodies at times	Caseating necrosis, ill-formed granuloma with intense inflammatory reaction and may be positive for acid-fast bacilli
Response to treatment		
Response to antituberculosis treatment	No response although spontaneous resolution in sarcoidosis is known	Good except in case of primary multidrug resistance
Dramatic clinicoradiologic response to steroids	Usual	No response or may worsen
(PCR: polymerase chain reaction; SACE: serum angiotensin converting enzyme; TB: tuberculosis)		

are considered to coexist, the so-called tuberculous sarcoidosis.[249] However, by definition, sarcoidosis indicates a granulomatous disease that is of an unknown cause. Thus, diagnosing tuberculous sarcoidosis is technically incorrect. This field requires further scientific work.

Necrotizing Sarcoid Granulomatosis and Nodular Sarcoidosis

Necrotizing sarcoid granulomatosis (NSG) is a rare but distinct entity which shows sarcoid-like granulomas, large areas of infarct-like necrosis, and granulomatous vasculitis that is often destructive with few inclusions. Nodular sarcoidosis, again a rare form, is a differential diagnosis of NSG. It manifests with pulmonary nodules 1–8 cm in diameter, either multiple and bilateral simulating metastases or solitary simulating lung cancer. According to some experts, NSG is the late stage of nodular sarcoidosis. Histologically, it consists of coalescent sarcoid granulomas without necrosis or vasculitis.[250]

TREATMENT

For two decades, the only available international expert statement/guideline on the treatment of sarcoidosis was the statement by the ATS, European Respiratory Society (ERS), and World Association of Sarcoidosis and Other Granulomatous Disorders (WASOG) published in 1999.[251] Recently, the ERS and the British Thoracic Society (BTS) have published their guiding documents on treating sarcoidosis.[252,253] Herein, we will discuss the treatment of sarcoidosis focusing on pulmonary sarcoidosis and covering only briefly the important aspects of treating extrapulmonary sarcoidosis.

When to Treat?

Pulmonary Sarcoidosis

Not all patients diagnosed with sarcoidosis need pharmacological therapy, as the disease is often self-limiting. Moreover, most therapeutic options are not without significant adverse effects. Pulmonary disease is treated, if there is lung function impairment with a significant future risk of mortality or permanent disability, or if there are significant and persistent symptoms causing impaired quality of life (QoL).[252,253] Traditionally, stage I disease and stage II disease with minimal lung abnormalities on chest radiograph, in the absence of significant symptoms, are not treated with immunosuppression. Patients have a good outcome with disease remission or resolution even without pharmacologic treatment. Patients with stage II and III disease on the chest radiograph with significant lung abnormalities usually require immunosuppression as it is known to be persistent or progressive and can evolve into fibrotic (stage IV) sarcoidosis. Fibrotic sarcoidosis is challenging to treat as sometimes, it is difficult to identify whether there is significant active inflammation in the lungs that could respond to anti-inflammatory treatment. Symptoms in this stage may be due to advanced lung fibrosis, PH, or other complications. Moreover, the structurally damaged lungs in this stage are susceptible to infections such as pulmonary mycosis, especially when immunosuppression is used. Thus, the decision to treat fibrotic pulmonary sarcoidosis with immunomodulation is difficult and needs to be based on clinical and radiologic clues to activity, previous therapy, response to therapy, and risk of infections. The role of PET-CT in this regard needs to be defined by further research.

Chest CT may be the preferred radiologic modality to better characterize the radiologic changes and forms part of multicomponent criteria for therapeutic decision-making. Sometimes, marked radiologic burden of the lung disease on CT, represented by extensive septal thickening or nodules, may trigger prescription of immunosuppressive treatment. Such disease, even if initially asymptomatic, might end up in significant fibrotic sequelae in the future, if the radiologic abnormalities remain unresolved over months to years. We use a systematic approach in our clinic to classify disease severity, disease evolution, and treatment response in pulmonary sarcoidosis **(Table 5)**.[254]

Extrapulmonary Sarcoidosis

Extrapulmonary disease that may require immunosuppressive treatment includes that affecting the skin and soft tissues, eye, upper airway, calcium metabolism, liver, spleen, heart, central or peripheral nervous systems, kidneys, joints, bones, or, rarely, other organs (such as the pituitary and muscles) The dictum is that mild disease of any organ with little potential to cause permanent organ dysfunction, organ damage, disability, or death may not be treated; close observation for spontaneous resolution is a good initial strategy. Examples include mild and nondestructive joint disease, hepatic sarcoidosis without architectural changes and only mild enzyme elevation, splenic lesions without hematologic abnormalities, asymptomatic and nondestructive bone lesions, and so on. Sometimes, short-term or symptomatic treatment may be offered. Milder disease of certain organs such as involvement of the anterior chamber of the eye and superficial, small, and nondisfiguring skin lesions can be treated with topical therapy. Extensive or disfiguring skin lesions, severe inflammation of the anterior chamber of the eye or posterior chamber involvement, hypercalcemia, hepatic sarcoidosis with significant biochemical cholestasis or imaging abnormalities, splenic enlargement with/without hypersplenism, significant parotid enlargement with/without salivary abnormalities, significant joint and bone disease, and so on need to be treated with systemic immunosuppression. Involvement of the heart, nervous system, kidneys, and any other organ- or life-threatening manifestation uniformly requires systemic immunosuppression. Severe or critical involvement of vital structures may initially need intense immunosuppression, such as using high-dose GC pulses.

Drugs Used to Treat Sarcoidosis

Glucocorticoids

Glucocorticoids are the first-line systemic pharmacologic agents for treating sarcoidosis.[255] A Delphi consensus reiterated them as the preferred agents.[256] They suppress inflammation by deactivating several proinflammatory genes (by repressing nuclear factor kappa B) and activating multiple anti-inflammatory genes. The aim of GC use in sarcoidosis is to suppress granulomatous inflammation in the target organ to restore the structural and functional

TABLE 5: Classification of disease severity, disease evolution, treatment response, and other treatment-related behavior in pulmonary sarcoidosis used in our clinic.

Terminology	Disease behavior
Disease severity	
Mild disease	Self-limited, not requiring systemic immunosuppression
Moderate disease	Causes significant organ dysfunction or quality of life impairment requiring systemic immunosuppressive drugs
Severe active disease	Threatens organ function or life requiring urgent and intense immunosuppression (prednisolone equivalent ≥ 40 mg/day or ≥0.75 mg/kg/day)
Advanced disease	Shows severe sequalae, such as pulmonary fibrosis, pulmonary hypertension, and/or others; may have residual activity
Disease evolution	
Resolution	No symptoms due to the disease with normal lung function and chest radiograph
Improvement	Respiratory symptoms improved by ≥50%, with either decreased radiologic abnormalities, or improved lung function (≥5-point increase in the %pred FVC or FEV_1), or both, without any worsening on imaging or spirometry
Stabilization	Reduction in symptoms with stable imaging and spirometry
Worsening	≥25% increase in respiratory symptoms with worsening of lung function (≥5-point reduction in %pred FVC or FEV_1), or worsened chest radiograph due to sarcoidosis
Treatment response	
Good response	Resolution or improvement of disease
Fair response	Disease stabilization
No response or treatment failure	Worsening during therapy or within 12 weeks of stopping it
Other treatment-related disease behavior	
Treatment-refractory disease	Worsening despite intense systemic immunosuppression (prednisolone equivalent ≥ 40 mg/day or ≥0.75 mg/kg/day)
Treatment-dependent disease	Worsening while tapering treatment or within 12 weeks of stopping it on two or more occasions
Relapse	Worsening after 12 weeks of stopping treatment

(FEV_1: forced expiratory volume in the first second; FVC: forced vital capacity)

Source: Adapted from Dhooria et al.[254]

states closer to normal. For example, the goal of treating pulmonary sarcoidosis with GCs is to achieve resolution (or improvement) in the imaging abnormalities reflecting restoration of the normal lung structure and to improve the measurable lung function testing parameters aiming to restore normal respiratory function. In a Cochrane database systematic review of available trials on the efficacy of GCs in pulmonary sarcoidosis, it was concluded that oral GCs mitigated imaging abnormalities, without statistically improving lung function.[257] The GC agents, dose, duration, and regimens are important considerations.

Agents and dose: Prednisone or prednisolone is the most common GC used to treat sarcoidosis; most reported studies have used this agent. Methylprednisolone is more potent than prednisone, while deflazacort is less potent. Deflazacort, in an equipotent dose, is considered to cause lesser adverse effects on glucose and calcium metabolism.[258] The initial dose of GCs to be used for treating pulmonary sarcoidosis depends on the extent and severity of the disease. If a decision has been made to use GCs, lower doses such as 5–10 mg/day have been suggested if only symptomatic relief is required to achieve better QoL.[253] Trying nonsteroidal agents for such a purpose before opting for GC is a good clinical practice. If GCs are required to treat significant lung structural and functional abnormalities, higher doses are required. Recently, the SARCORT study, a randomized controlled trial from our center found that high-dose (40 mg/day initial dose) prednisolone was not superior to a lower dose (20 mg/day initial dose) in improving outcomes or the health-related quality of life (HRQoL) in pulmonary sarcoidosis and was associated with similar adverse effects.[259] Therefore, the lower dose should be preferred as it was associated with numerically lesser adverse effects and lower cumulative dose. Choosing a 40 mg initial prednisolone dose is still an option as it was not inferior to 20 mg/day in terms of both efficacy and safety in this trial. Also, higher doses may be required for patients with critical organ involvement, such as severe uveitis or cardiac sarcoidosis, subsets which were excluded from the SARCORT study. A previous Delphi study suggested a 40 mg of daily prednisone equivalent as the maximum dose recommended for treating pulmonary sarcoidosis.[256]

Duration

The duration of GC treatment depends upon initial disease severity, initial treatment response, and disease course observed on tapering GCs. For mild disease, treated for symptoms alone, 8–12 weeks of low-dose (5–10 mg/day) prednisolone may be sufficient. If treatment is begun for significant organ dysfunction, the minimum duration of GC treatment is 6 months. In the SARCORT study, in which all subjects were initially treated for 6 months, 55% of subjects improved and remained relapse-free in the year following the end of treatment. A 45% incidence of treatment failure or relapse was observed during 18 months from treatment initiation. Thus, a significant proportion of patients need to be treated for longer than 6 months. The duration is mostly guided by the patient's disease behavior when the GCs are tapered to lower doses (5–10 mg/day). For patients who remain well at smaller doses, treatment can be stopped at 6 months, and they can be observed closely at least for the following year. For those who start worsening at small doses of GCs, long-term treatment, ranging from 9 to 24 months, or longer may be required. In most such cases, adding a GC-sparing agent may help reduce the adverse effects associated with long-term GC use. Significantly better results were observed in patients who had received prolonged treatment for 4 years or more in the BTS study.[260]

Some experts suggest a six-phase treatment for sarcoidosis.[261] Treatment is started at a dose of 20–40 mg/day of prednisolone administered for around 4-6 weeks (phase 1).[3] This is followed by tapering (phase 2) to a daily dose of 5–10 mg over a period of 1–6 months. The maintenance (phase 3) dosing is continued for 3–9 months followed by tapering off (phase 4) and stoppage of GCs after a total duration of 12 months. The patient should then be observed (phase 5) and treated for a relapse if it occurs (phase 6). Administration of GCs every other day is equally effective as daily dosing and may be used for patients developing significant adverse effects.[262-264]

Inhaled Corticosteroids

Some studies of inhaled corticosteroids (ICS) in pulmonary sarcoidosis have demonstrated slight improvements in pulmonary function or improved symptoms.[265-267] A meta-analysis found inconclusive evidence to support ICS use.[257] We suggest the use of ICS after completing oral GC treatment in patients having an obstructive defect on spirometry.

Adverse Effects

Glucocorticoid treatment is associated with significant adverse effects **(Table 6)**. Latent TB may get reactivated with GC therapy. It is challenging to explain the origin of active TB during the follow-up of a sarcoidosis patient. If it occurs early during follow-up, it might be due to an initial misdiagnosis implying that the disease was TB right from the start and was mistaken as sarcoidosis. Active TB might also occur during immunosuppressive therapy due to reactivation or new infection, anytime during the course. However, the usual recommendation by the ATS to undertake skin testing for LTBI before initiation of GC therapy is not practical for India for two reasons:[268] One, there is a high prevalence of TB infection in the population and a vast majority of our patients with sarcoidosis would be infected and two, as already discussed, the TST is likely to be negative in active sarcoidosis.

Another major complication of chronic GC therapy is osteoporosis. Cotrimoxazole prophylaxis should be used according to standard guidelines to prevent *Pneumocystis jirovecii* infection. Osteoporosis prevention requires use of calcium, vitamin D, and bisphosphonates, and other such drugs according to standard recommendations.

TABLE 6: Important adverse effects of drugs used in the management of sarcoidosis.

Drug	Adverse effects
Glucocorticoids	Weight gain, skin thinning, acne, mood changes, increased risk of infection, hypertension, diabetes, cataracts, and osteoporosis
Methotrexate	Hepatitis, hepatic fibrosis, interstitial pneumonia, pulmonary fibrosis, leucopenia, gastrointestinal intolerance, teratogenicity
Azathioprine	Myelosuppression, opportunistic infections, hepatitis, teratogenicity
Leflunomide	Rash, alopecia, peripheral neuropathy, interstitial pneumonia, gastrointestinal intolerance, teratogenicity
Mycophenolate mofetil	Hyperglycemia, hypercholesterolemia, gastrointestinal intolerance, bone marrow suppression, hepatitis, teratogenicity
Cyclophosphamide	Myelosuppression, opportunistic infections, hemorrhagic cystitis, bladder malignancy, cardiomyopathy, infertility, teratogenicity
Chloroquine, hydroxychloroquine	Retinopathy, corneal changes, muscle weakness, gastrointestinal intolerance
TNF-α antagonists	Infections (especially reactivation of tuberculosis), infusion reactions, gastrointestinal intolerance, headache
Rituximab	Infusion reactions, lymphopenia, opportunistic infections, asthenia

(TNF: tumor necrosis factor)

Glucocorticoid-sparing Agents

Alternatives to GCs are required due to the following reasons: (1) GC treatment causes unacceptable side effects, (2) the disease may relapse after stopping or tapering GCs, and (3) occasionally extrapulmonary disease may be refractory to GCs.[3,256,269] The options for nonsteroidal treatment are cytotoxic drugs, antimalarials, biologics, and other agents.[270] Barring the anti-TNF-α agents, most of these drugs take a few weeks to months to be effective. Therefore, GC treatment should not be tapered for at least 1–2 months after adding an alternative agent.[271]

Cytotoxic Drugs

These include methotrexate, azathioprine, leflunomide, mycophenolate mofetil, and cyclophosphamide.[272-275] Methotrexate is the preferred second-line drug.[256,276-278] Occasionally, it is used as a first-line agent in combination with GCs.[278] The ongoing PREDMETH study is testing methotrexate monotherapy against prednisone as a first-line agent for sarcoidosis.[279] The recommended initial dose is 10–15 mg once a week along with folic acid 5 mg weekly or 1 mg daily. If gastrointestinal adverse effects occur, splitting the dose may be useful. Response is relatively slower in onset. Methotrexate may take up to 6 months to be effective.[278] Azathioprine (2 mg/kg/day) may also be used as a GC-sparing agent.[280,281] It is equally efficacious as methotrexate but may result in a higher risk of infections.[282] Leflunomide (20 mg/day) is a less toxic alternative to methotrexate with a lower risk of hepatotoxicity and interstitial pneumonitis.[283,284] Data on mycophenolate mofetil are limited, but it may also be considered as a GC-sparing option in pulmonary and extrapulmonary sarcoidosis.[285-287] Cyclophosphamide is mostly reserved for use in GC-refractory cases of severe cardiac or neurosarcoidosis.[288,289] Careful monitoring is required for toxicity using liver and renal function tests and hematological assessment.

Antimalarial Drugs

Antimalarials such as chloroquine and hydroxychloroquine act as immunomodulators and have been successfully used for sarcoidosis involving the skin or paranasal sinuses, hypercalcemia, and neurosarcoidosis.[290-293] Hydroxychloroquine is the preferred agent and has also been used for chronic pulmonary sarcoidosis; the efficacy remains unknown.[294] The usual dose of hydroxychloroquine is 200–400 mg (6 mg/kg) daily. Retinopathy is an important adverse effect that is significantly more likely with chloroquine than hydroxychloroquine. An annual eye examination is required. Rare side effects include agranulocytosis and myopathy; therefore, periodic complete blood counts and neuromuscular strength assessment are recommended.

Biologic Therapy

TNF-α antagonists are the third-line agents for treating sarcoidosis. TNF-α is believed to play a central role in granuloma formation; thus, its inhibition might effectively control the disease.[271,295-304] Of all the agents in this class, infliximab is the most studied. It is typically administered as an intravenous infusion of 3–5 mg/kg on weeks 0 and 2, with repeat dosing every 4–8 weeks thereafter.[297,304] In one of the trials of infliximab in pulmonary sarcoidosis, there was an improvement in lung function while the other study did not find any significant improvement.[301,302] For extrapulmonary sarcoidosis, although there was improvement after 24 weeks of therapy, this benefit was not sustained after a 24-week washout.[296] More than half of the patients relapsed after discontinuing treatment.[305] Trials demonstrating long-term safety and efficacy of infliximab therapy are lacking. Adalimumab can be given subcutaneously and being a fully humanized antibody has a lower allergic reaction rate than infliximab.[306] It has been shown to be efficacious in a few small studies.[307-309] Etanercept and golimumab have been found to be ineffective and are not recommended for the treatment of sarcoidosis.[310,311]

One of the major concerns while using TNF-α inhibitors is the increased risk of reactivation of LTBI and other opportunistic infections. Screening for LTBI and its treatment is recommended for all patients planning to start therapy with a TNF-α inhibitor.[312] Other known side effects include a possible increase in the risk of malignancies, such as lymphoma, congestive heart failure, and demyelinating diseases. Paradoxical sarcoidosis-like granulomatous reactions may develop during TNF-α antagonist use due to cytokine disequilibrium.[313]

Rituximab, an antibody directed against CD20+ cells, has been reported to be efficacious in a few case reports and small studies.[314-317] Several other drugs have been reportedly tried in sporadic cases or small studies including thalidomide, colchicine, pentoxifylline, Acthar gel (repository corticotropin injection), and cyclosporin A.[306] These remain available options that can be used if the previously described agents are ineffective or not tolerated. Antifibrotic agents, pirfenidone and nintedanib, can be used to treat stage IV sarcoidosis in the presence of progressive pulmonary fibrosis.[318-321]

Acute Pulmonary Exacerbation of Sarcoidosis

Acute pulmonary exacerbation of sarcoidosis (APES) may be defined as worsening of pulmonary symptoms (present for at least 1 month) in a patient with sarcoidosis that are not explained by another cause, along with a decline in spirometry [≥10% decrease from previous baseline forced vital capacity (FVC) and/or forced expiratory volume in 1 second (FEV_1)].[322] It usually occurs after tapering or stopping immunosuppressive treatment. A suggested treatment is using 20 mg/day prednisone for a median of 21 days followed by tapering to a level at which the patient remains symptom-free.[323] Some experts have questioned equating the reappearance of symptoms in sarcoidosis to "exacerbations", as we understand with respect to diseases such as asthma, chronic obstructive pulmonary disease, or ILD. In contrast to the latter diseases, sarcoidosis is characterized by granulomatous inflammation that takes time to appear and resolve.[324] Therefore, symptom reappearance in sarcoidosis is better termed a relapse and treated accordingly. Relapses are generally treated with a regimen similar to the initial treatment except that GC treatment is tapered more rapidly. GC-sparing agents are added early to avoid GC-related adverse effects.

Treatment of Extrapulmonary Disease

A detailed discussion is outside the scope of this chapter. Localized skin lesions are treated with topical GCs and other topical drugs. Extensive or severe lesions require systemic therapy including oral GCs, hydroxychloroquine, cytotoxic drugs, and biologics. Locally delivered or systemic GCs are the mainstay of treatment of ocular sarcoidosis. Similar GC-sparing drugs are used to treat ocular disease as pulmonary disease. GCs are the first-line pharmacologic agents used to treat cardiac sarcoidosis. Treatment of LV dysfunction is based on angiotensin receptor II blockers, aldosterone inhibitors, and diuretics. Ventricular arrhythmias and heart block may require appropriate implantable devices apart from initial intense treatment with pulse methylprednisolone.[133] Similarly, neurosarcoidosis, hepatic, and renal sarcoidosis are treated using GCs and other immunosuppressants, as indicated.

Managing Symptoms and Complications

Managing symptoms, complications, treatment-emergent adverse events, and comorbid conditions is important. Cough can be treated with antitussives such as dextromethorphan, levodropropizine, levocloperastine, benzonatate, or others. Sometimes, codeine-based preparations or thalidomide may be required. Body aches and joint pains, if bothersome, can be tackled using paracetamol or nonsteroidal anti-inflammatory drugs. An important aspect of sarcoidosis is fatigue. Regardless of disease activity, patients often report fatigue, sleep disturbance, and impaired QoL.[325] Methylphenidate can be used to treat sarcoidosis-associated fatigue.[326] Sarcoidosis patients should be appropriately screened, clinically or with laboratory tests, for comorbidities such as hypertension, diabetes, coronary artery disease, osteoporosis, depression, obstructive sleep apnea, and others and should be treated accordingly.

Clinicians should consider calcium and vitamin D supplementation, after excluding hypercalcemia and hypercalciuria and monitoring for the same thereafter. Use of bisphosphonates has been recommended by the American College of Rheumatology in patients receiving >5 mg of prednisone per day or its equivalent for >3 months.[327] Gastrointestinal bleeding risk is low in ambulatory patients treated with GCs.[328] Proton-pump inhibitors or histamine H2 receptor antagonists should be considered if patients have significant dyspepsia due to GCs.

Bronchiectasis, fibrocavitary disease, aspergillomas, and chronic pulmonary aspergillosis (CPA) can complicate fibrotic sarcoidosis **(Figs. 10A and B)**. Bronchiectasis is treated with anti-inflammatory therapy, mucociliary clearance, and appropriate antimicrobials for exacerbations.[329] Systemic antifungal agents are used to treat CPA; intracavitary instillation of antifungal agents has also been tried.[330] Bronchial artery embolization or lung resection surgery may be required to manage massive, uncontrolled hemoptysis. Bronchoscopic balloon dilation has been tried in bronchial stenosis following sarcoidosis.[331] Extensive fibrosis causing hypoxemia requires supplemental long-term oxygen therapy. With severe functional impairment and patient disability, PH and right heart failure may supervene for which the patient will require oxygen and

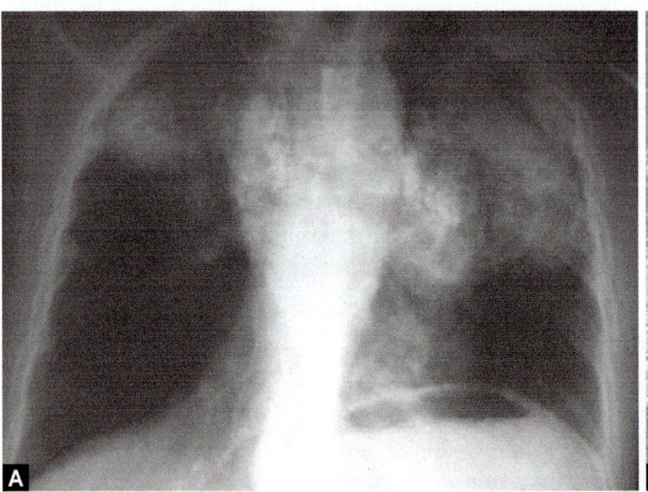

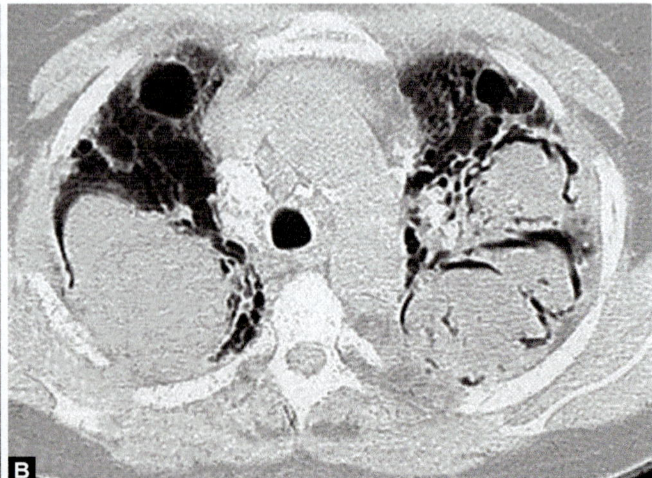

FIGS. 10A AND B: Bilateral upper lobe aspergillomas in sarcoidosis.

diuretics. When lung fibrosis and PH are present at the same time, there is a sharp increase in symptoms that should alert the clinician to this serious complication.[332] Pulmonary vasodilators may be used with caution for sarcoidosis-associated pulmonary hypertension (SAPH) when the degree of PH is disproportionate to lung fibrosis.[333] Cor pulmonale secondary to lung disease may paradoxically worsen with pulmonary vasodilators. Decongestive therapy is required for heart failure due to sarcoid cardiomyopathy. A pacemaker or implantable cardioverter defibrillator (ICD) may also be indicated.[334] Elderly sarcoidosis patients often present with unusual clinical features of sarcoidosis. Occasionally, these features resemble malignancy, malignant cells can induce a sarcoidosis-like reaction in the draining lymph nodes, and, rarely, sarcoidosis and malignancy may coexist.[335] Additional treatments for complications due to extrapulmonary organ involvement are needed as appropriate.

Immunization against pneumococcal disease and influenza are a must for patients with sarcoidosis; other guideline-concordant vaccines should also be considered. Pulmonary rehabilitation is an important modality to improve the functional capacity and QoL, especially in advanced disease. Supplemental oxygen is prescribed for advanced disease with hypoxemia. Lung transplantation is the only way to improve and prolong life when there is end-stage lung fibrosis or severe PH. Survival rates following lung transplantation for sarcoidosis are generally comparable to other indications. Sarcoidosis can recur in lung allografts but does not affect survival adversely.

PROGNOSIS AND MORTALITY

Sarcoidosis is a benign process. Many patients remain asymptomatic and spontaneous remission is common. The disease, however, follows a chronic course in 10–30% of the cases, sometimes leading to significant deterioration in lung function. Mortality rates of 1–6% have been reported.[336] Signs of fibrosis on the chest radiograph and a FVC < 1.5 L predict increased mortality due to respiratory failure.[337] The prognosis of sarcoidosis is mainly linked to organ involvement and disease severity. Sarcoidosis is associated with better survival at 5 years (91.6%) compared to other diffuse ILDs such as nonspecific or desquamative interstitial pneumonia (85.5%), HP (84.1%), collagen-related diffuse ILD (69.7%), undefined forms of pulmonary fibrosis (69.5%), and IPF (35.4%).[337-339]

FUTURE DIRECTIONS

Despite extensive research, sarcoidosis remains an enigmatic disease. We need to further explore genetic factors, delineate the immunopathogenesis using human tissue and animal models, find new approaches to diagnose and manage disease, and conduct randomized controlled trials to assess existing and new treatments.[340] The remarkable similarity of sarcoidosis to TB and the continued inter-relationship of the two conditions is of special interest to clinicians and researchers from high TB burden countries. Developing definitive tests for differentiating the two conditions is vital.

SUMMARY

Sarcoidosis is a multisystem granulomatous disorder of unknown etiology that occurs worldwide and affects young and middle-aged adults. The hallmark of sarcoidosis pathology is the presence of non-necrotic, compact, 'naked' granulomas. Pulmonary sarcoidosis commonly presents in a tuberculosis-like or interstitial lung disease-like manner, or as part of well-defined constellations of symptoms such as the Löfgren syndrome. Symmetric bihilar and mediastinal lymphadenopathy is characteristic of sarcoidosis on chest radiograph. Chest CT classically reveals symmetric, multistation, and bulky intrathoracic adenopathy devoid of hypodense areas with upper-mid predominant peribronchovascular septal thickening with a perilymphatic distribution of nodules. Conventional bronchoscopic techniques (TBNA plus TBLB plus EBB) achieve a high sensitivity for diagnosing pulmonary sarcoidosis. Apart from lungs and thoracic lymph nodes, the skin, eye, joints, liver, spleen, kidney, the heart, and the nervous system may be involved. Not all patients diagnosed with sarcoidosis need pharmacological therapy, as the disease is often self-limiting. Treatment is required if there is organ dysfunction or compromised quality-of-life. GCs are the first-line systemic pharmacologic agents for treating sarcoidosis. Alternatives to GCs are required if the treatment causes unacceptable side effects, the disease relapses after tapering GCs, or if extrapulmonary disease is GC refractory. The prognosis of sarcoidosis is mainly linked to organ involvement and disease severity.

REFERENCES

1. Hutchinson J. Case of livid papillary psoriasis. In: Illustrations of Clinical Surgery, Vol. 1. London: J & A Churchill; 1877. pp. 42-3.
2. Boeck C. Multiple benign sarkoid of the skin. J Cutan Genitourinary Dis. 1899;17:543-50.
3. Statement on sarcoidosis. Joint Statement of the American Thoracic Society (ATS), the European Respiratory Society (ERS) and the World Association of Sarcoidosis and Other Granulomatous Disorders (WASOG) adopted by the ATS Board of Directors and by the ERS Executive Committee, February 1999. Am J Respir Crit Care Med. 1999;160(2):736-55.
4. James DG. Descriptive definition and historic aspects of sarcoidosis. Clin Chest Med. 1997;18(4):663-79.
5. Baughman RP, Lower EE, Judson MA. Update on Sarcoidosis. Clin Chest Med. 2024;45(1):xiii.

6. Rossides M, Darlington P, Kullberg S, et al. Sarcoidosis: Epidemiology and clinical insights. J Intern Med. 2023;293(6):668-80.
7. Spagnolo P, Bernardinello N. Sarcoidosis. Immunol Allergy Clin North Am. 2023;43(2):259-72.
8. Dhooria S, Agarwal R, Sehgal IS, et al. Spectrum of interstitial lung diseases at a tertiary center in a developing country: A study of 803 subjects. PLoS One. 2018;13(2):e0191938.
9. Dhooria S, Sehgal IS, Agarwal R, et al. Incidence, prevalence, and national burden of interstitial lung diseases in India: Estimates from two studies of 3089 subjects. PLoS One. 2022;17(7):e0271665.
10. Arkema EV, Cozier YC. Sarcoidosis epidemiology: recent estimates of incidence, prevalence and risk factors. Curr Opin Pulm Med. 2020;26(5):527-34.
11. Yeager H, Rossman MD, Baughman RP, et al. Pulmonary and psychosocial findings at enrollment in the ACCESS study. Sarcoidosis Vasc Diffuse Lung Dis. 2005;22(2):147-53.
12. Hofmann S, Franke A, Fischer A, et al. Genome-wide association study identifies ANXA11 as a new susceptibility locus for sarcoidosis. Nat Genet. 2008;40(9):1103-06.
13. Franke A, Fischer A, Nothnagel M, et al. Genome-wide association analysis in sarcoidosis and Crohn's disease unravels a common susceptibility locus on 10p12.2. Gastroenterology. 2008;135(4):1207-15.
14. Moller DR, Rybicki BA, Hamzeh NY, et al. Genetic, Immunologic, and Environmental Basis of Sarcoidosis. Ann Am Thorac Soc. 2017;14(Supplement 6):S429-36.
15. McGrath DS, Daniil Z, Foley P, et al. Epidemiology of familial sarcoidosis in the UK. Thorax. 2000;55(9):751-4.
16. Rybicki BA, Iannuzzi MC, Frederick MM, et al. Familial aggregation of sarcoidosis. A case-control etiologic study of sarcoidosis (ACCESS). Am J Respir Crit Care Med. 2001;164(11):2085-91.
17. Becker ML, Martin TM, Doyle TM, Rose CD. Interstitial pneumonitis in Blau syndrome with documented mutation in CARD15. Arthritis Rheum. 2007;56(4):1292-1294.
18. Schurmann M, Valentonyte R, Hampe J, Muller-Quernheim J, Schwinger E, Schreiber S. CARD15 gene mutations in sarcoidosis. Eur Respir J. 2003;22(5):748-754.
19. du Bois RM, Beirne PA, Anevlavis SE. Genetics of sarcoidosis. Eur Resp Mon. 2005;32:64-81.
20. Rossman MD, Thompson B, Frederick M, et al. HLA-DRB1*1101: a significant risk factor for sarcoidosis in blacks and whites. Am J Hum Genet. 2003;73(4):720-35.
21. Iannuzzi MC, Maliarik MJ, Poisson LM, et al. Sarcoidosis susceptibility and resistance HLA-DQB1 alleles in African Americans. Am J Respir Crit Care Med. 2003;167(9):1225-31.
22. Schurmann M, Reichel P, Muller-Myhsok B, et al. Results from a genome-wide search for predisposing genes in sarcoidosis. Am J Respir Crit Care Med. 2001;164(5):840-6.
23. Rybicki BA, Maliarik MJ, Poisson LM, et al. The major histocompatibility complex gene region and sarcoidosis susceptibility in African Americans. Am J Respir Crit Care Med. 2003;167(3):444-9.
24. Sharma SK, Balamurugan A, Pandey RM, et al. Human leukocyte antigen-DR alleles influence the clinical course of pulmonary sarcoidosis in Asian Indians. Am J Respir Cell Mol Biol. 2003; 29(2):225-31.
25. Lin NW, Maier LA. Occupational exposures and sarcoidosis: current understanding and knowledge gaps. Curr Opin Pulm Med. 2022;28(2):144-51.
26. Huntley CC, Patel K, Mughal AZ, et al. Airborne occupational exposures associated with pulmonary sarcoidosis: a systematic review and meta-analysis. Occup Environ Med. 2023;80(10):580-9.
27. Izbicki G, Chavko R, Banauch GI, et al. World Trade Center "sarcoid-like" granulomatous pulmonary disease in New York City Fire Department rescue workers. Chest. 2007;131(5):1414-23.
28. Reich JM. Sarcoidosis and World Trade Center disaster. J Occup Environ Med. 2012;54(1):2; author reply 2-3.
29. Reich JM. The Curious Omission of Treatment as a Predictor of Pulmonary Sarcoidosis Mortality. Chest. 2018;153(6):1507.
30. Barnard J, Rose C, Newman L, et al. Job and industry classifications associated with sarcoidosis in A Case-Control Etiologic Study of Sarcoidosis (ACCESS). J Occup Environ Med. 2005;47(3):226-34.
31. Douglas JG, Middleton WG, Gaddie J, et al. Sarcoidosis: a disorder commoner in non-smokers? Thorax. 1986;41(10):787-91.
32. Gupta D, Singh AD, Agarwal R, et al. Is tobacco smoking protective for sarcoidosis? A case-control study from North India. Sarcoidosis Vasc Diffuse Lung Dis. 2010;27(1):19-26.
33. Ungprasert P, Crowson CS, Matteson EL. Smoking, obesity and risk of sarcoidosis: A population-based nested case-control study. Respir Med. 2016;120:87-90.
34. Mayer AS, Hamzeh N, Maier LA. Sarcoidosis and chronic beryllium disease: similarities and differences. Semin Respir Crit Care Med. 2014;35(3):316-29.
35. Gerke AK, Tangh F, Yang M, et al. An analysis of seasonality of sarcoidosis in the United States veteran population: 2000-2007. Sarcoidosis Vasc Diffuse Lung Dis. 2012;29(2):155-8.
36. Demirkok SS, Basaranoglu M, Coker E, et al. Seasonality of the onset of symptoms, tuberculin test anergy and Kveim positive reaction in a large cohort of patients with sarcoidosis. Respirology. 2007;12(4):591-3.
37. Gupta D. Seasonality of Sarcoidosis: the 'heat' is on. Sarcoidosis Vasc Diffuse Lung Dis. 2013;30(3):241-3.
38. Newman LS. Aetiologies of sarcoidosis. Eur Resp Mon. 2005; 32:23-48.
39. Vidal S, de la Horra C, Martin J, et al. Pneumocystis jirovecii colonisation in patients with interstitial lung disease. Clin Microbiol Infect. 2006;12(3):231-5.
40. Drake WP, Newman LS. Mycobacterial antigens may be important in sarcoidosis pathogenesis. Curr Opin Pulm Med. 2006;12(5):359-63.
41. Ishige I, Eishi Y, Takemura T, et al. Propionibacterium acnes is the most common bacterium commensal in peripheral lung tissue and mediastinal lymph nodes from subjects without sarcoidosis. Sarcoidosis Vasc Diffuse Lung Dis. 2005;22(1):33-42.
42. Oswald-Richter KA, Drake WP. The etiologic role of infectious antigens in sarcoidosis pathogenesis. Semin Respir Crit Care Med. 2010;31(4):375-9.
43. Gupta D, Agarwal R, Aggarwal AN, et al. Molecular evidence for the role of mycobacteria in sarcoidosis: a meta-analysis. Eur Respir J. 2007;30(3):508-16.
44. Mootha VK, Agarwal R, Aggarwal AN, et al. The Sarcoid-Tuberculosis link: evidence from a high TB prevalence country. J Infect. 2010;60(6):P501-3.
45. Perez RL, Rivera-Marrero CA, Roman J. Pulmonary granulomatous inflammation: From sarcoidosis to tuberculosis. Semin Respir Infect. 2003;18(1):23-32.

46. Kent DC, Houk VN, Elliott RC, et al. The definitive evaluation of sarcoidosis. Am Rev Respir Dis. 1970;101(5):721-7.
47. Hatzakis K, Siafakas NM, Bouros D. Miliary sarcoidosis following miliary tuberculosis. Respiration. 2000;67(2):219-22.
48. Vanek J, Schwarz J. Demonstration of acid-fast rods in sarcoidosis. Am Rev Respir Dis. 1970;101(3):395-400.
49. Cantwell AR, Jr. Variably acid-fast bacteria in a case of systemic sarcoidosis and hypodermitis sclerodermiformis. Dermatologica. 1981;163(3):239-48.
50. Cantwell AR, Jr. Histologic observations of variably acid-fast pleomorphic bacteria in systemic sarcoidosis: a report of 3 cases. Growth. 1982;46(2):113-25.
51. Mitchell DN, Rees RJ. A transmissible agent from sarcoid tissue. Lancet. 1969;2(7611):81-4.
52. Mitchell DN, Rees RJ. An attempt to demonstrate a transmissible agent from sarcoid material. Postgrad Med J. 1970;46(538):510-4.
53. Mitchell DN, Rees RJ, Goswami KK. Transmissible agents from human sarcoid and Crohn's disease tissues. Lancet. 1976;2(7989):761-5.
54. Mitchell DN. The nature and physical characteristics of a transmissible agent from human sarcoid tissue. Ann N Y Acad Sci. 1976;278:233-48.
55. Song Z, Marzilli L, Greenlee BM, et al. Mycobacterial catalase-peroxidase is a tissue antigen and target of the adaptive immune response in systemic sarcoidosis. J Exp Med. 2005;201(5):755-67.
56. Oswald-Richter K, Sato H, Hajizadeh R, et al. Mycobacterial ESAT-6 and katG are recognized by sarcoidosis CD4+ T cells when presented by the American sarcoidosis susceptibility allele, DRB1*1101. J Clin Immunol. 2010;30(1):157-66.
57. Agarwal R, Gupta D, Srinivas R, Verma I, Aggarwal AN, Laal S. Analysis of humoral responses to proteins encoded by region of difference 1 of *Mycobacterium tuberculosis* in sarcoidosis in a high tuberculosis prevalence country. Indian J Med Res. 2012;135(6):920-3.
58. Goyal B, Kumar K, Gupta D, et al. Utility of B-cell epitopes based peptides of RD1 and RD2 antigens for immunodiagnosis of pulmonary tuberculosis. Diagn Microbiol Infect Dis. 2014;78(4):391-7.
59. Dubaniewicz A. *Mycobacterium tuberculosis* heat shock proteins and autoimmunity in sarcoidosis. Autoimmun Rev. 2010;9(6):419-24.
60. Almenoff PL, Johnson A, Lesser M, et a;. Growth of acid fast L forms from the blood of patients with sarcoidosis. Thorax. 1996;51(5):530-3.
61. Rybicki BA, Hirst K, Iyengar SK, et al. A sarcoidosis genetic linkage consortium: the sarcoidosis genetic analysis (SAGA) study. Sarcoidosis Vasc Diffuse Lung Dis. 2005;22(2):115-22.
62. Schurmann M. Genetics of sarcoidosis. Semin Respir Crit Care Med. 2003;24(2):213-22.
63. Grunewald J, Eklund A. Role of CD4+ T cells in sarcoidosis. Proc Am Thorac Soc. 2007;4(5):461-4.
64. Agostini C, Adami F, Semenzato G. New pathogenetic insights into the sarcoid granuloma. Curr Opin Rheumatol. 2000;12(1):71-6.
65. Hunninghake GW, Crystal RG. Pulmonary sarcoidosis: a disorder mediated by excess helper T-lymphocyte activity at sites of disease activity. N Engl J Med. 1981;305(8):429-34.
66. Semenzato G, Pezzutto A, Chilosi M, et al. Redistribution of T lymphocytes in the lymph nodes of patients with sarcoidosis. N Engl J Med. 1982;306(1):48-9.
67. Silver RF, Crystal RG, Moller DR. Limited heterogeneity of biased T-cell receptor V beta gene usage in lung but not blood T cells in active pulmonary sarcoidosis. Immunology. 1996;88(4):516-23.
68. Konishi K, Moller DR, Saltini C, et al. Spontaneous expression of the interleukin 2 receptor gene and presence of functional interleukin 2 receptors on T lymphocytes in the blood of individuals with active pulmonary sarcoidosis. J Clin Invest. 1988;82(3):775-81.
69. Robinson BW, McLemore TL, Crystal RG. Gamma interferon is spontaneously released by alveolar macrophages and lung T lymphocytes in patients with pulmonary sarcoidosis. J Clin Invest. 1985;75(5):1488-95.
70. Baughman RP, Strohofer SA, Buchsbaum J, et al. Release of tumor necrosis factor by alveolar macrophages of patients with sarcoidosis. J Lab Clin Med. 1990;115(1):36-42.
71. Moller DR, Forman JD, Liu MC, et al. Enhanced expression of IL-12 associated with Th1 cytokine profiles in active pulmonary sarcoidosis. J Immunol. 1996;156(12):4952-60.
72. Agostini C, Trentin L, Facco M, et al. Role of IL-15, IL-2, and their receptors in the development of T cell alveolitis in pulmonary sarcoidosis. J Immunol. 1996;157(2):910-8.
73. Kreipe H, Radzun HJ, Heidorn K, et al. Proliferation, macrophage colony-stimulating factor, and macrophage colony-stimulating factor-receptor expression of alveolar macrophages in active sarcoidosis. Lab Invest. 1990;62(6):697-703.
74. Girgis RE, Basha MA, Maliarik M, et al. Cytokines in the bronchoalveolar lavage fluid of patients with active pulmonary sarcoidosis. Am J Respir Crit Care Med. 1995;152(1):71-5.
75. Shigehara K, Shijubo N, Ohmichi M, et al. IL-12 and IL-18 are increased and stimulate IFN-gamma production in sarcoid lungs. J Immunol. 2001;166(1):642-9.
76. Pinkston P, Bitterman PB, Crystal RG. Spontaneous release of interleukin-2 by lung T lymphocytes in active pulmonary sarcoidosis. N Engl J Med. 1983;308(14):793-800.
77. Hunninghake GW, Bedell GN, Zavala DC, et al. Role of interleukin-2 release by lung T-cells in active pulmonary sarcoidosis. Am Rev Respir Dis. 1983;128(4):634-8.
78. Bingisser R, Speich R, Zollinger A, et al. Interleukin-10 secretion by alveolar macrophages and monocytes in sarcoidosis. Respiration. 2000;67(3):280-6.
79. Dhooria S, Gupta D. Oxidative stress in sarcoidosis. In: Ganguly NK (Ed). Studies on Respiratory Disorders. New York: Springer; 2014. pp. 191-201.
80. Rizzi L, Sabbà C, Suppressa P. Sarcoidosis and autoimmunity: In the depth of a complex relationship. Front Med (Lausanne). 2022;9:991394.
81. Song M, Manansala M, Parmar PJ, et al. Sarcoidosis and autoimmunity. Curr Opin Pulm Med. 2021;27(5):448-54.
82. d'Alessandro M. Editorial: Sarcoidosis and autoimmunity: From bench to bedside. Front Med (Lausanne). 2023;10:1147529.
83. Papadopoulos KI, Hallengren B. Autoimmunity in sarcoidosis: the tip of the Iceberg. Clin Exp Med. 2023;23(3):951-3.
84. Miyara M, Amoura Z, Parizot C, et al. The immune paradox of sarcoidosis and regulatory T cells. J Exp Med. 2006;203(2):359-70.
85. Hudspith BN, Flint KC, Geraint-James D, Brostoff J, Johnson NM. Lack of immune deficiency in sarcoidosis: compartmentalisation of the immune response. Thorax. 1987;42(4):250-5.
86. Mathew S, Bauer KL, Fischoeder A, et al. The anergic state in sarcoidosis is associated with diminished dendritic cell function. J Immunol. 2008;181(1):746-55.

87. Takemura T, Matsui Y, Saiki S, et al. Pulmonary vascular involvement in sarcoidosis: a report of 40 autopsy cases. Hum Pathol. 1992;23(11):1216-23.
88. Perry A, Vuitch F. Causes of death in patients with sarcoidosis. A morphologic study of 38 autopsies with clinicopathologic correlations. Arch Pathol Lab Med. 1995;119(2):167-72.
89. Longcope WT, Freiman DG. A study of sarcoidosis; based on a combined investigation of 160 cases including 30 autopsies from The Johns Hopkins Hospital and Massachusetts General Hospital. Medicine (Baltimore). 1952;31(1):1-132.
90. Iwai K, Takemura T, Kitaichi M, et al. Pathological studies on sarcoidosis autopsy. II. Early change, mode of progression and death pattern. Acta Pathol Jpn. 1993;43(7-8):377-85.
91. Kitaichi M. Pathology of pulmonary sarcoidosis. Clin Dermatol. 1986;4(4):108-15.
92. Rosen Y. Pathology of sarcoidosis. Semin Respir Crit Care Med. 2007;28(1):36-52.
93. Sheffield EA. Pathology of sarcoidosis. Clin Chest Med. 1997;18(4):741-54.
94. Ma Y, Gal A, Koss MN. The pathology of pulmonary sarcoidosis: update. Semin Diagn Pathol. 2007;24(3):150-61.
95. Churg A, Carrington CB, Gupta R. Necrotizing sarcoid granulomatosis. Chest. 1979;76(4):406-13.
96. Hoang DQ, Nguyen ET. Sarcoidosis. Semin Roentgenol. 2010; 45(1):36-42.
97. Sones M, Israel HL. Course and prognosis of sarcoidosis. Am J Med. 1960;29:84-93.
98. Wurm K. The significance of stage classification of sarcoidosis (Boeck's disease). Dtsch Med Wochenschr. 1960;85:1541-8.
99. Mana J, Salazar A, Manresa F. Clinical factors predicting persistence of activity in sarcoidosis: a multivariate analysis of 193 cases. Respiration. 1994;61(4):219-25.
100. Winterbauer RH, Belic N, Moores KD. Clinical interpretation of bilateral hilar adenopathy. Ann Intern Med. 1973;78(1):65-71.
101. Judson MA. Sarcoidosis: clinical presentation, diagnosis, and approach to treatment. Am J Med Sci. 2008;335(1):26-33.
102. Nishino M, Lee KS, Itoh H, et al. The spectrum of pulmonary sarcoidosis: variations of high-resolution CT findings and clues for specific diagnosis. Eur J Radiol. 2010;73(1):66-73.
103. Dawson WB, Muller NL. High-resolution computed tomography in pulmonary sarcoidosis. Semin Ultrasound CT MR. 1990; 11(5):423-9.
104. Nakatsu M, Hatabu H, Morikawa K, et al. Large coalescent parenchymal nodules in pulmonary sarcoidosis: "sarcoid galaxy" sign. AJR Am J Roentgenol. 2002;178(6):1389-93.
105. Handa A, Dhooria S, Sehgal IS, et al. Primary cavitary sarcoidosis: A case report, systematic review, and proposal of new diagnostic criteria. Lung India. 2018;35(1):41-6.
106. Marchiori E, Zanetti G, Hochhegger B, et al. Sarcoid cluster sign and the reversed halo sign: Extending the spectrum of radiographic manifestations in sarcoidosis. Eur J Radiol. 2011;80(2):567-8.
107. Nishimura K, Itoh H, Kitaichi M, et al. Pulmonary sarcoidosis: correlation of CT and histopathologic findings. Radiology. 1993;189(1):105-9.
108. Desai SR, Sivarasan N, Johannson KA, et al. High-resolution CT phenotypes in pulmonary sarcoidosis: a multinational Delphi consensus study. Lancet Respir Med. 2024;12(5):409-18
109. Winterbauer RH, Hutchinson JF. Use of pulmonary function tests in the management of sarcoidosis. Chest. 1980;78(4): 640-7.
110. Madan K, Sryma PB, Pattnaik B, et al. Clinical Profile of 327 patients with Sarcoidosis in India: An Ambispective Cohort Study in a Tuberculosis (TB) Endemic Population. Lung India. 2022;39(1):51-7.
111. Baydur A, Pandya K, Sharma OP, et al. Control of ventilation, respiratory muscle strength, and granulomatous involvement of skeletal muscle in patients with sarcoidosis. Chest. 1993;103(2):396-402.
112. Baydur A, Alsalek M, Louie SG, et al. Respiratory muscle strength, lung function, and dyspnea in patients with sarcoidosis. Chest. 2001;120(1):102-8.
113. Huang CT, Heurich AE, Rosen Y, et al. Pulmonary sarcoidosis: roentgenographic, functional, and pathologic correlations. Respiration. 1979;37(6):337-45.
114. Gupta D, Jorapur V, Bambery P, et al. Pulmonary sarcoidosis: spirometric correlation with transbronchial biopsy. Sarcoidosis Vasc Diffuse Lung Dis. 1997;14(1):77-80.
115. Bergin CJ, Bell DY, Coblentz CL, et al. Sarcoidosis: correlation of pulmonary parenchymal pattern at CT with results of pulmonary function tests. Radiology. 1989;171(3):619-24.
116. Shorr AF, Helman DL, Davies DB, et al. Pulmonary hypertension in advanced sarcoidosis: epidemiology and clinical characteristics. Eur Respir J. 2005;25(5):783-8.
117. Handa T, Nagai S, Miki S, et al. Incidence of pulmonary hypertension and its clinical relevance in patients with sarcoidosis. Chest. 2006;129(5):1246-52.
118. Huggins JT, Doelken P, Sahn SA, et al. Pleural effusions in a series of 181 outpatients with sarcoidosis. Chest. 2006;129(6): 1599-604.
119. Salerno D. Sarcoidosis pleural effusion: a not so common feature of a well known pulmonary disease. Respir Care. 2010;55(4): 478-80.
120. Soskel NT, Sharma OP. Pleural involvement in sarcoidosis. Curr Opin Pulm Med. 2000;6(5):455-68.
121. Jarman PR, Whyte MK, Sabroe I, et al. Sarcoidosis presenting with chylothorax. Thorax. 1995;50(12):1324-5.
122. Rockoff SD, Rohatgi PK. Unusual manifestations of thoracic sarcoidosis. AJR Am J Roentgenol. 1985;144(3):513-28.
123. Szwarcberg JB, Glajchen N, Teirstein AS. Pleural involvement in chronic sarcoidosis detected by thoracic CT scanning. Sarcoidosis Vasc Diffuse Lung Dis. 2005;22(1):58-62.
124. Lemay V, Carette MF, Parrot A, et al. Hemoptysis in sarcoidosis. Apropos of 6 cases including 4 with fatal outcome. Rev Pneumol Clin. 1995;51(2):61-70.
125. Koss MN, Hochholzer L, Feigin DS, et al. Necrotizing sarcoid-like granulomatosis: clinical, pathologic, and immunopathologic findings. Hum Pathol. 1980;11(5 Suppl):510-9.
126. Gordonson J, Trachtenberg S, Sargent EN. Superior vena cava obstruction due to sarcoidosis. Chest. 1973;63(2):292-3.
127. Hietala SO, Stinnett RG, Faunce HF 3rd, et al. Pulmonary artery narrowing in sarcoidosis. JAMA. 1977;237(6):572-3.
128. Miller A. The vanishing lung syndrome associated with pulmonary sarcoidosis. Br J Dis Chest. 1981;75(2):209-14.
129. Sharma SK, Mohan A. Uncommon manifestations of sarcoidosis. J Assoc Physicians India. 2004;52:210-4.
130. Sharma OP. Fatigue and sarcoidosis. Eur Respir J. 1999;13(4): 713-4.
131. Caplan A, Rosenbach M, Imadojemu S. Cutaneous Sarcoidosis. Semin Respir Crit Care Med. 2020;41(5):689-99.
132. Sève P, Jamilloux Y, Tilikete C, et al. Ocular Sarcoidosis. Semin Respir Crit Care Med. 2020;41(5):673-88.

133. Stievenart J, Le Guenno G, Ruivard M, et al. Cardiac sarcoidosis: systematic review of the literature on corticosteroid and immunosuppressive therapies. Eur Respir J. 2022;59(5):2100449.
134. Patel R, Mistry AM, Mulukutla V, et al. Cardiac Sarcoidosis: A Literature Review of Current Recommendations on Diagnosis and Management. Cureus. 2023;15(7):e41451.
135. Sharma OP, Sharma AM. Sarcoidosis of the nervous system. A clinical approach. Arch Intern Med. 1991;151(7):1317-21.
136. Stern BJ, Aksamit A, Clifford D, et al. Neurologic presentations of sarcoidosis. Neurol Clin. 2010;28(1):185-98.
137. Chen RC, McLeod JG. Neurological complications of sarcoidosis. Clin Exp Neurol. 1989;26:99-112.
138. Stern BJ. Neurological complications of sarcoidosis. Curr Opin Neurol. 2004;17(3):311-6.
139. Gupta D, Gupta ML, Ghosh D, et al. Sarcoidosis presenting as multifocal remitting and relapsing neurological illness: A diagnostic dilemma. Neurol India. 1995;43:219-21.
140. Sharma OP. Hypercalcemia in granulomatous disorders: a clinical review. Curr Opin Pulm Med. 2000;6(5):442-7.
141. Burke RR, Rybicki BA, Rao DS. Calcium and vitamin D in sarcoidosis: how to assess and manage. Semin Respir Crit Care Med. 2010;31(4):474-84.
142. Bell NH, Stern PH, Pantzer E, et al. Evidence that increased circulating 1 alpha, 25-dihydroxyvitamin D is the probable cause for abnormal calcium metabolism in sarcoidosis. J Clin Invest. 1979;64(1):218-25.
143. Conron M, Young C, Beynon HL. Calcium metabolism in sarcoidosis and its clinical implications. Rheumatology (Oxford). 2000;39(7):707-13.
144. Zeimer HJ, Greenaway TM, Slavin J, et al. Parathyroid-hormone-related protein in sarcoidosis. Am J Pathol. 1998;152(1):17-21.
145. Muller-Quernheim J. Sarcoidosis: immunopathogenetic concepts and their clinical application. Eur Respir J. 1998;12(3):716-38.
146. Gupta D, Agarwal R, Singh A, et al. A "respiratory" cause of abdominal pain. Eur Respir J. 2006;27(2):430-3.
147. Rizzato G, Montemurro L. The clinical spectrum of the sarcoid peripheral lymph node. Sarcoidosis Vasc Diffuse Lung Dis. 2000;17(1):71-80.
148. Giovinale M, Fonnesu C, Soriano A, et al. Atypical sarcoidosis: case reports and review of the literature. Eur Rev Med Pharmacol Sci. 2009;13(Suppl 1):37-44.
149. Sharma OP. Sarcoidosis of the upper respiratory tract. Selected cases emphasizing diagnostic and therapeutic difficulties. Sarcoidosis Vasc Diffuse Lung Dis. 2002;19(3):227-33.
150. Sarnaik RM, Nair N, Guleria R, et al. Sarcoidosis in two brothers, manifesting in one with vocal cord palsy. Lung India. 1992;11(4):147-8.
151. Vatti R, Sharma OP. Course of asymptomatic liver involvement in sarcoidosis: role of therapy in selected cases. Sarcoidosis Vasc Diffuse Lung Dis. 1997;14(1):73-6.
152. James DG, Sherlock S. Sarcoidosis of the liver. Sarcoidosis. 1994;11(1):2-6.
153. Ebert EC, Kierson M, Hagspiel KD. Gastrointestinal and hepatic manifestations of sarcoidosis. Am J Gastroenterol. 2008;103(12):3184-92; quiz 3193.
154. Karagiannidis A, Karavalaki M, Koulaouzidis A. Hepatic sarcoidosis. Ann Hepatol. 2006;5(4):251-6.
155. Kahi CJ, Saxena R, Temkit M, et al. Hepatobiliary disease in sarcoidosis. Sarcoidosis Vasc Diffuse Lung Dis. 2006;23(2):117-23.
156. Warshauer DM. Splenic sarcoidosis. Semin Ultrasound CT MR. 2007;28(1):21-7.
157. Perez-Grueso MJ, Repiso A, Gomez R, et al. Splenic focal lesions as manifestation of sarcoidosis: Characterization with contrast-enhanced sonography. J Clin Ultrasound. 2007;35(7):405-8.
158. Kessler A, Mitchell DG, Israel HL, et al. Hepatic and splenic sarcoidosis: ultrasound and MR imaging. Abdom Imaging. 1993;18(2):159-63.
159. Kataria YP, Whitcomb ME. Splenomegaly in sarcoidosis. Arch Intern Med. 1980;140(1):35-7.
160. Yanardag H, Pamuk ON. Bone cysts in sarcoidosis: what is their clinical significance? Rheumatol Int. 2004;24(5):294-6.
161. Mana J, Gomez-Vaquero C, Montero A, et al. Lofgren's syndrome revisited: a study of 186 patients. Am J Med. 1999;107(3):240-5.
162. Grigor RR, Hughes GR. Chronic sarcoid arthritis. Br Med J. 1976;2(6043):1044.
163. Torralba KD, Quismorio FP, Jr. Sarcoid arthritis: a review of clinical features, pathology and therapy. Sarcoidosis Vasc Diffuse Lung Dis. 2003;20(2):95-103.
164. Crouser ED, Maier LA, Wilson KC, et al. Diagnosis and Detection of Sarcoidosis. An Official American Thoracic Society Clinical Practice Guideline. Am J Respir Crit Care Med. 2020;201(8):e26-e51.
165. Teirstein AS, Judson MA, Baughman RP, et al. The spectrum of biopsy sites for the diagnosis of sarcoidosis. Sarcoidosis Vasc Diffuse Lung Dis. 2005;22(2):139-46.
166. Jindal SK, Gupta D. Incidence and recognition of interstitial pulmonary fibrosis in developing countries. Curr Opin Pulm Med. 1997;3(5):378-83.
167. Gupta D, Behera D, Joshi K, et al. Role of fiberoptic bronchoscopy (transbronchial lung biopsy) in diagnosis of parenchymatous lung diseases J Assoc Physicians India. 1997;45:371-3.
168. Jindal SK, Gupta D, Aggarwal AN. Sarcoidosis in developing countries. Curr Opin Pulm Med. 2000;6(5):448-54.
169. Gilman MJ. Transbronchial biopsy in sarcoidosis. Chest. 1983;83(1):159.
170. Oki M, Saka H, Kitagawa C, et al. Prospective study of endobronchial ultrasound-guided transbronchial needle aspiration of lymph nodes versus transbronchial lung biopsy of lung tissue for diagnosis of sarcoidosis. J Thorac Cardiovasc Surg. 2012;143(6):1324-9.
171. Goyal A, Gupta D, Agarwal R, Bal A, et al. Value of different bronchoscopic sampling techniques in diagnosis of sarcoidosis: a prospective study of 151 patients. J Bronchology Interv Pulmonol. 2014;21(3):220-6.
172. Gupta D, Dadhwal DS, Agarwal R, et al. Endobronchial Ultrasound Guided TBNA vs. Conventional TBNA in the diagnosis of sarcoidosis. Chest. 2014;146(3):547-56.
173. Sehgal IS, Bal A, Dhooria S, et al. A Prospective Randomized Controlled Trial Comparing the Efficacy and Safety of Cup vs Alligator Forceps for Performing Transbronchial Lung Biopsy in Patients with Sarcoidosis. Chest. 2016;149(6):1584-6.
174. Sehgal IS, Bal A, Dhooria S, et al. Predictors of Successful Yield of Transbronchial Lung Biopsy in Patients with Sarcoidosis. J Bronchology Interv Pulmonol. 2018;25(1):31-6.
175. Gupta D, Mahendran C, Aggarwal AN, et al. Endobronchial vis a vis transbronchial involvement on fiberoptic bronchoscopy in sarcoidosis. Sarcoidosis Vasc Diffuse Lung Dis. 2001;18(1):91-2.
176. Dhooria S, Sehgal IS, Bal A, et al. Utility of Narrow-band Imaging Bronchoscopy in the Diagnosis of Endobronchial Sarcoidosis. J Bronchol Interv Pulmonol. 2023;30(4):346-53.

177. Dhooria S, Rathi K, Agarwal R, et al. A randomised controlled trial of narrow-band imaging vs. white light bronchoscopy-guided endobronchial biopsy in suspected sarcoidosis (NABS). Eur Respir J. 2023;62:PA5222;
178. Dhooria S, Bal A, Sehgal IS, et al. Transbronchial lung biopsy with a flexible cryoprobe: First case report from India. Lung India. 2016;33(1):64-8.
179. Dhooria S, Sehgal IS, Aggarwal AN, et al. Diagnostic Yield and Safety of Cryoprobe Transbronchial Lung Biopsy in Diffuse Parenchymal Lung Diseases: Systematic Review and Meta-Analysis. Respir Care. 2016;61(5):700-12.
180. Dhooria S, Sehgal IS, Bal A, et al. Transbronchial lung biopsy with a flexible cryoprobe during rigid bronchoscopy: Standardizing the procedure. Lung India. 2016;33(2):248-9.
181. Dhooria S, Sehgal IS, Prasad KT, et al. Transbronchial Lung Cryobiopsy with 2 Bronchoscopes: nec novum nec magna. J Bronchol Interv Pulmonol. 2018;25(1):e11-2.
182. Dhooria S, Agarwal R, Sehgal IS, et al. Bronchoscopic lung cryobiopsy: An Indian association for bronchology position statement. Lung India. 2019;36(1):48-59.
183. Dhooria S, Mehta RM, Srinivasan A, et al. The safety and efficacy of different methods for obtaining transbronchial lung cryobiopsy in diffuse lung diseases. Clin Respir J. 2018;12(4):1711-20.
184. Aragaki-Nakahodo AA, Baughman RP, Shipley RT, et al. The complimentary role of transbronchial lung cryobiopsy and endobronchial ultrasound fine needle aspiration in the diagnosis of sarcoidosis. Respir Med. 2017;131:65-9.
185. Khan A, Agarwal R, Aggarwal AN, et al. Blind transbronchial needle aspiration without an on-site cytopathologist: experience of 473 procedures. Natl Med J India. 2011;24(3):136-9.
186. Sehgal IS, Dhooria S, Gupta N, et al. Factors Determining Successful Diagnostic Yield of Conventional Transbronchial Needle Aspiration in the Diagnosis of Sarcoidosis. J Bronchology Interv Pulmonol. 2016;23(1):e1-3.
187. Sehgal IS, Dhooria S, Gupta N, et al. Impact of Endobronchial Ultrasound (EBUS) Training on the Diagnostic Yield of Conventional Transbronchial Needle Aspiration for Lymph Node Stations 4R and 7. PLoS One. 2016;11(4):e0153793.
188. Agarwal R, Aggarwal AN, Gupta D. Efficacy and safety of conventional transbronchial needle aspiration in sarcoidosis: a systematic review and meta-analysis. Respir Care. 2013;58(4):683-93.
189. von Bartheld MB, Dekkers OM, Szlubowski A, et al. Endosonography vs conventional bronchoscopy for the diagnosis of sarcoidosis: the GRANULOMA randomized clinical trial. JAMA. 2013;309(23):2457-64.
190. Dhooria S, Agarwal R, Gupta D. Conventional bronchoscopic techniques in sarcoidosis: not too far behind. Thorax. 2015;70(6):587.
191. Muthu V, Gupta N, Dhooria S, et al. A Prospective, Randomized, Double-Blind Trial Comparing the Diagnostic Yield of 21- and 22-Gauge Aspiration Needles for Performing Endobronchial Ultrasound-Guided Transbronchial Needle Aspiration in Sarcoidosis. Chest. 2016;149(4):1111-3.
192. Dhooria S, Sehgal IS, Gupta N, et al. A Randomized Trial Evaluating the Effect of 10 versus 20 Revolutions Inside the Lymph Node on the Diagnostic Yield of EBUS-TBNA in Subjects with Sarcoidosis. Respiration. 2018;96(5):464-71.
193. Dhooria S, Sehgal IS, Prasad KT, et al. Diagnostic yield and safety of the ProCore versus the standard EBUS-TBNA needle in subjects with suspected sarcoidosis. Expert Rev Med Devices. 2021;18(2):211-6.
194. Mohapatra DS, Gupta P, Gupta N, et al. Evaluation of the Utility of Liquid-based Cytology, Cell-blocks, and Flow Cytometric Immunophenotyping on Endobronchial Ultrasound-guided Transbronchial Needle Aspiration Samples in the Diagnosis of Sarcoidosis. J Bronchology Interv Pulmonol. 2022;29(4):260-8.
195. Gupta D, Chetty M, Kumar N, et al. Anergy to tuberculin in sarcoidosis is not influenced by high prevalence of tuberculin sensitivity in the population. Sarcoidosis Vasc Diffuse Lung Dis. 2003;20(1):40-5.
196. Lieberman J. Elevation of serum angiotensin-converting-enzyme (ACE) level in sarcoidosis. Am J Med. 1975;59(3):365-72.
197. Gupta SK. Markers of activity in sarcoidosis with a special reference to serum angiotensin converting enzyme (SACE). Indian J Chest Dis Allied Sci. 1993;35(3):117-27.
198. Sainani GS, Mahbubani V, Trikannad V. Serum angiotensin converting enzyme activity in sarcoidosis and pulmonary tuberculosis. J Assoc Physicians India. 1996;44(1):29-30.
199. Shorr AF, Torrington KG, Parker JM. Serum angiotensin converting enzyme does not correlate with radiographic stage at initial diagnosis of sarcoidosis. Respir Med. 1997;91(7):399-401.
200. Silverstein E, Brunswick J, Rao TK, et al. Increased serum angiotensin-converting enzyme in chronic renal disease. Nephron. 1984;37(3):206-10.
201. Studdy PR, Bird R. Serum angiotensin converting enzyme in sarcoidosis--its value in present clinical practice. Ann Clin Biochem. 1989;26(Pt 1):13-8.
202. Brice EA, Friedlander W, Bateman ED, et al. Serum angiotensin-converting enzyme activity, concentration, and specific activity in granulomatous interstitial lung disease, tuberculosis, and COPD. Chest. 1995;107(3):706-10.
203. Kruit A, Ruven HJ, Grutters JC, et al. Angiotensin-converting enzyme 2 (ACE2) haplotypes are associated with pulmonary disease phenotypes in sarcoidosis patients. Sarcoidosis Vasc Diffuse Lung Dis. 2005;22(3):195-203.
204. Kruit A, Grutters JC, Gerritsen WB, et al. ACE I/D-corrected Z-scores to identify normal and elevated ACE activity in sarcoidosis. Respir Med. 2007;101(3):510-5.
205. Floe A, Hoffmann HJ, Nissen PH, et al. Genotyping increases the yield of angiotensin-converting enzyme in sarcoidosis--a systematic review. Dan Med J. 2014;61(5):A4815.
206. Schimmelpennink MC, Quanjel M, Vorselaars A, et al. Value of serum soluble interleukin-2 receptor as a diagnostic and predictive biomarker in sarcoidosis. Expert Rev Respir Med. 2020;14(7):749-56.
207. Qin D, Fan LL, Zhong Y, Shen Y, et al. Diagnostic accuracy of interleukin-2 receptor in sarcoidosis: a systematic review and meta-analysis. Expert Rev Respir Med. 2023;17(6):495-505.
208. Winterbauer RH, Lammert J, Selland M, et al. Bronchoalveolar lavage cell populations in the diagnosis of sarcoidosis. Chest. 1993;104(2):352-61.
209. Costabel U, Bonella F, Ohshimo S, et al. Diagnostic modalities in sarcoidosis: BAL, EBUS, and PET. Semin Respir Crit Care Med. 2010;31(4):404-8.
210. Munro CS, Mitchell DN. The K veim response: still useful, still a puzzle. Thorax. 1987;42(5):321-31.
211. Siltzbach LE, Ehrlich JC. The Nickerson-Kveim reaction in sarcoidosis. Am J Med. 1954;16(6):790-803.
212. Siltzbach LE. The Kveim test in sarcoidosis. A study of 750 patients. JAMA. 1961;178:476-82.

213. Siltzbach LE. Qualities and behavior of satisfactory Kveim suspensions. Ann N Y Acad Sci. 1976;278:665-9.
214. Costabel U, Ohshimo S, Guzman J. Diagnosis of sarcoidosis. Curr Opin Pulm Med. 2008;14(5):455-61.
215. Treglia G, Taralli S, Giordano A. Emerging role of whole-body 18F-fluorodeoxyglucose positron emission tomography as a marker of disease activity in patients with sarcoidosis: a systematic review. Sarcoidosis Vasc Diffuse Lung Dis. 2011; 28(2):87-94.
216. Jung RS, Mittal BR, Maturu NV, et al. Ocular sarcoidosis: does (18)F-FDG PET/CT have any role? Clin Nucl Med. 2014;39(5): 464-6.
217. Sobic-Saranovic D, Artiko V, Obradovic V. FDG PET imaging in sarcoidosis. Semin Nucl Med. 2013;43(6):404-11.
218. Maturu VN, Agarwal R, Aggarwal AN, et al. Dual time point whole body 18F-FDG PET/CT in undiagnosed mediastinal lymphadenopathy-A prospective study of 117 patients with sarcoidosis and tuberculosis. Chest. 2014;146(6):e216-20.
219. Kaira K, Oriuchi N, Otani Y, et al. Diagnostic usefulness of fluorine-18-alpha-methyltyrosine positron emission tomography in combination with 18F fluorodeoxyglucose in sarcoidosis patients. Chest. 2007;131(4):1019-27.
220. Keir G, Wells AU. Assessing pulmonary disease and response to therapy: which test? Semin Respir Crit Care Med. 2010;31(4): 409-18.
221. Costabel U, Du Bois RD, Eklund A. Consensus conference: activity of sarcoidosis. Sarcoidosis. 1994;11(1):27-33.
222. Muller-Quernheim J. Serum markers for the staging of disease activity of sarcoidosis and other interstitial lung diseases of unknown etiology. Sarcoidosis Vasc Diffuse Lung Dis. 1998; 15(1):22-37.
223. Drent M, Jacobs JA, de Vries J, et al. Does the cellular bronchoalveolar lavage fluid profile reflect the severity of sarcoidosis? Eur Respir J. 1999;13(6):1338-44.
224. Costabel U, Teschler H. Biochemical changes in sarcoidosis. Clin Chest Med. 1997;18(4):827-42.
225. Keijsers RG, van den Heuvel DA, Grutters JC. Imaging the inflammatory activity of sarcoidosis. Eur Respir J. 2013;41(3): 743-51.
226. Sharma OP. Murray Kornfeld, American College of Chest Physician, and sarcoidosis: a historical footnote: 2004 Murray Kornfeld Memorial Founders Lecture. Chest. 2005;128(3): 1830-5.
227. Hadley GD, Emanuel RW. Diagnostic problems. No. 3. Tuberculosis and sarcoidosis? Arch Middx Hosp. 1951;1(4):288-91.
228. Lees AW. Tuberculin-negative tuberculosis presenting as sarcoidosis. Lancet. 1956;271(6944):656-8.
229. Editorial: Sarcoidosis and tuberculosis. Br Med J. 1974;4(5937): 124-5.
230. Gupta D, Agarwal R, Aggarwal AN, et al. Sarcoidosis and tuberculosis: the same disease with different manifestations or similar manifestations of different disorders. Curr Opin Pulm Med. 2012;18(5):506-16.
231. Hosoda Y, Hiraga Y, Odaka M, et al. A cooperative study of sarcoidosis in Asia and Africa: analytic epidemiology. Ann N Y Acad Sci. 1976;278:355-67.
232. Gupta D, Vinay N, Agarwal R, et al. Socio-demographic profile of patients with sarcoidosis vis-a-vis tuberculosis. Sarcoidosis Vasc Diffuse Lung Dis. 2013;30(3):186-93.
233. Woodring JH, Vandiviere HM, Fried AM, et al. Update: the radiographic features of pulmonary tuberculosis. AJR Am J Roentgenol. 1986;146(3):497-506.
234. Dhooria S, Agarwal R, Aggarwal AN, et al. Differentiating tuberculosis from sarcoidosis by sonographic characteristics of lymph nodes on endobronchial ultrasonography: A study of 165 patients. J Thorac Cardiovasc Surg. 2014;148(2):662-7.
235. Gupta N, Muthu V, Agarwal R, et al. Role of EBUS-TBNA in the Diagnosis of Tuberculosis and Sarcoidosis. J Cytol. 2019;36(2):128-30.
236. DeRemee RA. The roentgenographic staging of sarcoidosis. Historic and contemporary perspectives. Chest. 1983;83(1): 128-33.
237. Chugh IM, Agarwal AK, Arora VK, et al. Bilateral miliary pattern in sarcoidosis. Indian J Chest Dis Allied Sci. 1997;39(4):245-9.
238. Gupta D, Kumar S, Jindal SK. Bilateral miliary mottling without hilar lymphadenopathy: a rare presentation of sarcoidosis. Lung India. 1996;14:87-8.
239. Sharma SK, Mohan A, Pande JN, et al. Clinical profile, laboratory characteristics and outcome in miliary tuberculosis. QJM. 1995;88(1):29-37.
240. Israel HL, Sones M. Sarcoidosis, tuberculosis, and tuberculin anergy. A prospective study. Am Rev Respir Dis. 1966;94(6): 887-95.
241. Tuberculosis Prevention Trial. Trial of BCG vaccines in south India for tuberculosis prevention. Indian J Med Res. 1979;70: 349-63.
242. Tuberculosis Prevention Trial. Trial of BCG vaccines in south India for tuberculosis prevention: first report—Tuberculosis Prevention Trial. Bull World Health Organ. 1979;57(5):819-27.
243. Gupta D, Saiprakash BV, Aggarwal AN, et al. Value of different cut-off points of tuberculin skin test to diagnose tuberculosis among patients with respiratory symptoms in a chest clinic. J Assoc Physicians India. 2001;49:332-5.
244. Lee SS, Liu YC, Huang TS, et al. Comparison of the interferon-gamma release assay and the tuberculin skin test for contact investigation of tuberculosis in BCG-vaccinated health care workers. Scand J Infect Dis. 2008;40(5):373-80.
245. Gupta D, Kumar S, Aggarwal AN, et al. Interferon gamma release assay (QuantiFERON-TB Gold In Tube) in patients of sarcoidosis from a population with high prevalence of tuberculosis infection. Sarcoidosis Vasc Diffuse Lung Dis. 2011;28(2):95-101.
246. Gupta D, Kumar S, Verma I, et al. Interferon Gamma Release Assay (IGRA) in Sarcoidosis Patients from A High Tuberculosis (TB) Prevalence Country. Am J Respir Crit Care Med. 2010; 181:A2366.
247. Muthu V, Gupta N, Dhooria S, et al. Role of cytomorphology in differentiating sarcoidosis and tuberculosis in subjects undergoing endobronchial ultrasound-guided transbronchial needle aspiration. Sarcoidosis Vasc Diffuse Lung Dis. 2019; 36(3):209-16.
248. Tabak L, Agirbas E, Yilmazbayhan D, et al. The value of labial biopsy in the differentiation of sarcoidosis from tuberculosis. Sarcoidosis Vasc Diffuse Lung Dis. 2001;18(2):191-5.
249. Smith-Rohrberg D, Sharma SK. Tuberculin skin test among pulmonary sarcoidosis patients with and without tuberculosis: its utility for the screening of the two conditions in tuberculosis-endemic regions. Sarcoidosis Vasc Diffuse Lung Dis. 2006; 23(2):130-4.
250. Karpathiou G, Batistatou A, Boglou P, et al. Necrotizing sarcoid granulomatosis: A distinctive form of pulmonary granulomatous disease. Clin Respir J. 2018;12(4):1313-9.
251. Costabel U, Hunninghake GW. ATS/ERS/WASOG statement on sarcoidosis. Sarcoidosis Statement Committee. American Thoracic Society. European Respiratory Society. World

Association for Sarcoidosis and Other Granulomatous Disorders. Eur Respir J. 1999;14(4):735-7.
252. Baughman RP, Valeyre D, Korsten P, et al. ERS clinical practice guidelines on treatment of sarcoidosis. Eur Respir J. 2021;58(6):34140301.
253. Thillai M, Atkins CP, Crawshaw A, et al. BTS Clinical Statement on pulmonary sarcoidosis. Thorax. 2021;76(1):4-20.
254. Dhooria S, Sehgal IS, Agarwal R. Reply: A suggested classification of disease behaviour and treatment response in sarcoidosis trials. Eur Respir J. 2024;63(1):2302208.
255. Israel HL, Sones M, Harrell D. Cortisone treatment of sarcoidosis: experience with thirty-six cases. J Am Med Assoc. 1954;156(5):461-6.
256. Schutt AC, Bullington WM, Judson MA. Pharmacotherapy for pulmonary sarcoidosis: A Delphi consensus study. Respir Med. 2010;104(5):717-23.
257. Paramothayan NS, Lasserson TJ, Jones PW. Corticosteroids for pulmonary sarcoidosis. Cochrane Database Syst Rev. 2005;(2):CD001114.
258. Gonzalez-Perez O, Luquin S, Garcia-Estrada J, et al. Deflazacort: a glucocorticoid with few metabolic adverse effects but important immunosuppressive activity. Adv Ther. 2007;24(5):1052-60.
259. Dhooria S, Sehgal IS, Agarwal R, et al. High-dose (40 mg) versus low-dose (20 mg) prednisolone for treating sarcoidosis: a randomised trial (SARCORT trial). Eur Respir J. 2023;62(3):2300198.
260. Gibson GJ, Prescott RJ, Muers MF, et al. British Thoracic Society Sarcoidosis study: effects of long term corticosteroid treatment. Thorax. 1996;51(3):238-47.
261. Judson MA. An approach to the treatment of pulmonary sarcoidosis with corticosteroids: the six phases of treatment. Chest. 1999;115(4):1158-65.
262. Block AJ, Light RW. Alternate day steroid therapy in diffuse pulmonary sarcoidosis. Chest. 1973;63(4):495-504.
263. Selroos O, Sellergren TL. Corticosteroid therapy of pulmonary sarcoidosis. A prospective evaluation of alternate day and daily dosage in stage II disease. Scand J Respir Dis. 1979;60(4):215-21.
264. Spratling L, Tenholder MF, Underwood GH, et al. Daily vs alternate day prednisone therapy for stage II sarcoidosis. Chest. 1985;88(5):687-90.
265. Erkkila S, Froseth B, Hellstrom PE, et al. Inhaled budesonide influences cellular and biochemical abnormalities in pulmonary sarcoidosis. Sarcoidosis. 1988;5(2):106-10.
266. Alberts C, van der Mark TW, Jansen HM. Inhaled budesonide in pulmonary sarcoidosis: a double-blind, placebo-controlled study. Dutch Study Group on Pulmonary Sarcoidosis. Eur Respir J. 1995;8(5):682-8.
267. Pietinalho A, Tukiainen P, Haahtela T, et al. Early treatment of stage II sarcoidosis improves 5-year pulmonary function. Chest. 2002;121(1):24-31.
268. Targeted tuberculin testing and treatment of latent tuberculosis infection. American Thoracic Society. MMWR Recomm Rep. 2000;49(RR-6):1-51.
269. Lower EE, Broderick JP, Brott TG, et al. Diagnosis and management of neurological sarcoidosis. Arch Intern Med. 1997;157(16):1864-8.
270. Korsten P, Mirsaeidi M, Sweiss NJ. Nonsteroidal therapy of sarcoidosis. Curr Opin Pulm Med. 2013;19(5):516-23.
271. Beegle SH, Barba K, Gobunsuy R, et al. Current and emerging pharmacological treatments for sarcoidosis: a review. Drug Des Devel Ther. 2013;7:325-38.
272. Gibson GJ. Sarcoidosis: old and new treatments. Thorax. 2001;56(5):336-9.
273. Baughman RP, Lower EE. Alternatives to corticosteroids in the treatment of sarcoidosis. Sarcoidosis Vasc Diffuse Lung Dis. 1997;14(2):121-30.
274. Kataria YP. Chlorambucil in sarcoidosis. Chest. 1980;78(1):36-43.
275. Pacheco Y, Marechal C, Marechal F, et al. Azathioprine treatment of chronic pulmonary sarcoidosis. Sarcoidosis. 1985;2(2):107-13.
276. Lynch JP 3rd, McCune WJ. Immunosuppressive and cytotoxic pharmacotherapy for pulmonary disorders. Am J Respir Crit Care Med. 1997;155(2):395-420.
277. Baughman RP, Winget DB, Lower EE. Methotrexate is steroid sparing in acute sarcoidosis: results of a double blind, randomized trial. Sarcoidosis Vasc Diffuse Lung Dis. 2000;17(1):60-6.
278. Cremers JP, Drent M, Bast A, et al. Multinational evidence-based World Association of Sarcoidosis and other Granulomatous Disorders recommendations for the use of methotrexate in sarcoidosis: integrating systematic literature research and expert opinion of sarcoidologists worldwide. Curr Opin Pulm Med. 2013;19(5):545-61.
279. Kahlmann V, Janssen Bonás M, Moor CC, et al. Design of a randomized controlled trial to evaluate effectiveness of methotrexate versus prednisone as first-line treatment for pulmonary sarcoidosis: the PREDMETH study. BMC Pulm Med. 2020;20(1):271.
280. Muller-Quernheim J, Kienast K, Held M, et al. Treatment of chronic sarcoidosis with an azathioprine/prednisolone regimen. Eur Respir J. 1999;14(5):1117-22.
281. Lewis SJ, Ainslie GM, Bateman ED. Efficacy of azathioprine as second-line treatment in pulmonary sarcoidosis. Sarcoidosis Vasc Diffuse Lung Dis. 1999;16(1):87-92.
282. Vorselaars AD, Wuyts WA, Vorselaars VM, et al. Methotrexate vs azathioprine in second-line therapy of sarcoidosis. Chest. 2013;144(3):805-12.
283. Baughman RP, Lower EE. Leflunomide for chronic sarcoidosis. Sarcoidosis Vasc Diffuse Lung Dis. 2004;21(1):43-8.
284. Raj R, Nugent K. Leflunomide-induced interstitial lung disease (a systematic review). Sarcoidosis Vasc Diffuse Lung Dis. 2013;30(3):167-76.
285. Androdias G, Maillet D, Marignier R, et al. Mycophenolate mofetil may be effective in CNS sarcoidosis but not in sarcoid myopathy. Neurology. 2011;76(13):1168-72.
286. Brill AK, Ott SR, Geiser T. Effect and safety of mycophenolate mofetil in chronic pulmonary sarcoidosis: a retrospective study. Respiration. 2013;86(5):376-83.
287. Zaidi AA, Devita MV, Michelis MF, et al. Mycophenolate mofetil as a steroid-sparing agent in sarcoid-associated renal disease. Clin Nephrol. 2015;83(1):41-4.
288. Demeter SL. Myocardial sarcoidosis unresponsive to steroids. Treatment with cyclophosphamide. Chest. 1988;94(1):202-3.
289. Doty JD, Mazur JE, Judson MA. Treatment of corticosteroid-resistant neurosarcoidosis with a short-course cyclophosphamide regimen. Chest. 2003;124(5):2023-6.
290. Siltzbach LE, Teirstein AS. Chloroquine therapy in 43 patients with intrathoracic and cutaneous sarcoidosis. Acta Med Scand Suppl. 1964;425:302-8.
291. Hassid S, Choufani G, Saussez S, et al. Sarcoidosis of the paranasal sinuses treated with hydroxychloroquine. Postgrad Med J. 1998;74(869):172-4.

292. Barre PE, Gascon-Barre M, Meakins JL, et al. Hydroxychloroquine treatment of hypercalcemia in a patient with sarcoidosis undergoing hemodialysis. Am J Med. 1987;82(6):1259-62.
293. Sharma OP. Effectiveness of chloroquine and hydroxychloroquine in treating selected patients with sarcoidosis with neurological involvement. Arch Neurol. 1998;55(9):1248-54.
294. Baltzan M, Mehta S, Kirkham TH, et al. Randomized trial of prolonged chloroquine therapy in advanced pulmonary sarcoidosis. Am J Respir Crit Care Med. 1999;160(1):192-7.
295. Zissel G, Muller-Quernheim J. Sarcoidosis: historical perspective and immunopathogenesis (Part I). Respir Med. 1998;92(2):126-39.
296. Judson MA, Baughman RP, Costabel U, et al. Efficacy of infliximab in extrapulmonary sarcoidosis: results from a randomised trial. Eur Respir J. 2008;31(6):1189-96.
297. Baughman RP, Costabel U, du Bois RM. Treatment of sarcoidosis. Clin Chest Med. 2008;29(3):533-48, ix-x.
298. Rosen T, Doherty C. Successful long-term management of refractory cutaneous and upper airway sarcoidosis with periodic infliximab infusion. Dermatol Online J. 2007;13(3):14.
299. Kahler CM, Heininger P, Loeffler-Ragg J, et al. Infliximab therapy in pulmonary sarcoidosis. Am J Respir Crit Care Med. 2007;176(4):417; author reply 417-418.
300. Denys BG, Bogaerts Y, Coenegrachts KL, et al. Steroid-resistant sarcoidosis: is antagonism of TNF-alpha the answer? Clin Sci (Lond). 2007;112(5):281-9.
301. Rossman MD, Newman LS, Baughman RP, et al. A double-blinded, randomized, placebo-controlled trial of infliximab in subjects with active pulmonary sarcoidosis. Sarcoidosis Vasc Diffuse Lung Dis. 2006;23(3):201-8.
302. Baughman RP, Drent M, Kavuru M, et al. Infliximab therapy in patients with chronic sarcoidosis and pulmonary involvement. Am J Respir Crit Care Med. 2006;174(7):795-802.
303. Doty JD, Mazur JE, Judson MA. Treatment of sarcoidosis with infliximab. Chest. 2005;127(3):1064-71.
304. Drent M, Cremers JP, Jansen TL, et al. Practical eminence and experience-based recommendations for use of TNF-alpha inhibitors in sarcoidosis. Sarcoidosis Vasc Diffuse Lung Dis. 2014;31(2):91-107.
305. Vorselaars AD, Verwoerd A, van Moorsel CH, et al. Prediction of relapse after discontinuation of infliximab therapy in severe sarcoidosis. Eur Respir J. 2014;43(2):602-9.
306. Baughman RP, Nunes H, Sweiss NJ, et al. Established and experimental medical therapy of pulmonary sarcoidosis. Eur Respir J. 2013;41(6):1424-38.
307. Sweiss NJ, Noth I, Mirsaeidi M, et al. Efficacy Results of a 52-week Trial of Adalimumab in the Treatment of Refractory Sarcoidosis. Sarcoidosis Vasc Diffuse Lung Dis. 2014;31(1):46-54.
308. Pariser RJ, Paul J, Hirano S, et al. A double-blind, randomized, placebo-controlled trial of adalimumab in the treatment of cutaneous sarcoidosis. J Am Acad Dermatol. 2013;68(5):765-73.
309. Milman N, Graudal N, Loft A, et al. Effect of the TNF-alpha inhibitor adalimumab in patients with recalcitrant sarcoidosis: a prospective observational study using FDG-PET. Clin Respir J. 2012;6(4):238-47.
310. Field S, Regan AO, Sheahan K, et al. Recalcitrant cutaneous sarcoidosis responding to adalimumab but not to etanercept. Clin Exp Dermatol. 2010;35(7):795-6.
311. Utz JP, Limper AH, Kalra S, et al. Etanercept for the treatment of stage II and III progressive pulmonary sarcoidosis. Chest. 2003;124(1):177-85.
312. Centers for Disease Control and Prevention (CDC). Tuberculosis associated with blocking agents against tumor necrosis factor-alpha--California, 2002-2003. MMWR Morb Mortal Wkly Rep. 2004;53(30):683-6.
313. Massara A, Cavazzini L, La Corte R, et al. Sarcoidosis appearing during anti-tumor necrosis factor alpha therapy: a new "class effect" paradoxical phenomenon. Two case reports and literature review. Semin Arthritis Rheum. 2010;39(4):313-9.
314. Sweiss NJ, Lower EE, Mirsaeidi M, et al. Rituximab in the treatment of refractory pulmonary sarcoidosis. Eur Respir J. 2014;43(5):1525-8.
315. Lower EE, Baughman RP, Kaufman AH. Rituximab for refractory granulomatous eye disease. Clin Ophthalmol. 2012;6:1613-8.
316. Bomprezzi R, Pati S, Chansakul C, et al. A case of neurosarcoidosis successfully treated with rituximab. Neurology. 2010;75(6):568-70.
317. Belkhou A, Younsi R, El Bouchti I, et al. Rituximab as a treatment alternative in sarcoidosis. Joint Bone Spine. 2008;75(4):511-2.
318. Dhooria S, Agarwal R, Gupta D. Is pirfenidone ready for use in non-idiopathic pulmonary fibrosis interstitial lung diseases? Lung India. 2015;32(1):4-5.
319. Acharya N, Sharma SK, Mishra D, et al. Efficacy and safety of pirfenidone in systemic sclerosis-related interstitial lung disease-a randomised controlled trial. Rheumatol Int. 2020;40(5):703-10.
320. Dhooria S, Agarwal R, Sehgal IS, et al. A real-world study of the dosing and tolerability of pirfenidone and its effect on survival in idiopathic pulmonary fibrosis. Sarcoidosis Vasc Diffuse Lung Dis. 2020;37(2):148-57.
321. Flaherty KR, Wells AU, Cottin V, et al. Nintedanib in Progressive Fibrosing Interstitial Lung Diseases. N Engl J Med. 2019;381(18):1718-27.
322. Panselinas E, Judson MA. Acute pulmonary exacerbations of sarcoidosis. Chest. 2012;142(4):827-36.
323. McKinzie BP, Bullington WM, Mazur JE, et al. Efficacy of short-course, low-dose corticosteroid therapy for acute pulmonary sarcoidosis exacerbations. Am J Med Sci. 2010;339(1):1-4.
324. Moller DR. Negative clinical trials in sarcoidosis: failed therapies or flawed study design? Eur Respir J. 2014;44(5):1123-6.
325. Wirnsberger RM, de Vries J, Breteler MH, et al. Evaluation of quality of life in sarcoidosis patients. Respir Med. 1998;92(5):750-6.
326. Lower EE, Harman S, Baughman RP. Double-blind, randomized trial of dexmethylphenidate hydrochloride for the treatment of sarcoidosis-associated fatigue. Chest. 2008;133(5):1189-95.
327. Recommendations for the prevention and treatment of glucocorticoid-induced osteoporosis: 2001 update. American College of Rheumatology Ad Hoc Committee on Glucocorticoid-Induced Osteoporosis. Arthritis Rheum. 2001;44(7):1496-503.
328. Narum S, Westergren T, Klemp M. Corticosteroids and risk of gastrointestinal bleeding: a systematic review and meta-analysis. BMJ Open. 2014;4(5):e004587.
329. O'Donnell AE. Bronchiectasis. Chest. 2008;134(4):815-23.
330. Sehgal IS, Dhooria S, Muthu V, et al. Efficacy of 12-months oral itraconazole versus 6-months oral itraconazole to prevent relapses of chronic pulmonary aspergillosis: an open-label, randomised controlled trial in India. Lancet Infect Dis. 2022;22(7):1052-61.
331. Teo F, Anantham D, Feller-Kopman D, et al. Bronchoscopic management of sarcoidosis related bronchial stenosis with adjunctive topical mitomycin C. Ann Thorac Surg. 2010;89(6):2005-7.

332. Sulica R, Teirstein AS, Kakarla S, et al. Distinctive clinical, radiographic, and functional characteristics of patients with sarcoidosis-related pulmonary hypertension. Chest. 2005;128(3):1483-9.
333. Palmero V, Sulica R. Sarcoidosis-associated pulmonary hypertension: assessment and management. Semin Respir Crit Care Med. 2010;31(4):494-500.
334. Chapelon-Abric C. Cardiac sarcoidosis. Curr Opin Pulm Med. 2013;19(5):493-502.
335. Tachibana T, Iwai K, Takemura T. Sarcoidosis in the aged: review and management. Curr Opin Pulm Med. 2010;16(5):465-71.
336. Chappell AG, Cheung WY, Hutchings HA. Sarcoidosis: a long-term follow up study. Sarcoidosis Vasc Diffuse Lung Dis. 2000;17(2):167-73.
337. Thomeer MJ, Vansteenkiste J, Verbeken EK, et al. Interstitial lung diseases: characteristics at diagnosis and mortality risk assessment. Respir Med. 2004;98(6):567-73.
338. Askling J, Grunewald J, Eklund A, et al. Increased risk for cancer following sarcoidosis. Am J Respir Crit Care Med. 1999;160 (5 Pt 1):1668-72.
339. Romer FK, Hommelgaard P, Schou G. Sarcoidosis and cancer revisited: a long-term follow-up study of 555 Danish sarcoidosis patients. Eur Respir J. 1998;12(4):906-12.
340. Martin WJ 2nd, Iannuzzi MC, Gail DB, et al. Future directions in sarcoidosis research: summary of an NHLBI working group. Am J Respir Crit Care Med. 2004;170(5):567-71.

Pulmonary Eosinophilic Disorders

CHAPTER 117

Aditya Jindal, Subhash Varma

INTRODUCTION

Eosinophils are normal host defense cells against certain parasitic infections but take a pathogenic rather than a protective role, i.e., "eosinophilic immune dysfunction" in some conditions characterized with elevated eosinophil counts in blood and/or tissues.[1]

Association between pulmonary infiltrates and eosinophilia was labeled as "pulmonary infiltrates with eosinophilia" (PIE) by Reeder and Goodrich in 1952.[2] The role of these cells in the etiopathogenesis of systemic disease, including that of the lungs, is now better understood and defined. "Eosinophilia and lung disease" includes conditions in which lung involvement occurs either with eosinophilic infiltration or with peripheral eosinophilia.

EOSINOPHILS

Eosinophils originate from CD34+ myeloid progenitor cells; they share a common immediate precursor with basophils that points toward the eosinophilic lineage under the influence of various cytokines, mainly interleukin-5 (IL-5), granulocyte-macrophage colony-stimulating factor (GM-CSF), and IL3. Expression of high-affinity IL-5 receptors is a prerequisite and an early lineage-specific event in this process. Interleukin-5 gene knockout mice produce basal levels of eosinophils but fail to mount expected blood and/or tissue eosinophilia in response to various stimuli. IL-5 is produced by T cells and endothelial cells in the bone marrow, and T cells and parenchymal cells in the lung. Along with the differentiation of eosinophils, it also promotes the release of eosinophils into the bloodstream.

The mature eosinophil is of 12–17 μm in diameter and has a bilobed nucleus and an eosinophilic cytoplasm.[3] On electron microscopy, one can see primary granules as rounded structures with Charcot–Leyden crystal protein and secondary granules in the cytoplasm, which are oval and consist of a dense core formed by major basic protein (MBP) in a less dense matrix, which contains a few other enzymes such as eosinophil-derived neurotoxin (EDN), eosinophil cationic protein (ECP), and eosinophil peroxidase. In addition, there are dense lipid bodies that are not membrane bound and contain enzymes for metabolizing arachidonic acid.

After a brief intravascular stay of 3–8 hours following its release, the mature eosinophil enters various tissues, predominantly those having an epithelial–environment interface such as the respiratory, gastrointestinal, and genitourinary tracts. Once in tissues, survival depends upon the local production of cytokines regulating eosinophil apoptosis. It is eventually phagocytosed by tissue macrophages after a few days.[3] Eosinophils show a diurnal variation to the endogenous steroids with higher levels in the morning. Eosinophilia is commonly seen in parasitic infestations and drug toxicities, while eosinopenia is seen in pyogenic infections as well as in response to exogenous steroids, estrogens, and epinephrine.[4]

Circulating eosinophils, like other leukocytes, first move to the margins of the bloodstream where, by the process of rolling, they adhere to the vascular endothelium. They enter the interstitium by passing in between the endothelial cells by diapedesis and then migrate to the site of inflammation under the influence of various cytokines and chemokines. After their arrival, they are primed by cytokines, especially IL-5, platelet activating factor and complement fragment of C5a that through piecemeal degranulation results in the release of various mediators such as MBP, ECP, EDN, erythropoietin (EPO), substance P and also oxygen radicals, lipid mediators, and cytokines such as IL-1, IL-3, IL-5, IL-6, IL-8, GM-CSF, transforming growth factor (TGF)-α and -β, eotaxin, prostaglandins, leukotrienes, and platelet-activating factor. These contribute to the inflammatory actions of the eosinophils.

Eosinophils play an important role in the defense against helminthic infestations, allergic disorders, and parasitic and neoplastic diseases. They possess proinflammatory and cytotoxic effects which seem to relate to the release of preformed granules and inducible lipid mediators, cytokines, and oxidative products.

Eosinophilia, defined as mild, moderate, and severe **(Box 1)**, may occur in a large number of conditions which range from respiratory disorders such as phenotypic

BOX 1 Defining limits of eosinophilia.

Normal counts: Differential: ≤5%

AEC: ≤0.5×10^9/L

Eosinophilia:

- *Mild*: AEC 0.5–1.5 × 10^9/L
- *Moderate*: AEC 1.5–5.0 × 10^9/L
- *Severe*: AEC > 5.0 × 10^9/L
- Hypereosinophilic syndrome:
    - AEC: >1.5 × 10^9/L lasting for 6 months
    - Lack of evidence for known causes of:
        - Eosinophilia
    - Signs and symptoms of organ:
        - Involvement/Dysfunction

(AEC: absolute eosinophil count)

BOX 2 Pulmonary eosinophilic disorders.

- *Primary pulmonary eosinophilia*:
    - Predominant involving lung:
        - Acute eosinophilic pneumonia
        - Chronic eosinophilic pneumonia
    - *Systemic disease with lung disease*:
        - Eosinophilic granulomatosis with polyangiitis (Churg–Strauss syndrome)
        - Idiopathic hypereosinophilic syndrome
- *Secondary pulmonary eosinophilia*:
    - Infections:
        - Parasitic infestations
- Transient passage (Löffler's syndrome): Ancylostoma, ascaris, strongyloides
- *Tissue resident*: Paragonimiasis, echinococcosis
- *Heavy hematogenous seeding*:
    - Trichinella
    - Visceral larva migrans
    - Disseminated strongyloidiasis
    - Schistosomiasis:
        - Fungal infections: Coccidiomycosis, Histoplasmosis
        - Other infections: Tuberculosis, Brucellosis
    - Tropical pulmonary eosinophilia
    - Allergic bronchopulmonary aspergillosis
    - Hypersensitivity pneumonia
    - Drugs, toxins and radiation
- *Lung disorders with associated eosinophilia*:
    - Interstitial lung disease, sarcoidosis, idiopathic pulmonary fibrosis, Langerhans cell histiocytosis, connective tissue disease
    - Asthma
    - Bronchiolitis obliterans—organizing pneumonia
    - Neoplastic disorders, hematological malignancies, solid organ tumors
    - Postlung transplant

subsets of asthma, chronic obstructive pulmonary disease (COPD), and chronic rhinosinusitis with nasal polyposis to systemic diseases such as eosinophilic granulomatosis with polyangiitis (EGPA) and hypereosinophilic syndrome (HES) **(Box 2)**. Though secondary causes of eosinophilia are more likely (allergic disorders in the West and parasitic infections in the rest of the world), in many cases an underlying myeloid malignancy may be detected (clonal eosinophilia); the search may be inconclusive in several instances and lead to a diagnosis of idiopathic HES.

PULMONARY EOSINOPHILIC DISORDERS

Eosinophilic disorders are broadly classified into HESs, organ-restricted eosinophilic syndromes, syndromes where eosinophil-associated pathogenesis is central to the diagnosis [Churg-Strauss syndrome (CSS)], and hereditary disorders characterized by eosinophilia.[5]

Pulmonary eosinophilic disorders may occur with or without a known cause or as an association of known lung disease **(Box 2)**. Since many of these disorders have been dealt with elsewhere in this book, he focus in this chapter will be restricted to primary pulmonary eosinophilic disorders [acute eosinophilic pneumonia (AEP), idiopathic chronic eosinophilic pneumonia (ICEP), CSS, and HES] and those related to drugs and toxins. AEP and ICEP are only occasionally associated with extrapulmonary involvement, and predominant systemic symptoms suggest the possibility of systemic vasculitis, idiopathic HES, or other causes.

Löffler Syndrome

Löffler syndrome, first described by Löffler in 1932, is characterized with transitory pulmonary infiltrates, peripheral eosinophilia, and no to minimal respiratory symptoms. It is a self-limiting disease with low-grade fever, dry cough, and dyspnea. Eosinophils may be raised in respiratory secretions besides the presence of moderate to marked eosinophilia in the peripheral blood. Nonsegmental interstitial or alveolar infiltrates seen on chest radiology are often transient and migratory. The symptoms typically resolve within 1–2 weeks.[3,6]

Acute Eosinophilic Pneumonia

Acute eosinophilic pneumonia is a rapidly progressive condition in an otherwise healthy young individual which may sometimes cause severe respiratory failure.[7-9] The exact etiology is not known but may sometimes be associated with unusual activities such as cave exploring and wood working.[10] Hypersensitivity reaction to fungal antigens has been therefore suggested. AEP is also reported in subjects who have recently taken up smoking as well as those exposed to e-cigarettes and to environmental (passive) tobacco smoke.[11,12]

The patient may generally present with fever, cough, and dyspnea, with rapid progression to acute respiratory distress syndrome (ARDS).[13] Characteristically, there is no multisystem involvement even though there is severe respiratory failure.[12] AEP should always be considered in the differential diagnosis of any ARDS patient.

Laboratory investigations show leukocytosis with or without peripheral blood eosinophilia. IgE levels may show some increase. Up to 28% of patients may have peripheral blood eosinophilia at presentation; also, it may be associated with a better prognosis as compared to patients without initial eosinophilia. Plain chest X-ray may show bilateral patchy infiltrates soon progressing to an ARDS-like picture. The computed tomography (CT) scan shows ground-glass opacities and/or consolidation.[14] Bilateral pleural effusions may also be seen. Eosinophil count in the pleural fluid is often high. Bronchoalveolar lavage (BAL) shows marked eosinophilia along with variably elevated levels of beta-D-glucan and many cytokines such as IL-5 and IL-18. Pulmonary function tests during the acute phase show a restrictive defect with reduced DLCO.

Diffuse alveolar damage with marked eosinophilic infiltration is seen on pathological examination. Mucus plugging and fibrinous membrane formation are commonly seen; there is no formation of granulomas or alveolar hemorrhage. Pleural eosinophilic infiltration has been seen in 10% of cases.[13]

Acute eosinophilic pneumonia shows marked response to corticosteroids. Mechanical ventilation may be needed in severe cases and those with ARDS. A high index of suspicion is important to make an early diagnosis.

Idiopathic Chronic Eosinophilic Pneumonia

Idiopathic chronic eosinophilic pneumonia was first described by Carrington in 1969.[15,16] Though it may occur at any age, the peak incidence of the disease is seen between the ages of 30 and 40 years with a female preponderance. Patients with CEP are generally nonsmokers; a history of antecedent atopy, allergic rhinitis, or nasal polyps is present in one-third to half of the patients and that of asthma in about two-third of the patients. The asthma is adult onset and may arise spontaneously or precede ICEP by some time.

Idiopathic chronic eosinophilic pneumonia has an indolent course and an insidious onset.[17] Symptomatology consists of low-grade fever, night sweats, productive or nonproductive cough, dyspnea, wheezing, and weight loss. Dyspnea, which is generally mild, may sometimes progress to severe, necessitating mechanical ventilation.[17] Extrapulmonary manifestations are generally sparse and may include arthralgias, joint pains, and heart failure. ICEP is known to progress to interstitial pulmonary fibrosis in the long run.[18]

Diagnosis

Chronic eosinophilic pneumonia is diagnosed by the presence of a triad of clinical pulmonary symptoms, eosinophilia, and typical radiographic abnormalities.[19] Moderate leukocytosis and an elevated eosinophil and platelet count may be present. Absence of peripheral eosinophilia does not exclude the diagnosis of CEP. Differential cell counts of BAL along with more specific diagnostic tests such as polymerase chain reaction (PCR) or enzyme-linked immunosorbent assay, special cytopathologic stains, or specific microscopic findings are quite helpful.[20] Serum IgE levels are moderately elevated in about half of the cases. Pulmonary function testing may either be normal or show an obstructive or a restrictive defect. The obstructive defect may occur in patients with asthma though patients without asthma may also develop the same. The restrictive pattern occurs due to eosinophil infiltration into the interstitium. DLCO is mildly reduced.

The radiographic findings are quite variable and include the presence of dense and patchy infiltrates. Characteristically, the infiltrates are bilateral, peripherally located in subpleural regions and most commonly involving the upper and mid zones.[21] The radiographic appearance is sometimes described as the characteristic "photographic negative of pulmonary edema" which is seen in less than 25% of cases. Pleural effusion is uncommonly reported.[22] High-resolution computed tomography (HRCT) may show bilateral involvement with areas of ill-defined patchy consolidation, ground-glass opacities, areas of atelectasis, and septal thickening. Mediastinal lymphadenopathy and nodular infiltrates may be sometimes seen.[23]

Histopathologic examination of lung biopsy may show interstitial and alveolar infiltration by eosinophils, along with other inflammatory cells and disruption of the local architecture. Proliferative bronchiolitis obliterans, microangiitis, and microabscesses may also be seen. The diagnosis is suggested by appropriate investigations in the presence of a suitable clinical background. The differential diagnosis includes tuberculosis, fungal infections (like cryptococcosis), sarcoidosis, Löffler syndrome, desquamative interstitial pneumonia (DIP), and organizing pneumonia (OP), among others.

Management

Chronic eosinophilic pneumonia dramatically responds to corticosteroids in a dose ranging from 0.5 to 1 mg/kg/day. Symptoms resolve within a few hours, while radiological clearing may occur within about 2 months. Oral steroids are administered for about 6 months to 1 year or longer. Relapse may occur in half to two thirds of patients after discontinuation of steroids.[16,17] Steroids are readministered for relapses generally for prolonged periods of time.[16,23] Inhaled corticosteroids have also been used to bring down the dose of oral steroids.[3,23] The use of treatment with anti-IgE antibody such as omalizumab has also shown good results as a steroid-sparing agent.[24]

Eosinophilic Granulomatosis with Polyangiitis (Churg–Strauss Syndrome)

Eosinophilic granulomatosis with polyangiitis, originally described as CSS,[25-29] is an eosinophil-rich and necrotizing granulomatous inflammation which often involves the respiratory tract, with asthma and eosinophilia.[26] It is characterized by necrotizing vasculitis which predominantly affects small-to-medium vessels. The diverse clinical presentation and the difficulty in differentiating the disease often lead to a delay in the diagnosis. It is 2 to 10 times less common than the other antinuclear cytotoxic antibody (ANCA)-associated vasculitis with an incidence of 0.5–3.7 per million and a prevalence of 2–22 per million population.[28]

The patients are divided into two subgroups based on the presence or absence of ANCA. The ANCA-positive patients have more frequent manifestations of mononeuritis multiplex, glomerulonephritis, purpura, and alveolar hemorrhage while cardiomyopathic features and lung infiltrates are more frequently present in the ANCA-negative patients.[27-30]

Eosinophilic granulomatosis with polyangiitis has been also described with the use of leukotriene inhibitors, montelukast more than zafirlukast.[31] The disease can occur as early as 2 days to as late as 12 months after the initiation of therapy, almost exclusively when corticosteroids are being tapered off. It is more likely considered as an unmasking of the underlying disease rather than the side effect of the drug. EGPA has been occasionally described after the use of omalizumab.[29]

Clinical Features

The lung in systemic vasculitides presents with heterogeneous clinical, radiological, and histopathological features.[32] EGPA is most commonly diagnosed in the presence of long-standing asthma, peripheral eosinophilia, and lung infiltrates with features suggestive of vasculitis (i.e., mononeuritis multiplex, purpura, and others).

Three stages have been described clinically:

1. *Prodromal stage:* This can last for months to years. The patient usually presents with late-onset atopic states such as allergic rhinitis, nasal polyposis, and asthma in the absence of any family history.
2. *Eosinophilic stage:* This stage is characterized by the infiltration of various tissues by eosinophils, especially the skin, gastrointestinal tract (GIT), and lungs.
3. *Vasculitic stage:* It is characterized clinically by the onset of constitutional symptoms and microscopically by eosinophilic infiltration, vasculitis, and granulomatous infiltration.

The clinical course can be variable and may not strictly adhere to the mentioned stages. The respiratory system involvement includes upper respiratory tract disease, asthma, pleural effusions, and Löffler-like syndrome. Allergic rhinitis, sinusitis, and nasal polyposis are present in about 75–85% of cases. No necrosis is seen unlike in Wegener's granulomatosis.[33]

Asthma is the most significant clinical feature which may antedate the diagnosis of EGPA for many years. It is predominantly seen in the prodromal and eosinophilic stages. It may subside with the onset of the vasculitic phases. A short interval between the onset of asthma and that of vasculitis may indicate an increased disease severity. Pulmonary manifestations also include a Löffler-like syndrome (40%) and unilateral or bilateral pleural effusions or pleurisy without effusions in up to one-third of patients.

Patients may also develop cardiovascular complications such as coronary vasculitis leading to myocardial infarction, ischemic cardiomyopathy, or congestive cardiac failure secondary to eosinophilic myocardial infiltration. Cardiovascular disease is the leading cause of mortality in these patients while development of coronary vasculitis is associated with a mortality of up to 60%.[34] There may also occur acute and chronic constrictive pericarditis and pericardial tamponade.

Other prominent systemic manifestations of fever, weight loss, arthralgias, and arthritis are commonly present. Extrapulmonary disease includes the presence of lymphadenopathy, splenomegaly, and urological and ocular disease. Neurological manifestations of mononeuropathy and polyneuropathy are common in about two-thirds of patients. Cranial neuropathy may include optic neuritis, mononeuritis multiplex, seizures, cerebrovascular accidents, and subarachnoid hemorrhage.

Gastrointestinal tract involvement may be present in the form of eosinophilic gastroenteritis or vasculitis responsible for abdominal symptoms of pain, bleeding, and diarrhea. Occasionally, there may be more serious complications of intestinal obstruction, bowel perforation, and gastric ulcers. Liver function test abnormalities may indicate the presence of hepatic involvement. Dermatologic manifestations may occur in the form of palpable purpura, nodules, ulcers, maculopapular rashes, and livedo reticularis. Renal involvement includes interstitial nephritis or focal segmental glomerulosclerosis. Hematuria and hypertension may follow renal infarction. Chronic renal failure is unusual in EGPA unlike in other forms of vasculitides.

Diagnosis

Laboratory examination shows normocytic–normochromic anemia, normal platelet counts, and a high erythrocyte sedimentation rate (ESR). Leukocytosis with variable eosinophilia is commonly noted. Immunoglobulin E (IgE) and IgG levels are elevated, and there is hypergammaglobulinemia with rheumatoid factor seropositivity. IgE levels may parallel the disease activity. About 40% of patients have ANCA positivity which is generally perinuclear (pANCA) with specificity against myeloperoxidase. ANCA positivity is seen in only 25% of patients with EGPA who have no renal disease. Titers of ANCA do not have utility as a marker of disease activity on follow-up examinations.[27-29]

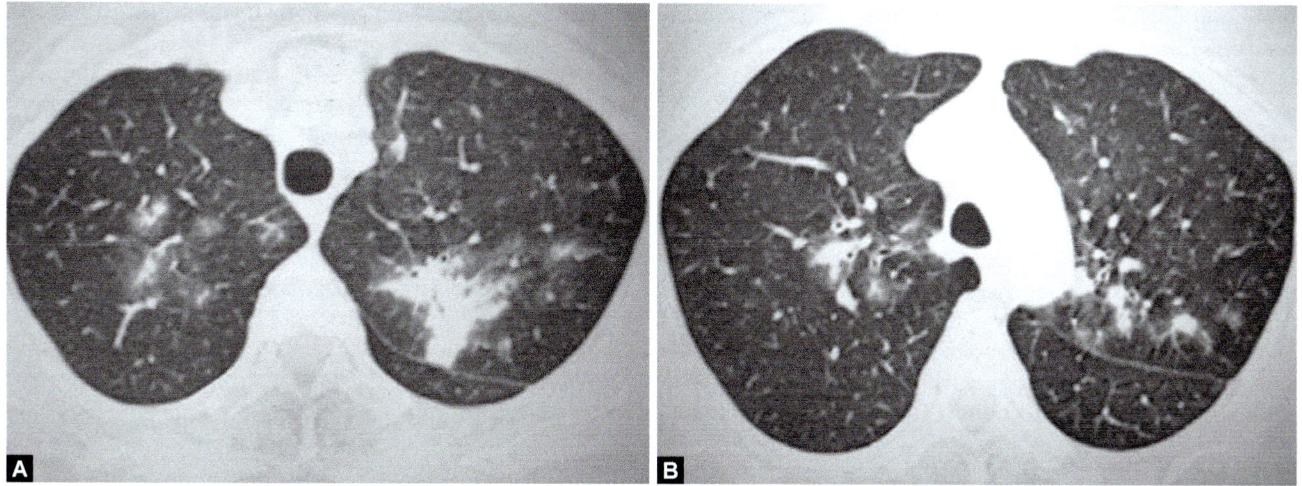

FIGS. 1A AND B: HRCT of a patient with EGPA with pulmonary infiltrates.
(EGPA: eosinophilic granulomatosis with polyangiitis; HRCT: high-resolution computed tomography)

The chest X-ray is either normal or nonspecific. Pulmonary infiltrates similar to those seen in Löffler syndrome may be present in up to 40% of individuals **(Figs. 1A and B)**, while pleural effusions are seen in one third. Other radiological features may include the presence of noncavitatory nodules, patchy areas of consolidation or ground-glass opacification, septal thickening, pulmonary artery enlargement, and peribronchial thickening. Pleural fluid is acidic with low glucose levels and high eosinophil count. The imaging findings are not specific to EGPA and should be interpreted in the overall clinical context.[32]

Pulmonary function tests show an obstructive physiology, while BAL shows variable eosinophilia. Positron emission tomography (PET) may show cardiac involvement. Histopathological examination of various tissues, including the lungs, pleura, skin, GIT, and nervous tissue, reveals both intravascular and extravascular noncaseating granulomas with eosinophilic infiltration accompanied by vasculitis of the small- and medium-sized arteries, veins, venules, and capillaries. Peripheral nerves are more commonly involved in EGPA as compared to other ANCA-associated vasculitides.[28] The inflammation may resolve with time and treatment or further lead to fibrous scarring.

In the absence of universally accepted diagnostic criteria, the diagnosis of EGPA is challenging. There are several diagnostic criteria that rely on symptoms of asthma, eosinophilia, and evidence of organ involvement secondary to medium- and small-vessel vasculitis. The American College of Rheumatology criteria published in 1990 require the presence of at least four out of the six given criteria, which give a sensitivity and specificity of 85% and 99.7%, respectively.[35] These include (1) asthma, (2) paranasal sinusitis, (3) monoarthropathy or polyarthropathy, (4) migratory or transient pulmonary infiltrates, (5) peripheral blood eosinophilia > 10%, and (6) extravascular eosinophils in a blood vessel on a biopsy specimen.

The differential diagnosis includes other ANCA-associated vasculitis such as granulomatosis with polyangiitis or Wegener's granulomatosis, polyarteritis nodosa, tuberculosis, fungal infections, allergic bronchopulmonary aspergillosis, chronic eosinophilic pneumonia, asthma, and Hodgkin's disease.

Treatment

There is no stratified treatment schedule available in EGPA as in other ANCA-associated vasculitis.[36] The choice of treatment is based on the presence of systemic involvement. The five factor score (FFS) is the most commonly used guide for treatment initiation. The five factors are: (1) proteinuria >1 g/24 h, (2) serum creatinine level > 140 mmol/L, (3) myocardial involvement, (4) severe gastrointestinal involvement, and (5) central nervous system involvement.[37] Presence of ≥1 of these factors is indicative of a higher risk of morbidity and mortality, if the FFS is ≥1, treatment is started with both steroids and immunosuppressive agents while steroids alone would suffice with a FFS of 0. Oral prednisolone started at a dose of 1 mg/kg/day is continued for 6–12 weeks followed by a gradual tapering. Maintenance dose is continued for about a year or more. Disease activity should be followed by the disappearance of constitutional symptoms and other clinical manifestations of different systems involvement. Laboratory markers of disease activity which include ESR, IgE levels, and leukocyte counts are also used to assess the disease; pANCA is not useful for follow-up evaluation.

Cytotoxic chemotherapy is indicated when there is nonresponsiveness to steroids and/or presence of severe systemic disease including cardiac, GIT, and renal (proteinuria > 1 g/day or renal insufficiency) involvement. In the acute phase, pulse cyclophosphamide is the immunosuppressive treatment of choice while azathioprine or mycophenolate is useful for maintenance therapy. Pulse steroids may also be used in acute settings. Other immunomodulators include the use of high-dose intravenous immunoglobulin and interferon-alpha in standard dose. Plasma exchange is sometimes tried in severe disease. There have been recent case reports of treatment with rituximab and mepolizumab.[37-40] With better understanding of the disease pathogenesis and its management, it is now proposed that steroid-sparing treatment plans with novel biological agents are more effective and better tolerated.[41-43]

The prognosis of EGPA is very poor without treatment. However, the use of corticosteroids has dramatically reduced the mortality rate. Long-term remissions are usually achieved, though relapses may occur. The use of steroids and immunosuppressive agents may cause significant morbidity though, in the form of infections, osteoporosis, solid-organ malignancies, etc.

Hypereosinophilic Syndrome

Also known as Löffler's endocarditis and eosinophilic leukemia, HES is a disorder characterized by multisystem involvement and a variable presentation.[44] It predominantly affects males and is more common from ages of 20–50 years, though it can occur at any age. There has been a significant confusion in the past over the terminology and at times it was thought that HES constitutes a spectrum of illness with minimal involvement on one hand and eosinophilic leukemia on the other extreme.

The cause of this disorder is unknown, and the various hypotheses propose it as a disorder ranging from a primary disturbance of myelopoiesis to a monoclonal expansion of T lymphocytes producing cytokines to an immune hypersensitivity reaction. The organ damage is the result of eosinophilic infiltration and/or thromboembolic phenomena.

Clinical Features

Three major clinical variants of HES are recognized,[45] i.e., myeloproliferative, lymphoproliferative, and familial HES. The myeloproliferative variant has been shown to be associated with *FIP1LI-PDGFR* α fusion gene. Since these patients have a clonal abnormality, these may also be classified by some as chronic eosinophilic leukemia. The lymphoproliferative variant is associated with monoclonal expansion of T cells that result in increased IL-5 secretion and hypereosinophilia. Familial HES is secondary to a genetic defect that results in increased IL-5 and eosinophilia. Currently, even after detailed investigations, a subset of patients may not reveal any cause, termed true idiopathic HES.

Clinical manifestations of HES are highly variable. Respiratory system is involved in about 40% of cases and generally manifests predominantly with nocturnal cough.[45] Wheezing and dyspnea may also occur. Occasionally, the disease can progress to ARDS. The disease may be complicated with pleural effusion, pulmonary hypertension, and thromboembolism. The cardiovascular system is commonly involved[44,46] with eosinophilic infiltration of the endocardium and myocardium responsible for restrictive cardiomyopathy, endocardial fibrosis, and mitral regurgitation. Peripheral arterial or venous thrombosis has been also reported.[47,48]

Neurological involvement in HES may present with encephalopathy, neuropsychiatric disturbances, memory loss, visual changes, and cerebrovascular accidents which may occur secondary to thromboembolism. Other systems are involved less frequently; the symptomatology varies according to the system involved **(Table 1)**.

Diagnosis

Blood examination shows anemia and leukocytosis (10,000–50,000/mm^3) with 30–70% eosinophils; associated may be blood and/or bone marrow neutrophilia, basophilia, and eosinophilic dysplasia.[49] Erythrocyte sedimentation rate, serum IgE, and gamma globulins are elevated. Also noted are elevated levels of serum B_{12} and leukocyte alkaline phosphatase. Circulating immune complexes are occasionally found. There is an increase in eosinophils and eosinophil precursors in the bone marrow and other organs **(Figs. 2 and 3)**. Eosinophilic blast transformation has been observed in 28–51% of patients.

Chest X-ray may show the presence of focal or diffuse nonspecific infiltrates and pleural effusions. An obstructive pattern is seen on pulmonary function tests. Intracardiac thrombi may be seen on echocardiography which should be done at 6 monthly follow-up of cardiovascular disease.[48]

The differential diagnosis includes the different eosinophilic disorders like CEP, CSS, AEP, tropical pulmonary eosinophilia, fungal infections, and parasitic infestations. Different laboratory criteria are used for the differential diagnosis of lymphoproliferative and myeloproliferative variants **(Box 3)**.

TABLE 1: End-organ damage in HES and hypereosinophilic disorders.

Cardiac	Pericarditis, EMF, cardiomyopathy, myocarditis, intramural thrombi, regurgitation
Neurologic	Thromboemboli, peripheral neuropathy, dementia/psychosis, meningitis, epilepsy
Dermatologic	Angioedema, urticaria, papulonodular lesions, mucosal ulcers, vesiculobullous, microthrombi, Raynaud's phenomenon, digital necrosis
Pulmonary	Infiltrates, fibrosis, effusion, emboli
Ocular	Microthrombi, vasculitis, retinal arteritis
Joints	Arthralgia, effusions, polyarthritis
Gastrointestinal	Ascites, diarrhea, gastritis, colitis, pancreatitis, cholangitis, Budd–Chiari syndrome

(EMF: endomyocardial fibrosis; HES: hypereosinophilic syndrome)

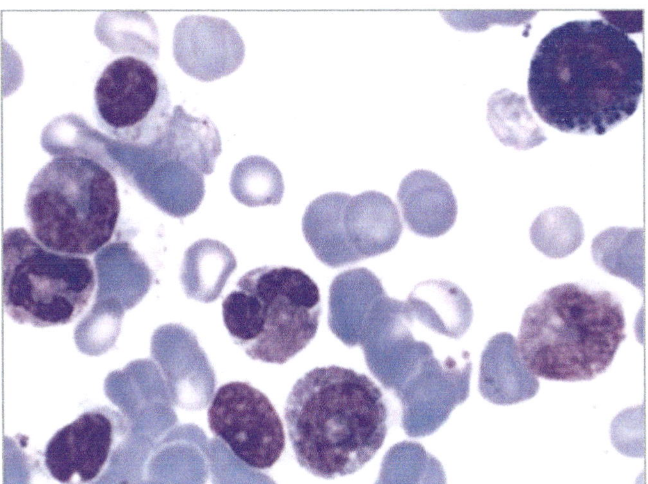

FIG. 2: BM smear in HES patient showing two metamyelocytes, one basophil, and two eosinophils (one has a ring nucleus).
(BM: bone marrow; HES: hypereosinophilic syndrome)

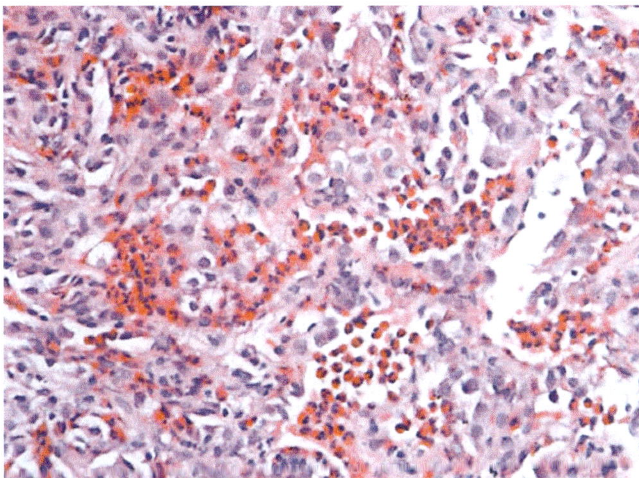

FIG. 3: Extensive eosinophilic infiltration of tissues on histopathological examination.

Treatment

Treatment is directed at both symptomatic management and prevention of end-organ damage. Presence of asymptomatic peripheral eosinophilia does not usually require any treatment. Oral corticosteroids (prednisone, 1 mg/kg/day) constitute the first line of treatment for the first 1–2 months, tapered to a maintenance dose for a year or more. Other immunosuppressants such as hydroxyurea, vincristine, chlorambucil, or cyclosporine are tried for the treatment of poor or nonresponsiveness to steroids.[44,50] Biological agents such as mepolizumab (monoclonal anti-IL-5 antibodies) have been found effective in patients with high IL-5 levels.[50,51]

The French guidelines provide practical recommendations for management and follow-up of the full spectrum of eosinophilic disorders including idiopathic HES.[52] Even though steroids had been the mainstay of treatment in the past, it is now realized that patients with myeloproliferative variant do not respond well to steroids and in case of *FIP1L1-PDGFRA* positive patients, use of tyrosine-kinase inhibitors such as imatinib[53] and dasatinib results in a gratifying response. The initial dose for a rapid cytogenetic response should be 400 mg/day with a lower maintenance dose. Whereas this variant is associated with exquisite sensitivity to imatinib even at a dose of 100 mg/day, other variants may require higher dosage and have variable response. Steroids should be added to imatinib in patients with evidence of myocarditis on echocardiography, electrocardiography, or biochemical parameters (elevated serum troponin). The anti-CD-52 antibody alemtuzumab has been tried in refractory cases, especially those of lymphoproliferative variant.[54] There are several reports of successful treatment using hematopoietic stem cell transplant in refractory cases.[55-57]

The causes of mortality in HES include refractory congestive cardiac failure, renal failure, hepatic failure, venous thromboembolism, gut perforation, and infections. Appropriate treatment leads to a mean survival of >10 years.[58]

BOX 3 **Laboratory diagnosis of myeloproliferative and lymphoproliferative variants of HES.**

Myeloproliferative variant

Definitive evidence:
- FIP1L1–PDGFRA fusion
- Eosinophil clonality

Supportive evidence: ≥4 of
- Increased serum tryptase
- Increased serum B12
- Splenomegaly
- Anemia, thrombocytopenia
- Increased circulating myeloid precursors
- Dysplastic eosinophils
- Myelofibrosis
- Increased spindle-shaped mast cells in BM

Lymphoproliferative variant
- Definitive evidence
- Phenotypically aberrant T cells
- TCR rearrangement
- Increased eosinophilopoietic cytokines
- Supportive evidence
- Increased serum TARC
- Increased serum IgE
- Predominantly cutaneous manifestations
- History of atopy
- Steroid responsive

(BM: bone marrow; TARC: thymus and activation-regulated chemokine; TCR: T-cell receptor)

Other Eosinophilic Lung Diseases

Langerhans Cell Granulomatosis

Histiocytosis X consists of three closely related disorders, occurring at different ages: (1) Langerhans cell histiocytosis, (2) Letterer-Siwe disease, and (3) Hand-Schüller-Christian disease.[59] Histiocytosis refers to a unifying concept for diseases characterized by pathogenetic myeloid cells that share histologic features with macrophages or dendritic cells.[60] Primary pulmonary histiocytosis X, earlier known as eosinophilic granuloma of the lung, is almost exclusively found in smokers. The male to female ratio is 1:1; patients in the third and fourth decades of life are commonly affected.

The disease presents with common respiratory symptoms and episodes of recurrent, sometimes bilateral pneumothorax. Diabetes insipidus and bone disease are other common features. On chest radiography, reticulonodular or cystic lesions and bullae are seen, more commonly in the upper and middle zones with sparing of the costophrenic angles. Bullae may often rupture to cause recurrent pneumothorax. Histopathologically, a granulomatous infiltrate of histiocytes, eosinophils, and other cells can be seen. The histiocyte is a large cell with an indented nucleus that has Birbeck granules on electron microscopy. S-100 antibody can also be found **(Fig. 3 and Flowchart 1)**. Treatment depends on the disease severity. Smoking cessation is important as a part of treatment. Drug therapy consists of corticosteroids and/or other agents such as vincristine, cyclophosphamide, and fludarabine.

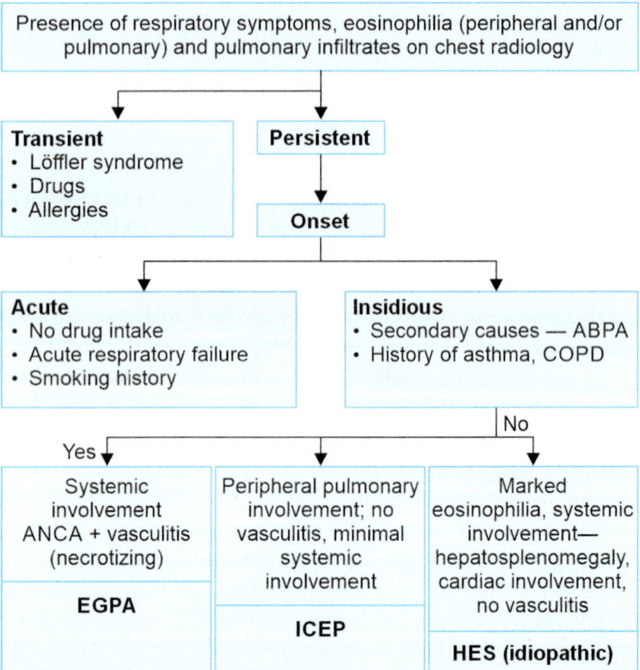

FLOWCHART 1: Proposed diagnostic algorithm for pulmonary eosinophilic disorders.

(ABPA: allergic bronchopulmonary aspergillosis; AEP: acute eosinophilic pneumonia; COPD: chronic obstructive pulmonary disease; EGPA: eosinophilic granulomatosis with polyangiitis; HES: hypereosinophilic syndrome; ICEP: idiopathic chronic eosinophilic pneumonia)

Sarcoidosis

Sarcoidosis is a multisystem disorder with pulmonary involvement in the majority of cases is discussed elsewhere in a separate chapter. Patients may present with fever, weight loss, mediastinal lymphadenopathy, and lung infiltrates. Histopathological examination reveals noncaseating epithelioid granulomas. Other granulomatous diseases such as tuberculosis, nontuberculous infections, and others constitute close differential diagnosis.[61] The incidence of eosinophilia in sarcoidosis ranges from 10 to 67%.[62]

Neoplastic Disorders

Peripheral blood eosinophilia can also occur in many hematological and solid organ malignancies.[63-65] Eosinophilia is sometimes considered as an adverse prognostic sign. This, however, is not always so and depends upon the type of malignancy. Chronic eosinophilic leukemia along with others is one of the three main types of the World Health Organization (WHO)-defined eosinophilia-associated myeloid neoplasms. Large-cell bronchogenic carcinoma, squamous cell cancer of cervix, skin, nasopharynx, and transitional cell carcinoma of urinary bladder are important solid organ malignancies associated with eosinophilia.

Tropical Pulmonary Eosinophilia

Tropical pulmonary eosinophilia is an important cause of marked eosinophilia, and hence, an important differential diagnosis (see Chapter on Tropical Lung Infections).

Infections

Eosinophilia may also occur in different bacterial, fungal, and parasitic diseases.[66] An undulating pattern of eosinophilia is also reported in tuberculosis and chronic brucellosis. Coccidiomycosis, *Histoplasmosis*, and cryptococcosis are important fungal infections in which eosinophilia has been reported.

Drug- and Toxin-induced Pulmonary Eosinophilia

Eosinophilic lung disease is also reported in association with or as a toxic reaction to administration of several drugs and toxins **(Box 4)**.[67,68] Clinical manifestations may appear within a few minutes after exposure but may take weeks in some cases. Nitrofurantoin is one of the most common drugs causing acute, subacute, and chronic reactions.

Eosinophilic phenotypes of chronic airway diseases and some types of interstitial lung diseases are important causes of peripheral and lung eosinophilia.[69,70] The subject has been discussed in greater details in separate chapters.

BOX 4 Drugs causing eosinophilic lung disease.

- *Antimicrobials*:
  - Para-amino salicyclic acid
  - Nitrofurantoin
  - Penicillin
  - Tetracycline
  - Streptomycin
  - Isoniazid
  - Sulfonamides
  - Tetracycline
  - Minocycline
  - Dapsone + pyrimethamine
- *Antineoplastic and immunosuppressives*:
  - Bleomycin
  - Methotrexate
  - Melphalan
  - Gold salts
  - Azathioprine
  - Penicillamine
  - Beclomethasone
- *Nonsteroidal anti-inflammatory drugs (NSAIDs)*:
  - Aspirin
  - Naproxen
  - Piroxicam
  - Nimesulide
  - Phenylbutazone
- *Cardiovascular and antidiabetics*:
  - Amiodarone
  - Hydralazine
  - Thiazides
  - Clofibrate
  - Sulfonylureas
- *Miscellaneous*:
  - Carbamazepine
  - Phenytoin
  - Dantrolene
  - Methylphenidate
  - Imipramine
  - Cocaine or heroin exposure
  - Iodinated contrast media
  - L-tryptophan

SUMMARY

Eosinophilic lung diseases are heterogeneous disorders that require a meticulous history taking, painstaking examination, and judicious use of investigations to reach a definite diagnosis. A simplified algorithmic approach is important to reach a diagnosis. Most of the causative illnesses have different courses and complications and thus involve important treatment decisions.

REFERENCES

1. Jackson DJ, Akuthota P, Roufosse F. Eosinophils and eosinophilic immune dysfunction in health and disease. Eur Respir Rev. 2022;31(163):210150.
2. Reeder WH, Goodrich BE. Pulmonary infiltration with eosinophilia (PIE syndrome). Ann Intern Med. 1952;36(5):1217-40.
3. Savani DM, Sharma OP. Eosinophilic lung disease in the tropics. Clin Chest Med. 2002;23(2):377-96, ix.
4. Beeson PB, Bass DA. The eosinophil. In: Smith LH Jr (Ed). Major Problems in Internal Medicine, Vol. 14. Philadelphia: Elsevier; 1977.
5. Wechsler ME, Fulkerson PC, Bochner BS, et al. Novel targeted therapies for eosinophilic disorders. J Allergy Clin Immunol. 2012;130(3):563-71.
6. Son BBB, Phu NM, Nam-Anh ND. Loeffler's syndrome mimicking lung tumor and pneumonia in a child: A case report. Respir Med Case Rep. 2022;37:101638.
7. Giacomi FD, Yi ES, Ryu JH. Acute Eosinophilic Pneumonia. Causes, Diagnosis, and Management. Am J Respir Crit Care Med. 2018;197:728-36.
8. Allen JN, Pacht ER, Gadek JE, et al. Acute eosinophilic pneumonia as a reversible cause of noninfectious respiratory failure. New Engl J Med. 1989;321(9):569-74.
9. Wechsler ME. Pulmonary eosinophilic syndromes. Immunol Allergy Clin North Am. 2007;27(3):477-92.
10. Allen J. Acute eosinophilic pneumonia. Semin Respir Crit Care Med. 2006;27(2):142-7.
11. Thota D, Latham E. Case report of electronic cigarettes possibly associated with eosinophilic pneumonitis in a previously healthy active duty sailor. J Emerg Med. 2014;47(1):15-7.
12. Natarajan A, Shah P, Mirrakhimov AE, et al. Eosinophilic pneumonia associated with concomitant cigarette and marijuana smoking. BMJ Case Reports. 2013;2013.
13. Vahid B, Marik PE. An 18-year-old woman with fever, diffuse pulmonary opacities, and rapid onset of respiratory failure: idiopathic acute eosinophilic pneumonia. Chest. 2006;130(6):1938-41.
14. Daimon T, Johkoh T, Sumikawa H, et al. Acute eosinophilic pneumonia: Thin-section CT findings in 29 patients. Eur J Radiol. 2008;65(3):462-7.
15. Carrington CB, Addington WW, Goff AM, et al. Chronic eosinophilic pneumonia. New Engl J Med. 1969;280(15):787-98.
16. Naughton M, Fahy J, FitzGerald MX. Chronic eosinophilic pneumonia. A long-term follow-up of 12 patients. Chest. 1993;103(1):162-5.
17. Allen JN, Davis WB. Eosinophilic lung diseases. Am J Respir Crit Care Med. 1994;150(5 Pt 1):1423-38.
18. Teixeira N, Santos MI, Pedro F, et al. Idiopathic Chronic Eosinophilic Pneumonia. Cureus. 2021;13(3):e14047.

19. Crowe M, Robinson D, Sagar M, et al. Chronic eosinophilic pneumonia: clinical perspectives. Ther Clin Risk Manag. 2019;15: 397-403.
20. Baqir M, Peikert T, Johnson TF, et al. Idiopathic Chronic Eosinophilic Pneumonia Evolving to Pulmonary Fibrosis: A Retrospective Analysis. Sarcoidosis Vasc Diffuse Lung Dis. 2022;39(2):e2022020.
21. Gaensler EA, Carrington CB. Peripheral opacities in chronic eosinophilic pneumonia: the photographic negative of pulmonary edema. AJR Am J Roentgenol. 1977;128(1):1-13.
22. Samman YS, Wali SO, Abdelaal MA, et al. Chronic eosinophilic pneumonia presenting with recurrent massive bilateral pleural effusion: case report. Chest. 2001;119(3):968-70.
23. Marchand E, Cordier JF. Idiopathic chronic eosinophilic pneumonia. Orphanet J Rare Dis. 2006;1:11.
24. Kaya H, Gumus S, Ucar E, et al. Omalizumab as a steroid-sparing agent in chronic eosinophilic pneumonia. Chest. 2012;142(2):513-6.
25. Keogh KA, Specks U. Churg-Strauss syndrome. Semin Respir Crit Care Med. 2006;27(2):148-57.
26. Jennette JC, Falk RJ, Bacon PA, et al. 2012 revised International Chapel Hill Consensus Conference Nomenclature of Vasculitides. Arthritis Rheum. 2013;65(1):1-11.
27. Vaglio A, Buzio C, Zwerina J. Eosinophilic granulomatosis with polyangiitis (Churg-Strauss): state of the art. Allergy. 2013;68(3): 261-73.
28. Mahr A, Moosig F, Neumann T, et al. Eosinophilic granulomatosis with polyangiitis (Churg-Strauss): evolutions in classification, etiopathogenesis, assessment and management. Curr Opin Rheumatol. 2014;26(1):16-23.
29. Mouthon L, Dunogue B, Guillevin L. Diagnosis and classification of eosinophilic granulomatosis with polyangiitis (formerly named Churg-Strauss syndrome). J Autoimmun. 2014;48-49: 99-103.
30. Vaglio A, Moosig F, Zwerina J. Churg-Strauss syndrome: update on pathophysiology and treatment. Curr Opin Rheumatol. 2012;24(1):24-30.
31. Wechsler ME, Pauwels R, Drazen JM. Leukotriene modifiers and Churg-Strauss syndrome: adverse effect or response to corticosteroid withdrawal? Drug Saf. 1999;21(4):241-51.
32. Makhzoum JP, Grayson PC, Ponte C, et al.; DCVAS Collaborators. Pulmonary involvement in primary systemic vasculitides. Rheumatology (Oxford). 2021;61(1):319-30.
33. Antunes T, Barbas CS. Wegener's granulomatosis. J Bras Pneumol. 2005;31(Suppl 1):S21-6.
34. Conron M, Beynon HL. Churg-Strauss syndrome. Thorax. 2000;55(10):870-7.
35. Masi AT, Hunder GG, Lie JT, et al. The American College of Rheumatology 1990 criteria for the classification of Churg-Strauss syndrome (allergic granulomatosis and angiitis). Arthritis Rheum. 1990;33(8):1094-100.
36. Mukhtyar C, Guillevin L, Cid MC, et al. EULAR recommendations for the management of primary small and medium vessel vasculitis. Ann Rheum Dis. 2009;68(3):310-7.
37. Moosig F, Gross WL, Herrmann K, et al. Targeting interleukin-5 in refractory and relapsing Churg-Strauss syndrome. Ann Intern Med. 2011;155(5):341-3.
38. Koukoulaki M, Smith KG, Jayne DR. Rituximab in Churg-Strauss syndrome. Ann Rheum Dis. 2006;65(4):557-9.
39. Kim S, Marigowda G, Oren E, et al. Mepolizumab as a steroid-sparing treatment option in patients with Churg-Strauss syndrome. J Allergy Clin Immunol. 2010;125(6):1336-43.
40. Herrmann K, Gross WL, Moosig F. Extended follow-up after stopping mepolizumab in relapsing/refractory Churg-Strauss syndrome. Clin Exp Rheumatol. 2012;30(1 Suppl 70):S62-5.
41. Mkorombindo T, Dransfield MT. Mepolizumab in the treatment of eosinophilic chronic obstructive pulmonary disease. Int J Chron Obstruct Pulmon Dis. 2019;14:1779-87.
42. Thiel J, Hassler F, Salzer U, et al. Rituximab in the treatment of refractory or relapsing eosinophilic granulomatosis with polyangiitis (Churg-Strauss syndrome). Arthritis Res Ther. 2013;15(5):R133.
43. Umezawa N, Kohsaka H, Nanki T, et al. Successful treatment of eosinophilic granulomatosis with polyangiitis (EGPA; formerly Churg-Strauss syndrome) with rituximab in a case refractory to glucocorticoids, cyclophosphamide, and IVIG. Mod Rheumatol. 2014;24(4):685-7.
44. Weller PF, Bubley GJ. The idiopathic hypereosinophilic syndrome. Blood. 1994;83(10):2759-79.
45. Klion AD, Bochner BS, Gleich GJ, et al. Approaches to the treatment of hypereosinophilic syndromes: a workshop summary report. J Allergy Clin Immunol. 2006;117(6):1292-302.
46. Cottin V, Cordier JF. Eosinophilic pneumonias. Allergy. 2005; 60(7):841-57.
47. Ogbogu PU, Rosing DR, Horne MK, 3rd. Cardiovascular manifestations of hypereosinophilic syndromes. Immunol Allergy Clin North America. 2007;27(3):457-75.
48. Varma N, Varma S, Marwaha N, Dash S. Hypereosinophilic syndrome: the spectrum of clinical, haematological and morphological features. J Assoc Physicians India. 1994;42(3):242-4.
49. Gotlib J. World Health Organization-defined eosinophilic disorders: 2014 update on diagnosis, risk stratification, and management. Am J Hematol. 2014;89(3):325-37.
50. Thomsen GN, Christoffersen MN, Lindegaard HM, et al. The multidisciplinary approach to eosinophilia. Front Oncol. 2023; 13:1193730.
51. Rothenberg ME, Klion AD, Roufosse FE, et al. Treatment of patients with the hypereosinophilic syndrome with mepolizumab. N Engl J Med. 2008;358(12):1215-28.
52. Groh M, Rohmer J, Etienne N, et al. French guidelines for the etiological workup of eosinophilia and the management of hypereosinophilic syndromes. Orphanet J Rare Dis. 2023;18(1):100.
53. Cools J, DeAngelo DJ, Gotlib J, et al. A tyrosine kinase created by fusion of the *PDGFRA and FIP1L1* genes as a therapeutic target of imatinib in idiopathic hypereosinophilic syndrome. New Engl J Med. 2003;348(13):1201-14.
54. Sefcick A, Sowter D, DasGupta E, et al. Alemtuzumab therapy for refractory idiopathic hypereosinophilic syndrome. British J Haematol. 2004;124(4):558-9.
55. Ueno NT, Anagnostopoulos A, Rondon G, et al. Successful non-myeloablative allogeneic transplantation for treatment of idiopathic hypereosinophilic syndrome. British J Haematol. 2002;119(1):131-4.
56. Cooper MA, Akard LP, Thompson JM, et al. Hypereosinophilic syndrome: long-term remission following allogeneic stem cell transplant in spite of transient eosinophilia post-transplant. Am J Hematol. 2005;78(1):33-6.
57. Halaburda K, Prejzner W, Szatkowski D, et al. Allogeneic bone marrow transplantation for hypereosinophilic syndrome: long-term follow-up with eradication of FIP1L1-PDGFRA fusion transcript. Bone Marrow Transplant. 2006;38(4):319-20.
58. Podjasek JC, Butterfield JH. Mortality in hypereosinophilic syndrome: 19 years of experience at Mayo Clinic with a review of the literature. Leukemia Res. 2013;37(4):392-5.

59. Lichtenstein L. Histiocytosis X; integration of eosinophilic granuloma of bone, Letterer-Siwe disease, and Schuller-Christian disease as related manifestations of a single nosologic entity. AMA Arch Pathol. 1953;56(1):84-102.
60. McClain KL, Bigenwald C, Collin M, et al. Histiocytic disorders. Nat Rev Dis Primers. 2021;7(1):73.
61. Valeyre D, Brauner M, Bernaudin JF, et al. Differential diagnosis of pulmonary sarcoidosis: a review. Front Med (Lausanne). 2023;10:1150751.
62. Renston JP, Goldman ES, Hsu RM, et al. Peripheral blood eosinophilia in association with sarcoidosis. Mayo Clinic Proc. 2000;75(6):586-90.
63. Grisaru-Tal S, Itan M, Klion AD, et al. A new dawn for eosinophils in the tumour microenvironment. Nature Rev Cancer. 2020;20:594-607.
64. Zalewska E, Obołończyk Ł, Sworczak K. Hypereosinophilia in Solid Tumors-Case Report and Clinical Review. Front Oncol. 2021;11:639395.
65. Hu G, Wang S, Zhong K, et al. Tumor-associated tissue eosinophilia predicts favorable clinical outcome in solid tumors: a meta-analysis. BMC Cancer. 2020;20:454.
66. O'Connell EM, Nutman TB. Eosinophilia in Infectious Diseases. Immunol Allergy Clin North Am. 2015;35(3):493-522.
67. Rauscher C, Freeman A. Drug-induced eosinophilia. Allergy Asthma Proc. 2018;39(3):252-6.
68. Carmi B, Iftach S, Leonid B. Drug-induced eosinophilic pneumonia: A review of 196 case reports. Medicine. 2018;97(4):p e9688.
69. George L, Brightling CE. Eosinophilic airway inflammation: role in asthma and chronic obstructive pulmonary disease. Ther Adv Chronic Dis. 2016;7(1):34-51.
70. Mormile M, Mormile I, Fuschillo S, et al. Eosinophilic Airway Diseases: From Pathophysiological Mechanisms to Clinical Practice. Int J Mol Sci. 2023;24(8):7254.

SECTION

11

Disorders of Pulmonary Circulation

SECTION OUTLINE

CHAPTER 118

Diffuse Alveolar Hemorrhage

F Karakontaki, E Stagaki, V Polychronopoulos

INTRODUCTION

Alveolar hemorrhage (AH) is a potentially life-threatening clinical-pathological syndrome characterized by diffuse intra-alveolar bleeding originating from the pulmonary microcirculation. Bleeding is caused by disruption of the pulmonary capillary lining due to a variety of conditions.[1,2] Diffuse alveolar hemorrhage (DAH) should be distinguished from other causes of localized pulmonary hemorrhage originating from the bronchial circulation caused by airway disorders such as bronchiectasis, infection, and tumors.[3]

Hemoptysis, diffuse alveolar infiltrates, and a significant drop in hematocrit constitute the characteristic triad of DAH manifestations, although in many cases the clinical picture is not typical. Hemoptysis may be absent in up to one third of patients even in severe AH; expectorated blood is disproportionately small, compared to the total blood in alveoli. Hematocrit drop should be considered in comparison with the value that the patient used to have before the episode of DAH and not with the normally considered hematocrit values.

DIAGNOSTIC EVALUATION

Diffuse alveolar hemorrhage is generally acute in onset but occasionally can be more subacute and recurrent.

The identification of the underlying cause and prompt implementation of appropriate therapy are crucial for a patient presenting with DAH. The differential diagnosis of DAH includes diseases associated with the pathologic finding of capillaritis, those associated with normal vessels, or otherwise bland hemorrhage, and those associated with diffuse alveolar damage (DAD) **(Box 1)**.[4]

The goals of the clinicolaboratory evaluation are first to establish the diagnosis of DAH and second to identify the underlying cause. The causes of AH can be broadly divided into immune and nonimmune **(Table 1)**.[3] The most frequent immune cause of AH is small-vessel vasculitis, a potentially organ-/life-threatening manifestation.[5] Recent evidence suggests that many cases of AH are of nonimmune origin and these causes should not be overlooked. The more frequent nonimmune causes of AH are heart diseases, especially left ventricular failure, mitral stenosis, infections, drugs, coagulation disorders, and malignancies.[3]

Clinical Features

Diffuse alveolar hemorrhage appears at any age and often with an established associated disease but may also appear as the initial manifestation of an underlying systemic disease. The medical history should include all the preexisting conditions that can cause AH. In addition, it should include a review of exposures and inhaled agents, smoking history, medication, and illicit drugs as well as exposure to infected animals or their urine, immersion in contaminated water (swimming, fishing, and floods), bites, and recent stay in tropical areas.

The severity of symptoms depends on the acuity and severity of DAH and on the extent of underlying disease. Symptoms of DAH other than hemoptysis are nonspecific and include chest pain, cough, and dyspnea. Hypoxemic respiratory failure is of variable severity and results from both ventilation/perfusion mismatch secondary to alveolar filling and anemia. Admission to the intensive care unit is required in up to 50% of cases.

Clinical evaluation should include the following for the assessment of the systemic disorders:

- General symptoms (fever, asthenia, weight loss) and recurrence of symptoms (fever, hemoptysis, dyspnea)
- Nasal symptoms (crusty rhinitis, septal erosions, sinusitis)
- Ocular symptoms (episcleritis, retinal vasculitis, iridocyclitis)
- Skin changes (palpable purpura, subcutaneous nodules, erythema, livedo)
- Musculoskeletal symptoms (arthralgias, myalgias, synovitis)
- Neurological symptoms (mono- or multineuritis)
- Signs of glomerulonephritis (glomerular erythrocytes in urine examination)

BOX 1 Histology and causes of diffuse alveolar hemorrhage.

- *Pulmonary capillaritis*:
  - ANCA-associated granulomatous vasculitis
  - Microscopic polyangiitis
  - Isolated pulmonary capillaritis (ANCA positive and negative)
  - SLE
  - Rheumatoid arthritis
  - Mixed connective tissue disorder
  - Scleroderma
  - Polymyositis
  - Primary antiphospholipid antibody syndrome
  - Henoch–Schönlein purpura
  - Behçet syndrome
  - IgA nephropathy
  - Goodpasture syndrome
  - Idiopathic glomerulonephritis (pauci-immune or immunocomplex-related)
  - Acute lung transplant rejection
  - Idiopathic pulmonary fibrosis
  - Diphenylhydantoin
  - Retinoic acid toxicity
  - Autologous bone marrow transplantation
  - Myasthenia gravis
  - Cryoglobulinemia
  - Ulcerative colitis
  - Propylthiouracil
- *Bland pulmonary hemorrhage*:
  - IPH
  - Goodpasture syndrome
  - SLE
  - Coagulation disorders
  - Trimellitic anhydride, isocyanate exposure, penicillamine, amiodarone, nitrofurantoin
  - Mitral stenosis
  - Subacute bacterial endocarditis
  - Polyglandular autoimmune syndrome
  - Multiple myeloma
- *Diffuse alveolar damage*:
  - Bone marrow transplantation
  - Crack cocaine inhalation
  - Cytotoxic drug therapy
  - SLE
  - Radiation therapy
  - ARDS

(ANCA: antineutrophil cytoplasmic antibody; ARDS: acute respiratory distress syndrome; IPH: idiopathic pulmonary hemosiderosis; SLE: systemic lupus erythematosus)

TABLE 1: Etiology of alveolar hemorrhage (AH) syndromes.

Diagnostic category	Common causes of AH	Rare causes of AH systemic
Systemic vasculitis*	GPA, microscopic polyangiitis†	Henoch–Schöenlein purpura, EGPA, Behcet syndrome, mixed cryoglobulinemia due to hepatitis C virus, pauci-immune pulmonary capillaritis (with or without antineutrophil cytoplasmic antibodies), polyarteritis nodosa related to hepatitis B virus, Takayasu disease
Connective tissue diseases*	Systemic lupus erythematosus†	Rheumatoid arthritis, systemic sclerosis, idiopathic inflammatory myopathies mixed connective tissue disease
Other immune causes*	Antibasement membrane antibody disease†	Pauci-immune glomerulonephritis, immune complex glomerulonephritis, hemolytic uremic syndrome, immunoglobulin A nephropathy, celiac disease, inflammatory bowel diseases, cows' milk intolerance
Infections	Leptospirosis*,†	• Invasive aspergillosis, systemic candidiasis, strongyloidiasis, staphylococci (including *Staphylococcus aureus* producing) • Panton–Valentine leukocidin), legionellosis, mycoplasma, cytomegalovirus, herpes simplex virus, Hantavirus, AIDS, H1N1 influenza, malaria, *Strongyloides stercoralis*, *Stachybotrys chartarum*
Drugs	Propylthiouracil*	Alemtuzumab, abciximab, transretinoic acid, aminoglutethimide, amiodarone, azathioprine, carbamazepine, carbimazole, cyclosporine, clomifene, cytarabine, dextran, dihydralazine, dimethylsulfoxide, D-penicillamine, everolimus, fludarabine, gemcitabine, glibenclamide, methotrexate, mitomycin, moxalactam, nitrofurantoin, nitric oxide, phenytoin, quinidine, rituximab, sirolimus, sunitinib, tirofiban; see also hemostasis disorders
Toxic	Cocaine*	Trimellitic anhydride, pyromellitic dianhydride, isocyanates, hydrocarbon derivatives

Continued

Continued

Diagnostic category	Common causes of AH	Rare causes of AH systemic
Intravascular metastasis		Angiosarcoma, Kaposi sarcoma, choriocarcinoma, epithelioid hemangioendothelioma, multiple myeloma, renal cell carcinoma
Transplantation	Bone marrow transplant	Solid organ transplantation
Hemostasis disorders		Disseminated intravascular coagulation, thrombocytopenia, antiphospholipid syndrome, thrombotic thrombocytopenic purpura, hemophilia, drugs (oral anticoagulants, antiaggregants, antiglycoprotein IIb/IIIa, fibrinolytic agents)
Pulmonary vascular disease		Idiopathic and thromboembolic pulmonary hypertension, pulmonary veno-occlusive disease, pulmonary capillary hemangiomatosis
Heart disease		Mitral stenosis, left heart failure, left atrial myxoma
Other		Acute respiratory distress syndrome, idiopathic pulmonary hemosiderosis, amyloidosis, lymphangioleiomyomatosis, sarcoidosis, idiopathic pulmonary fibrosis, barotrauma, fat embolism

*Causes with definite or suspected immunological mechanism.
†Pulmonary–renal syndromes.
(AIDS: acquired immunodeficiency syndrome; EGPA: eosinophilic granulomatosis with polyangiitis; GPA: granulomatosis with polyangiitis)

Chest Imaging

The chest radiograph [chest X-ray (CXR)] or high-resolution computed tomography (HRCT) is nonspecific and indicates air space disease that can be either patchy or diffuse in appearance. Pulmonary apices and costodiaphragmatic angles may be relatively spared. When AH is mild, the chest radiograph may be almost normal. Pleural effusion is uncommon. The presence of Kerley B lines on the chest radiograph suggests another cause of DAH such as pulmonary veno-occlusive disease, mitral stenosis, or possibly pulmonary edema due to myocarditis, which can potentially complicate a systemic vasculitis or collagen vascular disease.

Laboratory Investigations

Initial blood testing should include routine hematology, biochemistry, coagulation status, and baseline markers of inflammation [erythrocyte sedimentation rate (ESR) and C-reactive protein (CRP)]. A urinalysis should always be ordered, because renal involvement is very often associated with pulmonary capillary disease even if symptoms from renal disease may be subtle. In these cases, the typical finding is the presence of glomerular erythrocytes (usually in abundance) often associated with proteinuria. The underlying pathology either may be a segmental necrotizing glomerulonephritis rapidly progressing to renal failure or other syndromic manifestations such as granulomatous polyangiitis [GPA, earlier Wegener's granulomatosis (WG)], microscopic polyangiitis (MPA), and other systemic vasculitides, e.g., systemic lupus erythematosus (SLE), or may be pauci-immune idiopathic glomerulonephritis (Goodpasture syndrome). Testing for both proteinase 3 antineutrophil cytoplasmic antibody (PR3-ANCA) and myeloperoxidase (MPO)-ANCA using a high-quality antigen-specific assay as the primary method of testing is recommended.[5]

The test battery should include the following:
- Anti-glomerular basement membrane (GBM) (Goodpasture disease)
- Antibodies associated with connective tissue diseases including antinuclear antibodies (ANA), anti-ds DNA antibodies, rheumatoid factor (RF), anticyclic citrullinated peptide, antinucleoproteins, and antiphospholipids [SLE, rheumatoid arthritis (RA)]
- Creatinine kinase and complement levels (myositis)

The results should be available as soon as possible, ideally within 24 hours.

Pulmonary Function Tests

Most patients with DAH are too ill to undergo pulmonary function testing. When performed, lung function tests usually show a restrictive ventilatory defect. An increase in diffusing capacity of the lung for carbon monoxide (DLCO) has been reported in AH and attributed to increased carbon monoxide uptake by intra-alveolar red blood cells.[6-9] However, recent studies showed that DLCO was increased in only a quarter of cases and was reduced in half of them, probably as a result of ventilation/perfusion mismatching.[10]

Bronchoscopy—Bronchoalveolar Lavage

Bronchoscopy with bronchoalveolar lavage (BAL) serves two purposes: Documentation of AH and exclusion of infection. Progressively hemorrhagic BAL found in serial samples is diagnostic of DAH but not of the underlying cause. Subacute AH can be diagnosed if hemosiderin-laden macrophages represent 20–30% of the total macrophage count. This finding may be absent in DAH of <72-hour duration, as it takes 48–72 hours for macrophages to accumulate. BAL specimens should also be sent for routine bacterial cultures and especially in immune-compromised hosts to look for fungi, *Pneumocystis jirovecii*, and viruses.

Histopathology

Although diagnostic biopsy remains the gold standard, a confident diagnosis can be made without tissue biopsy in a sufficient number of patients. So, the decision to obtain a biopsy specimen (renal, lung, other sites—skin, upper airway, etc.) should be made taking into consideration the risk of the procedure and the likelihood of biopsy findings to alter the therapeutic approach. Lung biopsy is only rarely performed in DAH, although it almost always provides definitive pathological evidence when the lung is clinically involved. Transbronchial biopsies are usually insufficient. Video-assisted thoracoscopic surgery is preferred than open lung biopsy as it is associated with less morbidity and mortality. In general, surgical lung biopsy is considered if DAH is associated with negative serology and negative urine examination, and not as a part of a systemic disease.[4] Three characteristic patterns, which reflect the nature of the underlying vascular injury, can be detected:

1. *Vasculitis or capillaritis*, which is the most frequent underlying histologic lesion, characterized by interstitial neutrophilic predominant infiltration, fibrinoid necrosis of the alveolar and capillary walls, and leukocytoclasis
2. *Bland hemorrhage* without any evidence of inflammation or destruction of the alveolar capillaries
3. *DAD* characterized by intra-alveolar hyaline membrane and interstitial edema with minimal inflammation

It should be kept in mind that DAH recurrence may lead to interstitial fibrotic lesions; pathology may also reveal areas of organizing pneumonia, but this does not exclude DAH diagnosis. When a pulmonary-renal syndrome is suspected, renal biopsy is usually more informative and less invasive than lung biopsy. In typical cases with multiple organ involvement, the biopsy site could be skin or nose for GPA or can even be avoided if serology is compatible (ANCA for MPA or GPA, ANA for SLE, anti-GBM for Goodpasture syndrome). Because of the variety of tests performed on the samples, the processing should be closely coordinated among the physicians and surgeons involved, and the pathologist should be alerted that vasculitis is in the differential diagnosis.

The clinician should not wait for the laboratory or biopsy results to start treatment, when vasculitis is highly suspected on the basis of:

- Clinical findings (dyspnea, pale face, highly desaturated patient) and recurrence of "pneumonia-like" or ENT symptoms [elevated CRP, white blood cell (WBC), fever, otitis]
- Simple laboratory tests (significant drop of hematocrit and glomerular erythrocytes in urine), significant hypoxemia
- HRCT (alveolar filling disease, rapidly moving consolidations)
- BAL (hemorrhagic sequential BAL)

ANTINEUTROPHIL CYTOPLASMIC ANTIBODY

Antineutrophil cytoplasmic antibody detection is an important tool for diagnosing small-vessel vasculitis, and new data suggest a pathophysiologic role of ANCA in their development.[11] The main target antigen for cytoplasmic ANCA (c-ANCA) is serine PR3 located in azurophilic granules and for perinuclear ANCA (p-ANCA) is MPO, an enzyme from azurophilic granules that catalyzes peroxidation of chloride to hypochlorite.[12] In contrast to c-ANCA, a variety of antibodies can cause a perinuclear immunofluorescence pattern (p-ANCA) on ethanol-fixed neutrophils.

Only the PR3-ANCA with c-ANCA combination and the MPO-ANCA with p-ANCA combination are sensitive and specific for ANCA-associated vasculitis (AAV).[13]

Positive and negative predictive values of ANCA testing for GPA and MPA are critically dependent on the pretest probability of the disease in the patient tested as well as on the analytical accuracy of the test method. It is also emphasized that ANCA testing should always be done in experienced and specialized laboratories.[14]

It is important to recognize that most patients with active severe disease are ANCA positive; about 25% with limited GPA have no detectable ANCA. c-ANCA is highly sensitive (90–95%) in active, systemic GPA, with a specificity of approximately 90%. In the proper clinical setting (i.e., with a very high pretest probability of disease), a positive C-ANCA/anti-PR3 has sufficient positive predictive value (PPV) that biopsy may be deferred. False-positive ANCA test results have been reported. Particularly, subacute bacterial endocarditis has been reported with positive c-ANCA/PR3.[15] MPO antibodies are more typically found in MPA and eosinophilic granulomatosis with polyangiitis (EGPA) but are much less specific.

The clinical utility of serial measurements of ANCA levels in follow-up is less well established. Although there is an association between ANCA titers and disease activity, if the only finding is the elevation of ANCA levels, this does not always predict disease relapse, but requires close follow-up of the patient with clinical and laboratory examinations.[16]

CLASSIFICATION OF SYSTEMIC VASCULITIS

Classification generally reflects dominant vessel size and ANCA status **(Fig. 1 and Box 2)**.

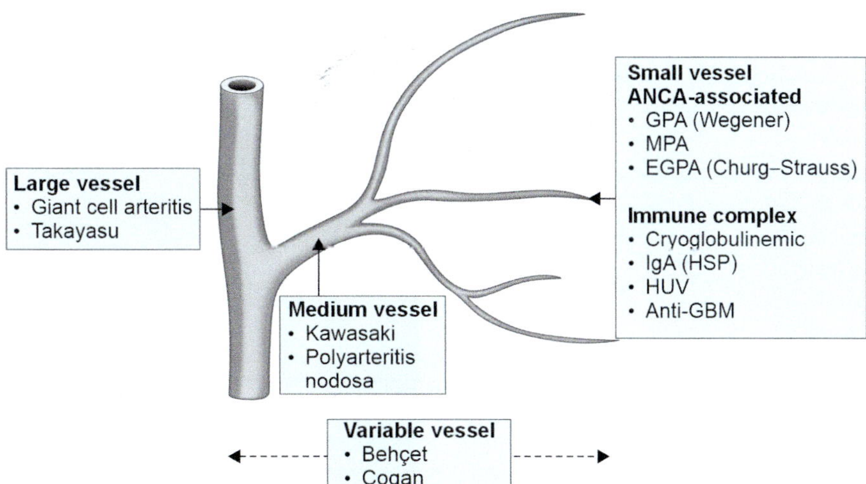

FIG. 1: Classification of systemic vasculitis based on vessel size and ANCA status.

(ANCA: antineutrophil cytoplasmic antibody; EGPA: eosinophilic granulomatosis with polyangiitis; GBM: glomerular basement membrane; GPA: granulomatosis with polyangiitis; HSP: Henoch–Schönlein purpura; HUV: hypocomplementemic urticarial vasculitis; IgA: immunoglobulin A; MPA: microscopic polyangiitis)

Source: Reports on Rheumatic Diseases, Series 7, Autumn 2012. Topical Reviews No 1.

GRANULOMATOSIS WITH POLYANGIITIS

Granulomatosis with polyangiitis, previously known as Wegener's granulomatosis, is the most common vasculitis characterized by necrotizing granulomatous inflammation, usually involving the upper and lower respiratory tracts, affecting predominantly small-to-medium vessels.[17]

About 90% of GPA patients present upper or lower airway involvement or both. In many patients, ear and nose or sinus symptoms are usually the predominant features which make them seek ENT consultation for a long time before AH ensues. Presence of fever, malaise, anemia, and high sedimentation rates should warn the clinician for the possibility of GPA. Serous otitis, chronic or subacute otitis, and/or mastoiditis are the main manifestations of ear involvement. Hearing loss is the result of either serous otitis or nerve involvement. Nose involvement is characterized by epistaxis, necrotizing inflammation with crusting, chondritis, septum perforation, and saddle-nose deformity.[18] Oropharynx may present ulcerations; "strawberry" gingival hyperplasia due to petechiae caused from interdental papillae is a rare but almost pathognomonic manifestation of GPA.[19] Subglottic stenosis causes wheezing which mimics asthma.[20]

Flow/volume loop associated with failure of improvement with correct asthma treatment may help the diagnosis. Bronchoscopy may reveal nonspecific findings as mucosal edema and erythema, ulceration, cobble-stone mucosa, and polypoid lesions **(Fig. 2)**. Necrotic mass (pseudotumor), stenosis, and trachea bronchomalacia may be found.[21] These findings are usually nonspecific for GPA, so biopsy does not reveal the diagnosis, except if the lesion is a necrotic mass, which may be mistaken as a tumor with necrosis (pathologists should be correctly informed by clinicians to look for granulomatosis with necrosis and not make the diagnosis of cancer, before considering the patient's data).

The lungs may be involved by GPA in two ways: Pulmonary nodules/masses or diffuse consolidations (due to AH/pulmonary capillaritis). Nodules are usually multiple and may cavitate **(Figs. 3 and 4)**. As they heal, the cavities become thin walled before disappearing. Relapses of disease as reappearance of nodules occur at the area of first location. Usually, the nodules are asymptomatic but when they appear in a patient with ENT and/or general symptoms (fever, malaise, anemia), physicians should think of the possibility of GPA.

Patients presenting with acute respiratory failure and acute respiratory distress syndrome (ARDS) should always be evaluated for the possibility of DAH, provided that cardiogenic pulmonary edema and infection are excluded. They usually have coexisting hematuria due to the presence of glomerular erythrocytes in urine, severe desaturation and remarkable fall of hemoglobin. Mortality is high and renal failure occurs in a very short time (few days or even hours). Treatment has to be started immediately, even if the diagnosis has not been confirmed.

Renal involvement is the most serious manifestation along with alveolar capillaritis. Up to 80% of the patients develop necrotizing glomerulonephritis as first or late manifestation of their disease which rapidly progresses to renal failure if not early recognized and treated.[22] Immunofluorescence shows no or only scant immune deposits in GPA and MPA, in contrast to the linear distribution of immune deposits along the basement membranes in Goodpasture syndrome or the granular immune complex deposits in SLE.

Heart involvement is often asymptomatic and underdiagnosed. Granulomatous infiltration of the myocardium is common with wall motion abnormalities. Complete

BOX 2 Classification of the vasculitides.

International Chapel Hill Consensus Conference on the Nomenclature of Vasculitides 2012

- *Large-vessel vasculitis (LVV)*:
  - Takayasu arteritis (TAK)
  - Giant cell arteritis (GCA)
- *Medium-vessel vasculitis (MVV)*:
  - Polyarteritis nodosa (PAN)
  - Kawasaki disease (KD)
- *Small-vessel vasculitis (SVV)*:
  - Antineutrophil cytoplasmic antibody (ANCA)-associated vasculitis (AAV):
    - Microscopic polyangiitis (MPA)
    - Granulomatosis with polyangiitis (Wegener's) (GPA)
    - Eosinophilic granulomatosis with polyangiitis (Churg–Strauss) (EGPA)
  - Immune complex SVV:
    - Antiglomerular basement membrane (anti-GBM) disease
    - Cryoglobulinemic vasculitis (CV)
    - IgA vasculitis (Henoch–Schönlein) (IgAV)
    - Hypocomplementemic urticarial vasculitis (HUV) (anti-C1qvasculitis)
- *Variable-vessel vasculitis (VVV)*:
  - Behcet's disease (BD)
  - Cogan's syndrome (CS)
- *Single-organ vasculitis (SOV)*:
  - Cutaneous leukocytoclastic angiitis
  - Cutaneous arteritis
  - Primary central nervous system vasculitis
  - Isolated aortitis
  - Others
- *Vasculitis associated with systemic disease:*
  - Lupus vasculitis
  - Rheumatoid vasculitis
  - Sarcoid vasculitis
  - Others
- *Vasculitis associated with probable etiology*:
  - Hepatitis C virus-associated cryoglobulinemic vasculitis
  - Hepatitis B virus-associated vasculitis
  - Syphilis-associated aortitis
  - Drug-associated immune complex vasculitis
  - Drug-associated ANCA-associated vasculitis
  - Cancer-associated vasculitis
  - Others

heart block may represent the first disease manifestation. Pericardial effusion and increased frequency of coronary artery disease with ischemic events have been referred.[23] About 20–50% of GPA patients may develop skin involvement. Leukocytoclastic vasculitis (palpable purpura with or without petechial lesions) is the most common manifestation.[24]

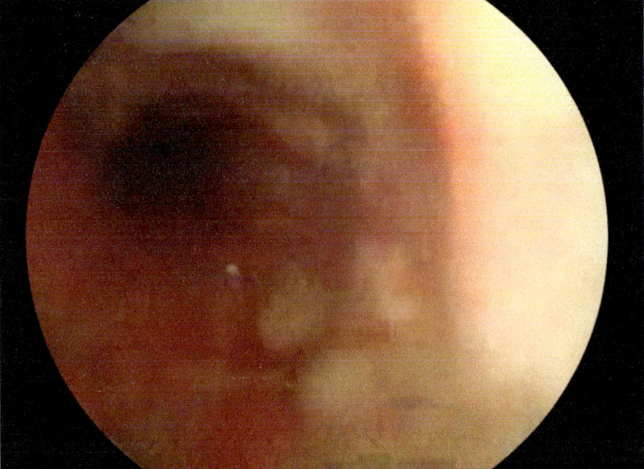

FIG. 2: Bronchoscopic appearance in granulomatous polyangiitis (Wegener's) showing diffuse erythema and plaques.

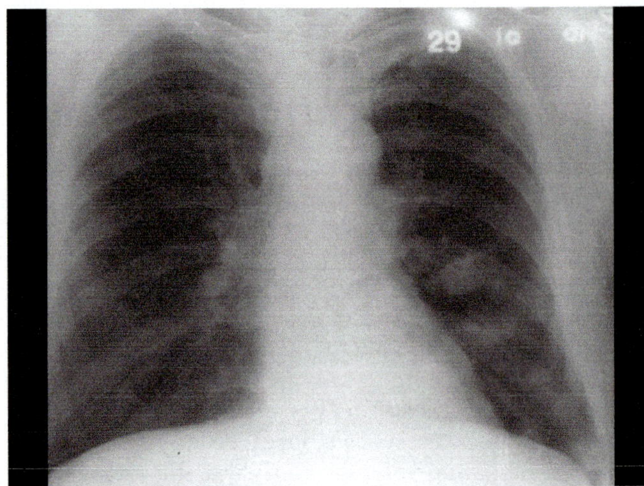

FIG. 3: Chest roentgenogram showing multiple nodular lesions in a patient of granulomatous polyangiitis (Wegener's).

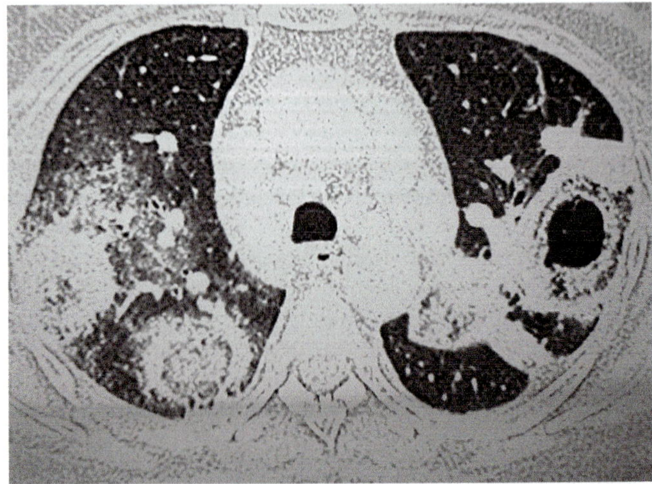

FIG. 4: Chest computed tomogram in a patient of granulomatous polyangiitis (Wegener's) with bilateral nodular lesion and cavities with intracavitary exudation.

The nervous system is rarely involved as the initial presentation of the disease, but later, it occurs during the course of the disease in up to 40% of patients.[22] The most common abnormality is multiple peripheral mononeuropathy, which is thought to be caused by vasculitis of vasa nervorum. Granulomatous infiltrations of the pituitary gland can cause diabetes insipidus. Ocular disease occurs in 50% of patients, usually as keratitis, conjunctivitis, scleritis, episcleritis, retro-orbital pseudotumor, or optic neuritis. Musculoskeletal symptoms are common, with most patients experiencing arthralgias and myalgias.[22]

Laboratory Testing

Laboratory test results may show mild-to-moderate normochromic normocytic anemia, mild leukocytosis, mild thrombocytosis, positive RF, elevated ESR, and CRP. It is important to emphasize that asymptomatic proteinuria may be present for weeks or even months before renal failure. Glomerular erythrocytes in urine and red cell casts are indicative of severe renal involvement in generalized disease. c-ANCA presents very high specificity for GPA (PR3 positive), but the diagnosis should not be made on ANCA serology alone, as ANCA can be found in other inflammatory diseases and infections or may be drug induced.[5] If the immunoassay is negative, but the clinical suspicion is still high, a second test is advised. A negative ANCA does not rule out a diagnosis of GPA, as a small proportion of patients with disease limited to the respiratory tract or with renal-limited vasculitis are ANCA negative.[5]

Diagnosis

Prolonged fever and persistent consolidations not responding completely to antibiotics, along with low saturations, low hematocrit and urine with glomerular erythrocytes, red cells casts, and proteinuria, make the diagnosis of GPA suspicious.

Clinicians should be concerned in cases of recurrent or nonresponding pneumonia.

Cytoplasmic ANCA PR3 are usually positive in this stage of GPA. If all of the above are present, diagnosis of GPA is already made and there is no need for biopsy specimen if the patient is too ill; treatment has to be started immediately.[22] In all other cases where GPA is suspected on strong clinical grounds, tissue biopsy is vitally important to confirm the diagnosis. Nasal septum biopsy in ENT disease is preferred, renal biopsy is preferred in patients with glomerular urine erythrocytes and prolonged proteinuria, and video-assisted thoracic surgery (VATS) is preferred for pulmonary nodules or masses.

The American College of Rheumatology (ACR) Board of Directors and the European Alliance of Associations for Rheumatology (EULAR) Executive Committee have recently approved new classification criteria for GPA in order to differentiate cases of GPA from similar types of vasculitis. The criteria should only be applied when a diagnosis of small- or medium-vessel vasculitis has been made and all potential "vasculitis mimics" have been excluded **(Table 2)**.[25]

TABLE 2: 2022 American College of Rheumatology/European Alliance for Rheumatology classification criteria for granulomatosis with polyangiitis.

Clinical criteria:	
Nasal involvement: Bloody discharge, ulcers, crusting, congestion, blockage, or septal defect/perforation	+3
Cartilaginous involvement (inflammation of ear or nose cartilage, hoarse voice or stridor, endobronchial involvement, or saddle nose deformity)	+2
Conductive or sensorineural hearing loss	+1
Laboratory, imaging, and biopsy criteria:	
Positive test for c-ANCA or anti-PR3 antibodies	+5
Pulmonary nodules, mass or cavitation on chest imaging	+2
Granuloma, extravascular granulomatous inflammation or giant cell on biopsy	+2
Inflammation, consolidation or effusion of nasal/paranasal sinuses or mastoiditis on imaging	+1
Pauci-immune glomerulonephritis on biopsy	+1
Positive test for p-ANCA or anti-MPO antibodies	−1
Blood eosinophils count > 1×10^9/L	−1
Sum the score for 10 items, if present. A score ≥ 5 is needed for classification of *granulomatosis with polyangiitis*	

(c-ANCA: cytoplasmic antineutrophil cytoplasmic antibody; MPO: myeloperoxidase; p-ANCA: peripheral ANCA; PR3: proteinase 3)

Source: Modified by Robson et al.[25]

Treatment

The treatment of GPA depends on the disease severity. For induction of remission in patients with new-onset GPA with organ /life threatening manifestations [AH, focal necrotizing glomerulonephritis, sensorineural hearing loss, mononeuritis multiplex, central nervous system (CNS) and cardiac involvement, leukocytoclastic vasculitis of the skin], the recommended treatment is a combination of corticosteroids and either rituximab (RTX) or cyclophosphamide (CYC).[5,26] RTX may be preferred, since it is considered less toxic and better tolerated than CYC and has been shown to provide similar benefits.[26] Retrospective studies suggest that the two remission induction regimens for RTX used in adults (375 mg/m^2 every week for 4 weeks and 1,000 mg on days 1 and 15) are equally efficacious. It remains controversial whether CYC should be preferred for certain types of severe disease, such as acute renal failure.

Although pharmacokinetics of RTX do not suggest inferior efficacy in patients with renal failure or DAH, some task force members prefer CYC over RTX in this setting.[5] Plasma exchange should not be initiated in patients with active glomerulonephritis or AH but can be considered for patients at a higher risk of progression to end-stage renal disease (ESRD) with a serum creatinine >300 μmol/L.[5,26]

For nonsevere disease without life- or organ-threatening manifestations (rhinosinusitis, uncomplicated cutaneous disease, noncavitating pulmonary nodules), treatment with a combination of glucocorticoids (GCs) and RTX is recommended. Methotrexate (MTX) or mycophenolate mofetil (MMF) can be considered as alternatives in patients with intolerance or contraindications to RTX.[5]

The recommended treatment with oral GCs is a starting dose of 50–75 mg prednisolone equivalent/day, depending on body weight and a stepwise reduction in GCs to 0.5 mg/kg after the first week and then a reduction of 5 mg every 2 weeks until achieving a dose of 5 mg prednisolone equivalent per day by 4–5 months.[5] High IV doses of corticosteroids (three daily pulses for a maximum total dose of 3 g) should be limited to treatment of severe organ-threatening manifestations, particularly either active renal involvement with a documented estimated glomerular filtration rate of <50 mL/min/1.73/m^2, or DAH.

As part of a strategy to substantially reduce exposure to GCs, avacopan (an oral C5aR inhibitor) may be considered for induction of remission in GPA in combination with RTX or CYC. It is recommended especially in patients who are at risk of developing GC-related adverse effects and complications or in patients with active glomerulonephritis and rapidly deteriorating kidney function who had better recovery of kidney function with avacopan.[5]

Time to a treatment response varies individually in the early treatment phase (weeks 0–4). Refractory disease is rare and needs to be distinguished from infections, other comorbidities, and alternative diagnoses. Raising the GC dose for some time can be a reasonable strategy, particularly if only minor symptoms persist. The combination of RTX and CYC is used in patients with refractory organ-threatening or life-threatening disease by many centers, but data on this approach are lacking. These patients should be referred to a center with expertise in vasculitis.[5]

For maintenance of remission, RTX (500 mg every 6 months) is the recommended treatment, with a lower relapse rate compared with azathioprine (AZA). AZA or MTX may be considered as alternatives.[5] Therapy to maintain remission for GPA must be continued for 24–48 months. Longer duration of therapy should be considered in relapsing patients or those with an increased risk of relapse but should be balanced against patient preferences and risks of continuing immunosuppression. Measurement of serum immunoglobulin concentrations prior to each course of RTX to detect secondary immunodeficiency is necessary. In addition, for patients receiving RTX, CYC, and/or high doses of GCs, the use of trimethoprim/sulfamethoxazole (T/S) as prophylaxis against *P. jirovecii* pneumonia (PJP) and other infections is recommended. The prophylaxis with T/S should be continued for the estimated duration of the biological effect of CYC and RTX of around 3 and 6 months after the last dose or B-cell reconstitution, respectively. For patients treated with GCs in combination with immunosuppressants other than CYC or RTX, T/S may be stopped once GC doses have been tapered to 15 mg/day, but that strong consideration should be given to continuing it until lower doses are achieved if other risk factors, such as pulmonary disease or hypogammaglobulinemia, are present.[5]

MICROSCOPIC POLYANGIITIS

Patients with MPA share some features with GPA patients; in early disease, distinction may be difficult. The typical histologic appearance is a pauci-immune focal segmental necrotizing glomerulonephritis, similar to that seen in GPA.[22] The majority of MPA patients has p-ANCA with specificity for MPO. Renal involvement is the most frequent organ manifestation occurring in 79% of patients, followed by skin (63%), peripheral nerve (58%), and gastrointestinal involvement (30%), while lung is involved in only 25% of patients (half of these present with AH).[27] Occasionally, MPA may be associated with pulmonary fibrosis, either as acute interstitial pneumonia or, more commonly, resembling idiopathic pulmonary fibrosis.[28] The ACR Board of Directors and the EULAR Executive Committee have recently approved new classification criteria for MPA in order to differentiate MPA from similar types of vasculitis **(Table 3)**.[29] Guidelines for the therapy of MPA are similar to those for GPA therapy; remission occurs in up to 93% of patients, while the relapse rate varies between 8 and 30%.[5] The overall 5-year survival is about 75%.[27]

TABLE 3: 2022 American College of Rheumatology/European Alliance for Rheumatology classification criteria for microscopic polyangiitis.

Clinical criteria:	
Nasal involvement: Bloody discharge, ulcers, crusting, congestion, blockage, or septal defect/perforation	–3
Laboratory, imaging, and biopsy criteria:	
Positive test for p-ANCA or anti-MPO antibodies	+6
Fibrosis or interstitial lung disease on chest imaging	+3
Pauci-immune glomerulonephritis on biopsy	+3
Positive test for c-ANCA or anti-PR3 antibodies	–1
Blood eosinophils count > 1 × 10^9/L	–4
Sum the score for 6 items, if present. A score ≥ 5 is needed for classification of microscopic polyangiitis	

(c-ANCA: cytoplasmic antineutrophil cytoplasmic antibody; MPO: myeloperoxidase; p-ANCA: peripheral ANCA; PR3: proteinase 3)
Source: Modified by Suppiah et al.[29]

EOSINOPHILIC GRANULOMATOSIS WITH POLYANGIITIS (CHURG–STRAUSS SYNDROME)

Eosinophilic granulomatosis with polyangiitis is a rare, eosinophilic-rich, and necrotizing granulomatous inflammation often involving the respiratory tract. It affects predominantly the small-to-medium vessels, associated with asthma and eosinophilia. Asthma especially distinguishes EGPA from GPA and MPA.[22] Asthma with or without allergic rhinitis and nasal polyps usually precedes vasculitis for several years and is usually refractory to standard therapy; its onset is late in life and becomes more severe when the vasculitis starts. Chest X-ray reveals transient peripheral alveolar-type infiltrates in >70% of the cases. DAH is extremely rare, in contrast to GPA and MPA.

Cardiac disease is common and is an important cause of mortality due to congestive heart failure, pericardial effusion, and restrictive cardiomyopathy. The peripheral nervous system may also be involved. Renal involvement is less common than in GPA and MPA.

The ACR Board of Directors and the EULAR Executive Committee have recently approved new classification criteria for EGPA in order to differentiate EGPA from similar types of vasculitis **(Table 4)**.[30]

Laboratory findings include peripheral blood eosinophilia, elevation of serum immunoglobulin E (IgE), and markers of inflammation (CRP, ESR). ANCA are detected in 40–70% of the patients, 75% of which are p-ANCA reacting with MPO and 25% c-ANCA. Only 25% of patients with EGPA who have no renal disease are ANCA positive, whereas 75% with any renal disease and 100% with documented necrotizing glomerulonephritis are ANCA positive.[31]

TABLE 4: 2022 American College of Rheumatology/ European Alliance for Rheumatology classification criteria for eosinophilic granulomatosis with polyangiitis.

Clinical criteria:	
Obstructive airway disease	+3
Nasal polyps	+3
Mononeuritis multiplex	+1
Laboratory and biopsy criteria:	
Blood eosinophils count > 1 × 10⁹/L	+5
Extravascular eosinophilic-predominant inflammation on biopsy	+2
Positive test for c-ANCA or anti-PR3 antibodies	−3
Hematuria	−1
Sum the score for 7 items, if present. A score ≥ 6 is needed for classification of *eosinophilic granulomatosis with polyangiitis*	

(c-ANCA: cytoplasmic antineutrophil cytoplasmic antibody; MPO: myeloperoxidase; p-ANCA: peripheral ANCA; PR3: proteinase 3)

Source: Modified by Crayson et al.[30]

BOX 3 Revised 2011 five-factor score.

1. Age > 65 years
2. Cardiac insufficiency
3. Renal insufficiency (creatinine 1.7 mg/dL)
4. Gastrointestinal involvement
5. Absence of ear, nose, and throat manifestations

CT scans are compatible with peripheral infiltrations with BAL eosinophilia, like chronic eosinophilic pneumonia.

Diagnosis needs a histological specimen from peripheral nerve or lung and compatible clinical and serological findings and should not be based only on peripheral and BAL eosinophilia.

The Five Factor Score (FFS) is used for prognostic assessment of EGPA **(Box 3)**. For patients with EGPA without risk factors for worse outcome with FFS = 0, corticosteroids are the recommended treatment with doses similar to those used for GPA.[5]

In cases of refractory or relapsing EGPA, the interleukin 5 (IL-5) inhibitor mepolizumab is recommended at a dose of 300 mg subcutaneously every 4 weeks. In patients with life-threatening manifestation of the disease, such as cardiac, nervous system, kidneys, and gastrointestinal tract involvement, CYC should be added to high-dose corticosteroids. RTX may be considered as an alternative.[5]

The ANCA-associated small-vessel diseases account for the major pulmonary vasculitic disorders. Other vasculitis are better associated with extrapulmonary disease and rarely cause AH.

IMMUNOGLOBULIN A VASCULITIS (HENOCH–SCHÖNLEIN PURPURA)

Henoch–Schönlein purpura is a vasculitis with IgA1-dominant immune deposits, affecting small vessels. Immunoglobulin A vasculitis (IgAV) often involves the skin and gastrointestinal tract and causes arthritis.[17] Glomerulonephritis indistinguishable from IgA nephropathy may occur. DAH has been reported in patients with IgA immune complexes which are present in the serum, lungs, and kidney. Corticosteroids and immunosuppressive drugs are the recommended therapy.

ISOLATED PULMONARY CAPILLARITIS

Isolated pulmonary capillaritis is a small-vessel vasculitis that is confined to the lung and without clinical or serologic features of an associated systemic disease. Some cases are associated with serum p-ANCA positivity, but most are pauci-immune. Patients with isolated pulmonary capillaritis have a better prognosis when compared with DAH occurring in the setting of a systemic vasculitis or collagen vascular disease.[4] Therapeutically, these patients should be approached in the same way as MPA and GPA.

VASCULITIS ASSOCIATED WITH SYSTEMIC DISEASE

Systemic Lupus Erythematosus

Diffuse alveolar hemorrhage due to pulmonary capillaritis with prominent immune complex deposits or due to bland hemorrhage in SLE occurs in approximately 4% of patients.[32] It must be distinguished from acute lupus pneumonitis and infectious pneumonia. Almost always the onset is abrupt with pulmonary infiltrates, fever, dyspnea, and hemoptysis (although the latter may be absent in 50%). Glomerulonephritis is usually present. Methylprednisolone and CYC remain the most commonly used therapies. Plasmapheresis and RTX are other beneficial treatment options.[33]

Diffuse alveolar hemorrhage has also occasionally been reported in other connective tissue diseases such as rheumatoid arthritis, mixed connective tissue disease, systemic sclerosis, polymyositis, and antiphospholipid antibody syndrome.[34]

Drug-associated Vasculitis

Several drugs can cause AH due to capillaritis, caused by immune mechanism—D-penicillamine, propylthiouracil, phenytoin, and transretinoic acid. D-penicillamine can cause AH and glomerulonephritis with granular deposits of immune complexes in glomerular capillaries. There are anecdotal reports of propylthiouracil-associated p-ANCA positive vasculitis with DAH.[35]

Other drugs (amiodarone and, less frequently, nitrofurantoin) may cause DAH associated with underlying bland hemorrhage or DAD (without evidence of capillaritis).[36]

ANTI-GLOMERULAR BASEMENT MEMBRANE DISEASE

Anti-GBM disease is a rare autoimmune disorder (one case per 1,000,000 population per year) characterized by rapidly progressive glomerulonephritis and AH. It is caused by autoantibodies directed against the NC1 domain of the a3 chain of the basement membrane collagen type 4 located on alveolar and glomerular basement membranes. Around 85% of patients with anti-GBM disease are active smokers, and exposure to another inhaled agent has been reported in up to one-third of patients.[10] The disease mainly affects young males in their third decade, but can also occur in females, older subjects, and nonsmokers. In approximately half of cases, pulmonary and renal involvement are both clinically apparent. In the other half, there is only renal impairment and fewer than 10% of patients have a disease that is limited to the lungs. Active cigarette smoking increases the risk of DAH.

The diagnosis is established by the detection of anti-basement membrane antibodies either in serum (in 80% of cases) or as linear deposits along glomerular basement membranes revealed by immune fluorescence staining on renal or sometimes lung biopsy. In about 20% of patients, p-ANCA (MPO) positivity is detected and DAH is more likely to develop in these patients. The standard treatment includes a combination of plasmapheresis, corticosteroids, and CYC. Plasmapheresis aims at rapid removal of circulating antibodies and immunosuppressive therapy at stopping antibody synthesis. Plasma exchanges are usually administered every 2–3 days until the disappearance of circulating antibodies. Treatment is continued for a median duration of 6 months.[36]

OTHER CAUSES OF DIFFUSE ALVEOLAR HEMORRHAGE

More than half of cases of AH are of nonimmune origin, such as mitral stenosis and left ventricular failure, infections, drugs, and coagulation disorders.

Hemodynamics Causes

Mitral stenosis can cause AH. The elevated hydrostatic pressure in pulmonary capillaries and/or bronchial veins at the surface of bronchial mucosa may lead to capillary rupture in the alveolar spaces and/or airway lumen. Besides mitral stenosis, nonvalvular systolic or diastolic left heart disease, mitral regurgitation, and pulmonary veno-occlusive disease may also cause AH.[37]

Infections

Pulmonary infections are rarely reported in association with DAH, but they should be considered in the diagnostic workup because of the obvious therapeutic implications. In immunocompromised patients, the main infectious diseases that cause DAH are cytomegalovirus, adenovirus, invasive aspergillosis, mycoplasma, legionella, and strongyloides. In immunocompetent patients, the infectious diseases that most frequently cause DAH are leptospirosis, influenza A (H1N1), dengue, malaria, and *Staphylococcus aureus* infection [especially strains producing Panton-Valentine leukocidin (PVL)]. Hantaviruses, cytomegalovirus (CMV), and tuberculosis (TB) may also cause AH, although such cases are rare. Certain angioinvasive bacteria and fungi may cause vasculitis. DAD and immune mechanisms may play a role in the manifestation of DAH due to pulmonary infections.[38]

Coagulation Disorders

Thrombocytopenia, either drug induced or secondary to idiopathic thrombocytopenic purpura, and hemolytic uremic syndrome are well-recognized causes of DAH. Oral anticoagulants, heparin, thrombolytic agents, and antiplatelet agents including have also been incriminated in the occurrence of AH.[39]

Diffuse Alveolar Damage

Diffuse alveolar damage complicating bone marrow and stem cell transplantation, cytotoxic drug therapy, sirolimus, nitrofurantoin, crack cocaine inhalation, severe viral infections, radiation therapy, and acute interstitial pneumonia, either idiopathic or associated with collagen vascular disease, can produce the syndrome of DAH.[40]

Diffuse alveolar hemorrhage has also been reported after the inhalation of fumes or dry powders of trimellitic anhydride. Antibodies to this compound may be found in the serum of affected workers, but DAH develops only following a latent period of 1–3 months. The treatment consists of removal from exposure.

CT scan may help the diagnosis since the DAD pattern is more likely to overshadow the alveolar filling pattern of DAH due to capillaritis (GPA origin), and the drop of hematocrit is not as impressive as in GPA disease.

Idiopathic Pulmonary Hemosiderosis

Idiopathic pulmonary hemosiderosis (IPH) is a rare disease characterized by recurrent episodes of AH resulting in chronic anemia and pulmonary fibrosis. Around 80% of cases occur in childhood and the remaining 20% occur in adults usually before the age of 30 years. The histology lacks evidence of capillaritis. Airspaces contain abundant hemosiderin-laden macrophages and red blood cells. The diagnosis of IPH is made by exclusion of other causes of AH. The cause is unknown, but an immune process may be involved as IPH appears to respond to immunosuppressant therapy. Corticosteroids may control the acute phase and prevent recurrences. In patients who have severe initial disease or have recurrent episodes of AH that limit tapering of oral corticosteroids, an immunosuppressive agent may be added.[41]

SUMMARY

Alveolar hemorrhage is a life-threatening syndrome which in 50% of cases is due to nonvasculitic causes, cardiogenic pulmonary edema, drugs, and infections. In GPA vasculitis, which is the most common one, ENT and constitutional symptoms predominate for months or years the acute phase of AH.

Very simple tests such as HRCT, low hematocrit, low saturation, glomerular erythrocytes in urine, and siderophages in BAL may give the diagnosis of vasculitis, especially if accompanied by positive ANCA. Early treatment is mandatory and has to be started immediately when these tests along with a compatible history may indicate GPA, accompanied by careful surveillance of the patient; these prolong the survival in most patients.

REFERENCES

1. Collard HR, Schwarz M. Diffuse alveolar hemorrhage. Clin Chest Med. 2004;25(3):583-92.
2. Specks U. Diffuse alveolar hemorrhage syndromes. Curr Opin Rheumatol. 2001;13(1):12-7.
3. Lazor R. Alveolar haemorrhage syndromes. Eur Respir Mon. 2011;54:15-31.
4. Lara AR, Schwarz MI. Diffuse Alveolar Hemorrhage. Chest. 2010, 137(5):1164-71.
5. Hellmich B, Sanchez-Alamo B, Schirmer JH, et al. EULAR recommendations for the management of ANCA-associated vasculitis: 2022 update. Ann Rheum Dis. 2023;83:1-18.
6. Addleman M, Logan AS, Grossman RF. Monitoring intrapulmonary hemorrhage in Goodpasture's syndrome. Chest. 1985;87:119-20.
7. Ball JA, Young KR Jr. Pulmonary manifestations of Goodpasture's syndrome. Antiglomerular basementmembrane disease and related disorders. Clin Chest Med. 1998;19:777-91.
8. Bowley NB, Steiner RE, Chin WS. The chest X-ray in antiglomerular basement membrane antibody disease (Goodpasture's syndrome). Clin Radiol. 1979;30:419-29.
9. Bowley NB, Hughes JM, Steiner RE. The chest X-ray in pulmonary capillary haemorrhage: correlation with carbon monoxide uptake. Clin Radiol. 1979;30:413-7.
10. Lazor R, Bigay-Gamé L, Cottin V, et al. Alveolar hemorrhage in anti-basement membrane antibody disease: a series of 28 cases. Medicine. 2007;86:181-93.
11. Kallenberg CGM. Pathogenesis of ANCA-associated vasculitides. Ann Rheum Dis. 2011;70:59-63.
12. Hoffman GS, Specks U. Anti-neutrophil cytoplasmic antibodies. Arthritis Rheum. 1998;41:1521-37.
13. Russell KA, Wiegert E, Schroeder DR, et al. Detection of anti-neutrophil cytoplasmic antibodies under actual clinical testing conditions. Clin Immunol. 2002;103:196-203.
14. Specks U. Controversies in ANCA testing. Cleve Clin J Med. 2012;79(Suppl 3):8 11.
15. Choi HK, Lamprecht P, Niles JL, et al. Subacute bacterial endocarditis with positive antineutrophil cytoplasmic antibodies and anti-proteinase 3 antibodies. Arthritis Rheum. 2000;43(1):226-31.
16. Finkielman JD, Merkel PA, Schroeder D, et al. Antiproteinase 3 antineutrophil cytoplasmic antibodies and disease activity in Wegener granulomatosis. Ann Intern Med. 2007;147(9):611-9.
17. Jennette JC, Falk RJ, Bacon PA, et al. 2012 Revised International Chapel Hill Consensus Conference Nomenclature of Vasculitides. Arthritis Rheum. 2013;65:1-11.
18. Langford C. Clinical features and diagnosis of small-vessel vasculitis. Cleve Clin J Med. 2012;79(3):3-7.
19. Specks U. Pulmonary vasculitis: In: Schwartz M, King T (Eds). Interstitial Lung Disease, 5th edition. Ontario: BC Decker; 2011. pp. 765-805.
20. Lynch J, Fishbein M, White E. Pulmonary vasculitis. In: Costabel U, Du Bois RM, Egan J (Eds). Diffuse Parenchymal Lung Disease. Basel: Karger Publishers; 2007. pp. 196-211.
21. Polychronopoulos VS, Prakash U, Golbin JM, et al. Airway involvement in Wegener's granulomatosis. Rheum Dis Clin North Am. 2007;33(4):755-75.

22. Watts R, Dharmapalaiah C. ANCA-associated vasculitis. Top Rev. 2012;1:1-10.
23. Faurschou M, Mellemkjaer L, Sorensen IJ, et al. Increased morbidity from ischemic heart disease in patients with Wegener's granulomatosis. Arthritis Rheum. 2009;60(4):1187-92.
24. Daoud MS, Gibson LE, DeRemee RA, et al. Cutaneous Wegener's granulomatosis: clinical, histopathologic, and immunopathologic features of thirty patients. J Am Acad Dermatol. 1994;31(4):605-12.
25. Robson JC, Grayson PC, Ponte C, et al. 2022 American College of Rheumatology/European Alliance of Associations for Rheumatology Classification Criteria for Granulomatosis with Polyangiitis. Arthritis Rheumatol. 2022;74(3):393-9.
26. Chung SA, Langford C, Maz M, et al. 2021 American College of Rheumatology/Vasculitis Foundation Guideline for the Management of Antineutrophil Cytoplasmic Antibody–Associated Vasculitis. Arthritis Rheumatol. 2021;73(8):1366-83
27. Guillevin L, Durand-Gasselin B, Cevallos R, et al. Microscopic polyangiitis: Clinical and laboratory findings in 85 patients. Arthritis Rheum. 1999;42:421-30.
28. Tzelepis GE, Kokosi M, Tzioufas A, et al. Prevalence and outcome of pulmonary fibrosis in microscopic polyangiitis. Eur Respir J. 2010;36(1):116-21.
29. Suppiah R, Robson J, Grayson P, et al. 2022 American College of Rheumatology/European Allianceof Associations for Rheumatology Classification Criteria for Microscopic Polyangiitis. Arthritis Rheumatol. 2022;74(3):400-6.
30. Grayson P, Ponte C, Suppiah R, et al. 2022 American College of Rheumatology/European Allianceof Associations for Rheumatology Classification Criteria for Eosinophilic Granulomatosis with Polyangiitis. Arthritis Rheumatology. 2022;74(3):386-92.
31. Sablé-Fourtassou R, Cohen P, Mahr A, et al. Antineutrophil Cytoplasmic Antibodies and the Churg–Strauss Syndrome. Ann Intern Med. 2005;143(9):632-8.
32. Kwok SK, Moon SJ, Ju JH, et al. Diffuse alveolar hemorrhage in systemic lupus erythematosus: risk factors and clinical outcome. Results from affiliated hospitals of Catholic University of Korea. Lupus. 2011;20:102-7.
33. Santos-Ocampo AS, Mandell BF, Fessler BJ. Alveolar hemorrhage in systemic lupus erythematosus: presentation and management. Chest. 2000;118:1083-90.
34. Schwarz MI, Zamora MR, Hodges TN, et al. Isolated pulmonary capillaritis and diffuse alveolar hemorrhage in rheumatoid arthritis and mixed connective tissue disease. Chest. 1998;113: 1609-15.
35. Ohtsuka M, Yamashita Y, Doi M, et al. Propylthiouracil-induced alveolar haemorrhage associated with antineutrophil cytoplasmic antibody. Eur Respir J. 1997;10:1405-7.
36. Tanawuttiwat T, Harindhanavudhi T, Hanif S, et al. Amiodarone-induced alveolar haemorrhage: a rare complication of a common medication. Heart Lung Circ. 2010;19:435-7.
37. Schwartz R, Myerson RM, Lawrence T, et al. Mitral stenosis, massive pulmonary hemorrhage, and emergency valve replacement. N Engl J Med. 1966;275:755-8.
38. Ranke FM, Zanetti G, Hochhegger B, et al. Infectious diseases causing diffuse alveolar hemorrhage in immunocompetent patients: a state-of-the-art review. Lung. 2013;191(1):9-18.
39. Ali A, Hashem M, Rosman HS, et al. Use of platelet glycoprotein IIb/IIIa inhibitors and spontaneous pulmonary hemorrhage. J Invasive Cardiol. 2003;15:186-8.
40. Lara A, Frankel S, Schwarz I. Diffuse alveolar hemorrhage: In: Schwartz M, King T (Eds). Interstitial Lung Disease, 5th edition Ontario: BC Decker; 2011. pp. 805-32.
41. Ioachimescu OC, Sieber S, Kotch A. Idiopathic pulmonary haemosiderosis revisited. Eur Respir J. 2004;24(1):162-70.

CHAPTER 119

Pulmonary Hypertension: Etiology and Classification

Radha Munje, Gyanshankar Mishra, Nikhil Rathod

INTRODUCTION

The history of pulmonary artery hypertension (PAH) can be traced back to the late 19th century when Ernst von Romberg, a renowned German physician, made pioneering observations on autopsies, exploring the pathological aspects of pulmonary vasculature. In 1901, Dr Abel Ayerza from Argentina conducted an autopsy on a cyanotic patient and provided a detailed explanation of the condition, naming it "Cardíaco Negro" to describe the state of the heart. Ayerza also proposed that chronic lung disorders caused damage to the pulmonary artery, leading to right heart hypertrophy, which became known as Ayerza's disease. In the 1940s, Dr Oscar Brenner challenged the prevailing belief that syphilis was the main cause of pulmonary hypertension (PH) by studying histopathological changes in 100 patients.

The introduction of cardiac catheterization by Dickinson W Richards and Andre F Cournand in the 1930s and 1940s was a significant milestone. These advancements allowed for improved right-heart catheterization techniques, resulting in the Nobel Prize in Physiology and Medicine in 1956. In the late 1960s, an outbreak of PH associated with the appetite suppressant aminorex occurred in Austria, the Federal Republic of Germany, and Switzerland. In response, the World Health Organization (WHO) convened a crucial meeting in Geneva in 1973 to evaluate PH as a rare disease. During this meeting, a mean pulmonary artery pressure (PAP) of 25 mm Hg was arbitrarily designated as the defining criterion for pulmonary hypertension. This definition persisted until the Sixth World Symposium on Pulmonary Hypertension (WSPH) in 2018, where the condition was redefined as a mean PAP exceeding 20 mm Hg, with a pulmonary vascular resistance of ≥3 Woods units, encompassing all forms of precapillary PH.[1,2]

DEFINITION OF PULMONARY HYPERTENSION

In recent times, the collaborative effort of the task force responsible for assessing the diagnosis and management of PH, comprising the European Society of Cardiology and the European Respiratory Society, laid down guidelines that impart a refined perspective on the condition. Here, the guidelines significantly lowered the threshold for pulmonary vascular resistance, now established at 2 Woods units, drawing from comprehensive data elucidating the uppermost bounds of pulmonary vascular resistance in individuals devoid of any pathological manifestations.[3]

The current updated definition of PH **(Table 1)** hemodynamically characterizes PH as well as allows understanding its pathophysiology using pulmonary vascular resistance (PVR) and pulmonary arterial wedge pressure (PAWP). The addition of PVR and PAWP to the definition, though may make it seem more complex, is crucial to include these parameters to differentiate elevated PAP caused by pulmonary vascular disease from that caused by left heart disease, or increased pulmonary blood flow, or increased intrathoracic pressure.

TABLE 1: Hemodynamic definitions of pulmonary hypertension.[3]

Definition	Hemodynamic characteristics
PH	mPAP > 20 mm Hg
Precapillary PH	mPAP > 20 mm Hg PAWP ≤15 mm Hg PVR > 2 WU
IpcPH	mPAP > 20 mm Hg PAWP > 15 mm Hg PVR ≤2 WU
CpcPH	mPAP > 20 mm Hg PAWP > 15 mm Hg PVR > 2 WU
Exercise PH	mPAP/CO slope between rest and exercise > 3 mm Hg/L/min

Note: Some patients present with elevated mPAP (0.20 mm Hg) but low PVR (≤2 WU) and low PAWP (≤15 mm Hg); this hemodynamic condition may be described by the term 'unclassified'.

(CO: cardiac output; CpcPH: combined post- and precapillary pulmonary hypertension; IpcPH: isolated post-capillary pulmonary hypertension; mPAP: mean pulmonary arterial pressure; PAWP: pulmonary arterial wedge pressure; PH: pulmonary hypertension; PVR: pulmonary vascular resistance; WU: Wood units)

CLASSIFICATION

In the past, the classification of PH revolved around the dichotomy of primary and secondary PH, with categorization based on discernible causative factors and associated risk elements. However, the Second WSPH held in 1998 brought forth a significant evolution in the clinical classification of this condition. This updated framework sought to individualize distinct categories of PH that showcased analogous pathological characteristics, shared hemodynamic profiles, and called for similar therapeutic approaches.[4] The Fifth WSPH proposed a comprehensive classification system, intended to be applicable to both adult and pediatric populations. Recent advancements in knowledge and understanding led to revision of the classification during the Sixth WSPH.

This updated classification entailed notable alterations, such as the repositioning of vasoreactive patients diagnosed with idiopathic pulmonary arterial hypertension (IPAH) and the reassessment of group 5 PH, resulting in the repositioning of PH associated with lymphangioleiomyomatosis within group 3. Additionally, within group 4 PH, the terminology chronic thromboembolic pulmonary disease (CTEPD), with or without PH, was introduced. It is important to note that while the World Health Organization (WHO) group system serves to identify the specific type of PH afflicting a patient, the WHO functional class system provides valuable insight into the extent to which the disease impacts their overall functionality.[5,6]

Pulmonary hypertension is intricately classified into five distinct groups based on clinical manifestations and etiology **(Table 2)**:

- *Group 1*: Pulmonary arterial hypertension
- *Group 2*: Pulmonary hypertension arising from left heart disease
- *Group 3*: Pulmonary hypertension induced by lung diseases or hypoxia, or a combination thereof

TABLE 2: Clinical classification of pulmonary hypertension.[3]

Group 1: Pulmonary arterial hypertension (PAH)	1.1 Idiopathic: 1.1.1 Nonresponders at vasoreactivity testing 1.1.2 Acute responders at vasoreactivity testing 1.2 Heritable 1.3 Associated with drugs and toxins 1.4 Associated with: 1.4.1 Connective tissue disease 1.4.2 HIV infection 1.4.3 Portal hypertension 1.4.4 Congenital heart disease 1.4.5 Schistosomiasis 1.5 PAH with features of venous/capillary (PVOD/PCH) involvement 1.6 Persistent PH of the newborn
Group 2: PH associated with left heart disease	2.1 Heart failure: 2.1.1 With preserved ejection fraction 2.1.2 With reduced or mildly reduced ejection fraction 2.2 Valvular heart disease 2.3 Congenital/acquired cardiovascular conditions leading to postcapillary PH
Group 3: PH associated with lung diseases and/or hypoxia	3.1 Obstructive lung disease or emphysema 3.2 Restrictive lung disease 3.3 Lung disease with mixed restrictive/obstructive pattern 3.4 Hypoventilation syndromes 3.5 Hypoxia without lung disease (e.g., high altitude) 3.6 Developmental lung disorders
Group 4: PH associated with pulmonary artery obstructions	4.1 Chronic thromboembolic PH 4.2 Other pulmonary artery obstructions
Group 5: PH with unclear and/or multifactorial mechanisms	5.1 Hematological disorders 5.2 Systemic disorders 5.3 Metabolic disorders 5.4 Chronic renal failure with or without hemodialysis 5.5 Pulmonary tumor thrombotic microangiopathy 5.6 Fibrosing mediastinitis

TABLE 3: World Health Organization classification of functional status of patients with pulmonary hypertension.[3]

Class	Description
WHO-FC I	Patients with pulmonary hypertension but without resulting limitation of physical activity. Ordinary physical activity does not cause undue dyspnea or fatigue, chest pain or near syncope
WHO-FC II	Patients with pulmonary hypertension resulting in a slight limitation of physical activity. They are comfortable at rest. Ordinary physical activity causes undue dyspnea or fatigue, chest pain or near syncope
WHO-FC III	Patients with pulmonary hypertension resulting in marked limitation of physical activity. They are comfortable at rest. Less than ordinary activity causes undue dyspnea or fatigue, chest pain or near syncope
WHO-FC IV	Patients with pulmonary hypertension with inability to carry out any physical activity without symptoms. These patients manifest signs of right heart failure. Dyspnea and/or fatigue may even be present at rest. Discomfort is increased by any physical activity

(WHO-FC: World Health Organization functional class)

- *Group 4*: Chronic thromboembolic pulmonary hypertension and pulmonary hypertension associated with obstructions in the pulmonary arteries,
- *Group 5*: Pulmonary hypertension with ambiguous or multifactorial origins

Among these groups, the highest proportion of patients worldwide is observed in group 2, which comprises PH resulting from left heart disease, closely followed by group 3, characterized by PH associated with chronic lung diseases. The WHO classification is based on the functional class system **(Table 3)**.[2]

PATHOPHYSIOLOGY

The pulmonary circulation, which refers to the blood flow within the lungs, normally exhibits low resistance, with the blood pressure in the pulmonary arteries being about one tenth of that in the rest of the body. PH is diagnosed when the mean PAP exceeds 20 mm Hg. In the case of PAH, the primary issue lies in a progressive and profound dysfunction of the pulmonary blood vessels. This condition is characterized by the narrowing of the vessels, remodeling of all layers of their walls, and the formation of blood clots within them. In the advanced stages, patients may develop complex vascular formations called plexiform lesions, originating from the remodeled pulmonary arteries.[2]

On the other hand, group 2 PH arises due to left heart disease, which leads to increased pressure in the pulmonary veins and subsequently PH. Although vascular remodeling does occur as a consequence of increased venous pressure and shear stress in this context, it is typically less pronounced compared to PAH.[2]

Group 3 PH is associated with chronic obstructive or interstitial lung diseases, which result in the destruction of lung tissue and a subsequent reduction in the density of the small blood vessels surrounding the air sacs. This reduction in density, known as alveolar-capillary density, contributes to the development of group 3 PH. In this group, vascular remodeling is further influenced by processes such as hypoxic pulmonary vasoconstriction, fibrosis, and inflammation.[2] The various lung diseases related to group 3 PH are listed as under:

- Chronic obstructive pulmonary disease (COPD)
- Diffuse interstitial lung diseases:
  - Idiopathic interstitial pneumonias
  - Environmental and occupational exposures
  - Multisystem diseases
  - Other rare lung diseases
- Mixed restrictive and obstructive diseases
- Sleep disordered breathing
- Alveolar hypoventilation syndrome
- Chronic exposure to high altitude
- Developmental lung diseases

Role of Tobacco Smoke in Pulmonary Hypertension Development

Tobacco smoke as a harmful factor and contributor to pulmonary vascular disease is particularly significant in Group 3 PH. Smoking has been observed to cause intimal hyperplasia, reduced expression of endothelial nitric oxide synthase (eNOS), increased expression of vascular endothelial growth factor (VEGF), infiltration of inflammatory cells, and an imbalance in mitochondrial fission and fusion, resulting in oxidative stress and dysfunction of mitochondria. Cigarette smoking is believed to play a central role in the vascular changes that lead to the development of PH in COPD. In laboratory studies, human pulmonary artery endothelial cells exposed to cigarette smoke have demonstrated decreased activity and expression of eNOS, as well as reduced expression of prostacyclin synthase mRNA and protein, in a dose- and time-dependent manner. Vascular remodeling caused by cigarette smoke exposure may occur before clinically detectable emphysema or airflow obstruction, as observed in animal models.[7]

Group 4 PH arises from the presence of pulmonary emboli or obstructions in the pulmonary arteries. These blockages cause a decrease in the functional area available for blood flow in the lungs, leading to an increase in resistance within the pulmonary blood vessels. As a result, unaffected vessels are overloaded with blood, triggering remodeling processes that further contribute to the development of PH.[2]

In the case of group 5 PH, the underlying causes are diverse and not yet fully comprehended. Conditions that are uncommon, such as Takayasu arteritis, have been observed to be linked with PH. Takayasu arteritis-associated PH is classified under group 5 PH.[8] However, they often involve a combination of the aforementioned processes. Additionally, in situations where there is chronic breakdown of red blood cells, known as hemolytic anemias, a significant factor in the development of PH is the subsequent depletion of stores of nitric oxide (NO), an important molecule for blood vessel function.[2]

PAH may rarely occur without a known cause (idiopathic) or, more commonly, as a consequence of various underlying medical conditions. Despite the cause, patients experience similar changes in their lungs that lead to partial blockage of small pulmonary arteries, increased resistance in the pulmonary vascular system, and eventually, right ventricular failure and death. These changes include increased contraction of the pulmonary arterioles, dysfunction of the endothelial cells, proliferation and remodeling of both endothelial and smooth muscle cells, and formation of blood clots in the lungs.

In fact, initial vascular injuries lead to increase in cytokines in vascular cells. After secretion into the bloodstream, cytokines promote accumulation of circulating neutrophils and monocytes, and T and B lymphocytes, resulting in increased vascular proliferation and damage.

Impact on the Right Ventricle

In the early stages of the disease, the right ventricle undergoes compensatory changes, which include angiogenesis (formation of new blood vessels), hypertrophy (enlargement of cardiac muscle cells), and increased thickness of the ventricular walls. During initial period, the right ventricle and the pulmonary artery work together harmoniously. However, as PH progresses to advanced stages, the right ventricle experiences maladaptive changes. These changes involve a shift in the heart muscle cells' energy generation (metabolic reprogramming), a decrease in capillary density (capillary rarefaction), the development of fibrous tissue (fibrosis), cell death (apoptosis), inflammation, immune cell recruitment, increased oxidative stress, and dysregulation of the renin-angiotensin-aldosterone system (RAAS) and neurohormonal pathways.[2] Consequently, the right ventricle dilates, and the septum separating the left and right ventricles may protrude into the left ventricle. Additionally, the workload on the right ventricle and pulmonary artery becomes uncoupled, resulting in reduced efficiency. These changes signify the progressive decline in right ventricular function as PH advances.

Current Concepts in Endothelial Cell Dysfunction

In the current understanding of PAH, there is a proposed sequence of changes in the behavior of endothelial cells that contribute to the progression of the disease. In the early stages, these cells are subjected to various harmful factors such as abnormal blood flow patterns, low oxygen levels, and inflammation. This initial injury to the endothelial cells triggers a process called apoptosis, where the cells undergo programmed cell death, leading to a reduction in the number of pulmonary blood vessels. However, the remaining endothelial cells respond by becoming hyperproliferative, meaning they multiply excessively, and they also become resistant to apoptosis. This abnormal behavior of the endothelial cells contributes to the formation of plexiform lesions, which are complex abnormal blood vessel structures. In the later stages of pulmonary arterial hypertension, the endothelial cells undergo a state of senescence, meaning they become aged and lose their normal functioning. This state of senescence is thought to make the disease irreversible, highlighting the importance of early intervention in managing the condition.[2]

Abnormal Metabolic Remodeling

Let us explore the significant metabolic alterations that take place in PAH. Abnormal metabolic remodeling has emerged as a primary contributor to the development of PAH, with a key focus on the shift from oxidative phosphorylation to glycolysis, commonly known as the Warburg effect. In PAH, there is an increased emphasis on glycolysis, the breakdown of glucose for energy. Specifically, lung cells exhibit elevated activity of two important enzymes, namely 6-phosphofructo-2-kinase/fructose-2,6-biphosphatase 3 (PFKFB3) and lactate dehydrogenase-B (LDHB). The heightened LDHB activity impacts pyruvate dehydrogenase (PDH), an enzyme responsible for energy production in the mitochondria. LDHB inhibits PDH through pyruvate dehydrogenase kinase (PDK), leading to lactate accumulation in the cytoplasm and a decline in new mitochondria generation. This leads to reduction in ATP production through the tricarboxylic acid (TCA) cycle, a crucial energy-producing pathway. Additionally, a decrease in mitochondrial DNA (mtDNA) content and an increase in the production of harmful reactive oxygen species (ROS) are observed. The specific changes in fatty acid oxidation, another energy-generating process, are not yet fully understood in this context. These metabolic abnormalities have been identified in various cell types involved in PAH, including pulmonary artery endothelial cells, pulmonary artery smooth muscle cells, and the right ventricle of the heart.[2]

Key Affected Pathways

The disruptions to three key signaling pathways (nitric oxide, prostacyclin and thromboxane A2, and endothelin-1) are the underlying causes of these progressive pulmonary vascular defects **(Fig. 1)**. Specifically, PAH occurs due to reduced production of vasodilators (such as prostacyclin) and decreased function of NOS, while at the same time, there is increased signaling from the vasoconstrictive and mitogenic effects of endothelin-1. Researchers have a mechanistic understanding of these three pathways, which has led to the development of targeted pharmacological therapies for PAH that have shown great promise.[9]

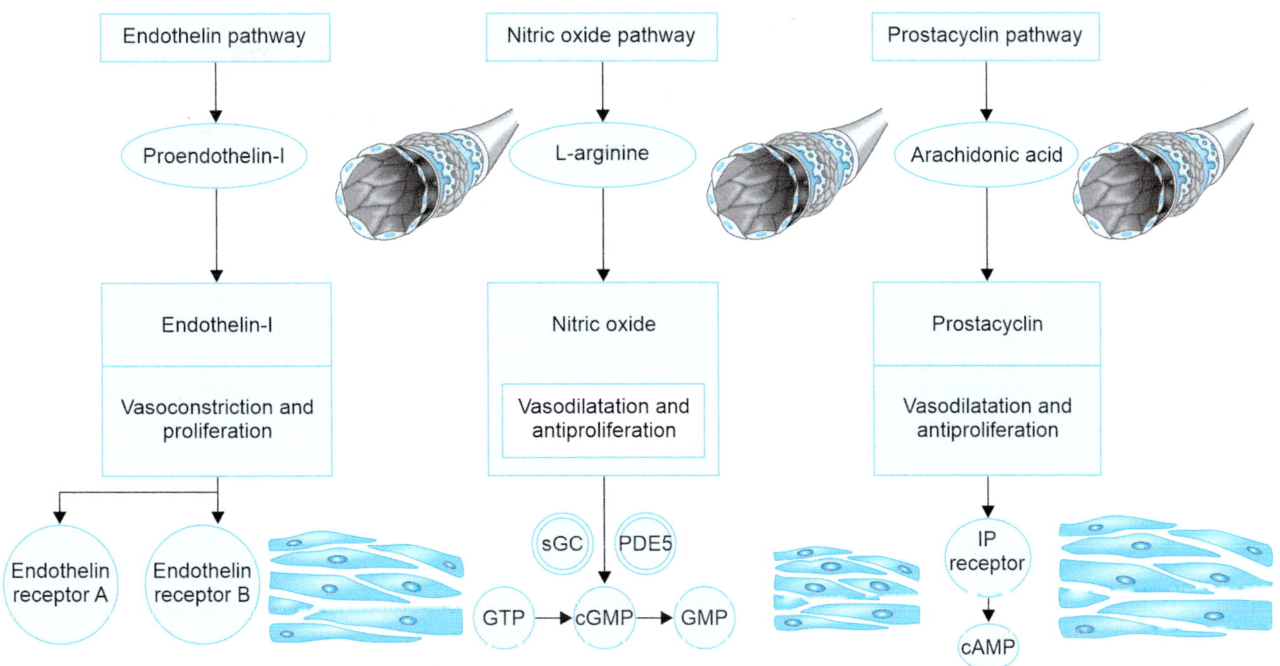

FIG. 1: Key signaling pathways involved in PAH.

(cAMP: cyclic adenosine monophosphate; cGMP: cyclic guanosine monophosphate; GMP: guanosine monophosphate; GTP: guanosine triphosphate; PAH: pulmonary artery hypertension; PDE5: phosphodiesterase type 5; sGC: soluble guanylate cyclase)

Nitric Oxide Pathway

Nitric oxide is a molecule produced by endothelial cells in blood vessels through the action of an enzyme called eNOS. In the presence of oxygen, NADPH, and other cofactors, eNOS converts l-arginine to l-citrulline, generating NO. This molecule diffuses into the smooth muscle cells of the pulmonary vasculature, where it binds to an enzyme called soluble guanylate cyclase. The binding triggers the conversion of guanosine triphosphate to cyclic guanosine monophosphate (cGMP). The activation of downstream cGMP-dependent protein kinases leads to pulmonary vasodilation. Nitric oxide also inhibits smooth muscle cell proliferation, platelet aggregation, and thrombosis, which help maintain healthy pulmonary blood vessels.[9]

In PAH, the availability of nitric oxide is reduced, leading to vasoconstriction, increased smooth muscle cell proliferation, inflammation, and thrombosis. Initially, reduced eNOS expression was thought to cause these pathological changes in PAH patients. However, recent studies have shown similar outcomes in animal and human models with persistent eNOS activation, suggesting a complex role. This apparent contradiction may be explained by the influence of reactive oxygen species, particularly tetrahydrobiopterin, on the dysfunction of eNOS. This dysfunction leads to endothelial dysfunction, vasoconstriction, and vascular remodeling in these models.[9]

Currently, there are two approved drug classes that target the NO pathway in PAH: Phosphodiesterase 5 inhibitors and guanylate cyclase stimulators. Phosphodiesterase 5 inhibitors prevent the degradation of cGMP, increasing its concentration in the bloodstream and promoting the vasodilatory and antiproliferative effects of nitric oxide. Guanylate cyclase stimulators directly act on soluble guanylate cyclase, even in the absence of nitric oxide, resulting in similar increases in cGMP concentration.[9]

Prostacyclin–Thromboxane A2 Pathway

The prostacyclin–thromboxane A2 pathway is crucial for maintaining healthy pulmonary vasculature. Prostacyclins, produced in endothelial cells, activate adenylate cyclase, which causes smooth muscle relaxation and vasodilation. They also inhibit platelet aggregation and smooth muscle proliferation and have anti-inflammatory and antithrombotic effects. However, in PAH, the pathway shifts toward thromboxane A2, which leads to platelet aggregation, vasoconstriction, and proliferation. Animal models have shown that IP knockout mice subjected to chronic hypoxia exhibit severe PAH and vascular remodeling. Furthermore, patients with PAH have reduced production of prostacyclins as well as reduced expression of prostacyclin receptor and synthase. Prostacyclin analogs and receptor agonists are the current clinical drugs developed for PAH therapy that act on the prostacyclin pathway.[9]

Endothelin-1 Pathway

The endothelin-1 (ET-1) pathway is a key regulator of vascular tone in the pulmonary circulation. ET-1 is a potent vasoconstrictor, which is produced by endothelial cells from the precursor big-ET-1. ET-1 binds to two G-protein-coupled receptors, ETA and ETB, which are expressed on vascular smooth muscle cells and endothelial cells. ETA promotes vasoconstriction, hypertrophy, proliferation, cell migration, and fibrosis, whereas activation of ETB on smooth muscle causes vasoconstriction, and on endothelial cells causes vasodilation and anti-proliferation. In PAH, there is an increase in expression of ETA and smooth muscle ETB, but reduced expression of endothelial ETB, leading to a shift toward vasoconstriction. This pathway is counteracted by endothelin receptor antagonists (ERAs), which are available as ETA selective or dual action on ETA and ETB receptors. PAH patients have increased ET-1 concentrations in their plasma and pulmonary vascular endothelial cells, and the use of ERAs has been shown to improve exercise capacity, hemodynamics, and overall quality of life in these patients.[9]

Genetic Factors

Heritable pulmonary arterial hypertension (hPAH) is a form of PAH that is inherited in an autosomal dominant manner, meaning that a person only needs to inherit one copy of the mutated gene from one parent to develop the condition. Mutations in several genes that encode proteins involved in the transforming growth factor β (TGF-β) receptor superfamily have been linked to hPAH. The most commonly mutated gene is *BMPRII*, which accounts for approximately 70% of hPAH cases and 10–40% of apparently sporadic cases. However, only 20% of individuals with disease-associated variants actually develop PAH, and the expression of these genes is influenced by various genetic, genomic, and environmental factors. Animal studies have demonstrated that reduced *BMPRII* activity leads to vascular remodeling and PAH, while improving *BMPRII* expression can limit endothelial dysfunction and attenuate PAH. Genetic testing is available but should be offered by trained individuals and according to ethical principles, as the incomplete penetrance and expressivity of these gene variants may lead to unnecessary anxiety.[10]

In children, PAH can manifest as a rare complication of some genetic syndromes. Although not always associated with congenital heart disease, PAH has been observed in genetic syndromes such as Down syndrome, DiGeorge syndrome, VACTERL, CHARGE syndrome, Noonan syndrome, Adams–Oliver syndrome, neurofibromatosis 1, long QT syndrome, hypertrophic cardiomyopathy, Cantu syndrome, Gaucher disease, and glycogen storage diseases. Extensive research indicates that individuals carrying variants in the *BMPR2* gene, when compared to non-carriers, tend to experience a more severe form of the disease. They present with an earlier age of onset, significant hemodynamic compromise at diagnosis, and a heightened likelihood of requiring lung transplantation. These findings underscore the impact of genetic factors on the clinical presentation and prognosis of PAH in pediatric patients.[10]

SUMMARY

The etiology and classification of PAH are complex and multifactorial. PAH can happen both as a primary idiopathic disease or secondary to a chronic disease. The classification is arbitrary but helps to understand the disease entity and etiology for a stratified management approach targeting the involved disease process.

REFERENCES

1. Butrous G. Pulmonary hypertension: From an orphan disease to a global epidemic. Glob Cardiol Sci Pract. 2020;2020(1):e202005.
2. Bousseau S, Sobrano Fais R, Gu S, et al. Pathophysiology and new advances in pulmonary hypertension. BMJ Med. 2023;2(1):e000137.
3. Humbert M, Kovacs G, Hoeper MM, et al. 2022 ESC/ ERS Guidelines for the Diagnosis and Treatment of Pulmonary Hypertension Developed by the Task Force for the Diagnosis and Treatment of (ESC) and the European Respiratory Society (ERS). Eur Heart J. 2022;00(43):3618-731.
4. Simonneau G, Gatzoulis MA, Adatia I, et al. Updated clinical classification of pulmonary hypertension. J Am Coll Cardiol. 2013;62(25):D34-41.
5. Condon DF, Nickel NP, Anderson R, et al. The 6th World Symposium on Pulmonary Hypertension: what's old is new. F1000Res. 2019;8.
6. Galiè N, McLaughlin VV, Rubin LJ, et al. An overview of the 6th World Symposium on Pulmonary Hypertension. Eur Resp J. 2019;53(1).
7. Singh N, Dorfmüller P, Shlobin OA, et al. Group 3 Pulmonary Hypertension: From Bench to Bedside. Circ Res [Internet]. 2022;130(9):1404-22.
8. Chung L, Kawut SM. Connective tissue disease-associated pulmonary arterial hypertension: "Beijing style." Eur Respir J. 2014;44(4):839-41.
9. Lan NSH, Massam BD, Kulkarni SS, et al. Pulmonary arterial hypertension: Pathophysiology and treatment. Diseases. 2018;6(2):38.
10. Del M, Castro-Mujica C, Abarca-Barriga H, et al. Genetic basis of pulmonary arterial hypertension. Revista de la Facultad de Medicina Humana [Internet]. 2020;20(4):670-81.

Pulmonary Hypertension: Clinical Features and Diagnostic Evaluation

CHAPTER 120

Aditya Jindal

INTRODUCTION

Pulmonary hypertension (PH), characterized by an increase in mean pulmonary artery pressure (mPAP), has almost turned "from an orphan disease to a global epidemic."[1] It is a complex condition which is often progressive, leads to right ventricular failure and premature death in due course of time. There is no apparent detectable cause in almost half the cases while the others are secondary to a chronic heart, lung, or other systemic disease. Early diagnosis is often difficult unless clinically suspected and investigated at time of patient presentation.

Historically, PH is defined hemodynamically by the presence of an increase in pulmonary artery pressure (PAP) (≥25 mm Hg).[2] A new threshold of mPAP >20 mm Hg was proposed at the Sixth World Symposium on Pulmonary Hypertension.[3,4] This was based on the results of right heart catheterization data of normal subjects in different studies reporting resting mPAP of 14 ± 3.3 mm Hg with a limit of 20 mm Hg using 2 SDs (standard deviations) above the normal values.[5] It was also reported that the risk for hospitalization as well as mortality for patients with mPAP 21–24 mm Hg was high.[6,7]

While left heart disease is the most common cause of PH worldwide, congenital heart disease and connective tissue disease (especially systemic lupus erythematosus) related PH are relatively more common in Asia.[8] There has been a lack of consensus about how to classify PH in view of the numerous differences in clinical, pathological, and hemodynamic characteristics, and treatment approaches for various underlying conditions. As per mutually agreed consensus between different international Societies, PH is classified into five different clinical groups (discussed in an earlier chapter) primarily based on etiological and hemodynamic differences; each group includes multiple conditions which also differ in prevalence and therapeutic approach.[2-4,9]

CLINICAL FEATURES

Patient may present with symptoms related to the underlying heart, lung, or systemic disease as well as symptoms of PH.[2,10] Symptoms of the underlying disease may include joint pains, skin rashes, daytime somnolence, and a history of blood clots. Fatigue, attributed to multiple associations is an important symptom.[11] There are few specific symptoms of PH but breathlessness on exertion is most commonly present. Other nonspecific symptoms may include wheezing, cough, mild hemoptysis, fatigue, chest pain early exhaustion, palpitations, and syncope. As the disease progresses, symptoms of right-sided heart failure manifest, such as weight gain, edema, abdominal distention, and ascites. Sometimes, there is hoarseness of voice (caused by compression of left recurrent laryngeal nerve)—Ortner syndrome.[12] With progression of disease, the right ventricle starts to fail and cardiac output than falls. This phase may manifest with worsening symptoms progressing to presyncope or even syncope. As this process progresses unabated, it may lead to right heart failure, shock, and death.

Physical signs are also either attributable to the underlying disease or to PH or common to both such as tachypnea and tachycardia. Various other physical examination findings may be present in patients with connective tissue disease (CTD) or chronic lung diseases, such as digital clubbing, telangiectasias, Raynaud's phenomenon, digital ulceration, symptoms related to gastroesophageal reflux, crackles/wheezing on lung auscultation, joint swelling/erythema. Signs of chronic lung disease such as those of chronic obstructive pulmonary disease (COPD) interstitial lung disease (ILD), or chest wall abnormalities (e.g., kyphoscoliosis) are present in cases of chronic cor pulmonale. Stigmata of collagen vascular disease (CVD) include skin changes of scleroderma (skin thickening/tightening, nailfold changes, telangiectasis), butterfly rash of lupus and heliotrope rash of dermatomyositis/polymyositis.

Pulmonary hypertension-specific signs will depend upon whether the patient is in a compensated or a decompensated cardiovascular state. In the early and compensated phase, the physical examination may be nonspecific. P2 (pulmonic) component of the second heart sound is usually loud on auscultation although masked in the presence of emphysema. Right ventricular enlargement and dysfunction (jugular venous distention in the neck and prominent 'a' wave and 'v-y collapse' signifying tricuspid regurgitation may be demonstrable). Chest and cardiac examination may reveal signs of emphysema and/or cardiomegaly, murmurs of tricuspid and pulmonary regurgitation depending upon the etiology. Presence of midsystolic murmur caused by turbulent flow across the pulmonary artery, left parasternal heave, and right-sided S4 gallop may be seen.

As disease progresses, hepatojugular reflex and inspiratory augmented tricuspid murmur (Caravallo's sign) may become apparent.[13] Signs of right heart failure include pulsatile liver, marked distention of jugular veins, ascites, and peripheral edema. Cold extremities and systemic hypotension may be present when cardiovascular collapse ensures. Full-blown picture of chronic cor-pulmonale may be present in an advanced case when edema may also be present.[14]

TABLE 1: Evaluation of a suspected case of pulmonary hypertension (PH).

Suspected cause of PH	Investigations
Left heart disease: Valvular, congenital, ischemic, cardiomyopathy	CXR, ECG, echo (cardiac catheterization)
Connective tissue disease: SLE, SSc, RA, MCTD	• Autoantibody testing • Radiology
Chronic lung disease: COPD, ILD, OSA, others	CXR, chest CT scan, PFT (spirometry), DLCO
Chronic pulmonary thromboembolism	CXR, CT scan, chest MRI, ventilation–perfusion scan
HIV infection	HIV testing
Chronic liver disease (portopulmonary hypertension): Cirrhosis and portal hypertension	LFT, liver ultrasound, abdomen CT scan

(COPD: chronic obstructive pulmonary disease; CT: computed tomography; CXR: chest X-ray; DLCO: diffusing capacity of the lungs for carbon monoxide; ECG: electrocardiogram; echo: echocardiogram; ILD: interstitial lung disease; LFT: liver function test; MCTD: mixed connective tissue disease; MRI: magnetic resonance imaging; OSA: obstructive sleep apnea; PFT: pulmonary function test; RA: rheumatoid arthritis; SSc: systemic sclerosis)

DIAGNOSTIC EVALUATION

The current diagnostic strategies stress upon the need for an early diagnosis of pulmonary hypertension, determination of its etiology, stratification of risk categories, recognition of comorbidities, and attempting phenotyping for early and appropriate therapeutic interventions.[15,16] Clinically, diagnostic evaluation is aimed at two components: (1) diagnosis of the presence and severity of pulmonary hypertension and (2) etiological diagnosis. Diagnosis of individual diseases and different groups of PH is discussed in separate chapters in this book. Some of the important tests to document PH and the underlying etiology **(Table 1)** include the following:

- *Imaging techniques*: Significant advances in imaging technologies have helped to make an early diagnosis even though their potential clinical utility in clinical practice is at least partly dependent on the availability of imaging procedure and expertise.[17,18]
  - *Chest X-ray (CXR)*: This may be normal or demonstrate the presence of enlarged main and hilar pulmonary arterial shadows with attenuated peripheral pulmonary vascular markings (pruning). There may be right ventricular enlargement, better seen on the lateral films as impingement of the anteriorly situated right ventricular silhouette into the retrosternal clear space. CXR is also helpful in the diagnosis of emphysema, ILD or of chest wall deformity in case of chronic cor pulmonale. A CXR creates pictures of the heart, lungs, and chest. CXR will also suggest the diagnosis of a valvular heart disease and congestive heart failure.
  - *Computerized tomography (CT) scan*: Advances in CT technology have led to improved imaging of heart and pulmonary vasculature.[19] Multidetector row CT with three-dimensional volume rendering can elucidate pulmonary vein anatomy in the thorax. Abnormalities in the pulmonary venous drainage can prompt evaluation for structural anomalies causing PH. On the helical CT chest, presence of right ventricular dysfunction after acute pulmonary embolism is suggested by the presence of right ventricular dilation and deviation of interventricular septum toward left ventricle (LV). Cardiac CT scan can show the size of the heart and any blockages in the pulmonary arteries. It can also help diagnose lung diseases that might lead to pulmonary hypertension such as COPD or pulmonary fibrosis.
  - *Magnetic resonance imaging (MRI)*: Thos uses magnetic fields and radio waves to create detailed images of the heart. It can show blood flow in the pulmonary arteries and determine how well the right lower heart chamber is working.[20]
- *Electrocardiogram (ECG or EKG) and echocardiogram (ECHO)*: ECG provides valuable information regarding the diagnosis **(Box 1)**. ECHO is the most commonly used screening tool for evaluating pulmonary hypertension **(Box 2)**.[21,22] It is a simple, non-invasive test that can provide detailed assessment of biventricular function and anatomy. Doppler echo can be used to calculate the right ventricle systolic pressure (RVSP) in the presence of tricuspid regurgitation jet. Presence of tricuspid jet is crucial to this measurement.
- Doppler echo can be used to calculate the RVSP in the presence of tricuspid regurgitation jet. Presence of tricuspid jet is crucial to this measurement. Sometimes,

BOX 1 ECG findings suggestive of pulmonary hypertension.

- Right-axis deviation
- rSR′ pattern in lead V1
- Tall R wave and small S wave with R/S ratio > 1 in lead V1
- qR complex in lead V1
- Large S wave and small R wave with R/S ratio < 1 in lead V5 or V6; or S1, S2, S3 pattern
- ST-T segment wave depression and inversion may be present in the right precordial leads
- Right atrial enlargement manifests as a tall P wave (>2.5 mm) in leads II, III, and aVF and frontal P-axis of 75°

(ECG: electrocardiogram)

BOX 2 Echocardiographic findings suggestive of pulmonary hypertension (PH).

- *Ventricular diameters and septum*:
  - Right ventricle/left ventricle: Basal diameter/area ratio > 1
  - Flattening of the inter ventricular septum
- *Pulmonary artery*:
  - RVOT AT < 105 ms and/or mid-systolic notching
  - Early diastolic pulmonary regurgitation velocity > 2.2 m/s
  - PA > AR diameter; PA diameter > 25 mm
- *Inferior vena cava and right atrium*:
  - IVC diameter > 21 mm with decreased inspiratory collapse (<50% with a sniff or <20% with quiet respiration)
  - RA area (end-systole) > 18 cm^2

(AR: aortic root; IVC: inferior vena cava; PA: pulmonary artery; RVOT AT: right ventricular outflow tract acceleration time; RA: right atrium)

an echo is done while exercising on a stationary bike or treadmill to learn how activity affects the heart.

- *Right heart catheterization (RHC)* remains the gold standard to diagnose of pulmonary hypertension. RHC provides accurate measurement of mPAP, right atrial pressure and cardiac output, and pulmonary capillary wedge pressure to determine the presence of pulmonary arterial versus pulmonary venous hypertension.[23-25] Pulmonary vascular reactivity can be also assessed during catheterization and presence of reactivity has important therapeutic and prognostic implications in the treatment of PAH. Pulmonary vasoreactivity is most commonly seen in idiopathic PAH, but <10% of patients elicit a positive vasodilator response. However, patients who show vasoreactivity appear to have a better prognosis when treated with long-term calcium channel blocker therapy than those who do not have a positive response.
- *Pulmonary function tests*:
  - *Spirometry* is helpful for functional assessment of lungs, especially in case of chronic lung diseases such as COPD and ILD.[26-28] It is also done to assess the presence of severity of airflow obstruction. Diffusion capacity of the lung for carbon monoxide (DLCO) is particularly helpful. Isolated reduction may strongly suggest of pulmonary vascular disease. Reduction in DLCO has been used to identify exercise PH in patients investigated for the cause of dyspnea.[29]
  - *Exercise stress tests* can show how the heart reacts to exercise. Exercise intolerance is an important feature of PH. Exercise capacity in a PH patient is assessed by cardiopulmonary exercise test and a 6-minute walk test (6MWT).[30,31] The test can be used as the primary end point to demonstrate efficacy of treatment of PAH. 6MWT is most commonly used as the primary endpoint in most studies for PAH treatments. It is a not only a measure of symptomatic improvement but also correlates well with variables of maximal cardiopulmonary exercise. It has decreased sensitivity in less severe disease but plays a key role in overall management of PH patients.
  - *Sleep study*: This is done in suspected cases of suspected sleep apnea, which can cause PH.[31] Details have been discussed elsewhere.
- *Ventilation/perfusion (V/Q) scan*: This is an important test to determine the presence of chronic thromboembolic disease.[32,33] V/Q scan has shown good sensitivity of 90–100% and specificity of 94–100% in differentiating between idiopathic PAH and chronic thromboembolic pulmonary hypertension (CTEPH). V/Q scan is also useful to look for the presence of an underlying lung disease that will be evident as ventilation defects.
- *Serological evaluation and biomarkers*: A complete serological evaluation should include testing for serological markers of systemic lupus erythematosus, scleroderma, rheumatoid arthritis, polymyositis/dermatomyositis, and mixed CTDs. Up to 40% of patients with PAH may have elevated antinuclear antibodies.

Right heart catheterization, the gold standard for diagnostic and prognostic evaluation of PAH, is invasive in nature and difficult to use for clinical practice and follow-up evaluations. There is a continued search for a noninvasive screening tool for early identification and classification of PH. Several different biochemical and metabolic biomarkers have been evaluated in different studies for both diagnosis and phenotyping.[15,16,34-37] An ideal biomarker is not yet available for clinical use.

Phenotyping of PH has also been tried for a more precise diagnosis and therapy for some of these patients. In one cohort study of idiopathic PH, it was found that patients with low DLCO and smoking-related form of PH more closely resembled patients with PH due to lung disease. These observations have pathogenetic, diagnostic, and therapeutic implications.[36] There is also an increased use of metabolomics to move forwards for a precision and personalized therapy.[38]

Several genes, some of distinct functional classes are now identified to predispose to the development of PAH.[39,40] It is now recommended that gene testing and genetic counseling should be offered to these patients with idiopathic, anorexigen-induced, congenital heart disease-associated PH, heritable PAH, and pulmonary veno-occlusive disease.[39]

SUMMARY

Diagnostic evaluation of PH remains inconclusive in view of the complex origin, manifestations, behavior, and natural history. It is difficult to describe PH as a single disease or a syndrome. Some authors have suggested a composite "snapshot" based on histopathology, developmental origin, associated clinical conditions, and potential for resolution.[41] Nonetheless, there remain wide gaps in our understanding of the disease—its pathophysiology, classification, and diagnostic and prognostic assessments.

REFERENCES

1. Butrous G. Pulmonary hypertension: From an orphan disease to a global epidemic. Glob Cardiol Sci Pract. 2020;2020(1):e202005.
2. Galiè N, Humbert M, Vachiery J-L, et al. 2015 ESC/ERS guidelines for the diagnosis and treatment of pulmonary hypertension: the joint task force for the diagnosis and treatment of pulmonary hypertension of the European Society of Cardiology (ESC) and the European Respiratory Society (ERS): endorsed by: Association for European Paediatric and Congenital Cardiology (AEPC), International Society for Heart and Lung Transplantation (ISHLT). Eur Respir J. 2015;46(4):903-75.
3. Simonneau G, Montani D, Celermajer DS, et al. Haemodynamic definitions and updated clinical classification of pulmonary hypertension. Eur Resp J. 2019;53(1):1801913.
4. Fukuda K, Date H, Doi S, et al. Guidelines for the treatment of pulmonary hypertension (JCS 2017/JPCPHS 2017). Circ J. 2019; 83(4):842-5.
5. Kovacs G, Avian A, Tscherner M, et al. Characterization of patients with borderline pulmonary arterial pressure. Chest. 2014;146(6):1486-93.
6. Maron BA, Hess E, Maddox TM, et al. Association of borderline pulmonary hypertension with mortality and hospitalization in a large patient cohort: insights from the Veterans Affairs clinical assessment, reporting, and tracking program. Circulation. 2016;133(13):1240-8.
7. Douschan P, Kovacs G, Avian A, et al. Mild elevation of pulmonary arterial pressure as a predictor of mortality. Am J Respir Crit Care Med. 2018;197(4):509-16.
8. Anderson JJ, Lau EM. Pulmonary Hypertension definition, classification, and epidemiology in Asia. JACC Asia. 2022;2(5): 538-46.
9. Condon DF, Nickel NP, Anderson R, et al. The 6th World Symposium on Pulmonary Hypertension: what's old is new. F1000Res. 2019;8:F1000.
10. Rich JD, Rich S. Clinical diagnosis of pulmonary hypertension. Circulation. 2014;130:1820-30.
11. Tartavoulle TM, Karpinski AC, Aubin A, et al. Multidimensional fatigue in pulmonary hypertension: prevalence, severity and predictors. ERJ Open Res. 2018;4(1):00079-2017.
12. Heikkinen J, Milger K, Alejandre-Lafont E, et al. Cardiovocal syndrome (Ortner's syndrome) associated with chronic thromboembolic pulmonary hypertension and giant pulmonary artery aneurysm: Case report and review of the literature. Case Rep Med. 2012;2012:230736.
13. Soto-Pérez-de-Celis E. José Manuel Rivero-Carvallo and the tricuspid valve. Clin Cardiol. 2011;34(3):E9-11.
14. Weitzenblum E. Chronic cor pulmonale. Heart. 2003;89(2):225-30.
15. Hewes JL, Lee JY, Fagan KA, et al. The changing face of pulmonary hypertension diagnosis: a historical perspective on the influence of diagnostics and biomarkers. Pulm Circ. 2020;10(1):2045894019892801.
16. Cullivan S, Gaine S, Sitbon O. New trends in pulmonary hypertension. Eur Respir Rev. 2023;32(167):220211.
17. Kiely DG, Levin D, Hassoun P et al. Statement on imaging and pulmonary hypertension from the Pulmonary Vascular Research Institute (PVRI). Pulm Circ. 2019;9(3):2045894019841990.
18. Sharma M, Burns AT, Yap K, et al. The role of imaging in pulmonary hypertension. Cardiovasc Diagn Ther. 2021;11(3):859-80.
19. Jaramillo FA, Gutierrez FR, Telli FGD, et al. Approach to pulmonary hypertension: From CT to clinical diagnosis. Radiographics. 2018;38(2):357-73.
20. Wessels JN, de Man FS, Noordegraaf AV. The use of magnetic resonance imaging in pulmonary hypertension: why are we still waiting? Eur Respir Rev. 2020;29:200139.
21. Topyła-Putowska W, Tomaszewski M, Wysokiński A, et al. Echocardiography in pulmonary arterial hypertension: Comprehensive evaluation and technical considerations. J Clin Med. 2021;10(15):3229.
22. Augustine DX, Coates-Bradshaw LD, Willis J, et al. Echocardiographic assessment of pulmonary hypertension: a guideline protocol from the British Society of Echocardiography. Echo Res Pract. 2018;5(3):G11-24.
23. Rosenkranz S, Preston IR. Right heart catheterisation: best practice and pitfalls in pulmonary hypertension. Eur Respir Rev. 2015;24:642-52.
24. Hansmann G, Rich S, Maron BA. Cardiac catheterization in pulmonary hypertension: doing it right, with a catheter on the left. Cardiovasc Diagn Ther. 2020;10(5):1718-24.
25. Manek G, Gupta M, Chhabria M, et al. Hemodynamic indices in pulmonary hypertension: a narrative review. Cardiovasc Diagn Ther. 2022;12(5):693-707.
26. Jing ZC, Xu XQ, Badesch DB, et al. Pulmonary function testing in patients with pulmonary arterial hypertension. Respir Med. 2009;103(8):1136-42.
27. Low AT, Medford ARL, Millar AB, et al. Lung function in pulmonary hypertension. Respir Med. 2015;109:1244-9.
28. Chaouat A, Naeije R, Weitzenblum E. Pulmonary hypertension in COPD. Eur Respir J. 2008;32:1371-85.

29. Farina S, Correale M, Bruno N, et al; "Right and Left Heart Failure Study Group" of the Italian Society of Cardiology. The role of cardiopulmonary exercise tests in pulmonary arterial hypertension. Eur Respir Rev. 2018;27:170134.
30. Demir R, Küçükoğlu MS. Six-minute walk test in pulmonary arterial hypertension. Anatol J Cardiol. 2015;15(3):249-54.
31. Kholdani C, Fares WH, Mohsenin V. Pulmonary hypertension in obstructive sleep apnea: is it clinically significant? A critical analysis of the association and pathophysiology. Pulm Circ. 2015;5(2):220-7.
32. Tunariu N, Gibbs SJR, Win Z, et al. Ventilation–perfusion scintigraphy is more sensitive than multidetector CTPA in detecting chronic thromboembolic pulmonary disease as a treatable cause of pulmonary hypertension. J Nucl Med. 2007;48(5):680-4.
33. Lang M, Plank C, Sadushi-Kolici R, et al. Imaging in Pulmonary Hypertension. JACC: Cardiovasc Imaging. 2010;3:1287-195.
34. Frost A, Badesch D, Gibbs JSR, et al. Diagnosis of pulmonary hypertension. Eur Respir J. 2019;53(1):1801904.
35. Santos-Gomes J, Gandra I, Adão R, et al. An Overview of Circulating Pulmonary Arterial Hypertension Biomarkers. Front Cardiovasc Med. 2022;9:924873.
36. Hoeper MM, Dwivedi K, Pausch C, et al. Phenotyping of idiopathic pulmonary arterial hypertension: a registry analysis. Lancet Respir Med. 2022;10(10):937-48.
37. García AR, Piccari L. Emerging phenotypes of pulmonary hypertension associated with COPD: a field guide. Curr Opin Pulm Med. 2022;28(5):343-51.
38. Bassareo PP, D'Alto M. Metabolomics in Pulmonary Hypertension-A Useful Tool to Provide Insights into the Dark Side of a Tricky Pathology. Int J Mol Sci. 2023;24(17):13227.
39. Rai N, Shihan M, Seeger W, et al. Genetic Delivery and Gene Therapy in Pulmonary Hypertension. Int J Mol Sci. 2021;22(3): 1179.
40. Eichstaedt CA, Belge C, Chung WK, et al; for PAH-ICON associated with the PVRI. Genetic counselling and testing in pulmonary arterial hypertension: a consensus statement on behalf of the International Consortium for Genetic Studies in PAH. Eur Respir J. 2023;61(2):2201471.
41. Kulik TJ, Austin ED. Pulmonary hypertension's variegated landscape: a snapshot. Pulm Circ. 2017;7(1):67-81.

Pulmonary Hypertension due to Left Heart Disease

CHAPTER 121

Mateus Fernandes, Erica Altschul

INTRODUCTION

Pulmonary hypertension due to left heart disease (PH-LHD), also known as group 2 pulmonary hypertension (PH), represents a significant proportion of cases within the broader spectrum of PH. The exact prevalence is difficult to determine due to varying definitions and heterogeneity in measuring pulmonary pressures over time, but it is generally recognized as the most common cause of PH, accounting for up to 80% of cases.[1,2] It is primarily driven by left ventricular dysfunction, including heart failure with reduced ejection fraction (HFrEF) or heart failure with preserved ejection fraction (HFpEF), and valvular heart disease **(Box 1)**.[3] PH-LHD confers substantial morbidity and mortality burdens, necessitating a thorough understanding of its underlying mechanisms and appropriate management strategies.

DEFINITION

The classification of PH is determined by hemodynamic criteria according to the 6th World Symposium on Pulmonary Hypertension **(Table 1)**.[4] PH is defined by a mean pulmonary arterial pressure (mPAP) >20 mm Hg. PH-LHD is further determined by measuring pulmonary arterial wedge pressure (PAWP) which is a surrogate for left atrial pressure representing postcapillary disease. A PAWP >15 mm Hg indicates elevated left-sided pressure and meets the definition for PH-LHD. Patients are then further classified into two groups: Isolated postcapillary pulmonary hypertension (IpcPH) and combined pre and postcapillary pulmonary hypertension (CpcPH) by calculating pulmonary vascular resistance (PVR). PVR is calculated by taking the difference between mPAP and PAWP divided by the cardiac output. Historically, patients with a PVR <3 Woods Units (WU) were considered to have normal resistance consistent with IpcPH, while those with elevated PVR >3 WU were considered to have CpcPH; however, recent guidelines from the European Respiratory Society and European Society of Cardiology have suggested adjusting the PVR cutoff to be 2 WU.

Most cases of PH-LHD are due to increased backflow from left heart disease (LHD), which passively increases pulmonary pressure without remodeling of the pulmonary vasculature or increasing pulmonary resistance.[4] However, PVR may be elevated by many intrinsic factors. The underlying mechanisms of increased resistance can be exacerbated by the presence of LHD suggesting PH due to multiple comorbidities (such as chronic hypoxia in the setting of lung disease). Alternatively, long-standing elevated left heart pressures resulting in chronic PH can lead to vascular remodeling similar to that seen in precapillary PH.[5]

Differentiating between combined and isolated PH-LHD is essential. IpcPH is more common, representing approximately 70% of cases.[6] However, CpcPH is associated with increased hospitalizations and higher mortality.[7] In general, for patients with PH-LHD, increasing PAWP

BOX 1 Group 2 pulmonary hypertension classification.

- *Heart failure*:
  - With preserved ejection fraction
  - With reduced or mildly reduced ejection fraction
- Valvular heart disease
- Congenital/acquired cardiovascular conditions leading to postcapillary pulmonary hypertension

TABLE 1: Hemodynamic classification of pulmonary hypertension due to left heart disease.

Classification	Hemodynamic characteristics
IpcPH	mPAP > 20 mm Hg PAWP > 15 mm Hg PVR ≤ 2 WU
CpcPH	mPAP > 20 mm Hg PAWP > 15 mm Hg PVR > 2 WU

(CpcPH: combined pre- and postcapillary pulmonary hypertension; IpcPH: isolated postcapillary pulmonary hypertension; mPAP: mean pulmonary arterial pressure; PAWP: pulmonary arterial wedge pressure; PVR: pulmonary vascular resistance) demonstrates a linear relationship with mortality. PVR, however, demonstrates a step-up in mortality when PVR is >2.5 WU, which highlights an important threshold for worse outcomes due to vascular resistance.[8] Individuals with CpcPH may also have a distinct genetic profile that predisposes them to increased PVR in the presence of environmental factors compared to patients with IpcPH.[5]

ETIOLOGY

Left heart disease encompasses a range of cardiac conditions that lead to PH due to increased pressure and dysfunction on the left side of the heart. The major types of LHD associated with PH include HFrEF, HFpEF, and valvular heart disease.[2,9] The underlying mechanism of LHD determines therapeutic targets for treatment.

Heart Failure with Reduced Ejection Fraction

Left ventricular systolic dysfunction refers to impaired contraction of the left ventricle, leading to reduced ejection fraction (EF) and compromised pumping ability. HFrEF is defined as an EF < 40%. Conditions such as ischemic heart disease, myocardial infarction, dilated cardiomyopathy, and genetic cardiomyopathies can cause left ventricular systolic dysfunction. Consequently, the weakened left ventricle fails to adequately pump blood forward, resulting in increased pressure and volume in the left atrium (LA) and subsequently elevated pulmonary venous pressure.[10] PH is common in individuals with HFrEF and is present in 50–80% of cases.[2] PH in HFrEF confers significantly increased morbidity and mortality, with a 5-year survival of <50%, compared to individuals with HFrEF without PH.[11,12] Patients may also have heart failure with mid-range ejection fraction (HFmrEF), defined by an EF of 41–49%. In these patients, a combination of factors contributes to the development of PH.

Atrial Fibrillation

Atrial fibrillation (AF), with or without valvular disease, leads to a loss of atrial pump function. When AF is present, the atria do not contract effectively, which leads to atrial dilation and increased left atrial volume. This can in turn impair the ability of the LA to relax and fill during ventricular diastole, ultimately leading to left atrial dysfunction and enlargement.

Heart Failure with Preserved Ejection Fraction

Heart failure with preserved ejection fraction occurs due to left ventricular diastolic dysfunction, which is characterized by impaired relaxation or increased stiffness of the left ventricle during diastole. Impaired relaxation leads to elevated diastolic ventricular pressure, which is transmitted to the LA, leading to increased left atrial pressure and subsequent pulmonary venous congestion. Over time, the increased pressure and volume overload lead to the development of PH. PH is present in approximately 52% of individuals with HFpEF and, like HFrEF, confers increased morbidity and mortality.[2,10]

Valvular Heart Disease

Valvular heart diseases, such as mitral stenosis (MS) or regurgitation, aortic stenosis (AS) or regurgitation, and tricuspid regurgitation (TR), can contribute to PH-LHD. In MS, narrowing of the mitral valve obstructs blood flow from the LA to the left ventricle, resulting in increased left atrial pressure, which is transmitted to the pulmonary circulation.[13] PH-LHD is present in approximately 70% of patients with MS. Similarly, AS leads to increased backflow to the left ventricle, LA, and pulmonary circulation. Approximately 50% of patients with symptomatic AS have PH-LHD. Identifying the type of valvular disease present determines the optimal treatment approach.[13]

Atrial fibrillation (AF), with or without valvular disease, leads to a loss of atrial pump function. When AF is present, the atria do not contract effectively, which leads to atrial dilation and increased left atrial volume. This can in turn impair the ability of the LA to relax and fill during ventricular diastole, ultimately leading to left atrial dysfunction and enlargement.[14]

Long-standing AF may also lead to atrial fibrosis which reduces compliance, leading to stiff left atrial syndrome (SLAS). In SLAS, atrial dysfunction occurs independent of left ventricle function, which can make the diagnosis elusive.[15] SLAS should therefore be considered when there is an increase in PAWP in the presence of normal left ventricle end diastolic pressure.

These different types of LHD can coexist. The presence of more than one risk factor increases the likelihood of developing PH. Determining the underlying etiology of LHD can identify potential therapeutic targets, which will be further discussed below.

PATHOPHYSIOLOGY

The pathophysiology of PH-LHD is multifactorial, involving mechanisms such as increased pulmonary venous pressure, endothelial dysfunction, neurohormonal activation, and vascular remodeling.

Endothelial Dysfunction

Endothelial dysfunction plays a significant role in the pathophysiology of PH-LHD.[15,16] In the presence of elevated pulmonary venous pressure, the endothelial cells that line the pulmonary arteries become activated and dysfunctional. This endothelial dysfunction is characterized by impaired production and release of vasodilators such as nitric oxide and prostacyclin and an increase in vasoconstrictors such as endothelin-1.[10] The imbalance results in net vasoconstriction, leading to increased PVR.

Vascular Remodeling

Vascular remodeling refers to structural changes in the pulmonary vessels that occur in response to chronic pressure overload and inflammation.[16] Endothelial dysfunction, as noted above, disrupts the balance of vasoactive substances, which also leads to proliferation of smooth muscle cells and fibroblasts within the pulmonary artery walls.[17] This results in vascular wall thickening, narrowing of the lumen, and progressive remodeling.[15] Remodeled pulmonary arteries are histologically similar to individuals with pulmonary arterial hypertension (PAH). Remodeled pulmonary arteries become less compliant and are more resistant to vasodilatory signals, which is compounded by endothelial dysfunction.

Additionally, the pulmonary veins undergo remodeling. Pulmonary veins usually contain a thin tunica intima with poorly organized thin tunica media. In PH-LHD, pulmonary veins exhibit increased thickness of the tunica intima and a more organized, thickened tunica media. These changes lead to a smaller lumen diameter and decreased compliance, both contributing to vascular resistance. The mediators of pulmonary vein remodeling, such as urokinase plasminogen activator, matrix metallopeptidase 9, interleukin 6, and hepatocyte growth factor, are different from the mediators of pulmonary artery remodeling.[17] This represents an important distinction from group 1 PH. These differences in mediators may in part explain why targeted group 1 PH therapies are not efficacious for group 2 PH, which will be further discussed below.

Increased Pulmonary Venous Pressure

In LHD, increased pressure within the LA and pulmonary veins leads to elevated pulmonary venous pressure, which occurs with any of the etiologies listed earlier. The elevated pressure is transmitted back to the pulmonary circulation, causing pulmonary venous congestion and a direct increase in hydrostatic pressure in the pulmonary capillaries.[16] This leads to fluid extravasation into the interstitium and alveoli, which decreases compliance and further increases the resistance of the capillary system. The pulmonary veins undergo remodeling over time, as noted above, which is compounded by the effects of endothelial dysfunction.

Neurohormonal Activation

Neurohormonal activation is a common feature in LHD and contributes to the development and progression of PH. The neurohormonal systems, including the renin–angiotensin–aldosterone system (RAAS) and the sympathetic nervous system, are activated as a compensatory response to reduced cardiac output, increased fluid volume, and elevated pulmonary venous pressure. However, sustained activation of these systems has detrimental effects. Angiotensin II, a potent vasoconstrictor, promotes vascular remodeling and endothelial dysfunction.[15] Increased sympathetic tone leads to vasoconstriction and increased heart rate, further exacerbating the workload on the left ventricle. Neurohormonal activation, therefore, contributes to the development of pulmonary vasoconstriction, remodeling, and increased PVR.

The natriuretic system also plays a key role in modulating metabolism, and dysfunction may contribute further to PH-LAD.[18] The natriuretic system is activated in response to high cardiac pressures, with release of brain natriuretic peptide (BNP) from the ventricles and atrial natriuretic peptide (ANP) from the atria, and primarily functions to reduce cardiac afterload.[19] Activation leads to increased natriuresis, diuresis, vasodilation, and inhibition of the RASS. N-terminal prohormone of brain natriuretic peptide (NTproBNP) and BNP are established prognostic indicators for cardiac outcomes, including PH, which has led to the development of targeted therapies such as neprilysin inhibitors. Chronic activation in response to high pulmonary and cardiac pressures leads to dysfunction of the natriuretic system and a relative deficiency of BNP and ANP.

Right Ventricular Remodeling

The right ventricle (RV) undergoes remodeling as it adapts to chronically elevated pulmonary pressures, including hypertrophy, dilatation, and impaired contraction.[20] Progressive TR further worsens RV overload and perpetuates maladaptive remodeling. RV–PA coupling refers to the relationship between right ventricular contractility and the ability for RV stroke volume to be transmitted to the PA. As the RV adapts, it can compensate for the increased afterload conferred by the PA in a stepwise manner, maintaining RV–PA coupling ratios. Over time, as remodeling worsens, the RV is no longer able to effectively pump against the high afterload of the PAs. This leads to RV–PA uncoupling, indicating the presence of RV failure. Patients with CpcPH, in particular, are more likely to have RV–PA uncoupling, ventricular interdependence, and reduced cardiac output.

The interplay between increased pulmonary venous pressure, endothelial dysfunction, neurohormonal activation, and vascular remodeling creates a complex pathophysiological cascade in PH-LHD. These mechanisms reinforce each other and contribute to elevated pulmonary arterial pressures, increased PVR, and, ultimately, the clinical manifestations associated with PH. Understanding these pathophysiological processes is crucial for developing targeted therapies to address the underlying mechanisms and improve outcomes in patients with PH-LHD.

CLINICAL PRESENTATION AND DIAGNOSIS

The diagnosis of PH-LHD relies on a comprehensive evaluation encompassing clinical assessment, echocardiography, right heart catheterization (RHC), and various imaging modalities **(Table 2)**. It is crucial to differentiate PH-LHD

TABLE 2: Clinical characteristics of patients at risk for group 2 pulmonary hypertension.

Characteristics	Probability of group 2 pulmonary hypertension		
	High	**Intermediate**	**Low**
Risk factors			
Age	>70 years	60–70 years	<60 years
Obesity, hypertension, dyslipidemia, diabetes	>2 present	1–2 present	Absent
History of heart disease			
Prior intervention	Yes	No	No
Atrial fibrillation	Persistent	Paroxysmal	Absent
Structural LHD	Present	Absent	Absent
Imaging			
ECG	LBBB or LVH	Mild LVH	Normal or signs of RV strain
Echocardiography	LA dilation; grade >2 mitral flow	No LA dilation; grade <2 mitral flow	No LA dilation
Cardiac MRI	LA strain or LA/RA ratio >1	No left heart abnormalities	No left heart abnormalities

(LA: left atrium; LBBB: left bundle branch block; LHD: left heart disease; LVH: left ventricular hypertrophy; MRI: magnetic resonance imaging; RA: right atrium; RV: right ventricle)

from other forms of PH to guide appropriate treatment strategies.

Risk factors for PH-PHD include obesity, hypertension, hyperlipidemia, and diabetes. Patients with PH-LHD may exhibit symptoms such as dyspnea, exercise intolerance, fatigue, and fluid retention. Physical examination may reveal signs of fluid overload, including elevated jugular venous pressure, hepatomegaly, peripheral edema, and pulmonary rales. Additionally, signs and symptoms of underlying LHD, such as murmurs or abnormal heart sounds, may be detected. The approach to the diagnosis of PH can be summarized using a three-step process:[21]

1. *Assess risk*: The first step is to raise suspicion of PH based on the patient's risk factors, symptoms, and imaging findings. This may be done by a first-line physician, such as a primary care physician.
2. *Detection*: The second step is to determine the probability of PH using noninvasive tests, with emphasis on echocardiography. Patients with intermediate to high suspicion should be referred to a PH center for additional workup. Patients with low probability should be evaluated for other etiologies.
3. *Confirmation*: A PH center performs a comprehensive workup to confirm the diagnosis of PH, determine the cause, and provide individual care. This may include invasive tests, such as RHC.

Echocardiography

Echocardiography plays a crucial role in the evaluation of patients with suspected PH-LHD. Left ventricular dilation and decreased ejection fraction may be observed. Valve morphology, gradients, and regurgitant volumes can be assessed to determine the severity of valvular lesions. Echocardiography provides an estimate of pulmonary artery pressures by assessing the tricuspid regurgitant jet velocity (TRV) using continuous wave Doppler. Overall, echocardiography can assist in estimating the probability of PH being present; however, it cannot be used by itself for diagnosis. Comprehensive assessment of the LHD is essential to facilitate the optimum treatment in PH-LHD.

Right Heart Catheterization

Right heart catheterization is the gold standard for diagnosing and evaluating PH. As mentioned above, PAWP reflects left atrial pressure and is elevated in LHD with PAWP >15 mm Hg signaling left-sided heart dysfunction. RHC should be performed in a patient at rest, ideally in the outpatient setting. The patient should not be in an acute exacerbation of heart failure.

The decision to perform RHC for diagnosing group 2 PH depends on the pretest probability of having LHD **(Table 1)** and the need for further prognostication to guide management.[21] Patients with established LHD and echocardiographic evidence of mild PH may not require RHC. Younger patients with variable risk factors in the absence of typical imaging findings have indeterminate risk, and RHC is needed to determine the PAWP. RHC may also be performed to differentiate between IpcPH and CpcPH, severe TR, and during evaluation for heart transplant.

Additional Maneuvers during Right Heart Catheterization

Exercise testing and fluid loading allow further characterization of PH-LHD using standard protocols. In general, the response to stress during exercise testing is more representative of the physiological and clinical performance of the cardiopulmonary system. The response to fluid loading provides a more objective, controlled evaluation of the cardiopulmonary system.[22,23] Both can be used to help elucidate diagnosis when the measured PAWP is borderline (13–15 mm Hg).[24]

Vasoreactivity testing is performed primarily for group 1 PH using compounds such as nitric oxide, iloprost, and epoprostenol. These treatment modalities are not routinely used in PH-LHD, so vasoreactivity is not usually performed except for evaluation prior to heart transplant.

Other Imaging Modalities

In addition to echocardiography and RHC, other imaging modalities can support the diagnosis. A chest radiograph or CT scan may show signs of pulmonary congestion, such as enlarged pulmonary arteries, interstitial edema, and pleural effusions. Chest radiographs may also show left atrial enlargement, with splayed carina sign, and left ventricle dilation. Vascular pruning, defined by the thinning out of markings, may also be observed, which is thought to be due to vascular remodeling. Although not routinely performed, cardiac MRI can assess ventricular function and myocardial tissue characterization and quantify pulmonary blood flow, providing additional insights into the structural and functional abnormalities of the heart. Patients with CpcPH should be referred to PH centers to evaluate for other risk factors that may lead to the development of precapillary PH for further characterization and individualized care.

MANAGEMENT

Management of PH-LHD requires a multidisciplinary approach involving the pulmonologist, cardiologist, and primary care physician. The tenets of management are as follows:

- Management of LHD
- Addressing underlying mechanisms driving PH
- Reversal of pulmonary vascular remodeling

Management of Left Heart Disease

Left heart disease encompasses functional (such as HFrEF and HFpEF) and anatomical (such as valvular disease) factors that contribute to PH. The management of LHD is based on guideline-directed therapy and is not comprehensively discussed here. The following sections provide a brief overview of LHD management with an emphasis on PH.

The key driver of PH-LHD results from the increased load on the LA that is transmitted to the pulmonary circulation. Thus, the treatment goal is to facilitate chronic offloading of the LA. This can be done with medications or intracardiac devices.

Heart Failure

Patients with HFrEF and HFmrEF require treatment based on stage and functional class defined by the New York Heart Association (NYHA). Symptomatic patients (NYHA class 2 and above) are managed with an angiotensin system inhibitor, preferably with an angiotensin receptor-neprilysin inhibitor (ARNi) as well as a beta blocker, mineralocorticoid receptor antagonist (MRA), and sodium–glucose cotransporter-2 inhibitor (SGLT-2i).[25] The etiology of HF should be confirmed, usually with left heart catheterization to evaluate for ischemic cardiomyopathy, which improves with revascularization.

HFpEF management centers on optimizing comorbidities and risk factors, which may lead to improved mPAP. SGLT-2is and MRAs, in particular, have been shown to improve HFpEF outcomes.[25]

Use of Heart Failure Medications in Group 2 Pulmonary Hypertension

A core principle in managing PH-LHD is chronic offloading of the LA. Medications that facilitate diuresis, such as furosemide and spironolactone, have favorable effects on improving PH hemodynamics. Medications that reduce LV remodeling, such as beta blockers, also facilitate improved cardiac output and LA offloading. As mentioned above, neurohormonal dysfunction of the RAAS system is a driver of PH, and the use of angiotensin inhibitors acts to reduce LV afterload and improve cardiac output. Overall, the use of guideline-directed medical therapy (GDMT) facilitates LA offloading.

Angiotensin receptor-neprilysin inhibitor: ARNi therapy has been shown to improve natriuretic peptide signaling, which is associated with improved hemodynamics, as noted above. By correcting the relative BNP and ANP deficiencies, PA pressure is reduced. ARNi therapy also reduces mediators of extracellular matrix fibrosis and may have a role in reversing pulmonary vascular remodeling.[26,27]

Sodium-glucose cotransporter-2 inhibitors: SGLT-2i therapy promotes osmotic diuresis by inducing glycosuria, which confers favorable metabolic effects, including weight loss, reduced insulin resistance, and improved heart failure outcomes.[28] The downstream effects lead to increased cardiac efficiency in glucose utilization, which may improve cardiac output, further offloading the pulmonary circulation. SGLT-2i therapy has also been shown to reduce PA diastolic pressures in small trials.

Glucagon-like peptide 1 agonists: GLP1 agonists are commonly used in the management of diabetes and obesity. They increase insulin secretion, decrease glucagon production, and delay gastric emptying, which leads to weight loss and improved glucose control. Semaglutide, a GLP1 agonist, was shown to improve symptoms in obese patients with HFpEF. Functional outcomes such as 6-minute walking distance (6MWD) were also improved. Given these findings, GLP1 agonists should be considered in the management of PH-LHD due to HFpEF.[29]

These medications demonstrate favorable hemodynamic effects for patients with group 2 PH, which reinforces the core management principle of treating LHD in line with guideline-directed therapy.

Use of Pulmonary Arterial Hypertension Medication in Heart Failure and Group 2 Pulmonary Hypertension

Several trials have evaluated the use of medications that are routinely used in group 1 PH for heart failure, which are reviewed here.

Endothelin receptor antagonists: In early trials assessing the use of PAH medication in patients with HF, endothelin-1 antagonists and vasodilators (such as tezosentan, bosentan, and darusentan) did not improve outcomes, and in some cases, were associated with worse outcomes.[30] Notably, most trials did not control for the presence of PH or optimize heart failure treatment prior to the use of endothelin receptor antagonists. More recent trials enrolling patients with HF and PH also showed no benefit with endothelin receptor antagonists.

Phosphodiesterase type 5 inhibitors: Early trials assessing the use of phosphodiesterase inhibitor patients with heart failure found no difference in outcomes. In small studies, sildenafil showed improvement in mPAP, PAWP, and PVR and was associated with improved quality of life in patients with CpcPH, but the effect was not seen in those with IpcPH.[31,32] A large retrospective study found that patients with severe CpcPH, as defined by PVR >5 WU, had the greatest benefit with sildenafil.[33] Given the significant morbidity and mortality conferred by CpcPH, guidelines recommend considering sildenafil in severe cases of CpcPH.[21]

Soluble guanylate cyclase inhibitors: Vericiguat was shown to reduce the risk of a composite outcome of death and hospitalizations in patients with symptomatic HFrEF. However, other studies targeting change in proBNP showed no difference with vericiguat in HFreF and HFpEF. Notably, these studies did not control for the presence of PH or group of PH.

Recently, small trials showed that riociguat was associated with a reduction in PVR and improved cardiac output in patients with both HFrEF and HFpEF.[34,35] However, the benefit was not reproduced in follow-up studies.[36]

Prostacyclin inhibitor: The prostacyclin inhibitor epoprostenol was assessed for treatment of advanced heart failure. However, the study was terminated early due to worse outcomes, including increased mortality.[37]

It is important to note that many trials evaluating the use of PAH medication in LHD that controlled for the presence and subtype of PH were small (fewer than 300 patients), while the trials evaluating these medications for PAH were large (more than 3,000 patients). As mentioned earlier, the mediators of remodeling in PH-LHD are different from the mediators of PAH. Additionally, in patients with uncontrolled or worsening heart failure, in which chronic LA offloading has not been achieved, the introduction of vasodilatory agents may be harmful. Vasodilation, in the setting of nonoptimized heart failure, reduces PVR, which increases preload delivery to remodeled pulmonary arteries and veins. Optimizing LHD may be essential prior to attempting reversal of pulmonary vasculature remodeling. Several studies have shown that phosphodiesterase 5 inhibitors (PDE5is) had favorable outcomes following left ventricular assist device (LVAD) placement and optimizing of LHD.[38,39]

Due to this gap in evidence, guidelines recommend against using PAH therapies in IpcPH. However, in patients with CpcPH, the use of PAH medications may be considered in consultation with an expert center, specifically for severe cases.

Interventional Treatment for Left Heart Unloading

Left Ventricular Assist Device or Left Atrium Pump

Patients on maximum GDMT who continue to have elevated pulmonary pressures and poor functional status may benefit from the placement of a LVAD or LA pump. These devices lead to improved cardiac output and further facilitate offloading of the pulmonary circulation.[40] A subset of patients may have normalization of mPAP following LVAD placement.

Interatrial Shunt Devices

Placement of an interatrial shunt device (ISD) is a recently developed intervention for treating heart failure in patients who continue to be functionally limited (NYHA class III/IV) despite optimal GDMT. ISDs are used to create a left-to-right shunt between the LA and RA to facilitate LA decompression.[41,42]

In the initial trial (REDUCE-LAP I), patients had improved NYHA class and quality of life following placement.[41] Notably, patients with PVR >4 WU and those with significant chronic pulmonary diseases were excluded. However, there was a reduction in PAWP at the 1-month follow-up. A phase III trial of ISDs (REDUCE-LAP II), which excluded patients with resting PVR >3.5 WU, failed to show benefit in reducing hospitalizations or major adverse cardiac events (MACE). Furthermore, patients with exercise PVR >1.7 WU had significantly worse outcomes.[42] More studies are needed on ISD use in PH; however, these trials signal that ISDs may be harmful for patients with increased PVR. This may be explained by increased loading of the remodeled RV and pulmonary vascular systems in PH. Additionally, increasing blood flow through the right heart in the setting of endothelial and neurohormonal dysfunction may perpetuate PA remodeling.

Valvular Heart Disease

Valvular heart disease is a common driver of PH-LHD. The management of valvular heart disease generally depends on the presence of symptoms and the grade of valve dysfunction.[43,44] Interventions directed at correcting valvular disease have been shown to improve hemodynamics, but a subset of patients continue to have residual PH-LHD. Management of residual PH-LHD is complex, and the use of vasodilators such as sildenafil are associated with worse outcomes. This is likely due to chronic left atrial remodeling and loss of compliance, which may be further worsened by the presence of AF. Following pulmonary vasodilation, the remodeled LA may not be able to accommodate the increased RV output, leading to volume overload and increased pulmonary pressures. Therefore, vasodilators such as sildenafil are not used in residual PH-PHD following valvular repair.

Mitral Valve Disease

Mitral stenosis and regurgitation are commonly associated with PH-LHD. Treatment is based on the severity of mitral regurgitation. Severe mitral regurgitation is managed with surgery when EF is between 30 and 60% regardless of symptoms. Patients with EF >60% are managed with surgery when symptomatic. Those with EF <30% may have irreversible LHD, and surgery is considered on a case-by-case basis. Whenever possible, repair is favored over replacement since replacement carries a high risk for thromboembolism and requires lifelong anticoagulation. Percutaneous balloon valvotomy is indicated for severe MS (mitral valve area <1.5 cm^2) in the presence of symptoms or elevated pulmonary artery systolic pressure (PASP) >50 mm Hg.

Guideline-based management of MR and MS has been shown to improve hemodynamics with reduced mPAP and PAWP, which is driven by increased cardiac output and offloading of the pulmonary circulation.[45]

Aortic Stenosis

Aortic valve replacement is indicated for severe, symptomatic AS (mean pressure gradient >40 mm Hg or aortic valve area <1 cm^2). Guideline-based surgical or catheter-based aortic valve repair can improve hemodynamics and quality of life in patients with AS.[46] However, the presence of PH is independently associated with worse outcomes in patients undergoing aortic valve repair or replacement.[47,48] Medical management of PH following valve repair is also complex and may be associated with worse outcomes. Notably, studies evaluating AS in PH did not control for the type of PH present; therefore, there is limited data to guide treatment.[9]

Tricuspid Regurgitation

The pathogenesis of PH in the presence of TR is discussed above. Primary TR is rare; however, both PH and LHD can confer functional TR due to tricuspid annular dilation. Tricuspid valve surgery carries high risk, which is further increased in PH and RV dysfunction.[49] Emerging treatment includes transcatheter tricuspid valve interventions (TTVIs), which may improve functional status and reduce the severity of TR. However, some patients have worse outcomes following TTVI repair, particularly those with RV–PA uncoupling.[50]

Functional TR is considered a compensatory mechanism that reduces RV strain by facilitating backflow into the right atrium. This is beneficial for patients with PH and right ventricular overload because it helps to prevent the RV from failing. However, if functional TR is repaired in a patient with PH and right ventricular overload, the RV may not be able to generate enough contractility to pump blood into the remodeled pulmonary vasculature, and there is loss of backflow into the RA to reduce RV pressure. This can lead to acute right ventricular failure. Patient selection is thus key when considering TR repair, particularly in those with advanced PH and RV–PA uncoupling.

Pulmonary Artery Denervation

Pulmonary artery denervation (PADN) is an advanced, transcatheter intervention that aims to ablate the baroreceptor reflex that mediates PH. In patients with PAH who failed medical therapy, PADN may improve hemodynamics and functional outcomes.[51] In patients with PH-LHD specifically, studies showed that PADN was associated with improved 6MWD and mPAP compared to sildenafil.[52] PADN offers a novel treatment option for PH-LHD. More studies are needed to assess long-term outcomes and determine ideal candidates.

MONITORING OF PH-LHD

Decompensated PH represents a late stage of the disease process. Clinically stable patients continue to have increased filling pressures over time, with presymptomatic congestion associated with maladaptive remodeling. As congestion increases, patients become symptomatic and decompensate, leading to hospitalization. The natural course of PH highlights the need for monitoring, which facilitates treatment intensification to prevent or reduce downstream congestion.

Right heart catheterization provides the most comprehensive reassessment. However, RHC is invasive, requires an in-person visit, and provides a snapshot of the hemodynamics at a single point in time when performed. The use of implantable pressure sensors has been implemented to address some of these shortcomings. Remote monitoring facilitates longitudinal assessment of PAP, which can refine treatment in the presymptomatic phase. This has been shown to improve heart failure outcomes and reduce hospitalizations in the CHAMPION and CardioMEMS studies, which included patients with HFpEF and HFrEF.[53,54] Although this trial was designed for heart failure, subgroup analysis identified patients who had IpcPH or CpcPH.[55] Similar reductions in hospitalizations and death were seen compared to those without PH.

PROGNOSIS AND FUTURE DIRECTIONS

Pulmonary hypertension due to left heart disease, in particular CpcPH, carries a worse prognosis than other forms of PH. Several ongoing clinical trials and research endeavors aim to enhance our understanding of the disease mechanisms and identify novel therapeutic approaches. Collaborative efforts between cardiologists, pulmonologists, and researchers will be instrumental in improving outcomes and refining treatment strategies.

Levosimendan

Levosimendan is a novel agent currently being evaluated for PH-LHD. It functions as a calcium sensitizer that increases myocardial contractility and vasodilation. This facilitates LA offloading and may reduce RV afterload and preload, which are key drivers of PH-LHD.[56] In small trials with patients with HFpEF, levosimendan use was associated with reductions in mPAP and PAWP, as well as functional outcomes such as 6MWD.[57] Clinical trials are currently in process to determine long-term effects.

Exogenous Nitrites

The physiological vasodilatory effects of endogenous nitrites are well established. Exogenous nitrites are currently being investigated as novel therapies in PH-LHD. They may address the imbalance of vasodilation and vasoconstriction due to endothelial and neurohormonal dysfunction seen in PH-LHD. Small phase II studies have shown improved hemodynamics with the use of oral and inhaled nitrites.[58,59] More trials are needed to delineate the role of exogenous nitrates in PH-LHD.

Mirabegron

Mirabegron is a β3 adrenergic receptor agonist currently approved for the treatment of overactive bladder. It was previously shown to decrease PVR and improve RV function in animal models.[60] The SPHERE-PH trial was the first to investigate the use of a β3 adrenergic agonist in treating CpcPH. The primary endpoint of reduced PVR was not met; however, mirabegron was associated with a significant improvement in RV ejection fraction.[61] Future studies may identify a subset of patients more likely to benefit from β3 adrenergic receptor agonists.

Sotatercept

Sotatercept is a first-in-class activin receptor ligand trap that was approved by the Food and Drug Administration (FDA) in 2022 for the treatment of PAH. It inhibits activins signaling, which are growth factors implicated in vascular remodeling in PAH. In the STELLAR phase 3 trial, sotatercept significantly improved the 6MWD in patients with PAH who were already receiving stable background therapy.[62] Sotatercept has also been shown to improve other important clinical outcomes in patients with PAH, such as PVR, proBNP levels, and World Health Organization (WHO) functional class.

Sotatercept is currently being studied in patients with PH-LHD due to HFpEF in the CADENCE trial (Combined Postcapillary and Precapillary Pulmonary Hypertension due to Heath Failure with Preserved Injection Fraction).

SUMMARY

Overall, PH due to LHD poses a significant clinical challenge, necessitating a comprehensive and multidisciplinary approach. This chapter has highlighted the pathophysiology, clinical presentation, diagnosis, and management strategies for PH-LHD. By advancing our understanding and implementing evidence-based interventions, we can strive to improve the outcomes and quality of life for individuals affected by PH-LHD.

REFERENCES

1. Weitsman T, Weisz G, Farkash R, et al. Pulmonary Hypertension with Left Heart Disease: Prevalence, Temporal Shifts in Etiologies and Outcome. Am J Med. 2017;130(11):1272-79.
2. Rosenkranz S, Gibbs JS, Wachter R, et al. Left ventricular heart failure and pulmonary hypertension. Eur Heart J. 2016; 37(12):942-54.
3. Strange G, Playford D, Stewart S, et al. Pulmonary hypertension: prevalence and mortality in the Armadale echocardiography cohort. Heart. 2012;98(24):1805-11.
4. Simonneau G, Montani D, Celermajer DS, et al. Haemodynamic definitions and updated clinical classification of pulmonary hypertension. Eur Respir J. 2019;53(1):1801913.
5. Miller WL, Grill DE, Borlaug BA. Clinical features, hemodynamics, and outcomes of pulmonary hypertension due to chronic heart failure with reduced ejection fraction: pulmonary hypertension and heart failure. JACC Heart Fail. 2013;1(4):290-9.
6. Hart SA, Krasuski RA, Wang A, et al. Pulmonary hypertension and elevated transpulmonary gradient in patients with mitral stenosis. J Heart Valve Dis. 2010;19(6):708-15.
7. Cappola TP, Felker GM, Kao WH, et al. Pulmonary hypertension and risk of death in cardiomyopathy: patients with myocarditis are at higher risk. Circulation. 2002;105(14):1663-8.
8. Gerges C, Gerges M, Lang MB, et al. Diastolic pulmonary vascular pressure gradient: a predictor of prognosis in "out-of-proportion" pulmonary hypertension. Chest. 2013;143(3): 758-66.
9. Bermejo J, González-Mansilla A, Mombiela T, et al. Persistent Pulmonary Hypertension in Corrected Valvular Heart Disease: Hemodynamic Insights and Long-term Survival. J Am Heart Assoc. 2021;10(2):e019949.
10. Vachiéry JL, Tedford RJ, Rosenkranz S, et al. Pulmonary hypertension due to left heart disease. Eur Respir J. 2019;53(1): 1801897.
11. Fang JC, DeMarco T, Givertz MM, et al. World Health Organization Pulmonary Hypertension group 2: pulmonary hypertension due to left heart disease in the adult—a summary statement from the Pulmonary Hypertension Council of the International Society for Heart and Lung Transplantation. J Heart Lung Transplant. 2012;31(9):913-33.
12. Ghio S, Gavazzi A, Campana C, et al. Independent and additive prognostic value of right ventricular systolic function and pulmonary artery pressure in patients with chronic heart failure. J Am Coll Cardiol. 2001;37(1):183-8.

13. Magne J, Pibarot P, Sengupta PP, et al. Pulmonary hypertension in valvular disease: a comprehensive review on pathophysiology to therapy from the HAVEC Group. JACC Cardiovasc Imaging. 2015;8(1):83-99.
14. Maeder MT, Nägele R, Rohner P, et al. Pulmonary hypertension in stiff left atrial syndrome: pathogenesis and treatment in one. ESC Heart Fail. 2018;5(1):189-92.
15. Zhang F, Chen A, Pan Y, et al. Research Progress on Pulmonary Arterial Hypertension and the Role of the Angiotensin Converting Enzyme 2-Angiotensin-(1-7)-Mas Axis in Pulmonary Arterial Hypertension. Cardiovasc Drugs Ther. 2022;36(2):363-70.
16. Kulik TJ. Pulmonary hypertension caused by pulmonary venous hypertension. Pulm Circ. 2014;4(4):581-95.
17. Hunt JM, Bethea B, Liu X, et al. Pulmonary veins in the normal lung and pulmonary hypertension due to left heart disease. Am J Physiol Lung Cell Mol Physiol. 2013;305(10):L725-36.
18. Kerkelä R, Ulvila J, Magga J. Natriuretic Peptides in the Regulation of Cardiovascular Physiology and Metabolic Events. J Am Heart Assoc. 2015;4(10):e002423.
19. Winquist RJ, Faison EP, Waldman SA, et al. Atrial natriuretic factor elicits an endothelium-independent relaxation and activates particulate guanylate cyclase in vascular smooth muscle. Proc Natl Acad Sci U S A. 1984;81(23):7661-4.
20. Melenovsky V, Hwang SJ, Lin G, et al. Right heart dysfunction in heart failure with preserved ejection fraction. Eur Heart J. 2014;35(48):3452-62.
21. Humbert M, Kovacs G, Hoeper MM, et al. 202. ESC/ERS Guidelines for the diagnosis and treatment of pulmonary hypertension. Eur Respir J. 2023;61(1). doi:10.1183/13993003.00879-2022
22. Fujimoto N, Borlaug BA, Lewis GD, et al. Hemodynamic responses to rapid saline loading: the impact of age, sex, and heart failure. Circulation. 2013;127(1):55-62.
23. D'Alto M, Romeo E, Argiento P, et al. Clinical Relevance of Fluid Challenge in Patients Evaluated for Pulmonary Hypertension. Chest. 2017;151(1):119-26.
24. Kovacs G, Herve P, Barbera JA, et al. An official European Respiratory Society statement: pulmonary haemodynamics during exercise. Eur Respir J. 2017;50(5):1700578.
25. Heidenreich PA, Bozkurt B, Aguilar D, et al. 2022 AHA/ACC/HFSA Guideline for the Management of Heart Failure: Executive Summary: A Report of the American College of Cardiology/American Heart Association Joint Committee on Clinical Practice Guidelines. J Am Coll Cardiol. 2022;79(17):1757-80.
26. Zile MR, O'Meara E, Claggett B, et al. Effects of Sacubitril/Valsartan on Biomarkers of Extracellular Matrix Regulation in Patients with HFrEF. J Am Coll Cardiol. 2019;73(7):795-806.
27. Pfau D, Thorn SL, Zhang J, et al. Angiotensin Receptor Neprilysin Inhibitor Attenuates Myocardial Remodeling and Improves Infarct Perfusion in Experimental Heart Failure. Sci Rep. 2019;9(1):5791.
28. Verma S, Rawat S, Ho KL, et al. Empagliflozin Increases Cardiac Energy Production in Diabetes: Novel Translational Insights Into the Heart Failure Benefits of SGLT2 Inhibitors. JACC Basic Transl Sci.;3(5):575-87.
29. Kayano H, Koba S, Hirano T, et al. Dapagliflozin Influences Ventricular Hemodynamics and Exercise-Induced Pulmonary Hypertension in Type 2 Diabetes Patients: A Randomized Controlled Trial. Circ J. 2020;84(10):1807-17.
30. Lteif C, Ataya A, Duarte JD. Therapeutic Challenges and Emerging Treatment Targets for Pulmonary Hypertension in Left Heart Disease. J Am Heart Assoc. 2021;10(11):e020633.
31. Lewis GD, Shah R, Shahzad K, et al. Sildenafil improves exercise capacity and quality of life in patients with systolic heart failure and secondary pulmonary hypertension. Circulation. 2007;116(14):1555-62.
32. Guazzi M, Vicenzi M, Arena R. Phosphodiesterase 5 inhibition with sildenafil reverses exercise oscillatory breathing in chronic heart failure: a long-term cardiopulmonary exercise testing placebo-controlled study. Eur J Heart Fail. 2012;14(1):82-90.
33. Kramer T, Dumitrescu D, Gerhardt F, et al. Therapeutic potential of phosphodiesterase type 5 inhibitors in heart failure with preserved ejection fraction and combined post- and pre-capillary pulmonary hypertension. Int J Cardiol. 2019;283:152-8.
34. Bonderman D, Ghio S, Felix SB, et al. Riociguat for patients with pulmonary hypertension caused by systolic left ventricular dysfunction: a phase IIb double-blind, randomized, placebo-controlled, dose-ranging hemodynamic study. Circulation. 2013;128(5):502-11.
35. Dachs TM, Duca F, Rettl R, et al. Riociguat in pulmonary hypertension and heart failure with preserved ejection fraction: the haemoDYNAMIC trial. Eur Heart J. 2022;43(36):3402-13.
36. Bonderman D, Pretsch I, Steringer-Mascherbauer R, et al. Acute hemodynamic effects of riociguat in patients with pulmonary hypertension associated with diastolic heart failure (DILATE-1): a randomized, double-blind, placebo-controlled, single-dose study. Chest. 2014;146(5):1274-85.
37. Califf RM, Adams KF, McKenna WJ, et al. A randomized controlled trial of epoprostenol therapy for severe congestive heart failure: The Flolan International Randomized Survival Trial (FIRST). Am Heart J. 1997;134(1):44-54.
38. Tedford RJ, Hemnes AR, Russell SD, et al. PDE5A inhibitor treatment of persistent pulmonary hypertension after mechanical circulatory support. Circ Heart Fail. 2008;1(4):213-9.
39. Salzberg SP, Lachat ML, von Harbou K, et al. Normalization of high pulmonary vascular resistance with LVAD support in heart transplantation candidates. Eur J Cardiothorac Surg. 2005;27(2):222-5.
40. Selim AM, Wadhwani L, Burdorf A, et al. Left Ventricular Assist Devices in Pulmonary Hypertension Group 2 with Significantly Elevated Pulmonary Vascular Resistance: A Bridge to Cure. Heart Lung Circ. 2019;28(6):946-52.
41. Shah SJ, Feldman T, Ricciardi MJ, et al. One-Year Safety and Clinical Outcomes of a Transcatheter Interatrial Shunt Device for the Treatment of Heart Failure with Preserved Ejection Fraction in the reduce Elevated Left Atrial Pressure in Patients with Heart Failure (REDUCE LAP-HF I) Trial: A Randomized Clinical Trial. JAMA Cardiol. 2018;3(10):968-77.
42. Shah SJ, Borlaug BA, Chung ES, et al. Atrial shunt device for heart failure with preserved and mildly reduced ejection fraction (REDUCE LAP-HF II): a randomised, multicentre, blinded, sham-controlled trial. Lancet. 2022;399(10330):1130-40.
43. Otto CM, Nishimura RA, Bonow RO, et al. 2020 ACC/AHA Guideline for the Management of Patients with Valvular Heart Disease: Executive Summary: A Report of the American College of Cardiology/American Heart Association Joint Committee on Clinical Practice Guidelines. Circulation. 2021;143(5):e35-e71.
44. Vahanian A, Beyersdorf F, Praz F, et al. 2021 ESC/EACTS Guidelines for the management of valvular heart disease. Eur Heart J. 2022;43(7):561-632.
45. Gaemperli O, Moccetti M, Surder D, et al. Acute haemodynamic changes after percutaneous mitral valve repair: relation to mid-term outcomes. Heart. 2012;98(2):126-32.

46. Zlotnick DM, Ouellette ML, Malenka DJ, et al. Effect of preoperative pulmonary hypertension on outcomes in patients with severe aortic stenosis following surgical aortic valve replacement. Am J Cardiol. 2013;112(10):1635-40.
47. Miyamoto J, Ohno Y, Kamioka N, et al. Impact of Periprocedural Pulmonary Hypertension on Outcomes after Transcatheter Aortic Valve Replacement. J Am Coll Cardiol. 2022;80(17):1601-13.
48. Iliuta L, Rac-Albu M, Rac-Albu ME, et al. Impact of Pulmonary Hypertension on Mortality after Surgery for Aortic Stenosis. Medicina (Kaunas). 2022;58(9):1231.
49. Lurz P, Orban M, Besler C, et al. Clinical characteristics, diagnosis, and risk stratification of pulmonary hypertension in severe tricuspid regurgitation and implications for transcatheter tricuspid valve repair. Eur Heart J. 2020;41(29):2785-95.
50. Brener MI, Lurz P, Hausleiter J, et al. Right Ventricular-Pulmonary Arterial Coupling and Afterload Reserve in Patients Undergoing Transcatheter Tricuspid Valve Repair. J Am Coll Cardiol. 2022; 79(5):448-61.
51. Chen SL, Zhang FF, Xu J, et al. Pulmonary artery denervation to treat pulmonary arterial hypertension: the single-center, prospective, first-in-man PADN-1 study (first-in-man pulmonary artery denervation for treatment of pulmonary artery hypertension). J Am Coll Cardiol. 2013;62(12):1092-100.
52. Zhang H, Zhang J, Chen M, et al. Pulmonary Artery Denervation Significantly Increases 6-Min Walk Distance for Patients with Combined Pre- and Post-Capillary Pulmonary Hypertension Associated with Left Heart Failure: The PADN-5 Study. JACC Cardiovasc Interv. 2019;12(3):274-84.
53. Abraham WT, Adamson PB, Bourge RC, et al. Wireless pulmonary artery haemodynamic monitoring in chronic heart failure: a randomised controlled trial. Lancet. 2011;377(9766):658-66.
54. Shavelle DM, Desai AS, Abraham WT, et al. Lower Rates of Heart Failure and All-Cause Hospitalizations during Pulmonary Artery Pressure-Guided Therapy for Ambulatory Heart Failure: One-Year Outcomes from the CardioMEMS Post-Approval Study. Circ Heart Fail. 2020;13(8):e006863.
55. Benza RL, Raina A, Abraham WT, et al. Pulmonary hypertension related to left heart disease: insight from a wireless implantable hemodynamic monitor. J Heart Lung Transplant. 2015; 34(3):329-37.
56. Hansen MS, Andersen A, Nielsen-Kudsk JE. Levosimendan in pulmonary hypertension and right heart failure. Pulm Circ. 2018;8(3):2045894018790905.
57. Burkhoff D, Rich S, Pollesello P, Papp Z. Levosimendan-induced venodilation is mediated by opening of potassium channels. ESC Heart Fail. 2021;8(6):4454-64.
58. Cosby K, Partovi KS, Crawford JH, et al. Nitrite reduction to nitric oxide by deoxyhemoglobin vasodilates the human circulation. Nat Med. 2003;9(12):1498-505.
59. Simon MA, Vanderpool RR, Nouraie M, et al. Acute hemodynamic effects of inhaled sodium nitrite in pulmonary hypertension associated with heart failure with preserved ejection fraction. JCI Insight. 2016;1(18):e89620.
60. García-Álvarez A, Pereda D, García-Lunar I, et al. Beta-3 adrenergic agonists reduce pulmonary vascular resistance and improve right ventricular performance in a porcine model of chronic pulmonary hypertension. Basic Res Cardiol. 2016; 111(4):49.
61. García-Álvarez A, Blanco I, García-Lunar I, et al. β3 adrenergic agonist treatment in chronic pulmonary hypertension associated with heart failure (SPHERE-HF): a double blind, placebo-controlled, randomized clinical trial. Eur J Heart Fail. 2023;25(3):373-85.
62. Hoeper MM, Badesch DB, Ghofrani HA, et al.; STELLAR Trial Investigators. Phase 3 Trial of Sotatercept for Treatment of Pulmonary Arterial Hypertension. N Engl J Med. 2023; 388(16):1478-90.

Pulmonary Hypertension due to Chronic Lung Disease (Group 3 Pulmonary Hypertension)

CHAPTER 122

Linda Benes, Himanshu Deshwal, Roxana Sulica

INTRODUCTION

Pulmonary hypertension (PH) is a heterogeneous disease of various etiologies that causes elevated pulmonary artery pressure and ultimately leads to right heart failure and death. A significant proportion of PH cases worldwide occur in the context of chronic lung disease (CLD) and/or hypoxia, classified as group 3 PH by the World Health Organization (WHO). Not only common, but with the most devastating prognosis, group 3 PH has recently attracted considerable research interest. This chapter discusses key aspects of the underlying pathophysiology, diagnosis, and management, highlighting recent advances in the understanding of this complex disease.

DEFINITION OF PULMONARY HYPERTENSION

Pulmonary hypertension is defined by a resting mean pulmonary artery pressure (mPAP) > 20 mm Hg measured during right heart catheterization (RHC). Further hemodynamic characterization by concomitant assessment of pulmonary vascular resistance (PVR) and pulmonary arterial wedge pressure (PAWP) is essential in order to differentiate between the various forms of PH. Precapillary PH is characterized by elevated PVR of >2 Wood units (WU) and PAWP of ≤15 mm Hg. The hemodynamic hallmark of postcapillary PH is an elevated PAWP of >15 mm Hg and can be divided into two groups based on PVR: Those with a significant precapillary component [PVR > 2 WU, combined pre- and post-capillary PH (CpcPH)] and those without [PVR ≤ 2 WU, isolated postcapillary PH (IpcPH)]. It is important to note the change in the most recent European Society of Cardiology/European Respiratory Society (ESC/ERS) guidelines in 2022, where the PVR threshold was lowered from 3 to 2 WU.[1] This was in line with new data that showed an increased risk of mortality and heart failure starting at a PVR of around 2.2 WU.[2]

DEFINITION OF GROUP 3 PULMONARY HYPERTENSION

The WHO classifies PH into five groups based on the predominant underlying pathophysiologic mechanism. Group 3 PH is characterized by a precapillary hemodynamic profile when CLD and/or hypoxia is the primary cause of elevated pulmonary pressures.[1]

Pulmonary hypertension can complicate a variety of CLDs, but this chapter focuses on PH associated with chronic obstructive pulmonary disease (COPD), various forms of interstitial lung disease (ILD), and combined pulmonary fibrosis and emphysema (CPFE). Other chronic hypoxic conditions complicated by PH development include sleep-disordered breathing, alveolar hypoventilation syndromes, and prolonged exposure to high altitude.[1]

Although the pathogenesis of group 3 PH is not fully understood, it is thought to be due to the interplay of several factors. Destruction of lung parenchyma results in loss of pulmonary vascular bed surface and decreased capacity to vasodilate in response to increased cardiac output. Impaired gas exchange leading to repeated or sustained hypoxic pulmonary vasoconstriction also contributes to vascular remodeling. However, the degree of hemodynamic impairment may be disproportionate to the lung involvement or hypoxia, and vascular remodeling has been reported in areas of normal lung. It is now increasingly recognized that other mechanistic pathways are involved in the development of PH in addition to the direct negative effects of the primary pulmonary process. In a similar fashion to pulmonary arterial hypertension (PAH), especially in severe forms of group 3 PH, there is evidence of pulmonary vascular disease due to endothelial dysfunction, and complex molecular, genetic, and cellular mechanisms are at play.[3,4]

Detecting PH in the setting of CLD can be challenging because the symptoms of PH and the underlying lung disease often overlap. Traditionally, there have been no standardized approaches to screening for PH outside of the evaluation for lung transplantation. The advent of new therapeutic options for PH related to ILD is changing the needs for timely diagnosis. A recent Delphi consensus concluded that early screening for PH in ILD patients is advisable, and the panel identified several parameters to raise suspicion of PH **(Box 1)**. Transthoracic echocardiography is the most useful noninvasive test for estimating right ventricular (RV) systolic pressure and assessing RV size and function. However, echocardiogram's sensitivity and specificity are limited, and RHC remains the gold standard for definitive diagnosis and risk stratification of these patients.[3-6] RHC is recommended to be performed in patients with CLD when significant PH is suspected and clinical management of the patient is potentially influenced by the results of the RHC: Transplantation referral, inclusion in clinical registries/trials, treatment of associated left heart disease or chronic thromboembolic PH (CTEPH), or specific therapy initiation.[7]

BOX 1 Findings that should raise suspicion for pulmonary hypertension in patients with chronic lung disease.

- *Symptoms and signs*:
  - Dizziness/syncope
  - Palpitations
  - Altered heart sounds (loud P2 or S2)
  - Jugular venous distention
  - Peripheral edema
  - Hepatomegaly/ascites
  - History of pulmonary embolism
- *Oxygen saturation and 6MWD*:
  - New or increased need for supplemental oxygen
  - Marked or worsening exertional oxygen desaturation
  - Markedly reduced or worsening 6MWD (especially with stable PFTs)
  - Impaired heart rate recovery after exercise (<13 bpm after 1 minute)
- *Echocardiography*:
  - Right ventricular dilation
  - Low TAPSE (<1.8 cm)
  - Elevated RVSP (>45 mm Hg)
- *PFTs*:
  - DLCO < 40% predicted
  - DLCO declines rapidly or by >15%
  - Disproportionately reduced DLCO (FVC%/DLCO% >1.6)
- *CT scan*:
  - Right ventricle enlargement (RV:LV > 1)
  - Pulmonary artery enlargement (PA:A > 1)
  - Flattening of the interventricular septum
- *Laboratory*:
  - Elevated BNP or NT-proBNP

(6MWD: 6-minute walk distance; BNP: brain natriuretic peptide; bpm: beat per minute; CT: computed tomography; DLCO: diffusing capacity of the lung for carbon monoxide; FVC: forced vital capacity; NT-proBNP: N-terminal pro-brain natriuretic peptide; PA:A: pulmonary artery to aorta ratio; PFTs: pulmonary function tests; RV:LV: right ventricle to left ventricle ratio; RVSP: right ventricular systolic pressure; TAPSE: tricuspid annular plane systolic excursion)

Because group 3 PH is indistinguishable from other types of precapillary PH based on hemodynamic assessment alone, it is important to rule out CTEPH, carefully screen for the presence of risk factors for PAH (e.g., connective tissue disease, HIV infection portopulmonary hypertension), and assess the degree of lung involvement by chest imaging and pulmonary function tests (PFTs). Features that favor group 3 PH over PAH include moderate-to-severe obstructive or restrictive impairment on PFTs [e.g., forced expiratory volume in 1 second (FEV1) < 60% predicted, forced vital capacity (FVC) < 70% predicted, and proportionally reduced diffusing capacity of the lung for carbon monoxide (DLCO)], advanced parenchymal abnormalities on computed tomography (CT) scan, and a predominantly ventilatory limitation during cardiopulmonary exercises testing (CPET).[7]

Scope of Problem

Group 3 PH is one of the leading causes of PH worldwide, second only to group 2 PH due to left heart disease. The development of PH in these patients is associated with significant morbidity and mortality, and patients are typically older with multiple comorbidities. According to the ASPIRE registry, patients with group 3 PH have the worst prognosis of all forms of PH, including patients with PAH. The 3-year survival rate was only 44% within this group and there were marked differences between subgroups, with patients suffering from ILD (16%) and COPD (41%) having the lowest survival rate, considerably worse compared to PH associated with sleep-disordered breathing/alveolar hypoventilation (90%). Furthermore, PH adversely affects symptoms with greater dyspnea, hypoxemia, reduced exercise capacity, and increased risk of exacerbations.[8,9]

The reported prevalence of PH in CLD varies depending on the definition of PH, the diagnostic technique used to identify PH, and the severity of the disease. Mild PH is common in COPD, with prevalence varying from 16–44% in mild cases to 59–84% in more advanced stages of the disease. However, only 1–5% of patients develop severe PH. Similarly, mild PH has been reported with a range of 3–86% in patients with ILD, while severe PH affects <10% of these patients. Patients with CPFE are at a particular risk of developing PH, with up to half of them experiencing a significant increase in pulmonary pressures. Several studies have shown that patients with severe PH have much worse outcomes than those with mild-to-moderate PH.[4,6]

Vasculopathic Phenotype and Clinical Evaluation

Patients with severe group 3 PH have a significantly worse prognosis than those with nonsevere PH, and this is independent of the degree of pulmonary involvement.[10] Thus, the hemodynamic distinction between these two forms is clinically relevant. While the previous ESC/ERS guidelines in 2015 defined severe PH as mPAP > 35 mm Hg or ≥25 mm Hg in the presence of a low cardiac index (CI < 2.5 L/min/m^2),[11] new data have demonstrated that PVR serves as a better predictor of prognosis. Recent studies showed that PVR > 5 WU is significantly associated with worse survival in patients with PH associated with COPD or ILD.[12,13] Therefore, the current guidelines have adopted the use of PVR to differentiate between nonsevere PH (PVR ≤ 5 WU) and severe PH (PVR > 5 WU). In addition to higher mortality, patients with severe PH often have different clinical characteristics, disease course, and response to treatment. The term "pulmonary vascular phenotype" has been proposed to describe a select group of PH associated with COPD (PH-COPD) patients with a unique clinical profile with less severe airflow limitation on spirometry, more pronounced hypoxemia, disproportionately low DLCO, significant dyspnea on exertion, and circulatory limitation to exercise.[14-16] In contrast, any level of PH in ILD is associated with increased mortality.[17] Clinical clues suggestive of a vasculopathic phenotype are included in **Table 1**.

Treatment

Optimal management of the underlying lung disease is the cornerstone of treatment for group 3 PH. Other adjunctive measures may include long-term supplemental oxygen, noninvasive ventilation, and participation in a pulmonary rehabilitation program. It is also important to treat comorbid conditions (e.g., cardiac problems, sleep-disordered breathing) that may contribute to worsening PH. Given the significantly increased mortality in these patients, the development of PH is an indication for lung transplantation evaluation and referral should be considered early.

There is limited and conflicting evidence regarding the use of pulmonary vasodilators in this patient population. Proponents of their use argue that there is increasing evidence that vascular remodeling resembles PAH, especially in severe forms. However, the potential benefits of these agents may be offset by concerns about adverse effects on hemodynamics and gas exchange due to ventilation-perfusion (VQ) mismatch. It is important to note, however, that any reduction in oxygenation due to reversal of hypoxic pulmonary vasoconstriction might be compensated for by an increase in the cardiac output induced by specific PH therapies. In effect, a recent systematic review and meta-analysis showed that treatment in both PH-COPD and PH-ILD did not worsen hypoxemia.[18]

The three main classes of drugs used to treat PAH target the prostacyclin, endothelin, and nitric oxide pathways. All have been studied in patients with COPD and ILD with varying degrees of success **(Tables 2 and 3)**. Despite the lack of conclusive evidence, the compassionate use of these drugs by clinicians has not been negligible. According to the results of a semiquantitative survey sent to PAH referral centers in the United States, 80% of specialists reported using PAH therapy for patients with group 3 PH, particularly when it was felt that the PH was severe or out of proportion to the lung disease.[19]

PH Associated with COPD or Emphysema

Studies on the use of PAH medications in patients with PH-COPD have produced conflicting results and are often limited by their small sample size, short duration, and poor patient selection. Bosentan failed to improve exercise tolerance and worsened hypoxemia and quality of life (QoL) in patients with advanced COPD and only modest pulmonary pressure elevation.[20] Conversely, in another study of patients with COPD and severe PH confirmed by RHC, bosentan showed significant improvements in invasive hemodynamics, exercise capacity, and dyspnea ratings, without deterioration of arterial oxygenation.[21]

TABLE 1: Features suggestive of vasculopathic versus nonvasculopathic phenotypes in group 3 pulmonary hypertension.

Nonvasculopathic phenotype	Test	Vasculopathic phenotype
Less severe dyspnea	Clinical	Significant exertional dyspnea
• Less severe hypoxemia • Normal or elevated CO_2	Blood gas	• More extensive hypoxemia • Mostly hypocapnia
More severe parenchymal changes	CT scan	Minimal parenchymal changes
• Moderate-to-severe airflow limitation or restriction • Proportionally reduced DLCO	PFTs	• Less severe airflow limitation or restriction • Very low DLCO (disproportional)
Ventilatory exercise limitation	CPET	Circulatory exercise limitation
Mild RV dysfunction	Echocardiogram	Significant RV dysfunction
• PVR ≤ 5 WU • Preserved CI	RHC	• PVR > 5 WU • Low CI

(CI: cardiac index; CO_2: carbon dioxide; CPET: cardiopulmonary exercise testing; DLCO: diffusing capacity of the lung for carbon monoxide; PVR: pulmonary vascular resistance; RHC: right heart catheterization; RV: right ventricle; WU: Wood units)

TABLE 2: Clinical trials of pulmonary vasodilators in COPD.

Study (First author, year)	Study drug	Study design	Study population (No. of participants)	PH definition	Results
Clinical trials primarily on COPD without significant PH					
Stolz et al., 2008[20]	Bosentan	Single-center RCT	Severe COPD ($n = 30$)	Echo: Mild PH, normal RV	• No improvement in 6MWD* • Worsened gas exchange and QoL
Lederer et al., 2012[22]	Sildenafil	Single-center, crossover RCT	Moderate-to-severe COPD without PH ($n = 10$)	RHC/Echo: Excluded if PH	• No improvement in 6MWD and peak VO_2 during cycle ergometry* • Worsened gas exchange and QoL
Blanco et al., 2013[23]	Sildenafil	Multicenter RCT	Severe COPD with mild PH ($n = 63$)	RHC/Echo: Mild PH	• No improvement in cycle endurance time*, 6MWD, and QoL • No difference in arterial oxygenation and adverse events
Goudie et al., 2014[24]	Tadalafil	Multicenter RCT	Moderate-to-severe COPD with mild PH ($n = 120$)	Echo: Mild PH, normal RV	• No improvement in 6MWD* or QoL • No difference in arterial oxygenation • More frequent dyspepsia and headache
Clinical trials primarily on PH-COPD with significant PH					
Valerio et al., 2009[21]	Bosentan	Single-center RCT	COPD with confirmed severe PH ($n = 32$)	RHC: mPAP ≥ 25 mm Hg	• Improved mPAP, PVR, 6MWD, and BODE index • Positive trend in arterial oxygenation • Mean PVR > 5 WU at baseline
SPHERIC-1 Vitulo et al., 2017[25]	Sildenafil	Multicenter RCT	Moderate COPD with confirmed severe PH (n = 28)	RHC: mPAP ≥ 35 mm Hg if FEV1 < 30%; mPAP ≥ 30 mm Hg if FEV1 > 30%	• Improvement in PVR*, BODE index, DLCO, and QoL • No difference in arterial oxygenation • Mean PVR > 5 WU at baseline

*Primary outcome.

(6MWD: 6-minute walking distance; BODE: body mass index, airflow obstruction, dyspnea, exercise capacity; COPD: chronic obstructive pulmonary disease; Echo: echocardiography; FEV1: forced expiratory volume in 1 second; mPAP: mean pulmonary arterial pressure; PH: pulmonary hypertension; PVR: pulmonary vascular resistance; RCT: randomized controlled trial; RHC: right heart catheterization; QoL: quality of life; VO_2: oxygen consumption)

TABLE 3: Clinical trials of pulmonary vasodilators in ILD.

Study (First author, year)	Study drug	Study design	Study population (No. of participants)	PH definition	Results
Clinical trials primarily on ILD without established PH					
BUILD-1 King et al., 2008[27]	Bosentan	Multicenter RCT	IPF ($n = 158$)	Not assessed (excluded if severe PH on echo)	• No improvement in 6MWD* • Trend in delayed time to death or disease progression, and improved QoL • No difference in gas exchange
BUILD-2 Seibold et al., 2010[29]	Bosentan	Multicenter RCT	SSc-related significant ILD ($n = 163$)	Not assessed (excluded if severe PH on echo)	• No improvement in 6MWD* • No difference in time to death or worsening PFTs
BUILD-3 King et al., 2011[28]	Bosentan	Multicenter RCT	IPF without extensive honeycombing ($n = 616$)	Not assessed	No difference in time to IPF worsening or death*, health-related QoL, or dyspnea
MUSIC Raghu et al., 2013[31]	Macitentan	Multicenter RCT	IPF without extensive honeycombing ($n = 178$)	Not assessed	No difference in PFTs* or time to IPF worsening or death
STEP-IPF Zisman et al. IPFnet, 2010[37]	Sildenafil	Multicenter RCT	Advanced IPF with DLCO < 35% predicted ($n = 180$)	Not assessed	• No improvement in 6MWD* • Small improvement in oxygenation, gas exchange, dyspnea, and QoL
INSTAGE Kolb et al., 2018[39]	Sildenafil (in addition to nintedanib)	Multicenter RCT	Advanced IPF with DLCO < 35% predicted ($n = 273$)	Not assessed	• No difference in health-related QoL* • No difference in oxygenation and gas exchange
Clinical trials primarily on ILD with assessment for PH					
ARTEMIS-IPF/PH Raghu et al., 2013[32]	Ambrisentan	Multicenter RCT	IPF without extensive honeycombing ($n = 492$)	RHC: Baseline PH (mPAP ≥ 25 mm Hg)	• Terminated early • Increased risk for disease progression* and respiratory hospitalizations • Only 10% in each group had precapillary PH
STEP-IPF substudy Han et al., 2013[38]	Sildenafil	Multicenter RCT	STEP-IPF cohort with echo available ($n = 119$)	Echo: Baseline RVSD	Better preservation of exercise capacity in patient with RVSD
INSTAGE subgroup Behr et al., 2019[40]	Sildenafil (in addition to nintedanib)	Multicenter RCT	INSTAGE cohort ($n = 273$)	Echo: Baseline RHD ($n = 117$)	• No difference in QoL • More pronounced BNP stabilization in patients with RHD
SP-IPF Behr et al., 2021[41]	Sildenafil (in addition to pirfenidone)	Multicenter RCT	Advanced IPF with DLCO ≤ 40% predicted, at risk of PH assess by echo or RHC ($n = 177$)	RHC (18%): precapillary PH (mPAP ≥ 20 mm Hg); or Echo (92%): intermediate-to-high probability of PH	No difference in disease progression defined as a composite endpoint*
iNO-PF Nathan et al., 2020[42]	Pulsed iNO	Multicenter RCT	Fibrotic ILD at risk of PH (n = 41)	Echo: intermediate-high probability of PH (71%)	Improvement in physical activity and oxygen saturation

Continued

Continued

Study (First author, year)	Study drug	Study design	Study population (No. of participants)	PH definition	Results
Clinical trials primarily on PH-ILD with assessment for PH					
BPHIT Corte et al., 2014[30]	Bosentan	Multicenter RCT	Fibrotic IIP with confirmed PH ($n = 60$)	RHC: mPAP ≥ 25 mm Hg	• No difference in PVRi reduction*, functional capacity, or symptoms • No difference in oxygen saturation • Mean PVR > 5 WU at baseline
Saggar et al., 2014[44]	Parenteral treprostinil	Open-label, prospective study	PF with advanced PH ($n = 15$)	RHC: mPAP ≥ 35 mm Hg	• Improvement in invasive hemodynamics, RV function, 6MWD, dyspnea, and BNP • No change in systemic oxygenation or blood pressure • Mean PVR > 8 WU at baseline
RISE-IIP Nathan et al., 2019[36]	Riociguat	Multicenter RCT	IIP with confirmed PH ($n = 147$)	RHC: mPAP ≥ 25 mm Hg	• Terminated early, no difference in 6MWD* • Increased serious adverse events and mortality • No difference in oxygen saturation
INCREASE Waxman et al., 2021[47]	Inhaled treprostinil	Multicenter RCT	ILD with confirmed PH ($n = 326$)	RHC: mPAP ≥ 25 mm Hg	• Improved 6MWD* • Reduction in NT-proBNP levels • Lower risk of clinical worsening • No difference in distance-saturation product

*Primary outcome.

(6MWD: 6-minute walking distance; IIP: idiopathic interstitial pneumonia; ILD: interstitial lung disease; iNO: inhaled nitric oxide; IPF: idiopathic pulmonary fibrosis; mPAP: mean pulmonary arterial pressure; NT-proBNP: N-terminal prohormone of brain natriuretic peptide; PF: pulmonary fibrosis; PVRi: pulmonary vascular resistance index; RCT: randomized controlled trial; RHC: right heart catheterization; RHD: right heart disease; RVSD: right ventricular systolic dysfunction; SSc: scleroderma)

To date, phosphodiesterase-5 inhibitors (PDEi) have been the most extensively studied agents in PH-COPD. Two early trials of sildenafil[22,23] and one of tadalafil[24] showed a negative result in patients with severe COPD and no or mild PH. While they did not improve exercise tolerance or QOL, there was a potential risk of adverse effects with impaired gas exchange. In a more recent randomized controlled trial, sildenafil significantly improved PVR, BODE index obstruction, dyspnea and general health perception without worsening gas exchange in patients with moderate COPD and significant PH 25. An important limitation of the study was its small size of only 28 participants. A subsequent meta-analysis of 9 RCTs with 579 patients showed a significant improvement in 6-minute walking distance (6MWD) and pulmonary artery systolic pressure with no difference in adverse events in patients treated with sildenafil versus placebo.[26] In the ASPIRE and COMPERA registries, patients with severe PH-COPD were predominantly treated with PDE5i monotherapy. Survival was found to be superior in patients arbitrarily defined as having a favorable response to treatment.[10,15] These findings suggest that sildenafil may be well tolerated and beneficial in the subset of patients with more severe PH and less advanced lung disease, possibly as a result of their distinct vasculopathic phenotype. However, in the absence of large clinical trials, the evidence is insufficient to support widespread use of these agents.

PH Associated with ILD

Endothelin Pathway: Endothelin Receptor Antagonists: Bosentan, Macitentan, Ambrisentan

Several studies have investigated the potential antifibrotic benefit of endothelin receptor antagonists (ERAs) in ILD, mostly with disappointing results. There is very limited data evaluating their direct effect on PH associated with lung disease.

The BUILD-1 study evaluated the effects of bosentan in 158 patients with idiopathic pulmonary fibrosis (IPF) without confirmed PH. While there was no improvement in exercise capacity, the treatment group showed a favorable trend toward a delay in time to death or disease progression and an improvement in QoL.[27] These effects were more pronounced in the subgroup of patients requiring surgical lung biopsy (SLB), leading to the hypothesis that they had less advanced fibrosis. Therefore, the BUILD-3 trial enrolled 616 patients with SLB-confirmed IPF and without extensive honeycombing, but failed to demonstrate superiority of bosentan in time to disease worsening or death, change in health-related QoL, or dyspnea.[28] Similarly, in 163 patents with scleroderma-related ILD and no PH, bosentan did not improve outcomes.[29] Only a small 60-patient RCT[30] evaluated bosentan in patients with RHC-confirmed PH and fibrotic idiopathic interstitial pneumonia (PH-IIP) and showed no difference in invasive pulmonary hemodynamics, functional capacity, or symptoms.

Macitentan, another dual ERA, yielded similarly negative results. The MUSIC trial of macitentan in patients with biopsy-proven IPF did not show a benefit in either the primary or the secondary endpoints.[31]

In addition, a large multicenter RCT in 492 IPF patients[32] comparing ambrisentan to placebo had to be stopped early due to lack of efficacy and a signal for harm, as the treatment group was associated with an increased risk of disease progression and respiratory hospitalizations. In this study, RHC was performed to stratify patients based on the presence of PH at baseline (defined as mPAP ≥ 25 mm Hg). Analysis of these results showed a relatively low prevalence of precapillary PH, with only 14% classified as group 3 PH in the entire cohort. In addition, 9% of patients had elevated left-sided filling pressures and another 30% had mPAP of 20–25 mm Hg, suggesting a potentially high incidence of subclinical left heart disease.[33] Thus, it could be speculated that the adverse effects seen in the ambrisentan group were due to a detrimental effect on patients with comorbid left heart disease and subsequent pulmonary edema.

In conclusion, given the repeatedly demonstrated lack of benefit and potential harm of ambrisentan, the use of ERAs for the treatment of PH-ILD is not currently supported.

Nitric Oxide Pathway: Soluble Guanylate Cyclase Stimulator: Riociguat

After a small pilot study[34] suggested a potential benefit, the RISE-IIP trial randomized 147 patients with PH-IIP to riociguat versus placebo and found no significant improvement in 6MWD.[35] The study was terminated early due to a higher incidence of serious adverse events and deaths in the treatment arm; therefore, riociguat should not be used in PH-ILD. It is important to note, however, that the negative signal in the study was likely driven by inclusion of a large number of patients with CPFE as demonstrated in a post hoc analysis of the trial.[36]

Phosphodiesterase 5 Inhibitor: Sildenafil, Tadalafil

Studies with the PDE5i sildenafil have shown some positive signals. One of the pivotal trials (STEP-IPF) enrolled 180 patients with advanced IPF and DLCO < 35% predicted. Although the primary endpoint of improvement in 6MWD was not met, there were some benefits in arterial oxygenation, gas exchange by DLCO, symptoms, and QoL in subjects treated with sildenafil.[37] PH was not a requirement for enrollment, but a post hoc analysis of the 119 patients with baseline echocardiograms suggested that sildenafil resulted in better preservation of exercise capacity and improved QoL in those with RV systolic dysfunction.[38] Subsequently, the INSTAGE trial evaluated the effect of sildenafil added to the antifibrotic agent nintedanib in a similar group of 274 patients.[39] Although it failed to show a significant difference in most outcomes, there was a possible benefit in disease progression (as defined by the risk of FVC decline), and a prespecified subgroup analysis[40] of patients with echocardiographic evidence of right heart disease suggested greater B-type natriuretic peptide (BNP) stabilization. Finally, the addition of sildenafil to the other antifibrotic pirfenidone in 177 patients with advanced IPF at risk of PH did not yield any positive results.[41]

An inhaled nitric oxide (iNO) pulse delivery system was studied in a small group of patients with fibrotic ILD at risk for PH and showed encouraging results with improvements in exercise capacity and oxygen saturation.[42] This inspired the design of the phase 3 REBUILD trial, which, after reduction of the target study size from 300 to 140 subjects, failed to meet its primary endpoint related to the change in moderate-to-vigorous physical activity.[43]

Prostacyclin Pathway: Parenteral Treprostinil

One of the main clinical dilemmas with the use of pulmonary vasodilators in ILD is worsening VQ mismatch and oxygenation, which could be of particular concern with the initiation and acute uptitration of parenteral prostanoids. This notion was challenged in a pilot study of 15 patients with pulmonary fibrosis referred for lung transplantation in the setting of an advanced PH phenotype with severely impaired hemodynamics and RV dysfunction.[44] With gentle chronic administration of parenteral treprostinil, the investigators demonstrated significant improvements in right heart hemodynamics, echocardiographic function, 6MWD, and dyspnea scores without altering systemic oxygenation. Conversely, a recent retrospective study of a heterogeneous group of nine patients with severe PH-ILD and multiple comorbidities suggested caution with parenteral prostanoids after failing to show improvement in functional class or exercise capacity, while there was a modest decrease in oxygen saturation.[45] While these agents may have a role in treating the most severe forms of PH-ILD, these results highlight the importance of careful patient selection, initiation, and monitoring and the need for further large controlled trials.

Inhaled Treprostinil

Small reports have suggested that inhaled prostacyclins may have a more selective pulmonary vasodilator effect on the well-ventilated portions of the lung, thereby optimizing VQ matching without significant effects on systemic oxygenation.[46] INCREASE was a multicenter, randomized trial of inhaled treprostinil, a prostacyclin analog.[47] The investigators found that it significantly improved 6MWD by a mean difference of 31.12 m over the 16-week treatment period, while there was a concomitant decline in exercise capacity in those taking placebo. In addition, the treatment group had a significant reduction in NT-proBNP levels, a lower risk of clinical worsening, and fewer exacerbations of an underlying lung disease. There was no difference in adverse events or adverse effects on PFTs.[47] In fact, a post hoc analysis[48] showed that inhaled treprostinil was associated with improvements in FVC, particularly in patients with underlying IPF. To date, inhaled treprostinil is the only Food and Drug Administration (FDA)-approved treatment for PH-ILD.

SUMMARY

Group 3 PH due to hypoxia and CLDs is a common condition globally as well as in India. The diagnosis is established by the demonstration of the underlying lung disease and evidence of PAH on clinical investigations. There is increasing evidence to suggest that the PAH pathogenesis has similarities to other groups, which may imply a more favorable response to pulmonary vasodilators.

Continued efforts to further characterize patients and identify relevant clinical phenotypes will be important. Refining our understanding of the "vasculopathic phenotype" may have implications for therapeutic decisions. With the emergence of new treatment options, there is increasing emphasis on early screening and diagnosis.

REFERENCES

1. Humbert M, Kovacs G, Hoeper MM, et al. 2022 ESC/ERS Guidelines for the diagnosis and treatment of pulmonary hypertension: Developed by the task force for the diagnosis and treatment of pulmonary hypertension of the European Society of Cardiology (ESC) and the European Respiratory Society (ERS). Endorsed by the International Society for Heart and Lung Transplantation (ISHLT) and the European Reference Network on rare respiratory diseases (ERN-LUNG). Eur Heart J. 2022;43(38):3618-731.
2. Maron BA, Brittain EL, Hess E, et al. Pulmonary vascular resistance and clinical outcomes in patients with pulmonary hypertension: a retrospective cohort study. Lancet Respir Med. 2020;8(9):873-84.
3. Singh N, Dorfmüller P, Shlobin OA, et al. Group 3 Pulmonary Hypertension: From Bench to Bedside. Circ Res. 2022;130(9): 1404-22.
4. King CS, Shlobin OA. The Trouble with Group 3 Pulmonary Hypertension in Interstitial Lung Disease: Dilemmas in Diagnosis and the Conundrum of Treatment. Chest. 2020;158(4):1651-64.
5. Rahaghi FF, Kolaitis NA, Adegunsoye A, et al. Screening Strategies for Pulmonary Hypertension in Patients with Interstitial Lung Disease: A Multidisciplinary Delphi Study. Chest. 2022;162(1):145-55.
6. Behr J, Nathan SD. Pulmonary hypertension in interstitial lung disease: screening, diagnosis and treatment. Curr Opin Pulm Med. 2021;27(5):396-404.

7. Nathan SD, Barbera JA, Gaine SP, et al. Pulmonary hypertension in chronic lung disease and hypoxia. Eur Respir J. 2019;53(1):1801914.
8. Hurdman J, Condliffe R, Elliot CA, et al. ASPIRE registry: Assessing the Spectrum of Pulmonary hypertension Identified at a referral centre. Eur Respir J. 2012;39(4):945.
9. King CS, Nathan SD. Pulmonary hypertension due to interstitial lung disease. Curr Opin Pulm Med. 2019;25(5):459-67.
10. Vizza CD, Hoeper MM, Huscher D, et al. Pulmonary Hypertension in Patients with COPD: Results from the Comparative, Prospective Registry of Newly Initiated Therapies for Pulmonary Hypertension (COMPERA). Chest. 2021;160(2):678-89.
11. Galie N, Humbert M, Vachiery JL, et al. 2015 ESC/ERS Guidelines for the diagnosis and treatment of pulmonary hypertension: The Joint Task Force for the Diagnosis and Treatment of Pulmonary Hypertension of the European Society of Cardiology (ESC) and the European Respiratory Society (ERS): Endorsed by: Association for European Paediatric and Congenital Cardiology (AEPC), International Society for Heart and Lung Transplantation (ISHLT). Eur Heart J. 2016;37(1):67-119.
12. Olsson KM, Hoeper MM, Pausch C, et al. Pulmonary vascular resistance predicts mortality in patients with pulmonary hypertension associated with interstitial lung disease: results from the COMPERA registry. Eur Respir J. 2021;58(2):2101483.
13. Zeder K, Avian A, Bachmaier G, et al. Elevated pulmonary vascular resistance predicts mortality in COPD patients. Eur Respir J. 2021;58(2):2100944.
14. Kovacs G, Agusti A, Barberà JA, et al. Pulmonary Vascular Involvement in Chronic Obstructive Pulmonary Disease. Is There a Pulmonary Vascular Phenotype? Am J Respir Crit Care Med. 2018;198(8):1000-11.
15. Hurdman J, Condliffe R, Elliot CA, et al. Pulmonary hypertension in COPD: results from the ASPIRE registry. Eur Respir J. 2013;41(6):1292-301.
16. Chaouat A, Bugnet AS, Kadaoui N, et al. Severe pulmonary hypertension and chronic obstructive pulmonary disease. Am J Respir Crit Care Med. 2005;172(2):189-94.
17. Piccari L, Wort SJ, Meloni F, et al. The Effect of Borderline Pulmonary Hypertension on Survival in Chronic Lung Disease. Respiration. 2022;101(8):717-27.
18. Prins KW, Duval S, Markowitz J, et al. Chronic use of PAH-specific therapy in World Health Organization Group III Pulmonary Hypertension: a systematic review and meta-analysis. Pulm Circ. 2017;7(1):145-55.
19. Trammell AW, Pugh ME, Newman JH, et al. Use of pulmonary arterial hypertension-approved therapy in the treatment of non-group 1 pulmonary hypertension at US referral centers. Pulm Circ. 2015;5(2):356-63.
20. Stolz D, Rasch H, Linka A, et al. A randomised, controlled trial of bosentan in severe COPD. Eur Respir J. 2008;32(3):619-28.
21. Valerio G, Bracciale P, Grazia D'Agostino A. Effect of bosentan upon pulmonary hypertension in chronic obstructive pulmonary disease. Ther Adv Respir Dis. 2009;3(1):15-21.
22. Lederer DJ, Bartels MN, Schluger NW, et al. Sildenafil for chronic obstructive pulmonary disease: a randomized crossover trial. COPD. 2012;9(3):268-75.
23. Blanco I, Santos S, Gea J, et al. Sildenafil to improve respiratory rehabilitation outcomes in COPD: a controlled trial. Eur Respir J. 2013;42(4):982-92.
24. Goudie AR, Lipworth BJ, Hopkinson PJ, et al. Tadalafil in patients with chronic obstructive pulmonary disease: a randomised, double-blind, parallel-group, placebo-controlled trial. Lancet Respir Med. 2014;2(4):293-300.
25. Vitulo P, Stanziola A, Confalonieri M, et al. Sildenafil in severe pulmonary hypertension associated with chronic obstructive pulmonary disease: A randomized controlled multicenter clinical trial. J Heart Lung Transplant. 2017;36(2):166-74.
26. Hao Y, Zhu Y, Mao Y, et al. Efficacy and safety of Sildenafil treatment in pulmonary hypertension caused by chronic obstructive pulmonary disease: A meta-analysis. Life Sci. 2020;257:118001.
27. King TE, Jr, Behr J, Brown KK, et al. BUILD-1: a randomized placebo-controlled trial of bosentan in idiopathic pulmonary fibrosis. Am J Respir Crit Care Med. 2008;177(1):75-81.
28. King TE Jr, Brown KK, Raghu G, et al. BUILD-3: a randomized, controlled trial of bosentan in idiopathic pulmonary fibrosis. Am J Respir Crit Care Med. 2011;184(1):92-9.
29. Seibold JR, Denton CP, Furst DE, et al. Randomized, prospective, placebo-controlled trial of bosentan in interstitial lung disease secondary to systemic sclerosis. Arthritis Rheum. 2010;62(7):2101-8.
30. Corte TJ, Keir GJ, Dimopoulos K, et al. Bosentan in pulmonary hypertension associated with fibrotic idiopathic interstitial pneumonia. Am J Respir Crit Care Med. 2014;190(2):208-17.
31. Raghu G, Million-Rousseau R, Morganti A, et al. Macitentan for the treatment of idiopathic pulmonary fibrosis: the randomised controlled MUSIC trial. Eur Respir J. 2013;42(6):1622-32.
32. Raghu G, Behr J, Brown KK, et al. Treatment of idiopathic pulmonary fibrosis with ambrisentan: a parallel, randomized trial. Ann Intern Med. 2013;158(9):641-9.
33. Raghu G, Nathan SD, Behr J, et al. Pulmonary hypertension in idiopathic pulmonary fibrosis with mild-to-moderate restriction. Eur Respir J. 2015;46(5):1370-7.
34. Hoeper MM, Halank M, Wilkens H, et al. Riociguat for interstitial lung disease and pulmonary hypertension: a pilot trial. Eur Respir J. 2013;41(4):853-60.
35. Nathan SD, Behr J, Collard HR, et al. Riociguat for idiopathic interstitial pneumonia-associated pulmonary hypertension (RISE-IIP): a randomised, placebo-controlled phase 2b study. Lancet Respir Med. 2019;7(9):780-90.
36. Nathan SD, Cottin V, Behr J, et al. Impact of lung morphology on clinical outcomes with riociguat in patients with pulmonary hypertension and idiopathic interstitial pneumonia: A post hoc subgroup analysis of the RISE-IIP study. J Heart Lung Transplant. 2021;40(6):494-503.
37. Zisman DA, Schwarz M, Anstrom KJ, et al. A controlled trial of sildenafil in advanced idiopathic pulmonary fibrosis. New Engl J Med. 2010;363(7):620-8.
38. Han MK, Bach DS, Hagan PG, et al. Sildenafil preserves exercise capacity in patients with idiopathic pulmonary fibrosis and right-sided ventricular dysfunction. Chest. 2013;143(6):1699-708.
39. Kolb M, Raghu G, Wells AU, et al. Nintedanib plus Sildenafil in Patients with Idiopathic Pulmonary Fibrosis. New Engl J Med. 2018;379(18):1722-31.
40. Behr J, Kolb M, Song JW, et al. Nintedanib and Sildenafil in Patients with Idiopathic Pulmonary Fibrosis and Right Heart Dysfunction. A Prespecified Subgroup Analysis of a Double-Blind Randomized Clinical Trial (INSTAGE). Am J Respir Crit Care Med. 2019;200(12):1505-12.

41. Behr J, Nathan SD, Wuyts WA, et al. Efficacy and safety of sildenafil added to pirfenidone in patients with advanced idiopathic pulmonary fibrosis and risk of pulmonary hypertension: a double-blind, randomised, placebo-controlled, phase 2b trial. Lancet Respir Med. 2021;9(1):85-95.
42. Nathan SD, Flaherty KR, Glassberg MK, et al. A Randomized, Double-Blind, Placebo-Controlled Study of Pulsed, Inhaled Nitric Oxide in Subjects at Risk of Pulmonary Hypertension Associated with Pulmonary Fibrosis. Chest. 2020;158(2):637-45.
43. NCT03267108. (2023). Bellerophon Pulse Technologies. A Study to Assess Pulsed Inhaled Nitric Oxide in Subjects with Pulmonary Fibrosis at Risk for Pulmonary Hypertension (REBUILD). ClinicalTrialsgov. [online] Available from https://trials.phassociation.org/trials/NCT03267108 [Last accessed July, 2024].
44. Saggar R, Khanna D, Vaidya A, et al. Changes in right heart haemodynamics and echocardiographic function in an advanced phenotype of pulmonary hypertension and right heart dysfunction associated with pulmonary fibrosis. Thorax. 2014;69(2):123-9.
45. Hinkamp CA, Shah T, Bartolome S, et al. Parenteral prostanoids for severe Group 3 pulmonary hypertension with right ventricular dysfunction. J Thorac Dis. 2021;13(3):1466-75.
46. Olschewski H, Simonneau G, Galiè N, et al. Inhaled iloprost for severe pulmonary hypertension. New Engl J Med. 2002;347(5):322-9.
47. Waxman A, Restrepo-Jaramillo R, Thenappan T, et al. Inhaled Treprostinil in Pulmonary Hypertension due to Interstitial Lung Disease. N Engl J Med. 2021;384(4):325-34.
48. Nathan SD, Waxman A, Rajagopal S, et al. Inhaled treprostinil and forced vital capacity in patients with interstitial lung disease and associated pulmonary hypertension: a post-hoc analysis of the INCREASE study. Lancet Respir Med. 2021;9(11):1266-74.

Management of Pulmonary Hypertension

CHAPTER 123

Trinath Dash, Karthik Tipparapu, K Arun Vishnu

INTRODUCTION

Management of pulmonary arterial hypertension (PAH) has significantly changed over the last few decades in the wake of more sensitive diagnostic tests and specialized clinical programs. Risk stratification using hemodynamic parameters and progressive nature of PAH drive management decisions. The cornerstone in the management of PAH is to treat the underlying etiology.

Therapy for PAH can be subdivided into:

- Supportive or conventional therapy
- Specific or targeted therapy

SUPPORTIVE THERAPIES

Physical Activity and Rehabilitation

Patients with PAH should be encouraged to be active within symptom limits. Several studies have shown the beneficial impact of exercise training on exercise capacity measured with 6-minute walking distance (6MWD) and quality of life (QoL).[1,2] A large, randomized controlled trial (RCT) in 11 centers across 10 European countries, including 116 patients with PAH/chronic thromboembolic pulmonary hypertension (CTEPH) on PAH drugs, showed a significant improvement in 6MWD of 34.1 ± 8.3 m, QoL, the World Health Organization functional class (WHO-FC), and peak VO_2 compared with standard of care.[1] Most of the studies included stable patients on medical treatment. The duration of such a supervised rehabilitation program is suggested to be 12–15 weeks.

Calcium Channel Blockers

Patients with PAH who respond favorably to acute vasoreactivity testing may respond to treatment with calcium channel blockers (CCBs). Less than 10% of patients are responders, while an acute vasodilator response does not predict a favorable long-term response to CCBs in patients with other forms of PAH. The CCBs that have predominantly been used in PAH are nifedipine, amlodipine, and diltiazem.[3] Amlodipine and felodipine are increasingly being used due to their long half-life and good tolerability. The daily doses that have shown efficacy in PAH are relatively high and they must be reached progressively. The most common adverse effects are systemic hypotension and peripheral edema. Patients who meet the criteria for a positive acute vasodilator response and treated with CCBs should be closely monitored for safety and efficacy, with a complete reassessment after 3–6 months of therapy, including RHC. Additional acute vasoreactivity testing should be performed at re-evaluation to detect persistent vasodilator response. In some cases, a combination of CCBs with approved PAH drugs is required because of clinical deterioration with CCB withdrawal attempts.

Oxygen Therapy

Oxygen administration reduces pulmonary vascular resistance (PVR) and improves exercise tolerance in patients with PAH associated with chronic obstructive pulmonary disease (COPD). There are no data to suggest that long-term oxygen therapy has sustained benefits over the course of time. Most patients with PAH, except those with congenital heart disease (CHD) and pulmonary-to-systemic shunts, have minor degrees of arterial hypoxemia at rest, exception is presence of persistent patent foramen ovale. The presence of more profound hypoxemia in a patient with PAH should raise suspicion for underlying parenchymal lung disease, systemic to pulmonary shunting, pulmonary veno-occlusive disease (PVOD), pulmonary capillary hemangiomatosis, or pulmonary arteriovenous malformations (PAVMs) as seen in pulmonary hypertension (PH) due to hereditary hemorrhagic telangiectasia (HHT).

Although oxygen is a pulmonary vasodilator, there are no long-term studies supporting its efficacy. There is general consensus that supplemental oxygen is indicated, if arterial PO_2 is < 60 mm Hg or systemic arterial O_2 saturation is <90% at rest. One exception to this approach is in patients with Eisenmenger syndrome, with hypoxemia due to right-to-left shunting; in this group, the use of supplemental oxygen may have negligible benefit.[4] Ambulatory oxygen may be considered when there is evidence of symptomatic benefit and correctable desaturation on exercise.[5] Nocturnal oxygen therapy should be considered in case of sleep-related desaturation.

Anticoagulation

There are several reasons to consider anticoagulation in patients with PAH. Histopathological specimens from PAH patients' lungs have shown in situ thrombosis of pulmonary vessels. Patients with CHD or pulmonary artery (PA) aneurysms may develop thrombosis of the central PAs. Abnormalities in the coagulation and fibrinolytic systems indicating a procoagulant state have been reported in patients with PAH.[6] Two recent meta-analyses also concluded that using anticoagulants may improve survival in patients with idiopathic pulmonary artery hypertension (IPAH); however, none of the included studies were methodologically robust.[7,8] In PAH associated with connective tissue disorder, registry data and meta-analyses uniformly indicated that anticoagulation may be harmful and not recommended in the absence of other comorbidities requiring anticoagulation.[7,8] In congenital heart disease associated with PAH, there are also no RCTs on anticoagulation. There is also no consensus about the use of anticoagulants in patients who have permanent intravenous lines for therapy with prostacyclin analogs. As anticoagulation is associated with an increased bleeding risk, and in the absence of robust data, no general recommendation has been made for or against the use of anticoagulants in patients with PAH; therefore, an individual decision-making is required.

Diuretics

Right heart failure (RHF) is associated with systemic fluid retention, reduced renal blood flow, and activation of the renin–angiotensin–aldosterone system. Increased right-sided filling pressures are transmitted to the renal veins, increasing interstitial and tubular hydrostatic pressure within the encapsulated kidney, which decreases net glomerular filtration rate and oxygen delivery.[9] Avoiding fluid retention is the key objective in managing patients with PH. Restricting fluid intake and using diuretics are recommended once the signs of RHF and edema set in. The three main classes of diuretics—loop diuretics, thiazides, and mineralocorticoid receptor antagonists— are used as monotherapy or in combination, as determined by the patient's clinical need and kidney function. Kidney function and serum electrolytes should be regularly monitored, and intravascular volume depletion must be avoided as it may cause a further decline in cardiac output and systemic blood pressure. Physicians should bear in mind that fluid retention and edema may not necessarily signal right-sided HF, but may also be a side effect of PAH therapy.[10]

Anemia

Iron deficiency is common in patients with PAH and is defined by serum ferritin < 100 μg/L, or serum ferritin 100–299 μg/L and transferrin saturation < 20%.[11] The underlying pathological mechanisms are complex. In patients with PAH, iron deficiency is associated with impaired myocardial function, aggravated symptoms, and increased risk of mortality. Regular monitoring of iron status (serum iron, ferritin, transferrin saturation, soluble transferrin receptors) is recommended in patients with PAH.

In patients with severe iron-deficiency anemia (Hb < 7–8 g/dL), intravenous supplementation is recommended.[12] Oral iron formulations containing ferrous (Fe^{2+}) sulfate, ferrous gluconate, and ferrous fumarate are often poorly tolerated, and drug efficacy may be impaired in patients with PAH.[13] Evidence comparing oral and IV iron supplementation in patients with PAH are limited.

Vaccination

As a general healthcare measure, patients with PAH are recommended to be vaccinated at least against SARS-CoV-2, influenza, and *Streptococcus pneumoniae*.

SPECIFIC OR TARGETED THERAPIES

The pathogenesis of PAH is complex and the implicated pathways remain central to modern medical therapy. The current approved medical therapies target three mechanistic pathways:

- Excess endothelin (ET) activity
- Abnormal nitric oxide (NO) activity
- Prostacyclin (PGi2) deficiency

Endothelin Receptor Antagonist

In PH, ET-1 serum concentrations are elevated and is found in higher amounts in pulmonary arterial smooth muscle cells.[14,15] All three currently approved endothelin receptor antagonists (ERAs) carry a risk of embryofetal toxicity and are likely to cause major birth defects based on animal studies. Pregnancy must be excluded before the initiation of treatment in women and prevented with two reliable forms of birth control during and up to at least 1 month after stopping therapy. A decrease in sperm counts have been observed in patients on ERA therapy.

Peripheral edema is common in the progression of PH, has been observed after initiation of ERA therapy, and may necessitate drug discontinuation if refractory to medical management.

Bosentan is an ERA with slight affinity for ETA over ET receptor B and was the first oral medication approved for the management of PAH. In BREATHE-1 trial, bosentan demonstrated improved PVR, patient exercise capacity by the 6-minute walk test (6MWT), and time to clinical worsening.[16] The approved target dose in adults is 125 mg bid. Dose-dependent increases in liver transaminases can occur in ~10% of treated patients (reversible after dose reduction or discontinuation).[17] Due to pharmacokinetic interactions, bosentan may render hormonal contraceptives unreliable and lower serum levels of warfarin, sildenafil, and tadalafil.[18] Bosentan, an ERA, is available for twice-daily dosing in both tablet form (62.5 and 125.0 mg) and oral suspension (32 mg), allowing for nasogastric administration.

Ambrisentan predominantly affects ETA and was approved in 2007 at 5 or 10 mg once daily dosing after the ARIES-1 and ARIES-2 randomized placebo-controlled trials demonstrated improvement in 6MWT and time to clinical worsening. Ambrisentan is contraindicated in patients with idiopathic pulmonary fibrosis after it demonstrated an increased risk of disease progression or death in patients with idiopathic pulmonary fibrosis, regardless of PH in the ARTEMIS-IPF study.[19] An increased incidence of peripheral edema was reported with ambrisentan use, while there was no increased incidence of abnormal liver function.

Macitentan is a dual ERA approved at 10 mg once daily dosing in 2013 after the SERAPHIN trial demonstrated a decrease in morbidity and mortality in patients with PAH.[20] Macitentan has been found to increase exercise capacity and reduce a composite endpoint of clinical worsening in patients with PAH.[20] While no liver toxicity has been shown, a reduction in Hb to ≤8 g/dL was observed in 4.3% of patients receiving 10 mg of macitentan.

Nitric Oxide Pathway Agents

Phosphodiesterase-5 inhibitors: Sildenafil and Tadalafil

Sildenafil is an approved drug for PAH at 20 mg based on improvement of exercise capacity by 6MWT in the SUPER trial. Most side effects of sildenafil are mild-to-moderate and mainly related to vasodilation (headache, flushing, and epistaxis). Sildenafil is available as a tablet, oral suspension, or for intravenous use.

Tadalafil is a longer-acting phosphodiesterase-5 (PDE-5) inhibitor approved for PAH in 2009. The PHIRST trial demonstrated that 40 mg once daily of tadalafil increased 6MWT after 16 weeks of therapy, even in patients already on background therapy with bosentan. Similar to sildenafil, tadalafil is contraindicated with the use of nitrates, and both medications carry similar adverse effect profiles. These include headache, flushing, myalgia, and dyspepsia, which typically improve or resolve over time and rarely result in the need for drug discontinuation. Transitions between sildenafil and tadalafil are generally well-tolerated.

Guanylate Cyclase Stimulator: Riociguat

Riociguat is typically started at 1 mg three times daily and increased every 2 weeks by 0.5 mg three times daily if systolic blood pressure remains greater than 95 mm Hg. When studied in combination with sildenafil, there was no evidence of a positive benefit-risk ratio and more pronounced hypotension. An RCT of 443 patients with PAH (44% and 6% on background therapy with ERAs or prostacyclin analogs, respectively) treated with riociguat up to 2.5 mg tid showed favorable results on exercise capacity, hemodynamics, WHO-FC, and time to clinical worsening.[21] The side effect profile was similar to that of PDE5is.

Prostacyclin Pathway Agents

The prostacyclin metabolic pathway is dysregulated in patients with PAH, with less prostacyclin synthase expressed in PAs and reduced prostacyclin urinary metabolites. Prostaglandin I2 (PGI2) is a potent vasodilator and inhibitor of platelet aggregation, with an important role in maintaining vascular homeostasis. Its actions are mediated by the IP receptor, causing cyclic adenosine monophosphate production, leading to marked vasodilation and inhibition of smooth muscle cell proliferation.[22] The most common adverse events observed with these compounds are related to systemic vasodilation and include headache, flushing, jaw pain, and diarrhea. Currently, there are three Food and Drug Administration (FDA)-approved PGI2 analogs: Epoprostenol, iloprost, and treprostinil, as well as an IP receptor agonist, selexipag.

Epoprostenol

Epoprostenol has a short half-life (3–5 minutes) and needs continuous IV administration via an infusion pump and a permanent tunneled catheter. A thermostable formulation is available to maintain stability up to 48 hours.[23] Infusions are typically initiated at 1–2 ng/kg/min and may be increased in small increments until dose-limiting effects are elicited. Pretreatment or aggressive treatment of transient side effects may improve tolerability during dose escalation. Its efficacy has been demonstrated in patients with IPAH (WHO-FC III and IV) and SSc-associated PAH.[24] Epoprostenol improved symptoms, exercise capacity, hemodynamics, and mortality. Serious adverse events related to the delivery system include pump malfunction, local site infection, catheter obstruction, and sepsis.

Iloprost

Iloprost is a shorter-acting inhaled PGI2 that requires six to nine inhalations of 2.5–5.0 µg each day, which may limit its widespread use despite also being shown to improve exercise capacity.[25] Inhaled therapy has theoretic advantages, including direct delivery to the site of action, ideally with fewer systemic side effects, although transient cough and throat irritation have been noted. Inhaled iloprost has been evaluated in one RCT, in which six to nine repetitive iloprost inhalations were compared with placebo in treatment-naïve patients with PAH or CTEPH.[25] The study showed an increase in exercise capacity and improvement in symptoms, PVR, and clinical events in the iloprost group compared with the placebo group.

Treprostinil

Treprostinil is available for SC, IV, inhaled, and oral administration. Treprostinil SC improved exercise capacity, hemodynamics, and symptoms in PAH.[26] Infusion-site pain was the most common adverse effect, which led to treatment discontinuation in 8% of cases. Based on its chemical stability, parenteral treprostinil may also be administered via implantable pumps, improving convenience and likely decreasing the occurrence of line infections.

Inhaled treprostinil improved the 6MWD, N-terminal pro b-type natriuretic peptide (NT-proBNP), and QoL measures in patients with PAH on background therapy with either bosentan or sildenafil.[27]

The recommended starting dose for oral treprostinil is 0.250 mg two times a day or 0.125 mg three times daily and is usually increased by either 0.25–0.50 mg two times a day or 0.125 mg three times daily every 3–4 days as tolerated. The maximum dose is determined by tolerability. Assuming a 70-kg patient, 1 mg two times a day of oral treprostinil is approximately equivalent to 10 ng/kg/min of infused treprostinil. Inhaled treprostinil is administered times times daily with a goal dose of nine inhalations (54 g) at each dose.

Selexipag

Selexipag is an orally available, selective, prostacyclin receptor agonist approved in 2015 based on the GRIPHON trial. Selexipag reduced PVR after 17 weeks.[28] Selexipag alone or on top of mono- or double therapy with an ERA and/or a PDE5i reduced the relative risk of composite morbidity/mortality events by 40%. The starting dose is 200 µg twice daily, increased by 200 µg at weekly intervals to a maximum of 1,600 µg twice daily as tolerated.

COMBINATION THERAPY STRATEGIES

The majority of patients with PAH will require combination therapy using agents targeting the ERA, PDE5i, and PG pathways. In all of the recent large trials, including SERAPHIN and GRIPHON, the majority of the patients were on background PAH therapy. Although these studies examined sequential combination therapy, the landmark AMBITION trial compared upfront combination oral therapy with monotherapy with favorable results, serving as key evidence for the recommendation for upfront dual oral therapy for most patients.[29]

Special Situations

Pregnancy

Pregnancy in women with PAH and other forms of severe PH has been associated with maternal mortality rates of up to 56% and neonatal mortality rates of up to 13%. With improved therapeutic options and management guidelines for women with PAH during pregnancy and the peripartum period, maternal mortality has declined significantly but still remains high, ranging about 11–25%.[30] The previous European Society of Cardiology/European Respiratory Society (ESC/ERS) guidelines for the diagnosis and treatment of PH have recommended that patients with PAH should avoid pregnancy. However, there are reports of favorable pregnancy outcomes in women with PH, including, but not limited to, women with IPAH who respond to CCB therapy.[31] Women with PH can deteriorate at any time during or after pregnancy. Therefore, physicians have a responsibility to inform patients about the risks of pregnancy, so that women and their families can make informed decisions.

Women with poorly controlled disease, indicated by an intermediate- or high-risk profile and signs of RV dysfunction, are at high risk of adverse outcomes; in the event of pregnancy, they should be carefully counseled and early termination should be advised. For patients with well-controlled disease, a low-risk profile, and normal or near-normal resting hemodynamics who consider becoming pregnant, individual counseling and shared decision-making are recommended. In such cases, alternatives such as adoption and surrogacy may also be explored. Preconception genetic counseling should also be considered in HPAH. Women with PH who become pregnant or present during pregnancy with newly diagnosed PAH should be treated, whenever possible, in centers with a multidisciplinary team experienced in managing PH in pregnancy. If pregnancy is continued, PAH therapy may have to be adjusted. It is recommended to stop ERAs, riociguat, and selexipag (prostacyclin receptor agonist) because of potential or unknown teratogenicity.[32] Despite limited evidence, CCBs, PDE5is, and inhaled/parenteral prostacyclin analogs are considered safe during pregnancy.[33]

Contraception

Women with PH of childbearing potential should be provided with clear contraceptive advice, considering the chances of contraceptive failure are high in PH. With appropriate use, many forms of contraception including oral contraceptives are highly effective. In patients of PAH treated with bosentan, reduced efficacy of hormonal contraceptives should be carefully considered. Using hormonal implants or an intrauterine device are alternative options with low failure rates. Surgical sterilization techniques can be considered but are associated with perioperative risks. Emergency postcoital hormonal contraception is safe in PH.

Travel and Altitude

Hypobaric hypoxia may induce arterial hypoxemia, hypoxic pulmonary vasoconstriction, and increase RV load in patients with PAH.[34] Cabin aircraft pressures are equivalent to altitudes up to 2438 m, at which the PaO_2 decreases to that of an inspired O_2 fraction of 15.1% at sea level.[34] However, evidence suggests that short-term (i.e., <1 day) normobaric hypoxia is generally well tolerated in clinically stable patients with PAH.[34] In-flight oxygen administration is advised for patients using oxygen at sea level and for those with PaO_2 < 8 kPa (60 mm Hg) or SaO_2 < 92%. A low oxygen flow of 2 L/min will raise inspired oxygen pressure to that of sea level. Patients who are already on oxygen therapy should increase the flow rate accordingly.

Surgical Procedures

Surgical procedures in patients with PH are associated with increased risk of right HF and mortality. In a prospective, multinational registry including 114 patients with PAH who underwent noncardiac and nonobstetric surgery, the perioperative mortality rate was 2% in elective procedures and 15% in emergency procedures.[35] The mortality risk is directly proportional to the severity of PH. The decision to perform surgery should be made by a multidisciplinary team.

OVERALL THERAPEUTIC STRATEGY

Supportive therapies including warfarin, diuretics, and oxygen are considered. An acute vasoreactivity test is recommended for patients with idiopathic PAH and, if a positive response is seen, CCB treatment is recommended. For patients with IPAH without acute vasoreactivity and for other PAH groups, the initial treatment decision is made based on PAH severity. Patients at highest risk for death or clinical worsening are treated with a systemic prostacyclin as the initial therapy, while lower risk patients may be offered therapy with an oral or in some cases an inhaled medication. There is no single prognostic marker that is sufficient in making this decision, but a combination of clinical impression, functional class, 6MWD, laboratory results, catheterization results, and assessment of right ventricular function by imaging can be used to assess risk.

Consideration of combination therapy is recommended for patients who have an inadequate response to a single agent, with response typically assessed at 3–6 months. Adding a second agent rather than switching from one class of medication to another is generally recommended.

Interventional Therapy in Pulmonary Arterial Hypertension

Balloon Atrial Septostomy and Potts Shunt

Balloon atrial septostomy by creating an interatrial shunt and Potts shunt, by connecting the left PA and descending aorta, aim to decompress the right heart and increase systemic blood flow, thereby improving systemic oxygen transport, despite arterial oxygen desaturation.[36,37] As these procedures are complex and associated with high risk, including substantial procedure-related mortality, they are rarely performed in patients with PAH and may only be considered in centers with experience in the techniques.

Pulmonary Artery Denervation

The rationale for performing a PA denervation (PADN) is based on the increased sympathetic overdrive characterizing PAH, which is associated with poor outcome. Although the contribution of this mechanism to developing PAH is not completely understood, it is associated with vasoconstriction and vascular remodeling through a baroreflex mediated by stretch receptors located at the bifurcation of the PAs. Applying radiofrequency at the latter acutely and chronically improves hemodynamic variables. A small multicenter study tested the feasibility of PADN using an intravascular ultrasound catheter in patients receiving dual or triple therapy for PAH;[38] the procedure was safe and associated with a reduction in PVR, and increases in 6MWD and daily activity. Although potentially promising, PADN is seldomly performed.

Lung and Heart–Lung Transplantation

Lung transplantation remains an important treatment option for patients with PAH refractory to optimized medical therapy or when they present with an intermediate-high or high risk of mortality. In patients with PAH, referral to a lung transplant center should be considered early.

Currently, most patients receive bilateral LTx, while combined heart-lung transplantation is reserved for patients who have additional non-correctable cardiac conditions.[39] Overall, posttransplantation survival after 1 year is approximately 75% and 5-year survival is 50%.

SUMMARY

Pulmonary arterial hypertension remains an incurable condition with a high mortality rate, despite use of PAH drugs mainly targeting imbalance of vasoactive factors. Many novel agents are currently in phase 3 development. It is a progressive disease with multiple complications that vary in severity and are influenced by the underlying cause. Regular monitoring and management are essential to minimize these complications and improve patient outcomes. Overall, the management requires a comprehensive approach that combines medical therapy, lifestyle modifications, and regular monitoring.

REFERENCES

1. Grünig E, MacKenzie A, Peacock AJ, et al. Standardized exercise training is feasible, safe, and effective in pulmonary arterial and chronic thromboembolic pulmonary hypertension: results from a large European multicentre randomized controlled trial. Eur Heart J. 2021;42(23):2284-95.
2. Mereles D, Ehlken N, Kreuscher S, et al. Exercise and respiratory training improve exercise capacity and quality of life in patients with severe chronic pulmonary hypertension. Circulation. 2006;114(14):1482-9.
3. Montani D, Savale L, Natali D, et al. Long-term response to calcium-channel blockers in non-idiopathic pulmonary arterial hypertension. Eur Heart J. 2010;31(15):1898-907.
4. He J, Fang W, Lv B, et al. Diagnosis of chronic thromboembolic pulmonary hypertension: comparison of ventilation/perfusion

scanning and multidetector computed tomography pulmonary angiography with pulmonary angiography. Nucl Med Commun. 2012;33(5):459-63.

5. Ulrich S, Saxer S, Hasler ED, et al. Effect of domiciliary oxygen therapy on exercise capacity and quality of life in patients with pulmonary arterial or chronic thromboembolic pulmonary hypertension: a randomised, placebo-controlled trial. Eur Resp J. 2019;54(2):1900276.
6. Johnson SR, Granton JT, Mehta S. Thrombotic arteriopathy and anticoagulation in pulmonary hypertension. Chest. 2006;130(2):545-52.
7. Khan MS, Usman MS, Siddiqi TJ, et al. Is anticoagulation beneficial in pulmonary arterial hypertension? a systematic review and meta-analysis. Circ Cardiovasc Qual Outcomes. 2018;11(9):e004757.
8. Wang P, Hu L, Yin Y, et al. Can anticoagulants improve the survival rate for patients with idiopathic pulmonary arterial hypertension? A systematic review and meta-analysis. Thromb Res. 2020;196:251-6.
9. Rosenkranz S, Howard LS, Gomberg-Maitland M, et al Systemic consequences of pulmonary hypertension and right-sided heart failure. Circulation. 2020;141(8):678-93.
10. Stickel S, Gin-Sing W, Wagenaar M, et al. The practical management of fluid retention in adults with right heart failure due to pulmonary arterial hypertension. Eur Heart J Suppl. 2019;21(Suppl K):K46-53.
11. McDonagh T, Damy T, Doehner W, et al. Screening, diagnosis and treatment of iron deficiency in chronic heart failure: putting the 2016 European Society of Cardiology heart failure guidelines into clinical practice. Eur J Heart Fail. 2018;20(12):1664-72.
12. Ruiter G, Manders E, Happé CM, et al. Intravenous iron therapy in patients with idiopathic pulmonary arterial hypertension and iron deficiency. Pulm Circ. 2015;5(3):466-72.
13. Ruiter G, Lankhorst S, Boonstra A, et al. Iron deficiency is common in idiopathic pulmonary arterial hypertension. Eur Resp J. 2011;37(6):1386-91.
14. Dupuis J, Hoeper MM. Endothelin receptor antagonists in pulmonary arterial hypertension. Eur Res J. 2008;31(2):407-15.
15. Giaid A, Yanagisawa M, Langleben D, et al. Expression of endothelin-1 in the lungs of patients with pulmonary hypertension. N Engl J Med. 1993;328(24):1732-9.
16. Rubin LJ, Badesch DB, Barst RJ, et al. Bosentan therapy for pulmonary arterial hypertension. N Engl J Med. 2002;346(12):896-903.
17. Humbert M, Segal ES, Kiely DG, et al. Results of European post-marketing surveillance of bosentan in pulmonary hypertension. Eur Resp J. 2007;30(2):338-44.
18. Wrishko RE, Dingemanse J, Yu A, et al. Pharmacokinetic interaction between tadalafil and bosentan in healthy male subjects. J Clin Pharmacol. 2008;48(5):610-8.
19. Raghu G, Behr J, Brown KK, et al. Treatment of idiopathic pulmonary fibrosis with ambrisentan: a parallel, randomized trial. Ann Intern Med. 2013;158(9):641-9.
20. Pulido T, Adzerikho I, Channick RN, et al. Macitentan and morbidity and mortality in pulmonary arterial hypertension. N Engl J Med. 2013;369:809-18.
21. Ghofrani HA, Galiè N, Grimminger F, et al. Riociguat for the treatment of pulmonary arterial hypertension. N Engl J Med. 2013;369:330-40.
22. Lang IM, Gaine SP. Recent advances in targeting the prostacyclin pathway in pulmonary arterial hypertension. Eur Resp Rev. 2015;24(138):630-41.
23. Sitbon O, Delcroix M, Bergot E, et al. EPITOME-2: An open-label study assessing the transition to a new formulation of intravenous epoprostenol in patients with pulmonary arterial hypertension. Am Heart J. 2014;167(2):210-7.
24. Barst RJ, Rubin LJ, Long WA, et al. A comparison of continuous intravenous epoprostenol (prostacyclin) with conventional therapy for primary pulmonary hypertension. N Engl J Med. 1996;334(5):296-301.
25. Olschewski H, Simonneau G, Galiè N, et al. Inhaled iloprost for severe pulmonary hypertension. N Engl J Med. 2002;347(5):322-9.
26. Simonneau GE, Barst RJ, Galiè NA, et al. Continuous subcutaneous infusion of treprostinil, a prostacyclin analogue, in patients with pulmonary arterial hypertension: a double-blind, randomized, placebo-controlled trial. Am J Respir Crit Care Med. 2002;165(6):800-4.
27. McLaughlin VV, Benza RL, Rubin LJ, et al. Addition of inhaled treprostinil to oral therapy for pulmonary arterial hypertension: a randomized controlled clinical trial. J Am Coll Cardiol. 2010;55(18):1915-22.
28. Simonneau G, Torbicki A, Hoeper MM, et al. Selexipag: an oral, selective prostacyclin receptor agonist for the treatment of pulmonary arterial hypertension. Eur Resp J. 2012;40(4):874-80.
29. Sitbon O, Channick R, Chin KM, et al. Selexipag for the treatment of pulmonary arterial hypertension. J Am Coll Cardiol. 2015;373(26):2522-33.
30. Luo J, Shi H, Xu L, et al. Pregnancy outcomes in patients with pulmonary arterial hypertension: A retrospective study. Medicine. 2020;99(23):e20285.
31. Corbach N, Berlier C, Lichtblau M, et al. Favorable pregnancy outcomes in women with well-controlled pulmonary arterial hypertension. Front Med. 2021;8:689764.
32. de Raaf MA, Beekhuijzen M, Guignabert C, et al. Endothelin-1 receptor antagonists in fetal development and pulmonary arterial hypertension. Reprod Toxicol. 2015;56:45-51.
33. DunnL, Greer R, Flenady V, et al. Sildenafil in pregnancy: a systemic review of maternal tolerance and obstetric and perinatal outcomes. Fetal Diagn Ther. 2017;41(2):81-8.
34. Burns RM, Peacock AJ, Johnson MK, et al. Hypoxaemia in patients with pulmonary arterial hypertension during simulated air travel. Resp Med. 2013;107(2):298-304.
35. Meyer S, McLaughlin VV, Seyfarth HJ, et al. Outcomes of noncardiac, nonobstetric surgery in patients with PAH: an international prospective survey. Eur Resp J. 2013;41(6):1302-7.
36. Khan MS, Memon MM, Amin E, et al. Use of balloon atrial septostomy in patients with advanced pulmonary arterial hypertension: a systematic review and meta analysis. Chest. 2019;156(1):53-63.
37. Grady RM, Canter MW, Wan F, et al. Pulmonary-to-systemic arterial shunt to treat children with severe pulmonary hypertension. J Am Coll Cardiol. 2021;78(5):468-77.
38. Rothman AM, Vachiery JL, Howard LS, et al. Intravascular ultrasound pulmonary artery denervation to treat pulmonary arterial hypertension (TROPHY1) multicenter, early feasibility study. Cardiovasc Interv. 2020;13(8):989-99.
39. Görzer I, Jaksch P, Strassl R, et al. Association between plasma Torque teno virus level and chronic lung allograft dysfunction after lung transplantation. J Heart Lung Transpl. 2017;36(3):366-8.

Pulmonary Thromboembolism

CHAPTER 124

Shona Arlin Christopher, Devasahayam J Christopher

INTRODUCTION

Pulmonary embolism (PE) is a common form of venous thromboembolism (VTE) which can frequently be fatal when acute. The evaluation of a patient with suspected PE should be done in a systematic and efficient manner. Early diagnosis and initiation of appropriate treatment are likely to reduce the morbidity and mortality associated with the disease.[1] PE is frequently misdiagnosed as its clinical signs and symptoms mimic several other respiratory and cardiac diseases.[2] Recent advances in the diagnostic strategies, pharmacotherapeutics, and surgical management have decreased mortality from venous thromboembolic disease significantly in the past few decades.[3]

EPIDEMIOLOGY

In a US population-based study, the incidence of VTE increased from 73 per 100,000 in 1985/1986 to 133 in 2009.[4] The increase could partly be explained by the introduction of computed tomography pulmonary angiogram.[4] Some studies show a higher prevalence in men, whereas other studies show a higher prevalence in women.[4-7] According to prospective cohort studies, the acute case fatality rate for PE ranges from 7 to 11%.[8] All-cause mortality due to PE has been declining.[9]

DEFINITION

Pulmonary embolism refers to obstruction of the pulmonary artery or one of its branches by material (e.g., thrombus, tumor, air, or fat) that originated elsewhere in the body. The nomenclature has been variously referred to as follows:

- *Based on the temporal pattern of presentation*:
  - Acute: Onset of symptoms and signs immediately after obstruction of pulmonary vessels
  - Subacute: Presentation within days or weeks following the initial event
  - Chronic: Symptoms of pulmonary hypertension over many years (i.e., chronic thromboembolic pulmonary hypertension)
- *Based on hemodynamic stability*: Acute PE can also be massive, submassive, and stable PE based on hemodynamic stability and the presence of right ventricular (RV) strain. Hemodynamically unstable PE is that which results in hypotension which in turn in defined as:
  - Systolic blood pressure < 90 mm Hg, or
  - A drop in systolic blood pressure of ≥ 40 mm Hg from baseline for a period > 15 minutes, or
  - Hypotension that requires vasopressors or inotropic support and is not explained by other causes such as sepsis, arrhythmia, left ventricular dysfunction from acute myocardial ischemia or infarction, or hypovolemia.

Hemodynamically unstable PE is usually a result of a large embolus (massive PE) or due to a small embolus in patients with underlying other cardiac and pulmonary diseases. Therefore, "massive PE" indicates hemodynamic instability and not the size of embolus. A patient with "submassive" PE may be hemodynamically stable or may have mild or borderline hypotension that stabilizes in response to fluid therapy or may present with right ventricle dysfunction. Those with hemodynamical instability are more likely to die from obstructive shock, i.e., due to severe RV failure.

Based on the anatomic location of embolus: PE can be unilateral or bilateral depending on whether arteries in one or both lungs are involved. Saddle embolus is an embolus that lodges at the bifurcation of the main pulmonary artery and may even extend to one or both main pulmonary artery branches and often presents with hemodynamic instability with a high risk of death. Obstruction distal to the bifurcation of the main pulmonary artery is more common. The obstruction could occur in the main pulmonary artery or its lobar, segmental, or subsegmental branches.

PATHOGENESIS AND PATHOPHYSIOLOGY

Pulmonary embolism pathogenesis is similar to that of thrombus formation based on Virchow's triad, i.e., venous stasis, endothelial injury, and hypercoagulable state.

The most common source of pulmonary emboli lies in the deep veins of the lower limbs, particularly between the knee and the inguinal ligament. PE is infrequently due to thrombosis of the pelvic veins or veins of the upper extremities or other organ systems (e.g., hepatic and renal veins). The thrombus dislodges and travels through the venous circulation and lodges in one of the pulmonary arteries. The embolism initially results in an area of the lung that is ventilated but underperfused, resulting in an alveolar dead space. Subsequently, there occurs elevation of pulmonary vascular resistance due to release of vasoactive substances such as serotonin from the platelets and the blockade of the pulmonary artery by the clot. This results in an increase in RV workload, leading to a redistribution of blood flow, which if excessive may result in RV failure **(Flowchart 1)**. Once this occurs, there is a fall in the pulmonary blood flow and reduction of left ventricular filling, causing systemic hypotension. Airway obstruction resulting from the reflex bronchoconstriction further contributes to the ventilation-perfusion (V/Q) mismatch. After about 24 hours, there is depletion of surfactant, which may result in atelectasis and edema in the affected area.

Pulmonary infarction itself is an uncommon consequence of PE, because pulmonary parenchyma has three potential sources of oxygen (namely, pulmonary arteries, bronchial arteries, and alveolar air). Generally, two of these sources need to be compromised before infarction develops and this usually happens only in patients with coexisting cardiopulmonary disease. Also, complete occlusion of the pulmonary artery is infrequent. However, pulmonary infarction may occur in 10% of patients secondary to obstruction in the segmental or sub-segmental arteries.[10]

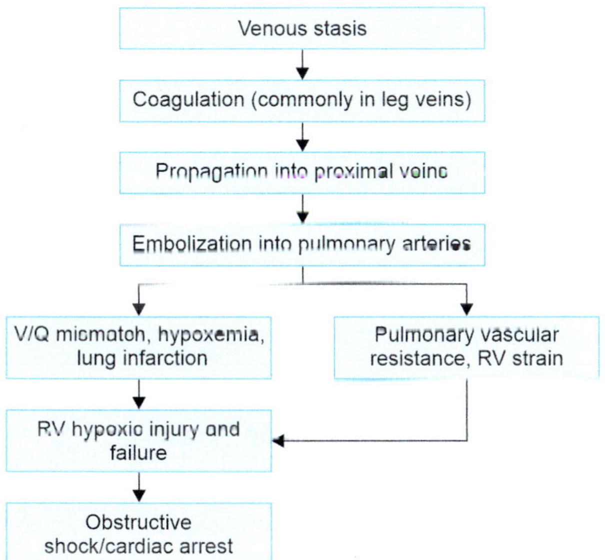

FLOWCHART 1: Pathophysiology of pulmonary embolism. Formation of DVT and embolization into pulmonary arteries leads to acute increase in pulmonary vascular resistance, which increases the demand on the right ventricle and may decrease the cardiac output. This combination of effects can lead to right ventricular dysfunction, infarction, and even cardiac arrest.

(DVT: deep venous thrombosis; RV: right ventricular; V/Q: ventilation/perfusion)

RISK FACTORS

The risk factors are broadly classified as inherited/genetic and acquired risk factors **(Flowchart 2)**. Some of the common genetic risk factors are factor V Leiden and prothrombin gene mutation.[11] Acquired risk factors can be further divided into provoking and nonprovoking risk factors.

Inherited/Genetic Causes

Factor V Leiden and prothrombin gene mutation are the two most common genetic causes for VTE (50–60%). Deficiencies of natural coagulation inhibitors, such as antithrombin, protein C, and protein S, are strong risk factors for VTE and account for the rest.[11]

Provoking Factors

Surgery and Fractures

Recent surgery and fractures, particularly of the femur and tibia, pose an increased risk. In surgical patients, the high-risk groups are those that have major high-risk operations performed for abdominal or pelvic malignancy and major orthopedic surgery, or any surgery requiring intensive care. The likely causative factors may decrease venous blood flow in the lower limbs, immobilization, reduction in fibrinolysis, release of tissue factor, and consumption of endogenous anticoagulants such as antithrombin.

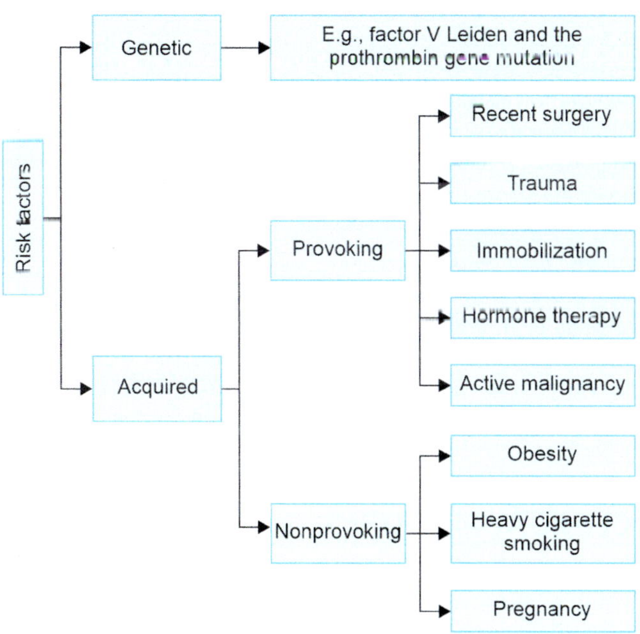

FLOWCHART 2: Various risk factors that cause pulmonary embolism.

Malignancy

Abnormalities of hemostasis occur in patients with neoplastic disease. A patient with malignancy tends to produce procoagulant substances such as tissue factor and cancer procoagulant, thus leading to a hypercoagulable state. A well-known example of this is the association of thrombophlebitis migrans with gastrointestinal tract malignant disease. The association of VTE is seen most often with lung cancer, followed in the order of frequency by carcinomas of the pancreas, colon and rectum, kidney and prostate.[12] There is an 18% attributable risk factor for the development of VTE due to malignancy.[13]

Immobilization

Immobilization for more than a week is an important risk factor. Diminished muscle activity in the lower limbs reduces venous return, facilitating accumulation of activated clotting factors.

Hormone Therapy

Most oral and transdermal contraceptives consist of a combination of estrogen and progestogen or progesterone alone. There is an increased risk of thrombosis the first 6–12 months after initiation of therapy.[14] A similar trend is seen in those receiving hormone replacement therapy as well.[15]

Pregnancy and Puerperium

Venous thromboembolism is one of the leading causes of maternal morbidity and mortality. About two-thirds of VTE cases occur during pregnancy and one-third during the postpartum period. The risk of VTE was increased 5-fold during pregnancy and increased 60-fold during the first 3 months following delivery compared with nonpregnant females.[16] The risk was highest in the third trimester of pregnancy and during the first 6 weeks after delivery. The thrombus formation is probably due to venous stasis in the lower limbs resulting from decreased venous return due to direct pressure from the enlarged uterus as well as the hypercoagulable state associated with pregnancy.

Obesity

Obesity is an important risk factor, especially in association with other risk factors such as smoking, use of hormonal therapy, and genetic causes.[17-19] *Smoking* is another important risk factor associated with an increased risk of VTE.[20]

CLINICAL FEATURES

The clinical presentation varies widely from one patient to another. Evaluating the likelihood of PE in an individual patient according to the clinical presentation is of utmost importance not only for the interpretation of the diagnostic test results but also for the selection of an appropriate diagnostic strategy.

Symptoms

Symptomatic PE refers to the presence of symptoms that usually lead to the radiologic confirmation of PE, while asymptomatic PE refers to patients who are incidentally detected on imaging done for some other purpose. Some of the important symptoms include the following:[10]

- Dyspnea at rest or with exertion (73%)
- Pleuritic pain (66%)
- Cough (37%)
- Orthopnea (28%)
- Calf or thigh pain and/or swelling (44%)
- Wheezing (21%)
- Hemoptysis (13%)

Less commonly, patients may present with transient or persistent arrhythmias (e.g., atrial fibrillation), presyncope, syncope, and hemodynamic collapse.[21-23] When the more distal segmental and subsegmental branches are involved, it may be associated with pleuritic chest pain and pulmonary infarction.

Some patients may have little or no symptoms at presentation even if the embolus is large[24] and some may manifest symptoms over weeks or days. Patients may become more symptomatic with time and rapidly deteriorate with evolution of hemodynamical instability which might be attributable to recurrent embolization or progressive pulmonary hypertension secondary to vasoconstriction.

Clinical Signs

Following are some of the common clinical signs with acute PE:[24]

- Tachypnea (54%)
- Tachycardia (24%)
- Calf or thigh swelling, erythema, edema, tenderness (47%)
- Rales (18%)
- Decreased breath sounds (17%)
- A loud pulmonic component of the second heart sound (15%)
- Jugular venous pressure (14%)
- Fever (3%)

Over 90% of patients present with either dyspnea or tachypnea, while 8% present with shock due to circulatory collapse or with cardiac arrest.[25,26]

Lower limb deep venous thrombosis (DVT) is the cause of PE in the majority of cases; it is prudent to look for features such as local pain, tenderness, redness, and warmth.

DIAGNOSIS

The diagnosis of PE requires the integration of a careful history and physical examination with laboratory testing and appropriate imaging modalities.

Routine and Ancillary Investigations

Routine investigations such as chest X-ray and ECG are of limited value for the diagnosis of PE. More importantly, they contribute to exclude many common conditions with similar clinical presentation like acute myocardial infarction, acute aortic dissection, pneumonia, pneumothorax, and cardiac failure. Most common chest radiographic findings were cardiomegaly, pleural effusion, elevated hemidiaphragm, atelectasis, and parenchymal pulmonary infiltrates. Some other important chest radiography signs include the following:

- *Fleischner sign*: Enlarged pulmonary artery
- *Hampton hump*: Peripheral wedge of airspace opacity which implies lung infarction
- *Westermark sign*: Regional oligemia
- *Knuckle sign*: Abrupt tapering off, of a pulmonary artery distal to an embolus
- *Palla sign*: Enlarged right descending pulmonary artery
- *Chang sign*: Dilated right descending pulmonary artery with sudden cutoff

Chest radiographic signs have both low sensitivity and specificity in the diagnosis of acute PE.[27,28]

The most common *ECG* changes seen in PE are sinus tachycardia and nonspecific ST and T-wave changes.[24] Other ECG patterns that may be seen and also predict poor outcomes are as follows:[29]

- Atrial arrhythmias (e.g., atrial fibrillation)
- Bradycardia (<50 beats/min) or tachycardia (>100 beats/min)
- New right bundle branch block
- Inferior Q waves (leads II, III, and aVF)
- Anterior ST-segment changes and T-wave inversion
- S1Q3T3 pattern

Other routine laboratory investigations include complete blood counts, liver function test, erythrocyte sedimentation rate (ESR), and serum creatinine. Leukocytosis, elevated aspartate aminotransferase (AST), and elevated ESR may be observed. Contrast imaging can be done only if serum creatinine is within normal limits.

Arterial blood gas (ABG) analysis often demonstrates hypoxemia and hypocapnia, but it may also be normal, especially in younger patients without an underlying cardiopulmonary disease.[10] In the setting of a normal or near-normal chest radiograph and significant unexplained hypoxemia, PE should be considered. A widened alveolar-arterial gradient for oxygen is also commonly seen in the ABG.

D-dimers formed because of fibrin degradation rise with intravascular coagulation. The levels in plasma reflect the fibrinolytic activity on pre-existing thrombi and not necessarily the rate of thrombus formation itself. D-dimer tests are nonspecific and may be elevated in conditions such as cancer, inflammation, and peripheral vascular disease and in hospitalized patients including obstetrics cases.[30,31] D-dimers, along with clinical probability scores, are useful in triaging patients for confirmatory tests such as computed tomography pulmonary arteriography (CTPA). A patient with a low clinical probability with D-dimer < 500 ng/mL does not warrant further testing due to its high negative predictive value. But a patient with an intermediate or high clinical probability will warrant further evaluation, especially if D-dimer is ≥500 ng/mL.[32-34] D-dimer levels tend to increase with age and there is reduced specificity when testing older individuals (>50 years), at a cutoff of 500 ng/mL. Hence, age-adjusted D-dimer levels are used.[35]

Age (if over 50 years) × 10 = Cutoff value in ng/mL (fibrinogen equivalent units)

Serum troponin may be elevated in acute PE, indicating RV ischemia or microinfarction.[36] Brain natriuretic peptide (BNP) levels may also be elevated in acute PE because of RV dilatation. These have more significance in prognostication and risk stratification than for the diagnosis of PE.[37]

Diagnostic Imaging for Suspected Pulmonary Embolism

Deep Venous Thrombosis Testing

Compression ultrasonography (CUS) is used as an indirect method for diagnosing PE **(Figs. 1A and B)**. CUS has a sensitivity of over 90% for proximal DVT and a specificity of about 95%.[38,39] It shows DVT in 30–50% of patients; finding a proximal DVT in patients suspected of PE is sufficient to warrant anticoagulant treatment without further testing.[40] The only validated diagnostic criterion for DVT is incomplete compressibility of the vein, which indicates the presence of a clot, whereas flow criteria are unreliable.[40] Proximal CUS can be performed when there are contraindications to contrast dye and/or irradiation.[40]

Echocardiogram

Echocardiography is best used in suspected or proven acute PE to assess the impact of acute PE on CTPA RV function. A regional pattern of RV dysfunction with akinesia of the basal and mid right ventricular free wall but normal apical contractility, i.e., McConnell's sign; acute RV infarction may also cause a similar appearance. Rarely, echocardiogram may identify emboli in-transit in the right atrium and if noted before lung imaging; may obviate the need for further confirmatory tests for PE.

Radioisotope Ventilation–Perfusion Scan

Ventilation–perfusion scintigraphy (V/Q scan) is a well-established diagnostic test for suspected PE **(Fig. 2)**. It is noninvasive and safe to use, barring few allergic reactions. The ventilation and perfusion phases of a V/Q lung scan are performed together and may include a chest X-ray for comparison or to look for other causes of lung disease. In the ventilation phase of the test, a gaseous radionuclide xenon ^{133}Xe or ^{99m}Tc-labeled aerosols or Tc-99 m-labeled carbon microparticles (Techne gas) are used. The perfusion phase of the test involves the intravenous injection of radioactive

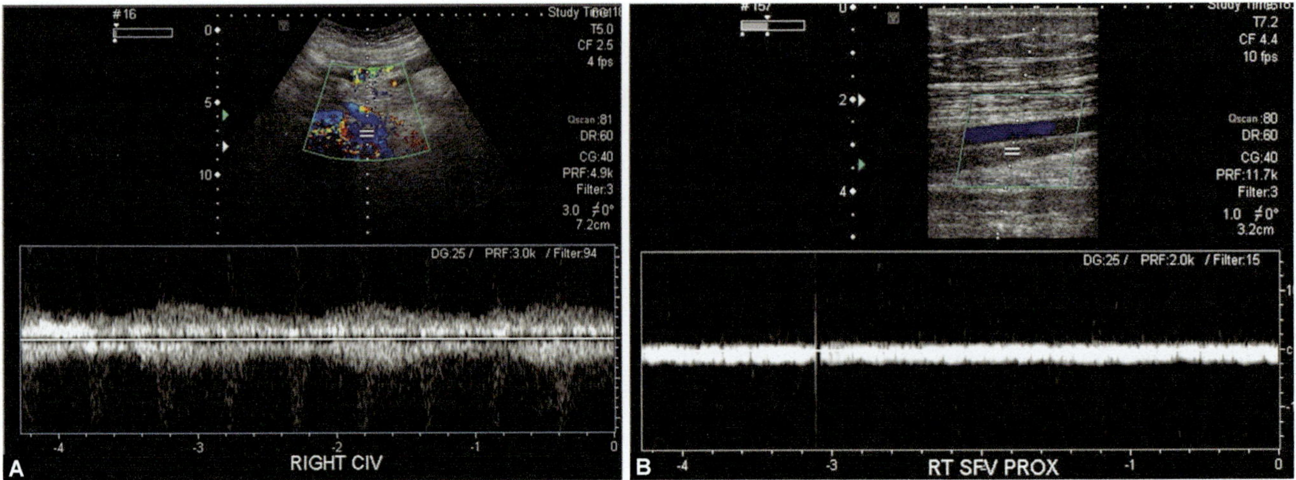

FIGS. 1A AND B: Color Doppler study of right lower limb. (A) Right common iliac vein shows normal color uptake with no thrombus within the lumen; (B) Superficial femoral vein is reduced in caliber, partially compressible with echogenic walls. Near-complete lumen filling flow is seen on augmentation suggesting recanalization.

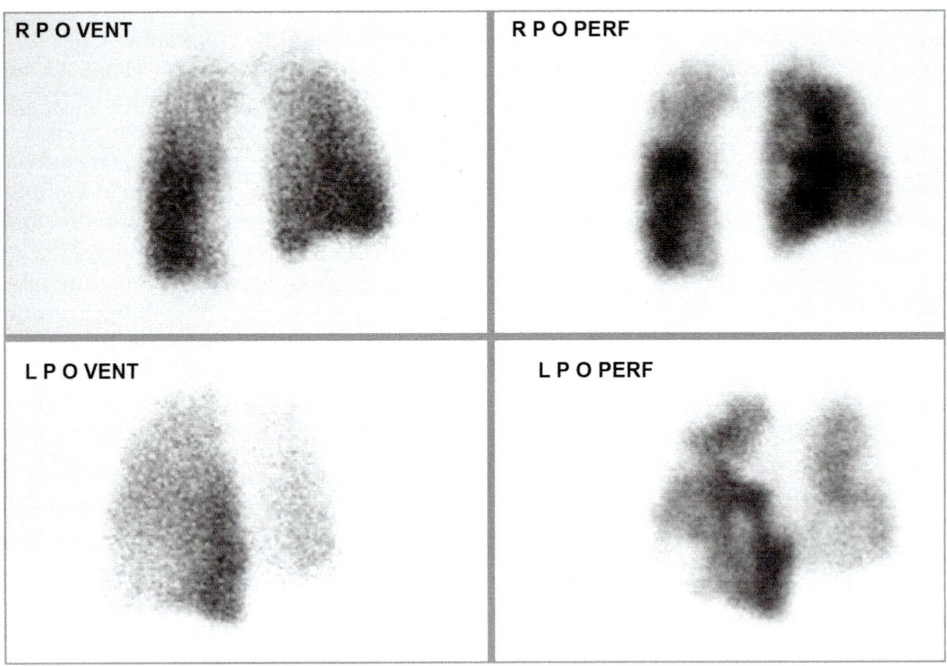

FIG. 2: Ventilation–perfusion lung scan shows several unmatched ventilation–perfusion defects, consistent with pulmonary emboli.

technetium macroaggregated albumin (Tc-99m-MAA), which blocks a small fraction of pulmonary capillaries and thereby enables scintigraphic assessment of lung perfusion at the tissue level. Where there is occlusion of pulmonary arterial branches, the peripheral capillary bed will not receive particles, rendering the area "cold" on subsequent images. A defect in the perfusion images with either normal or near-normal ventilation (mismatched defects) is indicative of PE.

Diagnostic accuracy of the V/Q scan is greatest when the test is combined with clinical probability:[41]

- Patients with high clinical probability of PE and a high-probability V/Q scan had a 95% likelihood of having PE.
- Patients with low clinical probability of PE and a low-probability V/Q scan had only a 4% likelihood of having PE.
- A normal V/Q scan virtually excludes PE.

- Strong clinical suspicion of PE in the presence of a nondiagnostic V/Q scan should lead to further evaluation [computed tomography pulmonary angiography (CTPA), pulmonary angiography, or lower limb DVT studies].

Computed Tomography Pulmonary Arteriography

Computed tomography pulmonary arteriography is both sensitive and specific for the diagnosis of PE and hence is the first-choice diagnostic imaging modality, when indicated as per clinical probability scores and diagnostic algorithms. CTPA involves obtaining thin section (≤2.5 mm) volumetric images of the chest after a bolus administration of intravenous contrast. The CT cuts are acquired in such a way that there is maximal contrast enhancement at the pulmonary arteries. A multidetector (≥16 detector rows) CT scanner is required to acquire good-quality accurate images and markedly improves visualization of segmental and subsegmental vessels **(Figs. 3 and 4)**.[42,43] In addition, both mediastinal and parenchymal structures are also evaluated, which may provide important alternate or additional diagnoses. The images should be acquired with the patient breath-holding for about 30 seconds to acquire images with optimum quality.

According to the Prospective Investigation of Pulmonary Embolism Diagnosis (PIOPED) II study, the multidetector computed tomography (MDCT) has positive predictive values of 96% with a concordantly high or low probability on clinical assessment and 92% with an intermediate probability on clinical assessment.[44]

Catheter-based Pulmonary Angiography

Pulmonary angiography is historically the gold standard investigation for the confirmation of PE **(Fig. 5)**.[45] It is an invasive procedure with potential risks. It is indicated in rare situations where there is a high clinical probability of PE, but CTPA or V/Q scanning is nondiagnostic. It is often done when a concurrent intervention such as catheter-directed embolectomy and/or thrombolysis may be required. The dye is injected into the pulmonary artery via a catheter inserted through the femoral, internal jugular, or subclavian vein. The features indicating the presence of an embolus include an intraluminal filling defect and an abrupt vascular cutoff in pulmonary arteries. This procedure, although tolerated reasonably well in hemodynamic stable patients, is also associated with 2% mortality and 5% morbidity.[46]

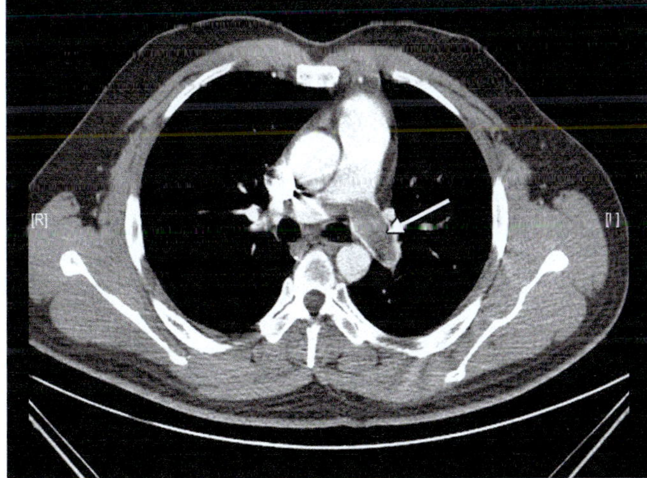

FIG. 3: CT pulmonary arteriography (CTPA) showing filling defect at the bifurcation of the main pulmonary artery and in the left main pulmonary artery (arrow) suggesting thromboembolism.

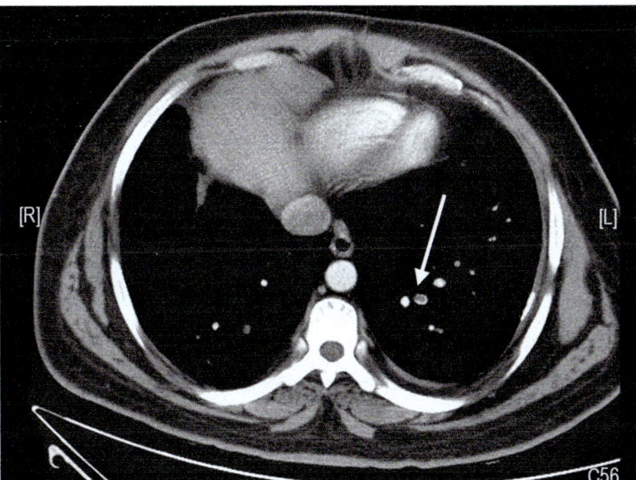

FIG. 4: CT pulmonary arteriography (CTPA) showing a filling defect (arrow) in the subsegmental branches of the left descending pulmonary artery suggesting thromboembolism.

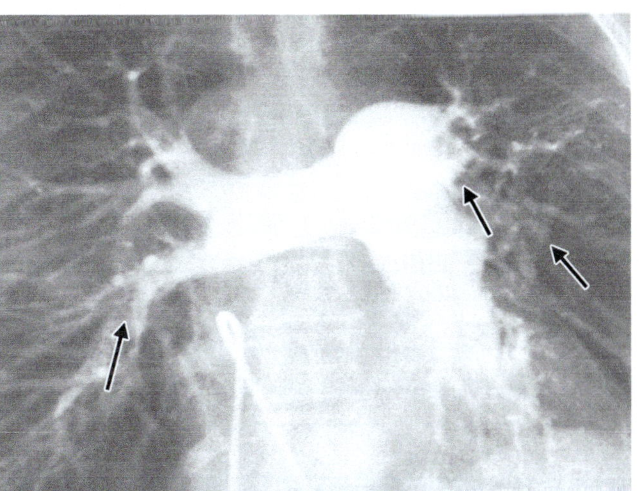

FIG. 5: This catheter-based pulmonary angiogram shows several small lucencies representing emboli obstructing the pulmonary arteries (arrows).

Clinical Probability Scores

The clinical pretest probability can be determined by considering a patient's clinical history, risk factors for VTE, clinical signs, and laboratory tests. The implicit evaluation of pretest probability was demonstrated to be relatively accurate in the PIOPED study.[41] The most widely used and validated scores are: Wells score; modified Wells score, and revised Geneva score **(Tables 1 and 2)**.[47-49] The Wells score categorizes patient as low, intermediate, and high probability of PE.

TABLE 1: Wells and modified Well's criteria.[47]

Variable	Points
Malignancy	+1
Hemoptysis	+1
Previous DVT or PE	+1.5
Heart rate > 100 beats/min	+1.5
Surgery or bed rest ≥ 3 days within 1 month	+1.5
Clinical signs of DVT	+3
No alternative diagnosis as more likely than PE	+3
Wells criteria	
Clinical probability	**Points**
Low	<2
Intermediate	2–6
High	≥7
Modified Wells criteria-simplified clinical probability	
Clinical probability	**Points**
PE unlikely	≤4
PE likely	>4

(DVT: deep venous thrombosis; PE: pulmonary embolism)

TABLE 2: Revised Geneva score.[49]

Variable	Points
Age > 65 years	+1
Active malignancy	+2
Hemoptysis	+2
Previous DVT or PE	+3
Surgery or lower limb fracture within 1 month	+2
Unilateral edema and pain at palpation	+4
Spontaneously reported calf pain	+3
Heart rate 75–94 beats/min	+3
Heart rate ≥ 95 beats/min	+5
Clinical probability	**Points**
Low	≤3
Intermediate	4–10
High	≥11

(DVT: deep venous thrombosis; PE: pulmonary embolism)

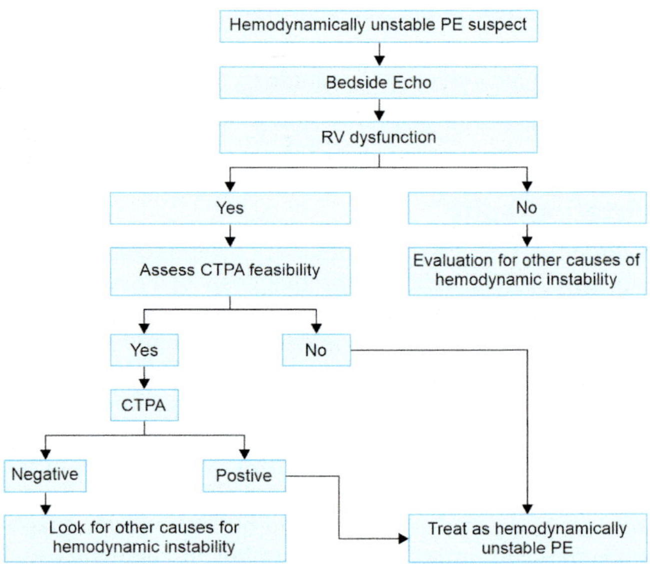

FLOWCHART 3: Diagnostic algorithm for hemodynamically unstable suspects with PE.

(CTPA: CT pulmonary arteriography; PE: pulmonary embolism; RV: right ventricular)

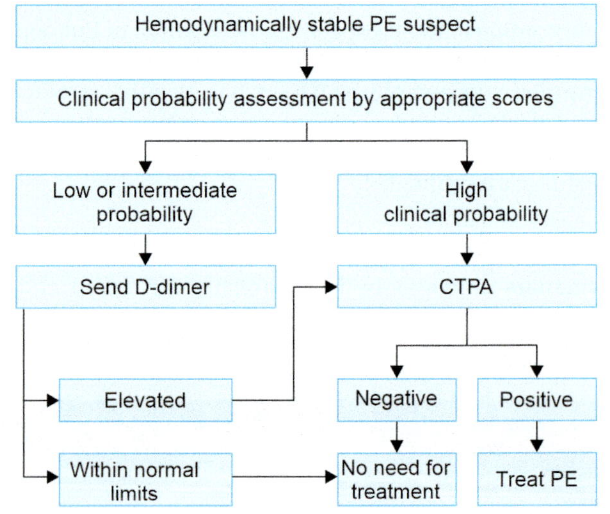

FLOWCHART 4: Diagnostic algorithm for hemodynamically stable suspects with PE.

(CTPA: CT pulmonary arteriography; PE: pulmonary embolism)

The diagnostic algorithm for PE is based on the presence or absence of hemodynamic instability **(Flowcharts 3 and 4)**.

MANAGEMENT

General Management

Available data are insufficient to recommend outpatient therapy for PE; inpatient therapy with initial bedrest for 24–48 hours is often recommended. The following general measures should be followed in all patients with acute PE:

- Secure IV access
- *Oxygen therapy*: It should be initiated in patients with respiratory failure.
- *Airway support*: Intubation and mechanical ventilation may be required in case hypoxia and respiratory distress are profound.
- *Empirical anticoagulation*: It is initiated in all patients with suspected PE unless otherwise contraindicated.
- *Inotropic support*: Use of vasopressors may be required for circulatory support.

Specific Treatment (Flowcharts 5 and 6)

- *Hemodynamically unstable patients*: These patients are usually not stable enough to undergo any imaging modality. Bedside echocardiography may be used to support the diagnosis. Lifesaving reperfusion therapy and other interventions such as surgical embolectomy, percutaneous catheter embolectomy, or catheter-directed thrombolysis may be planned.
- *Hemodynamically stable patients*: These patients are predominantly managed with therapeutic anticoagulation.

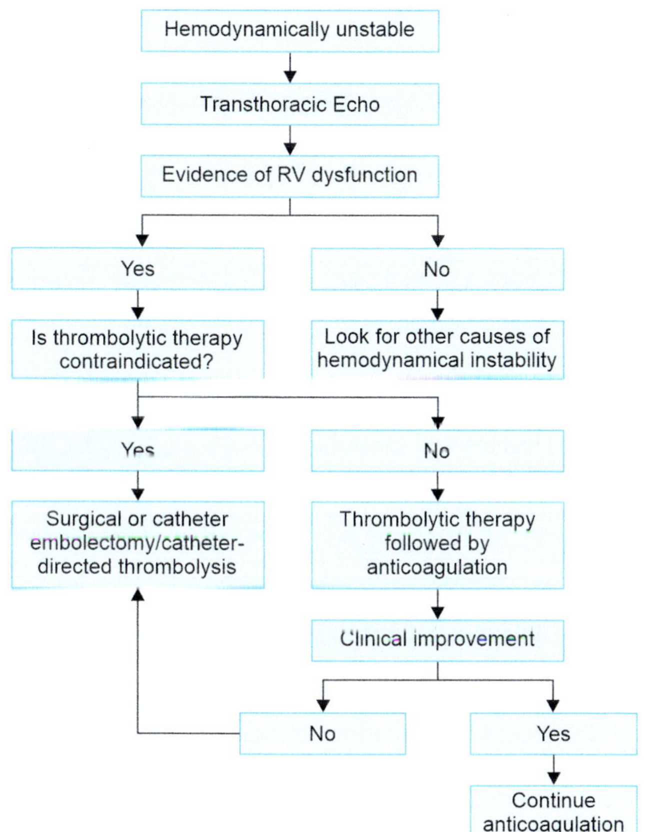

FLOWCHART 5: Management algorithm for patients with hemodynamically unstable PE.

(PE: pulmonary embolism; RV: right ventricular)

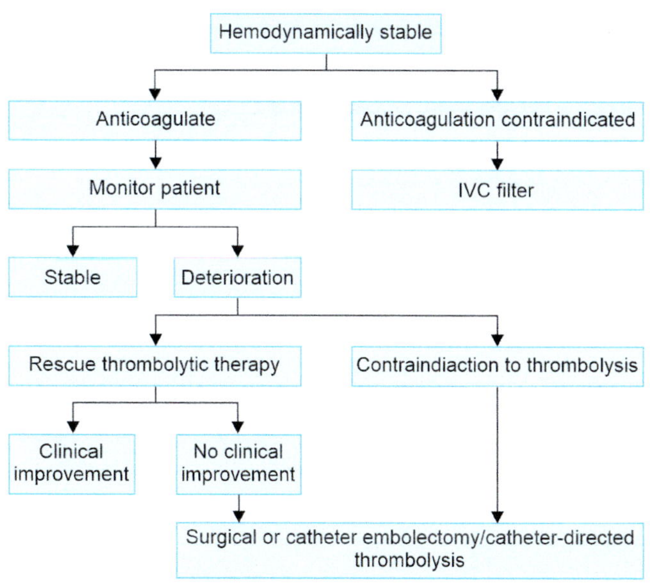

FLOWCHART 6: Management algorithm for patients with hemodynamically stable PE.

(IVC: inferior vena cava; PE: pulmonary embolism)

Anticoagulant Therapy

Anticoagulant treatment plays a critical role in the management of patients and is required universally regardless of whether the patient is hemodynamically stable or unstable. Anticoagulants help in preventing formation of new thrombus, death, and recurrent events with an acceptable rate of bleeding complications.

- *Agents used for initial anticoagulation (for the first 0–10 days)*:
  - Low-molecular-weight heparin (LMWH) derived from unfractionated heparin (UFH) by chemical or enzymatic depolymerization has more predictable pharmacokinetic and pharmacodynamic properties, a longer half-life than heparin, and a lower risk of nonhemorrhagic side effects. Trials have confirmed the efficacy of LMWH administered subcutaneously and have the advantages of a simple subcutaneous administration, without requiring laboratory monitoring. LMWH should be given with care in patients with renal failure. Intravenous UFH may be the preferred mode of initial anticoagulation for patients with severe renal impairment (creatinine clearance < 30 mL/min) and with severe risk of bleeding. Subcutaneous LMWH is generally recommended over standard UFH.[50] LMWH is the preferred anticoagulant in patients with active cancer and pregnancy. Therefore, in most cases of acute PE, LMWH is given subcutaneously at weight-adjusted doses without monitoring in preference to UFH **(Table 3)**.

TABLE 3: Subcutaneous regimens of low-molecular-weight heparins (LMWH) and fondaparinux.

Dosage of LMWH and Fondaparinux	
LMWH	**Dosage**
Enoxaparin	1.0 mg/kg every 12 hours Or 1.5 mg/kg once daily
Tinzaparin	175 U/kg once daily
Dalteparin	200 IU/kg once daily Or 100 IU/kg twice daily
Fondaparinux	• 5 mg (body weight ≤ 50 kg) once daily dosage • 7.5 mg (body weight 50–100 kg) once daily • 10 mg (body weight > 100 kg) once daily
Nadroparin	86 IU/kg every 12 hours Or 171 IU/kg once daily

BOX 1 Regimens of heparin therapy.

Intravenous route:
- 80 U/kg bolus (maximum 10,000 U) followed by 18 U/kg/h infusion (maximum 2,000 U/h)

OR
- 5,000 U bolus followed by 1,680 U/h infusion

Subcutaneous route:
- Initial dose of 333 U/kg subcutaneously followed by 250 U/kg twice daily

- Unfractionated heparin: UFH acts by binding to antithrombin and catalyzing the inactivation of thrombin factor Xa and other clotting factors. Besides, it also binds with other plasma proteins resulting in unpredictable pharmacokinetic and pharmacodynamic properties which can lead to nonhemorrhagic side effects, such as heparin-induced thrombocytopenia (HIT) and osteoporosis. Since the anticoagulant effect of UFH can be rapidly reversed, it is the agent of choice for patients with PE who are at high risk of bleeding and those with severe renal failure. Various regimens of heparin therapy have been recommended **(Box 1)**.[51,52]

For the intravenous regimen, the bolus dose followed by continuous infusion is titrated to a target activated partial thromboplastin time (APTT) of 1.5–2.5 times of control (approximately 60–80 seconds). The first measurement of APTT should be performed 4–6 hours after starting treatment to ensure adequate anticoagulation and repeated 3 hours after every change of dose and subsequently at least daily after the target therapeutic dose is reached. Dosing based on a patient's body weight is preferable to a standard regimen since it causes fewer fluctuations in APTT and achieves a therapeutic level more quickly with a shorter warfarin overlap. Subcutaneous heparin does not require frequent monitoring, unlike with intravenous dosing schedule, and is found to be as safe and effective as weight-adjusted LMWH.[53]

The important complications associated with heparin include bleeding, immune-mediated platelet activation leading to HIT, and osteoporosis. Sometimes, dermatological side effects such as necrosis, alopecia, and hypersensitivity are encountered. HIT is usually seen 4–14 days after heparin therapy and can lead to major bleeding and thrombotic complications. It does not respond to platelet transfusion, and heparin must be stopped. HIT may respond to plasmapheresis. There are several advantages of LMWH over UFH **(Box 2)**.

- Fondaparinux: It is a synthetic polysaccharide with anti-Xa activity. It has been shown to be as effective as heparin and is not associated with HIT. Dosage is required once daily and is weight related (5 mg once daily for <50 kg, 7.5 mg once daily for 50–100 kg, and 10 mg for >100 kg). It is contraindicated in renal failure (creatinine clearance < 30 mL/min). It is a preferred anticoagulant in nonpregnant patients with diagnosed acute PE. Its efficacy and safety are similar to those of LMWH.[50]

Treatment with parenteral anticoagulants alone followed by vitamin K antagonists (VKAs) or direct oral anticoagulants (DOACs) is a safe and effective therapeutic option. Parenteral anticoagulants should be given for ≥5 days and until the adequate maintenance anticoagulation with warfarin is achieved, i.e., international normalized ratio (INR) between 2 and 3 for >24 hours.[54]

- *Long-term anticoagulants*: Long-term anticoagulation to prevent clot recurrence is most crucial in the first 3 months of the acute event when there is a higher chance of recurrent thrombosis.
  - Direct thrombin and factor Xa inhibitors: The agents of choice for long-term anticoagulation are direct thrombin and factor Xa inhibitors for patients. These can be administered in fixed doses unlike VKAs **(Table 4)** without the need for close monitoring with no significant food-drug interactions. The peak

BOX 2 Advantages of low-molecular-weight heparin over standard unfractionated heparin.

Advantages:
- More bioavailability
- More effective in prophylactic settings—orthopedic surgeries, acute stroke, spinal cord injury, etc.
- No monitoring required—facilitates OPD treatment
- Less heparin-induced thrombocytopenia
- Better quality of life
- Fewer nosocomial infections

Disadvantage:
- Dose adjustment in patients with renal insufficiency

TABLE 4: Recommended dosage of direct oral anticoagulants.

Drug	Doses in patients with normal renal function
Rivaroxaban	15 mg BD for 21 days followed by 20 mg OD
Dabigatran	150 mg BD
Edoxaban	60 mg OD
Apixaban	10 mg BD for 7 days followed by 5 mg BD (2.5 mg BD for extended treatment beyond 6 months)

efficacy of these agents is between 1 and 4 hours of ingestion, so bridging anticoagulation is not required when switching from the initial anticoagulation therapy. It is not the preferred choice in pregnancy and in patients with active malignancy and severe renal failure.

Rivaroxaban and apixaban can be given both as extended anticoagulation therapy with or without prior parenteral anticoagulant, but endoxaban and dabigatran require a 5-day course of parenteral anticoagulation prior to initiation. Doses need to adjust as per creatinine clearance in patients with renal insufficiency. The efficacy of these agents is also questionable in patients with obesity, especially in those with body weight > 120 kg or body mass index (BMI) ≥ 40 kg/m^2.[55] There are lower rates of bleeding in DOACs as compared to VKAs.[56] In case of bleeding, reversal agents such as andexanet alfa and idarucizumab have been developed and are being studied but are not easily available.

- Vitamin K antagonists: VKAs such as warfarin or acenocoumarin are preferred agents in those with severe renal dysfunction and in whom therapeutic anticoagulation needs to be monitored closely. However, it should be initiated once PE has been reliably confirmed. Oral anticoagulation with warfarin is initiated with dose between 2 and 10 mg, preferably on the first treatment day, along with parenteral anticoagulants with subsequent dosing based on the INR response. In patients with high bleeding risk, the initial dose can be started at 2–5 mg/day.

If warfarin is used, a starting dose of 5 mg is preferred to be given for the first 2 days and then subsequently adjusted until the INR is within the target therapeutic range (2–3; target 2.5) for 2 consecutive days. Parenteral anticoagulation can be discontinued once optimal INR is achieved. INR should be monitored after the initial two or three doses of oral anticoagulation therapy. For patients who are receiving a stable dose of oral anticoagulants, monitoring should be done at an interval of no longer than every 4 weeks.[57]

Duration of Anticoagulation Therapy

The duration of anticoagulant treatment in a particular patient should be ascertained depending on the risk–benefit assessment between the estimated risk of recurrence after treatment discontinuation and the risk of bleeding complications while on treatment. As a rule, for a patient presenting with the first episode of PE, anticoagulation should be given for at least 3 months. Discontinuing anticoagulation after 3 months is recommended in patients who have transient reversible risk factors. The duration may be extended to 6–12 months if the persistent risk factor is present and if there was significant hemodynamic instability in the index event. Recurrent embolism in the absence of a recurrent or new risk factor should be treated with long-term anticoagulation. In patients with persisting underlying risk factors, such as deficiency of antithrombin III, protein C or protein S, and antiphospholipid antibody syndrome, the anticoagulation is usually prolonged to several years, possibly lifelong. Extended duration of anticoagulation is also considered in patients with VTE who have no identifiable risk factor.[57]

Thrombolytic Therapy

- *Systemic thrombolysis*: Thrombolytic therapy is recommended as the first-line treatment for patients with massive PE (hemodynamic compromise/imminent cardiac arrest). It should be instituted at the earliest in such patients provided there are no contraindications pertaining to risk of bleeding **(Box 3)**.[58] The therapy helps not only in achieving rapid resolution of PE, but also in rapid hemodynamic improvement. It has no role in the management of hemodynamically stable patients, except perhaps in the subgroup of patients with submassive PE (RV dysfunction but normal systemic arterial pressure), in which there is some evidence for its efficacy.

BOX 3 Contraindications for thrombolytic therapy.

Absolute:
- Previous intracranial hemorrhage
- Ischemic stroke in preceding 3 months
- Cerebral vascular lesion or intracranial neoplasm
- Recent head or facial trauma in last 3 months
- Active bleeding or bleeding diathesis
- Aortic dissection

Relative:
- Age > 75 years
- Previous ischemic stroke > 3 months prior
- Oral anticoagulant therapy
- Pregnancy
- Noncompressible vascular punctures
- Traumatic resuscitation (>10 minutes)
- Recent internal bleeding within 2–4 weeks
- Refractory or uncontrolled hypertension or systolic blood pressure > 180 mm Hg or diastolic blood pressure > 110 mm Hg
- Pericarditis and pericardial fluid
- Allergic reaction to any thrombolytic agents
- Diabetic retinopathy
- Infective endocarditis
- Active peptic ulcer

Thrombolytic treatment is usually administered within the first 24 hours of diagnosis. Thrombolysis may be withheld if the patient is clinically improved in the first 24 hours. On the other hand, if the patient has clinical worsening (borderline BP, worsening oxygenation) thrombolysis may be done even if the patient does not fit into the definition of massive PE. Systemic thrombolytic therapy leads to hemodynamic improvement and mortality benefit with an additional risk of bleeding.[59] There are several different thrombolytic agents available for use **(Table 5)**.

Drawbacks of thrombolytic therapy include high cost, risk of severe and often fatal bleeding, and allergic reactions (specifically to streptokinase).

- *Catheter-directed thrombolysis*: Thrombolytic agents can be administered systemically or directly into the pulmonary artery via a pulmonary arterial catheter. Lower doses of thrombolytic agents can be administered, and hence the risk of bleeding is reduced. This procedure can be done alone or along with clot removal.

TABLE 5: Thrombolytic agents and dosage schedule.

Thrombolytic agent	Dosage schedule	Advantages/ Disadvantages
Streptokinase	250,000 IU as a loading dose over 30 minutes, followed by 100,000 IU/h over 12–24 hours *Accelerated regimen*: 1.5 million IU over 2 hours	• Cheap • Antigenic and hypotensive • Risk of allergic/ anaphylactoid reaction on re-exposure
Urokinase	4,400 IU/kg as a loading dose over 10 minutes, followed by 4,400 IU/kg/h over 12–24 hours *Accelerated regimen*: 3 million IU over 2 hours	• Fewer complications • Unlike streptokinase, no risk of anaphylactoid reaction
Alteplase (rtPA)	No need for loading dose, 50 mg over 2 hours	• Short infusion time • Not associated with allergic reactions or hypotension • Expensive
Reteplase	No need for loading dose, 10 U IV bolus—twice with 30-minute interval	• Short infusion time • Not associated with allergic reactions or hypotension • Expensive
Tenecteplase	No loading dose needed, 10,000 U bolus single dose in 5–10 seconds	• Short infusion time • Not associated with allergic reactions or hypotension • Expensive

The pulmonary arteries are accessed via internal jugular and femoral veins. This modality is usually used in patients who have hemodynamic instability despite systemic thrombolysis.

Embolectomy

Embolectomy is reserved for those groups of hemodynamically unstable patients in whom thrombolysis in contraindicated or with failed systemic thrombolysis. Another indication for surgical embolectomy is the presence of thrombus in transit, i.e., in the right atrium, right ventricle, or patent foramen ovale. Thrombus in the main pulmonary artery branches may also be removed. An experienced surgeon and cardiac bypass facilities are required for surgical embolectomy.

Inferior Vena Caval Filters

Inferior vena cava (IVC) filter devices placed in the IVC protect the pulmonary circulation from emboli. The routine use of IVC filters is not recommended because of complications and late sequelae, such as recurrent DVT episodes, recurrent PE, and IVC thrombosis. Filters are used when there is absolute contraindication to anticoagulation because of high-risk bleeding and recurrence of PE despite being on anticoagulation. Retrievable IVC filters should be used and must be removed when the contraindication to anticoagulation has been resolved. If anticoagulation is contraindicated in a patient with acute PE, IVC should be placed even if there is no evidence of lower limb DVT.

Extracorporeal Membrane Oxygenation

The venoarterial extracorporeal membrane oxygenation (VA ECMO) can be used as a sole therapy or as a bride therapy prior to definitive intervention. Its use especially extends to those patients who need thrombolysis but have contraindications.

RISK STRATIFICATION IN ACUTE PULMONARY EMBOLISM

Risk stratification is important before appropriate management is instituted. There has been increasing interest in identifying low-risk patients who could be offered outpatient treatment or a short hospital stay. The commonly used prognostic scores are the PESI (pulmonary embolism severity index) score or sPESI score, which is a simplified version **(Table 6)**.[60] Patients classified as classes I and II are at low risk of mortality and those from classes 3–5 are at high risk. The sensitivity of this prediction model is >98% and specificity >48%.

In addition to this score, the presence of hemodynamic instability and RV dysfunction are important risk factors which affect long-term outcomes and mortality. The presence of clinical, radiological, or physiological evidence

TABLE 6: Pulmonary embolism severity index.[60]

Clinical feature	Points	
Age	In years	
Male gender	10	
History of cancer	30	
Heart failure	10	
Chronic lung disease	10	
Pulse ≥ 110/min	20	
Systolic blood pressure < 100 mm Hg	30	
Respiratory rate ≥ 30/min	20	
Temperature < 36°C	20	
Altered mental status	60	
Arterial oxygen saturation < 90%	20	
Total points		
Risk stratification		**Total score**
Class I	Low risk	<66
Class II		66–85
Class III	High risk	86–105
Class IV		106–125
Class V		>125

BOX 4 Markers of right ventricular dysfunction.[62-64]

Echocardiography:

- Increased RV size
- Decreased RV function
- RV/LV ratio ≥ 1
- Tricuspid regurgitation with jet velocity > 2.8 m/s
- Abnormal septal wall motion
- McConnell's sign

CT features suggestive of RV dysfunction:

- RV/LV ratio ≥ 1
- Main pulmonary artery diameter ≥ 29 mm

RV biomarkers:

- NTproBNP ≥ 300 pg/mL
- Troponin I ≥ 0.09 ng/mL

(LV: left ventricular; NTproBNP: N-terminal prohormone of brain natriuretic peptide; RV: right ventricular)

of RV dysfunction **(Box 4)** and the presence of elevated biomarkers, i.e., N-terminal prohormone of brain natriuretic peptide (NTproBNP) or troponin I, are also markers of poor outcomes.[61-64] In addition, the presence of RV thrombus had a higher 14-day and 3-month mortality[65] and the presence of DVT was associated with an increase in all-cause and PE-specific mortality at 3 months.[66]

PULMONARY EMBOLISM RESPONSE TEAM

Pulmonary embolism response team (PERT) is a multidisciplinary rapid response team which aims to engage experts from relevant fields to simultaneously generate a thoughtful, coordinated, and comprehensive treatment plan for each PE patient. This team is especially designed to rapidly initiate life-saving strategies at the earliest such as systemic thrombolysis, catheter-directed thrombectomy/thrombolysis, or others which may influence the short- and long-term outcomes.

SUMMARY

Pulmonary embolism is a medical emergency with a varied clinical picture. Diagnosis of PE is frequently missed, and therefore a high degree of suspicion is required. A systematic algorithmic approach is required for diagnosis. Anticoagulation constitutes the key to management. Thrombolytic therapy is needed in the presence of massive embolism and/or hemodynamic instability. Early diagnosis and initiation of appropriate treatment are crucial to reduce the morbidity and mortality. Early clinical suspicion along with advances in the diagnostic and treatment strategies have helped in reducing the mortality. Surgical treatment options are now also available for massive and recurrent embolism.

REFERENCES

1. Bělohlávek J, Dytrych V, Linhart A. Pulmonary embolism, part I: Epidemiology, risk factors and risk stratification, pathophysiology, clinical presentation, diagnosis and nonthrombotic pulmonary embolism. Exp Clin Cardiol. 2013;18(2):129-38.
2. Hendriksen JMT, Geersing GJ, Lucassen WAM, et al. Diagnostic prediction models for suspected pulmonary embolism: systematic review and independent external validation in primary care. BMJ. 2015;351:h4438.
3. Lilienfeld DE. Decreasing mortality from pulmonary embolism in the United States, 1979–1996. Int J Epidemiol. 2000;29(3): 465-9.
4. Huang W, Goldberg RJ, Anderson FA, et al. Secular trends in occurrence of acute venous thromboembolism: the Worcester VTE study (1985-2009). Am J Med. 2014;127(9):829-39.e5.
5. Naess IA, Christiansen SC, Romundstad P, et al. Incidence and mortality of venous thrombosis: a population-based study. J Thromb Haemost. 2007;5(4):692-9.
6. Silverstein MD, Heit JA, Mohr DN, et al. Trends in the incidence of deep vein thrombosis and pulmonary embolism: a 25-year population-based study. Arch Intern Med. 1998;158(6): 585-93.

7. Andersson T, Söderberg S. Incidence of acute pulmonary embolism, related comorbidities and survival; analysis of a Swedish national cohort. BMC Cardiovasc Disord. 2017;17(1): 155.
8. Stein PD, Kayali F, Olson RE. Estimated case fatality rate of pulmonary embolism, 1979 to 1998. Am J Cardiol. 2004;93(9): 1197-9.
9. Smith SB, Geske JB, Kathuria P, et al. Analysis of National Trends in Admissions for Pulmonary Embolism. Chest. 2016;150(1): 35-45.
10. Stein PD, Terrin ML, Hales CA, et al. Clinical, laboratory, roentgenographic, and electrocardiographic findings in patients with acute pulmonary embolism and no pre-existing cardiac or pulmonary disease. Chest. 1991;100(3):598-603.
11. Gohil R, Peck G, Sharma P. The genetics of venous thromboembolism. A meta-analysis involving approximately 120,000 cases and 180,000 controls. Thromb Haemost. 2009;102(2): 360-70.
12. Sørensen HT, Mellemkjær L, Olsen JH, et al. Prognosis of Cancers Associated with Venous Thromboembolism. N Engl J Med. 2000;343(25):1846-50.
13. Heit JA, O'Fallon WM, Petterson TM, et al. Relative impact of risk factors for deep vein thrombosis and pulmonary embolism: a population-based study. Arch Intern Med. 2002;162(11): 1245-8.
14. Bloemenkamp KW, Rosendaal FR, Helmerhorst FM, et al. Higher risk of venous thrombosis during early use of oral contraceptives in women with inherited clotting defects. Arch Intern Med. 2000;160(1):49-52.
15. Miller J, Chan BKS, Nelson HD. Postmenopausal estrogen replacement and risk for venous thromboembolism: a systematic review and meta-analysis for the U.S. Preventive Services Task Force. Ann Intern Med. 2002;136(9):680-90.
16. Pomp ER, Lenselink AM, Rosendaal FR, et al. Pregnancy, the postpartum period and prothrombotic defects: risk of venous thrombosis in the MEGA study. J Thromb Haemost. 2008; 6(4):632-7.
17. Ageno W, Becattini C, Brighton T, et al. Cardiovascular risk factors and venous thromboembolism: a meta-analysis. Circulation. 2008;117(1):93-102.
18. Severinsen MT, Overvad K, Johnsen SP, et al. Genetic susceptibility, smoking, obesity and risk of venous thromboembolism. Br J Haematol. 2010;149(2):273-9.
19. Pomp ER, le Cessie S, Rosendaal FR, et al. Risk of venous thrombosis: obesity and its joint effect with oral contraceptive use and prothrombotic mutations. Br J Haematol. 2007; 139(2):289-96.
20. Pomp ER, Rosendaal FR, Doggen CJM. Smoking increases the risk of venous thrombosis and acts synergistically with oral contraceptive use. Am J Hematol. 2008;83(2):97-102.
21. Liesching T, O'Brien A. Significance of a syncopal event. Pulmonary embolism. Postgrad Med. 2002;111(1):19-20.
22. Castelli R, Tarsia P, Tantardini C, et al. Syncope in patients with pulmonary embolism: comparison between patients with syncope as the presenting symptom of pulmonary embolism and patients with pulmonary embolism without syncope. Vasc Med. 2003;8(4):257-61.
23. Johnson JC, Flowers NC, Horan LG. Unexplained Atrial Flutter: A Frequent Herald of Pulmonary Embolism. Chest. 1971;60(1): 29-34.
24. Stein PD, Beemath A, Matta F, et al. Clinical characteristics of patients with acute pulmonary embolism: data from PIOPED II. Am J Med. 2007;120(10):871-9.
25. Courtney DM, Kline JA. Prospective use of a clinical decision rule to identify pulmonary embolism as likely cause of outpatient cardiac arrest. Resuscitation. 2005;65(1):57-64.
26. Courtney DM, Sasser HC, Pincus CL, et al. Pulseless electrical activity with witnessed arrest as a predictor of sudden death from massive pulmonary embolism in outpatients. Resuscitation. 2001;49(3):265-72.
27. Elliott CG, Goldhaber SZ, Visani L, et al. Chest radiographs in acute pulmonary embolism. Results from the International Cooperative Pulmonary Embolism Registry. Chest. 2000; 118(1):33-8.
28. Worsley DF, Alavi A, Aronchick JM, et al. Chest radiographic findings in patients with acute pulmonary embolism: observations from the PIOPED Study. Radiology. 1993;189(1): 133-6.
29. Shopp JD, Stewart LK, Emmett TW, et al. Findings From 12-lead Electrocardiography That Predict Circulatory Shock From Pulmonary Embolism: Systematic Review and Meta-Analysis. Acad Emerg Med. 2015;22(10):1127-37.
30. Miron MJ, Perrier A, Bounameaux H, et al. Contribution of noninvasive evaluation to the diagnosis of pulmonary embolism in hospitalized patients. Eur Respir J. 1999;13(6):1365-70.
31. Ghirardini G, Battioni M, Bertellini C, et al. D-dimer after delivery in uncomplicated pregnancies. Clin Exp Obstet Gynecol. 1999; 26(3-4):211-2.
32. Le Gal G, Righini M, Roy PM, et al. Value of D-dimer testing for the exclusion of pulmonary embolism in patients with previous venous thromboembolism. Arch Intern Med. 2006;166(2): 176-80.
33. Stein PD, Hull RD, Patel KC, et al. D-dimer for the exclusion of acute venous thrombosis and pulmonary embolism: a systematic review. Ann Intern Med. 2004;140(8):589-602.
34. Geersing GJ, Janssen KJM, Oudega R, et al. Excluding venous thromboembolism using point of care D-dimer tests in outpatients: a diagnostic meta-analysis. BMJ. 2009;339:b2990.
35. Righini M, Van Es J, Den Exter PL, et al. Age-adjusted D-dimer cutoff levels to rule out pulmonary embolism: the ADJUST-PE study. JAMA. 2014;311(11):1117-24.
36. Scridon T, Scridon C, Skali H, et al. Prognostic Significance of Troponin Elevation and Right Ventricular Enlargement in Acute Pulmonary Embolism. Am J Cardiol. 2005;96(2):303-5.
37. Vuilleumier N, Perrier A, Sanchez JC, et al. Cardiac biomarkers levels predict pulmonary embolism extent on chest computed tomography and prognosis in non-massive pulmonary embolism. Thromb Haemost; 2009;101(6):1176-8.
38. Perrier A, Bounameaux H. Ultrasonography of leg veins in patients suspected of having pulmonary embolism. Ann Intern Med. 1998;128(3):243; author reply 244-5.
39. Kearon C, Ginsberg JS, Hirsh J. The role of venous ultrasonography in the diagnosis of suspected deep venous thrombosis and pulmonary embolism. Ann Intern Med. 1998;129(12): 1044-9.
40. Torbicki A, Perrier A, Konstantinides S, et al. Guidelines on the diagnosis and management of acute pulmonary embolism: the Task Force for the Diagnosis and Management of Acute Pulmonary Embolism of the European Society of Cardiology (ESC). Eur Heart J. 2008;29(18):2276-315.

41. PIOPED Investigators. Value of the ventilation/perfusion scan in acute pulmonary embolism. Results of the prospective investigation of pulmonary embolism diagnosis (PIOPED). JAMA. 1990;263(20):2753-9.
42. Teigen CL, Maus TP, Sheedy PF, et al. Pulmonary embolism: diagnosis with contrast-enhanced electron-beam CT and comparison with pulmonary angiography. Radiology. 1995;194(2):313-9.
43. Remy-Jardin M, Remy J, Deschildre F, et al. Diagnosis of pulmonary embolism with spiral CT: comparison with pulmonary angiography and scintigraphy. Radiology. 1996;200(3):699-706.
44. Stein PD, Fowler SE, Goodman LR, et al. Multidetector computed tomography for acute pulmonary embolism. N Engl J Med. 2006;354(22):2317-27.
45. Gupta S, Gupta BMM. Acute pulmonary embolism advances in treatment. J Assoc Physicians India. 2008;56:185-91.
46. Hofmann LV, Lee DS, Gupta A, et al. Safety and hemodynamic effects of pulmonary angiography in patients with pulmonary hypertension: 10-year single-center experience. AJR Am J Roentgenol. 2004;183(3):779-86.
47. Wells PS, Anderson DR, Rodger M, et al. Derivation of a simple clinical model to categorize patients probability of pulmonary embolism: increasing the models utility with the SimpliRED D-dimer. Thromb Haemost. 2000;83(3):416-20.
48. Lucassen W, Geersing GJ, Erkens PMG, et al. Clinical decision rules for excluding pulmonary embolism: a meta-analysis. Ann Intern Med. 2011;155(7):448-60.
49. Klok FA, Mos ICM, Nijkeuter M, et al. Simplification of the revised Geneva score for assessing clinical probability of pulmonary embolism. Arch Intern Med. 2008;168(19):2131-6.
50. Büller HR, Davidson BL, Decousus H, et al. Fondaparinux or enoxaparin for the initial treatment of symptomatic deep venous thrombosis: a randomized trial. Ann Intern Med. 2004;140(11):867-73.
51. Cruickshank MK, Levine MN, Hirsh J, et al. A standard heparin nomogram for the management of heparin therapy. Arch Intern Med. 1991;151(2):333-7.
52. Raschke RA, Reilly BM, Guidry JR, et al. The weight-based heparin dosing nomogram compared with a "standard care" nomogram. A randomized controlled trial. Ann Intern Med. 1993;119(9):874-81.
53. Kearon C, Ginsberg JS, Julian JA, et al. Comparison of fixed-dose weight-adjusted unfractionated heparin and low-molecular-weight heparin for acute treatment of venous thromboembolism. JAMA. 2006;296(8):935-42.
54. Kearon C, Kahn SR, Agnelli G, et al. Antithrombotic therapy for venous thromboembolic disease: American College of Chest Physicians Evidence-Based Clinical Practice Guidelines (8th Edition). Chest. 2008;133(6 Suppl):454S-545S.
55. Martin KA, Beyer-Westendorf J, Davidson BL, et al. Use of direct oral anticoagulants in patients with obesity for treatment and prevention of venous thromboembolism: Updated communication from the ISTH SSC Subcommittee on Control of Anticoagulation. J Thromb Haemost. 2021;19(8):1874-82.
56. Wang X, Ma Y, Hui X, et al. Oral direct thrombin inhibitors or oral factor Xa inhibitors versus conventional anticoagulants for the treatment of deep vein thrombosis. Cochrane Database Syst Rev. 2023;4(4):CD010956.
57. Meyer G, Becattini C, Geersing GJ, et al. 2019 ESC Guidelines for the diagnosis and management of acute pulmonary embolism developed in collaboration with the European Respiratory Society (ERS). 2020;41(4):543-603.
58. Kearon C, Akl EA, Comerota AJ, et al. Antithrombotic therapy for VTE disease: Antithrombotic Therapy and Prevention of Thrombosis, 9th ed: American College of Chest Physicians Evidence-Based Clinical Practice Guidelines. Chest. 2012;141(2 Suppl):e419S-96S.
59. Chatterjee S, Chakraborty A, Weinberg I, et al. Thrombolysis for pulmonary embolism and risk of all-cause mortality, major bleeding, and intracranial hemorrhage: a meta-analysis. JAMA 2014;311(23):2414-21.
60. Aujesky D, Obrosky DS, Stone RA, et al. Derivation and validation of a prognostic model for pulmonary embolism. Am J Respir Crit Care Med. 2005;172(8):1041-6.
61. ten Wolde M, Söhne M, Quak E, et al. Prognostic value of echocardiographically assessed right ventricular dysfunction in patients with pulmonary embolism. Arch Intern Med. 2004;164(15):1685-9.
62. Kurnicka K, Lichodziejewska B, Goliszek S, et al. Echocardiographic Pattern of Acute Pulmonary Embolism: Analysis of 511 Consecutive Patients. J Am Soc Echocardiogr. 2016;29(9):907-13.
63. Osman AM, Abdeldayem EH. Value of CT pulmonary angiography to predict short-term outcome in patient with pulmonary embolism. Int J Cardiovasc Imaging. 2018;34(6):975-83.
64. Coutance G, Cauderlier E, Ehtisham J, et al. The prognostic value of markers of right ventricular dysfunction in pulmonary embolism: a meta-analysis. Crit Care. 2011;15(2):R103.
65. Torbicki A, Galié N, Covezzoli A, et al. Right heart thrombi in pulmonary embolism: results from the International Cooperative Pulmonary Embolism Registry. J Am Coll Cardiol. 2003;41(12):2245-51.
66. Jiménez D, Aujesky D, Díaz G, et al. Prognostic significance of deep vein thrombosis in patients presenting with acute symptomatic pulmonary embolism. Am J Respir Crit Care Med. 2010;181(9):983-91.

Pulmonary Arteriovenous Malformations

CHAPTER 125

Matthew Kheir, Erica Altschul, Joseph Parambil

INTRODUCTION

Pulmonary arteriovenous malformations (PAVMs) are abnormal connections between the pulmonary arteries and veins within the lung vasculature. These abnormal vascular structures bypass the normal lung capillary bed, leading to various clinical manifestations and potential complications. In this chapter, we will explore the etiology, pathophysiology, clinical and radiographic features, diagnosis, and management of PAVMs.

SIGNIFICANCE

Pulmonary arteriovenous malformations hold significant medical importance due to their potential impact on pulmonary circulation and overall health. These abnormal connections can disrupt normal blood flow, resulting in right-to-left shunting of deoxygenated blood directly into the systemic circulation. This condition can lead to hypoxemia, resulting in a variety of symptoms such as shortness of breath, fatigue, and cyanosis depending on the degree of blood shunting.[1] Furthermore, PAVMs can increase the risk of complications such as stroke, brain abscesses, and other systemic infections.[2] Early detection and proper management of PAVMs are crucial, even in the absence of symptoms, to prevent these potential complications and to optimize patients' overall health and quality of life.

ETIOLOGY

The etiology of PAVMs is multifactorial and can be either congenital or acquired. While the exact causes of PAVMs are not fully understood, several factors have been identified as potential contributors.

Congenital Pulmonary Arteriovenous Malformations

The majority of cases are congenital (up to 90%) and are associated with hereditary hemorrhagic telangiectasia (HHT), also known as Osler-Weber-Rendu syndrome.[3] HHT is an autosomal-dominant genetic disorder characterized by abnormal blood vessel formations throughout the body leading to telangiectasias and arteriovenous malformations (AVMs) in various organs, including the lungs. Mutations in genes such as *ENG* (endoglin) and *ACVRL1* (activin receptor-like kinase 1) have been associated with HHT and PAVMs.[4] In a study involving 199 patients with HHT, it was found that 58% of patients with *ENG* mutations had PAVMs visible on computed tomography (CT), whereas only 18% of patients with mutations in *ACVRL1/ALK1* had CT-evident PAVMs ($p < 0.001$).[5] On the other hand, pulmonary arterial hypertension and pulmonary venous hypertension are more frequently observed in patients with mutations in the *ACVRL1* gene.[6] Pulmonary hypertension is clinically significant in <5% of patients with HHT.[7]

Genetic factors besides HHT-related genetic mutations may contribute to the development of PAVMs. Studies have identified mutations in genes involved in angiogenesis and vascular development, such as *BMPR2* (bone morphogenetic protein receptor type 2) and *SMAD4* (mothers against decapentaplegic homolog 4), in individuals with PAVMs.[8] These mutations may disrupt normal vascular development and contribute to the formation of abnormal connections between the pulmonary arteries and veins. Interestingly, *BMPR2* gene mutations are also significantly associated with pulmonary hypertension.

Acquired Pulmonary Arteriovenous Malformations

Acquired PAVMs, on the other hand, can occur due to underlying conditions such as liver cirrhosis, penetrating chest trauma, and prior thoracic surgery.[9] Other less common causes include schistosomiasis, tuberculosis, Fanconi's syndrome, or as a complication after congenital heart disease surgical generation of a cavo-pulmonary shunt.[10] There are several case reports of other associations which are very low in frequency, while the remainder of the cases are deemed idiopathic.

EPIDEMIOLOGY

General Population

Pulmonary arteriovenous malformations are relatively rare vascular anomalies with a prevalence estimated to be around 1 in 2,600 to 1 in 14,000 individuals.[11] The exact incidence and prevalence of PAVMs may vary among different populations due to differences in genetic predisposition and diagnostic practices.

The condition can occur at any age, from infancy to late adulthood, but most commonly presents in individuals between the ages of 40 and 60 years.[12] There is a slight gender predilection, with PAVMs affecting females more frequently than males.[13]

In terms of geographic distribution, PAVMs have been reported worldwide, without any specific geographical clustering. The condition is observed across different ethnicities and races, suggesting a universal occurrence rather than a specific ethnic or racial association.[14]

The prevalence of PAVMs is notably higher in individuals with HHT. It is estimated that 15–50% of individuals with HHT have PAVMs. Among patients with PAVMs, up to 70–90% may have an underlying diagnosis of HHT.[15] The distribution of PAVMs in patients with HHT demonstrates a relatively equal occurrence between sexes with a slight increase in females (56% of cases).[16] These malformations tend to be more commonly multiple rather than solitary, and they are generally distributed evenly throughout the lungs without a specific predilection for any particular region.

PATHOLOGY

Pathophysiology

In a normal pulmonary circulation, deoxygenated blood from the right side of the heart flows into the lungs via the pulmonary artery. Within the lungs, the pulmonary arteries branch into smaller vessels, eventually reaching the capillary bed surrounding the alveoli, where gas exchange occurs. Oxygenated blood then returns to the left side of the heart through the pulmonary veins. In PAVMs, there is a direct connection between the pulmonary arteries and veins, bypassing the capillary bed. This results in a right-to-left shunt, leading to the mixing of deoxygenated blood with oxygenated blood and subsequent arterial desaturation.

Pulmonary arteriovenous malformations are classified as either simple or complex. Simple PAVMs are perfused by arteries arising from a single subsegmental artery and comprise up to 95% of cases of PAVM.[17] Complex PAVMs are perfused by more than one subsegmental artery and make up for the remaining 5% of cases. Small microvascular PAVMs are most commonly of the complex type. In addition, approximately 95% of cases of PAVMs are supplied by pulmonary arteries and 5% by systemic arteries (e.g., aorta, bronchial artery, or intercostal arteries).[18]

Pathogenesis

The exact pathogenesis is unknown; however, it is thought that PAVMs occur when the vascular septa, which normally separate the arterial and venous plexus during fetal development, are not fully resorbed.[10] As a result, the anastomosis between the arterial and the venous systems remains incomplete, leading to the formation of pulmonary AVMs.

The appearance of a PAVM may be a dilated and tortuous direct artery to vein anastomosis or a large, thin-walled, single or multiple vascular sac. Sometimes, it may appear as a plexiform-like mass of vascular channels as well.[19]

From a histological perspective, PAVMs typically exhibit thin walls, composed of a single layer of endothelium along with varying amounts of connective tissue stroma.[20] In some cases, there may be instances of calcification and mural thrombosis observed within the malformations.

CLINICAL MANIFESTATIONS

The clinical presentation of PAVMs can vary widely. Many individuals with small or asymptomatic PAVMs may remain undiagnosed until later in life. However, larger or multiple PAVMs can lead to significant clinical manifestations. Approximately 40% of patients with PAVMs present with symptoms,[21,22] with patients developing PAVM-related symptoms between the ages of 40 and 60 years.[12] The most common symptoms include: dyspnea, chest pain, cough, cyanosis, hemoptysis, platypnea and orthodeoxia, and clubbing. The most common symptoms are epistaxis (29–79%) followed by dyspnea (13–56%) and hemoptysis (7–30%).[2,21,22]

Evaluation for Hereditary Hemorrhagic Telangiectasia

In patients with PAVMS who have not been previously diagnosed with HHT, it is imperative to evaluate for clinical evidence of HHT, including patient signs and symptoms as well as a family history of typical manifestations. Most common symptoms include epistaxis, mucocutaneous telangiectasis, and symptoms arising from AVMs (e.g., gastrointestinal bleeding). HHT is typically diagnosed clinically based on the Second International Guidelines on HHT using the Curaçao criteria and/or identifying specific *HHT* genes **(Table 1)**.[23]

COMPLICATIONS OF PULMONARY ARTERIOVENOUS MALFORMATION

Notable Pulmonary Arteriovenous Malformations Complications

In patients with PAVMs, neurologic complications are not infrequent and can be present in up to 41% of patients.[6]

TABLE 1: Curaçao criteria for diagnosing HHT.

Criterion	Description	Diagnosis method
Epistaxis	Spontaneous or recurrent	Clinical
Telangiectasias	Multiple at characteristic sites: Lips, oral cavity, nose, and fingers	Skin examination
Visceral AVMs	Pulmonary, cerebral, spinal, hepatic, and gastrointestinal	Imaging
Family history	A first-degree relative with HHT according to these criteria	Clinical
HHT diagnosis		
Definite	3 or more criteria present	
Possible	2 criteria present	
Unlikely	1 or less criteria present	

(AVMs: arteriovenous malformations; HHT: hereditary hemorrhagic telangiectasias)

Most commonly, patients' neurologic complications include stroke and brain abscesses. Other neurologic complications associated with PAVMs include headaches, migraines, dizziness, syncope, diplopia, tinnitus, and seizures.[24]

Typically, a hemothorax occurs when a subpleural PAVM ruptures while hemoptysis is more likely to be due to rupture of a parenchymal PAVM or an endobronchial telangiectasia. Hemothorax, hemoptysis, and rarely massive hemoptysis can occur between 8 and 13% and can be life-threatening.[25,26]

Patients with PAVMs can also have secondary polycythemia or anemia, which is seen in approximately 25% and 17% of patients, respectively, based on an old case series.[26] Polycythemia is primarily attributed to chronic hypoxemia. Conversely, anemia is caused by blood loss resulting from complications associated with HHT patients (e.g., epistaxis and gastrointestinal bleeding).

Pulmonary hypertension can be seen in patients with PAVM. Typically, the etiology of the pulmonary hypertension is not directly attributable to PAVMs. Patients with HHT may have hepatic AVMs that lead to portopulmonary hypertension [PoPAH; World Health Organization (WHO) group I pulmonary hypertension]. Also due to the multiple AVMs, these patients may develop high output cardiac failure (WHO group II pulmonary hypertension) from significant shunting. A subset of HHT patients with mutations in the *ALK-1* (*HHT2*) gene can develop heritable pulmonary arterial hypertension.[27] These patients usually require genetic testing to differentiate from idiopathic PAH unless there is already confirmed evidence of hereditary PAH from prior genetic testing of family members. Of note, pulmonary hypertension may result following definitive treatment (embolization or surgical resection) of large or multiple PAVMs, although data is conflicting.[28-30] The theory is that the normal forward pulmonary arterial flow following PAVM treatment is redirected backward to residual pulmonary vasculature, thereby increasing pressure within the pulmonary artery, which is conceptually similar to that of a pulmonary embolism causing increased pulmonary hypertension. The normal pulmonary arteries are not accustomed to such increases in pulmonary blood flow, and this can lead to a significant rise in pulmonary artery pressures.

Miscellaneous Pulmonary Arteriovenous Malformations Complications

Additional complications arising from PAVMs include other types of non-neurologic paradoxical embolization (systemic thrombi, myocardial infarction, infectious endocarditis, etc.), congestive heart failure, and pregnancy-related deaths.[11] These complications are largely due to the paradoxical embolization of substances including but not limited to thrombi, air, fat, infectious vegetations, tumor, and amniotic fluid.

DIAGNOSTIC WORKUP

The diagnosis of PAVMs involves a combination of clinical evaluation, imaging studies, and confirmatory tests. Initial screening may include pulse oximetry to detect arterial desaturation. Further investigations may include the following testing modalities.

Transthoracic Contrast Echocardiography

The initial screening test of choice for patients with suspected PAVMs is a transthoracic contrast echocardiography (TTCE; referred to colloquially as "TTE bubble study") to evaluate for the presence and severity of a right-to-left shunt. The TTCE study involves injecting acoustically active particles (contrast), such as agitated saline, intravenously with the goal of producing opacification of the blood pool and microcirculation. The contrast, agitated saline, is injected into a peripheral vein while visualizing a four-chamber view on TTE. The bubbles are immediately seen in the right atrium and ventricle after injection. Typically, the contrast should not be seen on the left-sided chambers due to the microbubbles being filtered at the level of the pulmonary capillaries. When contrast is seen in the left-sided chambers, a right-to-left shunt is identified. TTCE has a sensitivity of 93–100% based on studies.[9,21,31] One study mentioned that TTCE may be too sensitive and may detect clinically insignificant PAVMs even after successful embolization of all visible PAVMs.[32]

The timing and the number of microbubbles seen in the left ventricle give guidance on the location of the shunt (i.e., intracardiac vs. extracardiac shunts) and the degree of

SECTION 11: DISORDERS OF PULMONARY CIRCULATION

severity of the shunt. In general, if microbubbles are seen in less than one cardiac cycle, then this is typically indicative of an intracardiac shunt, also known as "early bubbles". Intrapulmonary shunts are suspected when microbubbles are seen within four to eight cardiac cycles, known as "late bubbles".[33]

The degree, or grading, of the shunt is dependent on the quantity of bubbles seen in the left ventricle.[31] No appearance of bubbles implies no shunt and is classified as grade 0. When less than 30 bubbles are observed in the left ventricle, this is classified as a grade 1 shunt. Grade 1 shunts can be observed without further studies if there is low suspicion for PAVM. If there is a high suspicion for PAVM, a follow-up CT chest is recommended. If there are more than 30 bubbles (Grade 2 shunt: 30–100 bubbles; Grade 3 shunt: more than 100 bubbles), then a CT chest is recommended as the next step to evaluate for a PAVM.

100% Oxygen Shunt Fraction Measurement

The degree of right-to-left shunting can be estimated through a shunt fraction measurement. The normal amount of cardiac output that is shunted from left to right is considered to be <5%.[34] The shunt fraction measurement is performed by breathing 100% oxygen for 15–20 minutes and then measuring PaO_2 and SaO_2 from arterial blood gas. Individuals with shunt fractions > 5% warrant further investigation. In a group of 12 patients with PAVMs, using the 100% oxygen method with a shunt fraction > 5% demonstrated a sensitivity of 87.5% and a specificity of 71.4% of diagnosing PAVMs.[35] This method appears to be sensitive, but less specific in the diagnosis of PAVMs, as extrapulmonary shunts would have elevated shunt fractions as well.

Radionuclide Perfusion Scanning

The role of radionuclide perfusion scanning is limited as it only is able to identify the presence of any right-to-left shunt and is typically recommended for circumstances in which TTCE or 100% oxygen shunt fraction measurements are not available.[36] Essentially, technetium-99m (99mTc) labeled albumin is administered intravenously and in healthy individuals these particles are filtered by pulmonary capillaries. In patients with right-to-left shunts (e.g., intrapulmonary or intracardiac shunts), these particles are delivered systemically and are trapped in the brain and kidneys. The shunt fraction is determined by measuring the renal uptake as a percentage of the total administered dose. The disadvantages of this test are that it is unable to distinguish between intrapulmonary and intracardiac shunts as well as that it is an expensive test that is not readily available at most medical centers.

Computed Tomography of the Chest

CT Appearance of Pulmonary Arteriovenous Malformations

A CT with contrast enhancement of the chest is the test of choice for confirming and evaluating the location and anatomy of the PAVMs.[9-11,26,31] This is the most sensitive imaging modality to detecting PAVMs and can provide detailed information about the location, size, and number of PAVMs. As mentioned previously, CT chest is typically performed following a grade 2 or 3 shunt noted on TTCE or in patients with a grade 1 shunt and a high suspicion for PAVM. Enhancement with contrast shows the PAVM sac with both the feeding artery and draining veins **(Figs. 1A and B)**. If the feeding artery diameter (FAD) of the PAVM is

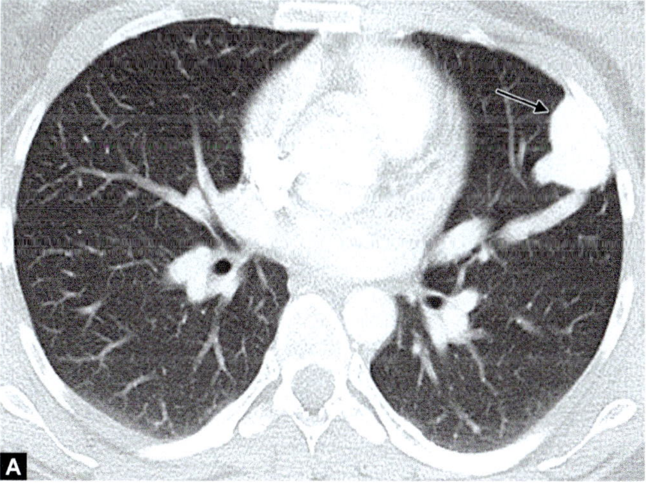

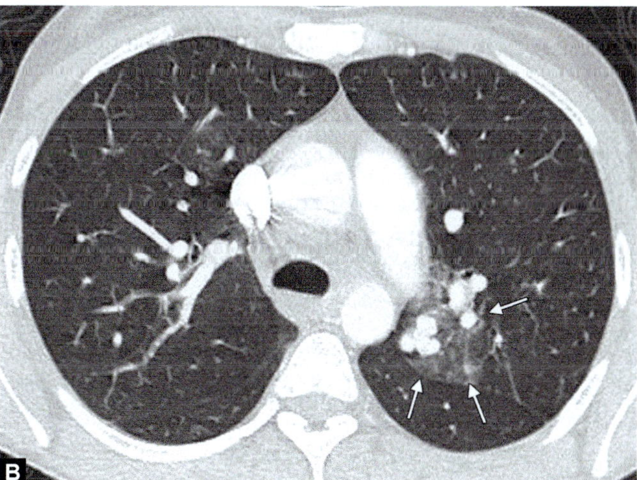

FIGS. 1A AND B: PAVMs on CTA chest. (A) A 35-year-old pregnant female presenting with pleuritic chest pain due to growing PAVM in the left upper lobe (black arrow); (B) A 26-year-old with HHT presenting with hemoptysis due to bleeding (ground-glass changes) from a pulmonary AVM (white arrows).

(CTA: computed tomography angiography; HHT: hereditary hemorrhagic telangiectasia; PAVMs: pulmonary arteriovenous malformations)

≥2–3 mm, then the patient should be referred to pulmonary angiography for definitive diagnosis and characterization of the PAVM as well as potential embolotherapy.[17]

If, however, the FAD < 2 mm, and the patient is asymptomatic, then pulmonary angiography may be deferred. Pulmonary angiography can be later performed when the patient develops symptoms (e.g., stroke, brain abscess). It can also be performed when the shunt worsens or FAD enlarges with annual observation, which may prompt a repeat TTCE and/or CT chest. The interval of repeating these studies is generally every 3–5 years unless the patient becomes symptomatic.[9,37]

Vascular and Nonvascular Mimickers of Pulmonary Arteriovenous Malformations

Occasionally, CT chest can demonstrate lesions that appear like PAVMs, which can be categorized as either a vascular or a nonvascular mimic. Vascular mimics include pulmonary artery pseudoaneurysms, hepatopulmonary vessels, arterial collaterals, venovenous collaterals, pulmonary vein varices, fibrosing mediastinitis, meandering pulmonary veins, and Sheehan vessels. Likewise, there can be nonvascular mimics, which include pulmonary hamartomas, primary lung cancer, metastasis, carcinoid tumor, granulomas, ground-glass opacities, atelectasis, bronchoceles, and mucoceles.[38] Examples of these mimics are illustrated in **Figures 2 to 4**.

Pulmonary Angiography

The gold standard for the diagnosis of PAVM is pulmonary angiography. Although it is not as sensitive at detecting all PAVMs as a CT scan, it can better characterize the PAVM vascular anatomy with contrast.[9,39] Contrast is typically injected into the feeding artery or a distal pulmonary arterial branch to determine if the lesion is appropriate for embolotherapy. It is also injected into the main left and right pulmonary arteries to detect other unsuspected lesions that may be suitable for embolotherapy.

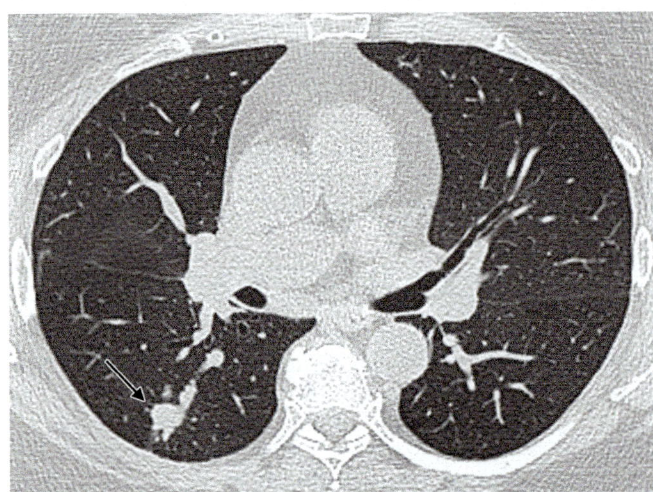

FIG. 3: Bronchocele, a nonvascular mimic of PAVM. A 75-year-old presenting with cough and on CT a tubular nodule is noted raising concerns for PAVM but did not show feeding or draining vessels on CT chest with contrast and was found to be a bronchocele (blue arrow).

(PAVM: pulmonary arteriovenous malformation)

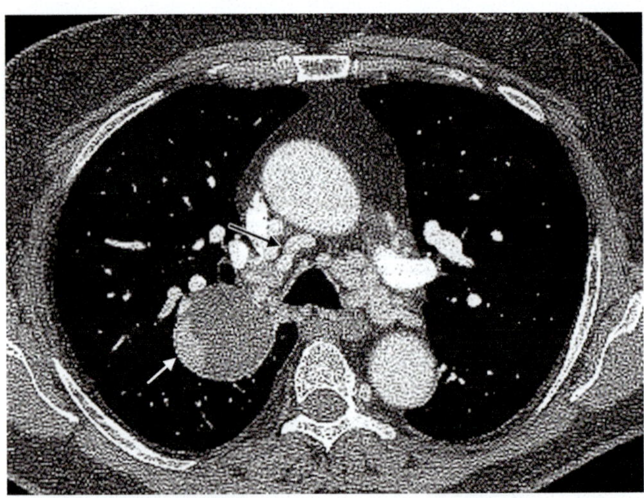

FIG. 2: Hemangioma, a vascular mimic of PAVM. A 69-year-old presenting with chest pain and CT shows a racemose hemangioma (white arrow) with feeding arteries arising (black arrow) from the aorta and draining into the right upper lobe pulmonary vein.

(PAVM: pulmonary arteriovenous malformation)

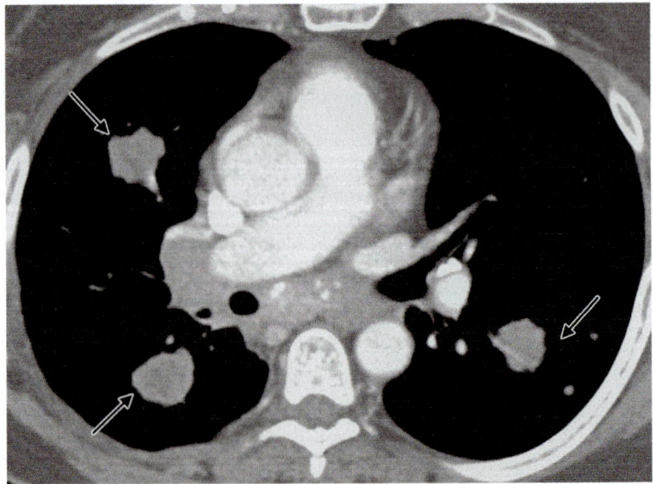

FIG. 4: Metastatic nodules, a nonvascular mimic of PAVM. A 67-year-old with renal cell cancer presenting with hemoptysis and found to have vascular enhancing nodules in the lungs concerning for PAVM but turned out to be metastatic deposits (black arrows).

(PAVM: pulmonary arteriovenous malformation)

Alternative Diagnostic Modalities

While CT remains the image modality of choice, contrast-enhanced MR angiography may be able to demonstrate PAVMs and may be considered in patients with a significant allergy to iodine contrast. MR angiography has a sensitivity of 92% and specificity between 62 and 97%, where CT was considered the reference standard.[40] Chest radiography is unable to detect small PAVMs but may be able to detect larger lesions or demonstrate typical radiographic findings of pulmonary hypertension. Basic laboratory workup includes complete blood count, comprehensive metabolic panel, and an arterial blood gas. It is recommended to perform pulmonary function tests. Typically, these patients will have a normal spirometry with mildly elevated diffusion capacity and an elevated resting minute ventilation.[41]

On a separate note, recommendations for screening for extrapulmonary AVMs are discussed in the 2020 International Guidelines on HHT.[42] These guidelines offer recommendations for screening cerebral AVMs, hepatic AVMs, and family members and make additional recommendations for special scenarios (anticoagulation, air travel, and more).

TREATMENT AND MANAGEMENT

Embolotherapy Candidates

Potential candidates for embolotherapy include patients with symptomatic PAVMs, abnormal FADs, and individuals who can tolerate the procedure.[43] As mentioned in the prior sections, symptomatic PAVMs are those individuals with complications [e.g., cerebrovascular accident (CVA), cerebral abscess, hemoptysis, etc.]. FAD $\geq$ 2–3 mm and should be referred for pulmonary angiography for definite treatment with embolotherapy regardless of the presence of symptoms.[17] In patients who are symptomatic with FAD < 2 mm, pulmonary angiography with embolotherapy is also recommended. The risk for developing complications for patients with FAD < 2 mm increases when individuals have grade 3 shunts noted on TTCE or multiple PAVMs noted on CT chest.[11] Lastly, patients with FAD < 2 mm without symptoms can be observed at least annually.[2,17,44]

Embolotherapy Overview

Embolotherapy, usually performed by an interventional radiologist, is done under fluoroscopy with the patient typically under conscious sedation. Contrast is first injected to confirm and characterize the feeding arteries in the PAVMs. Once confirmed, PAVMs are treated with catheter-directed placement of embolic material, which is usually either vascular plugs (detachable nitinol vascular plugs) or coils (metallic coils usually made of platinum).[45] Multiple PAVMs may be treated in one session and ideally all PAVMs should be treated if the patient is symptomatic, unless the PAVM is too small for embolization. The most common postprocedural complication is pleuritic chest pain, which is self-limiting and can be treated with a short course of nonsteroidal anti-inflammatory agents (NSAIDs) or corticosteroids.[3] Long-term complications involve persistence of PAVM.

Persistent Pulmonary Arteriovenous Malformations

Recurrent Pulmonary Arteriovenous Malformations following Initial Embolization

The procedural success rate is between 83 and 100% in the first 1–2 years based on recent small observational studies.[32,46,47] Persistent lesions may be identified in 8–25% of cases, where the PAVM demonstrates persistent perfusion (CT contrast enhancement of the sac or <70% decrease in sac size).[48,49] Common reasons for refractory PAVM after embolotherapy include: Recanalization within the embolic material, continued perfusion through missed feeding arteries, or reperfusion through new feeding arteries. Typically patients would have to undergo repeat embolotherapy, with one study demonstrating the success rate of repeat embolotherapy to be around 55% emphasizing the difficulty of treating recurrent PAVMs.[50]

Failed with Repeated Embolization

Patients that have failed one to two embolotherapy treatment options should be considered for surgical excision of individual PAVMs. This is becoming increasingly rare as many centers are gaining experience in embolotherapy, where surgery is becoming less employed.[47] Success rates of surgical excisions vary based on the quantity, size, and distribution of PAVMs necessitating surgeons to perform a more invasive procedure (e.g., local excision, wedge resection, lobectomy). In some cases, surgical resection may be necessary, especially for larger or complex PAVMs that are not amenable to embolization. Morbidity and mortality risk is present as with any thoracic surgery and varies between 0 and 9%.[26]

Refractory Pulmonary Arteriovenous Malformations to Embolization or Surgery

An overwhelming majority of patients will be successfully cured with embolization or surgical excision.[46] In the small population of patients with refractory PAVM, lung transplantation can be considered for patients with symptoms placing them at a high risk for death or for patients with diffuse bilateral PAVMs.[15] These individuals have a high risk of morbidity and mortality following lung transplantation as they are at a high risk for postoperative hemoptysis or hemothorax and fatal multiorgan failure.

Additional Management Considerations

In addition to definitive treatment with embolotherapy, surgical excision, or lung transplantation, there are extra therapies to consider while treating this patient population. Patients with PAVMs are at risk for air embolism, especially with administration of medications or fluids intravenously.[9,17] Extra caution should be placed to avoid the introduction of air bubbles intravenously. The use of in-line filters is recommended if available as they are able to filter a significant portion of macroscopic air bubbles. In a similar sense, patients should also be advised to avoid scuba diving as there is a theoretical risk of venous air embolism during rapid ascent as alveoli may rupture and air leak into the PAVM.[29] Patients diagnosed with PAVM should be administered antibiotic prophylaxis before undergoing dental procedures and other nonsterile procedures to mitigate the potential risk of developing a cerebral abscess.[51] Lastly, occasionally patients may require supplemental oxygen to alleviate hypoxemia and associated symptoms.

FOLLOW-UP

The International Guidelines for the Diagnosis and Management of Hereditary Haemorrhagic Telangiectasia can be used to direct follow-up for patients following embolotherapy.[23] Immediately following embolotherapy, patients are advised to monitor their symptoms and oxygen saturations. Some experts recommend a high-resolution CT chest with contrast 3–6 months following embolotherapy to confirm resolution of the PAVM (no CT contrast enhancement of the sac or ≥70% decrease in sac size). A TTCE is also done at this time to evaluate for persistence of right-to-left shunting as well as for grading the severity of the shunt.

According to the guidelines, if the initial postembolotherapy CT chest shows successful treatment of PAVM and the TTCE shows either a grade 0 or a 1 shunt, then it is recommended to follow-up with TTCE every 3–5 years (decreases ionizing radiation exposure). If the TTCE ever worsens to a grade 2 or 3 shunt, then it is recommended to repeat a CT chest to evaluate for new or persistent PAVMs. However, if the initial postembolotherapy CT does not show successful treatment of the PAVM or the TTCE shows a grade 2 or 3 shunt after treatment, then it is recommended to follow-up primarily with CT chest imaging with the addition of TTCE for persistent PAVMs to determine their clinical significance. Lastly, if symptoms worsen, TTCE worsens, or CT chest demonstrates larger or new PAVMs, then it is recommended to consider pulmonary angiography as the next step for better characterization of the PAVM and for potential embolization.

SUMMARY

Pulmonary arteriovenous malformations represent a complex and clinically significant condition that requires multidisciplinary collaboration between pulmonologists, interventional radiologists, and other specialists. Accurate diagnosis, appropriate management, and long-term follow-up are vital to preventing complications, improving patient outcomes, and enhancing our understanding of these rare vascular anomalies. Further research is needed to better elucidate the pathophysiology of PAVMs and develop more effective treatment strategies for affected individuals.

ACKNOWLEDGMENTS

We would like to thank Dr Joseph Parambil from the Cleveland Clinic Foundation for the CT scan images presented in this chapter.

REFERENCES

1. Gill SS, Roddie ME, Shovlin CL, et al. Pulmonary arteriovenous malformations and their mimics. Clin Radiol. 2015;70(1):96-110.
2. Wong HH, Chan RP, Klatt R, et al. Idiopathic pulmonary arteriovenous malformations: clinical and imaging characteristics. Eur Respir J. 2011;38(2):368-75.
3. Narsinh KH, Ramaswamy R, Kinney TB. Management of Pulmonary Arteriovenous Malformations in Hereditary Hemorrhagic Telangiectasia Patients. Semin Interv Radiol. 2013;30(4):408-12.
4. Bossler AD, Richards J, George C, et al. Novel mutations in ENG and ACVRL1 identified in a series of 200 individuals undergoing clinical genetic testing for hereditary hemorrhagic telangiectasia (HHT): correlation of genotype with phenotype. Hum Mutat. 2006;27(7):667-75.
5. van Gent MWF, Post MC, Snijder RJ, et al. Real prevalence of pulmonary right-to-left shunt according to genotype in patients with hereditary hemorrhagic telangiectasia: a transthoracic contrast echocardiography study. Chest. 2010;138(4):833-9.
6. Shovlin CL, Chamali B, Santhirapala V, et al. Ischaemic strokes in patients with pulmonary arteriovenous malformations and hereditary hemorrhagic telangiectasia: associations with iron deficiency and platelets. PLoS One. 2014;9(2):e88812.
7. Garcia-Rivas G, Jerjes-Sánchez C, Rodriguez D, et al. A systematic review of genetic mutations in pulmonary arterial hypertension. BMC Med Genet. 2017;18:82.
8. Ye F, Jiang W, Lin W, et al. A novel BMPR2 mutation in a patient with heritable pulmonary arterial hypertension and suspected hereditary hemorrhagic telangiectasia. Medicine (Baltimore). 2020;99(31):e21342.
9. Saboo SS, Chamarthy M, Bhalla S, et al. Pulmonary arteriovenous malformations: diagnosis. Cardiovasc Diagn Ther. 2018;8(3):325-37.
10. Martinez-Pitre PJ, Khan YS. Pulmonary Arteriovenous Malformation (AVMs). In: StatPearls [Internet]. Treasure Island (FL): StatPearls Publishing; 2023 [cited 2023 Jul 6]. Available from http://www.ncbi.nlm.nih.gov/books/NBK559289/ [Last accessed July, 2024].

11. Shovlin CL. Pulmonary Arteriovenous Malformations. Am J Respir Crit Care Med. 2014;190(11):1217-28.
12. Fuchizaki U, Miyamori H, Kitagawa S, et al. Hereditary haemorrhagic telangiectasia (Rendu-Osler-Weber disease). Lancet Lond Engl. 2003;362(9394):1490-4.
13. Mohammed MHA, Hrfi A, AlQwee AM, et al. Pulmonary arteriovenous malformation in a neonate: a condition commonly misdiagnosed. Sudan J Paediatr. 2018;18(2):56-60.
14. Kramdhari H, Valakkada J, Ayyappan A. Diagnosis and endovascular management of pulmonary arteriovenous malformations. Br J Radiol. 2021;94(1123):20200695.
15. Shovlin CL, Condliffe R, Donaldson JW, et al., British Thoracic Society. British Thoracic Society Clinical Statement on Pulmonary Arteriovenous Malformations. Thorax. 2017;72(12):1154-63.
16. Kroon S, van den Heuvel D, Vos JA, et al. Idiopathic and hereditary haemorrhagic telangiectasia associated pulmonary arteriovenous malformations: comparison of clinical and radiographic characteristics. Clin Radiol. 2021;76(5):394.e1-394.e8.
17. Danyalian A, Hernandez F. Pulmonary Arteriovenous Malformation. In: StatPearls [Internet]. Treasure Island (FL): StatPearls Publishing; 2023 [cited 2023 Jul 29]. Available from: http://www.ncbi.nlm.nih.gov/books/NBK560696/
18. Mottaghi H, Kahrom M, Nezafati MH, et al. Congenital pulmonary arteriovenous malformation: a rare cause of cyanosis in childhood. Pan Afr Med J. 2009;3:12.
19. Wert SE. 61 - Normal and Abnormal Structural Development of the Lung. In: Polin RA, Abman SH, Rowitch DH, Benitz WE, Fox WW (Eds). Fetal and Neonatal Physiology, 5th edition. Philadelphia: Elsevier; 2017. pp. 627-41.e3. Available from https://www.sciencedirect.com/science/article/pii/B9780323352147000615 [Last accessed August, 2024].
20. Durhan G, Ardali Duzgun S, Akpınar MG, et al. Imaging of congenital lung diseases presenting in the adulthood: a pictorial review. Insights Imaging. 2021;12(1):153.
21. Cottin V, Chinet T, Lavolé A, et al. Pulmonary arteriovenous malformations in hereditary hemorrhagic telangiectasia: a series of 126 patients. Medicine (Baltimore). 2007;86(1):1-17.
22. Angriman F, Ferreyro BL, Wainstein EJ, et al. Pulmonary arteriovenous malformations and embolic complications in patients with hereditary hemorrhagic telangiectasia. Arch Bronconeumol. 2014;50(7):301-4.
23. Faughnan ME, Palda VA, Garcia-Tsao G, et al. International guidelines for the diagnosis and management of hereditary haemorrhagic telangiectasia. J Med Genet. 2011;48(2):73-87.
24. Swanson KL, Prakash UB, Stanson AW. Pulmonary arteriovenous fistulas: Mayo Clinic experience, 1982-1997. Mayo Clin Proc. 1999;74(7):671-80.
25. White RI, Lynch-Nyhan A, Terry P, et al. Pulmonary arteriovenous malformations: techniques and long-term outcome of embolotherapy. Radiology. 1988;169(3):663-9.
26. Gossage JR, Kanj G. Pulmonary arteriovenous malformations. A state of the art review. Am J Respir Crit Care Med. 1998;158(2):643-61.
27. Walsh LJ, Collins C, Ibrahim H, et al. Pulmonary arterial hypertension in hereditary hemorrhagic telangiectasia associated with ACVRL1 mutation: a case report. J Med Case Reports. 2022;16:99.
28. Shimohira M, Iwata K, Ohta K, et al. Hemoptysis due to Pulmonary Arteriovenous Malformation after Coil Embolization during Long-Term Follow-Up. Case Rep Radiol. 2019;2019:4506253.
29. Hsu CC, Kwan GN, Evans-Barns H, et al. Embolisation for pulmonary arteriovenous malformation. Cochrane Database Syst Rev. 2018;2018(1):CD008017.
30. Shovlin CL, Tighe HC, Davies RJ, et al. Embolisation of pulmonary arteriovenous malformations: no consistent effect on pulmonary artery pressure. Eur Respir J. 2008;32(1):162-9.
31. Majumdar S, McWilliams JP. Approach to Pulmonary Arteriovenous Malformations: A Comprehensive Update. J Clin Med. 2020;9(6):1927.
32. Lee WL, Graham AF, Pugash RA, et al. Contrast echocardiography remains positive after treatment of pulmonary arteriovenous malformations. Chest. 2003;123(2):351-8.
33. Lau VI, Mah GD, Wang X, et al. Intrapulmonary and Intracardiac Shunts in Adult COVID-19 Versus Non-COVID Acute Respiratory Distress Syndrome ICU Patients Using Echocardiography and Contrast Bubble Studies (COVID-Shunt Study): A Prospective, Observational Cohort Study. Crit Care Med. 2023;51(8):1023-32.
34. Ming DKY, Patel MS, Hopkinson NS, et al. The "anatomic shunt test" in clinical practice; contemporary description of test and in-service evaluation. Thorax. 2014;69(8):773-5.
35. Haitjema T, Disch F, Overtoom TT, et al. Screening family members of patients with hereditary hemorrhagic telangiectasia. Am J Med. 1995;99(5):519-24.
36. Chokkappan K, Kannivelu A, Srinivasan S, et al. Review of diagnostic uses of shunt fraction quantification with technetium-99m macroaggregated albumin perfusion scan as illustrated by a case of Osler–Weber–Rendu syndrome. Ann Thorac Med. 2016;11(2):155-60.
37. Salibe-Filho W, de Oliveira FR, Terra-Filho M. Update on pulmonary arteriovenous malformations. J Bras Pneumol. 2023;49(2):e20220359.
38. Raptis DA, Short R, Robb C, et al. CT Appearance of Pulmonary Arteriovenous Malformations and Mimics. Radiogr Rev Publ Radiol Soc N Am Inc. 2022;42(1):56-68.
39. Khalid M, Malik N, Abbas S. Diagnosis: Pulmonary arteriovenous malformation (PAVM). Ann Saudi Med. 2005;25(6):518-20.
40. Van den Heuvel DAF, Post MC, Koot W, et al. Comparison of Contrast Enhanced Magnetic Resonance Angiography to Computed Tomography in Detecting Pulmonary Arteriovenous Malformations. J Clin Med. 2020;9(11):3662.
41. Sharma P, Kochar P, Sharma S, et al. A case of pulmonary arteriovenous malformation: role of interventional radiology in diagnosis and treatment. Ann Transl Med. 2017;5(17):345.
42. Faughnan ME, Mager JJ, Hetts SW, et al. Second International Guidelines for the Diagnosis and Management of Hereditary Hemorrhagic Telangiectasia. Ann Intern Med. 2020;173(12):989-1001.
43. Cartin-Ceba R, Swanson KL, Krowka MJ. Pulmonary arteriovenous malformations. Chest. 2013;144(3):1033-44.
44. Keinath K, Vaughn M, Cole N, et al. Exertional hypoxia in a healthy adult: a pulmonary arteriovenous malformation. BMJ Case Rep. 2019;12(10):e231981.
45. Schneider G, Massmann A, Fries P, et al. Safety of Catheter Embolization of Pulmonary Arteriovenous Malformations—Evaluation of Possible Cerebrovascular Embolism after Catheter Embolization of Pulmonary Arteriovenous Malformations in Patients with Hereditary Hemorrhagic Telangiectasia/Osler Disease by Pre- and Post-Interventional DWI. J Clin Med. 2021;10(4):887.

46. Andersen PE, Tørring PM, Duvnjak S, et al. Pulmonary arteriovenous malformations: a radiological and clinical investigation of 136 patients with long-term follow-up. Clin Radiol. 2018;73(11):951-7.
47. Lee DW, White RI, Egglin TK, et al. Embolotherapy of Large Pulmonary Arteriovenous Malformations: Long-Term Results. Ann Thorac Surg. 1997;64(4):930-40.
48. Latif MA, Bailey CR, Motaghi M, et al. Postembolization Persistence of Pulmonary Arteriovenous Malformations: A Retrospective Comparison of Coils and Amplatzer and Micro Vascular Plugs Using Propensity Score Weighting. Am J Roentgenol. 2023;220(1):95-103.
49. Trerotola SO, Pyeritz RE. Persistence of Pulmonary Arteriovenous Malformation after Embolization: Another Reason to Quit Smoking. Radiology. 2019;292(3):771-2.
50. Cusumano LR, Duckwiler GR, Roberts DG, et al. Treatment of Recurrent Pulmonary Arteriovenous Malformations: Comparison of Proximal Versus Distal Embolization Technique. Cardiovasc Intervent Radiol. 2020;43(1):29–36.
51. Shovlin C, Bamford K, Wray D. Post-NICE 2008: Antibiotic prophylaxis prior to dental procedures for patients with pulmonary arteriovenous malformations (PAVMs) and hereditary haemorrhagic telangiectasia. Br Dent J. 2008;205(10):531-3.

SECTION 12

Pleural Diseases

SECTION OUTLINE

CHAPTER 126

Pleura: Anatomy and Physiology

Srinivas Rajagopala

INTRODUCTION

To decrease the friction generated between the lung and thoracic wall during respiratory movements, the inner surface of the thoracic cage and the outer surface of the lungs and mediastinum are covered by a serous, elastic membrane with a smooth and lubricating surface: the pleura. The pleural cavity is like a sealed, wet, and stretchable elastic bag inserted between the lung and the thoracic wall.

ANATOMY OF THE PLEURA

The pleura (derived from Greek *Pleuron* for "side") is a serous membrane covering the lung, mediastinum, diaphragm, and rib cage. It can be divided into the visceral pleura and the parietal pleura; the former covers the lung parenchyma including the interlobar fissures and the latter lines the inside of the thoracic cavities. The parietal pleura is also arbitrarily classified into the costal, mediastinal, and diaphragmatic pleura according to the structure it invests. The visceral and the parietal pleura meet at the lung root. The surface area of the visceral pleura of one lung is similar to that of the parietal pleura of one hemithorax and is approximately 1,000 cm^2. The pleural pressure in humans is approximately –5 cm H_2O at mid-chest at functional residual capacity (FRC) and –30 cm H_2O at total lung capacity (TLC). This is generated by the balance of several forces; these include the elastic recoil pressures of the chest wall and the lung, the pressure of pleural fluid, the regional pleural surface deformation, and the weight of lung in dependent areas. The pleural space in health contains about 0.5–2 mL fluid on each side, allowing for close apposition of the visceral and parietal layers.

Surface Marking and Relevant Anatomic Considerations

The parietal pleura extends 2.5 cm above the medial end of the clavicle. It passes inferomedially behind the sternoclavicular joint at the 2nd costal cartilage and then vertically till the 6th costal cartilage on the right side. On the left side, it deviates to the lateral border of the sternum halfway till the apex of the heart. On either side, it turns laterally after the 6th costal cartilage to meet the 8th rib at the mid-clavicular line and 10th rib at the mid-axillary line. It moves posteriorly to the 12th rib, meeting the 12th vertebrae. At the left side, the upper pole of the kidney is just behind the parietal pleura as it dips into the costodiaphragmatic recess on either side. The pleural space can be injured in penetrating injuries directly at three unprotected sites: (1) Above the medial end of the first rib on either side, (2) below the xiphisternum on the right side, and (3) the costovertebral angles on either side. In other places, a penetrating injury in the intercostal spaces or injuries of the ribs themselves directly posteriorly can damage the pleural space.

DEVELOPMENT OF THE PLEURAL MEMBRANES[1]

The coelomic cavity in the fetus becomes partitioned into the pericardium and the pleural canals (cephalad portion) and into the peritoneal canals by the septum transversum (caudally) at 3 weeks of gestation. With further development at 9 weeks, the pleuropericardial membranes and the pleuroperitoneal membranes divide the pericardial and pleural cavities and unite with the septum transversum to complete the partition between each pleural cavity and the peritoneal cavity. This newly formed pleural cavity is separate on either side without communication and is fully lined by a mesothelial membrane that develops into the parietal pleura. The primordial lung buds bulging into the pleural cavities carry with them a covering of the lining mesothelium, which later develops into the visceral pleura.

HISTOLOGY OF THE PLEURA

The histology of the parietal pleura is fairly constant across species whereas that of the visceral pleura varies significantly. The parietal pleura has five layers and has a mean thickness of 20–25 μm. The layers include the innermost mesothelium, a submesothelial loose connective tissue layer, a superficial elastic layer, a subpleural highly vascularized loose connective tissue layer, and an outer fibroelastic layer. The visceral pleura is completely adherent to the lung. The parietal pleura is separated from the thoracic wall by an extrapleural connective tissue layer but this is densely adherent at the level of the fibrosus pericardium and diaphragm with no surgical plane at these sites. Mesothelial cells have a variety of functions important to pleural biology. Mesothelial cells can secrete extracellular matrix components and also organize them. They also secrete neutrophil and monocyte chemotactic factors. Mesothelial cells also produce several cytokines such as transforming growth factor-beta (TGF-β), epidermal growth factor (EGF), and platelet-derived growth factor (PDGF) that are important in pleural inflammation and fibrosis. Microvilli are present on the surface of mesothelial cells and serve to increase surface area for metabolic activity. The arterial supply of the parietal pleura is from the intercostal arteries or directly from the internal thoracic artery and its terminal branch, the musculophrenic artery. The venous drainage of the parietal pleura occurs into the brachiocephalic vein anteriorly and the azygos system posteriorly via the intercostal veins and the internal thoracic vein. The arterial supply and venous drainage of the visceral pleura is from the bronchial arteries, similar to the underlying lung. Lymphatic plexuses of the costal pleura drain along the intercostal nodes; those in the mediastinal pleura drain to the tracheobronchial and mediastinal nodes. The diaphragmatic pleura drains into the parasternal, middle phrenic, and posterior mediastinal nodes.

The visceral pleura may be thick (humans, sheep, cows, pigs, and horses) or thin (dogs, cats, and monkeys). This distinction is important physiologically because the blood supply is dependent on the thickness of the pleura. A thick visceral pleura is supplied by the bronchial circulation (systemic) while a thin visceral pleura depends on the lung parenchyma for nutrition. Only the parietal pleura contains sensory nerve fibers, supplied by the intercostal and phrenic nerves. Pain from pleural inflammation thus indicates involvement of the parietal pleura. The visceral pleura is only supplied by autonomic nerve fibers. Pleural pain can be perceived on the overlying skin or referred to shared thoracic spinal segments. Cervical pleurisy may be referred to inner aspect of the arms and mediastinal/central diaphragmatic pleurisy may be referred to C4 dermatome to the tip of ipsilateral shoulder by the phrenic nerve fibers.

PLEURAL FLUID: NORMAL VOLUME AND CELLULAR CONTENTS

The small amount of pleural fluid that is present physiologically is maintained by interplay of Starling's forces and lymphatic drainage. Fluid exchange across the pleural membranes is as follows:

$$\text{Fluid movement} = L \times S\,[(P_{cap} - P_{pl}) - \sigma(\Pi_{cap} - \Pi_{pl})],$$

where P and π are the hydrostatic and osmotic pressures, respectively, within the capillaries (cap) and pleural space (pl), L is the hydraulic conductivity of the membrane, S is the surface area, and Π is the osmotic coefficient for proteins.

Normal pleural fluid is a microvascular filtrate and is formed from the parietal pleura capillaries. It is drained predominantly via the parietal pleura lymphatic stoma; the absorptive gradient in the visceral pleural capillaries and the active transport across mesothelial cells play only a small role. The pleural fluid formed has characteristics of interstitial fluid (protein 1–2 g/100 mL and total leukocyte cell counts of 1,000–2,500/µL). Most of the protein is composed of albumin (50%), globulins (35%), and fibrinogen. This small amount of fluid is distributed uniformly along the pleural surface with an average thickness of 20 µm (thicker in dependent portions). The low pleural fluid protein (protein ratio 0.15–0.2) indicates a high degree of sieving of protein at the pleural microvasculature.

Two models have been proposed to explain the regional differences in pleural pressure. The *hydrostatic equilibrium model* states that the vertical pressure gradient is a consequence of the viscous flow, generating a continuous column of fluid throughout the pleural space, and generates a vertical gradient of 1 cm H_2O/cm height. The *viscous flow model* states that the pleural liquid pressure is always equal to pleural surface pressure. A thin layer of fluid generated by hydrostatic forces separates between the pleural surfaces; the pleural space is thus a "real" and not a potential space. As pleural fluid accumulates, the viscous resistance to flow falls rapidly and the gradient approaches the hydrostatic pressure gradient of 1 cm H_2O/cm height. The pleural space is 20 µm across and pressures (P_{pl}) cannot be accessed without creating deforming forces in health. As effusions accumulate, however, P_{pl} can be measured. While measuring P_{pl}, the zero-reference level is at the top of the effusion. Placement of the needle at the most dependent level will prevent damage to lungs and help remove the largest amount of pleural fluid.

PHYSIOLOGY AND PATHOPHYSIOLOGY OF PLEURAL FLUID TURNOVER[2,3]

Pleural fluid is formed at the parietal pleura capillaries. The constant pleural liquid production across species with differing visceral pleural thickness, the closer distance of parietal pleural microvessels (10–15 µm vs. 20–25 µm in visceral pleura) and the higher venous pressure in the parietal pleural side all favor a systemic (parietal pleural) origin of pleural fluid. Pleural fluid protein decreases as systemic blood pressure increases and also decreases with age (blood pressure increases and pulmonary resistance decreases with age), and these also favor the systemic circulation as the site of fluid formation. Fluid, thus, filtered enters the pleural space because of the leaky nature of the mesothelial surface and the strongly negative pleural pressures. In health, the pleural fluid production from parietal fluid capillaries in humans is about 0.01 mL/kg/hr or about 14.4 mL for a 60-kg person in a day.

Pleural fluid is absorbed by bulk flow at the lymphatic stoma (2–6 μm) in the parietal pleura. Diffusion, active transport, and transcytosis also contribute minimally to physiological turnover of pleural fluid. The importance of "bulk flow" as the mode of absorption is that pleural fluid protein remains constant with absorption (and does not increase as in diffusion). This permits the use of concentration of protein in the pleural fluid to differentiate between exudates and transudates. Pleural fluid formation is almost always due to a concurrent problem with the lungs or a systemic disease process. Often, this is the very first symptom or sign of such a process, leading to a new diagnosis. Transudative effusions result due to an imbalance between fluid formation at the parietal pleura capillaries and via visceral pleura in conditions of interstitial fluid excess and removal via parietal lymphatics. Exudative effusions result from an abnormality in the pleural surfaces and an exudation of protein-rich fluid in the pleura. Most of the parietal pleural stoma is distributed dorsocaudally and the visceral pleura is devoid of stoma. Parietal pleura lymphatics can absorb 0.28 mL/kg/hr, yielding a safety factor that is 28-fold before accumulation can occur in the presence of normal absorption.

Physiological Changes with a Pleural Effusion

When the pleural space is occupied by fluid, the pleural pressure becomes positive. The increase in volume must be compensated by an increase in size of thoracic cavity (distending pressure = $P_{atm} - P_{pleura}$) or a decrease in size of the heart or lungs (distending pressure = $P_{alv} - P_{pleura}$).

In experimental settings, decrease in lung volume with addition of saline was 30% at functional residual capacity and 20% at total lung capacity. Therapeutic thoracentesis has been shown to increase FEV1 and FVC by 200 mL for every 1,000 mL fluid removed. The increase in maximal inspiratory pressures post thoracocentesis is greater than the improvement in lung volume; relief of the downward displacement of the diaphragm is probably responsible for this finding. Pleural effusion leads to an ipsilateral intrapulmonary shunt and this does not change significantly post thoracocentesis. Consequently, PaO_2 does not increase post thoracocentesis and may actually paradoxically decrease. Exercise limitation in pleural effusions results from decline in lung volumes and cardiac function, as reflected by a reduced oxygen pulse. Therapeutic thoracocentesis, however, does not lead to any immediate improvement in exercise capacity as measured by VO_{2max}.

Physiological Changes with Pneumothorax

When a pneumothorax occurs, the pleural pressures become uniformly positive unlike a pleural effusion in which a gradient from bottom to top exists. As a result, with a pneumothorax, the upper lobe, which is more negative to begin with, is affected more than the lower lobe whereas with a pleural effusion, the lower lobes are more affected. With a pneumothorax, the increase in the volume of a hemithorax is four-fold less than the decrease in the volume of the lung. Hypoxemia occurs because of an intrapulmonary shunt and due to reduced cardiac output in tension pneumothoraces.

Pleural Manometry

Clinical application of pleural physiology begins with measurement of intrapleural pressures. Pleural manometry can be performed with both a vertical-column water manometer, an overdamped manometer with an interposed resistive element or a hemodynamic transducer connected to a standard physiologic system. Pleural manometry can be performed easily in the absence of complex equipment using central venous pressure (CVP) manometers connected to a thoracentesis catheter inserted in the most dependent portion of the pleural effusion.

There are three possible pleural elastance (change in pressure for volume removed) curves. These are (1) a large volume removed with minimal change in pressure (normal), (2) a normal initial elastance with a rapid drop in pressure (lung entrapment), and (3) an initial negative pressure with a rapid drop in pressure (trapped lung). In general, pressures of <-5 cm H_2O or pleural elastance (pressure change divided by the amount of fluid removed) >25 cm H_2O/L suggest trapped lung. An initial normal pressure with subsequent drop suggests pleural entrapment by malignancy or inflammation, extensive parenchymal disease, or endobronchial obstruction. Pleural elastance can also guide therapeutic thoracocentesis because reperfusion pulmonary edema does not occur till pleural pressures are <-20 cm H_2O. Also, an elastance >19 cm H_2O/L can predict the failure of pleurodesis as pleural opposition is unlikely if lung entrapment exists.

PLEURAL RADIOGRAPHY AND ULTRASOUND

Pleural fluid first accumulates in the subpulmonic space, between the inferior surface of the lungs and the diaphragm. About 500 mL of fluid is needed to obscure the diaphragm on an erect radiograph. On a lateral decubitus view, as low as 5–10 mL can be detected. Ultrasound has a very good sensitivity for diagnosing effusions and guiding thoracentesis when used in real-time. The presence of pleural fluid provides an excellent acoustic window that allows examination of the parietal and visceral pleura, as well as the effusion on ultrasound. Pleural fluid is usually hypoechoic (darker) and the air-filled lungs hyperechoic (brighter). It is nonionizing, can be performed bedside, and is easily repeated and is now an essential part of any pleural imaging and/or intervention.

SUMMARY

The pleural membranes (visceral and parietal) provide an excellent covering for the lungs for their smooth movement during respiration. The negative atmospheric pressure in the pleural cavity serves the purpose of keeping the lung expanded. Pleura gets involved in a number of diseases of lungs as well as other systemic diseases when fluid, inflammatory exudates, pus, blood, or air may accumulate in the pleural cavity.

REFERENCES

1. Charalampidis C, Youroukou A, Lazaridis G, et al. Physiology of the pleural space. J Thorac Dis. 2015;7(Suppl 1):S33-7.
2. Wang NS. Anatomy and physiology of the pleural space. Clin Chest Med 1985;6:3-16.
3. Lee KF, Olak J. Anatomy and physiology of the pleural space. Chest Surg Clin N Am. 1994;4:391-403.

CHAPTER 127

Pleural Disorders

Aditya Jindal

INTRODUCTION

Pleura can get involved either as the primary site or in diseases of the lungs and/or other systemic diseases. Pleural involvement may either be present as dry or manifest with presence of fluid/exudates or air in the pleural cavity, i.e., dry pleurisy, pleural effusion, and pneumothorax. The different clinical conditions may involve the pleura and pleural cavity with different mechanisms, symptoms, and complications. Although the general approach to pleural diseases is identical, different diagnostic investigations and treatments will be required for different clinical conditions. There is apparently an overall increase in the number of pleural diseases.[1] This is largely attributable to an increase in the incidence of infections and malignancies which are more frequent in an elderly and immunocompromised population with a larger number of comorbidities.[1,2]

TYPES OF PLEURAL DISEASES

There are several types of pleural diseases of various etiologies.[3] For purpose of simplicity, we can classify the pleural involvement in four broad categories depending upon the clinical and/or radiological appearances (**Box 1**). Most of pleural disorders will present with common symptoms of chest pain, shortness of breath, fatigue, and coughing. Symptoms may, however, differ depending upon the type, cause and severity of disorder. Some of the important types of pleural diseases are briefly discussed.

BOX 1 Types of pleural diseases.

- *Dry pleurisy*: Usually due to an infection of the pleural cavity—absence of any exudate in the pleural cavity
- *Pleural effusion*: Presence of fluid/pus (parapneumonic effusion or empyema), blood (hemothorax), chyle, or pseudochyle (chylothorax and pseudochylothorax)
- *Pneumothorax*: The presence of air or gas with or without fluid (hydro- or pyothorax) in the pleural cavity
- *Pleural tumors*: Primary or metastatic

Pleurisy

Pleurisy commonly recognized with presence of local chest pain, is defined as inflammation of the pleura which can occur following an infection, trauma, malignancy or other types of pleural injury.[4] Most commonly, it follows a viral or bacterial (including tubercular) infection. Other infections such as fungal or parasitic infections are uncommon. Blunt trauma to the chest which is frequently forgotten is a common cause of pleural inflammation. Malignancies such as lung cancer, primary pleural mesothelioma, and metastases from distal tumors as well as nonmalignant diseases such as granulomatous disorders (sarcoidosis), connective tissue diseases (rheumatoid arthritis), asbestosis, and lymphangioleiomyomatosis can also cause pleural involvement. Pleurisy can also occur over a site of pulmonary embolism and following heart surgery. It can sometimes occur following use of drugs such as procainamide, tobacco/electronic cigarettes, and illicit (intravenous) drug use.

Pleurisy is generally dry but may be accompanied with mild effusion and presents with usually severe and shooting localized chest pain which gets aggravated during deep breathing, coughing, or sneezing. Pleurisy may set in quickly (in minutes to hours) in certain acute conditions such as myocardial infarction, pulmonary embolism, acute pericarditis, and following chest wall injury. Tachypnea and dyspnea are other common features in acute and hyperacute pleurisy. Pleurisy due to infections (viral and bacterial pneumonia, tuberculosis), or when associated with rheumatoid arthritis, tumors, and other systemic causes can develop over hours to days.

Other symptoms of pleurisy may include shortness of breath, cough, fever and chills and other systemic features of the causative illness which may include fatigue, malaise, unexplained weight loss, joint pains, swelling, and soreness.

Pleural Effusion

Pleural effusion is defined as an abnormal collection of fluid in the pleural space which could be either inflammatory or noninflammatory in origin generally associated with different

BOX 2 Common causes of pleurisy and pleural effusion.

- *Noninfective, usually transudative effusion*:
  - Congestive heart failure
  - Hypotroteinemia
  - Liver cirrhosis
  - Nephrotic syndrome
  - Peritoneal dialysis
- *Infective disorders (exudative fluid)*:
  - Pneumonia
  - Tuberculosis
  - Other lung parenchymal and pleural infections
  - Pancreatitis
- *Malignancies*:
  - Lung cancer
  - Pleural tumors
  - Metastases from distal malignancies
  - Lymphomatous tumors
- Chest and lung trauma, chest or heart surgery
- *Connective tissue diseases*:
  - Rheumatoid arthritis
  - Systemic sclerosis
  - Systemic lupus erythematosus
- *Miscellaneous*:
  - Pulmonary thromboembolism
  - Asbestosis
  - Sarcoidosis
  - Chronic obstructive pulmonary disease
  - Rarely idiopathic
  - Drugs/iatrogenic: Beta-blockers, clozapine, dantrolene, nitrofurantoin, recreational drugs, electronic smoking (vaping)

lung, pleural, and systemic illnesses **(Box 2)**.[5,6] Congestive heart failure, infections, cancers, and pulmonary embolism are the common causes. The fluid volume and the underlying etiology determine the clinical manifestations.

Pleural effusion may not cause any symptom. Pleuritic chest pain, heaviness or chest discomfort, breathlessness, often dry and ineffective cough are more common symptoms. Symptoms suggestive of the underlying etiology may include the presence of fever, joint pains, malaise, weakness, weight loss, or other systemic symptoms.

Types of Pleural Effusion

Pleural effusion is normally classified depending upon the nature of the fluid into a transudate and an exudate or based upon the type of the fluid present in the pleural cavity.

Most of these conditions are subsequently discussed in separate chapters.

- *Parapneumonic effusion and empyema*: The accumulation of exudative fluid in the pleural cavity usually associated with bacterial or viral pneumonia is referred to as parapneumonic effusion. Presence of frank pus is called as empyema. It is generally accompanied with symptoms of chest pain, cough, fever and sometimes, shortness of breath. These symptoms may be absent in the elderly who present with nonspecific features of anemia, fatigue, and failure to thrive.
- *Hemothorax*: Presence of blood in the pleural cavity, commonly due to chest trauma, lung/pleural cancer, chest/heart surgery, pulmonary thromboembolism and sometimes, infections such as empyema or tuberculosis. Symptomatology is generally similar to other effusions, i.e., chest pain, cough, shortness of breath, and other systemic symptoms.

  Hemothorax due to malignancy is the second leading cause of exudative effusions. Around 15% of patients with lung cancer have malignant pleural effusion at presentation and about 50% are likely to develop during the course of their illness. Malignant pleural effusion is associated with a poor prognosis. Lung cancer and gastrointestinal cancers have the worst outcomes while mesothelioma and hematologic cancers have better survival of about 1 year.
- *Chylothorax*: This is defined with the presence of lymphatic fluid (chyle) in the pleural cavity, most frequently observed following thoracic surgery and in case of malignancies that block the thoracic duct or produce abnormal lymphatic flow. Leaks in the lymphatic channels are caused due to direct infiltration and obstruction to the flow.
- *Complicated transudative effusion*: Effusions associated with congestive heart failure, hepatic failure, and renal failure have poor survival rates, especially when recurrent and refractory to treatment.

Pneumothorax

Pneumothorax is the presence of air in the pleural cavity, which may occur either spontaneously or following a trauma.[7] Air enters the pleural cavity due to damage to the lung such as following rupture of a bleb or a bulla or following a severe lung infection (necrotizing pneumonia). Air can occur from outside through chest wall following an injury or a therapeutic intervention. It is often categorized as (1) primary pneumothorax, which develops without an obvious etiology and significant lung disease, or (2) secondary pneumothorax in the presence of an underlying lung disease. In the intensive care unit (ICU), mechanical ventilation causing barotrauma is a common cause for pneumothorax in critically ill patients.[8]

Pneumothorax generally presents with sudden sharp pain that worsens with deep breathing, shortness of breath, chest tightness, and cough. In some cases, there may be presence of both air and fluid/pus/blood, i.e., hydropneumothorax, pyothorax, and hemothorax, respectively.

Pleural Tumors

Pleura may be involved in a variety of malignant conditions arising from the pleura (e.g., mesothelioma) or spreading to the pleura from the lungs or metastatic from another site.[9] Occasionally, benign tumors may also arise from the pleura. Symptoms such as shortness of breath, chest pain, cough, and unexpected weight loss are generally slower in onset. Most patients of primary pleural tumor and mesothelioma are older adults who have worked around asbestos. Pleural mesothelioma patients commonly experience dyspnea, accompanied by dry cough, fatigue, chest pain, and weight loss.

DIAGNOSTIC APPROACH TO PLEURAL DISEASES

Pleural diseases are heterogeneous in presentation and etiology of the disease which require a thorough diagnostic approach including the imaging and invasive interventions for pleural fluid analysis and lung/pleural biopsies.[10,11] Pleural disease is suspected on the basis of clinical history and findings on physical examination. Presence of clinical findings on general physical examination may provide diagnostic clues to the underlying systemic disease.

Imaging

- *Chest X-ray (CXR):* A posteroanterior (PA) CXR is the first radiological investigation in most cases.[12] It will detect the presence of around 200 mL of fluid. Pneumothorax is confirmed with a CXR with the absence of lung marking.[13] CXR also provides a clue to the status of the lung parenchyma and chest wall such as a mass, consolidation, or cavity. CXR will also provide imaging of the mediastinum, heart, blood vessels, and bones and thus, help to diagnose lymphadenopathy, cardiomegaly, and/or vascular conditions, rib or other bone fractures, and lung parenchymal diseases such as pneumonia or tumors.
- *Computed tomography (CT) scan*: CXR findings, especially about the lung parenchyma and mediastinum, need detailed evaluation on CT scanning. CT is considered as the gold standard investigation for diagnosis of pneumothorax, bronchopleural fistulae, and esophageal leak. Vascular evaluation will require contrast-enhanced CT scan and/or CT pulmonary angiography with prior administration of iodinated intravenous contrast. CT scan can be used to distinguish simple from complicated parapneumonic effusions; the "split pleura" sign—visceral and parietal pleural thickening with separation—is often considered as diagnostic of empyema.[14]
- CT appearance may suggest malignant disease by the presence of pleural thickening (>10 mm), pleural nodularity, mediastinal thickening, or circumferential thickening.[15]
- *Magnetic resonance imaging (MRI):* This is costlier and not routinely required for pleural and lung parenchymal diseases. MRI may help to evaluate pulmonary vascular lesions and mediastinal structures as well as for soft-tissue tumors such as solitary pleural fibromas and lipomas. MRI is also useful as a substitute investigation in patients with contrast allergy.[16]
- *Positron emission tomography (PET) scan:* PET scan may help to differentiate between infections—benign and malignant lesions—whenever there is a doubt. This may show false-positive results in patients with previous talc pleurodesis.[17] Moreover, low-grade cancers may not be detected on PET-CT. PET-CT is useful in combination with other imaging modalities to highlight metabolically active targets for biopsy.[18,19]
- *Ultrasonography*: Medical sonography is a reliable, portable, and relatively cheap imaging technique helpful for both diagnostic and therapeutic purposes.[20,21] Transthoracic ultrasound can be used to distinguish between the presence of fluid, air, or solid material in the pleural cavity as well as to guide the site for diagnostic and therapeutic aspiration. It can help detect as little as 5 mL of pleural fluid and can be used to identify chest wall, pleural, and subpleural disease. Ultrasonographic finding such as increased B lines can help to distinguish between consolidation, interstitial edema, or thickening.

Pleural Fluid Examination

Examination of pleural fluid and/or pleural biopsy is the cornerstone of diagnosis unless the cause of the effusion is relatively straightforward (e.g., congestive heart failure, chronic renal or liver disease). Thoracocentesis is preferably done under ultrasound or CT guidance when fluid is loculated or small in quantity. In case of symptomatic effusions of moderate or large quantities, up to 1.5 L of pleural fluid can be removed for both diagnostics and temporary, microbiological (smear examination for acid-fast bacilli, culture, and sensitivity), immunological, and cytological investigations.

- *Pleural fluid biochemistry*: The first step involves the distinction between inflammatory (exudative) from noninflammatory (transudative) effusions based upon the traditional Light's criteria initially described in 1972 **(Table 1)**.[22] Typical exudative conditions include infections such as pneumonias, tuberculosis, sometimes connective tissue diseases and malignancy and transudative effusion broadly reflects systemic fluid overloaded states such as congestive heart failure, chronic renal or liver failure and hypoproteinemia. Misclassification of a transudate as an exudate is reported in elderly patients and those with fluid overloaded states such as congestive heart failure who are on diuretic therapy.[23]

  Pleural fluid level of N-terminal pro b-type natriuretic peptide (NT-proBNP) > 1,500 pg/mL identifies effusions

TABLE 1: Light's criteria for classification of pleural fluid.

Criterion	Exudative effusion	Transudative effusion
Ratio of pleural fluid protein to serum protein	>0.5	<0.5
Ratio of pleural fluid lactate dehydrogenase (LDH) level to serum LDH level	>0.6	<0.6
Pleural fluid LDH level	>200 IU/L or >67% of the upper limit of the normal range for serum LDH level	<200 IU

due to heart disease such as congestive heart failure. Pleural fluid pH and other biochemical tests may be required to define chylothorax, pseudochylothorax, and pancreatitis amongst others. Pleural fluid cholesterol level of >45 mg/dL is also suggestive of an exudative effusion.

Biomarkers in pleural infection: Other biomarkers such as C-reactive protein, procalcitonin (PCT), inflammatory cytokines, and enzymes have been evaluated but not *found* superior to traditional criteria.[24] Pleural fluid adenosine deaminase (ADA) is widely used in the diagnosis of pleural TB. A higher value of >40 IU/L is suggestive of pleural TB though false-positive results are seen in rheumatoid disease and pleural mesothelioma. On the other hand, a value of <40 IU/L is strongly against the diagnosis of pleural TB.[25]

- *Pleural fluid microbiology*: Microbiological smear and culture are essential diagnostic tests to determine organisms in pleural infections such as tuberculosis or parapneumonic effusions and empyema. Culture and sensitivity testing will also help to guide antibiotic treatment. Nucleic acid amplification testing, based on extracting and deep sequencing bacterial DNA, is used to improve diagnostic microbiological yield.[26] The point-of-care, Gene X-pert test is now commonly employed for pleural tuberculous infection.
- *Pleural fluid* cytology:[27,28] Cytological examination involves differential cell counts, sometimes, the sole parameter to achieve diagnosis. High lymphocyte count with >50% lymphocytes supports tubercular effusion while neutrophil predominance may typically suggest acute pathology, such as parapneumonic effusion, acute infections of lung and pleura or pulmonary embolism. Lymphocytic effusion may also be seen in congestive cardiac failure or hematological malignancy while eosinophilic effusions may suggest an underlying malignancy, allergic or inflammatory disorder or rarely and drug induced.

Presence of malignant cells in pleural fluid may depend upon the type of malignancy and can help to guide specific, personalized cancer treatment. Identification of molecular marker on tumor cells may help the choice of targeted immunomodulating treatment, e.g., for lung adenocarcinoma.[29]

Medical Thoracoscopy and Pleural Biopsy

Image-guided biopsy of a pleural/lung tumor is done in the presence of any suspicious mass. This can confirm the presence of a benign or malignant tumor in most cases. Thoracoscopic examination is of great help in cases of effusion as well as pneumothorax. It allows the visual examination of lung surface for any solid mass, bleb, bulla or an airleak. Thoracoscopy is helpful to obtain biopsy from the visceral pleural membrane. Closed pleural biopsies with the help of reversed-bevel closed needles (Abrams and Cope) are rarely employed because of the low yield and greater frequency of complications. Image-guided cutting needle biopsy or medical thoracoscopy is therefore preferred.[24,30]

Pleural biopsy is the gold standard in the diagnosis of malignant pleural effusions as well as increases the microbiological yield in both pleural infection and TB. It also helps to exclude benign asbestos-related pleural effusion and eosinophilic pleuritis. Image-guided needle biopsy should not be used to replace medical thoracoscopy, which allows biopsies under direct vision to assess the macroscopic appearance of the pleura, diaphragm, and lung and guide biopsy target.

Medical thoracoscopy is undertaken by pulmonary physicians under conscious sedation in a spontaneously breathing patient. On the other hand, surgical thoracoscopy [video-assisted thoracoscopic surgery (VATS)] is conducted under general anesthesia by a surgeon. The diagnostic yield of medical thoracoscopy for unexplained pleural effusion is above 90% in moist cases.[31]

Thoracoscopic approach is the method of choice in undiagnosed and recurrent effusion as well as in suspected malignant effusion and pleural mesothelioma. Thoracoscopy allows good sized and deeper biopsies.[32] It also allows simultaneous therapeutic interventions for fluid drainage and talc pleurodesis.[33]

Miscellaneous Investigations

Other investigations may be required for diagnosis of a systemic disease, especially in case of transudative effusions. Cardiac evaluation needs electrocardiography and echocardiography, sometimes additional stress testing and angiography. Hematological and biochemical investigations are required for evaluation of liver and renal function. Markers of connective tissue diseases are tested in suspected cases.

Pulmonary thromboembolism is another important cause of exudative pleural effusions, which should be considered if the initial evaluation is negative. Perfusion scanning and other investigations may be needed to establish the diagnosis. No apparent cause is detected in around 20% of patients of exudative effusion.

TREATMENT

Besides the standard medical/surgical treatment of the underlying etiology (such as the infection, tuberculosis, or malignancy), treatment of pleural disease involves two important components:

1. Drainage of pleural fluid, pus or blood with insertion of a needle or catheter (thoracentesis), or with an intercostal chest tube (thoracostomy). Sometimes, it is important to remove the diseased pleura (decortication) in the presence of thick and loculated exudates or pus. Pneumothorax is treated with a water-seal chest-tube insertion.
2. *Pleurodesis*: It involves adherence of the lung to the chest wall such as in case of recurrent pneumothorax or effusion. This is achieved by abrading the pleural surface with help of intrapleural administration of an irritant or chemical agent. This can be done either with help of the chest tube inserted for drainage or through thoracoscopy under direct visualization.

Transudative effusions do not generally require drainage of fluid or pleurodesis. Large-quantity symptomatic effusion which does not respond to standard medical treatment of the cause may, however, be drained. Pleurodesis may be done in case of repeated requirement for pleural aspiration. Bullectomy, i.e., surgical removal of a bulla, may be considered in a case of pneumothorax.

Parapneumonic effusion may be aspirated if there is significant amount of pleural fluid. Chest tube drainage is required if there is gross pus in the pleural cavity or if the Gram stain is positive. Chest tube drainage is also indicated if biochemical tests of the fluid show glucose level of <40 mg/dL, or pH < 7.00. Intrapleural administration of streptokinase or urokinase should be done if drainage with the chest tube is unsatisfactory.

Malignant effusions require treatment with chemotherapy and/or radiation depending upon the site and type of tumor. The three most common malignancies associated with pleural effusion are breast and lung carcinoma, lymphomas, and leukemias. Chemical pleurodesis or pleuroperitoneal shunt is done if a patient has dyspnea from a malignant effusion that responds to therapeutic thoracentesis.

SUMMARY

Presence of fluid, air, or other exudates in the pleural cavity can occur in a number of diseases of the pleura, lungs, or chest wall. Several systemic diseases may also be associated with unilateral or bilateral effusions. Imaging and pleural fluid examination are essential to establish the diagnosis. Several biochemical and immunological biomarkers have been identified for the diagnosis or infective or malignant etiology. Besides the symptomatic and palliative therapy with pleural aspiration and pleurodesis, treatment of the underlying disease is important.

REFERENCES

1. Bodtger U, Hallifax RJ. Epidemiology: why is pleural disease becoming more common? Sheffield, UK: European Respiratory Society monograph. pleural disease; 2020. pp. 1-12.
2. Maldonado F, Lentz RJ, Light RW. Diagnostic approach to pleural diseases: new tricks for an old trade. F1000Res. 2017;6:1135.
3. Feller-Kopman D. Light R. Pleural disease. N Engl J Med. 2018;378(8):740-51.
4. Reamy BV, Williams PM, Odom MR. Pleuritic chest pain: Sorting through the differential diagnosis. Am Fam Physician. 2017;96(5):306-12.
5. Light RW. Pleural diseases. Dis Mon. 1992;38(5):266-331.
6. Bedawi EO, Guinde J, Rahman NM, et al. Advances in pleural infection and malignancy. Eur Respir Rev. 2021;30(159):200002.
7. Bintcliffe O, Maskell N. Spontaneous pneumothorax. BMJ. 2014; 348:g2928.
8. Thachuthara-George J. Pneumothorax in patients with respiratory failure in ICU. J Thorac Dis. 2021;13(8):5195-204.
9. Sureka B, Thukral BB, Mittal MK, et al. Radiological review of pleural tumors. Indian J Radiol Imaging. 2013;23(4):313-20.
10. Sundaralingam A, Bedawi EO, Rahman NM. Diagnostics in pleural disease. Diagnostics (Basel). 2020;10(12):1046.
11. Addala DN, Denniston P, Sundaralingam A, et al. Optimal diagnostic strategies for pleural diseases and identifying high-risk patients. Expert Rev Respir Med. 2023;17(1):15-26.
12. Blackmore CC, Black WC, Dallas RV, et al. Pleural Fluid volume estimation: A chest radiograph prediction rule. Acad Radiol. 1996;3:103-9.
13. Chiles C, Ravin CE. Radiographic recognition of pneumothorax in the intensive care unit. Crit Care Med. 1986;14:677-80.
14. Porcel JM, Pardina M, Alemán C, et al. Computed tomography scoring system For discriminating between parapneumonic effusions eventually drained and those cured only with antibiotics: CT for parapneumonic effusions. Respirology. 2017;22:1199-204.
15. Waite RJ, Carbonneau RJ, Balikian JP, et al. Parietal pleural changes in empyema: appearances at CT. Radiology. 1990;175:145-50.
16. Hierholzer J, Luo L, Bittner RC, et al. MRI and CT in the differential diagnosis of pleural disease. Chest. 2000;118:604-9.
17. Brun C, Gay P, Cottier M, et al. Comparison of cytology, chest computed and positron emission tomography findings in malignant pleural effusion from lung cancer. J Thorac Dis. 2018;10:6903-11.

18. Porcel JM, Hernández P, Martínez-Alonso M, et al. Accuracy of fluorodeoxyglucose-PET imaging for differentiating benign from malignant pleural effusions: A meta-analysis. Chest. 2015;147:502-12
19. Treglia G, Sadeghi R, Annunziata S, et al. Diagnostic accuracy of 18F-FDG-PET and PET/CT in the differential diagnosis between malignant and benign pleural lesions: a systematic review and meta-analysis. Acad Radiol. 2014;21:11-20.
20. Asciak R, Hassan M, Mercer RM, et al. Prospective analysis of the predictive value of sonographic pleural fluid echogenicity for the diagnosis of exudative effusion. Respiration. 2019;97:451-6.
21. Ding W, Shen Y, Yang J, et al. Diagnosis of pneumothorax by radiography and ultrasonography: a meta-analysis. Chest. 2011;140:859-66.
22. Light RW, Macgregor MI, Luchsinger PC, et al. Pleural effusions: the diagnostic separation of transudates and exudates. Ann Intern Med. 1972;77:507-13.
23. Addala D, Mercer RM, Lu Q, et al. P102 discordant exudative pleural effusions: demographics and aetiology. Thorax. 2019;74: A146.
24. Hooper C, Lee GYC, Maskell NA. Investigation of a unilateral pleural effusion in adults: British Thoracic Society Pleural Disease Guideline 2010. Thorax. 2010;65(Suppl 2):ii4–ii17.
25. Sivakumar P, Marples L, Breen R, et al. The diagnostic utility of pleural fluid adenosine deaminase for tuberculosis in a low prevalence area. Int J Tuberc Lung Dis. 2017;21:697-701.
26. Kanellakis NI, Wrightson JM, Gerry S, et al. The bacteriology of pleural infection (TORPIDS): an exploratory metagenomics analysis through next generation sequencing. Lancet Microbe. 2022;3:e294-302.
27. Arnold DT, De Fonseka D, Perry S, et al. Investigating unilateral pleural effusions: the role of cytology. Eur Respir J. 2018;52(5):1801254.
28. Oba Y, Abu-Salah T. The prevalence and diagnostic significance of eosinophilic pleural effusions: a meta-analysis and systematic review. Respiration. 2012;83:198-208.
29. Ahmadzada T, Kao S, Reid G, et al. An update on predictive biomarkers for treatment selection in non-small cell lung cancer. J Clin Med. 2018;7:153.
30. Mei F, BoniFazi M, Rota M, et al. Diagnostic yield and safety of image-guided pleural biopsy: a systematic review and meta-analysis. Respiration. 2021;100:77-87.
31. Rahman NM, Ali NJ, Brown G, et al. Local anaesthetic thoracoscopy: British thoracic society pleural disease guideline 2010. Thorax. 2010;65:ii54–ii60.
32. Bibby AC, Dorn P, Psallidas I, et al. ERS/EACTS statement on the management of malignant pleural effusions. Eur Respir J. 2018;52:1800349.
33. Bhatnagar R, Laskawiec-Szkonter M, Piotrowska HEG, et al. Evaluating the efficacy of thoracoscopy and talc poudrage versus pleurodesis using talc slurry (TAPPS trial): protocol of an open-label randomised controlled trial. BMJ Open. 2014;4:e007045.

Parapneumonic Effusion and Empyema

CHAPTER 128

Devasahayam J Christopher, Priya N

INTRODUCTION

Parapneumonic effusion (PPE) is a pleural effusion that occurs due to bacterial pneumonia, lung abscess, or bronchiectasis.[1] PPEs occur in 20–40% of patients who are hospitalized with pneumonia. The mortality rate in patients with a PPE is higher than that in patients with pneumonia without a PPE. Some of the excess mortality is due to mismanagement of the PPE.[2]

DEFINITIONS

Empyema

Empyema is defined as pus within the pleural space. In its development, pleural fluid passes through stages of host's increasing defense activity and bacterial invasion. Not all infected pleural effusions progress to empyema.

Parapneumonic Effusion

Parapneumonic effusion is any pleural effusion occurring in association with bacterial pneumonia, lung abscess, or bronchiectasis

RISK FACTORS

The risk factors are as follows:

- Aspiration
- Poor dental hygiene
- Malnutrition
- Alcohol or intravenous drug abuse
- Gastroesophageal reflux disease (GERD)
- Partially treated pneumonia
- Immunosuppression

PATHOGENESIS

The formation of an infected pleural space is a complicated interaction between the host defense mechanisms and the organisms. There are three distinct pathophysiological stages in PPE reflecting the changing physiology within the pleural space **(Table 1)**. The distinctions between the stages are not sharply demarcated. Various characteristics of pleural fluid are seen during different stages of PPE **(Table 2)**.

TABLE 1: Stages of parapneumonic pleural effusion.[3]

Stages of parapneumonic effusion	Pathophysiology
Exudative	Increased capillary permeability causing neutrophil migration and release of proinflammatory cytokines
Fibrinopurulent	High fibrinolytic activity, increase in pleural tissue plasminogen activator inhibitors, fibrin deposition on parietal and visceral pleura causing loculations and adhesions
Organizational	Proliferation of fibroblasts causing pleural scarring and dense fibrous septations

Exudative Stage

This stage is characterized by the accumulation of sterile fluid within the pleural space. This is in response to inflammation induced by bacterial infection within the lung parenchyma and the pleural membranes. Proinflammatory cytokines, such as interleukin-8 (IL-8) and tumor necrosis factor-alpha (TNF-α), are released locally.[3] If appropriate antibiotic therapy is instituted, the effusion is likely to resolve and intercostal drainage is not required.

Fibrinopurulent Stage

The fibrinopurulent stage occurs in response to bacterial invasion, usually as a consequence of inadequate or inappropriate therapy. Early on, there is an increase in pleural fluid which contains polymorphs, bacteria, and cellular debris. Later, there is the formation of fibrin clots and fibrinous septae due to clotting factors from the serum entering the pleural space. This results in a loculated

TABLE 2: Classification of parapneumonic pleural effusion (PPE) based on pathophysiologic stage.[2]

Stages of PPE/ empyema	Classification scheme (Adapted from reference 2)[2]	pH	Glucose (mg/dL)	LDH (mg/dL)	Gram stain and/or culture	USG characteristics[4,5]
1	Uncomplicated PPE	>7.20	>40	<1,000/ or <2/3rd of upper limit of serum LDH	Negative	No loculations
2	Borderline complicated PPE	7.0 < pH < 7.20	>40	>1,000/ or < 2/3rd of upper limit of serum LDH	Negative	No loculations
	Simple complicated PPE	<7.0	<40	>1,000/ or >2/3rd of upper limit of serum LDH	Positive	• Anechoic and/or echoic • No loculations
3	Complex complicated PPE	<7.0	<40	>1,000/ or >2/3rd of upper limit of serum LDH	Positive	• Echoic • Multiloculated • Septations

(LDH: lactate dehydrogenase; USG: ultrasonography)

pleural space that may be resistant to drainage with a single intercostal tube. As infection progresses, the pleural fluid pH and glucose levels reduce and lactate dehydrogenase (LDH) level goes up. Pus is formed by the lysis of bacteria and inflammatory cells.

Organizational Stage

The last stage is characterized by fibroblast proliferation and deposition of fibrous tissue on both the visceral and the parietal pleural membranes—the inelastic "pleural peel." This results in the restriction of lung expansion and impairment of gas exchange. If untreated, there is potential for chronic infection resulting in penetration of fluid into the chest wall (empyema necessitans) or into the lung, resulting in a bronchopleural fistula.[4] The further course after the organization is variable, some individuals undergo spontaneous healing with the resolution of pleural thickening, while others are left with "pleural peel."[5]

EPIDEMIOLOGY

We do not have direct epidemiological data from India. In India, PPE accounts for 2–29% among all causes of pleural effusion in various studies.[6-9] PPEs and empyema are relatively common complications of pneumonia. Since the advent of antibiotics, their overall incidence has declined dramatically to approximately 2–3% of all pneumonias. However, epidemiologic studies suggest that rates are again slowly rising.[10,11] The overall yield of bacterial Gram stain or culture from pleural fluid ranged anywhere between 13 and 87%. Yield of polymicrobiological culture varied from 0.6 to 33%. *Pseudomonas aeruginosa* and *Staphylococcus aureus* were the most common gram-negative and gram-positive bacteria isolated from pleural fluid in these studies. In the study by Mohanty et al.,[12] *Acinetobacter* species was the predominant gram-negative bacilli (29%) isolated from pleural fluid. In an unpublished study conducted in Christian Medical College, Vellore by Vineet et al., among 64 patients with complicated para pneumonic pleural effusion, the overall culture yield for bacterial pathogens was 36%, with 78% of these growing aerobic and the rest growing anaerobic.

BACTERIOLOGY

Published reports of PPEs have shown substantial variations in the bacteriology of isolated aerobes. It is likely that the introduction of antibiotics may have at least partially contributed to this variation. Over the years, the most commonly isolated organisms have varied between *Strep. pneumoniae, Strep. hemolyticus, and S. aureus.*[13] Anaerobes require a stringent transport process to preserve viability. Probably the most thorough bacteriological evaluation occurred during the Multicenter Intrapleural Sepsis Trial (MIST I), which evaluated the role of streptokinase on a large number of (454) patients, with complicated PPEs.[14] Of the 434 patients who had pleural fluid cultures, 250 (58%) achieved a microbiological diagnosis using conventional methods.[14] In those with community-acquired infections, *Streptococcus* was the most common aerobe (52%), followed by *Staphylococcus* (10%), and gram-negative organisms (9%). Anaerobes were grown in 20% of cases. Of hospital-acquired cases, the most common aerobe was *Staphylococcus* (35%, nearly three quarters of which were methicillin-resistant) followed by gram-negative organisms (23%) and *Streptococcus* (18%). Bacteriological diagnosis in 16% of the total samples was made by molecular diagnostic methods only.[15] In a quarter of the patients, organism could not be isolated. These results have implications for empiric therapy and the choice of antibiotics. The important difference between the hospital and the community-acquired infections was that the predominant organism in the former was *Staphylococcus*, and in the later the *Streptococcus;* a large fraction being *methicillin-resistant S. aureus* (MRSA). The overall mortality was significantly higher in the hospital-acquired infections than in the community-acquired infections **(Table 3)**.

TABLE 3: Description of bacteriology of community and hospital-acquired pleural infection.

Community acquired		Hospital acquired
Organism	**Number (%)**	**Number (%)**
Aerobes		
Streptococcus	176 (52%)	11 (18%)
Streptococcus intermedius	80	4
Streptococcus anginosus–constellatus (milleri) group		
Streptococcus pneumoniae	71	3
Streptococcus pyogens	9	0
Other *Streptococcus* species	16	4
Staphylococcus	35 (10%)	21 (35%)
S. aureus	27	6
Methicillin-resistant *S. aureus*	7	15
S. epidermidis	1	
Enterococcus spp.	4 (1%)	7 (12%)
Gram negatives	29 (9%)	14 (23%)
Escherichia coli	11	2
Other coliforms	4	6
Proteus	6	2
Enterobacter species	5	1
Pseudomonas aeringosa	3	3
Anaerobes	67 (20%)	5 (8%)
Fusobacterium	19	1
Bacteroides	16	1
Peptostreptococcus	9	
Mixed anaerobes, unclassified	8	2
Prevotella species	13	1
Clostridium species	2	
Mycobacterium tuberculosis	2 (1%)	
Actinomyces species	4 (1%)	
Other*	17 (5%)	2 (3%)
Total	336	60

*Includes *Burkholderia anthina, Eikenella, Haemophilus influenzae*, oral bacterium, *Pasteurella multocida, Klebsiella* species.

Note: Both infections differ bacteriologically from pneumonia.

Source: Maskell NA, Batt S, Hedley EL, et al. The Bacteriology of Pleural Infection by Genetic and Standard Methods and its Mortality Significance. Am J Respir Crit Care Med. 2006;74(7):817-23.

CLINICAL FEATURES AND DIAGNOSIS

Patients with aerobic pleural infection usually present with features of pneumonia with an acute febrile illness, cough, purulent sputum, and dyspnea. Pleuritic chest pain (due to parietal pleural involvement) is present in around 60% of patients. Absence of pain does not exclude the diagnosis of pleural infection.[2] Anaerobic infections present often in an indolent manner with weight loss, anorexia, and malaise.[3]

There are no clinical criteria that could distinguish between pneumonia with or without PPE. Therefore, PPE should be considered while evaluating all patients with pneumonia, particularly those who are unresponsive to antimicrobial therapy. Furthermore, not all patients with PPE have an acute illness.

Radiological Investigations

Chest radiograph [posteroanterior (PA) view] **(Figs. 1A and B)** can detect significant effusion and is often the only required imaging for its detection. Effusion may be free or loculated, and may show evidence of air-fluid level. Empyema may give the appearance of pleural mass or tumor within the lung, when the collection occurs within a fissure. Computed tomography (CT) scan of the chest is used to detect and quantitate minimal effusion. In resource-limited settings, blunting of the costophrenic angle on a lateral chest radiograph or obscuration of the dome of the diaphragm are considered sufficient to detect the presence of pleural fluid. Decubitus views may complement the information obtained from the erect chest radiographs.

In the lateral decubitus film, the amount of fluid can be roughly quantitated by measuring the distance between the chest wall and the lower part of the adjacent lung. If the length is <10 mm, the effusion is deemed to be too small to be clinically significant. Such effusions resolve with antibiotics alone.[2] CT evidence of pleural thickening is present in 80–100% of the empyemas **(Figs. 2A and B)**, so, its presence would favor this diagnosis, when PPE is being evaluated. "Split pleura sign" on contrast CT enhancement of visceral and parietal pleura differentiates empyema from a peripherally situated lung abscess **(Fig. 3)**.[16]

Ultrasonography is an excellent method to assess pleural effusion. It can also help to quantify the amount of effusion by assessing the depth of fluid. It can also be used at the bedside, e.g., in the intensive care units (ICUs). Empyema results in dense echogenicity and loculations, which are detectable on ultrasonogram. It is also helpful in ensuring successful pleural fluid aspiration in as high as 97% of the cases **(Figs. 4 and 5)**.[16,17]

Clinical features and routine blood tests are poor predictors of the need for drainage; the delay in instituting adequate drainage increases the morbidity. It is, thus, recommended that diagnostic pleural aspiration should be performed in all patients with PPE.[18] The exception to this rule is a small pleural effusion (<10 mm on a lateral decubitus chest radiograph), which may resolve with antibiotics

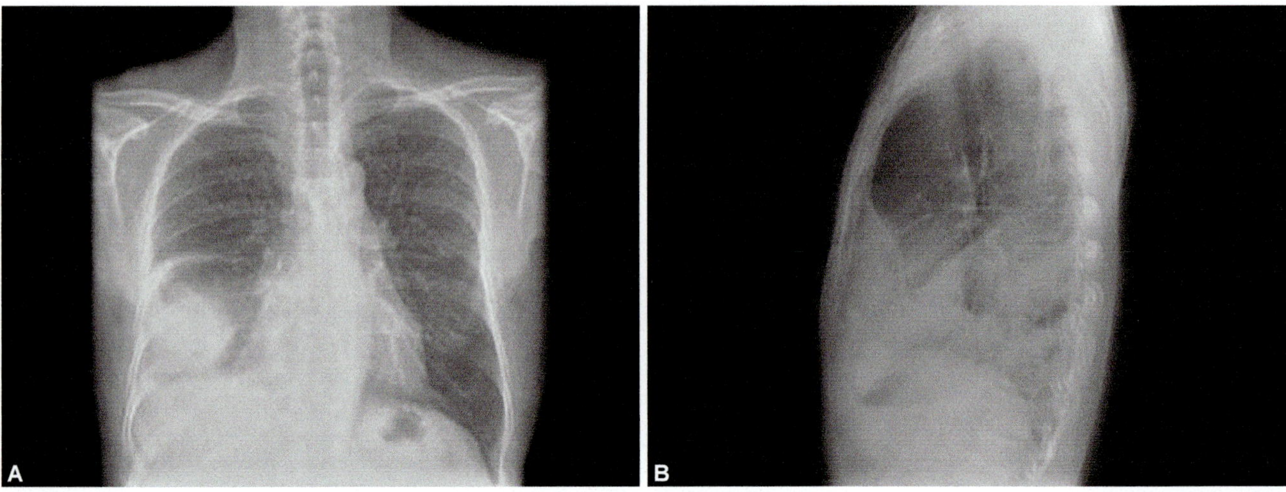

FIGS. 1A AND B: Chest radiograph posteroanterior (PA) and lateral views showing right sided loculated pleural effusion and fluid extending into the fissures.

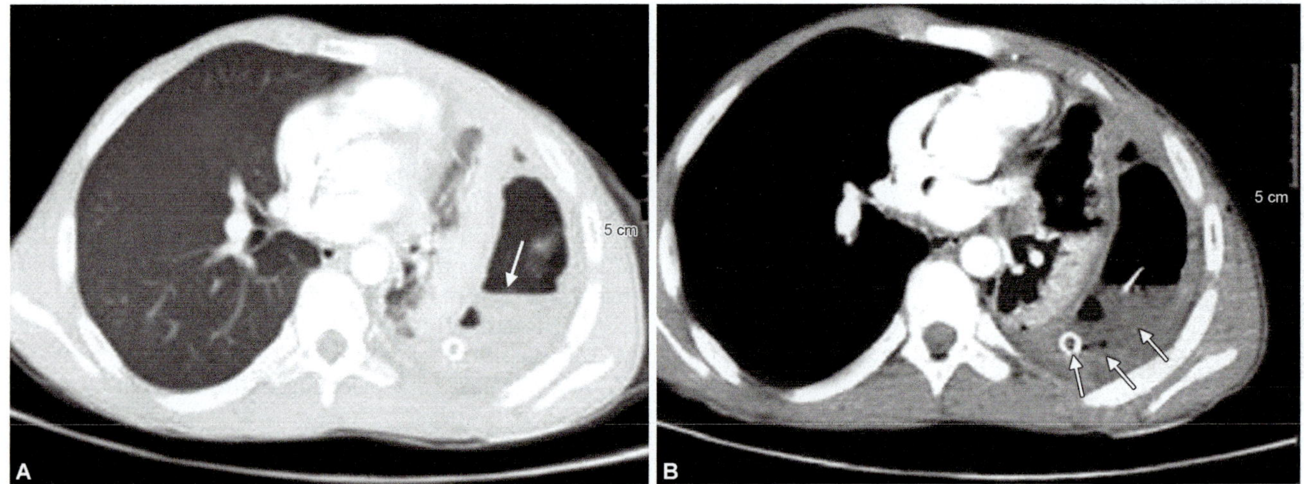

FIGS. 2A AND B: CT thorax (left-lung window, right-mediastinal window) showing left-sided loculated pleural effusion. (A) Single arrow shows the air fluid level with the intercostal tube within; (B) triple arrow shows the collapsed lung.

alone.[2,18,19] When the effusion is small and does not completely cover the dome of the diaphragm in a chest radiograph (PA view), it is safer to perform an ultrasound-guided aspiration. It is more accurate and reduces patient discomfort.[18] The presence of frank pus on thoracentesis is diagnostic of empyema; no further tests are needed to confirm the diagnosis. If not, the pleural fluid should be sent for microbiological and biochemical studies. Pus from empyema is also sent for microbiological cultures to aid in the choice of antibiotics. Tuberculous etiology should always be kept in mind while evaluating empyema in high-TB prevalence settings. It is our practice to perform pleural biopsy in all patients with exudative effusions or empyema, unless the effusion is of acute onset and preceded by a documented pneumonia.

PLEURAL FLUID ANALYSIS

In PPE, the fluid may vary between clear or straw colored and odorless to thick, purulent and foul smelling. Foul odor could indicate an anaerobic or mixed (aerobic and anaerobic) etiology. Absence of foul smell, however, does not rule out an anaerobic infection.[20] After gross examination, the pleural fluid is tested for proteins, LDH, glucose, and pH. The pleural fluid from PPEs and empyemas is an exudate; presence of a transudate on the basis of the light's criteria suggests an alternative diagnosis. The presence of a predominance of lymphocytes should raise the possibility of malignancy or tuberculosis. A sample is sent for microbiological studies—Gram stain, aerobic cultures, mycobacterial, and fungal cultures, as deemed necessary.

If the resources permit, anaerobic cultures too should be done on all exudative effusions of undetermined etiology. In countries, like India, with a high prevalence of tuberculosis, in addition to histopathology, pleural biopsy specimen should be sent for Xpert MTB/RIF test and for mycobacterial cultures, as also pleural fluid sample. The microbiologic diagnostic yield from tissue in tuberculosis is higher than from the pleural fluid.

In the absence of purulent fluid and positive microbiology, biochemical markers are used as surrogates for evidence of active pleural infection.

Fluid drainage is imperative in the presence of purulence of fluid. It is well understood that PPE with an acidic pH (<7.20) is more likely to run a complicated course with loculated fluid collections and empyema; when compared to an effusion with pH > 7.20. Intercostal drainage is instituted to avert this complication, antibiotic treatment alone may not suffice.[21,22] Furthermore, there is more likelihood of the need for surgical intervention in those with an acidic pH (<7.20).

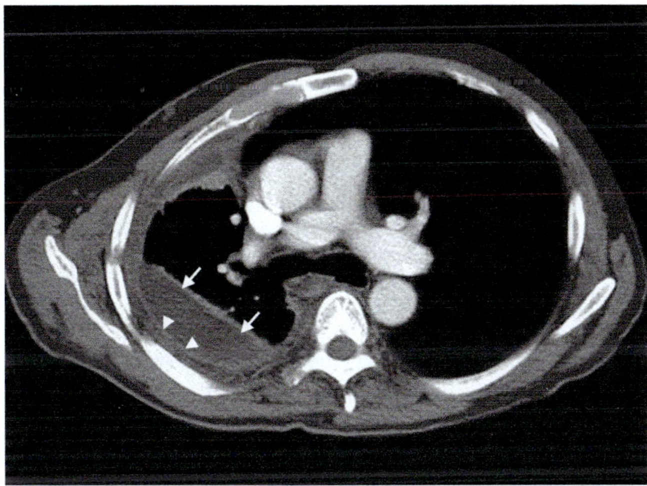

FIG. 3: CT thorax (mediastinal window) showing split-pleura sign. Arrowheads show thickened and enhanced parietal pleura and arrows show enhanced visceral pleura.

False-positive acidic pH measurement can be seen in malignant effusion, tuberculosis, rheumatoid, and lupus pleuritis. Since pleural fluid pH is crucial to decision-making, the fluid should be collected in a heparinized syringe, without contamination with lignocaine (which is acidic), and analyzed immediately using a blood gas analyzer. Measurement of pH should not be performed on obviously purulent pleural fluid, as it may damage the blood gas analyzer. Moreover, tube drainage should be instituted, regardless of the pH value in case of purulent effusion. The PPE caused by *Proteus* is known to present paradoxically with alkalotic pleural fluid pH, because the *Proteus* split urea to produce ammonia.[23,24]

It is well known that a significant proportion of bacterial pleural infection is caused by anaerobic bacteria which do not grow on aerobic culture media. The need to send anaerobic bacterial cultures on all exudative pleural effusions of undetermined etiology has been recommended by various authors. Availability of laboratory facilities, the logistics of suitable collection, and transport limits the implementation of this recommendation in resource-limited settings. In a study by Ferrer et al.,[25] there was a statistically (p = 0.03) superior bacteriological yield when pleural fluid was inoculated into blood culture vial, compared with inoculation by conventional method in suspected pleural infection. In a well-conducted study by Menzies et al.,[26] use of a blood culture bottle to culture pleural fluid in addition to conventional culture collected in a sterile tube, increased the proportion of patients with identifiable pathogens by 20.8%. This was true for both anaerobic and aerobic pathogens. In this study, the volume of culture inoculum (2, 5, or 10 mL) did not influence the yield. Thus, there is a case for direct blood culture bottle inoculation when infection is suspected.[21]

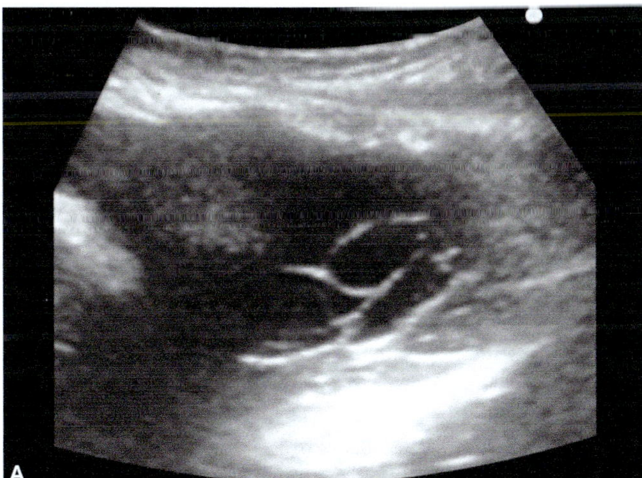

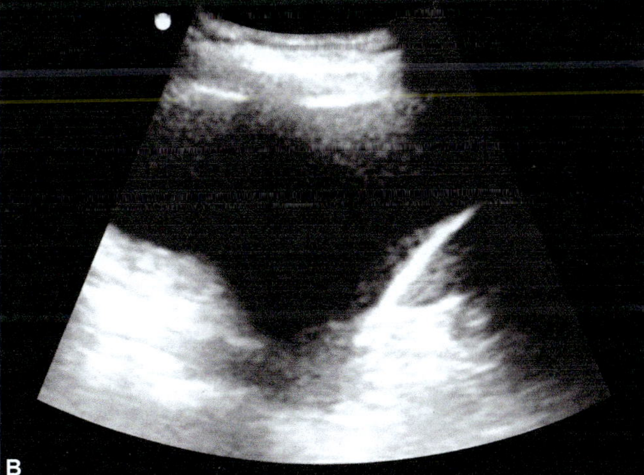

FIGS. 4A AND B: (A) Ultrasound image showing locules, septations, and echoic fluid of complex complicated parapneumonic effusion; (B) Ultrasound image showing anechoic pleural effusion of uncomplicated parapneumonic pleural effusion.

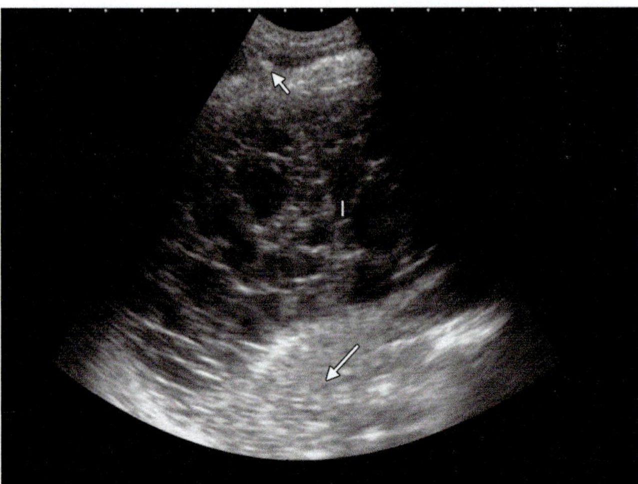

FIG. 5: Ultrasonogram chest showing multiple loculations. Short arrow indicates needle performing biopsy of the parietal pleura. Long arrow indicates collapsed lung.

Bad prognostic markers for PPEs and empyema are as follows:[27]

- Pus present in pleural space
- Gram stain of pleural fluid positive
- Pleural fluid glucose below 40 mg/dL
- Pleural fluid culture positive
- Pleura fluid pH 3× upper normal limit for serum
- Pleural fluid loculated

An expert panel from the American College of Chest Physicians has developed a new categorization of patients with PPEs.[24] This categorization is modeled on the tumor-node-metastasis (TNM) classification of tumors and is based upon the anatomy of the effusion, the bacteriology of the pleural fluid, and the chemistry of the pleural fluid **(Table 3)**.

TREATMENT

Prompt recognition is essential for optimal management of pleural infection. Antibiotic therapy and drainage of fluid collection constitute the cornerstone of management. The British Thoracic Society has drawn an excellent algorithm for the management of patients with pleural infection.[18]

Antibiotic Treatment

Antibiotics should be started as soon as possible whenever PPE or empyema is suspected or diagnosed. The empirical antibiotic should target anaerobic bacteria. Pleural pharmacokinetics in pleural infection are complex, due to the heterogeneity of patient presentation, with variable degrees of pleural thickening, pleural fluid characteristics and levels of inflammation, all of which are likely to influence penetration of antibiotics in the pleural space.[28]

Pleural penetration of aminoglycoside is poor and it gets inactivated in an acidic environment; hence, they should be avoided in empyema.[29,30] A study specifically addressing antibiotic levels in the empyema pleural fluid found that the equilibrium of serum and pleural fluid levels occurred most rapidly with penicillin and metronidazole;[28] guidelines also suggest these are an appropriate initial therapy.[29] Coamoxiclav is a reasonable option which can be considered with or without metronidazole; however, direct evidence for this is lacking. When risk for MRSA is low and highly resistant gram-negative infection is also low, a second-generation or a nonpseudomonal, third-generation cephalosporin (e.g., Ceftriaxone) or an Aminopenicillin with β-lactamase inhibitor (e.g., ampicillin/sulbactam) can be considered.[5] In case of hypersensitivity to penicillin, who cannot tolerate cephalosporins then respiratory Fluoroquinolone (Levofloxacin) plus Metronidazole, Monobactam (e.g., Aztreonam) plus Metronidazole, monotherapy with a Carbapenem can be considered. In significant proportion of MRSA infection alongwith resistant gram-negative bacteria and anaerobic bacteria infection, Vancomycin or Linezolid (for MRSA cover) + broad-spectrum anti-pseudomonas Cephalosporin (for gram-negative cover) + Metronidazole or Clindamycin (for anaerobic cover) can be considered. Risk factors for *Pseudomonas* infections (CAP and empyema) are: Immunocompromised states, chronic respiratory disease, enteral tube feeding, cerebrovascular disease, and other chronic neurological disorders. The presence of a pulmonary comorbidity (which included COPD, asthma, bronchiectasis, etc.) was the strongest predictor of *P. aeruginosa* pneumonia. Vancomycin + anti-pseudomonal, anti-beta-lactam/beta-lactamase inhibitor (Piperacillin + Tazobactum), Vancomycin + Carbapenems can be considered in such cases.[2] There is currently no role for intrapleural antibiotics in the routine treatment of pleural infection.[31] Intravenous antibiotics should be changed to oral therapy once there is clinical and objective evidence of improvement in sepsis.[29]

Cultures do not always grow pathogens, but may remain negative in up to 42% of the cases.[17] In community-acquired infection, the likely organisms include *Streptococcus milleri, Streptococcus pneumoniae,* staphylococci, and *Haemophilus influenzae.* Although the *Strep. milleri* group is highly sensitive, a substantial proportion of others are resistant to β-lactams.[27] "Atypical" bacteria constitute an exceedingly rare cause of pleural infection, although they can cause a simple PPE and anaerobic infection occurs in approximately 10%.[12] When cultures are negative, antibiotics should cover community-acquired or hospital-acquired pathogens as the case may be and anaerobes should be covered too. Antibiotic choice should be directed by the local policy guided by standard international and national recommendations; one such guideline is provided **(Table 4)**.

Empirical antibiotic regimen should be rationalized once culture results become available. Given the difficulty

TABLE 4: Illustrative antibiotic regimens for the initial treatment of culture negative pleural infection.

Origin of infection	Intravenous antibiotic treatment	Oral antibiotic treatment
Community-acquired culture negative pleural infection	Third-generation cephalosporin (e.g., *Ceftriaxone* or *Cefotaxime*) OR Single agent therapy with a beta-lactam/ beta-lactamase inhibitor combination (e.g., *Ampicillin–sulbactam*) *Note*: If allergic to penicillins, single-agent therapy with a carbapenem (e.g., *Imipenem, Meropenem) or* combine metronidazole with either a fluoroquinolone (e.g., *Levofloxacin*) or a monobactam (e.g., *Aztreonam*).	• Amoxycillin 1 g thrice daily + Clavulanic acid 125 mg thrice daily • Amoxycillin 1 g tds + Metronidazole 400 mg tds Clindamycin 300 mg qds
Hospital-acquired with culture negative pleural infection	• Piperacillin + Tazobactam 4.5 g qds IV • Ceftazidime 2 g tds IV • Meropenem 1 g tds IV ± Metronidazole 500 mg tds IV	Not applicable

in culturing anaerobic organisms, continuation of anti-anaerobic therapy is usually necessary. Direct data do not exist on how long to treat empyema. Antibiotics are often continued for at least 3 weeks,[29] based on clinical, biochemical, and radiological responses. Intravenous administration of antibiotics is often appropriate initially but should be changed to the oral route when objective clinical and biochemical improvement is seen.

Chest Drainage

There is consensus of opinion regarding the need of inter-costal tube drainage under the following circumstances:[2,21,27]

- Frank pus or turbid/cloudy fluid within the pleural space
- Presence of organisms identified by Gram stain or culture from (nonpurulent) effusion
- Effusion fluid with a pH < 7.2
- Large uncomplicated effusions for relief of dyspnea

Many experienced clinicians believe that a large-bore chest drain (>20 French) is necessary to treat empyema. However, studies with smaller-bore catheters (11–14 French) have shown equal success.[14,32,33] CT- or ultrasound-guided insertion of drain may be more optimal for an appropriate placement of the tube. In loculated effusions, the tube can be placed under guidance into the biggest locula. The role of suctioning and flushing the drainage tube with around 30 mL of sterile saline four times daily can be helpful, particularly when a small-bore chest tube is used. The optimal timing of drain removal is unknown, although clinical response is clearly the most important parameter. It is our practice to remove the drainage tube, when the drainage is <50 mL; provided the fluid is clear and non-turbid. If on the other hand the fluid is turbid, we remove it only after the drainage reduces to <10 mL.

Role of Medical Thoracoscopy in the Management of Parapneumonic Effusions

A few retrospective studies,[34-36] including a more recent study[37] with a review of existing literature, concluded that medical thoracoscopy is safe and effective in stage 1 and 2 thoracic empyema. Two of the studies[35,36] suggested the role of ultrasound in stratifying the patients amenable for medical thoracoscopy. In the study by Ravaglia et al.,[36] outcomes were described based on the stage of empyema. While stage 1 and 2 empyema had a success of 100% and 91%, respectively, the success in stage 3 empyema was only 50%. Since, stage 1 empyema is likely to do well even otherwise, thoracoscopy is likely unnecessary. The role of medical thoracoscopy appears to be more favorable in stage 2 empyema.

A prospective study[38] from Pakistan, recruited 160 patients with empyema including those with septations and loculations, with failure after initial therapy with chest drain and antibiotics. All of them were subjected to medical thoracoscopy and the documented success rate was 93.75% (complete resolution in 57.5%). The procedure contributed to the diagnosis of two thirds as of tuberculous etiology and 12.5% had adenocarcinoma. In addition to successful treatment of empyema, the role of medical thoracoscopy in establishing an etiologic diagnosis emerged from this study. The only randomized controlled trial (RCT)[39] on medical thoracoscopy in complicated PPE and empyema was from Egypt, with the comparator arm receiving treatment with chest drain and streptokinase. The medical thoracoscopy arm did well with significantly more clearance on CT and shorter hospital stay of 2 days. While medical thoracoscopy seems to be a reasonable option in stage 2 and 3 empyema patients, who are not fit for surgical intervention; more evidence is required before recommending its routine use. The availability and expertise needed for medical thoracoscopy in the country are likely to be limiting factors for its upfront use.

From the evaluation of available evidence, we feel medical thoracoscopy may have a role in stage 2 empyema. While in stage 3 empyema, it could fail half of the time and its role is not well established.

Intrapleural Fibrinolytics

Loculated pleural collections pose a challenge in the treatment, by hampering efforts at drainage which can also lead to failure of "medical treatment." While intrapleural fibrinolysis was used extensively, the MIST 1 study,[32]—a large trial conducted across 52 UK hospitals—showed no difference between intrapleural streptokinase and saline. The routine use of fibrinolytic agents alone at this point is not supported by evidence.

While there was only limited success with intrapleural fibrinolytic agents, the observation that DNA is the main cause of viscosity of empyema fluid has led to the hypothesis that intrapleural administration of the enzyme deoxyribonuclease (DNase) might reduce empyema fluid viscosity and thus, improve the drainage of pleural fluid. To examine the role of intrapleural DNase with and without concomitant tissue plasminogen activator (TPA) and to resolve the conflicting information about the utility of fibrinolytic agents, a clinical trial randomly assigned 210 patients with empyema to one of four intrapleural treatment groups, which were as follows: 10 mg intrapleural TPA twice daily for 3 days, 5 mg intrapleural DNase twice daily for 3 days, both TPA and DNase twice daily for 3 days, or double placebo. Tubes were clamped for 1 hour after each intrapleural dose administration. Combination TPA-DNase therapy resulted in a greater decrease in the radiographic pleural opacity, a lower rate of surgical referral [odds ratio 0.17; 95% confidence interval (CI) 0.03–0.87], and a shorter hospital stay (–6.7 days; 95% CI, –12.0 to –1.9) compared with placebo. Neither of the individual agents performed better than placebo, although the numbers were small. A systematic review and meta-analysis.[40] Subsequently published in CHEST, which included seven RCTs that compared fibrinolytic therapy and placebo, with a total number of 801 patients, concluded that there was insufficient evidence to support the routine use of this therapy for all PPEs/empyemas.

Overall, it may be concluded that there is no clear proven benefit of streptokinase or urokinase administered intrapleurally in the treatment of bacterial pleural infection. However, a combination of t-PA and DNase in patients with stage 2 bacterial pleural infection improves fluid drainage, and reduces the need for surgical referral and the duration of the hospital stay.

Surgical Treatment

Medical therapy fails in up to 30% of patients with empyema. No good-quality data exists on the optimum timing of surgery and indications for surgical referral. Patients who do not improve clinically and radiologically after 7 days of standard treatment, can derive benefit from surgical interventions.[41] Video-assisted thoracic surgery (VATS) is the next possible step in the treatment of empyema, when tube drainage has failed. The European Association of Cardio Thoracic Surgery (EACTS) in its position statement in 2015[42] and the American Association for Thoracic Surgery expert consensus guidelines[43] recommend that all stage 2 and 3 empyema should undergo a surgical intervention, claiming a benefit for surgical debridement over chest drain alone in terms of success and duration of hospital stay. However, the British Thoracic Society (BTS) guidelines of 2010[29] recommends referral to the thoracic surgeons only when there is failure or persistent sepsis after drainage and antibiotics in all empyemas. This is our practice also.

Nutrition

Patients with empyema enter a catabolic state; hence, good nutrition is vital. It has been observed that patients with low serum albumin have a worse outcome from empyema.[44] Although no trial has addressed this issue, an aggressive nutritional support is important for the patients.

Flowchart 1 demonstrates a proposed algorithm for the management of pleural infections.

SUMMARY

Parapneumonic effusion accompanies an infective illness such as bacterial pneumonia, lung abscess, or bronchiectasis. Its presence indicates greater degree of severity and the mortality rate in such patients is higher than in those patients without PPE. Medical management remains the same but aspiration may be needed if there is significant degree of effusion. Surgical management may be needed in the presence of empyema or other complications. Patients with empyema also need good nutrition because of a catabolic state. Outcomes are worse in patients with low serum albumin have a worse outcome from empyema. An aggressive nutritional support is important for the patients.

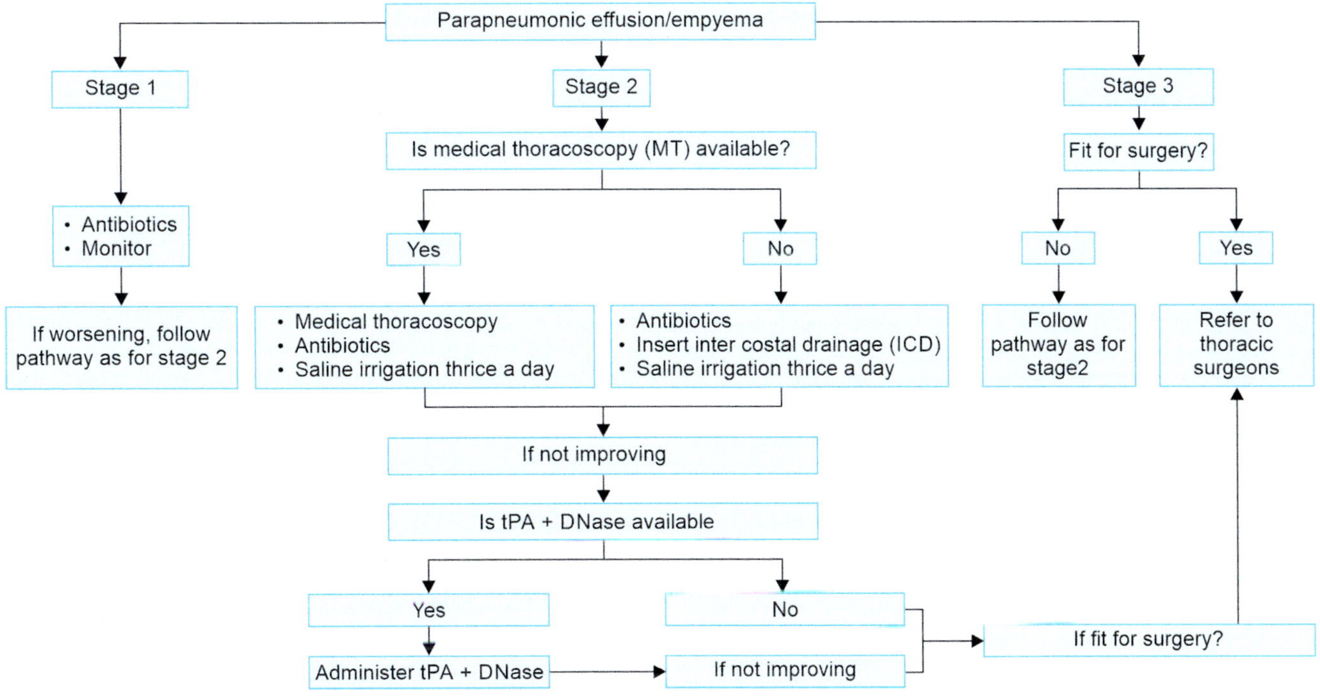

FLOWCHART 1: A proposed algorithm for the management of pleural infections.
(DNase: deoxyribonuclease; TPA: tissue plasminogen activator)

REFERENCES

1. Bye MR. Pleural Diseases, 3rd ed. By Richard W. Light. Baltimore: Williams & Wilkins Co., 1995, 361 pp. Pediatr Pulmonol. 1996;21(6):398-9.
2. Light RW. Parapneumonic effusions and empyema. Proc Am Thorac Soc. 2006;3(1):75-80.
3. Kroegel C, Antony VB. Immunobiology of pleural inflammation: Potential implications for pathogenesis, diagnosis and therapy. Eur Respir J. 1997;10(10):2411-8.
4. Hamm H, Light RW. Parapneumonic effusion and empyema. Eur Respir J. 1997;10(5):1150-6.
5. Neff CC, vanSonnenberg E, Lawson DW, et al. CT follow up of empyemas: pleural peels resolve after percutaneous catheter drainage. Radiology. 1990;176(1):195-7.
6. Reddy SI, Varaprasad K, Narahari N, et al. Clinical and etiological profile of an exudative pleural effusion in a tertiary care center. Indian J Respir Care. 2019;8(1):22.
7. Chinchkar NJ, Talwar D, Jain SK. A stepwise approach to the etiologic diagnosis of pleural effusion in respiratory intensive care unit and short-term evaluation of treatment. Lung India Off Organ Indian Chest Soc. 2015;32(2):107-15.
8. Parikh P, Odhwani J, Ganagajalia C. Study of 100 cases of pleural effusion with reference to diagnostic approach. Int J Adv Med. 2016;3(2):328-31.
9. Gupta R, Gupta A, Ilyas M. Spectrum of pleural effusion etiology revisited in 18–70 years of age group: A tertiary care center-based study of 1000 patients. CHRISMED J Health Res. 2018;5:110-3.
10. Finley C, Clifton J, Fitzgerald JM, et al. Empyema: An increasing concern in Canada. Can Respir J. 2008;15(2):85-9.
11. Grijalva CG, Zhu Y, Nuorti JP, et al. Emergence of parapneumonic empyema in the USA. Thorax. 2011;66(8):663-8.
12. Mohanty S, Kapil A, Das BK. Bacteriology of parapneumonic pleural effusions in an Indian hospital. Trop Doct. 2007;37(4):228-9.
13. Brook I, Frazier EH. Aerobic and anaerobic microbiology of empyema. A retrospective review in two military hospitals. Chest. 1993;103(5):1502-7.
14. Maskell NA, Davies CWH, Nunn AJ, et al. UK Controlled trial of intrapleural streptokinase for pleural infection. N Engl J Med. 2005;352(9):865-74.
15. Chen KY, Liaw YS, Wang HC, et al. Sonographic septation: a useful prognostic indicator of acute thoracic empyema. J Ultrasound Med Off J Am Inst Ultrasound Med. 2000;19(12):837-43.
16. Yang PC, Luh KT, Chang DB, et al. Value of sonography in determining the nature of pleural effusion: Analysis of 320 cases. AJR Am J Roentgenol. 1992;159(1):29-33.
17. Maskell NA, Batt S, Hedley EL, et al. The bacteriology of pleural infection by genetic and standard methods and its mortality significance. Am J Respir Crit Care Med. 2006;174(7):817-23.
18. Balfour-Lynn IM, Abrahamson E, Cohen G, et al. BTS guidelines for the management of pleural infection in children. Thorax. 2005;60(suppl 1):i1-21.
19. Sahn SA. Diagnosis and management of parapneumonic effusions and empyema. Clin Infect Dis Off Publ Infect Dis Soc Am. 2007;45(11):1480-6.
20. Shen KR, Bribriesco A, Crabtree T, et al. The American Association for Thoracic Surgery consensus guidelines for the management of empyema. J Thorac Cardiovasc Surg. 2017;153(6):e129-46.

21. Davies HE, Davies RJO, Davies CWH. Management of pleural infection in adults: British Thoracic Society pleural disease guideline 2010. Thorax. 2010;65(Suppl 2):ii41-53.
22. Jiménez Castro D, Díaz Nuevo G, et al. Pleural fluid parameters identifying complicated parapneumonic effusions. Respir Int Rev Thorac Dis. 2005;72(4):357-64.
23. Earasi K, Welch C, Zelickson A, et al. Proteus empyema as a rare complication from an infected renal cyst, a case report. BMC Pulm Med. 2020;20(1):314.
24. Pine JR, Hollman JL. Elevated pleural fluid pH in Proteus mirabilis empyema. Chest. 1983;84(1):109-11.
25. Ferrer A, Osset J, Alegre J, et al. Prospective clinical and microbiological study of pleural effusions. Eur J Clin Microbiol Infect Dis off Publ Eur Soc Clin Microbiol. 1999;18(4):237-41.
26. Menzies SM, Rahman NM, Wrightson JM, et al. Blood culture bottle culture of pleural fluid in pleural infection. Thorax. 2011;66(8):658-62.
27. Singh S, Singh SK, Tentu AK. Management of parapneumonic effusion and empyema. J Assoc Chest Physician. 2019;7(2):51-8.
28. Teixeira LR, Sasse SA, Villarino MA, et al. Antibiotic levels in empyemic pleural fluid. Chest. 2000;117(6):1734-9.
29. Davies HE, Davies RJO, Davies CWH; on behalf of the BTS Pleural Disease Guideline Group. Management of pleural infection in adults: British Thoracic Society pleural disease guideline 2010. Thorax. 2010;65(Suppl 2):ii41-53.
30. Vaudaux P, Waldvogel F. Gentamicin inactivation in purulent exudates: Role of cell lysis. J Infect Dis. 1980;142(4):586-93.
31. Bedawi EO, Hassan M, McCracken D, et al. Pleural infection: A closer look at the etiopathogenesis, microbiology and role of antibiotics. Expert Rev Respir Med. 2019;13(4):337-47.
32. Rahman NM, Maskell NA, West A, et al. Intrapleural Use of Tissue Plasminogen Activator and DNase in Pleural Infection. N Engl J Med. 2011;365(6):518-26.
33. Shen KR, Bribriesco A, Crabtree T, et al. The American Association for Thoracic Surgery consensus guidelines for the management of empyema. J Thorac Cardiovasc Surg. 2017;153(6):e129-46.
34. Solèr M, Wyser C, Bolliger CT. Treatment of early parapneumonic empyema by "medical" thoracoscopy. Schweiz Med Wochenschr. 1997;127(42):1748-53.
35. Brutsche MH, Tassi GF, Györik S, et al. Treatment of sonographically stratified multiloculated thoracic empyema by medical thoracoscopy. Chest. 2005;128(5):3303-9.
36. Ravaglia C, Gurioli C, Tomassetti S, et al. Is medical thoracoscopy efficient in the management of multiloculated and organized thoracic empyema? Respiration. 2012;84(3):219-24.
37. Hardavella G, Papakonstantinou NA, Karampinis I, et al. Hippocrates Quoted "If an empyema does not rupture, death will occur": Is medical thoracoscopy able to make it rupture safely? J Bronchol Interv Pulmonol. 2017;24(1):15-20.
38. Sumalani KK, Rizvi NA, Asghar A. Role of medical Thoracoscopy in the Management of Multiloculated Empyema. BMC Pulm Med. 2018;18(1):179.
39. Hewidy A, Elshafey M. Medical thoracoscopy versus intrapleural fibrinolytic therapy in complicated parapneumonic effusion and empyema. Egypt J Chest Dis Tuberc. 2014;63(4):889-96.
40. Janda S, Swiston J. Intrapleural fibrinolytic therapy for treatment of adult parapneumonic effusions and empyemas: a systematic review and meta-analysis. Chest. 2012;142(2):401-11.
41. Colice GL, Curtis A, Deslauriers J, et al. Medical and surgical treatment of parapneumonic effusions: an evidence-based guideline. Chest. 2000;118(4):1158-71.
42. Scarci M, Abah U, Solli P, et al. EACTS expert consensus statement for surgical management of pleural empyema. Eur J Cardio-Thorac Surg Off J Eur Assoc Cardio-Thorac Surg. 2015;48(5):642-53.
43. Shen KR, Bribriesco A, Crabtree T, et al. The American Association for Thoracic Surgery consensus guidelines for the management of empyema. J Thorac Cardiovasc Surg. 2017;153(6):e129-46.
44. Ferguson AD, Prescott RJ, Selkon JB, et al. The clinical course and management of thoracic empyema. QJM Mon J Assoc Physicians. 1996;89(4):285-9.

CHAPTER

129

Tuberculous Pleural Effusion

Dharmesh Patel, Radhika Banka

INTRODUCTION

Tuberculosis (TB) remains a serious health problem globally. While nearly a quarter of the global population is estimated to be infected with the bacteria, approximately 5–10% will develop active disease.[1] Extrapulmonary TB (EPTB) accounts for 15–20% of the total TB cases in immunocompetent hosts while this proportion may be as high as 50% in patients infected with human immunodeficiency virus (HIV).[2] Tuberculous pleural effusion (TPE) is the second most common manifestation of EPTB after lymph node TB.[2] According to the India TB Report, out of the 2.42 million notified TB cases in 2022, around 24% cases had EPTB; most common sites being lymph node (26.3%) and pleura (23.3%).[3] TPE is the leading cause of an effusion in our country. In the HIV-infected population, TPE is the most common cause of a lymphocytic effusion and the pleura is the primary site of infection in 30% of patients.[4]

PATHOPHYSIOLOGY

Traditionally, TPE is thought to develop secondary to rupture of a subpleural caseous focus in the lung into the pleural space. The subsequent pleural inflammation causes an increase in parietal pleural capillary permeability and occlusion of the lymphatic stoma leading to pleural fluid formation. The cellular component is initially dominated by polymorphonuclear leukocytes, particularly neutrophils followed by macrophage influx, peaking after 3 days, and thereafter a prolonged lymphocyte-driven intense T-helper type 1 (Th1) cell-mediated delayed hypersensitivity reaction. This leads to release of adenosine deaminase (ADA), gamma interferon (IFN-γ), interleukin 12 (IL-12), and various other cytokines. TPE have a markedly higher proportion of Th cells than serum or peripheral blood, a phenomenon known as "compartmentalization."

These factors have led to the conclusion that TPE is a delayed hypersensitivity reaction rather than true pleural infection and hence characterized by the paucibacillary nature of the effusion and low yield on TB culture. The role of a delayed hypersensitivity reaction is further evidenced by development of an exudative pleural effusion when tuberculous protein is injected into the pleural spaces of guinea pigs sensitized to purified protein derivative and suppression of the effusion when these sensitized guinea pigs are given antilymphocyte serum. Recent studies have shown increasing yield of TB bacilli from pleural fluid and pleural tissue suggesting direct infiltration of TB bacilli in the pleural space, also as a mechanism for development of TPE.[5]

CLINICAL FEATURES

Prior to the advent of antituberculous treatment, the natural course of TPE was spontaneous resolution within 2–4 months. In the past, 65% of these patients developed active pulmonary tuberculosis within 5 years—independent of the initial size of effusion and residual radiological abnormalities.[6] Patients with TPE in endemic countries tend to be younger in comparison to nonendemic countries, possibly because reactivation predominates over primary infection as the mechanism of development of disease in the latter.[7] TPE typically present as an acute-to-subacute illness with the most frequent symptoms being cough (~70%), which is usually nonproductive and chest pain (~70%), which is usually pleuritic in nature. If both cough and pleuritic pain are present, the pain usually precedes the cough. Most patients are febrile but approximately 15% will be afebrile.[8] TPE should be suspected when chest pain precedes cough, peripheral white blood cell count is not raised, purulent material in the cough is absent and the pleural fluid is clear.[9] Symptoms of TPE tend to be more pronounced in patients with HIV. These patients have a longer duration of illness, milder chest pain, and higher rates of systemic features such as night sweats, fatigue, and weight loss.[10]

DIAGNOSIS

Pleural Fluid Analysis

Cell Count

Tuberculous pleural effusion typically tends to be a lymphocytic predominant effusion, ranging from 50% to

90% of the total pleural fluid cell count. A neutrophilic response is seen within the first few days; but can remain persistently neutrophilic predominant in around 10% cases. In a single-center cohort, neutrophilic-predominant TPE was associated with higher rates of fever, higher rates of decortication, and a higher inflammatory effusion.[11] Pleural fluid loculations and tuberculous empyema are also associated with a neutrophilic predominance. TPE rarely has scattered mesothelial cells. Mesothelial cells are cells that cover both the visceral and parietal pleura. The intense lymphocytic infiltration in TPE covers both the pleural surfaces and prevents the mesothelial cells from entering the pleural space. Four different series have confirmed that patients with TPE rarely contain >5% mesothelial cells. Eosinophilia > 10% in the pleural fluid is also an uncommon finding in TPE.

Biochemistry

Pleural fluid with a TPE is invariably an exudate characterized by raised protein > 30 g/L seen in 60–77% of cases and elevated lactate dehydrogenase (LDH) levels are present in >75% of cases and often exceed 500 IU/L. Pleural fluid glucose concentration in TPE is usually in the range of 3.3–5.6 mmol/L, with glucose levels < 2.8 mmol/L seen in 7–20% cases, while extremely low glucose concentration (<1.7 mol/L) may suggest a tuberculous empyema. The pleural fluid pH is usually <7.40 with values below 7.30 in about 20% of cases; pH < 7.2 indicates a possible empyema.[4,12]

Adenosine Deaminase

Adenosine deaminase is a purine-degrading predominant T-lymphocyte enzyme that catalyzes the conversion of adenosine and deoxyadenosine to inosine and deoxyinosine, respectively. The enzyme has two isoforms: ADA1 which is found in all cells but particularly in lymphocytes and monocytes while ADA2 is found only in monocytes. ADA2 is the predominant isoform that is raised in patients with TPE.[13] Testing for ADA in pleural fluid is an inexpensive and rapid method for establishing the diagnosis of TPE, especially in resource-limited settings. The diagnostic utility of ADA is highly dependent on the local prevalence of TB. Its primary utility is in low-prevalence settings for its negative predictive value. In populations with a high prevalence of TB and clinical suspicion of TB effusion, elevated ADA level might be considered as a confirmatory test justifying treatment initiation.

In a recent meta-analysis involving more than 27,000 patients, pleural fluid ADA had a good sensitivity of 0.92 and specificity of 0.90 for diagnosis TPE.[14] Various other diseases can cause an increase in ADA; nearly one third of parapneumonic effusions and two thirds of empyemas have ADA levels > 40 U/L. Other causes of elevated ADA are HIV infection, lung cancer, mesothelioma, lymphoma, rheumatoid arthritis, brucellosis, Q fever, and hemorrhagic effusions.[15] ADA levels may be low in early pleural disease and repeat testing might be needed. Elderly patients and smokers may also have low ADA levels.[15]

The optimum pleural fluid ADA cutoff for diagnosing TPE has remained a subject of debate. In general, ADA levels >70 IU/L are highly suggestive of TPE, whereas levels <40 IU/L are more helpful in excluding disease. A cutoff of 40 U/L has a sensitivity and specificity of 0.93 and 0.90, respectively. When pleural fluid ADA is >250 IU/L, bacterial empyema or lymphoid malignancy should be considered.[16]

Adenosine deaminase has two molecular forms: ADA-1 and ADA-2. ADA-1 is found in all cells and has greatest activity in lymphocytes and monocytes, while ADA-2 is found only in monocytes. ADA-2 is raised in TPE which seems paradoxical as ADA-1 comes from lymphocytes and TPE are lymphocytic-rich effusions. However, ADA subtype assessment has shown to provide little diagnostic benefit and does not fare better than total ADA measurement and hence is not used routinely.[17] Various other markers such as LDH, carcinoembryonic antigen (CEA), and lymphocyte-to-neutrophil ratio have been studied in combination with ADA, but none of them has shown increased sensitivity for diagnosis of TPE as compared to ADA alone.[18,19]

Other Tests

Interferon Gamma (IFN)

IFN is released from activated CD4 + T lymphocytes, primarily functioning as an activator of macrophages that increases their mycobactericidal activity. Pleural fluid IFN has been studied as a marker to distinguish TPE from nontuberculous effusions. Similar to ADA, cutoff values and specificity for IFN have remained a matter of controversy. Similar to ADA, levels of IFN are sometimes elevated with hematologic malignancies and empyemas.[20] A meta-analysis of 67 eligible studies showed a high sensitivity of 0.93 and specificity of 0.96 for unstimulated IFN to diagnose TPE but there was wide heterogeneity.[20] ADA and IFN were compared in a recent meta-analysis that analyzed more than 4,000 evaluations of patients with TPE and nearly 5,000 evaluations of non-TPE.[21-23] The authors also concluded that for TPE diagnosis, IFN combined with ADA could improve specificity up to 100% by reducing sensitivity.[22] However, the biggest challenges are unavailability and high cost of IFN and hence is not used routinely.

Interferon Gamma-release Assays (IGRA)

IGRAs such as the QuantiFERON-TB Gold (QIAGEN) and T-SPOT.TB (Oxford Immunotec) are conventional tests to detect latent TB. In a meta-analysis analyzing IGRA on pleural fluid, the results were disappointing with pooled sensitivity and specificity at 75% and 79%, respectively, similar to findings of IGRA on blood. Hence, IGRA testing on pleural fluid for diagnosis of TPE is not recommended.[23]

Lysozyme (LP)

LP is a low-molecular-weight bacteriolytic protein present in various body fluids and passively enters the pleural space through blood. Activated macrophages in tuberculous granulomas secrete lysozyme and hence, pleural fluid lysozyme and pleural fluid to serum lysozyme (LP/LS) is raised in TPE and is useful in differentiating TPE from nontuberculous effusions.[24] Given its poor specificity, poorly automated and time-consuming assays, this test has not been widely adopted. High pleural LP levels are associated with residual pleural thickening in patients with TPE.[25]

Tumor Necrosis Factor (TNF)

TNF plays an important role in formation of granulomas and enhances mycobacterial killing by macrophages in patients with TPE. Data initially suggested that measurement of pleural fluid TNF could help distinguish TPE from nontuberculous effusions. Overall sensitivity and specificity of TNF to diagnose TPE was 79% and 82%, respectively.[26] Pleural fluid TNF is markedly raised in TPE and parapneumonic effusion as compared to malignant pleural effusion. TNF has poor diagnostic accuracy and is not routinely recommended for diagnosis of TPE.[26]

Microbiological Analysis

Acid-fast Bacilli Smear

Acid-fast bacilli (AFB) smear is rarely positive in TPE given its paucibacillary nature and for AFB smear to be positive, AFB density of >10,000/mL in the pleural fluid is needed. Less than 10% of patients with TPE have a positive AFB smear, increases to 20% in the HIV population, and TB empyema indicating higher bacillary loads in these cohorts.[27]

Mycobacterium tuberculosis Culture

Mycobacterium tuberculosis (M.tb) culture requires much less viable material and is more sensitive as compared to AFB smear. The yield of mycobacterial culture of pleural fluid depends on the culture medium used. Solid media such as Lowenstein-Jensen medium has a <30% yield and a longer time to culture positivity as compared to liquid media. Liquid media such as BACTEC-MGIT semiautomated system or Bactec 9120 Myco/F lytic blood culture system are preferred as they are associated with increased yield ranging from 40 to 70% and shorter turnaround time for culture positivity.[28]

Pleural Fluid *M.tb* Polymerase Chain Reaction

Cartridge-based polymerase chain reaction (PCR) tests such as Xpert MTB Rif (Cepheid California) have revolutionized diagnostics in pulmonary tuberculosis by increasing yield and providing information on rifampicin resistance within 2 hours of running the test. In 2014, the World Health Organization (WHO) endorsed Xpert MTB/RIF as the first line of testing for pulmonary tuberculosis. In a recent Cochrane review involving 25 studies on Xpert MTB/RIF for TPE diagnosis, pooled sensitivity and specificity against culture were 49.5% and 98.9%, respectively.[29] The Xpert MTB RIF Ultra assay was developed to increase diagnostic sensitivity as it has a limit of detection of 16 bacterial colony forming units (CFU) per milliliter compared to 114 CFU/mL for Xpert MTB/RIF. The pooled sensitivity and specificity of Xpert MTB/RIF Ultra based on four studies for diagnosis of TPE against culture were 75.0% and 87.0%, respectively, which is a significant improvement in sensitivity compared to the prior assay.[29] Given its easy availability, minimal technical assistance, rapid turnaround time, and improved sensitivity with Xpert MTB/RIF Ultra, these PCR-based tests are a useful addition to TPE diagnosis.

Sputum Examination

Sputum culture has a low yield but TB may be positive in up to 55% patients even in the absence of appreciable parenchymal infiltrates, hence should be obtained when possible.[30]

Pleural Biopsy

Pleural tissue can be obtained under direct vision by thoracoscopy or as closed biopsy (with or without ultrasound guidance). Thoracoscopic appearance of TPE includes random and diffuse involvement of the parietal pleura with nodules, pleural pustules, hyperemia, and increased vascularization, plaque-like appearances, rarely ulcerations, and miliary lesions **(Fig. 1)**. Appearance of small uniform pleural nodules, also called as pleural pustule have a 93% positivity on Xpert MTB/RIF **(Fig. 2)**.[31,32] TB empyemas are characterized by the presence of septations and pus formation. Thoracoscopy offers the advantage of direct visualization of the pleura, procurement of larger biopsy samples, can be performed in the outpatient setting with an excellent safety profile and increases the diagnostic sensitivity to nearly 100% when histology is used.[5,31] Diagnostic yield of pleural tissue Xpert MTB/RIF is reported to be as high as 85% with thoracoscopic biopsies.[33] However, it is limited

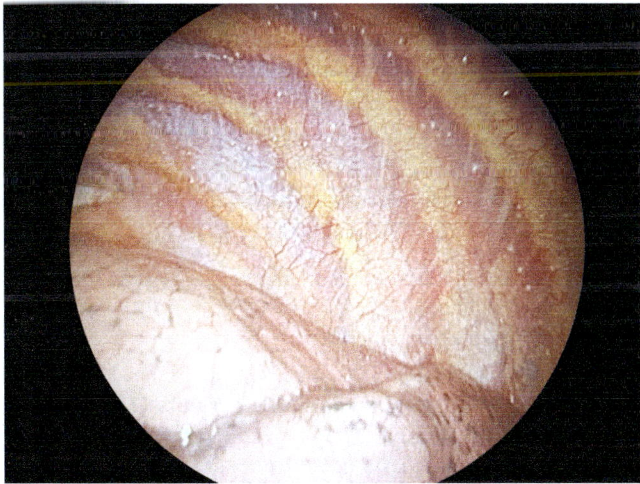

FIG. 1: Thoracoscopic pleural tuberculosis (TB) miliary lesions.

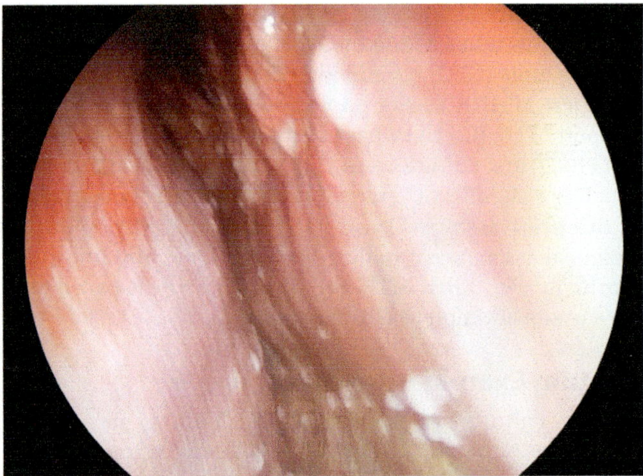

FIG. 2: Thoracoscopic pleural tuberculosis (TB) nodules.

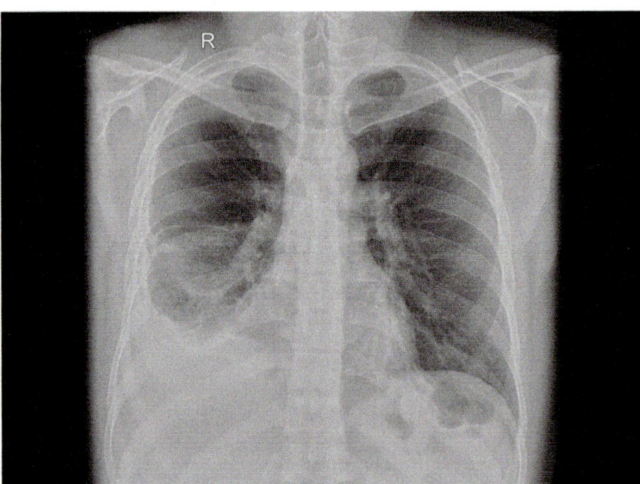

FIG. 4: Chest X-ray tuberculous effusion.

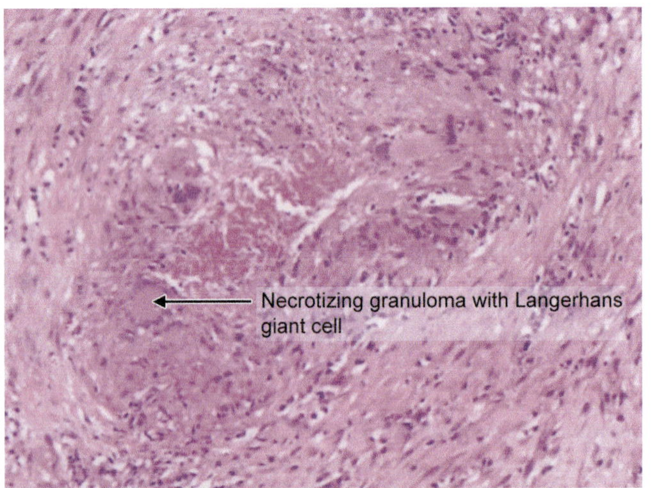

FIG. 3: Tuberculosis (TB) pleural biopsy histopathology.

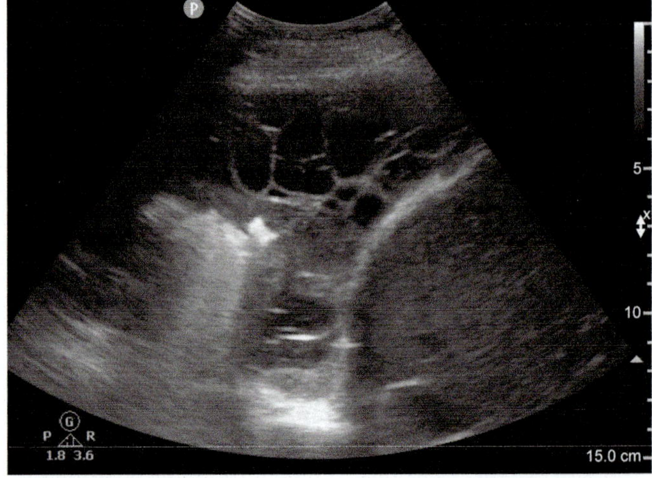

FIG. 5: Pleural ultrasound tuberculosis (TB) septation.

by its availability and hence, closed pleural biopsy also remains an option for TPE diagnosis. Closed pleural biopsy can be blind performed by Abrams needle which is simple to perform and is a cost-effective way to obtain pleural tissue. Sensitivity for histopathology varies from 40 to 70%.[34] Given the high sensitivity and specificity, thoracoscopy combined with histopathology and microbiological evaluation remains the gold standard for TPE diagnosis **(Fig. 3)**.

Radiology

Chest Radiograph

TPE are typically unilateral with a slightly higher right-sided predominance seen in around 55% patients **(Fig. 4)**. They tend to be small to moderate in size occupying around one third to two thirds of the hemithorax in nearly 80% of the cases. However, neither the side nor the size of the effusion has been reported to have a bearing on prognosis. There is likely a higher incidence of pleural effusion in drug-resistant TB than drug-sensitive TB.[35] Reported rates of concomitant parenchymal abnormalities on chest radiograph range from 20 to 50% in various studies and are usually seen on the ipsilateral side in the form of infiltrates or cavitary lesions.[7,36] Occasionally, transient parenchymal nodular infiltrates and increase in effusion may be seen during TPE treatment, and this may represent a paradoxical reaction due to enhanced immune response.[37]

Ultrasound

TPE on ultrasound can appear anechoic, echogenic, or septated **(Fig. 5)**. Septations appear as thin white strands, which could be freely moving within the pleural fluid or densely adhered. Data suggests that a complex septated effusion and a positive TB culture are associated with a higher risk (odds ratio: 145 and 20, respectively) of developing residual pleural thickening > 10 mm at the end

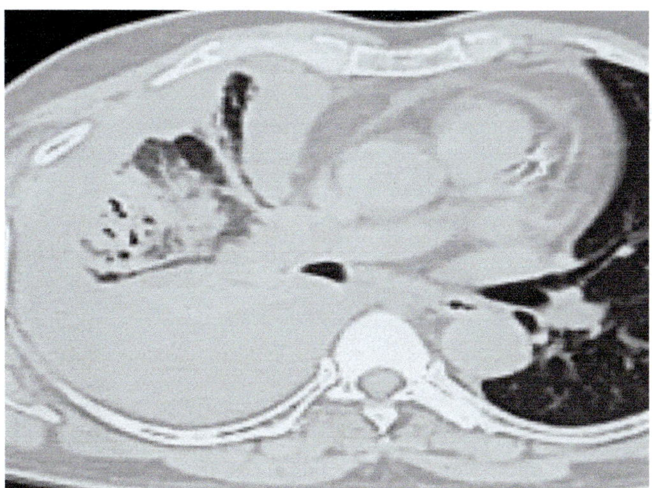

FIG. 6: CT chest in tuberculous effusion.

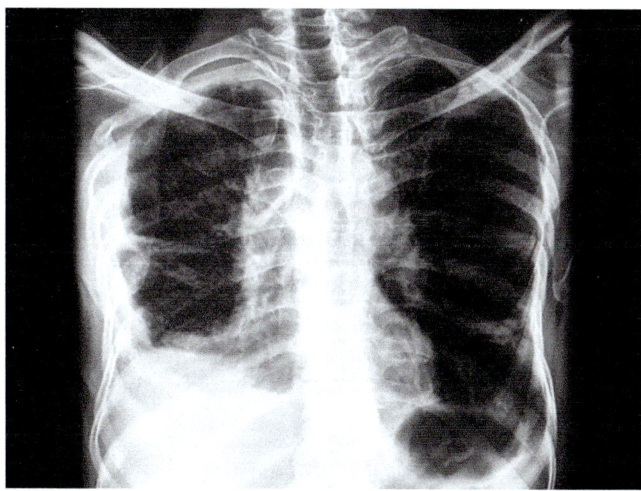

FIG. 7: Chest X-ray post-tuberculosis (TB) pleural thickening.

of 1 year.[38] Septated effusions are associated with a higher microbiological yield possibly due to a higher bacterial load.[39] Thoracic ultrasound has also become the standard of care while performing pleural procedures and can particularly help while performing pleural biopsies as can be done under direct vision or can assist the operator to select the optimum site.

Computed Tomography (CT) Chest

It improves visualization of parenchymal involvement in TPE. Studies have shown that parenchymal involvement can be as high as 80% when CT chest is concomitantly performed for TPE diagnosis. Most common findings include subpleural distribution of micronodules followed by interlobular septal thickening, consolidation, and cavitation **(Fig. 6)**.[40] CT chest is also more sensitive to diagnose residual pleural thickening as compared to thoracic ultrasound.

Positron Emission Tomography/CT (PET/CT)

The ^{18}F-fluorodeoxyglucose (FDG)-PET CT is an integrated metabolic and anatomical imaging technique, which may have some utility in differentiating TPE from malignant pleural effusion. Diffuse pleural uptake on PET is reported to have a sensitivity of 60% for TPE diagnosis.[41] There is no difference between SUVmax uptake between TPE and malignant effusions. PET-CT has also been used to differentiate active from inactive disease, and to monitor treatment.[41,42] However, given its cost it has limited utility in TPE diagnostics, especially in middle- and low-income countries.

TREATMENT

The management of TPE is identical to parenchymal TB and comprises pharmacotherapy that includes four drugs in a 6-month regimen. The drugs used are Isoniazid (H), Rifampicin (R), Pyrazinamide (Z), and Ethambutol (E). Based on the body weight of the patient, these four drugs are administered for the first 2 months in the intensive phase followed by three drugs (H, R, and E) in the continuation phase of 4 months. There is currently no convincing data to show that shorter regimens are effective or longer ones enhance cure. Most patients respond well with the effusion gradually resolving in 2–12 weeks.[13] HIV-positive patients are to be treated in an identical manner with some caveats of starting antiretroviral therapy (ART) within 2 weeks of initiating anti-TB drugs in those with CD4 count > 50 cells/μL, whereas in all others, a 6–8-week delay is recommended.[43]

Residual pleural opacities (RPO) in the form of varying degrees and extent of pleural thickening are seen in approximately 50% of patients (20% with >10-mm thickening to 40% in those with 2 mm) **(Figs. 6 and 7)**.[25] RPO is more commonly seen in males, those with low pleural fluid glucose levels and those with loculated effusions.[44] A few patients, after initiation of treatment, have a rebound increase in effusion reflecting immune reconstitution inflammatory syndrome (IRIS) wherein a combination of increased antigen load resulting from the lysis of the bacilli and improved immunity results in this paradoxical worsening of the effusion.[45] Corticosteroids help in ameliorating this paradoxical response.

Controversies in Management of Tuberculous Pleura Effusion

- *Should all TB effusions be treated?*
  Tuberculous effusions are likely to resolve spontaneously without treatment. However, patients frequently develop active TB at a later stage. A follow-up study in the past demonstrated that out of 2,816 untreated members of the Finnish Armed Forces who developed pleural effusion between 1939 and 1945, 43% developed TB after a period of 7 years.[46]

- *Should all TB effusions undergo complete therapeutic aspiration?*
  Attempting to completely remove all pleural fluid does not appear to reduce the amount of residual pleural thickening. In a study where 61 TB effusion patients were randomized to receive pigtail drainage until the drainage was <50 mL/day or until there was no drainage, the residual pleural thickening was identical in both groups.[47] It should, however, be noted that the duration of dyspnea was significantly shortened by the use of pigtail drainage by a median of 4 days versus 8 days. It, therefore, maybe more prudent to perform a therapeutic aspiration only in those symptomatic patients with large effusions.
- *Corticosteroids in TB effusion.*
  The use of adjuvant steroids in TB effusion is based on the premise that as the pathogenesis of TB effusion is secondary to host inflammatory reaction to pathogenic antigens, the use of anti-inflammatory may mitigate symptoms, enhance pleural fluid resolution, and reduce adhesions and pleural thickening. But no such long-term beneficial effect has been observed in a number of studies investigating the role of steroids in TB effusion; rapid improvements in clinical parameters were observed but this was not supported by any lasting improved outcomes.[48-50]

Complications of Tuberculosis Effusion and Management

Tuberculosis Empyema

Pleural tuberculosis can present as an empyema due to direct invasion of the pleural space by *M.tb* or rupture of a subpleural focus. This results in frank pyothorax, pyopneumothorax, bronchopleural fistula (BPF), or empyema necessitans when there is a communication to the chest wall **(Figs. 8 and 9)**. Management principles remain the same as in treating bacterial empyemas, namely routine pharmacotherapy (anti-TB drugs), intercostal chest drainage followed by surgical intervention in nonresponders in the form of decortication or lobectomy/pneumonectomy. Nonsurgical bronchoscopic intervention procedures have been successfully used in selected patients for BPF closure just as medical thoracoscopic adhesionolysis have been practiced in certain centers in early stages of empyema.

Pleural Thickening (Fibrothorax)

Tuberculous effusion, especially those complicated with empyema, bronchopleural fistula, or chronic persistent effusion, often lead to localized or diffuse pleural thickening, which may impact respiratory functions and cause symptoms of breathlessness and chest pain. Such patients often need surgical decortication.

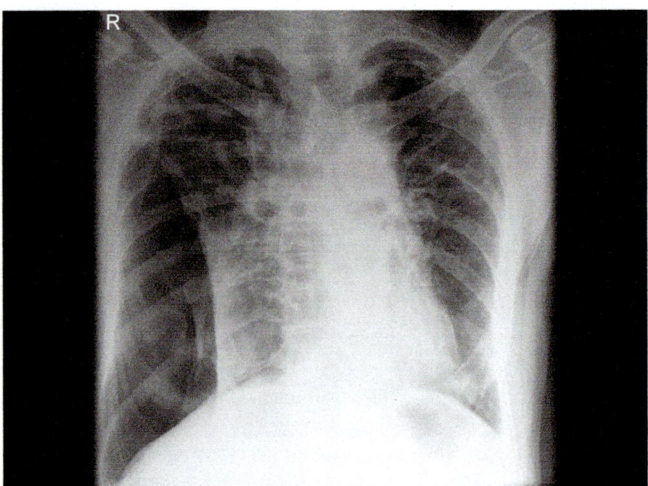

FIG. 8: Tuberculosis (TB) bronchopleural fistula (BPF).

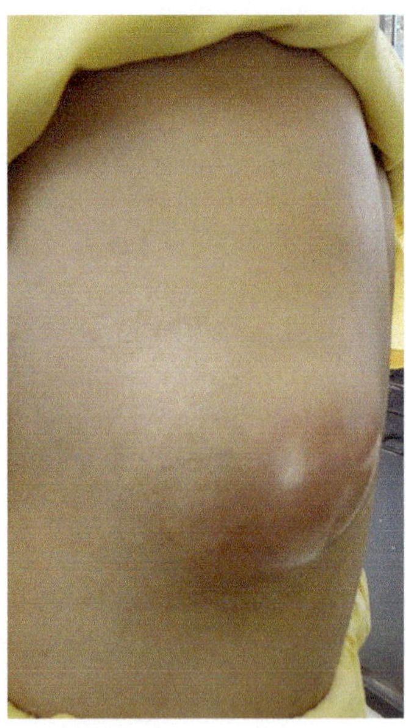

FIG. 9: Empyema necessitans.

SUMMARY

Tuberculous pleural effusion is the second most common manifestation of EPTB. The effusion is most commonly lymphocytic and exudative in character. The diagnosis is established with radiological investigations supplemented with biochemical and microbiological tests of the aspirated pleural fluid. Anti-Tb treatment is given as for other forms of TB. Therapeutic aspiration may be required only in large and symptomatic effusions.

REFERENCES

1. WHO. (2022). Global Tuberculosis Report 2022. [online] Available from https://www.who.int/teams/global-tuberculosis-programme/tb-reports/global-tuberculosis-report-2022. [Last accessed August, 2024].
2. Sharma SK, Mohan A. Extrapulmonary tuberculosis. Indian J Med Res. 2004;120(4):316-53.
3. India TB report 2023: Leading the way. (2023). [online] Available from https://static.pib.gov.in/WriteReadData/specificdocs/documents/2023/mar/doc2023324176101.pdf. [Last accessed August, 2024].
4. Vorster MJ, Allwood BW, Diacon AH, et al. Tuberculous pleural effusions: advances and controversies. J Thorac Dis. 2015; 7(6):981-91.
5. Christopher DJ, Dinakaran S, Gupta R, et al. Thoracoscopic pleural biopsy improves yield of Xpert MTB/RIF for diagnosis of pleural tuberculosis. Respirology. 2018;23(7):714-7.
6. Roper WH, Waring JJ. Primary serofibrinous pleural effusion in military personnel. Am Rev Tuberc. 1955;71:616-34.
7. Seibert AF, Haynes JJ, Middleton R, et al. Tuberculous pleural effusion. Twenty-year experience. Chest. 1991;994:883-6.
8. Berger HW, Mejia E. Tuberculous pleurisy. Chest. 1973;63:88-92.
9. Levine H, Szanto PB, Cugell DW. Tuberculous pleurisy. An acute illness. Arch Intern Med. 1968;122(4):329-32.
10. Richter C, Perenboom R, Mtoni I, et al. Clinical features of HIV-seropositive and HIV-seronegative patients with tuberculous pleural effusion in Dares Salaam, Tanzania. Chest. 1994;106: 1471-5.
11. Zhao T, Chen B, Xu Y, et al. Clinical and pathological differences between polymorphonuclear-rich and lymphocyte-rich tuberculous pleural effusion. Ann Thorac Med. 2020;15(2):76-83.
12. Shaw JA, Diacon AH, Koegelenberg CFN. Tuberculous pleural effusion. Respirology. 2019;24(10):962-71.
13. Light RW. Update on tuberculous pleural effusion. Respirology. 2010;15(3):451-8.
14. Aggarwal AN, Agarwal A, Sehgal IP, et al. Adenosine deaminase for diagnosis of tuberculous pleural effusion: a systematic review and meta-analysis. PLoS One. 2019;14(3):e0213728.
15. Lee SJ, Kim HS, Lee HS, et al. Factors influencing pleural adenosine deaminase level in patients with tuberculous pleurisy. Am J Med Sci. 2014;348(5):362-5.
16. Porcel M. Pearls and myths in pleural fluid analysis. Respirology. 2011;16:44-52.
17. Castro DJ, Neuvo GD, Perez-Rodriguez E, et al. Diagnostic value of adenosine deaminase in nontuberculous lymphocytic pleural effusions. Eur Respir J. 2003;21(2):220-4.
18. Saraya T, Ohkuma K, Koide T, et al. A novel diagnostic method for distinguishing parapneumonic effusion and empyema from other diseases by using the pleural lactate dehydrogenase to adenosine deaminase ratio and carcinoembryonic antigen levels. Medicine. 2019;98(13):e15003.
19. Wang J, Liu J, Xie X, et al. The pleural fluid lactate dehydrogenase/adenosine deaminase ratio differentiates between tuberculous and parapneumonic pleural effusions. BMC Pulm Med. 2017; 17(1):168.
20. Villena V, Lopez-Encuentra A, Pozo F, et al. Interferon gamma levels in pleural fluid for the diagnosis of tuberculosis. Am J Med. 2003;115:365-70.
21. Aggarwal AN, Agarwal R, Dhooria S, et al. Unstimulated pleural fluid interferon gamma for diagnosis of tuberculous pleural effusion: A systematic review and meta-analysis. J Clin Microbiol. 2021;59(5):e02112-20.
22. Aggarwal AN, Agarwal R, Dhooria S, et al. Comparative accuracy of pleural fluid unstimulated interferon-gamma and adenosine deaminase for diagnosing pleural tuberculosis: a systematic review and meta-analysis. PLoS One. 2021;16(6):e0253525.
23. Aggarwal AN, Agarwal R, Gupta D, et al. Interferon gamma release assays for diagnosis of pleural tuberculosis: A systematic review and meta-analysis. J Clin Microbiol. 2015;53(8):2451-9.
24. Aggarwal AN, Agarwal R, Dhooria S, et al. Pleural fluid lysozyme as a diagnostic biomarker of pleural tuberculosis: A systematic review and meta-analysis. Lung India. 2022;39(5):428-36.
25. de Pablo A, Villena V, Echave-Sustaeta J, et al. Are pleural fluid parameters related to the development of residual pleural thickening in tuberculosis? Chest. 1997;112:1293-7.
26. Aggarwal AN, Agarwal R, Dhooria S, et al. Pleural fluid tumor necrosis factor for diagnosis of pleural tuberculosis: a systematic review and meta-analysis. Cytokine. 2021;141:155467.
27. Gopi A, Mahdavan SM, Sharma SK, et al. Diagnosis and treatment of tuberculous pleural effusion in 2006. Chest. 2007;131(3): 880-9.
28. Ruan SY, Chuang YC, Wang JY, et al. Revisiting tuberculous pleurisy: Pleural fluid characteristics and diagnostic yield of mycobacterial culture in an endemic area. Thorax. 2012; 67(9):822-7.
29. Kohli M, Schiller I, Dendukuri N, et al. Xpert MTB/RIF Ultra and Xpert MTB/RIF assays for extrapulmonary tuberculosis and rifampicin resistance in adults. Cochrane Database Syst Rev. 2021;15;1(1):CD012768.
30. Conde MB, Loivos AC, Rezende VM, et al. Yield of sputum induction in the diagnosis of pleural tuberculosis. Am J Respir Crit Care Med. 2003;167:723-5.
31. Wang Z, Xu LL, Wu Y-B, et al. Diagnostic value and safety of medical thoracoscopy in tuberculous pleural effusion. Respir Med. 2015;109(9):1188-92.
32. Maturu VN, Prasad VP, Biradar M, et al. Pleural Pustule—a novel thoracoscopic appearance of pleural tuberculosis. J Bronchol Interv Pulmonol. 2023;30(4):354-62.
33. Gao S, Wang C, Yu X, et al. Xpert MTB/RIF Ultra enhanced tuberculous pleurisy diagnosis for patients with unexplained exudative pleural effusion who underwent a pleural biopsy via thoracoscopy: A prospective cohort study. Int J Infect Dis. 2021;106:370-5.
34. Diacon AH, Van de Wal BW, Wyser C, et al. Diagnostic tools in tuberculous pleurisy: A direct comparative study. Eur Respir J. 2003;22 (4):589-91.
35. Wang YXJ, Chung MJ, Skrahin A, et al. Radiological signs associated with pulmonary multi-drug resistant tuberculosis: An analysis of published evidences. Quant Imaging Med Surg. 2018;8:161-73.
36. Bielsa S, Acosta C, Pardina M, et al. Tuberculous pleural effusion: clinical characteristics of 320 patients. Arch Bronconeumol. 2019;55(1):17-22.
37. Choi YW, Jeon SC, Seo HS, et al. Tuberculous pleural effusion: new pulmonary lesions during treatment. Radiology. 2002;224(2):493-502.

SECTION 12: PLEURAL DISEASES

38. Lai Y, Su M, Weng H, et al. Sonographic septation: a predictor of sequelae of tuberculous pleurisy after treatment. Thorax. 2009;64:806-9.
39. Ko Y, Kim C, Chang B, et al. Loculated tuberculous pleural effusion: easily identifiable and clinically useful predictor of positive mycobacterial culture from pleural fluid. Tuberc Respir Dis. 2017;80(1):35-44.
40. Ko JM, Park HJ, Kim CH. Pulmonary changes of pleural TB: up-to-date CT imaging. Chest. 2014;146(6):1604-11.
41. Sun Y, Yu H, Ma J, et al. The role of 18F-FDG PET/CT integrated imaging in distinguishing malignant from benign pleural effusion. PLoS One. 2016;11(8):e0161764.
42. Du X, Zhu F, Yu C. The Value of 18F-FDG PET/CT in the diagnosis of tuberculous pleurisy and in the differential diagnosis between tuberculous pleurisy and pleural metastasis from lung adenocarcinoma. Contrast Media Mol Imaging. 2022;2022: 4082291.
43. Meintjes G, Moorhouse MA, Carmona S, et al. Adult antiretroviral therapy guidelines 2017. South Afr J HIV Med. 2017;18:776.
44. Rai DK, Thakur S. Study to identify incidence and risk factors associated residual pleural opacity in tubercular pleural effusion. Indian J Tuberc. 2021;68(3):374-8.
45. Al-Majed SA. Study of paradoxical response to chemotherapy in tuberculous pleural effusion. Respir Med. 1996;90:211-4.
46. Patalia J. Initial tuberculous pleuritis in the Finnish Armed Forces in 1939–1945 with special reference to eventual post pleuritic tuberculosis. Acta Tuberc Scand Suppl. 1954;36:1-57.
47. Lai YF, Chao TY, Wang YH, et al. Pigtail drainage in the treatment of tuberculous pleural effusions: a randomized study. Thorax. 2003;58:149-51.
48. Shuanshuan Xie, Lin Lu, Ming Li, et al. The efficacy and safety of adjunctive corticosteroids in the treatment of tuberculous pleurisy: a systematic review and meta-analysis. Oncotarget. 2017;8(47):83315-22.
49. Evans DJ. The use of adjunctive corticosteroids in the treatment of pericardial, pleural and meningeal tuberculosis: do they improve outcome. Respir Med. 2008;102(6):793-800.
50. Ryan H, Yoo J, Darsini P. Corticosteroids for tuberculous pleurisy. Cochrane Database Syst Rev. 2017;3(3):CD001876.

Malignant Pleural Effusions and Pleurodesis

CHAPTER 130

Srinivas Rajagopala

INTRODUCTION

Malignant pleural effusion (MPE) is the second most common cause of exudative pleural effusions in developing countries and the most common cause of exudative effusion in areas of low tuberculosis prevalence.[1] MPE most commonly is metastatic in origin secondary to cancer of the lung or breast. Not all patients with MPEs are symptomatic; many patients may have asymptomatic stable effusions that do not require management throughout their disease course.

ETIOLOGY OF MALIGNANT EFFUSIONS

About 15% of all patients with cancer develop a malignant pleural effusion and 50–65% of these MPEs are associated with lung and breast cancer.[2,3] Another 25% are associated with lymphoma, and gastrointestinal and genitourinary cancers.[4] Mesotheliomas, sarcomas (including melanomas), germ-cell tumors, and prostatic carcinoma together account for another 10% of all MPEs.[5] The primary cancer is unknown in 7–15% cases; the diagnosis of pleural malignancy is the first indication of cancer in about 10% of effusions.[6,7] Primary pleural malignancy is an uncommon cause of malignant pleural effusion; metastatic malignant pleural effusions are 25-fold common than mesothelioma even in areas where the latter is relatively common.[5] Pleural effusion in a patient with lung cancer is a poor prognostic marker and indicates metastatic dissemination. These patients are automatically staged IVA (M1a) in the 8th TNM (Tumor, Node, Metastasis) staging system for lung cancer and offered palliative therapy.[4,8]

Lung cancer is the most common cause of MPEs and 30–43% of all MPEs are related to lung cancer. Effusions are present in 15% of patients at diagnosis and 50% of patients during their disease course.[9] Adenocarcinomas are most frequently associated with MPEs; however, effusions may be seen with all histopathological types. Anti-p53 positivity increases the risk of pleural effusion in patients with carcinoma lung. Breast cancer is the second most common cause of MPEs. The time from the initial diagnosis to development of effusion is usually 2 years, but can be up to 20 years. The effusion is usually ipsilateral (70%) but can be contralateral (20%) or bilateral (10%).[10] About 40% of non-Hodgkin's lymphoma (NHL) and 16% of patients with Hodgkin's lymphoma (HL) have an associated effusion.[11]

PATHOGENESIS OF METASTASIS AND EFFUSIONS

Pleural metastases occur by several mechanisms **(Box 1)**: Pulmonary vascular invasion with tumor emboli to the visceral pleural surface with subsequent seeding of

BOX 1 Mechanisms for formation of pleural effusions in relation to malignancy.

Direct:

- Increased capillary permeability from direct pleural invasion
- Lymphatic obstruction due to malignant lymphadenopathy
- Disruption of thoracic duct or its major tributaries (chylothorax)*

Indirect (paramalignant):$

- Bronchial obstruction with atelectasis
- Bronchial obstruction with pneumonia
- Lung entrapment by malignancy (thick visceral pleural involvement)
- Hypoalbuminemia (serum albumin <1.5 g/dL)
- Pulmonary embolism
- Malignant pericardial involvement
- Superior vena cava syndrome
- *Radiation therapy*:
  - Early (<6 months): Pleuritis 6 weeks to 6 months after radiation
  - Late (>6 months):
    - Mediastinal fibrosis
    - Constrictive pericarditis
    - Superior vena cava obstruction
- Chemotherapy (methotrexate, cyclophosphamide, mitomycin, procarbazine and bleomycin) and immunotherapy

*Most commonly seen with lymphomas.

$Do not indicate nonoperability when seen with carcinoma lung.

the parietal pleura, direct tumor invasion, hematogenous metastases to the parietal pleura from extra-pulmonary primary, and lymphatic involvement.[12] In lung cancer, pulmonary artery emboli and ipsilateral visceral pleura invasion (invasion beyond the elastic layer including invasion to the visceral pleural surface) is the first step.[13] Tumor seeding of the parietal pleura always follows visceral pleural involvement.[14] Pleural metastases may be present without associated effusion.[12,14] MPEs (malignant cells identified in pleural fluid or pleural tissue with associated effusion) are formed by several mechanisms, which may be direct or indirect. Increased pleural permeability secondary to production of vascular endothelial growth factor (VEGF) is largely responsible for the development of MPE.[15,16] Lymphatic blockade in the parietal pleura stoma and at the lymph nodes also contribute to generation of MPE and pleural involvement and intrathoracic lymphadenopathy correlate with pleural effusions related to malignancy in autopsy studies.[14] In general, direct involvement of pleura by the malignancy makes it inoperable and the treatment approaches are predominantly palliative. "Paramalignant" causes of effusion result from indirect effects of the tumor on the pleural space such as especially bronchial obstruction, mediastinal lymph nodal obstruction, pneumonia, pulmonary embolism, heart failure, atelectasis and superior vena cava syndrome and may be operative in about 17% of cases. Paramalignant effusions are managed according to the etiology and careful consideration of these causes is important to prevent upstaging of the TNM category in lung cancer.[17]

CLINICAL PRESENTATION

Breathlessness is the most common presenting symptom in patients with MPEs, occurring in more than half of all effusions.[18] The pathogenesis of dyspnea from a large MPE appears to be related to decreased chest wall compliance, contralateral mediastinal shift, decreased ipsilateral lung volume, and reflex stimulation from the chest wall and lung parenchyma.[19] Nonproductive cough may also be caused by the presence of a MPE. Both dyspnea and cough are relieved promptly by thoracentesis; failure of improvement suggests atelectasis, pneumonia, lymphangitic carcinomatosa, pulmonary embolism, or another associated medical condition (congestive cardiac failure) as the etiology.

Patients with lung entrapment by the pleural malignancy will have an improvement in dyspnea without complete lung expansion; the inhibition of stretch receptors by the fluid removal is believed to mediate this. Patients may also have systemic manifestations such as malaise, anorexia, and weight loss that are related to the advanced stage of malignancy. A constant dull, aching chest pain may be seen in MPEs; however, this is more common in patients with mesothelioma.[5] Chest pain is related to malignant involvement of the parietal pleura, ribs, and other intercostal structures. Patients with benign causes of their effusions are more likely to describe "pleuritic" chest pain. The presence of hemoptysis suggests an endobronchial growth as the primary responsible for the MPE. A history of smoking and occupational exposure to asbestos may suggest the diagnosis of MPE. Symptoms for more than a month, absence of fever, massive effusion and serosanguineous fluid on thoracocentesis also favor the possibility of MPE.[20]

RADIOLOGICAL FINDINGS

At presentation, patients with a MPE typically have an effusion occupying half to two thirds of the hemithorax. While small effusions are seen in about 10%, an additional 10% present with a massive pleural effusion.[21] A massive effusion is associated with contralateral shift of the mediastinum. When there is an absence of contralateral mediastinal shift with an apparent large pleural effusion, bronchogenic carcinoma involving the ipsilateral mainstem bronchus malignant mesothelioma, fixation of the mediastinum due to malignant lymph nodes or lung entrapment by extensive pleural malignancy should be suspected **(Fig. 1)**. Multiloculation at presentation is unusual in malignant effusions (as opposed to parapneumonic effusions) because of the high fibrinolytic activity of the metastatic tumor lesions. Chest radiographs of patients with lung primary and an effusion often demonstrate associated abnormalities; these might sometimes be apparent after a therapeutic thoracocentesis.

Contrast-enhanced computerized tomography (CECT) of the chest should include upper abdomen to enable visualization of mediastinal lymphadenopathy and adrenal and/or hepatic metastasis. The diagnosis of malignant pleural thickening is favored by the presence of parietal pleural thickening > 1 cm, circumferential pleural thickening, nodular pleural thickening and mediastinal pleural thickening (specificity 94–100%).[22] CECT chest may be helpful in the evaluation of patients with a malignant effusion by demonstrating pleural abnormalities, mediastinal lymphadenopathy, parenchymal disease, distant metastases, chest wall and airway involvement that cannot be detected on standard chest radiograph **(Figs. 2 and 3)**. CT appearances of mesothelioma may be very similar to metastatic pleural effusion. Presence of concomitant pleural plaques (20%), asbestosis, extensive chest wall invasion, circumferential nodular lung encasement, pleural thickening with irregular pleura-pulmonary margins, interfissure thickening and pleural thickening with superimposed nodules should suggest mesothelioma.[23] About 3% of effusions related to HL and 20% of effusions related to NHL are chylothoraces **(Fig. 4)**. Magnetic resonance imaging is not commonly performed in patients with MPE; it may be helpful in evaluating chest wall involvement in mesothelioma. Positron emission tomography may be helpful in evaluating the extent of pleural involvement in malignant mesothelioma but does not offer additional information of routine use in patients with MPE **(Fig. 5)**.

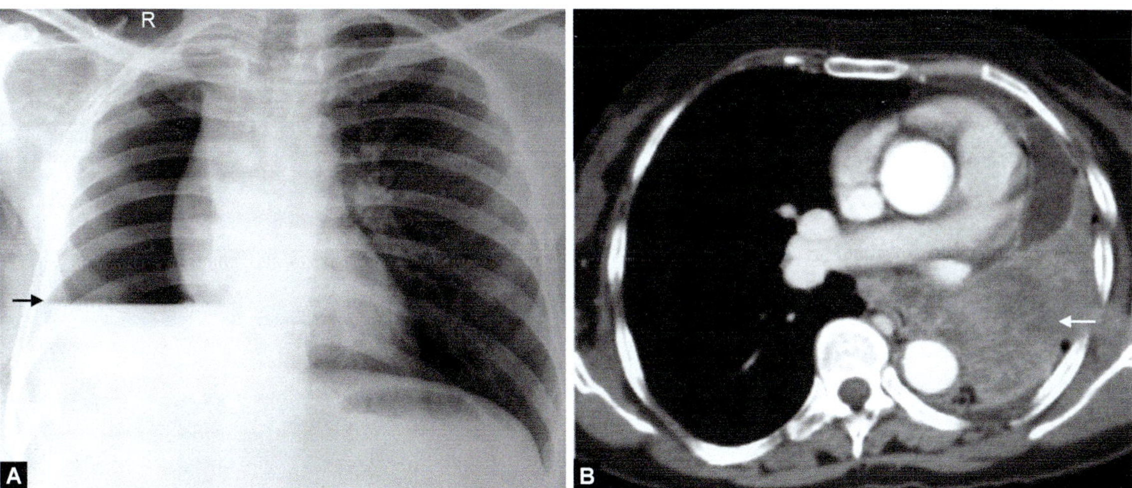

FIGS. 1A AND B: Composite image of chest radiograph (A) showing right-sided hydropneumothorax following thoracocentesis and lung entrapment due to a thick visceral pleural peel. The computed tomographic image (B) of another patient shows a large intrabronchial mass, loculated effusion and ipsilateral mediastinum.

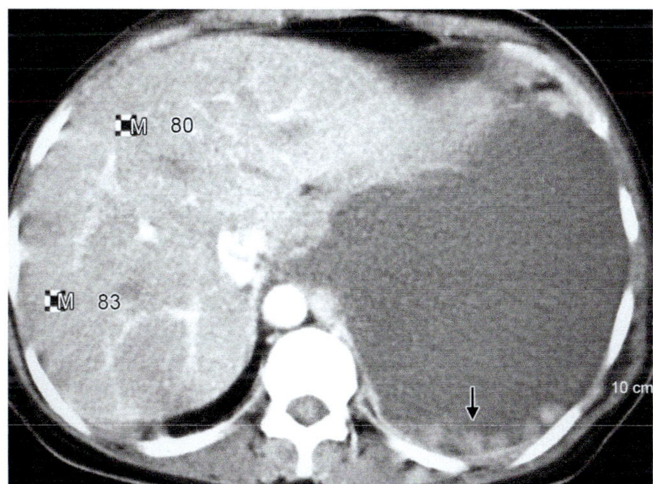

FIG. 2: Computed tomography showing left-sided effusion and multiple pleural nodules. Pleural biopsy showed adenocarcinoma.

DIAGNOSIS

Pleural Fluid Analysis

Malignant pleural effusions can be serous, hemorrhagic, or grossly bloody; and malignant disease is the most common cause of hemorrhagic effusion. However, about 50% of MPEs are nonhemorrhagic and have red blood cell counts of <10,000 cells/μL. The pleural fluid is almost always an exudate but these effusions may occasionally fulfill Light's criteria by an elevated lactate dehydrogenase (LDH) only. Nucleated cell count is typically low, generally <3,000/μL, composed mainly of lymphocytes, macrophages, and mesothelial cells. The lymphocyte differential mostly varies from 50 to 70% of all cells. The presence of pleural eosinophilia does not negate the possibility of pleural malignancy and the prevalence of malignancy is similar in both eosinophilic and noneosinophilic effusions.[24]

The pleural glucose concentration is lower than 60 mg/dL in approximately 20% of MPE. Impaired glucose transfer to pleural fluid and glucose utilization by tumor burden contributes to the observed low-glucose levels.[25] Lactic acid generated by anaerobic glycolysis in the pleural space and impaired carbon dioxide movement from the pleural space are responsible for low pH generation. A low pleural fluid pH (<7.30) and a low pleural fluid glucose (<60 mg/dL) are markers of advanced disease in the pleural space with increased tumor burden; this is also associated with a decreased survival, a higher sensitivity of diagnosis by initial cytology examination and less successful pleurodesis.[26,27] Increased amylase concentration is seen in 10–14% of patients with MPEs, especially adenocarcinoma lung and ovary, usually due to increased salivary isoenzyme concentration. The routine assay of amylase is unhelpful in the diagnosis of exudates of undetermined etiology and should be measured only if there is a pretest suspicion of acute pancreatitis, chronic pancreatic disease, or esophageal rupture.

Pleural Cytology

The diagnosis of MPE is established by demonstrating malignant cells in the pleural fluid or in the pleura tissue. Pleural fluid cytology is diagnostic in up to 55–60% of patients with MPEs depending on the tumor load and the histopathological type of the primary. Pleural cytology is rarely positive in squamous cell carcinoma because bronchial obstruction and lymphatic involvement are frequent causes of pleural effusion in this setting. At least two samples are submitted for cytology and these need not exceed 50 mL in quantity.[28] Use of a cellblock analysis increases the yield of positive tests and enables immunohistochemistry. A positive cytology establishes malignancy, but provides no information about the site of primary. This is evaluated by subsequent imaging, endoscopy or markers [thyroid

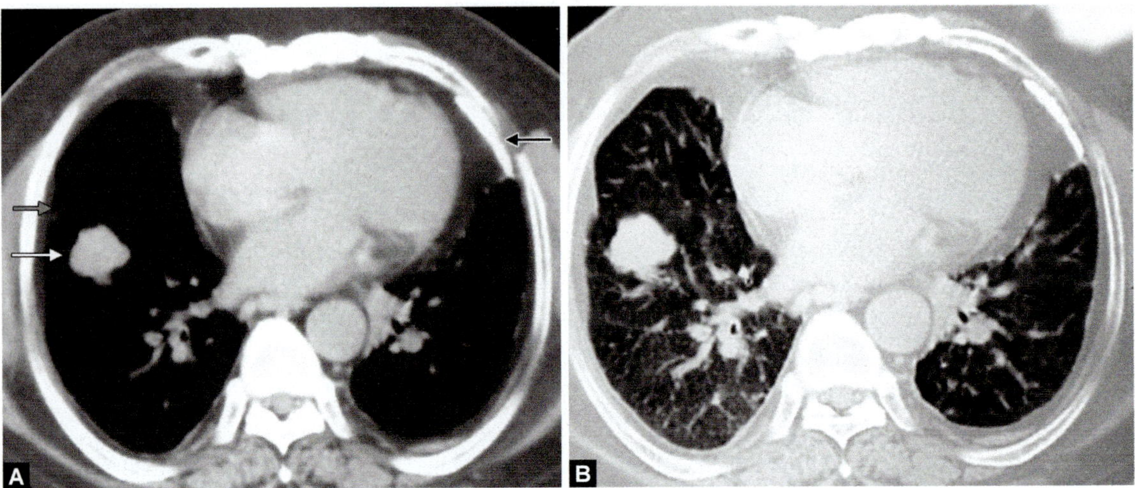

FIGS. 3A AND B: Composite image of computed tomography showing pleural calcification (A, black arrow) and a nodule (A, white arrow) along with pleural thickening (A, gray arrow) in the right lower lobe with a minimal right-sided effusion. Fine-needle aspiration and immunohistochemistry from the nodule confirmed adenocarcinoma.

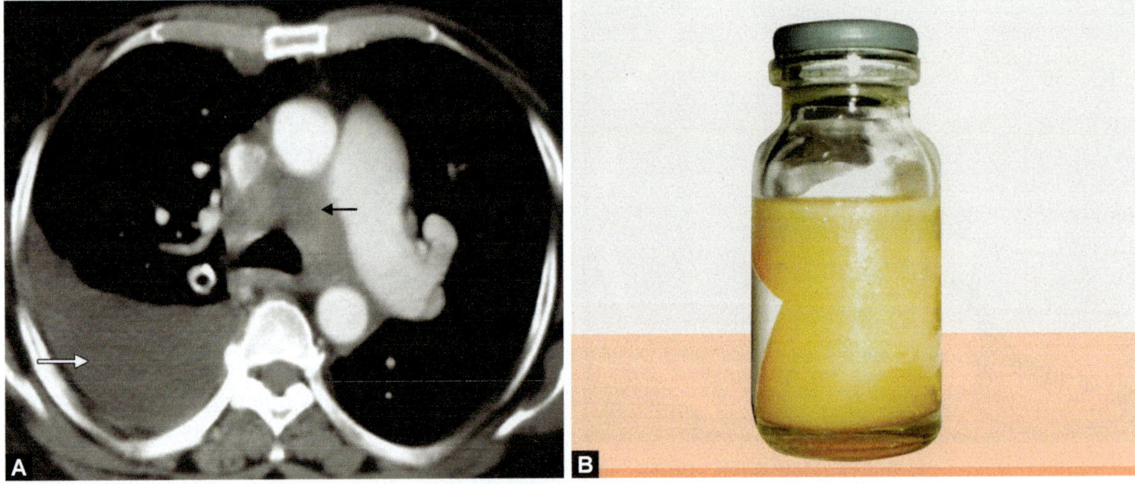

FIGS. 4A AND B: (A) Composite image of computed tomography showing right moderate pleural effusion (white arrow) and mediastinal lymphadenopathy (black arrow); (B) Thoracocentesis suggested a chylothorax (B, triglyceride 150 mg/dL and cholesterol of 45 mg/dL, and mediastinoscopy-guided biopsy confirmed lymphoma.

transcription factor-1 (TTF-1), prostate-specific antigen (PSA), cancer antigen 125 (CA-125), and others].

Pleural Biopsy

The sensitivity of percutaneous blind pleural biopsy using Abrams' biopsy needle varies between 40 and 75% depending on the extent of parietal pleural involvement, number, and adequacy of biopsies, and operator experience. If blind biopsy is performed without cytology, one third of patients who would otherwise be diagnosed will be missed. Currently, blind pleural biopsies are seldom performed.[29] CT-guided percutaneous pleural biopsy has a yield similar to thoracoscopic biopsy and may be performed when confirmation of the diagnosis (without the need for pleurodesis) is the dominant clinical problem or where thoracoscopy is unavailable.

Medical thoracoscopy has a yield exceeding 95% for malignancy; further, this can be combined with complete drainage of the effusions and talc poudrage with a greater percentage of successful pleurodesis. Medical thoracoscopy can be performed using local anesthesia with conscious sedation in an endoscopy suite using nondisposable rigid or semirigid instruments, making it less invasive and cheaper than video-assisted thoracoscopic surgery. It is also safe; major complications are seen in <2–3% of cases. Pleuroscopy may be performed with a rigid or semi-rigid pleuroscope. The use of rigid pleuroscope is associated with a greater need for sedation, analgesia and scar size but is associated with higher yield, bigger biopsy size, ease of biopsy and

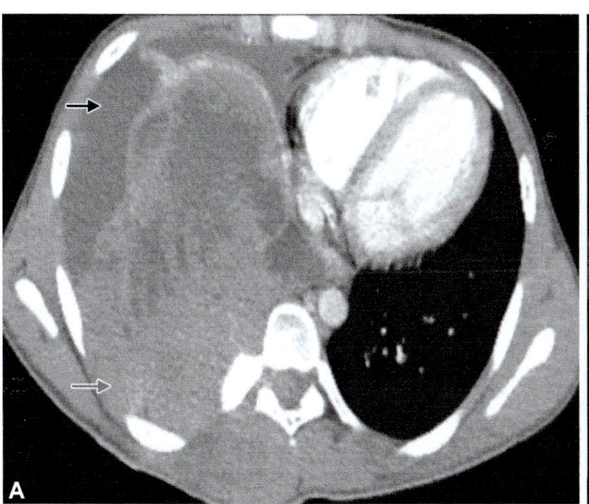

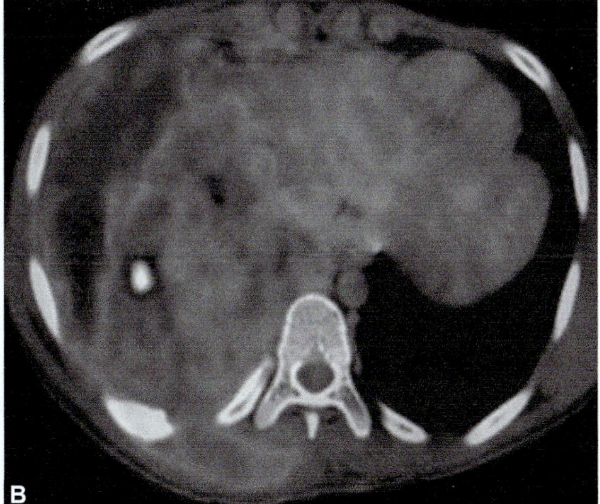

FIGS. 5A AND B: Composite image of computed tomography (A) showing right moderate pleural effusion (black arrow) and a large right lower lobe mass (gray arrow). CT-guided biopsy established the diagnosis of Askin's tumor. Positron emission tomography images; (B) Shows an area of increased uptake in the right lower lobe corresponding to the mass.

quality of imaging.[30] Either of these could be combined with therapeutic poudrage during the diagnostic procedure.

Pleural fluid levels of tumor markers such as carcino-embryonic antigen (CEA), carbohydrate antigens (CA) 15-3, 19-9, 549 and 72-4, neuron-specific enolase, squamous cell carcinoma (SCC) antigen, cytokeratin 19 fragments (CYFRA21-1), and sialyl stage-specific mouse embryonic antigen (SSEA-1) have been evaluated for separating benign and malignant effusions. In general, these markers are not specific enough and have no role in daily practice.[31] Clonality of lymphocytes demonstrated by flow cytometry on fluid samples establishes the diagnosis of lymphoma.

Immunohistochemistry is routinely used to differentiate adenocarcinomas from mesothelioma. Metastatic adeno-carcinomas stain positive with CEA, MOC-3.1, B72.3, Ber-EP4 and BG-8, whereas mesotheliomas (and benign mesothelial cells) stain positive with calretinin and cytokeratin. A panel of four markers is usually employed in clinical practice.[19] Staining for TTF-1 in fluid and tissue can help establish pulmonary or thyroid origin of adenocarcinomas.

MANAGEMENT

The presence of a MPE indicates advanced cancer and management is palliative without survival benefit. Step-wise treatment **(Flowchart 1)** should focus on patient-centered goals and priority given for treatment that accelerates symptom relief, improvement in quality of life, minimal invasiveness, affordability, and time spent out of hospital. The initial step is to establish malignancy and its primary site. This guides subsequent therapy which may include targeted therapy, immunotherapy, chemotherapy, hormonal therapy, and radiotherapy alone or in varying combinations. The major indication for palliative treatment in patients with a malignant pleural effusion is relief of dyspnea. The main considerations affecting management decisions include the patient's degree of breathlessness, functional status, duration of expected survival, type of primary tumor (and expected response to chemotherapy), and lung expansion following thoracentesis. The below modalities are used in isolation or combined as the clinical situation dictates.

Observation

Observation is appropriate when patients are asymptomatic and neither therapeutic thoracocentesis nor pleurodesis are indicated in patients with asymptomatic mild-moderate diagnosed MPEs.

Chemotherapy and Radiation

Malignant pleural effusions from small-cell lung cancer, breast carcinoma, and lymphoma may respond favorably to chemotherapy alone. If the effusion is mild to moderate, a trial of chemotherapy may be performed as a modality to control the effusion. In chylothorax from lymphoma, mediastinal radiation is effective. Chemotherapy is not useful in isolation to control the effusion, however, in most patients with MPEs secondary to carcinoma lung. Anti-VEGF antibody, bevacizumab, is used as a triplet-combination therapy in nonsquamous lung cancer. Pleurodesis should precede this treatment since VEGF is essential for successful pleurodesis. In patients undergoing systemic chemotherapy, pleural effusions should be aspirated before chemotherapy is given because the antineoplastic drugs may accumulate in the pleural space and lead to increased systemic toxicity. Pleurodesis always precedes chemotherapy because the intercostal drain may become a potential nidus of infection.

Therapeutic Thoracentesis

Ultrasound-guided therapeutic thoracentesis is performed in all symptomatic patients with MPEs for relief of

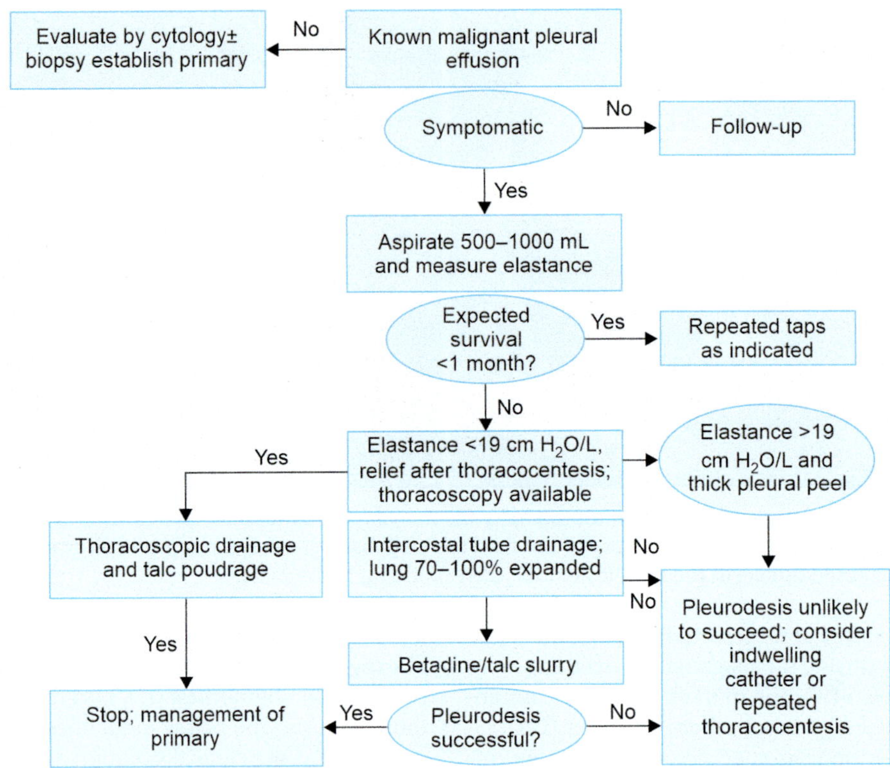

FLOWCHART 1: Evaluation and management of a patient with suspected malignant pleural effusion.

breathlessness. The initial therapeutic thoracocentesis should always be combined with pleural manometry and pleural elastance measurement if there is an imaging concern for lung entrapment on CT chest. Caution should be exercised when draining >1.5 L in a single session because of the potential of reperfusion pulmonary edema (REPO) **(Fig. 6)**. Pleural manometry is sometimes used to limit the procedure when pressure falls to <–20 cm H_2O can guide safe thoracentesis in this setting.[32] The amount of fluid evacuated by pleural aspiration should also be guided by the presence of cough or chest discomfort.

Mechanisms proposed for REPO include reperfusion injury of the underlying hypoxic lung, increased capillary permeability, and local production of neutrophil chemotactic factors such as interleukin-8. Caution must be exercised, especially when the underlying lung has been collapsed for more than a week and large (>1.5 L) are being drained without manometry and reperfusion edema complicates 2–7% such procedures. A recent trial has shown no benefit of routine pleural manometry in moderate effusions.[33] REPO can also complicate thoracoscopic drainage of effusions. Therapeutic thoracocentesis alone has a high rate of symptom recurrence at 1 month and alternate options must be explored in all symptomatic patients.[19] The main choices include thoracoscopic or tube drainage with pleurodesis versus an indwelling pleural catheter.

Thoracoscopic Poudrage versus Intercostal Tube Drainage and Pleurodesis

Thoracoscopic talc poudrage may be more effective when compared to talc slurry. However, the evidence-base of the superiority of talc poudrage is weak; several trials suggest that talc slurry is as efficacious as poudrage when there are no loculations in the pleural space.[34]

Pleurodesis

Pleurodesis is a treatment that aims to produce symphysis of the pleural surfaces by chemical or mechanical means for symptom relief. The aim of pleurodesis in patients with malignant pleural effusions is to prevent re-accumulation of the effusion and symptoms. Pleurodesis occurs through diffuse inflammation and local activation of coagulation with fibrin deposition. High intrapleural fibrinolytic activity, high tumor burden, and concomitant use of steroids and possibly nonsteroidal anti-inflammatory drugs (NSAIDs), reduce the effectiveness of pleurodesis. The initial event is injury to the pleural surfaces, followed by subsequent development of fibrosis with the obliteration of the pleural space. However, the mechanism of pleurodesis is highly complex, involves the intrapleural procoagulant-fibrinolytic milieu and angiogenesis pathways, and differs from agent to agent.[35]

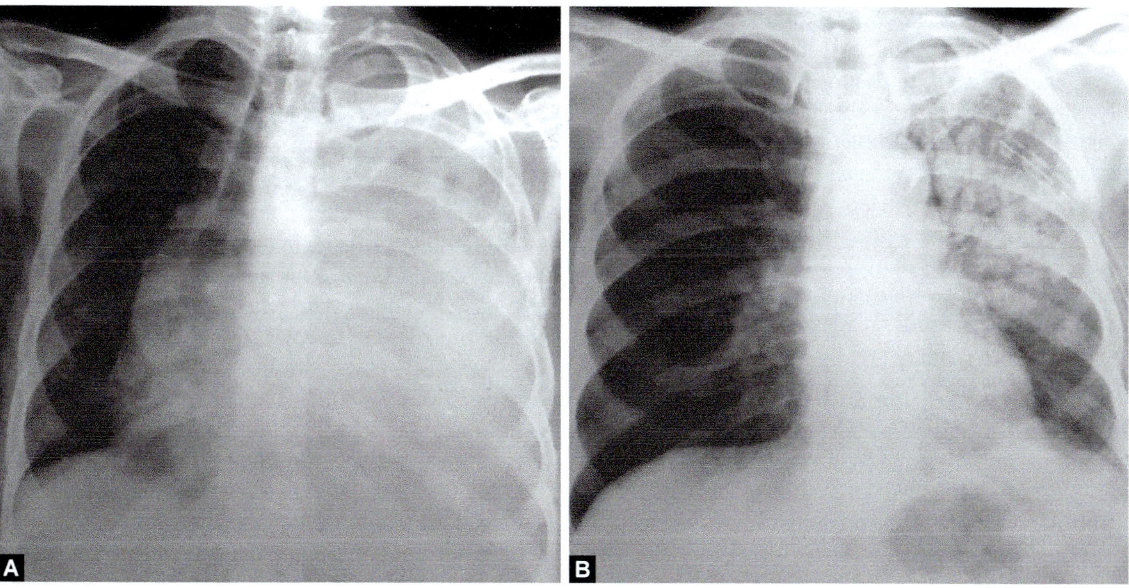

FIGS. 6A AND B: Composite image of chest radiographs of a patient with massive left-sided pleural effusion (A). Subsequent to thoracoscopy and intercostal tube drainage, the patient developed re-expansion pulmonary edema (B). The patient was managed with diuretics and oxygen and recovered at 48 hours.

Patient Selection, Initial Preparation, and Procedure

The *sine quo non* for successful pleurodesis is apposition of the pleural surfaces. While the exact amount of apposition required for a successful pleurodesis is unknown, it is usual to attempt pleurodesis after at least 50–70% apposition is visible on frontal radiographs. Suction may be applied if apposition does not occur; however, this is usually unnecessary and excessive use of suction may increase the risk of REPO. Lack of apposition may be due to a thick visceral peel ("lung entrapment"), pleural loculation, proximal large airway obstruction, or a persistent air leak. If thick visceral peel is evident on initial imaging, consideration is given to tunneled catheters as the definitive initial procedure. If pleural loculations are evident, thoracoscopic drainage, adhesiolysis, and pleurodesis are the procedure of choice. If this is unavailable, surgical pleurectomy or intercostal tube drainage, fibrinolysis, and subsequent slurry instillation after pleural apposition can be attempted. Presence of proximal airway obstruction is a relative contraindication for initial intercostal tube drainage; the endobronchial obstruction is first alleviated by airway interventions. Suction is attempted for incomplete lung expansion due to persistent air leak. When suction is applied, the use of high-volume low-pressure systems is recommended with a gradual increment in pressure to about –20 cm H_2O. Good analgesia and mild sedation with midazolam is achieved just prior to pleurodesis. 3 mg/kg (21 mL of 1% solution for a 70-kg male, maximum of 250 mg) lignocaine is instilled intrapleurally just prior to the sclerosant. This achieves good analgesia with safe peak serum levels of lignocaine. The chemical sclerosant is then instilled in the pleural space either through an intercostal tube as a solution or during thoracoscopy with an atomizer, following complete drainage of the effusion. The intercostal drain is clamped for an hour after the procedure. Position changes during this time may be advised but is unnecessary as pleurodesis is virtually instantaneous.[4,6]

Choice of Sclerosant

An ideal sclerosant must have high molecular weight and chemical polarity, low regional clearance, rapid systemic clearance, a steep dose-response curve and should be well tolerated with minimal or no side effects. The choice of a sclerosant will be determined by the efficacy, accessibility, safety, ease of administration, number of administrations to achieve a complete response, and cost. Despite the evaluation of a wide variety of agents, to date no ideal sclerosant exists. Graded talc as slurry or poudrage is the most widely used and the most effective agent for pleurodesis currently.[34] Acute respiratory distress syndrome using graded medical talc has been reported but is very uncommon using commercially available graded (<10 μm removed) medical talc. Iodopovidone is an iodine-based topical antiseptic and has been shown to be as efficacious as talc slurry from several trials in low-to-middle-income countries. Iodopovidone is extensively absorbed from mucosal surfaces with a 100-fold increase in serum iodine concentration and undergoes minimal metabolism. A solution containing a mixture of 20 mL 10% iodopovidone and 80-mL normal saline through the intercostal drain is used to create pleurodesis and is as efficacious as talc slurry.[36,37] Doxycycline and bleomycin are other commonly used agents in pleurodesis but their efficacy is lower than iodopovidone or talc. Nitrogen mustard and mitoxantrone are other antineoplastic agents, which have been used for successful pleurodesis. Silver nitrate causes caustic injury to the mesothelium and results in pleural adhesions and pleurodesis. Quinacrine is an antimalarial agent that has also been used for pleurodesis. The search for more effective and safe agents for pleurodesis is ongoing. Transforming growth factor-β is a unique cytokine with potent profibrotic as well as anti-inflammatory activity. It upregulates collagen production and does not cause any inflammatory pleural response in animal models. It appears to be a more effective pleurodesis agent than talc in animals and human trials are awaited.

Other issues in pleurodesis: Small-bore drain (10–14 Fr) insertion is generally easier to perform, causes less discomfort to the patient and are equally effective as larger drains (24–32 Fr); therefore, these drains should be the initial choice for effusion drainage and pleurodesis.[38] Traditionally, pleurodesis was performed once drain output was <150 mL/day and the lung fully expanded. The chest drain is removed once the output is <150 mL/day post pleurodesis. This leads to longer hospital stays and greater costs. Rapid pleurodesis involves placing a 9–14-Fr catheter under guidance, achieving complete drainage and then attempting pleurodesis immediately. If loculations or fluid re-accumulation is detected, sonographically guided thoracentesis and pleurodesis through the thoracentesis needle is performed. This has been shown to be effective and can be performed with small drains in <24 hours.

The amount and duration of fluid draining after sclerosant instillation does not indicate pleurodesis success, and the length of stay is significantly reduced when the chest drain is removed at 24 hours (4 vs. 8 days). In the absence of excessive fluid drainage (>250 mL/day), the intercostal tube is removed within 24–48 hours of pleurodesis. The use of rotation and position change to disperse sclerosant after instillation through the chest drain is not supported by evidence. Unlike mesothelioma, malignant seeding of biopsy sites and drain site is extremely uncommon in metastatic pleural effusions and routine radiation to these sites is not recommended.[4-6]

Indwelling Pleural Catheters

Indwelling pleural catheters are 15.5 F silicone rubber catheters, 66 cm in length, with fenestrations along the proximal 24 cm and are inserted into the pleural space using the Seldinger technique under local anesthesia (Rocket or PleurX). A one-way valve prevents air from entering and permits drainage into a vacuum bottle at regular intervals on an ambulatory basis by a trained nurse. Incomplete lung re-expansion due to a thick visceral pleural peel (lung entrapment) prevents pleural apposition and prevents successful pleurodesis. Unlike patients with "trapped lung", these effusions are exudative, associated with ongoing pleural malignancy or inflammation and may increase in size and the best management option for this situation is the insertion of a tunneled silicone pleural catheter.

Upfront Use of an IPC versus Pleurodesis in a MPE Recurring after a Therapeutic Thoracocentesis

Increasingly, an IPC inserted and managed on an ambulatory basis is becoming standard of care for a symptomatic MPE, especially in Western settings. The advantages include lower time spent in hospital, good symptom relief, lower need for a repeat pleural intervention, and concurrent chemotherapy while drainage is ongoing. IPCs cause autopleurodesis in 27–70% (typically 40–45%) within 2–12 weeks of insertion and can be removed once drainage is <50 mL for 3 consecutive days in the absence of a moderate effusion and lung sliding on ultrasound.[39] A hybrid-mode with ambulatory IPC insertion, rapid drainage, followed by talc slurry instilled through IPC on ambulatory basis can accelerate pleurodesis.[40] Complications of IPC include bleeding, catheter blockage, catheter fracture on removal, tract metastases and infection (tract and/or pleural space). Perception, lack of availability, costs (especially of the drainage bags), infection, and need for training nurses or caregivers to perform ongoing drainage in a large country have hindered use of IPCs as first-line in Indian settings.

Refractory Malignant Effusion

Patients who fail thoracoscopic pleurodesis and/or IPC can be managed with pleuroperitoneal shunt or pleurectomy but this is seldom performed in clinical practice.

Prognosis

The presence of a MPE signifies advanced-stage cancer with a median survival of 4–7 months from presentation. Approximately 25% of patients with a MPE are readmitted within 30 days of discharge after diagnosis; 17% die during readmission.[4] Predictors of survival in terms of decreasing importance include the performance status of the patient, the site of the primary cancer, and pleural fluid characteristics (pH and sugar). The performance status is significantly associated with mortality and the median survival is 1.1 months with a Karnofsky score < 30 and 13.2 months with a score >70. Several scoring systems exist to predict survival; these include the LENT score [pleural fluid LDH, ECOG (Eastern Cooperative Oncology Group) score, blood neutrophil-to-lymphocyte ratio and tumor type], PROMISE [eight variables—hemoglobin, CRP, total leukocyte count (TLC), ECOG, Cancer type, pleural fluid tissue inhibitor of matrix metalloproteinase 1 (TIMP1) and previous chemotherapy or radiotherapy] and BLESS (Breast and lung effusion survival score) scores have been proposed but require external validation.

SUMMARY

A malignant etiology is an important cause in the overall differential diagnosis of pleural effusion. Recognition of malignant nature of effusion is clinically significant to establish for both management and prognostication. In addition to cancer chemo- and/or immunotherapy, drainage of fluid is required for symptomatic palliative treatment. Pleurodesis is often preferred in view of the frequent recurrences of effusion.

REFERENCES

1. Marel M, Zrůstová M, Stasný B, et al. The incidence of pleural effusion in a well-defined region. Epidemiologic study in central Bohemia. Chest. 1993;104(5):1486-9.
2. Light R. Pleural Effusions Related to Metastatic Malignancies Pleural diseases, 5th edition. Lippincott Williams & Wilkins; 2007. pp. 133-61.
3. Bibby AC, Dorn P, Psallidas I, et al. ERS/EACTS statement on the management of malignant pleural effusions. Eur Respir J. 2018;52(1).
4. Feller-Kopman DJ, Reddy CB, DeCamp MM, et al. Management of malignant pleural effusions. An official ATS/STS/STR clinical practice guideline. Am J Respir Crit Care Med. 2018;198(7): 839-49.
5. BTS statement on malignant mesothelioma in the UK, 2007. Thorax. 2007;62 Suppl 2(Suppl 2):ii1-19.
6. Roberts ME, Neville E, Berrisford RG, et al. Management of a malignant pleural effusion: British Thoracic Society Pleural Disease Guideline 2010. Thorax. 2010;65(Suppl 2):ii32-40.
7. Light RW. The undiagnosed pleural effusion. Clin Chest Med. 2006;27(2):309-19.
8. Goldstraw P, Chansky K, Crowley J, et al. The IASLC lung cancer staging project: Proposals for revision of the TNM stage groupings in the forthcoming (eighth) edition of the TNM classification for lung cancer. J Thorac Oncol. 2016;11(1):39-51.
9. Naito T, Satoh H, Ishikawa H, et al. Pleural effusion as a significant prognostic factor in non-small cell lung cancer. Anticancer Res. 1997;17(6D):4743-6.
10. Banerjee AK, Willetts I, Robertson JF, et al. Pleural effusion in breast cancer: a review of the Nottingham experience. Eur J Surg Oncol. 199420(1):33-6.
11. Xaubet A, Diumenjo MC, Marín A, et al. Characteristics and prognostic value of pleural effusions in non-Hodgkin's lymphomas. Eur J Respir Dis. 1985;66(2):135-40.
12. Rodrîguez-Panadero F, Borderas Naranjo F, et al. Pleural metastatic tumours and effusions. Frequency and pathogenic mechanisms in a post-mortem series. Eur Respir J. 1989;2(4):366-9.
13. Travis WD, Brambilla E, Rami-Porta R, et al. Visceral pleural invasion: Pathologic criteria and use of elastic stains: Proposal for the 7th edition of the TNM classification for lung cancer. J Thorac Oncol. 2008;3(12):1384-90.
14. Meyer PC. Metastatic carcinoma of the pleura. Thorax. 1966; 21(5):437-43.
15. Light RW, Hamm H. Malignant pleural effusion: Would the real cause please stand up? Eur Respir J. 1997;10(8):1701-2.
16. Grove CS, Lee YCG. Vascular endothelial growth factor: The key mediator in pleural effusion formation. Curr Opin Pulm Med. 2002;8(4):294-301.
17. Marel M, Stastny B, Melínová L, et al. Diagnosis of pleural effusions. Experience with clinical studies, 1986 to 1990. Chest. 1995;107(6):1598-603.
18. Asciak R, Rahman NM. Malignant pleural effusion: From diagnostics to therapeutics. Clin Chest Med. 2018;39(1):181-93.
19. Kapp CM, Lee HJ. Malignant pleural effusions. Clin Chest Med. 2021;42(4):687-96.
20. Ferrer J, Roldán J, Teixidor J, et al. Predictors of pleural malignancy in patients with pleural effusion undergoing thoracoscopy. Chest. 2005;127(3):1017-22.
21. Jiménez D, Díaz G, Gil D, et al. Etiology and prognostic significance of massive pleural effusions. Respir Med. 2005; 99(9):1183-7.
22. Leung AN, Müller NL, Miller RR. CT in differential diagnosis of diffuse pleural disease. AJR Am J Roentgenol. 1990;154(3): 487-92.
23. Metintas M, Ucgun I, Elbek O, et al. Computed tomography features in malignant pleural mesothelioma and other commonly seen pleural diseases. Eur J Radiol. 2002;41(1):1-9.
24. Riantawan P, Bangpattanasiri K, Chaowalit P, et al. Etiology and clinical implications of eosinophilic pleural effusions. Southeast Asian J Trop Med Public Health. 1998;29(3):655-9.
25. Good JTJ, Taryle DA, Sahn SA. The pathogenesis of low glucose, low pH malignant effusions. Am Rev Respir Dis. 1985;131(5): 737-41.
26. Sahn SA, Good JTJ. Pleural fluid pH in malignant effusions. Diagnostic, prognostic, and therapeutic implications. Ann Intern Med. 1988;108(3):345-9.
27. Martínez-Moragón E, Aparicio J, Sanchis J, et al. Malignant pleural effusion: Prognostic factors for survival and response to chemical pleurodesis in a series of 120 cases. Respiration. 1998;65(2):108-13.
28. Abouzgheib W, Bartter T, Dagher H, et al. A prospective study of the volume of pleural fluid required for accurate diagnosis of malignant pleural effusion. Chest. 2009;135(4):999-1001.
29. Maskell NA, Gleeson FV, Davies RJO. Standard pleural biopsy versus CT-guided cutting-needle biopsy for diagnosis of malignant disease in pleural effusions: A randomised controlled trial. Lancet (London, England). 2003;361(9366):1326-30.
30. Casal RF, Eapen GA, Morice RC, Jimenez CA. Medical thoracoscopy. Curr Opin Pulm Med. 2009;15(4):313-20.
31. Alataş F, Alataş O, Metintaş M, et al. Diagnostic value of CEA, CA 15-3, CA 19-9, CYFRA 21-1, NSE and TSA assay in pleural effusions. Lung Cancer. 2001;31(1):9-16.
32. Echevarria C, Twomey D, Dunning J, et al. Does re-expansion pulmonary oedema exist? Interact Cardiovasc Thorac Surg. 2008;7(3):485-9.
33. Lentz RJ, Lerner AD, Pannu JK, et al. Routine monitoring with pleural manometry during therapeutic large-volume thoracentesis to prevent pleural-pressure-related complications: a multicentre, single-blind randomised controlled trial. Lancet Respir Med. 2019;7(5):447-55.

34. Dipper A, Jones HE, Bhatnagar R, et al. Interventions for the management of malignant pleural effusions: a network meta-analysis. Cochrane Database Syst Rev. 2020;4(4):CD010529.
35. Rodriguez-Panadero F, Montes-Worboys A. Mechanisms of pleurodesis. Respiration. 2012;83(2):91-8.
36. Agarwal R, Aggarwal AN, Gupta D. Efficacy and safety of iodopovidone pleurodesis through tube thoracostomy. Respirology. 2006;11(1):105-8.
37. Muthu V, Dhooria S, Sehgal IS, et al. Iodopovidone pleurodesis for malignant pleural effusions: an updated systematic review and meta-analysis. Support Care Cancer. 2021;29(8):4733-42.
38. Parulekar W, Di Primio G, Matzinger F, et al. Use of small-bore vs large-bore chest tubes for treatment of malignant pleural effusions. Chest. 2001;120(1):19-25.
39. Fysh ETH, Bielsa S, Budgeon CA, et al. Predictors of clinical use of pleurodesis and/or indwelling pleural catheter therapy for malignant pleural effusion. Chest. 2015;147(6):1629-34.
40. Yeung M, Loh E-W, Tiong T-Y, et al. Indwelling pleural catheter versus talc pleurodesis for malignant pleural effusion: a meta-analysis. Clin Exp Metastasis. 2020;37(4):541-9.

CHAPTER 131

Uncommon Pleural Effusions

MS Barthwal, Sachinkumar S Dole

INTRODUCTION

Pleural effusions can occur because of various etiologies, most commonly due to causes such as congestive heart failure, infections including tuberculosis, malignancy and pulmonary embolism.[1] There are some uncommon causes of pleural effusions, which present with distinct clinical and biochemical features. This chapter describes important uncommon pleural effusions such as chylothorax, pseudochylothorax, Meigs syndrome, yellow nail syndrome (YNS), and urinothorax (UT).

CHYLOTHORAX

Chylothorax refers to the presence of chyle in the pleural space which is caused due to disruptions of flow of chyle through the thoracic duct. Thoracic duct starts at the cisterna chili, formed by lymphatics from intraabdominal, lower extremities and retroperitoneal, which is located anterior to the second lumbar vertebra (T12 to L1) and ends at the junction of the left subclavian and jugular veins.[2] The thoracic duct carries chyle (which contains chylomicrons, T-lymphocytes, electrolytes, proteins, immunoglobulins, and fat-soluble vitamins) from the intestine to the bloodstream.

Etiology

Chylothorax can occur due to either nontraumatic or traumatic causes **(Box 1)**.[3,4] Malignancy is the most common cause of nontraumatic chylothorax. Lymphoma, lung cancer, chronic lymphocytic leukemia, Kaposi's sarcoma, and multiple myeloma are common malignancies responsible for chylothorax. Thoracic procedures involving esophagus, heart, and lung surgery are the major causes of traumatic chylothorax.[5]

BOX 1 Causes of chylothorax.

Nontraumatic

- *Malignant:*
  - Lymphomas
  - Lung cancers
  - Mediastinal cancers
  - Chronic lymphocytic leukemia
  - Multiple myeloma
  - Kaposi's sarcoma
  - Metastatic cancers
- *Nonmalignant:*
  - Lymphangioleiomyomatosis
  - Tuberculosis
  - Sarcoidosis
  - Amyloidosis
  - Filariasis
  - Idiopathic

Traumatic

- *Surgical:*
  - Cardiac surgery
  - Thoracic surgery
  - Neck surgery
  - Spine surgery
- *Nonsurgical:*
  - Trauma to the neck, thorax, and upper abdomen

Clinical Features

Dyspnea is the predominant symptom in majority of patients with chylothorax. Other symptoms include heaviness in the chest, loss of weight, and fatigue. Fever and chest pain are rare symptoms.[6] Onset of symptoms is insidious in patients with nontraumatic chylothorax while it is acute in traumatic chylothorax.

Diagnosis

Thoracic duct disruption below 5th thoracic vertebra usually results in a right-sided pleural effusion whereas disruption above this level gives rise to a left-sided effusion.[6] Unless the patient is severely malnourished, serum triglycerides, total protein, albumin, and immunoglobulin levels are generally normal despite the loss of these molecules into the pleural space.

Pleural Fluid Characteristics

Since milky appearance in chylothorax is seen in about 50% of cases, diagnosis of chylothorax should be considered in patients with predisposing conditions as mentioned earlier. The differential diagnosis of milky appearance of

BOX 2 Pleural fluid characteristics in chylothorax.

- Chylothorax is exudative with lymphocyte predominance
- Pleural fluid lactate dehydrogenase (LDH) levels are low with normal pleural fluid glucose levels
- Pleural fluid triglycerides level > 100 mg/dL
- Pleural fluid cholesterol level > 60 mg/dL but <200 mg/dL
- Detection of chylomicrons in pleural fluid by lipoprotein electrophoresis of pleural fluid

pleural fluid includes chylothorax, pseudochylothorax, and empyema. The pleural fluid when centrifuged, the supernatant become clear in case of empyema while it remains opaque in chylothorax and pseudochylothorax. On adding 1–2 mL ethyl ether in a test tube containing the fluid, the turbidity will be cleared in pseudochylothorax (due to cholesterol crystals) while the turbidity will remain as it is in chylothorax (due to chylomicrons). Chylothorax is exudative with lymphocyte predominance. Lactate dehydrogenase (LDH) levels are low with normal pleural fluid glucose levels. Chylothorax classically has high level of triglycerides (>110 mg/dL) and the cholesterol level is usually < 200 mg/dL **(Box 2)**. In patients with milky appearance, the cholesterol level > 200 mg/dL indicates pseudochylothorax (cholesterol effusion). The detection of chylomicrons by lipoprotein electrophoresis of pleural fluid is the confirmative test for diagnosis of chylothorax.

Imaging Studies

Chest X-ray usually shows unilateral pleural effusion. In addition, it may show features suggestive of underlying predisposing condition such as mediastinal and lung masses. Computed tomography (CT) of the chest, abdomen, and pelvis should be done to assess source of chyle leak, mediastinal masses or lymphadenopathy, and abdominal accumulation of chyle as well as thoracic duct and lymphatic abnormalities. Magnetic resonance (MR) lymphangiography may be indicated in a smaller proportion of patients.

Management

Management of chylothorax depends on the underlying cause (traumatic or nontraumatic), size of the effusion and the rate of accumulation. For small-to-moderate and stable pleural effusions, observation is usually sufficient. The goals of treatment in patients with chylothorax include relief of dyspnea by drainage of the chyle, reduction in the rate of chyle formation, and maintenance of nutrition.

Chest Tube Drainage

Chest tube drainage should be done in patients with large pleural effusion in the presence of dyspnea and rapid reaccumulation of chyle. In patients with underlying malignancy requiring palliative care indwelling pleural catheters may be used for relief of dyspnea.[7] Since prolonged drainage of chylothorax may lead to complications of malnutrition and immunocompromised state, attention should be paid for adequate nutritional support and infection control measures.

Nutritional Support

Patients with low volume chylothorax (<1 L/day) should be started on high-protein, low-fat (<10 g fat/day) oral or enteral diet so as to reduce the accumulation of chyle in the pleural space.[8] Long-chain triglycerols (LCTs) should be avoided since these are converted into monoglycerides and free fatty acids (FFA), and transported as chylomicrons to the intestinal lymph ducts. LCTs should be replaced with medium-chain triglycerols (MCTs) since these are absorbed directly into intestinal cells and transported directly to the liver via the portal vein, thus bypassing the thoracic duct. The common side effects of MCTs are nausea, vomiting, steatorrhea, and flatulence. In view of low-fat diet, supplementation of fat-soluble vitamins should be given parenterally. For patients with high-volume chylothorax (>1 L/day), total parenteral nutrition should be preferred. Fat intake should be increased gradually as the patient improves and the volume of pleural drainage decreases.

Somatostatin (Octreotide)

Somatostatin and octreotide reduces the chyle flow by inhibiting gastric, pancreatic, and biliary secretions, and inhibiting absorption of chyle from the intestine.[9] These drugs may be used as adjunct therapy in view of limited evidence regarding its efficacy.[9]

Surgical Management

Earlier surgical intervention is indicated when the daily pleural drainage continues to be in excess (e.g., >1.5 L/day). These interventions, which include pleurodesis, pleurectomy, thoracic duct repair or ligation, lymphovenous anastomosis, and pleuroperitoneal shunting, may be used singly or in combination. The choice of surgical approach (open thoracotomy vs. thoracoscopy) depends on the available expertise and requires a multidisciplinary approach involving pulmonologists, thoracic surgeons, and interventional radiologists.

PSEUDOCHYLOTHORAX

Pseudochylothorax (chyliform or cholesterol effusion) is less common than chylothorax. It is usually unilateral and is characterized by accumulation of turbid or milky white pleural fluid due to its high lipid content not resulting from disruption of the thoracic duct.

Etiology

The two most common causes of pseudochylothorax include rheumatoid pleuritis and tuberculosis, while other uncommon causes are chronic pneumothorax, chronic hemothorax, pleural paragonimiasis, echinococcosis, malignancy, or trauma.[10,11] Pseudochylothorax is usually seen in patients with long-standing pleural effusions and in patients with thickened or calcified pleura.[12] The high concentration of cholesterol in the pleural fluid is believed to originate from degraded erythrocytes and neutrophils and poorly absorbed through thickened pleural membranes.[12]

Clinical Features

Majority of patients are asymptomatic while some may have dyspnea on exertion. Pleural effusion is usually unilateral in pseudochylothorax.

Diagnosis

Chylothorax is acute in nature with normal pleural surfaces, while pseudochylothorax is usually a chronic condition with a thickened or calcified pleura.[13] On chest radiography, pseudochylothoraces are unilateral with no distinguishing features, except for ipsilateral pleural thickening in most cases.[14] Diagnosis is established by pleural fluid analysis. Pleural fluid is neutrophilic exudates in nature. Typically, the pleural fluid cholesterol level is 200 mg/dL or greater while the triglyceride level is <110 mg/dL. There are important differentiating features between chylothorax and pseudochylothorax **(Table 1)**. Triglycerides may be elevated in pseudochylothorax but the pleural fluid cholesterol to triglyceride ratio is always >1.0.[15]

Management

Majority of cases of pseudochylothorax have a benign course and do not require any specific therapy. Therapeutic thoracentesis should be done to relieve dyspnea in symptomatic patients. Treatment of underlying condition may lead to resolution of pseudochylothorax in some cases. Patients with recurrent symptomatic pseudochylothorax may require pleurodesis and decortication.

TABLE 1: Differentiating features between chylothorax and pseudochylothorax.

Characteristics	Chylothorax	Pseudochylothorax
Etiology	Traumatic, nontraumatic (lymphoma and other malignancies)	• Rheumatoid arthritis, tuberculosis • Chronic pneumothorax and hemothorax
Onset	Acute	Chronic
Pleural fluid cytology	Predominantly lymphocytes	Predominantly neutrophils
Pleural fluid cholesterol	>60 and <200 g/dL	>200 g/dL
Diagnosis	Presence of chylomicrons	• Presence of cholesterol crystals • Cholesterol/ triglycerides ratio > 1
Management	Treatment of underlying conditions, pleurodesis	• Observation • Decortication in some cases

MEIGS SYNDROME

Meigs syndrome is characterized by the presence of ascites and pleural effusion in patients with benign solid ovarian tumors. Although Meigs syndrome is classically associated with solid ovarian tumors, yet similar presentations can be seen in benign cystic ovarian tumors, benign tumors of the uterus, low-grade ovarian malignant tumors without evidence of metastases and with endometrioma.[16] Meigs-type syndromes which are not associated with benign solid ovarian tumors are sometimes known as pseudo-Meigs syndrome.[16]

Etiology

The pleural effusion in Meigs syndrome is due to translocation of ascites via diaphragmatic pores. The possible mechanism of ascites is due to release of inflammatory cytokines (IL-6) and growth factors (vascular endothelial growth factor and fibroblast growth factor) from ovarian tumor resulting in increased vascular permeability and capillary leakage.[16]

Clinical Features

Weight loss, pleural effusion, ascites, and a pelvic mass are common presenting symptoms in patients with Meigs syndrome.[17] The pleural effusion is right sided in approximately 70% of patients, left sided in 10%, and bilateral in 20%.[18] The pleural effusion is usually an exudates but in some cases has been reported as a transudate.[19] Serum cancer antigen 125 (CA-125) levels are raised in majority of the patients while raised pleural fluid CA-125 levels are seen in a few cases.[20]

Diagnosis and Management

Meigs syndrome should be considered in a patient who has pleural effusion, ascites, and a pelvic mass. The biochemical and cytological examination of the ascitic and pleural fluid does not reveal any diagnostic features apart from being exudative. Although elevated serum CA-125 is suggestive of ovarian cancer, its elevation in Meigs syndrome is not diagnostic since it is expressed by mesothelial cells and not by the tumor itself.[21] The complete resolution of ascitic and pleural fluid after surgical removal of tumor confirms the diagnosis of Meigs syndrome.

YELLOW NAIL SYNDROME

Yellow nail syndrome typically comprises a triad of yellow, thickened, deformed nails; lymphedema; and pleural effusion or other respiratory abnormality.[22]

Pathogenesis

Pathogenesis of YNS is not completely understood. Anatomic abnormality of the lymphatic ducts such as lymphatic hypoplasia has been demonstrated on lymphangiography in some patients while in other cases functional lymphatic abnormalities based on results of lymphoscintigraphy has also been observed.[23] Pleural effusions may develop when a lower respiratory tract infection or pleural inflammation damages impaired lymphatic vessels resulting in accumulation of pleural fluid.[24]

Clinical Features

Presentation of YNS is usually seen between fourth and sixth decades of life.[22] Nail abnormalities include slow growth, thickening, transverse ridging and excessive curvature from side to side, uneven pigmentation, and onycholysis.[22] Lymphedema presents as nonpitting edema and typically involves the lower extremities. It may also occurs in the upper extremities, face, and rarely in the peritoneal cavity with ascites. Respiratory abnormalities include bronchiectasis and recurrent lower respiratory tract infections (50%), followed by chronic sinusitis (40%), and pleural effusion (40%). Pleural fluid is usually bilateral, exudative with lymphocytic predominance and normal glucose level. Once pleural effusion has occurred, it persists and recurs rapidly after thoracentesis.[23]

Diagnosis and Management

The diagnosis is made when a patient has a chronic pleural effusion in conjunction with yellow nails or lymphedema. Pleurodesis should be considered in patients with symptomatic and recurrent effusion.[25,26] Respiratory manifestations such as bronchiectasis can be controlled with a combination of postural drainage and antimicrobial therapy. The nail manifestations improve along with better control of respiratory and lymphatic manifestations and do not require any specific treatment. Lymphedema responds often to decongestive therapy.

URINOTHORAX

Urinothorax, or accumulation of urine in the pleural space, is an uncommon cause of pleural effusion.

Etiology

Urinothorax can occur rarely in patients with obstructive uropathy. Obstruction of both ureters or at the level of the bladder or urethra is associated with urinary leak, ascites formation, and UT.[27] Other causes include trauma, surgical injury, malignancy of the urinary tract, failed tube nephrostomy, lithotripsy, renal transplantation, and kidney biopsy.[27] Direct movement of the leaked urine from abdomen into the pleural space via diaphragmatic defects appears to be a major cause of UT.[27]

Clinical Features

In majority of patients, UT is unilateral, transudate, and odor consistent with urine.[28] Pleural fluid protein level is <1.0 g/dL, glucose levels can be normal or markedly reduced, and LDH level is frequently high.[28] The pleural fluid pH is usually below 7.2 but can be normal. The pleural fluid to serum creatinine ratio is >1.0 in majority of the patients.[27]

Diagnosis and Management

Most of the time, the diagnosis of UT can be made from the presence of predisposing factors and characteristics features of pleural fluid. At times, renal scintigraphy may be helpful in establishing the diagnosis by demonstrating leakage of the tracer from the urinary tract into the pleural space.[29] The management of UT involves treatment of the underlying cause.

SUMMARY

It is important to be vigilant for rare causes of pleural effusion. In clinical practice, one should look for such an etiology in a patient which poses difficulties in the differential diagnosis or remains refractory to treatment.

REFERENCES

1. Light RW. Pleural Diseases, 6th edition. Philadelphia, PA: Lippincott Williams and Wilkins; 2013. p. 128.
2. Macfarlane JR, Holman CW. Chylothorax. Am Rev Respir Dis. 1972;105:287.
3. Valentine VG, Raffin TA. The management of chylothorax. Chest. 1992;102:586.
4. Doerr CH, Allen MS, Nichols FC 3rd, Ryu JH. Etiology of chylothorax in 203 patients. Mayo Clin Proc. 2005;80:867.
5. Prakash, UBS. Chylothorax and pseudochylothorax. Eur Respir Mon. 2002;7:249.
6. Doerr CH, Miller DL, Ryu JH. Chylothorax. Semin Respir Crit Care Med. 2001;22:617.
7. Jimenez CA, Mhatre AD, Martinez CH, et al. Use of an indwelling pleural catheter for the management of recurrent chylothorax in patients with cancer. Chest. 2007;132:1584-90.
8. Sriram K, Meguid RA, Meguid MM. Nutritional support in adults with chyle leaks. Nutrition. 2016;32:281.
9. Kalomenidis I. Octreotide and chylothorax. Curr Opin Pulm Med. 2006;12:264.
10. Garcia-Zamalloa A, Ruiz-Irastorza G, Aguayo FJ, et al. Pseudochylothorax. Report of 2 cases and review of the literature. Medicine. 1999;78:200-7.
11. Wrightson JM, Stanton AE, Maskell NA, et al. Pseudochylothorax without pleural thickening: Time to reconsider pathogenesis? Chest. 2009;136:1144-7.

12. Coe JE, Aikawa JK. Cholesterol pleural effusion. Arch Intern Med. 1961;108:763-74.
13. Song JW, Im JG, Goo J M, et al. Pseudochylous pleural effusion with far-fluid levels: Report of six cases. Radiology. 2000;21(6):478-80.
14. Garcia-Zamalloa A. Pseudochylothorax, an unknown disease. Chest. 2010;137(4):1004-5.
15. Agrawal V, Sahn SA. Lipid pleural effusions. Am J Med Sci. 2008;335:16-20.
16. Abramov Y, Anteby SO, Fasouliotis SJ, et al. Markedly elevated levels of vascular endothelial growth factor, fibroblast growth factor, and interleukin 6 in Meigs syndrome. Am J Obstet Gynecol. 2001;184:354-5.
17. Meigs JV. Fibroma of the ovary with ascites and hydrothorax. Meigs' syndrome. Am J Obstet Gynecol. 1954;67:962-87.
18. Majzlin G, Stevens FL. Meigs' syndrome: Case report and review of literature. J Int Coll Surg.1964;42:625-30.
19. O'Flanagan SJ, Tighe BF, Egan TJ, et al. Meigs' syndrome and pseudo-Meigs' syndrome. JR Soc Med. 1987; 80:252-3.
20. Patsner B . Meigs syndrome and "false positive" preoperative serum CA-125 levels: analysis of ten cases. Eur J Gynaecol Oncol. 2000;21:362-3.
21. Riker D, Goba D. Ovarian mass, pleural effusion, and ascites: revisiting Meigs syndrome. J Bronchol Interv Pulmonol. 2013;20(1):48-51.
22. Maldonado F, Tazelaar HD, Wang CW, et al. Yellow nail syndrome: analysis of 41 consecutive patients. Chest. 2008;134:375-81.
23. Bull RH, Fenton DA, Mortimer PS. Lymphatic function in the yellow nail syndrome. Br J Dermatol. 1996;134:307-12.
24. Emerson PA. Yellow nails, lymphoedema, and pleural effusions. Thorax. 1966;21:247-53.
25. Lewis M, Kallenbach J, Zalczman M, et al. Pleurectomy in the management of massive pleural effusion associated with primary lymphoedema: demonstration of abnormal pleural lymphatics. Thorax. 1983;38:637-9.
26. Jiva TM, Poe RH, Kallay MC. Pleural effusion in yellow nail syndrome: chemical pleurodesis and its outcome. Respiration. 1994;61:300-2.
27. Garcia-Pachon E, Romero S. Urinothorax: a new approach. Curr Opin Pulm Med. 2006;12:259-63.
28. Salcedo JR. Urinothorax: Report of 4 cases and review of the literature. J Urol. 1986;135:805-8.
29. Bhattacharya A, Venkataramarao SH, Kumar S, et al. Urinothorax demonstrated on 99mTc ethylene dicysteine renal scintigraphy. Nephrol Dial Transplant. 2007;22:1782-3.

CHAPTER 132

Pneumothorax

Uma Devaraj, Geroge D'Souza

INTRODUCTION

"Pneumothorax", defined as air in the pleural space, is one of the most common thoracic diseases affecting adolescents and young adults. Pneumothoraxes are classified as "spontaneous", which occur without antecedent trauma or another obvious cause, and "traumatic", which occur from direct or indirect trauma to the chest.

Spontaneous pneumothoraxes are subdivided into primary spontaneous pneumothorax (PSP) and secondary spontaneous pneumothorax (SSP). PSPs occur in otherwise healthy individuals. SSPs occur as a complication of an underlying lung disease. Many pneumothoraxes labeled as primary have an occult lung disease as evidenced by subpleural blebs on computed tomography (CT) scans. The bimodal distribution of the disease, with a peak in the 15-34-year age-group and another peak after 55 years of age, further suggests that there is an underlying predisposition that is different in the two groups.[1] Traumatic pneumothorax is further subcategorized as "iatrogenic" (consequence of a diagnostic or therapeutic procedure) and "noniatrogenic".

DEFINITIONS

Recurrent pneumothorax: A recurrent pneumothorax is one that occurs on the same side after 7 days of initial resolution. A pneumothorax is considered "persistent" if the air leak lasts for more than 5 days.

Closed pneumothorax: A closed pneumothorax[2] is one in which the alveolar pleural communication is sealed. The degree to which the lung collapses depends on the volume of air introduced during the air leak.

Tension pneumothorax: A tension pneumothorax is one in which the intrapleural pressure in the pleural cavity is above atmospheric pressure. The mediastinum is always shifted to the opposite side.

Open pneumothorax: An open pneumothorax[3] is when the pneumothorax communicates with the atmosphere and results in pendulum breathing (shunting of the physiological dead space between the two lungs) in addition to lung collapse.

PATHOPHYSIOLOGY

Normally, the pressure in the pleural space is negative with reference to the atmospheric pressure during the entire respiratory cycle. The negative pressure is due to the inherent tendency of the lungs to collapse and of the chest wall to expand. The resting volume of the lung, the functional residual capacity (FRC), is the volume at which the outward pull of the chest wall is equal, but opposite in direction, to the inward pull of the lung with the respiratory muscles relaxed. The pleural pressure is always less than the alveolar pressure and the atmospheric pressure owing to the elastic recoil of the lung. Therefore, if a communication develops between the pleural space and an alveolus or between the pleural space and the atmosphere, air will flow into the pleural space until a pressure gradient no longer exists or until the communication is sealed. Pneumothorax causes alteration of lung volume and other dynamics.

Most PSP are attributed to rupture of underlying blebs and bullae.[1] A *bleb* is a gas-containing space within the visceral pleura and is usually seen at the apex. A *bulla is* a space lined partly by thickened fibrotic pleura and partly by fibrous tissue within the lung itself.[2] The negative intrapleural pressure is not uniform throughout the pleural space; a gradient of 0.25 cm H_2O/cm exists from the base to the apex of the lung. This results in greater distension of the alveoli at the apex due to greater negative pressure at the apex. This also makes the blebs and bullae at the apex vulnerable to rupture due to greater swings in pressure during a respiratory cycle.

But blebs and bullae are seen in only 20% of patients with PSP. Peripheral pleural porosity has been observed by fluorescent-enhanced autofluorescence thoracoscopy (FEAT). This is another mechanism suggested for the leak of alveolar air into the pleural space. A third mechanism postulated is peripheral airway obstruction with air trapping causing the alveoli to distend and rupture.[2]

Air reaches the pleural space either due to (1) rupture of a subpleural bulla or bleb, (2) rupture of an overdistended alveoli into the adjacent bronchovascular sheath producing pneumomediastinum (Macklin effect), accompanied by subcutaneous emphysema or pneumothorax, or (3) rupture of overdistended alveoli with air dissecting from alveoli to the peripheral portion of the lung.[3]

At FRC, the thoracic cavity is below while the lung is above its resting volume. With pneumothorax, the thoracic cavity enlarges and the lung collapses toward the hilum. This results in the main physiologic consequences of decreased vital capacity and decreased arterial PO_2. The reduction in arterial PO_2 is a result of areas with low ventilation-perfusion (V/P) ratios, anatomic shunts, and, occasionally, alveolar hypoventilation.[4,5] The decreased vital capacity is usually well tolerated in patients with PSP, whereas it can precipitate respiratory failure in patients with SSP. The total lung capacity, FRC, and diffusing capacity are also reduced, although less than the vital capacity.[3]

When perfusion to the collapsed lung is preserved, there is an increase in the pulmonary shunt and substantial hypoxemia. If perfusion to the collapsed lung is reduced by hypoxic vasoconstriction, hypoxemia may be minimal. In general, pneumothoraxes occupying <25% of the hemithorax are not associated with significant shunts. Redistribution of pulmonary blood flow and improved V/P ratios usually result in improvement of hypoxemia within 24 hours, despite the extent of the pneumothorax.

Resolution of Pneumothorax

Normally, there is no air in the pleural space as the pressure in the capillary blood with a person breathing room air is about 706 mm Hg ($PN_2 + PO_2 + PH_2O + PCO_2 = 573 + 40 + 47 + 46 = 706$) which is less than atmospheric pressure. This favors absorption of air from the pleural space into the venous blood. The rate of gas resorption depends on (1) the pressure gradient between the gases in the pleural space and the venous blood, (2) the diffusion properties of the gases present in the pleural space, (3) the area of contact between the pleural gas and pleura, and (4) the permeability of the pleural surface (i.e., a fibrotic pleura absorbs less than a normal pleura).

The net gradient for gas absorption, from pleural space into capillary blood, is only 54 mm Hg 760–706), assuming that the pleural pressure is approximately zero when there is pneumothorax. The absorption of air from the pleural cavity is approximately 1.25% per day breathing room air. This can be hastened by breathing 100% oxygen. Breathing 100% oxygen, the sum of all the partial pressures in the capillary blood will fall to below 200 mm Hg [PN_2 approaches zero, PO_2 will remain under 100 mm Hg ($PN_2 + PO_2 + PH_2O + PCO_2 = 0 + 100 + 47 + 46 = 193$)]. Therefore, the net gradient for gas absorption is enhanced to >550 mm Hg or 10 times greater that when the patient is breathing room air. Oxygen is absorbed 62 times faster than nitrogen, the slowest gas to be reabsorbed. Carbon dioxide is absorbed 23 times faster than oxygen, and carbon dioxide and water equilibrate almost instantaneously. Hence, breathing 100% oxygen will accelerate the rate of absorption of the pneumothorax.

INCIDENCE

Primary spontaneous pneumothorax: It occurs more commonly in men between ages of 20–40 years. Women tend to develop PSP 2–5 years earlier than men though they have a much lower incidence. The incidence of PSP reported in the Western literature is 15.5–22.7 cases/100,000 population per year with a male-to-female ratio ranging from 3.3:1 to 5:1.[6-8]

Secondary spontaneous pneumothorax: It may be associated with a host of underlying lung diseases, chronic obstructive pulmonary disease (COPD) being the most common condition in the western world. In Olmsted County, Minnesota, the incidence of SSP was 6.3/100,000/year for males and 2.0/100,000/year for females.[9] On an average, patients with SSP are 15–20 years older than patients with PSP. The recurrence risk of 40–80% in SSP is higher than that for PSP.

Incidence in India

The reported incidence in India of PSP among all patients presenting with spontaneous pneumothorax shows wide variability in the few studies available ranging from 99 to 1,590 per lakh.[10,11] The annual incidence, respectively, for PSP and SSP was 20 to 37 and 80.0 to 1,553 per 100,000 hospital admissions respectively in a study from north India.[10] However, a study from south India showed a lower incidence of spontaneous pneumothorax—SSP was 61.7 per lakh and PSP was 16.6 per lakh hospital admissions.[12] This figure probably overestimates the true incidence of SP in the general population, as they are hospital based with the denominator being all hospitalized patients. Our experience is consistent with the finding that SSP is more common and tuberculosis is the most common cause. The incidence of SSP peaks a little earlier in the Indian population (40–50 years) compared to the west (60–65 years),[6-8] probably because tuberculosis is an important cause.

ETIOLOGY (BOX 1)

Primary Spontaneous Pneumothorax

Though PSP by definition occurs in people without an underlying lung disease, most often it is associated with the subpleural blebs or bullae in the apical portion of the upper lobes. Blebs can be found in more than 75% of patients undergoing thoracoscopy for the treatment of PSP. It is unclear how often these lesions are actually the site of air leakage as on thoracoscopy, ruptured blebs are seen in only a few. FEAT, a novel method involving a fluorescein aerosol administration, followed by sequential white and blue

BOX 1 Etiology of spontaneous secondary pneumothorax.

Infection:
- Tuberculosis (most common cause in India)
- *Pneumocystis jirovecii* pneumonia
- Acute bacterial pneumonia

Obstructive lung disease:
- Chronic obstructive lung disease (COPD)
- Asthma
- Interstitial lung disease
- Idiopathic pulmonary fibrosis [usual interstitial pneumonitis (UIP)]
- Nonspecific interstitial pneumonitis
- Eosinophilic granuloma
- Lymphangioleiomyomatosis
- Sarcoidosis
- Langerhans cell granulomatosis
- Radiation pneumonitis or fibrosis
- Histiocytosis X

Malignancy:
- Primary lung carcinoma
- Pulmonary metastasis (especially sarcomas)
- Complications of chemotherapy

Connective tissue disease:
- Rheumatoid arthritis
- Ankylosing spondylitis
- Marfan syndrome
- Ehlers–Danlos syndrome
- Polymyositis/dermatomyositis
- Scleroderma

Others:
- Catamenial pneumothorax
- Pulmonary infarction
- Pulmonary hemorrhage
- Pulmonary alveolar proteinosis
- Tuberous sclerosis
- von Recklinghausen's disease
- Wegener's granulomatosis

light thoracoscopy using a blue light, shows FEAT-positive lesions that are normal when viewed under normal white-light thoracoscopy (WLT).[13] Several areas of subpleural fluorescein accumulation, undetectable by normal WLT, were observed. This observation supports the concept that air leakage in PSP is not necessarily associated with blebs or bullae but could occur at areas that have a completely normal appearance during WLT. These lesions, called "pleural porosity", are areas of disrupted mesothelial cells on the visceral pleura, replaced by an inflammatory elastofibrotic layer with increased porosity, allowing air to leak into the pleural space.

The development of blebs, bullae, and areas of pleural porosity may be linked to a variety of factors. These include distal airway inflammation, hereditary predisposition, anatomical abnormalities of the bronchial tree, ectomorphic physiognomy with the more negative intrapleural pressures and the relative apical ischemia, low body mass index due to caloric restriction, and abnormal connective tissue.

There is a significantly increased risk of spontaneous pneumothorax in smokers. When four separate series of patients with PSP were combined, 91% (461 of 505 patients) with PSP were smokers or ex-smokers. The occurrence of a spontaneous pneumothorax is related to the severity of cigarette smoking. In men, there appears to be a dose effect with the relative risk of a pneumothorax 7 times higher in light smokers (1–12 cigarettes/day), 21 times higher in moderate smokers (13–22 cigarettes/day), and 102 times higher in heavy smokers (>22 cigarettes/day) than in nonsmokers.[14]

Marijuana smoking has been implicated with an increased risk of developing pneumothorax. It was associated with more frequent and severe emphysema than cigarette smoking alone. Lung histology shows inflammation, heavily pigmented macrophages, and emphysema. But most studies are limited by their small size and inability to distinguish between pure cannabis smokers and cannabis and tobacco smokers.[14]

Patients with PSP tend to be taller and thinner than control subjects. A study on military recruits who developed spontaneous pneumothorax found that they were, on average, 2 inches taller and 25 pounds lighter than the typical military recruit.[15] As pleural pressure drops by 0.20 cm H_2O/cm of vertical height, pleural pressure is more negative at the apex of lung in tall people; therefore, the alveoli at their lung apex are subjected to a greater mean distending pressure. In the long run, this could lead to the formation of subpleural blebs in those tall people who are genetically predisposed to bleb formation.

Change in atmospheric pressure has also been attributed to triggering the development of pneumothorax. One study showed that there was a significant fall in the atmospheric pressure 4 days prior to the development of symptoms.[15] A study from Turkey showed that PSP incidence increased on rainy days when the atmospheric pressure was low in the preceding 2 days.[16] This adds credence to the theory that pressure changes affecting the lung are important.

In women, smoking and body shape appear to be less relevant than in men. Catamenial pneumothorax is seen in about 3% of PSP in women.[16] There are few reports of pneumothorax in pregnancy.[17] Another cause exclusive to females is lymphangioleiomyomatosis.

Genetic factors: Studies have shown an important genetic contribution in the development of spontaneous pneumothorax. Some cases occur due to an autosomal-dominant gene[18] with incomplete penetrance, the penetrance being lower in women (21%) than in men (50%). There also appears to be an inheritance linked to an X-linked recessive gene.[19]

Birt-Hogg-Dubé (BHD) syndrome is an autosomal-dominant condition characterized by the presence of facial fibrofolliculomas and pulmonary cysts which may be associated with spontaneous pneumothorax and renal tumors. BHD is caused by loss-of-function mutations in the folliculin (FLCN) protein.[19] The molecular function of FLCN is still largely unknown and debated. There is opposite and conflicting evidence of the role of FLCN in the mammalian target of rapamycin signaling/phosphorylated ribosomal protein S6 (p-S6) activation.

Other genetic conditions associated with spontaneous pneumothorax are lymphangioleiomyomatosis,[20] alpha1-antitrypsin deficiency,[21] and cystic fibrosis (CF).[22] Pneumothorax also occurs with increased frequencies in Marfan syndrome,[23] Ehler-Danlos syndrome,[23] and homocystinuria.[24]

Though **Box 1** is fairly exhaustive, almost every other pulmonary disease has been associated with SSP. In a study of 60 patients in north India, the most common etiology for SSP was identified as pulmonary tuberculosis (41%) followed by COPD and pyogenic infections. Acquired immunodeficiency syndrome (AIDS)-associated pulmonary infections were seen in four (8.3%) patients with SSP.[10,11] This is similar to data from the author's center in south India, where tuberculosis accounted for 53.8% of SSP followed by COPD (34.6%).[12]

CLINICAL MANIFESTATIONS

Primary Spontaneous Pneumothorax

Primary spontaneous pneumothorax occurs most commonly between 20 and 40 years of age and rarely after 40 years. Most often, PSP occurs during rest rather than exertion. The main symptoms are chest pain and dyspnea. Chest pain is acute in onset, pleuritic in nature, and localized to the side of pneumothorax. Though onset is acute, there is a delay in seeking medical attention as the symptoms subside within the next 24 hours. In one series, 18% of patients waited more than 1 week after the development of symptoms before seeking medical help. Other uncommon manifestations due to a pneumothorax are cough, hemoptysis, orthopnea, and Horner syndrome.[2]

The physical findings depend on the size of the pneumothorax; small pneumothoraxes (occupying less than 20%) may have normal physical findings. In PSP, the vital signs are usually normal, except for moderate tachycardia. A tension pneumothorax should be suspected if the pulse rate exceeds 140 beats/min or if hypotension, cyanosis, or electromechanical dissociation is present.

On examination of the chest, the ipsilateral hemithorax is larger and has reduced movements on respiration. On the affected side, tactile fremitus is reduced or absent, the percussion note is hyper-resonant, and the breath sounds are reduced or absent. The lower edge of the liver may be shifted inferiorly with a right-sided pneumothorax. With a large pneumothorax, the trachea may be shifted toward the contralateral side. A crunching or clicking noise heard synchronous with the heartbeat may be auscultated with a pneumothorax (particularly on the left side) or pneumomediastinum (Hamman's sign) and is influenced by respiration and body position.[25,26]

Secondary Spontaneous Pneumothorax

Secondary spontaneous pneumothorax often presents as a potentially life-threatening condition, requiring immediate action because lung function in these patients is already compromised. Dyspnea is the most prominent clinical feature; chest pain, cyanosis, hypoxemia, and hypercapnia, sometimes resulting in acute respiratory failure, can also be present. Hence, it needs early diagnosis and urgent intervention.

LABORATORY INVESTIGATIONS AND DIAGNOSIS

Diagnosis can be confirmed in the majority of cases with an upright posteroanterior chest radiograph demonstrating a pleural line **(Figs. 1 and 2)**. Chest radiograph shows a collection of lucent gas, with absent pulmonary vascular markings, between the outer margin of visceral pleura (lung) and parietal pleura (chest wall). Expiratory radiographs add little and are no longer recommended in diagnosing pneumothorax. The lateral decubitus radiograph is superior to erect or supine chest radiograph and is as sensitive as CT scanning in pneumothorax detection.

High-resolution thoracic ultrasound (USG) is the standard of care, particularly in an emergency. It is more sensitive than the chest X-ray; the sensitivity and

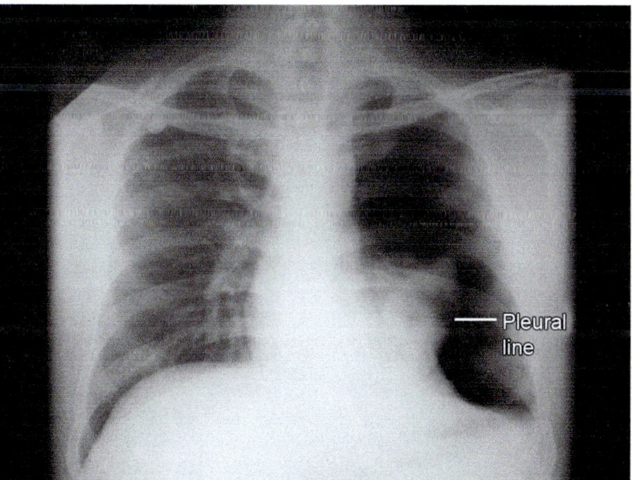

FIG. 1: Chest radiograph showing left-sided pneumothorax (primary spontaneous pneumothorax).

specificity of US as compared to CT were 95.5% and 100%, respectively.[27,28] It is also very useful in checking for post-procedural pneumothorax and following up patients with pneumothorax. On performing lung USG, "lung sliding" (movement of visceral pleura against parietal pleura), or "seashore sign" (sand like grainy image in M mode), indicates that the lung touches the chest wall.[29] Absence of lung sliding in B mode and "stratosphere" or "bar code sign" in M mode suggests the presence of pneumothorax. Identification of a "lung point" confirms the presence of pneumothorax with 100% certainty.[30]

CT thorax is the gold standard for the diagnosis of pneumothorax. However, the cost and radiation exposure and the availability of modalities like USG restrict its routine use. It is particularly useful in diagnosing associated underlying lung pathology and differentiating between a large bulla and a pneumothorax. The apparent pleural line with a large bulla is usually concave toward the lateral chest wall because it represents the medial border of the bulla, whereas the pleural line with a pneumothorax is usually oriented convexly toward the lateral chest wall **(Figs. 3A and B)**. High-resolution CT (HRCT) is more sensitive than a plain CT in identifying underlying lung pathology like blebs, bullae, and cysts.[31] CT scans are also useful in critically ill patients when decubitus films are not possible and in detecting small pneumothoraxes not evident on the chest radiograph.

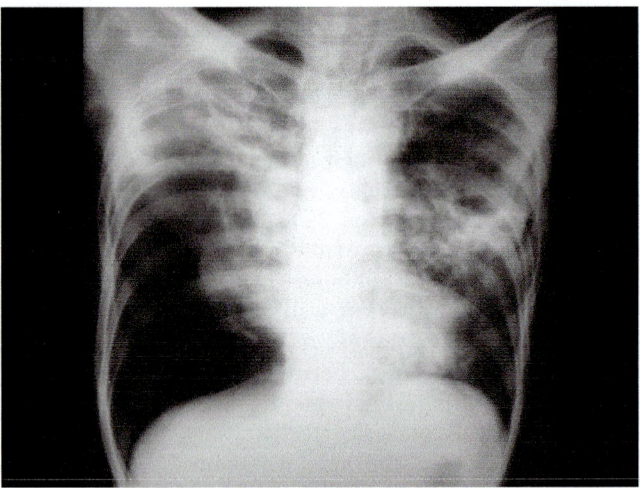

FIG. 2: Right spontaneous pneumothorax secondary to tuberculosis (secondary spontaneous pneumothorax).

Quantifying a Pneumothorax

The CT thorax is the best way to quantify a pneumothorax, but most often the chest X-ray is sufficient. The most commonly used method is the light index which is dependent on the proportional relationship between the collapsed lung and the hemithorax. The percentage pneumothorax is calculated with the formula: PNX% = 100 [1 – (lung diameter^3/hemithorax diameter^3)] **(Fig. 4)**.[32]

An alternate method to estimate the percentage of collapse, the distance between the apex of the partially collapsed lung and the apex of the thoracic cavity (distance A), the midpoints of the upper (distance B) and lower (distance C) halves of the collapsed lung and the lateral chest wall are measured in centimeters **(Fig. 5)**.[29] The percentage of the pneumothorax can be calculated by the formula: PNX% = 4.2 + [4.7 × (A + B + C)]. When the volume calculated from a helical CT scan was compared with the volume measured with this formula in 20 patients, the correlation coefficient was 0.98.

The British Thoracic Society prefers to group pneumothoraxes into "small" or "large" depending on the presence of a visible rim of <2 cm or ≥2 cm between lung margin and the chest wall.[33] This is a more practical way of calculating the size of a pneumothorax for therapeutic purposes. In contrast, the American College of Chest Physicians (ACCP) guidelines use the apex-to-cupola

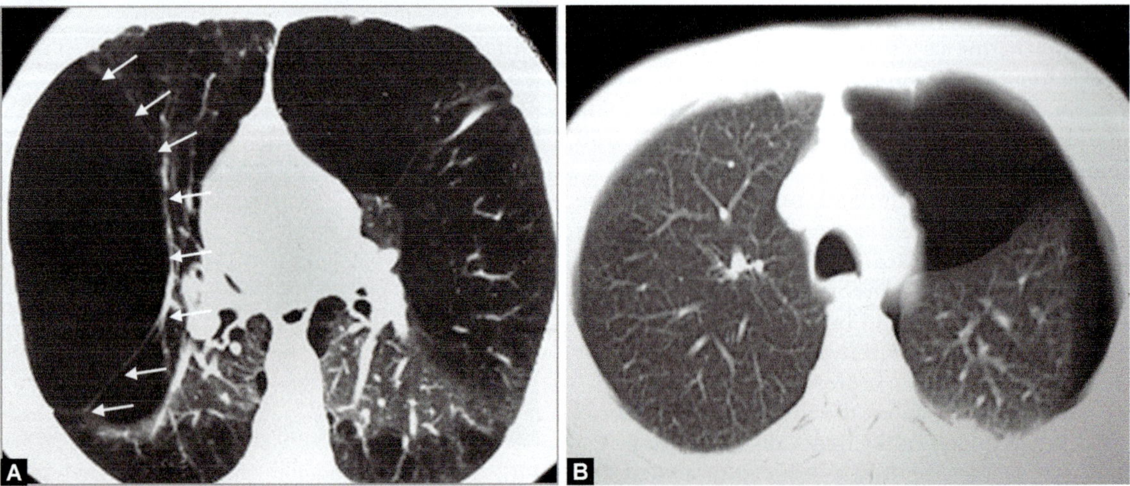

FIGS. 3A AND B: Comparison of (A) bullous emphysema and (B) pneumothorax.

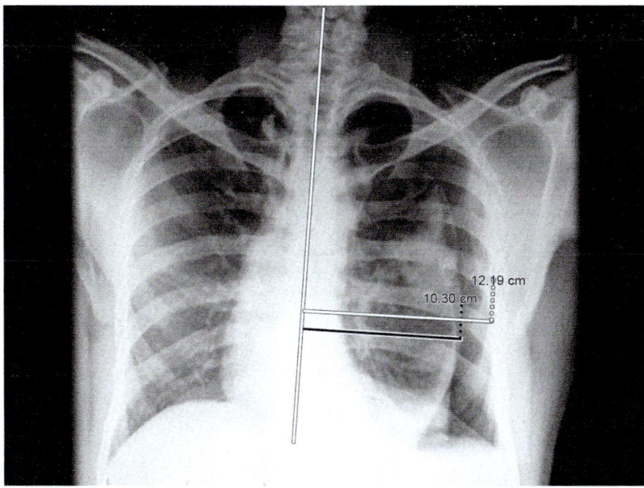

FIG. 4: Quantitation of pneumothorax by Light index: 100 ($12.19^3 - 10.3^3/12.19^3$).

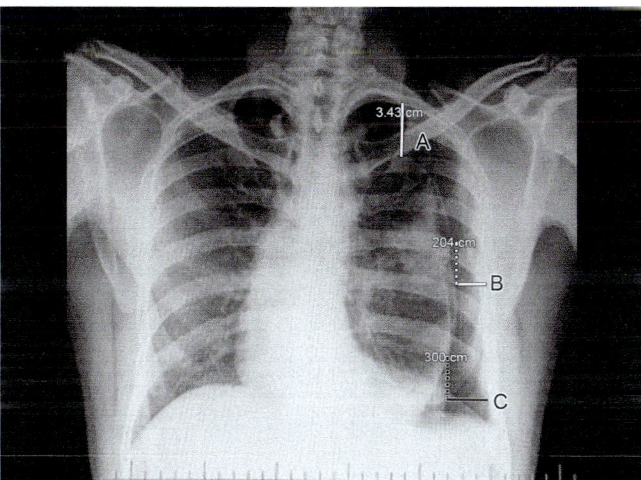

FIG. 5: Alternative formula for quantitation of pneumothorax by Collin et al.

distance to estimate the size of the pneumothorax (<3 cm distance is small and <3 cm is large pneumothorax). There is considerable discrepancy between classifications of large pneumothoraces between international guidelines.[1,12] Unfortunately, there is no evidence that measuring the size of a pneumothorax helps guide treatment. Treatment decisions are made based on how symptomatic the patient is and the presence of an underlying lung disease.

Pleural effusions may accompany pneumothorax in 20–25% of cases. Hemopneumothorax occurs in 2–3% of spontaneous pneumothoraxes. This is due to bleeding from rupture or tearing of vascular adhesions between the visceral and parietal pleura as the lung collapses.

Electrocardiographic changes may be seen due to the mechanical effects of a pneumothorax. A left-sided pneumothorax may mimic anterolateral myocardial infarction showing a rightward shift of the frontal QRS axis, diminution of precordial R voltage, decrease in QRS amplitude, and precordial T-wave inversion.[34] Absence of significant Q wave and ST segment elevation helps differentiate ECG changes due to pneumothorax from that due to myocardial infarction. With a right-sided pneumothorax, changes mimicking a posterior myocardial infarction may be seen: Diminution of precordial QRS voltage, right-axis deviation, and a prominent R wave in lead V2 with associated loss of S-wave voltage.

Arterial blood gas analysis is frequently abnormal in patients with pneumothorax with the PO_2 being <80 mm Hg in 75% of patients.[35] It needs to be done only if the resting saturation is <90%.

RECURRENCE RATES

There is a risk of recurrence of pneumothorax, particularly soon after the initial episode. In a follow-up study on 153 patients with PSP for a mean period of 54 months a 39% recurrence rate on the same side is reported, the majority within the first year.[36] Once a patient has a PSP, there is also an increased risk of having a pneumothorax on the contralateral side. In the same study, 15% developed a pneumothorax on the contralateral side.[36] The rate of recurrence increases with each successive pneumothorax. Recurrence is seen in a third of patients after the first PSP, but this may increase to 62% after the first recurrence and 83% after a third. The challenge in the management of pneumothorax is to anticipate and prevent recurrence.

TREATMENT

Primary Spontaneous Pneumothorax

The main goals of therapy are to clear the air from the pleural space and to prevent recurrence. A multitude of therapeutic options are available for the treatment of PSP, varying from conservative to an invasive approach **(Box 2)**. There are considerable differences among the international guidelines for the management of pneumothorax; clinical application and practice differ in the various regions of the world. An algorithmic approach can be employed for its management **(Flowchart 1)**.

BOX 2 **Treatment options for primary spontaneous pneumothorax.**

- Observation
- Oxygen treatment
- Simple manual aspiration
- Small catheter drainage
- Chest tube drainage
- Medical thoracoscopic talc poudrage or pleural abrasion
- Video-assisted thoracoscopic surgery (VATS) with bleb or bullectomy
- VATS with pleural abrasion or partial pleurectomy
- Axillary thoracotomy

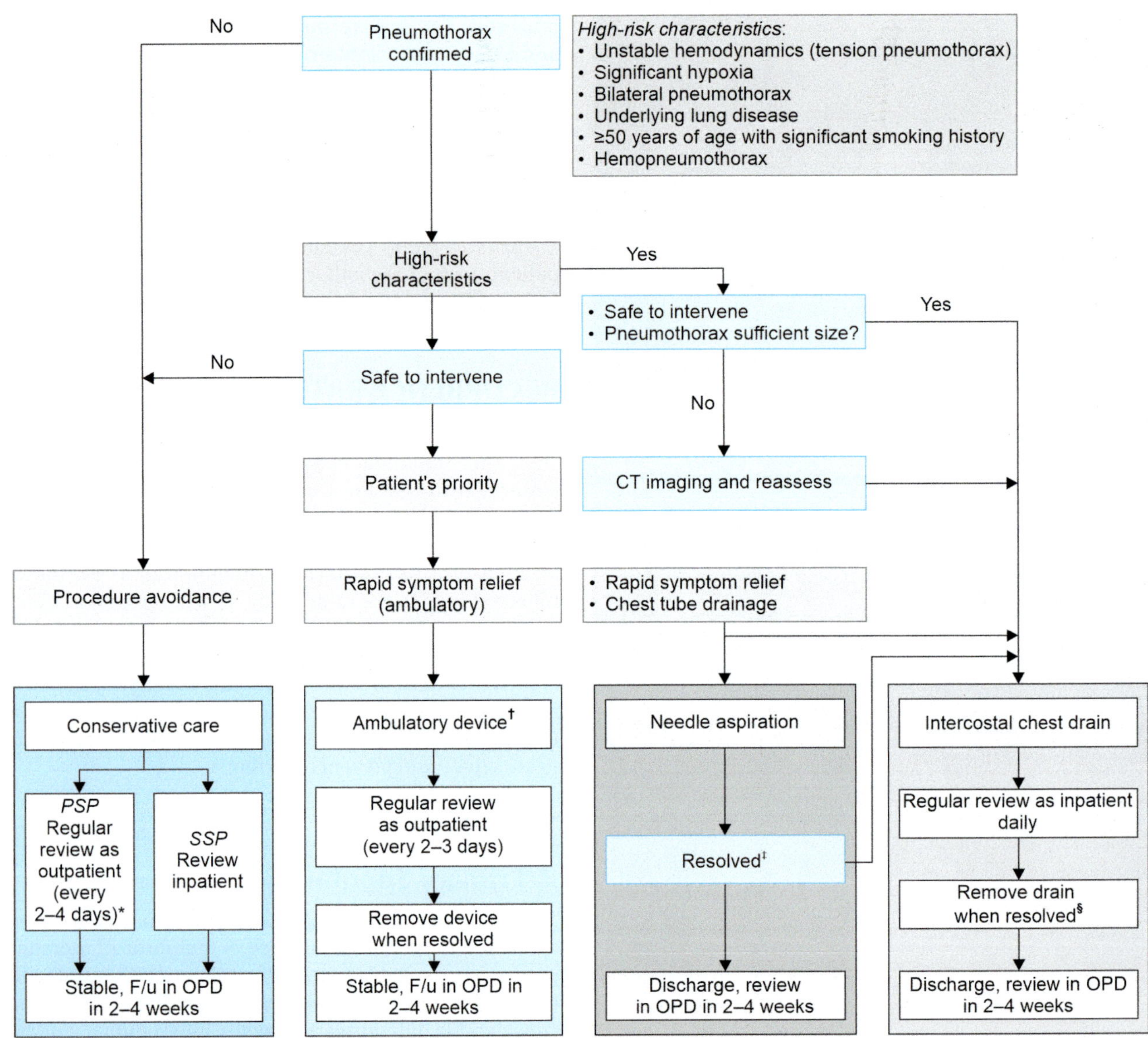

* At review, worsening symptoms or enlarging pneumothorax: Admission and intercostal drainage.

‡ Success: Radiological and clinical improvement.

† If an ambulatory device is available locally.

§ Pleurodesis to be considered on the first episode of pneumothorax in high-risk patients, where recurrence can be hazardous (e.g., COPD).

FLOWCHART 1: Algorithmic approach to manage pneumothorax.

(PSP: primary spontaneous pneumothorax; SSP: secondary spontaneous pneumothorax)

Observation or Conservative Management

Management of pneumothorax depends upon the presence of symptoms and clinical status. PSP patients with minimal symptoms are treated conservatively, regardless of the size of the pneumothorax. This is based on the fact that once the communication between the alveoli and the pleural space is sealed, the pleural space air is slowly but gradually reabsorbed at the rate of 1.25% per day.[34] In a patient with a 20% pneumothorax, it will take roughly 16 days for pleural air to be absorbed spontaneously. There is no evidence that intervention is better than observation in terms of outcomes like resolution and recurrence in PSP even in patients with a moderate-to-large pneumothorax.[37,38] A patient presenting with a first episode of PSP and not ill or significantly symptomatic is managed conservatively and followed up on an outpatient basis provided he/she is within the close reach of effective medical treatment.

Supplemental Oxygen

Administration of supplemental oxygen accelerates the rate of pleural air absorption. Administration of humidified 100% oxygen to rabbits with experimentally induced pneumothoraxes increased the rate of absorption sixfold.[38] Studies in patients with spontaneous pneumothorax have demonstrated that pleural air is absorbed about four times faster when given high concentrations of supplemental oxygen.[39] Supplemental oxygen at high concentrations is hence recommended in hospitalized patients with any type of pneumothorax who are not subjected to aspiration or tube thoracostomy.

Simple Aspiration

Simple manual aspiration should be the treatment approach in PSP patients not deemed suitable for conservative or ambulatory management.[33,37] The success rates vary between 50 and 70% of cases, averaging two thirds of cases and marginally lower than with intercostal tube drainage.[40] Complications are absent, pain and discomfort are minimized, and recurrence rates are similar to those seen after typical chest tube drainage. It can be done in the outpatient department with immediate discharge. Patients residing more than 15 minutes from the hospital should be considered for overnight observation in the hospital. Patients are reviewed in 24–72 hours with a chest radiograph.

Procedure: A 16- or 18-gauge plastic catheter is introduced, at the second anterior intercostal space in the mid-clavicular line, into the pleural space under local anesthesia using a sterile technique. The catheter is connected to a three-way stopcock and a large-volume syringe. Aspiration is performed until 2.5 L is aspirated or no further air can be withdrawn. Follow-up chest radiograph is performed. As there is a necessity for repeat aspiration or insertion of a catheter in a third of patients, placement of a small catheter attached to a Heimlich valve followed by immediate discharge has been proposed as an alternative mode of management.[1] The use of a flutter valve is advantageous in that it allows better ambulation and outpatient management, but care is required to ensure that it is connected correctly. Ambulatory care is possible subject to local availability and patients' preference.

Tube Thoracostomy

Tube thoracostomy is recommended if simple aspiration is ineffective **(Flowchart 2)**; it rapidly results in the re-expansion of the underlying lung and does not require prolonged hospitalization. A water seal is used with intercostal tube drainage which allows bubbling of air to be easily recognized.[33] Smaller intercostal tubes (sizes from 14 to 22 French) are usually recommended as they minimize the discomfort. Larger-sized tubes (24–28 French) are used if the patient is unstable and has a large pneumothorax or if the patient is suspected to have a large bronchopleural fistula (air leak), hemopneumothorax, or is in need of positive-pressure ventilation.

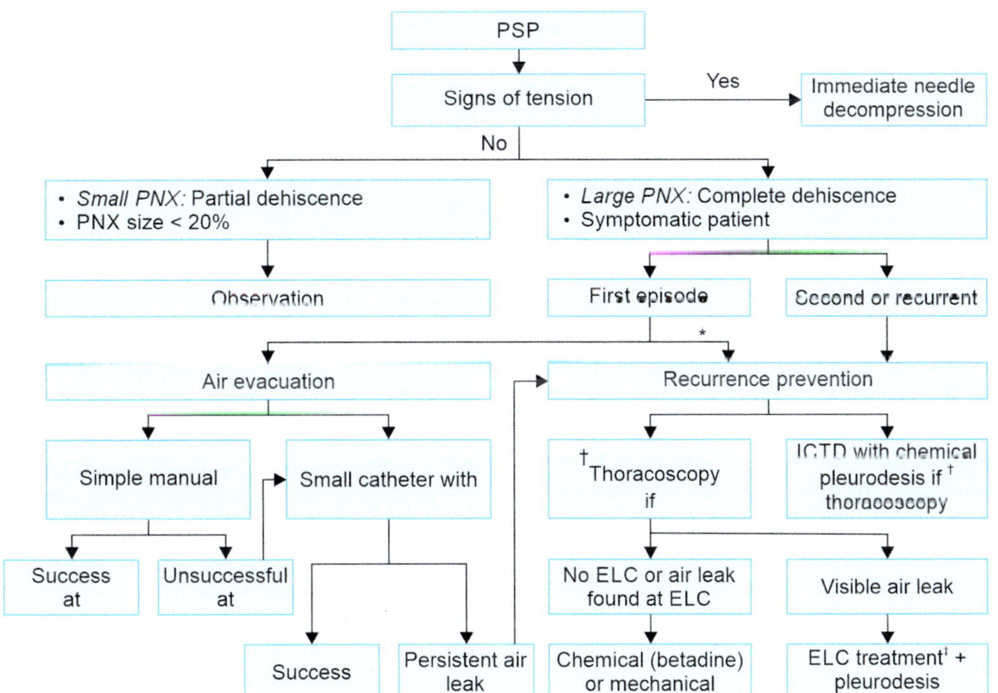

* After informed consent or in certain patient groups (aircraft personnel, divers).
† In resource-poor settings, pleurodesis without thoracoscopy is successful and cost effective.
‡ Staple bleb/bullectomy, electrocoagulation, ligation.

FLOWCHART 2: An algorithmic approach to the treatment of PSP.[5]
(ELCs: emphysema-like changes; ICTD: intercostal chest tube drainage; PNX: pneumothorax)

SECTION 12: PLEURAL DISEASES

Suction: It should be avoided for the first 24 hours of tube thoracostomy to reduce the risk of re-expansion pulmonary edema. There is also a theoretical risk of preventing the leak from closing due to suction. Randomized studies have shown varied results. Most guidelines do not recommend suction as a routine. If there is incomplete expansion after 24–48 hours, suction could be tried. Bubbling through the water seal chamber of the drainage system suggests persistent air leak. If there is no bubbling on quiet respiration, the patient should be asked to cough. The absence of bubbling indicates that there is no air leak. Clamping of the intercostal drain is not advised as it confers no advantage if the air leak has stopped. If it has not happened, a dangerous situation may develop, which may be unrecognized. After the lung has re-expanded and the air leak has ceased for 24 hours, the chest tube is removed.

Persistent Air Leak

In PSP, air leak would have already ceased in two thirds at the time of presentation and in 88% within the next week. Intervention with video-assisted thoracoscopy (VATS) or open thoracotomy should be considered when the air leak persists beyond 5 days in PSP.

Recurrence Prevention

This should be considered after the first recurrence as thereafter the rate of recurrence increases with each successive pneumothorax. Recurrence has been noted to be 20.3%[41] in PSP. Exceptions are patients at professional risk (aviation personnel, divers) and patients with a prolonged air leak (14 days) in whom a definitive procedure is indicated in the first instance. Intrapleural insertion of a catheter or tube has only a minimal (if any) effect on prevention of recurrence (34–36% observed recurrence rates after chest tube drainage only).[40]

Pleurodesis

The goal of pleurodesis is to prevent recurrence in both PSP and SSP. Pleurodesis is a procedure that causes the symphysis of the two pleural membranes. Medical or chemical pleurodesis consists of using agents such as quinacrine, silver nitrate, talc, or tetracycline to create an intense inflammatory reaction which obliterates the pleural space. Talc slurry (100 mg/kg) is the most effective agent for pleurodesis but may be associated with acute respiratory distress syndrome (ARDS), hypoxia, and hypotension in a small number of patients. ARDS is probably more common if smaller talc particles (<10 μm) are used. Talc pleurodesis should be avoided in the young because of delayed side effects including compromise on respiratory function and increased risk of developing malignancy.[40,42]

Parenteral preparation of tetracycline (35 mg/kg) or doxycycline (10 mg/kg), or 20 mL 10% iodopovidone and 80 mL normal saline solution are effective in producing pleurodesis in patients.[43,44] Since severe chest pain is a common side effect of tetracycline pleurodesis, adequate analgesia is indicated before and after the procedure. Recurrence rates can be reduced from approximately 40% to 25% by pleurodesis. Mechanical pleurodesis by thoracoscopic pleural abrasion along with stapling of pleural blebs can reduce the recurrence rates to <5%. But in many centers, it would not be available and chemical pleurodesis may be an acceptable alternative.

Thoracoscopy

Surgical procedure, either thoracoscopically or by open thoracotomy, is the definitive procedure for pneumothorax recurrence prevention. VATS is recommended by most guidelines because of less pain and shorter hospital stays. In a meta-analysis of 12 trials that randomized 670 patients, VATS was associated with shorter length of stay (reduced by 1.0–4.2 days) and less pain or use of pain medication than thoracotomy in five out of seven trials.[45] Indications for operative management are: (1) First recurrence, (2) high-risk professions/lifestyles, such as pilots or scuba divers, and (3) bilateral or tension pneumothorax.[33,46] Relative indications for VATS during the first occurrence include the presence of persistent air leak after 72 hours, and patients from remote areas without ready access to medical care.[47] VATS is also appropriate for SSP. The entire lung can be inspected and the cause of air leak identified. VATS with resection of large bullous lesions is associated with a recurrence rate of 2–14%. Pleural blebs responsible for pneumothorax are treated by a method called endo-stapling or suturing followed by pleurodesis by pleural abrasion.

Video-assisted thoracoscopic surgery was associated with substantially fewer recurrences than pleural drainage in two trials. In a study of 59 patients, pleuroscopy with insufflation of talc had a recurrence rate of 5% during a follow-up period of 5 years.[47] Even in the first episodes of PSP, thoracoscopic management reduced the length of hospital stay, recurrence rates, and days on intercostal chest tube drainage (ICTD).

Open Thoracotomy

Open thoracotomy with suturing of the blebs and pleural abrasion is a reasonable alternative when VATS is not available. A transaxillary minithoracotomy is preferred to minimize the trauma and the length of the scar. Persistent air leak after 5 days of intercostal drainage and patients with previous forms of therapy resulting in incomplete re-expansion of the lung are indications for surgical care. The other indications for surgical management are tension pneumothorax and in people in high-risk occupations. The recurrence rates with open thoracotomy are the lowest and four times less than even thoracoscopic procedures. Pain and hospital stay are longer.

Secondary Spontaneous Pneumothorax

Secondary spontaneous pneumothorax requires immediate air evacuation followed by prevention of recurrence at the first episode **(Figs. 6 and 7A and B)**. All patients with SSP should be hospitalized. Awaiting recurrence prevention treatment, air evacuation can be achieved by simple manual aspiration in young (<50 years old) patients with small pneumothoraces, but most authors and guidelines recommend immediate insertion of a chest tube.[33] The evacuation of even a small pneumothorax can lead to a rapid improvement in symptoms. If respiratory failure occurs, necessitating mechanical ventilation, a chest tube should be placed immediately because the pneumothorax is likely to enlarge during mechanical ventilation.

Small-bore chest tubes and even pigtail catheters are usually sufficient; large-bore chest tubes are recommended when large air leaks are suspected or when positive-pressure ventilation is required. Persistent air leak is more common in SSP, particularly in the elderly. Recurrence prevention should preferably use a thoracoscopic approach; in case a visible air leak is present (e.g., a ruptured emphysematous bulla), it should be closed by electrocautery or stapling. In all cases, pleurodesis should be done using talc poudrage, pleural abrasion, or partial pleurectomy. Most transplant teams do not consider pleurodesis as a contraindication for transplantation.

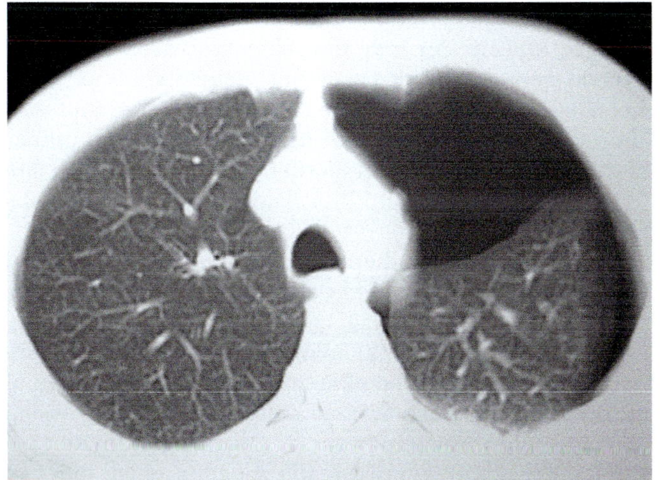

FIG. 6: Chest CT scan showing left pneumothorax.

Pneumothorax Secondary to Tuberculosis

Tuberculosis was the commonest etiology of SSP in India (41% and 53.8% for SSP in studies from north and south India, respectively). SSP associated with tuberculosis should be treated with tube thoracostomy and often requires prolonged periods of chest tube drainage. Surgery should be delayed if possible till he or she has received antituberculous therapy for at least 6 weeks.

Pneumothorax in Patients with Acquired Immunodeficiency Syndrome

Pneumothorax is not uncommon (around 5%) in patients with HIV and AIDS. It is associated with multiple etiologies: *Pneumocystis jirovecii*, pyogenic infections, Kaposi's sarcoma, cytomegalovirus, pulmonary cryptococcus, coccidiomycosis, and mycobacterial disease.[10] Most patients have a CD4+ count < 100 cells/mm^3. Approximately 5% of patients who receive prophylactic pentamidine develop a spontaneous pneumothorax. This population is also at a higher risk of contralateral pneumothorax and iatrogenic pneumothorax because of frequent pulmonary procedures or need for ventilation. SSP-associated with *P. jirovecii* is notoriously difficult to treat due to the necrotizing nature of the pneumonia. All patients with SSP due to associated AIDS should undergo tube thoracostomy. Heimlich valve or VATS is indicated if air leak persists for more than a few days.

Chronic Obstructive Pulmonary Disease and Asthma

Pneumothorax is a well-recognized, potentially lethal, and often hard to treat complication of emphysema.[48] COPD is the leading cause of SSP in the West, while it accounts for only 25% cases of SSP in India. Pneumothorax occurs

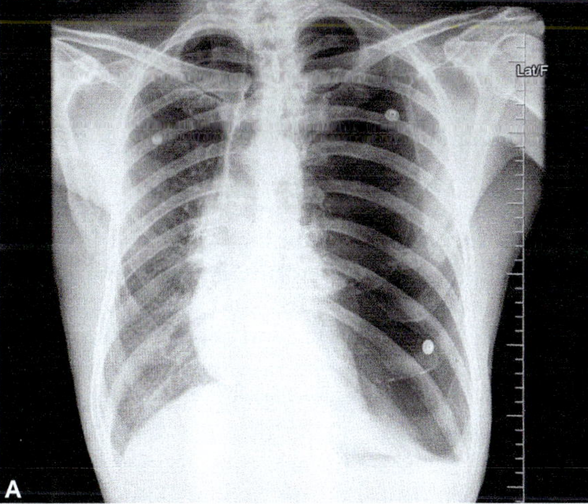

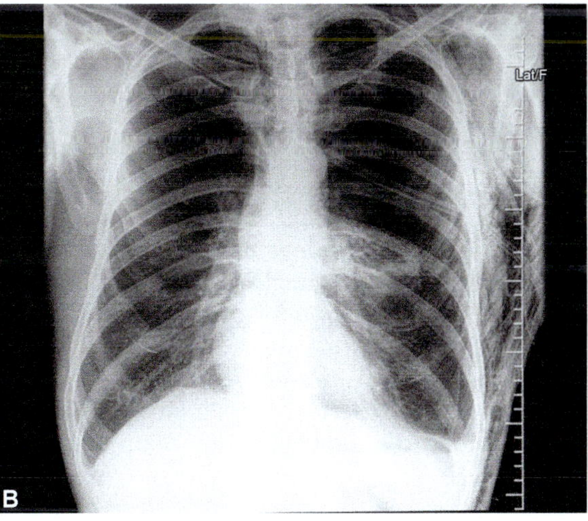

FIGS. 7A AND B: Intercostal tube drainage for left-sided pneumothorax.

in less than 2% of adults with acute asthma. In subjects with prolonged pulmonary air leaks, who are poor surgical candidates due to low pulmonary reserve, the use of autologous blood pleurodesis or endobronchial valves is an effective and minimally invasive intervention.[49,50]

Cystic Fibrosis

Pneumothorax is a serious complication in patients with CF. It is associated with a high rate of mortality and is an indicator of poor prognosis. The risk of developing a pneumothorax increases as age increases and pulmonary function [forced expiratory volume in 1 second (FEV1)] decreases. The presence of *Pseudomonas aeruginosa, Burkholderia cepacia*, and *Aspergillus* in the airways increases the risk of pneumothorax by causing increased inflammation, airway secretions, and air trapping. Recurrence rates are high, and hence recurrence preventive measures have to be taken with the first episode of pneumothorax.[22,51]

Catamenial Pneumothorax

Pneumothorax that occurs in conjunction with menstruation is called catamenial pneumothorax. Respiratory symptoms usually develop within 24–48 hours of the onset of the menstrual flow.[1] Catamenial pneumothoraxes are more common on the right side. This is due to transperitoneal migration of endometrial tissue from the pelvis through small defects in the right diaphragm. Left-sided and even bilateral pneumothoraxes have also been reported. Catamenial pneumothoraxes tend to be recurrent unless there is a therapeutic intervention.

The treatment of catamenial pneumothorax is aimed at treating endometriosis, by suppressing the ectopic endometrium. This is done by suppression of ovulation with oral contraceptives or by suppression of gonadotropins with danazol or gonadotropin-releasing hormone to produce a medical oophorectomy. But in a large series, there was a 50% recurrence and hence surgery is often required. This includes removal of endometrial implants, stapling of blebs, closure of diaphragmatic defects, parietal abrasion or pleurectomy, or chemical pleurodesis.[52]

IATROGENIC PNEUMOTHORAX

Iatrogenic pneumothoraxes are more common than PSP and SSP combined. The leading cause of iatrogenic pneumothorax is transthoracic needle aspiration. Pneumothorax is more likely if the patient has underlying COPD, if the lesion is deep within the lung, or if the angle of the needle route is wide. Other causes are transbronchial lung biopsy, thoracentesis, pleural biopsy, central vein catheterization, ventilation with high levels of positive end-expiratory pressure, tracheostomy, intercostal nerve block, mediastinoscopy, pacemaker insertion, liver biopsy, and cardiopulmonary resuscitation.[34]

Diagnosis of iatrogenic pneumothorax is often delayed. This delay can now be overcome with the application of immediate bedside USG after the procedure. Small and asymptomatic iatrogenic pneumothoraxes often do not need any treatment and resolve spontaneously. In larger or symptomatic pneumothoraxes, simple manual aspiration or placement of a small catheter or chest tube attached to a Heimlich valve is usually successful. Larger tubes may be necessary in emphysematous patients or when mechanical ventilation is indicated.

TRAUMATIC (NONIATROGENIC) PNEUMOTHORAX

Pneumothorax due to thoracic trauma is common: 40–50% are likely to have a pneumothorax. A traumatic pneumothorax can result from either penetrating or non penetrating chest trauma. In penetrating injuries, the object penetrating the chest disrupts the visceral pleural surface prompting air to enter from the lung or allows air entry through the breached chest wall. 80% of penetrating injuries are associated with pneumothorax. With blunt chest trauma, pneumothorax is either due to a rib fracture lacerating the visceral pleura or due to abrupt elevation in the alveolar pressure causing alveolar rupture. Air may then dissect toward either the visceral pleura or the mediastinum. Pneumothorax develops when either the visceral or the mediastinal pleura ruptures. The incidence increases with the increase in the number of ribs fractured; 6.7% with no rib fractures, 24.9% with one to two ribs fractured, and 81.4 % with more than two ribs fractured.[36]

Traumatic pneumothoraxes may be occult, not seen on chest radiograph but found by additional imaging. Although chest X-ray is the initial imaging modality used, the sensitivity is only 20.9%. Additional information obtained like rib fractures, hyperlucent hemithorax, inferior displacement of the diaphragm, and mediastinal shift are useful in diagnosing or suspecting a pneumothorax. A substantial number (29–72%) are occult, emphasizing the need for a high index of suspicion and early routine CT in all chest and multitrauma patients.[53,54] Thoracic ultrasonography, which can be done at the bedside as part of an extended focused assessment for trauma patients (BLUE protocol),[55] can detect most (92–100%) pneumothoraxes. It should be emphasized that these results are operator dependent, and hence adequate training is required. CT is the definitive procedure to rule out a pneumothorax. Occult pneumothorax seen on CT but not suspected clinically or on chest X-ray is seen in a significant number but may not require intervention. In one study, only 3.9% of such patients after blunt trauma with pneumothorax needed tube thoracostomy. Patients with subcutaneous emphysema, rib fractures, and pulmonary contusions are more likely to deteriorate and need tube thoracostomy.

Most traumatic pneumothoraxes should be treated initially with tube thoracostomy. If the patient has an occult pneumothorax or if the distance between the lung and the chest wall is <1.5 cm, tube thoracostomy is probably not indicated unless the patient is receiving mechanical ventilation. Fracture of the trachea or a major bronchus or traumatic rupture of esophagus are uncommon causes of traumatic pneumothorax, and an immediate thoracotomy is indicated. Rupture of the esophagus is accompanied by hydropneumothorax, and the pleural fluid amylase concentration is raised. Mortality approaches 100% if surgical treatment is not carried out promptly.[34]

TENSION PNEUMOTHORAX

Tension pneumothorax is present when the intrapleural pressure exceeds atmospheric pressure throughout expiration and frequently during inspiration. Most patients suffering a tension pneumothorax receive positive pressure to their airways, either during mechanical ventilation or during resuscitation.[34] Tension may also develop in spontaneously breathing patients, in the presence of a one-way valve process permitting air to enter the pleural space during inspiration but not exit during expiration.

Presentation is abrupt with sudden deterioration in the cardiopulmonary status of the patient. Decreased cardiac output due to impaired venous return and profound hypoxia due to V/P mismatch results in severe cardiopulmonary compromise. Patients with tension pneumothorax present with severe distress, displaying cyanosis, diaphoresis, tachycardia, hypotension, and labored breathing. Treatment should not be delayed pending radiographic confirmation, especially in a mechanically ventilated patient. When the diagnosis is suspected, the patient should immediately be given a high concentration of supplemental oxygen to alleviate the hypoxia. A large-bore (14- to 16-gauge) catheter with needle should be immediately inserted into the pleural space through the second anterior intercostal space. This confirms the diagnosis by usually eliciting an audible rush of air from the pressurized pleural space. Alternatively, the needle may be fitted with a partially sterile-water-filled syringe and introduced into the pleural space until air is aspirated. Marked bubbling after the syringe plunger is removed confirms the diagnosis. Placement of the needle through the anterior axillary line in the fifth intercoastal space may be safer and less likely to fail, particularly in those with an increased body mass index (BMI). Thereafter, an intercostal tube drainage should be placed immediately.

SUMMARY

Pneumothorax is defined as air in the pleural space. Pneumothoraxes are classified as primary or secondary spontaneous and traumatic. Smoking is an important risk factor for primary spontaneous pneumothorax, apart from genetic risk factors. In India, tuberculosis is the most common disease leading to secondary spontaneous pneumothorax.

The main symptoms of pneumothorax are pleuritic chest pain and dyspnea. The physical findings depend on the size of the pneumothorax. A chest X-ray showing lucent gas, with absent pulmonary vascular markings, between the lung and chest wall confirms the diagnosis. Based on the clinical setting, treatment of pneumothoraces ranges from simple observation, oxygen supplementation, intercoastal drainage and surgery.

REFERENCES

1. Bintcliffe OJ, Hallifax RJ, Edey A, et al. Spontaneous pneumothorax: time to rethink management? Lancet Respir Med. 2015;3(7):578-88.
2. Grippi MA, Fishman JA, Kotloff RM, et al. Pneumothorax. In: Grippi MA (Ed). Fishman's Pulmonary Diseases and Disorders, 5th edition. New York: McGraw-Hill Education; 2015.
3. Lumb AB, Thomas CR. Nunn's Applied Respiratory Physiology. 9th edition. Philadelphia: Elsevier; 2020.
4. Morioka H, Takada K, Matsumoto S, et al. Re-expansion pulmonary edema: Evaluation of risk factors in 173 episodes of spontaneous pneumothorax. Respir Investig. 2013;51(1):35-9.
5. Norris RM, Jones JG, Bishop JM. Respiratory gas exchange in patients with spontaneous pneumothorax. Thorax. 1968;23(4):427-33.
6. Kircher LT. Spontaneous pneumothorax and its treatment. J Am Med Assoc. 1954;155(1):24.
7. Noppen M, De Keukeleire T. Pneumothorax. Respiration. 2008;76(2):121-7.
8. Hallifax RJ, Goldacre R, Landray MJ, et al. Trends in the Incidence and Recurrence of Inpatient-Treated Spontaneous Pneumothorax, 1968-2016. JAMA. 2018;320(14):1471-80.
9. Melton LJ, Hepper NG, Offord KP. Incidence of spontaneous pneumothorax in Olmsted County, Minnesota: 1950 to 1974. Am Rev Respir Dis. 1979;120(6):1379-82.
10. Gupta D, Mishra S, Faruqi S, et al. Aetiology and clinical profile of spontaneous pneumothorax in adults. Indian J Chest Dis Allied Sci. 2006;48(4):261-4.
11. Gayatridevi Y, Usharani N, Premkumar A, et al. Clinical Profile of Spontaneous Pneumothorax in Adults: A Retrospective Study. Indian J Chest Dis Allied Sci. 2015;57(4):219-23.
12. Devaraj U, Ramachandran P, Krishnaswamy U, et al. Comparison of methods to quantitate spontaneous pneumothorax—A study from a tertiary care hospital. Egypt J Bronchol. 2019;13(3):388-93.
13. Noppen M, Dekeukeleire T, Hanon S, et al. Fluorescein-enhanced Autofluorescence Thoracoscopy in Patients with Primary Spontaneous Pneumothorax and Normal Subjects. Am J Respir Crit Care Med. 2006;174(1):26-30.
14. Bense L, Eklund G, Wiman L-GG. Smoking and the increased risk of contracting spontaneous pneumothorax. Chest. 1987;92(6):1009-12.
15. Light R. Pleural Diseases, 5th edition. Philadelphia: Lippincott, Williams and Wilkins; 2007.
16. Ozpolat B, Gözübüyük A, Koçer B, et al. Meteorological conditions related to the onset of spontaneous pneumothorax. Tohoku J Exp Med. 2009;217(4):329-34.
17. Jain P, Goswami K. Recurrent spontaneous pneumothorax during pregnancy: a case report. J Med Case Rep. 2009;3(1):81.

18. Khoo SK, Giraud S, Kahnoski K, et al. Clinical and genetic studies of Birt-Hogg-Dubé syndrome. J Med Genet. 2002;39(12):906-12.
19. Boone PM, Scott RM, Marciniak SJ, et al. The Genetics of Pneumothorax. Am J Respir Crit Care Med. 2019;199(11): 1344-57.
20. Glasgow CG, Steagall WK, Taveira-Dasilva A, et al. Lymphangioleiomyomatosis (LAM): molecular insights lead to targeted therapies. Respir Med. 2010;104(Suppl 1):S45-58.
21. Serapinas D, Obrikyte V, Vaicius D, et al. Alpha-1 antitrypsin deficiency and spontaneous pneumothorax: possible causal relationship. Pneumologia. 2014;63(1):32-5.
22. Flume PA, Mogayzel PJ, Robinson KA, et al. Cystic fibrosis pulmonary guidelines: pulmonary complications: hemoptysis and pneumothorax. Am J Respir Crit Care Med. 2010;182(3):298-306.
23. Hall JR, Pyeritz RE, Dudgeon DL, et al. Pneumothorax in the Marfan syndrome: prevalence and therapy. Ann Thorac Surg. 1984;37(6):500-4.
24. Bass HN, LaGrave D, Mardach R, et al. Spontaneous pneumothorax in association with pyridoxine-responsive homocystinuria. J Inherit Metab Dis. 1997;20(6):831-2.
25. Baumann MH, Sahn SA. Hamman's sign revisited. Pneumothorax or pneumomediastinum? Chest. 1992;102(4):1281-2.
26. Devaraj U, Ramachandran P, D'souza GAGA. Recurrent spontaneous pneumomediastinum in a young female: Hamman's crunch revisited. Oxf Med Case Rep. 2014;2014(2):18-20.
27. Alrajab S, Youssef AM, Akkus NI, et al. Pleural ultrasonography versus chest radiography for the diagnosis of pneumothorax: review of the literature and meta-analysis. Crit Care. 2013; 17(5):R208.
28. Ashton-Cleary DT. Is thoracic ultrasound a viable alternative to conventional imaging in the critical care setting? Br J Anaesth. 2013;111(2):152-60.
29. Collins CD, Lopez A, Mathie A, et al. Quantification of pneumothorax size on chest radiographs using interpleural distances: regression analysis based on volume measurements from helical CT. AJR Am J Roentgenol. 1995;165(5):1127-30.
30. Lichtenstein DA. Whole Body Ultrasonography in the Critically Ill, 4th edition, Vol. 21. London: Springer; 2020. vii. [online] Available from http://journal.um-surabaya.ac.id/index.php/JKM/article/view/2203 [Last accessed August, 2024].
31. Yarmus L, Feller-Kopman D. Pneumothorax in the critically ill patient. Chest. 2012;141(4):1098-105.
32. Hoi K, Turchin B, Kelly AM. How accurate is the Light index for estimating pneumothorax size? Australas Radiol. 2007;51(2): 196-8.
33. Roberts ME, Rahman NM, Maskell NA, et al. British Thoracic Society Guideline for pleural disease. Thorax. 2023;78(Suppl 3):s1-s42.
34. Courtney Broaddus V, Mason RJ, Gotway MB. Murray and Nadel's Textbook of Respiratory Medicine. Philadelphia: Elsevier; 2016. [online] Available from https://linkinghub.elsevier.com/retrieve/pii/C20111081237 [Last accessed August, 2024]
35. MacDuff A, Arnold A, Harvey J. Management of spontaneous pneumothorax: British Thoracic Society pleural disease guideline 2010. Thorax. 2010;65(Suppl 2):ii18-31.
36. Sadikot RT, Greene T, Meadows K, et al. Recurrence of primary spontaneous pneumothorax. Thorax. 1997;52(9):805-9.
37. Wakai A, O'Sullivan RG, McCabe G. Simple aspiration versus intercostal tube drainage for primary spontaneous pneumothorax in adults. Cochrane database Syst Rev. 2007;(1).
38. Brown SGA, Ball EL, Perrin K, et al. Conservative versus Interventional Treatment for Spontaneous Pneumothorax. N Engl J Med. 2020;382(5):405-15.
39. Vallee P, Sullivan M, Richardson H, et al. Sequential treatment of a simple pneumothorax. Ann Emerg Med. 1988;17(9):936-42.
40. Mendogni P, Vannucci J, Ghisalberti M, et al. Epidemiology and management of primary spontaneous pneumothorax: a systematic review. Interact Cardiovasc Thorac Surg. 2020; 30(3):337-45.
41. Yi E, Park JE, Chung JH, et al. Trends in recurrence of primary spontaneous pneumothorax in young population after treatment for first episode based on a nationwide population data. Sci Rep. 2023;13(1):13478.
42. Dubois L, Malthaner RA. Video-assisted thoracoscopic bullectomy and talc poudrage for spontaneous pneumothoraces: effect on short-term lung function. J Thorac Cardiovasc Surg. 2010;140(6):1272-5.
43. Hallifax RJ, Yousuf A, Jones HE, et al. Effectiveness of chemical pleurodesis in spontaneous pneumothorax recurrence prevention: A systematic review. Thorax. 2017;72(12):1121-31.
44. Agarwal R, Aggarwal AN, Gupta D. Efficacy and safety of iodopovidone pleurodesis through tube thoracostomy. Respirology. 2006;11(1):105-8.
45. Sedrakyan A, van der Meulen J, Lewsey J, et al. Video assisted thoracic surgery for treatment of pneumothorax and lung resections: systematic review of randomised clinical trials. BMJ. 2004;329(7473):1008.
46. Lin Z, Zhang Z, Wang Q, et al. A systematic review and meta-analysis of video-assisted thoracoscopic surgery treating spontaneous pneumothorax. J Thorac Dis. 2021;13(5):3093-104.
47. Barker A, Maratos EC, Edmonds L, et al. Recurrence rates of video-assisted thoracoscopic versus open surgery in the prevention of recurrent pneumothoraces: a systematic review of randomised and non-randomised trials. Lancet (London, England). 2007;370(9584):329-35.
48. Zhang Y, Jiang C, Chen C, et al. Surgical management of secondary spontaneous pneumothorax in elderly patients with chronic obstructive pulmonary disease: retrospective study of 107 cases. Thorac Cardiovasc Surg. 2009;57(6):347-52.
49. Ambrosino N, Ribechini A, Allidi F, et al. Use of endobronchial valves in persistent air leaks: a case report and review of the literature. Expert Rev Respir Med. 2013;7(1):85-90.
50. Hance JM, Martin JT, Mullett TW. Endobronchial valves in the treatment of persistent air leaks. Ann Thorac Surg. 2015;100(5):1780-6.
51. Flume PA, Strange C, Ye X, et al. Pneumothorax in cystic fibrosis. Chest. 2005;128(2):720-8.
52. Attaran S, Bille A, Karenovics W, et al. Videothoracoscopic repair of diaphragm and pleurectomy/abrasion in patients with catamenial pneumothorax: a 9-year experience. Chest. 2013;143(4):1066-9.
53. Ball CG, Kirkpatrick AW, Feliciano DV. The occult pneumothorax: what have we learned? Can J Surg. 2009;52(5):E173-9.
54. Ball CG, Kirkpatrick AW. Utility of c-spine and abdominal CT in diagnosing occult pneumothoraces. J Trauma Acute Care Surg. 2013;74(3):948.
55. Lichtenstein D. Lung ultrasound in the critically ill. Curr Opin Crit Care. 2014;20(3):315-22.

Tunneled Indwelling Pleural Catheter

George Mundanchira, Abhinav Agrawal, Viera Lakticova

CHAPTER 133

INTRODUCTION

Pleural effusions of any origin can cause significant dyspnea. Symptomatic patients who undergo thoracentesis with improvement in their symptoms with or without re-expansion of the lung may benefit from serial thoracentesis or chest tube placement. The decision for a particular intervention usually depends on the rate of reaccumulation and patient preference. In this chapter, we will discuss tunneled indwelling pleural catheters (TIPCs) which are smaller, semipermanent chest tubes that allow home drainage of pleural effusions. Serial drainage of pleural space by TIPC can results in space pleurodesis. Additionally, instillation of sclerosing agents via TIPC can be done to facilitate pleurodesis.

INDICATIONS

Tunneled indwelling pleural catheter is indicated for patients with recurrent symptomatic pleural effusions whose symptoms improve after fluid removal with initial thoracentesis and/or chest tube drainage.

Malignant Pleural Effusion

Many malignancies, most commonly of lung, lymphoma, and breast, can cause malignant pleural effusions (MPE).[1] Treatment of MPE should be directed at the underlying cause through oncologic medical management. However, pleural effusions can accumulate and cause significant dyspnea prior to initiation of such treatment and during the period of time when oncologic treatment is taking effect. A therapeutic, large-volume thoracentesis should initially be attempted to assess for symptom improvement. TIPC is indicated for those patients with recurrent MPE who improved with large-volume thoracentesis, regardless of lung re-expansion. Four common indications are described as below:[2]

1. As a bridge to initiation of oncological therapy
2. As a mode for more definitive management through auto or chemical assisted pleurodesis
3. As salvage therapy if pleurodesis fails
4. As a palliative measure when further cancer therapy is no longer offered

Improvement in dyspnea with TIPC is shown to be of comparable efficacy to talc pleurodesis.[3,4] Studies to assess efficacy of TIPC-assisted pleurodesis compared to video-assisted thoracoscopic surgery (VATS) pleurodesis are currently underway and their results may signify a large change in the current management strategies. Safety of TIPC in patients undergoing chemotherapy has been established. There is no significant rise in rate of infection despite the significant immune suppression in both solid and liquid malignancies group of patients.[5-8]

Nonmalignant Pleural Effusion

Although benign in nature, nonmalignant pleural effusions (NMPE) often cause significant morbidity and are also associated with an increase in mortality.[9,10] Four large categories of common NMPE have been described:

1. Heart failure (HF)-related pleural effusions
2. Hepatic hydrothorax (HH)
3. End-stage renal disease (ESRD)-related pleural effusions
4. Chylothorax

Tuberculous pleural effusion, being nonmalignant in etiology, is also included in this category.

Left ventricular (LV) systolic and diastolic dysfunction results in increased left atrial filling pressures leading to eventual fluid extravasation from the pulmonary capillaries. Pleural effusion occurs when the rate of fluid accumulation in pleural space exceeds the rate of removal by the lymphatics.[11] The standard management of pleural effusions in HF focuses on diuretics. TIPC for HF-related pleural effusions is currently indicated in patients with severe HF with symptomatic pleural effusions refractory to diuresis or for individuals who are prone to adverse reactions related to excessive diuresis (such as hypotension, electrolyte imbalance, and renal failure). Symptomatic improvement has been shown in these patients with minor complications.[12,13] TIPC can be performed in HF-related NMPE after a multiple disciplinary discussion in refractory/palliative care cases.

Hepatic hydrothorax occurs due to the translocation of ascitic fluid through the defects in the diaphragm into the associated pleural space with cirrhosis induced hypoalbuminemia playing a minimal role.[11] The mainstay of HH therapy consists of control of ascitic fluid production through medical optimization, diuretics, transjugular intrahepatic portosystemic shunt or liver transplantation, as necessary. Direct pleural fluid removal via thoracentesis, chest tube, or TIPC can be considered when patients have persistent and significant respiratory symptoms. Thoracentesis is always recommended preceding TIPS to prevent large fluid shifts and rapid reaccumulation of pleural fluid.

Tunneled indwelling pleural catheter is sometimes used palliatively in HH refractory to diuresis for patients who are not a candidate for transjugular intrahepatic portosystemic shunt or an early liver transplant. Serial thoracentesis is favored if a patient has an expeditious portosystemic shunt or liver transplant or if the projected time on hospice care is short. There are conflicting results of studies regarding rates of pleurodesis and infectious complications. It is reported in a recent meta-analysis that almost half of patients achieved pleurodesis. The rates of infectious complications were similar when compared to rates of infections reported with TIPC placed for MPE.[14] Other studies suggest an overestimation of both pleurodesis rates and infection rates.[15]

Patients with ESRD rely on dialysis for overall fluid balance. In addition to fluid overload due to inadequate dialysis, hypoproteinemia, uremia, and accompanying heart dysfunction contribute to accumulation of pleural effusions in this patient population.[16] TIPC is indicated for symptomatic and recurrent pleural effusions which are refractory to dialysis or as a palliative measure in those who cannot tolerate dialysis. Limited data are available for this patient population; improvement in dyspnea and achievement of pleurodesis have been observed.[17]

Chylothorax, the accumulation of chyle in the pleural space, occurs due to a disruption in the thoracic duct either because of trauma or due to malignancy among other reasons. TIPC should be considered in patients with persistent (>2 weeks) high-volume (>500 cc/day) chylothorax, despite medical treatment and dietary restriction and who are not candidate for VATS/thoracic duct ligation and interventional radiology (IR)-guided thoracic duct embolization.[18] TIPC has been used as a temporary measure to control persistent low-volume chylothorax prior to medical therapy. A few studies have suggested improvement in dyspnea and eventual pleurodesis.[19,20] Caution should be exercised as over drainage can lead to malnourishment and infection.

Tuberculous pleural effusion (TBPE): It can be seen as an extrapulmonary manifestation of tuberculosis both in primary and reactivation disease. The role of TIPC for this specific diagnosis has not been well elucidated although certain conclusion can be made regarding drainage strategies. Although TBPE causing dyspnea should undergo drainage, there is usually no long-term differences in dyspnea past 1 week of treatment initiation.[21,22] The use of a pigtail catheter for drainage did not lead to decreased amounts of residual pleural thickening post treatment but the addition of fibrinolytic agents may have some role in decreasing the amounts of residual pleural thickening.[23,24] Given that tuberculous pleural effusions will likely respond to standard medical therapy with good resolution of pleural effusion and dyspnea on its own without need for long term drainage, TIPC is not indicated in standard patient with TBPE.[25]

TUNNELED INDWELLING PLEURAL CATHETER PLACEMENT

Tunneled indwelling pleural catheter placement is an outpatient procedure performed under ultrasound guidance with or without sedation depending on the patient's needs. Some steps in the standard insertion of a TIPC may slightly differ depending on the brand of TIPC used. The pleural effusion is allowed to accumulate to be safely accessible for ideally anterior placement of catheter. Anterior placement is desired as it allows the patient to perform self-drainage. The procedure is usually performed with the patient lying in lateral decubitus position with instrumented pleural space up, but can be performed in other positions as well, e.g., sitting position.[26]

Placement of TIPC is a sterile procedure. Site is anesthetized using local anesthetics, most commonly lidocaine. Ultrasound examination confirms the appropriate site for accessing the pleural space, typically in mid-axillary line in the 6th or 7th intercostal space. The site may vary depending on fluid distribution, but catheter exit site should be always in mid axillary line or anteriorly from this plane. Needle is placed into pleural effusion and guidewire is passed into pleural space. Guidewire is confirmed with ultrasound. The catheter exit site is then identified, typically 5 cm anteriorly. Skin is cut and the catheter is tunneled subcutaneously from the exit site to the pleural access site. Peel-away catheter with dilator is advanced over the wire into the pleural space.[27] Dilator and guidewire are removed and pleural catheter is placed into the peel-away catheter. Peel-away catheter is then removed by peeling while TIPC is pushed in at the same time. Catheter is palpated within the insertion site to resolve any possible kinks. Both incision sites are then closed with sutures. The initial drainage is done intraoperatively with removal of as much fluid as the patient tolerates. Finally, the tube is capped and dressed appropriately.

Tunneled indwelling pleural catheter can also be placed after thoracoscopy if this is performed to collect additional tissue for diagnostic studies.[18]

DRAINAGE FREQUENCY

Drainage schedule should be individualized and depends on the rate of reaccumulation and severity of dyspnea. Studies have shown no difference in symptom improvement in patients who were aggressively drained everyday versus drainage driven by symptoms.[28] The current consensus guidelines recommend daily drainage for MPE when pleurodesis or removal of TIPC is the goal. However, in a trapped lung when pleurodesis or removal is not intended, drainage schedule should be based on symptoms.[29] For NMPE, drainage schedule is usually based on symptoms. Frequency interval between drainages can be extended if drainage amount is decreasing over time.

COMPLICATIONS

Complications such as pneumothorax, bleeding, and infection arising from the TIPC insertion are similar to those associated with thoracentesis or chest tube placement. Complications related to the indwelling catheter are well described, which include pleural infections, skin infections, catheter fracture during removal, catheter obstruction, catheter tract metastases/seeding, pericatheter leakage, dislodgment, and chest pain.[30,31]

Infection, a rare but mostly treatable complication of TIPC, occurs in about 5% of patients with an associated mortality risk of only 0.29%.[32] The guidelines recommend oral antibiotics against skin pathogens for simple exit-site infections, which can be treated on outpatient basis.[29] If an infection extends into the tunnel, removal of the TIPC should be considered with separate chest tube insertion as needed. As microbial colonization is common in indwelling pleural catheters, care must be taken to define a TIPC-related pleural infection. These infections occur when clinical signs and symptoms of pleural infection are present and either frank pus is drained, or Gram stain or cultures are positive or biochemical markers are indicative of infection. In clinical practice, these infections are best confirmed via direct thoracentesis. In some cases, fibrinolytics and DNAse via TIPC can be added to assist with continuous or daily drainage. Broad-spectrum antibiotics are recommended for these patients until further speciation and resistance panel of the causative infectious organism can be done. Finally, some cases require TIPC removal with or without new chest tube placement.[31]

The removal process is not without its own complications as tube fracture has been reported.[33] Tube fracture can be prevented if the cuff is no more than 1 cm distance from catheter exit site. Even if the tube is fractured and retained products are suspected within pleural cavity, aggressive retrieval measures are not indicated as the patients usually remain asymptomatic.[32,34]

Fibrinous material within the pleural space usually from an exudative effusion can cause impending catheter blockage. Initially, sterile normal saline should be flushed through the TIPC to see if flow returns. If drainage is not resumed, fibrinolytics can be administered. Targeted radiation or intrapleural chemotherapy may be required when the source of the obstruction is secondary to metastases, as reported in mesothelioma.

If the accumulated pleural fluid is under pressure and catheter is malfunctioning requiring removal, thoracentesis prior to removal of catheter is recommended. With regards to the pericatheter leakage, firm securing of the tube may prevent this complication as well as prevent dislodgement. Cachectic patients undergoing chemotherapy are at higher risk for this complication.[30]

Postprocedural chest pain resolves within 3–5 days and can be managed by oral analgesics. Chest pain associated with drainage can be experienced by some and is similar in nature to the discomfort experienced during thoracentesis due to the negative pressure created during drainage in patients with trapped lung. This can often be mitigated by slowing the drainage or stopping altogether. Removal of the TIPC may be the only option in those patients with severe chest pain that is refractory to cessation of drainage and uncontrolled by analgesics.[30]

Pleurodesis, or the obliteration of the pleural space, is a welcome result of long-term TIPC drainage. Historically, pleurodesis has been performed either through mechanical irritation of the pleura during VATS, or through chemical irritation of pleural surfaces. Substances such as talc, bleomycin, doxycycline, or povidone-iodine have been used. Although these methods work, they often induce significant pain and require short hospitalization to manage the pain. TIPC itself can induce pleurodesis over time likely due to catheter-related pleural irritation combined with apposition of pleural surfaces occurring with frequent, daily drainage as observed in up to almost 60% of cases.[35,36] Process of pleurodesis can be augmented with the addition of chemicals mentioned earlier.[37,38]

REMOVAL

Removal of the TIPC is indicated in a few scenarios. Pleurodesis, either caused by the TIPC itself over time or successfully through chemical agents, can obviate the need for TIPC which should then be removed. In MPE, a response to oncologic treatment can lead to decreased production of pleural fluid, ultimately fluid resolution, which would also indicate removal of the TIPC. Removal of TIPC is once again indicated in malfunctioning TIPC where an accumulation of pleural fluid is causing symptoms while there is no longer output from the TIPC which does not respond to treatment or is caused by mechanical failure of the tube itself. Finally, the indications of TIPC removal in pleural infections (when benign bacterial colonization is not suspected) has not been well studied and is not clearly defined. The current consensus guidelines should be followed.[31]

COST

In general, TIPC usage is found to be a cost-effective alternative to symptom-guided drainage when combined with talc pleurodesis.[39] Patients undergoing active treatment for malignancy had also shown greater improvement.[40]

SUMMARY

Tunneled indwelling pleural catheter allows for patient-derived control over pleural effusions and should be considered in recurrent pleural effusion causing dyspnea. Placement under ultrasound guidance and local anesthesia makes it a useful and a cost-effective tool. Pleurodesis can occur spontaneously but can be enhanced with talc insertion via TIPC. With minimal complications of infections, TIPC can safely remain in patients for extended period of time.

REFERENCES

1. Awadallah SF, Bowling MR, Sharma N, et al. Malignant pleural effusion and cancer of unknown primary site: A review of literature. Ann Transl Med. 2019;7(15):353.
2. Feller-Kopman DJ, Reddy CB, DeCamp MM, et al. Management of malignant pleural effusions. An official ATS/STS/STR clinical practice guideline. Am J Respir Crit Care Med. 2018;198(7):839-49.
3. Davies HE, Mishra EK, Kahan BC, et al. Effect of an indwelling pleural catheter vs chest tube and talc pleurodesis for relieving dyspnea in patients with malignant pleural effusion: the TIME2 randomized controlled trial. JAMA. 2012;307(22):2383-9.
4. Thomas R, Fysh ETH, Smith NA, et al. Effect of an indwelling pleural catheter vs talc pleurodesis on hospitalization days in patients with malignant pleural effusion: The AMPLE randomized clinical trial. JAMA. 2017;318(19):1903-12.
5. Chan Wah Hak C, Sivakumar P, Ahmed L. Safety of indwelling pleural catheter use in patients undergoing chemotherapy: a five-year retrospective evaluation. BMC Pulm Med. 2016;16:41.
6. Mekhaiel E, Kashyap R, Mullon JJ, et al. Infections associated with tunnelled indwelling pleural catheters in patients undergoing chemotherapy. J Bronchology Interv Pulmonol. 2013;20(4):299-303.
7. Faiz SA, Pathania P, Song J, et al. Indwelling pleural catheters for patients with hematologic malignancies. A 14-year, single-center experience. Ann Am Thorac Soc. 201;14(6):976-85.
8. Gilbert CR, Lee HJ, Skalski JH, et al. The use of indwelling tunneled pleural catheters for recurrent pleural effusions in patients with hematologic malignancies: A multicenter study. Chest. 2015;148(3):752-8.
9. DeBiasi E, Puchalski J. Pleural effusions as markers of mortality and disease severity: A state-of-the-art review. Curr Opin Pulm Med. 2016;22(4):386-91.
10. Walker SP, Morley AJ, Stadon L, et al. Nonmalignant pleural effusions: A prospective study of 356 consecutive unselected patients. Chest. 2017;151(5):1099-105.
11. Kinasewitz GT. Transudative effusions. Eur Resp J. 1997;10(3):714-8.
12. Majid A, Kheir F, Fashjian M, et al. Tunneled pleural catheter placement with and without talc poudrage for treatment of pleural effusions due to congestive heart failure. Ann Am Thorac Soc. 2016;13(2):212-6.
13. Srour N, Potechin R, Amjadi K. Use of indwelling pleural catheters for cardiogenic pleural effusions. Chest. 2013;144(5):1603-8.
14. Avula A, Acharya S, Anwar S, et al. Indwelling pleural catheter (IPC) for the management of hepatic hydrothorax: The known and the unknown. J Bronchology Interv Pulmonol. 2022;29(3):179-85.
15. Baltaji S, Shojaee S. Indwelling pleural catheters for refractory hepatic hydrothorax? A call for prospective studies and randomized controlled trials. J Bronchology Interv Pulmonol. 2022;29(3):161-3.
16. Kumar AP, Pathrudu BMS, Rani NU, et al. A study on etiology and profile of pleural effusion in chronic kidney disease. J Evol Med Dent Sci. 2015;4(68):11785.
17. Potechin R, Amjadi K, Srour N. Indwelling pleural catheters for pleural effusions associated with end-stage renal disease: a case series. Ther Adv Respir Dis. 2015;9(1):22-7.
18. Agrawal A, Chaddha U, Kaul V, et al. Multidisciplinary management of chylothorax. Chest. 2022;162(6):1402-12.
19. DePew ZS, Iqbal S, Mullon JJ, et al. The role for tunneled indwelling pleural catheters in patients with persistent benign chylothorax. Am J Med Sci. 2013;346(5):349-52.
20. Jimenez CA, Mhatre AD, Martinez CH, et al. Use of an indwelling pleural catheter for the management of recurrent chylothorax in patients with cancer. Chest. 2007;132(5):1584-90.
21. Lai Y-F, Chao T-Y, Wang Y-H, et al. Pigtail drainage in the treatment of tuberculous pleural effusions: a randomised study. Thorax. 2003;58(2):149-51.
22. Bhuniya S, Arunabha DC, Choudhury S. Role of therapeutic thoracentesis in tuberculous pleural effusion. Ann Thorac Med. 2012;7(4):215-9.
23. Viedma EC, Dus MJL, González-Molina A, et al. A study of loculated tuberculous pleural effusions treated with intrapleural urokinase. Respir Med. 2006;100(11):2037-42.
24. Cao G-Q, Li L, Wang Y-B, Shi Z-Z, et al. Treatment of free-flowing tuberculous pleurisy with intrapleural urokinase. Int J Tuberc Lung Dis. 2015;19(11):1395-400.
25. Chen B, Zhang J, Ye Z, et al. Outcomes of video-assisted thoracic surgical decortication in 274 patients with tuberculous empyema. Ann Thorac Cardiovasc Surg. 2015;21(3):223-8.
26. Health, Iskus; YouTube, (2017). PleurX® pleural catheter placement video. [online] Available from www.youtube.com/watch?v=3WrYDhOetbY. [Last accessed September, 2024].
27. Abhinav A, Murgu S. Multimodal approach to the management of malignant pleural effusions: role of thoracoscopy with pleurodesis and tunneled indwelling pleural catheters. J Thorac Dis. 2020;12(5):2803-11.
28. Muruganandan S, Azzopardi M, Fitzgerald DB, et al. Aggressive versus symptom-guided drainage of malignant pleural effusion via indwelling pleural catheters (AMPLE-2): An open-label randomised trial. Lancet Respir Med. 2018;6(9):671-80.

29. Miller RJ, Chrissian AA, Lee YCG, et al. AABIP Evidence-informed Guidelines and Expert Panel Report for the Management of Indwelling Pleural Catheters. J Bronchol Interv Pulmonol. 2020;27(4):229-45.
30. Chalhoub M, Saqib A, Castellano M, et al. Indwelling pleural catheters: Complications and management strategies. J Thorac Dis. 2018;10(7):4659-66.
31. Gilbert CR. Interventional Pulmonary Outcomes Group. Management of indwelling tunneled pleural catheters: A modified Delphi consensus statement. Chest. 2020;158(5):2221-8.
32. Fysh ETH, Tremblay A, Feller-Kopman D, et al. Clinical outcomes of indwelling pleural catheter-related pleural infections: an international multicenter study. Chest. 2013;144(5):1597-1602.
33. Grosu HB, Eapen GA, Morice RC, et al. Complications of removal of indwelling pleural catheters. Chest. 2012;142(4):1071.
34. Fysh ETH, Wrightson JM, Lee YCG, et al. Fractured indwelling pleural catheters. Chest. 2012;141(4):1090-4.
35. Suzuki K, Servais EL, Rizk NP, et al. Palliation and pleurodesis in malignant pleural effusion: the role for tunneled pleural catheters. J Thorac Oncol. 2011;6(4):762-7.
36. Schneider T, Reimer P, Storz K, et al. Recurrent pleural effusion: who benefits from a tunneled pleural catheter? Thorac Cardiovasc Surg. 2009;57(1):42-6.
37. Bhatnagar R, Keenan EK, Morley AJ, et al. Outpatient talc administration by indwelling pleural catheter for malignant effusion. N Engl J Med. 20185;378(14):1313-22.
38. Reddy C, Ernst A, Lamb C, et al. Rapid pleurodesis for malignant pleural effusions: a pilot study. Chest. 2011;139(6):1419-23.
39. Shafiq M, Simkovich S, Hossen S, et al. Indwelling pleural catheter drainage strategy for malignant effusion: A cost-effectiveness analysis. Ann Am Thorac Soc. 2020;17(6):746-53.
40. Ost DE, Jimenez CA, Lei X, et al. Quality-adjusted survival following treatment of malignant pleural effusions with indwelling pleural catheters. Chest. 2014;145(6):1347-56.

SECTION

13

Mediastinum, Chest Wall and Diaphragm Disorders

SECTION OUTLINE

Mediastinal Anatomy and Disorders

CHAPTER 134

Arjun Srinivasan, Surinder K Jindal

INTRODUCTION

Mediastinum is thoracic cavity sans the lungs. It is bound laterally by the parietal pleurae, anteriorly by the sternum, posteriorly by the vertebral column and paravertebral gutters, superiorly by the thoracic inlet, and inferiorly by the diaphragm. Interest in mediastinum stems from myriad of vital structures it encloses and their associated diseases with classical clinical as well as radiological presentations. The lack of distinct anatomical planes between compartments, similar clinical manifestations due to spectrum of diseases, and relative inaccessibility of the structures makes evaluation of mediastinal disorders a daunting task.

MEDIASTINAL ANATOMY AND COMPARTMENTS

Subdivision of mediastinum has been attempted by clinicians, radiologists, and surgeons resulting in numerous classifications and a lot of confusion. The classification proposed by Shields in 1972 divides mediastinum into three compartments: Anterior, middle (visceral), and posterior (paravertebral sulcus). This is a simple and useful classification as further subdivisions in the absence of distinct anatomical planes are redundant because neither disease nor air can be contained within the compartments. The only resistance to spread of either is the mediastinal pleural reflections laterally; superior communication with neck and inferiorly with retroperitoneum ensures free dissemination. The boundaries of the anterior compartment consist of the sternum, the first rib, and an imaginary curved line along the anterior heart border and brachiocephalic vessels from the diaphragm to the thoracic inlet. The middle (visceral) compartment extends from the posterior limit of the anterior compartment to the anterior surface of the vertebral columns and then to the thoracic inlet. The posterior compartment (paravertebral sulcus) extends from the anterior surface of the vertebral column to the anterior surface of the paravertebral ribs. Recently, the International Thymic Malignancy Interest Group (ITMIG) proposed a more organized classification mainly based on computerized tomography (CT) which consists of three similar compartments with subtle differences. The contents of the compartments are summarized in **Box 1**.

BOX 1 Contents of mediastinal compartments.

Anterior	Middle	Posterior
Pericardial fat	Heart and pericardium	Azygos and hemiazygos veins
Thymus gland	Trachea, main bronchus, and hila	Esophagus
Substernal extensions of thyroid and parathyroid glands	Innominate veins and superior vena cava	Azygos and hemiazygos veins
	Aortic arch and great vessels	Descending aorta
	Phrenic and vagus nerves	Sympathetic trunk
Lymph nodes	Lymph nodes	Intercostal nerves
		Thoracic duct
Connective tissue	Connective tissue	Connective tissue

Lymphatics

As with the compartments of mediastinum, the lymphatics are interconnected and involvement of adjacent stations is extremely common in disease. Separation to distinct stations forms the cornerstone in the management of bronchogenic carcinoma. Naruke's division into 14 stations is widely used for this purpose.

IMAGING OF MEDIASTINUM

Conventional Chest Radiograph

Conventional chest radiograph is the first step in the evaluation of any chest symptom and mediastinal disease. In fact, as many as 40% of mediastinal masses may be detected during routine chest radiograph.[1] Radiographs with posteroanterior (PA) and laterolateral (LL) views represent the basic imaging modality in the study of the chest and mediastinum. Chest radiography allows localization of the pathological process: Orthogonal projections can demonstrate site, size, density and the presence of calcifications, thereby narrowing the range of differential diagnoses. Additional views (oblique or lordotic) may be useful for distinguishing true images from composition images. Moreover, fluoroscopic examination and opacification of the esophagus will provide valuable complementary information.

Radiologically, a line is formed when certain conditions are met: There is a difference in density between two adjacent tissues; the two tissues are separated by a curved surface; the beam hits this surface tangentially. These conditions occur often in chest radiography where the reflections of the lungs (ventilated and therefore radiolucent) on the mediastinum (radiopaque) form several "lines", known as mediastinal lines. If the line has a double interface (air–mediastinum–air), it may be called a "stripe".[2] In the anterior mediastinum, PA view reveals the anterior junction line and LL view the retrosternal line.[3] Normal morphology of these lines is a reliable indication of normality of single mediastinal compartments: The presence of space-occupying lesions will cause their displacement, distortion, or cancellation. A mass on the other hand may be plainly visible protruding from either side of mediastinum. Chest radiography is almost always able to indicate the presence and site of mediastinal disease, but apart from a few exceptions, it cannot define its nature, organ of origin, or the presence of possible infiltrative features. Further investigations are therefore needed to characterize the disease.

Computerized Tomography

Axial imaging avoids the problem of overlapping tissues with similar density: Demonstration of mediastinal spaces with their lymph nodes and relations with surrounding structures and blood vessels represent the most important contributions of CT. Indications include characterization of lesions previously identified on standard X-ray and assessment of the mediastinum in patients with a clinical suspicion of disease but negative X-ray.[4,5] Improved resolution ensures better delineation of structures including point of origin, extension, and relation to adjacent organs. This also helps in directing diagnostic procedures like fine needle aspiration or biopsy.

Magnetic Resonance Imaging

Magnetic resonance imaging (MRI) is used less frequently than the CT in the evaluation of mediastinal masses, mainly because of its lesser availability and higher cost; however, MRI has a capacity for multiplanar imaging and the ability to image vessels, and it can provide better tissue characterization than CT. MRI provides excellent soft-tissue resolution and is better for differentiation between solid and cystic components even in the absence of IV contrast.[6] Additionally, MRI is excellent in the evaluation of regions of complex anatomy such as the thoracic inlet and the perihilar, paracardiac, and peridiaphragmatic regions, and for the assessment of posterior mediastinal or paravertebral masses.[7] Several new advances in thoracic MRI have now expanded its applications, in particular for assessment of pulmonary and mediastinal tumors.[8]

Ultrasonography

Traditional ultrasonography (US) has its role in evaluation of anterior mediastinal masses in children, especially thymic masses. Esophageal ultrasonography (eUS) and endobronchial ultrasonography (EBUS) are increasingly being used to detect mediastinal involvement in bronchogenic and esophageal carcinoma and guiding diagnostic aspiration of lymph nodes that would otherwise not be possible by conventional methods. EBUS-TBNA (transbronchial needle aspiration) specimens are also found useful for rapid diagnosis of tubercular mediastinal lymphadenopathy.[9]

Radionuclide Imaging

Positron emission tomography (PET) with or without CT has almost become a prerequisite in the preoperative evaluation of bronchogenic carcinoma to assess for resection. Radioactive iodine scans are useful in detecting mediastinal extension of suspected thyroid neoplasms. Technetium-99m (Tc-99) sestamibi can be used to detect parathyroid tissue.

PNEUMOMEDIASTINUM

Free air in the mediastinum detected on a chest X-ray or chest CT test is pneumomediastinum.[7] It is "spontaneous" when it occurs without surgical or medical procedures, chest trauma or mechanical ventilation, and in the absence of an underlying lung disease. Secondary pneumomediastinum, though a rare entity, is far more common, especially in recent times with mechanically ventilated patients. Both the entities are distinct in pathophysiology and clinical presentations. The key to understanding the distribution of extra-alveolar air lies in the recognition of common fascial planes that unite these areas. Anatomical continuity may lead to extensive subcutaneous emphysema over the head and neck area; interstitial emphysema, pneumoperitoneum, or air may dissect the pleural layers/pericardium leading to associated pneumothorax/pneumopericardium. The source of air includes alveolar in spontaneous pneumomediastinum (SPM) and that associated with mechanical ventilation. Other areas of origin include head and neck where it could be secondary to infection by gas-producing organisms or dental procedures requiring use of compressed gas at high pressures. Upper respiratory tract, tracheobronchial tree, and extrathoracic gas are the source in trauma patients; uncommon sources include pneumoperitoneum and pneumoretroperitoneum in postsurgical patients.

Spontaneous Pneumomediastinum

This entity was first recognized in 1939 by Hamman with the demonstration of crepitations synchronous with heart which is classically described as "Hamman's crunch". Idiopathic SPM is rare with a reported incidence of 0.001–0.01% among all adult inpatients.[10] Most cases are young males; the age is distributed roughly from 18 to 25 years old and males account for 73.1%.[11] SPM has also been reported in patients with interstitial lung disease associated with connective tissue disorders, more specifically dermatomyositis[12] and in COVID-19-associated pneumonia and lung damage.[13] These carry distinctly worse prognosis than idiopathic SPM.

No relation is reported with either smoking or other environmental exposures. Pressure differences across the alveolar membrane that resulted from rapid increments of airway pressure cause terminal alveolar rupture. A recent analysis of 600 patients over 22 years revealed that SPM results from straining against a closed glottis, as during vomiting, coughing, exercising, or in the presence of associated asthma.[14] Other factors, such as direct toxic effects of heat induced by inhalation of illegal drugs and the thinner alveolar wall due to malnutrition, are also responsible for the rupture.[15] This rupture occurs without pleural dissection, which causes air to enter the lung interstitium and then migrate toward the mediastinum, occasionally the pericardium and the retropharyngeal and the retroperitoneal space, along the bronchovascular bundle by the pressure gradient between the peripheral part and the hilum of the lung, the so-called Macklin effect.[16]

The common presenting symptoms are chest pain and dyspnea. Pain typically radiates to the neck or back and is aggravated by bending forward, swallowing, or deep inspiration. Other symptoms include cough and dysphonia. Differential diagnosis in any young person presenting with acute chest symptoms should include SPM. Severity of symptoms is usually moderate; patients tend to present within 24 hours of onset of symptoms. History regarding trigger events may help in clinching the diagnosis, but no trigger can be identified in up to 40% of cases. Subcutaneous emphysema detected in up to 62% of reported cases is the most common physical finding and is usually restricted to the head and neck region. Hamman's crunch is reported in 30% of cases; careful auscultation with placement in left lateral position improves the chances.[17]

RADIOLOGICAL FINDINGS

Common findings in chest radiograph's PA view are air streaks in the superior mediastinum (sometimes they reach to the neck), the prominent silhouette of the heart (especially on the left), and subcutaneous emphysema of the shoulder and neck. All the above findings may not be identified in a given patient. The double-bronchial-wall sign (bronchial wall sandwiched between inner and outer air) and the continuous diaphragm sign (the diaphragm of both sides appearing connected by leaked air between the inferior surface of heart and diaphragm) are uncommon but characteristic signs when present.[11] Lateral views are more sensitive in detecting air and must be used when clinical suspicion is high and frontal radiographs are unrevealing. One must resort to CT when strong clinical suspicion is present with normal chest radiograph. CT is also informative regarding additional lung disease and in complicated pneumomediastinum like Boerhaave syndrome.

DIFFERENTIAL DIAGNOSIS

Differential diagnosis includes pneumothorax, pulmonary thromboembolism, pericarditis, and acute coronary syndrome. While SPM is detected, one should be careful to rule out Boerhaave syndrome as it carries a high mortality unlike SPM.

TREATMENT AND CLINICAL COURSE

Symptoms tend to subside in 24–48 hours with complete radiological resolution. Symptomatic therapy with analgesics is all that is required in most cases. Antibiotics may be considered in the presence of signs of inflammation like fever after ruling out other differentials. Subcutaneous emphysema is drained using a tunneled intravenous catheter if extensive. The most common complication is tension pneumothorax which needs prompt recognition and appropriate management. Recovery is total and recurrence uncommon (1.2%), unlike in spontaneous pneumothorax.[11]

Pneumomediastinum in Mechanically Ventilated Patients

Mechanically ventilated patients, especially those who are subjected to high tidal volumes, high peak inspiratory pressures, and high positive end expiratory pressures (PEEP) and are fighting the ventilator, are at high risk for developing pneumomediastinum.[18] Air trapping (auto-PEEP) due to high frequency or underlying obstructive lung disease may also lead to an increase in peak inspiratory pressures. Unlike SPM, pneumomediastinum in mechanically ventilated patients can be life-threatening due to continuous positive pressure increasing the likelihood of associated tension pneumothorax. This may be incidentally detected on chest radiograph, but once detected serial screening with chest radiograph is required to monitor pneumothorax. Chest tube drainage is needed if pneumothorax occurs regardless of how small it is if the patient continues to require positive pressure ventilation. In the presence of only pneumomediastinum, steps to curb increase in peak inspiratory pressures are taken if the patient cannot be safely taken off the ventilator. Patient-triggered pressure-limited ventilation (e.g., inspiratory pressure support) or low-rate intermittent mandatory ventilation would probably be preferable to mandatory volume-limited ventilation if clinically feasible.[19]

Prophylactic bilateral chest tube insertion is not recommended in the absence of sudden deterioration.

MEDIASTINITIS

Inflammation of the mediastinal structures is defined as mediastinitis. Based on the duration and severity of symptoms, mediastinitis may be broadly classified into acute and chronic. Clinical presentation is dramatic and is often life-threatening in acute mediastinitis whereas chronic tends to present as a mediastinal mass.

Acute Mediastinitis

Infection is the most common cause of acute mediastinitis, but predominant inflammation could also occur with secondary infection as in esophageal rupture. Based on etiology, specific compartments may be more commonly involved in the beginning. With the advent of invasive endoscopic therapeutic procedures, esophageal perforation is the most common cause of acute mediastinitis. Other common causes include infection following sternotomy, descending necrotizing mediastinitis following neck infections, infection from tracheobronchial tree and, rarely, direct involvement as in anthrax mediastinitis.

Patients are usually gravely ill. A high index of suspicion is the key to diagnosis, especially in postprocedure patients as in esophageal manipulation or cardiac surgery. The patients may deteriorate rapidly developing multiorgan dysfunction within few hours. CT of the chest with contrast enhancement is the investigation of choice in these patients. Treatment of these patients requires appropriate antibiotics and surgical debridement. Management of acute mediastinitis is summarized in **Table 1**.

Chronic Mediastinitis

The active form of chronic mediastinitis encompasses granulomatous disease, while mediastinal fibrosis represents the sequalae. The former tends to be asymptomatic, whereas the latter presents as a mass. Symptoms depend upon the part of mediastinum which is involved. Histoplasmosis or tuberculosis are important examples of chronic mediastinitis. Either begins as an infection in the lung with mediastinal adenitis secondary to regional drainage. There can be associated perinodal inflammation in a subset of individuals with a residual breakdown of conglomerate of lymph nodes akin to matting seen in the periphery. This mass gets covered by a fibrous capsule and tends to calcify as it is usually seen on chest radiograph as a sequalae. In some individuals, the fibrous capsule tends to increase in thickness with compression and invasion of adjacent organs. The reason for its occurrence in certain individuals and not in others is unclear. Goodwin and associates postulated that prolonged gradual seepage of some soluble antigen or other substance from the involved lymph nodes, at least in patients with histoplasmosis, causes fibrosis.[20] In some patients with concomitant retroperitoneal fibrosis, autoimmune phenomena might be responsible.

CLINICAL MANIFESTATIONS

Predominant symptoms are manifestations of mass effect on the adjacent organs. Primary symptoms include cough, chest pain, hemoptysis, and dyspnea secondary to airway involvement. Trachea or any of the major bronchi can be involved. Compression or erosion of the right middle lobe is most common which may present as right middle lobe syndrome. Right paratracheal region involvement may lead to compression of superior vena cava (SVC), leading to SVC syndrome (SVCS). Though malignancy accounts for up to 95% of SVCSs encountered in clinical practice; fibrosing mediastinitis is an important nonmalignant cause. Extrinsic esophageal compression presents as dysphagia and perforation as hematemesis or trachea-esophageal fistula. Mediastinal nerve compression leads to hoarseness of voice. Pulmonary vascular involvement can lead to pulmonary hypertension and cor pulmonale.[21] Mediastinal fibrosis is occasionally reported to mimic sarcoidosis.[22]

TABLE 1: Management of acute mediastinitis.

Etiology	Investigation	Antibiotics	Surgical procedure
Descending necrotizing mediastinitis	Contrast-enhanced CT of neck and chest	Anaerobic and gram-negative organisms	Surgical drainage
Esophageal manipulation	Contrast esophagogram, contrast-enhanced CT of chest	Gram-negative organisms, methicillin-resistant *Staphylococcus aureus* (MRSA)	Debridement and closure of perforation
Boerhaave syndrome	Contrast esophagogram, contrast-enhanced CT of chest	Gram-negative organisms	Debridement and closure of perforation
Poststernotomy	Contrast-enhanced CT of chest	*Pseudomonas* and MRSA	Extensive sternal and mediastinal debridement
Tracheobronchial perforation	Contrast-enhanced CT of chest	Gram-negative organisms, MRSA	Stenting/open surgical repair
Anthrax mediastinitis	Chest radiograph, contrast-enhanced CT	Ciprofloxacin or doxycycline + clindamycin	

MANAGEMENT

Diagnosis is established by clinical features. Chest radiology reveals mediastinal enlargement. Definite diagnosis requires mediastinal sampling by exploratory laparotomy to exclude malignancy. Debulking of mediastinum should be attempted while being careful to avoid injury to the surrounding structures. Antitubercular or antifungal can be given if specific infections are identified. Anti-inflammatory agents like steroids have been used with equivocal results but may be considered in an individual patient. Mechanical compression can be relieved by endovascular, esophageal, or endobronchial stenting, where appropriate.

Tumors and Cysts of Mediastinum

A mediastinal mass may be congenital or acquired in origin, the contents of the mediastinal compartments serve as points of origin. Hence, localization of the mass in mediastinum gives a clue toward etiology but can be confirmed only by tissue sampling. The contents of the respective compartments have been summarized in **Box 1**. Anterior mediastinal mass most commonly arises from thymus, lymph nodes, thyroid, or primitive germ cells. The middle compartment which mostly comprises tracheobronchial tree, heart, and esophagus is the site for duplication cysts. Posterior mediastinum abuts the vertebral body, enclosing the sympathetic trunk and vagal nerve; a mass arising from this region is likely to be of neural origin.

Location of the mass, age of presentation, and presence of symptoms are the three major determinants of whether the mass is benign or malignant in etiology. Although majority of mediastinal masses are benign (2/3rd), anterior mediastinal (59%) and symptomatic lesions (85%) are more likely to be malignant. Symptoms are broadly classified into: (1) Local, secondary to the mass effect and comprised of surrounding structures [cough (60%), chest pain (30%), and dyspnea (16%)], and (2) systemic manifestations due to the release of excess hormones, antibodies, or cytokines and are typically seen in malignant neoplasm as a part of paraneoplastic syndrome. These include cachexia, anorexia, fever, neurologic, and endocrine manifestations.

The initial workup of a suspected mediastinal mass involves obtaining PA and LL chest radiographs. This can provide information pertaining to the size, anatomic location, density, and composition of the mass. CT scanning is used to characterize mediastinal masses and their relationship to the surrounding structures as well as to identify cystic, vascular, and soft-tissue structures.[23] Multidetector-row CT scanning is shown to be helpful to determine different characteristics of enlarged mediastinal lymph nodes caused by tuberculosis and chronic lymphocytic leukemia.[24] The role of MRI is primarily in ruling out or evaluating a neurogenic tumor. MRI is also valuable to evaluate the extent of vascular invasion or cardiac involvement.[25]

Mediastinal Sampling

Tissue diagnosis of mediastinal lesions can be performed using surgical techniques such as thoracoscopy, cervical mediastinoscopy, extended cervical mediastinoscopy, and anterior mediastinotomy. Needle biopsy techniques include image-guided percutaneous needle biopsy, transbronchial needle biopsy, including endobronchial ultrasound-guided transbronchial needle aspiration (EBUS-FNA), transesophageal endobronchial ultrasound-guided fine-needle aspiration (EUS-B-FNA), and transesophageal endoscopic ultrasound-guided fine-needle aspiration biopsy (EUS-FNA). Minimally invasive transcutaneous or transpulmonary image-guided fine needle aspiration or biopsy is preferred over open surgical techniques as the diagnostic yield is comparable with a dramatic reduction in complication rates. The choice of the procedure is also dictated by its local availability, institutional and physician preference, patient's condition, and location as well as size of the lesion.

Transbronchial needle aspiration through a flexible bronchoscope is the time-tested method for sampling enlarged subcarinal and hilar lymph nodes. This is limited by the absence of real-time imaging; hence, it can be used only in the presence of lymph nodes of at least 1.5–2 cm in diameter. The reported sensitivity when used to stage nonsmall-cell carcinoma is 25–81%.[26] EBUS-FNA, which was developed recently, has been documented to have high diagnostic value, with sensitivities of more than 90% in the staging of non-small-cell lung cancer.[27] Recent attempts to increase the size of sample obtained using EBUS scope by use of biopsy forceps and cryo probe have significantly expanded the scope of EBUS even for etiologies like lymphoma.[28] Transesophageal EUS-guided needle biopsy allows access to the lower paratracheal, subcarinal, aortopulmonary, and paraesophageal regions. The reported sensitivity of EUS-guided biopsy in the mediastinum is 02–90%.[26] However, anterior lymph nodes, including those in the pretracheal and high right paratracheal regions, are not accessible because of the interposition of the air-filled trachea.

Before the advent of minimally invasive techniques, all patients of bronchogenic carcinoma planned for resection were subjected to cervical mediastinoscopy. Even now, this is the procedure of choice when multiple lymph node stations need to be sampled for accurate staging. It allows direct visualization and sampling of pretracheal, paratracheal, and anterior subcarinal lymph nodes and is reported to yield a diagnosis in 83–89% of patients with lung cancer.[29,30] It is done under general anesthesia with 1–3% risk of major complications. Aortopulmonary, retrotracheal, posterior subcarinal, and inferior mediastinal lymph nodes are inaccessible. Extended cervical mediastinoscopy, anterior mediastinotomy, and thoracoscopy are alternative surgical techniques, which can be used to assess mediastinal regions not accessible by standard mediastinoscopy.

Rapid on-site evaluation (ROSE) of EBUS-FNA samples is widely used to diagnose malignant lesions. Bioevaluator, a device to determine whether the tissues obtained by EBUS-TBNA are appropriate for pathological diagnosis, has been useful to enhance the value of ROSE.[31] Since its initial description, ROSE has undergone several modifications as per the preferences and logistics of institutions including those being done by a pulmonologist on site (P-ROSE)[32] and done by a pulmonologist through WhatsApp confirmation by a cytologist (WHOSE).[33] Percutaneous transthoracic needle biopsy using image guidance under local anesthesia and conscious sedation allows access to virtually all mediastinal regions, including those that are inaccessible by mediastinoscopy, transbronchial biopsy, and EUS-guided biopsy. The accuracy of transthoracic biopsy for the diagnosis of mediastinal lesions ranges from 75 to 90%.[29,30] A major limitation of this technique is the risk of pneumothorax, reported to occur in 10–60% of cases. If encountered, this can be managed by percutaneous single-time aspiration or by chest tube drainage.

Anterior Mediastinal Masses

Thymoma

They account for 20% of anterior mediastinal neoplasms in adults.[34] Systemic syndromes like myasthenia gravis (30–50%), hypogammaglobulinemia (10%), and pure red cell aplasia (PRCA) may present as primary manifestations, and the mediastinal mass may be picked up incidentally during evaluation. Thymomas as a group have a wide spectrum of histologic diversity and are classified based on cell-type predominance as lymphocytic, epithelial, or spindle cell variants. There is a strong association between histologic subtype and invasiveness as well as prognosis. Thymomas are usually solid tumors but may have cystic areas due to degeneration, necrosis, or hemorrhage. Thirty-four percent of thymomas invade through their own capsules, extending into the surrounding structures.[35,36] There can be transdiaphragmatic or pleural extension, but distal lymphatic or hematogenous spread is rare. The classification system proposed by the World Health Organization is based on cytologic differences, which is helpful in determining treatment regimens and predicting survival.[37]

The Masaoka clinical staging system is based on the degree of invasion of tumor through the capsule into the surrounding structures, which has important implications for prognosis.[38] In one study, the Masaoka staging system was shown to be useful as an independent predictor of survival in patients with thymoma.[39] Most recently, thymic tumors are divided into thymomas, thymic carcinomas, and neuroendocrinal tumors.[40] Diagnosis is easily established by percutaneous image-guided fine needle aspiration, but capsular invasion can only be made out on histopathologic examination of excision biopsy. Surgical excision is the standard of care for both invasive and noninvasive thymomas as it is the only potentially curative option. Adjunctive chemotherapy and radiation treatment are used for locally invasive or metastatic disease or inoperable tumors.

Tumors and cysts of the thymus are summarized in **Table 2**.

Mediastinal Germ Cell Tumors

Speculations regarding etiology have ranged from the opinion that these tumors are of true gonadal origin which represent spread from an occult or "burned-out" primary tumor to the view that the tumors are extragonadal in origin with separate clinical and biological behaviors. Primitive germ cells that fail to migrate completely during early embryonic development is the currently accepted theory regarding the origin of GCTs. They constitute about 15% of anterior mediastinal masses. GCTs are classified into the following three groups based on cell type: Benign teratomas, seminomas, and embryonal tumors/malignant teratomas/nonseminomatous GCTs.

TABLE 2: Tumors and cysts of thymus.

Tumor	Incidence	Association	Poor prognostic markers	Treatment
Thymoma	20% of anterior mediastinal mass	Myasthenia gravis, hypogammaglobulinemia, PRCA	Metastasis, size > 10 cm, tracheal/vascular compression, age > 30 years, epithelial or mixed histology, PRCA	Surgical resection, palliative chemotherapy, and radiation
Thymic carcinoma	Rare	–	Tumor margin infiltration, absence of a lobular growth pattern, high-grade atypia and necrosis, >10 mitoses per high-power field	Surgical resection, palliative chemotherapy, and radiation
Thymic carcinoid	8% of MEN1 syndrome	Cushing and MEN syndromes	Regional and distant metastasis	Surgical resection, chemotherapy, and radiation not effective
Thymolipoma	Rare	–	Benign	Surgical resection
Thymic cysts	Rare	Inflammation, Hodgkin's disease, or other congenital abnormality	Acquired or congenital, benign	Surgical resection

(MEN1: multiple endocrine neoplasia type 1; PRCA: pure red cell aplasia)

Teratomas: They are derived from at least two of the three primitive germs layers. They are subclassified into mature and immature (malignant) teratomas based on the cell of origin. Mature teratomas are more common and are histologically well-defined. Ectodermal tissues, which usually predominate, include skin, hair, sweat glands, and tooth-like structures. Mesodermal tissues, such as fat, cartilage, bone, and smooth muscle are less common, as are endodermal structures like respiratory and intestinal epithelium.[41] Malignant teratomas contain fetal or neuroendocrine tissue and have a favorable prognosis in children but can recur or metastasize.

Mature teratomas tend to be silent or may present with cardinal mediastinal symptoms. Occasionally, the presentation may be dramatic with expectoration of hair or sebum due to endobronchial rupture of teratoma. Rarely malignant transformation may occur. A typical radiological picture is a well-defined round or lobulated mass with up to 26% showing calcification due to the presence of bone or teeth elements. CT or MRI may reveal sebaceous elements or fat, which may further support the diagnosis and help in assessing resectability. Complete surgical resection is the treatment of choice and adjuvant chemotherapy is preferred, if resection is incomplete.

Mediastinal seminoma: Approximately 40% of mediastinal GCTs are seminomas, occurring most commonly in males between the second and the fourth decade. Apart from the usual presenting features of mediastinal mass, gynecomastia and weight loss may occur as paraneoplastic manifestations. Beta human chorionic gonadotropin (β-HCG) is elevated in up to 10% of patients, but an elevated alpha fetoprotein (AFP) suggests an alternate diagnosis. Radiographically, seminomas are bulky, lobulated, homogenous masses. Local invasion is rare, but metastasis to lymph nodes and bones may occur.[42] CT and gallium scanning is used to evaluate the extent of disease. Unlike other mediastinal tumors, seminomas are highly radiosensitive. Management may involve only radiotherapy or chemotherapy and radiotherapy or a neoadjuvant chemotherapy followed by surgery. 5 year survival ranges between 54% with radiotherapy alone and >90 % with chemotherapy with or without radiation.[43,44]

Nonseminomatous germ cell tumors: The nonseminomatous malignant germ cell tumors (GCTs) include embryonal cell carcinoma, endodermal sinus tumor, choriocarcinoma, or mixed GCTs composed of multiple histologic features. These are malignant and typically cause symptoms in young adult men. Unlike seminomas, lactate dehydrogenase and serologic markers such as AFP and β-HCG are frequently positive. Another unique association is with hematologic malignancies with up to 20% of patients having Klinefelter syndrome.[42]

Radiologically, these are large, irregular, anterior mediastinal masses, often with extensive, central, irregular, and heterogeneous areas of low attenuation due to necrosis, hemorrhage, and/or cyst formation. Invasion of adjacent structures with associated pleural and pericardial effusions is common. The tumor may protrude through the chest wall and distal metastasis is not uncommon. Chemotherapy with bleomycin, etoposide, and cisplatin is the current standard of care for patients with nonseminomatous malignant GCTs. Complete response is rare, with most patients requiring resection of residual tumor. As compared to seminomas, nonseminomatous GCTs have a poor long-term survival with only 46% alive at 5 years in contrast to 86%.[45]

A recent study of on 54 patients of primary malignant GCTs reports favorable long-term survival with surgical resection after chemoradiotherapy; patients with pure seminomas had a better prognosis than with nonseminomatous GCTs.[46]

Mediastinal Goiter

Clinically, mediastinal extension of goiter is detected by the inability to identify the lower border of thyroid during examination. The incidence is in the range of 1–15% among patients undergoing thyroidectomy. Most patients are euthyroid, appear as lobulated, encapsulated, and heterogenous tumors with classic cervicomediastinal continuity seen on CT. Radioiodine will show avid uptake if there is functional thyroid tissue. Due to retrosternal position, diagnostic sampling is difficult and exploratory thoracotomy with complete surgical excision is recommended as malignancy develops in a significant number of patients.

Mediastinal Lymphomas

Mediastinal involvement as a part of systemic disease is a common manifestation of lymphomas and figures among the top differentials while evaluating mediastinal lymphadenopathy. Primary mediastinal lymphoma is relatively a rare entity accounting for around 10% of all mediastinal lymphomas. Nodular sclerosing type of Hodgkin's lymphoma, large B-cell lymphoma, and lymphoblastic lymphoma are the three most common lymphomas with mediastinal involvement. Presentation is similar to other mediastinal masses with constitutional symptoms (B symptoms) which predominate especially in Hodgkin's lymphoma. They can present as mediastinal emergencies with SVCS or pericardial tamponade leaving little time for establishing diagnosis. Diagnosis is achieved by sampling peripheral or mediastinal lymph nodes. Ann Arbor staging system is based on the number of lymph node regions and/or other organ systems involved by the disease process. The treatment of mediastinal lymphomas is no different from lymphomas elsewhere; it primarily involves appropriate chemotherapy. Adjuvant radiotherapy may be justified in stage I or IIa disease or in the presence of SVCS. Relapsed disease is usually treated with high-dose chemotherapy followed by bone marrow transplantation.

Tumors of Middle Mediastinum

Mediastinal Cysts

Mediastinal cysts are congenital anomalies resulting from defects during embryonic development. They occur most commonly in the middle mediastinum, but neural-derived cysts are found in the posterior mediastinum. The presentation can be insidious due to compression of adjacent structures or acute due to infection or rupture. They comprise 12–20% of mediastinal masses. The most common type of mediastinal cysts are foregut cysts, with enterogenous cysts (50–70%) and bronchogenic cysts (7–15%) being the major subtypes.

Bronchogenic Cyst

Approximately 40% of bronchogenic cysts are symptomatic with cough, dyspnea, or chest pain, whereas the rest are picked up during routine chest radiographs.[47] The lung bud develops caudally from the laryngotracheal tube, beginning in the fourth week of gestation. By the fifth week, the single bud has divided into right and left main bronchi, which grow into the surrounding splanchnic mesenchyme and are destined to become bronchial cartilage and smooth muscle as well as visceral pleura. Dichotomous branching of the primitive bronchi continues until about the 24th week, when the terminal bronchioles begin to give rise to primitive alveoli. Throughout this period of embryogenesis, abnormal bronchi and bronchioles may form larger saccular structures, which are clinically recognized as bronchogenic cysts and are lined with ciliated, pseudostratified, columnar epithelium and contain bronchial glands and cartilaginous plates.

Anomalies that occur early are contained within the mediastinum and are mostly commonly seen abutting the trachea, carina, or hila. Less frequently, errors occurring late in embryogenesis may result in intraparenchymal bronchogenic cysts. They are seen as well-defined, rounded masses on chest radiographs and on CT have a similar Hounsfield unit to water. Air fluid level signifies either bronchial communication or secondary infection. Diagnosis is confirmed by image-guided or endobronchial needle aspiration. Endobronchial needle aspiration of cyst with EBUS scope carries a risk of infection and mediastinitis.[48] Symptomatic cysts are managed by either surgical resection or therapeutic aspiration with or without instillation of a sclerosing agent (ethanol or bleomycin), but controversy exists regarding the management of asymptomatic cysts. Subjecting such patients to a major surgery must be weighed against potential long-term complications including malignancy when observation is planned.

Enterogenous Cyst

Enterogenous cysts arise from the dorsal foregut. They are lined by squamous or enteric (alimentary) epithelium and may contain gastric or pancreatic tissue. It is also known as esophageal duplication cyst and represents the failure of esophagus to separate from the respiratory tract, a process which normally occurs around the fifth week during embryogenesis. Communication to the alimentary tract is rare. Twelve percent may have associated malformations of the gastrointestinal tract. Majority of patients present in early childhood. There is a potential for hemorrhage or rupture due to the presence of gastric or pancreatic tissue. There is predilection for the right side, and symptomatically dyspnea is rare. In asymptomatic patients, the most common clue leading to this diagnosis is the coexistence of other gastrointestinal duplications.

Radiological manifestations are similar to bronchogenic cysts, have slightly thicker walls, and are nearer to esophagus. Barium meal study may show indentation along the posterior wall. Technetium pertechnetate nuclear scan may suggest the presence of ectopic gastric mucosa within the chest. The potential for rupture mandates surgical resection of all enterogenous cysts after confirming diagnosis. The presence of gastric lining mucosa also predisposes these patients to the development of adenocarcinoma; hence, it needs long-term follow-up following surgery.

Pericardial Cysts

Unlike other cystic lesions of the middle mediastinum, pericardial cysts are often detected in the fourth to fifth decade. Therefore, the case for at least some of them being an acquired cyst is strong, but majority of them seem to be from the persistence of parietal recess during embryogenesis. Most are asymptomatic but can present with hemodynamic compromise secondary to cardiac compression or arrythmia. Their estimated incidence is 1 in 1,00,000.[47] The most common presenting site is the cardiophrenic angle on the right side and can be mistaken for foramen of Morgagni hernia or thickened pericardial fat. They are also called "spring water cysts" because of their characteristic radiologic picture showing low-density clear serous fluid content. Pericardial cysts have no malignant potential and can therefore be followed up after diagnosis is established. Symptomatic cysts are resected by either an open or an endoscopic approach.

Lymphangiomas

Lymphangiomas classically present as cervical swelling and are clinically identified by the presence of fluctuation and transluminescence. In up to 10% of patients, there can be a mediastinal extension with associated chylothorax and hemangioma. They are congenital malformation of the lymphatics leading to saccular dilatation and cyst formation. Cervical lymphangiomas typically present in early childhood, but isolated mediastinal lesions may present during adult life with symptoms of mediastinal compression. Radiographically, the lesions appear cystic and can be confused with pericardial cysts, though lymphangiomas are more likely to have a loculated appearance.[49] The use of lymphangiographic contrast media combined with CT scanning can also differentiate these lesions. Complete surgical resection is the treatment of choice; however, adjuvant radiotherapy may be used in complicated cases.[50] Lymphangiomatosis (LAM), a type of cystic interstitial lung disease seen almost exclusively in women, may be an advanced form of lymphangioma of chest.

Tumors of Posterior Mediastinum

Neuroenteric Cysts

Enterogenous cysts that are in continuation of or adjacent to vertebral anomalies are called neuroenteric cysts. Neuroenteric cysts are very rare congenital anomalies and result due to failure or incomplete separation of notochord from primitive foregut. Associated vertebral anomalies include butterfly vertebrae, hemivertebrae, and anterior spina bifida. These cysts present early in life, often before the first year of life with a triad of respiratory symptoms, mediastinal mass, and vertebral anomaly. Evaluation should include imaging of the chest with CT scan and a complete spinal imaging using MRI spine. Treatment usually requires cooperation between the neurosurgical and the thoracic surgical teams for spinal decompression, vertebral reconstruction, and mediastinal resection. Given the complexity of the procedures, a staged approach is preferred. Residual neurologic deficit may be present after surgery.

Neurogenic Tumors

Neurogenic tumors arise from various neural elements such as (1) peripheral nerve roots (neurofibroma, schwannoma, neurogenic sarcoma), (2) sympathetic ganglia (ganglioneuroma, ganglioneuroblastoma, and neuroblastoma), (3) aorticosympathetic paraganglia (paravertebral paraganglioma), or, rarely, (4) intrathoracic spinal canal (e.g., meningocele or meningomyelocele).[51] They constitute about 20% of all mediastinal masses; roughly 95% of them lie in the posterior mediastinum. Nearly three fourths of them are benign and half are asymptomatic; they can occasionally cause compressive or neurologic symptoms.[52]

Nerve Sheath Tumors

Nerve sheath tumors constitute about half to two thirds of the neural tumors of posterior mediastinum. They are benign and extremely slow-growing tumors such as the neurilemoma or schwannomas and neurofibromas. The former are encapsulated, firm masses consisting of Schwann cells, whereas the latter are soft, friable, nonencapsulated, and associated with neurofibromatosis. They appear as sharply marginated spherical masses on radiographs often with signs of erosion of adjacent spine. The classic dumbbell appearance due to growth of tumor through the intervertebral foramina is seen in only 10% of tumors. Complete surgical resection is the standard of care. Adjuvant chemotherapy or radiotherapy may be considered if resection is incomplete. Paraparesis and Horner's syndrome are potential complications of surgery.

Malignant nerve sheath tumors are the spindle sarcomas of posterior mediastinum and include malignant neurofibromas, malignant schwannomas, and neurogenic fibrosarcomas. They are generally symptomatic, with pain and nerve deficits being the predominant symptoms. Complete surgical resection with or without adjuvant chemotherapy or radiotherapy is the treatment of choice.

Tumors of Autonomic Nervous System

These tumors arise from neuronal cells rather than the nerve sheath. They are either benign and encapsulated (ganglioneuroma) but can be fast growing, malignant, and nonencapsulated (neuroblastoma). They arise from either the adrenals or the sympathetic ganglia of posterior mediastinum. Surgery is the treatment of choice for benign tumors. Localized malignant tumors can also be excised completely. If the resection is incomplete, treatment regimen includes postoperative chemotherapy and radiotherapy.

Superior Vena Cava Syndrome

No review of mediastinum would be complete without an overview of this dramatic syndrome which once seen in clinical practice remains etched in the memory of any clinician. SVCS is a common complication of lung cancer and non-Hodgkin's lymphoma (NHL). About 2–4% of lung cancer and NHL patients develop SVCS; together, they constitute about 90% of cases of SVCS seen in modern practice.[47] Benign causes constitute around 5–10% of cases, usually due to smoldering infections such as tuberculosis or fungus. Thrombosis of SVC due to iatrogenic procedures like central venous or Swan–Ganz catheter or insertion of pacemaker leads is another important cause of SVCS.

The severity of the complaints depends on the site of occlusion (site distal to azygos vein is more symptomatic than proximal) and the rate of onset of occlusion. If the occlusion is slowly progressive, the collaterals effectively decompress the system; hence, the symptoms are minimal. The collateral channels include azygos, intercostal, mediastinal, paravertebral, hemiazygos, thoracoepigastric, internal mammary, thoracoacromioclavicular, and anterior chest wall veins. Collaterals often take several weeks to dilate and accommodate the diverted blood from SVC. Clinically, the site of obstruction at the level of SVC is identified by the direction of flow in the collaterals from above downward, both above and below the umbilicus. Patients present with symptoms of dyspnea, orthopnea, chest pain, hemoptysis, swelling of neck, upper limbs and face, dilated veins in the upper chest wall, headaches, confusion, and rarely seizures due to raised intracranial tension. Radiologic examination with a contrast-enhanced CT will identify the mass lesion, and the presence of collaterals on CT is highly sensitive and specific for presence of SVCS.[53] If suspected, CT angiography can detect the site and extent of the thrombus.

Evaluation of these patients should be quick as they can deteriorate rapidly. Careful general examination should be carried out to look for peripheral lymphadenopathy. Patients often have pleural effusions which are often secondary to venous hypertension and unlikely to yield the diagnosis. Patient having significant orthopnea may face difficulty in undergoing image-guided sampling of the mediastinal mass since these procedures require the patient to lie down. Under such circumstances, endoscopic stenting of the SVC is the treatment of choice in relieving the symptoms when diagnosis is not established. Stenting provides near-total relief of symptoms within 24–72 hours; subsequently, the patient is able to undergo mediastinal sampling.[54] Once the diagnosis is established, the patients may undergo chemotherapy in cases of lung cancer and lymphoma or radiotherapy in cases of small-cell carcinoma of lung.

All patients should receive supportive care with oxygen supplementation, head-end elevation, and restriction of fluids and diuretics. Use of steroids before the tissue diagnosis is established should be discouraged; it may lead to architectural distortion making subsequent biopsies difficult to interpret. Median life expectancy in patients with SVCS is approximately 6 months with a range of 1.5–9.5 months; estimates vary widely, depending on the underlying malignant condition.

SUMMARY

Mediastinum contains the vital components of thoracic cavity other than the lungs. These structures get involved in various infective, congenital, inflammatory and malignancy pathologies due to presence of rich lymphatics. The recent advances in the field of imaging and sampling technology has improved our ability to diagnose and treat these pathologies with more conviction.

REFERENCES

1. Carter BW, Marom EM, Detterbeck FC. Approaching the patient with an anterior mediastinal mass: a guide for clinicians. J Thorac Oncol. 2014;9(9 Suppl 2):S102-9.
2. Davis RD Jr, Oldham HN Jr, Sabiston DC Jr. Primary cysts and neoplasms of the mediastinum: recent changes in clinical presentation, methods of diagnosis, management, and results. Annals Thorac Surg. 1987;44(3):229-37.
3. Priola SM, Priola AM, Cardinale L, et al. The anterior mediastinum: anatomy and imaging procedures. Radiol Med. 2006;111(3): 295-311.
4. Proto AV. Mediastinal anatomy: emphasis on conventional images with anatomic and computed tomographic correlations. J Thorac Imaging. 1987;2(1):1-48.
5. Tecce PM, Fishman EK, Kuhlman JE. CT evaluation of the anterior mediastinum: spectrum of disease. Radiographics. 1994;14(5):973-90.
6. Nakazono T, Yamaguchi K, Egashira R, et al. MRI Findings and Differential Diagnosis of Anterior Mediastinal Solid Tumors. Magn Reson Med Sci. 2023;22(4):415-33.
7. Naidich DP, Web WR, Muller NL, et al. Mediastinum. Computed Tomography and Magnetic Resonance of the Thorax. Philadelphia: Lippincott Williams and Wilkins; 1999. pp. 37-159.
8. Ohno Y. New applications of magnetic resonance imaging for thoracic oncology. Semin Respir Crit Care Med. 2014;35(1): 27-40.
9. Senturk A, Arguder E, Hezer H, et al. Rapid diagnosis of mediastinal tuberculosis with polymerase chain reaction evaluation of aspirated material taken by endobronchial ultrasound-guided transbronchial needle aspiration. J Investig Med. 2014;62(6):885-9.
10. Naidich DP. Helical computed tomography of the thorax. Clinical applications. Radiol Clin North Am. 1994;32(4):759-74.
11. Takada K, Matsumoto S, Hiramatsu T, et al. Management of spontaneous pneumomediastinum based on clinical experience of 25 cases. Respir Med. 2008;102(9):1329-34.
12. Okamoto S, Tsuboi H, Noma H, et al. Predictive Factors for Pneumomediastinum during Management of Connective Tissue Disease-related Interstitial Lung Disease: A Retrospective Study. Intern Med. 2021;60(18):2887-97.
13. Chowdhary A, Nirwan L, Abi-Ghanem AS, et al. Spontaneous Pneumomediastinum in Patients Diagnosed with COVID-19: A Case Series with Review of Literature. Acad Radiol. 2021; 28(11):1586-98.
14. Takada K, Matsumoto S, Hiramatsu T, et al. Spontaneous pneumomediastinum: an algorithm for diagnosis and management. Ther Adv Respir Dis. 2009;3(6):301-7.
15. van Veelen I, Hogeman PH, van Elburg A, et al. Pneumomediastinum: a rare complication of anorexia nervosa in children and adolescents. A case study and review of the literature. Eur J Pediatr. 2008;167(2):171-4.
16. Macklin MT MC. Malignant interstitial emphysema of the lung and mediastinum as an important occult complication in many respiratory diseases and other conditions. Medicine. 1944;23: 281-358.
17. Miura H, Taira O, Hiraguri S, et al. Clinical features of medical pneumomediastinum. Ann Thorac Cardiovasc Surg. 2003;9(3): 188-91.
18. Gammon RB, Shin MS, Buchalter SE. Pulmonary barotrauma in mechanical ventilation. Patterns and risk factors. Chest. 1992;102(2):568-72.
19. Kacmarek RM. Management of the patient-ventilator system. In: Kacmarek RM, Pierson DJ (Eds). Foundations of Respiratory Care. New York: Churchill Livingstone; 1992. pp. 973-98.
20. Goodwin RA, Nickell JA, Des Prez RM. Mediastinal fibrosis complicating healed primary histoplasmosis and tuberculosis. Medicine. 1972;51(3):227-46.
21. Arbra CA, Valentino JD, Martin JT. Vascular sequelae of mediastinal fibrosis. Asian Cardiovasc Thorac Ann. 2015;23(1):36-41.
22. Ferrer Galvan M, Rodriguez Portal JA, Serrano Gorarredona MP, et al. Fibrosing mediastinitis mimicking sarcoidosis. Clin Respir J. 2015;9(1):125-8.
23. Silverman NA, Sabiston DC Jr. Mediastinal masses. Surg Clin North Am. 1980;60(4):757-77.
24. Zhang S, Yang ZG, Liu X, et al. Tuberculosis vs. chronic lymphocytic leukaemia in mediastinal lymph nodes using computed tomography. Int J Tuberc Lung Dis. 2014;18(2):211-5.
25. Grillo HC, Ojemann RG, Scannell JG, et al. Combined approach to "dumbbell" intrathoracic and intraspinal neurogenic tumors. Ann Thorac Surg. 1983;36(4):402-7.
26. Ahrar K, Wallace M, Javadi S, et al. Mediastinal, hilar, and pleural image-guided biopsy: current practice and techniques. Semin Respir Crit Care Med. 2008;29(4):350-60.

27. Wiersema MJ, Vazquez-Sequeiros E, Wiersema LM. Evaluation of mediastinal lymphadenopathy with endoscopic US-guided fine-needle aspiration biopsy. Radiology. 2001;219(1):252-7.
28. Zhang J, Guo JR, Huang ZS, et al. Transbronchial mediastinal cryobiopsy in the diagnosis of mediastinal lesions: a randomised trial. Eur Respir J. 2021;58(6).
29. Yasufuku K, Chiyo M, Koh E, et al. Endobronchial ultrasound guided transbronchial needle aspiration for staging of lung cancer. Lung Cancer. 2005;50(3):347-54.
30. Protopapas Z, Westcott JL. Transthoracic hilar and mediastinal biopsy. Radiol Clin North Am. 2000;38(2):281-91.
31. Minami D, Takigawa N, Inoue H, et al. Rapid on-site evaluation with BIOEVALUATOR((R)) during endobronchial ultrasound-guided transbronchial needle aspiration for diagnosing pulmonary and mediastinal diseases. Ann Thorac Med. 2014;9(1):14-7.
32. Bonifazi M, Sediari M, Ferretti M, et al. The role of the pulmonologist in rapid on-site cytologic evaluation of transbronchial needle aspiration: a prospective study. Chest. 2014;145(1):60-5.
33. Damaraju V, Gupta N, Saini M, et al. The utility of WhatsApp-based off-site evaluation for rapid cytology of EBUS-TBNA samples. Cytopathology. 2023;34(1):43-7.
34. Toloza EM, Harpole L, Detterbeck F, et al. Invasive staging of non-small cell lung cancer: a review of the current evidence. Chest. 2003;123(1 Suppl):157S-66S.
35. Mullen B, Richardson JD. Primary anterior mediastinal tumors in children and adults. Ann Thorac Surg. 1986;42(3):338-45.
36. Lattes R. Thymoma and other tumors of the thymus: analysis of 107 cases. Cancer. 1962;15:1224-60.
37. Verstandig AG, Epstein DM, Miller WT Jr, et al. Thymoma–report of 71 cases and a review. Crit Rev Diagn Imaging. 1992;33(3): 201-30.
38. Wilkins EW Jr, Edmunds LH Jr, Castleman B. Cases of thymoma at the Massachusetts General Hospital. J Thorac Cardiovasc Surg. 1966;52(3):322-30.
39. Shamji F, Pearson FG, Todd TR, et al. Results of surgical treatment for thymoma. J Thorac Cardiovasc Surg. 1984;87(1):43-7.
40. Ruffini E, Venuta F. Management of thymic tumors: a European perspective. J Thorac Dis. 2014;6(Suppl 2):S228-37.
41. Okumura M, Ohta M, Tateyama H, et al. The World Health Organization histologic classification system reflects the oncologic behavior of thymoma: a clinical study of 273 patients. Cancer. 2002;94(3):624-32.
42. Gonzalez-Crussi F. Extragonadal teratomas. In: Hartmann WH, Cowan WR (Eds). Atlas of Tumor Pathology. Washington, DC: Armed Forces Institute of Pathology; 1982. pp. 77-94.
43. Strollo DC, Rosado de Christenson ML, Jett JR. Primary mediastinal tumors. Part 1: tumors of the anterior mediastinum. Chest. 1997;112(2):511-22.
44. Bush SE, Martinez A, Bagshaw MA. Primary mediastinal seminoma. Cancer. 1981;48(8):1877-82.
45. Bokemeyer C, Droz JP, Horwich A, et al. Extragonadal seminoma: an international multicenter analysis of prognostic factors and long term treatment outcome. Cancer. 2001;91(7):1394-401.
46. Liu Y, Wang Z, Peng ZM, et al. Management of the primary malignant mediastinal germ cell tumors: experience with 54 patients. Diagn Pathol. 2014;9:33.
47. International Germ Cell Consensus Classification: a prognostic factor-based staging system for metastatic germ cell cancers. International Germ Cell Cancer Collaborative Group. J Clin Oncol. 1997;15(2):594-603.
48. Takeda S, Miyoshi S, Minami M, et al. Clinical spectrum of mediastinal cysts. Chest. 2003;124(1):125-32.
49. Nakazato Y, Ohno Y, Nakata Y, et al. Cystic lymphangioma of the mediastinum. Am Heart J. 1995;129(2):406-9.
50. Johnson DW, Klazynski PT, Gordon WH, et al. Mediastinal lymphangioma and chylothorax: the role of radiotherapy. Ann Thorac Surg. 1986;41(3):325-8.
51. Khanlou H, Khanlou N, Eiger G. Schwannoma of posterior mediastinum: a case report and concise review. Heart Lung. 1998;27(5):344-7.
52. Duwe BV, Sterman DH, Musani AI. Tumors of the mediastinum. Chest. 2005;128(4):2893-909.
53. Ostler PJ CD, Watkinson AF, et al. Superior vena cava obstruction: a modern management strategy. Clin Oncol (R Coll Radiol). 1997;9(2):83-9.
54. Rowell NP GF. Steroids, radiotherapy, chemotherapy and stents for superior vena caval obstruction in carcinoma of the bronchus: a systematic review. Clin Oncol (R Coll Radiol). 2002;14(5):338-51.

Diseases of the Chest Wall

CHAPTER 135

Balamugesh T

INTRODUCTION

The chest wall plays a crucial role in the respiratory pump which consists of the rib cage, rib cage muscles, and the diaphragm. Disorders involving the chest wall may affect ventilation and eventually lead to respiratory failure. The thoracic cage abnormalities in childhood may also influence the growth of the lungs.[1] The disorders of the diaphragm are discussed in a separate section. The important nonmuscular diseases of the chest wall are discussed in the following text.

KYPHOSCOLIOSIS

Kyphoscoliosis is a group of conditions in which patients have scoliosis (lateral curvature of the spine) and kyphosis (backward curvature of spine) **(Fig. 1)**. Based on the etiology, the curvature abnormalities can be considered in three groups:

1. *Congenital*: Neurofibromatosis, Friedreich's ataxia, muscular dystrophy, Ehlers–Danlos syndrome, Marfan syndrome, etc.
2. *Paralytic*: Poliomyelitis, muscular dystrophy, cerebral palsy, Friedreich's ataxia
3. Idiopathic

Kyphoscoliosis is idiopathic in approximately 80%, with a female predominance (4:1). The severity of kyphoscoliosis is determined radiologically using the Cobb angle. Two lines are drawn parallel to the upper border of the highest and the lower border of the lowest vertebral body of the curvature as seen on an anteroposterior radiograph of the spine, respectively. The angle made by two lines drawn perpendicular to these lines at the intersection point is measured **(Fig. 2)**. An angle $>10°$ defines scoliosis while >40 is indicative of severe scoliosis with a higher risk of progression to respiratory failure.

Pulmonary Functions Tests

Predicted values for lung function in patients with kyphoscoliosis should be calculated on the basis of arm span measurements because of reduction in height due to spinal deformity.[2] Restrictive ventilatory pattern is seen in patients

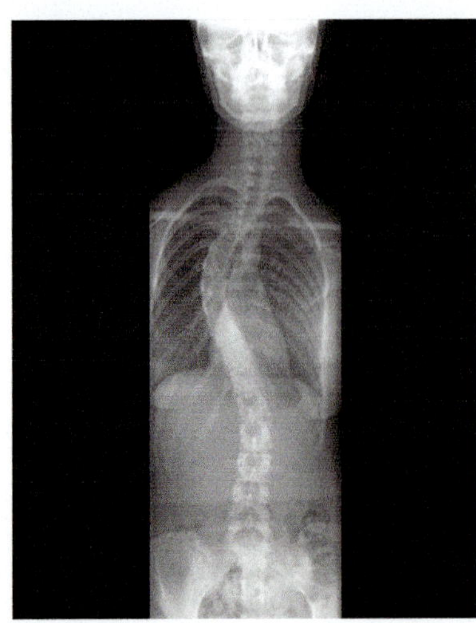

FIG. 1: X-ray spine showing scoliosis.

Courtesy: With permission from Dr Frank Gaillard. www.radiopaedia.org

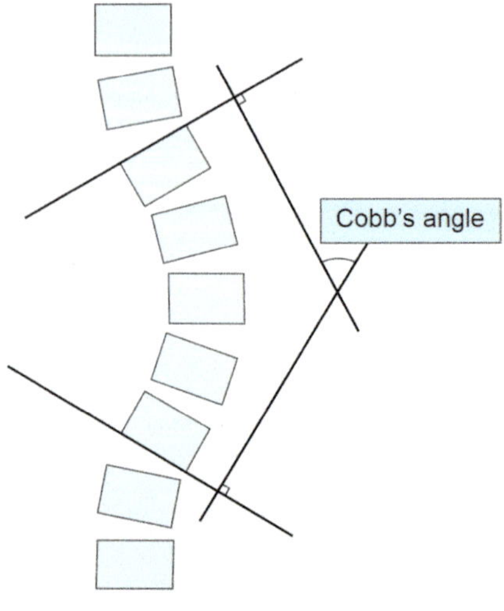

FIG. 2: Cobb's angle.

with severe kyphoscoliosis with reduction in vital capacity (VC) and total lung capacity (TLC).[3] This is due to reduction in chest-wall compliance. In order to reduce the work of breathing, the patients adopt a pattern of rapid shallow breathing. This in turn leads to reduction in lung compliance due to microatelectasis and increases the deadspace ventilation. The pulmonary function tests significantly correlate with the degree of scoliotic angle and the number of involved vertebrae.[4] Those with paralytic kyphoscoliosis have pronounced reduction in inspiratory muscle strength and have greater reduction in VC. In those with Cobb's angle > 50°, there is significant reduction in inspiratory and expiratory muscle strength attributed to altered chest wall geometry and resultant mechanical disadvantage of the respiratory muscles.

Some patients have airway obstruction in addition to lung restriction; this is due to bronchial torsion and compression of central airways.[5] The increase in oxygen cost of breathing may place these patients at high risk of respiratory muscle fatigue. The residual volume (RV) is normal leading to increase in RV/TLC ratio. Diffusing capacity for carbon monoxide (DLCO) is reduced in proportion to the reduction in lung volumes, giving normal values for transfer factor (KCO).[6] In some patients, DLCO is reduced disproportionately and it is attributed to failure of alveolar development and pulmonary hypertension. The maximum oxygen consumption during exercise is reduced with normal ventilatory performance during exercise. Exercise intolerance may be due to deconditioning.[7] The discrepancy between desired and achieved tidal volume may result in afferent-efferent dissociation and cause sensation of dyspnea. The neural drive for breathing as measured by mouth occlusion pressure at 100 ms ($p = 0.1$) is normal or increased. But the ventilatory response to carbon dioxide (CO_2) is reduced by the reduced mobility of the stiffened chest wall.[6]

Sleep Disordered Breathing

The most common abnormality in patients with kyphoscoliosis during sleep is hypoventilation. In awake state, the intercostal and accessory muscles are recruited to assist the diaphragm in displacing the stiff chest wall. When sleeping, these patients may hypoventilate due to hypotonia of the intercostal and accessory muscles and decreased neural drive to diaphragm.[8] Since chest wall movement is compromised, any degree of diaphragmatic dysfunction can aggravate hypoventilation during sleep. Untreated nocturnal desaturation can further worsen the respiratory muscle function leading to respiratory failure and cor pulmonale. The prevalence of obstructive sleep apnea is same as in general population, but if present can further worsen the nocturnal hypoventilation.[9]

Prognosis

Prognosis is worse in those with a greater Cobb's angle and curvature at a higher level in the spine. In congenital and paralytic kyphoscoliosis, there can be chances of progressively worsening skeletal deformity leading to respiratory failure. Individuals with idiopathic kyphoscoliosis have a more benign course. Pulmonary hypertension develops due to persistent hypoxia or due to nocturnal hypoventilation. Once cor pulmonale develops, there is a rapid downhill course unless treatment is started. Death usually occurs as a result of respiratory failure or cardiac diseases and the risks are highest in juvenile and post-polio scoliosis.[10] Pregnancy is poorly tolerated if the VC is <1 L.

Medical Management

Mild kyphoscoliosis has a good prognosis, while more severe kyphoscoliosis can result in progressive respiratory failure and cor pulmonale. General measures include immunization against pneumococci and influenza, prompt treatment of respiratory infections, smoking cessation, avoidance of sedatives, maintenance of ideal body weight, and prevention of physical deconditioning by exercise. Supplemental oxygen may be required during activity or exercise.

Specific treatment of nocturnal hypoventilation is by noninvasive positive-pressure ventilation by a nasal or full-face mask. Volume-preset and pressure-preset ventilators have equivalent physiological benefits. The Consensus Conference 1999 has laid down indications for noninvasive ventilation (NIV) for kyphoscoliosis **(Box 1)**.[11] The benefits of noninvasive nocturnal ventilation in patients with kyphoscoliosis include improvements in quality of life, gas exchange, sleep architecture, and reduction in pulmonary artery pressure.[12-14] Long-term NIV also reduces the number of hospitalizations due to respiratory failure. However, there are no remarkable changes in VC and respiratory muscle strength. The improvement in respiratory failure is due to increased ventilatory response to CO_2, prevention of respiratory muscle fatigue, and reversal of microatelectasis. Negative-pressure ventilation by cuirass, body wrap ventilators, or tank ventilators can aggravate upper airway obstruction during sleep and are not recommended.

Surgery for Kyphoscoliosis

Surgery plays an important role in those with kyphoscoliosis secondary to neurological disorders among children and

BOX 1 Indication of noninvasive ventilation (NIV) (Consensus Conference Report, 1999).[11]

Symptoms (e.g., fatigue, morning headaches, dyspnea)

OR

Signs of cor pulmonale

AND one of the following:

- Daytime arterial $PCO_2 \geq 45$ mm Hg
- Nocturnal oxygen saturation ≤ 88% for 5 consecutive minutes
- Progressive neuromuscular disease with maximal inspiratory pressure (Pi_{max}) < 60 cm H_2O or forced vital capacity (FVC) < 50% of predicted

adolescents.[15] Operative treatment traditionally consists of spinal fusion and/or insertion of Harrington rods, which may result in short-term improvement in lung function. However, surgery can sometimes result in chronic back pain or further spinal deformities. Initial results from further refinements in surgical techniques are promising.[16]

Thoracoplasty

Thoracoplasty is a surgical technique that was used to collapse the lungs affected by tuberculosis, prior to the advent of antitubercular drugs **(Fig. 3)**. It consists of various combinations of rib removal, artificial pneumothorax, phrenic nerve resection, and compression of lung by foreign material. The patients who underwent thoracoplasty subsequently developed restrictive lung disease and chronic respiratory failure as they aged.

The severity of dysfunction was related to the number of ribs removed, presence of fibrothorax, degree of fibrosis of the underlying lung, phrenic nerve damage, and degree of scoliosis. There are significant associations between the development of cardiorespiratory or respiratory failure and a preoperative contralateral artificial pneumothorax, older age at operation, the presence of cavities before operation, and male sex.[17] Currently, thoracoplasty is used in rare situations such as postpneumonectomy complications, persistent tubercular bronchopleural fistula, and sputum-positive drug-resistant tuberculosis.[18]

In a series of 139 patients who underwent thoracoplasty in India, the indications for surgery were tubercular empyema (84 patients), pyogenic empyema (33 patients), postoperative empyema with bronchopleural fistula (8 patients), drug-resistant pulmonary tuberculosis (2 patients), and recurrent hemoptysis (2 patients).[18] Successful outcome in the form of control of sepsis, closure of bronchopleural fistula, sputum conversion, and control of hemoptysis was achieved in the majority. There were four deaths in the entire series. In another series of 37 patients who underwent thoracoplasty and intrathoracic muscle transposition, the most common indication was postpneumonectomy/lobectomy empyema.[19]

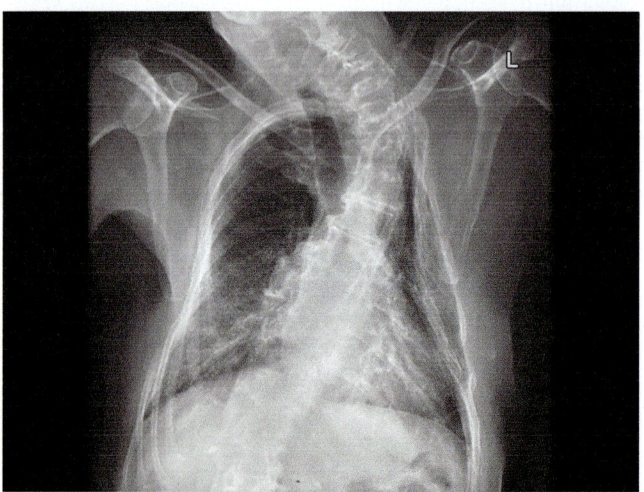

FIG. 3: Thoracoplasty.
Courtesy: With permission from Dr Frank Gaillard. www.radiopaedia.org

Thoracoplasty is still relevant in developing countries as pulmonary tuberculosis continues to be a challenging and persisting problem. Treatment of respiratory failure in post-thoracoplasty patients is the same as for those with kyphoscoliosis.[20] Pulmonary rehabilitation significantly improves the dyspnea score and 6-minute walk distance in such patients.[21]

PECTUS EXCAVATUM

Pectus excavatum, also known as "funnel chest", is characterized by excessive depression of sternum. It is the most common chest deformity seen by pediatricians. It is present in 0.4% of school children.[22] It is more common among boys than girls. The etiology is not clear but a defect in connective tissue surrounding sternum and imbalance of forces counteracting the inward pull of diaphragm on xiphisternum during development has been implicated.[23] Upper airway obstruction due to enlarged tonsils and adenoids predisposes to pectus excavatum.[24] Marfan syndrome has a higher incidence of pectus excavatum. Incidence of congenital heart disease is also higher among those with pectus excavatum.

Most individuals with pectus excavatum remain asymptomatic. The most common complaint is cosmesis. Dyspnea out of proportion to the mild restrictive ventilatory defect is seen. Majority of them have cardiac murmurs mimicking pulmonary stenosis caused by cardiac displacement. Chest radiograph frequently shows right paracardiac opacity due to parasternal soft tissues and should not be mistaken for middle lobe infiltrate **(Fig. 4)**.[24] Similarly, electrocardiogram may show abnormalities like T inversion in right chest leads, right axis deviation, P wave inversion in V1, and a QR pattern.[25]

More than 3 cm distance between anterior chest wall and the sternal depression and <10 cm distance between the posterior border of the sternum and the anterior border of the thoracic vertebra as seen on the lateral chest radiograph suggests severe deformity **(Fig. 5)**. The degree of the deformity is measured by the computerized tomography (CT) scan as the ratio of transverse to anteroposterior diameter at the level of deepest sternal depression **(Fig. 6)**. A ratio (pectus index) > 3.25 is considered severe excavatum.

Pulmonary function tests are usually normal or mildly reduced in those with severe excavatum.[26,27] The reduced exercise tolerance out of proportion to lung function can be attributed to reduced venous return secondary to right ventricular compression by the depressed sternum. Patients with minimal deformity can benefit from a program of physical therapy to improve posture and the appearance of the chest. Surgery is necessary only in severe situations or

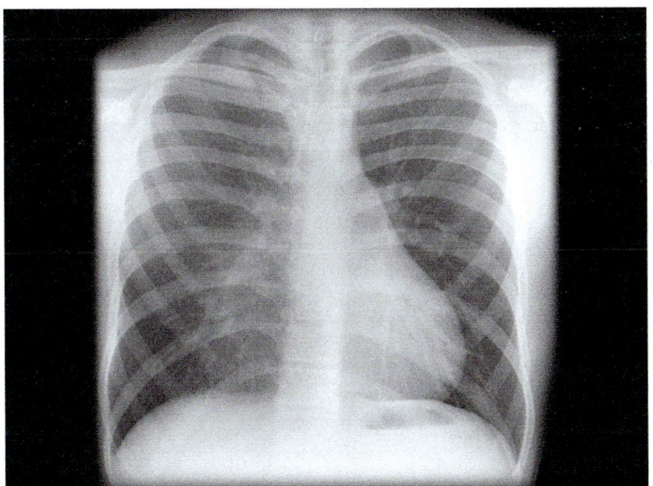

FIG. 4: Pectus excavatum: Chest radiograph posteroanterior (PA) view—right paracardiac opacity due to parasternal soft tissue, could be mistaken for middle-lobe infiltrate.

Courtesy: With permission from Dr Frank Gaillard. www.radiopaedia.org

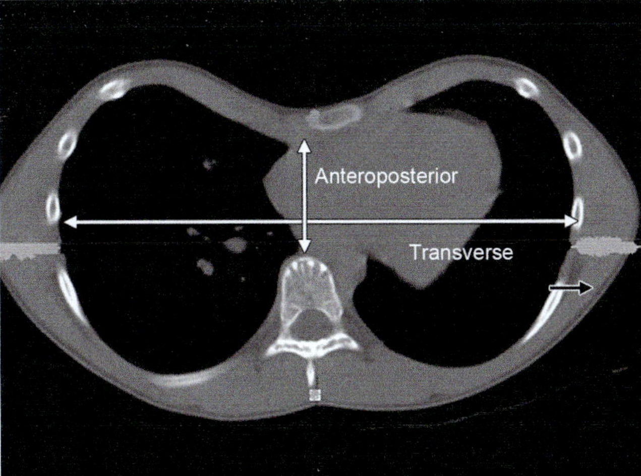

FIG. 6: Pectus excavatum: Ratio of transverse to anteroposterior diameter at the level of deepest sternal depression > 3.25 suggests severe deformity.

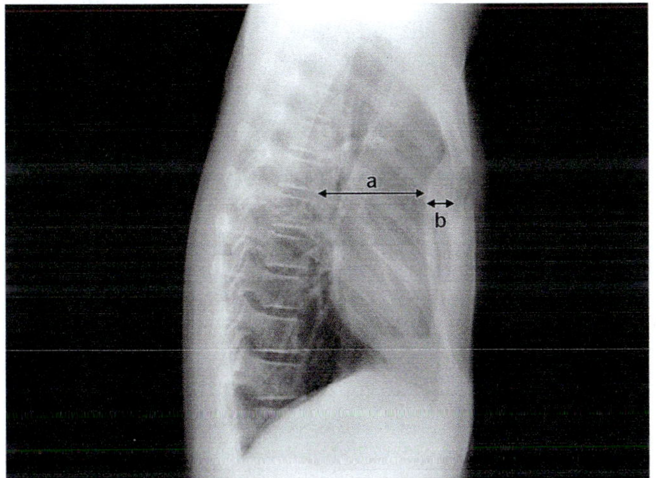

FIG. 5: Pectus excavatum: Chest radiograph—lateral view <10 cm distance between the posterior border of the sternum and the anterior border of the thoracic vertebra (a) and >3 cm distance between anterior chest wall and the sternal depression (b) suggest severe deformity.

Courtesy: With permission from Dr Frank Gaillard. www.radiopaedia.org

for cosmetic purposes. The indications for surgery include pectus index of >3.25 (measured on CT scan), cardiac compression, displacement, mitral valve prolapse, murmurs, or conduction abnormalities, pulmonary function testing showing severe restrictive abnormalities and failed previous repair of pectus excavatum.[28]

The earlier surgeries like the Ravitch repair are associated with many complications.[28] Less-invasive procedures like the Nuss procedure and sternochondroplasty have been developed in the last decade which are safer.[29-31] In the Nuss procedure, a curved bar in inserted behind the sternum to displace the sternum ventrally. These procedures are not always associated with improvement in pulmonary function or exercise capacity.

PECTUS CARINATUM

In this condition (also called "pigeon breast"), the sternum excessively protrudes anteriorly. It may be associated with other congenital anomalies, especially cardiac lesions and coarctation of aorta.[32] Pectus carinatum may result from premature obliteration of the sternal sutures due to inadequate segmentation during fetal life or due to malattachment of diaphragm.[33] There is no functional defect with pectus carinatum, surgery is indicated for cosmetic reasons.

ANKYLOSING SPONDYLOSIS

Ankylosis spondylosis (AS) belongs to a group of conditions with strong association with human leukocyte antigen B27 (HLA-B27) in which there is inflammation of axial skeleton. There is inflammation and bony ankylosis of vertebral structures, costovertebral and sternoclavicular joints. This leads to reduction in chest expansion. Chest expansion at the level of 4th intercostal space < 2.5 cm in a young adult with back pain should raise the suspicion of AS. Exercise intolerance and dyspnea are uncommon, unless there is associated underlying lung fibrosis, diaphragmatic dysfunction, or cardiac disease.

The degree of restrictive ventilatory defect correlates with spinal mobility. Since the rib cage is fixed in the inspiratory position, the RV is increased leading to increase in RV/TLC ratio.[34] The modest decrease in respiratory muscle strength is observed and it is attributed to intercostal muscle atrophy secondary to decreased rib cage mobility. There will be exercise limitation with reduced maximal oxygen consumption, especially with those with VC < 70% of predicted.[35] Other factors such as deconditioning and inspiratory muscle fatigue also contribute to exercise limitation.[36,37]

About 1–4% of patients, especially men with chronic disease of >15 years' duration, develop fibrobullous upper lobe disease.[38] Apical fibrosis can be detected in high-resolution CT scan in about 9%.[39] The cause of apical fibrobullous changes is unknown. Various theories have been postulated which include, diminished upper-lobe ventilation due to chest wall rigidity, altered apical mechanical stress due to rigid thoracic spine, recurrent pulmonary infection due to impaired cough, and respiratory mechanics as a result of thoracic rigidity.[40] Aspergillomas may form in the cavities or bullae. Other rare complications include pleural effusion, pneumothorax, airway obstruction by cricoarytenoid joint ankylosis, and amyloidosis of the lung.[41,42] About 20% of patients who were on sulfasalazine have been found to have asymptomatic interstitial lung disease detected by high-resolution CT scanning.[43]

Treatment is focused on symptom relief and maintenance of posture and mobility. Physiotherapy to improve chest wall movements and breathing exercises are important. Tumor necrosis factor (TNF) antagonists have revolutionized the management of patients with AS.[44]

OBESITY

The prevalence of obesity is increasing worldwide. The body mass index (BMI) is positively associated with morbidity and mortality. An individual with a BMI between 18.5 and 24.9 kg/m^2 is normal, a BMI between 25 and 29.9 kg/m^2 is overweight, and a BMI > 30 kg/m^2 is obese. Those with a BMI > 40 kg/m^2 (morbid obesity) are especially predisposed to develop restrictive lung disease. Some investigators have concluded that Indians are more predisposed to obesity-related complications due to different body, genetic, and metabolic composition.[45] In India, based on morbidity and prevalence of cardiovascular risk factors, a cut-off BMI for overweight is 23 kg/m^2 and for obesity is 25 kg/m^2.[46]

The respiratory morbidity due to obesity is considered under three categories: (1) Simple obesity (SO) with minimal effects on respiration, (2) morbid obesity (MO) eucapnic individuals with compromised pulmonary function, and (3) obesity hypoventilation syndrome (OHS) with hypercapnia during awake state. Obstructive sleep apnea can coexist with any of these.

Pulmonary Function Test

Both the thoracoabdominal pattern and lung function tests are altered during spontaneous respiration.[47] FVC and TLC are usually preserved in SO but reduced in OHS. The fat in the chest wall and abdomen causes reduction in functional reserve capacity (FRC) with near-normal RV **(Fig. 7)**. This

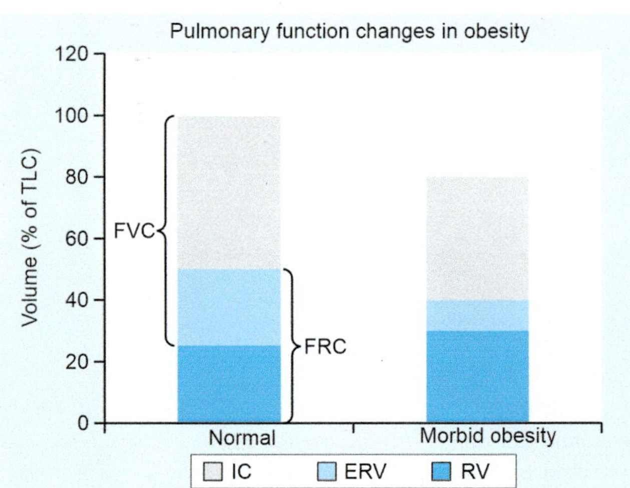

FIG. 7: Pulmonary function changes in obesity: Reduction in expiratory reserve volume (ERV) with preservation of residual volume (RV) and reduction in forced vital capacity (FVC).

results in markedly reduced expiratory reserve volume (ERV).[48] Similar degrees of obesity in SO and OHS can cause much more reduction in ERV in OHS due to difference in distribution of body fat. Even if FEV1/FVC ratio is normal, the specific conductance of airways is reduced to 50–70%, which is more evident in supine position.[48] The cause of increased airway resistance in obesity appears to lie in lung tissue and small airways. This leads to expiratory flow limitation and orthopnea. Patients with OHS adapt to increased elastic and resistive loads by adopting rapid, shallow breathing pattern. The diameter of small airways is reduced at lower lung volumes. The chest wall compliance is reduced to adipose tissue in the chest wall and abdomen. The lung compliance is also reduced due to increased pulmonary blood volume and early airway closure. Expiratory flow limitation and intrinsic positive end-expiratory pressure (auto-PEEP) can occur in morbidly obese individuals, and these are worsened in supine position.[49]

The work of breathing and oxygen cost of breathing are markedly increased in OHS.[50] The increased oxygen consumption required for quiet breathing might place obese patients at risk for respiratory failure during conditions characterized by increased ventilatory demands such as an intercurrent illness. Respiratory muscle strength is preserved in SO, but reduced in OHS due to deconditioning and fatty infiltration of muscle. This along with disordered respiratory control and blunted respiratory drive contributes to hypercapnia in OHS.

Severely obese patients tend to have a widened alveolar-arterial oxygen tension gradient and hypoxia. The mechanism responsible for hypoxemia is primarily a ventilation-perfusion mismatch that results from airway closure.[51] Hypoxia is also contributed by hypoventilation and venous admixture occurring in lung bases due to alveolar collapse.[52]

Treatment

Weight loss induced by either diet or surgery helps in improvement of ERV and improvement of hypoxia in patients with OHS. But there is difficulty in losing weight and maintaining it in the majority. In patients with OHS, noninvasive ventilation helps improving gas exchange and daytime symptoms.

FLAIL CHEST

This is a condition in which fractures of ribs produce a segment of rib cage that moves paradoxically during respiration. Generally, double fractures of three or more contiguous ribs or a combination of sternal and rib fractures are required to produce a flail segment. The most common cause of flail chest is trauma due to fall or automobile accidents. Rarely, pathological fractures of ribs can cause a flail segment.

During inspiration, the negative intrapleural pressure causes the flail segment to be displaced inward instead of expanding outward **(Figs. 8A and B)**. The most common site of flail segment is lateral chest wall, posteriorly. Respiratory failure caused by flail chest is multifactorial:

1. Hypoventilation caused by paradoxical movement of flail segment and restricted chest wall movements due to pain. The VC and FRC may be reduced to 50% of predicted
2. Regional atelectasis caused by ineffective cough reflex and hypoventilation
3. Pulmonary contusion, hemothorax, or pneumothorax, which is frequently associated with flail chest
4. Inspiratory muscle dysfunction due to muscle spasm and altered recruitment pattern causing increased work of breathing

Treatment consists of adequate pain relief to prevent atelectasis and improve tidal volume. It can be achieved with medications, intercostal nerve blocks, and epidural anesthesia. Stabilizing the flail segment by external strappings is not very successful. Positive-pressure ventilation can provide effective stabilization by eliminating the negative intrapleural pressure. Earlier mechanical ventilation was used to provide the ventilation. But recently noninvasive continuous positive airway ventilation together with regional anesthesia has been found to reduce morbidity and avoid complications.[53] In severe injuries, a variety of surgical procedures are described for fracture fixation and improvement of respiratory mechanics.

MISCELLANEOUS CONDITIONS

Cervical Ribs

Cervical ribs occur in about 0.5% of the population.[54] They arise from the seventh cervical vertebra and are bilateral in 80%.[55,56] They are usually asymptomatic **(Fig. 9)** but rarely can cause thoracic outlet syndrome due to compression of subclavian vessels or cervical nerve roots. The presence of symptoms is not dependent on the size of the rib, since the fibrous attachment itself may cause compression. Neurological complications can be managed by shoulder muscle-strengthening exercises; rib resection may be needed for vascular complications.

Tietze's Syndrome or Costochondritis

The etiology of this condition is unknown. It presents with pain, swelling of one or more of the upper six costal cartilages. It is more common in young adults with no sex predisposition and affects predominately second costal cartilage. Coughing or deep breathing may exacerbate the pain. The condition may persist for weeks, months, or years. Biopsy may show normal cartilage and there are

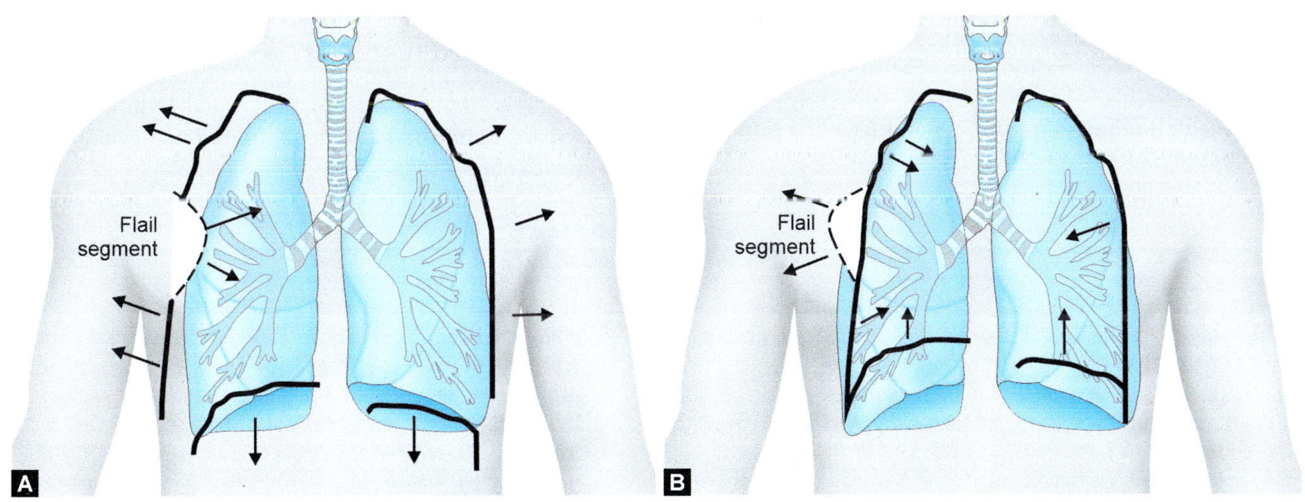

FIGS. 8A AND B: Flail chest. (A) During inspiration the flail segment paradoxically moves inward; (B) During expiration the flail segment moves outward.

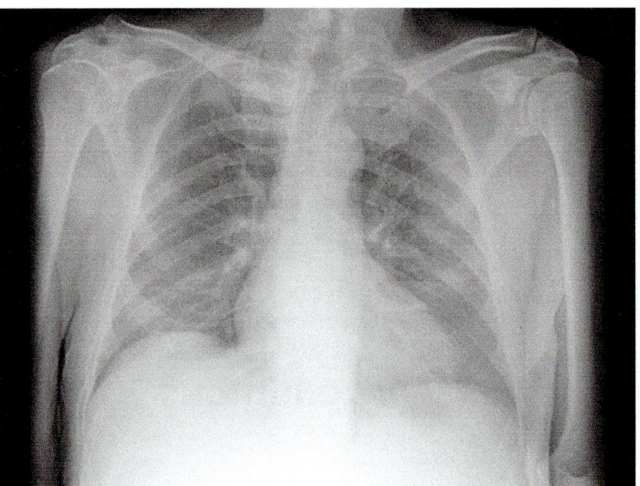

FIG. 9: Right cervical rib.
Courtesy: With permission from Dr Jeremy Jones. www.radiopaedia.org

no X-ray changes.[57] Ultrasonography will show thickened cartilage with inhomogeneously increased echogenicity, and hypoechoic halo.[58] A CT scan will show thickened hypodense cartilage with blurred outline.[59] Recently, magnetic resonance imaging has been claimed to be the investigation of choice to evidence the cartilage and bone abnormalities.[60] The main treatment is reassurance with or without administration of analgesics, to which the majority respond. In those with severe pain, local steroid injection may be required.

Rib Notching

Erosion of the inferior border of ribs (inferior rib notching) is most commonly seen in patients with coarctation of aorta. It is due to the enlarged intercostal arteries, which cause erosion of ribs by pulsating. The first two and last three ribs are never involved.[61] The other causes include subclavian artery obstruction, Takayasu's arteritis, pulmonary arteriovenous fistula, and intercostal neuroma. Superior notching of third to sixth ribs is reported in patients with poliomyelitis and in patients with connective tissue disorders.[62]

Chest Wall Hernias

Lung herniation through the chest wall can occur after thoracotomy, trauma, violent coughing and sneezing.[63,64] Chronic obstructive pulmonary disease, steroid use, and diabetes were also reported as risk factors for lung herniation. Prosthetic herniorrhaphy was successfully performed in these patients without any complications.

Tumors of the Chest Wall

Metastatic tumors of the chest wall are more common that the primary tumors. Breast is the most site of primary malignancy in these cases. Lipoma and fibrosarcoma are the most common benign and malignant soft-tissue tumors of the chest wall, respectively. Osteochondroma and chondrosarcoma are the most common benign and malignant tumors of the bony thoracic skeleton.

Tuberculosis of the Thoracic Cage

Costal cartilages and sternoclavicular and acromioclavicular joints can rarely be involved by tuberculosis. Multiple lesions of costovertebral portions of the ribs may accompany tuberculosis of the spine with paravertebral abscess formation. Cold abscess of the chest wall, which originates from tuberculosis of the intercostal lymph glands can present in three sites: (1) near the erector spinae muscles when pus tracks along the posterior primary division of the intercostal nerve, (2) lateral chest wall, when pus tracks along the anterior division, and (3) near-costal cartilages. It presents as painless fluctuant swelling. Diagnosis is made by aspiration of pus and it responds well to conventional antitubercular chemotherapy.

SUMMARY

The important non muscular diseases of the chest wall discussed in this chapter include thoracic cage abnormalities such as kyphoscoliosis, pectoral deformities, obesity and ankylosing spondylitis which are likely to impair respiratory pump function and affect ventilation. Eventually it may lead to respiratory failure due to prolonged hypoventilation. Thoracic cage abnormalities in childhood may also influence the growth of the lungs.

REFERENCES

1. Koumbourlis AC. Chest wall abnormalities and their clinical significance in childhood. Paediatr Respir Rev. 2013; pii: s1526-0542(13)00156-5.
2. Hepper NG, Black LF, Fowler WS. Relationships of lung volume to height and arm span in normal subjects and in patients with spinal deformity. Am Rev Respir Dis. 1965;91:356-62.
3. Lin MC, Liaw MY, Chen WJ, et al. Pulmonary function and spinal characteristics: their relationships in persons with idiopathic and postpoliomyelitic scoliosis. Arch Phys Med Rehabil. 2001; 82:335-41.
4. Xue X, Shen J, Zhang J, et al. An analysis of thoracic cage deformities and pulmonary function tests in congenital scoliosis. Eur Spine J. 2015;24(7):1415-21.
5. Al-Kattan K, Simonds A, chung KF, et al. Kyphoscoliosis and bronchial torsion. Chest. 1997;111:1134.
6. Siegler D, Zorab PA. The influence of lung volume on gas transfer in scoliosis. Br J Dis Chest. 1982;76:44-50.
7. Kesten S, Garfinkel SK, Wright T, et al. Impaired exercise capacity in adults with moderate scoliosis. Chest. 1991;99:663

8. Sawicka EH, Branthwaite MA. Respiration during sleep in kyphoscoliosis. Thorax. 1987;42:801-8.
9. Guilleminault C, Kurlan G, Wirkle R. Severe kyphoscoliosis, breathing, and sleep. Chest. 1981;79:626-30.
10. Pehrsson K, Larsson S, Oden A, et al. Long-term follow-up of patients with untreated scoliosis. A study of mortality, causes of death, and symptoms. Spine (Phila Pa 1976). 1992;17:1091-6.
11. Consensus Conference. Clinical indications for noninvasive positive pressure ventilation in chronic respiratory failure due to restrictive lung disease, COPD, and nocturnal hypoventilation - a Consensus conference report. Chest. 1999;116:521-34.
12. Chailleux E, Fauroux B, Binet F, et al. Predictors of survival in patients receiving domiciliary oxygen therapy or mechanical ventilation. A 10-year analysis of ANTADIR Observatory. Chest. 1996;109:741-9.
13. Gonzalez C, Ferris G, Diaz J, et al. Kyphoscoliotic ventilatory insufficiency: effects of long-term intermittent positive-pressure ventilation. Chest. 2003;124:857-62.
14. Annane D, Orlikowski D, Chevret S, et al. Nocturnal mechanical ventilation for chronic hypoventilation in patients with neuromuscular and chest wall disorders. Cochrane Database Syst Rev. 2007;(4):CD001941.
15. Shneerson JM, Edgar MA. Cardiac and respiratory function before and after spinal fusion in adolescent idiopathic scoliosis. Thorax. 1979;34:658-61.
16. Kim YJ, Lenke LG, Cho SK, et al. Comparative analysis of pedicle screw versus hook instrumentation in posterior spinal fusion of adolescent idiopathic scoliosis. Spine (Phila Pa 1976). 2004; 29:2040-8.
17. Phillips MS, Kinnear WJ, Shneerson JM. Late sequelae of pulmonary tuberculosis treated by thoracoplasty. Thorax. 1987; 42:445-51.
18. Dewan RK, Singh S, Kumar A, et al. Thoracoplasty: an obsolete procedure? Indian J Chest Dis Allied Sci. 1999;41:83-8.
19. Peppas G, Molnar TF, Jeyasingham K, et al. Thoracoplasty in the context of current surgical practice. Ann Thorac Surg. 1993; 56(4):903-9.
20. Krassas A, Crima R, Bagan P, et al. Current indications and results for thoracoplasty and intrathoracic muscle transposition. Eur J Cardiothorac Surg. 2010;37(5):1215-20.
21. Ando M, Mori A, Esaki H, et al. The effect of pulmonary rehabilitation in patients with post-tuberculosis lung disorder. Chest. 2003;123(6):1988.
22. Guller B, Hable K. Cardiac findings in pectus excavatum in children: review and differential diagnosis. Chest. 1974;66: 165-71.
23. Wooler GH, Mashhour YA, Garcia JB, et al. Pectus excavatum. Thorax. 1969;24:557-62.
24. Fan L, Murphy S. Pectus excavatum from chronic upper airway obstruction. Am J Dis Child. 1981; 135:550-2.
25. Martins DOJ, Sambhi MP, Zimmerman HA. The electrocardiogram in pectus excavatum. Br Heart J. 1958;20:495-501.
26. Fink A, Rivin A, Murray JF. Pectus excavatum. An analysis of twenty-seven cases. Arch Intern Med. 1961;108:427-37.
27. Kaguraoka H, Ohnuki T, Itaoka T, et al. Degree of severity of pectus excavatum and pulmonary function in preoperative and postoperative periods. J Thorac Cardiovasc Surg. 1992;104: 1483-8.
28. Nuss D, Kelly RE Jr. Indications and technique of Nuss procedure for pectus excavatum. Thorac Surg Clin. 2010;20(4):583.
29. Luu TD, Kogon BE, Force SD, et al. Surgery for recurrent pectus deformities. Ann Thorac Surg. 2009;88:1627-31.
30. Coelho Mde S, Silva RF, Bergonse Neto N, et al. Pectus excavatum surgery: sternochondroplasty versus Nuss procedure. Ann Thorac Surg. 2009;88:1773-9.
31. Robicsek F, Hebra A. To Nuss or not to Nuss? Two opposing views. Semin Thorac Cardiovasc Surg. 2009;21:85-8.
32. Robicsek F, Cook JW, Daugherty HK, et al. Pectus carinatum. J Thorac Cardiovasc Surg. 1979;78:52-61.
33. Currarino G, Silverman FN. Premature obliteration of the sternal sutures and pigeon-breast deformity. Radiology. 1958;70: 532-40.
34. Miller JM, Sproule BJ. Pulmonary function in ankylosing spondylitis. Am Rev Respir Dis. 1964;90:376-82.
35. Hsieh LF, Wei JC, Lee HY, et al. Aerobic capacity and its correlates in patients with ankylosing spondylitis. Int J Rheum Dis. 2016;19(5):490-9.
36. Elliott CG, Hill TR, Adams TE, et al. Exercise performance of subjects with ankylosing spondylitis and limited chest expansion. Bull Eur Physiopathol Respir. 1985;21:363.
37. Grassino A, Gross D, Macklem PT, et al. Inspiratory muscle fatigue as a factor limiting exercise. Bull Eur Physiopathol Respir. 1979;15:105.
38. Fenlon HM, Casserly I, Sant SM, et al. Plain radiographs and thoracic high-resolution CT in patients with ankylosing spondylitis. Am J Roentgenol. 1997;168:1067-72.
39. El Maghraoui A. Pleuropulmonary involvement in ankylosing spondylitis. Joint Bone Spine. 2005;72:496-502.
40. Thai D, Ratani RS, Salama S, et al. Upper lobe fibrocavitary disease in a patient with back pain and stiffness. Chest. 2000;118:1814-6.
41. Libby DM, Schley WS, Smith JP. Cricoarytenoid arthritis in ankylosing spondylitis. A cause of acute respiratory failure and cor pulmonale. Chest. 1981;80:641-2.
42. Blavia R, Toda MR, Vidal F, et al. Pulmonary diffuse amyloidosis and ankylosing spondylitis. A rare association. Chest. 1992;102: 1608-10.
43. Ayhan-Ardic FF, Oken O, Yorgancioglu ZR, et al. Pulmonary involvement in lifelong non-smoking patients with rheumatoid arthritis and ankylosing spondylitis without respiratory symptoms. Clin Rheumatol. 2006;25(2):213.
44. Goh L, Samanta A. A systematic MEDLINE analysis of therapeutic approaches in ankylosing spondylitis. Rheumatol Int. 2009; 29:1123-35.
45. Snehalatha C, Viswanathan V, Ramachandran A. Cutoff values for normal anthropometric variables in Asian Indian adults. Diabetes Care. 2003;26:1380-4.
46. Misra A, Chowbey P, Makkar BM, et al; Concensus Group. Consensus statement for diagnosis of obesity, abdominal obesity and the metabolic syndrome for Asian Indians and recommendations for physical activity, medical and surgical management. J Assoc Physicians India. 2009;57:163-70.
47. Barcelar Jde M, Aliverti A, Melo TL, et al. Chest wall regional volumes in obese women. Respir Physiol Neurobiol. 2013;189(1): 167-73.
48. Sahebjami H, Gartside PS. Pulmonary function in obese subjects with a normal FEV1/FVC ratio. Chest. 1996;110:1425-9.
49. Pankow W, Podszus T, Gutheil T, et al. Expiratory flow limitation and intrinsic positive end-expiratory pressure in obesity. J Appl Physiol (1985). 1998;85:1236.
50. Kress JP, Pohlman AS, Alverdy J, et al. The impact of morbid obesity on oxygen cost of breathing (VO(2RESP)) at rest. Am J Respir Crit Care Med. 1999;160:883-6.

51. Farebrother MJ, McHardy GJ, Munro JF: Relation between pulmonary gas exchange and closing volume before and after substantial weight loss in obese subjects. Br Med J. 1974;3:391-3.
52. Hurewitz AN, Susskind H, Harold WH. Obesity alters regional ventilation in lateral decubitus position. J Appl Physiol. 1985;59:774-83.
53. Gunduz M, Unlugenc H, Ozalevli M, et al. A comparative study of continuous positive airway pressure (CPAP) and intermittent positive pressure ventilation (IPPV) in patients with flail chest. Emerg Med J. 2005;22:325-9.
54. Fisher MS: Eve's rib (letters to the editor). Radiology. 1981; 140:841.
55. Dick R. Arteriography in neurovascular compression at the thoracic outlet, with special reference to embolic patterns. Am J Roentgenol Radium Ther Nucl Med. 1970;110:141-7.
56. Scher LA, Veith FJ, Haimovici H, et al. Staging of arterial complications of cervical rib: guidelines for surgical management. Surgery. 1984;95:644-9.
57. Carabasi RJ, Christian JJ, Brindley HH. Costosternal chondrodynia: A variant of Tietze's syndrome? Dis Chest. 1962;41: 559-62.
58. Martino F, Ettorre GC, Macarini L, et al. Diagnostic imaging of Tietze's syndrome. Comparison of computerized tomography and ultrasonography. Radiol Med. 1993;86:208-12.
59. Salomon MI. Thoracochondralgia (Tietze's syndrome); report of three cases. NY State J Med. 1958;58:530-3.
60. Volterrani L, Mazzei MA, Giordano N, et al. Magnetic resonance imaging in Tietze's syndrome. Clin Exp Rheumatol. 2008;26: 848-53.
61. Boone ML, Swenson BE, Felson B. Rib notching: Its many causes. Am J Roentgenol Radium Ther Nucl Med. 1964;91:1075-88.
62. Sargent EN, Turner AF, Jacobson G. Superior marginal rib defects. An etiologic classification. Am J Roentgenol Radium Ther Nucl Med. 1969;106:491-505.
63. Sedar CW, Allen MS, Nichols FC, et al. Primary and prosthetic repair of acquired chest wall hernias: A 20-year experience. Ann Thorac Surg. 2014;pii: s0003-4975(14)00599-2.
64. Bhardwaj H, Bhardwaj B, Youness HA. A painful sneeze: spontaneous thoracic lung herniation induced by vigorous sneeze. J Bronchology Interv Pulmonol. 2014;21(1): 61-4.

Diseases of Diaphragm

CHAPTER 136

Balamugesh T

INTRODUCTION

The diaphragm is a musculotendinous sheet that separates the thoracic and abdominal contents into two compartments. It has three anatomic components:

1. Sternal portion—arising from the xiphoid process of sternum
2. Costal portion—arising from lower six ribs
3. Crural portion—arising from external and internal arcuate ligaments attached to vertebrae

The muscle fibers from all three components insert into the boomerang-shaped central tendon. Excursion of the diaphragm is estimated to account for 60–75% of vital capacity (VC), the remaining contributed by the intercostal and accessory muscles.[1] During quiet respiration, the mean right and left hemidiaphragmatic excursions are 53 ± 16 and 46 ± 12 mm, respectively.[2] The diaphragm receives its nerve supply solely from the phrenic nerve, which originates predominantly from the fourth cervical ramus with contributions from third and fifth ramus. Any damage to the phrenic nerve along its long course through the neck and mediastinum can affect its function.

SIGNS AND SYMPTOMS OF DIAPHRAGMATIC DISORDERS

The onset of presentation depends greatly on the etiology of diaphragmatic dysfunction. Unilateral diaphragmatic paralysis is generally asymptomatic. Exertional dyspnea is present when there is concomitant pulmonary parenchymal or airway disease. However, bilateral diaphragmatic paralysis presents severe exertional dyspnea and orthopnea. Poor-quality sleep and daytime fatigue are also frequent.

Physical examination will reveal rapid shallow breathing. There will be paradoxical abdominal wall retraction during inspiration. Percussion will suggest a raised diaphragm and reduced diaphragmatic excursion during inspiration. The intensity of breath sounds will be reduced on the affected side. The compressed lung may give rise to crackles on auscultation, just above the area of paralyzed diaphragm.

CAUSES

The causes of diaphragmatic disorders can be classified based on anatomical and neurological causes.

- *Anatomical*:
  - *Congenital*: Bochdalek hernia, Morgagni hernia, eventration of the diaphragm, and diaphragmatic agenesis
  - *Acquired*: Traumatic
- *Neurological*:
  - *Central nervous system*: Brainstem stroke
  - *Spinal cord*: Syringomyelia, anterior horn cell diseases, poliomyelitis, Arnold–Chiari malformation, tetanus, Strychnine poisoning
  - *Nerves*: Guillain–Barre syndrome, neuropathy due to a variety of causes, invasion of phrenic nerve by neoplasm (most common cause), damage to nerve by surgery or trauma, infectious neuritis [e.g., herpes zoster, poliomyelitis, severe acute respiratory syndrome coronavirus 2 (SARS-COV-2)]
  - *Muscles*: Myasthenia gravis, myopathy (muscular dystrophy, Duchenne muscular dystrophy, metabolic myopathy, connective tissue disorders [e.g., polymyositis, "shrinking lung syndrome" in systemic lupus erythematosus (SLE)], acid maltase deficiency

DIAGNOSIS

Chest Radiography

Posteroanterior radiographs show the dome of right hemidiaphragm to project into a plane ranging from the anterior end of the fifth rib to the sixth anterior interspace in about 95% of normal individuals.[3] In most people, the right hemidiaphragm projects half an interspace higher than the left, being at the same level as or lower than the left hemidiaphragm in only about 10%.[4] Diaphragmatic paralysis manifests as elevated hemidiaphragm. Linear atelectasis may be present at the lung bases. X-ray may also reveal a thoracic mass lesion, which is responsible for phrenic nerve paralysis or a congenital diaphragmatic hernia.

Fluoroscopy

Paradoxical upward movement of diaphragm by >2 cm on deep inspiratory effort against a closed airway ("sniff test") is suggestive of diaphragmatic paralysis.[5] However, in 6% of normal population, this can be found without any apparent reason. The cephalad movement of the paralyzed diaphragm during inspiration is accompanied by outward chest wall and inward abdominal wall motion, a phenomenon known as *thoracoabdominal paradox*.[6] Mediastinal swing found during respiration can be found in recent unilateral diaphragmatic palsy. In bilateral paralysis, sniff test may be misleading because the cephalad movement of ribs may produce a false appearance of downward movement of diaphragm. Also, recruitment of abdominal expiratory muscles can cause a false-negative sniff test result. **Figures 1A to H** show the movement of the diaphragm in normal, unilateral, and bilateral diaphragmatic palsy.

Ultrasonography

Ultrasound scanning has been found to be more reliable than fluoroscopy in evaluation of diaphragmatic movements.[7] It is widely available, is portable, allows visualization of structure above and below diaphragm, and can be done in uncooperative patients. Ultrasound allows the study of the muscular posterior and lateral aspects of diaphragm, while fluoroscopy visualizes only the anterior tendinous portion. Ultrasound measurements of thickness of diaphragm can be used to determine if a diaphragm is paralyzed.[8] A diaphragmatic thickness < 0.2 cm measured at end expiration is suggestive of atrophy. Although many views are described, the anterior subcostal view is the preferred view to study diaphragmatic excursions.

In a normal diaphragm, the muscle fibers shorten and thicken during inspiration. A paralyzed diaphragm does not contract during contraction, and this can be detected during

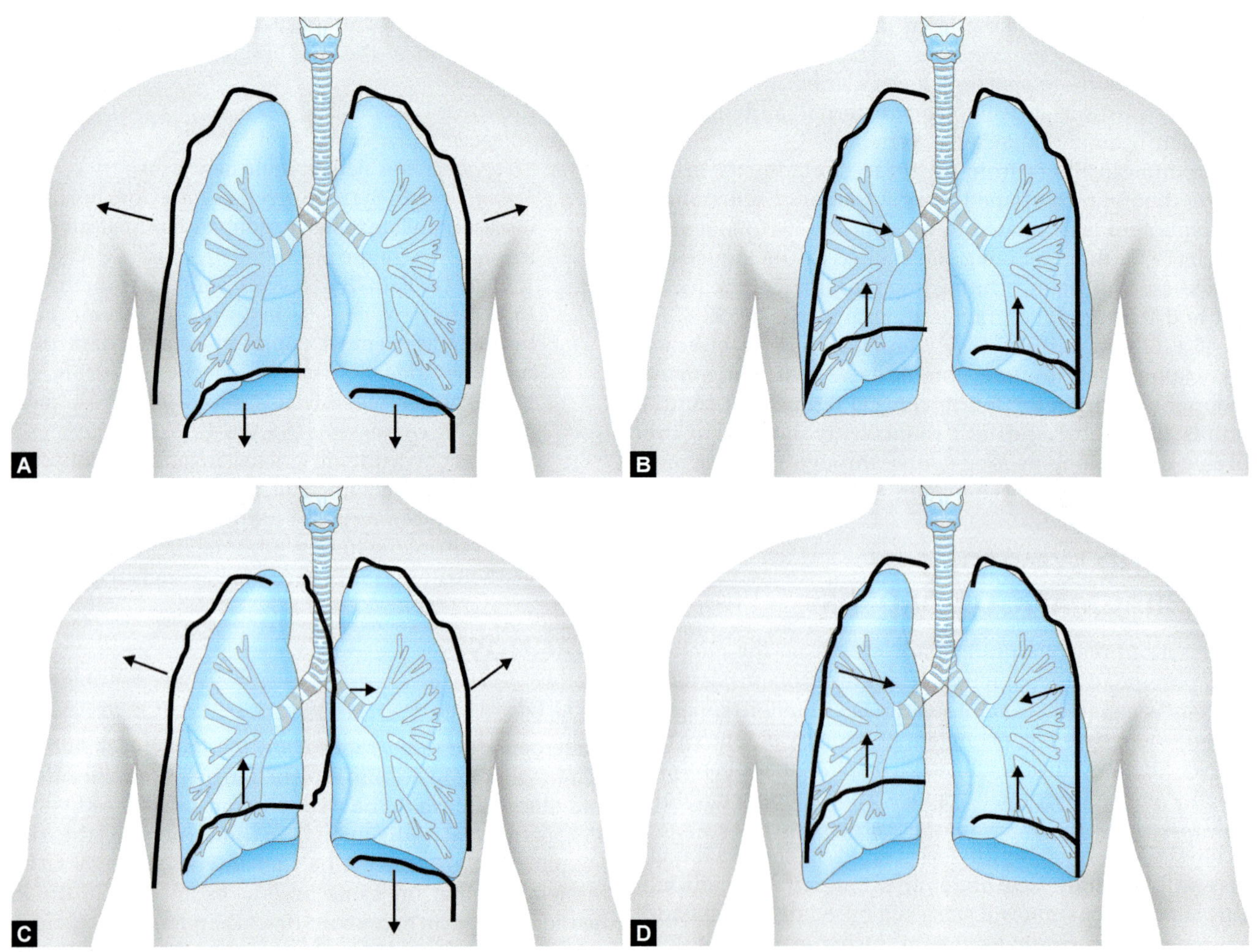

FIGS. 1A TO H: *Continued*

Continued

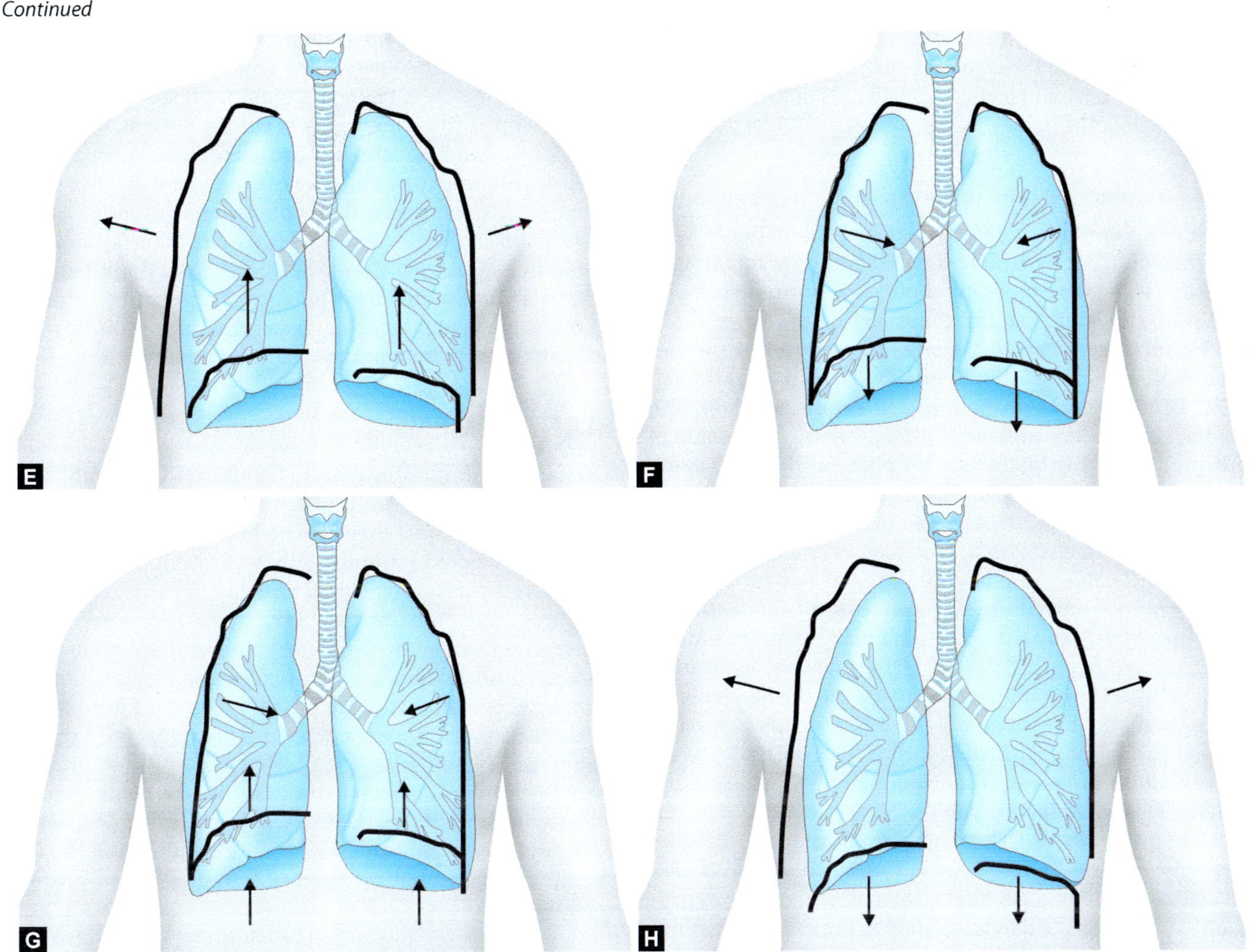

FIGS. 1A TO H: (A) Normal inspiration. Chest wall moves outward and diaphragm moves downward. (B) Normal expiration. Chest wall moves inward and diaphragm moves upward. (C) Right diaphragmatic palsy during inspiration: Paralyzed right diaphragm passively elevates in response to the more negative intrapleural pressure. The mediastinum shifts toward left. (D) Right diaphragmatic palsy during expiration: On full expiration, a rise in intra-abdominal pressure causes an even greater elevation. (E) Bilateral diaphragmatic palsy on inspiration: On inspiration, the increased negative intrapleural pressure "sucks" both the diaphragms up and draw the abdominal wall in. (F) Bilateral diaphragmatic palsy on expiration to functional residual capacity (FRC): Diaphragm descends and the abdomen protrudes. (G) Bilateral diaphragmatic palsy on expiration to right ventricle (RV): On deeper expiration, there is active contraction of abdominal muscles and the diaphragm rises. (H) Bilateral diaphragmatic palsy early inspiration to FRC: Abdominal muscles relax associated with descent of the flaccid diaphragm, creating the false impression of active contraction.

sonography. Diaphragmatic thickening of <20% is suggestive of paralysis. Diaphragmatic excursions can be measured during respiration and values >2.5 cm rule out diaphragmatic palsy. Similarly, lesser diaphragmatic excursion has been found to predict weaning failure after mechanical ventilation. CT scan is helpful to identify any mass lesion along the course of phrenic nerve causing the paralysis.

Ultrasound assessment has been found to be useful to evaluate co-existing neuromuscular respiratory weakness in chronic obstructive pulmonary disease (COPD).[9]

The thickness of diaphragm measured by ultrasonography may also help to study lung hyperinflation and loss of fat-free mass as indicators of COPD progression.[10]

Computerized Tomography Scan

Computerized tomography (CT) scan may reveal other mimics of raised diaphragm such as subpulmonic effusion or a mediastinal lesion which caused phrenic nerve paralysis. Diaphragmatic paralysis can result in atrophy of the crus of the diaphragm. One retrospective study showed that on coronal CT, crus thinning to ≤2.5 mm at the L1 vertebral level identified paralysis of the hemidiaphragm with a sensitivity of 100% and a specificity of 88% on the right and with a sensitivity of 100% and a specificity of 77% on the left.[11]

Pulmonary Function Tests

Restrictive ventilatory defects are seen in patients with diaphragmatic paralysis. In unilateral paralysis, forced vital capacity (FVC) is reduced to about 75% of predicted and total lung capacity (TLC) is about 85% of predicted.[12] Up to 10% decrease in VC in the supine position can present in normal individuals. In diaphragmatic weakness, the fall in VC is much more pronounced in supine position. The maximal inspiratory pressure (MIP) decreases to a value of 60% predicted.[13] In patients with bilateral diaphragmatic paralysis, FVC is reduced by 50% and TLC by 55%. The MIP is <60 cm H_2O. Rarely, the MIP can be near normal because of adequate compensation by the accessory muscles.

Low MIP values could be due to poor patient effort or poor technique, and hence quality control for testing is very important. Standards for testing for respiratory muscle strength have been published.[14] The maximal expiratory pressure (MEP) is usually normal but may be slightly reduced. An elevated MEP to MIP ratio (MEP/MIP) > 1.5 is suggestive of the diaphragmatic dysfunction.[15] A MEP/MIP of 1.5 had a sensitivity of 87% and a specificity of 45% for detecting unilateral diaphragmatic paralysis.

Hyperinflation in COPD can falsely reduce MIP due to diaphragmatic flattening resulting in mechanical disadvantage of the muscle fibers. In such situations, appropriate corrections need to be applied to the predicted values of MIP depending on the degree of hyperinflation. A MIP of less than one-third the predicted normal indicates a risk for hypercarbic respiratory failure. A MEP < 60 cm H_2O indicates weak cough reflex and risk for aspiration.

Electrophysiological Studies

Unilateral diaphragmatic paralysis can be diagnosed with confidence using combination of chest radiography, pulmonary function tests (PFTs), sniff test, and respiratory muscle strength testing. If the findings are equivocal, specific electrophysiological studies can be done. However, some of them are invasive and technically demanding.

Phrenic nerve conduction studies are useful in detecting neurological causes of paralysis. The phrenic nerve is stimulated at the level of the neck where it passes over the scalene muscle. Reduced amplitude and prolongation of phrenic nerve conduction may support neuropathy. Electromyograph of diaphragm studies help in the diagnosis of myopathic conditions involving the diaphragm. It is recorded with either esophageal or surface electrodes placed bilaterally below the lower ribs.

Transdiaphragmatic pressure measurements can accurately quantify the degree of diaphragmatic weakness by measuring the difference between intragastric and intrapleural pressure. This test is performed via the transnasal placement of two thin-walled balloon-tipped catheters. One is placed in the lower third of the esophagus above the diaphragm to assess changing pleural pressure; the second balloon is placed in the stomach. During normal inspiration, gastric pressure becomes more positive and esophageal pressure becomes more negative. In unilateral diaphragmatic paralysis, gastric pressure becomes more negative during inspiration, although to a lesser extent than the negative swing in esophageal pressure. In bilateral diaphragmatic paralysis, during tidal breathing, gastric pressure decreases to the same extent as esophageal pressure resulting in no active transdiaphragmatic pressure generation.[16]

MANAGEMENT

Treatment of diaphragmatic dysfunction depends on etiology. If patients with unilateral diaphragmatic paralysis had mild symptoms, they can be followed up periodically. Carefully selected patients with severe symptoms can be considered for surgical plication to prevent paradoxical diaphragmatic movement. Surgery is indicated in the management of anatomic defects in the diaphragm. Most patients with bilateral diaphragmatic paralysis ultimately develop progressive ventilatory failure resulting from fatigue of the accessory muscles. These patients usually require noninvasive ventilation (NIV). **Box 1** lists the indications for NIV in neuromuscular disease.[17,18] NIV helps in many ways to improve the patient's symptoms and gas exchange. NIV rests the respiratory muscles and help to reset the CO_2 sensitivity of the central chemoreceptors. It also reverses microatelectasis.

Other possible indications include repeated hospitalizations for respiratory failure and cor pulmonale. Phrenic nerve or diaphragmatic pacing is a useful treatment modality when the phrenic nerve is intact, and the problem lies in the actual transmission of nerve impulse.[19]

DISORDERS IN THE STRUCTURE OF DIAPHRAGM

Eventration of Diaphragm

Eventration is a condition in which all or part of the diaphragm is largely composed of fibrous tissue with only a few

BOX 1 Indications for noninvasive ventilation in neuromuscular disease.[17,18]

Symptoms (fatigue, dyspnea, morning headache, etc.)

And

One of the following physiological abnormalities:

- Daytime hypercapnia (arterial pCO_2 > 45)
- Nocturnal hypoventilation (O_2 sat < 88% for >5 consecutive minutes) or
- Forced vital capacity < 50% predicted or maximal inspiratory pressure < 60 cm H_2O

interspersed muscle fibers. It is usually congenital. Complete eventration mostly occurs on the left side and is characterized by elevation of left diaphragm. This hemidiaphragm may move paradoxically during "sniff test". The adult patients are usually asymptomatic, but occasionally they have dyspeptic symptoms. Dyspnea is common if eventration is associated with other lung diseases. In infants, eventration may occur on either side and can give rise to severe respiratory distress. Plication of the diaphragm is performed to keep the diaphragm in its normal position.[20]

Partial eventration occurs exclusively on the right side. It manifests as an anteromedial bulge of the diaphragm that moves downward during inspiration with normal portions of the hemidiaphragm, but with some delay.[21] There is usually an accessory lobe of liver, which occupies the bulge.[22]

Diaphragmatic Hernias

Hernias can occur at various sites of the diaphragm **(Fig. 2)**.

- *Hiatus hernia*: Herniation through the esophageal hiatus is the most common type of diaphragmatic hernia. It may predispose to gastroesophageal reflux disease and can appear as a retrocardiac opacity with a fluid level on chest radiograph **(Figs. 3A and B)**.

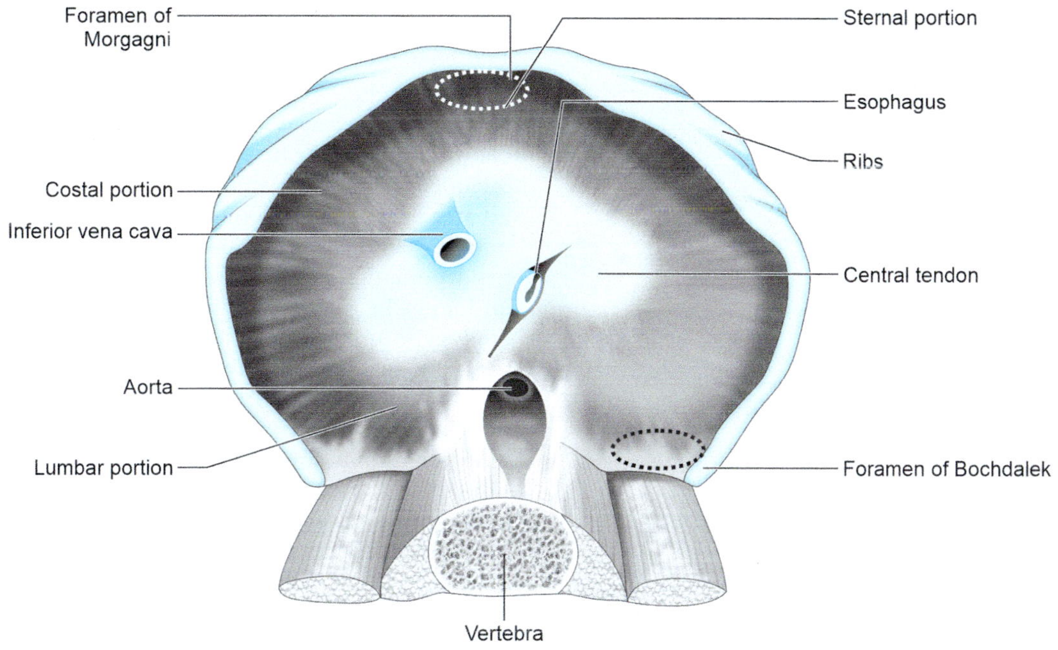

FIG. 2: Anatomy of diaphragm viewed from below.

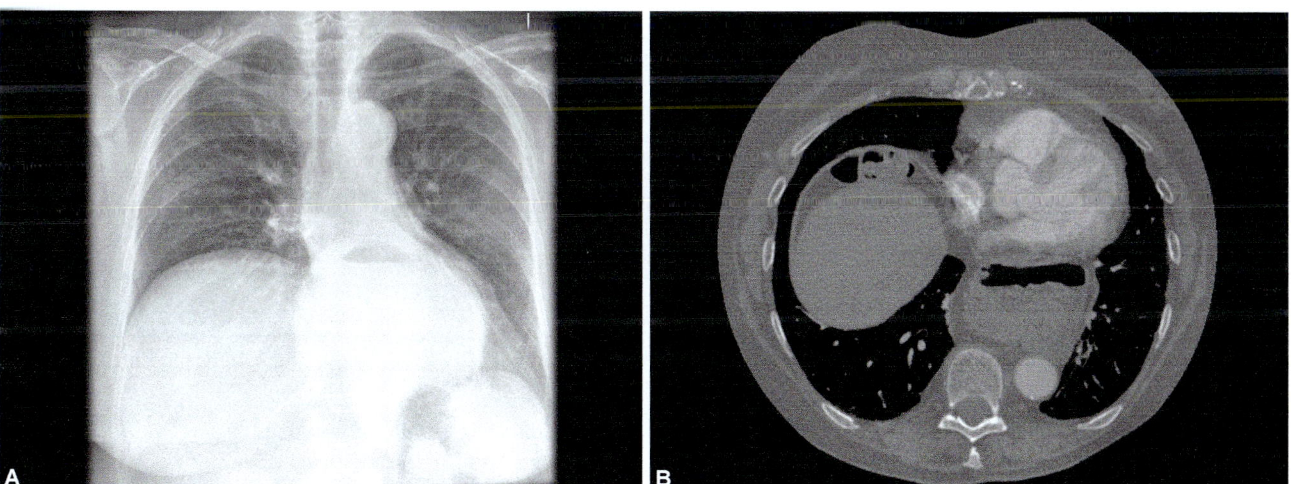

FIGS. 3A AND B: Hiatus hernia. (A) Chest radiograph showing retrocardiac fluid level; (B) CT scan of the same patient showing stomach in the posterior mediastinum.

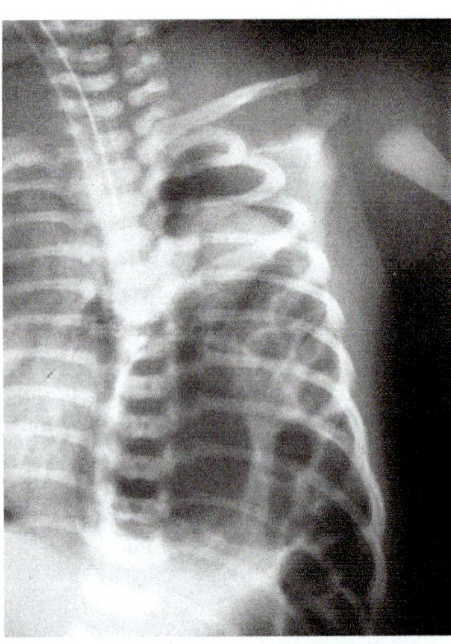

FIG. 4: Congenital diaphragmatic hernia. Absent diaphragm on the left side with presence of abdominal contents in the thorax.
Courtesy: Dr Pradeep A Wijayagoonawardana, www.radiopaedia.org, used with permission.

- *Bochdalek hernia*: The hernia is at the posterolateral part of the diaphragm and is the most common site for congenital diaphragmatic hernia.[23] The majority present immediately after birth with respiratory distress. The mortality rate is 45–50%. It is more common on the left side and may be associated with central nervous system anomalies and lung hypoplasia. X-ray reveals absence of diaphragm on the affected side and presence of abdominal contents in the thorax **(Fig. 4)**. Presentation in adulthood is uncommon.[24]
- *Morgagni hernia*: Foramen of Morgagni is present anteromedially and is usually filled with loose connective tissue, but abdominal contents may herniate through the foramen, more commonly on the right **(Fig. 2)**. Presentation in childhood is rare.[25] Chest X-ray shows as a rounded opacity in the cardiophrenic angle that may or may not contain gas.

Symptomatic diaphragmatic herniation is sometimes reported following open and minimally invasive surgery for the mediastinal structures, such as esophagectomy.[26]

Postpolio Syndrome

Postpolio syndrome (PPS) is a neurological disorder that produces a cluster of symptoms occurring in 22–64% of patients, 30–50 years after an attack of acute paralytic poliomyelitis.[27] The symptoms include progressive weakness, fatigue, and less commonly muscle atrophy, breathing, swallowing difficulties, and sleep disorders. The criteria for diagnosis of PPS include documentation of paralytic polio, partial recovery of function followed by a period of stabilization, and progressive neurologic deterioration.[28]

Respiratory insufficiency, which occurs in about 40%, is more common in those who had respiratory failure during the acute stage.[29] It results usually from respiratory muscle weakness with central hypoventilation and scoliosis contributing to it.[30] Risk factors, which contribute to PPS, include severe initial episode, older age at initial episode, greater recovery from the first episode, and overuse of muscles.[31] Initially, respiratory failure manifests as nocturnal hypoventilation and then it progresses. Electromyography and muscle biopsy show characteristic findings. The etiology is unknown, although premature exhaustion of the new sprouts that develop after acute poliomyelitis and of their motor neurons are important factors.[32] Other possible contributory factors include persistent poliovirus infection and an immune-mediated process. Treatment is primarily supportive and NIV when required. Nonfatiguing strengthening exercises can improve strength and provide short-term benefit.

TABLE 1: Syndromes of inappropriate respiratory muscle contraction.

Syndrome	Type of respiratory muscle involvement
Hiccups	Spasmodic contraction of diaphragm, other inspiratory muscles
Respiratory myoclonus (tic, flutter of diaphragm)	Spasmodic contraction of diaphragm
Respiratory dyskinesia	Abnormal asynchronous pattern of breathing associated with neurocirculatory asthenia
Convulsive disorders	Status epilepticus, tetanus, strychnine poisoning

Syndromes of Inappropriate Respiratory Muscle Contraction

These disorders share some common features like inappropriate timing, asynchronous activity, or excessive contraction of respiratory muscles **(Table 1)**.

Hiccups

Hiccups are produced by short, sharp contractions of the diaphragm and inspiratory intercostal muscles, coupled with transient closure to the glottis, which can occur 10–30 times per minute.[33]

Causes

Central nervous system: Multiple sclerosis, meningitis, encephalitis, cerebrovascular causes, brain tumor, postcranial surgery.

- *Metabolic*: Uremia, hyponatremia
- *Drugs*: Alcohol intoxication, dexamethasone
- *Nerve irritation (vagus or phrenic nerve)*: Herpes zoster infection, inflammatory or neoplastic lesions of the mediastinum

- *Gastrointestinal*: Esophageal irritation (neoplasm/stent/infection), stimulation of the diaphragm, stomach by heat, cold, spasm, dilation, and distention

The pathogenesis of hiccups is unclear but seems to be related to supraspinal mechanism and reflex arcs. Numerous treatments for hiccups have been described **(Table 2)**.[34,35] For those with persistent hiccup, pharmacological therapy should be tried.

Respiratory myoclonus (Leeuwenhoek's disease) is a rhythmic repetitive contraction of respiratory muscles, at a frequency of 30-300/min.[36] The pathogenesis is not clear, though some nervous system dysfunction at the level of the brain, spinal cord, or phrenic nerve has been postulated. It is associated with palatal myoclonus.

TABLE 2: Treatment of hiccups.

General measures	Drugs
Stimulate the throat: • Quickly swallow two heaped teaspoons of sugar, drink cold water or eat crushed ice, or rub with a clean cloth inside the top of the mouth • Rapid pharyngeal stimulation with a nasogastric tube *Interrupt normal breathing*: • Hold breath or breathe into paper bag Pull knees to chest and lean forward (compress the chest)	• The choice of drug should depend on the probable cause of hiccup • Metoclopramide • Haloperidol • Baclofen • Chlorpromazine • Anticonvulsants (carbamazepine, gabapentin) • Calcium channel blocker

SUMMARY

A variety of disorders can affect the functioning of diaphragm. A systematic evaluation is necessary to find out the cause and plan management. Noninvasive ventilation has an important role in managing those with respiratory failure due to bilateral diaphragmatic palsy.

REFERENCES

1. Lasser EC. Some aspects of pulmonary dynamics revealed by concurrent roentgen kymography of spirometric movements and diaphragmatic excursions. Radiology. 1961;77:434-44.
2. Houston JG, Morris AD, Howie CA, et al. Technical report: Quantitative assessment of diaphragmatic movement: A reproducible method using ultrasound. Clin Radiol. 1992;46:705-7.
3. Lennon EA, Simon G. The height of the diaphragm in the chest radiograph of normal adults. Br J Radiol. 1965;38:937-43.
4. Felson B. Chest Roentgenology. Philadelphia: WB Saunders; 1973.
5. Gierada DS, Slone RM, Fleishman MJ. Imaging evaluation of the diaphragm. Chest Surg Clin N Am. 1998;8:237-80.
6. Ch'en IY, Armstrong JD 2nd. Value of fluoroscopy in patients with suspected bilateral hemidiaphragmatic paralysis. AJR Am J Roentgenol. 1993;160:29-31.
7. Sarwal A, Walker FO, Cartwright MS. Neuromuscular ultrasound for evaluation of the diaphragm. Muscle Nerve. 2013;47(3):319-29.
8. Gottesman E, McCool FD. Ultrasound evaluation of the paralyzed diaphragm. Am J Respir Crit Care Med. 1997;155:1570-4.
9. Baria MR, Shahgho Li, Ghahfaroskhi LS, et al. B-mode ultrasound assessment of diaphragm structure and function in patients with COPD. Chest. 2014;146(3):680-5.
10. Smargiassi A, Inchingolo R, Tagliaboschi L, et al. Ultrasonographic assessment of the diaphragm in chronic obstructive pulmonary disease patients: relationships with pulmonary function and the influence of body composition—a pilot study. Respiration. 2014;87:364-71.
11. Sukkasem W, Moftah SG, Kicska G, et al. Crus atrophy: Accuracy of Computed Tomography in Diagnosis of Diaphragmatic Paralysis Thorac Imaging. 2017;32(6):383-90.
12. Easton PA, Fleetham JA, de la Rocha A, et al. Respiratory function after paralysis of the right hemidiaphragm. Am Rev Respir Dis. 1983;127:125-8.
13. Gibson GJ. Diaphragmatic paresis: pathophysiology, clinical features, and investigation. Thorax. 1989;44:960-70.
14. American Thoracic Society/European Respiratory Society. ATS/ERS Statement on respiratory muscle testing. Am J Respir Crit Care Med. 2002;166(4):518-624.
15. Koo P, Oyieng'o DO, Gartman EJ, et al. The Maximal Expiratory-to-Inspiratory Pressure Ratio and Supine Vital Capacity as Screening Tests for Diaphragm Dysfunction. Lung. 2017;195(1):29-35.
16. Davis J, Goldman M, Loh L, et al. Diaphragm function and alveolar hypoventilation. Q J Med. 1976;45:87-100.
17. Hill NS. Ventilator Management for Neuromuscular Disease. Semin Respir Crit Care Med. 2002;23(3).293-305.
18. Consensus Conference. Clinical indications for noninvasive positive pressure ventilation in chronic respiratory failure due to restrictive lung disease, COPD, and nocturnal hypoventilation—a Consensus conference report. Chest. 1999;116:521-34.
19. DiMarco AF, Onders RP, Kowalski KE, et al. Phrenic nerve pacing in a tetraplegic patient via intramuscular diaphragm electrodes. Am J Respir Crit Care Med. 2002;166:1604-6
20. Tiryaki T, Livanelioglu Z, Atayurt H. Eventration of the diaphragm. Asian J Surg. 2006;29:8-10.
21. Larson RK, Evans BH. Eventration of the diaphragm. Am Rev Respir Dis. 1963;87:753.
22. Spencer RP, Spackman TJ, Pearson HA. Diagnosis of right diaphragmatic eventration by means of liver scan. Radiology. 1971;99:375-6.
23. Bock HB, Zimmennann JH. Study of selected congenital abnormalities in Pennsylvania. US Public Health Rep. 1967;82:446-50.
24. Ahrend RT, Thomson BW. Hernia of the foramen of Bochdalek in the adult. Am J Surg. 1971;122:612-5.
25. Cohen MD. Intermittent cyanotic attacks in an infant: an unusual presentation of a congenital anterior diaphragmatic (Morgagni) hernia. Br J Radiol. 1981;54:260-1.

26. Messenger DE, Higgs SM, Dwerryhouse SJ, et al. Symptomatic diaphragmatic herniation following open and minimally invasive oesophagectomy: experience from a UK specialist unit. Surg Endosc. 2015;29(2):417-24.
27. Windebank AJ, Litchy WJ, Daube JR, et al. Late effects of paralytic poliomyelitis in Olmsted County, Minnesota. Neurology. 1991; 41:501-7.
28. Mulder DW, Rosenbaum RA, Layton DD. Late progression of poliomyelitis or forme fruste amyotrophic lateral sclerosis? Mayo Clin Proc. 1972;47:756-61.
29. Jubelt B, Drucker J. Post-polio syndrome: an update. Semin Neurol. 1993;13(3):283-90.
30. Bach JR, Alba AS, Bohatiuk G, et al. Mouth intermittent positive pressure ventilation in the management of postpolio respiratory insufficiency. Chest. 1987;91:859-64.
31. Klingman J, Chui H, Corgiat M, et al. Functional recovery: a major risk factor for the development of postpoliomyelitis muscular atrophy. Arch Neurol. 1988;45:645-7.
32. Jubelt B, Drucker J. Poliomyelitis and the post-polio syndrome. In: Younger DS (Ed). Motor Disorders. Philadelphia: Lippincott Williams & Wilkins; 1999.
33. Lewis JH. Hiccups: Causes and cures. J Clin Gastroenterol. 1985; 7:539-52.
34. Engleman EG, Lankton J, Lankton B. Granulated sugar as treatment for hiccups in conscious patients (letter). N Engl J Med. 1971;285:1489.
35. Salem RM, Baraka A, Rattenborg CC, et al. Treatment of hiccups by pharyngeal stimulation in anesthetized and conscious subjects. JAMA. 1967;202:126-30.
36. Phillips JR, Eldridge FL. Respiratory myoclonus (Leeuwenhoek's disease). N Engl J Med. 1973;289:1390-5.

SECTION

14

Systematic Diseases and Pregnancy

SECTION OUTLINE

CHAPTER 137

Rare Lung Diseases

Sanjeev Mehta, Bineet Ahluwalia

INTRODUCTION

A rare disease is difficult to define in strict epidemiological terms. For clinical purposes, it is usually a chronic disease of such low prevalence that the diagnosis is frequently missed, and special combined efforts and investigations are needed to address the diagnosis. Some such important pulmonary syndromes are discussed in the following text.

PULMONARY ALVEOLAR PHOSPHOPROTEINOSIS

Introduction

Pulmonary alveolar proteinosis (PAP) is a rare, idiopathic, diffuse lung disease, characterized by accumulation of large amounts of surfactant within the alveolar spaces. Only 2% of the intra-alveolar content is protein; the rest is constituted by dipalmitoyl lecithin. Hence, pulmonary alveolar phospholipoproteinosis is considered a more appropriate term for this condition.

Epidemiology

First described by Rosen et al. in 1958, PAP is characterized by bilateral diffuse pulmonary infiltrates and varying degrees of hypoxemia.[1] The epidemiological data is scarce and variable due to underestimation of the disease owing to its rarity. A US retrospective study attributed the annual prevalence of PAP to be 6.87 ± 0.33 per million.[2]

Pulmonary alveolar proteinosis is more commonly seen in men (male:female ratio 2:1). Although knowledge on a causal relationship between tobacco use and environmental dust is lacking, it is reported higher among smokers and individuals with significant dust exposure, which may explain the gender predisposition.[3,4] A bimodal age distribution is seen with the first and second peaks reported in fourth and seventh decades, respectively.[2]

Pathophysiology and Clinical Classification

Pulmonary alveolar proteinosis is considered a common phenotypic response to a number of biochemical or molecular abnormalities, resulting in altered surfactant homeostasis, i.e., excessive production and/or reduced clearance of surfactant by defective function of the alveolar macrophage and the growth factor necessary for its maturation, the granulocyte macrophage-colony stimulating factor (GM-CSF), leading to intra-alveolar accumulation of surfactant protein. Production of antibodies against GM-CSF or GM-CSF receptor gene mutations (*CSF2RA*, *CSF2RB*) are responsible for 90–95% of causes of PAP, labeled as primary PAP.[5] Secondary PAP (5–10%) develops in conditions involving functional impairment or reduced numbers of alveolar macrophages.[3] These are being increasingly recognized, and PAP-like pathology is noted in several conditions **(Box 1)**. Rarely, secondary PAP has been described following exogenous exposure to dust or in association with Hermansky–Pudlak syndrome.[6,7] An interesting association has been described with squamous cell lung carcinoma wherein PAP increased with development of lung cancer and disappeared after resection of the tumor.[8] Congenital PAP contributes to <1% of

BOX 1 Causes of secondary pulmonary alveolar proteinosis.

- Hematological conditions (myeloid leukemias, neutropenia, lymphomas, Fanconi's anemia, plasma cell disorders)
- Infections (atypical mycobacteria, *Pneumocystis jirovecii* pneumonia, HIV, mycoses, SARS-CoV-2)
- Drug induced (chlorambucil, busulfan, imatinib, mycophenolate)
- Immunosuppression (status post hematopoietic stem-cell transplantation, bone marrow transplantation)
- Toxic dust inhalation (volcanic ash, aluminum dust, titanium, silica dust)

the cases, attributed to abnormal surfactant production due to mutations in surfactant synthesis genes (*SFTPA, SFTPB, SFTPC, ABCA3, TTF1*).[9]

Diagnosis

Clinical Features

The disease involves only the lungs. Clinically, nearly one-third are asymptomatic or minimally symptomatic.[10] Most patients with acquired PAP present with progressive exertional dyspnea of insidious onset and cough. Less frequently, fever, chest pain or hemoptysis occurs, especially if secondary infection is present.[4]

In some patients, PAP may begin with an initial febrile episode, followed later by progressive dyspnea, productive cough, low-grade fever, chest pain, and loss of weight. Cough is minimally productive with gelatinous white "chunky" expectoration. Physical examination may be unremarkable, but crackles are present in about 50%, cyanosis in 25%, and clubbing in a smaller number of patients.[4]

Radiology

The extent of radiographic abnormalities is often disproportionate to the severity of the symptoms and physical findings. The chest X-ray **(Fig. 1)** reveals bilateral airspace infiltrates with ill-defined acinar nodules, ground-glass opacification or confluent pattern, more dense in the lower lobes. The classic perihilar "batwing" or "reverse pulmonary edema" pattern is seen in about 50% cases.[11] Air bronchograms are not a predominant feature. As the disease progresses, the alveolar infiltrates become denser. High-resolution computed tomography (HRCT) scan of the chest reflects the alveolar filling process as patchy airspace consolidation (ground-glass opacity) with thickened interlobular septae, which are predominantly perihilar, with relative sparing of the peripheral lung. Accentuation of the interlobular septa is usually caused by presence of the proteinaceous material in the septal interstitium. There is a sharp transition between the normal and the abnormal lung, described as "crazy paving" appearance, that is characteristic but not specific for PAP **(Box 2)**.[12]

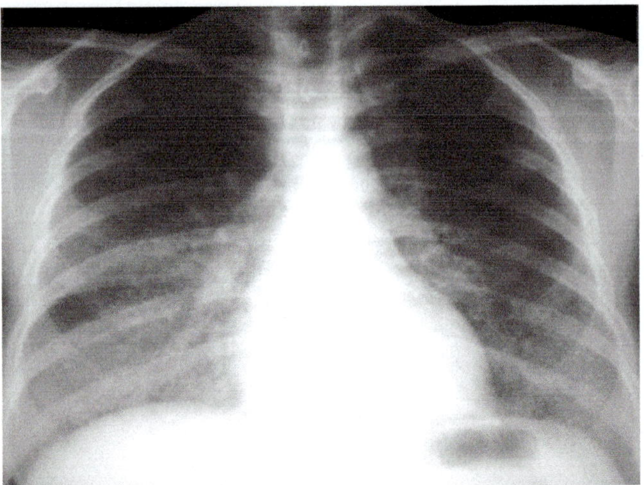

FIG. 1: Chest roentgenograph of pulmonary alveolar proteinosis (PAP) showing bilateral air space infiltrates, acinar nodules and ground-glass opacification.

Laboratory Tests

Routine laboratory tests are generally unremarkable. There may be mild leukocytosis. Elevated serum lactate dehydrogenase (LDH) is a useful marker but has limited specificity.[3,4] Primary PAP patients have shown antibodies to GM-CSF in both serum and bronchoalveolar lavage (BAL) fluid; however, it has limited availability at various centers.[4,13] Elevated serum levels of carcinoembryonic antigen, cytokeratin 19, mucin KL-6, and surfactant proteins A, B and D have been reported but of unclear value.

Pulmonary function tests usually reveal a restrictive ventilatory defect, with reduced lung volumes and a disproportionate reduction in diffusing capacity of carbon monoxide (DLCO). Hypoxemia caused by ventilation-perfusion inequality and intrapulmonary shunting is common, resulting in a widened alveolar-arteriolar diffusion gradient.[4]

Bronchoscopy and Histopathology

Open lung biopsy has been the gold standard for diagnosis, but bronchoscopic lung biopsy generally suffices. Aspiration of opaque, milky or sandy, light-brown fluid from an affected segment during BAL is characteristic. The cellular component of PAP in the BAL fluid consists predominantly of enlarged, foamy macrophages with numerous complex phospholipoprotein inclusions. Under light microscopy, the BAL fluid stains deep pink with periodic acid Schiff (PAS) stain and negative with alcian blue stain, which allows the differentiation of the phospholipoprotein aggregates from mucins.[3,14] The alveolar architecture is well preserved in the "primary" form of PAP **(Fig. 2)**. In secondary PAP, septal thickening, edema, and lymphocytic and neutrophilic infiltration can be seen **(Fig. 3)**.

BOX 2 **Conditions having "crazy paving" appearance on high-resolution CT (HRCT) scan of chest.**

- Pulmonary alveolar proteinosis
- Acute respiratory distress syndrome
- Cardiogenic pulmonary edema
- Infections (Pneumocystis pneumonia)
- Diffuse alveolar hemorrhage
- Bronchoalveolar carcinoma
- Lymphangitic carcinomatosis
- Radiation- or drug-induced lung injury

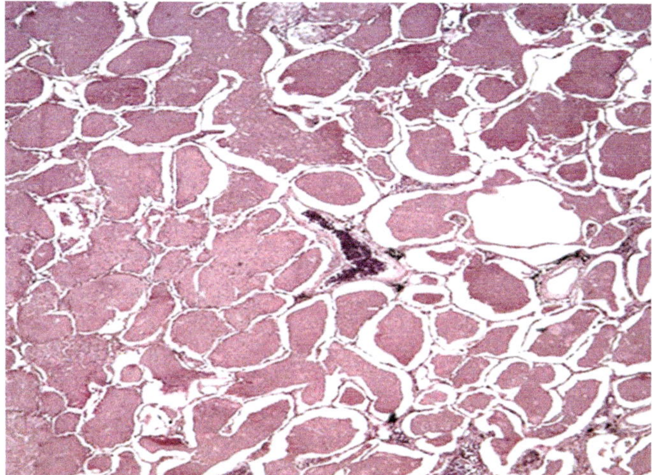

FIG. 2: Alveolar eosinophilic material filling the alveolar lumina with preserved architecture in primary alveolar proteinosis.

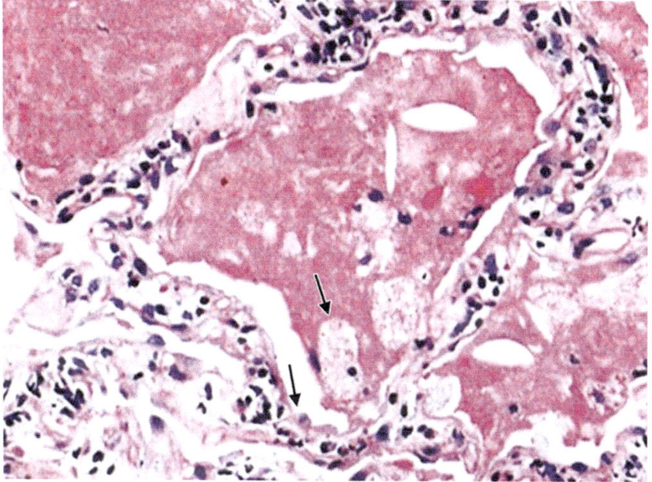

FIG. 3: Secondary pulmonary alveolar proteinosis (PAP): Septal thickening, edema and inflammatory infiltration of alveoli.

Treatment

Treatment decision essentially depends on the severity of the disease. There is no validated criterion to assess the clinical severity of the disease; the therapeutic decisions thus depend on combined subjective and objective assessment of symptom severity, pulmonary function tests, radiology, and worsening hypoxemia as assessed by the arterial blood gas level.

Whole lung lavage remains the mainstay of therapy for primary and secondary PAP. Done under general anesthesia, this invasive procedure lavages one lung at a time with selective ventilation of the other lung using a double-lumen endotracheal tube. Serial aliquots of warmed normal saline are used, often followed by chest physiotherapy and retrieval of the lavaged saline in an external fluid collector. On average, 12–15 L of normal saline is used per lung. The interval between the lavage of the two lungs varies among centers. Evidence from China and France suggests a relapse rate of 30–56% following the procedure. Procedural-related morbidities include fever, worsened hypoxemia, spillage of lavage fluid in the opposite lung, superinfections, and pneumothorax.[15]

Whole lung lavage does not alter the underlying pathogenetic mechanisms revolving around defective GM-CSF signaling. Hence, the role of exogenous administration of recombinant human GM-CSF (rhGM-CSF) has been assessed. The available literature is scarce, limited by some case series and few prospective trials albeit on a small sample population. A recent meta-analysis favored its use in autoimmune PAP. Inhaled treatment was deemed better than subcutaneously administered rhGM-CSF due to a higher response rate [better PaO_2 and $P(A\text{-}a)O_2$ values].

Steroids have not shown to be beneficial. Strategies targeting autoimmunity-like plasmapheresis and rituximab have limited evidence supporting their use.[16]

Treatment of infection and supportive care, such as the use of oxygen, should be administered as appropriate. Lung transplantation is rarely indicated for an advanced disease. Treatment of the underlying cause should be undertaken, wherever possible. Aggressive attempts should be made at cessation of smoking.

Progress and Complications

Progressive respiratory failure occurs from disease persistence. Interstitial fibrosis develops in chronic cases. Infections with unusual organisms, such as *Nocardia* species, *Aspergillus* species, *Mycobacteria*, *Pneumocystis*, *Cryptococcus neoformans*, and other organisms, are known to occur.

PULMONARY CALCIFICATION AND OSSIFICATION SYNDROMES

Pulmonary calcification commonly seen on chest X-ray is usually an incidental finding. It may be metastatic, benign or malignant, or dystrophic in origin. The list of causes is rather exhaustive.[17] Frequency-wise, the dystrophic causes of infectious etiology are more common **(Box 3)**. The condition depends on abnormalities in serum calcium and phosphate concentration, alkaline phosphatase activity, and local physicochemical conditions, such as pH. It is most common after about 10 years of hemodialysis.

Pathophysiology

Metastatic calcification is usually seen at an elevated calcium-phosphate product of 70 mg^2/dL^2 (normal < 40). When it occurs at normal or even at low serum calcium, it may be attributed to azotemia (previous or current), elevated parathyroid hormone levels, and/or exogenous vitamin D administration.

BOX 3 Causes of pulmonary calcification.

- *Dystrophic calcification*:
  - Tuberculosis
  - Sarcoidosis
  - Histoplasmosis and other fungal infections
  - Postvaricella pneumonia
  - Smallpox handler's lung
  - Parasitic infections: Paragonimiasis
  - Amyloidosis
  - Silicosis
  - Coal worker's pneumoconiosis
  - Pulmonary vascular calcification
  - Idiopathic: Pulmonary alveolar microlithiasis
- *Metastatic:*
  - Chronic renal insufficiency on hemodialysis
  - Primary hyperparathyroidism
  - Hypervitaminosis D
  - Excess exogenous administration of calcium and vitamin D (milk-alkali syndrome)
  - Osteopetrosis
  - Osteitis deformans (Paget's disease)
  - Malignant causes: Parathyroid carcinoma, multiple myeloma, lymphoma/ leukemia, choriocarcinoma

BOX 4 Causes of pulmonary ossification.

- *Pre-existing pulmonary disorder:*
  - Tuberculosis
  - Sarcoidosis
  - Pulmonary amyloidosis
  - Idiopathic pulmonary fibrosis
  - Metastatic breast cancer
  - Histoplasmosis
  - Chronic busulfan therapy
  - Pulmonary metastases of osteogenic sarcoma
  - Metastatic melanoma
- *Other systemic causes*:
  - Primary and secondary hyperparathyroidism
  - Hypervitaminosis D
  - Mitral stenosis
  - Chronic left ventricular failure
  - Pyloric stenosis with alkalosis
  - Idiopathic hypertrophic subaortic stenosis
- Idiopathic pulmonary ossification

Calcium salts get precipitated in an alkaline environment. Blood pH in the lung is more alkalotic than in other organs because of the CO_2 removal. The upper lobe predilection of some pulmonary calcific disorders may occur due to a higher blood pH (approximately 7.51) and lower $PaCO_2$ (approximately 30 mm Hg) at the apex due to the higher ventilation-perfusion (V/Q) ratio (about 3.3 vs. 0.63, respectively). Hypercalcemia and alkalosis most likely act synergistically to predispose to ectopic calcification, when other risk factors are present.

Dystrophic calcification occurs with normal serum calcium levels in the injured or the abnormal tissues. It is typically seen in granulomas and in lymphadenopathy associated with fungal diseases, tuberculosis, and sarcoidosis. It has also been described in amyloidosis and after inhalation exposures in coal workers pneumoconiosis and silicosis. Injury results in caseation, necrosis, or fibrosis. The calcification is most likely due to the production of 1, 25-vitamin D in the macrophages within the granulomas and increased intestinal absorption of calcium and phosphate, which provides an additive or a synergistic factor that promotes calcification in these tissues.

Sarcoidosis-related calcification could be dystrophic or metastatic, secondary to hypercalcemia or both. It may sometimes mimic pulmonary alveolar microlithiasis (PAM) with a calcified micronodular pattern. Pulmonary vascular calcification (PVC) is dystrophic due to shear stress. PAM is a unique idiopathic calcific disorder with distinct histologic and radiographic features that do not fit into either metastatic or dystrophic calcification.[18,19]

Pulmonary ossification is more complex attributable to various mechanisms, such as angiogenesis, chronic venous congestion, lung fibrosis, and/or the influence of various growth factors. It can be idiopathic in origin or result from a variety of underlying pulmonary, cardiac, or extracardiac pulmonary disorders **(Box 4)**. Pulmonary metastatic malignant lesions can become calcified or ossified.

PULMONARY ALVEOLAR MICROLITHIASIS

Introduction

Pulmonary alveolar microlithiasis is a rare disorder, characterized by bilateral intra-alveolar deposition of minute calcific concretions uniformly throughout the lungs. First reported in 1918 as occurrence of extensive calcification of the lungs, the condition was labeled as pulmonary alveolar microlithiasis in 1933.[20,21]

Etiopathology

Pulmonary alveolar microlithiasis is caused by mutation in *SLC34A2* gene resulting in a defective sodium phosphate-2b transporter protein which is involved in regulating phosphate uptake by type II alveolar cells. Insufficient alveolar phosphate uptake leads to luminal accumulation of phosphate which precipitates with calcium in extracellular fluid to form intra-alveolar calcium-phosphate stones.[22,23]

Diagnosis

The cases have been reported in the age group of 20–30 years, with a female predilection. A familial incidence has been observed with a tendency to appear in siblings.[24,25]

Clinical Features

Although the condition presents with an abnormal chest radiograph in an asymptomatic patient, the advanced cases may present with cough, dyspnea, and respiratory failure. Hemoptysis may occasionally occur, and very rarely calcified bodies may be coughed.[26] Physical examination of the chest often does not reveal any abnormality. In advanced stages, the disease may show the presence of inspiratory crackles and ultimately the signs of cor pulmonale. Extrapulmonary calcification of pericardium, aortic valves, testicles, nephrocalcinosis, and nephrolithiasis has been reported.[27]

Radiology

The chest radiograph gives widespread snowstorm appearance from minute calcified mottled shadows (also known as "sandstorm appearance"). The dense, diffusely distributed microliths may conglomerate to make the lung appear diffusely white, especially in mid and lower lung zones obscuring the cardiac borders **(Fig. 4A)**. A subpleural strip of hyperlucency between the pleura and dense calcified lung parenchyma gives the "black pleura" sign.[28] The radiological appearance of stenosis, talc granulomatosis, and calcified miliary histoplasmosis may simulate microlithiasis, but the lesions in those conditions are larger and have different distribution.

Computed tomography demonstrates extensive microcalcific deposits in the posterior and inferior subpleural spaces and along bronchovascular bundles, interstitial fibrosis, and bronchiectasis. Calcified nodules > 1 mm (up to 5 mm) are visible on HRCT scans **(Fig. 4B)**.

Histopathology

The lungs appear solid containing sand-like grains, i.e., multiple intra-alveolar spherical calcium and phosphate deposits (known as calcospherite or microlith). Under a microscope, the microliths, containing hydroxyapatite crystals, form concentric lamellae appearing as "onion-skin" bodies in the alveoli. Usually 1 mm in size, microliths up to 5 mm have been reported. Biopsy findings of inflammation, fibrosis, and calcification of the lung interstitium and pleura have also been reported.[29,30]

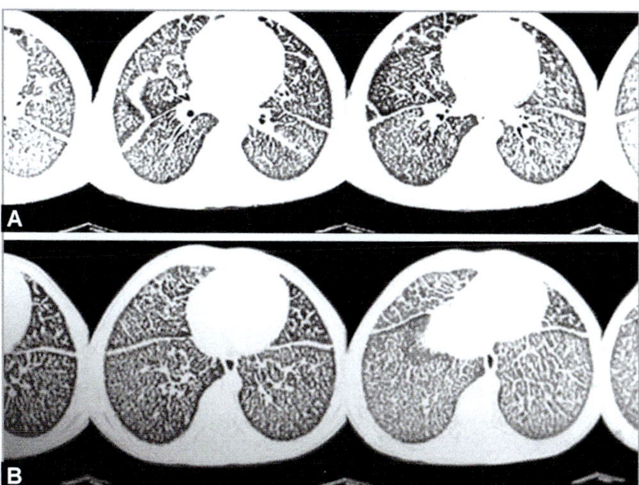

FIGS. 4A AND B: Chest CT scan in pulmonary alveolar microlithiasis, showing bilateral, diffuse, distinct micronodular, sand-like mottling of lungs giving the appearance of a white lung. *Courtesy*: Dr Sanjeev Mehta.

Lung Function Tests

Lung function tests are normal initially. A restrictive lung defect is seen in advanced cases with reduced lung volumes and diffusion capacity.[31]

Treatment

Therapeutic strategies with corticosteroids, sodium etidronate, and whole lung lavage have been proven to be ineffective.[32-34] PAM has a variable clinical course with studies suggesting a slowly progressive disease course in some while being stable in others. Treatment is mainly supportive (oxygen therapy, vaccination, smoking cessation, etc.).[35] Lung transplant may prove to be a favorable alternative with studies suggesting no recurrence of the disease in recipients.[36]

SUMMARY

Rare lung diseases are often missed owing to their low prevalence. It is imperative for clinicians to be aware of these uncommon diseases often presenting with common symptoms. Diagnosis can be challenging due to the universal unavailability or costs of the tests. Histopathology holds the gold standard for diagnosis, though it is not always feasible. Thus, a thorough clinical evaluation in conjunction with imaging patterns and laboratory tests help clinch the diagnosis.

REFERENCES

1. Rosen SH, Castleman B, Liebow AA, et al. Pulmonary alveolar proteinosis. New England J Med. 1958;258(23):1123-42.
2. McCarthy C, Avetisyan R, Carey BC, et al. Prevalence and healthcare burden of pulmonary alveolar proteinosis. Orphanet J Rare Dis. 2018;13(1):1-5.
3. Seymour JF, Presneill JJ. Pulmonary alveolar proteinosis: progress in the first 44 years. Am J Respir Crit Care Med. 2002;166(2):215-35.
4. Inoue Y, Trapnell BC, Tazawa R, et al. Characteristics of a large cohort of patients with autoimmune pulmonary alveolar proteinosis in Japan. Am J Respir Crit Care Med. 2008;177(7):752-62.
5. Tanaka N, Watanabe J, Kitamura T, et al. Lungs of patients with idiopathic pulmonary alveolar proteinosis express a factor which neutralizes granulocyte-macrophage colony stimulating factor. FEBS Lett. 1999;442(2-3):246-50.
6. Hisata S, Moriyama H, Tazawa R, et al. Development of pulmonary alveolar proteinosis following exposure to dust after the Great East Japan Earthquake. Respir Investig. 2013;51(4):212-6.
7. Ozyilmaz E, Gunasti S, Kuyuku Y, et al. Hermansky Pudlak syndrome and pulmonary alveolar proteinosis at the same patient: first case report in the world literature. Sarcoidosis Vasc Diffuse Lung Dis. 2013;30(3):217-20.
8. Liu H, Wang Y, He W, et al. Lung squamous cell carcinoma in pulmonary alveolar proteinosis. Ann Thorac Cardiovasc Surg. 2014;20(Suppl):650-3.
9. Nogee LM. Genetic mechanisms of surfactant deficiency. Neonatology. 2004;85(4):314-8.
10. Shah PL, Hansell D, Lawson PR, et al. Pulmonary alveolar proteinosis: clinical aspects and current concepts on pathogenesis. Thorax. 2000;55(1):67-77.
11. Swensen SJ, Aughenbaugh GL, Douglas WW, et al. High-resolution CT of the lungs. AJR Am J Roentgenol. 2001;158(5):971-9.
12. Mehrian P, Homayounfar N, Karimi MA, et al. Features of idiopathic pulmonary alveolar proteinosis in high resolution computed tomography. Polish J Radiol. 2014;79:65.
13. Lin FC, Chang GD, Chern MS, et al. Clinical significance of anti-GM-CSF antibodies in idiopathic pulmonary alveolar proteinosis. Thorax. 2006;61(6):528-34.
14. Burkhalter A, Silverman JF, Hopkins III MB, et al. Bronchoalveolar lavage cytology in pulmonary alveolar proteinosis. Am J Clin Pathol. 1996;106(4):504-10.
15. Kumar A, Abdelmalak B, Inoue Y, et al. Pulmonary alveolar proteinosis in adults: pathophysiology and clinical approach. Lancet Respir Med. 2018;6(7):554-65.
16. Sheng G, Chen P, Wei Y, et al. Better approach for autoimmune pulmonary alveolar proteinosis treatment: inhaled or subcutaneous granulocyte-macrophage colony-stimulating factor: a meta-analysis. Respir Res. 2018;19(1):1-1.
17. Chan ED, Morales DV, Welsh CH, et al. Calcium deposition with or without bone formation in the lung. Am J Respir Crit Care Med. 2002;165(12):1654-69.
18. Mariotta S, Guidi L, Papale M, et al. Pulmonary alveolar microlithiasis: review of Italian reports. Eur J Epidemiol. 1997;13:587-90.
19. Prakash UBS. Pulmonary alveolar microlithiasis. Semin Respir Crit Care Med. 2002;23:103-13.
20. Harbitz F. Extensive calcification of the lungs as a distinct disease. Arch Int Med. 1918;21(1):139-46.
21. Puhr I. Microlithiasis alveolaris pulmonum. Virchows Arch A Patho. Anat Histopathol. 1933;290:156.
22. Corut A, Senyigit A, Ugur SA, et al. Mutations in SLC34A2 cause pulmonary alveolar microlithiasis and are possibly associated with testicular microlithiasis. Am J Hum Genet. 2006;79(4): 650-6.
23. Traebert M, Hattenhauer O, Murer H, et al. Expression of type II Na-pi cotransporter in alveolar type II cells. Am J Physiol. 1999;277(5):L868-73.
24. Sosman MC, Dodd GD, Jones WD, et al. The familial occurrence of pulmonary alveolar microlithiasis. Am J Roentgenol. 1957;77:947.
25. Mitra S, Ghoshal AG. A family of pulmonary alveolar microlithiasis. Lung India. 2000;18:87-100.
26. Thind GS, Bhatia JL. Pulmonary alveolar microlithiasis. Br J of Dis Chest. 1978;72:151-4.
27. Jönsson ÅL, Hilberg O, Bendstrup EM, et al. SLC34A2 gene mutation may explain comorbidity of pulmonary alveolar microlithiasis and aortic valve sclerosis. Am J Respir Crit Care Med. 2012;185(4):464.
28. Alkhankan E, Yamin H, Bukamur H, et al. Pulmonary alveolar microlithiasis diagnosed with radiography, CT, and bone scintigraphy. Radiology Case Rep. 2019;14(6):775-7.
29. Hira HS, Singh T, Chowdhary V. Pulmonary alveolar microlithiasis: role of transbronchial lung biopsy. J Assoc Phys India. 2000;48(8):832-3.
30. Khan KA, Gilmartin JJ. Bilateral micronodular pulmonary infiltrate: is it important to make a histological diagnosis? Respir Care. 2013;58(7):e69-71.
31. Jönsson ÅL, Simonsen U, Hilberg O, et al. Pulmonary alveolar microlithiasis: two case reports and review of the literature. Eur Respir Rev. 2012;21(125):249-56.
32. Tachibana T, Hagiwara K, Johkoh T. Pulmonary alveolar microlithiasis: review and management. Curr Opin Pulm Med. 2009;15(5):486-90.
33. Ozcelik U, Yalcin E, Arıyurek M, et al. Long-term results of disodium etidronate treatment in pulmonary alveolar microlithiasis. Pediatr Pulmonol. 2010;45(5):514-7.
34. Pracyk JB, Simonson SG, Young SL, et al. Composition of lung lavage in pulmonary alveolar microlithiasis. Respiration. 1996;63(4):254-60.
35. Enemark A, Jönsson ÅLM, Bendstrup E, et al. Pulmonary alveolar microlithiasis – a review. Yale J Biol Med. 2021;94:637-44.
36. Alrossais NM, Alshammari AM, Alrayes AM, et al. Pulmonary hypertension and polycythemia secondary to pulmonary alveolar microlithiasis treated with sequential bilateral lung transplant: a case study and literature review. Am J Case Rep. 2019;20:1114.

Diabetes Mellitus and Respiratory Disease

CHAPTER 138

Rajneesh Mittal

INTRODUCTION

Diabetes mellitus (DM) and respiratory diseases are two common noncommunicable diseases (NCD) that significantly impact global health. Understanding the relationship between these two conditions is important for clinicians to provide comprehensive care. Both influence the outcome of each other and significantly affect the quality of life and can lead to higher incidence of mortality. Many of the respiratory diseases have a bidirectional relationship with DM. Individuals with DM are at an increased risk of developing respiratory infections including coronavirus disease 2019 (COVID-19) and tuberculosis (TB) as well as noninfectious diseases such as chronic obstructive pulmonary disease (COPD), bronchial asthma, and obstructive sleep apnea (OSA). On the other hand, respiratory diseases can worsen glycemic control and further complicate DM management. Shared risk factors including obesity, inflammation, oxidative stress, and impaired immune function contribute to the development and progression of both conditions. This chapter examines this adverse association between DM and respiratory diseases, their clinical implications, and challenges in the management.

PATHOPHYSIOLOGY OF LUNG DYSFUNCTION IN PATIENTS WITH DIABETES MELLITUS

The pathophysiology of pulmonary symptoms in DM is complex and multifactorial. It involves various mechanisms such as hyperglycemia,[1] hyperinsulinemia,[2] autonomic neuropathy,[3] oxidative stress, micro-/macroangiopathy,[4] tissue protein glycosylation,[5] collagen and elastin changes,[6] connective tissue alteration,[7] surfactant dysfunction,[8] and respiratory muscle dysfunction.[9] Hyperglycemia can lead to interstitial fibrosis, alveolar capillary microangiopathy, and both restrictive and obstructive lung function impairment. The molecular mechanisms underlying this association involve proinflammatory pathways and vascular inflammation such as the involvement of the receptor for advanced glycation end products (RAGE) and interleukin-6. Persistent hyperglycemia can directly damage lung tissues through glycosylation, inflammation, fibrosis, and impaired muscle strength. Hyperglycemia also affects elastic proteins in the lungs, leading to chronic airflow limitation and increased susceptibility to chronic obstructive pulmonary disease (COPD).

Diabetes mellitus, as a chronic inflammatory state, contributes to oxidative stress and changes in the pulmonary vasculature, resulting in decreased lung diffusion capacity and thickening of capillaries and arteriolar walls. DM also worsens interstitial lung diseases (ILD) and increases breathlessness and parenchymal fibrosis. Autonomic neuropathy affects the control of ventilation and bronchial innervation, impairing pulmonary function and increasing vulnerability to lung infections. Respiratory muscle strength is reduced in DM due to defective muscle metabolism and neuropathy, leading to lung volume reduction and restrictive complications. Chronic inflammation, oxidative stress, and loss of antioxidant capacity can cause lung endothelial dysfunction and thickening of the lung interstitium.

LUNG INFECTIONS

Patients living with DM are more susceptible to lung infections because of impaired immune system and poor glycemic control. Several impairments in neutrophil and macrophage functions have been described in individuals with DM.[10] There is impaired chemotaxis, adherence, phagocytosis, and the ability to kill microorganisms. In addition, the reduced complement system C4 and humoral immunity, along with decreased T-cell response, further increase the vulnerability of diabetic patients to infections.[11]

Hyperglycemia and insulin resistance in type 2 diabetes mellitus (T2DM) specifically impair the collective surfactant D-mediated host defenses of the lung. Loose junctions between airway epithelial cells, combined with increased glucose concentration in the airway surface liquid due to hyperglycemia, may weaken the airway's defense against infection, leading to bacterial overgrowth in the lungs. Various pathogens such as *Staphylococcus aureus*, *Streptococcus pneumoniae*, influenza virus, *Klebsiella pneumoniae*, *Pseudomonas aeruginosa*; and fungal species such as *Mucorales* and *Aspergillus* are frequently implicated in lung infections among individuals with DM.[12]

Diabetic patients have a higher risk of pneumonia-related hospitalization and poor prognosis, particularly when glycemic control is inadequate. Timely administration of appropriate antibiotics has been associated with improved outcomes in diabetic patients with pneumonia. Some pharmacological studies have suggested that treatment with angiotensin-converting-enzyme inhibitors[13] or statins[14] may reduce the risk of pneumonia in both type 1 and type 2 diabetic patients, although the underlying mechanisms are not yet fully understood.

Although vaccination against pneumococcal infection is recommended, the higher rate of lung infections in diabetic patients persists, possibly due to low vaccine uptake or reduced vaccine effectiveness in this population. Hyperglycemia plays a significant role in increasing the risk of lung infections in diabetic patients by adversely affecting immune system function, leading to higher morbidity and mortality.

PULMONARY TUBERCULOSIS

The risk of developing active tuberculosis (TB) is approximately three times higher in individuals with DM.[15] Additionally, a significant proportion of TB patients (10–30%) also suffer from DM. The impaired immune response associated with DM plays a role in the increased susceptibility to TB. Alveolar macrophages, which are important in the pathogenesis of TB, exhibit reduced opsonization, binding, and phagocytotic activity in diabetic patients. This weakened immune response may contribute to the increased susceptibility of diabetic patients to TB. The role of other immune cells, such as neutrophils, natural killer T cells, and dendritic cells, in the context of DM and TB is not well understood. Studies on the adaptive immune system in diabetic patients with TB have yielded conflicting results. There are some reports that there is reduced T-cell proliferation and cytokine production, while others have found higher numbers of T helper type 1 and 17 cells but lower frequencies of T regulatory cells.[16] Type 1 and 17 cytokine production was positively correlated with HbA1c levels in diabetic patients with TB.

Type 2 diabetes mellitus does not appear to have a significant effect on the numbers or subset distribution of CD8+ T and natural killer (NK) cells, but it alters their response to *Mycobacterium tuberculosis*. T2DM patients with active TB show higher frequencies of mycobacterial antigen-stimulated CD8+ T cells and NK cells expressing type 1 and type 17 cytokines, but cytotoxic markers are decreased in these cells.

Diabetic patients with TB are more prone to developing drug-resistant strains of the disease. This increased susceptibility to drug resistance can lead to treatment failure, relapse of the disease even after completing treatment, and higher mortality rates. The suboptimal immune response in diabetic patients allows TB bacteria to persist and replicate, increasing the likelihood of mutations that confer resistance to common anti-TB drugs. This drug resistance makes the treatment of TB more challenging, as standard medications may no longer be effective against the resistant strains. Proper management and close monitoring of both DM and TB are crucial in improving outcomes for individuals affected by this dual burden.

COVID-19 INFECTION

The association between DM and coronavirus disease 2019 (COVID-19) has been a topic of significant interest since the emergence of the pandemic. Numerous studies have highlighted that individuals with DM are at higher risk of severe illness and worse outcomes, if they contract COVID-19.

Firstly, individuals with DM are more likely to experience complications from viral infections in general. The virus responsible for COVID-19, severe acute respiratory syndrome-coronavirus-2 (SARS-CoV-2), primarily targets the respiratory system, but it can also affect other organs, including the pancreas. The presence of DM, particularly uncontrolled or poorly managed DM, can weaken the immune response, making it more difficult to fight off the infection.

Secondly, DM is often associated with several comorbidities, such as obesity, hypertension, and cardiovascular disease, which are known risk factors for severe COVID-19. These underlying health conditions can further exacerbate the impact of the virus on the body and increase the likelihood of complications.

Thirdly, the inflammatory response and cytokine dysregulation seen in severe cases of COVID-19 can be more pronounced in individuals with DM. This heightened inflammation, often referred to as a cytokine storm, can contribute to the development of acute respiratory distress syndrome (ARDS) and multiorgan dysfunction, which are associated with worse outcomes in COVID-19.

Moreover, the use of certain medications for DM management, such as corticosteroids or some classes of antidiabetic drugs, has been a subject of investigation in relation to COVID-19. These medications can affect the immune system and potentially influence the course of the infection. It is important to note that not all individuals with DM are equally at risk. Factors such as glycemic control, duration of DM, age, and the presence of other comorbidities play a role in determining the individual's vulnerability to severe COVID-19. It is important for individuals with DM to be vigilant in their preventive measures and DM management to reduce the impact of COVID-19.

CHRONIC OBSTRUCTIVE PULMONARY DISEASE

Increased levels of C-reactive protein (CRP), tumor necrosis factor-alpha (TNF-α) interleukin 1 (IL-1), IL-6, and fibrinogen as well as chronic inflammation are common features in COPD and DM.[17] Several studies have shown a higher incidence of COPD in diabetic patients, particularly those with higher body mass index and elevated hemoglobin A1c (HbA1c) levels.[18] The pulmonary function of diabetic patients with a history of smoking is often reduced compared to nondiabetic smokers, leading to decreased activity-related quality of life and exercise capacity. DM may also increase the risk of COPD exacerbation and mortality, with hyperglycemia being associated with poor outcomes and increased COPD-related morbidity and mortality.

While the role of COPD as a risk factor for DM remains controversial, some studies have reported a higher risk of DM in patients with COPD. However, others have not found a significant association between the two conditions. Treatment with corticosteroids, both by inhalation and systemically, is commonly used in COPD patients to improve quality of life and reduce exacerbations. Inhaled corticosteroids in COPD patients have not been associated with an increased risk of new-onset DM or significant changes in HbA1c levels. On the other hand, metformin treatment in patients with coexisting DM and COPD has shown benefits in reducing emergency room visits and hospitalization.

While it is understood that DM may increase the risk of COPD and worsen the quality of life, exacerbation rates, and mortality in COPD patients, further research is needed to investigate the complex interaction. Prospective population-based studies considering the order of disease appearance, type and duration of DM, severity of COPD, glycemic condition, smoking status, and treatment strategies are necessary to gain a more detailed understanding of this relationship.

BRONCHIAL ASTHMA

Relationship between DM and asthma has been quiet intriguing as there are contrasting immune mechanisms involved in these conditions, with asthma mediated by T-helper type 2 (Th2) cells and T1DM mediated by Th1 cells.[10] Previous findings have suggested a negative association between T1DM and asthma, while recent studies have shown an increased risk of subsequent development of T1DM in individuals with previously diagnosed asthma.[20] There is growing evidence of a positive correlation between T1DM and asthma symptoms at the population level. The interplay between the sequential appearance of these diseases suggests a distinct relationship between them, influenced by genetic and/or early environmental factors. Common immune-pathogenetic mechanisms and shared environmental factors have been proposed to contribute to the simultaneous occurrence of autoimmune diseases such as T1DM and allergic diseases such as asthma. Some studies have reported a positive correlation between HbA1c levels and asthma occurrence in individuals with T1DM.

In the case of T2DM, the relationship with asthma prevalence is inconsistent across different study designs and populations. However, T2DM and obesity have been associated with an increased risk of asthma, with obesity also impacting the effectiveness of asthma therapy and increasing the rate of hospitalizations due to exacerbations. Insulin has been found to have various effects on the respiratory system, including inhibiting surfactant production, shifting T-cell responses, promoting mast cell activity, activating inflammatory macrophages, and affecting airway smooth muscle cells.[21] These mechanisms contribute to the multiple links between DM and asthma.

OBSTRUCTIVE SLEEP APNEA

Obstructive sleep apnea is a sleep disorder characterized by the repetitive obstruction of the upper airway during sleep, leading to intermittent cerebral hypoxia, sleep fragmentation, and a failure to achieve deeper stages of sleep. OSA has been linked to systemic inflammation, increased oxidative stress, insulin resistance, and cardiovascular disease. Studies, including the Sleep Heart Health Study, have demonstrated a bidirectional association between OSA and DM, independent of age, gender, and body mass index (BMI). OSA patients are more likely to develop DM, and individuals with DM are more prone to sleep-disordered breathing. The estimated prevalence of DM among OSA patients ranges from 15 to 30%.

Symptoms of OSA such as snoring, daytime somnolence, and witnessed sleep apnea are associated with elevated fasting plasma glucose levels. However, the impact of continuous positive airway pressure (CPAP) treatment on glucose metabolism remains uncertain, with conflicting results from different studies. Some studies have shown a relationship between OSA severity and worsened glycemic control, with greater OSA severity correlating with poorer glucose control. The International Diabetes Federation and the American Diabetes Association recognize OSA as an important comorbidity in patients with DM. While short-term CPAP therapy may not significantly improve glucose metabolism and insulin resistance, long-term CPAP therapy has been associated with better control of fasting blood glucose levels. CPAP therapy remains the mainstay of treatment for OSA, regardless of glycemic levels, as it has been proven to improve hypertension, quality of sleep, and overall quality of life.

LUNG CANCER

It is postulated that hyperglycemia, along with hyperinsulinemia, may further contribute to cancer cell growth, imbalances in pro-/anti-inflammatory cytokines, chronic inflammation, oxidative stress, and suppression of anticancer immunity. While the relationship between DM and lung cancer has not been extensively studied, recent research from Sweden, Denmark, and Taiwan suggests that DM significantly increases the risk of lung cancer.[22,23] There are a number of mixed studies either supporting or negating the link between the two. Further, well-designed prospective population-based studies are needed to compare the incidence of lung cancer among individuals with high insulin levels and/or hyperglycemia with or without DM, as well as nondiabetic individuals with normal insulin sensitivity and/or normal blood sugar levels. These studies should consider various common risk factors, including the type and duration of DM, body weight, physical activity, age, sex, ethnicity, diet, therapy, degree of glycemic control, and tobacco smoke and alcohol consumption, to reduce heterogeneity across studies. Diabetic patients are more vulnerable to radiation pneumonitis in lung cancer patients who receive radiotherapy.

The antineoplastic effects of certain antidiabetic medications, particularly metformin, have been suggested to contribute to a reduced incidence and progression of lung cancer in diabetic patients. The underlying biological mechanisms are not yet fully understood, and the results of studies in this area are contradictory.

CYSTIC FIBROSIS

Cystic fibrosis is a monogenic autosomal inherited disorder due to mutation in cystic fibrosis transmembrane conductance regulator (*CFTR*) gene. It primarily affects the functions of the exocrine glands and commonly involves respiratory and digestive systems leading to frequent pulmonary infections and pancreatic enzyme insufficiency. Bronchiectasis is one of the major complications and can have an effect in diabetics. Cystic fibrosis-related diabetes (CFRD) is the most common and life-threatening complication in CF due to pancreatic insufficiency and abnormal insulin secretion. It is found to reduce survival and increase mortality in CF patients compared to those without DM. CFRD has a negative effect on lung function, with CF patients with DM having a lower average forced expiratory volume in 1 second compared to those without DM. Lung function decline can be observed for several years prior to the diagnosis of CFRD, and the severity of pulmonary dysfunction correlates with the degree of insulin deficiency in CFRD patients. Insulin treatment has shown to improve lung function and increase forced expiratory volume in 1 second in patients with CFRD. Coinfections with *Staphylococcus aureus* and *Pseudomonas aeruginosa* are associated with CFRD and can accelerate pulmonary deterioration and lung function decline in these patients.[24] Further research, both basic and clinical, is needed to investigate the relationships between hyperglycemia, insulin deficiency, long-term insulin therapy, and pulmonary function in CFRD.

ACUTE LUNG INJURY/ACUTE RESPIRATORY DISTRESS SYNDROME

While T2DM does not appear to affect the lung physiopathology in patients with ARDS, studies have shown that both type 1 diabetes mellitus (T1DM) and T2DM may prevent the development of ARDS in patients with predisposing risk factors.[25] However, the protective effect of DM against ARDS development does not reduce mortality among patients who develop ARDS.

The underlying mechanisms of how DM prevents ARDS development are not fully understood. Experimental studies suggest that DM may lead to decreased neutrophil numbers and function, impaired activation of nuclear factor κ-light-chain-enhancer of activated B-cells, reduced superoxide generation, insulin growth factor and its receptor deficiency, leptin resistance, and lower concentrations of inflammatory cytokines.[26] Insulin therapy has shown beneficial effects in clinical studies, including shortened time of mechanical ventilation and decreased mortality and morbidity rates in hyperglycemic patients with prolonged intensive care unit stays.[27]

IDIOPATHIC PULMONARY FIBROSIS

Aging, DM, and obesity are considered contributing factors that may affect the initiation and/or progression of pulmonary fibrosis.[28] Autopsied lungs from diabetic patients have shown increased thickness of alveolar capillary walls, alveolar walls, and pulmonary arteriolar walls, indicating fibrotic histopathological changes.[29] However, studies have shown inconsistent findings regarding the presence of fibrotic changes in the lungs of diabetic individuals compared to controls. Comorbidities such as hypertension, cardiovascular disease, and other malignancies are more prevalent in idiopathic pulmonary fibrosis (IPF) patients with DM compared to those without DM. DM has also been shown to increase mortality in IPF patients. The mechanisms underlying the association between DM and IPF are not fully understood and require further clinical and experimental research. Accumulation of advanced glycation end product-modified proteins in lung macrophages has been suggested as a potential mechanism. Recognition and management of comorbidities, including DM, in IPF patients may help limit disease progression and improve survival.

LUNG DISEASES AND ANTIDIABETIC DRUGS

Interestingly, antidiabetic drugs have been found to play a role beyond their primary function of DM control. Traditionally, their role is believed to lower blood sugar levels to control hyperglycemia while managing respiratory infections (including TB). But the anti-DM drug may also serve as a modulator of airway glucose homeostasis, influencing the exacerbation or prevention of lung disease **(Table 1)**.

TABLE 1: Antidiabetic drugs and their effects on lung.[30]

Oral antidiabetic drug	Possible mechanism	Outcome on lung
Metformin	Promote macrophage bactericidal activity	Enhanced life expectancy in lung infections
	Antifibrotic	Reduction in lung fibrosis
	Anti-inflammatory	Reduction in asthma attacks
	Antiproliferative	Better life expectancy in lung cancer
		Protective against radiation- and chemotherapy-induced lung injury
PPAR-γ agonists	Reduced airway inflammation/mucus production	Asthma/COPD
	Antifibrotic	Lung fibrosis
	Antitumor and antiproliferative	Lung cancer
DDP-4 inhibitors	Mediates allergic airway inflammation and regulate common immunological pathways (in vitro)	?Asthma
Sulfonylurea	Airway muscle relaxation in mice , inhibits cytokine mediated eosinophil survival and superoxide production	?Asthma protection
GLP-1 agonists	Anti-inflammatory	Reduced COPD exacerbation
SGLT-2 inhibitors	Human pulmonary artery smooth muscle cell relaxation in an NO-dependent manner	?Pulmonary artery hypertension
Insulin (negative correlation)	Modifies mast cell activity, increases bronchoconstriction, and oncogenic activity	Higher the risk of asthma, higher the prevalence of lung cancer

(COPD: chronic obstructive pulmonary disease; DDP-4: dipeptidyl peptidase 4; GLP-1: glucagon-like peptide-1; NO: nitric oxide; PPAR-γ: peroxisome proliferator-activated receptor gamma; SGLT-2: sodium-glucose cotransporter-2)

SUMMARY

Diabetes mellitus affects multiple organs but the lungs have been relatively overlooked in this context. Hyperglycemia's proinflammatory, proliferative, and oxidative effects play a significant role in affecting the pulmonary vasculature, airways, and lung tissue. New emerging evidence also suggests that DM and certain oral antidiabetic drugs can impact the development, progression, prognosis, and clinical outcome of various lung diseases. While optimizing glycemic control is important, further research is needed to clarify this bidirectional bond between lungs and DM.

REFERENCES

1. Lange P, Groth S, Kastrup J, Mortensen J, et al. Diabetes mellitus, plasma glucose and lung function in a cross-sectional population study. Eur Respir J. 1989;2:14-9.
2. Singh S, Prakash YS, Linneberg A, et al. Insulin and the lung: connecting asthma and metabolic syndrome. J Allergy (Cairo). 2013;2013:627384.
3. Bottini P, Scionti L, Santeusanio F, et al. Impairment of the respiratory system in diabetic autonomic neuropathy. Diabetes Nutr Metab. 2000;13:165-72.
4. Forgiarini LA Jr, Kretzmann NA, Porawski M, et al. Experimental diabetes mellitus: oxida oxidative stress and changes in lung structure. J Bras Pneumol. 2009;35:788-91.
5. Soulis T, Thallas V, Youssef S, et al. Advanced glycation end products and their receptors co-localise in rat organs susceptible to diabetic microvascular injury. Diabetologia. 1997;40:619-28.
6. Cavan DA, Parkes A, O'Donnell MJ, et al. Lung function and diabetes. Respir Med. 1991;85:257-8.
7. Ofulue AF, Thurlbeck WM. Experimental diabetes and the lung. II. In vivo connective tissue metabolism. Am Rev Respir Dis. 1988;138:284-9.
8. Foster DJ, Ravikumar P, Bellotto DJ, et al. Fatty diabetic lung: altered alveolar structure and surfactant protein expression. Am J Physiol Lung Cell Mol Physiol. 2010;298:392-403.
9. Kolahian S, Leiss V, Nürnberg B. Diabetic lung disease: fact or fiction?. Reviews in Endocrine and Metabolic Disorders. 2019;20:303-19.
10. Bhargava P, Lee CH. Role and function of macrophages in the metabolic syndrome. Biochem J. 2012;442:253-62.
11. Peleg AY, Weerarathna T, McCarthy JS, et al. Common infections in diabetes: pathogenesis, management and relationship to glycaemic control. Diabetes Metab Res Rev. 2007;23:3-13.
12. Muller LM, Gorter KJ, Hak E, et al. Increased risk of common infections in patients with type 1 and type 2 diabetes mellitus. Clin Infect Dis. 2005;41:281-8.
13. van de Garde EM, Souverein PC, Hak E, et al. Angiotensin-converting enzyme inhibitor use and protection against pneumonia in patients with diabetes. J Hypertens. 2007;25:235-9.
14. van de Garde EM, Hak E, Souverein PC, et al. Statin treatment and reduced risk of pneumonia in patients with diabetes. Thorax. 2006;61:957-61.

15. Harries AD, Lin Y, Satyanarayana S, et al. The looming epidemic of diabetes-associated tuberculosis: learning lessons from the HIV-associated tuberculosis. Inter J Tuberc Lung Dis. 2011;15: 1436-45.
16. Al-Attiyah RJ, Mustafa AS. Mycobacterial antigen-induced T helper type 1 (Th1) and Th2 reactivity of peripheral blood mononuclear cells from diabetic and non-diabetic tuberculosis patients and *Mycobacterium bovis* bacilli Calmette-Gue rin (BCG)–vaccinated healthy subjects. Clin Exp Immunol. 2009; 158:64-73.
17. Forgiarini LA Jr, Kretzmann NA, Porawski M, et al. Experimental diabetes mellitus: oxida oxidative stress and changes in lung structure. J Bras Pneumol. 2009;35:788-91.
18. Ehrlich SF, Quesenberry CP Jr, Van Den Eeden SK, et al. Patients diagnosed with diabetes are at increased risk for asthma, chronic obstructive pulmonary disease, pulmonary fibrosis, and pneumonia but not lung cancer. Diabetes Care. 2010;33:55-60.
19. Fahy JV. Type 2 inflammation in asthma—present in most, absent in many. Nat Rev Immunol. 2015;15:57-65.
20. Cardwell CR, Shields MD, Carson DJ, et al. A metaanalysis of the association between childhood type 1 diabetes and atopic disease. Diabetes Care. 2003;26:2568-74.
21. Viardot A, Grey ST, Mackay F, et al. Potential anti-inflammatory role of insulin via the preferential polarization of effector T cells toward a T helper 2 phenotype. Endocrinology. 2007;148: 346-53.
22. Lee CT, Mao IC, Lin CH, et al. Chronic obstructive pulmonary disease: a risk factor for type 2 diabetes: a nationwide population-based study. Eur J Clin Investig. 2013;43:1113e1119.
23. Carstensen B, Witte DR, Friis S. Cancer occurrence in Danish diabetic patients: Duration and insulin effects. Diabetologia. 2012;55:948-58.
24. Limoli DH, Yang J, Khansaheb MK, et al. *Staphylococcus aureus* and *Pseudomonas aeruginosa* co-infection is associated with cystic fibrosis-related diabetes and poor clinical outcomes. Eur J Clin Microbiol Infect Dis. 2016;35:947-53.
25. Singla A, Turner P, Pendurthi MK, et al. Effect of type II diabetes mellitus on the outcomes in patients with acute respiratory distress syndrome. J Crit Care. 2014;29:66e69.
26. Alba-Loureiro TC, Munhoz CD, Martins JO, et al. Neutrophil function and metabolism in individuals with diabetes mellitus. Braz J Med Biol Res. 2007;40:1037-44.
27. Van den Berghe G, Wouters P, Weekers F, et al. Intensive insulin therapy in critically ill patients. N Engl J Med. 2001;345:1359-67.
28. Alakhras M, Decker PA, Nadrous HF, et al. Body mass index and mortality in patients with idiopathic pulmonary fibrosis. Chest. 2007;131:1448-53.
29. Matsubara T, Hara F. The pulmonary function and histopathological studies of the lung in diabetes mellitus. Nippon Ika Daigaku Zasshi. 1991;58:528-36.
30. Khateeb J, Fuchs E, Khamaisi M. Diabetes and lung disease: an underestimated relationship. Rev Diabet Stud. 2019;15(1):1-5.

Pulmonary Disease in Pregnancy

CHAPTER 139

Umesh N Jindal

INTRODUCTION

With the changing lifestyle and modern medical practice, pregnancies are more likely to be associated with challenging medical and respiratory conditions. Pregnancies at advanced age, improved survival of hereditary diseases such as cystic fibrosis (CF) and malignancies, and increased use of assisted reproduction techniques in otherwise low fertility women are now common. Pulmonary diseases are common in occurrence, and therefore the pulmonary specialists may face the dilemmas of managing such pregnancies and deciding diagnostic evaluation and management. They may be also consulted for preconception advice for or against conceiving in serious long-standing conditions which have a potential of decompensation during pregnancy or childbirth. Shared decision-making with obstetricians is required in certain difficult situations requiring consideration of termination of pregnancy in many life-threatening situations. Pregnant women may require critical care for many preexisting conditions which may aggravate. In addition, there are conditions which are unique to pregnancy but require intensive care for management.

MATERNAL RESPIRATORY ADAPTATION

Pregnancy is a physiological state of increased demand on almost all organ systems of a woman's body. The cardiovascular, respiratory, gastrointestinal, renal, hematological, and all systems undergo extensive changes to fulfil the metabolic and nutritional requirements of the developing fetus. Marked changes occur in the musculoskeletal system to accommodate space requirements of an enlarging uterus. These changes begin immediately with conception and start resolving during lactation and slowly come back to normal in prepregnancy state. Most of these changes are hormone mediated which are secreted by corpus luteum and growing placenta.

Besides the physiological changes, pregnancy may also alter the values of many laboratory parameters, imaging and other functional tests leading to entirely different interpretation and validity. It is also a state which tests the reserve capacity of all systems, and many diseases may manifest for the first time during pregnancy. Furthermore, any drug treatment has to be considered and modified very carefully, keeping in view the teratogenicity and pharmacodynamic and pharmacokinetic changes which occur during pregnancy.

RESPIRATORY PHYSIOLOGY DURING PREGNANCY[1]

The respiratory tract undergoes major anatomical and physiological changes to meet increased oxygen demands of mother and baby and accommodate the space required for the growing uterus. It takes almost 24 weeks for the chest wall changes to return to prepregnancy levels.

Anatomical Changes

Changes in Rib Cage and Respiratory Muscles

The progressive uterine enlargement is the main factor for anatomical changes in chest wall. The lower rib cage widens leading to (1) increased anteroposterior and transverse diameter and almost 5–7 cm increase in chest diameter; (2) widening of subcostal angle by about 50% from 68.5° to 103.5°; (3) impaired chest wall compliance in late pregnancy, however lung compliance remains same; (4) upward displacement of diaphragm by 5 cm; (5) respiratory muscle strength is preserved, and (6) compensatory stretching and changes in abdominal and spinal muscle actions.

In addition, there is bronchodilatory effect of progesterone due to relaxation of smooth muscles.

Implications:

- Rib flare pain during late pregnancy and postpartum period due to altered biomechanics and compensatory increased lumber lordosis and back pain.
- Impaired total lung compliance [decreased functional residual capacity (FRC) and expiratory reserve volume (ERV)] due to earlier closure of lower airways due to increased intra-abdominal pressure and raised diaphragm.

- Total lung capacity (TLC) remains the same because a decrease in thoracic height is compensated by increased cage diameter.
- Reduced diaphragmatic movements in supine position.
- Intubation and laryngoscopy may be more difficult and preoxygenation may be less effective.
- Any preexisting chest wall deformities or muscle weakness of chest wall may interfere with this adaptation and compromise lung function during pregnancy.

Respiratory Tract

There is a lot of capillary edema, hyperemia, glandular hypersecretion, and engorgement of the upper airways including nasal, oral cavity, pharynx, vocal cords, and arytenoids. Nasal congestion begins early in pregnancy. There are higher chances of snoring, and there may sleep-disordered breathing. These conditions may be associated with hyperventilation and preeclampsia. Upper airway obstruction and bleeding are more likely during intubation or mask anesthesia and make intubation difficult. Increase in chest diameter, weight of enlarged breasts, and smaller laryngeal diameter require skill in intubation with appropriate size of tube and blades.

Hormonal Changes

Increased progesterone has a significant effect on pulmonary physiology. Increased estrogen acts mainly by upregulation of the progesterone receptors in the respiratory center in the central nervous system.

- It is the main mediator of bronchial and smooth muscle relaxation. As a result, there is no change in airway resistance or conductance despite mucosal congestion.
- The respiratory center also becomes hypersensitive to CO_2 and increases the minute ventilation.
- Progesterone may have direct stimulatory effect on the respiratory center independent of CO_2 levels.
- The upward displacement of diaphragm and widening of rib cage occur much earlier than the mechanical effect of enlarging uterus. This effect is attributed the effect of progesterone on relaxin which relaxes all ligaments and muscles.
- It also causes hyperemia and edema of mucosal surfaces.
- Progesterone also increases the carbonic anhydrase in red blood cells (RBCs) which facilitates gas exchange across RBCs.

Physiological Functional Measurements

There are no major changes in spirometry during pregnancy. Flow rates including the forced vital capacity (FVC), forced expiratory volume in 1 second (FEV1), peak expiratory flow (PEF), and FEV1/FVC essentially remain unchanged. The major effects of physiological changes occur in lung volumes.

- Tidal volume increases by up to 50% (from 350 to 500 to 650 mL).
- Respiratory rate (RR) remains the same, and any increase in RR is pathological.
- Minute volume (MV) increases by 50%.
- Both residual volume (RV) and FRC) decrease by 20–30% due to raised diaphragm and decreased recoil of chest wall.
- Inspiratory capacity, defined as maximum inhaled volume, is increased by 10%, thus making TLC (inspiratory capacity + FRC) unchanged.
- Inspiratory and expiratory maximum pressure values remain unchanged despite all anatomical changes.

These changes may increase the risk of hypoxemia during general anesthesia. They do not differ between singleton and twin pregnancies. Lung volume changes return to normal within 48 hours postpartum.

LUNG PERFUSION

There occurs an increase in cardiac output, blood volume, and lower peripheral resistance in order to increase placental circulation. Similar to systemic circulation, pulmonary vascular resistance decreases but pulmonary arterial pressure remains unchanged. There is increased lung perfusion and increased ventilation/perfusion matching and diffusion of gases in order to meet increased oxygen demands.

VENTILATION

To meet the excess demands of pregnancy, minute ventilation increases by about 40% due to increase mainly in tidal volume. RR remains essentially unchanged.

BLOOD GASES

There is no significant change in diffusion capacity during pregnancy. The gas exchange during pregnancy occurs at two places: The maternal lungs cater to the needs of both the mother and the fetus in utero while placenta maintains gas transfer to fetus.

- *Carbon dioxide (CO_2)*: $PaCO_2$ reduces from 35–40 to 30 mm Hg. There is a proportionate increase in renal bicarbonate excretion and lower plasma bicarbonate levels.
    - Plasma pH remains the same, but buffering capacity is reduced and increases the risk of acidosis.
    - These changes are further marked at high altitude to compensate for lower atmospheric oxygen. Low PaO_2 further increases the risk of intrauterine growth restriction and preeclampsia.
- *Oxygen (O_2)*: At sea level, maternal alveolar oxygen pressure (PAO_2) increases to 100–105 mm Hg. This is an important adaptation to facilitate O_2 transfer across placenta. The alveolar-arterial gradient (alveolar PO_2–arterial PO_2) increases from 15 to about 20 mm Hg. In supine position, there may be a decrease in PO_2 and an

increase in the alveolar-arterial gradient due to effect of position on cardiac output and airway closure.

- O_2 consumption is increased by about 20%, of which nearly one third is required for the fetus and placenta and the rest for increased maternal metabolism. There is a further increase in labor and delivery to almost 60% of baseline value. There is a shift in the oxyhemoglobin curve to the right to meet the requirement of increased oxygen diffusion across the placenta.

CARDIOVASCULAR SYSTEM[1]

Many major changes in the cardiovascular system (CVS) which occur during pregnancy are intimately related to respiratory physiology. The apex of heart is tilted toward left. There is mild tachycardia, peripheral edema, and slight distension of jugular veins. The first heart sound is louder, and third sound may be heard. A physiological systolic flow murmur may be heard in over 90% of women. Cardiac output increases by 45%. Increased blood volume and stroke volume are both responsible for an increase in cardiac output. In addition, there is increased extravascular fluid. In total, 6–9 L of fluid is increased. Supine hypotension is quite common during pregnancy because of the pressure of the gravid uterus on inferior vena cava.

The CVS is particularly vulnerable during labor and postpartum period. At delivery, during expulsion of placenta, maternal cardiac output increases by 10–15% above late pregnancy levels and further 40–50% at delivery due to pumping of blood from placental circulation into systemic circulation. In addition, there is increased catecholamine release, anxiety, pain, exertion, and stress of labor. Careful hemodynamic monitoring is essential in patients with cardiac and pulmonary diseases with significant compromised lung function. This autotransfusion of 300–500 mL of blood increases preload and poses a risk of acute heart failure in patients who have underlying cardiac problems, especially pulmonary arterial hypertension (PAH) or cor pulmonale. Avoidance of strong uterotonics and pain, use of diuretics, and intensive monitoring can be life saving.

Fetal Lung

The lung development and maturation are critical for extrauterine survival of fetus. The four stages of anatomical lung development (pseudoglandular 6–16 weeks, canalicular stage 16–26 weeks, terminal sac stage 26–32 weeks, and alveolar stage 32 weeks to 8 years of life) have a fixed timeline which is not modified by time of delivery or any therapy.[2] Moreover, many unfavorable stage-specific events during pregnancy may have adverse effects on this process and have long-term sequalae. Oligohydramnios, premature rupture of membranes, preterm delivery, low birth weight, birth asphyxia, hyperoxia, artificial ventilation, etc., have a profound impact on pediatric and adult diseases. Maternal nutrition, smoking, alcohol, and drugs may have significant effects on lung developments.[3]

Fetal Oxygenation

Low PO_2 in fetal umbilical vein, high oxygen affinity, and high oxygen-carrying capacity of fetal blood and hemoglobin together ensure preferential O_2 diffusion to fetus and adequate O_2 content of fetal blood. The dramatic events at first breath after delivery are crucial in the transition from 100% maternal dependence to neonatal respiratory and cardiovascular systems.

COMMON CLINICAL SYMPTOMS AND OTHER ISSUES

Dyspnea

Breathlessness is a common symptom during pregnancy. Nearly half of the women notice change in their breathing in first and second trimesters itself and another quarter by mid third trimester. Women with dyspnea have a higher hyperventilatory response to CO_2 and hypoxia. These changes are related more to the congestion and other anatomical changes in the respiratory tract, effect of progesterone, mechanical effect of growing uterus, increasing weight, and increased intra-abdominal pressure. There is no increase in RR. In the absence of any underlying disease, most women are able to carry out their daily routine. Physical examination and O_2 saturation are normal both at rest and at exertion.

Rhinitis of Pregnancy

Rhinitis of pregnancy is a common condition characterized by nasal congestion in the last 6 weeks of pregnancy without evidence of any allergies or infection which disappears completely within 2 weeks of delivery. Nasal congestion and rhinorrhea are common symptoms during pregnancy reported by almost 30% of women. Increased vascularity and mucosal edema may be responsible. There are increased chances in smokers, underlying nasal allergies, and polyps. Allergic rhinitis may be associated with asthma in up to 40% of women which may worsen during pregnancy. In some women, sinusitis may develop. The symptoms of headache, purulent discharge, or fever signify infective pathology. Antibiotics would be required to treat these women.

Exercise during Pregnancy

There is a beneficial effect of exercise during pregnancy to improve circulation and carbohydrate metabolism and improvement in glycemic control. Most healthy women are able to take moderate exercise. The ventilation increases during moderate weight-bearing exercises such as walking and treadmill. There is also an increase in cardiac output, mainly because of an increase in stroke volume. Thus, moderate exercise helps to increase oxygen delivery to the fetus. Fetal heart rate also increases after maternal exercise. Core body temperature of mother may increase by 1–1.5°C. On the whole, moderate exercise is beneficial to both the mother and the child. Restriction of activity is required in women with compromised lung function.

Imaging during Pregnancy

Ionizing radiation during imaging or accidentally is a common concern. The risk-benefit ratio of various diagnostic procedures requires to be weighed whenever ordering a test. Birth defects, mental retardation, growth restriction, and miscarriages have been reported with exposure to high doses of ionizing radiation. These are highly unlikely with doses given for diagnostic purposes. The dose of radiation and the gestation period are important determinants. Pulmonary imaging does not involve direct exposure to uterus or the fetus. Moreover, shielding of abdomen with lead shield gives added protection against any scatter radiation. Most abdominal or pelvic imaging studies expose the fetus to less than 10 rads (<0.1 Gy), while the detrimental effects have been shown with over 150 rads (>1.5 Gy) dose in experimental animal studies.

There are no risks of imaging during the first 2 weeks of pregnancy, i.e., before ovulation. In the next 2 weeks, i.e., before the missed period, the embryo usually follows all-or-none law—the embryo will either not implant or not be affected at all. The first 12–18 weeks are more crucial for exposure.

During pregnancy, restricting and limiting the exposure to the minimum remain the general principle. Whenever indicated, ultrasound examination and magnetic resonance imaging (MRI) do not involve any ionizing radiation and should be preferred over computed tomography (CT scan). Any radioisotope imaging is contraindicated.

Interventional Procedures during Pregnancy

Bronchoscopic and/or pleural intervention for diagnostic or therapeutic purposes required for a variety of malignant or nonmalignant lung or pleural diseases has been safely performed during pregnancy. There are no large studies to serve as guidelines. A multidisciplinary team along with intensive care facilities should be preferably available. Intervention should be postponed to second trimester or postpartum period, if possible.

Vaccination during Pregnancy

Pregnant women are disproportionately prone to severe morbidity and mortality in case they contract many common viral and bacterial respiratory infections. The shift from cell-mediated to humoral immunity helps a woman to develop immune tolerance to an allogenic fetus. Physiological adaptation in cardiorespiratory systems also makes women more susceptible to respiratory complications. The increased risk was observed during several pandemics; after 2009, influenza vaccination was introduced in the antenatal schedule in UK and USA.[4]

Vaccinations and postexposure prophylaxis (in case of any significant exposure) are done both before pregnancy and during pregnancy as well as in the postpartum period. There are three main purposes of vaccination during pregnancy: (1) Prevention of severe maternal morbidity and mortality; (2) prevention of congenital malformations in the baby due to teratogenicity of certain infections occurring during critical phases of pregnancy; (3) conferring passive immunity to the newborn; vaccination for special categories and immune-compromised individuals; and (4) opportunistic vaccination for long-term health of female. However, there should be adequate proof of safety and efficacy before any vaccination can be introduced in the immunization program for pregnant women. As a rule of thumb, all live vaccines are contraindicated during pregnancy because of the potential risk of viremia or disease in the mother and consequences for the fetus. The Global Alignment of Immunization Safety Assessment in Pregnancy (GAIA), constituted by the World Health Organization (WHO), monitors various aspects of immunization during pregnancy.[5]

Routine Vaccination during Pregnancy[6]

Maternal vaccination boosts both cell-mediated and humoral immunity in mother and protects both mother and fetus against common diseases which can have serious consequences. Antibodies of the class immunoglobin (Ig) G are transferred to the neonate and give passive immunity to fetus during the early neonatal period. In addition, IgA and IgM antibodies are secreted in maternal milk. Universal immunization against tetanus has virtually reduced the global burden of neonatal tetanus by 95%. Universal immunization program recommends routine vaccination of all pregnant women against tetanus, diphtheria, pertussis, and influenza.

Vaccination in the Presence of Comorbidities or High Risk

This category of vaccines is of special importance to physicians who deal with women with comorbidities and immune-deficiencies due to various causes. Common examples are women suffering from malignancies, HIV, splenic deficiencies, transplant recipients, cochlear implants, and chronic airway diseases. These include polysaccharide and conjugate vaccine for *Haemophilus influenzae B*, *Neisseria meningitidis* and *Streptococcus pneumoniae* (PCV13, 13-valent pneumococcal conjugate vaccine; PPSV23, 23-valent pneumococcal polysaccharide vaccine). These vaccines are safe during pregnancy.

Respiratory Infections

Presentation, immune response, and recovery from respiratory tract infections (RTIs) may vary during pregnancy.

Limitations of choice of drugs because of risk of teratogenicity and also risk of vertical transmission of infection to the baby are important considerations. The physiological changes during pregnancy involving rib cage and respiratory tract may impair clearance of secretions. The immune response to various organisms also may be altered which make women more prone to severe infections.

- *Acute bronchitis*: It is mostly viral in origin. Some atypical bacterial infections, e.g., *Bordetella pertussis, Chlamydia pneumoniae, Streptococcus pneumoniae,* and *Mycoplasma pneumoniae,* are other important infections. Treatment is largely symptomatic. Antibiotics (azithromycin, erythromycin, or co-amoxiclav) are given if bacterial infection is suspected. Antiviral agents prescribed for influenza have very low safety data during pregnancy.
- *Influenza virus infection*: It is characterized by sudden-onset fever, marked rhinitis, body aches, malaise, and dry cough. It is usually self-limiting and requires symptomatic treatment. The complicated course is more likely in the third trimester. In India, influenza vaccine is recommended for all pregnant women. The safety of antiviral agents during pregnancy has not been proven. These drugs may only be given in the third trimester in very severe cases.
- *Community-acquired pneumonia*: Pregnant women are no more susceptible to pneumonias than normal age-matched women.[7] However, the course can get serious, especially in the presence of an underlying disease, and is one of the common causes of indirect maternal deaths.[8,9] Raised diaphragm, suppressed cough reflex, and increased fluid volume put women at a higher risk for severe complications. Pregnant women in the third trimester are more prone to respiratory failure as they are less likely to tolerate hypoxia due to reduced functional lung capacity and increased oxygen requirement. Maternal anemia, asthma, antepartum corticosteroids, postpartum period, smoking, and use of tocolytics are other risk factors. The baby also has a higher chance of preterm birth or having low birth weight.

Increasing prevalence of many respiratory viruses like swine flu and severe acute respiratory syndrome (SARS) infections and other immunodeficiency states (HIV, renal transplants) is also responsible for contributing to maternal morbidity and mortality due to pneumonia.[10] The prognosis for mother has improved in recent years because of availability and use of effective antibiotic therapy.

Aspiration pneumonia was the cause of almost 2% of maternal deaths in the past. The physiological alterations in chest wall diameters, raised diaphragm, loose gastroesophageal sphincter, and suppression of cough reflex due to anesthesia and analgesia contribute to this important cause of maternal death. Awareness of the problem and strategies to prevent aspiration have greatly reduced the incidence in recent years.[11]

The common organisms causing pneumonia in pregnancy are similar to those seen in nonpregnant women. The most commonly reported are: *S. pneumoniae, Haemophilus influenzae, Mycoplasma pneumoniae* or common viruses like *influenza A* or *varicella* which can cause severe infections. Severe atypical pneumonias may be caused by *Legionella* species, *M. pneumoniae* and *C. pneumoniae, S. aureus* (including methicillin-resistant strains), and *P. aeruginosa* which may complicate bronchiectasis and CF. Fungal pneumonia due to Coccidioidomycosis and *Pneumocystis jirovecii* (with HIV infection) may be seen uncommonly.[12]

Certain organisms have higher hazard during pregnancy and carry a risk of severe morbidity and mortality. Primary varicella infection during pregnancy may be complicated by pneumonia in almost 9% as compared to 0.3–1.8% in nonpregnant women.[13] Influenza A is a common infection and carries a very high mortality rate during pregnancy. Most notable among these were H1N1 and SARS infection caused by a coronavirus. All these infections when occur in the third trimester are more serious and associated with intensive care admissions and obstetric complications.

Other dreaded forms of community-acquired pneumonia may occur due to antibiotic resistance strains of *S. pneumoniae* (drug-resistant *S. pneumoniae*) and methicillin-resistant *S. aureus* (MRSA) [community-acquired (CA) MRSA]. These strains may be acquired from community outbreaks in children in daycare centers or in patients on prolonged antibiotics.[10]

The diagnosis of pneumonia during pregnancy can be challenging. The symptoms are common and similar to a nonpregnant state. Distinguishing dyspnea and cough from physiological symptoms or mild upper RTIs may delay the diagnosis. However, sudden onset of symptoms with fever may raise suspicion. Reluctance of getting a chest X-ray by both physician and patient may also delay the diagnosis and may be the cause of increased morbidity and mortality in severe cases. Other investigations include assessment of oxygenation or blood gases as indicated and other blood chemistry and counts. Appropriate microbiological studies should be done. Every effort should be done to establish etiological diagnosis including a bronchoscopy if needed.

Community-acquired pneumonias can be treated on an outpatient basis depending upon the severity of symptoms. The guidelines for the recommendations for admission to critical care have not been specifically tailored to pregnant women. These need to be individualized and liberalized because of the reduced ability of pregnant women to tolerate hypoxemia. Various warning signs include coexisting diseases like diabetes, chronic obstructive pulmonary disease (COPD), asthma, other systemic diseases, or signs of impending respiratory failure. The choice of antibiotics remains largely empirical based on local microbial susceptibility, disease severity, and safety during pregnancy. In addition, the supportive therapy includes hydration, and oxygen. Noninvasive and invasive ventilation need to be assessed and provided as per requirement. An obstetric consultant should be part of the treating team since there is a high risk of associated obstetric complications such as miscarriages and preterm labor.

Chronic Airway Diseases and Pregnancy

The outlook for young women with chronic respiratory airway disease has changed in recent years. Many of these women are in their reproductive years and have moderate-to-severe impairment of lung functions. A significant proportion of them wants to complete their desires for pregnancy and childbirth. The common diseases include asthma, CF, and non-CF bronchiectasis. These women require careful prepregnancy assessment and counseling, advice regarding contraception, and specialized care through pregnancy, childbirth, and postpartum period. These women should be advised to complete their family early. There is no contraindication to oral contraceptives for contraception.

Asthma and Pregnancy

The incidence of asthma during pregnancy is reported from 2 to 8% in different countries.[14] Asthma may worsen in nearly 18.8% of cases during pregnancy.[15] Maternal asthma may contribute to increased risks for the mother for pregnancy complications such as preeclampsia, gestational diabetes, prematurity, upper and lower respiratory infections, and increased anesthesia risks. There is a higher risk of low birth weight, prematurity, congenital malformations, and perinatal mortality. The risks are higher in severe and uncontrolled asthma. In addition to physiological factors, severity of asthma, common viral infections, and avoidance of medicines are important factors which determine severity. Obesity, rhinitis, and eosinophilic phenotypes are more prone to deterioration during pregnancy.

Diagnosis of Asthma

A careful history of nasobronchial allergy and use of inhaled corticosteroids (ICS) in past should alert the obstetrician of the possibility of asthma. Symptoms during pregnancy are similar to those in nonpregnant state, and diagnosis remains clinical. Common symptoms include wheeze, variable cough episodes, and breathlessness. The symptoms may worsen after viral infection, after exercise, and during night, cold, or allergen exposure. However, dyspnea during pregnancy is a common symptom and one has to be very careful about the new-onset diagnosis of asthma.

Assessment and Monitoring

Basic assessment includes assessment of severity and possible risk of aggravation. A minimum of once-a-month visit is required. Correct inhaler technique and adherence should be confirmed. The target peak expiratory flow rate (PEFR) should be between 380 and 550 L/min or 80–100% of personal best. Blood eosinophil counts and exhaled nitric oxide (FeNO) test are other useful tests to monitor control.

There is a higher incidence of early onset asthma in children born to mothers with uncontrolled asthma. Vitamin D levels also need to be monitored in asthmatic women since low maternal levels are associated with childhood asthma in babies and supplementation may provide protection.[16]

Management of Asthma

Although there is a general concern regarding the use of medicines during pregnancy, the advantages of actively treating asthma clearly outweigh any risks (Level A).[17,18] The goals of management of asthma are (1) good symptom control, (2) to minimize the risk of acute attacks, (3) to prevent irreversible damage to lungs, (4) to maintain normal activity, (5) and to avoid drug-related side effects on mother and baby. A written asthma control plan should be prescribed for every patient so as to avoid any delays in treatment. There is no restriction of normal physical activity.

Pharmacological Management

Asthma during pregnancy is managed similar to that in the nonpregnant state. Most of the antiasthma drugs are generally safe **(Table 1)**. The main difference is that the control assessment is done every month instead of 3 months and no step-down is attempted to avoid the risk of acute exacerbations. Step-up treatment is done in case of worsening of symptoms. There is no increased risk with the use of ICS, beta-2 agonists, montelukast, and theophylline. Anti-immunoglobulin E (IgE) monoclonal antibodies and specific immunotherapy should not be initiated during pregnancy.[16-18] Inhaled glucocorticoids remain the mainstay of treatments and reduce the incidence of acute attacks. The side effects of uncontrolled asthma are more severe than those of drugs for both the mother and the baby. Avoidance of triggers and early treatment of acute exacerbations remain the priority.

Education

All pregnant asthmatic women need guidance and education regarding the importance of asthma control medicines in appropriate doses and with the correct technique. Most women need reassurance regarding safety of medicines for the baby. They also need guidance on avoiding triggers and recognizing early warning signs. Some home management practical tips for self-management and titration of ICS should be given. Infections, especially viral infections, are most common triggers and every effort should be made to avoid these. Asthmatics are strongly recommended vaccination against influenza. They are also advised to control comorbidities like rhinitis, obesity, and sleep disorders.

Managing Acute Attack of Asthma

Asthma may worsen in 8%, 47%, and 65% in mild, moderate, or severe disease, respectively, during pregnancy, most commonly in the second trimester. Major triggers are viral infections and avoidance of controlling medicines by the patient. Worsening of symptoms, requirement of increased dose of controlling medicines, or worsening PEF are indicative of an acute attack. The management of an acute attack remains the same as in the nonpregnant state. Hospitalization should be done early if there is any indication of hypoxia or if symptoms are not relieved. These patients may require OCS or intravenous therapy for relief.

TABLE 1: Common medicines used for asthma during pregnancy and their safety.

Group	Drug	Pregnancy safety category
Inhaled glucocorticoids (ICS)	Budesonide, beclomethasone, fluticasone, ciclesonide, mometasone	• A and B • Placenta can metabolize; usually does not affect baby
Oral corticosteroids (OCS)	Prednisolone and methyl prednisolone, hydrocortisone dexamethasone, and betamethasone	• A and C • Majority drug does not cross placental barrier • Dexa and beta methasone not recommended as cross placental barrier
Beta-2 agonists	All categories	• Suitable for all stages of pregnancy • Safe
Short-acting beta-2-agonist (SABA)	Salbutamol, terbutaline, and pirbuterol	Safe
Long-acting beta-2-agonist (LABA)	Salmeterol, formoterol	Safe but data less than for SABA
Ultra-LABAs	• Olodaterol • Vilanterol	• B and C • Possibly safe • No human data Animal data suggest low risk
Anticholinergics [short-acting muscarinic antagonists (SAMAs) and long-acting muscarinic antagonists (LAMAs)]	Ipratropium bromide, tiotropium bromide	• Possibly safe • Experience very less
Methylxanthines	Theophylline	A and C
	Aminophylline	A
Leukotriene receptor antagonists (LTRAs)	Zafirlukast and montelukast	Limited data but probably safe
5-Lipoxygenase pathway inhibitors	Zileuton	• Not recommended • No data
Anti-IgE monoclonal antibody	Omalizumab	B
Other monoclonal antibodies	• Benralizumab • Dupilumab • Mepolizumab • Reslizumab	Probably safe

Management during Labor

Majority of asthmatics undergo labor and delivery without acute exacerbation. They may require inhaled bronchodilators. Women on chronic oral steroids (more than 2 weeks) should be watched for any evidence for adrenal insufficiency. If suspected, injection hydrocortisone 100 mg 6–8 hourly can be given. Babies of women who have used high doses of short-acting beta-agonist (SABA) may need monitoring for hypoglycemia. There is no contraindication for use of oxytocin or prostaglandin E2. Prostaglandin F2 alpha and methyl ergometrine should not be used for prevention of postpartum hemorrhage (PPH) as these may trigger an acute attack. Narcotic analgesics like morphine or meperidine should be avoided, but fentanyl is not contraindicated. Adequate pain relief by epidural labor analgesia is recommended.

For operative delivery, epidural rather than general anesthesia should be used. In women with severe asthma, there could be a higher risk of respiratory failure as hyperventilation, pain, and anxiety act as triggers. These women need close monitoring of oxygen saturation and expert care by the pulmonologist. The decision for operative delivery is entirely dependent on obstetric indications. The second stage of labor should be cut short to reduce expulsive efforts. Maintenance of hydration, blood sugars, and oxygen saturation is of utmost importance. The women should be closely monitored for at least 24 hours for any possible exacerbation after delivery which may be triggered by sudden hemodynamic changes during delivery or anesthesia.

Breastfeeding

Most women are able to breastfeed the baby without any problems. The medications used for asthma control also do not have any side effects for the breastfed babies.

Cystic Fibrosis and Bronchiectasis

Women with CF who live up to adulthood wish to enjoy motherhood. These women need careful prepregnancy evaluation and counseling in addition to multidisciplinary specialist care during and after pregnancy.[19]

Prepregnancy Considerations

There is a higher incidence of subfertility (35%) in women with CF. The pregnancy rate in these women is improving. The options of intrauterine insemination (IUI) and in vitro fertilization (IVF-ET) can also be given. In case of IVF, single-embryo transfer should be done to avoid risk of multiple pregnancy. Males affected with CF also have congenital absence of vas deference (CABVD). The children of women with CF (homozygous) are obligatory carriers of *CFTR* mutation. The partner of a CF woman also needs to be tested. If the partner is also a carrier of *CFTR* mutation, genetic counseling is required. The options of preimplantation genetic testing or ovum donation or surrogacy need to be discussed to avoid the birth of affected children (50% chance). Women, who are doing well on mucolytic therapy, have good nutrition status and need advice on contraception.

Prepregnancy Evaluation for Health Risks

Pregnancy and neonatal complications depend upon health status at the time of conception.

Severely compromised lung function [percent predicted FEV1 (ppFEV1) < 50–60%] and PAH constitute absolute contraindications to pregnancy because of a very high risk of maternal mortality.[20] Severe maternal morbidity consequent to destabilization of disease and fetal morbidity because of low birth weight and prematurity are also higher. Colonization of lungs with bacteria constitutes a major risk. Poor control of CF-related diabetes is another factor which affects maternal and perinatal outcome.

Women with CF often suffer from nutritional deficiencies. Good body mass index (BMI) at the start of pregnancy is associated with good maternal and fetal outcome and also indicates a better prognosis phenotype and pulmonary status. Aggressive nutritional intervention with adequate calories, proteins, and fat supplements along with vitamins and mineral should be done.

Risk of Long-term Deterioration of CF

Pregnancy does not alter the course of CF in women. The deterioration in lung functions and survival is similar to women who did not conceive. These women are likely to belong to a better prognosis group. Experience is very limited about the prognosis in women with severe disease.

Considerations during Pregnancy

The major reason for improvement in survival of CF patients is the use of medicines. Inhaled antibiotics (Tobramycin, Aztreonam, Colistin, Levofloxacin) and mucolytic agents (dornase alfa and hypertonic saline) have very little systemic absorption. Oral pancreatic and fat-soluble vitamin supplementation is also very safe in therapeutic doses. Chronic administration of oral azithromycin is the cornerstone of treatment and has proven safety. CFTR modulators (ivacaftor, ezacaftor/ivacaftor, lumacaftor/ivacaftor, elexacaftor/tezacaftor/ivacaftor) are the newer category of drugs about which the safety data does not exist. However, animal studies indicate safety. Few reports in humans also indicate no major incidence of congenital malformations.[16]

The harm of discontinuation of therapy far outweighs any risk to the baby and all treatments have to be continued during pregnancy. For the management of diabetes, insulin is the first-line treatment with close monitoring of sugars and dietary therapy. These women need to be monitored more closely with more frequent visits. The third stage of labor after delivery of the placenta is the period of maximum risk. The cardiorespiratory function has to be very closely monitored because of the risk of autotransfusion of nearly 300–500 mL of blood from placental circulation. Cesarean delivery is done only for obstetric indications and epidural analgesia is preferred for pain relief. To prevent thrombotic complications, early mobilization, chest physiotherapy and deep vein thrombosis prophylaxis are indicated. There is no contraindication for lactation; most drugs are secreted in breast milk in subtherapeutic doses.

Maternal and Fetal Outcome

The risk of serious morbidity and mortality can be minimized with expert care, and outlook has improved in recent years. The incidence of maternal deaths is higher in CF cases, especially with significant lung damage. The infants are more likely to have low birth weight, prematurity, and slightly higher risk of congenital malformation (14.3%), particularly cardiac anomalies (3.9%).[21]

Pulmonary Arterial Hypertension

Pulmonary arterial hypertension is a rare debilitating disorder with poor prognosis and limited life expectancy. The disease is more common in young females. Many therapeutic modalities have evolved in recent years leading to improved survival and quality of life and so has the demand for childbearing. There is a universal agreement that the disease is an absolute contraindication for pregnancy because of the high mortality of nearly 36% which has recently been reported to decline to still unacceptable 12%. In addition to the mother, there is a risk to the baby also which is mainly because of prematurity.[21] A higher risk of congenital malformations has also been reported. Despite this knowledge, some women will still opt to take a risk and choose to become pregnant and choose to continue with pregnancy.

The etiology of PAH is related to cardiac lesions, lung conditions, thrombotic phenomenon, hereditary, idiopathic, and many other miscellaneous causes. Genetic diagnosis and counseling are required in women suspected to having hereditary PAH. During pregnancy, there are major changes in respiratory and cardiovascular physiology. The blood volume, heart rate, and cardiac output increase by 40–50%. There is a higher risk of thromboembolism because of a hypercoagulable state. The right heart can easily decompensate because of the compromised vascular bed. During labor and delivery, there is a more pronounced sudden shift in blood volume from placental circulation to maternal circulation. Common reasons for mortality are right heart failure, cardiac arrest, cardiac arrhythmias, pulmonary hypertension crisis, thromboembolism, preeclampsia, and sepsis.[22]

Women should be advised to use contraception to avoid pregnancy. Permanent surgical sterilization can be done and there is no contraindication for emergency contraception. If patient does conceive, it is a clear indication for medical termination of pregnancy (MTP). Planned surgical method under controlled conditions is preferred over medical methods. If a patient decides to continue, then appropriate counseling regarding risks, treatment modalities, pregnancy, and labor care should be done. These pregnancies have to be very closely monitored by a multidisciplinary team having a pulmonologist, cardiologist, and high-risk obstetric care expert. The pregnancy and delivery should be supervised in a well-equipped center with cardiac and pulmonary critical care units.

Of the newer PAH-specific drugs, the endothelin receptor antagonists and Riociguat are contraindicated during pregnancy. Low-molecular-weight heparin should be given prophylactically during pregnancy and postpartum period. In worse situations, intensive care support or even extracorporeal membrane oxygenation may be life saving for some women. Venous thromboembolism and amniotic fluid embolism (AFE) may cause acute PAH and need to be managed by thrombolysis or thrombectomy. Both these conditions are at high risk for mortality.

The long-term impact of pregnancy on the course of PAH is not clear at the moment. Patients willing to build their families can be given the choice of adoption or surrogacy which are much safer for the mother. The future appears better for these patients. More experience with newer modalities of treatment and improved survival will widen the horizon for these patients.

Critical Care in Obstetric Patients

Most healthy women can undergo the physiological changes in respiratory and circulatory systems which are required to accommodate the increased demands of growing fetus and pregnancy. There are certain conditions specific to pregnancy which may unexpectedly appear or there may be underlying pulmonary or other health conditions which may destabilize and require intensive care **(Table 2)**. The intensivist has to be well conversant with the fundamental knowledge of physiological adaptation of pregnancy, specific aspects of obstetric care, and critical care in obstetric patients.[23]

TABLE 2: Common conditions requiring critical care in pregnancy.

Medical problem	Pregnancy-related precipitating factors
Acute respiratory distress syndrome	Chorioamnionitis, sepsis, placental abruption
Pulmonary edema	Preeclampsia, tocolytics induced, fluid overload, severe edema
Acute lung injury	Gastric acid aspiration, transfusion-related acute lung injury
Embolism	Amniotic fluid, venous embolism, trophoblastic embolism
Heart conditions	Peripartum cardiomyopathy, underlying stenotic heart disease
Underlying diseased lung	Asthma, pulmonary arterial hypertension, cystic fibrosis, severely damaged lungs
Acute pneumonia	Bacterial, viral, fungal, others
Miscellaneous	Drugs, toxins, trauma, pancreatitis

Postpartum Hemorrhage

Postpartum hemorrhage can be defined as blood loss of >1,000 mL at the time of delivery. It is the leading cause of maternal mortality and morbidity. The common etiologies include atonic PPH, traumatic PPH, and coagulation disorders. The treatment remains that of the cause. Massive hemorrhage and blood replacement itself may trigger disseminated intravascular coagulation (DIC). The patient can go into hypovolemic shock or suffer from fluid overload due to replacement with too much inotropes. There is a need to monitor fluid replacement under central line monitoring and maintenance of renal and cardiac function. Oxygen or ventilatory support may be required. The patient is at risk of developing multiorgan failure, ARDS, and sepsis. The management of these conditions remains as that in nonpregnant state except that one has to take into consideration certain changes which may occur in the postpartum period, e.g., fluid shift from third space, lactation, and risk of deep vein thrombosis.

Hypertensive Emergencies, Preeclampsia, and Eclampsia

Hypertensive emergencies are second in frequency requiring intensive care unit (ICU) admissions and also a cause of maternal mortality worldwide. Preeclampsia is defined if blood pressure is >140/90 mm Hg at >20 weeks' pregnancy with proteinuria and pedal edema. Blood pressure > 160/110 mm Hg defines severe preeclampsia. If accompanied by convulsions, it is labeled eclampsia. The main pathophysiological changes are intravascular volume restriction and creation of third space. For this reason, these patients tolerate blood loss very poorly. There should be a lower threshold for blood transfusion in these patients. If required, diuretics should only be given after ensuring adequate intravascular volume expansion. The initial drug of choice for hypertension is labetalol, hydralazine, or nifedipine. For imminent eclampsia and eclampsia, anticonvulsive therapy with magnesium sulfate is the first-line treatment. In resistant cases, other anticonvulsants can be used. The specific treatment is termination of pregnancy. Steroid prophylaxis is given for fetal lung maturity in preterm cases. The patient requires management for hypertension, coagulation disorders, maintenance of critical blood volume, and perfusion of vital organs.[24] Patients with severe respiratory, cardiovascular, renal, or central nervous system (CNS) complications need to be cared in a critical care setup and multidisciplinary team. They may require ventilator support or even extracorporeal membrane oxygenation (ECMO).

Amniotic Fluid Embolism

Amniotic fluid embolism (AFE) is a very rare entity but a dreaded complication with a mortality rate of 20–60%. The underlying mechanisms include emboli of amniotic fluid entering in maternal circulation resulting in an anaphylactoid reaction most commonly occurring during labor or delivery. There is sudden dyspnea/hypoxia followed by cardiovascular collapse, altered sensations, seizures, and severe coagulopathy. Treatment includes supportive, blood replacement, and tranexamic acid.

Peripartum Cardiomyopathy

Peripartum cardiomyopathy is defined as left ventricular systolic dysfunction (ejection fraction < 45%) in the absence of any known heart condition, usually at the end of pregnancy or after delivery.[25]

Older and hypertensive women are at a higher risk. Echocardiography is the only diagnostic test. Management is of heart failure with diuretics, beta blockers, and sometimes inotropes are required. Anticoagulation is recommended to prevent thromboembolic complications. In severe cases, mechanical ventilation or ECMO support may be required.

Pulmonary Embolism

During pregnancy, there is venous stasis, hypercoagulability, and vascular injury which is an ideal combination for thromboembolic phenomenon. Pulmonary embolism (PE) is reported to occur in about 0.6–2 per 1,000 deliveries. PE is a leading cause of maternal mortality. Massive and submassive PE needs aggressive management. Treatment with anticoagulants, thrombectomy, and thrombolysis and support with ECMO may be required.

Pulmonary Edema

Preexisting heart disease is an important predisposition for pulmonary edema, the highest risk at the time of delivery or early postpartum period due to massive shift of fluid in the intravascular compartment. Other causes include peripartum cardiomyopathy, severe preeclampsia or fluid overload for replacement, tocolysis with B2 agonists, or tocolysis with calcium channel blockers.

Acute Respiratory Distress Syndrome

Pregnant women are at risk of developing ARDS in cases of increased circulating blood volume, reduced serum albumin levels, infections, or gastric content aspiration. Transfusion-related acute lung injury (TRALI) is related to blood component therapy. Management is similar to that of any nonpregnant patient. Good recovery can be anticipated with appropriate management since the patients are young and usually without underlying comorbidities.

Chronic Restrictive Lung Disease[26]

Interstitial lung diseases (ILD) such as lymphangioleiomyomatosis and systemic lupus erythematosus (SLE) may be uncommonly encountered during pregnancy. Women with ILD may suffer from hypoxemia and may be unable to meet the increased oxygen demands of pregnancy. Similarly, women with chest wall deformities (e.g., kyphoscoliosis, neuromuscular weakness, marked obesity) are at high risk. Although the lungs may be healthy, there may be marked reduction in lung volumes. Successful pregnancies have been described with even severe reduction in vital capacity of up to 40%. These women require a detailed prepregnancy risk assessment, counseling, and close monitoring during pregnancy. Pregnancy is contraindicated if there is associated PAH. Respiratory decompensation is most likely to occur near-term, during delivery and the postpartum phase.

SUMMARY

The presence of a respiratory disease during pregnancy is likely to present a complex picture with increased risks to both the mother and the fetus. The general diagnostic and therapeutic principles remain similar to those in the nonpregnant state. Whether to continue or to terminate pregnancy requires critical assessment made jointly by the pulmonary physician and the obstetrician in consultation with the patient and her family.

REFERENCES

1. Hegewald MJ, Crapo RO. Respiratory physiology in pregnancy. Clin Chest Med. 2011;32(1):1-13.
2. Burri PH. Fetal and Postnatal Development of the Lung. Annu Rev Physiol. 1984;46:617-28.
3. Britt RD Jr, Faksh A, Vogel E, et al. Perinatal factors in neonatal and pediatric lung diseases. Expert Rev Respir Med. 2013;7(5):515-31.

4. Mackin DW, Walker SP. The historical aspects of vaccination in pregnancy. Best Pract Res Clin Obstet Gynaecol. 2021;76:13-22.
5. Bonhoeffer J, Kochhar S, Hirschfeld S, et al.; GAIA project participants. Global alignment of immunization safety assessment in pregnancy—The GAIA project. Vaccine. 2016;34(49): 5993-7.
6. Arora M, Lakshmi R. Vaccines-safety in pregnancy. Best Pract Res Clin Obstet Gynaecol. 2021;76:23-40.
7. Lim WS, Macfarlane JT, Colthorpe CL. Treatment of Community-Acquired Lower Respiratory Tract Infections during Pregnancy. Am J Respir Med. 2003;2(3):221-33.
8. Benedetti TJ, Valle R, Ledger WJ. Antepartum pneumonia in pregnancy. Am J Obstet Gynecol. 1982;144:413-7.
9. Richey SD, Roberts SW, Ramin KD, et al. Pneumonia complicating pregnancy. Obstet Gynecol. 1994;84:525-8.
10. Brito V, Niederman MS. Pneumonia complicating pregnancy. Clin Chest Med. 2011;32(1):121-32.
11. Engelhardt T, Webster NR. Pulmonary aspiration of gastric contents in anaesthesia. Br J Anaesth. 1999;83:453-60.
12. Khan S, Niederman MS. Pneumonia in the pregnant patient. In: Rosene-Montela K, Bourjeily G (Eds). Pulmonary Problems in Pregnancy. New York: Humana Press; 2009. p. 177-96.
13. Haake DA, Zakowski PC, Haake DL, et al. Early treatment with acyclovir for varicella pneumonia in otherwise healthy adults: retrospective controlled study and review. Rev Infect Dis. 1990;12:788-98.
14. Wang H, Li N, Huang H. Asthma in Pregnancy: Pathophysiology, Diagnosis, Whole-Course Management, and Medication Safety. Can Respir J. 2020;2020:9046842.
15. Grosso A, Locatelli F, Gini E, et al. The course of asthma during pregnancy in a recent, multicase-control study on respiratory health. Allergy Asthma Clin Immunol. 2018;14:16.
16. Middleton PG, Gade EJ, Aguilera C, et al. ERS/TSANZ Task Force Statement on the management of reproduction and pregnancy in women with airways diseases. Eur Respir J. 2020;55:1901208.
17. Levy ML, Bacharier LB, Bateman E, et al. Key recommendations for primary care from the 2022 Global Initiative for Asthma (GINA) update. NPJ Prim Care Respir Med. 2023;33(1):7.
18. Global Initiative for Asthma. (2023). 2023 GINA Report, Global Strategy for Asthma Management and Prevention[online] Available from www.ginasthma.org [Last accessed September, 2024].
19. Jain R, Kazmerski TM, Zuckerwise LC, et al. Pregnancy in cystic fibrosis: Review of the literature and expert recommendations. J Cyst Fibros. 2022;21(3):387-95.
20. Sliwa K, van Hagen IM, Budts W, et al. Pulmonary hypertension and pregnancy outcomes: data from the registry of pregnancy and cardiac disease (ROPAC) of the European Society of Cardiology. Eur J Heart Fail. 2016;18(9):1119-28.
21. Jelin AC, Sharshiner R, Caughey AB. Maternal co-morbidities and neonatal outcomes associated with cystic fibrosis. J Matern Fetal Neonatal Med. 2017;30(1):4-7.
22. Barańska-Pawełczak K, Wojciechowska C, Jacheć W. Pregnancy in Patients with Pulmonary Arterial Hypertension in Light of New ESC Guidelines on Pulmonary Hypertension. Int J Environ Res Public Health. 2023;20(5):4625.
23. Lapinsky SE. Management of Acute Respiratory Failure in Pregnancy. Semin Respir Crit Care Med. 2017;38(2):201-7.
24. Gestational hypertension and preeclampsia. Obstet Gynecol 2020;135(6):e237-60.
25. Griffin KM, Oxford-Horrey C, Bourjeily G. Obstetric Disorders and Critical Illness. Clin Chest Med. 2022;43(3):471-88.
26. Lapinsky SE, Tram C, Mehta S, et al. Restrictive lung disease in pregnancy. Chest. 2014;145:394-8.

Respiratory Drugs during Pregnancy

CHAPTER 140

Manishi Mittal

INTRODUCTION

Pulmonary disorders can affect pregnant women with an incidence proportional to that of the general population within the same age group. Managing common conditions during pregnancy largely mirrors their treatment in non-pregnant individuals. However, it is crucial to recognize that the pharmacokinetics of drugs used in these cases can be influenced by the physiological changes that occur during pregnancy. A steady rise in renal function and volume of distribution during pregnancy can lead to low concentration of drug in maternal circulation. Additionally, the fall in protein binding leads to higher free fraction of drug.

SAFETY CONCERNS

Drugs used in the periconceptional period may have no effect or lead to early miscarriage or biochemical pregnancy. A primary concern when using drugs during pregnancy is the risk of teratogenicity. Teratogenesis can occur when drugs are used during the period of organogenesis, which spans from the third to the eighth week of gestation when the embryo undergoes significant cellular growth and differentiation. Teratogenic effect depends on fetal genetic composition, time and duration of exposure, and concentration of the drug or metabolites. Drugs given later in pregnancy can affect the development and functioning of morphologically normal fetal organs; for example, use of nonsteroidal anti-inflammatory drugs (NSAIDs) in the third trimester can lead to oligohydramnios and patent ductus arteriosus in the fetus.[1]

Given these considerations, it is advisable to use drugs during pregnancy that have a well-established history of use and safety data. Drugs that have been labeled as safe after extensive large cohort studies or meta-analyses are preferred choices. Moreover, drugs should only be administered for specific indications, at the minimum effective dose, and for the shortest necessary duration to minimize fetal exposure. To aid in drug selection, various classification systems are available.

The Food and Drug Administration (FDA) of the USA earlier employed a labeling system categorizing drugs based on their safety during pregnancy **(Table 1)**. In 2015, the FDA introduced the Pregnancy and Lactation Labeling Rule. This rule mandates that prescribing information for drugs includes a narrative summary of both animal and human gestational safety data, as well as clinical considerations. Nonetheless, the previous FDA classification remains a valuable starting point for prescribing clinicians. Notably, the majority of drugs used for pulmonary disorders was typically categorized as either class B or class C, indicating that they are considered safe for use during pregnancy.

During lactation, drugs cannot affect organogenesis, but they are secreted in breast milk; therefore, they can lead to neonatal sedation, hyperactivity, jaundice, and hematologic or respiratory disorders. The WHO has classified drugs according to their safety during lactation **(Table 2)**.[2]

TABLE 1: FDA classification of teratogenicity of drugs.

Category	Characteristics
A	Adequate, well-controlled studies in pregnant women, have failed to demonstrate fetal risk
B	No evidence of risk in humans: • Animal studies show risk but human studies do not • No human studies available but animal studies show no risk
C	Risk cannot be ruled out. Potential benefit may outweigh potential risk: • Human studies are not available and animal studies not available or show risk
D	Positive evidence of risk. Investigation or postmarketing data show risk to the fetus. Still, potential benefit may outweigh potential risk
X	Contraindicated in pregnancy. Human or animal studies or investigation and postmarketing data show fetal risk that clearly outweighs any potential benefit

(FDA: Food and Drug Administration)

TABLE 2: WHO classification of drug use during breastfeeding.

Category	Characteristics
Compatible with breastfeeding	• No known or theoretical contraindications for drug use • Considered safe for the mother to take the drug and continue to breastfeed
Compatible with breastfeeding. Monitor infant for side effects	Drugs could theoretically cause side effects in the infant but either have not been observed to do so or have only occasionally caused mild side effects
Avoid if possible. Monitor infant for side effects	• Drugs that have been reported to cause side effects in the infant • Use these drugs only when they are really essential for the mother's treatment and when no safer alternative is available
Avoid if possible. May inhibit lactation	• Drugs that may reduce breast milk production • Decrease can be prevented by frequent suckling
Avoid	• Drugs with dangerous side effects on the baby • Breastfeeding to be completely avoided when these drugs are given

(WHO: World Health Organization)

Medications used for Upper Respiratory Tract Disorders (Table 3)

Antihistamines

Antihistamines, or specific H1 receptor antagonists, represent the primary line of treatment for upper respiratory tract disorders such as allergic rhinitis and the common cold. Both first-generation (e.g., brompheniramine, clemastine, chlorpheniramine, diphenhydramine, and triprolidine) and second- or third-generation (e.g., loratadine, cetirizine, fexofenadine, levocetirizine, desloratadine, astemizole, terfenadine, ebastine, and rupatadine) antihistamines are generally considered safe for use during pregnancy.[3] While isolated reports of teratogenicity exist, comprehensive retrospective studies have not established any association between first trimester use of antihistamines and congenital anomalies.[4] A meta-analysis of 24 studies, encompassing over 200,000 first-trimester exposures to various antihistamines, did not identify any teratogenic risks.[5]

First-generation antihistamines such as chlorpheniramine are often preferred during pregnancy due to their long history of use with no significant adverse effects. In cases where sedation or anticholinergic side effects become problematic for the pregnant woman, second-generation agents can be considered. Drugs such as loratadine, cetirizine, and fexofenadine have been widely used with demonstrated safety during pregnancy.[6] Many clinicians favor loratadine, primarily because it does not induce sedation.

Antihistamine nasal sprays such as azelastine and olopatadine have reassuring data in animal studies, but data in human pregnancy is not available. Given their negligible systemic absorption, these nasal sprays can be cautiously used under close observation.[7] Newer agents such as acrivastine and mizolastine have not been adequately studied. Regarding ebastine, animal studies have not discovered any teratogenicity, but human studies are awaited.[8] Phenothiazines, such as promethazine, are typically prescribed for nausea and vomiting during pregnancy. They are considered to have a low teratogenic potential but may induce extrapyramidal side effects, which are usually self-limiting, in both the mother and newborn, particularly when used in the last trimester.

The use of antihistamines during breastfeeding is generally discouraged, as most of these drugs are excreted into breast milk in small amounts. Exposure to these drugs in infants may result in irritability, tachycardia, feeding refusal, and, rarely, convulsions, especially in premature infants. Nevertheless, it remains unclear what dose and duration of exposure may lead to these issues. Additionally, the anticholinergic properties of antihistamines can potentially decrease breast milk production. Dexbrompheniramine and triprolidine are considered safer choices during lactation.[9]

Decongestants

Oral or nasal decongestants such as Oxymetazoline and Xylometazoline, commonly used for nasal congestive symptoms in upper respiratory tract infections (URTIs), are sympathomimetics that stimulate alpha-1-adrenergic receptor leading to vasoconstriction of small vessels in the nose, throat, and paranasal sinuses. Even though the drugs are used locally, there is systemic absorption through the nasal vessels. The degree to which they are absorbed and cross the placenta is not defined.

Use of intranasal decongestants in the first trimester was associated with pyloric stenosis, while use of oxymetazoline in the second trimester was associated with renal collecting system abnormalities.[10] Other studies showed no teratogenic effects of use of xylometazoline and oxymetazoline in the first trimester.[11] Still, these drugs should be avoided in the first trimester. In addition, the risk of rebound with overuse of these drugs should be explained to the patients.

Oral decongestants such as pseudoephedrine (banned in India), phenyl propanolamine, and phenylephrine are used as part of combinations for symptomatic relief in URTI. Their use should be curtailed, especially in the first trimester. Though it is not known whether these drugs can cross the placenta, their vasoconstrictive action can act on uterine vessels (which selectively express alpha-1-adrenergic receptors), leading to hypoxia-induced oxidative stress, which can affect the fetus. The dose at which this effect is seen is more than the therapeutic dose.[12] Still, they should not be used in women with hypertension and placental disorders.

Pseudoephedrine has been linked with limb reduction defects in a few studies, though seen more often when used

TABLE 3: Safety of drugs used for upper respiratory tract disorders.

Drug	Safety in first trimester	Safety in second and third trimesters	Safety in breastfeeding	Special considerations
Antihistamines				
First generation: • Brompheniramine • Chlorpheniramine • Clemastine • Diphenhydramine • Triprolidine	Safe	Safe	May cause irritability, tachycardia, refusal to feed in infant. May decrease milk production	Chlorpheniramine preferred as proven safe over many years of experience
Second generation: • Loratadine • Cetirizine • Astemizole • Terfenadine • Ebastine • Rupatadine	Safe	Safe	May cause irritability, tachycardia, refusal to feed in infant. May decrease milk production	Loratadine and cetirizine are most commonly used in pregnancy, hence preferred
Third generation: • Desloratadine • Fexofenadine • Levocetirizine	Safe	Safe	Less likely to cause CNS side effects	
Decongestants				
Intranasal spray: • Oxymetazoline • Xylometazoline	Possibly safe but should be avoided	Safe	Safe	Risk or rebound with overuse
Oral: • Pseudoephedrine • Phenylpropanolamine • Phenylephrine	Possibly safe but should be avoided	Safe	Safe	Vasoconstrictive effect on uterine blood vessels, so should be avoided in women with hypertension or placental disorders
Corticosteroids				
Intranasal: • Budesonide • Ciclesonide • Fluticasone • Mometasone	Safe	Safe	Safe	Budesonide is the agent of choice. Preparations should be used in low dose as there is significant systemic absorption
Antitussives				
Dextromethorphan	Safe	Safe	Safe	
Benzonatate	Possibly safe	Safe	Safe	
Expectorants: • Guaifenesin • Bromhexine • Ambroxol	Possibly safe but should be avoided	Possibly safe but should be avoided	Possibly safe but should be avoided	Iodine-containing agents contraindicated
Analgesics				
Paracetamol	Safe	Safe	Safe	Excessive use should be avoided as it has been linked to neurodevelopmental, reproductive, and urogenital disorders in the fetus
NSAIDs	Contraindicated	Contraindicated	Contraindicated	
Mast cell stabilizers				
• Sodium cromoglycate • Lodoxamide	Safe	Safe	Safe	

(CNS: central nervous system; NSAIDs: nonsteroidal anti-inflammatory drugs)

in combination with acetaminophen.[10] Use of pseudoephedrine and phenylpropanolamine was linked to gastroschisis in few studies.[13] On the other hand, a large prospective study on pregnant women who used decongestants (mainly phenylpropanolamine or pseudoephedrine) did not report any teratogenic effects.[14] Phenylephrine is less effective for treatment of nasal congestion and may cause significant reduction of uterine blood flow. Moreover, there have been reports of endocardial cushion defect with use of phenylephrine in pregnancy.[10] Pseudoephedrine is secreted into breast milk, though considered as safe to use during lactation.[9] Data on other decongestants is not available.

Intranasal Corticosteroids

Glucocorticoid nasal sprays are quite safe and useful during pregnancy, considered treatment of choice in moderate-to-severe rhinitis. Studies have not shown any adverse effects or malformations with use of intranasal corticosteroids such as budesonide, fluticasone, and mometasone during pregnancy in any trimester.[15] Inhalational steroids have been exhaustively studied for use in asthma during pregnancy, and this reassuring data can be extrapolated to intranasal steroids for allergic rhinitis. There are few reports of use of triamcinolone leading to respiratory system abnormalities in the fetus, but association is not clearly established.[16] Intranasal budesonide is preferred as first choice for use during pregnancy.[4] It should be kept in mind that there is significant systemic absorption of corticosteroids used in conventional dosage. Hence, they should be given in the lowest possible dose.[17]

Antitussives

Cough can be quite debilitating and troublesome during pregnancy. A variety of home remedies and combinations are used for cough relief. Several honey-based cough syrups are available in the market whose safety in pregnancy has not been studied. Though no obvious congenital malformations have been noted with their use, minor anomalies or growth defects cannot be ruled out.

Of the other drugs available, dextromethorphan which is the methyl ether of d-isomer of levorphanol, an opiate analgesic, is the most commonly used cough suppressant. Data regarding its use in pregnancy is reassuring, showing no teratogenic effects, even when used in the first trimester.[18] Cough syrups containing codeine are less frequently available and not recommended in pregnancy as codeine use may lead to respiratory depression and withdrawal symptoms in the neonate.[19] It is also excreted in breast milk in small amounts. Benzonatate is considered safe during pregnancy as well as lactation.[19] Levocloperastine has not shown any teratogenic effects in animal studies. Still, caution is advised regarding its use in pregnancy and lactation, as it is known to cross the placental barrier.[20]

Among expectorants, guaifenesin, ambroxol and bromhexine are commonly used to treat productive cough. Use of guaifenesin and bromhexine has not been associated with any teratogenic effects.[21] Ambroxol is labeled as category C. Iodines such as potassium iodide and iodinated glycerol are expectorants, which are no more used in cough syrups, are contraindicated in pregnancy. Iodides used for long duration have been seen to cause large fetal goiters, tracheal obstruction, congenital hypothyroidism, and even fetal death.[22] Iodides also result in a higher iodine level in breast milk.

Analgesics

Analgesics are the second most common drugs used during pregnancy after vitamins. Paracetamol, ibuprofen, and acetylsalicylic acid are the most frequently used analgesics, alone or in combination. Paracetamol has been for long labeled as the safest analgesic in pregnancy. However, indiscriminate use of this drug should be avoided. Paracetamol is an endocrine disruptor and its use during pregnancy can cause particular neurodevelopmental, reproductive and urogenital disorders in the fetus.[23] Therefore, it should be used for a short time, in minimum dose.

Paracetamol, aspirin, and ibuprofen are weak acids and lipid soluble; therefore, they can cross the placenta.[24] Ibuprofen, naproxen, indomethacin, and diclofenac are potent, nonselective inhibitors of the enzyme cyclo-oxygenase. In the fetus, cyclo-oxygenase causes dilatation of the ductus arteriosus and pulmonary vessels. Therefore, its suppression by NSAIDS could cause premature closure of these vessels leading to pulmonary hypertension. Consequently, NSAIDs should not be used after 30 weeks of gestation.[25] Furthermore, use of NSAIDs in the last trimester can decrease fetal urine output due to hypoperfusion of fetal kidneys. This in turn causes oligohydramnios. Use of NSAIDs in the first trimester can lead to pregnancy loss due to downregulation of prostaglandin synthesis, affecting implantation.[26] This effect was not seen with paracetamol.

Topical NSAIDs are considered safe to use, but their absorption is increased with use over larger surface area and application of heat. Aspirin is rarely used for pain or fever but is commonly used for prevention of preeclampsia or management of thrombophilia and is not associated with teratogenicity.

Opioids such as codeine, oxycodone, hydromorphone, hydrocodone and morphine, pethidine, and tramadol are not associated with any congenital malformations. However, their chronic use can cause dependance and withdrawal symptoms in the neonate. During lactation, all NSAIDs are considered safe. Regarding paracetamol, only 6% of the maternal dose is excreted into the breast milk. This quantity is 0.65% and 1% for ibuprofen and diclofenac, respectively.[27]

Mast Cell Stabilizers

Mast cell stabilizers, such as sodium cromoglycate and lodoxamide, are categorized as FDA category B. Intranasal sodium cromoglycate is a preferred treatment for allergic rhinitis during pregnancy, and its use has not been linked to an increase in the incidence of congenital anomalies.[28]

It is minimally absorbed into systemic circulation when used locally. Its use is less preferred because of more frequent dosing requirement of up to six times daily. Moreover, its efficacy is less when compared to intranasal corticosteroids and decongestants.

Immunotherapy

Allergen immunotherapy is used in patients with chronic allergies. There are case reports of miscarriage with used of desensitization vaccines.[29] At the same time, few studies have shown the beneficial effect of immunotherapy on allergic rhinitis, without an adverse effect on the fetus.[30] Nonetheless, the risk of anaphylactic reaction cannot be ruled out.

In brief, allergic rhinitis during pregnancy should not be ignored as it may precipitate underlying asthma and worsen the pregnancy outcome. Avoidance of allergens such as house dust mites, pollens, and grasses should be stressed besides the use of effective and safe pharmacological agents.

Medications used for Lower Respiratory Tract Disorders

Bronchial Asthma (Table 4)

Most women have been seen to stop or decrease the dose of treatment as soon as they get pregnant, due to fear of fetal side effects and inadequate education about asthma. This leads to precipitation of severe events which is a major issue during pregnancy. Uncontrolled asthma can adversely affect the fetus, especially during a period of embryogenesis. A 50% rise in the incidence of congenital malformations has been recorded in women with uncontrolled asthma while use of medication is shown to decrease the incidence.[31,32] Moreover, it has been documented that active control of asthma helps to decrease chances of preterm labor and delivery.[33] Therefore, apt management of asthma is more important for fetal and maternal health, as compared to perceived risk of the drugs.

Pregnant women with asthma should be apprised of the risk of uncontrolled asthma to the fetus and the safety of medications used.[34] The management remains the same as in a nonpregnant state, with emphasis on maintenance of normal pulmonary function, control of symptoms, and prevention of exacerbation. Treatment should be individualized according to the patient's requirement. In general, inhalational treatment is preferred as it has negligible systemic adverse effects. However, if symptoms are not controlled, oral or parenteral medication should be added. Drugs used for asthma include anti-inflammatory medication, bronchodilators, and a recent addition, biologics.

Anti-inflammatory Medications

Corticosteroids

Glucocorticoids are the most potent and efficacious anti-inflammatory drugs presently available. They are available in inhalational, oral, and parenteral forms. Inhalational corticosteroids (ICS) are the most effective and convenient long-term therapy for asthma of any severity. Moreover, they have minimal adverse effects on the fetus because of low plasma concentration seen after systemic absorption. Systemic adverse effects are mostly seen if the dose requirement crosses 2,000 µg/day.[19] However, local reactions such as dysphonia and oral candidiasis may occur. Inhaled budesonide is the most widely used ICS during pregnancy with no reports of congenital anomalies or still births.[35,36]

If the patient is already taking another ICS, the same is continued, as changing may sometimes lead to loss of control. Other ICS such as flunisolide, fluticasone, and triamcinolone have also not shown teratogenicity or association with fetal growth restriction, preterm labor, or gestational hypertension. In higher doses though, these complications may be seen.[37] Moreover, the association with premature deliveries and fetal growth restriction can be blamed on the effects of asthma itself.[38] ICS may be continued during lactation, as the dose used is not seen to achieve a significant level in breast milk.[39]

Systemic corticosteroids such as short-acting prednisone, prednisolone, and methylprednisolone or long-acting agents (dexamethasone and betamethasone) are only used as a short-term measure for controlling uncontrolled persistent asthma, prior to starting long-term therapy and occasionally for long-term regulation of severe persistent asthma. Prednisone and prednisolone have been found in cord blood after systemic use in pregnant woman, but in 8–10 times lower concentration than in maternal blood.[40] On the other hand, fluorinated preparations such as dexamethasone and betamethasone are not much broken down in the placenta and can reach the fetus in greater quantity; therefore, they are beneficial for treating fetal diseases. On the other hand, prednisone and prednisolone are preferred for maternal problems.

Recent evidence has not shown any association between the use of systemic corticosteroids and congenital anomalies, even when used in the first trimester.[41] An increased risk of preterm delivery, low birth weight, gestational hypertension, preeclampsia, and gestational diabetes was found with the use of systemic steroids in pregnancy, but it may be due to an underlying maternal disease.[42] Pathological changes in the body can lead to bronchial muscle hyper-reactivity as well as vascular hyper-reactivity, hence predisposing asthma patients to hypertension and other complications.

Systemic corticosteroids are documented to result in cleft palate, internal hydrocephaly, and skeletal defects in some rodent studies, but there is no such association documented in human studies with their use in the first trimester or periconceptional period.[43] The current guidelines recommend that oral corticosteroids should be continued in case of severe asthma during pregnancy as their benefits outweigh the risks.[44]

In case a woman on corticosteroids during pregnancy undergoes prolonged labor or caesarean section, the stress

TABLE 4: Safety of drugs used in bronchial asthma.

Drugs	Safety in first trimester	Safety in second and third trimesters	Safety in lactation	Special considerations
Bronchodilators				
SABA: • Salbutamol • Terbutaline	Safe	Safe	Safe	• Salbutamol preferred • Systemic administration may cause cardiovascular and metabolic adverse effects
LABA: • Salmeterol • Formoterol	Safe	Safe	Safe	Salmeterol preferred
Ultra LABA: • Olodaterol • Vilanterol	Possibly safe	Possibly safe	Possibly safe	Human studies lacking
Theophylline	Safe	Safe	Safe	Blood levels should be monitored
Tiotropium bromide	Possibly safe	Possibly safe	Safe	Human studies lacking but may cause defects in higher doses
Anti-inflammatory medication				
• Inhalational corticosteroids • Budesonide • Beclomethasone • Fluticasone • Triamcinolone	Safe	Safe	Safe	Budesonide and beclomethasone preferred and most widely used
Inhalational corticosteroids: • Ciclesonide • Mometasone	Possibly safe	Possibly safe	Possibly safe	Human studies lacking
Systemic corticosteroids: • Prednisolone • Prednisone • Hydrocortisone	Possibly safe	Possibly safe	Possibly safe	Major benefit of systemic corticosteroids in severe asthma exceeds the possible fetal risk. It is advisable to delay breastfeeding for 3–4 hours after the dose to minimize transfer to breast milk
Leukotriene receptor antagonists				
Montelukast	Possibly safe	Safe	Safe	Can be used if asthma not controlled standard medication
Monoclonal antibodies				
• Omalizumab • Benralizumab • Dupilumab • Mepolizumab • Reslizumab	Possibly safe	Possibly safe	Possibly safe	Monoclonal antibodies cross the placenta, with transfer rising as pregnancy progresses; therefore, potential fetal adverse effects may be more in later pregnancy. More human studies required

(LABA: long-acting beta-2 agonist; SABA: short-acting beta-2 agonist)

dose of corticosteroids (intravenous 100 mg hydrocortisone sodium succinate 8 hourly) can be used in the peripartum period.[19] In addition, one should remain watchful for adrenal insufficiency in the neonate. Only 10% of prednisone and prednisolone are secreted into breast milk; therefore, they are considered safe during lactation.[21] For prolonged and high-dose treatment (>20 mg/day), a 4-hour gap between ingestion of drug and nursing can be given, as temporary loss of milk supply may occur.[45]

Mast Cell Stabilizers

Cromolyn sodium and nedocromil sodium are anti-inflammatory agents that can be used for prophylaxis before unavoidable exposure to known immune triggers. No adverse reactions have been reported during pregnancy.[46] When used as in inhalational form, less than 10% Cromolyn is absorbed systemically. Secretion in breast milk has not been assessed.

Leukotriene Modifiers

This group includes selective competitive inhibitors of leukotriene D4 (LTD4) and leukotriene E4 (LTE4) receptors, such as montelukast and zafirlukast, and 5-lipoxygenase inhibitors, such as zileuton. Montelukast has been widely used for treatment of allergic disorders and not found to be associated with an increased risk of congenital malformations.[47,48] Moreover, use of leukotriene modifiers does not increase chances of stillbirth, first-trimester miscarriage, preterm delivery, and low birth weight.[49,50] The American College of Obstetricians and Gynecologists (ACOG) and the American College of Allergy, Asthma and Immunology recommend use of Montelukast as an adjuvant for management of asthma during pregnancy, which is resistant to other treatment.[51] When used in standard dose during lactation, very low levels of these drugs are achieved in breast milk.[52] Zileuton is not advocated in pregnancy because of insufficient data regarding its use.

Bronchodilators

Beta-2-adrenergenic Agonists

Inhaled short-acting beta-2 agonists (SABAs), e.g., salbutamol (albuterol), are safe for managing acute bronchospasm. Inhaled forms of long-acting beta-2 agonists (LABA), such as salmeterol and formoterol, are used along with corticosteroids for chronic management of symptoms. Beta-2 agonists are especially useful for nocturnal symptoms and prevention of exercise-induced bronchospasm.

Salbutamol and other SABAs do not pose teratogenic risks. Even though a few case-control studies had shown a modest increase in the risk of anomalies such as cardiac defects, cleft lip, cleft palate, gastroschisis, esophageal atresia, and omphalocele,[53] recent evidence has refuted these observations.[54] Beta-2 agonists may cause symptoms in the fetus and mother consequent to cardiovascular and metabolic effects of these drugs, such as tremors, anxiety, inhibition of uterine contractions, fetal and maternal tachycardia, maternal hypotension, transient fetal and maternal hyperglycemia, and neonatal hypoglycemia. However, these effects are negligible with use of inhalational preparations. Moreover, there is no evidence of complications such as perinatal mortality, congenital malformations, preterm births, low-birth-weight infants, neonatal distress, peripartum problems, or postpartum hemorrhage.[55] In fact, beta-2 agonists are uterine relaxants; intravenous terbutaline and salbutamol had been used in the past to inhibit preterm labor. This action is not seen with inhaled preparations.[46] Metaproterenol and isoetharine have not been studied in pregnant women.

Available evidence does not associate LABAs with any congenital malformations or other pregnancy complications.[56] LABA can cause uterine relaxation when taken in the third trimester. Furthermore, beta mimetic effects such as tachycardia, tremors, and hypoglycemia may be seen in the newborn. When used along with ICS, their benefits outweigh the risks and should be continued if the patient was controlled on ICS–LABA combination prior to pregnancy. The National Institute of Health of USA has reiterated safety of beta-2 agonists for asthma in pregnancy.[57] Indacaterol and vilanterol are new ultra LABAs used once a day in combination with ICS. Animal studies have shown low chances of congenital malformations; hence, they are not preferred during pregnancy.

Epinephrine is a rapid-acting adrenergic agent which is avoided during pregnancy and is reserved for use in anaphylaxis. Subcutaneous terbutaline is sometimes used for acute exacerbation of asthma during pregnancy.

Methylxanthines

Methylxanthines are purine derivatives that have bronchodilatory action. Theophylline can be used as a long-acting sustained-release oral preparation for nocturnal asthma. It is also used as intravenous preparation (aminophylline) for control of acute episodes. Theophylline has a narrow therapeutic window with high interpersonal variability of dose requirement. Due to liver metabolism, serum levels are affected by various physiological conditions such as pregnancy. Use of theophylline during pregnancy is restricted because of the risk of toxicity and drug interactions (like with beta agonists). Severe effects are seen after serum levels cross 20 μg/mL; therefore, if used during pregnancy, theophylline levels should be assessed regularly and maintained between 10 and 20 μg/mL.[58] It may exacerbate nausea, reflux, and vomiting of pregnancy. Regarding fetal effects, it is not associated with still births or birth defects,[59] but increased fetal respiratory movements may be seen in mothers taking theophylline.[60] Newborns of mothers with high serum theophylline concentration may experience temporary toxicity in the form of vomiting, tachycardia, and jitteriness.[61]

Anticholinergics

Ipratropium and tiotropium are anticholinergic agents that cause bronchial muscle relaxation relieving bronchospasm. They are used through the inhalational route and have negligible systemic absorption and minimal side effects. Not much data is available for their use during pregnancy and lactation, though these are considered safe due to low serum concentration.[62]

Biologics

Use of omalizumab [anti-immunoglobulin E (IgE) monoclonal antibody] and allergen immunotherapy during pregnancy are still under investigation. Few studies have shown that use of omalizumab during pregnancy does not increase the risk of congenital malformations, preterm delivery, or low birth weight.[63] Omalizumab during pregnancy may be continued if the woman was taking it prior to pregnancy.[64] It is given as subcutaneous injection once or twice a month and should be used only at a place with adequate facilities to handle medical emergencies and anaphylaxis. Sublingual and subcutaneous administration of allergen immunotherapy, touted as targeting etiology of asthma, is safe during pregnancy.[65] While Global Initiative for Asthma (GINA)[34] supports its use, the British guidelines do not.[44]

Anti-interleukin (IL)-5 antibody biological therapies reduce inflammation by specifically inhibiting eosinophil recruitment, activation, and survival. They are used in severe eosinophilic asthma not responding to other treatment. Animal studies have not shown teratogenic effects, but no human data is available for Mepolizumab (anti-IL-5 receptor), Reslizumab (anti-IL-5 receptor), and Benralizumab (anti-IL-5 receptor).[66] Dupilumab binds to IL-4 receptor and inhibits action of IL-4 and IL-13, both involved in type 2 airway inflammation. It is used in severe oral steroid-dependent asthma. Anti-IL-5 biologics and dupilumab are found as safe in pregnancy.[67] Regarding lactation, these molecules are large proteins; hence, they would be most likely destroyed in the infant's gastrointestinal tract.

Thymic stromal lymphopoietin (TSLP) is a cytokine produced early in the inflammatory pathway by the epithelium, after exposure to allergens. Tezepelumab is an immunoglobulin that binds to human TSLP arresting its action. Animal studies have not shown teratogenic effects, but human studies are lacking. Asthma is a hyper-reactive condition with higher reactive oxygen species' formation in pregnancy. Consequently, adding antioxidants, such as beta-carotene and lycopene, may help to decrease asthma severity.[68]

Most clinical trials do not include pregnant women during trials, leading to fear in the minds of both patients and treating physicians regarding continuation of treatment. At the same time, we need to realize that risk of medication to fetus may be overestimated. Furthermore, majority of studies available are from western nations. Indian chest physicians and obstetricians should put more of an effort to document use and response of asthma medication in pregnant women.

Medications used for Infectious Pulmonary Diseases

Antibiotics

Pneumonia, the most common infection during pregnancy unrelated to obstetric changes, remains a significant cause of morbidity and mortality. Typically bacterial in nature, pneumonia is primarily treated with antibiotics. In cases where the causative organism is not identified, the choice of antibiotic is influenced by several factors, including the severity of symptoms, age, antimicrobial intolerance, comorbidities, concomitant medications, gestational age, and epidemiological context. The general approach is to prioritize well-established drugs, employ the lowest effective dose for the shortest necessary duration, and use a single antibiotic whenever feasible.

In nonpregnant individuals, preferred antibiotics include macrolides, doxycycline, fluoroquinolones, amoxicillin–clavulanate, or second-generation cephalosporins. During pregnancy, a more cautious approach is warranted. Macrolides such as azithromycin, beta-lactams such as amoxicillin, or second-generation cephalosporins are preferred choices for outpatient treatment. In cases with severe symptoms requiring hospitalization, injectable antibiotics like third-generation cephalosporins, in conjunction with macrolides (erythromycin or azithromycin), are administered.[69] Guidelines recommend that community-acquired pneumonia should be treated with a combination of drugs that cover pneumococcus and atypical pathogens.[70] If there is a risk of pseudomonal infection, beta-lactamase inhibitors such as imipenem, meropenem, or piperacillin–tazobactam, combined with aminoglycosides and macrolides, may be considered.

Various antibiotics have been studied for their safety during pregnancy:

- Penicillins are highly effective and considered safe during pregnancy, provided there is no known allergy. No fetal side effects have been documented, but maternal allergic reaction may lead to fetal problems.
- First- and second-generation cephalosporins are proven to be safe during pregnancy and are widely used.[71] Third-generation cephalosporins are less commonly employed and should be reserved for cases where other treatments have been ineffective.
- Macrolides such as erythromycin and azithromycin are sparingly transported across the placenta and not been associated with teratogenic effects. They can be an alternative for women allergic to penicillin. Azithromycin, in particular, is favored due to its minimal gastrointestinal side effects and absence of teratogenicity.[72] Erythromycin estolate is seen to predispose to intrahepatic cholestasis and is avoided in pregnancy. Clarithromycin was not associated with congenital defects when used in the first trimester, but there was a higher incidence of spontaneous abortions; hence, it is not preferred.
- Aminoglycosides are generally avoided during pregnancy but may be considered for severe gram-negative infections. Streptomycin and Kanamycin have been linked to congenital deafness, although this has not been reported with gentamicin and tobramycin. Gentamicin is generally preferred during pregnancy due to extensive study on its use and favorable safety profile.
- Tetracyclines are contraindicated in pregnancy as they freely cross the placenta and get deposited in fetal teeth and long bones as calcium complex. This produces permanent yellow-brown staining and hypoplasia of deciduous teeth and suppression of growth of long bones. These effects are most prominent in the second and third trimesters, while first-trimester use is considered safe. There is up to 40% reduction in growth rate of long bones, particularly the fibula.[73] In preterm neonates,

this effect may be more pronounced. Doxycycline may be given during pregnancy if no alternative is available, as no teratogenic effect has been documented with it.[74] Tetracyclines in high doses have also been associated with maternal hepatotoxicity and acute fatty liver.

- Cotrimoxazole, sulfamethoxazole, and trimethoprim alone are some of the earliest antibiotics and are quite safe to use. Sulfonamides have a theoretical risk of promoting neonatal hyperbilirubinemia; hence, they are avoided if the mother is at risk of premature delivery. Sulfonamides are contraindicated in glucose-6-phosphate dehydrogenase (G6PD)-deficient women.
- Clindamycin is quite efficacious for management of both aerobic and anaerobic infections. No teratogenic or otherwise common side effects have been reported. However, it may cause pseudomembranous enterocolitis.
- Metronidazole has been associated with mutagenesis and carcinogenesis in rodents, better avoided in the first trimester. On the other hand, large human studies have not shown evidence of teratogenicity or fetal growth restriction.[75]
- Fluoroquinolones have an affinity for bone tissue, leading to arthralgia and tendonitis. They were not found to be embryotoxic or teratogenic in human studies. They are contraindicated in pregnancy due to reports of arthropathy and cartilage erosion in young animals.[69]
- Vancomycin use during pregnancy has not been linked to birth defects, ototoxicity, or nephrotoxicity.[76]
- Chloramphenicol is contraindicated in pregnancy, as it can cause bone marrow suppression in fetus. Its use in the last trimester can cause gray baby syndrome, which includes gray facies, flaccidity, and cardiovascular disorders.[77]
- Linezolid, a protein synthesis inhibitor, is typically avoided in pregnancy due to limited evidence regarding its use.

During lactation, use of antibacterials can lead to alteration of the neonate's bowel flora, allergy or sensitization in the baby, and interference with investigations of the neonate. Neonates, especially when premature, have immature digestive and excretory functions; hence, they are at a higher risk from accretion of drugs in breast milk.

Antiviral Drugs

The WHO and various other associations endorse early empirical use of antiviral drugs, based on clinical suspicion, in pregnant and postpartum women with influenza.[78-80] Neuraminidase inhibitors are preferred during pregnancy, with oseltamivir as the first choice, and zanamivir if oseltamivir is not available. Use of antivirals within 48 hours of onset of symptoms helps to decrease morbidity and mortality. Physiological changes of pregnancy can change the pharmacokinetics of antivirals drugs lowering the serum concentration of oseltamivir and its metabolites. Moreover, the levels of oseltamivir were seen to vary in different trimesters, being higher in the third trimester.[81] These findings suggest that higher dosage of drug may be required. Oseltamivir has been documented to cross placenta in both human and animal models. But recent evidence has shown that neuraminidase inhibitors, especially oseltamivir, are not associated with abnormal maternal or fetal outcome.[82,83] They may cause nausea and vomiting, which could be amplified in pregnancy.

The incidence of congenital anomalies was similar to that in general population with use of oseltamivir.[84] However, its use should be restricted to the third trimester, in which mortality due to influenza is highest. Postexposure antiviral chemoprophylaxis with oseltamivir (75 mg once daily for 10 days) or zanamivir (two inhalations once daily for 10 days, if oseltamivir is unavailable) is recommended during pregnancy and up to 2 weeks after delivery or miscarriage.[78] Regarding other neuraminidase inhibitors, less evidence is available. Long-acting inhaled laninamivir, used to treat influenza, has no association with adverse pregnancy or fetal outcome.[85] Intravenous peramivir and zanamivir were approved for emergency use during the 2009 H1N1 pandemic in the USA, in patients not responding to oseltamivir.[86] Oseltamivir and zanamivir are secreted in breast milk, though levels are around 1% of levels in maternal serum; hence, they are considered safe during lactation. Animal studies have reiterated their safety during lactation.[87]

M2 ion channel inhibitors such as amantadine and rimantadine may cause neurological side effects. Animal studies on amantadine have not shown harmful effects on fetus even at 25 times the dose given in humans.[88] However, there are case reports documenting cardiac anomalies and tibial hemimelia, with antenatal exposure to amantadine.[89] Amantadine is secreted in breast milk; therefore, it should be used with caution in lactating women.

Acyclovir is a DNA polymerase inhibitor widely used for varicella pneumonia in pregnancy. It has not been associated with any maternal or fetal adverse effects. No increase of congenital anomalies was seen, even after first-trimester use.[90] Oral acyclovir may be used for pregnant women presenting with chicken pox so that they do not progress to pneumonia. No congenital malformations have been seen with use of famciclovir and valacyclovir also.[91]

Management of COVID-19 infection in pregnancy is still not well-defined. Remdesivir is now recommended for treatment of admitted patients with severe symptoms.[92] Most common side effects seen are nausea, transaminitis, and respiratory failure. Its use should be accompanied with regular surveillance of side effects and transaminase enzyme levels.[93] Most studies on efficacy and safety of remdesivir in COVID-19 have been done in second and third trimesters of pregnancy; thus, first-trimester use is still under debate. Remdesivir has previously been safely used for Ebola virus in pregnancy, with no maternal or fetal adverse effects.[94] Favilavir, Lopinavir, and Ritonavir have also been used in COVID-19, but their safety in pregnancy is not established. Ribavirin is another antiviral used for viral pneumonia.

It has teratogenic or lethal effect in all animal studies done; therefore, it is contraindicated in pregnancy.[95]

Antifungal Drugs

Antifungal drugs active against *Coccidioides* species are polyenes like amphotericin B and azoles like fluconazole, itraconazole, posaconazole, voriconazole, and isavuconazole. Amphotericin B is the only antifungal drug approved for use in pregnancy. Azoles are proven to be teratogenic in the first trimester. Amphotericin B has been effectively used for the treatment of disseminated coccidioidomycosis and other fungal infections such as Aspergillosis and cryptococcal pneumonia. Amphotericin B has low teratogenic potential, though maternal toxicity may be seen in the form of anemia, hypokalemia, nephrotoxicity, azotemia, fever, thrombophlebitis, and electrolyte disorders.[96] Adequate monitoring should be done for timely management.

Isolated fungal pneumonia in pregnant women without comorbidities may recover without any active treatment. Amphotericin B is useful in severe pneumonia with multilobar disease, resting hypoxemia, or clinical instability and should not be delayed.[97] Nonmeningeal coccidiodal infection in the first trimester of pregnancy can be managed with intravenous amphotericin B, no therapy with close monitoring or an azole, after informing the mother about the risk of congenital anomalies.[98] After the first trimester, azoles such as fluconazole and itraconazole can be given or amphotericin B can be continued. In case the patient becomes pregnant while on azole treatment, it should be discontinued. Breastfeeding is contraindicated in mothers taking azoles other than fluconazole, as they are secreted in breast milk.[99]

Treatment with intravenous amphotericin B should be followed with oral fluconazole postpartum. Single-dose oral fluconazole is considered safe in pregnancy,[100] but use in higher dose (400–800 mg/day) or for longer duration in the first trimester has been linked with brachycephaly, abnormal facies, abnormal calvarial development, craniosynostosis, skeletal abnormalities, congenital heart defects, and cleft palate.[101] More observation is necessary before we can rule out association of congenital heart defects and skeletal defects with fluconazole, and fetal eye defects with itraconazole.[102] Animal studies have shown similar abnormalities with use of other azoles in the first trimester.[103] There is very less evidence available for voriconazole, posaconazole, or isavuconazole use in pregnancy. A single case report documents safe use of voriconazole for 5 months after 19 weeks, in a patient with invasive Aspergillosis treated initially with liposomal amphotericin B.[104] Isavuconazole has also been used to treat invasive fungal lung infection in late pregnancy, without any adverse effects.[105]

Pneumocystis jirovecii pneumonia is a leading cause of AIDS-related death, especially in pregnant women, with mortality rate of up to 50%. Women taking trimethoprim-sulfamethoxazole for treatment and prophylaxis should be monitored for preterm delivery, and newborns should be assessed for neonatal jaundice and kernicterus. Immune reconstitution inflammatory syndrome may be seen after delivery, so women need to be monitored. In the first trimester, aerosolized pentamidine may be used as it is minimally absorbed systemically and thus has lesser teratogenic potential.[106]

Antitubercular Therapy (Table 5)

Tuberculosis (TB) is still a major health problem, with India having the highest number of new cases, in the world.[107] It is a major cause of maternal morbidity and mortality. Treatment of TB in pregnancy follows the guidelines given by Revised National Tuberculosis Program of India (RNTCP), now revised as National Tuberculosis Elimination Program

TABLE 5: ATT in pregnancy.[111]

Antitubercular drug	Side effects in pregnancy	Recommendation
Isoniazid	Hepatotoxicity	Monitoring of liver function every 14 days
Rifampicin	• Maternal and neonatal • Hypoprothrombinemia	Vitamin K for both mother and baby
Ethambutol	Retrobulbar neuritis	
Pyrazinamide	Less studies	
Fluoroquinolones—levofloxacin, moxifloxacin	Risk to cartilage and joints as seen in animal studies	Can be given if benefits outweigh risks
Streptomycin	Fetal nephrotoxicity and ototoxicity	Contraindicated in pregnancy
Capreomycin, ethionamide, PAS	Animal studies show teratogenic effects	
Bedaquiline, clofazimine, terizidone, cilastatin, meropenem	No data available	
Linezolid, cycloserine		Can be given if benefits outweigh risks
Delamanid, prothionamide		Contraindicated in pregnancy

(ATT: antitubercular therapy; PAS: para-amino salicylic)

(NTEP) wherein Directly Observed Treatment Short course (DOTS) is endorsed. Pregnant women are treated under category 1 of DOTS similar to the protocol in nonpregnant women.

Pyridoxine 10–25 mg/day is added to combat fetal neuropathy caused by isoniazid. Use of pyrazinamide is considered safe in pregnancy by the WHO and National Tuberculosis Elimination Programme (NTEP).[108] Isoniazid, rifampicin, and ethambutol all cross the placenta, but are considered safe, even in first trimester, with no evidence of increased risk of congenital malformations.[109] Maternal surveillance is necessary to assess side effects and compliance. Isoniazid is hepatotoxic, which is especially worrisome in the peripartum period. Rifampicin, especially in the last trimester, may cause hypoprothrombinemia in both mother and baby. Drug interactions are also a concern during pregnancy; hence, treatment should be carefully monitored by an expert.

Streptomycin is avoided in pregnancy as it can potentially cause fetal ototoxicity. A retrospective study in mothers who were given streptomycin did not find any significant deafness in neonates.[110] Other drugs contraindicated in pregnancy are kanamycin, amikacin, capreomycin, fluoroquinolones, ethionamide, and para-amino salicylic (PAS) acid.[111]

Evidence regarding safety of drugs used for multidrug-resistant TB (MDR-TB) in pregnancy is lacking; hence, patients can be given the option of termination of pregnancy, if detected early **(Flowchart 1)**.[112] If a patient wishes to continue, second-line drugs such as kanamycin, levofloxacin, ethionamide, cycloserine, PAS, and capreomycin can be added, though judiciously with monitoring. Reports of a successful outcome in MDR-TB are available with use of second-line drugs. In fact, morbidity of untreated MDR-TB is more as compared to the potential side effects of drugs used.[113] PAS combined with isoniazid is considered safe in pregnancy. These drugs can be postponed till after first trimester is over to reduce teratogenic side effects. The safety of bedaquiline, a newer drug for MDR-TB, in pregnancy is not known.

All first-line antitubercular drugs are considered safe in breastfeeding, as they are secreted into breast milk in very low concentration.[111] Effects on the nursing infant can be further decreased by intake of drugs just after breastfeeding. In case the patient has severe symptoms or MDR-TB, expressed breast milk may be given, although both WHO and RNTCP do not recommend separation of mother and baby.[108,112]

Management of TB in HIV-infected pregnant women is a big challenge. Rifampicin interacts with both non-nucleoside reverse transcriptase inhibitors and protease inhibitors. This leads to low levels of antiretroviral therapy (ART) drugs, such as nevirapine. Rifabutin may be used instead of rifampicin to reduce this interaction.[114] Pregnant women with HIV are at a high risk for progression from latent to active TB. However, the efficacy and safety of isoniazid prophylaxis during pregnancy are still under question. There is conflicting evidence, but the incidence of stillbirth, spontaneous abortion, low birth weight, preterm delivery, and birth defects was found to be higher with use of 28 weeks of isoniazid-preventive therapy.[115]

Drugs for Cystic Fibrosis and Bronchiectasis

Pregnancy does not cause accelerated loss of pulmonary function in women with cystic fibrosis or bronchiectasis, but more pulmonary exacerbations and infections have been seen in pregnant women. There are reports of continuing use of cystic fibrosis transmembrane conductance regulators, such as ivacaftor and lumacaftor during pregnancy and breastfeeding. No congenital anomalies were seen with these drugs.[116] The modulators are secreted into breast milk. Inhaled mucolytics such as hypertonic saline, mannitol, and dornase alfa have limited systemic absorption, considered safe to use during pregnancy and lactation.[116] Inhaled anti-

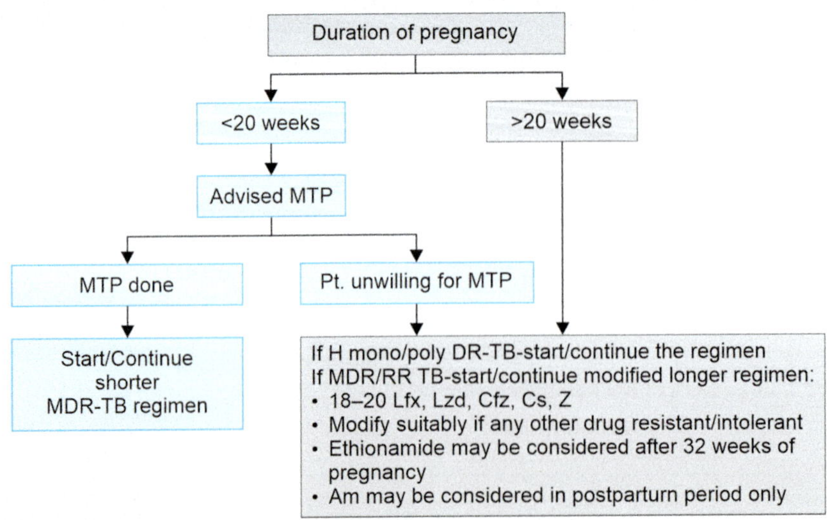

FLOWCHART 1: MDR-TB in pregnancy.[112]
(MDR-TB: multidrug-resistant TB; MTP: medical termination of pregnancy)

biotics, tobramycin, colistimethate, or aztreonam used in cystic fibrosis are thought to be safe because of minimal systemic absorption.[116] Safety of oral antibiotics and antifungals has already been discussed. Pancrelipase, a combination of porcine-derived pancreatic enzymes, is widely used for cystic fibrosis in pregnancy, though limited human studies are available.[116]

Antithrombotic Therapy

Anticoagulants are used for prevention of deep vein thrombosis and pulmonary embolism during pregnancy, in high-risk patients. They are also widely used in patients with a history of recurrent abortions having thrombophilia. Hence, there is extensive experience of safe and effective use of heparin during pregnancy. Unfractionated heparin was initially preferred during pregnancy, but has now been replaced by low-molecular-weight heparin (LMWH), which is easier to use with more reliable pharmacokinetics. It is also safer and as effective as unfractionated heparin.

Unfractionated heparin does not cross the placenta and therefore does not affect the fetus.[117] It has a beneficial effect of decreasing the incidence of pregnancy loss. Maternal side effects seen with heparin are hemorrhage, heparin-induced thrombocytopenia (HIT), and heparin-associated osteopenia. Anticoagulant effect of heparin may last for 24 hours after the last subcutaneous injection. Therefore, injections need to be stopped at least 24 hours prior to planned delivery. In case less time is available, epidural analgesia should not be given. Partial thromboplastin time (PTT) should be regularly checked in later pregnancy so that protamine sulfate may be given in case of excessive anticoagulation. A PTT value of 1.5 times control value shows adequate anticoagulation. Heparin-associated osteopenia has been reported in pregnancy, but it is more often seen with a higher dose, that is, 20,000 IU/day for more than 6 months.[19] A 2% risk of symptomatic vertebral fractures is present.[118] HIT may be seen in 5–30% of patients receiving unfractionated heparin.[117] Heparin is safe during lactation as it is not secreted into breast milk.

Low-molecular-weight heparins have a longer plasma half-life, better bioavailability, and a more predictable dose response than unfractionated heparin. They also have lesser risk of HIT, hemorrhage, and osteoporosis.[119] Spinal anesthesia or planned delivery should be scheduled at least 12 hours after the last prophylactic dose of LMWH and 24 hours after the therapeutic dose. LMWH may be restarted 24 hours after delivery. The incidence of HIT is <0.1% in patients on LMWH. There is no recommendation for monitoring of a platelet count or PTT while the patient is exclusively on LMWH.[120] Also, no difference was reported in bone density, with only 0.04% risk of osteoporosis.[121]

Low-molecular-weight heparin is considered the anticoagulant of choice in pregnancy, for both prevention and treatment of venous thromboembolism (VTE). In acute management of pulmonary embolism, LMWH should be used in standard dose according to body weight. Moreover, clearance of LMWH is increased in pregnancy; therefore, twice-daily dose is recommended for treatment. For prophylaxis, a single dose may be given as it is more patient friendly. Monitoring with anti-Xa levels and subsequent dose adjustment has not proven to be helpful in improving patient outcome during prophylaxis; however, it may be monitored during treatment of acute VTE.[122] Current guidelines recommend low-dose LMWH for thromboprophylaxis during pregnancy and postpartum, with a 1.2% risk of recurrent VTE.[122] Allergic skin reactions may be occasionally seen with LMWH and are more common with dalteparin and nadroparin than enoxaparin.[122] It is important to differentiate allergic reaction from bruising due to a faulty technique. In case all LMWH preparations cause intolerable allergic reaction, Danaparoid or Fondaparinux may be considered.

Oral coumarins such as warfarin can cross the placenta and have been associated with congenital malformations. They can also cause hemorrhagic complications in the mother; hence, they should not be used peripartum.[123] Warfarin if used in the first trimester can lead to miscarriage or anomalies encompassing midface hypoplasia, stippled chondral calcification, scoliosis, short proximal limbs, and short phalanges in the fetus. Fetal warfarin syndrome or warfarin embryopathy is seen in 4–5% of women having a history of taking warfarin between 6 and 9 weeks of gestation.[123] Furthermore, the risk increases with a dose >5 mg/day. Fetal cerebral hemorrhage may occur at the time of delivery. Coumarins have also been associated with neurological deficit and low intelligence quotient in young children, if their mothers were exposed during pregnancy.[124] Warfarin is not secreted into breast milk; hence, it can be used safely during lactation. Other oral anticoagulants are contraindicated during lactation. Phenindione may cause hemorrhage in the infant.

Heparinoids such as Danaparoid are effective anticoagulants with lesser potential to cause recurrent HIT; therefore, Danaparoid is the treatment of choice in pregnant women with HIT. It does not cross the placenta.[122] Dextran is contraindicated in pregnancy due to chances of anaphylactoid reaction, leading to uterine hypertonus, fetal distress, and intrauterine fetal demise or profound neurologic damage.[125] Hirudin is a direct thrombin inhibitor and is avoided in pregnancy as it crosses the placenta. It can be used during lactation for HIT as it is not detected in breast milk.[126] Fondaparinux is a synthetic penta-saccharide with no HIT or allergic reactions. It is effective for thromboprophylaxis. Though nominal transplacental passage is seen, evidence suggests its safety in pregnancy. Still, it should be avoided in the first trimester.[122]

Danaparoid and Fondaparinux are not secreted into breast milk and are safe during lactation. Preliminary evidence has shown safety in second and third trimesters of pregnancy, so they may be used in women with history of HIT or heparin allergy. Aspirin has been widely used in pregnancy for obstetric reasons and is proven to be safe in low doses.[127]

It has been found to be useful in prevention of deep venous thrombosis, but its efficacy is probably less than LMWH. Direct oral anticoagulants such as apixaban, dabigatran, edoxaban, and rivaroxaban are recent additions to the drug armamentarium for management of VTE. Animal studies have shown that they cross the placenta and are secreted into breast milk. Case reports of congenital malformations are there, and these are not recommended during pregnancy.[122]

Thrombolytic therapy using lytic agents such as streptokinase, urokinase, or alteplase has been employed in massive pulmonary embolism with severe hemodynamic instability. The drugs are justified in pregnancy in case of a life-threatening event. There is no increase in risk of preterm delivery, preterm rupture of membranes, or placental abruption. Poor fetal outcome may occur due to pulmonary embolism rather than effect of drugs.[128] However, more evidence regarding risks and benefits of these drugs during pregnancy is required.

Vaccination for Influenza

Influenza vaccination is recommended for all pregnant women. A single dose is given in any trimester taking into account seasonal strain of influenza.[129] Influenza vaccine is produced from highly purified egg-grown viruses, which have been inactivated. In India, two vaccines are commercially available and recommended for use in pregnant women—standard-dose trivalent inactivated influenza vaccine and standard-dose quadrivalent inactivated influenza vaccine. Both are safe to use in all trimesters of pregnancy and during breastfeeding.[130] Both vaccines are avoided in women who are allergic to eggs or other components of the vaccine, those with acute febrile illness, and those who have a history of Guillain-Barré syndrome within 6 weeks of a previous influenza vaccination.

Individuals who previously only experienced hives with vaccine can be given the vaccine during pregnancy. Live attenuated nasal vaccine is not recommended in India as its safety and efficacy in pregnancy are not known. Peak antibody levels are seen within 2 weeks of administration of the vaccine. Cord blood levels of antibodies to influenza A were found to be higher in babies whose mother received influenza vaccine or were infected with influenza A.[131] Furthermore, the onset of respiratory symptoms was later and less severe in these babies at the time of seasonal onset of the disease.

SUMMARY

Any drug given for a pulmonary disease during pregnancy needs to balance the maternal and fetal risk of giving versus withholding treatment. The decision for managing the disease should be individualized considering the severity of disease, patient characteristics, period of gestation, and effect on fetus.

REFERENCES

1. Antonucci R, Zaffanello M, Puxeddu E, et al. Use of non-steroidal anti-inflammatory drugs in pregnancy: impact on the fetus and newborn. Curr Drug Metab. 2012;13(4):474-90.
2. World Health Organization. Breastfeeding and maternal medication: recommendations for drugs in the eleventh WHO model list of essential drugs. [online] Available from https://www.who.int/publications/i/item/55732 [Last accessed September, 2024].
3. Kar S, Krishnan A, Preetha K, et al. A review of antihistamines used during pregnancy. J Pharmacol Pharmacother. 2012;3(2):105-8.
4. Mazzotta P, Loebstein R, Koren G. Treating allergic rhinitis in pregnancy. Safety considerations. Drug Saf. 1999;20(4):361-75.
5. Seto A, Einarson T, Koren G. Pregnancy outcome following first trimester exposure to antihistamines: meta-analysis. Am J Perinatol. 1997;14(3):119-24
6. Källén B. Use of antihistamine drugs in early pregnancy and delivery outcome. J Matern Fetal Neonatal Med. 2002;11(3):146-52.
7. Somoskövi Á, Bártfai Z, Tamási L, et al. Population-based case–control study of allergic rhinitis during pregnancy for birth outcomes. Eur J Obstet Gynecol Reprod Biol. 2007;131(1):21-7.
8. Aoki Y, Funabashi H, Terada Y, et al. Reproductive and developmental toxicity studies of ebastine. II: Teratogenicity study in rats. Yakuri to Chiryo. 1994;22(3):89-111.
9. Committee on Drugs. The transfer of drugs and other chemicals into human milk. Pediatrics. 2001;108(3):776-89.
10. Yau WP, Mitchell AA, Lin KJ, et al. Use of decongestants during pregnancy and the risk of birth defects. Am J Epidemiol. 2013; 178(2):198-208.
11. Werler MM. Teratogen update: pseudoephedrine. Birth Defects Res A Clin Mol Teratol. 2006;76(6):445-52.
12. Hornby PJ, Abrahams TP. Pulmonary pharmacology. Clin Obstet Gynecol. 1996;39(1):17-35.
13. Werler MM, Mitchell AA, Shapiro S. First trimester maternal medication use in relation to gastroschisis. Teratology. 1992; 45(4):361-7.
14. Källén BA, Olausson PO. Use of oral decongestants during pregnancy and delivery outcome. Am J Obstet Gynecol. 2006; 194(2):480-5.
15. Namazy JA, Schatz M. The safety of intranasal steroids during pregnancy: a good start. J Allergy Clin Immunol. 2016;138(1): 105-6.
16. Bérard A, Sheehy O, Kurzinger ML, et al. Intranasal triamcinolone use during pregnancy and the risk of adverse pregnancy outcomes. J Allergy Clin Immunol. 2016;138(1):97-104.
17. Lipworth BJ, Seckl JR. Measures for detecting systemic bioactivity with inhaled and intranasal corticosteroids. Thorax. 1997;52:476-82.
18. Einarson A, Lyszkiewicz D, Koren G. The safety of dextromethorphan in pregnancy: results of a controlled study. Chest. 2001;119(2):466-9.
19. Fabre E, Tajada M, de Agüero RG. Use of drugs in pulmonary medicine in pregnant women. Clin Pulm Med. 2002;9(1):20-32.
20. Aliprandi P, Cima L, Carrara M. Therapeutic use of levocloperastine as an antitussive agent: an overview of preclinical data and clinical trials in adults and children. Clin Drug Invest. 2002;22:209-20.

21. Briggs GG, Freeman RK, Yaffe SJ. Drugs in Pregnancy and Lactation: A Reference Guide to Fetal and Neonatal Risk. Philadelphia: Lippincott Williams & Wilkins; 2012.
22. Mehta PS, Mehta SJ, Vorherr H. Congenital iodide goiter and hypothyroidism: a review. Obstet Gynecol Surv. 1983;38(5): 237-47.
23. Bauer AZ, Swan SH, Kriebel D, et al. Paracetamol use during pregnancy—a call for precautionary action. Nature Rev Endocrinol. 2021;17(12):757-66.
24. Adams SS, Bough RG, Cliffe EE, et al. Absorption, distribution and toxicity of ibuprofen. Toxicol Appl Pharmacol. 1969;15(2): 310-30.
25. Koren G, Florescu A, Costei AM, et al. Nonsteroidal antiinflammatory drugs during third trimester and the risk of premature closure of the ductus arteriosus: a meta-analysis. Ann Pharmacother. 2006;40(5):824-9.
26. Li DK, Liu L, Odouli R. Exposure to non-steroidal anti-inflammatory drugs during pregnancy and risk of miscarriage: population based cohort study. BMJ. 2003;327(7411):368.
27. Malhotra S, Khanna S. Safety of analgesics in pregnancy. Int J Obstet Gynaecol Res. 2016;3(1):208-12.
28. Wilson J. Use of sodium cromoglycate during pregnancy. J Pharm Med. 1982;8:45-51.
29. Francis N. Abortion after grass pollen injection. J Allergy. 1941; 12:559-63.
30. Shaikh WA. A retrospective study on the safety of immunotherapy in pregnancy. Clin Exp Allergy. 1993;23:857-60.
31. Blais L, Forget A. Asthma exacerbations during the first trimester of pregnancy and the risk of congenital malformations among asthmatic women. J Allergy Clin Immunol. 2008;121(6):1379-84.
32. Yland JJ, Bateman B, Huybrechts KF, et al. Fetal outcomes among women with asthma during pregnancy: evidence from a large healthcare database in the United States. J Allergy Clin Immunol. 2019;143(2):AB422.
33. Murphy VE, Namazy JA, Powell H, et al. A meta-analysis of adverse perinatal outcomes in women with asthma. BJOG. 2011;118(11):1314-23.
34. Global Initiative for Asthma. (2022). Global strategy for asthma management and prevention. [online] Available from www.ginasthma.org. [Last accessed September, 2024].
35. Norjavaara E, de Verdier MG. Normal pregnancy outcomes in a population-based study including 2968 pregnant women exposed to budesonide. J Allergy Clin Immunol. 2003;111(4):736-42.
36. Gluck PA, Gluck JC. A review of pregnancy outcomes after exposure to orally inhaled or intranasal budesonide. Curr Med Res Opin. 2005;21(7):1075-84.
37. Rahimi R, Nikfar S, Abdollahi M. Meta-analysis finds use of inhaled corticosteroids during pregnancy safe: a systematic meta analysis review. Hum Exp Toxicol. 2006;25:447-52.
38. Mabie WC. Asthma in pregnancy. Clin Obstet Gynecol. 1996;39: 56-69.
39. Schatz M. Asthma during pregnancy: interrelationships and management. Ann Allergy. 1992;68:123-8.
40. Guidelines for the Diagnosis and Management of Asthma. Expert Panel Report 2. National Institute of Health. National Heart, Lung and Blood Institute. NIH Publications. No 97-4051. July 1997.
41. Skuladottir H, Wilcox AJ, Ma C, et al. Corticosteroid use and risk of orofacial clefts. Birth Def Res A Clin Mol Teratol. 2014;100: 499-506.
42. Bandoli G, Palmsten K, Forbess Smith CJ, et al. A review of systemic corticosteroid use in pregnancy and the risk of select pregnancy and birth outcomes. Rheum Dis Clin North Am. 2017;43:489-502.
43. Carmichael SL, Shaw GM. Maternal corticosteroid use and risk of selected congenital anomalies. Am J Med Genet. 1999;86:242-4.
44. Scottish Intercollegiate Guidelines Network, British Thoracic Society, Scotland. Healthcare Improvement Scotland. British guideline on the management of asthma: a national clinical guideline. Edinburgh: Healthcare Improvement Scotland; 2019.
45. McGuire E. Sudden loss of milk supply following high-dose triamcinolone (Kenacort) injection. Breastfeed Rev. 2012;20: 32-4.
46. Burdon JG, McDonald CF, Burdon JG. Asthma in pregnancy and lactation: a position paper for the Thoracic Society of Australia and New Zealand. Med J Aust. 1996;165(9):485-8.
47. Koren G, Sarkar M, Einarson A. Safety of using montelukast during pregnancy. Can Fam Physician. 2010;56(9):881-2.
48. Sarkar M, Koren G, Kalra S, et al. Montelukast use during pregnancy: a multicentre, prospective, comparative study of infant outcomes. Eur J Clin Pharmacol. 2009;65:1259-64.
49. Hatakeyama S, Goto M, Yamamoto A, et al. The safety of pranlukast and montelukast during the first trimester of pregnancy: A prospective, two-centered cohort study in Japan. Congenit Anom. 2022;62(4):161-8.
50. Bakhireva LN, Jones KL, Schatz M, et al., Organization of Teratology Information Specialists Collaborative Research Group. Safety of leukotriene receptor antagonists in pregnancy. J Allergy Clin Immunol. 2007;119(3):618-25.
51. American College of Obstetricians and Gynecologists and The American College of Allergy, Asthma and Immunology (ACAAI). The use of newer asthma and allergy medications during pregnancy. Ann Allergy Asthma Immunol. 2000;84(5):475-80.
52. Datta P, Rewers-Felkins K, Baker T, et al. Transfer of montelukast into human milk during lactation. Breastfeed Med. 2017;12: 54-7.
53. Garne E, Hansen AV, Morris J, et al. Use of asthma medication during pregnancy and risk of specific congenital anomalies: a European case-malformed control study. J Allergy Clin Immunol. 2015;136(6):1496-502.
54. Eltonsy S, Kettani FZ, Blais L. Beta2-agonists use during pregnancy and perinatal outcomes: a systematic review. Respir Med. 2014;108(1):9-33.
55. Schatz M, Dombrowski MP, Wise R, et al. The relationship of asthma medication use to perinatal outcomes. J Allergy Clin Immunol. 2004;113(6):1040-5.
56. Eltonsy S, Forget A, Beauchesne MF, Blais L. Risk of congenital malformations for asthmatic pregnant women using a long-acting β2-agonist and inhaled corticosteroid combination versus higher-dose inhaled corticosteroid monotherapy. J Allergy Clin Immunol. 2015;135(1):123-30.
57. National Heart, Lung, and Blood Institute, National Asthma Education and Prevention Program. (2004). Managing asthma during pregnancy: recommendations for pharmacologic treatment-2004 update. 2004;1-57. https://www.nhlbi.nih.gov/files/docs/resources/lung/astpreg_full.pdf
58. Barnes PJ. Theophylline. Am J Respir Crit Care Med. 2013;188(8): 901-6.
59. Stenius-Aarniala B, Riikonen S, Teramo K. Slow-release theophylline in pregnant asthmatics. Chest. 1995;107:642-7.

60. Ishikawa M, Yoneyama Y, Power GG, et al. Maternal theophylline administration and breathing movements in late-gestation human fetuses. Obstet Gynecol. 1996;88:973-8.
61. Yeh TF, Pildes RS. Transplacental aminophylline toxicity in a neonate. Lancet. 1977;1:910.
62. Chambers CD, Krishnan JA, Alba L, et al. The safety of asthma medications during pregnancy and lactation: Clinical management and research priorities. J Allergy Clin Immunol. 2021; 147(6):2009-20.
63. Namazy J, Cabana MD, Scheuerle AE, et al. The Xolair Pregnancy Registry (EXPECT): the safety of omalizumab use during pregnancy. J Allergy Clin Immunol. 2015;135(2):407-12.
64. Namazy JA, Blais L, Andrews EB, et al. Pregnancy outcomes in the omalizumab pregnancy registry and a disease-matched comparator cohort. J Allergy Clin Immunol. 2020;145(2):528-36.
65. Wang H, Li N, Huang H. Asthma in pregnancy: pathophysiology, diagnosis, whole-course management, and medication safety. Can Respir J. 2020;2020:9046842.
66. Cusack RP, Whetstone CE, Gauvreau GM. Use of Asthma Medication during Gestation and Risk of Specific Congenital Anomalies. Immunol Allergy Clin. 2023;43(1):169-85.
67. Bravo-Solarte DC, Garcia-Guaqueta DP, Chiarella SE. Asthma in pregnancy. In: Allergy and Asthma Proceedings 2023 Jan (Vol. 44, No. 1, p. 24). United States: OceanSide Publications.
68. Wood LG, Garg ML, Powell H, Gibson PG. Lycopene-rich treatments modify noneosinophilic airway inflammation in asthma: proof of concept. Free Radic Res. 2008;42(1):94-102.
69. Lim WS, Macfarlane JT, Colthorpe CL. Treatment of community-acquired lower respiratory tract infections during pregnancy. Am J Respir Med. 2003;2:221-33.
70. Mandell LA, Wunderink RG, Anzueto A, et al. Infectious Diseases Society of America/American Thoracic Society consensus guidelines on the management of community-acquired pneumonia in adults. Clin Infect Dis. 2007;44(Suppl 2):S27-72.
71. Czeizel AE, Rockenbauer M, Sørensen HT, et al. Use of cephalosporins during pregnancy and in the presence of congenital abnormalities: a population-based, case-control study. Am J Obstet Gynecol. 2001;184(6):1289-96.
72. Laopaiboon M, Panpanich R, Swa Mya K. Azithromycin for acute lower respiratory tract infections. Cochrane Database Syst Rev. 2015;2015(3):CD001954.
73. Rendle-Short TJ. Tetracycline in teeth and bone. Lancet. 1962; 279(7240):1188.
74. Czeizel AE, Rockenbauer M. Teratogenic study of doxycycline. Obstet Gynecol. 1997;89(4):524-8.
75. Piper JM, Mitchel EF, Ray WA. Prenatal use of metronidazole and birth defects: no association. Obstet Gynecol. 1993;82(3): 348-52.
76. Reyes MP, Ostrea Jr EM, Cabinian AE, et al. Vancomycin during pregnancy: does it cause hearing loss or nephrotoxicity in the infant? Am J Obstet Gynecol. 1989;161(4):977-81.
77. Khan S, Niederman MS. Pneumonia in the pregnant patient. Pulm Probl Pregn Clin Res Aspects. 2009:177-96.
78. ACOG Committee Opinion No. 732. Summary: Influenza Vaccination during Pregnancy. Obstet Gynecol. 2018;131(4):752-3.
79. World Health Organization. WHO guidelines for pharmacological management of pandemic (H1N1) 2009 influenza and other influenza viruses.
80. Uyeki TM, Bernstein HH, Bradley JS, et al. Clinical practice guidelines by the Infectious Diseases Society of America: 2018 update on diagnosis, treatment, chemoprophylaxis, and institutional outbreak management of seasonal influenza. Clin Infect Dis. 2019;68(6):e1-47.
81. Greer LG, Leff RD, Rogers VL, et al. Pharmacokinetics of oseltamivir according to trimester of pregnancy. Am J Obstet Gynecol. 2011;204(6):S89-93.
82. Chow EJ, Beigi RH, Riley LE, et al. Clinical effectiveness and safety of antivirals for influenza in pregnancy. Open Forum Infect Dis. 2021;8(6):ofab138.
83. Donner B, Niranjan V, Hoffmann G. Safety of oseltamivir in pregnancy: a review of preclinical and clinical data. Drug Saf. 2010;33:631-42.
84. Wollenhaupt M, Chandrasekaran A, Tomianovic D. The safety of oseltamivir in pregnancy: an updated review of post-marketing data. Pharmacoepidemiol Drug Saf. 2014;23(10):1035-42.
85. Minakami H, Kubo T, Nakai A, et al. Pregnancy outcomes of women exposed to laninamivir during pregnancy. Pharmacoepidemiol Drug Saf. 2014;23(10):1084-7.
86. Chan-Tack KM, Kim C, Moruf A, et al. Clinical experience with intravenous zanamivir under an emergency IND program in the United States (2011–2014). Antiviral Ther. 2015;20(5):561-4.
87. Brito V, Niederman MS. Pneumonia complicating pregnancy. Clin Chest Med. 2011;32(1):121-32.
88. Laibl VR, Sheffield JS. Influenza and pneumonia in pregnancy. Clin Perinat. 2005;32(3):727-38.
89. Nora J, Nora A, Way G. Cardiovascular maldevelopment associated with maternal exposure to amantadine. Lancet. 1975; 306(7935):607.
90. Stone KM, Reiff-Eldridge R, White AD, et al. Pregnancy outcomes following systemic prenatal acyclovir exposure: conclusions from the international acyclovir pregnancy registry, 1984–1999. Birth Defects Res A Clin Mol Teratol. 2004;70(4):201-7.
91. Lamont RF, Sobel JD, Carrington D, et al. Varicella-zoster virus (chickenpox) infection in pregnancy. BJOG. 2011;118(10): 1155-62.
92. Singh V, Trigunait P, Majumdar S, et al. Managing pregnancy in COVID-19 pandemic: A review article. J Fam Med Primary Care. 2020;9(11):5468.
93. Budi DS, Pratama NR, Wafa IA, et al. Remdesivir for pregnancy: A systematic review of antiviral therapy for COVID-19. Heliyon. 20228(1):e08835.
94. Mulangu S, Dodd LE, Davey Jr RT, et al. A randomized, controlled trial of Ebola virus disease therapeutics. New Engl J Med. 2019;381(24):2293-303.
95. Kochhar DM, Penner JD, Knudsen TB. Embryotoxic, teratogenic, and metabolic effects of ribavirin in mice. Toxicol Appl Pharmacol. 1980;52(1):99-112.
96. King CT, Rogers PD, Cleary JD, Chapman SW. Antifungal therapy during pregnancy. Clin Infect Dis. 1998;27(5):1151-60.
97. Ely EW, Peacock Jr JE, Haponik EF, et al. Cryptococcal pneumonia complicating pregnancy. Medicine. 1998;77(3):153-67.
98. Galgiani JN, Ampel NM, Blair JE, et al. 2016 Infectious Diseases Society of America (IDSA) clinical practice guideline for the treatment of coccidioidomycosis. Clin Infect Dis. 2016; 63(6):e112-46.
99. Committee on Drugs. The transfer of drugs and other chemicals into human milk. Pediatrics. 2001;108(3):776-89.
100. Jick SS. Pregnancy outcomes after maternal exposure to fluconazole. Pharmacotherapy. 1999;19(2):221-2.
101. Lopez-Rangel E, Van Allen MI. Prenatal exposure to fluconazole: an identifiable dysmorphic phenotype. Birth Defects Res A Clin Mol Teratol. 2005;73(11):919-23.

102. Liu D, Zhang C, Wu L, et al. Fetal outcomes after maternal exposure to oral antifungal agents during pregnancy: A systematic review and meta-analysis. Int J Gynecol Obstet. 2020;148(1):6-13.
103. Tiboni GM, Giampietro F. Murine teratology of fluconazole: evaluation of developmental phase specificity and dose dependence. Pediatr Res. 2005;58(1):94-9.
104. Shoai Tehrani M, Sicre de Fontbrune F, Roth P, et al. Case report of exposure to voriconazole in the second and third trimesters of pregnancy. Antimicrob Agents Chemother. 2013;57(2):1094-5.
105. Johnson JA, Pearson JC, Kubiak DW, et al. Treatment of Chronic Granulomatous Disease–related Pulmonary Aspergillus Infection in Late Pregnancy. Open Forum Infect Dis. 2020;710:ofaa447.
106. Ahmad H, Mehta NJ, Manikal VM, Lamoste TJ, Chapnick EK, Lutwick LI, Sepkowitz DV. Pneumocystis carinii pneumonia in pregnancy. Chest. 2001;120(2):666-71.
107. World Health Organization. (2009). Global tuberculosis control: epidemiology, strategy, financing: WHO report 2009. World Health Organization; 2009. [online] Available from https://iris.who.int/handle/10665/44035 [Last accessed September, 2024].
108. World Health Organization. WHO recommendations on antenatal care for a positive pregnancy experience: screening, diagnosis and treatment of tuberculosis disease in pregnant women. Evidence-to-action brief: Highlights and key messages from the World Health Organization's 2016 global recommendations. World Health Organization; 2023 Feb 7. [online] Available from https://www.who.int/publications/i/item/9789240057562 [Last accessed September, 2024].
109. Jana N, Barik S, Arora N, et al. Tuberculosis in pregnancy: the challenges for South Asian countries. J Obstet Gynaecol Res. 2012;38(9):1125-36.
110. Donald PR, Doherty E, Van Zyl F. Hearing loss in the child following streptomycin administration during pregnancy. Cent Afr J Med. 1991;37(8):268-71.
111. Yadav V, Sharma JB. Tuberculosis in pregnancy. Indian Obstet Gynaecol. 2023;10(3). [online] Available from https://iog.org.in/journal/index.php/iog/article/view/102 [Last accessed September, 2024].
112. Ministry of Health and Family Welfare. Government of India. Collaborative Framework for Management of Tuberculosis in Pregnant Women. Ministry of Health and Family Welfare; February 2021.
113. Nguyen HT, Pandolfini C, Chiodini P, et al. Tuberculosis care for pregnant women: a systematic review. BMC Infect Dis. 2014;14(1):617.
114 Centers for Disease Control and Prevention. (2013). Managing drug interactions in the treatment of HIV-related tuberculosis. [online] Available from https://stacks.cdc.gov/view/cdc/25866. [Last accessed September, 2024].
115. Gupta A, Montepiedra G, Aaron L, et al. Isoniazid preventive therapy in HIV-infected pregnant and postpartum women. New Engl J Med. 2019;381(14):1333-46.
116. Middleton PG, Gade EJ, Aguilera C, et al. ERS/TSANZ Task Force Statement on the management of reproduction and pregnancy in women with airways diseases. Eur Respir J. 2020;55(2):1901208.
117. Sellman JS, Holman RL. Thromboembolism during pregnancy: risks, challenges, and recommendations. Postgrad Med. 2000;108(4):71-84.
118. Greer IA. Thrombosis in pregnancy: maternal and fetal issues. Lancet. 1999;353(9160):1258-65.
119. Hull RD, Pineo GF, Valentine KA. Treatment and prevention of venous thromboembolism. Semin Thromb Hemost. 1998;24:21-31.
120. Warkentin TE, Greinacher A. Heparin-induced thrombocytopenia: recognition, treatment, and prevention: the Seventh ACCP Conference on Antithrombotic and Thrombolytic Therapy. Chest. 2004;126(3):311S-37S.
121. Greer IA, Nelson-Piercy C. Low-molecular-weight heparins for thromboprophylaxis and treatment of venous thromboembolism in pregnancy: a systematic review of safety and efficacy. Blood. 2005;106(2):401-7.
122. Wiegers HM, Middeldorp S. Contemporary best practice in the management of pulmonary embolism during pregnancy. Ther Adv Respir Dis. 2020;14:1753466620914222.
123. Bates SM, Ginsberg JS. 5 Anticoagulants in pregnancy: fetal effects. Baillière's Clin Obstet Gynaecol. 1997;11(3):479-88.
124. Greer IA. Prevention and management of venous thromboembolism in pregnancy. Clin Chest Med. 2003;24(1):123-37.
125. Barbier P, Jonville AP, Autret E, et al. Fetal risks with dextrans during delivery. Drug Saf. 1992;7:71-3.
126. Lindhoff-Last E, Willeke A, Thalhammer C, et al. Hirudin treatment in a breastfeeding woman. Lancet. 2000;355(9202):467-8.
127. CLASP Collaborative Group. CLASP: a randomised trial of low-dose aspirin for the prevention and treatment of pre-eclampsia among 9364 pregnant women. Lancet. 1994;343(8898):619-29.
128. Sousa Gomes M, Guimarães M, Montenegro N. Thrombolysis in pregnancy: a literature review. J Matern Fetal Neonatal Med. 2019;32(14):2418-28.
129. Dhar R, Ghoshal AG, Guleria R, et al. Clinical practice guidelines 2019: Indian consensus-based recommendations on influenza vaccination in adults. Lung India. 2020;37(Suppl 1):S4.
130. Harper SA, Fukuda K, Uyeki TM, Cox NJ, Bridges CB. Prevention and control of influenza: recommendations of the Advisory Committee on Immunization Practices (ACIP). MMWR Recomm Rep. 2005;54(8):1-41.
131. Englund JA. Maternal immunization with inactivated influenza vaccine: rationale and experience. Vaccine. 2003;21(24):3460-4.

Oxygen Therapy in Critically Ill Pregnant Women

CHAPTER 141

Mohankumar Thekkinkattil

DEFINITION

Any medical condition during pregnancy that poses a risk to the mother's life or the life of the fetus and necessitates immediate medical intervention is referred to as a critical illness.[1] It can be brought on by a number of conditions, including infections, pregnancy difficulties, and preexisting medical disorders. The common causes of critical illness in pregnant women are obstetric hemorrhage, preeclampsia, sepsis, and respiratory failure.[2] Obstetric hemorrhage is the most common cause of critical illness in pregnant women. Multiple organ dysfunction syndrome (MODS) is a condition that can be brought on by a number of different diseases.[3] MODS is associated with high mortality and morbidity rates. To enhance mother and fetal outcomes, serious illness in pregnancy must be identified and managed early. Oxygen therapy is one of the main interventions used in the management of critically ill pregnant women.[4]

IMPORTANCE OF OXYGEN THERAPY IN CRITICALLY ILL PREGNANT WOMEN

Oxygen treatment is an essential component of the management of critically sick pregnant patients because it can improve the delivery of oxygen to key organs and avoid hypoxia, both of which have the potential to have a severe influence on the outcomes for both the mother and the unborn child.[5] Oxygen treatment can also lessen the risk of maternal death.[6]

Oxygen treatment can enhance oxygen delivery while also lessening the strain on the respiratory system and enhancing respiratory performance, both of which might be affected in critically sick pregnant women due to altered lung mechanics and elevated oxygen demand.[7] Due to the fact that severe nausea is a common side effect of pregnancy, knowing this information is essential in circumstances involving respiratory failure. The severity of the sickness as well as the patient's present clinical status will determine the treatment strategy that is implemented. It is crucial to monitor oxygen treatment to make sure it is working properly and not having any negative side effects.

Physiology of Oxygen Transport in Pregnancy

During pregnancy, there is a significant shift in both demand for and supply of oxygen, a change that is essential for the growth and development of the fetus. The increasing and more metabolically active organs of the fetus bring an increase in the requirement for oxygen throughout the duration of the pregnancy. The increased metabolic demands of pregnancy cause a concurrent increase in the amount of oxygen that a pregnant woman needs to breathe.[8]

In order to adapt to the higher need for oxygen, the cardiovascular and respiratory systems of the mother undergo a variety of changes during pregnancy. There is a 30–50% increase in the maternal cardiac output, most of which may be attributed to an increase in stroke volume. Because of the rise in cardiac output, both the placenta and the developing baby get a greater supply of oxygen. In addition, there is a 40–50% increase in the volume of the mother's blood, which results in an increase in the blood's capacity to carry oxygen.

Alterations in respiratory physiology during pregnancy include an increase in both tidal volume and minute ventilation.[9] The need to cut down on the amount of carbon dioxide that is produced as a result of the increased metabolic activity and the increased demand for oxygen are the factors that have led to these changes. It is possible for the respiratory rate to remain the same or even slightly decrease due to the compensatory rise in tidal volume.[9]

The pathophysiology of oxygen supply to the mother and the developing fetus involves a complex interplay between the circulatory and respiratory function of the mother, the function of the placenta, and the routes that the developing fetus uses to transfer oxygen.[10] In order to meet the increased oxygen demand of the mother's tissues as well as those of the developing fetus, the oxygen-carrying capacity of the mother's blood increases during pregnancy as a result of an increase in both the mass of the red blood cells and the volume of the plasma.[11]

The placenta is absolutely necessary for the transfer of oxygen from the mother to the developing child. After passing through the placenta and diffusing from the maternal blood into the fetal blood, oxygen is brought to the fetal blood through the processes of diffusion and aided diffusion. The placenta is responsible for removing carbon dioxide and other waste products from the fetal blood and transferring them to the circulation of the mother, where they may be eliminated.[12]

Fetal hemoglobin concentration, heart rate, blood pressure, and the level of placental perfusion also affect fetal oxygen transfer. Conditions including placental insufficiency, fetal growth limitation, and maternal hypoxemia can all affect how much oxygen is delivered to the fetus.[13] Reduced prenatal oxygen delivery caused by these factors may cause fetal discomfort, hypoxia, and even fetal death. In some situations, including preeclampsia, ARDS, and sepsis, the transport of oxygen to the mother may be hampered. Maternal oxygen demand may exceed maternal oxygen supply in these circumstances, leading to hypoxemia and possible organ dysfunction.

Overall, intricate interactions between maternal cardiovascular and respiratory function, placental function, and fetal oxygen transport pathways are involved in the pathophysiology of maternal and fetal oxygen delivery. In order to manage severe disease during pregnancy and prevent negative effects for the mother and the fetus, it is crucial to comprehend these connections.

Oxygen supply to the mother and fetus might be significantly impacted by critical sickness during pregnancy. Both underlying ailment causing the serious sickness and the fetus' gestational age affect the severity of the impact. Critical illness during pregnancy often increases the risk of hypoxemia, decreased oxygen transport to the tissues, and probable organ dysfunction in both the mother and fetus.[14] ARDS can cause hypoxemia, decreased lung compliance, and ventilation-perfusion mismatch, which reduces the amount of oxygen delivered to the maternal tissues.[15] Decreased placental perfusion and oxygen supply to the fetus can be caused by preeclampsia, a disease marked by hypertension and proteinuria, and may result in fetal hypoxia and distress.[16]

The goal of managing a serious illness during pregnancy should be to ensure that the mother and fetus receive enough oxygen. To enhance maternal cardiovascular performance and placental perfusion, this may entail measures such as more oxygen, mechanical breathing, and inotropic support.[17] To increase fetal oxygenation and stop further maternal decompensation in extreme situations, delivery may be indicated.

Oxygen Therapy

Depending on the underlying disease causing the severe illness, there are several indications for oxygen treatment in critically sick pregnant women. However, maintaining adequate tissue perfusion and oxygenation is a crucial component of managing these patients, and supplemental oxygen therapy can be a crucial intervention in achieving this goal. The following are some typical indications for oxygen treatment in seriously sick pregnant women:

- Hypoxemia
- *ARDS*: It is possible for critically unwell pregnant women to develop ARDS, a severe form of respiratory failure.[18] Supporting sufficient oxygenation is critical to stop additional lung damage, and oxygen treatment is a crucial component of controlling ARDS.
- *Sepsis*: Tissue hypoxia and organ failure can occur from sepsis, a potentially fatal illness brought on by a dysregulated immunological response to infection.[19] Additional oxygen therapy can enhance tissue oxygenation and stop further organ deterioration.
- *Preeclampsia*: This is a disorder that only affects pregnant women that is characterized by proteinuria and hypertension. This condition can result in impaired placental perfusion and fetal hypoxia.[20] The oxygenation of the fetus and placenta can both be enhanced by oxygen treatment.
- *Pulmonary embolism*: It is an important cause of morbidity, hypoxia, and death in pregnant women.[21] While further management is being implemented, additional oxygen therapy can enhance oxygenation.

Overall, oxygen therapy is an essential treatment for treating critically sick pregnant patients, particularly those who have respiratory, septic, or cardiovascular impairment. The results for the mother and fetus can be improved with prompt and efficient therapy of tissue hypoxia and hypoxemia.

Oxygen Delivery Systems

The selection of an oxygen treatment technique depends on the patient's state, the underlying cause of hypoxemia, and the advantages and disadvantages of each possible intervention.

- *Nasal cannula*: The most popular oxygen delivery technique for severely unwell pregnant patients is a nasal cannula. It includes inserting two tiny prongs into the nose to supply oxygen, and it has a flow rate range of 1–6 L/min. In mild-to-moderate episodes of hypoxemia, nasal cannulas can be employed since they are often well tolerated.
- *Face mask*: Patients who require higher oxygen flow rates can use face mask oxygen delivery. For patients with moderate-to-severe hypoxemia, face masks can supply oxygen at flow rates of up to 15 L/min. They can be either straightforward face masks or non-rebreather masks.
- *Noninvasive positive pressure ventilation (NIPPV)*: NIPPV is a technique for administering oxygen while also providing positive-pressure ventilation to support breathing using a face mask or nasal mask. Patients with respiratory failure or those unable to tolerate invasive mechanical ventilation can use NIPPV. In pregnant women experiencing respiratory distress, NIPPV has been demonstrated to be successful in treating hypoxemia.[22]

- *Invasive mechanical ventilation*: Endotracheal tubes are inserted into the trachea during invasive mechanical ventilation in order to support breathing and distribute oxygen. Patients with severe respiratory failure who do not respond to noninvasive therapies are often the only ones who get it. In order to prevent problems such aspiration and alterations in uterine blood flow during mechanical breathing in pregnant women, extra precautions must be taken.[23]

When deciding how best to treat a patient with oxygen, it is important to take into account both the patient's current clinical status and how well they respond to treatment. In order to provide a therapy that is successful, it is necessary to carefully monitor the patient's respiratory rate, levels of oxygen saturation, and general clinical state. To guarantee efficient oxygen therapy and avoid problems related to hypoxemia, monitoring oxygen levels in critically sick pregnant patients is crucial. Some commonly employed techniques for oxygen monitoring include the following:

- *Pulse oximetry*: A noninvasive technique for tracking blood oxygen saturation levels is pulse oximetry. It entails applying a tiny sensor to the patient's finger, toe, or earlobe to gauge the blood's level of oxygen-bound hemoglobin. In order to monitor oxygen saturation levels and spot changes in oxygenation status in severely unwell pregnant women, continuous pulse oximetry monitoring is frequently performed.[24]
- *Arterial blood gas (ABG) analysis*: Drawing an arterial blood sample for an ABG study allows the measurement of many parameters, including the partial pressures of oxygen and carbon dioxide (PaO_2 and $PaCO_2$). The patient's acid–base state, breathing, and oxygenation are evaluated using an ABG analysis. Patients with severe hypoxemia or those receiving mechanical ventilation are often the only ones who have an ABG analysis.[25]
- *Transcutaneous oxygen monitoring*: A sensor that detects how much oxygen diffuses through the skin is applied for transcutaneous oxygen monitoring. In some circumstances, it can be employed as an alternative to ABG analysis and provides continuous monitoring of oxygenation status.
- *End-tidal carbon dioxide ($EtCO_2$) monitoring*: When monitoring $EtCO_2$, carbon dioxide levels in exhaled air are counted. It is used to monitor the patient's breathing and it also has the potential to offer data on the patient's oxygenation. Monitoring of $EtCO_2$ is frequently used in patients who are undergoing mechanical ventilation.

When deciding on an oxygen monitoring strategy, it is important to take into account both the clinical condition of the patient and the required level of monitoring. In order for oxygen therapy to be effective, it is necessary to pay close attention to the patient's respiratory rate as well as their clinical status and to continuously check their oxygen saturation levels.

Oxygen Toxicity

- Oxygen poisoning can develop after prolonged exposure to high concentrations of oxygen, which can be detrimental to the health of the lungs and other organs. It is possible that pregnant women have an increased risk of oxygen poisoning due to changes in their lung function as well as an increased susceptibility to the damage caused by free radicals.
- *Retinopathy of prematurity*: Prematurity-related retinopathy, a disorder that can result in blindness or visual loss, can be brought on by high oxygen exposure levels in preterm newborns. Infants born prematurely who are at risk of having this illness may be more common among pregnant mothers who get high doses of oxygen treatment.[26]
- *Absorption atelectasis*: Absorption atelectasis, a condition in which alveoli collapse because of low nitrogen levels, can result with high oxygen treatment doses. Gas exchange may be hampered and lung capacity may decrease as a result.[27]
- *Hypercapnia*: Reduced respiratory drive caused by oxygen treatment can result in hypercapnia, a condition where blood carbon dioxide levels rise. Acidosis, respiratory failure, and other problems might result from hypercapnia.[28]
- *Fire hazard*: When utilized improperly, oxygen, which is extremely flammable, can raise the danger of fire. All safety measures should be taken to prevent fires around pregnant women receiving oxygen therapy, and they should be closely monitored.

In general, the advantages of oxygen treatment for severely sick pregnant patients outweigh any possible dangers.

EVIDENCE FOR OXYGEN THERAPY DURING PREGNANCY

The efficacy of oxygen treatment in seriously unwell pregnant women has been the subject of a great interest. In the randomized controlled trial, high-flow oxygen therapy for pregnant women with hypoxemia (HOT-TOHP), pregnant women with hypoxemia were given either high-flow oxygen treatment or conventional oxygen therapy, and the results were compared to see whether type of oxygen therapy was more effective. It was concluded that high-flow oxygen therapy had a decreased risk of intubation or mortality when compared to regular oxygen therapy.[29]

It was demonstrated that in an evaluation of the effectiveness of noninvasive positive-pressure ventilation in pregnant women with acute respiratory distress syndrome that noninvasive positive-pressure ventilation was preferable to invasive mechanical ventilation in terms of higher oxygenation and lower mortality.[30] The authors of a systematic review and meta-analysis evaluated the efficacy of oxygen treatment in pregnant women who were diagnosed with preeclampsia or eclampsia and concluded that oxygen therapy improved the oxygenation of the mother and reduced the risk that the baby would experience discomfort.[31]

In another retrospective study on evaluation of the effectiveness of a multidisciplinary obstetric critical care team (MOCCI) in reducing the risk of maternal death and morbidity among critically ill pregnant women, it was concluded that the utilization of oxygen therapy as part of the MOCCI protocol was an essential component that was associated with a reduced likelihood of maternal mortality and morbidity.[32]

These studies collectively imply that oxygen treatment is useful in enhancing oxygenation and lowering mortality in critically unwell pregnant patients. In general, oxygen treatment is regarded as safe for fetuses and pregnant mothers.

Overall, these studies indicate that oxygen therapy is typically safe for expectant mothers and developing fetuses, but high-dose oxygen therapy may be linked to a higher risk of problems from hyperoxia in some groups. In order to prevent hyperoxia, it is crucial to monitor oxygen saturation levels and modify oxygen treatment as necessary. In severely sick pregnant patients, the potential advantages of supplementary oxygen typically exceed the risks, although high-dose oxygen treatment should be administered carefully and titrated to prevent hyperoxemia and oxygen toxicity.

SUMMARY

Oxygen treatment is crucial to maintain sufficient oxygenation and prevent hypoxemia in severely sick pregnant women. ABG analysis and pulse oximetry should be used to monitor oxygen levels in severely unwell pregnant patients. Oxygen toxicity, hyperoxemia, and carbon dioxide retention are potential side effects of oxygen treatment in critically unwell pregnant women.

The efficacy of oxygen treatment in severely sick pregnant women is supported by data from clinical trials and observational research. Supplemental oxygen can increase fetal and maternal oxygenation and lower the risk of newborn problems, but it should be administered carefully to prevent any potential risks. In severely sick pregnant patients, the advantages of supplementary oxygen therapy often exceed the dangers, although oxygen therapy needs to be adjusted to prevent hyperoxemia and oxygen toxicity.

It is important to undertake large-scale randomized controlled studies evaluating various ways of oxygen administration and to understand how oxygen treatment may affect mother and fetal outcomes throughout the long term. One needs to understand its role to treat or prevent pre-eclampsia and other pregnancy-related problems as well as to examine how oxygen treatment affects the microbiomes of the mother and fetus.

REFERENCES

1. Lapinsky SE, Kruczynski K, Slutsky AS. Critical care in pregnancy. In: Vincent JL, Abraham E, Kochanek P, Moore FA, Fink MP (Eds). Textbook of Critical Care, 6th edition. Philadelphia, PA: Elsevier; 2011.
2. Bauer ME, Bateman BT, Bauer ST, et al. Maternal sepsis mortality and morbidity during hospitalization for delivery: Temporal trends and independent associations for severe sepsis. Anesth Analg. 2013;117(4):944-50.
3. Kissoon N, Carcillo JA, Espinosa V, et al. World Federation of Pediatric Intensive Care and Critical Care Societies: Global Sepsis Initiative. Pediatr Crit Care Med. 2011;12(5):494-503.
4. Eslami V, Saadati M, Mohammadpoorasl A, et al. Oxygen therapy in critically ill pregnant women: systematic review and meta-analysis. J Matern Fetal Neonatal Med. 2021;34(14):2346-54.
5. Kacmar RM, Wong J, Glantz JC, et al. Oxygen therapy and outcomes in critically ill pregnant women: a retrospective cohort study. J Matern Fetal Neonatal Med. 2018;31(1):71-5.
6. Chandraharan E, Arulkumaran S. Management of critically ill obstetric patients: a structured approach. Best Pract Res Clin Obstet Gynaecol. 2013;27(6):877-91.
7. Shennan AH, Crawshaw S, Briley A, et al. The administration of oxygen in women presenting with acute severe asthma:a randomized controlled trial. Am J Obstet Gynecol. 2011;204 (6 Suppl 1): S27-8.
8. Madden LA, Vinall LE, Oliver E, et al. Oxygen consumption and uterine artery blood flow in non-pregnant, pregnant and postpartum women. Am J Physiol Regul Integr Comp Physiol. 2014;306(12): R908-15.
9. Hegewald MJ, Crapo RO. Respiratory physiology in pregnancy. Clin Chest Med. 2011;32(1):1-13.
10. Mayhew TM, Charnock-Jones DS, Kaufmann P. Aspects of human fetoplacental vasculogenesis and angiogenesis. III. Changes in complicated pregnancies. Placenta. 2004;25(2-3):127-39.
11. Kechichian T, Budak K, Togal T, et al. Pathophysiology of maternal-fetal oxygenation and related perinatal outcomes. J Obstet Gynaecol Res. 2018;44(9):1574-85.
12. Burton GJ, Jauniaux E. Placental oxygen transport: how does the human placenta compare with others? Placenta. 2015;36(4): 319-28.
13. De Koninck P, Moutquin JM. Fetal oxygen delivery. Paediatr Anaesth. 2014;24(1):56-68
14. Kechichian T, Budak K, Togal T, et al. Pathophysiology of maternal-fetal oxygenation and related perinatal outcomes. J Obstet Gynaecol Res. 2018;44(9):1574-85.
15. Matthay MA, Zemans RL. The acute respiratory distress syndrome: pathogenesis and treatment. Annu Rev Pathol. 2011;6:147-63.
16. Sibai BM. Diagnosis and management of gestational hypertension and preeclampsia. Obstet Gynecol. 2003;102(1): 181-92.
17. Wong CA, McCarthy RJ. Critical care obstetrics. Int J Obstet Anesth. 2010;19(4):38292.
18. Aissaoui N, Larcher R, Marcoux A, et al. acute respiratory distress syndrome during pregnancy: a systematic review and meta-analysis. Obstet Gynecol. 2016;128(5):1157-66.

19. Singer M, Deutschman CS, Seymour CW, et al. The Third International Consensus Definitions for Sepsis and Septic Shock (Sepsis-3). JAMA. 2016;315(8):801-10.
20. Sibai BM. Diagnosis and management of gestational hypertension and preeclampsia. Obstet Gynecol. 2003;102(1): 181-92.
21. Pomp ER, Lenselink AM, Rosendaal FR, et al. Pregnancy, the postpartum period and prothrombotic defects: risk of venous thrombosis in the MEGA study. J Thromb Haemost. 2008;6(4):632-7.
22. Aly H, Hammad TA, Essa R, et al. Non-invasive ventilation for respiratory distress syndrome in preterm infants. Cochrane Database Syst Rev. 2021;1:CD013457.
23. Wilson JG, Balki M. Anesthetic management of critically ill pregnant patients. Curr Opin Anaesthesiol. 2020;33(3):366-73.
24. Duran-Crane A, Stevens TP. Noninvasive monitoring of oxygenation in infants and children: practical considerations and areas of concern. Respir Care. 2013;58(12):2137-50.
25. Hess DR. How to read a blood gas. Respir Care. 2019;64(1): 78-91.
26. Chen ML, Guo L, Smith LEH, et al. Complications and challenges of oxygen therapy in the neonatal intensive care unit. Neurol Res. 2017;39(7):663-72.
27. Smit B, Smulders Y. Absorption atelectasis and anesthesia-induced hypoxemia. Open Anesthesiol J. 2009;3:33-6.
28. Kallet RH. Physiology and management of hypercapnia. Respir Care. 2013;58(1):49-60.
29. Sultan P, Dickinson M, McKeen D, et al. High-flow nasal cannula oxygen therapy versus standard oxygen therapy in pregnant women with suspected hypoxemia: a randomized controlled trial. Obstet Gynecol. 2018;132(2):281-9.
30. Chen H, Qian X, Tang Z, et al. Comparison of noninvasive positive pressure ventilation with invasive mechanical ventilation in pregnant women with acute respiratory distress syndrome: a retrospective cohort study. J Thorac Dis. 2017;9(5):1344-52.
31. Wang Y, Zhang Y, Qian X, et al. Oxygen therapy for pre-eclampsia or eclampsia: A systematic review and meta-analysis. BMC Pregnancy Childbirth. 2017;17(1):44.
32. Mhyre JM, Tsen LC, Einav S, et al. Cardiac arrest during hospitalization for delivery in the United States: a 10-year population-based study. Anesthesiology. 2014;120(4):810-8.

SECTION

15

Respiratory Sleep Disorders

SECTION OUTLINE

Sleep-related Respiratory Disorders

CHAPTER 142

Sean Michael Duenas, Harly Greenberg

INTRODUCTION

Sleep-related respiratory disorders refer to a large group of conditions characterized with one or the other breathing anomaly ranging from chronic or habitual snoring to frank obstructive sleep apnea (OSA). Diagnosis of a sleep disorder is frequently missed due to late recognition of symptoms and delayed investigations. We discuss here some of the common sleep disorders seen in clinical practice.

OBSTRUCTIVE SLEEP APNEA

Definitions

Obstructive sleep apnea is the most prevalent form of sleep-disordered breathing and is characterized by periods of partial to complete upper airway collapse during sleep. As a result of airflow limitation, patients with OSA often experience symptoms of snoring, sleep disruption, daytime somnolence, nocturnal hypoxemia, and intermittent increases in sympathetic tone. While not required for diagnosis, classic features associated with an increased risk for OSA include obese body habitus, increased neck circumference, crowded oropharynx, and craniofacial abnormalities such as micrognathia and retrognathia. However, OSA may also be present in the absence of classic body habitus and symptom phenotypes. Comorbid conditions that have been shown to be independently associated with OSA include cardiovascular, cerebrovascular, and metabolic diseases as well as functional impairments including impaired vigilance, memory, cognition, and mood.[1] Population-based studies also demonstrate an independent association of OSA with increased all-cause mortality.[2]

Epidemiology

The worldwide prevalence of OSA is estimated at approximately 936 million people with over 425 million diagnosed with moderate-to-severe OSA.[3] Furthermore, it is estimated that more than 80% of those with OSA are undiagnosed.[4] Countries most affected by OSA include China, the United States, Brazil, and India.[3] Estimated rates of OSA in India range from 3.7 to 11% with higher prevalence in those living in urban environments.[5-7] Furthermore, males tend to be disproportionately affected compared to females in the age range of 30–70 years with reported prevalence of 14% compared to 6%, respectively.[7,8]

Prevalence in Disease-specific and Ethnic Cohorts

Increased prevalence of OSA can also be seen among different disease-specific cohorts. For example, approximately 50% of patients with hypertension are estimated to have OSA, whereas those with chronic kidney disease are estimated to have a prevalence of approximately 40%.[9,10] The presence of OSA has also been associated with increases in coronary artery disease, hypertension, atrial fibrillation, and cerebrovascular accidents.[11] OSA prevalence may also vary based on ethnicity with higher rates of OSA in African-American and Asian populations compared to Caucasians.[12,13]

Upper Airway Physiology

Upper airway anatomy plays a critical role in determining the presence and severity of OSA. One of the greatest risk factors for upper airway obstruction is a narrow luminal cross-sectional area. When compared to non-OSA subjects, patients with OSA show smaller upper airway area independent of body mass index (BMI) and overall body habitus.[14] In addition, tongue size can contribute significantly to airway narrowing with increased tongue fat at the base of the tongue also reducing the size of the retroglossal airway.[15] Modifiable factors may also influence total luminal area including airway edema, positionally dependent rostral fluid shifts, and snoring induced soft tissue inflammation.[16,17]

In addition to upper airway cross-sectional area, susceptibility to dynamic collapse is another prominent risk factor for upper airway obstruction. Patency of the airway is maintained through a balance between the collapsing forces of the pharynx and surrounding tissues and the opposing opening forces of the upper airway dilator muscles.[18]

Areas most susceptible to collapse in the upper airway include the retropalatal, retroglossal, hypopharyngeal, and epiglottic areas. Dynamic collapse occurs most frequently in the retropalatal region due to a narrow lumen and high compliance. The retroglossal region is also a major site of upper airway obstruction during sleep. The epiglottic region, which experiences reduced elasticity during aging, can be the area of greatest collapse in approximately 30% of patients with OSA and portends poor response to positive airway pressure therapy and mandibular advancement devices.[19] Increased total upper airway length from mandibular plane to hyoid bone may also reflect increased collapsibility as this portion of the airway is not supported by bony structures.[20]

Mechanisms of Upper Airway Flow Limitation

Flow through the upper airway can be affected by intrinsic properties of the airway, including compliance and elasticity, as well as the function of the upper airway dilator muscles. During inhalation, pressure within the pharyngeal lumen becomes increasingly negative relative to atmospheric pressure and continues to decrease as inspiratory effort increases. The intraluminal pressure at which the upper airway narrows with resulting inspiratory flow limitation is known as the *critical closing pressure* (P_{crit}). While normal subjects have a negative P_{crit} in the range of −10 to −15 cm of water pressure, OSA patients have a less negative P_{crit} that can even exceed atmospheric pressure in those with severe OSA.[21] In these instances, upper airway patency is maintained primarily through the action of upper airway dilators. Patients may also experience further reduction in flow throughout inspiration, as inspiratory effort may be insufficient to overcome increasing upper airway resistance, resulting in further reductions in inspiratory flow, a phenomenon known as *negative effort dependence (NED)*.

While anatomic properties of the upper airway that determine its P_{crit} are a major contributing factor to OSA in many individuals, other physiologic traits or endotypes have been shown to influence the development of OSA. These include the following:

- *Loop gain*, which is defined as the ratio of the ventilatory response to a ventilatory disturbance, a metric which reflects the degree of increase in ventilation occurring in response to a hypopnea or apnea. When the ventilatory response is equivalent to the magnitude of the prior decrement in ventilation, breathing is stabilized. However, if the magnitude of the ventilatory response is greater than that of the preceding decrement, loop gain is said to be high, and ventilatory instability ensues that affects ventilatory drive to the upper airway dilators as well as the respiratory muscles and contributes to further episodes of apnea/hypopnea.
- The *arousal threshold* describes the likelihood of cortical arousal in response to varying degrees of ventilatory disturbances. Individuals with a low arousal threshold can experience frequent sleep disruption due to hypopneas and apneas, while those with a higher arousal threshold can restore upper airway patency during periods of partial or complete obstruction without the sleep destabilizing effect of cortical arousals.
- *Upper airway dilator responsiveness and effectiveness* is another endotype with interindividual variability which can affect the propensity to upper airway obstruction and OSA severity.[22]

Signs and Symptomatology

Classic symptoms of OSA include snoring, nocturnal gasping, paradoxical respiratory efforts, witnessed apneas, frequent nocturnal awakenings, unrefreshing sleep, and dry mouth. Coexisting symptoms, such as morning headaches, may also suggest the presence of nocturnal hypoventilation leading to cerebral vasodilation causing transient morning headaches. It is important to note that while snoring occurs through flow limitation, it can also be present in those without significant degrees of OSA. Impaired sleep quality that results from chronic fragmentation of sleep due to recurrent arousals associated with sleep-disordered breathing may result in daytime somnolence. Poor sleep quality resulting from sleep apnea may also lead to cognitive deficits (e.g., reduced concentration, vigilance, memory and executive function), chronic fatigue, mood disorders, and overall impaired functional capacity. In addition to the classic symptoms indicated above, large population-based studies have identified different symptom subtypes of OSA. These include disturbed sleep and insomnia, minimal symptoms, moderate somnolence, and excessive somnolence. Recognition of the variability of symptom subtypes is important for clinical identification of individuals at risk for sleep apnea. It has also been shown that the phenotype of excessive sleepiness has been associated with the greatest incidence of adverse cardiovascular outcomes.[23,24]

Diagnostic Testing

Screening for OSA should be performed in the setting of suggestive clinical features or high-risk comorbidities. Questionnaire-based assessments, such as the Epworth Sleepiness Scale (ESS) and the STOP-BANG questionnaire, can be used to assist with pretest probability. However, the Epworth has a low sensitivity for detecting OSA (sensitivity 49.9% and specificity for moderate-to-severe OSA 61.1%)[25] with the STOP-BANG having the highest sensitivity (87% sensitivity and 31% specificity for moderate-to-severe OSA).[26] Once clinical suspicion for OSA is confirmed, diagnostic testing should be pursued for confirmation and determination of disease severity. The decision whether to pursue in-center polysomnography (PSG) or home sleep testing should be based on the presence of comorbid cardiopulmonary conditions, considerations for associated nonrespiratory sleep disorders, patient preference, practicality, and insurance coverage concerns.

In-Center Polysomnography

In-center PSG is the gold standard for the diagnosis of OSA. The in-center PSG measures a multitude of physiologic parameters that can assist with sleep staging and sleep-related respiratory events. Scoring of sleep is performed by measurements of electroencephalography (EEG), electrooculogram (EOG), and electromyogram (EMG). Apneas are evaluated by oronasal thermistor and hypopneas, and flow-limited events are assessed by nasal pressure measurements via a nasal cannula. Respiratory effort is determined by thorax and abdomen total compartmental displacement as assessed by inductance plethysmography. Pulse oximetry assesses oxygen saturation (SpO_2) and provides a plethysmography signal that provides additional information on peripheral vasoconstriction. A single-channel ECG is also recorded. Body position and continuous video are also recorded. Transcutaneous or end-tidal CO_2 monitoring may be used when nocturnal hypoventilation is suspected.

An apnea is defined as >90% reduction of airflow for a minimum duration of 10 seconds. Criteria for hypopneas may vary based on different societies and insurance organizations. The *American Academy of Sleep Medicine* (*AASM*) defines a hypopnea as a period of at least 10 seconds with 30–90% reduction in airflow and an accompanying 4% desaturation (AHI4) or a desaturation of at least 3% and/or an associated cortical arousal (AHI3A). Severity of OSA in adults (age > 18 years) is defined by the total number of apnea and hypopnea events per hour with 5–14.9, 15–29.9, and 30 or more indicating mild, moderate, and severe sleep apnea, respectively. Children (at least 1 year old) require lower thresholds with apnea–hypopnea indexes (AHIs) of 1–4.9, 5–9.9, and 10/hr or more correlating with mild, moderate, and severe sleep apnea, respectively. Other polysomnographic findings are helpful to assess the severity of sleep-disordered breathing. The oxygen desaturation index (ODI), sleep time spent less than 90% saturation (T90), and the recently described hypoxic burden index (HBI), an index measuring degree and duration of oxygen desaturation associated with apneas or hypopneas, may be reported. The HBI is an emerging biomarker that may be more closely correlated with cardiovascular outcomes of OSA than AHI.[27] Other metrics to better define the severity of OSA and its relationship with cardiovascular and cerebrovascular risk are under investigation and include the pulse rate response to apneas, which may reflect apnea-associated sympathetic activation[28] and variability in plethysmographic pulse wave amplitude.[29] Other reported measures include respiratory effort-related arousals (RERAs) which quantify arousals associated with periods of inspiratory flow limitation as well as the frequency of arousals that are not related to respiratory events (including periodic limb movements and spontaneous arousals).

Home Sleep Testing

While the in-center polysomnogram provides a wealth of information to assess sleep quality, respiratory events, and other abnormalities that occur during sleep, there may be insufficient availability of in-center testing for assessment of the large population of suspected OSA (**Fig. 1**). Home

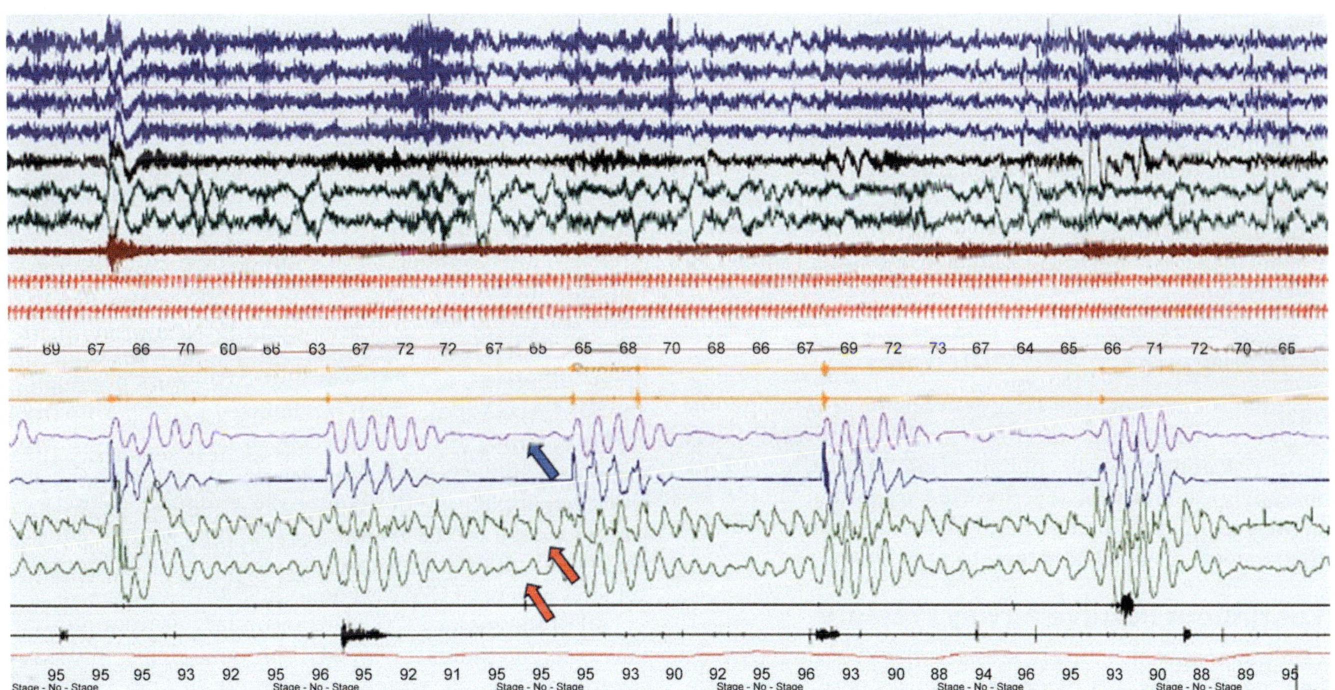

FIG. 1: Polysomnogram depicting obstructive sleep apnea. Blue arrow indicates greater than 90% reduction of inspiratory flow with red arrows demonstrating associated thoracic and abdominal effort.

sleep apnea testing (HSAT) uses fewer physiologic variables to measure the presence and severity of sleep-disordered breathing. There exists a wide variety of HSATs and they can differ based on the ways in which they measure sleep-disordered breathing events. A type 3 HST measures four or more channels including nasal airflow, chest and abdominal respiratory effort, and oximetry. Type 4 devices measure two or more parameters and most commonly utilize peripheral arterial tonometry (PAT), photoplethysmography (PPG), and SpO_2 to assess disordered breathing events. Some of these devices also include actigraphy and use movement along with variability in the above signals to estimate sleep staging. Emerging technology using machine learning and artificial intelligence is beginning to provide more information on sleep derived from home test variables.[30]

When selecting patients for HSAT, clinicians should consider key criteria that may preclude or limit the utility of home testing. As a result of the lack of EEG on most home sleep test devices, total sleep time may be overestimated when compared to measurements obtained from a PSG. Thus, for patients with mild-to-moderate OSA, HSAT may result in underestimation of overall severity. A 2019 review of home sleep testing noted false-negative rates for OSA between 13 and 20% with greatest rates in those with mild-to-moderate OSA.[31] HSAT is best utilized for those with a high clinical suspicion of moderate-to-severe OSA. Patients in whom comorbid sleep disorders are suspected, such as periodic limb movement disorder, parasomnias, or seizures, should avoid HSAT due to lack of EEG assessment and limb evaluation. The suspicion of central sleep apnea (CSA) alone is not a contraindication for HSAT, although the testing device should have the capability to accurately assess respiratory effort to distinguish obstructive from central apneas. Evaluation of hypoventilation is also limited in HSAT, and patients who require transcutaneous CO_2 monitoring (obesity/OHS, neuromuscular disorders, chronic cardiopulmonary conditions) should be referred for in-center testing. Due to the unattended nature of the study, patients who have limited cognitive ability or who are otherwise unable to perform the test in a home environment should be referred for in-center PSG.

Management and Outcomes

Optimal management of OSA depends on a combination of patient symptoms, comorbid conditions, overall long-term risk reduction, likelihood of adherence to various therapeutics, and OSA severity. OSA treatment should be viewed as long-term chronic disease management rather than a single diagnosis and therapy prescription.[32]

Continuous Positive Airway Pressure

Continuous positive airway pressure (CPAP) is the current gold standard for OSA treatment and uses positive pressure to maintain upper airway patency. Therapy can be initiated through in-center PSG with CPAP titration or at-home auto-titrating positive airway pressure (APAP) devices. While APAP therapy has been shown to be noninferior to CPAP in terms of adherence and effects on daytime somnolence, it should be avoided in those with nocturnal hypoventilation or comorbid CSA.[33,34] Initial treatment with CPAP therapy may result in the emergence of CSA, though this will often resolve and should be monitored for at least 3 months prior to change in therapy.

Comparison between OSA patients on CPAP versus placebo therapy has demonstrated subjective improvements in daytime somnolence as well as quality of life and mood.[35,36] The optimal duration for CPAP usage in regard to improvements in functional outcomes and daytime sleepiness is unclear. However, a multicenter study of 149 patients demonstrated greater improvements in subjective and objective daytime somnolence and quality of life outcomes in patients with longer CPAP use up to 7 hours a night.[1] It is important to note that patients in this study demonstrated variability in treatment response, with many subjects showing improvement with less than 4 hours a night usage, highlighting the importance of patient-specific management.

Most, but not all, studies have shown an improvement in systemic arterial pressure with CPAP therapy.[37] Further, most studies have shown that CPAP therapy reduces the rate of recurrence of atrial fibrillation after cardioversion or ablation therapy.[38]

The effect of CPAP therapy on major adverse cardiovascular events (MACEs) has been studied in several secondary prevention randomized controlled trials (RCTs). The large multicenter SAVE study failed to demonstrate reduction in cardiovascular-related mortality, myocardial infarction, stroke, or progression to heart failure with CPAP therapy in patients with OSA and a previous history of cardiovascular disease, despite improvements in daytime somnolence and functional status. However, results are confounded by poor adherence to CPAP therapy (average 3.3 hours per night) as well as exclusion of higher risk patients with severe somnolence (ESS > 15) or hypoxemia (<80%).[39] Similarly, the International Study of Asthma and Allergies in Childhood (ISAAC) study showed no association between CPAP usage and cardiovascular risk reduction in nonsleepy patients with a history of acute coronary syndrome, though mean adherence to CPAP was only 2.78 hours per night.[40] The RICCADSA trial, which randomized patients with prior coronary artery disease and OSA to CPAP or usual care, excluding subjects with daytime sleepiness, also did not show an impact on the composite endpoint of incident cardiovascular events. However, a subgroup analysis showed significant reduction in cardiovascular event incidence in subjects who used CPAP > 4 hours/night.[41]

All of the major RCTs were secondary prevention trials that excluded patients with daytime somnolence and more severe hypoxemia, which are features of OSA that have been associated with an increased risk for cardiovascular disease.[24,42] Further, reversing existing cardiovascular disease may be more difficult than primary prevention. As a result, real-world observational studies, inclusive of all patients, may better reflect the impact of CPAP on cardiovascular outcomes. A large French national database analysis using propensity matching demonstrated a reduced mortality over 3 years [hazard ratio (HR) 0.61, 95% confidence interval (CI) 0.47–0.65] in those who continued CPAP (n = 88,007) compared with those who discontinued therapy (n = 88,007).[43] Another real-world observational study of 5,138 patients in France using propensity matching and adjustment for healthy user bias examined the effects of CPAP on MACEs. The study demonstrated that continued CPAP use resulted in reduction in MACE (HR 0.75–0.78) at a median follow up of 6.6 years for those using CPAP at least 6 hours a night compared to those using CPAP for 0–4 hours.[44]

Oral Appliance Therapy

Mandibular advancement devices may be used as an alternative treatment for those intolerant of CPAP therapy or as primary treatment for patients with mild-to-moderate OSA. These devices maintain upper airway patency through protrusion of the mandible and associated advancement of the tongue base, which increases the dimensions of the airway in both anterior–posterior and lateral dimensions. While less effective in the improvement of AHI compared to CPAP, oral appliances have been demonstrated to have similar efficacy in reducing blood pressure and improving functional outcomes.[45,46] Predictive factors for oral appliance therapy success are lower initial AHI and BMI.[47] Side effects of mandibular advancement therapy include alteration of dental occlusion and temporal–mandibular joint pain which necessitate dental follow-up.

Hypoglossal Nerve Stimulation

Hypoglossal nerve stimulation (HGNS) is an emerging form of therapy for OSA and is reserved for those with AHI 15–65 per hour and BMI < 35 kg/m^2 who are intolerant of CPAP therapy. However, these criteria may be broadened as this modality evolves. This form of therapy uses a surgically implanted electronic device, with electrodes placed on the hypoglossal nerve, to provide electrical stimulation, timed to inspiration, and to augment genioglossal activity and upper airway dilation. Candidacy for HGNS also requires anterior–posterior collapse of the airway determined through direct endoscopic visualization during drug-induced sleep endoscopy (DISE). Clinical studies show an approximate 70% response rate, defined by reduction of AHI < 50% and overall AHI < 20 events per hour, with most common side effects being discomfort from stimulation.[48]

CENTRAL SLEEP APNEA

Definitions

Central sleep apnea is defined as 90% reduction in airflow that lasts for 10 seconds or more without accompanying thoracoabdominal effort. CSA is often associated with Hunter–Cheyne–Stokes respiration (HCSR/CSR), which refers to periodic breathing that is characterized by three or more central apneas with an interspersed crescendo-decrescendo flow pattern that lasts for a cycle length of at least 40 seconds **(Fig. 2)**.[49] Clinical signs and symptoms of CSA can often overlap with OSA and can present with features of sleep fragmentation and resulting daytime somnolence and fatigue. Patients may also present with complaints of insomnia and difficulty maintaining sleep.

Pathophysiology

Clinical conditions associated with CSA include heart failure, atrial fibrillation, cerebrovascular disease, exposure to high altitude, and opiates. CSA often occurs as a result of instability of respiratory drive with fluctuation of the $PaCO_2$ above and below the apneic threshold, which is unmasked during sleep with withdrawal of the wakefulness drive to breath. Thus, chemoreceptor activity is an important contributing factor to CSA, at least during nonrapid eye movement (NREM) sleep. Elevated controller gain (ventilatory response to CO_2 $\Delta VE/\Delta PCO_2$), elevated plant gain ($\Delta PCO_2/\Delta VE$), and circulatory delay all contribute to periodic breathing in CSA.[50] Chemical drive to breath plays less of a role during REM sleep, and therefore CSA/CSR occurs less frequently during REM than during NREM sleep.

Central Sleep Apnea and Heart Failure

Heart failure is a highly prevalent comorbid condition in patients with CSA with an estimated prevalence of approximately 25–40%.[51] Approximately 50% of patients with left ventricular ejection fraction < 40% demonstrate CSA, with the prevalence of CSA increasing with worsening systolic dysfunction.[52,53] Diastolic dysfunction with moderately reduced ejection fraction has also been associated with an increased prevalence of CSA.[54-56] Patients with CSA have been shown to have a lower peak $\dot{V}O_2$, worse New York Heart Association (NYHA) functional class, and decreased 6-minute walk distance compared to those with OSA.[57] In a retrospective study of over 2,900 US veterans with CSA, comorbid CSA and heart failure were associated with an overall increased mortality (HR 7.4; 95% CI 6.67, 8.21) compared to patients with heart failure and OSA (HR 4.3; 95% CI 4.26, 4.34) independent of associated comorbidities.[58] CSA is also associated with atrial fibrillation.[59]

Treatment

Treatment of CSA is highly dependent on the underlying etiology and comorbid conditions associated with CSA. Optimized treatment of any underlying cardiac disease is paramount. If CSA is related to opioid use, consideration should be given toward alternative options or dose reduction as this can lead to improvement in or resolution of CSA.[60]

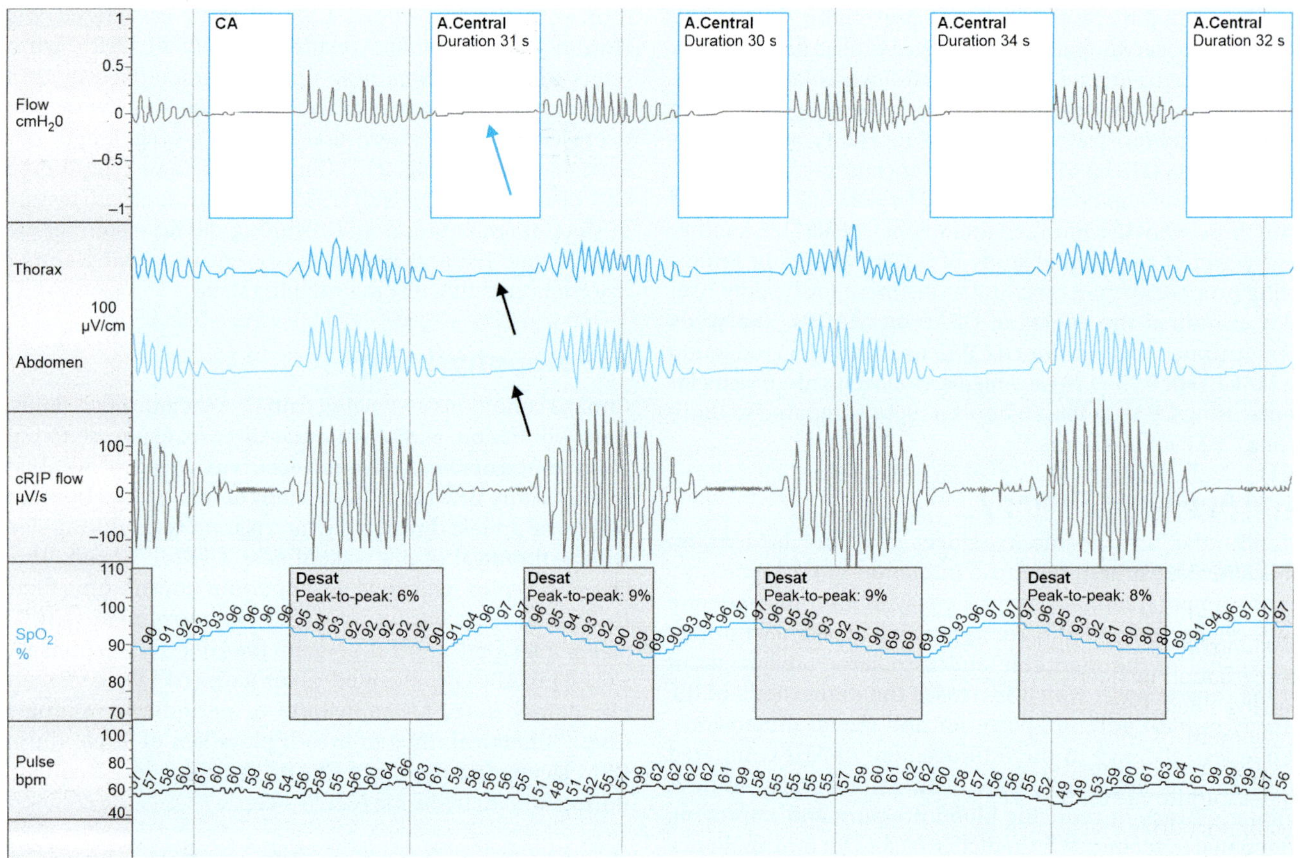

FIG. 2: Respiratory channels from home polygraphy demonstrating central sleep apnea and periodic breathing (Hunter–Cheyne–Stokes respiration). Blue arrow indicates cessation of inspiratory flow with black arrows indicating associated lack of thoracoabdominal effort.

Oxygen Therapy

Supplemental oxygen may be beneficial in CSA-CSR. Short-term randomized trials of nocturnal oxygen therapy for less than 1 month duration have demonstrated reduction in AHI by approximately 50% in those with comorbid heart failure with reduce ejection fraction (HFrEF). However, nocturnal oxygen use did not have a significant effect on daytime somnolence or quality of life in these groups.[61,62] Limited data has shown improvement in systolic function and NYHA functional class after oxygen use for CSA.[63] However, usage of nocturnal O_2 has been limited due to concern for increased oxidative stress, free radical generation, and cardiac stress that can occur from hyperoxia. At this time, use of supplemental O_2 in patients with comorbid CSA/CSR remains an unproven therapeutic modality.

Positive Airway Pressure Therapy

Various modalities of positive airway pressure therapy may be used in patients with CSA. Continuous positive airway pressure has been demonstrated to be beneficial in patients with CSA-CSR and heart failure by reducing left ventricular afterload and improving alveolar clearance of fluid. The multicenter randomized CANPAP study evaluated the use of CPAP versus usual care in those with systolic heart failure and CSA-CSR. Improvements in mean nocturnal oxygen saturation, LV ejection fraction, 6-minute walk distance, and lower norepinephrine levels were demonstrated in the CPAP group. However, CPAP had no significant effects on hospitalization, quality of life, or overall long-term survival.[64] However, CSA-CSR only improved in some of the CPAP-treated patients. A post hoc analysis of the CANPAP trial showed that the subset of patients whose CSA improved with CPAP did achieve a survival benefit.[65] However, CPAP is not effective in most patients with CSA. Bilevel PAP with a backup rate (bilevel ST) is often used in CSA-CSR. However, it is important to note that bilevel PAP even with a backup rate may worsen periodic breathing as it provides pressure support not only for apneas and hypopneas but also for hyperpneas that can worsen ventilatory instability and drive the $PaCO_2$ below the apneic threshold. Adaptive servo-ventilation (ASV) is a form of bilevel PAP therapy that can autoadjust inspiratory pressures to provide pressure support for hypopneas and apneas and automatically reduce or eliminate pressure support during hyperpneas. However, the SERVE-HF trial, which assessed the effects of ASV in patients with comorbid CSA/CSR and systolic heart failure, detected an increase in all-cause mortality and cardiovascular mortality in patients with LV ejection fraction < 45% and ASV therapy.[66] While current studies are re-examining these outcomes, ASV is presently contraindicated in systolic heart failure with ejection fraction below 45%.

Phrenic Nerve Stimulation

Phrenic nerve stimulation via a transvenous implantable neuro stimulator (remede® system) is a newer modality for treatment of CSA and HCSR. Studies of phrenic nerve stimulation in patients with CSA–HCSR and comorbid heart failure demonstrated improvements in AHI, quality of life, daytime sleepiness, 6-minute walk distance, nocturnal hypoxemic burden, and systolic function, without demonstrable change in overall cardiovascular-related mortality.[67,68]

NOCTURNAL HYPOVENTILATION SYNDROMES

Overview and Physiology

Nocturnal hypoventilation syndromes encompass a broad array of conditions that can lead to the presence or exacerbation of sleep-related hypercarbia and hypoxemia. During sleep, relaxation of thoracic muscles and cephalad movement of the diaphragm in the recumbent position lead to a reduction in functional residual capacity and end-expiratory lung volumes.[69,70] In addition, diminished respiratory drive that occurs during sleep leads to a reduction in overall minute ventilation compared to wakefulness. REM sleep is associated with the greatest degree of hypoventilation due to atonia of the accessory muscles of respiration as well as a further decrease in inspiratory drive secondary to reduced chemosensitivity, ultimately leading to further reduction in minute ventilation relative to NREM sleep.[71] Conditions that restrict thoracic expansion, impair diaphragmatic excursion, or limit inspiratory flow can exacerbate sleep-related hypoventilation to a pathologic level. Common causes of nocturnal hypoventilation include neuromuscular disorders, obesity hypoventilation syndrome (OHS), diseases of the chest wall such as kyphoscoliosis, and severe chronic obstructive pulmonary disease (COPD). Patients with comorbid OSA and COPD, termed "overlap syndrome," experience a higher degree of nocturnal desaturations with an associated increase in conditions such as atrial fibrillation, right heart failure, pulmonary hypertension, and mortality.[72] Comprehensive assessment of baseline lung function including pulmonary function testing, arterial blood gas measurements, and determination of respiratory muscle strength with maximal inspiratory and expiratory pressures should be performed for diagnosis and severity assessment as well as to monitor disease progression and therapeutic efficacy. When nocturnal hypoventilation is suspected, in-center PSG with transcutaneous CO_2 measurement may be helpful to assess comorbid OSA or CSA and to determine the severity of nocturnal hypoxemia and hypercapnia. This information can guide subsequent therapy.

Management

Management of nocturnal hypoventilation syndromes often involves the use of positive airway pressure to augment tidal volume and overall minute ventilation. In patients with neuromuscular-related hypoventilation, the use of noninvasive positive-pressure ventilation (NIPPV) has led to improvements in overall quality of life and mortality.[73,74] However, due to the paucity of data in patients with neuromuscular-related hypoventilation, the timing and form of NIV are left to the clinician's discretion.

Several modalities of noninvasive positive airway pressure ventilation are available. The two most common forms are bilevel positive airway pressure and volume-assured pressure support (VAPS). The latter relies on algorithmic adjustment of inspiratory and expiratory pressures to deliver a targeted tidal volume or minute ventilation. The goal for NIV should be to improve or normalize CO_2 levels as eucapnia has been associated with improvement, in gas exchange, respiratory function, sleep architecture, quality of life, and survival.[75-82] When configuring NIV, settings should be personalized to address the underlying disease process and patient physiology. In patients with OHS and OSA (OHS–OSA), CPAP is usually sufficient to improve overall nocturnal hypoventilation, although some patients may require NIV. However, patients with neuromuscular or chest wall disease may require greater degrees of pressure support to improve nocturnal hypoventilation.[83] These patients may benefit from NIV delivered via bilevel PAP, VAPS, or assist-control ventilation delivered via open circuit or closed circuit ventilatory systems. Mask interface fit is crucial to optimize comfort and minimize leaks. Further, the type of NIV must be personalized to individual patient needs. It is important to recognize that patients with neuromuscular weakness may have difficulty triggering or sustaining inspiration on the ventilator. This requires adjustment of variables such as trigger sensitivity and cycle threshold (defined as the decrement of inspiratory flow at which the ventilator cycles from inspiratory to expiration). Duration of usage should be continually reexamined not only to assess adherence but also to recognize that increased usage beyond nocturnal hours may suggest progression of the underlying neuromuscular disease. Last, contraindications for NIV should be examined and weighed against potential therapeutic benefit. Weak cough and recurrent aspiration can be worsened through the use of NIV. Adjunct airway clearance regimens including cough assist devices or secretion management with anticholinergics may be beneficial.[73]

SUMMARY

Sleep is associated with withdrawal of the wakefulness drive to breath with reduction in overall minute ventilation. REM sleep is associated with further variability in ventilation and reduced chemoreceptor regulation of ventilation. Sleep also results in reduced tonic and phasic drive to the upper airway dilator muscles increasing the propensity for upper airway narrowing and collapse. Thus, sleep is a time of vulnerability for the respiratory system. Challenges to ventilation during sleep may take the form of OSA or CSA, periodic breathing or HCSR, and sleep-related hypoventilation due to neuromuscular disorders and concomitant pulmonary disorders. In many cases, recognition and treatment of sleep-disordered breathing may result in improvement in quality of life, associated medical comorbid conditions, and overall survival.

REFERENCES

1. Weaver TE, Maislin G, Dinges DF, et al. Relationship between hours of CPAP use and achieving normal levels of sleepiness and daily functioning. Sleep. 2007;30(6):711-9.
2. Xie C, Zhu R, Tian Y, Wang K. Association of obstructive sleep apnoea with the risk of vascular outcomes and all-cause mortality: A meta-analysis. BMJ Open. 2017;7(12):e013983.
3. Benjafield AV, Ayas NT, Eastwood PR, et al. Estimation of the global prevalence and burden of obstructive sleep apnoea: A literature-based analysis. Lancet Respir Med. 2019;7(8):687-98.
4. Chen L, Pivetta B, Nagappa M, et al. Validation of the stop-bang questionnaire for screening of obstructive sleep apnea in the general population and commercial drivers: A systematic review and meta-analysis. Sleep Breath. 2021;25(4):1741-51.
5. Pinto AM, Devaraj U, Ramachandran P, et al. Obstructive sleep apnea in a rural population in South India: Feasibility of health care workers to administer level III sleep study. Lung India. 2018;35(4):301-6.
6. Devaraj U, Maheswari K U, Balla S, et al. Prevalence and risk factors for OSA among urban and rural subjects in Bengaluru District, South India: A cross-sectional study. Indian J Sleep Med. 2021;16(1):5-9.
7. Suri TM, Ghosh T, Mittal S, et al. Prevalence of obstructive sleep apnea in India: A systematic review and meta-analysis. C74. Do Not Miss: Sleep Disorders in Vulnerable Populations. Am J Respir Crit Care Med. 2023;207:A5840.
8. Young T, Peppard PE, Gottlieb DJ. Epidemiology of obstructive sleep apnea. Am J Respir Crit Care Med. 2002;165(9):1217-39.
9. Konecny T, Kara T, Somers VK. Obstructive sleep apnea and hypertension. Hypertension. 2014;63(2):203-9.
10. Nicholl DDM, Ahmed SB, Loewen AHS, et al. Declining kidney function increases the prevalence of sleep apnea and nocturnal hypoxia. Chest. 2012;141(6):1422-30.
11. Faria A, Macedo A, Castro C, et al. Impact of sleep apnea and treatments on cardiovascular disease. Sleep Sci. 2022;15(2):250-8.
12. Chen X, Wang R, Zee P, et al. Racial/ethnic differences in sleep disturbances: The multi-ethnic study of atherosclerosis (MESA)'. Sleep. 38(6):877-88.
13. Dudley KA, Patel SR. Disparities and genetic risk factors in obstructive sleep apnea. Sleep Med. 2016;18:96-102.
14. Ciscar MA, Juan G, Martínez V, et al. Magnetic resonance imaging of the pharynx in OSA patients and healthy subjects. Eur Respir J. 2001;17(1):79-86.
15. Kim AM, Keenan BT, Jackson N, et al. Tongue fat and its relationship to obstructive sleep apnea', Sleep. 2014;37(10):1639-48.
16. Boyd JH, Petrof BJ, Hamid Q, et al. Upper airway muscle inflammation and denervation changes in obstructive sleep apnea. Am J Respir Crit Care Med. 2004;170(5):541-6.
17. Redolfi S, Yumino D, Ruttanaumpawan P, et al. Relationship between overnight rostral fluid shift and obstructive sleep apnea in nonobese men. Am J Respir Crit Care Med. 2009;179(3):241-6.
18. Horner RL, Targets for obstructive sleep apnea pharmacotherapy: Principles, approaches, and emerging strategies. Exp Opin Therap Targets. 2023;27(7):609-26.
19. Irvine LE, Yang Z, Kezirian EWJ, et al. Hyoepiglottic ligament collagen and elastin fiber composition and changes associated with aging. Laryngoscope. 2018;128(5):1245-8.
20. Schwab RJ, Pasirstein M, Pierson R, et al. Identification of upper airway anatomic risk factors for obstructive sleep apnea with volumetric magnetic resonance imaging. Am Ji Respir Crit Care Med. 2003;168(5):522-30.
21. Isono S, Remmers JE, Tanaka A, et al. Anatomy of pharynx in patients with obstructive sleep apnea and in normal subjects. J Appl Physiol. 1997;82(4):1319-26.
22. Sands SA, Edwards BA, Terrill PI, et al. Phenotyping pharyngeal pathophysiology using polysomnography in patients with obstructive sleep apnea. Am J Respir Crit Care Med. 2018;197(9):1187-97.
23. Keenan BT, Kim J, Singh B, et al. (2018) Recognizable clinical subtypes of obstructive sleep apnea across international sleep centers: A cluster analysis. Sleep. 2018;41(3):zsx214.
24. Mazzotti DR, Keenan BT, Lim DC, et al. Symptom subtypes of obstructive sleep apnea predict incidence of cardiovascular outcomes. Am J Respir Crit Care Med. 2019;200(4):493-506.
25. Ulasli SS, Gunay E, Koyuncu T, et al. Predictive value of Berlin Questionnaire and Epworth Sleepiness Scale for obstructive sleep apnea in a sleep clinic population. Clin Respir J. 2014;8(3):292-6.
26. Chung F, Yang Y, Brown R, et al. Alternative scoring models of stop-BANG questionnaire improve specificity to detect undiagnosed obstructive sleep apnea. J Clin Sleep Med. 2014;10(9):951-8.
27. Chen F, Chen K, Zhang C, et al. Evaluating the clinical value of the hypoxia burden index in patients with obstructive sleep apnea. Postgrad Med. 2018;130(4):436-41.
28. Azarbarzin A, Sands SA, Younes M, et al. The sleep apnea–specific pulse-rate response predicts cardiovascular morbidity and mortality. Am J Respir Crit Care Med. 2021;203(12):1546-55.
29. Solelhac G, Sánchez-de-la-Torre M, Blanchard M, et al. Pulse Wave Amplitude Drops Index: A biomarker of cardiovascular risk in obstructive sleep apnea. Am J Respir Crit Care Med. 2023;207(12):1620-32.
30. Ross M, Fonseca P, Overeem S, et al. Autonomic arousal detection and cardiorespiratory sleep staging improve the accuracy of home sleep apnea tests. Front Physiol. 2023;14:1254679.
31. Rosenberg R, Hirshkowitz M, Rapoport DM, et al. The role of home sleep testing for evaluation of patients with excessive daytime sleepiness: Focus on obstructive sleep apnea and narcolepsy. Sleep Med. 2019;56:80-9.
32. Pack AI. Dealing with a paradigm shift. J Clin Sleep Med. 2015;11(8):925-9.

33. Rosen CL, Auckley D, Benca R, et al. A multisite randomized trial of portable sleep studies and positive airway pressure autotitration versus laboratory-based polysomnography for the diagnosis and treatment of obstructive sleep apnea: The HOMEPAP study. Sleep. 2012;35(6):757-67.
34. Kuna ST, Gurubhagavatula I, Maislin G, et al. Noninferiority of functional outcome in ambulatory management of obstructive sleep apnea. Am J Respir Crit Care Med. 2011;183(9):1238-44.
35. Patil SP, Ayappa IA, Caples SM, et al. Treatment of adult obstructive sleep apnea with positive airway pressure: An American Academy of Sleep Medicine Systematic Review, meta-analysis, and grade assessment. J Clin Sleep Med. 2019;15(2):301-34.
36. Weaver TE, Mancini C, Maislin G, et al. Continuous positive airway pressure treatment of sleepy patients with milder obstructive sleep apnea. Am J Respir Crit Care Med. 2012;186(7):677-83.
37. Bratton DJ, Gaisl T, Wons AM, et al. CPAP vs mandibular advancement devices and blood pressure in patients with obstructive sleep apnea. JAMA. 2015;314(21):2280-93.
38. Shukla A, Aizer A, Holmes D, et al. Effect of obstructive sleep apnea treatment on atrial fibrillation recurrence. JACC. 2015; 1(1-2):41-51.
39. McEvoy RD, Antic NA, Heeley E, et al. CPAP for prevention of cardiovascular events in obstructive sleep apnea. N Engl J Med. 2016;375(10):919-31.
40. Sánchez-de-la-Torre M, et al. Effect of obstructive sleep apnoea and its treatment with continuous positive airway pressure on the prevalence of cardiovascular events in patients with acute coronary syndrome (ISAACC study): A randomised controlled trial. Lancet Respir Med. 2020;8(4):359-67.
41. Peker Y, Glantz H, Eulenburg C, et al. Effect of positive airway pressure on cardiovascular outcomes in coronary artery disease patients with nonsleepy obstructive sleep apnea. the RICCADSA randomized controlled trial. Am J Respir Crit Care Med. 2016;194(5):613-20.
42. Azarbarzin A, Sands SA, Stone KL, et al. The hypoxic burden of sleep apnoea predicts cardiovascular disease-related mortality: The osteoporotic fractures in men study and the Sleep Heart Health Study. Eur Heart J. 2019;40(14):1149-57.
43. Pépin JL, Bailly S, Rinder P, et al. Relationship between CPAP termination and all-cause mortality. Chest. 2022;161(6):1657-65.
44. Gervès-Pinquié C, Bailly S, Goupil F, et al. Positive airway pressure adherence, mortality, and cardiovascular events in patients with sleep apnea. Am J Respir Crit Care Med. 2022;206(11):1393-404.
45. Phillips CL, Grunstein RG, Ali Darendeliler M, et al. Health outcomes of continuous positive airway pressure versus oral appliance treatment for obstructive sleep apnea. Am J Respir Crit Care Med. 2013;187(8):879-87.
46. de Vries GE, Wijkstra PJ, Houwerzijl EJ, et al. Cardiovascular effects of oral appliance therapy in obstructive sleep apnea: A systematic review and meta-analysis. Sleep Med Rev. 2018;40:55-68.
47. Ferguson KA, Cartwright C, Rogers R, et al. Oral appliances for snoring and obstructive sleep apnea: A Review. Sleep. 2006;29(2):244-62.
48. Thaler E, Schwab R, Maurer J, et al. Results of the adhere upper airway stimulation registry and predictors of therapy efficacy. Laryngoscope. 2020;130(5):1333-8.
49. Berry RB, Budhiraja R, Gottlieb DJ, et al. Rules for scoring respiratory events in sleep: Update of the 2007 AASM Manual for the scoring of sleep and associated events. J Clin Sleep Med. 2012;8(5):597-619.
50. Javaheri S, Badr MS. Central sleep apnea: Pathophysiologic Classification. Sleep. 2023;46(3):zsac113.
51. Randerath W, Verbraecken J, Andreas S, et al. Definition, discrimination, diagnosis and treatment of central breathing disturbances during sleep. Eur Respir J. 2017;49(1):1600959.
52. Sleep–related breathing disorders in adults: Recommendations for syndrome definition and measurement techniques in clinical research. Sleep. 1999;22(5):667-89.
53. Tamisier R, Damy T, Davy JM, et al. Cohort profile: Face, prospective follow-up of chronic heart failure patients with sleep-disordered breathing indicated for adaptive servo ventilation. BMJ Open. 2020;10(7):e038403.
54. Bitter T, Faber L, Hering D, et al. Sleep-disordered breathing in heart failure with normal left ventricular ejection fraction. Eur J Heart Fail. 2009;11(6):602-8
55. Borrelli C, Gentile F, Sciarrone P, et al. Central and obstructive apneas in heart failure with reduced, mid-range and preserved ejection fraction. Front Cardiovasc Med. 2019;6:125.
56. Ponikowski P, Voors AV, Anker SD, et al. 2016 ESC guidelines for the diagnosis and treatment of acute and chronic heart failure. Eur Heart J. 2016;37(27):2129-2200.
57. Oldenburg O, Lamp B, Faber L, et al. Sleep-disordered breathing In patients with symptomatic heart failure a contemporary study of prevalence in and characteristics of 700 patients. Eur J Heart Fail. 2007;9(3):251-7.
58. Agrawal R, Sharafkhaneh A, Gottlieb DJ, et al. Mortality patterns associated with central sleep apnea among veterans: A large, retrospective, longitudinal report. Ann Am Thorac Soc. 2023;20(3):450-5.
59. Sanchez AM, Germany R, Lozier MR, et al. Central sleep apnea and atrial fibrillation: A review on pathophysiological mechanisms and therapeutic implications. Int J Cardiol Heart Vasc. 2020;30:100527.
60. Davis MJ, Livingston M, Scharf SM. Reversal of central sleep apnea following discontinuation of opioids. J Clin Sleep Med. 2012;8(5):579-80.
61. Javaheri S, Ahmed M, Parker TJ, et al. Effects of nasal O_2 on sleep-related disordered breathing in ambulatory patients with stable heart failure. Sleep. 1999;22(8):1101-6.
62. Hanly PJ. The effect of oxygen on respiration and sleep in patients with congestive heart failure. Ann Int Med. 1989;111(10):777.
63. Nakao YM, Ueshima K, Yasuno S, et al. Effects of nocturnal oxygen therapy in patients with chronic heart failure and central sleep apnea: CHF-hot study. Heart Vessels. 2016;31(2):165-72.
64. Bradley TD, Logan AG, Kimoff RJ, et al. Continuous positive airway pressure for central sleep apnea and heart failure. N Engl J Med. 2005;353(19):2025-33.
65. Arzt M, Floras JS, Logan AG, et al. Suppression of central sleep apnea by continuous positive airway pressure and transplant-free survival in heart failure. Circulation. 2007:115(25):3173-80.
66. Cowie MR, Woehrle H, Wegscheider K, et al. Adaptive servo-ventilation for central sleep apnea in systolic heart failure. N Engl J Med. 2015;373(12):1095-105.
67. Costanzo MR, Ponikowski P, Coats A, et al. Phrenic nerve stimulation to treat patients with central sleep apnoea and heart failure. Eur J Heart Fail. 2018;20(12):1746-54.
68. Oldenburg O, Costanzo MR, Germany R, et al. Improving nocturnal hypoxemic burden with transvenous phrenic nerve stimulation for the treatment of central sleep apnea. J Cardiovasc Transl Res. 2021;14(2):377-85.

69. Koo P, Gartman EJ, Sethi JM, et al. End-expiratory lung volume decreases during REM sleep despite continuous positive airway pressure. Sleep Breath. 2020;24(1):119-25.
70. Patel N, Chong K, Baydur A. Methods and applications in respiratory physiology: Respiratory mechanics, drive and muscle function in neuromuscular and chest wall disorders. Front Physiol. 2022;13:838414.
71. Wiegand L, Zwillich CW, Wiegand D, et al. Changes in upper airway muscle activation and ventilation during phasic REM sleep in normal men. J Appl Physiol. 1991;71(2):488-497.
72. Singh S, Kaur H, Singh S, et al. The overlap syndrome. Cureus. 2018;10(10):e3453.
73. Khan A, Frazer-Green L, Amin R, et al. Respiratory management of patients with neuromuscular weakness. Chest. 2023;164(2): 394-413.
74. Hess DR. Noninvasive ventilation for neuromuscular disease. Clin Chest Med. 2018;39(2):437-47.
75. Nugent A-M, Smith IE, Shneerson JM. Domiciliary-assisted ventilation in patients with myotonic dystrophy. Chest. 2002;121(2):459-64.
76. Bourke SC, et al. Effects of non-invasive ventilation on survival and quality of life in patients with amyotrophic lateral sclerosis: A randomised controlled trial. Lancet Neurol. 2006;5(2):140-7.
77. Toussaint M, Chatwin M, Soudon P. Review article: Mechanical ventilation in Duchenne patients with chronic respiratory insufficiency: Clinical implications of 20 years published experience. Chronic Respir Dis. 2007;4(3):167-77.
78. Barbé F, Quera-Salva MA, de Lattre J, et al. Long-term effects of nasal intermittent positive-pressure ventilation on pulmonary function and sleep architecture in patients with neuromuscular diseases. Chest. 1996;110(5):1179-83.
79. Schonhofer B. Effect of non-invasive mechanical ventilation on sleep and nocturnal ventilation in patients with chronic respiratory failure. Thorax. 2000;55(4):308-13.
80. Simonds AK, Muntoni F, Heather S, et al. Impact of nasal ventilation on survival in hypercapnic Duchenne muscular dystrophy. Thorax. 1998;53(11):949-52.
81. Kung SC, Shen YC, Chang ET, et al. Hypercapnia impaired cognitive and memory functions in obese patients with obstructive sleep apnoea. Sci Rep. 2018;8(1):17551.
82. Kleopa KA, Sherman M, Neal B, et al. BiPAP improves survival and rate of pulmonary function decline in patients with ALS. J Neurol Sci. 1999;164(1):82-8.
83. Dreher M, Storre JH, Schmoor C, et al. High-intensity versus low-intensity non-invasive ventilation in patients with stable hypercapnic COPD: A randomised crossover trial. Thorax. 2010;65(4):303-8.

Obstructive Sleep Apnea–Hypopnea Syndrome

CHAPTER 143

Harmanjit Singh Hira, Naresh Kumar

INTRODUCTION

Obstructive sleep apnea-hypopnea (OSAH) is a common disease but under-recognized by most primary care physicians in India. Historically, the disease can be traced to the 19th century when Charles Dickens' detailed literacy description of a sleepy red-faced fat boy "Joe."[1] Burwell et al.[2] described a medical description of Pickwickian syndrome as "obesity, somnolence, cyanosis, polycythemia, right heart failure" in 1956. In 1964, Gastaut et al.[3] provided the polygraphic recording of Pickwickian patients "presence of apneas during sleep" and introduction of the term "sleep apnea syndrome (SAS)" in patients presenting clinical picture.

DEFINITION

Obstructive sleep apnea-hypopnea is characterized by recurrent episodes of upper airway collapse and obstruction during sleep. The episodes of obstruction are associated with recurrent oxyhemoglobin desaturations and arousals from sleep. OSAH associated with excessive daytime sleepiness (EDS) is commonly called obstructive sleep apnea-hypopnea syndrome (OSAHS), different from the Pickwickian syndrome, was coined by Guilleminault in 1976.[4]

An apnea is a period of time during which breathing stops, or <25% of a normal breath for a period that lasts 10 seconds or more. A hypopnea is a decrease in breathing to 69–26% and is associated with a 4% or greater drop in the saturation of oxygen in the blood. SAS is defined when these frequent interruptions (apneas) occur up to 30 times or more in overnight sleep. Natural history of SAS may be depicted as:

Pure snoring → snoring with occasional apneas → overt SAS→ sleep apnea with daytime hypoventilation → Pickwickian syndrome.

Also, an estimated 80% of Americans with OSAHS are not diagnosed.[5] Central apnea syndrome occurs when the brain fails to signal the diaphragm and chest muscles to breathe. It is more common in the elderly. The past decade has seen a rapid increase in the number of patients being referred for investigation for the OSAHS. OSAHS is a common disease globally and in India.[6]

PATHOPHYSIOLOGY

Conceptually, the upper airway is a compliant tube and therefore subject to collapse.[6] Most patients with OSAHS demonstrate upper airway obstruction at either the level of the soft palate (nasopharynx) or the level of the tongue (oropharynx), which normally are dilated as open airways. Both anatomic and neuromuscular factors are important. Anatomic factors (enlarged tonsils, volume of the tongue, soft tissue, or lateral pharyngeal walls), length of the soft palate, and abnormal positioning of the maxilla and mandible decrease the cross-sectional area of the upper airway and/or increase the pressure surrounding the airway, both of which predispose the airway to collapse.[7,8]

Upper airway neuromuscular activity, including reflex activity, decreases with sleep, and this decrease may be more evident in patients with OSAHS. Reduced ventilatory motor output to upper airway muscles is believed to be the critical initiating event leading to upper airway obstruction; this effect is most evident in patients with an upper airway predisposed to collapse for anatomical reasons.

Central breathing instability is a well-established factor contributing to the development of central sleep apnea, particularly in patients with severe congestive heart failure. Evidence also indicates that central breathing instability contributes to the development of OSAHS. First, evidence of upper airway obstruction in the absence of ventilatory motor output (central sleep apnea) has been present.[9-11] Second, reduction in pharyngeal dilator activity has been associated with periodic breathing and hypocapnia in subjects with evidence of inspiratory flow limitation. Third, men seems to be more susceptible to the development of central sleep apnea and have a decreased responsiveness to carbon dioxide compared with women, a result consistent with the increased prevalence of OSAHS in men compared with women.

Systemic hypertension is present in 50–70% of patients with OSAHS. It has been shown that patients with OSAHS had increased glucose levels and increased insulin resistance.[12] OSAHS has been associated with increased production of reactive oxygen species and other oxidative stress biomarkers, uric acid, and lactate. Plasma levels of xanthine/hypoxanthine were significantly elevated in patients of OSAS, and these were positively correlated with age, serum triglyceride levels, apnea–hypopnea index (AHI), and severity of the disease.[13]

CLINICAL FEATURES

The estimated prevalence of OSAHS is 2% for women and 4% for men. The male-to-female ratio in community-based studies is 2–3:1. The large epidemiologic studies have demonstrated that the prevalence of OSAHS in women appears to increase after menopause. The prevalence of OSAHS increases with age,[16] with an estimated rate as high as 65% in a community sample of people older than 65 years.[14]

The symptoms of OSAHS generally begin insidiously and are often present for years before the patient is referred for evaluation.

Nocturnal symptoms:

- Snoring, usually loud, habitual, and bothersome to others
- Witnessed apneas, which often interrupt the snoring and end with a snort
- Gasping and choking sensations that arouse the patient from sleep
- Restless sleep, with patients often experiencing frequent arousals and tossing or turning during the night
- Increased frequency of micturition

Daytime symptoms:[15]

- Not feeling refreshed upon awakening
- Morning headache, dry and/or sore throat
- Excessive daytime sleepiness (EDS) that usually begins during quiet activities (reading and watching television). As the severity worsens, the patient begins to feel sleepy during activities that generally require alertness (school, work, and driving). It is the experience of the author that these patients commonly sleep while waiting for their turn for examination in outpatient department.
    - The Epworth Sleepiness Scale (ESS) is useful to help determine how frequently the patient is likely to doze off in eight frequently encountered situations.
    - An ESS score ≥ 10 is generally considered sleepy. However, a 2003 study showed that an ESS score of 12 is associated with a greater propensity to fall asleep on the Multiple Sleep Latency Test (MSLT) suggesting that 12 would be a better cutoff.[17] The ESS is useful for evaluating responses to treatment; the ESS score should decrease with effective treatment.
- *Daytime fatigue/tiredness*: Most patients who do not report EDS do report being fatigued, having a lack of energy, or getting tired during the day. In one study of 190 patients with OSAHS, patients were more likely to report lack of energy (62%), fatigue (57%), and tiredness (61%) than sleepiness (47%).[16] When asked to choose their most significant symptom, 40% of patients chose lack of energy, compared with 22% for sleepiness.[18]
- Problems with memory, concentration, and cognitive function, particularly executive functioning
- Impotence
- History of motor vehicle accident(s)

PHYSICAL EXAMINATION

The general physical examination is frequently normal other than the presence of obesity [defined as body mass index (BMI) > 30 kg/m^2], an enlarged neck circumference, and hypertension. On evaluation of the upper airway in all patients, particularly in nonobese adults with symptoms consistent with OSAHS, the following features have been associated with the presence of OSAHS:

- A neck circumference ≥ 43 cm (17 in) in men and 37 cm (15 in) in women has been associated with an increased risk of OSAHS.
- The modified Mallampati classification[19] is a simple scoring system that relates the amount of mouth opening to the size of the tongue and provides an estimate of space available for oral intubation by direct laryngoscopy. According to the Mallampati scale, class I is present when the soft palate, uvula, and pillars are visible; class II when the soft palate and the uvula are visible; class III when only the soft palate and base of the uvula are visible; and class IV when only the hard palate is visible

    A 2006 study showed that for each 1-unit increase in the Mallampati score, the odds ratio of having OSAHS (defined by an AHI > 5) is increased by 2.5. In addition, the AHI increased by 5 events per hour.[20]
- Narrowing of the lateral airway walls, which is an independent predictor of the presence of OSAHS in men but not women.
- Enlarged ("kissing") tonsils (3+ to 4+)
- Retrognathia or micrognathia
- Large degree of overjet
- High-arched hard palate

CAUSES

Following are the risk factors for sleep apnea:

- Obesity
- Male sex
- Age
- Adenotonsillar hypertrophy, particularly in children and young adults
- Alcohol use
- Craniofacial skeletal abnormalities, particularly in nonobese adults and children

- *Family history*: Risk increases with each additional close family relative with OSAHS.[21]

Other diseases associated with the development of OSAHS are as follows:

- *Hypothyroidism*: This has been associated with the development of OSAHS;[15] however, evidence indicates that the prevalence of hypothyroidism in patients with OSAHS is no higher than in the general population, and patients with OSAHS needs no screening for hypothyroidism, except possibly elderly women.
- Neurologic syndromes such as postpolio syndrome, muscular dystrophies, and autonomic failure syndromes such as Shy-Drager syndrome.
- *Stroke*: The obstructive sleep apnea syndrome is significantly associated with the risk of stroke or death from any cause, and this association is independent of other risk factors, including hypertension. Increased severity of the syndrome is associated with an incremental increase in the risk of this composite outcome.[22]
- Acromegaly
- OSA promotes metabolic dysfunction, increases the incidence of diabetes and impaired glucose control.[23.]

LABORATORY INVESTIGATIONS

Patient with possible OSAHS has other signs or symptoms of hypothyroidism. An arterial blood gas determination should be carried out in patients presenting with cor pulmonale, in order to rule out daytime hypoxemia or hypercapnia. Pulmonary function tests are performed if the patient has evidence of cor pulmonale or if symptoms are suggestive of nocturnal asthma (patient wakes up with shortness of breath that does not immediately resolve or is associated with wheezing).

An overnight sleep study, or polysomnography, is required to diagnose OSAHS. During polysomnography, multiple body functions are monitored with multiple sensors in the sleep laboratory. Guidelines for the indications and performance of polysomnography include the following:[24]

- Sleep stages are recorded via an electroencephalogram, electrooculogram, and chin electromyogram **(Figs. 1 and 2)**.
- Heart rhythm is monitored with a single-lead electrocardiography (ECG).
- Leg movements are recorded via an anterior tibialis electromyogram.
- Breathing is monitored, including airflow at the nose and mouth (using both thermal sensor and nasal pressure transducer), effort (using inductance plethysmography), and oxygen saturation.
- The breathing pattern is analyzed, as indicated in the following text, for the presence of apneas and hypopneas. Definitions have been standardized by the American Academy of Sleep Medicine (AASM).[21]
- Obstructive apnea is the cessation of airflow for at least 10 seconds with persistent respiratory effort **(Figs. 1 and 2)**
- *Central apnea* is the cessation of airflow for at least 10 seconds with no respiratory effort.
- *Mixed apnea*: A complete absence of nasal and airflow. A total absence of respiratory effort at the beginning of the event (black thick arrow) is followed by gradual increase in effort (red thick arrow) which eventually breaks the apnea with an oxygen desaturation ≥ 3%.
- The recommended definition of a hypopnea is a 30% or greater decrease in flow lasting for at least 10 seconds and associated with a 4% or greater oxyhemoglobin desaturation. An alternative definition is a 50% or greater reduction in flow lasting at least 10 seconds and associated with either a 3% or greater oxyhemoglobin desaturation or an arousal.
- Respiratory event-related arousal is an event in which a patient has a series of breaths with increasing respiratory effort or flattening of the nasal pressure waveform leading to an arousal from sleep that does not otherwise meet the criteria for an apnea or hypopnea.
- The AHI is derived from the total number of apneas and hypopneas divided by the total sleep time in hours.
- A normal cutoff for AHI has never been defined in an epidemiological study of healthy people. Most sleep centers use a cutoff of 5–10 episodes per hour.[10]
- The severity of OSAHS is arbitrarily defined and differs widely between centers. Recommendations for cutoff levels on AHI include 5–15 episodes per hour for mild, 15–30 episodes per hour for moderate, and ≥ 30 episodes per hour for severe.

The use of portable monitors for the in-home diagnosis of OSAHS is becoming more common. The AASM has published guidelines on the use of portable monitors. These guidelines recommend the use only in patients with a high probability of disease and those without comorbidities (particularly congestive heart failure), and that negative studies be followed by a full, attended study.[21]

Multiple sleep latency test: Polysomnography can be followed by MSLT considered an objective measurement of EDS. The MSLT consists of four to five naps of 20-minute duration every 2 hours during the day. The latency to sleep onset for each nap is averaged to determine the daytime sleep latency. Normal daytime sleep latency is ≥10–15 minutes. OSAHS is generally associated with latencies of ≤10 minutes. The routine use of the MSLT in the evaluation of OSAHS has significantly decreased because sleep physicians generally treat OSAHS based on the subjective symptoms reported by the patient. The MSLT is generally used to confirm the diagnosis of narcolepsy in patients in whom narcolepsy is a consideration. As opposed to people without narcolepsy, narcoleptic patients have rapid eye movement sleep on at least two of the four to five naps during the day.

When to do polysomnography is still unclear. The results of studies and guideless to conduct sleep study is undetermined.[25] Authors suggested that polysomnography to conduct on those patients who shave loud snoring along with excessive daytime sleepiness.

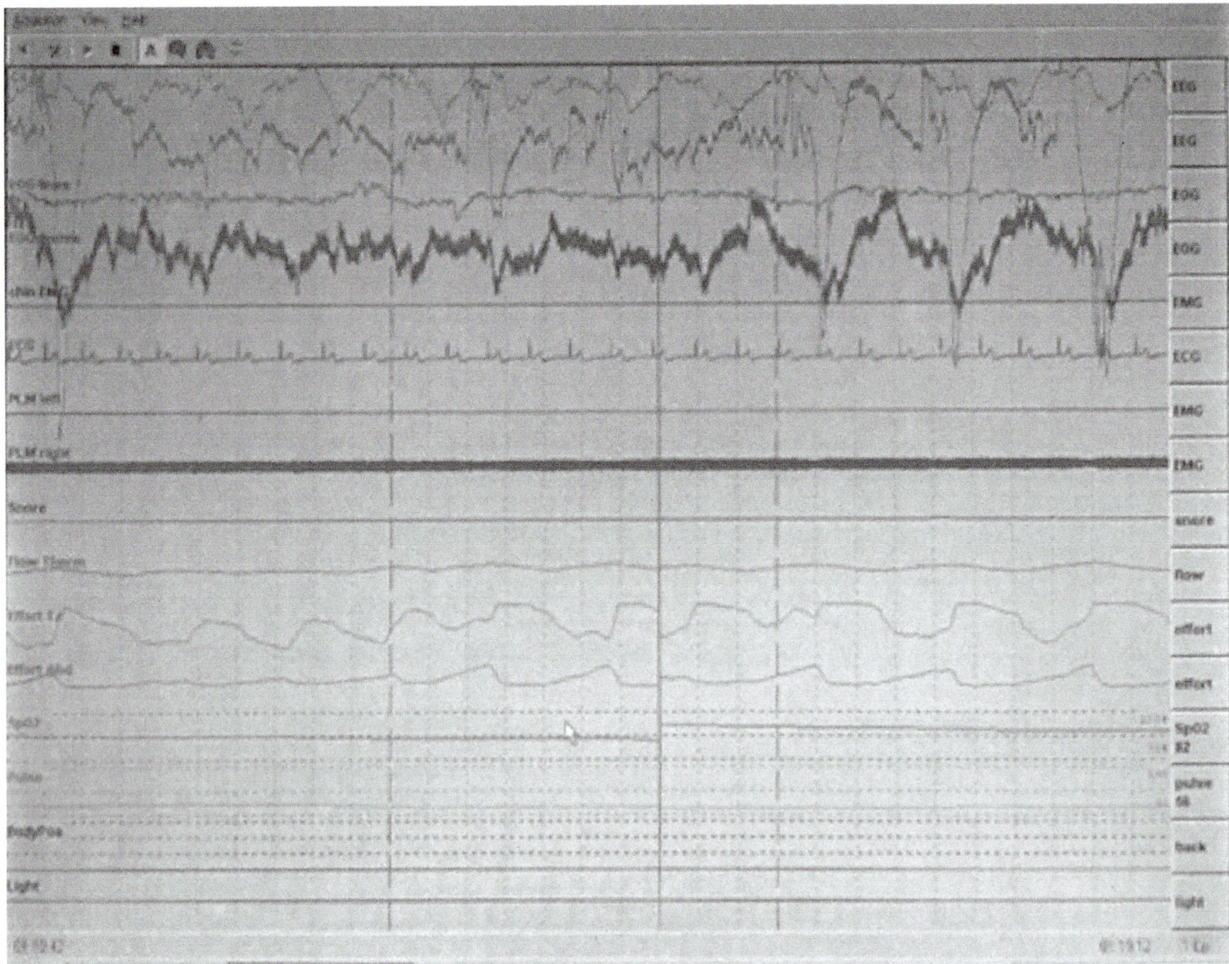

FIG. 1: Demonstrated parameters during running polysomnography.

TREATMENT

The treatment of OSAHS in part depends on the severity of the sleep-disordered breathing. People with mild apnea have a wider variety of options, while people with moderate-to-severe apnea need treatment with nasal continuous positive airway pressure (CPAP).

Conservative measures include weight loss, avoidance of alcohol for 4–6 hours prior to bedtime, and sleeping on one's side rather than on the stomach or back. Include these measures in the treatment of all patients with OSAHS, but use them only in patients with very mild apnea whose main symptom is snoring. In a 2006 practice parameter, both weight loss and positional therapy were rated as "guidelines," indicating a patient care strategy with a moderate degree of evidence.[26]

Nasal CPAP: CPAP is the most effective treatment for OSAHS, and has become the standard of care. CPAP works by splinting the upper airway, preventing the soft tissues from collapsing. By this mechanism, it effectively eliminates the apneas and/or hypopneas, decreases the arousals, and normalizes the oxygen saturation.

Most sleep physicians prefer to titrate the CPAP level during a sleep study. This can be done during a second night of study or during the second half of the diagnostic study, which is termed a split-night polysomnography. Guidelines for positive-pressure titration studies have been available.[27-29]

Currently, CPAP devices are available that automatically change pressures based on the presence and/or absence of OSAHS (autopositive airway pressure, or auto-PAP), where the need of titration is not required.[30,31] The rationale for autotitrating devices is that the pressure required to treat OSAHS may vary over the course of the night and between different nights, sleep stages, and body positions, with the variations not captured by a one-night titration study.[32] In theory, the mean pressure delivered by auto-PAP devices is lower than that delivered with fixed CPAP; however, no studies have shown increased patient compliance with auto-PAP devices.[34]

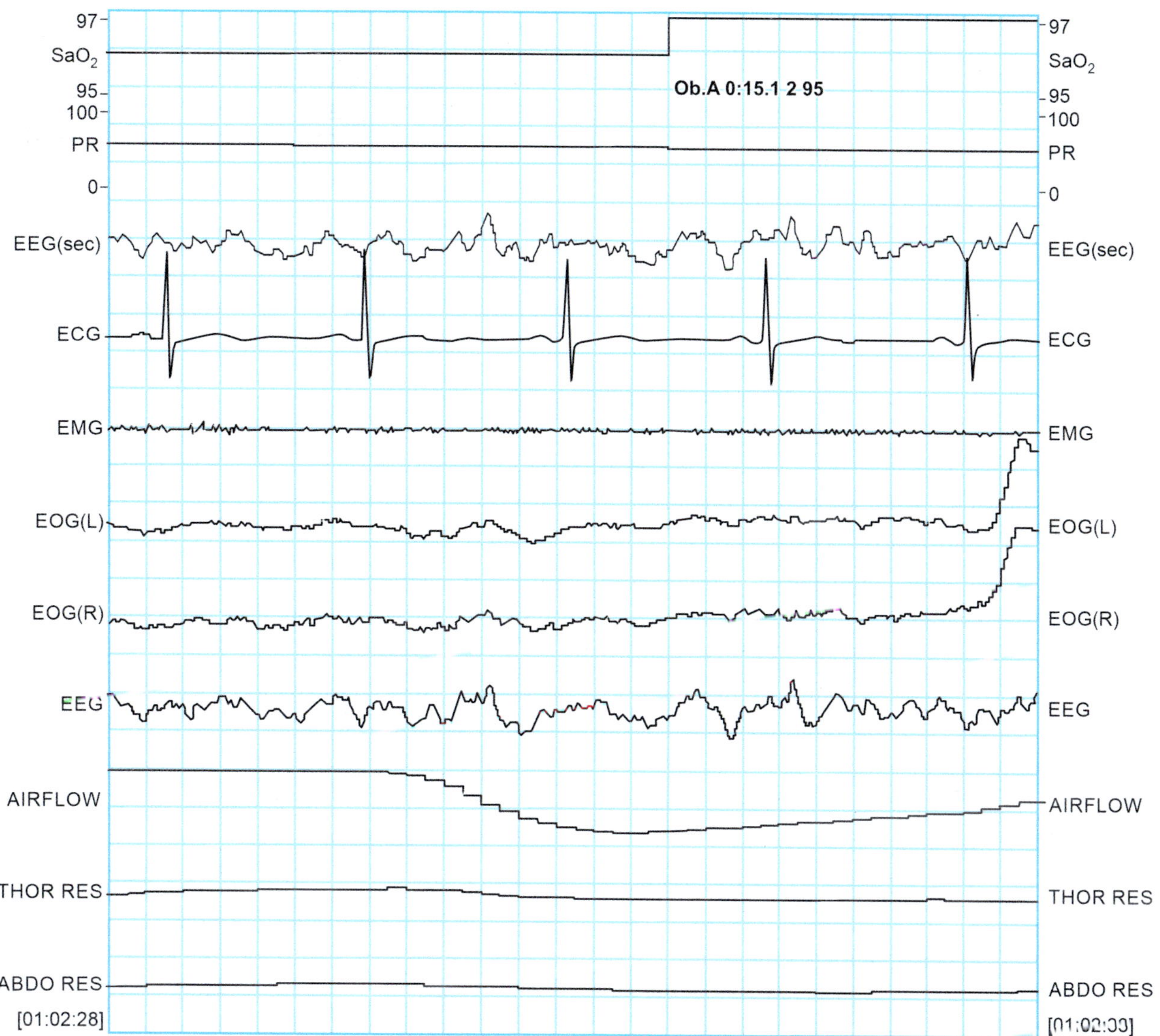

FIG. 2: Polysomnograph in a case of OSAHS.
(ECG: electrocardiogram; EEG: electroencephalogram; EMG: electromyogram; EOG: electrooculogram; OSAHS: obstructive sleep apnea–hypopnea syndrome)

All patients with an AHI ≥ 15 are eligible for CPAP, regardless of symptoms. For patients with an AHI of 5–14.9, CPAP is useful only if the patient has EDS, hypertension, cardiovascular disease, or combination of them.

CPAP improves daytime sleepiness, mood, and cognitive function in people with both mild and moderate apnea.[35,36] CPAP has also been shown to improve the quality of life.[37] CPAP decreases blood pressure, primarily in patients with severe OSAHS. Evidence also indicates that it may improve the left ventricular ejection fraction in patients with congestive heart failure and OSAHS.[3]

The most common adverse effects of CPAP are dry mouth, rhinitis, and sinus congestion. These can be treated effectively with humidification and antihistamines and/or nasal steroids.

Many patients do not accept (or even initiate) CPAP therapy and that up to 25% do not regularly follow up with a sleep physician,[31] most of these patients being no adherent to therapy. CPAP compliance may be determined as early as 2 weeks after initiation of CPAP. Patients who consistently use their positive airway pressure device at 6 months were, on average, using the device for more than 2 hours more per night during the first 2 weeks and were more ready and confident to continue use. On the other hand, intermittent users were more likely to report adverse effects from the device, general discomfort, and that the device was too inconvenient. Compliance can be objectively measured.[36] Most modern positive airway pressure machines measure both "machine-on" and "mask-on" times, with the mask-on time used to measure compliance.

Some patients require the use of bilevel positive airway pressure (BiPAP). In BiPAP, a higher inspiratory pressure and a lower expiratory pressure are used. In patients with sleep apnea, the levels are set such that the expiratory pressure eliminates apneas and the inspiratory pressure eliminates hypopneas. BiPAP is generally used in patients who cannot tolerate high CPAP pressures (patients who experience difficult exhalations) or who have barotrauma complications (ear infections and bloating). Many laboratories automatically place a patient on BiPAP if the critical CPAP level is ≥15 cm H_2O. Compliance with BiPAP has not been demonstrated to be better than with CPAP.[37]

Follow-up of Patients on CPAP Therapy

Once diagnosed OSAHS and started on nasal CPAP, patients require regular follow-up with a sleep specialist. Most patients are seen within 2 months of initiating CPAP to determine if it has been effective in alleviating symptoms, to troubleshoot problems preventing regular use of the CPAP, and to reinforce the importance of daily use. Further follow-up depends on whether the CPAP has been effective.

- If effective, the patient is generally seen at 6–12-month intervals to troubleshoot new problems, to reinforce daily use, and to be certain the CPAP remains effective.
- If CPAP has not been effective, problems preventing use are identified, steps are taken to eliminate problems, and the patient is seen at 2–3-month intervals until use is regular and the CPAP is alleviating symptoms. Repeat titration may be necessary.
- Routine repeat polysomnography is generally not indicated for patients who report improved symptoms. Repeat CPAP titrations are usually performed in patients without effective relief of their symptoms despite intervention or in patients who had relief of symptoms but present months to years later reporting the return of symptoms, generally in association with weight gain.
- Advances in mask interfaces, the use of humidification, the downloading of usage information, the development of pressure delivery modifications, and reductions in the size and noise of the machines have improved the devices over the past decade. Nevertheless, the basic premise of positive pressure delivery to splint the airway remains the primary driver of efficacy.

Oral Appliances

These devices act by moving the tongue or mandible forward, enlarging the posterior airspace. Multiple different devices are available. In 2006, the AASM published practice parameters and a review of the use of oral appliances in persons with OSAHS.[38,39]

Multiple small cohort studies have shown that these devices effectively lower the AHI influenced the efficacy of oral appliances: (1) mild-to-moderate disease (AHI < 30), (2) lower BMI, (3) increased mandibular protrusion with the device, and (4) the presence of positional OSAHS.

Guidelines recommend that oral appliances be indicated for: (1) patients with mild-to-moderate OSAHS who prefer oral appliances to CPAP devices, (2) patients with mild-to-moderate OSAHS who do not respond to CPAP therapy, and (3) patients with mild-to-moderate OSAHS in whom treatment attempts with CPAP devices fail. Oral appliances are effective therapy for patients with severe OSAHS. Among the newer therapies, transnasal insufflation and nasal expiratory resistance clearly have promise, again for patients with mild to moderate OSA.[40]

Surgical Treatment

Surgical correction of the upper airway is still performed but is not considered primary therapy for OSAHS. The theoretic advantage of surgery is that if the patient improves compliance with CPAP or an oral appliance is no longer an issue. However, a primary reason that surgery has not become a standard therapy is the lack of long-term outcome studies that show that the surgical correction continues to be effective 5 or more years after it is performed.

Factors that increase the likelihood of successful surgery include: (1) lower AHI, (2) lower BMI, (3) the location of collapse (surgeries targeted specifically to collapse at either the nasopharynx or oropharynx improve outcome), (4) the degree of mandibular protrusion (better outcomes are achieved in patients with clear deficiencies), and (5) the presence of fewer comorbidities.

Patients should be considered for surgery primarily if multiple attempts at therapy with CPAP have failed and if an oral appliance is not an option. If the patient opts for surgery, ensure that a qualified ear, nose, and throat surgeon should perform it and the patient should be willing to undergo combination or multiple surgeries. Guidelines for the surgical treatment of OSAHS were last published in 1995.[41] Surgery procedures include the following:

- Uvulopalatopharyngoplasty (UPPP) is the resection of the uvula and soft palate. It is effective in approximately 40% of patients, but predicting which patients will benefit from the procedure is problematic. Patients with treatment success often present with a recurrence of symptoms, especially if they continue to gain weight.
- Craniofacial reconstruction involves advancement of the tongue [geniohyoid advancement with hyoid myotomy (GAHM0 or maxillomandibular bones) maxillomandibular osteotomy (MMO)]. These procedures should be performed only at centers with expert personnel. Short-term success rates are approximately 70% for GAHM and 95% for MMO. No good long-term studies have been performed to evaluate the success for either GAHM or MMO.
- Tracheostomy provides definitive correction because it bypasses the obstruction. It is recommended for patients

with very severe OSAHS, especially if the patient does not tolerate CPAP or has cor pulmonale. In the author's experience, patients in India do not opt for tracheostomy.
- Because the jaws and related structures influence the development of this syndrome, dentists play an important role in both identifying patients who should be assessed by sleep specialists and instituting treatment in selected cases.[37]
- Bariatric surgery as therapy for OSAHS has been investigated in several nonrandomized, uncontrolled studies, with most showing a decrease in the AHI with weight loss.
- *Upper airway stimulation (UAS)*:[42] This is a system of unilateral hypoglossal nerve stimulation, consisting of an implantable pulse generator, stimulation lead placed on the hypoglossal nerve and respiratory sensing electrode.[42] This modality may be used for selected patients with moderate-to-severe OSA who failed or were intolerant to positive airway pressure therapy. The device detects breathing patterns and, when necessary, stimulates the nerve that controls movement of the tongue.

Follow-up of Patient with Surgery/Oral Devices

If a patient chooses upper airway surgery or an oral appliance, he or she requires repeat polysomnography after surgery or with the device in place to be sure the OSAHS has improved.

Diet: All patients who are obese should be counseled about the importance of diet and exercise and should be referred to a dietitian and/or a weight loss program.

Drug therapy: The drugs have been used but no demonstrable effect is generally seen. The recently published AASM practice parameters can be summarized as below:
- Use of protriptyline as a patient care strategy; based on level 2 or 3 evidence[43]
- The use of modafinil is recommended for the treatment of residual sleepiness in persons with OSAHS and is considered a standard treatment (generally accepted patient care strategy with level 1 or excellent level 2 evidence).
- Selective serotonin reuptake inhibitors, methylxanthines, and estrogen replacement therapy should not be considered for the treatment of OSAHS.
- Central nervous system stimulants and nonamphetamine are used for treatment of fatigue without interfering with normal sleep architecture. They promote wakefulness.
- Concern exists that the use of modafinil (or other stimulants) in the management of OSAHS may result in decreased CPAP usage. This is important because stimulants do not control the sleep-disordered breathing, resulting in worsening symptom control and potentially increasing the risk of cardiovascular morbidity. The dose of modafil used is 100–200 mg PO qd; some patients may require as much as 300 mg PO qd. This is not recommended for the children.

PROGNOSIS

The short-term prognosis, in relation to symptoms such as daytime sleepiness and snoring, ranges from good to excellent with regular use of CPAP. The long-term prognosis is unknown because no randomized treatment studies investigating the effect of CPAP on preventing the development of cardiovascular squeal have been conducted.

PATIENT EDUCATION

All patients should receive education about sleep and proper sleep hygiene, OSAHS, and the risks of driving while sleepy. They also should receive education regarding the role of nasal CPAP and the importance of daily use.

SPECIAL CONCERNS

Motor Vehicle Accident Risk

Predicting accident risk in patients with OSAHS is difficult because many individuals with OSAHS do not accurately perceive their level of drowsiness.[44] A large body of work has been compiled on the influence of OSAHS on driving-simulator performance, with the majority of the studies indicating poor performance, similar to that seen with alcohol impairment while driving.[45] Evidence indicates that CPAP improves driving performance. At least two studies have shown improvement on a driving simulator after CPAP use.[46,47] Specifically, in one study, the number of off-road events decreased from 17.8 to 9 after 1 month of effective CPAP therapy, but no change was noted after a month of ineffective pressure set at 1 cm H_2O.

Geriatric Populations

The prevalence of OSAHS increases with age. However, the clinical significance of OSAHS in healthy, community-dwelling people has been questioned because these people do not show significant squeal (sleepiness). Elderly patients presenting to sleep centers for evaluation have similar symptomatology (including EDS) and polysomnographic results compared with patients who are not elderly, except those elderly patients under-report snoring as a chief complaint, they tend to be less obese, and they are less objectively sleepy based on MSLT results. Thus, all elderly people, particularly if overweight, should be questioned about snoring, witnessed apneas, and daytime sleepiness, and should be referred for evaluation if necessary.

Age does not appear to influence compliance to CPAP therapy. Thus, all elderly patients with significant and symptomatic OSAHS should be offered therapy.

Pediatric Populations

Obstructive sleep apnea-hypopnea syndrome in children has an estimated prevalence of 2%, affecting boys and girls in equal numbers. Children most often present with loud snoring and symptoms and signs of adenotonsillar hypertrophy. EDS is not a common symptom in children with OSAHS. Instead, school-aged children often report problems with schoolwork. Studies have shown improvement in cognitive function and/or grades after adenotonsillectomy in children with OSAHS.[48]

Pregnancy

Several case reports associate intrauterine growth restriction in pregnant women with concomitant untreated OSAHS. A study from Sweden reports that hypertension, preeclampsia, low Apgar scores, and intrauterine growth restriction were more common in habitually snoring pregnant women compared with nonsnoring pregnant women.[49] Habitual snoring was independently predictive of hypertension and growth restriction after correction for other factors (weight, age, and smoking status).[50]

SUMMARY

Obstructive sleep apnea-hypopnea syndrome is a common but frequently missed clinical condition which is potentially serious and sometimes a cause of sudden death. Diagnosis can be made on clinical history and examination and confirmed on polysomnography. Other investigations are usually required for concomitant conditions and comorbidities. CPAP therapy remains the standard of care for moderate-to-severe OSAHS.

REFERENCES

1. Dickens C. The Posthumous Papers of the Pickwick Club. London: Chapman & Hall; 1837.
2. Burwell C, Robin E, Whaley R, et al. Extreme obesity associated with alveolar hypoventilation: a Pickwickian syndrome. Am J Med. 1956;358-60.
3. Gastaut H, Tassinari C, Duron B. Etude polygraphique des manifestations episodiques (hypniques et respiration), du syndrome de Pickwick. Rev Neurol. 1964;112:568.
4. Guilleminault C, Tilkian A, Dement WC. The sleep apnea syndromes. Annu Rev Med. 1976;27:465-84.
5. Young T, Evans L, Finn L, et al. Estimation of the clinically diagnosed proportion of sleep apnea syndrome in middle-aged men and women. Sleep 1997;20:705-6.
6. Patil SP, Schneider H, Schwartz AR, et al. Adult obstructive sleep apnea: pathophysiology and diagnosis. Chest. 2007;132:325-37.
7. Schwab RJ, Pasirstein M, Pierson R, et al. Identification of upper airway anatomic risk factors for obstructive sleep apnea with volumetric magnetic resonance imaging. Am J Respir Crit Care Med. 2003;168:522-30.
8. White DP. Sleep apnea. Proc Am Thorac Soc. 2006;3:124-8.
9. Badr MS, Toiber F, Skatrud JB, et al. Pharyngeal narrowing/occlusion during central sleep apnea. J Appl Physiol. 1995;78:1806-15.
10. Hira HS, Arora S, Chauhan MR. Oxygen saturation, breathing pattern and arrhythmias in patients of chronic obstructive pulmonary disease and bronchial asthma during sleep. Lung India. 1994;12:186-91.
11. Young T, Palta M, Dempsey J, et al. The occurrence of sleep-disordered breathing among middle-aged adults. N Engl J Med. 1993;328:1230-5.
12. Ip MS, Lam B, Ng MM, et al. Obstructive sleep apnea is independently associated with insulin resistance. Am J Respir Crit Care Med. 2002;165:670-76.
13. Hira HS, Samal P, Kaur A, et al. Plasma level of hypoxanthine/xanthine as markers of oxidative stress with different stages of obstructive sleep aea syndrome Ann Saudi Med. 2014;34:308-13.
14. Young T, Shahar E, Nieto FJ, et al. Predictors of sleep-disordered breathing in community-dwelling adults: the Sleep Heart Health Study. Arch Intern Med 2002;162:893-900.
15. Hira HS, Arora S. Sleep Apnea Syndrome: An Indian Experience. Ind J Chest Dis & Allied Sci. 1995;37:119-25.
16. Ancoli-Israel S, Kripke DF, Klauber MR, et al. Sleep-disordered breathing in community-dwelling elderly. Sleep. 1991;14:486-95.
17. Punjabi NM, Bandeen-Roche K, Young T. Predictors of objective sleep tendency in the general population. Sleep. 2003;26:678-83.
18. Chervin RD. Sleepiness, fatigue, tiredness, and lack of energy in obstructive sleep apnea. Chest. 2000;118:372-9.
19. Samsoon GL, Young JR. Difficult tracheal intubation: A retrospective study. Anaesthesia. 1987;42:487.
20. Nuckton TJ, Glidden DV, Browner WS, et al. Physical examination: Mallampati score as an independent predictor of obstructive sleep apnea. Sleep. 2006;29:903-8.
21. Redline S, Tishler PV, Tosteson TD, et al. The familial aggregation of obstructive sleep apnea. Am J Respir Crit Care Med. 1995;151:682-7.
22. Yaggi H K, Concatoto J, Kernan WN, et al. Obstructive sleep apnea as a risk factor for stroke and death. N Eng J Med. 2005;353: 2034-42.
23. Drager LF, Heno ML, Maki-Nunes C, et al. The impact of obstructive sleep apnea on metabolic and inflammatory markers in consecutive patients with metabolic syndrome. PLoS One. 2010;5:e12065.
24. Iber C, Ancoli-Israel S, Chesson AL, et al. The AASM Manual for the Scoring of Sleep and Associated Events. Westchester, IL: American Academy of Sleep Medicine; 2007.
25. Kapur VK, Auckley DH, Chowdhuri S, et al. Clinical practice guideline for diagnostic testing for adult obstructive sleep apnea: An American Academy of Sleep Medicine Clinical Practice Guideline. J Clinic Sleep Med. 2017;13:479-504.
26. Collop NA, Anderson WM, Boehlecke B, et al. Clinical guidelines for the use of unattended portable monitors in the diagnosis of

obstructive sleep apnea in adult patients. Portable Monitoring Task Force of the American Academy of Sleep Medicine. J Clin Sleep Med. 2007;3:737-47.

27. Morgenthaler TI, Kapen S, Lee-Chiong T, et al. Practice parameters for the medical therapy of obstructive sleep apnea. Sleep. 2006;29:1031-5.
28. Kushida CA, Chediak A, Berry RB, et al. Clinical guidelines for the manual titration of positive airway pressure in patients with obstructive sleep apnea. J Clin Sleep Med. 2008;4:157-71.
29. Kushida CA, Littner MR, Hirshkowitz M, et al. Practice parameters for the use of continuous and bi-level positive airway pressure devices to treat adult patients with sleep-related breathing disorders. Sleep. 2006;29:375-80.
30. Gay P, Weaver T, Loube D, et al. Evaluation of positive airway pressure treatment for sleep related breathing disorders in adults. Sleep. 2006;29:381-401.
31. Smith I, Lasserson TJ. Pressure modification for improving usage of continuous positive airway pressure machines in adults with obstructive sleep apnoea. Cochrane Database Syst Rev. 2009;CD003531.
32. Morgenthaler TI, Aurora RN, Brown T, et al. Practice parameters for the use of autotitrating continuous positive airway pressure devices for titrating pressures and treating adult patients with obstructive sleep apnea syndrome: an update for 2007. An American Academy of Sleep Medicine report. Sleep. 2008;31:141-7.
33. Engleman HM, Martin SE, Deary IJ, et al. Effect of continuous positive airway pressure treatment on daytime function in sleep apnoea/hypopnoea syndrome. Lancet. 1994;343:572-5.
34. Bennett LS, Barbour C, Langford B, et al. Health status in obstructive sleep apnea: relationship with sleep fragmentation and daytine sleepiness, and effects of continuous positive airway pressure treatment. Am J Respir Crit Care Med. 1999;159:1884-90.
35. Kaneko Y, Floras JS, Usui K, et al. Cardiovascular effects of continuous positive airway pressure in patients with heart failure and obstructive sleep apnea. N Engl J Med. 2003;348:1233-41.
36. Lin HS, Zuliani G, Amjad EH, et al. Treatment compliance in patients lost to follow-up after polysomnography. Otolaryngol Head Neck Surg. 2007;136:236-40.
37. Kribbs NB, Pack AI, Kline LR, et al. Objective measurement of patterns of nasal CPAP use by patients with obstructive sleep apnea. Am Rev Respir Dis. 1993;128.
38. Reeves-Hoche MK, Hudgel DW, Meck R, Et al. Continuous versus bilevel positive airway pressure for obstructive sleep apnea. Am J Respir Crit Care Med. 1995;151:443-9.
39. Kushida CA, Morgenthaler TI, Littner MR, et al. Practice parameters for the treatment of snoring and Obstructive Sleep Apnea with oral appliances: an update for 2005. Sleep. 2006;29:240-3.
40. Collop NA. Advances in treatment of obstructive sleep apnea syndrome. Curr Treat Options Neurol. 2009;11:340-8.
41. Goodday RHB, Precious DS, Morrison AD, et al. Obstructive sleep apnea syndrome: Diagnosis and management. J Can Dent Assoc. 2001;67:652-8.
42. Heiser C, Thaler E, Soose RJ, et al. Technical tips during implantation of selective upper airway stimulation. Laryngoscope. 2018;128:756-62.
43. Ferguson KA, Cartwright R, Rogers R, et al. Oral appliances for snoring and obstructive sleep apnea: a review. Sleep. 2006;29:244-62.
44. Sher AE, Schechtman KB, Piccirillo JF. The efficacy of surgical modifications of the upper airway in adults with obstructive sleep apnea syndrome. Sleep 1996;19:156-77.
45. Veasey SC, Guilleminault C, Strohl KP, et al. Medical therapy for obstructive sleep apnea: a review by the Medical Therapy for Obstructive Sleep Apnea Task Force of the Standards of Practice Committee of the American Academy of Sleep Medicine. Sleep. 2006;29:1036-44.
46. Risser MR, Ware JC, Freeman FG. Driving simulation with EEG monitoring in normal and obstructive sleep apnea patients. Sleep. 2000;23:393-8.
47. Hack M, Davies RJ, Mullins R, et al. Randomised prospective parallel trial of therapeutic versus subtherapeutic nasal continuous positive airway pressure on simulated steering performance in patients with obstructive sleep apnoea. Thorax. 2000;55:224-31.
48. Turkington PM, Sircar M, Saralaya D, et al. Time course of changes in driving simulator performance with and without treatment in patients with sleep apnoea hypopnoea syndrome. Thorax. 2004;59:56-9.
49. Gozal D, Pope DW. Snoring during early childhood and academic performance at ages thirteen to fourteen years. Pediatrics. 2001;107:1394-9.
50. Franklin KA, Holmgren PA, Jonsson F, et al. Snoring, pregnancy-induced hypertension, and growth retardation of the fetus. Chest 2000;117:137-41.

Obstructive Sleep Apnea Syndrome Comorbidities

CHAPTER 144

Dipti Gothi, Sunil Kumar

INTRODUCTION

Obstructive sleep apnea syndrome (OSA) is frequently associated with systemic, metabolic, respiratory, and neuropsychiatric comorbidities.[1] There is a growing evidence that these comorbidities have a bidirectional relationship with OSA.[1] OSA leads to intermittent hypoxia, fluctuating intrathoracic pressure, and recurring microarousals which generate sympathetic excitation, systemic inflammation, and oxidative stress, in addition to metabolic and endothelial dysfunction.[2,3] Thus, these mechanisms lead to systemic, metabolic, respiratory, and neuropsychiatric comorbidities in a patient with OSA. On the other hand, fluid retention due to heart failure (HF) and end-stage renal redistribution can result in OSA. Metabolic syndrome (obesity) and stroke can also lead to OSA.[1] Similarly, chronic obstructive pulmonary disease (COPD) and asthma can also contribute to OSA due to rising intrathoracic pressure.[4,5] Neuropsychiatric complications like insomnia can also be a contributor to OSA.

According to some studies, the comorbidity burden progressively increases with OSA severity.[6-8] The distribution of comorbidities also differs between men and women. Diabetes mellitus and ischemic heart disease (IHD) are more prevalent in men with OSA, whereas hypertension and depression are more prevalent in women with OSA compared to non-OSA subjects.[9] As far as mortality related to comorbidities is concerned, age and occurrence of comorbidities predict mortality in OSA patients.[10] In patients aged > 50 years, the protective effect of continuous positive airway pressure (CPAP) treatment is seen only in patients with comorbidities.[10] In patients with moderate-to-severe obesity and OSA, treatment with CPAP or noninvasive ventilation is associated with fewer cardiovascular events only in patients with a high number of comorbidities.[11] Therefore, occurrence of comorbidities can identify the subgroups of OSA patients at high risk, who might show benefit from CPAP treatment.

Obstructive sleep apnea similarly can adversely affect respiratory disorders like asthma and COPD and vice versa. Respiratory failure may be precipitated due to coexisting OSA in patients with COPD. Similarly, the control of respiratory disorders may be jeopardized because of the presence of OSA. Thus, it is important to identify the presence of OSA in bronchial asthma and COPD patients.[1,8] OSA association with other sleep disorders like insomnia and restless leg syndrome (RLS) may also lead to adverse metabolic outcomes. Treatment of only OSA in patients who have insomnia and RLS can lead to poor compliance and incomplete treatment leading to poor quality of life (QoL). Like metabolic disorders and respiratory disorders, presence of comorbid sleep disorders can adversely affect the patient's management. Last, though obesity hypoventilation syndrome association with OSA is more of a spectrum of OSA than comorbidity, management of OSA with comorbidity is incomplete if hypoventilation is not evaluated. This chapter entails association of OSA with metabolic and systemic comorbidities, respiratory comorbidities, sleep comorbidities, and obesity hypoventilation syndrome **(Flowchart 1)**.

METABOLIC AND SYSTEMIC COMORBIDITIES

The combination of metabolic syndrome and OSA has been termed "syndrome Z." The frequent association of OSA with metabolic and cardiovascular diseases has been recognized since the early studies, but the role of OSA as an independent risk factor has long remained controversial due to the presence of powerful confounders, such as hypertension and obesity.[12] The evidence is greater for some comorbidities than others. In cardiovascular disease, the association is strongest for hypertension and atrial fibrillation (AF).[13] Furthermore, there is an evidence of a bidirectional relationship between OSA and several comorbidities that include HF as a result of nocturnal fluid accumulation in the neck, in addition to stroke and metabolic syndrome.[13] The relationship between OSA and metabolism is highly complex since nocturnal intermittent hypoxia has been shown to affect glucose metabolism, and OSA could independently contribute to the pathogenesis of metabolic disorders.[14]

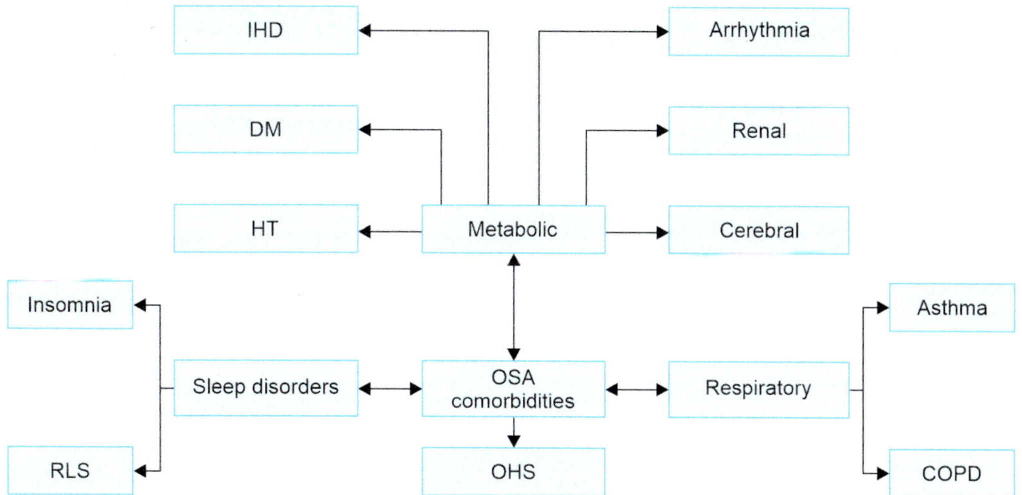

FLOWCHART 1: Obstructive sleep apnea (OSA) with metabolic and systemic comorbidities.

Note: There are bidirectional arrows with metabolic, respiratory, and sleep disorders. However, with OHS there is a unidirectional arrow because OHS is more of OSA spectrum and there is no bidirectional relationship unlike the other comorbid disorders.

(COPD: chronic obstructive pulmonary disease; DM: diabetes mellitus; HT: hypertension; IHD: ischemic heart disease; OHS: obesity hypoventilation syndrome; OSA: obstructive sleep apnea; RLS: restless leg syndrome)

Hypertension

There is large evidence of OSA association with hypertension, cardiovascular disease, and all-cause mortality.[15-18] The largest prospective follow-up Wisconsin Sleep Cohort Study demonstrated a dose–response relationship between baseline OSA severity and development of hypertension with 4 years of follow-up, showing 2.9 times higher odds of developing hypertension in those with moderate-to-severe OSA compared with those without OSA.[19,20] It has been established with reasonable certainty that OSA leads to hypertension. It is thus recommended that OSA should be ruled out in patients suspected with secondary hypertension or malignant hypertension.[21] The treatment with CPAP therapy has shown to improve blood pressure in different studies and meta-analyses.[22,23]

Cardiovascular Comorbidities

There is a high cardiovascular risk in patients with severe OSA as well as increased overall and cardiovascular mortality in untreated OSA.[16,24] The cardiovascular risk has been shown to normalize after treatment.[24] A prospective, observational study on the incidence of coronary artery disease (CAD) in patients with and without OSA who were free of cardiovascular disease at baseline has also shown an increased relative risk for the development of CAD in patients with OSA after 7 years of follow-up.[16] More recent analyses pointed to sleep fragmentation and hypoxia as risk factors for cardiovascular events or death, and regular CPAP use appeared to exert a protective effect.[11]

On the other hand, a meta-analysis of randomized controlled trials (RCTs) on the effects of CPAP in patients with known coronary or cerebrovascular disease has failed to show any protective effect of CPAP treatment on cardiovascular risk.[25] A similar finding was observed in a recently concluded ISAAC study too.[26] The discrepancy between data obtained from observational studies described earlier and RCTs is possibly attributable to inclusion of patients without excessive daytime sleepiness in RCTs; the compliance to CPAP treatment is low (<4 hours) in nonsleepy patients. There is also a possibility that chronic intermittent hypoxia due to OSA could activate some protective mechanisms, for example, through the development of coronary vessel collaterals in patients with IHD which is why CPAP has failed to show protective effect.[27] The results of observational studies have confirmed the association of ischemic heart disease (IHD) with untreated OSA. Also, a trial with multivariable analysis corrected for sociodemographic factors, comorbidities, and cardiovascular risk factors including depression, which included excessive daytime sleepiness, did show that there is 2.85-times greater risk of cardiovascular death in those with daytime sleepiness.[28]

Cardiac Arrhythmias

Obstructive sleep apnea is known to cause AF.[29] Thus, AF is considered a clinical feature suggestive of OSA like excessive daytime sleepiness in the diagnostic algorithm of OSA. Conversely, the literature on ventricular arrhythmias is relatively scarce and heterogeneous.[30]

Cerebrovascular Disease

The Sleep Heart Health Study, a community-based, prospective cohort study showed a three-fold increased risk of ischemic stroke in men with OSA who were followed up for a median of 8.7 years.[31] But most studies have used a composite cardiovascular outcome including stroke, rather than reporting data for each type of event. Available RCTs on the effects of CPAP in patients with stroke and OSA have also reported improvement in neurological function in CPAP users.[32,33]

Diabetes Mellitus

There is a bidirectional relationship between OSA and diabetes mellitus.[34] Treatment of OSA may help to prevent severe consequences of diabetes mellitus like neuropathy, peripheral arterial disease, diabetic retinopathy, optic nerve atrophy, and diabetic nephropathy.[34-37] The SAVE trial showed a higher risk of adverse outcomes in diabetic compared to nondiabetic patients, and a protective effect of CPAP on recurrent cardiovascular events only in diabetic patients with OSA showing a good adherence to CPAP treatment, i.e., at least 4 hours/night, in the first 2 years of the study.[38]

In summary, OSA appears as a potential trigger for metabolic disorders and worse prognosis by worsening chronic organ damage, justifying the hypothesis of a dangerous liaison between OSA and metabolic/systemic comorbidities. Although the possible protective role of OSA treatment is still uncertain, it could differ among different clinical phenotypes of OSA patients.

Renal Disorder

The evidence on OSA with renal disorders suggests that there is a bidirectional relationship between sleep apnea and chronic kidney disease (CKD). The presence of OSA in CKD is associated with more rapid progression of the disease and increased cardiovascular mortality. Also, the presence of OSA is often clinically not apparent in CKD patients. It is thus recommended that diagnostic testing for sleep apnea in all patients with CKD should be considered, particularly in those with more advanced stages of disease. The results of ongoing RCTs are needed to provide definitive evidence to delineate the role of CPAP in slowing renal function decline in select populations who are at risk of CKD. However, it is clear that fluid overload plays an important role in the pathogenesis of sleep apnea in end-stage renal disease. Further studies designed to better understand the effect of fluid overload on key pathophysiological mechanisms such as airway collapsibility and ventilator instability and the role of uremia are needed. There is a scope for a personalized approach to treatment of sleep apnea in end-stage renal disease, as an alternative to CPAP, by optimizing fluid volume status and guiding tailored renal replacement therapies.[39]

OBSTRUCTIVE SLEEP APNEA AND RESPIRATORY COMORBIDITY

Obstructive Sleep Apnea and Chronic Obstructive Pulmonary Disease

The co-occurrence of OSA and COPD is termed "overlap syndrome". COPD has a spectrum of clinical phenotypes ranging from the predominant emphysema to the predominant chronic bronchitis phenotype. The predominant emphysema patients having hyperinflation are less likely to develop OSA while higher body mass index (BMI) and right-sided HF in the predominant chronic bronchitis phenotype predispose to the development of OSA.[40] The presence of low BMI is protective for OSA.

Patients with overlap syndrome have a worse prognosis compared with COPD or OSA alone. During sleep, patients with overlap syndrome suffer more frequent episodes of nocturnal oxygen desaturation. They also have greater daytime hypoxemia and hypercapnia than those who have isolated COPD or OSA.[41] These patients are also more prone to developing cardiac arrhythmias and pulmonary arterial hypertension, 16% of those with OSA had pulmonary hypertension, compared with 86% of those with overlap syndrome.[42] Overlap syndrome patients also tend to develop severe respiratory failure requiring noninvasive ventilator during acute exacerbation. The life expectancy of untreated overlap syndrome is much worse than COPD alone with the same lung function.[43] Snoring and normal to high BMI (>25 kg/m^2) are considered to be risk factors for OSA. Even in patients with COPD, these predisposing factors can be considered the risk factors and patients should be investigated with polysomnography if the patient is obese or has snoring.

Overlap syndrome should not be mistaken with COPD leading to hypoventilation. The patients having overlap syndrome have preserved lung functions and higher BMI.[44] It is important to differentiate between COPD hypoventilation and overlap syndrome because patients with overlap syndrome require CPAP or higher expiratory pressure if bilevel positive airway pressure (PAP) is given. It is thus best to do a titration study in wards with arterial blood gas (ABG) monitoring or in a polysomnography laboratory if there is a doubt regarding overlap syndrome versus hypoventilation. The guidelines also suggest that one should rule out overlap syndrome/OSA before prescribing bilevel PAP to patients suspected of having hypoventilation disorder.[45]

Obstructive Sleep Apnea and Bronchial Asthma

The association between asthma and OSA can be coincidental or causal, or both. OSA is associated with increased bronchial hyper-responsiveness and inflammation.[46] Asthma patients may have poor sleep due to nocturnal symptoms. Two diseases share risk factors like obesity, rhinitis, and gastroesophageal reflux.[47] It is debatable whether they are distinct diseases or are pathophysiologically associated. Even if they are not pathophysiologically linked, the association can decrease the QoL and lead to significant medical comorbidities.

The significant medical comorbidities when the two diseases coexist are because OSA promotes inflammatory responses by means of hypoxia, hypercapnia, and sleep fragmentation, resulting in a reversible increase in C-reactive protein (CRP). Production of tumor necrosis factor α (TNF-α), a proinflammatory cytokine, is also elevated in OSA patients which can adversely affect asthma control. Both proinflammatory factors tend to decrease following CPAP treatment, thereby improving asthma symptoms, bronchodilator use, morning peak expiratory flow, lung function, and QoL.[48] Proportion of adult asthmatic patients suffering from uncontrolled asthma as well as acute exacerbation of asthma decreased in response to CPAP treatment.[49] Also, OSA treatment in asthma patients decreases the cardiovascular risk.

SLEEP COMORBIDITIES

Insomnia and RLS are two common sleep disorders that can coexist with OSA.

Insomnia

Obstructive sleep apnea and insomnia are among the most common disorders presenting to sleep clinics with increasing burden on health care resources.[50] Insomnia presents with symptoms of difficulty in sleep initiation, sleep maintenance, or early morning awakening. When the nocturnal symptoms are associated with significant distress or daytime dysfunction and last for a minimum of 3 months, the condition is known as chronic insomnia disorder.[51] There is increasing evidence of association between OSA and insomnia. The Comorbid Insomnia OSA (COMISA) overlap is also known as "sleep-insomnia apnea syndrome" and "sleep apnea plus".[52] The association, first reported in 1973, seemed as a paradox since OSA and insomnia have opposing spectrums.[53] Insomnia-OSA overlap relationship is bidirectional with one contributing to exacerbation of the other. Repeated nocturnal apneas and awakenings in OSA may lead to insomnia. Similarly, insomnia may lead to nocturnal arousals and superficial sleep increasing upper airway instability. The prevalence of insomnia among OSA varies from 6.4 to 84%.[54,55] The consequences of this dual threat are serious. Insomnia-OSA overlap patients have greater daytime impairment and poorer QoL as compared to either disease alone. It also constitutes a cumulative risk factor for psychiatric and cardiovascular diseases.

The insomnia-OSA overlap has significant diagnostic and therapeutic implications. The history pertaining to insomnia should be taken prior to polysomnography as it will help in deciding which type of study the patient should undergo. As per the American Academy of Sleep Medicine (AASM) guidelines, patients with high pretest probability of moderate-to-severe uncomplicated OSA, type III study is recommended. But in patients with comorbidities and other sleep disorders including severe insomnia, type I study is indicated.[56] This is because total recording time and total sleep duration are not the same in patients with insomnia-OSA overlap and may result in falsely low AHI. The compliance to CPAP, the first line of treatment for OSA, is also affected due to insomnia.[54] The optimal strategy for adequately treating coexisting insomnia and OSA remains unclear. Concurrent treatment for both sleep disorders may be the best treatment approach.[57] But the treatment options for insomnia and OSA present many challenges. Treatment of OSA in patients with insomnia may be difficult because CPAP therapy might increase awakenings, thus perpetuating insomnia symptoms. Additionally, patients with insomnia may be experiencing hyperarousal or anxiety, which may impede the initiation and continuation of CPAP therapy. The overlap patients may require a hypnotic drug as an add-on therapy to improve compliance with CPAP. The benzodiazepines are the preferred drugs for insomnia; however, they should be avoided for overlap patients because they might exacerbate OSA. The nonbenzodiazepine hypnotics such as zolpidem and eszopiclone are the ideal choice. Newer drugs for the treatment of insomnia, i.e., dual orexin receptor antagonists like suvorexant and daridorexant, look promising in the management of coexisting disorders as they do not appear to have any respiratory depressant effect.[58]

Restless Leg Syndrome

Restless leg syndrome, also known as Willis-Ekbom disease, is a common chronic sensorimotor neurological disorder. The diagnosis of RLS is clinical, which is based on URGES criteria (U = Urge to move the legs, R = Rest induces symptoms, G = Gets better with activity, E = Evening and night accentuation, S= Synonyms of RLS, i.e., RLS mimics are ruled out).[59] Sleep disorders are known to overlap with RLS. The overlap of OSA with RLS is called comorbid OSA with RLS (ComOSAR).[60] Though the co occurrence of these two conditions is likely to be coincidental and not causal, the comorbidities are likely to be higher because of increased sleep disturbance.[60] RLS is known to cause insomnia, whereas OSA can lead to frequent awakening. A significant number of ComOSAR patients have insomnia. Similarly, ComOSAR patients have a significantly higher prevalence of anxiety/depression compared to OSA alone.[61] The likelihood of metabolic complications is also higher in ComOSAR compared to OSA alone.

Due to more severe disruption of sleep in patients with ComOSAR as compared to OSA alone, it is imperative to identify RLS, because treating OSA alone will not relieve the patient's symptoms. Compliance with CPAP is also likely to be affected due to the co-occurrence. Management of RLS consists of evaluating iron deficiency. Those with iron deficiency require oral iron supplementation. Those without any iron deficiency may be treated with dopamine agonists and $\alpha 2\delta$ ligands.[62]

OBESITY HYPOVENTILATION SYNDROME

Diagnosis of OHS requires the following criteria to be satisfied: (1) obesity (BMI > 30 kg/m^2), (2) daytime hypercapnia ($PaCO_2 \geq 45$ mm Hg), (3) sleep disordered breathing (SDB) [apnea-hypopnea index (AHI) ≥ 5 or sleep hypoventilation], and (4) other known causes of hypoventilation are excluded[63,64] The AASM has defined sleep hypoventilation in adults as: $PaCO_2$ (or surrogate such as end-tidal carbon dioxide tension or transcutaneous carbon dioxide) > 55 mm Hg for >10 minutes or an increase in $PaCO_2$ (or surrogate) > 10 mm Hg compared to an awake supine value > 50 mm Hg for >10 minutes.[65] Although the definition of OHS requires presence of hypercapnia during the day, OHS is preceded by hypoventilation during sleep. So diurnal hypercapnia represents an advanced stage of OHS **(Table 1)**.[66]

TABLE 1: Obesity hypoventilation stages.

Stage	Name of disorder	Features
0	At risk	No hypercapnia
I	Obesity-associated sleep hypoventilation	• Hypercapnia during sleep—present • Daytime bicarbonate—<27 mmol/L • Daytime hypercapnia—absent • Cardiometabolic abnormality—absent
II	Obesity-associated sleep hypoventilation	• Hypercapnia during sleep—present • Daytime bicarbonate—≥27 mmol/L • Daytime hypercapnia—absent • Cardiometabolic abnormality—absent
III	Obesity hypoventilation	• Hypercapnia during sleep—present • Daytime bicarbonate—≥27 mmol/L • Daytime hypercapnia—present • Cardiometabolic abnormality—absent
IV	Obesity hypoventilation syndrome	• Hypercapnia during sleep—present • Daytime bicarbonate—≥27 mmol/L • Daytime hypercapnia—present • Cardiometabolic abnormality—present

The diagnosis of OHS requires a high index of suspicion. As per an Indian report, a BMI of 31 kg/m^2 also may lead to OHS.[67] Presence of high bicarbonate ≥27 mmol/L, baseline saturation of ≤95%, and severe OSA should alert the physician to order ABG for the diagnosis.[67] It is important to diagnose OHS in patients with OSA because OHS is associated with significant morbidity and mortality. OHS patients compared to eucapnic patients of SDB have lower QoL, greater risk of pulmonary hypertension and cor pulmonale, higher need of mechanical ventilation with longer hospital stay, and more healthcare expenses.[64,68] The management of OHS also differs in that OHS may often require bilevel positive airway pressure with or without oxygen. Recent recommendations have however suggested that CPAP rather than noninvasive ventilation be offered as the first-line treatment to stable ambulatory patients with OHS and coexistent severe obstructive sleep apnea.[66,69] Patients hospitalized with respiratory failure and those with mild-to-moderate OSA may require bilevel positive airway pressure therapy. It is imperative to use weight-loss interventions that produce sustained weight loss of 25–30% of body weight to achieve resolution of OHS with bariatric surgery or drugs.[70]

SUMMARY

The holistic approach to OSA includes evaluation of metabolic and systemic comorbidities. Respiratory comorbidities, especially obstructive airway disease like COPD and bronchial asthma, are important as the outcome of respiratory disorder and OSA combined is much worse than any of the diseases occurring individually. Sleep disorders like insomnia and RLS are also common and can coexist. The treatment of OSA will be incomplete without their management. Last, patients suspected to have OHS based on a high index of suspicion should undergo ABG evaluation and structured weight-loss program for optimal management.

Note: See **Appendix 1** which captures these details in terms of comorbidities; these should be filled in by each patient prior to doing polysomnography and prescribing CPAP.

REFERENCES

1. Abbasi A, Gupta SS, Sabharwal N, et al. Obstructive sleep apnoea syndrome (OSA) is frequently associated with systemic, metabolic, renal, respiratory and neuropsychiatric comorbidities. Sleep Sci. 2021;14:142-54.
2. Garvey JF, Taylor CT, McNicholas WT. Cardiovascular disease in obstructive sleep apnoea syndrome: the role of intermittent hypoxia and inflammation. Eur Respir J. 2009;33:1195-205.
3. Vgontzas AN, Gaines J, Ryan S, et al. CrossTalk proposal: metabolic syndrome causes sleep apnoea. J Physiol. 2016;594: 4687-90.
4. Prasad B, Nyenhuis SM, Imayama I, et al. Asthma and Obstructive Sleep Apnea Overlap: What has the Evidence Taught Us? Am J Respir Crit Care Med. 2020;201:1345-57.
5. Locke BW, Lee JL, Sundar KM. OSA and chronic respiratory disease: Mechanisms and epidemiology. Int J Environ Res Public Health. 2022;19:5473.
6. Appleton SL, Gill TK, Lang CJ, et al. Prevalence and comorbidity of sleep conditions in Australian adults: 2016 Sleep Health Foundation national survey. Sleep Health. 2018;4:13-9.
7. Tveit RL, Lehmann S, Bjorvatn B. Prevalence of several somatic diseases depends on the presence and severity of obstructive sleep apnea. PLoS One. 2018;13:e0192671.
8. Robichaud-Hallé L, Beaudry M, Fortin M. Obstructive sleep apnea and multimorbidity. BMC Pulm Med. 2012;12:60.
9. Mokhlesi B, Ham SA, Gozal D. The effect of sex and age on the comorbidity burden of OSA: an observational analysis from a large nationwide US health claims database. Eur Respir J. 2016;47:1162-9.
10. Marrone O, Lo Bue A, Salvaggio A, et al. Comorbidities and survival in obstructive sleep apnoea beyond the age of 50. Eur J Clin Invest. 2013;43:27-33.
11. Zinchuk AV, Jeon S, Koo BB, et al. Polysomnographic phenotypes and their cardiovascular implications in obstructive sleep apnoea. Thorax. 2018;73:472-80.
12. Patro M, Gothi D, Vaidya S, et al. Obstructive Sleep Apnea with Insomnia Overlap: An Under-recognized Entity. Indian J Chest Dis Allied Sci. 2022;64:207-11.
13. Wolk R, Shamsuzzaman AS, Somers VK. Obesity, sleep apnea, and hypertension. Hypertension. 2003;42:1067-74.
14. Anothaisintawee T, Reutrakul S, Van Cauter E, et al. Sleep disturbances compared to traditional risk factors for diabetes development: Systematic review and meta-analysis. Sleep Med Rev. 2016;30:11-24.
15. Logan AG, Perlikowski SM, Mente A, et al. High prevalence of unrecognized sleep apnoea in drug-resistant hypertension. J Hypertens. 2001;19:2271-7.
16. Peker Y, Hedner J, Norum J, et al. Increased incidence of cardiovascular disease in middle-aged men with obstructive sleep apnea: a 7-year follow-up. Am J Respir Crit Care Med. 2002;166:159-65.
17. Arzt M, Young T, Finn L, et al. Association of sleep-disordered breathing and the occurrence of stroke. Am J Respir Crit Care Med. 2005;172:1447-51.
18. Marshall NS, Wong KK, Liu PY, et al. Sleep apnea as an independent risk factor for all-cause mortality: the Busselton Health Study. Sleep. 2008;31:1079-85.
19. Young T, Finn L, Peppard PE, et al. Sleep disordered breathing and mortality: eighteen-year follow-up of the Wisconsin sleep cohort. Sleep. 2008;31:1071-8.
20. Peppard PE, Young T, Palta M, et al. Prospective study of the association between sleep-disordered breathing and hypertension. N Engl J Med. 2000;342:1378-84.
21. Unger T, Borghi C, Charchar F, et al. International Society of Hypertension Global Hypertension Practice Guidelines. Hypertension. 2020;75:1334-57.
22. Montesi SB, Edwards BA, Malhotra A, et al. The effect of continuous positive airway pressure treatment on blood pressure: a systematic review and meta-analysis of randomized controlled trials. J Clin Sleep Med. 2012;8:587-96.
23. Fava C, Dorigoni S, Dalle Vedove F, et al. Effect of CPAP on blood pressure in patients with OSA/hypopnea a systematic review and meta-analysis. Chest. 2014;145(4):762-71.
24. Marin JM, Carrizo SJ, Vicente E, et al. Long-term cardiovascular outcomes in men with obstructive sleep apnoea-hypopnoea with or without treatment with continuous positive airway pressure: an observational study. Lancet. 2005;365:1046-53.
25. Vakulin A, D'Rozario A, Kim JW, et al. Quantitative sleep EEG and polysomnographic predictors of driving simulator performance in obstructive sleep apnea. Clin Neurophysiol. 2016;127:1428-35.
26. Sánchez-de-la-Torre M, Sánchez-de-la-Torre A, Bertran S, et al. Spanish Sleep Network. Effect of obstructive sleep apnoea and its treatment with continuous positive airway pressure on the prevalence of cardiovascular events in patients with acute coronary syndrome (ISAACC study): a randomised controlled trial. Lancet Respir Med. 2020;8(4):359-67.
27. Al-Shawwa BA, Badi AN, Goldberg AN, et al. Defining common outcome metrics used in obstructive sleep apnea. Sleep Med Rev. 2008;12:449-61.
28. Jingen Li, Covassin N, Bock JM, et al. Excessive Daytime Sleepiness and Cardiovascular Mortality in US Adults: A NHANES 2005–2008 Follow-up Study. Nat Sci Sleep. 2021;13:1049-59.
29. Deng F, Raza A, Guo J. Treating obstructive sleep apnea with continuous positive airway pressure reduces risk of recurrent atrial fibrillation after catheter ablation: a meta-analysis. Sleep Med. 2018;46:5-11.
30. Raghuram A, Clay R, Kumbam A, et al. A systematic review of the association between obstructive sleep apnea and ventricular arrhythmias. J Clin Sleep Med. 2014;10:1155-60.
31. Redline S, Yenokyan G, Gottlieb DJ, et al. Obstructive sleep apnea-hypopnea and incident stroke: the sleep heart health study. Am J Respir Crit Care Med. 2010;182:269-77.
32. Brill AK, Horvath T, Seiler A, et al. CPAP as treatment of sleep apnea after stroke: A meta-analysis of randomized trials. Neurology. 2018;90:e1222-3.
33. Fox H, Bitter T, Horstkotte D, Oldenburg O. Sleep-disordered breathing and arrhythmia in heart failure patients. Sleep Med Clin. 2017;12(2):229-41.
34. Reutrakul S, Mokhlesi B. Obstructive Sleep Apnea and Diabetes: A State of the Art Review. Chest. 2017;152:1070-86.
35. Tahrani AA, Ali A, Raymond NT, et al. Obstructive sleep apnea and diabetic neuropathy: a novel association in patients with type 2 diabetes. Am J Respir Crit Care Med. 2012;186:434-41.

36. Altaf QA, Dodson P, Ali A, et al. Obstructive sleep apnea and retinopathy in patients with type 2 diabetes. A longitudinal study. Am J Respir Crit Care Med. 2017;196:892-900.
37. Leong WB, Jadhakhan F, Taheri S, et al. The Association between Obstructive Sleep Apnea on Diabetic Kidney Disease: A Systematic Review and Meta-analysis. Sleep. 2016;39:301-8.
38. Quan W, Zheng D, McEvoy RD, et al. High risk characteristics for recurrent cardiovascular events among patients with obstructive sleep apnoea in the SAVE study. EClinicalMedicine. 2018;2(3):59-65.
39. Lin C, Lurie RC, Lyons OD. Sleep Apnea and Chronic Kidney Disease: A State-of-the-Art Review. Chest. 2020;157(3):673-85.
40. Kim V, Han MK, Vance GB, et al. The chronic bronchitic phenotype of COPD: an analysis of the COPD Gene Study. Chest. 2011;140:626-33.
41. Singh S, Kaur H, Sigh S. The overlap syndrome. Cureus. 2018;10: e3453.
42. Owens RL, Malhotra A. Sleep-disordered Breathing and COPD: The Overlap Syndrome. Respir Care. 2010;55:1333-46.
43. McNicholas WT. Comorbid obstructive sleep apnoea and chronic obstructive pulmonary disease and the risk of cardiovascular disease. J Thorac Dis. 2018;10:S4253-61.
44. Vaidya S, Gothi D, Patro M. COPD sleep phenotypes: Genesis of respiratory failure in COPD. Monaldi Arch Chest Dis. 2022;92: 1776.
45. Macrea M, Oczkowski S, Rochwerg B, et al.; on behalf of the American Thoracic Society Assembly on Sleep and Respiratory Neurobiology. Long-term Noninvasive Ventilation in Chronic Stable Hypercapnic Chronic Obstructive Pulmonary Disease. An Official American Thoracic Society Clinical Practice Guideline. Am J Respir Crit Care Med. 2020;202:e75-e87.
46. Lin C-C, Lin C-Y. Obstructive sleep apnea syndrome and bronchial hyperreactivity. Lung. 1995;173:117-26.
47. Prasad B, Nyenhuis SM, Weaver TE. Obstructive sleep apnea and asthma: associations and treatment implications. Sleep Med Rev. 2014;18:165-71.
48. Deslypere G, Dupont L. Principal comorbidities in severe asthma: how to manage and what is their influence on asthma endpoints. EC Pulm Respir Med. 2017;3:162-74.
49. Serrano-Pariente J, Plaza V, Soriano JB, et al. Asthma outcomes improve with continuous positive airway pressure for obstructive sleep apnea. Allergy Eur J Allergy Clin Immunol. 2017;72:802-12.
50. Bouscoulet LT, Vazquez-Garcia JC, Muino A, et al. Prevalence of sleep related symptoms in four Latin American cities. J Clin Sleep Med. 2008;4:579-85.
51. American Academy of Sleep Medicine. International Classification of Sleep Disorders, 3rd edition. Darien, IL: American Academy of Sleep Medicine; 2014.
52. Al-Jawder SE, BaHammam AS. Comorbid insomnia in sleep-related breathing disorders: an under-recognized association. Sleep Breath. 2012;16:295-304.
53. Krell SB, Kapur VK. Insomnia complaints in patients evaluated for obstructive sleep apnoea. Sleep Breath. 2005;9:104-10.
54. Zhang Y, Ren R, Lei F, et al. Worldwide and regional prevalence rates of co-occurrence of insomnia and insomnia symptoms with obstructive sleep apnoea: A systematic review and meta-analysis. Sleep Med Rev. 2019;45:1-17.
55. Gupta MA, Knapp K. Cardiovascular and Psychiatric Morbidity in Obstructive Sleep Apnoea (OSA) with Insomnia (Sleep Apnoea Plus) versus Obstructive Sleep Apnoea without Insomnia: A Case-Control Study from a Nationally Representative US Sample. PLoS One. 2014;9:e90021.
56. Kapur VK, Auckley DH, Chowdhuri S, et al. Clinical practice guideline for diagnostic testing for adult obstructive sleep apnoea: an American Academy of Sleep Medicine clinical practice guideline. J Clin Sleep Med. 2017;13:479-504.
57. Luyster FS, Buysse DJ, Strollo PJ. Comorbid Insomnia and Obstructive Sleep Apnea: Challenges for Clinical Practice and Research. J Clin Sleep Med. 2010;6:95.
58. Mogavero MP, Silvani A, Lanza G, et al. Targeting Orexin Receptors for the Treatment of Insomnia: From Physiological Mechanisms to Current Clinical Evidence and Recommendations. Nat Sci Sleep. 2023;15:17-38.
59. Allen RP, Picchietti DL, Garcia-Borreguero D, et al. Restless legs syndrome/Willis-Ekbom disease diagnostic criteria: updated International Restless Legs Syndrome Study Group (IRLSSG) consensus criteria--history, rationale, description, and significance. Sleep Med. 2014;15:860-73.
60. Pistorius F, Geisler P, Wetter TC, et al. Sleep apnea syndrome comorbid with and without restless legs syndrome: differences in insomnia specific symptoms. Sleep Breath. 2020;24:1167-72.
61. Gupta R, Lahan V, Goel D. Prevalence of restless leg syndrome in subjects with depressive disorder. Indian J Psychiatry. 2013; 55:70-3.
62. Romero-Peralta S, Cano-Pumarega I, Garcia-Malo C, et al. Treating restless legs syndrome in the context of sleep disordered breathing comorbidity. Eur Respir Rev. 2019;28: 190061.
63. Al Dabal L, Bahammam AS. Obesity hypoventilation syndrome. Ann Thorac Med. 2009;4:41-9.
64. Mokhlesi B. Obesity hypoventilation syndrome: A state-of-the-art review. Respir Care. 2010;55:1347-62.
65. Berry RB, Budhiraja R, Gottlieb DJ, et al. Rules for scoring respiratory events in sleep: update of the 2007 AASM Manual for the Scoring of Sleep and Associated Events. Deliberations of the Sleep Apnea Definitions Task Force of the American Academy of Sleep Medicine. J Clin Sleep Med. 2012;8:597-619.
66. Randerath W, Verbraecken J, Andreas S, et al. Definition, discrimination, diagnosis and treatment of central breathing disturbances during sleep. Am J Respir Crit Care Med. 2019;200:1325-6.
67. Patro M, Gothi D, Ojha UC, et al. Predictors of obesity hypoventilation syndrome among patients with sleep-disordered breathing in India. Lung India. 2019;36:499-505.
68. Berg G, Delaive K, Manfreda J, et al. The use of health-care resources in obesity-hypoventilation syndrome. Chest. 2001; 120:377-83.
69. Randerath W, Verbraecken J, Andreas S, et al. Definition, discrimination, diagnosis and treatment of central breathing disturbances during sleep. Eur Respir J. 2017;49:1600959.
70. Deng Y, Park A, Zhu L, et al. Effect of semaglutide and liraglutide in individuals with obesity or overweight without diabetes: a systematic review. Ther Adv Chronic Dis. 2022;13: 20406223221108064.

Appendix 1

Proforma for Evaluation of Comorbidities Prior to Prescribing CPAP.

Name:
Age/sex:
Phone No:
Occupation:
Shift duty (how many times/week):
Smoking:

Nocturnal Symptoms

- *Snoring*:
  - Is it loud and habitual (more than 3 nights/week)?
  - Is it audible in the other room?
  - Is it crescendo-decrescendo?
  - Does the individual wake up with his/her own snoring?
- *Witnessed apnea*: Has the relative witnessed apneas or sudden interruption in the loud snoring sound?
- *Nocturnal choking*: Does he/she wake up with gasping or choking sensation?
- *Nocturia*: How many times does he/she wake up due to nocturia?
- *Sleep quality*:
  - Is the sleep disturbed with tossing and turning?
  - Are there frequent sleep fragmentation and difficulty in maintaining sleep leading to insomnia?
  - What is the total duration of sleep?
  - Is there a feeling of unrefreshing sleep or early morning headache or dryness of throat?

Daytime Symptoms

- *Excessive daytime sleepiness (EDS)*: Does the patient feel sleepy during quiet activities like reading and watching television or during activities that generally require alertness like school, work, and driving?
- *Lethargy*: Does he/she have daytime fatigue/tiredness or decreased alertness?
- *Cognitive deficits*: History of memory, concentration, and intellectual impairment
- *Psychiatry symptoms*: Personality, mood changes, depression, anxiety, sexual dysfunction like impotence and decreased libido
- *Systemic complaints*: Gastroesophageal reflux, hypertension, diabetes mellitus

Stop Bang

- S—Snoring
- T—Tiredness
- O—Observed apnea
- P—Blood pressure
- B—BMI > 35 kg/m^2
- A—>50 years
- N—> 40 cm
- G—Gender, male

RLS Symptoms

- U—Unpleasant sensation in leg
- R—Rest induced
- G—Gets relived on exercise
- E—Evening or night symptom

Insomnia Symptoms

- Difficulty in falling asleep: Yes/no
- Difficulty in sleep maintenance: Yes/no
- Early morning awakening: Yes/no
- Duration
- Excessive sleepiness in day: Yes/no

Epworth Sleepiness Score

- 0 = Would never doze
- 1 = Slight chance of dozing
- 2 = Moderate chance of dozing
- 3 = High chance of dozing

Situation Chance of Dozing

Situation	
1. Sitting and reading	________________
2. Watching TV	________________
3. Sitting inactive in a public place (e.g., a theater or a meeting)	________________
4. As a passenger in a car for an hour without a break	________________
5. Lying down to rest in the afternoon when circumstances permit	________________
6. Sitting and talking to someone	________________
7. Sitting quietly after a lunch without alcohol	________________
8. In a car, while stopped for a few minutes in traffic	________________
Total (max. 24)	

Examination

P: Sat:
BP:
Weight: Height:
Neck circumference:
Waist circumference:
RS:

Comorbid Diseases

Investigations

Hb: TLC: DLC:
BUN: CREAT:
BSF/R:
ABG:
Lipid profile:
T3, T4, TSH:
XRC (PA):
Spirometry:

	Pre (%)	Post (%)
FVC (L):		
FEV1:	(L)	
FEV1/FVC (%):		

ECG:
2D echo:

Final Diagnosis

Nocturnal Limb Movement Disorders

CHAPTER 145

Kevin Shayani, Jacob Schwartz, Margarita Oks

INTRODUCTION

Nocturnal limb movements during sleep encompass a large umbrella of pathology and make up a subset of disease under what is known as sleep-related movement disorders. Limb movement disorders themselves can most simply be divided into events that are simple or periodic/rhythmic. This group of disorders is heterogeneous, and the pathophysiology and subsequent management vary depending on the underlying etiology. Some phenomena are benign in nature and require no intervention, while others can be more dramatic and require intervention and possible pharmacotherapy. The International Classification of Sleep Disorders (ICSD-3) includes a variety of clinically identifiable disorders, with simple behaviors including hypnic jerks, exploding head syndrome, propriospinal myoclonus, epileptic myoclonus, and nocturnal leg cramping, whereas periodic behaviors include sleep-related rhythmic disorder, hypnagogic foot tremor, and periodic limb movements in sleep (PLMS), which can subsequently be diagnosed as periodic limb movement disorder (PLMD) if other diagnoses have been excluded.[1]

EPIDEMIOLOGY AND RISK FACTORS

It is challenging to determine the exact prevalence of nocturnal limb movement disorder owing to its large heterogeneity and spectrum of disease and given the fact that it can often be comorbid with restless leg syndrome (RLS), a sleep-related movement disorder which despite its association with sleep impairment does not occur during sleep. The reported prevalence of RLS is believed to be around 5–15%, but the actual number may be higher given that the disease can be underdiagnosed and that not all cases are clinically significant.[2] It can be comorbid with PLMS in nearly 80% of the cases, and in cases where RLS is absent, the prevalence of PLMD itself is thought to be in the range of 4–11%.[3]

Given the comorbid association with RLS and PLMS, workup of PLM typically involves concomitant evaluation for RLS. The most common risk factors associated with RLS are depleted central nervous system (CNS) iron stores, most often reflected in low serum ferritin.[4] Other risk factors for RLS would be uremia, and this is most commonly seen in patients with end-stage kidney disease on dialysis. Additional associations with RLS include peripheral neuropathies (which can be secondary to many conditions including diabetes mellitus, chronic alcohol use, amyloidosis, and others), spinal cord injury (whether transient or permanent), and pregnancy (owing to a relative iron deficiency).[4]

Family history is also important in the evaluation of nocturnal limb movements, as a family history of RLS specifically has a strong association with the development of PLMS. Congruent with family history, there appears to be a genetic component to PLMS as well as certain genes such as *MEIS1* and *BTBD9* that appear to be implicated in the pathogenesis.[5] A careful medication history must be taken when evaluating for PLMS, as certain drugs such as serotonin selective reuptake inhibitors, dopamine blockers, and tricyclic antidepressants may increase the risk of PLMS. Other independent risk factors for PLMS include age (with higher age being associated with PLMS), male sex, obesity, active smoking, physical inactivity, and diabetes.[6]

PATHOPHYSIOLOGY

The pathophysiology of nocturnal limb movements varies depending on the underlying etiology, and in the case of PLMS and PLMD, the exact mechanism itself is unknown. Broadly, the pathophysiology can be divided into issues of the peripheral nervous system versus primary issues of the CNS. Given the strong association with RLS, the underlying pathology can also be related to metabolic disturbances.

In cases where the peripheral nervous system is involved, there is postulated to be a regional iron deficiency affecting the neurotransmission of dopamine in the subcortical area of the brain, which may be augmented by genetic factors affecting the iron metabolism in the brain.[4] Given that the pathways involved are dopaminergic, this also explains the association with neurotropic medications, specifically dopamine blockers, and PLMS. In cases of RLS (especially those associated with iron deficiency and low ferritin states), this is believed to be the core cause of the disease and it is not uncommon for this disease state to be comorbid with PLMS. There is also evidence that peripheral neuropathy, whether from long-standing diabetes mellitus or otherwise, increases the risk for PLMS and this association may be multifactorial as impaired carbohydrate metabolism may be implicated in sleep fragmentation, which results in lower nonrapid eye movement (NREM) sleep, lower sleep efficiency, and higher arousals.[4]

In cases where the CNS is involved, there is debate as to whether the neurologic impairment that manifests as PLMS arises in the cortical regions of the brain or the spinal cord. In early studies, there was found to be an association between polysomnography (PSG) cortical activity and subsequent PLMS.[7] Subsequent studies have shown an association between spinal cord reflexes and periodic limb movements as reflected in spinal flexor reflexes.

CLINICAL FEATURES

Features of nocturnal limb movement disorders vary depending on the phenotypic syndrome that most closely correlates with the patient's symptoms. In the event of PLMS, there is a direct correlation with age, where increased age is highly associated with an increase in the number of nocturnal limb movements.[6] It is also often highly comorbid with multiple other conditions including obstructive sleep apnea, Parkinson's disease, rapid eye movement behavior sleep disorder (RBD), and narcolepsy. In cases where nocturnal limb movements exist and are either out of proportion to the underlying comorbidity, or occur in the absence of any of the above disease processes, the entity is then referred to as PMLD.[1]

DIAGNOSIS AND DIFFERENTIAL DIAGNOSIS

The diagnosis of nocturnal limb movement disorder varies depending on the underlying disorder. In the case of PLMS, the American Academy of Sleep Medicine (AASM) has explicit diagnostic criteria which combine clinical criteria in addition to PSG to make a definitive diagnosis.[8] Clinically, patients must have a history of sleep disturbance or daytime fatigue. On PSG, patients must display the following:[9]

- The minimum number of consecutive limb movement events needed to define a PLMS series is 4 limb movements.
- The minimum period length between limb movement (defined as the time between the onsets of consecutive LMs) to include them as part of a PLMS series is 5 seconds.
- The maximum period length between limb movements to include them as part of a PLM series is 90 seconds.
- Limb movements on two different legs separated by <5 seconds between movement onsets are counted as a single movement.

In addition, patients must have exclusion of other causes of their sleep complaints as PLMD itself is a diagnosis of exclusion. The requirement for a PSG will help capture patients with undiagnosed OSA and narcolepsy.

On the other hand, RLS is a clinical diagnosis and should be thought of in the context of a patient who complains of an urge to move their legs when lying in bed accompanied by an unpleasant sensation in the legs which worsens during periods of inactivity and improves or is relieved by movement. Patients will typically complain that this sensation is worse in the evenings or at night. Alternative diagnosis should be considered if the symptoms are not fully accounted for by another medical condition or if the index of clinical suspicion for an alternative diagnosis remains high such as a situation in which there is concern for another sleep disorder, such as when a patient is noted to have arousals or if there is concern for sleep apnea. In this situation, it would be appropriate to pursue further workup with a PSG.

Restless leg syndrome and PLMS must be distinguished from other conditions which may cause abnormal movements of the legs or abnormal movements during sleep **(Box 1)**. These include volitional movements such as foot tapping which typically do not have any circadian rhythm associations. Patients with akathisia, unlike RLS patients, do not complain of unpleasant sensations. Nocturnal leg cramps are of acute onset, short in duration, and are associated with a palpable muscle contraction. Alternating leg muscle activation (ALMA) characterizes a series of EMG bursts in one leg after the other during sleep; unlike in PLMS, these bursts approximate the frequency of muscle activation seen in human locomotion as opposed to PLMS which are usually separated by 20–40-second intervals. Patients may experience hypnagogic foot tremor, a rhythmic movement of the feet occurring at the transition between wake and sleep. Additionally, patients may exhibit normal physiologic jerks associated with sleep. These include partial myoclonic jerks of the distal muscles, hypnic jerks which may affect the trunk. Lastly, patients may also exhibit movements such

BOX 1 Simple versus periodic/rhythmic behaviors.

- *Simple:*
  - Hypnic jerks
  - Bruxism
  - Propriospinal
  - Myoclonus at sleep onset
  - Nocturnal leg cramps
  - Exploding head syndrome
- *Complex:*
  - Periodic limb movement
  - Hypnagogic
  - Foot tremor
  - Sleep-related rhythmic movement disorder
  - Alternating leg muscle activation

as sleep-related bruxism which refers to repetitive jaw-muscle activity, and sleep-related rhythmic movements characterized by repetitive, stereotyped, rhythmic motor behaviors with a defined frequency range of 0.5–2.0 Hz with at least four defined movements. Patients may also exhibit propriospinal myoclonus at sleep onset which is characterized by jerks involving the abdominal and truncal muscles occurring during the transition from wakefulness to sleep or excessive fragmentary myoclonus which is characterized by small movements of the corners of the mouth, fingers, or toes during NREM sleep.

TREATMENT (TABLE 1)

Nonpharmacologic Therapy

In cases of nocturnal limb movement disorder with mild symptom burden, nonpharmacologic approaches can be trialed which typically include some level of behavioral and lifestyle modification to reduce the incidence of nocturnal events.[10] These include mental alerting activities (such as puzzles), regular exercise, and refraining from caffeine and alcohol. Additionally, patients are encouraged to avoid aggravating factors such as getting insufficient sleep.

In cases with comorbid RLS, and especially in cases where there is an underlying etiology to the RLS, correcting this deficiency would be a reasonable first step and may include iron supplementation in those with deficient ferritin or hemodialysis for those with elevated blood urea nitrogen. Iron replacement should be considered for those with a ferritin level < 75 ng/mL (and transferrin saturation level < 45%). There are no direct comparisons for the supplementation of intravenous versus oral iron in patients with RLS, because oral iron is easier and safer and an appropriate initial therapy while IV iron may be appropriate for patients with severe symptoms or those who need a rapid response.

Pharmacologic Therapy

In patients with persistent or troublesome symptoms interfering with sleep, a large array of pharmacotherapies exist for RLS which concomitantly can also be used for PLMS. First line therapy for RLS is the gabapentinoid class of medications including gabapentin and pregabalin. Gabapentin enacarbil, a prodrug of gabapentin, is often preferred as it can be timed for early evening administration so that the peak action of the drug can take effect at bedtime, where most of the symptoms will occur in patients. While the exact mechanism of action is unknown, it is believed to be due to alpha-2-delta calcium channel agonism.[11] Dopamine agonists such as pramipexole and ropinirole serve as second-line options; however, there is a risk of long-term augmentation with prolonged use which carries an array of side effects that are unpleasant for patients including a risk of withdrawal syndrome as well. In cases where gabapentinoids pose an increased risk to patients (those with obesity, depression, or gait instability), dopamine agonists would be preferred.

TABLE 1: Nonpharmacologic versus pharmacologic management of periodic limb movement disorder (PLMD).

Nonpharmacologic treatment options	Pharmacologic
Mental alerting activities	Iron replacement
Exercise	Gabapentinoids: Gabapentin, pregabalin
Avoid caffeine and alcohol	Dopamine agonists: Pramipexole, ropinirole
Avoid insufficient sleep	Benzodiazepines, opiates

While there is no evidence on the exact mechanism of action for dopamine agonists, it is postulated that its effect is due to enhancement of dopamine neurological pathways as loss of dopaminergic neurons is believed to play some role in the potential etiology of RLS.[10] Multiple randomized controlled trials have displayed the efficacy of gabapentinoids and dopamine agonists versus placebo in the treatment of RLS. In cases of refractory RLS, combination therapy may be considered versus the addition of benzodiazepines or substituting therapy to a low-dose opiate. In situations where opiates are required, high-potency opiates such as oxycodone or methadone are often required.[12] Opiates are typically reserved for the patients with the most severe symptoms and require close follow-up for monitoring on potential adverse events and response to therapy. While an abundance of evidence exists for pharmacologic intervention in RLS, there is no strong data or recommendations by the AASM in regards to intervention for PLMD.[9] In nonrandomized trials, the use of clonazepam, melatonin, and valproate has been associated with a statistically significant improvement subjectively in daytime alertness and fatigue and objectively in sleep parameters including sleep efficiency and stages 1, 3, and 4 sleep.[13]

Investigational Therapies

Other drugs may be helpful in the management of nocturnal leg movement disorders; however, little data exist and the surrounding literature involves mostly small studies. These drugs include carbamazepine,[14] clonidine,[15] and amantadine.[16] Few other therapies are also currently being investigated but have little supporting data such as magnesium supplementation, dipyridamole,[17] and vitamin D supplementation.[18] Lastly, cannabis has been described as being helpful in the management of RLS,[19] but no large systemic trials have evaluated this.

SUMMARY

There are multiple conditions characterized with nocturnal limb movements during sleep which can be divided into events that are simple or periodic/rhythmic. This group of disorders is heterogeneous and the management varies according to the underlying etiology. It is challenging to determine the exact prevalence owing to the complexity of clinical manifestations. While some of the conditions are benign in nature, others may require therapeutic intervention and possible pharmacotherapy.

REFERENCES

1. Sateia MJ. International classification of sleep disorders-third edition: highlights and modifications. Chest. 2014;146(5): 1387-94.
2. Allen RP, Walters AS, Montplaisir J, et al. Restless legs syndrome prevalence and impact: REST general population study. Arch Intern Med. 2005;165(11):1286-92.
3. Hornyak M, Feige B, Riemann D, et al. Periodic leg movements in sleep and periodic limb movement disorder: prevalence, clinical significance and treatment. Sleep Med Rev. 2006;10: 169-77.
4. Vlasie A, Trifu SC, Lupuleac C, Kohn B, Cristea MB. Restless legs syndrome: An overview of pathophysiology, comorbidities and therapeutic approaches (Review). Exp Ther Med. 2022;23(2):185.
5. Tilch E, Schormair B, Zhao C, et al. Identification of Restless Legs Syndrome Genes by Mutational Load Analysis. Ann Neurol. 2020;87(2):184-93.
6. Leary EB, Moore HE 4th, Schneider LD, et al. Periodic limb movements in sleep: Prevalence and associated sleepiness in the Wisconsin Sleep Cohort. Clin Neurophysiol. 2018;129(11): 2306-14.
7. Iriarte J, Urrestarazu E, Alegre M, et al. Oscillatory cortical changes during periodic limb movements. Sleep. 2004;27(8):1493-8.
8. Stefani A, Högl B. Diagnostic Criteria, Differential Diagnosis, and Treatment of Minor Motor Activity and Less Well-known Movement Disorders of Sleep. Curr Treat Options Neurol. 2019;21(1):1.
9. American Academy of Sleep Medicine. International Classification of Sleep Disorders, 3rd edition. Illinois: American Academy of Sleep Medicine; 2023.
10. Silber MH, Buchfuhrer MJ, Earley CJ, et al.; Scientific and Medical Advisory Board of the Restless Legs Syndrome Foundation. The Management of Restless Legs Syndrome: An Updated Algorithm. Mayo Clin Proc. 2021;96(7):1921-37.
11. Kushida CA, Becker PM, Ellenbogen AL, et al.; XP052 Study Group. Randomized, double-blind, placebo-controlled study of XP13512/GSK1838262 in patients with RLS. Neurology. 2009;72(5):439-46.
12. Silber MH, Becker PM, Buchfuhrer MJ, et al.; Scientific and Medical Advisory Board, Restless Legs Syndrome Foundation. The Appropriate Use of Opioids in the Treatment of Refractory Restless Legs Syndrome. Mayo Clin Proc. 2018;93(1):59-67.
13. Aurora RN, Kristo DA, Bista SR, et al.; American Academy of Sleep Medicine. The treatment of restless legs syndrome and periodic limb movement disorder in adults—an update for 2012: practice parameters with an evidence-based systematic review and meta-analyses: an American Academy of Sleep Medicine Clinical Practice Guideline. Sleep. 2012;35(8):1039-62.
14. Telstad W, Sørensen O, Larsen S, et al. Treatment of the restless legs syndrome with carbamazepine: a double blind study. Br Med J (Clin Res Ed). 1984;288(6415):444-6.
15. Wagner ML, Walters AS, Coleman RG, et al. Randomized, Double-blind, Placebo-controlled Study of Clonidine in Restless Legs Syndrome. Sleep. 1996;19(1):52-8.
16. Evidente VG, Adler CH, Caviness JN, et al. Amantadine is beneficial in restless legs syndrome. Mov Disord. 2000;15(2): 324-7.
17. Garcia-Borreguero D, Garcia-Malo C, Granizo JJ, et al. A Randomized, Placebo-Controlled Crossover Study with Dipyridamole for Restless Legs Syndrome. Mov Disord. 2021; 36(10):2387-92.
18. Wali S, Alsafadi S, Abaalkhail B, et al. The Association between Vitamin D Level and Restless Legs Syndrome: A Population-Based Case-control Study. J Clin Sleep Med. 2018;14(4): 557-64.
19. Ghorayeb I. Cannabis for Restless Legs Syndrome. Adv Exp Med Biol. 2021;1297:173-81.

Rapid Eye Movement Behavior Sleep Disorder

CHAPTER 146

Kevin Shayani, Margarita Oks

INTRODUCTION

Rapid eye movement (REM) sleep is a phase of sleep characterized by atonia, where typically there is a loss of skeletal muscle tone (with the exception of the ocular muscles and diaphragms).[1] This is due to direct inhibition of alpha motor neurons, which is reflected in electromyography (EMG) monitoring. REM sleep accounts for nearly 25% of total sleep time, and brain activity during this period is closest to that of brain activity during waking periods. It is also the stage of sleep where dreaming happens. In REM behavior sleep disorder (RBD), there is a loss of REM sleep atonia and it is characterized by dream enactment which can range from benign gestures to violent thrashing leading to self-induced harm and/or harm to the bed partner. RBD is characterized as a parasomnia, which can be subcategorized into REM, non-REM, and wake disorders.[2] In addition to RBD, two other REM parasomnias exist—nightmares and recurrent isolated sleep paralysis.

EPIDEMIOLOGY

Per the latest Diagnostic and Statistical Manual of Mental Disorders (DSM-V), the prevalence of RBD is reported in the range of approximately 0.5% of the general population, although this number can be significantly higher as many cases can go unrecognized.[3] Its prevalence is also higher in the older adult population, totaling nearly 2%, with a predilection toward males. The distribution of the disease, however, is not homogenous amongst the population and can be seen in higher proportions in those with comorbid psychiatric illnesses, thought to be related to prescribed medications to treat said psychiatric conditions. This is especially true in those aged 40 years or below. In the older adult population, RBD is most commonly viewed as a prodromal event in alpha-synuclein neuropathology as the disease is comorbid with Parkinson's disease (PD), multiple system atrophy (MSA), and Lewy body dementia (DLB).[4]

PATHOGENESIS

From a physiologic perspective, muscle atonia during REM sleep is an adaptive measure as it prevents individuals from acting out their dreams, thus preventing injurious behavior to both self and the bed partner. There is also some data to suggest the near-absent motor function during REM sleep is a key component in memory consolidation.[5]

The neurologic pathway for normal REM sleep originates in the pons and follows multiple neuronal circuits which ultimately terminate in the spinal cord motor neurons, which in turn innervate the skeletal muscles. The exact location of neuronal dysfunction culminating in RBD is unknown, but evidence suggests that it originates in the subcoeruleus complex in the rostral pons, irrespective of the underlying etiology as this is the part of the brain responsible for paralysis during REM sleep.[6] In animal studies, cats who have had brainstem lesions in the locus coeruleus display normal NREM sleep with impaired REM sleep where they are viewed walking around chasing figures which are not present, believed to be dream enactment.[7] In cases where RBD is associated with narcolepsy, an orexin deficiency is believed to instigate wake, REM and non-REM instability resulting in frequent transitioning between states.

ETIOLOGY

- *Alpha-synuclein neurodegeneration:* Alpha-synuclein pathology is the most common cause of RBD, especially in the absence of an underlying neurodegenerative comorbidity or inciting psychiatric medication. It is the presumed cause for almost all isolated cases of RBD. Given the normal neuronal pathways controlling REM sleep and muscle atonia, the pathogenesis of alpha synucleinopathies involves degeneration of pontine and medullary nuclei which are implicated in REM sleep.[8] It often predates the declaration of a neurodegenerative disorder such as Parkinson's disease (PD), multiple system atrophy (MSA), and dementia with Lewy bodies (DLB) outright. There is large variability between the onset of RBD and manifestation of neurodegenerative disease, and not all cases of RBD will phenotypically convert per se. In one large multicenter study, the annual conversion rate in 1,000 RBD patients to outright neurodegenerative disorder was found to be 6%, with a total of 74% of patients converting within 12 years of diagnosis.[9] Amongst the remainder of patients who did not progress, diffuse Lewy body disease was still seen on postmortem analysis indicating underlying and advanced alpha-synucleinopathy.[9]

- *Nonsynuclein disorders*: Nonsynuclein disorders, which include neurodegenerative diseases such as Alzheimer's, progressive supranuclear palsy, amyotrophic lateral sclerosis, frontotemporal dementia, spinocerebellar ataxia, Huntington disease, and myotonic dystrophy, may present comorbid with RBD. Similar to alpha-synucleinopathies, there appears to be a link between these neurodegenerative diseases and some level of pontine pathology. There is also some data to suggest that even in nonsynuclein disorders, some level of alpha-synuclein pathology exists and this can be evident on postmortem analysis.[8] Clinically, the progression compared to alpha-synuclein disorders differs in that the neurologic deficits predate RBD in those with non-synuclein pathology.
- *Narcolepsy and orexin deficiency*: Perhaps, the most pathologically distinct group of RBD is seen in narcolepsy as the exact mechanism of RBD in these patients is related to orexin deficiency as opposed to direct pontine pathology. Orexin plays a key role in mediating wake, REM and non-REM stability, and its absence causes instability between these phases resulting in daytime sleepiness, sleep fragmentation, sleep paralysis, cataplexy, and hallucinations.[10] There is an absence of alpha-synuclein biomarkers in this group of patients, and they do not have increased risk of neurodegeneration.
- *Others:* Any pontine lesion, whether traumatic or atraumatic, can manifest as RBD. In cases with suspected pontine damage, neuroimaging such as magnetic resonance imaging (MRI) can help determine the location of the lesion and support pontine damage as the etiology to RBD. Encephalitis, usually associated with *Caspr2* and *LGI1*, have also been implicated in the development of RBD, likely owing to some level of pontine dysfunction.[11] Perhaps most prominently associated with RBD is medication-induced RBD. Typically, any serotonergic modulating agent can be implicated in the development of RBD, and this is the most common form of RBD seen in young adults aged under 40 years.[12] The mechanism is believed to be due to serotonergic nuclei in the pons having an activating effect on REM-off nuclei, wherein excess serotonergic output can result in dream enactment. Given that this phenomenon is not seen in all individuals who initiate these medications, there may also be a link between medication associated-RBD as a prognostic marker of the development of alpha-synuclein pathology.

CLINICAL FEATURES

The clinical hallmark of RBD is the presence of dream enactment behaviors, which presents as a large spectrum of activity ranging from simple vocalizations to violent thrashing resulting in harm to self and/or the bed partner.[13] The actions are short lasting (typically <60 seconds) and purposeful, such as throwing a punch or winding up to throw a baseball. The patient is not always aware of these actions, and in one cohort study nearly half of the patients were unaware that they were enacting their dreams.[13] Nearly all patients in this cohort reported vocalizations, and a majority (over 80%) reported physical enactments of their dreams. Symptoms will most commonly manifest during the second half of the sleep cycle, where REM sleep is predominant. Symptoms can manifest as frequently as nightly to as infrequently as annually, owing to the heterogeneity of the disease.

Symptoms often do not present until late adulthood, typically in the sixth and seventh decades of life.[14] Diagnosis will often be delayed by several years, as patients will not seek care or workup until an injurious behavior has happened. Beyond dream enactment, patients will also display findings consistent with early neurodegeneration given the predominant etiology of the disease lies in alpha-synuclein pathology. In cases where RBD is related to PD or DLB, gait abnormalities, postural instabilities, dysarthria, limb bradykinesia and progressive cognitive decline. In patients with known alpha-synucleinopathy (i.e., PD or DLB), comorbid RBD is often associated with a rapid decline in mental faculties, resistance to treatment, and more widespread neurologic dysfunction compared to those without comorbid RBD.[9]

DIAGNOSIS

The international classification of sleep disorders (ICSD3) lists four criteria for RBD:[2]

1. Repeated episodes of sleep-related vocal and/or complex motor behaviors
2. Sleep-related behaviors are recorded during polysomnography (PSG) as happening during REM sleep
3. PSG demonstrates REM sleep without atonia (RSWA)
4. The sleep disturbance is not explained by another sleep disorder, mental disorder, or medication or substance abuse

Polysomnography is the key diagnostic test in RBD, and should be pursued in patients who have a history of dream enactment behavior **(Figs. 1A and B)**. PSG is necessary to confirm the diagnosis of RBD, as well as ruling out other sleep disorders which may mimic RBD. RSWA is the key finding in those with suspected RBD. RSWA has little night-to-night

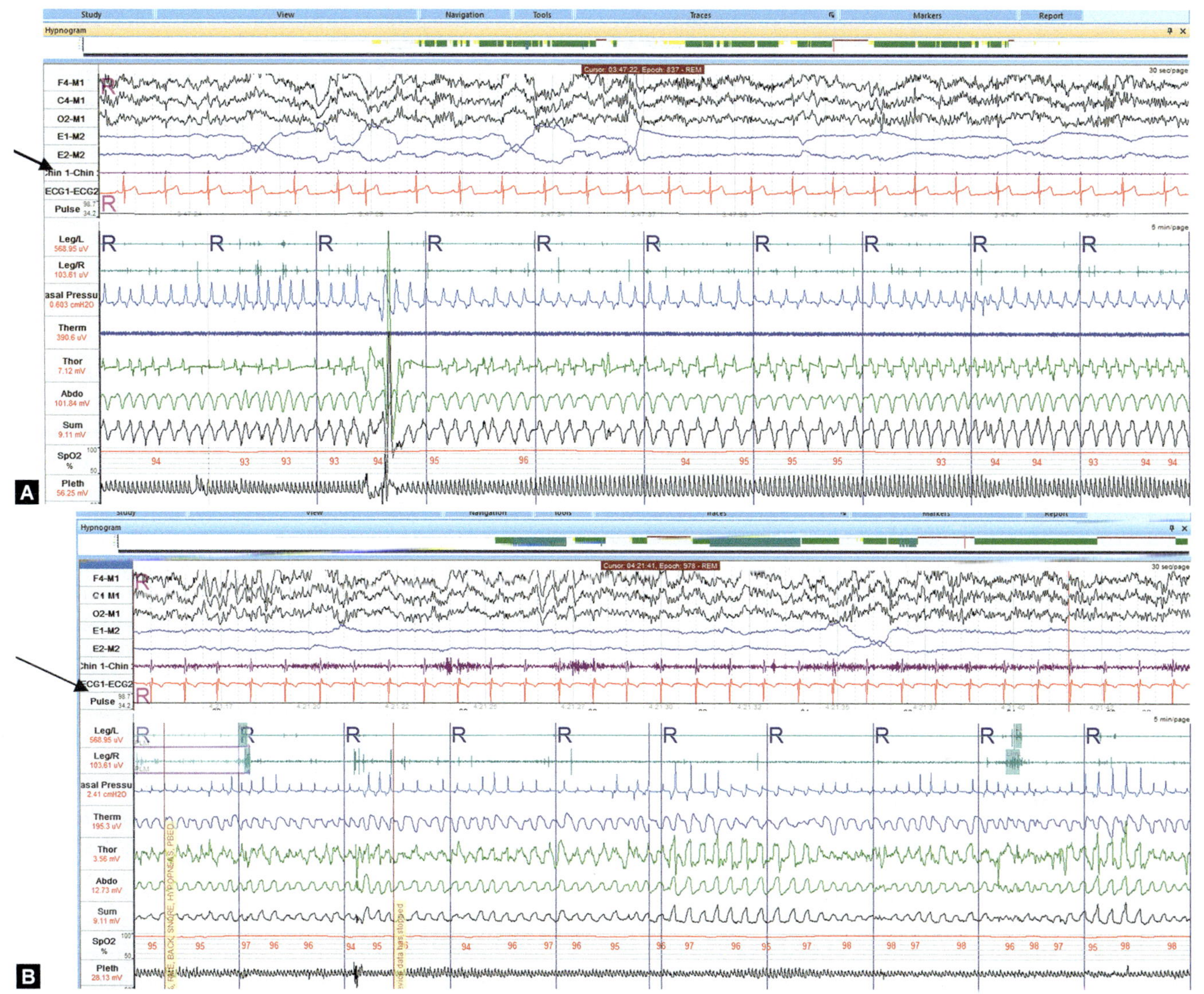

FIGS. 1A AND B: (A) Normal PSG with evidence of atonia as evidenced by lack of EMG activity during REM sleep (black arrow) versus RSWA; (B) PSG displaying excessive muscle tone during REM sleep (black arrow).

(EMG: electromyography; PSG: polysomnography; REM: rapid eye movement; RSWA: REM sleep without atonia)

variability, and therefore can reliably be used in testing for RBD.[15]

The American Academy of Sleep Medicine (AASM) defines RSWA as a 30-second epoch of REM sleep when any of the following are present:[16]

- Excessive sustained muscle activity (tonic activity) in the chin EMG. Excessive sustained activity exists when chin amplitude is at least two times greater than the stage R atonia level (or the minimum amplitude during NREM sleep if no stage R atonia is present) for at least half of the epoch
- Excessive transient muscle activity (phasic activity) in the chin or limb EMG. Excessive transient activity exists when amplitude is at least two times higher than the stage R atonia level (or lowest amplitude in NREM, if no stage R atonia is present) during 0.1–5.0-second bursts in at least 5 of 10 3-second mini-epochs
- At least half of 3-second mini-epochs contain any chin activity with amplitude at least two times greater than the stage R atonia level (or lowest amplitude in NREM, if no stage R atonia is present), without regard to the duration of the activity (including bursts of 5–15 seconds)
- At least half of 3-second mini-epochs contain limb activity, defined as bursts of EMG activity 0.1–5 seconds in duration and at least two times as high in amplitude as the stage R atonia level (or lowest amplitude in NREM, if no stage R atonia is present)

While PSG is required in the diagnosis of RBD, multiple screening tools including questionnaires have been created to screen for the condition. Several questionnaires, including the Hong Kong questionnaire, Mayo Sleep questionnaire, and Innsbruck RBD Inventory, have been developed as possible screening tools for RBD.[17] While not all of these questionnaires exclusively rule in or out RBD, they can be used as a risk stratification tool in the appropriate setting. Caution must be taken, however, as the false-negative and false-positive rates in these questionnaires can be as high as 16%, most often seen in cases where the questionnaires are completed without the presence of the bed partner.[17]

While data is limited, the use of artificial intelligence and machine algorithms has emerged as a potential screening tool for RBD. This is of particular interest as RBD can be the herald of neurodegenerative disease, and early identification can assist in the establishment of care and potential reduction in mortality and morbidity in this patient population.

In one study using the Cyclic Alternating Pattern (CAP) Sleep Database, a machine algorithm was created to increase the detection of RWSA and RBD in patients undergoing PSG. This was subsequently compared to a private database (the TURIN database) as a measure of robustness and reproducibility.[18] The key value used in this determination was the REM atonia index (RAI), a value which ranges from 0 to 1 and machine calculated to assess the level of muscle atonia at the submental EMG. Values below 0.8 are strongly indicative of altered muscle atonia, while values greater than 0.9 are normal. Values between 0.8 and 0.9 suggest slightly altered atonia. Within this data set, healthy subjects on average have an RAI of 0.93 ±0.14, whereas RBD subjects have an average RAI of 0.44 ±0.37. While the baseline RAI is significantly lower in the RBD group, there is a larger amount of intragroup variability supporting the notion that the dissociation of REM sleep is diverse and occurs heterogeneously in the RBD population.[18]

Given the robustness of available PSG data, artificial intelligence can also potentially serve as a powerful tool for data analysis in this population. This is of particular importance as the rise in use of antidepressant medication has complicated RBD diagnosis as it pertains to predicting neurodegeneration given that these medications increase muscle tone during REM sleep. There have been computer-designed algorithms to assist in this distinction between alpha-synucleinopathy RBD and medication induced; however, they are not widely used in clinical practice.[19] The goal is for this technology to eventually identify which patients with RBD have a predilection for neurodegeneration and benefit from neuroprotective agents.

DIFFERENTIAL DIAGNOSIS

REM behavior sleep disorder is characterized as a REM parasomnia. REM parasomnias themselves can be subcategorized into one of three groups—RBD, nightmares and recurrent isolated sleep paralysis. RBD is typically easily separated from its REM parasomnia counterparts given that recurrent isolated sleep paralysis is an event that occurs during the wake period, and nightmares typically do not have a motor component associated with them.[2]

In addition to REM parasomnias, there exists a spectrum of non-REM parasomnias, which must be distinguished from RBD. Non-REM parasomnias include confusional arousals, sleep walking, sleep terrors, and sleep-related eating disorders. They typically occur in childhood, although sleepwalking can persist into adulthood and may also be a prognosticator of neurodegeneration.[20] In contrast to RBD, these typically manifest in the earlier portions of the sleep cycle, most often in the first third and during N3 sleep. N3 sleep time naturally declines with age; hence, the increased incidence in childhood, although in sleep deprivation N3 sleep is increased and this may trigger a non-REM parasomnia. PSG can easily distinguish RBD from non-REM parasomnias, given this distinction—by definition—RBD must occur during REM sleep whereas the non-REM parasomnias will not.[21]

Despite the physiologic and diagnostic distinctions between RBD and non-REM parasomnias, there exists a phenomenon known as overlap parasomnia where RBD can coexist with a non-REM parasomnia.[22] Again, this often manifests earlier in age and many times will be comorbid with concurrent psychiatric illness or narcolepsy.

While not a parasomnia per se, obstructive sleep apnea (OSA) must also be ruled out as part of the work up for RBD. Patients with severe sleep apnea may have behaviors which mimic RBD, likely owing to fragmented sleep as a consequence of untreated OSA. This will resolve with treatment of the underlying sleep apnea. OSA itself can be diagnosed via PSG, which will be required as part of the workup of RBD.

MANAGEMENT

Management of RBD can be divided into nonpharmacologic and pharmacologic therapies. Most often, patients will start with nonpharmacologic therapies, although some will require a combination of both modalities for optimal therapy. No large clinical trials or placebo-controlled trials exist, and recommendations are based on case series and small uncontrolled trials. It is important to note that all recommendations are considered "conditional" by the AASM, and no "strong" recommendations exist.[23] "Strong" recommendations are ones that should be followed for all patients, whereas "conditional" ones have a lower degree of certainty in regards to benefit across the entire patient population.

- *Nonpharmacologic therapies*: In patients where there is believed to be a drug-induced form of RBD, as seen in those on antidepressant class of medications, the first option that exists is to stop the offending medication. In cases where this is not feasible or poses a greater harm to the patient in stopping the medication, management can be catered to symptom severity. Modification of the sleep environment may often be the only intervention required in patients who display mild symptoms and are at low risk for harm to themselves or their bed partner. In cases where injurious behavior has occurred, sleeping alone is recommended so as to protect the bed partner. Any harmful objects should also be removed from the immediate sleeping area and patients may need to resort to using padded bed rails or sleeping in sleeping bags to limit harm. Other novel therapies are currently in development, including the use of bed alarms with customized messages which will play in instances where the dream enactment behavior occurs to prevent the patient from getting out of bed.[24]

- *Pharmacologic therapies:* The AASM has conditional recommendations for several pharmacotherapies in instances where nonpharmacologic therapies fail or are not feasible. This is particularly the case in patients with evidence of injurious behavior either to themselves or the bed partner. Clonazepam, melatonin, pramipexole, and rivastigmine all have conditional recommendations for use in RBD by the AASM.[25] The only condition against recommendation was for the use of deep brain stimulation (DBS). Given the lower side effect profile, fewer medication interactions, ease of access, and tolerability, melatonin is often given as first-line therapy, although clonazepam is a suitable alternative. While melatonin's mechanism of action in treating RBD is unclear, the proposed benefit is believed to be due to its known actions on stabilizing circadian rhythm variability, increasing sleep efficiency, and promoting REM sleep atonia.[26]

Similar to melatonin, the exact mechanism of action for clonazepam is unclear, but may be due to its effect on serotonergic modulation.[27] In the elderly population, there is an associated increased risk in falls and confusion with clonazepam and melatonin would be a safer alternative. Cholinergic agents also reduce the frequency of RBD behaviors, and may be especially efficacious in patients with comorbid dementia such as those with Alzheimer's, mild cognitive impairment, or even PD and DLB. The mechanism of action with cholinergic agents is believed to be related to cholinergic neurons in the pedunculopontine nuclei and their role in producing REM sleep and the associated atonia of REM sleep.[25] Per the latest AASM guidelines, the variability in pharmacotherapy may lay in the different phenotypic variants of RBD and future directions may benefit from the development of studies assessing optimal pharmacotherapy as a function of the phenotype.[1,23,25]

PROGNOSIS

The largest concern with RBD is the progression to a neurodegenerative disorder, specifically an alpha-synucleinopathy. As previously mentioned, RBD has a strong association with PD, MSA, and DLB, and RBD often predates the presentation of these neurodegenerative disorders outright.[28] The opposite is also true, and RBD can be unmasked in the workup of a neurodegenerative disorder itself. Despite this association, no single test exists with sufficient sensitivity and specificity to promote routine clinical use as a screening device for patients diagnosed with RBD.[29] While a diagnosis of RBD does not guarantee progression to a neurodegenerative disorder, open discussions between physician and patient should be had and keen detail to the development of psychomotor symptoms should be paid attention to.[30]

SUMMARY

Rapid eye movement behavior sleep disorder, reported in approximately 0.5% of the general population, is characterized with a loss of REM sleep atonia and dream enactment, which can range from benign gestures to violent thrashing. Other REM parasomnias such as nightmares and recurrent isolated sleep paralysis may also be present. RBD may manifest with presence of dream enactment behaviors with a large spectrum of activities which are typically short lasting and purposeful. RBD may progress to a neurodegenerative disorder, specifically an alpha-synucleinopathy and may often predate the presentation of these neurodegenerative disorders. Modification of the sleep environment may often help patients with mild symptoms and are at low risk for harm to themselves or their bed partner. In cases where injurious behavior has occurred, sleeping alone is recommended so as to protect the bed partner. Any harmful objects should also be removed from the immediate sleeping area and patients may need to resort to using padded bed rails or sleeping in sleeping bags to limit harm. Novel therapies are currently in development especially to prevent harm to the sleep partner.

REFERENCES

1. Berry RB, Quan SF, Abreu AR, et al.; American Academy of Sleep Medicine. The AASM Manual for the Scoring of Sleep and Associated Events: Rules, Terminology and Technical Specifications, Version 2.6. Darien, IL: American Academy of Sleep Medicine; 2020.
2. Sateia MJ. International classification of sleep disorders-third edition: highlights and modifications. Chest. 2014;146(5): 1387-94.
3. American Psychiatric Association. Diagnostic and statistical manual of mental disorders (5th ed.). Indian J Psychiatry. 2013; 55(3):220-3.
4. Miglis MG, Adler CH, Antelmi E, et al. Biomarkers of conversion to α-synucleinopathy in isolated rapid-eye-movement sleep behaviour disorder. Lancet Neurol. 2021;20(8):671-84.
5. Rasch B, Born J. About sleep's role in memory. Physiol Rev. 2013;93(2):681-766.

6. Figorilli M, Lanza G, Congiu P, et al. Neurophysiological Aspects of REM Sleep Behavior Disorder (RBD): A Narrative Review. Brain Sci. 2021;11(12):1588.
7. Mahowald MW, Schenck CH. Rem sleep without atonia–from cats to humans. Arch Ital Biol. 2004;142(4):469-78.
8. Boeve BF. REM sleep behavior disorder: Updated review of the core features, the REM sleep behavior disorder-neurodegenerative disease association, evolving concepts, controversies, and future directions. Ann NY Acad Sci. 2010;1184:15-54.
9. Postuma RB, Iranzo A, Hu M, et al. Risk and predictors of dementia and parkinsonism in idiopathic REM sleep behaviour disorder: a multicentre study. Brain. 2019;142(3):744-59.
10. Nevsimalova S, Pisko J, Buskova J, et al. Narcolepsy: clinical differences and association with other sleep disorders in different age groups. J Neurol. 2013;260(3):767-75.
11. Sabater L, Gaig C, Gelpi E, et al. A novel non-rapid-eye movement and rapid-eye-movement parasomnia with sleep breathing disorder associated with antibodies to IgLON5: a case series, characterisation of the antigen, and post-mortem study. Lancet Neurol. 2014;13(6):575-86.
12. Teman PT, Tippmann-Peikert M, Silber MH, et al. Idiopathic rapid-eye-movement sleep disorder: associations with antidepressants, psychiatric diagnoses, and other factors, in relation to age of onset. Sleep Med. 2009;10(1):60-5.
13. Fernández-Arcos A, Iranzo A, Serradell M, et al. The Clinical Phenotype of Idiopathic Rapid Eye Movement Sleep Behavior Disorder at Presentation: A Study in 203 Consecutive Patients. Sleep. 2016;39(1):121-32.
14. Olson EJ, Boeve BF, Silber MH. Rapid eye movement sleep behaviour disorder: demographic, clinical and laboratory findings in 93 cases. Brain. 2000;123(Pt 2):331-9.
15. Högl B, Stefani A. REM sleep behavior disorder (RBD): Update on diagnosis and treatment. Somnologie (Berl). 2017;21(Suppl 1): 1-8.
16. Cesari M, Heidbreder A, St Louis EK, et al. Video-polysomnography procedures for diagnosis of rapid eye movement sleep behavior disorder (RBD) and the identification of its prodromal stages: guidelines from the International RBD Study Group. Sleep. 2022;14;45(3).
17. Boeve BF, Molano JR, Ferman TJ, et al. Validation of the Mayo Sleep Questionnaire to screen for REM sleep behavior disorder in a community-based sample. J Clin Sleep Med. 2013;9(5):475-80.
18. Rechichi I, Iadarola A, Zibetti M, et al. Assessing REM Sleep Behaviour Disorder: From Machine Learning Classification to the Definition of a Continuous Dissociation Index. Int J Environ Res Public Health. 2021;19(1):248.
19. Goldstein CA, Berry RB, Kent DT, et al. Artificial intelligence in sleep medicine: background and implications for clinicians. J Clin Sleep Med. 2020;16(4):609-18.
20. Irfan M, Schenck CH, Howell MJ. NonREM Disorders of Arousal and Related Parasomnias: an Updated Review. Neurotherapeutics. 2021;18(1):124-39.
21. Castelnovo A, Lopez R, Proserpio P, et al. NREM sleep parasomnias as disorders of sleep-state dissociation. Nat Rev Neurol. 2018;14(8):470-81.
22. Schenck CH, Howell MJ. Spectrum of rapid eye movement sleep behavior disorder (overlap between rapid eye movement sleep behavior disorder and other parasomnias). Sleep Biol Rhythm. 2013;11:27-34.
23. Howell M, Avidan AY, Foldvary-Schaefer N, et al. Management of REM sleep behavior disorder: An American Academy of Sleep Medicine systematic review, meta-analysis, and GRADE assessment. J Clin Sleep Med. 2023;19(4):769-810.
24. Howell MJ, Arneson PA, Schenck CH. A novel therapy for REM sleep behavior disorder (RBD). J Clin Sleep Med. 2011;7(6): 639-44A.
25. Howell M, Avidan AY, Foldvary-Schaefer N, et al. Management of REM sleep behavior disorder: an American Academy of Sleep Medicine clinical practice guideline. J Clin Sleep Med. 2023;19(4):759-68.
26. McGrane IR, Leung JG, St Louis EK, et al. Melatonin therapy for REM sleep behavior disorder: a critical review of evidence. Sleep Med. 2015;16(1):19-26.
27. Aurora RN, Zak RS, Maganti RK, et al. Best practice guide for the treatment of REM sleep behavior disorder (RBD). J Clin Sleep Med. 2010;6(1):85-95.
28. Schenck CH, Boeve BF, Mahowald MW. Delayed emergence of a parkinsonian disorder or dementia in 81% of older men initially diagnosed with idiopathic rapid eye movement sleep behavior disorder: a 16-year update on a previously reported series. Sleep Med. 2013;14(8):744-8.
29. Wang C, Chen F, Li Y, et al. Possible predictors of phenoconversion in isolated REM sleep behaviour disorder: a systematic review and meta-analysis. J Neurol Neurosurg Psychiatry. 2022;93: 395-403.
30. Teigen LN, Sharp RR, Hirsch JR, et al. Specialist approaches to prognostic counseling in isolated REM sleep behavior disorder. Sleep Med. 2021;79:107-12.

CHAPTER 147

Insomnia

Eby Thekkedath, Margarita Oks

INTRODUCTION

Insomnia is a common sleep disorder characterized with difficulty in falling or staying asleep. The International Classification of Sleep Disorders (ICSD) defines insomnia as a persistent difficulty with sleep initiation, duration, or consolidation that occurs despite adequate opportunity and circumstances for sleep and results in concern, dissatisfaction, or perceived daytime impairment, such as fatigue, decreased mood or irritability, general malaise, or cognitive impairment.[1]

CLASSIFICATIONS

The insomnia nosology presented in the 3rd edition of the ICSD is markedly different from prior definitions. Previous iterations have classified insomnia based on presumed pathophysiology and duration. Historically, insomnia has been classified as primary or secondary (or comorbid). ICSD 1 and ICSD-2 had further subtyped primary insomnia as psychophysiological, idiopathic, and paradoxical.[2] However, the diagnostic reliability and validity of primary insomnia and its subtypes have been challenged in recent years on the basis of several studies warranting the reclassification of insomnia disorders in the most recent ICSD-3 guidelines. The current classification of insomnia falls into three broad categories: Chronic insomnia disorder, short-term insomnia disorder, and other insomnia disorders.

Chronic Insomnia Disorder

Chronic insomnia disorder is defined as a report of sleep initiation or maintenance problems, adequate opportunity and circumstances to sleep, and daytime consequences. The frequency and duration criterion for chronic insomnia disorder is at least 3 days per week for at least 3 months.

Short-term Insomnia Disorder

Short-term insomnia disorder is also referred to as acute insomnia or adjustment insomnia, and it is defined by symptoms like chronic insomnia but are present for less than 3 months. Short-term insomnia is often linked to an identifiable stressor. These stressors can be physical, psychological, psychosocial, or interpersonal. Symptoms of short-term insomnia disorder are temporary and often resolve once the identified stressor is eliminated or resolved; however, some patients progress to developing chronic insomnia disorder.

Other Insomnia Disorders

Fatal familial insomnia (FFI) is a rare autosomal-dominant condition characterized by a missense mutation at codon 178 of the *PRNP* gene located on chromosome 20p13 coupled with methionine at codon 129 on the mutated allele. The pathophysiology of FFI is thought to be secondary to neuronal loss and gliosis most pronounced in the thalamus but often with involvement of other brain regions. Symptoms of insomnia in addition to other neuropsychiatric symptoms often develop during midlife and continue to progress as patients age with no known cure or effective treatment currently.[3]

EPIDEMIOLOGY AND ETIOLOGY

Prevalence

The exact prevalence of insomnia is difficult to quantify as numerous studies over the years have examined this but often with differing diagnostic criteria. When using Diagnostic and Statistical Manual of Mental Disorders (DSM) or ICSD criteria, prevalence rates are estimated to be between 6 and 10% in the general population. When looking at general population data, at least one third of patients report one nocturnal insomnia symptom (difficulty initiating or maintaining sleep, nonrestorative sleep), but this rate falls to 10–15% when daytime effects are added to the definition. Insomnia is a chronic problem in 31–75% of patients. The lack of concrete and consistent data on the prevalence of insomnia in the population underscores the necessity for more standardized diagnostic criteria.[4]

Risk Factors

Risk factors associated with developing insomnia include demographic factors such as female sex and older age as well as a personal or familial history of insomnia. Women tend to have a higher risk, particularly during and after menopause, and this has been attributed to hormonal changes. Psychological and biological factors have also been shown to play a role. Specifically, patients with an anxiety disorder and those with increased hypothalamic-pituitary-axis (HPA) activity have been shown to have increased risk.[5]

Comorbidities

Insomnia has been associated with a host of comorbid conditions from psychological to cardiovascular consequences. Cross sectional studies have demonstrated that patients with insomnia have higher rates of hypertension and diabetes as well as metabolic syndrome compared to those without. There is also evidence that insomnia is an independent risk factor for future cardiac events such as acute myocardial infarction and coronary artery disease even in patients with no history of cardiovascular disease.[4,5] However, results from other studies with shorter time frames and additional variables have not corroborated these findings.[4,5]

Insomnia in the South Asian Population

Insomnia is a common yet often neglected problem, especially in the Indian population. In one study examining elderly primary care patients, clinical insomnia was detected in 11.8% of patients with subclinical insomnia detected in 30.4% of patients.[6] In another review of the global Indian population, the prevalence of insomnia varied widely from 18% to more than 50% with higher rates seen in patients with comorbidities such as diabetes and chronic kidney disease. Rates were also significantly higher in patients with underlying psychiatric conditions with the most common being depression and anxiety.[7,8]

SIGNS AND SYMPTOMS

All patients diagnosed with an insomnia disorder have two features: Difficulty initiating or maintaining sleep and daytime consequences secondary to poor quality or duration of sleep. It is important to understand that many patients with insomnia may have comorbidities and/or be on medications that may impact the quality and duration of their sleep, but this does not preclude them from a diagnosis of insomnia disorder.

Difficulty Initiating or Maintaining Sleep

Patients with clinically diagnosed insomnia often complain of difficulty initiating or maintaining sleep and/or early awakenings despite having adequate opportunity and circumstances. This is an important distinction as patients with sleep deprivation do not have the opportunity or circumstances for adequate sleep. Patients' sleep patterns may be variable with several nights of poor-quality or duration of sleep followed by one or two nights of improved sleep. The time to sleep onset in healthy individuals is usually within 30 minutes and often within 20 minutes. In contrast, patients with insomnia report taking longer than 30 minutes for sleep initiation. Patients who have issues with sleep maintenance also have prolonged periods of nighttime awakening that last longer than 30 minutes. Similarly, many patients also report early morning awakening, which is defined as the termination of sleep 30 minutes before the desired wake-up time. These symptoms on their own or in combination are the most common symptoms reported by patients with insomnia disorder.

The second feature necessary for diagnosis of an insomnia disorder is compromised daytime function secondary to poor-quality sleep. Patients with chronic insomnia often develop psychological and behavioral adaptations that can worsen their symptoms. Patients frequently report that they may worry about the effect their poor sleep has on their professional and personal lives. This increased distress, especially during scheduled hours of sleep, may worsen their ability to fall and stay asleep leading to a vicious cycle that can worsen their insomnia.[1]

PATHOPHYSIOLOGY

Genetic Factors

Regulation of the sleep-wake cycle, such as sleep duration and timing, has been shown to be heritable and regulated by numerous genes. Genes linked to cognitive functioning, arousal regulation, and sleep-wake processes have been most consistently found to be associated with insomnia.[9] The circadian rhythms are modulated endogenously by clock-related genes such as *Per1* and *Per2* (and, to a lesser degree, *Per3*) and externally by external cues such as light, food, and temperature. The *Per* genes, part of the Period family of genes, is primarily expressed in the central nervous system (CNS) including the suprachiasmatic nuclei (SCN), the primary circadian pacemaker.[10] The various interactions of these genes and their variable expression may, in part, be responsible for the heterogeneity seen in insomnia symptoms and severity.

Sleep–Wake Regulation

At a global level, sleep is regulated by the interactions between both the wake and sleep brain networks. The two-process model of sleep regulation has been used to describe the delicate balance between sleep-wake regulation. According to the two-process model, sleep propensity is regulated by the interactions of the wake-dependent process (Process S) and relatively wake-independent circadian process (Process C). Process S dictates that greater brain activity during wakefulness promotes sleep need. In addition, accumulation of extracellular adenosine during wakefulness has been theorized to be a homeostatic accumulator of the need for sleep. Process C, governed by the circadian rhythm, is regulated by intrinsic circadian oscillations governed by the SCN of the hypothalamus. Process C can be influenced by external factors such as exogenous light, melatonin, and social factors. Optimal sleep is hypothesized to be achieved by a coordinated balance between both processes.[9]

Theories for Insomnia

At a neural level, sleep onset is driven by activation of GABAergic and galanin neurons in the ventrolateral preoptic area (VLPO) and median preoptic area (MnPO), with accumulated adenosine being the primary input into these systems. During initiation of normal sleep, arousal systems are downregulated by inhibition from the VLPO and MnPO. One of the more widely accepted theories is that insomnia is a disorder of excessive activation of the arousal systems of the brain (hyperarousal). Hyperarousal of physiologic, emotional, and cognitive networks is believed to dysregulate the natural sleep–wake cycle in patients with insomnia. However, there is data to suggest that hyperarousal alone is insufficient for the development of chronic insomnia. Future studies examining the complex interplay between the sleep–wake cycle may provide more insight on the pathophysiology behind insomnia.[9]

EVALUATION AND DIAGNOSIS

Laboratory Workup

Routine laboratory workup is not necessary for the evaluation and diagnosis of insomnia. It may be indicated when assessing for comorbidities that may be contributing to insomnia symptoms.[11]

Sleep Logs/Diary

Sleep logs and sleep diaries are usually the first step in evaluating insomnia. Providers should ask patients to record sleep times, duration of sleep, and subjective sleep quality. Detailed descriptions of the sleep problem such as duration until sleep initiation, number of awakenings, durations of awakenings, and daytime consequences have been recommended.[12] However, some argue that encouraging patients to be more cognizant of their sleeping difficulties may cause them to be more anxious and worried which in turn can worsen their symptoms.[13] Sleep logs/diaries that examine sleep behavior over a short period of time (1–2 weeks) may provide valuable insight into any contributing/reversible factors such as poor sleep hygiene and use of stimulants.[14]

Actigraphy

Actigraphy is a noninvasive method that records and integrates the occurrence and degree of limb movement activity over the course of several days to several weeks. It is normally worn like a watch on the nondominant hand but can also be worn on the ankle or waist.[15] Actigraphy is not routinely indicated in the evaluation of chronic insomnia. However, it is useful when objective measurements of sleep parameters are important in clinical decision-making, particularly in patients not responsive to cognitive behavioral therapy or for patients requesting escalating doses of medication to treat their insomnia. It is less invasive than attended polysomnography and provides similar clinical data.[16]

Polysomnography

Polysomnography is only indicated in the evaluation and management of insomnia if another comorbid sleep disorder such as sleep apnea is suspected. Patients with chronic, treatment-refractory insomnia and daytime sleepiness should be evaluated for another sleep disorder. In these patients, the prevalence of sleep apnea may be as high as 90%.[16] However, PSG may play a role in the diagnosis of paradoxical insomnia. Paradoxical insomnia, previously called sleep state misperception, is a phenomenon characterized by a complaint of severe insomnia disproportional to the presence of objective sleep disturbance or daytime impairment. PSG has played a role in the diagnostic criteria for paradoxical insomnia including a difference from self-report of 60 minutes or more for total sleep time or a difference of at least 15% for sleep efficiency,[17] and Turcotte et al. suggested that an individual could be diagnosed with paradoxical insomnia if they meet both of these criteria on two of four nights.[18] Paradoxical insomnia is a controversial topic as it was previously diagnosed as a subset of insomnia in the ICSD-2 criteria but was removed due to lack of robust evidence in distinguishing it from a chronic insomnia disorder. Further research is warranted to clarify the pathophysiology of paradoxical insomnia as a subset of insomnia.

Artificial Intelligence

There is increasing evidence that supports the use of artificial intelligence (AI) technology in the diagnosis and even management of insomnia. Particularly, machine-learning algorithms have been shown to accurately predict sleep disorders with both sensitivity and specificity > 75%.[19] In addition, the use of these machine-learning algorithms has been shown to classify sleep stages in PSG data with accuracy comparable to human interrater variability.[20] The use of AI and machine learning in the identification, classification, and interpretation of sleep studies and disorders will only continue to grow over the coming decade.

Diagnostic Criteria

According to the third edition of the ICSD, the diagnosis of insomnia is confirmed when all four of the following criteria are met:[1]

1. The patient reports difficulty initiating asleep, difficulty maintaining sleep, or waking up too early. In children or individuals with dementia, sleep disturbances may manifest as resistance to going to bed at the appropriate time or difficulty in sleeping without caregiver assistance.
2. Sleep difficulties occur despite adequate opportunity and circumstances for sleep.
3. The patient describes daytime impairment that is attributable to sleep difficulties. This may include fatigue or malaise; attention, concentration, or memory impairment; social dysfunction, vocational dysfunction, or poor school performance; mood disturbance or irritability; daytime sleepiness; motivation, energy, or initiative reduction; errors or accidents at work or while driving; and concerns or worries about sleep.
4. The sleep-wake difficulty is not better explained by another sleep disorder.

MANAGEMENT

Nonpharmacologic

Sleep Hygiene

Most patients that complain of poor quality or inadequate sleep have unhealthy sleep habits. Often, proper sleep hygiene can improve and resolve insomnia in most people. Optimal sleep hygiene includes having a regular bedtime and rise time and having a consistent bedtime and wake-up time allowing for a more regular sleep schedule. Naps should be avoided, particularly for longer than 1 hour or later in the day, as they may make it more difficult to fall asleep at night. Limiting caffeine intake and avoidance of caffeine intake after lunch allow for two half-lives of caffeine to be metabolized prior to bedtime. Avoiding alcohol near bedtime is important as it is sedating at first but is activating as it becomes metabolized. In addition, alcohol has been shown to lead to poor quality of sleep due to its effects on sleep architecture. Similarly, nicotine should be avoided near bedtime as it also acts as a stimulant. Daytime physical exercise 4–6 hours can promote sleep onset, but rigorous exercise should be avoided 2 hours prior to bedtime due to its awakening effect. Maintaining a sleep environment that is dark and quiet while also avoiding screen time before bed has been shown to improve sleep onset. It is also recommended to not have a television or entertainment devices in the bedroom. This is because the brain needs to maintain the psychological association of the bedroom as a place of sleep and rest. Building on this association, patients who wake up in the middle of the night and are unable to fall back asleep within 20 minutes should leave the bedroom and only partake in lightly stimulating activities (reading, meditation, listening to music) until they are sleepy again. Use of white noise, ear plugs, blackout shades, and eye masks is also recommended as adjuncts to promote sleep onset and maintenance in the bedroom. Patients should also avoid checking the time during hours of sleep, especially on devices such as a smart phone as this increases cognitive arousal. Finally, patients should avoid eating large meals close to bedtime as well as late-night snacks.[21] Many of the components of sleep hygiene are addressed in various insomnia treatment methods such as cognitive behavioral therapy for insomnia (CBT-I), sleep restriction therapy, and stimulus control therapy. Proper sleep hygiene can have a profound difference in the sleep duration and quality of most patients in those with and without insomnia.

Cognitive Behavioral Therapy

Cognitive behavioral therapy for insomnia is the preferred form of treatment for chronic insomnia in adults and has been endorsed as a first-line therapy by multiple societies and guideline panels. There is ample evidence that demonstrates that CBT is as effective if not more effective over the long term in the management of insomnia when compared to pharmacologic therapy. A meta-analysis examined five randomized controlled trials that compared CBT-I against pharmacologic therapy and found that CBT-I was at least as effective as medications for treating insomnia and may be more durable over the long term.[22] CBT-I is a multimodal approach to chronic insomnia that is characterized by face-to-face therapy in an individual or group setting, but remote delivery (telephone or online) is also effective. Many of the principles of CBT-I are addressed in proper sleep hygiene with some differences and more attention to detail. CBT-I addresses behavioral and cognitive components of chronic insomnia. The behavioral components of sleep include establishing a regular bedtime and wakeup time, reducing the time in bed for only hours of sleep (time in bed restriction), use of the bed for only sleep and sex, and sleep hygiene.[23] The cognitive components consist of addressing anxiety associated with insomnia, managing expectations about hours of sleep and the effects of sleeplessness, and relaxation techniques.

Sleep Restriction Therapy

Sleep restriction therapy has been used as a modality for the management of insomnia for over 30 years and has been shown to be an effective component of CBT-I. As mentioned previously, sleep restriction therapy or time in bed restriction is meant to reduce the time spent awake in bed and effectively to only be in bed for the expected hours of sleep.[24,25] This is meant to improve the association of the bedroom for sleep and not for any stimulating activities (outside of sex).

Pharmacologic

Pharmacologic treatment for insomnia is only indicated for patients with refractory insomnia not responsive to conservative approaches such as sleep hygiene and CBT-I. The choice of pharmacotherapy should be individualized based on comorbidities, side effects, and patient tolerance. In a systematic review and meta-analysis on the pharmacologic management of acute and chronic insomnia, the nonbenzodiazepine receptor agonist eszopiclone and dual orexin antagonist Lemborexant had the best overall efficacy profiles; however, data on adverse events and safety profiles are lacking.[26] Medications with regulatory approval for treatment of insomnia fall into four categories based on the mechanism of action: Benzodiazepine receptor agonists, dual orexin receptor antagonists, melatonin agonists, and histamine receptor antagonists.

Benzodiazepine Receptor Agonists

Benzodiazepine receptor agonists have fallen out of favor for the management of insomnia due to their increased side-effect profile and duration of action, especially in the elderly.[27] The five drugs used in this class are estazolam, flurazepam, temazepam, triazolam, and quazepam.

Nonbenzodiazepine Receptor Agonists

Nonbenzodiazepine receptor agonists are the first-line pharmacotherapy due to their more favorable side-effect profile and reduced residual effects compared to their benzodiazepine analogs. It is important to note that although the drugs in this category are not technically benzodiazepines, they fall into the category of benzodiazepine receptor agonists due to their action on the family of benzodiazepine receptor subunits. The drugs in this class include zolpidem, eszopiclone, and zaleplon and are the most prescribed medications for the management of chronic insomnia.[28,29] However, these medications do not come without their fair share of pitfalls. Zolpidem is the most commonly prescribed drug in this class and widely used to treat chronic insomnia. However, there is data to suggest that it increases the risk of reversible dementia in the elderly population even when controlled for confounders such as age, sex, and other comorbidities.[30] With the approval of newer generation drugs for the management of chronic insomnia, drugs like zolpidem are increasingly falling out of favor, particularly in the elderly population.

Melatonin Agonists

Melatonin is one of the most commonly used over-the-counter supplements as a sleep aid. It is produced endogenously by the pineal gland and plays an important role regulating the sleep–wake cycle and circadian rhythm. Several studies have demonstrated the benefit of melatonin therapy in circadian rhythm sleep-wake disorders (CRSWDs) and REM sleep behavior disorder (RBD). Several studies have shown that exogenous melatonin supplementation may reduce time to sleep onset, improve sleep efficiency, and increase total sleep time, although the margin of benefit is narrower than other prescription medications when compared to placebo.[31-34] Currently, Ramelteon (a melatonin receptor agonist) is the only Food and Drug Administration (FDA) approved drug in this class used for the treatment of insomnia. Melatonin may be a safer alternative for adults > 55 years due to its minimal sedating and neuropsychiatric effects in addition to reduced risk of dependency when compared to other prescription medications.[31-34]

Dual Orexin Receptor Antagonists

The orexinergic system was first described over 30 years ago and research since that time has described the role of orexins (aka hypocretins) as wake-promoting neurotransmitters. The pathophysiology of narcolepsy detailing the relative deficiency of orexin further supports its role in wakefulness. Although single orexin receptor antagonists (SORAs) have been studied, they have not been shown to be as effective as dual orexin receptor antagonists (DORAs) in promoting sleep in animal studies. The effects of DORAs are much more targeted and restricted to the orexin system of the brain compared to the widespread CNS effects of most other medications. This may result in a more favorable side-effect profile, and early studies have been encouraging. In contrast to other sedating hypnotics used for insomnia, DORAs have been shown to promote REM sleep as well as NREM sleep.[28,31,35] Current DORAs approved for treatment of insomnia by the FDA include daridorexant, lemborexant, and suvorexant. Data thus far has demonstrated the overall efficacy and improved side-effect profile of DORAs for the management of insomnia, but they are significantly more expensive which is a major barrier to entry. In addition, studies examining long-term effects are lacking due to their relative novelty.

Histamine-1 Receptor Antagonists

Histamine-1 receptor antagonists have fallen out of favor and are not routinely recommended for the treatment of insomnia, and large randomized controlled trials are lacking that support their use. Previous trials have shown mixed results in terms of efficacy and side-effect profile.[28,31] Within this class of medications, low-dose doxepin may have a limited role in the management of insomnia in the elderly due to its reported efficacy, tolerability, and lack of significant adverse events.

Off-label Drugs

Antidepressants

Several antidepressant medications have modest sedating effects, but they are not routinely recommended for the treatment of insomnia. The only approved antidepressant for the treatment of insomnia is doxepin, a tricyclic antidepressant with strong antihistamine-1 effects, and even this is at low doses. Despite these recommendations, medications such as trazodone, mirtazapine, and amitriptyline are some of the most prescribed off-label drugs for the management of primary insomnia. There is a paucity of peer-reviewed data and RCTs supporting the use of these medications for primary insomnia so they should be used with caution.[28,31] However, an argument can be made for use in patients with comorbid depression. Sleep disturbances are an integral part of depressive disorders and teasing out primary insomnia from sequalae secondary to depressive disorders can be difficult.

Atypical Antipsychotics

Atypical antipsychotics are not generally recommended for the treatment of insomnia unless there is a comorbid psychiatric condition (schizophrenia, bipolar disorder, etc.). Quetiapine is by far the most widely prescribed antipsychotic for sleep disorders. Data on its efficacy in the treatment of primary insomnia is scarce, and the existing literature is limited to small nongeneralizable trials.[36] This in combination with its unfavorable side-effect profile does not make it a recommended treatment for primary insomnia in the absence of another psychiatric condition.

Anticonvulsants

There is limited evidence for the use of anticonvulsants for the treatment of insomnia and it is not recommended. However, there is adequate data to support the use of gabapentin in the treatment of insomnia in patients with comorbid conditions such as fibromyalgia, neuropathic pain, and other chronic pain syndromes. Initially designed for use in epilepsy, gabapentin is now one of the most used drugs to treat neuropathic pain. There is some evidence to suggest that gabapentin may enhance slow wave sleep, reduce nocturnal arousals, and improve sleep efficiency in primary insomnia, but further studies with larger sample sizes are needed.[37,38]

OTHER DISEASE ASSOCIATIONS

Restless Leg Syndrome

Restless leg syndrome (RLS) is a common neurological disorder characterized by an irresistible urge to move one's legs. It is often accompanied by an uncomfortable sensation or even pain in the legs that is relieved with movement. RLS can be idiopathic or a secondary sequalae of a comorbid underlying medical condition.[39] Patients with RLS will often complain of trouble falling and staying asleep, and it is important to differentiate these patients from those with primary insomnia.

Periodic Limb Movement Disorder

Periodic limb movement disorder is characterized by periodic movements of the arms and/or legs during sleep that usually interfere with sleep quality and duration. It is highly associated with RLS, and it is rare for patients to have PMLD without RLS. The pathophysiology is poorly understood, and treatment options are limited.

Sleep-related Breathing Disorders

Historically, insomnia has been cited as a common symptom of sleep-related breathing disorders (SRBDs) such as obstructive sleep apnea (OSA) or central sleep apnea. However, increasing data has shown that patients with SRBDs may have comorbid primary insomnia as a distinct clinical entity.[40] Differentiating between the two may pose difficult as there is a large overlap in symptoms warranting PSG testing for further evaluation.

Psychiatric Disorders

Insomnia is a common symptom in patients with psychiatric conditions such as depression, anxiety disorders, attention-deficit/hyperactivity disorder (ADHD), and schizophrenia. In fact, insomnia or hypersomnia is part of the diagnostic criteria for the diagnosis of major depressive disorder based on the DSM-5 criteria. In addition, it is seen in more than 90% of patients with depression and has been found to be an independent marker for an increased risk of suicidal ideations. Epidemiologic studies have found that approximately 40% of patients with primary insomnia have a comorbid psychiatric condition, most notably depression. There is also a high prevalence of insomnia in patients with anxiety disorders that vary widely based on subtype. Several anxiety disorders include insomnia as a component of their diagnostic criteria as well. Other psychiatric disorders not discussed here have also been shown to have a bidirectional relationship with insomnia.[41,42] The prudent clinician should screen patients with primary insomnia for a comorbid psychiatric condition and vice versa.

Dementia

The prevalence of insomnia in patients with dementia ranges from 20 to 35% and may be exacerbated by an array of factors from the underlying pathophysiology to medications used in treatment. In addition, changes in sleep architecture are a normal part of aging demonstrated by decreased delta (slow wave) sleep and increased nocturnal awakenings. These normal physiologic changes further confound the assessment of insomnia in this patient population. Careful attention to detail to the patient's sleep schedule and sleep habits that can be confirmed with a caregiver provides valuable insight into possible lifestyle interventions.[43] It is important to minimize sedating medications as much as possible, particularly in this patient group as it may worsen cognitive impairment and daytime functioning.

EFFECTS ON OTHER PHYSIOLOGIC SYSTEMS

Role in Cardiovascular Disease

The far-reaching effects of insomnia on overall physiology have been well-documented, and there is ample data documenting the negative consequences of insomnia on numerous organ systems. Insomnia has been shown to be associated with an increased risk of hypertension, chronic heart disease, acute coronary disease, and heart failure. The pathophysiology behind this is not fully understood; however, it is thought to be secondary to a combination of a dysregulated HPA, increased sympathetic nervous system activity, increased inflammation, and increased atherogenesis. The dysregulated HPA in addition to the increased adrenergic activity and proinflammatory state is also theorized to be responsible for an increased risk in insulin resistance, diabetes, and mental health disorders such as depression and anxiety.[44]

Role in Pulmonary Disease

The impact insomnia has on pulmonary disease is not limited to SRBDs. Patients with chronic obstructive pulmonary disease (COPD) also have an increased prevalence of insomnia and sleep-related disorders.[45] The pathophysiology of sleep disorders in COPD seems to be complex and multifactorial.

Role in Renal Disease

Approximately half of patients with chronic kidney disease have insomnia, and that number is even higher for patients on some form of dialysis. However, kidney transplantation in patients receiving hemodialysis or peritoneal dialysis significantly reduced the prevalence of insomnia suggesting the underlying renal pathology or consequences of treatment that may play a large role in insomnia symptoms.[46]

Role in Pregnancy

Physiologic changes in pregnancy may also promote insomnia and other sleep disorders. The prevalence of insomnia in pregnancy ranges from 44% in the first trimester to as high as 64% in the third trimester. These sleep disturbances have been shown to worsen over the course of the pregnancy and are not limited to insomnia. There are higher rates of SRBDs and sleep movement disorders in pregnancy.[47-49] Collectively, these findings have been termed pregnancy-associated sleep disorder by the American Academy of Sleep Medicine (AASM).

Role in Menopause

Women are more likely to develop sleep disorders with advancing age compared to men, especially after menopause. The incidence of sleep disorders in women ranges from 16% to 47% at perimenopause, but it increases significantly to 35–60% postmenopause. Rates of RLS, PLMD, depression, and anxiety also show an increase postmenopause. The pathophysiology behind this increase in sleep-related disorders is complex and attributed to be multifactorial. Endogenous production of melatonin has been shown to decrease as you age, but there is a significant drop in production in women postmenopause. This in combination with reductions in progesterone and estrogen, both of which have been shown to promote sleep quality and duration, also has been shown to contribute to this increase in sleep-related disorders.[48,50]

SUMMARY

Insomnia is a common sleep disorder that often coexists with various other health conditions. A comprehensive diagnostic evaluation should focus on gathering a detailed history, particularly regarding sleep hygiene habits and any daytime impairments linked to insomnia. In the Indian population, insomnia remains underdiagnosed and frequently overlooked, highlighting the need for further research in this area. Most patients can be effectively treated through conservative measures, including strict adherence to sleep hygiene and cognitive behavioral therapy. However, pharmacologic therapy may be warranted for those with resistant or severe cases. It is also crucial to identify and address any comorbid conditions, especially psychiatric disorders, that may contribute to insomnia symptoms.

REFERENCES

1. American Academy of Sleep Medicine. International Classification of Sleep Disorders, 3rd edition. Illinois: American Academy of Sleep Medicine; 2014.
2. Hauri PJ (Ed). The International Classification of Sleep Disorders, Diagnostic and Coding Manual, 2nd edition. Westchester: American Academy of Sleep Medicine; 2005.
3. Cracco L, Appleby BS, Gambetti P. Fatal familial insomnia and sporadic fatal insomnia. Handb Clin Neurol. 2018;153: 271-99.
4. Morin CM, Jarrin DC. Epidemiology of Insomnia: Prevalence, Course, Risk Factors, and Public Health Burden. Sleep Med Clin. 2022;17(2):173-91.

5. Vgontzas AN, Bixler EO, Lin HM, et al. Chronic insomnia is associated with nycthemeral activation of the hypothalamic-pituitary-adrenal axis: clinical implications. J Clin Endocrinol Metab. 2001;86:3787-94.
6. Dahale AB, Jaisoorya TS, Manoj L, et al. Insomnia Among Elderly Primary Care Patients in India. Prim Care Companion CNS Disord. 2020;22(3):19m02581.
7. Bhaskar S, Hemavathy D, Prasad S. Prevalence of chronic insomnia in adult patients and its correlation with medical comorbidities. J Family Med Prim Care. 2016;5(4):780-4.
8. Bhattacharya D, Sen MK, Suri JC. Epidemiology of insomnia: A review of the global and Indian scenario. Indian J Sleep Med. 2013;8.3:100-10.
9. Levenson JC, Kay DB, Buysse DJ. The pathophysiology of insomnia. Chest. 2015;147(4):1179-92.
10. Kim M, de la Peña JB, Cheong JH, et al. Neurobiological Functions of the Period Circadian Clock 2 Gene, Per2. Biomol Ther (Seoul). 2018;26(4):358-67.
11. Partinen M, Kaprio J, Koskenvuo M, et al. Genetic and environmental determination of human sleep. Sleep. 1983;6(3):179-85.
12. Johns MW. Sleepiness in different situations measured by the Epworth Sleepiness Scale. Sleep. 1994;17(8):703-10.
13. Buysse DJ, Reynolds CF, Monk TH, et al. Quantification of subjective sleep quality in healthy elderly men and women using the Pittsburgh Sleep Quality Index (PSQI). Sleep. 1991;14(4):331-8.
14. Carney CE, Buysse DJ, Ancoli-Israel S, et al. The consensus sleep diary: standardizing prospective sleep self-monitoring. Sleep. 2012;35(2):287-302.
15. Smith MT, McCrae CS, Cheung J, et al. Use of Actigraphy for the Evaluation of Sleep Disorders and Circadian Rhythm Sleep-Wake Disorders: An American Academy of Sleep Medicine Clinical Practice Guideline. J Clin Sleep Med. 2018;14(7):1231-7.
16. Littner M, Hirshkowitz M, Kramer M, et al.; American Academy of Sleep Medicine. Standards of Practice Committee. Practice parameters for using polysomnography to evaluate insomnia: an update. Sleep. 2003;26(6):754-60.
17. Edinger JD, Bonnet MH, Bootzin RR, et al.; American Academy of Sleep Medicine Work Group. Derivation of research diagnostic criteria for insomnia: report of an American Academy of Sleep Medicine Work Group. Sleep. 2004;27(8):1567-96.
18. Turcotte I, St-Jean G, Bastien CH. Are individuals with paradoxical insomnia more hyperaroused than individuals with psychophysiological insomnia? Event-related potentials measures at the peri-onset of sleep. Int J Psychophysiol. 2011;81(3):177-90.
19. Huang AA, Huang SY. Use of machine learning to identify risk factors for insomnia. PLoS One. 2023;18(4):e0282622.
20. Goldstein CA, Berry RB, Kent DT, et al. Artificial intelligence in sleep medicine: background and implications for clinicians. J Clin Sleep Med. 2020;16(4):609-18.
21. Qaseem A, Kansagara D, Forciea MA, et al.; Clinical Guidelines Committee of the American College of Physicians. Management of Chronic Insomnia Disorder in Adults: A Clinical Practice Guideline from the American College of Physicians. Ann Intern Med. 2016;165(2):125-33.
22. Mitchell MD, Gehrman P, Perlis M, et al. Comparative effectiveness of cognitive behavioral therapy for insomnia: a systematic review. BMC Fam Pract. 2012;13:40.
23. Praharaj SK, Gupta R, Gaur N. Clinical Practice Guideline on Management of Sleep Disorders in the Elderly. Indian J Psychiatry. 2018;60(Suppl 3):S383-96.
24. Miller CB, Espie CA, Epstein DR, et al. The evidence base of sleep restriction therapy for treating insomnia disorder. Sleep Med Rev. 2014;18(5):415-24.
25. Morin CM, Bootzin RR, Buysse DJ, et al. Psychological and behavioral treatment of insomnia: update of the recent evidence (1998-2004). Sleep. 2006;29(11):1398-414.
26. Sateia MJ, Buysse DJ, Krystal AD, et al. Clinical Practice Guideline for the Pharmacologic Treatment of Chronic Insomnia in Adults: An American Academy of Sleep Medicine Clinical Practice Guideline. J Clin Sleep Med. 2017;13(2):307-49.
27. Pottie K, Thompson W, Davies S, et al. Deprescribing benzodiazepine receptor agonists: Evidence-based clinical practice guideline. Can Fam Physician. 2018;64(5):339-51. [Erratum in: Medicine (Baltimore). 2016;94(24):1]
28. De Crescenzo F, D'Alò GL, Ostinelli EG, et al. Comparative effects of pharmacological interventions for the acute and long-term management of insomnia disorder in adults: a systematic review and network meta-analysis. Lancet. 2022;400(10347):170-84.
29. Becker PM, Somiah M. Non-Benzodiazepine Receptor Agonists for Insomnia. Sleep Med Clin. 2015;10(1):57-76.
30. Shih HI, Lin CC, Tu YF, et al. An increased risk of reversible dementia may occur after zolpidem derivative use in the elderly population: a population-based case-control study. Medicine (Baltimore). 2015;94(17):e809.
31. Atkin T, Comai S, Gobbi G. Drugs for Insomnia beyond Benzodiazepines: Pharmacology, Clinical Applications, and Discovery. Pharmacol Rev. 2018;70(2):197-245.
32. Scheer FA, Morris CJ, Garcia JI, et al. Repeated melatonin supplementation improves sleep in hypertensive patients treated with beta-blockers: a randomized controlled trial. Sleep. 2012;35:1395-402.
33. Fatemeh G, Sajjad M, Niloufar R, et al. Effect of melatonin supplementation on sleep quality: a systematic review and meta-analysis of randomized controlled trials. J Neurol. 2022;269(1):205-16.
34. Duffy JF, Wang W, Ronda JM, et al. High dose melatonin increases sleep duration during nighttime and daytime sleep episodes in older adults. J Pineal Res. 2022;73:e12801.
35. Janto K, Prichard JR, Pusalavidyasagar S. An Update on Dual Orexin Receptor Antagonists and Their Potential Role in Insomnia Therapeutics. J Clin Sleep Med. 2018;14(8):1399-408.
36. Modesto-Lowe V, Harabasz AK, Walker SA. Quetiapine for primary insomnia: Consider the risks. Cleve Clin J Med. 2021; 88(5):286-94.
37. Liu GJ, Karim MR, Xu LL, et al. Efficacy and Tolerability of Gabapentin in Adults with Sleep Disturbance in Medical Illness: A Systematic Review and Meta-analysis. Front Neurol. 2017;8:316.
38. Lo HS, Yang CM, Lo HG, et al. Treatment effects of gabapentin for primary insomnia. Clin Neuropharmacol. 2010;33(2):84-90.
39. Bogan RK. Effects of restless legs syndrome (RLS) on sleep. Neuropsychiatr Dis Treat. 2006;2(4):513-9.
40. Wickwire EM, Collop NA. Insomnia and sleep-related breathing disorders. Chest. 2010;137(6):1449-63.
41. Khurshid KA. Comorbid Insomnia and Psychiatric Disorders: An Update. Innov Clin Neurosci. 2018;15(3-4):28-32.
42. Ford DE, Kamerow DB. Epidemiologic study of sleep disturbances and psychiatric disorders. An opportunity for prevention? JAMA. 1989;262(11):1479-84.
43. Molano J, Vaughn BV. Approach to insomnia in patients with dementia. Neurol Clin Pract. 2014;4(1):7-15.

44. Javaheri S, Redline S. Insomnia and Risk of Cardiovascular Disease. Chest. 2017;152(2):435-44.
45. Budhiraja R, Siddiqi TA, Quan SF. Sleep disorders in chronic obstructive pulmonary disease: etiology, impact, and management. J Clin Sleep Med. 2015;11(3):259-70.
46. Tan LH, Chen PS, Chiang HY, et al. Insomnia and Poor Sleep in CKD: A Systematic Review and Meta-analysis. Kidney Med. 2022;4(5):100458.
47. Román-Gálvez RM, Amezcua-Prieto C, Salcedo-Bellido I, et al. Factors associated with insomnia in pregnancy: A prospective Cohort Study. Eur J Obstet Gynecol Reprod Biol. 2018;221:70-5.
48. Shechter A, Lesperance P, Ng YKN, et al. Nocturnal polysomnographic sleep across the menstrual cycle in premenstrual dysphoric disorder. Sleep Med. 13(8):1071-8.
49. Silvestri R, Aricò I. Sleep disorders in pregnancy. Sleep Sci. 2019;12(3):232-9.
50. Tandon VR, Sharma S, Mahajan A, et al. Menopause and Sleep Disorders. J Midlife Health. 2022;13(1):26-33.

Pediatric Obstructive Sleep Apnea

CHAPTER 148

Unnati Desai, Jyotsna M Joshi

INTRODUCTION

Pediatric sleep-disordered breathing consists of a heterogenous spectrum similar to that in adults. Obstructive sleep apnea syndrome (OSAS) in children was described by Osler in 1892 and the first case series was published in 1976.[1] Thereafter, many studies have elaborated on pediatric OSAS, but there still remain many areas of debate. Habitual snoring is reported in 8–12% of children, but only 1–3% show associated OSAS.[2]

Pediatric OSAS is most commonly caused by anatomical abnormalities such as adenoid and tonsillar hypertrophy, which is correctable by surgery. A spectrum of pediatric OSAS is encountered with obesity, syndromes associated with obesity, and orofacial abnormalities in children. These have an inherited and genetic cause. It is a serious condition that can adversely affect the child's growth, emotional and cognitive development, and cardiovascular health. OSA in children is a distinct disorder form that occurs in adults with respect to clinical manifestations, polysomnography (PSG) diagnostic criteria, treatment approaches, and genetic counseling.

DEFINITION

The American Association of Pediatrics (AAP) guidelines define OSAS in children as a "disorder of breathing during sleep characterized by prolonged partial upper airway obstruction and/or intermittent complete obstruction (obstructive apnea) that disrupts normal ventilation during sleep and normal sleep patterns," accompanied by characteristic symptoms or signs **(Table 1)**.[3] It includes primary snoring, upper airway resistance syndrome, obstructive hypoventilation, and OSAS.

ETIOLOGY

Adenoid and tonsillar hypertrophy is the most common cause of pediatric OSAS **(Box 1)**. Children experiencing neuromuscular diseases are also at an increased risk of OSAS in addition to more common hypoventilation and central sleep apneas. The pathophysiology of childhood OSAS is poorly understood.[5] It is proposed to be caused by a combination of anatomic and neuromotor factors, i.e., by the superimposition of structural aberrations upon an integrally more collapsible upper airway. The most important contributory anatomic factor is adenotonsillar hypertrophy, particularly in the preschool age group, the other being craniofacial abnormalities. Obesity leading to changes of upper airway anatomy is more important in the older children and adolescents, most likely attributable to upper airway neuromotor tone as well as imbalance of the pharyngeal dilator and constrictor muscles. Subtle abnormalities in the ventilator responses are also suggested. Nasal and oropharyngeal inflammation might contribute to

TABLE 1: Symptomatology and clinical signs of OSAS.[4]

History	Frequent snoring (≥3 nights/week), labored breathing during sleep, gasps/snorting noises/observed episodes of apnea, sleep enuresis (especially secondary enuresis), sleeping in a seated position or with the neck hyperextended, cyanosis, headaches on awakening, daytime sleepiness, attention-deficit/hyperactivity disorder, learning problems
Physical examination	Underweight or overweight, tonsillar hypertrophy, adenoidal facies, micrognathia/retrognathia, high-arched palate, failure to thrive, hypertension

BOX 1 Causative factors for pediatric obstructive sleep apnea (OSA).

- Adenotonsillar hypertrophy
- Obesity
- Allergic rhinitis
- Craniofacial malformations
- Neuromuscular diseases
- Genetic syndromes
- Metabolic syndromes

TABLE 2: Complications of obstructive sleep apnea (OSA) in children.

Effects on growth	• Obesity • Lethargy • Abnormalities related to syndromic association
Neurocognitive	• Hyperactivity, inattention, aggression • Impaired school performance • Daytime sleepiness • Depression
Cardiovascular consequences	• Pulmonary hypertension • Atherosclerosis, peripheral artery disease (PVD) • Cor pulmonale • Systemic hypertension • Atrial fibrillation and arrhythmias
Metabolic problems	• Thyroid associated abnormalities • Insulin resistance and diabetes mellitus (DM) • Hyperlipidemia

the pathogenesis of breathing disturbances during sleep.[6] Inflammatory hypothesis suggests the role of leukotrienes.[7]

Neuromuscular diseases cause OSAS owing to weakness of pharyngeal muscles and adenotonsillar hypertrophy. They are at an increased threat for developing pulmonary hypertension, cor pulmonale, and neurocognitive dysfunction. Sleep-related hypoventilation/hypoxemia because of neuromuscular diseases might be aggravated in the presence of OSAS. In addition, some of these children have reduced central neural chemoresponsiveness.[8,9] Pediatric OSAS can lead to various complications, some of which may prove to be serious **(Table 2)**.

HISTORY AND CLINICAL EXAMINATION

History and physical examinations are essential to diagnose OSAS in children. The AAP guidelines recommend that clinicians as a part of routine health-maintenance visits should ask whether the child or adolescent snores and look for other clinical effects of OSA.[10,11] Audiotapes or videotapes of the sleeping child recorded by the parents can occasionally be used by healthcare teams to hear and watch for noticeable apneic episodes.[12,13] The regular healthcare visits and school clinic visits should comprise sleep history screening for snoring. In children, OSAS is very unlikely with the lack of habitual snoring. More thorough history concerning labored breathing during sleep, observed apnea, restless sleep, diaphoresis, enuresis, cyanosis, excessive daytime sleepiness, and behavior or learning problems should be acquired.

Physicians should keep in mind that certain syndromes are associated with OSA in children **(Box 2)**. Findings such as malnutrition (under or overweight), adenoid facies, nasal obstruction, adenotonsillar hypertrophy, micro/retrognathia, and hypertension may be present on clinical examination. Systemic hypertension, an enhanced pulmonic component of the second heart sound representing pulmonary hypertension, and reduced growth may be observed as complications of underlying OSA. Adenotonsillar hypertrophy is graded as follows: Grade I, less than 25% space between pillars; grade II, less than 50% space between pillars; grade III, less than 75% space between pillars; and grade IV, tonsils in direct contact. Numerous studies have established that there is no connection between the size of the tonsils and adenoids and occurrence of OSAS.[14,15]

BOX 2 Syndromes associated with obstructive sleep apnea (OSA) in children.

- Prader–Willi, Teacher–Collins, Bardet–Biedl, Beckwith–Wiedemann syndromes
- Achondroplasia
- Crouzon and Apert syndromes
- Duchenne muscular dystrophy, spinal muscular atrophy
- Myelomeningocele
- Pierre–Robbin syndrome
- Cerebral palsy
- Down syndrome
- Sickle cell disease
- Choanal stenosis
- Osteopetrosis
- Klippel–Feil and Hallerman–Streiff syndromes
- Mucopolysaccharidosis

Sleep Questionnaires

Sleep questionnaires were developed to (1) diagnose pediatric OSAS and (2) assess quality of life and response to OSAS therapy. These questionnaires and clinical scoring scales are not completely accurate and standardized. They could be used as per the clinic/institute/sleep physician practice preferences to triage management in children. Some of these questionnaires include Pediatric Sleep Questionnaire (PSQ),[16] "BEARS" sleep screening score,[17] OSA 18,[18] OSD 6,[19] and the questionnaire I'M SLEEPY.[20]

Alternate Diagnostics other than Polysomnography

The 2002 AAP guidelines recommended that a single-channel system, such as overnight oximetry, could aid in suggesting a history of uncomplicated OSAS by showing positive results. Nonetheless, a normal study could not eliminate OSAS and PSG continued to be the gold standard analysis.[21] However, OSAS in children is usually effectively treated by adenotonsillectomy, and the procedure may have postoperative complications in a subgroup of patients. Various easy algorithms have been evaluated to diagnose OSA and prioritize for adenotonsillar surgery. The McGill Oximetry

Score[22] (MOS), which facilitated logical prioritization of the adenotonsillectomy surgical list and also predicted risk of postoperative complications, was not very sensitive and specific. The updated 2012 AAP guidelines stated: "*Although polysomnography is the gold standard for diagnosis of OSAS, there is a shortage of sleep laboratories with pediatric expertise. Hence, polysomnography may not be readily available in certain regions of the country. Alternative diagnostic tests have been shown to have weaker positive and negative predictive values than polysomnography, but nevertheless, objective testing is preferable to clinical evaluation alone. If an alternative test fails to demonstrate OSAS in a patient with a high pretest probability, full polysomnography should be sought.*"[3]

Home Respiratory Polygraphy

Home respiratory polygraphy (HRP), also known as level 3 PSG, involves unsupervised home-based recording of cardiorespiratory channels, i.e., oronasal flow, snoring, O_2 saturation, heart rate, thoracoabdominal movements, and body position during sleep. This technique has been validated in adults.[23-25] Studies in pediatric population also provide the same results.[5,26] Studies on results of continuous positive airway pressure (CPAP) treatment prescribed based on diagnosis by PSG and HRP yielded similar improvements in terms of apnea-hypopnea index (AHI), quality of life, clinical symptoms, and adherence to CPAP therapy.[27,28]

Polysomnography

Overnight PSG evaluation in sleep laboratory is the gold standard to diagnose OSA at all levels of severity. Pediatric AHI severity criteria for children over < 12 years of age are as follows: AHI 1 to <5 is mild, 5 to ≤10 is moderate, and >10 is severe **(Table 3)**. PSG is costly and time consuming, requires specialized expertise, has limited accessibility, and may entail long waiting periods. There are other challenges in carrying out and interpreting PSG in children compared with a supportive adult. The laboratory technician must show a friendly approach and be comfortable with the child while not too childish to discourage adolescents. Children reveal shorter and lesser respiratory events than adults and an increased proportion of hypopneas; hence, the studies must be recorded and studied with great caution. In adults, obstructive apneas of 10s or longer are scored, but in children, apnea is scored if the decrease in oronasal flow more than 90% is for at least two respiratory cycles in the presence of respiratory effort. For a long time, an adult model has been incorrectly used for the diagnosis and therapy of affected children. Hence, the diagnostic algorithm needs revision to appropriately triage; integrate use of screening tools, questionnaires, and alternative tests for OSAS; and selective referral for PSG in resource-limited situations.

The AAP guidelines[3] recommend that clinicians as a part of regular health-maintenance visits should ask about snoring, i.e., whether the child or adolescent snores. If a child snores on a regular basis and reveals any of the problems or findings given in **Table 1**, clinicians should either get a polysomnogram (level A) or refer the child to a sleep specialist or otolaryngologist for a more wide-ranging evaluation (level D). If PSG is not obtainable, then clinicians may direct for other diagnostic tests, such as nocturnal video recording, nocturnal oximetry, daytime nap PSG, or ambulatory PSG (level C).

Adenotonsillectomy can be suggested as the first-line therapy if the child detected as experiencing OSAS shows a clinical inspection consistent with adenotonsillar hypertrophy and does not have a contraindication. A clinical decision is mandatory to examine the benefits of adenotonsillectomy compared with other therapies in obese children with different degrees of adenotonsillar hypertrophy (level B).[3]

TABLE 3: OSA severity criteria in children[7] versus adults.

OSA severity	AHI in children	AHI in adults
None	0	0–5
Mild	1–5	5–15
Moderate	5–10	15–30
Severe	>10	>30

(AHI: apnea–hypopnea index; OSA: obstructive sleep apnea)

MANAGEMENT OF OBSTRUCTIVE SLEEP APNEA IN CHILDREN

Obstructive sleep apnea in children is a distinct disorder from that which occurs in adults with respect to clinical manifestations, PSG diagnostic criteria, and treatment approaches. A simplified multimodality diagnostic algorithm is needed for early diagnosis and treatment. In particular, when availability of PSG is an issue, a protocol-based assessment avoids unnecessary evaluation in selected children and referring them for ambulatory adenotonsillectomy while further assessing high risk **(Box 3)** children with inconclusive HRP for definitive tests such as PSG.

Box 3 High-risk conditions for postoperative respiratory complications in children with obstructive sleep apnea syndrome (OSAS) undergoing adenotonsillectomy.[29]

- Younger than 3 years
- Severe OSAS
- Cardiac complications
- Failure to thrive
- Obesity
- Craniofacial anomalies
- Neuromuscular disorders
- Recent respiratory tract infection

Adenotonsillectomy is the therapy of choice in typical cases. High-risk patients should be monitored as inpatient postoperatively for 24 hours. Adenoid regrowth may occur after surgical intervention, which may be associated with persistent symptoms.[21]

Treatment with montelukast results in a significant decrease in adenoid size and in respiratory-related sleep parameters.[29] Anti-inflammatory therapy of childhood OSA in the form of intranasal corticosteroid is an encouraging method that might substitute surgical treatment in children with mild OSA.[3] CPAP is suggested as therapy if OSAS persists postoperatively and weight loss does not help in addition to other treatments in pediatric patients who are overweight or obese. It is important for clinicians to keep in mind that children symptomatic for OSA may exhibit typical PSG results, but PSG parameters may be atypical in relatively asymptomatic children. A holistic evaluation and management for endocrinopathies, obesity, and metabolic disorders is necessary, as OSA is often an accompaniment of syndromes common in childhood, especially those causing obesity.

SUMMARY

Pediatric OSA is a distinct disorder with some similarities with the adult disease but with different clinical features and complications. It requires a different algorithmic approach to diagnosis and treatment. It is important to undertake an early and more aggressive treatment approach including the surgical options as appropriate.

REFERENCES

1. Guilleminault C, Eldridge FL, Simmons FB, et al. Sleep apnea in eight children. Pediatrics. 1976;58:23-30.
2. Teplitzky TB, Zauher A, Isaiah A. Evaluation and diagnosis of pediatric obstructive sleep apnea—An update. Front Sleep. 2023;2:1127784.
3. Marcus CL, Brooks LJ, Draper KA, et al. Diagnosis and management of childhood obstructive sleep apnea syndrome. Pediatrics. 2012;130:576-84.
4. Desai U, Karkhanis VK, Joshi JM. Pediatric sleep apnea—a simplified approach. Indian J Sleep Med. 2015;10(1):1-10.
5. Marcus CL. Pathophysiology of childhood obstructive sleep apnea: current concepts. Respir Physiol. 2000;119:143-54.
6. Goldbart AD, Tal A. Inflammation and sleep disordered breathing in children: a state-of-the-art review. Pediatr Pulmonol. 2008;43: 1151-60.
7. Goldbart AD, Goldman JL, Li RC, et al. Differential expression of cysteinyl leukotriene receptors 1 and 2 in tonsils of children with obstructive sleep apnea syndrome or recurrent infection. Chest. 2004;126:13-8.
8. Alves RS, Resende MD, Skomro RP, et al. Sleep and neuromuscular disorders in children. Sleep Med Rev. 2009;13:133-48.
9. Hull J, Aniapravan R, Chan E, et al. British Thoracic Society guideline for respiratory management of children with neuromuscular weakness. Thorax. 2012;67(Suppl 1):i1-40.
10. Brouillette RT, Hanson D, David R, et al. A diagnostic approach to suspected obstructive sleep apnea in children. J Pediatr. 1984;105:10-4.
11. Carroll JL, McColley SA, Marcus CL, et al. Inability of clinical history to distinguish primary snoring from obstructive sleep apnea syndrome in children. Chest. 1995;108:610-8.
12. Brietzke SE, Katz ES, Roberson DW. Can history and physical examination reliably diagnose pediatric obstructive sleep apnea/hypopnea syndrome? A systematic review of the literature. Otolaryngol Head Neck Surg. 2004;131:827-32.
13. Lamm C, Mandeli J, Kattan M. Evaluation of home audiotapes as an abbreviated test for obstructive sleep apnea syndrome (OSAS) in children. Pediatr Pulmonol. 1999;27:267-72.
14. Laurikainen E, Erkinjuntti M, Alihanka J, et al. Radiological parameters of the bony nasopharynx and the adenotonsillar size compared with sleep apnea episodes in children. Int J Pediatr Otorhinolaryngol. 1987;12:303-10.
15. Brooks LJ, Stephens BM, Bacevice AM. Adenoid size is related to severity but not the number of episodes of obstructive apnea in children. J Pediatr. 1998;132:682-6.
16. Chervin RD, Weatherly RA, Garetz SL, et al. Pediatric Sleep Questionnaire. Prediction of sleep apnea and outcomes. Arch Otolaryngol Head Neck Surg. 2007;133:216-22.
17. Owens JA, Dalzell V. Use of the "BEARS" sleep screening tool in a pediatric residents' continuity clinic: a pilot study. Sleep Med. 2005;6:63-9.
18. Franco RA Jr, Rosenfeld RM, Rao M. First place—resident clinical science award 1999. Quality of life for children with obstructive sleep apnea. Otolaryngol Head Neck Surg. 2000;123:9-16.
19. de Serres LM, Derkay C, Astley S, et al. Measuring quality of life in children with obstructive sleep disorders. Arch Otolaryngol Head Neck Surg. 2000;126:1423-9.
20. Kadmon G, Chung SA, Shapiro CM. I'M SLEEPY: A short pediatric sleep apnea questionnaire. Int J Pediatr Otorhinolaryngol 2014;78:2116-20.
21. Section on Pediatric Pulmonology, Subcommittee on Obstructive Sleep Apnea Syndrome, American Academy of Pediatrics. Clinical practice guideline: diagnosis and management of childhood obstructive sleep apnea syndrome. Pediatrics. 2002;109:704-12.
22. Nixon GM, Kermack AS, Davis GM, et al. Planning adenotonsillectomy in children with obstructive sleep apnea: the role of overnight oximetry. Pediatrics. 2004;113:e19-25.
23. Masa JF, Corral J, Pereira R, et al. Effectiveness of home respiratory polygraphy for the diagnosis of sleep apnoea and hypopnoea syndrome. Thorax. 2011;66:567-73.
24. Calleja JM, Esnaola S, Rubio R, et al. Comparison of a cardiorespiratory device versus polysomnography for diagnosis of sleep apnoea. Eur Respir J. 2002;20:1505-10.
25. Tan HL, Gozal D, Ramirez HM, et al. Overnight polysomnography versus respiratory polygraphy in the diagnosis of pediatric obstructive sleep apnea. Sleep. 2014;37:255-60.

26. Alonso-Álvarez ML, Terán-Santos J, Ordax Carbajo E, et al. Reliability of home respiratory polygraphy for the diagnosis of sleep apnea in children. Chest. 2015;147:1020-8.
27. Mulgrew AT, Fox N, Ayas NT, et al. Diagnosis and initial management of obstructive sleep apnea without polysomnography: a randomized validation study. Ann Intern Med. 2007;146:157-66.
28. Whitelaw WA, Brant RF, Flemons WW. Clinical usefulness of home oximetry compared with polysomnography for assessment of sleep apnea. Am J Respir Crit Care Med. 2005;171:188-93.
29. Goldbart AD, Goldman JL, Veling MC, et al. Leukotriene modifier therapy for mild sleep-disordered breathing in children. Am J Respir Crit Care Med. 2005;17:364-70.

SECTION 16

Lung Neoplasms

SECTION OUTLINE

Epidemiology and Risk Factors of Lung Cancer

CHAPTER 149

Deepak Aggarwal, Komaldeep Kaur

INTRODUCTION

Lung cancer has become the leading cause of cancer-related deaths in both men and women worldwide.[1,2] The tumor originates in bronchial or alveolar epithelial cells and presents with significant molecular and histological heterogeneity. The last decade has seen a major change in the predominant histological type (adenocarcinoma) of lung cancer in many countries including India. Active tobacco smoking has the most dependable association with lung cancer risk. Changes in smoking behavior, presence of other risk factors, and use of better diagnostic tests including molecular studies have contributed to varied as well as changing profile of this pulmonary neoplasm. With the better understanding of the molecular alterations and genetics involved in its pathogenesis, the diagnosis and treatment of this potentially fatal disease have markedly improved. But despite this and improved treatment options, 5-year survival of the patients has generally remained poor.[3] Understanding of the current epidemiological aspects and risk factors of lung cancer is essential for its better control and prevention.

EPIDEMIOLOGY OF LUNG CANCER

Lung cancer is the second most commonly diagnosed malignancy worldwide representing 11.4% of the all new cancer cases. In terms of mortality, it still remains the leading cause of cancer-related deaths (18.0% of all cancer-related deaths) in both the genders worldwide.[4] In simple terms, lung cancer is responsible for 1 in 10 cancers diagnosed and 1 in 5 cancer-related deaths. The average incidence of lung cancer over the last four decades was 59.0/100,000 person-years with its peak around 1992 when its incidence was 65.9/100,000 person-years. Gradual decline in tobacco smoking globally has led to an overall decrease in its incidence with 48.9/100,000 person-years being reported in 2015.[5]

Conventionally, lung cancer is divided into two broad groups: Small-cell carcinomas and non-small-cell lung carcinomas (NSCLC) which include squamous cell, adenocarcinoma, large cell, and other less common types. Squamous cell carcinoma and small-cell carcinoma are the two smoking-associated lung cancers that each constitutes 20% and slightly more than 10% of all lung cancers, respectively.[6] Till the 1990s, squamous cell carcinoma was the most prevalent histological pattern but now, it has been superseded by adenocarcinoma which comprises 40% of all lung cancers.[6] The reasons behind this change are decrease in tobacco smoking prevalence, change in smoking behavior, differences in the composition of cigarettes, and possible effect of other/unknown risk factors.[7-9] Other histological subtypes include large cell and adeno-squamous that constitute less than 5% of all lung cancers.[6]

In terms of molecular epidemiology, the number of targetable driver mutations in lung cancer has expanded in the last decade with at least four mutations [*EGFR*, *BRAF*, *MET*, *ERBB2* (HER2)] and four fusions or rearrangements (ALK, ROS1, RET, NTRK). Out of these, *EGFR* mutations are the most common actionable mutations that are more commonly detected in Asians (40–50%) as compared to the Western patients (10–16%). Overall, *KRAS* is the most common mutation with an estimated prevalence of 30–40% in NSCLC.[10]

Cancer-related mortality has been reported to be the highest in black men and lowest in Asian Americans. This racial and ethnic difference is largely attributed to the variation in cigarette-smoking habits and the advanced stage at presentation in black men. In Asia, Japan has a high incidence and mortality rates from lung cancer. In contrast, India and few other countries in south central Asia have shown a relatively higher mortality due to cancers involving other sites such as oral cavity, reflecting the popularity of betel nut chewing in these regions.[11,12]

LUNG CANCER EPIDEMIOLOGY IN INDIA

According to the GLOBOCAN 2020 report, age-standardized incidence and mortality rates of lung cancer in India stand at 97.1 and 63.1 per lakh population, respectively.[4] Nearly 75% of lung cancers have a strong association with smoking.[13,14] Variations in local cultural and lifestyle factors across different parts of the country contribute to differences in the cancer incidence pattern among different states. The highest cancer incidence in the country has been reported from the north-east region with Aizawl district of the Mizoram state ranking first in terms of figures (38.8 cases per 100,000 males and 37.9 cases per 100,000 females).[15]

Historically, males have been more commonly affected by lung cancer as compared to females, though this gender difference has narrowed down in recent years. The mean age at presentation is reported to be lower in India as compared to the European and American figures. In a recent Indian study, the median age at disease diagnosis was lesser in females as compared to males (56 vs. 60 years, $p < 0.0001$).[16] Similar to other parts of globe, adenocarcinoma is the most common subtype of lung cancer in India.[14] The prevalence of *EGFR* mutations and ALK rearrangements has been found to be around 25–30% and 11% among adenocarcinoma patients, respectively.[14,17]

India being a tuberculosis endemic country poses a great challenge in the diagnosis of lung cancer. Many a time, lung cancer is misdiagnosed as tuberculosis and patients are initiated on antitubercular treatment.[18] A diagnostic delay of 3 months' duration was observed in a study from a tertiary care institute from north India. Lack of awareness and tendency of Indian population to seek other forms of treatment are some of the reasons that cause a delay in diagnosis and treatment.[16]

LUNG CANCER IN NEVER SMOKERS

Lung cancer in the individuals who have never smoked is considered as a distinct entity because of its unique biological and epidemiological perspective. The term nonsmokers or never smokers refer to individuals who have smoked less than 100 cigarettes in their lives.[19] Worldwide, 20% of men and up to 50% of women who develop lung cancer are never smokers.[20] Moreover, it is the seventh leading cause of cancer deaths among such individuals. Adenocarcinoma is the major histopathological type seen in these patients. Common risk factors of lung cancer among nonsmokers include age, second-hand smoke (SHS), environmental and occupational exposures (like radon, PM2.5, cooking oil fumes), genetic factors, underlying lung disease, oncogenic viruses, and estrogens.[21] Data on lung cancer in nonsmokers are scarce form India. In the two recent studies, out of all lung cancer patients, it was seen that 23.6% and 40.9% were nonsmokers. These patients were more likely to be younger, females, and had better survival as compared to smokers with lung cancer.[13,22]

RISK FACTORS OF LUNG CANCER

Smoking has been the most important risk factor for the development of lung cancer. Besides, with the increase in adenocarcinoma and its gender and geographical variations, there has been a continuum of efforts to identify other etiological risk factors of lung cancer. **Box 1** enumerates common factors that have been linked with an increased incidence of lung cancer. Some of these factors are amenable to change and can be managed by adopting a healthy lifestyle, avoiding the use of tobacco and alcohol and addressing occupational exposures.

BOX 1 Risk factors with proven or possible association with lung cancer.

Behavioral:
- Tobacco smoking—active, passive, e-cigarettes, smokeless tobacco
- Dietary factors and alcohol intake

Environmental:
- Outdoor and indoor air pollution (particulate matter, diesel exhaust, solid fuels, etc.)
- Radon exposure

Occupational exposures:
- Asbestos, silica
- Chemicals like pesticides
- Heavy metals (arsenic, nickel, chromium, beryllium, cadmium)
- Exposure to mineral fibers, irritants

Pulmonary diseases:
- Chronic obstructive pulmonary disease (COPD)
- Interstitial lung disease
- Pneumoconiosis

Systemic infections:
- HIV infection
- *Chlamydia pneumoniae* infections

Genetic factors:
- Familial (hereditary)
- Specific genetic mutations (nonhereditary)

Others: Hormone therapy

Tobacco Smoking

Active Tobacco Smoking

Tobacco smoking, undoubtedly, has the most plausible causal relationship with the lung cancer so much so that almost 90% of cancer deaths are attributable to it.[23] The detrimental effects of tobacco smoking were unnoticed until the 1950s when two landmark studies depicting the strong connection between tobacco smoking and lung cancer were published. In 1964, a report of the advisory to the surgeon general documented that smoking was responsible for 9–10-fold increased risk for developing lung cancer. This report became the turning point as it made a significant impact on decreasing the tobacco consumption in US.[24-26]

The risk of lung cancer generally increases with the duration and intensity of cigarette smoking and is more common in current smokers as compared to reformed smokers. The risk of lung cancer in smokers exists beyond racial and ethnic boundaries, though certain variations do exist due to differences in smoking behavior, environmental exposures, type of smoking devices (pipes, cigar, cigarette, *bidis*, etc.), and ingredients in tobacco products. In terms of histology, smoking has a strong association with squamous cell and small-cell carcinoma and a weaker one with large-cell carcinoma and adenocarcinoma. "Quit smoking" is the single-most important intervention for the prevention of lung cancer. It is said that more than 15 years of abstinence from smoking reduces the risk of lung cancer in former smokers by 80–90%.

Based on nearly 100 years of observations of cigarette use in developed countries, a model of smoking epidemic was established in 1994 which depicted the four stages of smoking epidemic in any country. The transition through various phases is dependent upon three variables, namely prevalence of smoking, consumption of tobacco, and mortality due to smoking. According to the model, there is a three to four decades lag between the peak of tobacco prevalence and the subsequent peak of smoking-related mortality.[27]

Indian scenario: In contrast to the smoking epidemic model which was suitable to all the developed countries, India experienced a compressed tobacco epidemic. The prevalence of tobacco consumption increased and decreased simultaneously in a relatively short span of time.[28] Overall, India is home to almost 11% of the world's total tobacco users. The report of Global Adult Tobacco Survey-II (GATS-II) conducted in 2016–2017 stated that the overall prevalence of tobacco use in India is 10.38% in smoking form and 21.38% in the form of smokeless products.[29] The National Family Health Survey 2019–2021 reported that 38% and 8.9% of men and women above 15 years of age, respectively, have a history of consuming any form of tobacco.[30]

Bidi smoking and smokeless forms are the common forms of tobacco consumed in India and frequently responsible for cancer.[31] *Bidi* smoke contains higher concentration of carcinogenic chemicals including hydrogen cyanide, carbon monoxide, ammonia, benz[a]anthracene, and benzopyrene as compared to conventional cigarettes, thus posing a higher risk for lung cancer. Although the overall prevalence of smoking has decreased in many Indian states, there has been an upward trend in certain states like Sikkim, Goa, Bihar, Gujrat, Himachal Pradesh, and Mizoram among male tobacco users and in Mizoram and Sikkim among female tobacco users.[32]

Mechanism of carcinogenesis: Tobacco smoke contains more than 7,000 chemicals among which 73 have been proven to be carcinogens to either humans or laboratory animals by the International Agency for Research of Cancer (IARC).[33] Most of these carcinogens are substrates for drug metabolizing enzymes like cytochrome p450, glutathione S-transferase, and UDP-glucuronosyl transferases which convert them into more water-soluble forms. But during this process, various electrophilic reactive intermediates like carbocations or epoxides are formed which can react with DNA bases. This formation of DNA adducts if go unrepaired can put a person at risk for carcinogenesis.[34,35]

Second-hand Smoke

Second-hand smoke is the sum of tobacco smoke exposures in the multiple microenvironments where a person spends time. This constitutes both mainstream smoke, i.e. smoke released from the burning end of a smoldering cigarette/pipe/cigar, and side-stream smoke that is exhaled from the lungs of an active smoker. The risk of developing lung cancer increases up to 25% in individuals exposed to SHS as compared to those who are not.[36,37] The presence of DNA adducts has also been noticed in never smokers who are exposed to SHS. SHS contains the same carcinogens as that are inhaled by active smokers.

Generally, females, children, and elderly individuals, sharing the space at home with the active smoker, are more vulnerable to SHS. Occupations involved at places like bars, betting establishments, bowling alleys, etc., where smoking is permitted also pose the risk to their employees.[38] In order to control the detrimental effects of active and passive smoking, India implemented the Cigarettes and Other Tobacco Products Act (COTPA) in 2003 banning smoking at workplace and public places. The effect of this law reflected in the recent GATS-II report where the proportion of nonsmokers exposed to SHS decreased to 35% and 25.7% at home and at public places, respectively, as compared to the previous report (2009–2010).[29]

Electronic cigarettes: Electronic cigarette or e-cigarette is a battery-operated device that produces aerosol by heating a mixture of liquid nicotine, flavorings, and other chemical solvents in a replaceable cartridge. The vapors contain different toxic and carcinogenic compounds such as formaldehyde, acetaldehyde, acetone, and acrolein that can cause inflammation, increased membrane permeability, and cytotoxicity of the bronchial epithelium.[39] According to the GATS-II report, the prevalence of vapors or e-cigarettes use in India stands at 0.02%.[29] Although human evidence of its association with lung cancer is lacking, animal evidence showed development of lung adenocarcinoma in exposed mice exposed to e-cigarette smoke for 12 weeks.[40] Beside a potential risk of lung cancer, e-cigarettes are also associated with an increased risk of addiction to conventional cigarettes. Considering the potential harms associated with e-cigarettes, the Indian government implemented a total ban on the import and sale of these products in the year of 2013.

Outdoor and Indoor Air Pollution

Air pollution is an important though often under-recognized risk factor for lung cancer. Based on the evidence from human and animal studies, outdoor air pollution and particulate matter (PM) in outdoor air pollution were classified as Group 1 human carcinogens by the IARC in 2013.[41] The risk of developing lung cancer increases as the level of particulate matter (PM2.5) increases in the air. Mining and other industries, municipal waste sites, inadequate incineration, and stubble burning of the crop are the major sources of

PM2.5. In urban areas motor vehicular emission, particularly, diesel exhaust and nitrogen dioxide (NO_2) exposure, has been linked with an increased risk of lung cancer.[42]

Household combustion of solid fuel like coal and biomass fuel (primarily wood) is also a major contributor to indoor and outdoor air pollution, particularly in rural India. Numerous cancer trigger factors such as benzene, carbon monoxide, formaldehyde, and polycyclic aromatic hydrocarbons are produced by burning coal indoors. Both coal and biomass combustion for cooking/heating and other activities have been found to increase the risk of lung cancer.[43]

Occupational Hazards

Asbestos: These are naturally occurring fibrous silicates that are largely used in acoustical and thermal energy. All types of asbestos have been labeled as carcinogenic to humans and can cause lung cancer and mesothelioma.[44] The Environmental Protection Agency has also classified asbestos as group A carcinogen to humans. Carcinogenicity with asbestos is directly related to the length of fiber. Most of the fibers related to malignancy have a length of 8 mm. Not only the worker, but also his family members are also at risk from the asbestos dust brought on the clothes from the workplace. In addition to natural exposure from the erosion of asbestos or asbestiform rocks, residential exposure results from asbestos mining or manufacturing in the nearby places.

Chemical exposures (pesticides): India, being the second-largest agro-economy, a good percentage of population is exposed to pesticides during various stages of handling, dilution, and application. Agriculturists get exposure mainly via direct contact through skin and via the inhalational route. Chlorophenols, dioxin compounds, and related phenoxy-acetic acids are certain pesticide groups that have been found to have a carcinogenic effect on lungs.[45,46]

Heavy metals: Use of heavy metals such as arsenic, beryllium, cadmium, chromium, and nickel in different occupations like alloy, smelting, and production of other commercial products have been linked to the development of lung cancer.[47-49] Out of these, arsenic is both an environmental and an occupational lung carcinogen which commonly exists in the form of arsenite and arsenate.[49]

Silica exposure: Long-term silica exposure in the form of crystalline silica dust leads to irreversible lung disease called silicosis. Professions like mining, construction, stone works/quarries, pottery manufacturing, and denim sandblasting are usually involved with exposure to silica dust. Heavy exposure to silica has also been associated with lung cancer, mainly via a nongenetic pathway possibly due to long-term chronic inflammation and damage to the lung tissue.[50]

Other occupations and lung cancer: Occupations like coal gasification, construction and rubber industry, glass factory, sandblasting, uranium mining, masons, painters, truck drivers, and traffic police involve exposure to various airborne chemicals, mineral fibers, irritants, and persistent organic pollutants that can elevate lung cancer risks in these professions. Besides, occupational exposures, simultaneous nonoccupational exposures and change in sleep pattern due to night shifts may increase or decrease the strength of association of these risk factors with lung cancer. All occupation exposures pose significant public health implications and highlight the importance of strict occupational safety regulations at the government level.[51,52]

Radon Exposure

Radon is considered the most important cause of lung cancer among nonsmokers.[53] In 1987, indoor radon was labeled as human carcinogen by the World Health Organization (WHO). It is found to be responsible for 3–14% of lung cancer cases depending on the national average radon level and smoking prevalence.[54] Radon is a radioactive gas that arises naturally in the decay process of uranium-238. Before decaying further to short-lived radioactive particles, namely polonium-218 and polonium-214, it gets diffused through the soil into the air and water. As the pressure inside the buildings is low as compared to that of subsoil, radon gets its entry through diffusion via the cracks, crevices, and leaks of the buildings. Though epidemiologic studies have encountered challenges in the assessment of residential radon concentration, limited evidence from different parts of India have found a wide variation in its levels with majority being lower than that labeled as carcinogenic by the WHO.[55]

Genetic Factors and Family History

A positive family history is associated with an increased risk of development of lung cancer to the tune of 1.7-fold.[56] This risk is found to further increase two to four times in the first-degree relatives. Although genetic susceptibility could explain some of the association, common environmental and lifestyle risk factors as well as gene–environment interactions are also important contributors to this relationship.[57] Tumors acquire intrinsic genetic driver mutations which involve cell signaling pathways including ErbB protein family (EGFR/HER1-4) and GTP-ase Kirsten rat sarcoma virus (*K-ras*) gene. Other genetic and epigenetic changes cause inactivation of tumor suppressor genes *p53*, *p16*, and *PTEN* leading to development of cancer. Various genome-wide association studies have linked chromosome regions *5p15*, *15q25-26*, and *6q21* with an increased risk of lung cancer. The *5p15* region encodes telomerase reverse transcriptase (TERT) that is involved in cell replication, the mutation of which leads to uncurbed proliferation of cells. Mutation in the 15q25-26 region has also been found in association with nicotine dependence which highlights the role of gene–environment interactions in increasing the susceptibility to lung cancer. Variants of chromosome locus 6q21 confers misregulation of G-protein signaling leading to an increased cancer risk in never smokers.[58]

Diet and Alcohol

The relationship between dietary intake and lung cancer risk is inconclusive. Limited evidence suggests that diet rich in vegetables and fruits may have protective effect against the development of lung cancer. On the contrary, diet rich in red meat and high intake of coffee consumption and total carotenoids have been linked to the development of lung cancer. The association between low levels of vitamin D and lung cancer risk is not clear.[59,60] Many times, a positive correlation between smoking and alcohol intake makes it difficult to rule out the potential confounding effect of tobacco. However, a pooled analysis of seven cohort studies found high alcohol consumption to be a risk factor for the development of lung cancer after adjusting for smoking.[61]

Chronic Inflammatory Conditions

Patients with persistent structural damage to the lungs due to inflammatory conditions like interstitial lung disease, asthma, chronic obstructive pulmonary diseases, sequelae to pulmonary tuberculosis, and *Chlamydia pneumoniae* infection have been found to be at an increased risk of lung cancer.[62-64] Discussed previously, occupational lung diseases like asbestosis and silicosis are also considered risk factors of lung cancer. Lung cancer is the most common non-AIDS defining malignancy in people living with HIV infection and accounts for nearly 30% of such patients. Immunosuppression has been implicated in oncogenesis in these patients along with increased prevalence of smoking in this population.[65]

SUMMARY

The last decade saw significant changes in the epidemiology, etiological factors, and prognosis of lung cancer worldwide. Better diagnostic services, advances in molecular and genetic understanding of lung cancer, changes in smoking practices and behavior, and new legislative laws pertaining to smoking and occupational exposures are some of the reasons for these changes. New prediction tools and equations are being developed using these risk factors to predict lung cancer risk and plan cancer screening accordingly.

REFERENCES

1. Miller KD, Siegel RL, Lin CC, et al. Cancer treatment and survivorship statistics, 2016. CA Cancer J Clin. 2016;66:271-89.
2. Kocher F, Hilbe W, Seeber A, et al. Longitudinal analysis of 2293 NSCLC patients: a comprehensive study from the TYROL registry. Lung Cancer. 2015;87:193-200.
3. Thomas A, Chen Y, Yu T, et al. Trends and characteristics of young non-small cell lung cancer patients in the United States. Front Oncol. 2015;5:113.
4. Sung H, Ferlay J, Siegel RL, et al. Cancer statistics 2020: GLOBOCAN estimates of incidence and mortality worldwide for 36 cancers in 185 countries. CA Cancer J Clin. 2021;71:209-49.
5. Lu T, Yang X, Huang Y, et al. Trends in the incidence, treatment, and survival of patients with lung cancer in the last four decades. Cancer Manag Res. 2019;11:943-53.
6. Lewis DR, Check DP, Caporaso NE, et al. US lung cancer trends by histologic type. Cancer. 2014;120(18):2883-92.
7. Thun MJ, Lally CA, Flannery JT, et al. Cigarette smoking and changes in the histopathology of lung cancer. J Natl Cancer Inst 1997;89:1580-6.
8. Travis W, Brambilla E, Noguchi M, et al. International Association for the Study of Lung Cancer/American Thoracic Society/ European Respiratory Society international multidisciplinary classification of lung adenocarcinoma. J Thorac Oncol. 2011; 6:244-85.
9. Lortet-Tieulent J, Soerjomataram I, Ferlay J, et al. International trends in lung cancer incidence by histological subtype: Adenocarcinoma stabilizing in men but still increasing in women. Lung Cancer. 2014;84:13-22.
10. Fois SS, Paliogiannis P, Zinellu A, et al. Molecular Epidemiology of the Main Druggable Genetic Alterations in Non-Small Cell Lung Cancer. Int J Mol Sci. 2021;22:612.
11. Ferlay J, Soerjomataram I, Ervik M, et al. GLOBOCAN 2012 v1.0. Cancer Incidence and Mortality Worldwide: IARC Cancer Base No. 11. 2013.
12. Youlden D, Cramb S, Baade P. The international epidemiology of lung cancer: Geographic distribution and secular trends. J Thorac Oncol. 2008;3:819-31.
13. Jindal SK, Malik SK, Datta BN. Lung cancer in Northern India in relation to age, sex and smoking habits. Europ J Respir Dis. 1987;70:23-8.
14. Mohan A, Garg A, Gupta A, et al. Clinical profile of lung cancer in North India: a 10-year analysis of 1862 patients from a tertiary care centre. Lung India. 2020;37:190-7.
15. Mathur P, Sathish kumar K, Chaturvedi M, et al. Cancer Statistics, 2020: Report From National Cancer Registry Programme, India. JCO Glob Oncol. 2020;6:1063-75.
16. Iyer H, Ghosh T, Garg A, et al. Lung cancer in Asian Indian females: Identification of disease-specific characteristics and outcome measures over a 12-year period. Lung India. 2023;40: 4-11.
17. Nakra T, Mehta A, Bal A, et al. Epidermal growth factor receptor mutation status in pulmonary adenocarcinoma: multi-institutional data discussion at national conference of "Lung Cancer Management in Indian context". Curr Probl Cancer. 2020;44:100561.
18. Garg A, Iyer H, Jindal V, et al. Evaluation of delays during diagnosis and management of lung cancer in India: A prospective observational study. Eur J Cancer Care (Engl). 2022;31: e13621.
19. Centers for Disease Control and Prevention. (2017). Glossary. General concepts. [online] Available from https://www.cdc.gov/nchs/nhis/tobacco/tobacco_glossary.htm#:~:text=Current smoker%3A [Last accessed September, 2024].
20. Parkin DM, Bray F, Ferlay J, et al. Global cancer statistics, 2002. CA Cancer J Clin. 2005;55:74-108.
21. Dubin S, Griffin D. Lung Cancer in Non-Smokers. Mo Med. 2020;117:375-9.

22. Vasudevan S, Krishna V, Mehta A. Lung Cancer in Non-Smokers: Clinicopathological and Survival Differences from Smokers. Cureus. 2022;14:e32417.
23. Siemiatycki J, Karp I, Sylvestre MP, et al. Estimating the proportion of cases of lung cancer legally attributable to smoking: a novel approach for class actions against the tobacco industry. Am J Public Health. 2014;104:e60-6.
24. Wynder EL, Graham EA. Tobacco smoking as a possible etiologic factor in bronchogenic carcinoma: a study of six hundred and eighty-four proved cases. JAMA. 1950;143:329-36.
25. Doll R, Hill A. Smoking and carcinoma of the lung: preliminary report. BMJ. 1950;2:739-48.
26. U.S. Department of Health, Education, and Welfare. Smoking and Health: Report of the Advisory Committee to the Surgeon General of the Public Health Service. Washington: U.S. Department of Health, Education, and Welfare, Public Health Service, Center for Disease Control; 1964. PHS Publication No. 1103.
27. Lopez AD, Collishaw N, Piha T. A descriptive model of the cigarette epidemic in developed countries. Tob Control. 1994; 3:242-7.
28. Shaikh R, Janssen F, Vogt T. The progression of the tobacco epidemic in India on the national and regional level, 1998-2016. BMC Public Health. 2022;22:317.
29. Tata Institute of Social Sciences (TISS), Mumbai and Ministry of Health and Family Welfare, Government of India. Global Adult Tobacco Survey GATS 2. India 2016-2017 Report. [online] Available from https://ntcp.nhp.gov.in/assets/document/surveys-reports-publications/Global-Adult-Tobacco-Survey-Second-Round-India-2016-2017.pdf. [Last accessed September, 2024].
30. Ministry of Health and Family Welfare, Government of India, Compendium of fact Sheets, Key indicators India and 14 States/UTs (Phase-II): National Family Health Survey (NFHS-5) 2019-2020. [online] Available from https://mohfw.gov.in/sites/default/files/NFHS-5_Phase-II_0.pdf
31. Gupta D, Boffetta P, Gaboriean V, et al. Risk factors of lung cancer in Chandigarh, India. Ind J Med Res. 2001;113:142-50.
32. Ladusingh L, Dhillon P, Narzary P. Why do the youths in Northeast India use tobacco? J Environ Public Health. 2017;2017:1391253.
33. Rodgman A, Perfetti T. The Chemical Components of Tobacco and Tobacco Smoke. Boca Raton, FL: CRC Press; 2009. pp. 1483-784.
34. Pleasance ED, Stephens PJ, O'Meara S, et al. A small-cell lung cancer genome with complex signatures of tobacco exposure. Nature. 2010;463:184-90.
35. Lee W, Jiang Z, Liu J, et al. The mutation spectrum revealed by paired genome sequences from a lung cancer patient. Nature. 2010;465:473-7.
36. Kim AS, Ko HJ, Kwon JH, et al. Exposure to Secondhand Smoke and Risk of Cancer in Never Smokers: A Meta-analysis of Epidemiologic Studies. Int J Environ Res Public Health. 2018;15:1981.
37. Rapiti E, Jindal SK, Gupta D, et al. Passive smoking and lung cancer in Chandigarh, India. Lung Cancer. 1999;23:183-9.
38. Siegel M, Skeer M. Exposure to secondhand smoke and excess lung cancer mortality risk among workers in the "5 B's": bars, bowling alleys, billiard halls, betting establishments, and bingo parlours. Tob Control. 2003;12:333-8.
39. Scheffler S, Dieken H, Krischenowski O, et al. Evaluation of E-cigarette liquid vapor and mainstream cigarette smoke after direct exposure of primary human bronchial epithelial cells. Int J Environ Res Public Health. 2015;12:3915-25.
40. Tang MS, Wu XR, Lee HW, et al. Electronic-cigarette smoke induces lung adenocarcinoma and bladder urothelial hyperplasia in mice. Proc Natl Acad Sci U S A. 2019;116:21727-31.
41. Outdoor air pollution. IARC Monographs on the Evaluation of Carcinogenic Risks to Humans. 2016;109. pp. 9-444.
42. Ge C, Peters S, Olsson A, et al. Diesel engine exhaust exposure, smoking, and lung cancer subtype risks: a pooled exposure–response analysis of 14 case–control studies. Am J Respir Crit Care Med. 2020;202:402-11.
43. IARC Working Group on the Evaluation of Carcinogenic Risks to Humans Household use of solid fuels and high-temperature frying. IARC Monogr Eval Carcinog Risks Hum 2010;95:1–430.
44. US Environmental Protection Agency. Integrated Risk Information System (IRIS) on Asbestos. Washington, DC: National Center for Environmental Assessment. Office of Research and Development. [online] Available from https://cfpub.epa.gov/ncea/iris/iris_documents/documents/subst/1026_summary.pdf. [Last accessed September, 2024].
45. Walker NJ, Yoshizawa K, Miller RA, et al. Pulmonary lesions in female Harlan Sprague-Dawley rats following two-year oral treatment with dioxin-like compounds. Toxicol Pathol. 2007; 35:880-9.
46. Singh NP, Singh UP, Guan H, et al. Prenatal exposure to TCDD triggers significant modulation of microRNA expression profile in the thymus that affects consequent gene expression. PLoS One. 2012;7:e45054.
47. Mosquin PL, Rothman KJ. Reanalysis of Reported Associations of Beryllium and Lung Cancer in a Large Occupational Cohort. J Occup Environ Med. 2017;59:274-81.
48. Sarlinova M, Majerova L, Matakova T, et al. Polymorphisms of DNA repair genes and lung cancer in chromium exposure. Adv Exp Med Biol. 2015;833:1-8.
49. Lubin JH, Moore LE, Fraumeni JF Jr, et al. Respiratory cancer and inhaled inorganic arsenic in copper smelter workers: a linear relationship with cumulative exposure that increases with concentration. Environ Health Perspect. 2008;116:1661-5.
50. Ge C, Peters S, Olsson A, et al. Respirable crystalline silica exposure, smoking, and lung cancer subtype risks: a pooled analysis of case–control studies. Am J Respir Crit Care Med. 2020;202:412-21.
51. Engholm G, Englund A. Mortality and cancer incidence in various groups of construction workers. Occup Med. 1995;10:453-81.
52. Pilidis GA, Karakitsios SP, Kassomenos PA, et al. Measurements of benzene and formaldehyde in a medium sized urban environment. Indoor/outdoor health risk implications on special population groups. Environ Monit Assess. 2009;150: 285-94.
53. Man-made mineral fibres and radon. IARC Monographs on the Evaluation of Carcinogenic Risks to Humans. 1988;43. pp. 39-171.
54. World Health Organization. Handbook on Indoor Radon: A Public Health Perspective. Geneva: World Health Organization; 2009.
55. Adithya VSP, Chidambaram S, Prasanna MV, et al. Health Risk Implication and Spatial Distribution of Radon in Groundwater

Along the Lithological Contact in South India. Arch Environ Contam Toxicol. 2021;80:308-18.
56. Lissowska J, Foretova L, Dabek J, et al. Family history and lung cancer risk: international multicentre case-control study in Eastern and Central Europe and meta-analyses. Cancer Causes Control. 2010;21:1091-104.
57. Kanwal M, Ding XJ, Cao Y. Familial risk for lung cancer. Oncol Lett. 2017;13(2):535-42.
58. Yokota J, Shiraishi K, Kohno T. Genetic basis for susceptibility to lung cancer: Recent progress and future directions. Adv Cancer Res. 2010;109:51-72.
59. Lam TK, Gallicchio L, Lindsley K, et al. Cruciferous vegetable consumption and lung cancer risk: a systematic review. Cancer Epidemiol Biomark Prev. 2009;18:184-95.
60. Herr C, Greulich T, Koczulla RA, et al. The role of vitamin D in pulmonary disease: COPD, asthma, infection, and cancer. Respir Res. 2011;12:31.
61. Freudenheim JL, Ritz J, Smith-Warner SA, et al. Alcohol consumption and risk of lung cancer: a pooled analysis of cohort studies. Am J Clin Nutr. 2005;82:657-67.
62. Mizushima Y, Kobayashi M. Clinical characteristics of synchronous multiple lung cancer associated with idiopathic pulmonary fibrosis. A review of Japanese cases. Chest. 1995;108:1272-7.
63. Wu AH, Fontham ET, Reynolds P, et al. Previous lung disease and risk of lung cancer among lifetime nonsmoking women in the United States. Am J Epidemiol. 1995;141:1023-32.
64. Littman AJ, Jackson LA, Vaughan TL. Chlamydia pneumoniae and lung cancer: epidemiologic evidence. Cancer Epidemiol Biomark Prev. 2005;14:773-8.
65. Grulich AE, van Leeuwen MT, Falster MO, et al. Incidence of cancers in people with HIV/AIDS compared with immunosuppressed transplant recipients: a meta-analysis. Lancet. 2007;370:59-67.

Lung Cancer: Clinical Manifestations

CHAPTER 150

Javid Ahmad Malik

INTRODUCTION

There is a rapid change in the current scene of clinical manifestations of lung cancer all over the world. Because of the recent advances in the diagnostic and treatment modalities, there have occurred significant variations of clinical features than those described in the past in the earlier medical literature. Commonly, lung cancer is recognized late in its natural history and only 20% may proceed to curative resection.[1] The number of potentially resectable tumors at the time of diagnosis is much less in India. Lung cancer produces more symptoms in adults than any other cancer, which includes both respiratory and constitutional symptoms.[2]

The symptoms and signs of bronchogenic carcinoma may be caused by the local tumor, invasion of the tumor into the adjacent structures, regional lymph node enlargement, growth at anatomically discontiguous sites after dissemination. and effects of tumor products. Accordingly, the spectrum of clinical presentation of lung cancer can be divided into: (1) local manifestations, (2) metastatic manifestations, and (3) nonmetastatic systemic manifestations (also called paraneoplastic syndromes). Most of the lung cancer patients in developing countries like India have lower mean age and advanced disease at diagnosis with 52% patients having evidence of metastases.[3-5]

LOCAL MANIFESTATIONS

Hemoptysis

Although the cardinal symptom of lung cancer, particularly in an elderly smoker, hemoptysis, is neither the most common feature nor diagnostic of cancer. Hemoptysis is one specific symptom that prompts rapid consultation from the physician.[6] It is usually caused by bronchial mucosal ulceration; thus, it tends to be scanty. If the tumor erodes the bronchial or the pulmonary artery **(Fig. 1)**, hemoptysis may be massive resulting in potentially fatal hemodynamic or airway compromise. Chest radiograph in a small percentage of patients may be normal. In the developing countries, tuberculosis is a competing diagnosis at all ages.

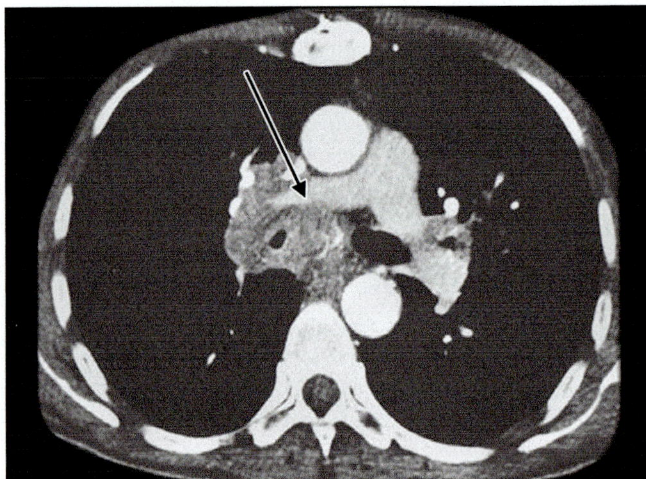

FIG. 1: Contrast computed tomography scan showing a large right hilar mass causing invasion and narrowing of the right pulmonary artery (arrow).

Cough

Cough is the most common presenting symptom of lung cancer, but it does not per se alarm the physician to look for malignancy, hence the delay in the diagnosis.[7,8] The development of new cough or a recent increase in the preexisting chronic productive cough in a middle-aged smoker raises suspicion of lung cancer. In smokers of more than 35 years of age, any new cough that persists for more than 2 weeks should be taken as suspicious of malignancy and investigated accordingly. Among the initial symptoms of lung cancer, cough is present in more than 65% patients and productive cough in more than 25% of patients and is more likely among patients with tumor originating in the airways. In patients with chronic lung disease, a change in the character of an established cough may actually herald the development of lung cancer. Other conditions that can contribute to cough in these patients include esophageal reflux, coexisting chronic obstructive pulmonary disease (COPD), or congestive heart failure.[9]

Bronchorrhea, i.e., expectoration of large amounts of mucoid sputum, occurs in 10% of patients with some variants of invasive adenocarcinoma (formerly known as BAC or bronchioloalveolar carcinoma). Endobronchial tumors cause cough either by airway obstruction and its associated postobstructive pneumonia or by bronchial mucosal ulceration, whereas peripheral tumors cause cough primarily by pleural involvement.

Breathlessness

Like cough, dyspnea is the other most commonly reported symptom, more commonly in men, older patients, and those with lower quality of life scores. The incidence of dyspnea is higher when pain and anxiety predominate.[10] Various causes of dyspnea in patients with lung cancer include the following:

- Direct involvement of the respiratory system by the tumor (major airway obstruction, consolidation, carcinomatous lymphangitis)
- Indirect respiratory complications (postobstructive pneumonia, pleural effusion, phrenic nerve paralysis)
- Treatment-related causes (anemia or radiation and chemotherapy-induced lung toxicity)
- Respiratory complications that occur more frequently in these patients (pulmonary embolism and lung infections)
- Comorbid conditions (COPD, asthma, heart failure, prior lung resection, pericardial effusion, and malnutrition)
- No obvious cause of breathlessness but the patient may have significant respiratory muscle weakness, due to general weight loss and the muscle deconditioning of advanced illness

Chest Pain

An ill-defined chest discomfort which is intermittent and aching in quality is common in bronchogenic carcinoma, occurring in up to 50% of patients at diagnosis. Definite pleuritic pain is the result of direct spread of the tumor to the pleural surface and is usually a manifestation of peripheral neoplasms (adenocarcinoma or large-cell carcinoma) because of their tendency to seed pleura. It is the invasion of pain receptors in the parietal pleura by the tumor that produces typical pleuritic pain which frequently disappears with accumulation of pleural fluid. Once the malignancy spreads beyond the pleura into the chest wall, it produces continuous pain that usually interferes with sleep. Shoulder pain that typically radiates along the ulnar distribution of arm may originate from local extension of tumor growing in the apex of the lung involving eighth cervical and first and second thoracic nerves (Pancoast's or superior sulcus tumor).

METASTATIC MANIFESTATIONS

Intrathoracic Metastasis

Superior Vena Cava Syndrome

The thin vessel wall coupled with low intravascular pressure and surrounding lymph nodes makes superior vena cava (SVC) vulnerable to extrinsic compression and obstruction by the malignant tumor, leading to increased venous pressure in the head, neck, and upper thorax producing a clinically unique entity known as superior vena cava syndrome (SVCS). Bronchogenic carcinoma accounts for 46–75% of all cases of SVC obstruction; the most common histological subtype associated with SVCS is small-cell carcinoma.[11] At the time of diagnosis, SVC obstruction is present in 10% of patients with small-cell lung cancer (SCLC) and 1.7% with non-small-cell lung cancer (NSCLC).[12] Malignancies other than lung cancer that are responsible for obstruction of SVC in 20% of the cases include lymphoma, mesothelioma, and metastatic mediastinal lymphadenopathy and the remaining 20% patients can have benign etiologies like granulomatous mediastinitis, mediastinal fibrosis, intrathoracic goiter or aneurysm, placement of pacemakers or thrombosis complicating central venous catheterization. SVC obstruction may occur due to direct compression by the primary tumor, compression by enlarged right paratracheal metastatic lymph nodes, or intraluminal thrombosis **(Fig. 2)**.

Symptoms of SVCS are often debilitating, tend to get exacerbated in supine position, include progressive swelling of neck, face, eyelids, arms and upper chest, conjunctival congestion, epistaxis, tinnitus, headache, disturbances in vision, and sensorium.[11] Neck veins are distended and non-pulsatile, well-developed collaterals are usually obvious on neck and anterior chest wall. SVC obstruction may get

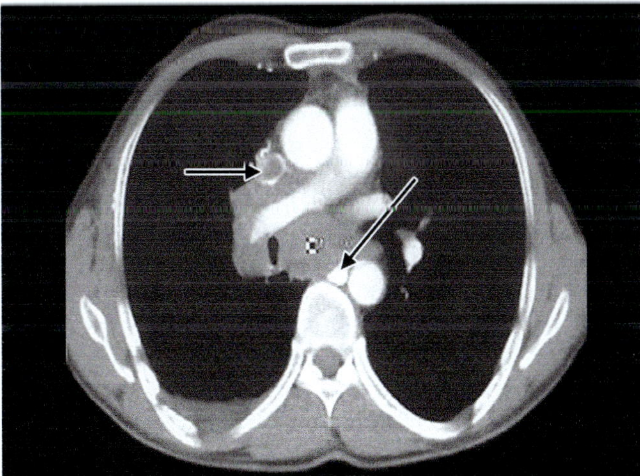

FIG. 2: Contrast CT scan chest of a patient of small-cell carcinoma showing a thrombus in superior vena cava (short arrow). Enlargement of right hilar, subcarinal, and azygoesophageal recess lymph nodes is also seen. Note pleural effusion on right side and dilated azygos vein (long arrow) due to blood diversion.

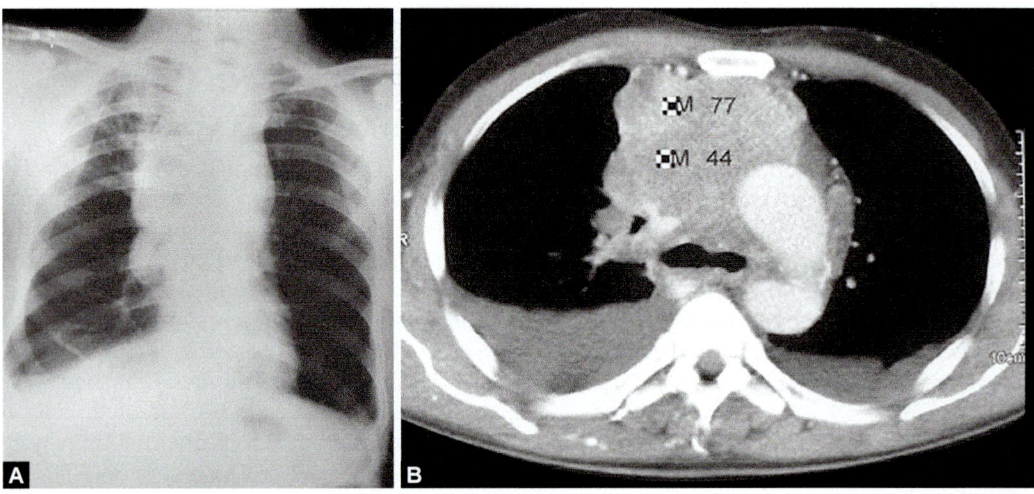

FIGS. 3A AND B: (A) Chest radiograph showing massive mediastinal adenopathy with right pleural effusion in superior vena cava obstruction in a 65-year-old male who presented with rapidly progressive swelling of neck, face, and neck vein distension. (B) Contrast CT scan showing a huge mediastinal mass causing posterior displacement and invasion of the aortic arch and superior vena cava with bilateral pleural effusion. The diagnosis of small-cell carcinoma was confirmed by bronchoscopic biopsy.

complicated with jugular venous and cerebrovascular thrombosis. Although the radiograph of chest may show nonspecific mediastinal widening, diagnosis is usually confirmed by a contrast CT scan **(Figs. 3A and B)** which not only demonstrates the blockage of SVC with collateral formation but also suggests the most likely underlying etiology.

Malignant Pleural Effusion

Pleural effusions that occur due to direct pleural involvement by bronchogenic carcinoma occur in 7–15% of lung cancer patients. Paramalignant pleural effusions may be due to postobstructive pneumonia complicated by parapneumonic effusion, pulmonary embolism and infarction, chylothorax due to obstruction of the thoracic duct, radiation therapy, and chemotherapy.[13] Lung cancer patients may also have pleural effusions that are due to concurrent nonmalignant disorders like congestive heart failure, renal disease, or hypoproteinemia.

Dyspnea, the most common presenting symptom of malignant pleural effusion, is reported by more than 50% of patients. Although the exact mechanism of dyspnea in pleural effusions is unclear, various mechanical factors influencing the chest wall, depression of the ipsilateral diaphragm, mediastinum and its contents, pleural space, and the lung itself, all may contribute to dyspnea. Malignant pleural effusion if massive **(Figs. 4A and B)** may also produce other symptoms such as orthopnea, cough, and chest discomfort.

Recurrent Laryngeal Nerve Palsy

Patients of lung cancer may develop hoarseness of voice because of vocal cord paralysis due to recurrent laryngeal nerve involvement. It produces cough that lacks explosive quality of a normal cough resulting in ineffectual expiratory noise (bovine cough). Recurrent laryngeal nerve palsy occurs in 2–18% of lung cancer patients, is associated with poor expectoration of tracheobronchial secretions, and has an increased risk of aspiration.[14] Left recurrent laryngeal nerve is more commonly involved due to entrapment by the tumor or by the metastatic mediastinal lymph nodes, as it passes over the left main bronchus and loops around the aortic arch. Right recurrent laryngeal nerve loops around the right subclavian artery at the root of neck and may be involved by thoracic inlet tumor or metastatic cervical nodes.

Phrenic Nerve Paralysis

Diaphragmatic paralysis may complicate lung cancer due to phrenic nerve entrapment by the tumor in the mediastinum.[14] In unilateral phrenic nerve dysfunction, the patient may not have any specific symptom; it may be incidentally discovered on the chest radiograph from the presence of an elevated hemidiaphragm. In bilateral phrenic nerve paralysis, patients are severely symptomatic and have orthopnea and a downhill disease course.

Pancoast Syndrome

Pancoast tumor (also known as thoracic inlet or superior sulcus tumor), first reported in 1924 by Henry Pancoast, is a complication of local extension of an apical lung cancer.[15] It is usually associated with squamous cell lung cancer, but any histological type of bronchogenic carcinoma can produce this syndrome. Pancoast tumors comprise fewer than 5% of all lung cancers and result from the involvement of the lower part of brachial plexus by the tumor producing

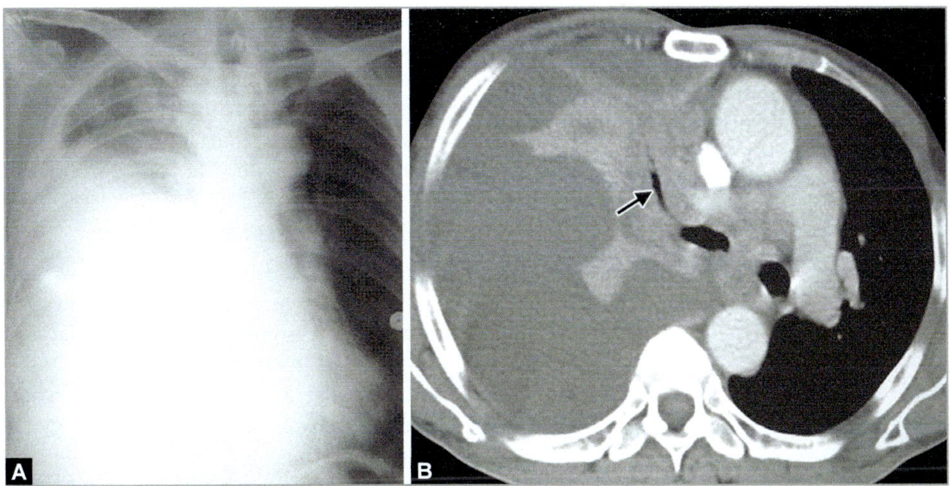

FIGS. 4A AND B: Malignant pleural effusion. (A) Chest X-ray showing massive pleural effusion on the right side. (B) Contrast-enhanced CT scan chest showing massive pleural effusion causing compression of the right upper lobe bronchus (arrow) and collapse of the underlying lung along with displacement of mediastinal structures to the left. Bronchoscopy in this 70-year-old male revealed an endobronchial growth and pleural fluid cytology confirmed metastatic non-small-cell lung cancer.

pain in the lower part of shoulder and inner aspect of arm along C8, T1, and T2 distribution that may be associated with sensory loss, weakness, and wasting of the small muscles of hand. Incomplete forms of Pancoast syndrome are also seen in clinical practice. Radiologically, in addition to the apical lung mass, Pancoast tumor is often characterized by the destruction of first and second ribs posteriorly and sometimes of the transverse process or vertebral body. In the anterior superior sulcus tumor, the predominant complaint is chest pain; the imaging studies reveal destruction of anterior ends of the first and second ribs and invasion of subclavian vessels. In order to determine the extent of involvement of neurovascular structures, a magnetic resonance imaging (MRI) scan is often required in addition to a CT scan in the evaluation of Pancoast tumor.[16]

Horner Syndrome

Horner syndrome is a consequence of invasion by the apical lung cancer of the lower cervical and first thoracic ganglia, which frequently fuse into a single ganglion, the stellate ganglion. It may be observed in 20–50% of bronchogenic carcinoma patients at presentation. Its clinical components include ipsilateral ptosis, miosis, enophthalmos, and lack of facial sweating (anhidrosis). Application of topical cocaine to the miotic eye fails to cause pupillary dilatation, while appropriate dilatation is noted in the unaffected eye. Horner syndrome is usually a complication of superior sulcus lung tumor but may very rarely complicate spontaneous pneumothorax that produces mediastinal shift and consequent mechanical traction of the sympathetic ganglion.[17,18]

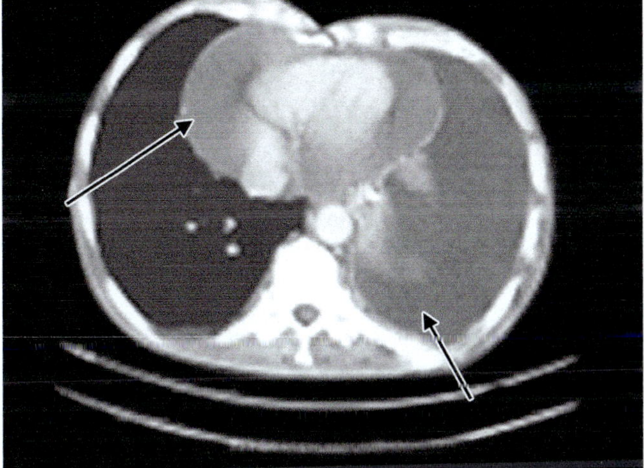

FIG. 5: Malignant pericardial effusion. A 65-year-old male patient had signs of pleural effusion and volume loss on left hemithorax. Contrast CT scan chest showing pericardial effusion (long thin arrow) and volume loss on the left side with massive pleural effusion (short thick arrow) on the same side. Bronchoscopy revealed an endobronchial growth that completely occluded the left main bronchus. The patient subsequently developed cardiac tamponade that needed pericardial catheter drainage.

Involvement of Heart and Pericardium

Cardiac and pericardial metastases from bronchogenic carcinoma usually occur by direct lymphatic spread. In lung cancer, cardiac involvement is reported in 15% of the cases at autopsy.[19] Pericardium is the most common site of cardiac involvement in lung cancer **(Fig. 5)**. Some patients may even develop cardiac tamponade.

Involvement of Esophagus

Dysphagia due to esophageal compression by massively enlarged metastatic hilar and mediastinal nodes is an unusual clinical feature of lung cancer and is generally a late symptom.

Extrathoracic Metastasis

Metastases from lung cancer may occur in virtually every organ system but are more common in brain, bones, liver, adrenal glands, and lymph nodes. Extrathoracic spread of bronchogenic carcinoma makes a patient clearly inoperable. Metastatic disease in general is more common with SCLC than with NSCLC.

Brain Metastases

Intracranial metastases constituted the first clinical problem in 10% of SCLC patients; the cumulative incidence at 2 years is more than 50%.[20] Brain metastases are more common from lung cancer than from any other primary site, lung being the primary site of 70% of cancers that initially present with symptomatic brain metastases.[21] Squamous cell lung cancer metastasizes to brain less often than adenocarcinoma and large-cell carcinomas. Sometimes, brain metastases form the only extrathoracic site of spread of lung cancer.

Intracranial metastatic lung cancer usually presents with headache, nausea, and vomiting and rarely with impaired intellectual function or personality changes. Seizures and motor or sensory neurological deficits may occur. Progressive neurological symptoms in cerebral metastases usually complicate the widespread disease. Rarely, brain metastases are detected when primary bronchogenic carcinoma is asymptomatic and radiological examination of the chest is normal. If the patient with brain metastases is not treated, neurologic deterioration occurs quickly.[22] Lung cancer can metastasize to any part of the brain **(Figs. 6A and B)** and cause devastating neurological complications.

Skeletal Metastases

Bronchogenic carcinoma frequently metastasizes to vertebrae **(Figs. 7A and B)** and ribs; however, any bone in the body may be involved. Bony metastases usually produce pain which is invariably progressive. If the ribs are involved, pain gets aggravated by coughing and body movement. Skeletal metastases may also lead to pathological fractures. When bone marrow is invaded by metastatic lung cancer, it leads to cytopenias or leukoerythroblastosis.

Radiograph of the affected bone may reveal lytic lesions, but it is not as sensitive as isotope bone scanning in detecting skeletal metastases. Though sensitive, bone scan lacks specificity; up to 50% of the scans may be false positive, mostly due to benign metabolic bone disorders. Bone scan is more useful in small-cell carcinoma, because of the higher incidence of skeletal metastases with SCLC than with NSCLC.[23] Rarely, bone biopsy is required to confirm the metastatic spread of bronchial tumor.

Spinal Cord Compression

Epidural or vertebral metastases may complicate lung cancer producing an oncologic emergency.[24] Such patients need immediate assessment by a neurologist. Spinal cord metastases are less common and tend to occur in patients with cerebral metastases.

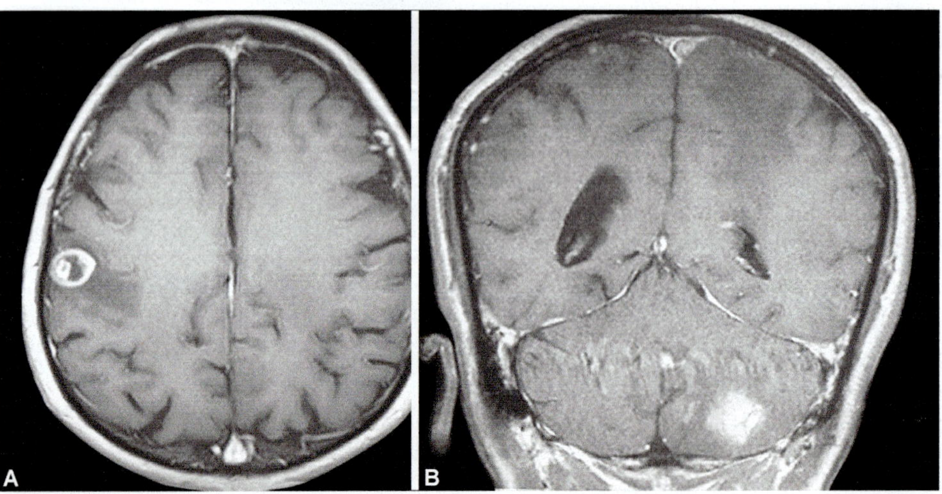

FIGS. 6A AND B: Brain metastasis from bronchogenic carcinoma. (A) Postgadolinium T1W MRI of the brain in a patient of small-cell carcinoma lung showing a ring-enhancing lesion with a central nodule and thick walls surrounded by vasogenic edema in the right parietal lobe. (B) Coronal postgadolinium MRI in a 55-year-old male patient showing metastatic deposits in the cerebellum with avid enhancement of the lesion.

Courtesy: Dr Irfan Rubani, Radiologist, SKIMS.

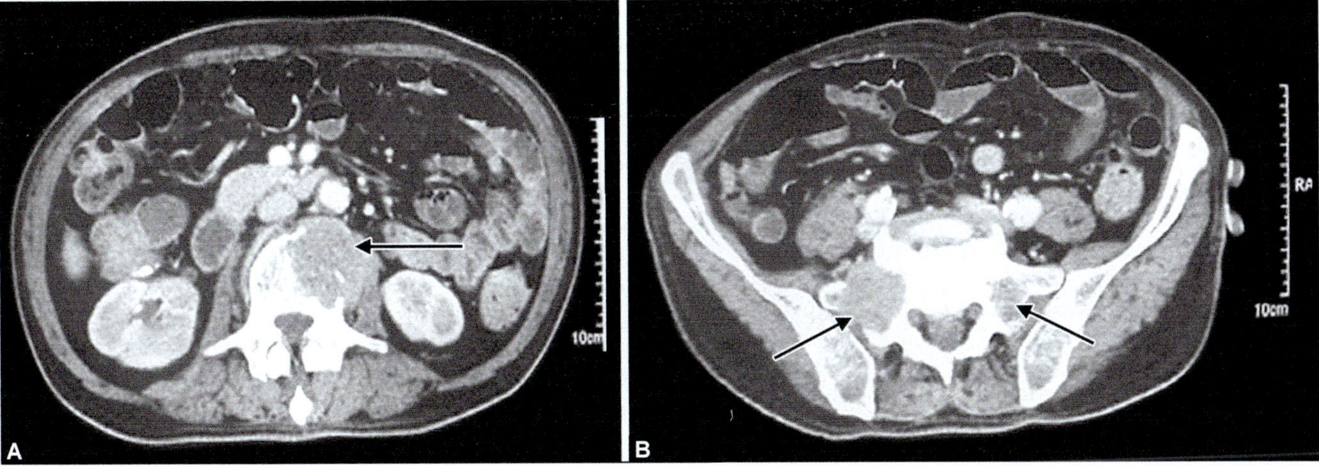

FIGS. 7A AND B: Spinal metastasis from bronchogenic carcinoma. CT scan showing lumbar (A) vertebral body deposits and (B) multiple sacral deposits.

Courtesy: Dr Naseer Choh, Radiologist, SKIMS Soura.

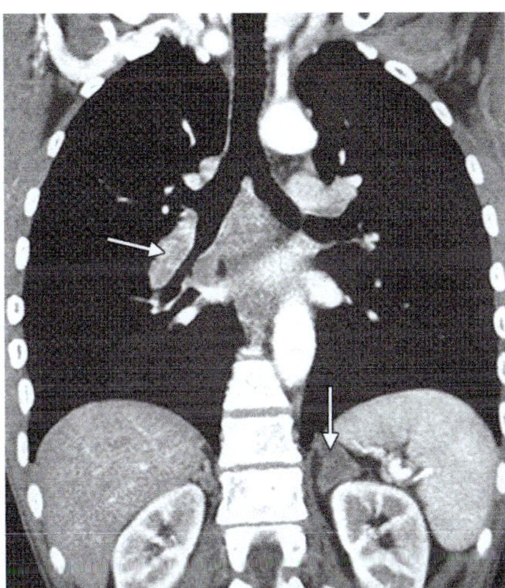

FIG. 8: Coronal contrast CT scan revealing a right hilar bronchogenic carcinoma (short arrow) with metastasis in the left adrenal gland (long arrow).

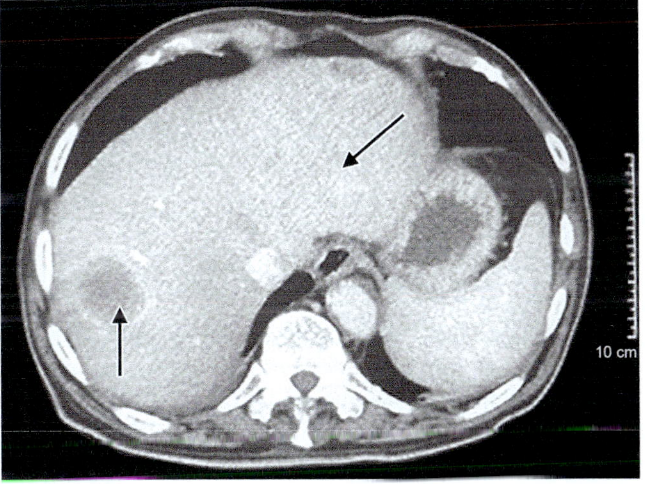

FIG. 9: Hepatic metastasis in lung cancer. Contrast CT scan of a 65-year-old male with small-cell carcinoma of lung showing multiple ring enhancing lesions in liver (arrows). These lesions on fine needle aspiration cytology (FNAC) were found to be metastatic deposits.

Adrenal Metastases

Involvement of adrenal glands **(Fig. 8)** by metastatic lung cancer, usually by small-cell carcinoma, is common but rarely produces adrenal insufficiency.[14] Solitary adrenal metastasis if resected along with primary lung tumor has a better prognosis with a 3-year survival rate of 38%.[25] Surgical resection for solitary adrenal metastases, in comparison to chemotherapy alone for usual disseminated metastatic disease, prolongs the median survival, resulting in survival rate of 17% at 15 years.

Lymph Node Metastases

An enlarged lymph node due to metastatic lung cancer is extremely helpful in facilitating both diagnosis and staging. Supraclavicular lymph nodes are the more common sites of palpable lymphadenopathy in lung cancer, involved in 15–20% of patients during the course of the disease.[14] Fine needle aspiration of the enlarged lymph node has high sensitivity and little morbidity. Biopsy of these metastatic lymph nodes is frequently preferred by many oncologists in clinical practice.

Hepatic Metastases

Liver metastases occur commonly with lung cancer **(Fig. 9)**; their presence carries a very poor prognosis.[14] The patient usually complains of fatigue and weight loss; on physical examination, the liver is hard and irregularly enlarged. However, liver function test results are seldom abnormal until the metastases are numerous and large. Both ultrasonography and CT scan are equally good in picking up hepatic metastases, a finding that makes the patient inoperable.

Paraneoplastic Syndromes

A group of clinical disorders that are associated with malignant diseases, not directly related to the physical effects of primary or metastatic tumors, are known as paraneoplastic syndromes.[26] These syndromes occur in about 10% of patients with lung cancer, more frequently associated with small-cell cancers. The pathogenetic mechanisms by which paraneoplastic syndromes occur are not fully understood in all cases, but in many, they appear to relate to either the production of biologically active substances by the tumor itself (e.g., polypeptide hormones or cytokines) or in response to the tumor (e.g., antibodies).[27] The size of the primary tumor has no impact on the extent of paraneoplastic symptoms. These paraneoplastic syndromes can precede the diagnosis of malignant disease by months, or even years, may occur late in the course of the illness, or herald the first sign of recurrence of lung cancer. Paraneoplastic syndromes may simulate metastatic cancer, thereby leading to inappropriate palliation rather than curative treatment of the underlying tumor. With successful treatment of lung cancer, the paraneoplastic phenomena usually resolve.

ENDOCRINE SYNDROMES

Cushing Syndrome

Lung cancer is the most common source of ectopic secretion of adrenocorticotropic hormone (ACTH) among non-pituitary neoplasms. Biologically active ACTH resulting in adrenal gland hyperplasia and hyperfunction is usually produced by small-cell carcinoma (85%), uncommonly by carcinoid tumors (10%) and adenocarcinoma (5%) of the lung. Cushing syndrome has been described in 1–5% of patients with SCLC. Paraneoplastic Cushing syndrome may rarely be caused by ectopic production of corticotropin-releasing hormone (CRH) which leads to excessive ACTH secretion from the pituitary gland.

Because of the short natural history of SCLC, these patients usually do not develop the classical features of Cushing syndrome. Diagnosis is usually suggested by features of acute hypercortisolism such as hypertension, hyperglycemia, and hypokalemic alkalosis. Muscle weakness associated with hypokalemia may be profound. Proximal myopathy and edema are commonly found on physical examination.[28] However, full-blown Cushing syndrome may be caused by certain slow-growing cancers like pulmonary carcinoids and tumorlets.[29] The clinical course of Cushing syndrome may be complicated by devastating fungal infections.

Though the biochemical abnormalities of cortisol metabolism including the raised ACTH levels, loss of diurnal variation, and failure of cortisol levels to suppress after dexamethasone administration are found in 50% patient's with SCLC, the clinical syndrome is obvious in <5%.[27,30] Diagnosis is confirmed by demonstration of plasma ACTH level of >22 pmol/L, plasma cortisol of >600 nmol/L, and 24-hour urinary-free cortisol of >400 nmol/day, which do not suppress after a high-dose dexamethasone.

In addition to the effective treatment of the underlying lung malignancy, hypercortisolism needs to be addressed early to reduce the morbidity. Chemotherapy with or without irradiation for small-cell carcinoma and surgical resection for carcinoid tumors should be offered to the patient as early as possible. When the tumor cannot be resected or ectopic ACTH secretion cannot be controlled, bilateral adrenalectomy may be effective in some patients. Ketoconazole, metyrapone, aminoglutethimide, or octreotide may be used to induce effective steroid synthesis inhibition.[31] Ectopic ACTH production by small-cell carcinoma of lung is associated with aggressive tumor behavior, hence poor prognosis.[30]

Hypercalcemia

Overall, 10% patients of lung cancer have hypercalcemia, which usually complicates squamous cell carcinoma that secretes parathyroid hormone-related peptide (PTH-rP).[32] Hypercalcemia may also be seen with adenocarcinoma, but it is extremely rare in patients with small-cell carcinoma of lung. Although bone metastases may be found in patients with lung cancer and hypercalcemia, most commonly humoral mechanisms account for the hypercalcemia.[33] Bronchogenic carcinoma causes hypercalcemia primarily by ectopic production of PTH-rP, uncommonly by osteolytic metastatic deposits, and very rarely by ectopic secretion of PTH.[33]

The diagnosis of PTH-rP-associated paraneoplastic syndrome is considered if serum calcium level exceeds 10.5 mg/dL. Hypercalcemia initially produces nausea, vomiting, constipation, polyuria, and nocturia resulting in hypovolemia and renal failure. As serum calcium goes up, the patient may become confused and drowsy and ultimately, coma may supervene misleading the physician toward intracranial metastases. The clinical behavior of PTH-rP associated paraneoplastic syndrome is highly unpredictable; the patient may present with subtle symptoms or as medical emergency. Bone scan should be obtained to exclude skeletal metastases. An elevated PTH-rP level confirms the diagnosis in the absence of bone metastases. Other causes of hypercalcemia (sarcoidosis, hyperthyroidism, and drugs like thiazides, lithium, and vitamin D) should also be considered in the differential diagnosis. Primary hyperparathyroidism should be excluded by PTH radioimmunoassay.

Parathyroid hormone-related peptide-associated hypercalcemia usually develops in patients with advanced lung cancer; treatment may not be always required. Control or treatment of underlying lung cancer constitutes the most effective method of managing hypercalcemia. Intravenous saline, usually with furosemide diuresis, is often sufficient in symptomatic mild-to moderate hypercalcemia. In severe hypercalcemia, calcitonin is used because of its rapid onset of action. Bisphosphonates are used for long-term control of hypercalcemia and may cause a dramatic fall in serum calcium.[34] Glucocorticoids though frequently used have an unreliable calcium-lowering effect in this syndrome. Similarly, mithramycin, a cytotoxic antibiotic, is rarely used because of its toxicity.

SYNDROME OF INAPPROPRIATE ANTIDIURETIC HORMONE

Elevated antidiuretic hormone (ADH) levels and impaired water handling are found in 30–70% of patients with lung cancer, but the production of excess ADH does not always produce symptoms.[35] Only 1–5% of lung cancer patients have symptoms that are attributable to the syndrome of inappropriate antidiuretic hormone (SIADH) production. The SIADH production is mainly associated with SCLC, although other malignant tumors of the lung may rarely be associated with this syndrome.[36] The excess levels of ADH have been reported to originate from either ectopic production by lung cancer cells or inappropriate peripheral baroreceptor stimulation of ADH release from the hypothalamus.[37] Excess of ADH leads to abnormal water retention resulting in hyponatremia and low plasma osmolality. Urinary loss of sodium continues at a level inappropriate for plasma sodium concentration resulting in urinary osmolality twice as high as concomitant plasma osmolality. The exact role of atrial natriuretic peptide (ANP) in hyponatremia of malignancy is not known, though it is also ectopically secreted by the lung tumors. ANP also affects renal salt and water handling. In an individual patient, increased levels of ANP may contribute to hyponatremia by inducing natriuresis.[37] If plasma sodium concentration is marginally low, the patient may be asymptomatic or may have confusion, headache, nausea, and vomiting. A sodium level of <115 mmol/L can produce convulsions, coma, and death. However, more often than not, lung cancer-associated hyponatremia is only a laboratory abnormality.

Like for any other paraneoplastic phenomenon, the treatment of SIADH consists that of the underlying tumor. The syndrome resolves within 3 weeks after the initiation of combination cytotoxic chemotherapy in 80% of SCLC patients, but commonly recurs with tumor progression. Clinicians should keep in mind that some of the drugs like cisplatin, vincristine, melphalan, and cyclophosphamide used to treat these cancers can themselves produce SIADH.[38]

Other measures which may be effective to counter hyponatremia while awaiting the effects of chemotherapy include strict fluid restriction (i.e., 500 mL/day), which alone may be sufficient to maintain serum sodium above 128 mEq/L. If a patient does not comply with fluid restriction or if it does not prove effective, demeclocycline, which blocks the action of vasopressin in the renal tubule, is used in a daily oral dose of 600–1200 mg.[39] Severe symptomatic hyponatremia is treated with hypertonic saline (3%) along with intravenous loop diuretic that enhances net free-water clearance. The sodium level should not be raised by >2 mEq/hr because it may lead to central pontine myelinolysis, an acute neurologic catastrophe. Unlike ectopic ACTH production, SIADH does not worsen the prognosis of small-cell cancer.

Acromegaly

Carcinoid tumor is the most common cause of acromegaly associated with lung malignancy. Small-cell carcinoma can also produce this syndrome. Paraneoplastic acromegaly is commonly caused by secretion of growth hormone-releasing hormone (GHRH) and rarely by growth hormone (GH) into the blood. These patients develop thick leathery skin, prominent skin folds, hypertrophy of face and extremities, and sometimes diabetes and hypertension. Increased plasma levels of GHRH and insulin-like growth factor-1 (IGF-1) in the presence of a lung tumor virtually establish the diagnosis. Lung cancer-related acromegaly promptly responds to surgical resection as well as to radiotherapy. Patients who are not eligible for resection or irradiation should receive octreotide, which inhibits GHRH secretion from the tumor and decreases GH and IGF-1 levels in the serum.

NEUROLOGICAL SYNDROMES

A variety of poorly understood neurological syndromes including Lambert–Eaton myasthenic syndrome (LEMS), limbic encephalopathy, polyneuropathy, cerebellar degeneration, retinopathy, opsoclonus–myoclonus, and autonomic neuropathy have been reported.[40,41] Paraneoplastic neurologic syndromes affect 5% of lung cancer patients, associated almost exclusively with small-cell carcinoma. The severity of neurologic symptoms is unrelated to the tumor bulk, more often seen in patients with limited disease; in some patients, a primary malignant lesion may be undetected before death despite the disabling symptoms.[41-43] The syndromes develop through autoimmune mechanisms as nearly all are associated with the presence of type 1 antineuronal nuclear antibodies (also known as anti-Hu antibodies). Up to 20% of patients with SCLC have detectable circulating levels of anti-Hu antibodies, but paraneoplastic neurologic syndromes may not develop in all of these patients.[41,44]

The diagnosis of a neurologic syndrome should be made only after other causes such as electrolyte imbalance, metastatic disease, cerebral and spinal vascular disease, infections, and treatment toxicity are carefully excluded. These neurological phenomena progress rapidly and cause significant disability. The response of the neurologic syndrome to an effective chemotherapy in patients with small-cell cancer is variable.[28,45] Sustained improvements, particularly in patients with motor or sensory neuropathies, have been reported. The overall prognosis is more favorable in SCLC patients with LEMS than in those without it.[46]

Eaton–Lambert Syndrome

Eaton–Lambert myasthenic syndrome affects up to 5% of patients with SCLC and uncommonly complicates NSCLC. It is caused by the formation of IgG autoantibodies directed at voltage-gated P/Q calcium channels involved in the release of acetylcholine at nerve terminals, thereby producing a functional blockade at the neuromuscular junction.[28,47]

These patients usually present with fatigue, dysphagia, dysarthria, visual blurring, muscle aches, and weakness of pelvic girdle muscles. Unlike in myasthenia gravis, muscle weakness in LEMS improves with exercise and not with anticholinesterases. The syndrome is worse in the morning and improves during the day. Although extraocular muscle involvement is uncommon, ptosis is often seen.[48] There is increased muscle action potential with repeated nerve stimulation on electromyography. Demonstration of IgG autoantibodies in the serum of patients with SCLC confirms the diagnosis of Eaton–Lambert syndrome. Eaton–Lambert syndrome usually resolves with chemotherapy of small-cell carcinoma. If treatment of lung tumor does not improve neuromuscular weakness, remission may be induced with azathioprine, intravenous gamma globulin, diaminopyridine, or plasma exchange.

Encephalomyelitis and Sensory Neuropathy

This syndrome is associated with SCLC, and the neuronal damage is mediated by IgG anti-Hu antibody.

These patients may present with progressive sensory loss in hands and feet, myelopathy, brainstem involvement or features of limbic encephalopathy including behavioral changes, memory loss, or convulsions. Autonomic neuropathy resulting in postural hypotension or gastrointestinal motility disturbances may also occur. Diagnosis of encephalomyelitis is suggested by the MRI images which show an increased T2 signal in the affected areas of the brain and is confirmed by demonstration of anti-Hu antibody in the serum. Removal of culprit IgG by plasmapheresis and corticosteroids' administration is effective in only 15% of these patients.

Paraneoplastic Cerebellar Degeneration

Some patients of SCLC develop cerebellar degeneration leading to nystagmus, impaired coordination, and ataxia. These patients have anti-Hu antibodies in serum and frequently tend to develop encephalitis or sensory neuropathy.

Cancer-associated Retinopathy

Cancer-associated retinopathy is a rare paraneoplastic syndrome that occurs as the first sign of occult small-cell carcinoma of lung. Ganglion cells of retina are characteristically damaged by binding of autoantibodies to recoverin, a photoreceptor-specific protein. Clinically, these patients have photosensitivity, rapid loss of vision, night blindness, visual field defects, and arteriolar narrowing. In a given clinical setting, demonstration of antirecoverin antibody establishes the diagnosis of cancer-associated retinopathy. Cancer-associated retinopathy responds to systemic steroids but not to the chemotherapy for primary tumor.

Opsoclonus and Myoclonus

This rare paraneoplastic syndrome is associated with both SCLC and NSCLC. The patient shows rapid involuntary conjugate eye movements in both the horizontal and the vertical directions. Some SCLC patients with this syndrome have anti-Hu antibody in serum.

HEMATOLOGICAL SYNDROMES

Granulocytosis

Granulocytosis with an absolute white cell count of 10,000–25,000 occurs in 20% patients of NSCLC. The specific ectopic hormone responsible for paraneoplastic granulocytosis has not been characterized, although some non-small-cell tumors may produce various cytokines like interleukin-6 (IL-6), granulocyte colony-stimulating factor (G-CSF), or granulocyte–monocyte colony-stimulating factor (GM-CSF). The increase in total white cell count may also be associated with neutrophilia and eosinophilia.[49] Bone marrow biopsy is usually normal. Diagnosis is made on exclusion; granulocytosis per se does not produce any symptom in these patients.

Thrombocytosis

Paraneoplastic thrombocytosis is a common phenomenon observed in 40% patients of both small-cell and non-small-cell carcinomas. The exact pathogenetic mechanism of lung cancer-associated thrombocytosis is not known; it is most likely linked to a megakaryocyte cytokine, i.e., IL-6. Like granulocytosis, lung cancer-associated thrombocytosis is asymptomatic, diagnosed if bone marrow biopsy is normal and platelet count exceeds 500,000/mm.[2]

Thromboembolism

The pathogenetic basis of lung cancer-associated venous thromboembolism is not known, no proteins or cytokines have been linked to it. It can complicate both NSCLC and SCLC. Trousseau syndrome or recurrent migratory venous thrombophlebitis is more commonly associated with bronchogenic carcinoma than pancreatic or other gastrointestinal cancers. Isolated venous thrombosis is treated with oral warfarin, but long-term heparin is more effective than warfarin in recurrent thrombosis (Trousseau syndrome).[50]

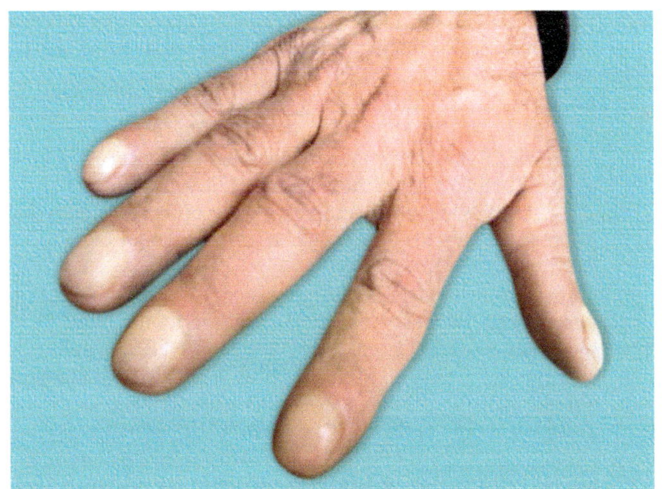

FIG. 10: Digital clubbing in a 56-year-old patient of squamous cell carcinoma of lung.

SKELETAL

Digital Clubbing and Hypertrophic Osteoarthropathy

Digital clubbing **(Fig. 10),** which is more common among women than men (40% vs. 19%), is observed in 30% patients and hypertrophic pulmonary osteoarthropathy (HPOA) in 10% patients of NSCLC.[51] Quantitative indexes of the nail profile angle, hyponychial angle, and phalangeal depth ratio can be determined to assist in identifying clubbing.[52] Hypertrophic pulmonary osteoarthropathy may be present in up to 5% of patients with squamous and adenocarcinoma of lung and 1% patients with small-cell carcinoma. HPOA is a systemic disorder, which involves both a painful symmetrical arthropathy, usually of the ankles, wrists and knees, and periosteal new bone formation in the distal long bones of the limbs.

The exact mechanism responsible for the development of clubbing and HPOA is not known. The past explanations included neurogenic, hormonal, and vascular mechanisms.[53] Overexpression of vascular endothelial growth factor (VEGF) has been implicated in the pathogenesis. Bone scans show active deposition of new bone along the inner aspect of periosteum. Clinically, HPOA responds well to surgical resection of the primary lung tumor. In unresectable tumors, corticosteroids and nonsteroidal anti-inflammatory drugs are used for symptomatic relief. For symptom relief, vagotomy can also be done, if thoracotomy is undertaken with an attempt to cure.

MISCELLANEOUS SYNDROMES

There are various other unusual paraneoplastic syndromes known to be associated with bronchogenic carcinoma: Renal (glomerulonephritis, nephrotic syndrome), vasculitic (systemic lupus erythematosus), systemic (fever, anorexia, cachexia), and metabolic (hypouricemia, lactic acidosis).[1,54] Several other endocrinal, neurological, and hematological syndromes, in addition to those listed earlier, can rarely occur.

Cutaneous manifestations of lung cancer are rare, which include dermatomyositis-polymyositis, scleroderma, acanthosis nigricans, papillary dermatosis, erythema gyratum repens, erythema multiforme, exfoliative dermatitis, Sweet syndrome, pruritus, and urticaria.[55] Adenocarcinoma and large-cell bronchogenic carcinoma are known to be associated with gynecomastia due to tumor cell production of human chorionic gonadotropin, which results in overproduction of testicular estrogen.[56]

SUMMARY

There are significant variations in clinical features of lung cancer than those described in the past. Lung cancer produces more symptoms in adults than any other cancer. The symptoms and signs of bronchogenic carcinoma may be caused by the local tumor, invasion into the adjacent structures, regional lymph node enlargement, growth at anatomically discontiguous sites after dissemination and effects of tumor products. There are various other unusual endocrinal, neurological, and haematological paraneoplastic syndromes known to be associated with bronchogenic carcinoma. Cutaneous manifestations of lung cancer are rare but significant. Clubbing and osteoarthropathy are frequently characteristic of lung cancer. Adenocarcinoma and large-cell bronchogenic carcinoma are in particular known to be associated with gynecomastia due to tumor cell production of human chorionic gonadotropin.

REFERENCES

1. Scagliotti G. Symptoms, signs and staging of lung cancer. Eur Respir Mon. 2001;17:86-119.
2. Cooley ME. Symptoms in adults with lung cancer: A systematic research review. J Pain Symptom Manage. 2000;19:137-53.
3. Jindal SK, Malik SK, Dhand R, et al. Bronchogenic carcinoma in Northern India. Thorax. 1982;37:343-7.
4. Sharma CP, Behera D, Aggarwal AN, et al. Radiographic patterns in lung cancer. Indian J Chest Dis Allied Sci. 2002;44:25-30.
5. Behera D, Balamugesh T. Lung Cancer in India. Indian J Chest Dis Allied Sci. 2004;46:269-81.
6. Corner J, Hopkinson J, Fitzsimmons D, et al. Is late diagnosis of lung cancer inevitable? Interview study of patients' recollections of symptoms before diagnosis. Thorax. 2005;60:314-9.
7. Buccheri G, Ferrigno D. Lung cancer: clinical presentation and specialist referral time. Eur Respir J. 2004;24:898-904.

8. Hamilton W, Peters TJ, Round A, et al. What are the clinical features of lung cancer before the diagnosis is made? A population based case-controlled study. Thorax. 2005;60:1059-65.
9. Kvale PA. Chronic cough due to lung tumors: ACCP evidence-based clinical practice guidelines. Chest. 2006;129:147S-53S.
10. Smith EL, Hann DM, Ahles TA, et al. Dyspnea, anxiety, body consciousness, and quality of life in patients with lung cancer. J Pain Symptom Manage. 2001;21:323-9.
11. Yellin A, Rosen A, Reichert N, et al. Superior vena cava syndrome. Am Rev Respir Dis. 1990;141:1114-8.
12. Rowell NP, Gleeson FV. Steroids, radiotherapy, chemotherapy and stents for superior vena caval obstruction in carcinoma of the bronchus: a systematic review. Clin Oncol (R Coll Radiol). 2002;14:338-51.
13. Anthony VB, Lodden Kemper R, Astoul P, et al. Management of malignant pleural effusions. Am J Respir Crit Care Med. 2000;162:1987-2001.
14. Beckles MA, Spiro SG, Colice GL, et al. Initial Evaluation of the Patient with Lung Cancer. Chest. 2003;123:97S-104S.
15. Pancoast HK. Importance of careful roentgen ray investigations of apical chest tumors. JAMA. 1924;83:1407-11.
16. Balcer LJ, Galetta SL. Images in clinical medicine. Pancoast's syndrome. N Engl J Med. 1997;337:1359.
17. Aston SJ, Rosove M. Horner's syndrome occurring with spontaneous pneumothorax. N Engl J Med. 1972;287:1098.
18. Campbell P, Neil T, Wake PN. Horner's syndrome caused by an intercostal drain. Thorax. 1989;44:305-6.
19. Mukai K, Shinkai T, Tominaga K, et al. The incidence of secondary tumors of the heart and pericardium. Jpn J Clin Oncol. 1988;18:195-201.
20. Hirsch FR, Paulson OB, Hansen HH, et al. Intracranial metastases in small cell carcinoma of the lung: prognostic aspects. Cancer. 1983;51:529-33.
21. Merchut MP. Brain metastases from undiagnosed systemic neoplasms. Arch Intern Med. 1989;149:1076-80.
22. Kelly K, Bunn PA. Is it time to reevaluate our approach to the treatment of brain metastases in patients with non-small cell lung cancer? Lung Cancer. 1998;20:85-91.
23. Levenson RM, Sauerbrunn BJL, Ihde DC, et al. Small cell lung cancer: radionuclide bone scans for assessment of tumor extent and response. Am J Roentgenol. 1981;137:31.
24. Baldini EH. Palliative radiation therapy for non-small cell lung cancer. Hematol Oncol Clin North Am. 1997;11:303-19.
25. Luketich JD, Burt ME. Does resection of adrenal metastases from non-small cell lung cancer improve survival? Ann Thorac Surg. 1996; 62:1614-6.
26. Patel AM, Davila DG, Peters SG. Paraneoplastic syndromes associated with lung cancer. Mayo Clin Proc. 1993;68:278-87.
27. Spiro SG, Gould MK, Colice GL; American College of Chest Physicians. Initial evaluation of the patient with lung cancer: symptoms, signs, laboratory tests, and paraneoplastic syndromes: ACCP evidenced-based clinical practice guidelines (2nd edition). Chest. 2007;132(3 Suppl):149S-160S.
28. Eisen T, Hickish T, Smith IE, et al. Small cell lung cancer. Lancet. 1995;345:1285.
29. Arioglu E, Doppman J, Gomes M, et al. Cushing's syndrome caused by corticotropin secretion by pulmonary tumorlets. N Engl J Med. 1998;339:883-6.
30. Sheppard F, Laskey J, Evans W, et al. Cushing's syndrome associated with ectopic corticotrophin production and small cell lung cancer. J Clin Oncol. 1992;10:21-7.
31. Hoffman D, Brigham B. The use of ketoconazole in ectopic adrenocorticotrophic hormone syndrome. Cancer. 1991;67: 1447.
32. Takai E, Yano T, Iguchi H, et al. Tumor induced hypercalcemia and parathyroid- related protein in lung carcinoma. Cancer. 1996;78:1384-7.
33. Mazzone PJ, Arroliga AC. Endocrine paraneoplastic syndromes in lung cancer. Curr Opin Pulm Med. 2003;9:313-20.
34. Ralston SH. Pathogenesis and management of cancer associated hypercalcaemia. Cancer Surv. 1994;21:179-96.
35. Moses AM, Scheinman SJ. Ectopic secretion of neurohypophyseal peptides in patients with malignancy. Endocrinol Metab Clin North Am. 1991;20:489-506.
36. Sorensen JB, Andersen MK, Hansen HH. Syndrome of in appropriate secretion of antidiuretic hormone (SIADH) in malignant disease. J Intern Med. 1995;238:97-110.
37. Johnson BE, Chute JP, Rushin J, et al. A prospective study of patients with lung cancer and hyponatremia of malignancy. Am J Respir Crit Care Med. 1997;156:1669-78.
38. Littlewood TJ, Smith AP. Syndrome of inappropriate antidiuretic hormone secretion due to treatment of lung cancer with cisplatin. Thorax. 1984;39:636-7.
39. Schrier RW. Treatment of hyponatremia. N Engl J Med. 1985; 312:1121.
40. Swash M, Schwartz MS. Paraneoplastic syndromes. In: Johnson RT (Ed). Current Therapy in Neurologic Disease. Philadelphia, PA: BC Decker; 1990. pp. 236-43.
41. Martina T, Clay AS. A 50-year-old woman with bilateral vocal cord paralysis and hilar mass. Chest. 2005;128:1028-31.
42. Elrington GM, Murray NM, Spiro SG, et al. Neurological paraneoplastic syndromes in patients with small cell lung cancer: a prospective survey of 150 patients. J Neurol Neurosurg Psychiatry. 1991;54:764-7.
43. Seute T, Leffers P, ten Velde GP, et al. Neurologic disorders in 432 consecutive patients with small cell lung carcinoma. Cancer. 2004;100:801-6.
44. Darnell RB, Posner JB. Para-neoplastic syndromes involving the nervous system. N Engl J Med. 2003;349:1543-4.
45. Levin KH. Paraneoplastic neuromuscular syndromes. Neurol Clin. 1997;15:597-614.
46. Croteau D, Owainati A, Dalmau J, et al. Response to cancer therapy in a patient with a paraneoplastic choreiform disorder. Neurology. 2001;57:719-22.
47. Nakao YK, Motomura M, Suenaga A, et al. Specificity of omega-conotoxin MV11C-binding and –blocking calcium channel antibodies in Lambert-Eaton myasthenic syndrome. J Neurol. 1999;246:38-44.
48. Mareska M, Gutmann L. Lambert-Eaton myasthenic syndrome. Semin Neurol. 2004;24:149-53.
49. Knox AJ, Johnson CE, Page RL. Eosinophilia associated with thoracic malignancy. Br J Dis Chest. 1986;80:92.
50. Zuger M, Demarmels-Biasiutti F, Wuillemin WA, et al. Subcutaneous low molecular weight heparin for treatment of Trousseau's syndrome. Ann Hematol. 1997;75:165-7.
51. Sridhar KS, Lobo CF, Altman RD. Digital clubbing and lung cancer. Chest. 1998;114:1535-7.
52. Myers KA, Farquhar DR. Does this patient have clubbing? JAMA. 2001;286:341-7.
53. Shneerson JM. Digital clubbing and hypertrophic osteoarthropathy. Br J Dis Chest. 1981;75:113-31.
54. Carbone PP, Frost JK, Feinstein AR, et al. Lung cancer: perspectives and prospects. Ann Intern Med. 1970;73:1003-24.
55. Barnes BE. Dermatomyositis and malignancy. Ann Intern Med. 1976;84:68-76.
56. Rabson AS, Rosen SW, Tashjian AH, et al. Production of human chorionic gonadotrophin in vitro by a cell line derived from a carcinoma of the lung. J Natl Cancer Inst. 1973;50:669-74.

Staging and Management Decisions of Lung Cancer

CHAPTER

151

Pawan Singh, Aman Ahuja

INTRODUCTION

In India, lung cancer is the most frequently diagnosed cancer overall (10.6%) followed by breast and esophagus.[1] Majority of the mortality linked with lung cancer is due to an advanced stage at presentation, age, and added comorbidities. Establishing the clinical stage helps in explaining prognosis, deciding on therapy, and taking management decisions. Uniform staging of the disease also helps in harmonizing the research and communications regarding individual cases. The International Association on Study of Lung Cancer (IASLC) is the leading organization working on staging project for lung cancer.[2] Currently, the 8th TNM version of staging is being practiced whereas the 9th TNM staging project is near its completion. The primary aim of the TNM project is to predict the prognosis as close as to the real-world figures in the paradigm of advancements in management.

Staging is done with the help of clinical examination, radiology, and nuclear scans.[3] In surgically resected cases, pathological staging is also done although the TNM descriptors remain the same. We deliberate upon the current descriptors, types, and pitfalls of staging as well as a brief overview of management decisions according to stages.

DESCRIPTORS

The most used descriptors for clinical staging are T (tumors characteristics), N (nodal involvement), and M (metastasis) **(Table 1)**. Additional descriptors employed in pathological staging include m, y, r, a, L, V, and Pn.[4] Details of additional descriptors of pathological staging and the overall staging summary are provided **(Table 2)**.

Tumor Descriptors

T: Primary tumor size and invasion are measured under the T descriptor. Greatest dimension of the tumor is considered while accounting for the T. Presence of ipsilateral satellite nodules around the same tumor is also considered in the T. Additionally, invasion into nearby structures such as mediastinum, phrenic nerve, diaphragm, chest wall, or pericardium also impact T **(Table 1)**.

N: Short-axis diameters of the draining lymph nodes are measured for the N descriptor. During clinical staging, using radiology or endosonography, a size > 1 cm in the short axis is considered to be significant. Nondraining lymph nodes like abdominal or axillary lymph nodes are considered in the M descriptor. The IASLC has provided labels to the lymph node group in the form of stations. These stations are based on drainage of the lymph node.

M: Metastasis descriptor has undergone major changes in the recent past given the advancement in the available treatment options. It is subdivided into intrathoracic and extrathoracic and further subclassified based on the number of lesions.

PATHOLOGICAL STAGING

The IASLC recommends the use of physical examination, imaging, endoscopy, and surgical exploration for the categorization of TNM categories. The ideal method of staging involves histopathological documentation of tumor cells which is not commonly available or feasible, for all suspected lesions. In cases where curative surgical resection is planned, mediastinal staging with the use of endobronchial ultrasound/endoesophageal ultrasound (EBUS/EUS)-guided transbronchial needle aspiration (TBNA) or mediastinoscopy is recommended to confirm the TNM staging.

Definitions of postresection descriptors specific for pathological staging are provided below:

- *m*: Presence of multiple primary tumors in the surgical site
- *Y*: If the staging is performed after multimodality therapy
- *R*: Used to describe recurrent tumor after disease-free period
- *A*: Used if the staging is performed at the time of autopsy
- *L*: To describe the presence of lymphatic invasion in the surgical specimen
- *V*: Used to describe the presence of microscopic or macroscopic venous invasion
- *Pn*: To describe the presence of perineural invasion

TABLE 1: 8th TNM staging of lung cancer.

- **Tx**: Primary tumor cannot be assessed, or tumor proven by the presence of malignant cells in sputum or bronchial washings but not visualized by imaging or bronchoscopy
- **T0**: No evidence of a primary tumor
- **Tis**: Carcinoma in situ—tumor measuring 3 cm or less and has no invasive component at histopathology

T1		Tumor measuring 3 cm or less in greatest dimension surrounded by lung or visceral pleura without bronchoscopic evidence of invasion more proximal than the lobar bronchus
	T1mi	Minimally invasive adenocarcinoma
	T1a	Tumor ≤ 1 cm in greatest dimension
	T1b	Tumor > 1 cm but ≤2 cm in greatest dimension
	T1c	Tumor > 2 cm but ≤3 cm in greatest dimension
T2		Tumor > 3 cm but ≤5 cm or tumor with any of the following features: • Involves the main bronchus without the involvement of the carina • Invades visceral pleura • Associated with atelectasis or obstructive pneumonitis
	T2a	Tumor > 3 cm but ≤4 cm in greatest dimension
	T2b	Tumor > 4 cm but ≤5 cm in greatest dimension
T3		Tumor > 5 cm but ≤7 cm in greatest dimension or associated with separate tumor nodule(s) in the same lobe as the primary tumor OR Directly invades chest wall, phrenic nerve, or parietal pericardium
T4		Tumor > 7 cm in greatest dimension or associated with separate tumor nodule(s) in a different ipsilateral lobe than that of the primary tumor OR Invades any of the following structures: Diaphragm/mediastinum/great vessels/trachea/recurrent laryngeal nerve/esophagus/vertebra
N: Regional lymph node involvement		
Nx		Regional lymph nodes cannot be assessed
N0		No regional lymph node metastasis
N1		Metastasis in ipsilateral peribronchial and/or ipsilateral hilar lymph nodes and intrapulmonary nodes, including involvement by direct extension
N2		Metastasis in ipsilateral mediastinal and/or subcarinal lymph node(s)
N3		Metastasis in contralateral mediastinal, contralateral hilar, ipsilateral or contralateral scalene, or supraclavicular lymph node(s)
M: Distant metastasis		
M0		No distant metastasis
M1		Distant metastasis present
M1a		Separate tumor nodule(s) in a contralateral lobe; tumor with pleural or pericardial nodule(s) or malignant pleural or pericardial effusions
M1b		Single extrathoracic metastasis in a single organ or in a nonregional node
M1c		Multiple extrathoracic metastases in one or more organs

Modalities Used in Staging

It is recommended to use all feasible diagnostic modalities to confirm the extent of tumor burden to reach a definite staging opinion. For T descriptor, the use of imaging is most commonly employed. Contrast-enhanced computed tomography (CECT) or 18-FDG positron emission tomography (PET) is used for describing the extent of the tumor as well as invasiveness. 18-FDG PET has a marginal edge over CECT to provide the information about a metabolically active segment of the tumor. In certain cases of endobronchial tumors, where the distal segment is collapsed, it is

TABLE 2: Staging grid.

	N0	N1	N2	N3
T1a	IA1	IIB	IIIA	IIIB
T1b	IA2	IIB	IIIA	IIIB
T1c	IA3	IIB	IIIA	IIIB
T2a	IB	IIB	IIIA	IIIB
T2b	IIA	IIB	IIIA	IIIB
T3	IIB	IIIA	IIIB	IIIC
T4	IIIA	IIIA	IIIB	IIIC
M1a	IVA	IVA	IVA	IVA
M1b	IVA	IVA	IVA	IVA
M1c	IVB	IVB	IVB	IVB

difficult to differentiate between tumor and lung **(Figs. 1A to D)**. Similarly in tumors with a necrotic component, PET-CT offers an advantage over CT, to identify areas from where the biopsy can be taken.[5]

Apart from tissue diagnosis, bronchoscopy is also useful to document the involvement of carina. Invasion into carina is staged as T4, whereas involvement of the main bronchi (with spared carina), irrespective of the distance from carina, is labeled as T2. EBUS-guided assessment for the involvement of lymph nodes is a routine procedure for accurate mediastinal staging. An EBUS-guided description of lymph nodes at predefined stations (size, homogeneity, architecture) has been shown to differentiate between benign and malignant causes of involvement.[6] EBUS-guided TBNA has high concordance with surgical mediastinoscopy. Currently staging EBUS is an accepted preoperative

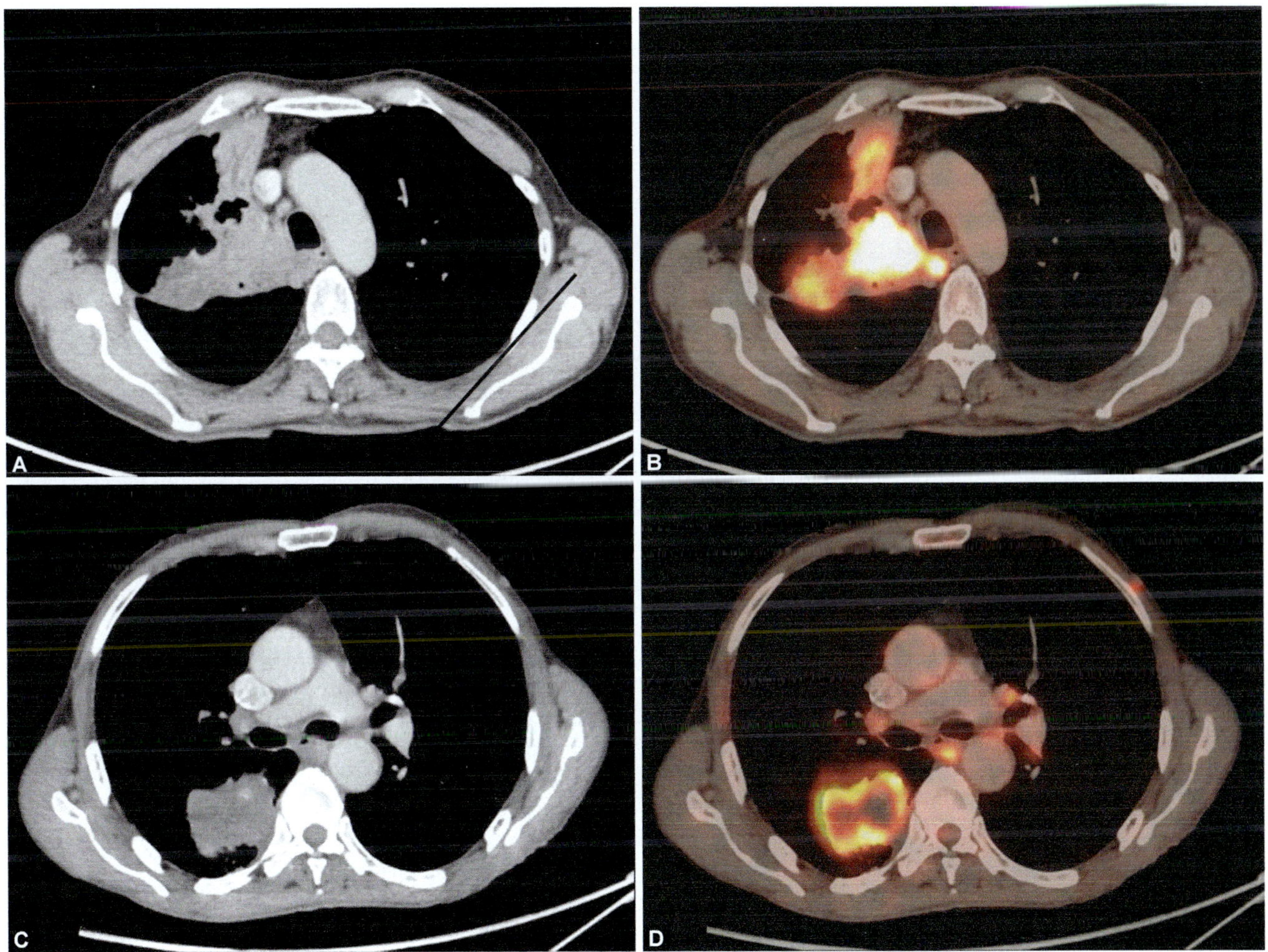

FIGS. 1A TO D: Comparison of utility of 18-FDG PET-CT scans in different settings. (A) Contrast-enhanced computed tomography image showing paratracheal mass with adjacent upper lobe segmental collapse and breakdown; (B) PET-CT image of the same section delineating the tumor component; (C) Computed tomography axial image of thorax showing a mass lesion in the right lower lobe; (D) PET-CT image of the section demonstrating activity only in the periphery of the lesion whereas rest of the lesion is necrotic.

procedure to confirm the nodal involvement for the lung cancer. Mediastinoscopy after negative EBUS does not add significantly to the treatment algorithm due to high NNT (numbers needed to treat).[7] For evaluation of supraclavicular nodes, physical examination is sufficient when features are suggestive of metastasis (hard, fixed), though ultrasound neck carries a higher sensitivity.[8]

For metastasis evaluation, imaging is recommended. Among imaging, PET-CT had added advantage over CT except for the involvement of brain. Whenever brain metastasis is suspected, contrast-enhanced MRI of brain is recommended.[9]

Alternative Staging Methods

Small-cell lung cancer (SCLC) is staged using the 8th TNM version by the IASLC but historically and even currently it has been classified into extensive disease (ED) and limited diseases (LD) as per Veterans Administration Lung Study Group (VALG).[10] LD is defined as tumor burden which is limited one hemithorax and is amenable to one radiotherapy (RT) portal. Extrathoracic involvement, opposite lung involvement, and effusions are classified as ED. The IASLC and National Comprehensive Cancer Network (NCCN) recommend the use of TNM staging for SCLC as well, but LD and ED are still commonly used for making management decisions.

Based on resectability, non-small-cell lung cancer (NSCLC) is classified into early-stage and advanced-stage lung cancer whereas advanced stage is further subdivided into locally advanced and metastatic. Stages I to IIIA (resectable tumors) are grouped into early stage, whereas stages IIIB and IIIC are labeled as locally advanced.[11] This terminology is commonly used for identifying cases where surgery can be offered as a curative attempt. Definitive chemoradiotherapy is also considered to be standard of care for the locally advanced stages of lung cancer.

PITFALLS OF CURRENT STAGING

Despite the accuracy in predicting the prognosis, there are several lacunae in the 8th TNM staging. Some of the important factors contributing to the overall prognosis are performance status, histology, and constitutional symptoms. Additionally, immunotherapy and targetable treatment options have significantly improved the prognosis of selected cases even in advanced diseases. The current staging system does not account for these factors and hence the overall prognosis remains a gray area. Also, management decisions for stages IIIA and IIIB have remained a complicated issue. The new evidence supporting the use of immunotherapy and epidermal growth factor receptor tyrosine kinase inhibitor (EGFR-TKI) in early-stage lung cancer has also influenced the overall treatment algorithm.[12]

To account for the complex issues which influence the treatment as well as prognosis, along with the 8th TNM guidelines, the IASLC has also proposed a *prognostic factors grid*. Prognostic grid includes tumor-related factors, host-related factors, and environmental factors and is classified according to resectability and histology (NSCLC and SCLC).

With an increase in the availability and use of lung cancer screening, subsolid nodules are more commonly picked up. Adenocarcinoma histology has high propensity to present as a subsolid nodule (part solid or completely ground-glass opacity), especially in never smokers. The same has not been captured adequately in the 8th TNM system.[13]

MANAGEMENT OPTIONS

In the past two decades, lung cancer management landscape has witnessed gigantic advancements. In selected cases, the overall survival has moved from below 1 year to over 5–10 years. In brief, the management options include the following:

- *Surgery*: For early-stage resectable lung cancer, surgery with curative intent remains the standard of care. Surgery encompasses removal of the tumor and the surrounding tissue with draining N1 and N2 lymph nodes. Surgical resection has moved from pneumonectomies to lung-sparing surgeries like wedge resection and segmentectomies. The interface and access have also been updated to video-assisted thoracic surgeries (VATS) and robotic surgeries. VATS have an added advantage of less chest wall trauma and a shortened postoperative recovery period. Despite the superior pulmonary functions in the postoperative period, wedge resection and segmentectomies are associated with a high risk of disease relapse and hence require careful case selection. Based upon the postoperative staging (T and N), decisions of further therapy (adjuvant therapy or postoperative RT) are taken.[14]
- *Radiotherapy*: This has remained a major part of the lung cancer management armamentarium, in both definitive and palliative settings. High accuracy of the external beam RT has transformed care by better target definition which has subsequently led to intense tissue targeting and accurate sparing of the healthy tissues. Improved accuracy has also led to testing of hypofractionation which reduces the number of fractions by increasing the dose per fraction. Hypofractionation is currently being investigated for its noninferiority to conventional fractionation as it is estimated to reduce the treatment burden and cost of care.

  Newer techniques of RT include intensity-modulated radiotherapy (IMRT), image-guided radiotherapy (IGRT), stereotactic body radiotherapy (SBRT), and stereotactic radiosurgery (SRS). Alternate delivery agents in the form of charged particles like proton instead of conventional photons are also being studied. Proton beam RT is believed to improve target definition with better safety, but the same is yet to be proven in a randomized controlled trial. Further, the utility of proton beam RT is limited by cost and availability. IGRT is becoming the new gold standard for RT delivery.

IGRT is commonly linked with CT scan (in cases of lung cancer) but for brain tumors or metastasis, MRI is used. SBRT is delivered over one to five fractions only through a high-intensity device which has a steep fallout in the surrounding healthy tissue.[15]

- *Chemotherapy*: Despite the advances, a larger proportion of lung cancer cases are dependent on conventional chemotherapy as they might be ineligible for the newer therapies, or the cost could be prohibitive. Platinum-based doublet therapy is standard of care. Nanoparticle albumin-bound drugs like nab-paclitaxel and lipid emulsified forms of drugs like docetaxel have been developed which allow optimal dose delivery with reduced adverse effects.
- *Immunotherapy*: Reactivation of host immune cells against tumor cells is the main mechanism of immunotherapy. There are several types of immunotherapies which have been developed and investigated, but immune checkpoint inhibitors (ICIs) have the maximum evidence. Programmed cell death protein-1/ programmed death ligand-1 (PD1-PDL1) axis and cytotoxic T-lymphocyte-associated protein 4 (CTLA4) axis inhibitors have been investigated both individually and in combination with chemotherapy for all stages and histology of lung cancer. Currently used and approved ICIs include nivolumab, durvalumab, pembrolizumab, atezolizumab, and ipilimumab.
- *Targeted therapy*: Driver genetic alterations have been identified in tumor cells against which drugs have been developed and tested. Especially in the nonsquamous histology (mainly adenocarcinoma), the prevalence of these genetic alterations is high. *EGFR* mutation and *ALK* and *ROS1* genetic rearrangements are the most common targets. Major advancements and options for these and other genetic alterations have come up with ever increasing progression-free survival.

MANAGEMENT DECISIONS BASED ON STAGING

One of the most important purposes of staging is to decide on the management options. Apart from staging, other factors which influence management decisions include the type of histology, patient's performance status, genetic alterations, and status of biomarkers of immunotherapy. With increasing options of treatment including ICIs as well as targeted therapy, the management algorithm for lung cancer has become increasingly complex and beyond the scope of this book. A preliminary approach is presented below. Majority of content has been derived from NCCN or American Society of Clinical Oncology (ASCO) guidelines.[16-20]

- *Nonsquamous NSCLC*: It accounts for the most common histology among lung cancers.
  - *Earlystage tumors (Stages IA–IIIA)*: These are the tumors where resection is feasible. In later stages (IIB and IIIA), neoadjuvant chemotherapy (with or without immunotherapy) is recommended prior to surgery. In the postoperative period, adjuvant therapy is offered in selected cases based upon the pathological staging as well as overall performance status of the patient. In recent updates, targeted adjuvant therapy is being evaluated in oncogenic gene-addicted tumors, but choosing the appropriate subject and positioning the intervention in the management algorithm still remain a debatable topic. Similarly, ICIs have been found to be effective in improving disease-free and event-free survivals when used in neoadjuvant settings. In subjects where surgery is not an option due to patient characteristics and comorbidities, stereotactic ablative radiotherapy (SABR) can be used with or without immune check point inhibitors.
  - *Locally advanced (IIIB and selected IIIC)*: Conventionally, definitive concurrent chemotherapy RT (CCRT) has been considered the standard of care in subjects with performance status 0 or 1. In some selected cases with single N2 node resection has been considered with or without neoadjuvant therapy. Following CCRT, maintenance or consolidation therapy with Durvalumab is recommended. The role of targeted therapy and immunotherapy in the IIIB and IIIC stages is evolving as these cases have formed a minority of the study population in clinical trials.
  - *Metastatic disease (IVA and IVB)*: Systemic therapy is recommended in metastatic disease. Upfront testing for targetable genetic alterations is mandatory for cases with nonsquamous histology. The method of testing varies significantly depending upon the availability of resources, tissue, and affordability. *EGFR*, *ALK*, and *ROS1* are commonly considered to be bare minimum testing. Targeted next-generation sequencing is being increasingly available and commonly used. In patients where the tissue is exhausted and the patient is unwilling for a repeat procedure, blood can be used as a surrogate for the tissue (liquid biopsy). In cases where the tumor is negative for any targetable genetic alteration, immunotherapy is recommended. ICIs have become an integral part of the treatment regimen for this subgroup of cases. The biomarker commonly used for choosing the treatment regimen is the tumor proportion score for the PD-L1 on tumor cells. Different immunohistochemistry platforms have been approved by the Food and Drug Administration (FDA) for PD-L1 testing. Details of treatment options are considered in separate chapters. The utility of isolated chemotherapy remains limited in the current era except for subjects unresponsive or intolerant to ICI.

Metastatic diseases where the disease burden is limited and thoracic primary is resectable and metastatic sites are amenable for local therapy in the form of radio-ablation or surgery can still be considered for definitive treatment. With the availability of stereotactic radio-ablation, unresectable tumors and inoperable patients can be taken up for definitive management.

- *Squamous NSCLC*: The treatment options for squamous cell lung carcinoma are largely similar to those in non-squamous cell lung cancer, but testing for genetic alterations is not routinely recommended. In some scenarios where the patient is young, or female, or a never smoker, testing for genetic alterations can be considered.
- *SCLC*: Though TNM staging is recommended for SCLC, classification according to disease extent is commonly used for determining management.
  - *Limited disease*: In patients with proven N_0 status, surgical resection followed by subsequent systemic therapy is the standard of care. But in subjects with any N positive status, systemic chemotherapy is recommended with concurrent RT. Irrespective of the performance status, systemic therapy should be offered to all cases of SCLC.
  - *Extensive disease*: ICIs have recently been approved for their use in ED SCLC cases. Atezolizumab with chemotherapy is the standard of care for first-line therapy. Metastatic disease also requires locally ablative therapies for symptoms' management. Prophylactic cranial irradiation for cases with no brain metastasis is also recommended in cases with acceptable performance status. In subjects with symptomatic brain metastasis, cranial irradiation is offered first before systemic therapy. SCLC cases are prone to frequent and early relapse, which indicates close disease monitoring and in such cases follow-up systemic therapy is recommended.

SUMMARY

Lung cancer management has gone through rapid and transformative changes in the management algorithm. Parallel to the same, the IASLC has been updating the TNM staging system for lung cancer. Despite the shortcoming, staging remains an integral part of diagnostic and management algorithm. Multidisciplinary involvement of a pulmonologist, radiologist, pathologist, and oncologist is vital for an appropriate and accurate staging. Staging is a dynamic exercise which needs revision on temporal grounds or after therapy administration. Awareness about the current advances in staging methods and descriptors is indispensable for a pulmonologist.

REFERENCES

1. Kulothungan V, Sathishkumar K, Leburu S, et al. Burden of cancers in India—estimates of cancer crude incidence, YLLs, YLDs and DALYs for 2021 and 2025 based on National Cancer Registry Program. BMC Cancer. 2022;22(1):527.
2. Goldstraw P, Chansky K, Crowley J, et al. The IASLC Lung Cancer Staging Project: Proposals for Revision of the TNM Stage Groupings in the Forthcoming (Eighth) Edition of the TNM Classification for Lung Cancer. J Thoracic Oncol. 2016;11(1): 39-51.
3. Rami-Porta R. Staging Manual in Thoracic Oncology. North Fort Myers, FL: International Association for the Study of Lung Cancer; 2016.
4. Rami-Porta R, Call S, Dooms C, et al. Lung cancer staging: a concise update. Eur Respir J. 2018;51(5):1800190.
5. Kandathil A, Kay FU, Butt YM, et al. Role of FDG PET/CT in the Eighth Edition of TNM Staging of Non-Small Cell Lung Cancer. Radiographics. 2018;38(7):2134-49.
6. Agrawal S, Goel AD, Gupta N, et al. Diagnostic utility of endobronchial ultrasound (EBUS) features in differentiating malignant and benign lymph nodes—A systematic review and meta-analysis. Respir Med. 2020;171:106097.
7. Sanz-Santos J, Almagro P, Malik K, et al. Confirmatory Mediastinoscopy after Negative Endobronchial Ultrasound-guided Transbronchial Needle Aspiration for Mediastinal Staging of Lung Cancer: Systematic Review and Meta-analysis. Ann Am Thoracic Soc. 2022;19(9):1581-90.
8. van Overhagen H, Brakel K, Heijenbrok MW, et al. Metastases in supraclavicular lymph nodes in lung cancer: assessment with palpation, US, and CT. Radiology. 2004;232(1):75-80.
9. Krüger S, Mottaghy FM, Buck AK, et al. Brain metastasis in lung cancer. Comparison of cerebral MRI and 18F-FDG-PET/CT for diagnosis in the initial staging. Nuklearmedizin. 2011;50(3): 101-6.
10. Ganti AKP, Loo BW, Bassetti M, et al. Small Cell Lung Cancer, Version 2.2022, NCCN Clinical Practice Guidelines in Oncology. J Natl Compr Canc Netw. 2021;19(12):1441-64.
11. Crinò L, Weder W, van Meerbeeck J, et al. Early stage and locally advanced (non-metastatic) non-small-cell lung cancer: ESMO Clinical Practice Guidelines for diagnosis, treatment and follow-up. Ann Oncol. 2010;21(Suppl 5):v103-15.
12. Vlahos I. Dilemmas in Lung Cancer Staging. Radiol Clin North Am. 2018;56(3):419-35.
13. Kim YW, Kwon BS, Lim SY, et al. Lung cancer probability and clinical outcomes of baseline and new subsolid nodules detected on low-dose CT screening. Thorax. 2021;76(10):980-8.
14. Udelsman BV, Blasberg JD. Advances in Surgical Techniques for Lung Cancer. Hematol Oncol Clin North Am. 2023;37(3):489-97.
15. Zhu Z, Ni J, Cai X, et al. International consensus on radiotherapy in metastatic non-small cell lung cancer. Transl Lung Cancer Res. 2022;11(9):1763-95.
16. Network NCC. Non-Small Cell Lung Cancer. NCCN Clinical Practice Guidelines in Oncology (NCCN Guidelines®). Plymouth Meeting, PA2023.
17. Owen DH, Singh N, Ismaila N, et al. Therapy for Stage IV Non–Small-Cell Lung Cancer With Driver Alterations: ASCO Living Guideline, Version 2023.2. J Clin Oncol. 2023;41(24): e.1-e.22.
18. Singh N, Jaiyesimi IA, Ismaila N, et al. Therapy for Stage IV Non–Small-Cell Lung Cancer Without Driver Alterations: ASCO Living Guideline, Version 2023.1. J Clin Oncol. 2023;41(15):e51-e62.
19. Pisters K, Kris MG, Gaspar LE, et al. Adjuvant Systemic Therapy and Adjuvant Radiation Therapy for Stage I-IIIA Completely Resected Non–Small-Cell Lung Cancer: ASCO Guideline Rapid Recommendation Update. J Clin Oncol. 2022;40(10):1127-9.
20. Daly ME, Singh N, Ismaila N, et al. Management of Stage III Non–Small-Cell Lung Cancer: ASCO Guideline. J Clin Oncol. 2022;40(12):1356-84.

Approach to Management of Lung Cancer in India

CHAPTER 152

Sudhir Kumar, Neha Pathak

INTRODUCTION

Lung cancer is among the top five common malignancies in India, fourth in incidence and overall mortality. It is the leading cause of cancer among males.[1] The initial presentation of lung cancer in India is at an advanced stage in about half of all cases due to delays in diagnosis, lack of established screening programs, prevalence of tuberculosis as a confounder, and difficulties in access to appropriate care.[2-4] The median age of diagnosis is about 58 years,[5] which is a decade younger as compared to the Western countries.[6] Histologically, 80–85% are non-small-cell lung cancer (NSCLC) and 15–20% are small-cell lung cancer (SCLC). Among NSCLCs, we have shifted from tobacco-driven squamous cell lung cancer (SqCC) to adenocarcinoma, the most common subtype, in the last 10 years.[2]

Etiologically, SCLC and SqCC are strongly linked with smoking.[7,8] Moreover, molecular pathways underlying lung cancer have been elucidated in the last few decades, and some somatic genetic alterations have been identified as driver mutations. For SCLC, loss of the tumor suppressor genes *p53* and *Rb* are characteristic. SCLC has a high tumor mutational burden (TMB), rendering it susceptible to immunotherapy. For NSCLC, precision oncology has managed to target a number of genetic alterations such as mutations [Exon 21, L858R, epidermal growth factor receptor (EGFR)], skipping mutations (MET exon skipping mutations), fusions [anaplastic lymphoma kinase (ALK) and ROS1 fusions], and deletions (Exon 19 deletion of EGFR) with specific drugs.[9] The evolution of such therapy has changed the treatment paradigms in nonmetastatic and metastatic lung cancer.

CLINICAL PRESENTATION

In a large database of over 1,800 patients published from India recently, most lung cancer patients are male (80%), with a median age of 58 years, presenting at an advanced stage (90% in NSCLC with stage III/IV and 75% of SCLC with extensive stage), and the majority are smokers (70%).[10] Similar findings were echoed in a large study from southern India.[5] Paraneoplastic manifestations associated with lung cancer are varied and can occur in about 20% of patients. These include but are not limited to anemia (15%), leukocytosis (10%), thrombocytosis (20%), deep venous thrombosis (5%), and syndrome of inappropriate secretion of antidiuretic hormone (SIADH) (5%), and rarely hypercalcemia.[11]

DIAGNOSIS AND STAGING (TABLES 1 AND 2)

Imaging

The first step in evaluating a suspected case of lung cancer is a contrast-enhanced computed tomography (CECT) of the chest.[12] This scan assesses the size, location, and extent of the primary tumor, involvement of the pleura, and mediastinum including the lymph nodes, thoracic vertebrae, at least the upper sections of the liver and adrenal glands, and the lower sections of the neck. It also helps plan the most appropriate route to obtain a biopsy. The contrast is an important part of this study to delineate the involvement of structures such as the pleura, pericardium, lymph nodes, and soft tissues.[12]

The drawbacks of the CECT chest are that it has low sensitivity (50–71%) and specificity (66–89%) to assess for lymph node involvement, can miss occult metastases and will not be able to assess distant metastases, for which we need more extensive imaging.[13]

Systematic assessment for distant metastases can be a symptomatic or lab-directed suspicion of involvement, for example, a CECT abdomen and pelvis in view of abnormal liver function tests or all-inclusive imaging performed such as a whole-body positron emission tomography (WBPET)-CT, for example, to rule out distant metastases in a stage II NSCLC planned to undergo curative surgery. Even if a WBPET-CT is performed, it is worth getting a CECT chest and dedicated brain imaging (vide infra) as the CT of a WBPET-CT is more commonly a noncontrast study. A WBPET-CT helps assess the tumor's metabolic activity, looking for occult metastases and mediastinal staging; its sensitivity and specificity in mediastinal staging are higher than those of a CECT chest.

TABLE 1: Role of different tests for the management of lung cancer.[12,14,17]

Test	Role
CECT chest	Tumor size, site, extent and extensions, pleura, pericardium, lymph nodes, and mediastinum. Also gives an idea about the dorsal column, soft tissues, liver, and adrenals
CECT abdomen and pelvis	Part of comprehensive staging for distant metastases, can be used in place of WBPET-CT
Bone scan	To evaluate presence of bone metastases. Nowadays supplanted by use of WBPET-CT
Brain imaging (MRI brain with gadolinium contrast preferred over CECT head)	To evaluate the presence of brain metastases, leptomeningeal involvement, and neurological paraneoplastic syndromes
WBPET-CT	For comprehensive staging; can be used in place of CECT abdomen and pelvis and a bone scan. Also helps in mediastinal staging
EBUS-TBNA	For mediastinal staging in case of resectable/potentially resectable cases For diagnostic sampling in case of centrally located mass
Pulmonary function tests, transthoracic echocardiography	These tests, along with others, may be used in resectable cases to assess medical fitness for surgery
Complete blood count, Liver function test, Kidney function test, and LDH, INR	Baseline tests for organ function and fitness for treatment

(CECT: contrast-enhanced computed tomography; EBUS-TBNA: endobronchial ultrasound-guided transbronchial needle aspiration; LDH: lactate dehydrogenase; INR: international normalized ratio; WBPET-CT: whole-body positron emission computed tomography)

TABLE 2: Role of histocytological material for diagnosis and management of lung cancer.[12,14,17]

Histopathology • Morphology • Immunohistochemistry • Molecular study and identification of potential targets for therapy	• *Morphology of lung cancer*: o SCLC versus NSCLC: SCLC typically has a high nuclear cytoplasmic ratio, salt and pepper chromatin, "blue cell tumor", hyperchromatic with rosette cells o NSCLC subtype: - Adenocarcinoma: Gland formation and intracytoplasmic mucin - SqCC: Keratin production by cancer cells, intracellular desmosomes/bridges - Adenosquamous: Composed of ≥10% malignant glandular and squamous components. - Large-cell carcinoma: Poorly differentiated, no features suggestive of adenocarcinoma/SqCC - NSCLC not otherwise specified (NOS): When IHC is uninformative or ambiguous • *Immunohistochemistry*: o Adenocarcinoma is generally positive for TTF-1, napsin A, cytokeratin (CK) 7 o SqCC is p40, p63 and CK 5/6 positive and CK7 negative o Adenosquamous will have combination of both the above o SCLC will have synaptophysin, CD56, chromogranin and neuron-specific enolase positive; TTF-1 can also be positive • *Molecular testing*: o For all metastatic nonsquamous NSCLC and nonsmoker SqCC o Broad-based panel (using NGS) testing preferred, which can test for multiple alterations at once o Important to test EGFR and ALK for stages I–III NSCLC, to decide for adjuvant therapy options/ maintenance therapy options PDL1 testing by IHC for immunotherapy related decisions
Bone marrow test	In case of SCLC if the LDH is elevated or there are cytopenias

Continued

Continued

Cytology studies • Pleural fluid cytology • Cerebrospinal fluid cytology	• To confirm involvement of pleura, especially if only site of involvement qualifying the disease as stage 4. Three cytologies repeated to confirm. Can be considered involved if hemorrhagic fluid aspirated even in the absence of positive cytology report • May also be performed as the only accessible site for diagnosis; cell block preparation may aid in further testing • To check for meningeal involvement, if clinically suspected
Liquid biopsy	Cannot diagnose lung cancer alone. Can be used to test for EGFR mutations/deletions. If positive, considered positive. If negative, need to repeat on tissue sample. Can also be used to detect T790M mutation as a resistance mechanism for patients on anti-EGFR tyrosine kinase inhibitors
(ALK: anaplastic lymphoma kinase; EGFR: epidermal growth factor receptor; IHC: immunohistochemistry; NGS: next-generation sequencing; NSCLC: non-small-cell lung cancer; PDL1: programmed cell death ligand 1; SCLC: small-cell lung cancer; SqCC: squamous cell lung cancer)	

In addition, brain imaging is warranted in all SCLC patients, as 10–15% of asymptomatic patients may have brain metastases.[14] For NSCLC cases, brain imaging is considered in all symptomatic patients and patients with a higher burden of disease (stage III/IV), while it is controversial in the early stage (stages I and II). While there is a support for brain imaging in all NSCLC patients from one prospective study with up to 21% of patients having brain metastases and brain imaging resulting in an upgraded stage in 7%, other studies have shown no survival benefit in patients who undergo upfront brain imaging versus those who do not.[15,16]

The preferred method of brain imaging is magnetic resonance imaging (MRI) with gadolinium contrast, but if that is not possible, a CECT head should be done.[17]

HISTOPATHOLOGY

The diagnosis of lung cancer needs histopathological proof of malignancy. This is commonly obtained through a biopsy or, when a biopsy is not feasible, a fluid cytology and cell block from effusion or a fine needle aspiration cytology (FNAC), with or without a cell block.[12]

The decision for the best site from where to conduct a biopsy should be from a multidisciplinary discussion in a Tumor Board. A histopathology specimen confirms the diagnosis and the morphology helps to identify the subtype of lung cancer, which is supplemented by tests of immune histochemical markers. Molecular testing to help identify targetable mutations is essential for managing NSCLC. Most guidelines recommend broad-based panel testing by next-generation sequencing (NGS) to identify relevant driver alterations in metastatic NSCLC. In addition, with the entry of immunotherapy and EGFR inhibitors into the curative setting, it is also recommended to test for EGFR, ALK, and programmed cell death ligand 1 (PDL1) in nonmetastatic lung cancer.

The known targetable drivers include an ever-evolving list of EGFR, ALK, ROS1, RET, MET, BRAF, NTRK, KRAS, and HER2.[18] In addition, immunohistochemistry (IHC) for PDL1 is important for making decisions regarding immunotherapy.[17,18] The lack of availability of NGS in India, its high cost, and the lack of drugs that can target rarer alterations like RET, KRAS, and HER2, for example, limit the extent to which molecular tests can occur and how they can guide therapy. An Indian expert panel recommends at least *EGFR*, *ALK*, *ROS1* genes, and PDL1 protein as first-line biomarkers for molecular testing.[19]

Liquid Biopsy

Liquid biopsy is a method to assess circulating tumor DNA (ctDNA) or circulating tumor cells (CTCs), which are shed by lung cancer into the bloodstream.[20] It is also being studied in pericardial, pleural, and cerebrospinal fluid. The method of this assessment involves use of specialized polymerase chain reaction techniques and NGS.[9] Liquid biopsy can detect targetable alterations in NSCLC and is currently an approved test for EGFR alteration testing.[21] Liquid biopsy can detect many other alterations as well. However, it is not yet approved for screening diagnosis or response to treatment assessment in lung cancer. In addition, they are easy to obtain, noninvasive if blood is used, and can reflect the overall state and current state in time of a tumor.[20]

The main concern with this test is its high chance of a false negative, as the quantity of genetic material in such samples is usually quite low, and some tumors do not have the propensity to shed DNA or cells into the bloodstream. This test has a sensitivity of 60–80% across assays and, thus, if negative, needs confirmation by testing in a tissue sample.[22]

Role of the Clinician

A systematic assessment of symptoms and signs of a patient who is suspected to have lung cancer can lead a clinician toward a proper assessment of metastatic disease. Evaluation includes a good clinical history and examination focused on the possibility of metastatic involvement and paraneoplastic syndromes, laboratory investigations such as a complete blood count and kidney and liver function tests, electrolytes such as calcium and sodium, albumin, and lactate dehydrogenase (LDH). Imaging studies can then be directed as per the results of the assessment; for example, an elevated alkaline phosphatase should raise the suspicion of liver and/or bone metastases, resulting in gamma-glutamyl transferase test (abnormal in case of liver metastases), a bone scan, and/or MRI of spine or a WBPET-CT.

The benefit of this approach was demonstrated in a meta-analysis that showed a high negative predictive value of an expanded clinical examination for metastases of the brain (95%), abdomen (94%), and bone (89%).[23]

In addition, it is important to assess the performance status, organ function, and presence of comorbidities to determine the fitness of the patient and tolerance to therapy.

Mediastinal Staging

Staging of the mediastinum, i.e., assessment of the mediastinal lymph node involvement, is an important part of the workup of resectable lung cancer. Current guidelines recommend that all patients with resectable NSCLC undergo invasive mediastinal staging, barring the very small (≤3 cm) peripherally located tumor with no nodal involvement on imaging.[24]

The first step of this process is to do an imaging test, usually a CECT chest or WBPET-CT; however, in most cases, a confirmatory test for pathological proof of involvement is employed. A WBPET-CT can have a false-negative rate of about 7–15% and a false-positive rate of 45–48%.[25,26] Once confirmed, involvement of the hilar (N1) or the mediastinal (N2 and N3) generally indicates that either we need neoadjuvant chemotherapy or the patient needs chemoradiation.

Historically, mediastinoscopy has been the gold standard of assessment of nodal staging. The mediastinoscopy targets specific nodal stations in the chest, including 2R, 2L (right and left upper paratracheal, respectively), 4R, 4L (right and left lower paratracheal, respectively), and 7 (subcarinal). Despite a high sensitivity of about 80% and a negative predictive value of 91%, mediastinoscopy (even if done by a video-assisted technique) has significant complications of hemorrhage, tracheal or esophageal injury, and recurrent nerve injury.[12,27]

The endobronchial ultrasound (EBUS)-guided lymph node sampling can address the same stations as mediastinoscopy and access 10 and 11 stations (hilar and interlobar, respectively). The sensitivity of EBUS ranges from 70% to 99% and specificity of 99% to detect N2 disease.[28] It is also less invasive and has more adaptability. The ASTER trial reported that EBUS alone had a sensitivity of 85% versus 79% in the comparator arm, which increased to 94% with EBUS + mediastinoscopy.[29] There was no difference in 5-year survival in both arms.[30]

In addition, the risk of an unforeseen N2 disease at surgery remains the same with EBUS + mediastinoscopy versus EBUS alone in another study.[31] Therefore, EBUS has emerged as the modality of choice for mediastinal staging in the current era.

ROLE OF THE MULTIDISCIPLINARY APPROACH

A multidisciplinary discussion in tumor (MDT) board for every lung cancer patient helps optimize individualized decision-making.[32] An MDT board is useful for deciding the best approach for biopsy, choosing between two therapies like stereotactic body radiation (SBRT) and surgery for stage I lung cancer, decision on mediastinal staging, addressing borderline resectable cases, incorporating biomarker-driven strategies, enrolment in clinical trials, and many more.[33]

STAGE-WISE MANAGEMENT OF LUNG CANCER *(SEE CHAPTER ON LUNG CANCER STAGING)*

Non-small-cell Lung Cancer: Early Stage

Patients with NSCLC who have a disease limited to a single lobe of a lung without involvement of mediastinum are considered to have earlystage disease. This corresponds to stages I and II of American Joint Committee on Cancer (AJCC) 8th edition staging and comprise about 30% of all cases of NSCLC. Surgery is the treatment of choice in such cases. This may need a multidisciplinary discussion to consider neoadjuvant therapy/resectability for centrally located tumors.[34] For peripherally located tumors, surgery is generally feasible. Centers that perform more lung cancer resections tend to have better outcomes and less mortality.[35] Video-assisted thoracic surgery (VATS) and robot-assisted thoracic surgery (RATS) have become prominent in recent years, and oncologic outcomes are considered as good as open surgery.[36]

The most common surgical extent is a lobectomy. That may be difficult for central tumors, and a pneumonectomy may be needed; however, this surgery is quite morbid and has worse outcomes.[37] Instead, a sleeve resection can get adequate margins with lesser postoperative burden.[38] SBRT is an alternative for medically inoperable or declined surgery. After surgery, unless the margins are positive, there is no role for postoperative radiation. Systematic lymph node dissection is recommended over sampling, except in small peripherally located T1 tumors.[39]

Adjuvant therapy is required after surgery for stage II NSCLC to improve overall survival (OS) and decrease recurrence.[40] The standard option was platinum doublet chemotherapy, which can include regimens like cisplatin with vinorelbine, docetaxel, or gemcitabine and cisplatin-pemetrexed in cases of adenocarcinoma.[41] These are given for four cycles. Stage IB may be considered for adjuvant chemotherapy if other higher-risk features, like lymphovascular invasion, high grade, and high WBPET-CT avidity, are present. Stage IA tumors do well even without adjuvant chemotherapy.[41]

With the advent of precision oncology, detecting driver mutations has become important in management. In patients with EGFR exon 19 deletion and exon 21 L858R mutation, osimertinib, an EGFR inhibitor, has been approved as extended adjuvant therapy (for 3 years), preferably after adjuvant chemotherapy, as it showed a disease-free survival (DFS) and OS benefit in a phase III study.[42]

There is also an emerging role of immunotherapy as adjuvant treatment added on after adjuvant chemotherapy, with two drugs approved in this domain: Atezolizumab in adult patients with stages II to III NSCLC with at least 5 cm size primary or positive lymph nodes and with PDL1 expression on ≥1% of tumor cells[43] and adjuvant pembrolizumab, Food and Drug Administration (FDA)-approved for patients with resected stages II to III NSCLC, which is at least 4 cm or lymph node-positive, independent of PDL1 expression.[44]

Neoadjuvant chemotherapy is a consideration in cases of node-positive tumors or in those with borderline general status who need optimization. There is no survival outcome difference between using neoadjuvant therapy and adjuvant chemotherapy.[45] The regimens remain the same as those of adjuvant chemotherapy.

Recently, neoadjuvant therapy in the form of chemotherapy plus immunotherapy (nivolumab) and perioperative therapy (pembrolizumab) has gained approval based on two important studies[46,47] that have demonstrated improvement with event-free survival (EFS) and pathological complete remission (pCR) and are becoming the new standard of care. Peri-operative durvalumab, a PDL1 inhibitor, was also approved for resectable stage IIA- IIIB NSCLC, in combination with neoadjuvant chemotherapy, based on pCR and EFS benefits.[48]

Locally Advanced NSCLC

Locally advanced NSCLC should be evaluated by a detailed history, physical examination, and a CECT of the chest and upper abdomen. Additionally, brain imaging should be done to complete the staging workup,[49] and if available and feasible, a WBPET-CT should be included. A WBPET-CT can upstage a stage III NSCLC in up to 24% of cases.[50] A biopsy site should be selected to confirm the highest stage and yield enough tissue for molecular testing.[51] Mediastinal staging (see above) is required before any definitive treatment.

A multidisciplinary team should evaluate all patients with stage III NSCLC to decide the best approach to management.[52] A single treatment modality is insufficient for locally advanced disease, and patients need various combinations of surgery, chemotherapy, and radiation for optimal survival. Resectability needs to be decided by the surgeon. Cases expected to be completely (negative margins or an R0 resection) resected have a very low chance of N3 disease on multidisciplinary discussion, and cases with low mortality risk (≤5% in 90 days) are those that should undergo curative surgery.[51] Heavy mediastinal burden may also be considered to exclude surgery. Other than these important considerations, surgery in stage III NSCLC needs to be determined by expert consensus. Multimodal therapy with and without surgery has yielded similar results in many randomized controlled trials (RCTs). Additionally, medical fitness and pulmonary reserve need to be addressed.

Systemic therapy for patients planned for surgery has been neoadjuvant platinum-based doublet chemotherapy, based on the strong trial-based evidence of OS benefit over surgery alone. Radiotherapy as a part of neoadjuvant therapy (chemoradiation) did not improve survival and is not routinely recommended.[53] The exception is superior sulcus tumors, which require trimodality therapy, namely neoadjuvant chemoradiotherapy followed by surgery, due to the difficulty in obtaining local control in this region, as these tumors have a predisposition of early infiltration into the brachial plexus, bone, blood vessels, and chest wall. Trimodality therapy in these patients has demonstrated a better OS.[54]

The stage III patient subgroup especially benefitted from the chemoimmunotherapy regimen in the trials testing this combination in the neoadjuvant setting (see above).[46,47,55] The patients who do not receive neoadjuvant chemotherapy should receive platinum-based adjuvant chemotherapy, based on a 5% OS benefit in 5 years from the landmark LACE meta-analysis.[40] There is also an option of adding adjuvant immunotherapy (discussed above) and, in select patients, Osimertinib as adjuvant therapy in the current era.

Concurrent chemoradiation is the standard recommendation for patients who are not candidates for surgery but are otherwise fit.[56] Sequential chemotherapy and radiation are better than radiation alone in those who are not fit.[57] Improvement in radiotherapy techniques over the years has lowered the toxicity of this therapy, in particular cardiovascular and oesophageal toxicity. The standard dose for concurrent chemoradiation is at least 60 Gy, although studies have used various doses of 60–70 Gy with similar results.[51] The chemotherapy backbone in concurrent chemoradiation is a platinum doublet, with various regimens usually followed by two to four cycles of chemotherapy alone.[51] After concurrent chemoradiation, if the patient does not progress, they should receive durvalumab for 1 year, based on the PACIFIC study, which has demonstrated reliable OS benefit over a 3-year follow-up (estimated 5-year OS rates: 43% for durvalumab vs. 33% for placebo).[58]

Postoperative radiation is no longer recommended; exceptional cases that merit consideration include positive margins postsurgery and extracapsular nodal extension.[59]

Metastatic NSCLC

The approach to stage IV NSCLC in today's age relies on biomarker testing. A panel of targets now exists against which targetable drugs exist in the first and subsequent lines of therapy. These include, but are not limited to, driver alterations in EGFR, ALK, ROS1 fusions, BRAF V600e mutations, RET fusions, MET exon 14 skipping mutations, NTRK fusions, KRAS G12C and HER2 exon 20 insertion mutations.[60] The details of each target and its inhibitors are beyond the scope of this chapter and can be found elsewhere.[9,61] Most oncogenic drivers were believed to be common in nonsmokers; however, some, like KRAS, HER2, and BRAF, are seen in patients with a smoking history. In addition, PDL1 testing should be done to guide immunotherapy discussions.[17]

Underlying this is the economic feasibility of extensive testing and the availability and cost of new drugs that can inhibit potential targets (see above). European guidelines recommend testing for those markers for which appropriate medication is available to avoid futility.[61]

In those without oncogenic drivers, PDL1 helps guide the discussion for immunotherapy. Single-agent immunotherapy has shown promise in those with PDL1 ≥ 50% and is considered standard first-line therapy.[62] Chemoimmunotherapy is the gold standard for any other expression of PDL1; other options include those of dual immunotherapy or chemotherapy alone.[63] The caveat is that the patient should be fit, as most trials only included patients with Eastern Cooperative Oncology Group (ECOG) 0–1 and do not have a contraindication to immunotherapy (e.g., uncontrolled autoimmune disease).[62] The patient's fitness, as judged by the performance status, is important for deciding therapy in nononcogene-driven metastatic NSCLC, as while a poor performance status does not preclude administration of oral tyrosine kinase inhibitors, chemotherapy ± immunotherapy becomes a challenge. Limited data does suggest the feasibility of low-dose chemotherapy[64] and single-agent immunotherapy[65] in carefully selected patients, but more research is warranted in this domain.

Small Cell Lung Cancer

Small-cell lung cancer is characterized by its strong association with smoking, aggressive behavior, rapid growth, high chemo- and radiation sensitivity, a high propensity of recurrence, and poor survival outcomes.[66] SCLC presents as a centrally located tumor accessed via bronchoscopy for biopsy. Workup of SCLC includes brain imaging via MRI and a bone marrow examination (in case of clinical suspicion based on elevated LDH and/or abnormal complete blood counts).[8] Invasive mediastinal staging is mandatory for limited-stage disease. Due to abnormal humoral immunity activation, SCLC is associated with various paraneoplastic syndromes. These include SIADH, Cushing syndrome, Lambert-Eaton syndrome, encephalomyelitis, sensory neuropathy syndromes, dermatomyositis, hyperglycemia, hypoglycemia, hypercalcemia, and gynecomastia.[67]

Although SCLC can be staged using the TNM like NSCLC,[68] conventionally for all practical purposes, it is divided into two stages: Limited stage (confined to one hemithorax and can be covered in a single tolerable radiation field) and extensive stage based on the Veterans' Affairs Lung Study Group (VALSG).[69]

Most (70%) cases present with extensive-stage SCLC; among limited stage, <5% present as a peripheral nodule with negative mediastinal staging that can undergo surgery.[70] However, the data supporting surgery and the option of adjuvant therapy after it is sparse due to the rarity of this presentation. In most cases, limited-stage SCLC undergoes chemoradiation with four cycles of platinum and etoposide-based chemotherapy. This is known to improve OS versus chemotherapy alone.[70] There is a role of prophylactic cranial irradiation in patients who respond to chemoradiation, as it has been shown to improve OS.[71]

For extensive-stage SCLC, two studies revolutionized first-line therapy by adding the anti-PDL1 monoclonal antibodies atezolizumab and durvalumab to platinum-based chemotherapy followed by immunotherapy maintenance.[72,73] Both studies demonstrated an improvement in PFS and OS with similar incidence of side effects. Second-line therapies for SCLC include the use of lurbinectedin, topotecan, irinotecan, paclitaxel, and temozolomide.[8] The molecular subtypes of SCLC have been defined (SCLC-A, N, P, and I).[74] However, as of now, they do not determine management in patients; research is ongoing.

Role of Palliative Care and Early Palliative Care

In lung cancer, early palliative care is essential to comprehensive patient management. Early palliative care entails a patient-centered approach that focuses on symptom management, psychosocial support, and communication about values and goals of care. It does not equate to end-of-life care but complements curative or life-prolonging treatments.[75]

Studies have shown that early integration of palliative care in NSCLC results in improved symptom control, enhanced quality of life, and better communication between healthcare providers and patients.[76] It addresses the complex physical and emotional burdens often accompanying cancer, providing patients with the support they need to navigate their treatment journey. Furthermore, early palliative care discussions foster open dialogues about goals of care, advance directives, and treatment preferences, ensuring that patients receive treatments aligned with their values.[77]

Palliative care can entail a variety of approaches to address a patient's needs. These can include but are not limited to palliative radiation such as whole brain radiation for multiple brain metastases, palliative systemic therapy given to prolong life, relieving symptoms while maintaining the quality of life in stage IV SCLC and NSCLC, medications, nonpharmacologic interventions and lifestyle modifications to help manage symptoms of disease (e.g., dyspnea), pain management, psychosocial support to the patient and their caregivers, nutritional optimization, hospice support, advanced care planning and directives, social support with better-shared decision-making, rehabilitation, spiritual support, and many more.[78]

Palliative care is not just about end-of-life care but focuses on enhancing the patient's comfort, dignity, and overall quality of life throughout their cancer journey. The interventions and services provided may vary depending on the patient's needs, preferences, and disease stage. The goal is to provide comprehensive, holistic care that addresses the physical, emotional, and spiritual dimensions of living with lung cancer.[78,79]

SUMMARY

There have been remarkable developments in the management of lung cancer. Different modalities of treatment are based on the clinical staging as well as genetic mutations. There are different treatment paradigms in nonmetastatic and metastatic lung cancer. It is important to follow the MDT decisions of the Tumor Board for the best treatment outcomes. Lastly, palliative care has also come to be viewed as an effective treatment modality to enhance patient's comfort and quality of life.

REFERENCES

1. Sung H, Ferlay J, Siegel RL, et al. Global Cancer Statistics 2020: GLOBOCAN Estimates of Incidence and Mortality Worldwide for 36 Cancers In 185 Countries. CA Cancer J Clin.2021;71(3): 209-49.
2. Singh N, Agrawal S, Jiwnani S, et al. Lung Cancer in India. J Thorac Oncol. 2021;16(8):1250-66.
3. Ramachandran K, Thankagunam B, Karuppusami R, et al. Physician Related Delays in the Diagnosis of Lung Cancer in India. J Clin Diagn Res. 2016;10(11):OC05-8.
4. Mathur P, Sathishkumar K, Chaturvedi M, et al. Cancer Statistics, 2020: Report From National Cancer Registry Programme, India. JCO Glob Oncol. 2020;(6):1063-75.
5. Murali AN, Radhakrishnan V, Ganesan TS, et al. Outcomes in Lung Cancer: 9-Year Experience From a Tertiary Cancer Center in India. J Glob Oncol. 2017;3(5):459-68.
6. Ganti AK, Klein AB, Cotarla I, et al. Update of Incidence, Prevalence, Survival, and Initial Treatment in Patients With Non–Small Cell Lung Cancer in the US. JAMA Oncol. 2021;7(12): 1824-32.
7. Molina JR, Yang P, Cassivi SD, et al. Non–Small Cell Lung Cancer: Epidemiology, Risk Factors, Treatment, and Survivorship. Mayo Clin Proc. 2008;83(5):584-94.
8. Rudin CM, Brambilla E, Faivre-Finn C, et al. Small-cell lung cancer. Nat Rev Dis Primers. 2021;7(1):3.
9. Pathak N, Chitikela S, Malik PS. Recent advances in lung cancer genomics: Application in targeted therapy. In: Advances in Genetics. Cambridge: Academic Press; 2021
10. Mohan A, Garg A, Gupta A, et al. Clinical profile of lung cancer in North India: A 10-year analysis of 1862 patients from a tertiary care center. Lung India. 2020;37(3):190
11. Darling HS, Viswanath S, Singh R, et al. A clinico-epidemiological, pathological, and molecular study of lung cancer in Northwestern India. J Cancer Res Ther. 2020;16(4):771.
12. Silvestri GA, Gonzalez AV, Jantz MA, et al. Methods for staging non-small cell lung cancer: Diagnosis and management of lung cancer, 3rd ed: American College of Chest Physicians evidence-based clinical practice guidelines. Chest. 2013;143 (5 Suppl):e211S-50S.
13. Gould MK, Kuschner WG, Rydzak CE, et al. Test performance of positron emission tomography and computed tomography for mediastinal staging in patients with non-small-cell lung cancer: a meta-analysis. Ann Intern Med. 2003;139(11):879-92.
14. Kalemkerian GP. Staging and imaging of small cell lung cancer. Cancer Imaging. 2011;11(1):253-8.
15. Naresh G, Malik PS, Khurana S, et al. Assessment of Brain Metastasis at Diagnosis in Non–Small-Cell Lung Cancer: A Prospective Observational Study From North India. JCO Glob Oncol. 2021;(7):593-601.
16. Bizzi A, Pascuzzo R. Is Brain MRI Unnecessary for Early-Stage Non–Small Cell Lung Cancer? Radiology. 2022;303(3):644-5.
17. Ettinger DS, Wood DE, Aisner DL, et al. NCCN Guidelines Insights: Non-Small Cell Lung Cancer, Version 2.2021. J Natl Compr Canc Netw. 2021;19(3):254-66.
18. IASLC. (2023). IASLC Atlas of Molecular Testing for Targeted Therapy in Lung Cancer. [online] Available from https://www.iaslc.org/iaslc-atlas-molecular-testing-targeted-therapy-lung-cancer [Last accessed September, 2024].
19. Prabhash K, Advani SH, Batra U, et al. Biomarkers in Non-Small Cell Lung Cancers: Indian Consensus Guidelines for Molecular Testing. Adv Ther. 2019;36(4):766-85.
20. Li W, Liu JB, Hou LK, et al. Liquid biopsy in lung cancer: significance in diagnostics, prediction, and treatment monitoring. Mol Cancer. 2022;21(1):25.
21. Kwapisz D. The first liquid biopsy test approved. Is it a new era of mutation testing for non-small cell lung cancer? Ann Transl Med. 2017;5(3):46.
22. Sacher AG, Paweletz C, Dahlberg SE, et al. Prospective Validation of Rapid Plasma Genotyping for the Detection of EGFR and KRAS Mutations in Advanced Lung Cancer. JAMA Oncol. 2016;2(8):1014–22.
23. Silvestri GA, Littenberg B, Colice GL. The clinical evaluation for detecting metastatic lung cancer. A meta-analysis. Am J Respir Crit Care Med. 1995;152(1):225-30.
24. Agrawal A, Ghori U, Chaddha U, et al. Combined EBUS-IFB and EBUS-TBNA vs EBUS-TBNA Alone for Intrathoracic Adenopathy. A Meta-Analysis. Ann Thorac Surg. 2022;114(1):340-8.
25. Li S, Zheng Q, Ma Y, et al. Implications of false negative and false positive diagnosis in lymph node staging of NSCLC by means of ^{18}F-FDG PET/CT. PLoS One. 2013;8(10):e78552.
26. Kim KY, Park HL, Kang HS, et al. Clinical Characteristics and Outcome of Pathologic N0 Non-small Cell Lung Cancer Patients With False Positive Mediastinal Lymph Node Metastasis on FDG PET-CT. In Vivo. 2021;35(3):1829-36.
27. Czarnecka-Kujawa K, Yasufuku K. The role of endobronchial ultrasound versus mediastinoscopy for non-small cell lung cancer. J Thorac Dis. 2017;9(Suppl 2):S83-97.
28. Crombag LMM, Dooms C, Stigt JA, et al. Systematic and combined endosonographic staging of lung cancer (SCORE study). Eur Respir J. 2019;53(2):1800800.

29. Annema JT, van Meerbeeck JP, Rintoul RC, et al. Mediastinoscopy vs endosonography for mediastinal nodal staging of lung cancer: a randomized trial. JAMA. 2010;304(20):2245-52.
30. Kuijvenhoven JC, Korevaar DA, Tournoy KG, et al. Five-Year Survival After Endosonography vs Mediastinoscopy for Mediastinal Nodal Staging of Lung Cancer. JAMA. 2016;316(10):1110-2.
31. Bousema JE, van Dorp M, Noyez VJJM, et al. Unforeseen N2 Disease after Negative Endosonography Findings with or without Confirmatory Mediastinoscopy in Resectable Non-Small Cell Lung Cancer: A Systematic Review and Meta-Analysis. J Thorac Oncol. 2019;14(6):979-92.
32. Berghmans T, Lievens Y, Aapro M, et al. European Cancer Organisation Essential Requirements for Quality Cancer Care (ERQCC). Lung Cancer. 2020;150:221-39.
33. Popat S, Navani N, Kerr KM, et al. Navigating Diagnostic and Treatment Decisions in Non-Small Cell Lung Cancer: Expert Commentary on the Multidisciplinary Team Approach. Oncologist. 2021;26(2):e306-15.
34. O'Reilly D, Botticella A, Barry S, et al. Treatment Decisions for Resectable Non–Small-Cell Lung Cancer: Balancing Less With More? Am Soc Clin Oncol Educ Book. 2023;(43):e389950.
35. Lüchtenborg M, Riaz SP, Coupland VH, et al. High procedure volume is strongly associated with improved survival after lung cancer surgery. J Clin Oncol. 2013;31(25):3141-6.
36. Yan TD, Black D, Bannon PG, et al. Systematic review and meta-analysis of randomized and nonrandomized trials on safety and efficacy of video-assisted thoracic surgery lobectomy for early-stage non-small-cell lung cancer. J Clin Oncol. 2009;27(15):2553-62.
37. Albain KS, Swann RS, Rusch VR, et al. Radiotherapy plus Chemotherapy with or without Surgical Resection for Stage III Non-Small Cell Lung Cancer. Lancet. 2009;374(9687):379-86.
38. Ferguson MK, Lehman AG. Sleeve lobectomy or pneumonectomy: optimal management strategy using decision analysis techniques. Ann Thorac Surg. 2003;76(6):1782-8.
39. Lardinois D, De Leyn P, Van Schil P, et al. ESTS guidelines for intraoperative lymph node staging in non-small cell lung cancer. Eur J Cardiothorac Surg. 2006;30(5):787-92.
40. Pignon JP, Tribodet H, Scagliotti GV, et al. Lung Adjuvant Cisplatin Evaluation: A Pooled Analysis by the LACE Collaborative Group. J Clin Oncol. 2008;26(21):3552-9.
41. Pisters KMW, Evans WK, Azzoli CG, et al. Cancer Care Ontario and American Society of Clinical Oncology adjuvant chemotherapy and adjuvant radiation therapy for stages I-IIIA resectable non small-cell lung cancer guideline. J Clin Oncol. 2007;25(34): 5506-18.
42. Herbst RS, Wu YL, John T, et al. Adjuvant Osimertinib for Resected EGFR-Mutated Stage IB-IIIA Non–Small-Cell Lung Cancer: Updated Results From the Phase III Randomized ADAURA Trial. J Clin Oncol. 2023;41(10):1830-40.
43. Felip E, Altorki N, Zhou C, et al. Adjuvant atezolizumab after adjuvant chemotherapy in resected stage IB-IIIA non-small-cell lung cancer (IMpower010): a randomised, multicentre, open-label, phase 3 trial. Lancet. 2021;398(10308):1344-57.
44. O'Brien M, Paz-Ares L, Marreaud S, et al. Pembrolizumab versus placebo as adjuvant therapy for completely resected stage IB-IIIA non-small-cell lung cancer (PEARLS/KEYNOTE-091): an interim analysis of a randomised, triple-blind, phase 3 trial. Lancet Oncol. 2022;23(10):1274-86.
45. Provencio M, Calvo V, Romero A, et al. Treatment Sequencing in Resectable Lung Cancer: The Good and the Bad of Adjuvant Versus Neoadjuvant Therapy. Am Soc Clin Oncol Educ Book. 2022;(42):711-28.
46. Forde PM, Spicer J, Lu S, et al. Neoadjuvant Nivolumab plus Chemotherapy in Resectable Lung Cancer. New Engl J Med. 2022;386(21):1973-85.
47. Wakelee H, Liberman M, Kato T, et al. Perioperative Pembrolizumab for Early-Stage Non–Small-Cell Lung Cancer. New Engl J Med. 2023;389(6):491-503.
48. Heymach JV, Harpole D, Mitsudomi T, et al. Perioperative Durvalumab for Resectable Non–Small-Cell Lung Cancer. New England Journal of Medicine [Internet]. 2023;389(18): 1672–84.
49. Diaz ME, Debowski M, Hukins C, et al. Non-small cell lung cancer brain metastasis screening in the era of positron emission tomography-CT staging: Current practice and outcomes. J Med Imaging Radiat Oncol. 2018;62(3):383-8.
50. Sharma R, Tripathi M, D'Souza M, et al. The importance of 18F-FDG PET/CT, CT and X-rays in detecting primary stage III A lung cancer and the incidence of extra thoracic metastases. Hell J Nucl Med. 2009;12(1):22–5.
51. Daly ME, Singh N, Ismaila N, et al. Management of Stage III Non–Small-Cell Lung Cancer: ASCO Guideline. J Clin Oncol. 2022;40(12):1356-84.
52. Pan CC, Kung PT, Wang YH, et al. Effects of multidisciplinary team care on the survival of patients with different stages of non-small cell lung cancer: a national cohort study. PLoS One. 2015;10(5):e0126547.
53. Chen Y, Peng X, Zhou Y, et al. Comparing the benefits of chemoradiotherapy and chemotherapy for resectable stage III A/N2 non-small cell lung cancer: a meta-analysis. World J Surg Oncol. 2018;16(1):8.
54. Rusch VW, Giroux DJ, Kraut MJ, et al. Induction Chemoradiation and Surgical Resection for Superior Sulcus Non–Small-Cell Lung Carcinomas: Long-Term Results of Southwest Oncology Group Trial 9416 (Intergroup Trial 0160). J Clin Oncol. 2007;25(3):313-8.
55. Singh N, Daly ME, Ismaila N, et al. Management of Stage III Non–Small-Cell Lung Cancer: ASCO Guideline Rapid Recommendation Update. J Clin Oncol. 2023;41(27). https://ascopubs.org/doi/full/10.1200/JCO.23.01261
56. Aupérin A, Le Péchoux C, Rolland E, et al. Meta-Analysis of Concomitant Versus Sequential Radiochemotherapy in Locally Advanced Non–Small-Cell Lung Cancer. J Clin Oncol. 2010; 28(13):2181-90.
57. Hung MS, Wu YF, Chen YC. Efficacy of chemoradiotherapy versus radiation alone in patients with inoperable locally advanced non-small-cell lung cancer: A meta-analysis and systematic review. Medicine (Baltimore). 2019;98(27):e16167.
58. Spigel DR, Faivre-Finn C, Gray JE, et al. Five-Year Survival Outcomes From the PACIFIC Trial: Durvalumab After Chemoradiotherapy in Stage III Non–Small-Cell Lung Cancer. J Clin Oncol. 2022;40(12):1301-11.
59. Pechoux CL, Pourel N, Barlesi F, et al. Postoperative radiotherapy versus no postoperative radiotherapy in patients with completely resected non-small-cell lung cancer and proven mediastinal N2 involvement (Lung ART, IFCT 0503): an open-label, randomised, phase 3 trial. Lancet Oncol. 2022;23(1): 104-14.

60. Hanna NH, Robinson AG, Temin S, et al. Therapy for Stage IV Non–Small-Cell Lung Cancer With Driver Alterations: ASCO and OH (CCO) Joint Guideline Update. J Clin Oncol. 2021;39(9): 1040-91.
61. Hendriks LE, Kerr K, Menis J, Mok TS, Nestle U, Passaro A, et al. Oncogene-addicted metastatic non-small-cell lung cancer: ESMO Clinical Practice Guideline for diagnosis, treatment and follow-up. Ann Oncol 2023;34(4):339-57.
62. Hendriks LE, Kerr KM, Menis J, et al. Non-oncogene-addicted metastatic non-small-cell lung cancer: ESMO Clinical Practice Guideline for diagnosis, treatment and follow-up. Ann Oncol. 2023;34(4):358-76.
63. Singh N, Temin S, Baker S, et al. Therapy for Stage IV Non–Small-Cell Lung Cancer Without Driver Alterations: ASCO Living Guideline. J Clin Oncol. 2022;40(28):3323-43.
64. Pathak N, Garg R, Khurana S, et al. Improving the performance status in advanced non-small cell lung cancer patients with chemotherapy (ImPACt trial): a phase 2 study. J Cancer Res Clin Oncol. 2023;149(9):6399-409.
65. Lee SM, Schulz C, Prabhash K, et al. IPSOS: Results from a phase III study of first-line (1L) atezolizumab (atezo) vs single-agent chemotherapy (chemo) in patients (pts) with NSCLC not eligible for a platinum-containing regimen. Ann Oncol. 2022; 33(suppl_7):S808-69.
66. Thai AA, Solomon BJ, Sequist LV, et al. Lung cancer. Lancet. 2021;398(10299):535-54.
67. van Meerbeeck JP, Fennell DA, De Ruysscher DKM. Small-cell lung cancer. Lancet. 2011;378(9804):1741-55.
68. Lababede O, Meziane MA. The Eighth Edition of TNM Staging of Lung Cancer: Reference Chart and Diagrams. Oncologist. 2018;23(7):844-8.
69. Davis S, Stanley KE, Yesner R, et al. Small-cell carcinoma of the lung--survival according to histologic subtype: a Veterans Administration Lung Group Study. Cancer. 1981;47(7):1863-6.
70. Hiddinga BI, Raskin J, Janssens A, et al. Recent developments in the treatment of small cell lung cancer. Eur Respir Rev. 2021;30(161):210079.
71. Xu J, Yang H, Fu X, et al. Prophylactic Cranial Irradiation for Patients with Surgically Resected Small Cell Lung Cancer. J Thorac Oncol. 2017;12(2):347-53.
72. Horn L, Mansfield AS, Szczęsna A, et al. First-Line Atezolizumab plus Chemotherapy in Extensive-Stage Small-Cell Lung Cancer. N Engl J Med. 2018;379(23):2220-9.
73. Antonia SJ, Villegas A, Daniel D, et al. Durvalumab after Chemoradiotherapy in Stage III Non–Small-Cell Lung Cancer. New Engl J Med. 2017;377(20):1919-29.
74. Gay CM, Stewart CA, Park EM, et al. Patterns of transcription factor programs and immune pathway activation define four major subtypes of SCLC with distinct therapeutic vulnerabilities. Cancer Cell. 2021;39(3):346-60.e7.
75. Pieniążek M, Pawlak P, Radecka B. Early palliative care of non-small cell lung cancer in the context of immunotherapy. Oncol Lett. 2020;20(6):396.
76. Temel JS, Greer JA, Muzikansky A, et al. Early Palliative Care for Patients with Metastatic Non–Small-Cell Lung Cancer. New Engl J Med. 2010;363(8):733-42.
77. Temel JS, Petrillo LA, Greer JA. Patient-Centered Palliative Care for Patients With Advanced Lung Cancer. J Clin Oncol. 2022;40(6):626-34.
78. Ferrell B, Koczywas M, Grannis F, et al. Palliative Care in Lung Cancer. Surg Clin North Am. 2011;91(2):403-ix.
79. Harding R, Murtagh FE. Palliative care for management of small-cell lung cancer. Lancet. 2006;367(9509):474.

Targeted Therapy in Lung Cancer

CHAPTER 153

Puneet Saxena, Itishree Singh, Pawan Singh, Anvesh Rathore

INTRODUCTION

Lung cancer, especially stage IV or metastatic disease, continues to be the harbinger of bad prognosis. Metastatic lung cancer has historically been treated with systemic cytotoxic chemotherapy. Molecular research in early 2000s brought about the understanding of driver mutations and paved way for development of molecules that could target such genetic alterations. As per National Cancer Institute (NCI), the term "targeted therapy" has been defined as a treatment type using drugs or other substances, targeting specific molecules essential for the growth and survival of cancer cells.

DRIVER VERSUS PASSENGER MUTATIONS

Terminologies like driver mutations or passenger mutations are often used in oncology practice. Mutations that occur in cancer cells encoding genes for cell growth and survival are driver mutations. Driver mutations are significantly transforming, i.e., not only do they convert the normal cells to tumor cells but also provide signal to the mutated cells for survival. The feedback inhibition loop and stimulator that regulate cellular division are compromised in driver mutation.[1] Driver mutations are more common in non-small cell lung cancer (NSCLC) and have been the target of several candidate drugs aimed at "personalized" therapy. In comparison to squamous cell carcinoma, adenocarcinoma is more often associated with targetable driver mutations. Opposed to driver mutations, passenger mutations contribute indirectly and are facilitated by mutagenic process exposure and lack of repair. These are often termed as "mini drivers" or neutral mutations.

Figure 1 shows the relative distribution of various driver mutations in NSCLC. Targeted drug to the driver mutation in individual patients with NSCLC showed improved therapeutic efficacy and decreased toxicity. Screening for driver mutations as a standard protocol aids in decision-making for therapeutic intervention, i.e., choosing between standard chemotherapy (or/with immune checkpoint inhibitors) when driver mutation is absent and upfront targeted therapy in the presence of the same.

The Lung Cancer Mutation Consortium conducted a multicentric study to determine the prevalence of oncogenic drivers among patients with lung adenocarcinoma, collated the data on targeted therapies received, and measured survival. Among 733 patients tested for 10 genes, 64% patients had targetable driver mutation. Moreover, patients with driver mutation undergoing a targeted therapy had a median survival of 3.5 years and 5% better performance status when compared to those without targeted therapy who had a median survival of 2.4 years. The study highlights the immense potential of molecular-profiling-guided treatment strategies and prognostication in lung cancer.[2]

EPIDERMAL GROWTH FACTOR RECEPTOR MUTATIONS

The epidermal growth factor receptor (*EGFR*) gene encodes for ErbB1/HER1, a receptor tyrosine kinase. Exons 18–24 encode EGFR kinase, although mutations primarily occur at exons 18–21, which in turn enhance *EGFR*'s kinase activity.[3] Further, due to activation of downstream survival pathway, NSCLC tumorigenesis occurs via three pathways, namely, phosphatidylinositol 3-kinase (PI3K)/AKT/mammalian target of rapamycin (mTOR), mitogen-activated protein kinases (MAPK)/extracellular signal-regulated kinases (ERK), and interleukin 6 (IL-6)/Janus kinase (JAK)/signal transducer and activator of transcription 3 (STAT3) signaling pathways **(Fig. 2)**.[4-6]

The prevalence of EGFR alterations in NSCLC varies with ethnicity and race, ranging from 5 to 15% in Caucasians, 35 to 40% in Indian patients, and from 40 to 55% in East Asians.[7,8]

The EGFR tyrosine kinase inhibitors (TKI) have been used for the patients having activating mutations in the *EGFR* kinase domain. Response may be better with lesser metastatic sites and presence of particular activating mutations in the tyrosine kinase domain of the EGFR (exon 19 deletions

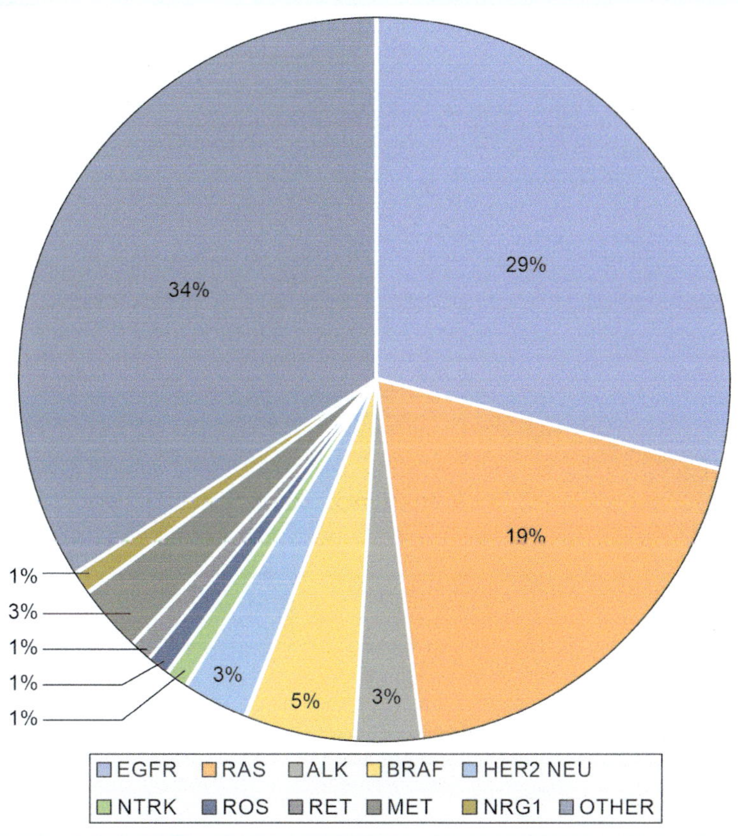

FIG. 1: Distribution of mutations in nonsmall cell lung carcinoma.

(ALK: anaplastic lymphoma kinase; BRAF: v-raf murine sarcoma viral oncogene homolog B1; EGFR: epidermal growth factor receptor; HER2 NEU: human epidermal growth factor receptor 2; MET: mesenchymal epithelial transition factor; NRG1: neuregulin 1; NTRK: neurotrophic tropomyosin receptor kinase; RAS: rat sarcoma; ROS: ROS Proto-Oncogene 1; RET: rearranged during transfection)

or L858R point mutation in exon 21 rather than mutations in exons 20 or 18).[9]

EGFR TKIs are divided into three generations:

1. *First generation:* Gefitinib[10,11] and Erlotinib[12,13] (reversible inhibitors)
2. *Second generation:* Afatinib[14,15] and dacomitinib (irreversible inhibitors)
3. *Third generation:* Osimertinib[11] (irreversible inhibitor)

The first generation TKIs are reversible inhibitors that bind to EGFR and block binding of ATP to the tyrosine kinase domain, whereas the second generation TKIs are irreversible inhibitors that additionally target HER2 and HER4 as well. Although afatinib was able to demonstrate positive preclinical results against substitution mutation of methionine for threonine at residue 790 (*T790M*), it was unable to show clinical efficacy in NSCLC patients with *T790M* mutation and was also accompanied by serious adverse effects.[16,17]

To address resistance caused due to the *T790M* mutation of EGFR, third-generation TKIs came into play and got further approved after benefits were reported in phase 1 and phase 2 trials in patients with *T790M*-positive NSCLC, pretreated with first- or second-generation EGFR TKIs.[18] Osimertinib is the first third-generation TKI approved for management of metastatic NSCLC patients with *T790M* mutation.[19] Its potency to cross the blood-brain barrier is higher and bestows better selectivity and lesser toxicity. Subsequent trials have compared osimertinib's efficacy with standard chemotherapy and first-generation TKIs in patients with metastasized NSCLC and *T790M* mutation. Osimertinib was able to demonstrate better efficacy by prolonging the progression-free survival (PFS) and overall survival (OS) with lower toxicity incidence.[20,21] Based on results from osimertinib's clinical trials, two other third-generation TKIs were developed; aumolertinib and furmonertinib, which also showed improved efficacy.

The details of these drugs are elucidated in **Table 1**.

Treatment-naïve tumors with a sensitizing EGFR mutation should be managed with upfront EGFR TKIs including osimertinib, erlotinib, gefitinib, or afatinib. However, osimertinib is considered to be the preferred first-line option. In EGFR-mutated NSCLC with central nervous system (CNS) disease, osimertinib shows greater efficacy.

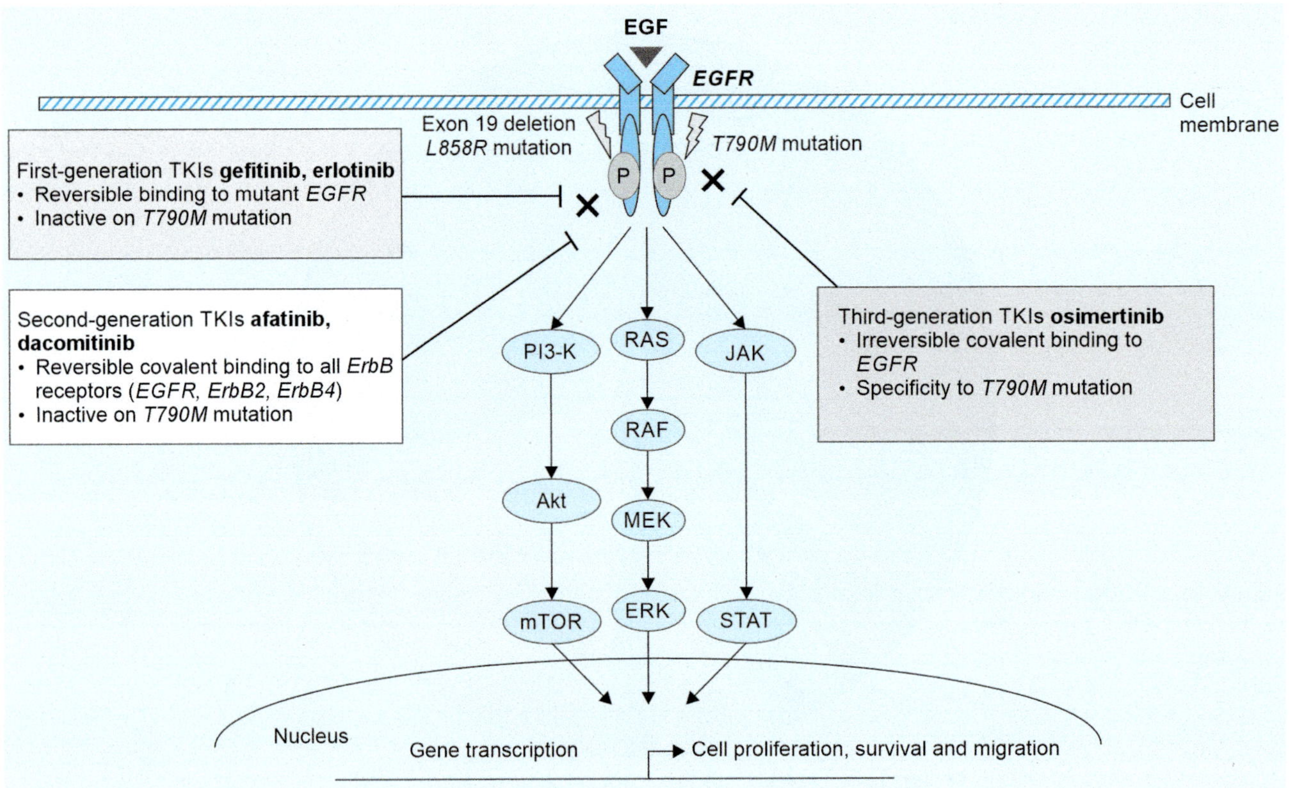

FIG. 2: EGFR signaling pathways.

(EGF: epidermal growth factor; ERK: extracellular signal-regulated kinases; EGFR: epidermal growth factor receptor; JAK: Janus kinase; mTOR: mammalian target of rapamycin; RAS: rat sarcoma; STAT: signal transducer and activator of transcription; TKI: tyrosine kinase inhibitor)

TABLE 1: EGFR TKIs.

Name	Trial	Design	Median PFS (month)	ORR (%)	Median OS (months)
First-generation TKI					
Gefitinib	IPASS[11]	Gefitinib (*n* = 132) versus carboplatin + paclitaxel (*n* = 129)	9.8 versus 6.4	71.2 versus 47.3	21.6 versus 21.9
	WJT0G3405[10]	Gefitinib versus cisplatin + docetaxel	9.2 versus 6.3	62.1 versus 32.2	36.0 versus 39.0
Erlotinib	OPTIMAL[13]	Erlotinib (*n* = 82) versus carboplatin + gemcitabine (*n* = 72)	13.1 versus 4.6	83.0 versus 36.0	22.8 versus 27.2
	EURTAC[12]	Erlotinib (*n* = 86) versus cisplatin + docetaxel (*n* = 87)	9.7 versus 5.2	64.0 versus 18.0	19.3 versus 19.5
Second-generation TKI					
Afatinib	LUX-Lung 3[14]	Afatinib (*n* = 230) versus cisplatin + pemetrexed (*n* = 115)	11.1 versus 6.9	56.1 versus 22.6	28.2 versus 28.2
	LUX-Lung 6[15]	Afatinib (*n* = 242) versus gemcitabine + cisplatin (*n* = 122)	11.0 versus 5.6	66.9 versus 23.0	23.1 versus 23.5
Third-generation TKI					
Osimertinib	AURA 3[20]	Osimertinib versus platinum-based chemotherapy	10.1 versus 4.4	26.8 versus 22.5	NA

(EGFR: epidermal growth factor receptor; ORR: objective response rate; OS: overall survival; PFS: progression-free survival; TKI: tyrosine kinase inhibitor)

ANAPLASTIC LYMPHOMA KINASE REARRANGEMENTS

Anaplastic lymphoma kinase (*ALK*) is another tyrosine kinase that shows aberrant expression in NSCLC. Chromosome rearrangements that involve *ALK* gene loci are found in 3–5% of NSCLC tumors. [22] These patients are relatively younger, having an associated history of never or light smoking (<10 pack-years). Majority of lung tumors harboring the *ALK* fusion oncogene are adenocarcinomas (97%) and rare in squamous cell carcinoma.[23] Other studies have reported abundance of signet ring cell histology among *ALK*-positive tumors. Brain metastasis is a common finding among patients with *ALK*-positive NSCLC compared to patients with NSCLC lacking *EGFR* or *ALK* driver.

The TKIs have been developed to treat *ALK*-positive NSCLC since it is a gene fusion-driven cancer. Fluorescence in situ hybridization (FISH), next-generation sequencing (NGS), or immunohistochemistry (IHC) are utilized to identify these abnormalities, and treatment modalities are decided according to the detected mutation. Details of various generations of *ALK* inhibitors are shown in **Table 2**. Newer drugs like brigatinib and ensartinib have also been developed. These *ALK* inhibitors have shown statistically significant OS benefits over chemotherapy and are associated with better health-related quality-of-life measure.[19,24-27]

Lorlatinib is a third-generation *ALK* inhibitor having a wider coverage of *ALK*-resistant mutations, particularly designed to cross the blood–brain barrier in order to achieve high exposure in CNS. Based on previous phase 1 and phase 2 trials, the antitumor potential of lorlatinib was highlighted, after comparing to failed treatment by generation 1, generation 2 or combination of *ALK* inhibitors.[28] Initial and updated results from an ongoing large, multicentric, phase 3 trial have confirmed the superiority of lorlatinib in patients with or without CNS metastasis.[29,30] Hence, lorlatinib is considered as a standard treatment modality for *ALK*-positive patients for whom other lines of therapies have failed.

Other preferred options also include alectinib,[31] brigatinib,[24,27] ceritinib,[32,33] and crizotinib.[34,35] Brigatinib targets a wide range of *ALK* mutations and also shows improved efficacy when compared to crizotinib as a first-line treatment of *ALK*-positive advanced NSCLC. Pulmonary toxicity is an observed side effect of brigatinib that can be mitigated through step-up dosing. Ceritinib although superior to combination chemotherapy in a first-line setting, is less preferred to alectinib or brigatinib due to poorer efficacy in cross-trial comparisons. Crizotinib is advised to be used in absence of next-generation *ALK* inhibitor. Previous randomized trials have demonstrated greater efficacy of crizotinib over chemotherapy in both first-line and subsequent-line settings in patients with *ALK* rearrangement.

TABLE 2: Anaplastic lymphoma kinase (ALK) inhibitors.

Name	Trial	Design	Median PFS (month)	ORR (%)	Median OS (months)
First-generation					
Crizotinib	PROFILE-1007[34]	Crizotinib versus chemotherapy for patients who failed at least one prior platinum-containing regimen	7.7 versus 3.0	65 versus 20	
	PROFILE 1014[35]	Crizotinib versus chemotherapy in patients with no previous treatment for advanced NSCLC	10.9 versus 7.0	74.4 versus 45	Not estimable versus 47.5
Second-generation					
Ceritinib	ASCEND-4[33]	Ceritinib versus platinum-based chemotherapy	16.6 versus 8.1	72.5 versus 26.7	
	ASCEND-5[32]	Ceritinib versus single-agent chemotherapy	5.4 versus 1.6	45 versus 8	
Alectinib	ALEX trial[31]	Alectinib versus Crizotinib in first line	Reduction in risk of progression or death of 53% median PFS not reached versus 11.1 months		Median OS was not reached versus 57 months
Third-generation					
Lorlatinib	CROWN trial[29]	Lorlatinib versus Crizotinib	Median PFS not evaluable versus 9.3 months	75.8 versus 57.8	Insufficient events to estimate the median OS time

(NSCLC: nonsmall cell lung carcinoma; ORR: objective response rate; OS: overall survival; PFS: progression-free survival)

ROS1 REARRANGEMENTS

ROS proto-oncogene 1 (*ROS1*) belongs to the insulin receptor subfamily encoding for tyrosine kinase. *ROS1* rearrangements affect 1–2% of NSCLC patients, with 10,000–15,000 new cases reported each year. These alterations are identified using a FISH break-apart platform as well as NGS and have clinical characteristics overlapping with *ALK*-rearranged NSCLC, despite the fact that genetic rearrangements in *ROS1*, *EGFR*, and *ALK* are usually mutually exclusive.[36,37] Patients with adenocarcinoma histology, absence of history of smoking, and younger age are more likely to have ROS1 rearrangements.

There are two TKIs validated and approved as a first-line therapy for *ROS1*-positive NSCLCs, i.e., crizotinib and entrectinib **(Table 3)**. Phase I PROFILE 1001 trial results demonstrated crizotinib efficacy in a patient population having metastatic *ROS1*-positive NSCLC.[38] The drug efficacy was further validated through subsequent retrospective trials, prospective phase II trials, and extended phase I trials.[39-43] Further research in pursuit of creating *ROS1*-targeting molecules with better cerebral penetration, led to the development of entrectinib. In vitro studies demonstrated better potency of entrectinib against ROS-1 activity compared to crizotinib. Further phase I/II trials displayed not only its anti-tumoral activity but also better tolerability. An integrated analysis of three clinical trials (ALKA-372-001, STARTRK-1, and STARTRK-2) reported entrectinib's high clinical efficacy in patients having ROS1-fusion-positive NSCLC, including those with CNS metastasis.[44,45] The treatment-related side-effects were similar to those seen with *ALK*-positive NSCLC, and it has resulted in improved quality of life relative to patients on chemotherapy in a randomized trial in that setting. Most patients tolerate the drug well, but dose modifications maybe required considering the associated side effects such as congestive heart failure, hepatotoxicity, fractures, CNS toxicity, and QT prolongation.

Lorlatinib is another TKI inhibitor that has shown anti-tumor activity in *ROS1*-positive NSCLC that has acquired resistance to crizotinib. A phase I/II trial showed that lorlatinib was effective in patients with *ROS1*-positive NSCLC. Not only did it lead to a positive response in crizotinib-naïve patients [objective response rate (ORR): 62%] but also in those with prior crizotinib exposure (ORR: 35% among those who received crizotinib as their only prior TKI).[28,46,47] Although further studies are required to confirm the exploratory observations demonstrating lorlatinib's response to tumor-resistance behavior developed through crizotinib.[28]

Other TKIs like cabozantinib and ceritinib have demonstrated efficacy in *ROS1*-positive NSCLC whereas alectinib and brigatinib have limited role in these patients. Repotrectinib is another next-generation TKI, undergoing phase I/II clinical trial, with properties enabling it to pass through the blood–brain barrier, that stays as a main resistance mechanism.[48]

MESENCHYMAL-EPITHELIAL TRANSITION FACTOR ABNORMALITIES

Mesenchymal-epithelial transition (*MET*) is a tyrosine kinase receptor for hepatocyte growth factor (HGF). Three types of *MET* TKIs have been developed and tested in trials and referred to as Type I, II, and III MET TKIs. Type I and II are ATP-competitive but Type I binds to *MET* in its catalytically active conformation whereas Type II binds to inactive *MET* conformation. Type I is further classified as Ia (crizotinib), which interacts with the solvent front G1163, and Ib (capmatinib, tepotinib, and savolitinib), which functions independent of G1163 interaction. Type II inhibitors (cabozantinib, merestinib, and glesatinib) bind to *MET* in its inactive conformation. Type III (Tivantinib) is noncompetitive allosteric inhibitor and failed in clinical trials.

There are two abnormalities of *MET* that make them oncogenic-drivers and potentially targetable.

1. *MET exon-14 skipping mutation:* This mutation drives the tumor growth by minimizing the MET protein breakdown. Detected mostly by deoxyribonucleic acid

TABLE 3: ROS-1 inhibitors.

Name	Trial	Design	Median PFS (month)	ORR (%)	Median 12-month OS rate (%)
Crizotinib	Crizotinib in ROS1-rearranged non-small-cell lung cancer[38] and phase I PROFILE 1001 study with updated results	*ROS1/MET inhibitor:* Open-label interventional study, included 53 patients, 87% of whom had received one or more prior chemotherapy regimens	19.3	72	79
Entrectinib	ALKA-372-001, STARTRK-1, and an integrated analysis of three clinical trials [ALKA-372-001 (phase I), STARTRK-1 and STARTRK-2 (phase I/II)]	*ROS1/tropomyosin receptor kinase (TRK) inhibitor:* Pooled analysis of three phase I or II trials including 161 patients	15.7	67	81

(NSCLC: nonsmall cell lung carcinoma; ORR: objective response rate; OS: overall survival; PFS: progression-free survival)

(DNA) or ribonucleic acid (RNA) NGS, this mutation occurs in 3–4% of lung adenocarcinomas and may be detected in almost 20% of sarcomatoid variants of NSCLC. Targeted therapy with TKIs is recommended in the presence of this mutation, in the first-line setting (preferable to immunotherapy or chemotherapy) as well as after failure of one or more lines of therapy. Currently, capmatinib and tepotinib are approved for use in *MET* exon-14 skipping mutation, based on safety profile and efficacy. Crizotinib and cabozantinib have shown efficacy in trials but are currently less preferred, as compared to capmatinib and tepotinib.

2. *MET gene amplification*: This abnormality is linked to 2–4% of treatment-naive NSCLC and 5–20% of *EGFR*-mutated tumors that have developed resistance to *EGFR* inhibitors.[49,50] This *MET* abnormality has been associated with overall worse prognosis. It is detected by FISH or NGS panels[51] MET-TKIs, like crizotinib and capmatinib, may be used after failure of initial line of therapy, when *MET* gene amplification is found.

The *EGFR* TKIs in combination with *MET* TKIs have also elicited antitumor activities and the combination is considered a promising therapy line specifically beneficial to patients with *MET*-driven, *EGFR*-TKI acquired resistance. Osimertinib in combination with savolitinib demonstrated acceptable tolerability and safety profile for patients with advanced NSCLC having *MET*-driven *EFGR* mutation positivity.[52]

In a randomized phase II trial, where cabozantinib was compared with erlotinib, alone and in combination, it showed significant improvement in PFS for cabozantinib arm as well as the combination therapy arm opposed to erlotinib alone.[53]

V-RAF MURINE SARCOMA VIRAL ONCOGENE HOMOLOG B1 MUTATIONS

V-raf murine sarcoma viral oncogene homolog B1 (*BRAF*) is a signaling mediator of the Kirsten rat sarcoma (*KRAS*) viral oncogene homolog pathway that stimulates the MAPK pathway. BRAF mutations are found in 1–3% of NSCLC patients and may appear either at the V600 site of exon 15 (known as *V600 BRAF mutations*), or elsewhere (*non-V600 BRAF* mutations). The former may have a superior survival. These mutations are more commonly associated with a history of smoking and are identified with polymerase chain reaction (PCR) or NGS.[54]

Dabrafenib and vemurafenib are novel-generation *BRAF* inhibitors that specifically target *BRAF V600E* mutations. Vemurafenib's antitumor activity and its efficacy against *BRAF-V600* mutants have been demonstrated in several studies. In an initial basket study that included multiple nonmelanoma cancers with *BRAF V600* mutants, NSCLC patients showed positive results (ORR: 42% and PFS: 7.3 months).[55] Another study also demonstrated vemurafenib specifically targeting *BRAF-V600* and showing no activity in *BRAF non-V600* mutants.[56] These findings helped in corroborating vemurafenib as an optional regimen for NSCLC patients with *BRAF-V600* mutation. Other inhibitor, lifirafenib (BGB-283), has also shown promising results, although activity of such single *BRAF* inhibitors is restricted, and hence combination therapy requires exploration.[57]

Currently, a combination of *BRAF* inhibitor (dabrafenib) and MEK inhibitor (trametinib) is approved for use in NSCLC harboring *BRAF V600* mutations, and this therapy is preferred over chemotherapy and immunotherapy in such patients.[58]

NEUROTROPHIC TROPOMYOSIN RECEPTOR KINASE FUSIONS

Neurotrophic tropomyosin receptor kinase (*NTRK*) gene fusion is a rare oncogenic driver of NSCLC. Downstream signaling pathway required for tumor growth and proliferation is tenaciously activated due to the fusion oncogene expressed when 3' sequence of *NTRK* gene merges with 5' sequence of a fusion partner gene. Multicontinental studies have shown the prevalence of *NTRK* fusions varying from 0.1 to 3.3%. Nucleic acid-based sequencing is usually done for identifying *NTRK* fusions, which could be further followed by IHC, FISH, and RT-PCR. First-generation NTRK-TKIs, larotrectinib and entrectinib, have shown antitumor activities that provided them approval for being used as a first-line treatment modality among patients with *NTRK* fusion with advanced or metastatic NSCLC. The efficacy of larotrectinib has been studied in three clinical trials with Hong et al. reporting a pooled analysis of all the three trials (ORR: 75% in NSCLC population and PFS: 28.3 months for the overall population) that further led to approval of larotrectinib.[59] Additionally, entrectinib is another inhibitor that is being studied currently for its role as a neoadjuvant therapy in patients with resectable stage II–III NSCLC. Other second-generation TRK inhibitors such as selitrectinib, repotrectinib, and taletrectinib are also being studied with the aim to overcome resistance acquired to the first-generation inhibitors.

RAT SARCOMA MUTATIONS

Rat sarcoma (*RAS*) is one of the most frequently mutated oncogenes with *KRAS* being the most mutated isoform of *RAS*.[60] Detected in 20–35% of adenocarcinomas, activating *KRAS* mutations are able to trigger several downstream pathways leading to tumorigenesis. It has been seen that molecular alterations involving *KRAS* and *BRAF* are more responsive to immunotherapy than NSCLC with other oncogenic drivers.[56]

Sotorasib, and later, adagrasib have been approved for KRAS G12C-mutated NSCLC, in the subsequent-line setting.

HER2 MUTATIONS AND AMPLIFICATIONS

Human epidermal growth factor receptor 2 [HER2 (ERBB2)], a receptor tyrosine kinase of the *EGFR* family, has been found in nearly 1–3% of NSCLC tumors using PCR or NGS.[61] These tumors are prevalent among nonsmokers and women and are associated predominantly with adenocarcinomas.

Fam-trastuzumab deruxtecan is a trastuzumab-based antibody-drug conjugate approved for patients with unresectable or metastatic NSCLC with *HER2* exon-20-insertion mutation, in the subsequent-line setting. The efficacy of this conjugate was shown in the DESTINY-Lung01 study in 91 patients harboring the *HER2* mutation who had progressed on systemic chemotherapy.[62]

Evidence is emerging in favor of ado-trastuzumab emtansine and other trastuzumab-based regimens that have shown effectiveness in numerous phase II trials but have yet to receive approval.

TARGETED THERAPY IN EARLY-STAGE LUNG CANCER

Encouraged with success of targeted therapy in metastatic NSCLC, there has been a keen interest in exploring the potential of targeted therapy in management of early-stage NSCLC harboring driver mutations. The emerging evidence is primarily in the role of targeted therapy in the adjuvant and neoadjuvant setting, in resectable NSCLC. The prevalence of *EGFR* mutations is much higher as compared to other targetable mutations in this group. Use of TKIs, especially osimertinib, has shown an unequivocal benefit in disease-free survival in adjuvant settings.[63] Osimertinib is now approved for this indication, though it is still not clear whether the combination of TKI with chemotherapy is superior to TKI alone in the adjuvant setting. Evidence is similarly emerging for use of TKI in neoadjuvant setting, and phase II trials have been promising.

SUMMARY

Advances in genomics and translational research are increasingly opening up novel avenues for personalized treatment of lung cancer, particularly in NSCLC. Targeted therapies have proven their potential to remarkably transform the clinically relevant outcomes, and thus it is mandatory now for thoracic oncologists to explore all possible potential targets for personalized therapy before resorting to conventional chemotherapy and immunotherapy. Future research will focus not only on newer targets and molecules but also in trials of combination therapies involving targeted therapies tailored to produce the best efficacy with the least adverse effects.

REFERENCES

1. He B, Li T, Guan L, et al. *CTNNA3* is a tumor suppressor in hepatocellular carcinomas and is inhibited by miR-425. Oncotarget. 2016;7(7):8078-89.
2. Kris MG, Johnson BE, Berry LD, et al. Using multiplexed assays of oncogenic drivers in lung cancers to select targeted drugs. Jama. 2014;311(19):1998-2006.
3. Yoneda K, Imanishi N, Ichiki Y, et al. Treatment of non-small cell lung cancer with EGFR-mutations. J UOEH. 2019;41(2):153-63.
4. Sharma SV, Bell DW, Settleman J, et al. Epidermal growth factor receptor mutations in lung cancer. Nat Rev Cancer. 2007;7(3):169-81.
5. Herbst RS. Review of epidermal growth factor receptor biology. Int J Radiat Oncol Biol Phys. 2004;59(2 Suppl):21-6.
6. Hynes NE, Lane HA. ERBB receptors and cancer: The complexity of targeted inhibitors. Nat Rev Cancer. 2005;5(5):341-54.
7. Ha SY, Choi SJ, Cho JH, et al. Lung cancer in never-smoker Asian females is driven by oncogenic mutations, most often involving EGFR. Oncotarget. 2015;6(7):5465-74.
8. Kaler AK, Patel K, Patil H, et al. Mutational Analysis of EGFR Mutations in Non-Small Cell Lung Carcinoma: An Indian Perspective of 212 Patients. Int J Environ Res Public Health. 2022;20(1):758.
9. Garg A, Batra U, Choudhary P, et al. Clinical predictors of response to EGFR-tyrosine kinase inhibitors in EGFR-mutated non-small cell lung cancer: A real-world multicentric cohort analysis from India. Curr Probl Cancer. 2020;44(3):100570.
10. Mitsudomi T, Morita S, Yatabe Y, et al. Gefitinib versus cisplatin plus docetaxel in patients with non-small-cell lung cancer harbouring mutations of the epidermal growth factor receptor (WJTOG3405): An open label, randomised phase 3 trial. Lancet Oncol. 2010;11(2):121-8.
11. Mok TS, Wu YL, Thongprasert S, et al. Gefitinib or carboplatin-paclitaxel in pulmonary adenocarcinoma. N Engl J Med. 2009;361(10):947-57.
12. Rosell R, Carcereny E, Gervais R, et al. Erlotinib versus standard chemotherapy as first-line treatment for European patients with advanced EGFR mutation-positive non-small-cell lung cancer (EURTAC): A multicentre, open-label, randomised phase 3 trial. Lancet Oncol. 2012;13(3):239-46.
13. Zhou C, Wu YL, Chen G, et al. Final overall survival results from a randomised, phase III study of erlotinib versus chemotherapy as first-line treatment of EGFR mutation-positive advanced non-small-cell lung cancer (OPTIMAL, CTONG-0802). Ann Oncol. 2015;26(9):1877-83.
14. Sequist LV, Yang JC, Yamamoto N, et al. Phase III study of afatinib or cisplatin plus pemetrexed in patients with metastatic lung adenocarcinoma with EGFR mutations. J Clin Oncol. 2013;31(27):3327-34.
15. Wu YL, Zhou C, Hu CP, et al. Afatinib versus cisplatin plus gemcitabine for first-line treatment of Asian patients with advanced non-small-cell lung cancer harbouring EGFR mutations (LUX-Lung 6): An open-label, randomised phase 3 trial. Lancet Oncol. 2014;15(2):213-22.
16. Park K, Tan EH, O'Byrne K, et al. Afatinib versus gefitinib as first-line treatment of patients with EGFR mutation-positive non-small-cell lung cancer (LUX-Lung 7): A phase 2B, open-label, randomised controlled trial. Lancet Oncol. 2016;17(5):577-89.

17. Wu YL, Cheng Y, Zhou X, et al. Dacomitinib versus gefitinib as first-line treatment for patients with EGFR-mutation-positive non-small-cell lung cancer (ARCHER 1050): A randomised, open-label, phase 3 trial. Lancet Oncol. 2017;18(11):1454-66.
18. Sankar K, Gadgeel SM, Qin A. Molecular therapeutic targets in non-small cell lung cancer. Expert Rev Anticancer Ther. 2020; 20(8):647-61.
19. Greig SL. Osimertinib: First global approval. Drugs. 2016;76(2): 263-73.
20. Mok TS, Wu Y-L, Ahn M-J, et al. Osimertinib or platinum–pemetrexed in EGFR T790M–positive lung cancer. N Engl J Med. 2017;376(7):629-40.
21. Ramalingam SS, Vansteenkiste J, Planchard D, et al. Overall survival with osimertinib in untreated, EGFR-mutated advanced NSCLC. N Engl J Med. 2020;382(1):41-50.
22. Chevallier M, Borgeaud M, Addeo A, et al. Oncogenic driver mutations in non-small cell lung cancer: Past, present and future. World J Clin Oncol. 2021;12(4):217-37.
23. Shaw AT, Yeap BY, Mino-Kenudson M, et al. Clinical features and outcome of patients with non-small-cell lung cancer who harbor EML4-ALK. J Clin Oncol. 2009;27(26):4247-53.
24. Camidge DR, Kim HR, Ahn MJ, et al. Brigatinib versus crizotinib in ALK-positive non-small-cell lung cancer. N Engl J Med. 2018;379(21):2027-39.
25. Horn L, Infante JR, Reckamp KL, et al. Ensartinib (X-396) in ALK-positive non-small cell lung cancer: Results from a first-in-human phase I/II, multicenter study. Clin Cancer Res. 2018;24(12): 2771-9.
26. Horn L, Wang Z, Wu G, et al. Ensartinib vs crizotinib for patients with anaplastic lymphoma kinase-positive non-small cell lung cancer: A randomized clinical trial. JAMA Oncol. 2021;7(11): 1617-25.
27. Kim DW, Tiseo M, Ahn MJ, et al. Brigatinib in patients with crizotinib-refractory anaplastic lymphoma kinase–positive non–small-cell lung cancer: A randomized, multicenter phase II trial. J Clin Oncol. 2017;35(22):2490-8.
28. Shaw AT, Solomon BJ, Chiari R, et al. Lorlatinib in advanced ROS1-positive non-small-cell lung cancer: A multicentre, open-label, single-arm, phase 1-2 trial. Lancet Oncol. 2019;20(12): 1691-701.
29. Shaw AT, Bauer TM, de Marinis F, et al. First-line lorlatinib or crizotinib in advanced ALK-positive lung cancer. N Engl J Med. 2020;383(21).2018-29.
30. Solomon BJ, Bauer TM, Mok TSK, et al. Efficacy and safety of first-line lorlatinib versus crizotinib in patients with advanced, ALK-positive non-small-cell lung cancer: Updated analysis of data from the phase 3, randomised, open-label CROWN study. Lancet Respir Med. 2023;11(4):354-66.
31. Peters S, Camidge DR, Shaw AT, et al. Alectinib versus crizotinib in untreated ALK-positive non-small-cell lung cancer. N Engl J Med. 2017;377(9):829-38.
32. Shaw AT, Kim TM, Crinò L, et al. Ceritinib versus chemotherapy in patients with ALK-rearranged non-small-cell lung cancer previously given chemotherapy and crizotinib (ASCEND-5): A randomised, controlled, open-label, phase 3 trial. Lancet Oncol. 2017;18(7):874-86.
33. Soria JC, Tan DSW, Chiari R, et al. First-line ceritinib versus platinum-based chemotherapy in advanced ALK-rearranged non-small-cell lung cancer (ASCEND-4): A randomised, open-label, phase 3 study. Lancet. 2017;389(10072):917-29.
34. Shaw AT, Kim DW, Nakagawa K, et al. Crizotinib versus chemotherapy in advanced ALK-positive lung cancer. N Engl J Med. 2013;368(25):2385-94.
35. Solomon BJ, Mok T, Kim DW, et al. First-line crizotinib versus chemotherapy in ALK-positive lung cancer. N Engl J Med. 2014; 371(23):2167-77.
36. Balduzzi PC, Notter MF, Morgan HR, et al. Some biological properties of two new avian sarcoma viruses. J Virol. 1981; 40(1):268-75.
37. Roskoski R Jr. ROS1 protein-tyrosine kinase inhibitors in the treatment of ROS1 fusion protein-driven non-small cell lung cancers. Pharmacol Res. 2017;121:202-12.
38. Shaw AT, Ou SH, Bang YJ, et al. Crizotinib in ROS1-rearranged non-small-cell lung cancer. N Engl J Med. 2014;371(21):1963-71.
39. Landi L, Chiari R, Tiseo M, et al. Crizotinib in *MET*-deregulated or ROS1-rearranged pretreated non-small cell lung cancer (METROS): A phase II, prospective, multicenter, two-arms trial. Clin Cancer Res. 2019;25(24):7312-9.
40. Michels S, Massutí B, Schildhaus HU, et al. Safety and efficacy of crizotinib in patients with advanced or metastatic ROS1-rearranged lung cancer (EUCROSS): A European phase II clinical trial. J Thorac Oncol. 2019;14(7):1266-76.
41. Moro-Sibilot D, Cozic N, Pérol M, et al. Crizotinib in c-MET- or ROS1-positive NSCLC: Results of the AcSé phase II trial. Ann Oncol. 2019;30(12):1985-91.
42. Wu YL, Yang JC, Kim DW, et al. Phase II Study of crizotinib in east Asian patients with ROS1-positive advanced non–small-cell lung cancer. J Clin Oncol. 2018;36(14):1405-11.
43. Shaw AT, Riely GJ, Bang YJ, et al. Crizotinib in ROS1-rearranged advanced non-small-cell lung cancer (NSCLC): Updated results, including overall survival, from PROFILE 1001. Ann Oncol. 2019;30(7):1121-6.
44. Drilon A, Siena S, Ou SI, et al. Safety and antitumor activity of the multitargeted pan-TRK, ROS1, and ALK inhibitor entrectinib: Combined results from two phase I trials (ALKA-372-001 and STARTRK-1). Cancer Discov. 2017;7(4):400-9.
45. Dziadziuszko R, Krebs MG, De Braud F, et al. Updated integrated analysis of the efficacy and safety of entrectinib in locally advanced or metastatic ROS1 fusion-positive non-small-cell lung cancer. J Clin Oncol. 2021;39(11):1253-63.
46. Shaw AT, Felip E, Bauer TM, et al. Lorlatinib in non-small-cell lung cancer with ALK or ROS1 rearrangement: An international, multicentre, open-label, single-arm first-in-man phase 1 trial. Lancet Oncol. 2017;18(12):1590-9.
47. Solomon BJ, Besse B, Bauer TM, et al. Lorlatinib in patients with ALK-positive non-small-cell lung cancer: Results from a global phase 2 study. Lancet Oncol. 2018;19(12):1654-67.
48. Yun MR, Kim DH, Kim SY, et al. Repotrectinib exhibits potent antitumor activity in treatment-naïve and solvent-front-mutant ROS1-rearranged non-small cell lung cancer. Clin Cancer Res. 2020;26(13):3287-95.
49. Bean J, Brennan C, Shih JY, et al. MET amplification occurs with or without T790M mutations in EGFR mutant lung tumors with acquired resistance to gefitinib or erlotinib. Proc Natl Acad Sci USA. 2007;104(52):20932-7.
50. Sequist LV, Waltman BA, Dias-Santagata D, et al. Genotypic and histological evolution of lung cancers acquiring resistance to EGFR inhibitors. Sci Transl Med. 2011;3(75):75ra26.
51. Camidge DR, Ou SHI, Shapiro G, et al. Efficacy and safety of crizotinib in patients with advanced c-MET-amplified non-small cell lung cancer (NSCLC). J Clin Oncol. 2014;32(15_suppl):8001.

52. Hartmaier RJ, Markovets AA, Ahn MJ, et al. Osimertinib + savolitinib to overcome acquired MET-mediated resistance in epidermal growth factor receptor-mutated, MET-amplified non-small cell lung cancer: TATTON. Cancer Discov. 2023;13(1): 98-113.
53. Reckamp KL, Frankel PH, Ruel N, et al. Phase II trial of cabozantinib plus erlotinib in patients with advanced epidermal growth factor receptor (EGFR)-mutant non-small cell lung cancer with progressive disease on epidermal growth factor receptor tyrosine kinase inhibitor therapy: A California cancer consortium phase II trial (NCI 9303). Front Oncol. 2019;9:132.
54. Paik PK, Arcila ME, Fara M, et al. Clinical characteristics of patients with lung adenocarcinomas harboring BRAF mutations. J Clin Oncol. 2011;29(15):2046-51.
55. Hyman DM, Puzanov I, Subbiah V, et al. Vemurafenib in multiple nonmelanoma cancers with BRAF V600 mutations. N Engl J Med. 2015;373(8):726-36.
56. Mazieres J, Cropet C, Montané L, et al. Vemurafenib in non-small-cell lung cancer patients with BRAF(V600) and BRAF(nonV600) mutations. Ann Oncol. 2020;31(2):289-94.
57. Desai J, Gan H, Barrow C, et al. Phase I, open-label, dose-escalation/dose-expansion study of lifirafenib (BGB-283), an RAF family kinase inhibitor, in patients with solid tumors. J Clin Oncol. 2020;38(19):2140-50.
58. Planchard D, Besse B, Groen HJM, et al. Phase 2 study of dabrafenib plus trametinib in patients with BRAF V600E-mutant metastatic NSCLC: Updated 5-year survival rates and genomic analysis. J Thorac Oncol. 2022;17(1):103-15.
59. Hong DS, DuBois SG, Kummar S, et al. Larotrectinib in patients with TRK fusion-positive solid tumours: A pooled analysis of three phase 1/2 clinical trials. Lancet Oncol. 2020;21(4):531-40.
60. Kirsten WH, Mayer LA. Morphologic responses to a murine erythroblastosis virus. J Natl Cancer Inst. 1967;39(2):311-35.
61. Arcila ME, Chaft JE, Nafa K, et al. Prevalence, clinicopathologic associations, and molecular spectrum of ERBB2 (HER2) tyrosine kinase mutations in lung adenocarcinomas. Clin Cancer Res. 2012;18(18):4910-8.
62. Li BT, Smit EF, Goto Y, et al. Trastuzumab Deruxtecan in HER2-mutant non-small-cell lung cancer. N Engl J Med. 2022;386(3): 241-51.
63. de Scordilli M, Michelotti A, Bertoli E, et al. Targeted therapy and immunotherapy in early-stage non-small cell lung cancer: Current evidence and ongoing trials. Int J Mol Sci. 2022;23(13): 7222.

CHAPTER 154

Solitary Pulmonary Nodule

Alladi Mohan, B Vijayalakshmi Devi, Abha Chandra

INTRODUCTION

Solitary pulmonary nodules (SPNs) are small, focal, radiographic opacities that may be caused by a variety of benign and malignant disorders, which constitute a unique diagnostic problem faced by pulmonologists, radiologists, and thoracic surgeons.[1-6] In the earlier days of conventional radiography, these lesions used to be most commonly encountered as incidental findings on chest radiographs. In the present era, the widespread use of computed tomography (CT) has resulted in a significant increase in the detection of these lesions.[7,8] Many patients with early-stage lung cancer can present with an SPN. The overall 5-year survival rate in patients with lung cancer is poor (≤ 15%); in comparison, long-term survival in stage IA lesions that can be resected may be as high as 80%.[1,7,8] Therefore, it is important to distinguish whether the lesion is benign or malignant so that early intervention can be done in patients with lung cancer and unnecessary surgery can be avoided in patients with benign SPNs.

Advances in CT technology, such as multidetector row CT (MDCT) for the evaluation of lung and cardiovascular disease, computer-aided diagnosis (CAD), ^{18}F-fluorolabeled 2-deoxy-D-glucose positron emission tomography (FDG-PET), have markedly influenced the diagnostic workup of a patient presenting with an SPN.[1,7] Comprehensive evaluation of an SPN requires careful consideration of a variety of patient-related variables, imaging findings, appropriate use of invasive sampling, and logistics related to a meticulous follow-up schedule. This chapter attempts to provide an overview regarding the clinical approach to the diagnosis and management of a patient with an SPN.

TERMINOLOGY

It is preferred that the term *coin lesion* is not used to describe SPNs because coin lesion implies a flat two-dimensional structure.[9-12] The SPN is defined as a single, spherical, well-circumscribed, radiographic opacity that measures ≤3 cm in diameter, which is surrounded completely by aerated lung and is not associated with atelectasis, other parenchymal infiltrates, hilar or mediastinal lymphadenopathy, or pleural effusion.[9-12] Focal pulmonary lesions that are greater than 3 cm in diameter are called *lung masses* and these are commonly the manifestations of bronchogenic carcinoma. The lung nodules that measure <8–10 mm in diameter are called *subcentimeter* nodules; these are much less likely to be malignant, are difficult to accurately characterize by imaging modalities, and are often difficult to approach by needle biopsy.[9-12] For practical purposes, the term SPN is used in the context of lung nodules that are at least 8–10 mm, but ≤3 cm in diameter.

Considering the probability of malignancy, pulmonary nodules have been categorized into (i) small solid (<8 mm), (ii) larger solid nodules (≥8–30 mm), and (iii) subsolid nodules. Subsolid nodules have been further divided into ground-glass nodules (no solid component) and part-solid (both ground-glass and solid components).[1]

The SPN needs to be distinguished from multiple pulmonary nodules, the diagnostic significance and the algorithm for workup are different. Furthermore, up to 20% of SPNs observed on chest radiographs may in fact be nonpulmonary in origin, may represent nipple shadow, skin lesions (**Figs. 1A to C**), rib fracture, end-on view of blood vessels, composite shadows, or monitor leads.[13] This chapter describes the evaluation of a patient presenting with a single dominant pulmonary nodule (the largest or the most suspicious-appearing nodule is termed *dominant* nodule).[1] Evaluation of pulmonary nodules in patients with known malignancy and patients with multiple pulmonary nodules without a dominant pulmonary nodule are not dealt with in this chapter.

EPIDEMIOLOGY

The dutch language debbreviation for this is Nederlands-Leuvens Longkanker Screenings On-derzoek [NELSON].

WORLD SCENARIO

In an early study,[14] SPN was found in 1 of 500 (0.2%) chest radiographs that were obtained in community settings.

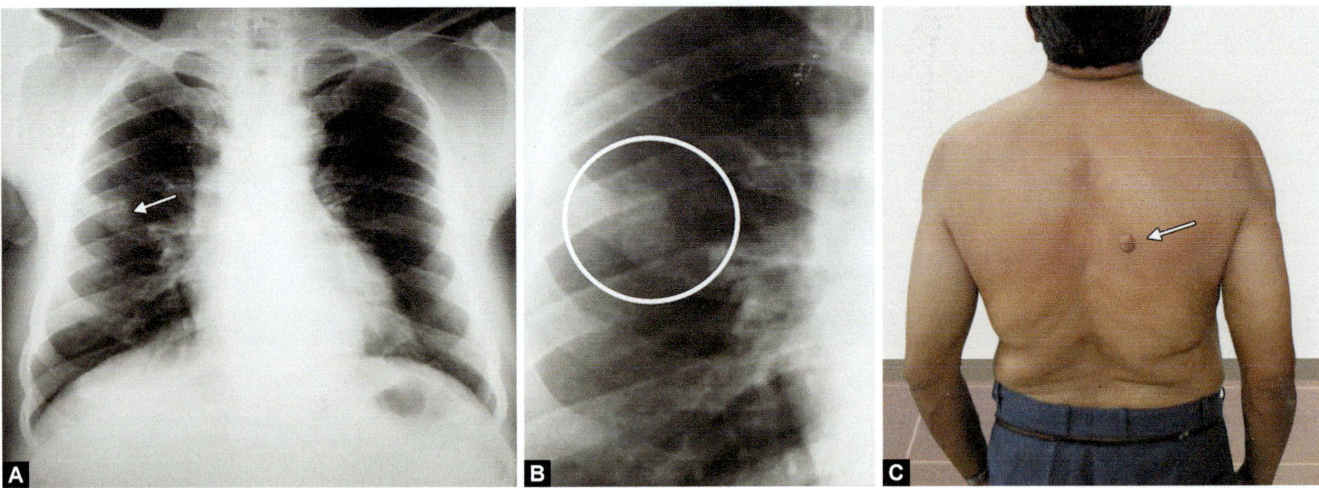

FIGS. 1A TO C: (A) Chest radiograph (posteroanterior view) of a patient referred for further evaluation showing a solitary pulmonary nodule (SPN) in the right mid-zone (arrow); (B) Close-up view (open circle) of the SPN; and (C) Clinical examination revealed that the lesion was a cutaneous papilloma mimicking an SPN.

In the Dutch-Belgian randomized lung cancer screening trial (Dutch acronym: NELSON study),[15] 147/6,309 (2.3%) patients undergoing screening for lung cancer had a nodule identified during baseline screening that grew at a concerning pace when measured 3 months later. In two studies[16,17] of screening chest X-rays (n = 103,500 participants), a pulmonary nodule was identified in 7.8–8.9% of the chest X-rays.

INDIA

Though there have been occasional case reports, reliable epidemiological data on the true incidence of SPN is lacking. Pulmonary tuberculosis (TB) uncommonly has been documented to present as an SPN in some studies.[6,18-20] At the Sri Venkateswara Institute of Medical Sciences (SVIMS), Tirupati, during the period 1994–2005, in the 82 patients with SPN, the etiological diagnosis was bronchogenic carcinoma (n = 31; 37.8%) and TB (n = 20; 24.4%), among others.[6]

The variations in the definitions used, differences in the population chosen for evaluation, and the radiological technique are important causes responsible for the wide range of prevalence observed. Because of lack of uniformity, comparison of data across various studies also becomes difficult.

ETIOLOGY

Various etiological causes that manifest as an SPN are listed in **Box 1**. The etiological spectrum varies depending on the age group, geographical location of the patient, and prevalence of risk factors for lung cancer. Common benign causes of SPN include active granulomatous infection (e.g., tuberculosis), hamartoma, lung abscess, round pneumonia, round atelectasis, bronchogenic cyst, hydatid cyst, healed pulmonary infarcts, focal hemorrhage, hemangiomas, and arteriovenous malformations. Most common causes of malignant SPN are adenocarcinoma, squamous cell carcinoma, solitary metastasis, undifferentiated non-small cell lung carcinoma (NSCLC), small cell lung cancer, and bronchioloalveolar cell carcinoma.[1-6]

CLINICAL EVALUATION

Majority of patients presenting with SPN are asymptomatic with the lesion being picked up incidentally in a chest radiograph or CT carried out for some other purposes. Clinical evaluation of a patient with SPN begins with a detailed history and thorough physical examination **(Box 2)**. This is followed by appropriate imaging investigations and interventions for procuring tissue for cytopathological or histopathological diagnosis. Experienced clinicians evaluating patients with SPN intuitively tend to acquire clinical information in order to estimate the clinical "pre-test" probability of the SPN being malignant before ordering imaging tests or biopsy procedures.

Age of the patient is an important clue and one of the independent factors predictive of malignancy in an SPN.[1-6,21] Malignancy is rarely a cause of SPN in patients under 30 years of age; older the patient, higher the likelihood that the SPN is caused by malignancy. A history of current or remote malignancy (especially lung cancer or head and neck cancer) significantly increases the probability of a malignant SPN.[21,22] The probability of the SPN being a metastatic lesion in the absence of a known prior malignancy is low.

History of tobacco smoking and other established exposures associated with an increased risk of lung cancer, such as silica, air pollution, arsenic, cadmium, chromium,

BOX 1 Etiological causes of a solitary pulmonary nodule.

- *Developmental*:
  - Bronchogenic cyst
  - Bronchial atresia with mucoid impaction
  - Sequestration
- *Infections*:
  - Tuberculosis
  - Fungal infections (e.g., coccidioidomycosis, histoplasmosis, cryptococcosis, and aspergillosis)
  - Organizing pneumonia
  - Lung abscess
  - Septic embolus
  - Round pneumonia
- *Neoplastic*:
  - Benign
  - Hamartoma
  - Chondroma
  - Teratoma
  - Leiomyoma
  - Endometriosis
- *Malignant*:
  - Carcinoma
  - Metastasis
  - Carcinoid tumor
- *Vascular*:
  - Arteriovenous malformation
  - Pulmonary infarction
  - Hematoma
  - Pulmonary artery aneurysm
- *Lymphatic*:
  - Intrapulmonary lymph node
  - Lymphoma
- *Inflammatory*:
  - Rheumatoid nodule
  - Wegener's granulomatosis
  - Sarcoidosis
- *Airway*:
  - Mucus impaction (e.g., bronchiectasis)
- *Others*:
  - Rounded atelectasis
  - Amyloidosis

and radiation (e.g., radon, X-rays, and gamma rays) should be obtained. Other important clinical factors in the evaluation of the etiology of SPN include a history of hemoptysis, fever, constitutional symptoms (tuberculosis), travel history (fungal and parasitic diseases), and human immunodeficiency virus (HIV) infection. Meticulous physical examination is helpful in identifying mimics of an SPN, such as nipple shadow, skin lesions, or monitor leads.

BOX 2 Parameters to be considered in the evaluation of a patient presenting with an incidentally-detected solitary pulmonary nodule.

- *Clinical*:
  - Age
  - Smoking history
  - Presence of other risk factors for lung cancer
  - Current or remote history of malignancy
- *Radiological*:
  - Size of the lesion
  - Site where it is located in the lung
  - Presence of calcification
  - Growth rate
  - Edge characteristics (smooth, spiculated, and lobulated)
  - Internal characteristics*
  - Contrast enhancement

*Include the attenuation, satellite nodules, presence of air bronchogram, halo sign, reverse halo sign, growth rate, and wall thickness in cavitary nodules.[1-8]

PREDICTING THE RISK OF MALIGNANCY IN SOLITARY PULMONARY NODULE

Some workers have developed models for predicting malignant etiology in a patient with SPN. Herder et al.[23] using multiple logistic regression analyses described older age, current or past tobacco-smoking history, and history of extrathoracic cancer more than 5 years before nodule detection as independent predictors of malignancy. Gould et al.,[24] using multivariate analysis, found current or former smoking status, increasing age, increasing nodule diameter, and decreasing interval since smoking cessation to be predictors of a malignant SPN. There have also been other attempts at predicting malignancy using the likelihood ratio form of Bayes' theorem[25] and neural networks.[26] Application of radiomics and deep learning technologies has been evaluated for diagnostic and prognostic purposes in solid SPN; both convolutional neural networks (CNN) models and random forest (RF) models performed comparably.[27] Further, several risk calculators have been developed and their performance has been validated. These include the Mayo Clinic model,[21] Herder model,[23] Veterans Affairs SNAP Cooperative Study Group model,[24] Brock University mode,[28] and Cleveland Clinic model.[29]

IMAGING STUDIES

Chest Radiograph

The evaluation of an SPN usually begins with a review of the chest radiograph. Use of nipple markers or apical lordotic projections may help to distinguish normal anatomic structures from lesions causing an SPN. SPNs are often missed on chest radiographs even by experienced chest radiologists, especially if they are located below the diaphragm or behind the clavicles, ribs, or heart. Availability of dual-energy subtraction digital chest radiograph systems is expected to improve the pickup rate of SPNs on chest radiographs. Sometimes, characteristic radiological patterns of calcification are suggestive of a presumptive diagnosis. Presence of diffuse, central, laminated, and popcorn patterns of calcification are considered to be benign. But stippled and eccentric patterns of calcification should prompt further workup to rule out malignant etiology.[1-6]

When available, the current chest radiograph should be compared with a previous chest film. This will also facilitate the estimation of the growth rate (doubling time) of the SPN.

Computed Tomography

Computed tomography is the primary imaging modality in the evaluation of a patient with an SPN. The CT, by identifying whether the lesion is single or multiple **(Fig. 2)** and by detecting atelectasis, other parenchymal infiltrates, hilar or mediastinal lymphadenopathy, or pleural effusion, helps in characterizing the lesion as a true SPN. The current multidetector row CT scanners that use 16–256 detector channels facilitate thin-section (0.6–2.0 mm) analysis of an SPN.[1-6]

Location of the Nodule

Some studies have suggested that the location of the lesion in the lung is an independent predictor of the lesion being a malignant SPN. While malignant lesions are more likely to be located in the right lung and in the upper lobes, benign lesions are equally distributed throughout the lung fields.[1-6]

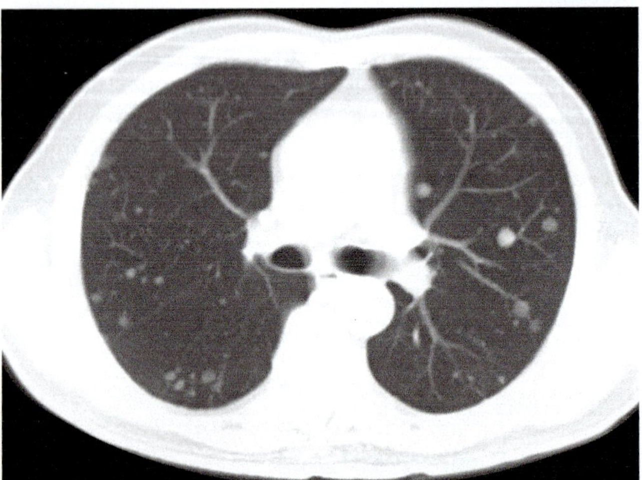

FIG. 2: Computed tomography (CT) of the chest (lung window) showing bilateral multiple nodules. Further workup confirmed metastatic malignancy.

This predilection for the upper lobes is probably related to the higher concentration of inhaled carcinogens that result from tobacco smoking.

Size

As described earlier, larger the SPN, higher is likelihood of malignancy; lesions greater than 3 cm in diameter should be considered malignant until proven otherwise **(Fig. 3)**. The likelihood ratio of malignancy in relation to the size of the SPN as described by Gurney[22] is shown in **Table 1**.

Shape and Margins

Assessment of the shape and margins of the SPN, even though not specific, provides useful clues for categorizing the lesion as benign or malignant.[1-6] In general, benign SPNs are round in shape and have smooth margins. Malignant SPNs may rarely present with smooth margins, as in the case of lung cancer **(Figs. 4A and B)**, solitary hematogenous metastases from colorectal, renal cell, or breast cancer, and peripheral carcinoid tumors. Presence of irregular spiculated margins (*corona radiata*) is highly suggestive of

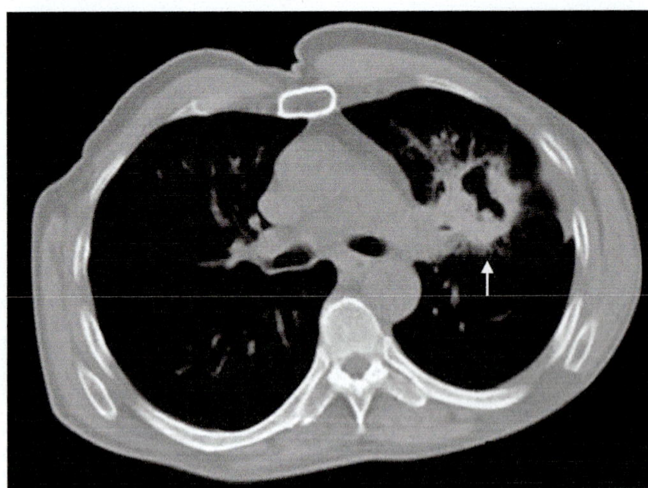

FIG. 3: Noncontrast enhanced CT of the chest (mediastinal window) showing a nodule measuring 41 mm suggestive of a mass lesion. Image-guided biopsy confirmed squamous cell carcinoma of the lung.

TABLE 1: The likelihood ratio of malignancy in lesions.[22]

Size (cm)	Likelihood ratio
<1.0	0.52
1.1–2.0	0.74
2.1–3.0	3.7
>3.0	5.2

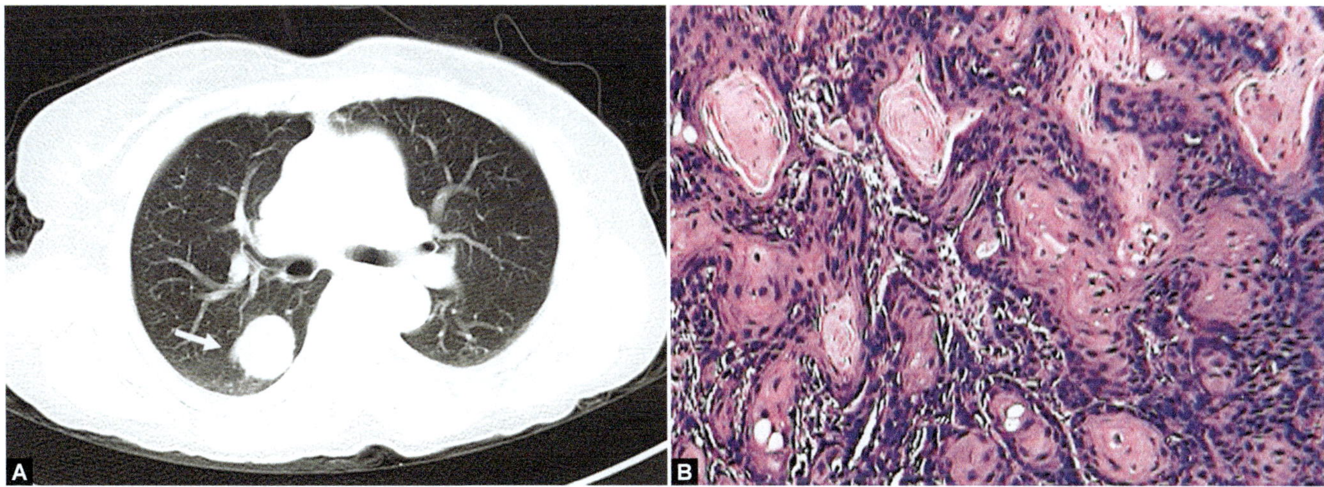

FIGS. 4A AND B: (A) CT of the chest (lung window) showing a solitary pulmonary nodule (SPN) with smooth rounded margins (arrow); (B) Photomicrograph of the image-guided fine needle aspiration cytology (FNAC) was suggestive of squamous cell carcinoma (Papanicolaou stain; ×400).

malignancy. Rarely, irregular margins can be observed even in benign lesions, such as lipoid pneumonia, focal atelectasis, tuberculoma, and progressive massive fibrosis. A lobulated margin is most often seen in hamartomas but can be observed in malignant conditions like peripheral carcinoid tumors, and adenocarcinomas. A ragged margin suggests growth pattern along the alveolar wall (lepidic pattern of adenocarcinoma). Presence of satellite lesions surrounding a larger central nodule is suggestive of granulomatous disease (e.g., tuberculosis). In pulmonary arteriovenous malformations presenting as an SPN, a feeding and draining pulmonary vessel extending from the hilum of the lung can be evident.

The *comet tail sign* is typically seen in rounded atelectasis and indicates a bundle of curvilinear bronchi and vessels extending into the hilar aspect of a peripherally located SPN that lies adjacent to pleural thickening.[1-6]

Fat

For practical purposes, presence of fat [attenuation value of between -40 and -120 Hounsfield units (HU)] within an SPN with smooth or rounded margins is suggestive of pulmonary hamartoma; nearly 60% of hamartomas contain fat. Rarely, lipoid pneumonia, pulmonary metastases from renal cell carcinoma, or liposarcoma presenting as an SPN may show fat.[1-6]

Ground-glass Attenuation

The use of MDCT has facilitated the detection of "subsolid" nodules that contain a component of ground-glass attenuation. These may be pure ground-glass SPNs, as well as partly solid lesions consisting of mixed solid and ground-glass lesions, which have been found to have a higher potential of being malignant. Atypical adenomatous hyperplasia, bronchioloalveolar carcinoma, and invasive adenocarcinoma can present as subsolid nodules.[1-6]

The *halo sign* **(Figs. 5A to D)** has been described in invasive aspergillus infection and bronchioloalveolar carcinoma and refers to a poorly defined rim of ground-glass attenuation around the SPN; the halo may represent hemorrhage, tumor infiltration, or perinodular inflammation. The *reverse halo sign* (a focal round area of ground-glass attenuation surrounded by a ring of consolidation) has been described in cryptogenic organizing pneumonia and paracoccidioidomycosis.[30]

Calcification

The presence and pattern of calcification within the lesion offer important clues to the etiology of SPN. Though the chest radiograph is useful in identifying calcification within the SPN, the diagnostic yield is low (sensitivity 50% and specificity 87%).[1-6] Nearly one-third of SPNs that do not manifest calcification within the lesion on the chest radiograph, may show calcification on chest CT.[3] Therefore, noncontrast chest CT (1–3 mm collimation) is considered to be the best technique to identify calcification within an SPN.[1-6] Certain patterns of calcification within the SPN, such as central, laminated, diffuse **(Fig. 6)**, and calcification within a smooth or lobulated nodule are suggestive of a benign lesion, such as a granuloma; popcorn calcification is suggestive of hamartoma. Rarely, presence of eccentric calcification may be indicative of calcified granuloma engulfed by malignancy, amorphous calcification can be present due to dystrophic malignant calcification.

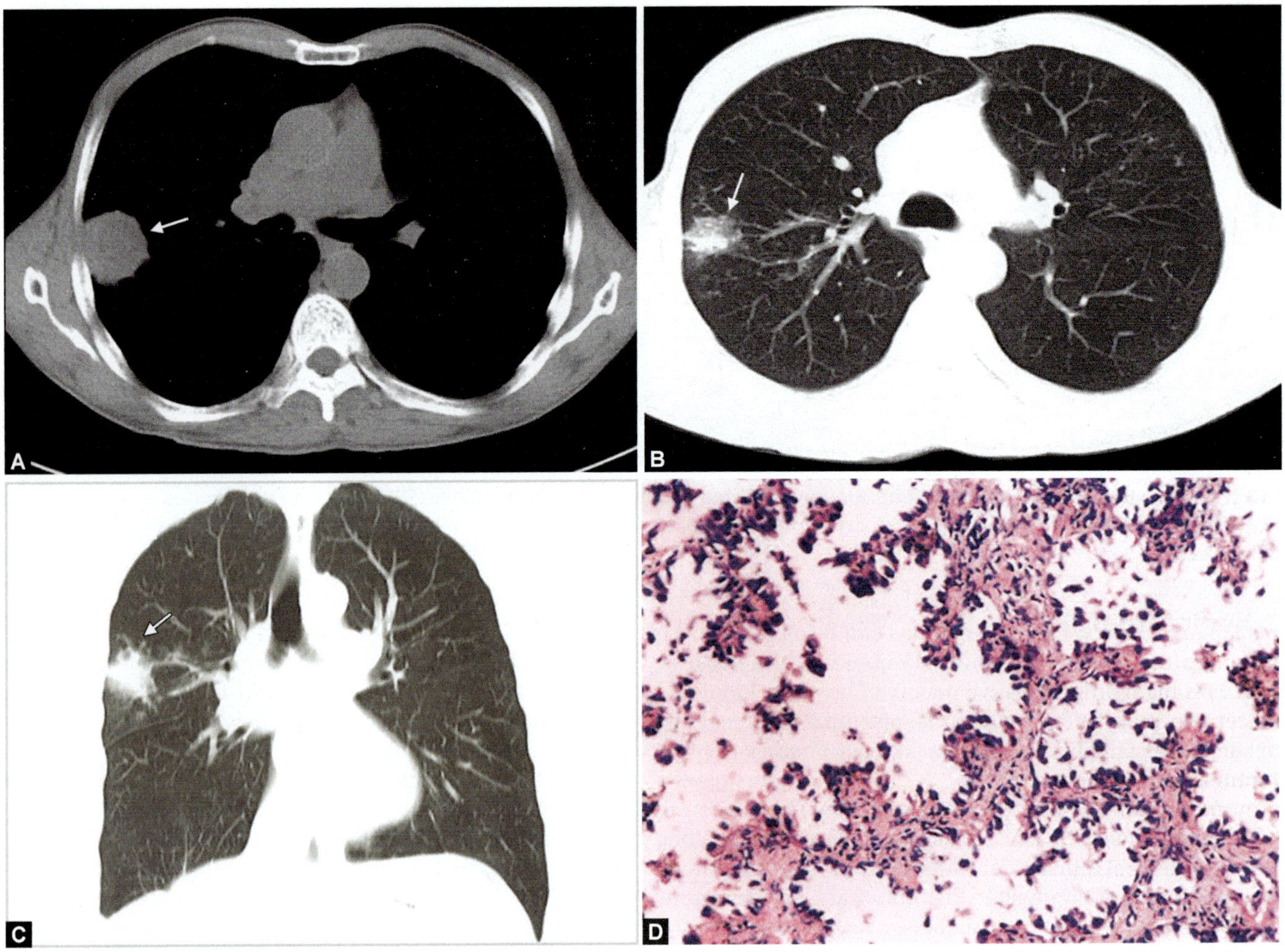

FIGS. 5A TO D: (A) Noncontrast enhanced CT of the chest (mediastinal window) showing a peripherally-located solitary pulmonary nodule; (B) CT of the chest (lung window); (C) and coronal reconstruction of the same patient showing ground-glass attenuation surrounding the nodule suggestive of *halo sign;* and (D) Photomicrograph of the excised lesion suggestive of bronchioloalveolar cell carcinoma (Hematoxylin and eosin; ×200).

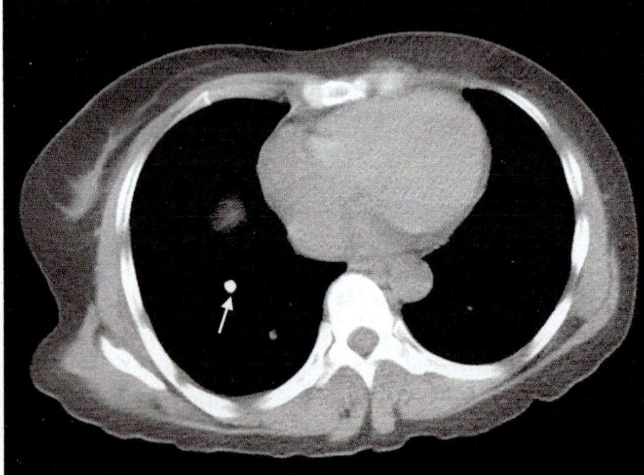

FIG. 6: Non-contrast enhanced CT of the chest (mediastinal window) showing a calcified nodule (arrow).

When calcification is not evident in the lesion, CT densitometry can be helpful. With the advent of modern MDCT, a reference CT phantom is no longer being used and the average attenuation of an SPN can be measured directly. Attenuation values of 200 HU or greater within a smoothly-marginated nodule are considered to be evidence of microscopic calcification and suggest benign etiology.[1-6]

Cavitation

Cavitation can be evident in necrotic malignant SPNs (e.g., squamous cell carcinoma) or conditions such as abscess, infectious granulomas (e.g., TB), vasculitides, early Langerhans cell histiocytosis, and pulmonary infarction.[1-6] Rarely, fluid-filled lesions from mucus impaction can present as a cavitating SPN. Estimating the cavity wall thickness can be helpful; wall thickness of 5 mm or less suggests a benign lesion, whereas wall thickness of 15 mm or more is suggestive of a malignant lesion.[1,31]

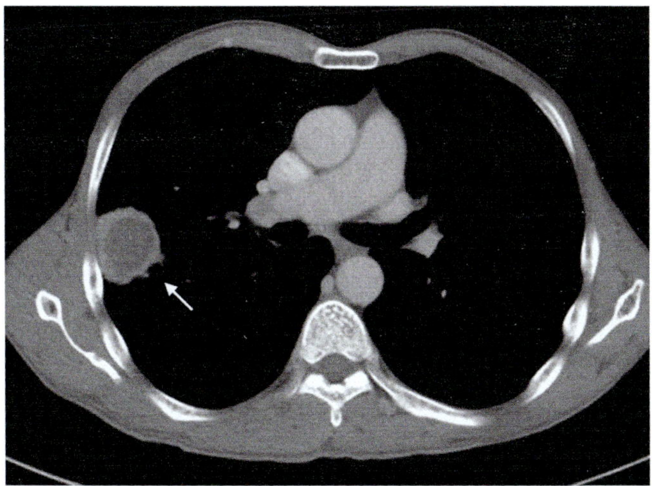

FIG. 7: Contrast-enhanced CT of the chest (mediastinal window) showing cystic lucency within the solitary pulmonary nodule (SPN) (arrow).

Other Internal Characteristics

Detection of cystic or "bubbly" lucencies within an SPN **(Fig. 7)** is highly suggestive of malignant etiology (e.g., lung cancer, especially adenocarcinomas with bronchioloalveolar cell features and pulmonary lymphoma). Occasionally, bubbly lucencies can also be evident in sarcoidosis, round pneumonia, and organizing pneumonia. Evidence of air bronchogram within an SPN is suggestive of malignant etiology (especially bronchioloalveolar carcinoma and rarely pulmonary lymphoma); sometimes, benign lesions, such as sarcoidosis and round pneumonia[32,33] may manifest an air bronchogram. Presence of subsolid SPNs, in which the nodule has a component of ground-glass attenuation, is suggestive of malignancy, especially bronchioloalveolar carcinoma.[1,34]

Contrast Enhancement

Contrast enhancement, also called "wash-in" (defined as an increase in attenuation of a lesion >15 HU after intravenous contrast), of an SPN can help in providing a clue to its etiological origins. The SPNs that enhance <15 HU are almost certainly benign (sensitivity 98%, specificity 58%, and accuracy 77%).[35] Malignant lesions, by virtue of increased vascularity, tend to enhance avidly with the administration of intravenous contrast; typically, malignant SPNs enhance >20 (HU).[1,35,36] Benign lesions like active granuloma, hamartoma, arteriovenous malformation, and organizing pneumonia can also manifest contrast enhancement.[37] Recently, "wash-out" or decrease in attenuation over the 15 minutes following contrast injection has also been found to be useful.[1-6]

Growth

Since an SPN is assumed to be a sphere and the volume of a sphere is given by the mathematical expression $\frac{4}{3}\pi r^3$ (where r = radius of the sphere) or $\pi dr^3/6$ (where d = diameter), an increase in nodule diameter by 26% corresponds approximately to one doubling in tumor volume.

The doubling time can be calculated by using the following formula:[9]

$$dt = (t \times \log 2)/\{3 \times [\log (d2/d1)]\}$$

where,

dt = doubling time (days)
t = time in days between the chest radiographs
d2 = diameter of the nodule at the time of the current CT/chest radiograph
d1 = diameter of the nodule at the time of the previous CT/chest radiograph

It has been estimated that the doubling time for majority of malignant nodules is between 20 and 300 days.[36-38] If the SPN has been stable for at least 2 years, it is likely to be benign and usually, does not require further evaluation.[1-6,38-40]

Magnetic Resonance Imaging

Magnetic resonance imaging (MRI), in spite of having the advantage of avoiding ionizing radiation, has been less frequently utilized than MDCT in evaluation of lung nodules because of its limited spatial resolution and effect of respiratory and cardiac motion on sequences with low temporal resolution. Half-Fourier acquisition single-shot turbo spin-echo (HASTE) imaging facilitates identification of malignant tissues that manifest high signal intensity (due to high T2 relaxivity) against a backdrop of surrounding air-filled, low-signal, lung parenchyma; vessels are identified as flow voids without any apparent signal. For SPNs of 5–10 mm in size, HASTE sequence has been found to have a sensitivity of close to 95%.[41,42]

The different turbo spin echo (TSE) and 3D gradient-echo [volume interpolated breath-hold (VIBE)] MRI sequences of the lung for detecting pulmonary metastases,[43] enhancement characteristics of nodules on MRI, such as maximal enhancement ratio and slope of contrast uptake are also explored as potential imaging modalities for SPNs. These issues merit further study.

Positron Emission Tomography—Computed Tomography

Positron emission tomography-CT (PET-CT) **(Figs. 8A to C)** using the radiopharmaceutical ^{18}F labeled 2-deoxy-D-glucose (FDG) has been used to characterize an SPN as malignant or benign.[1-6] The FDG standardized uptake

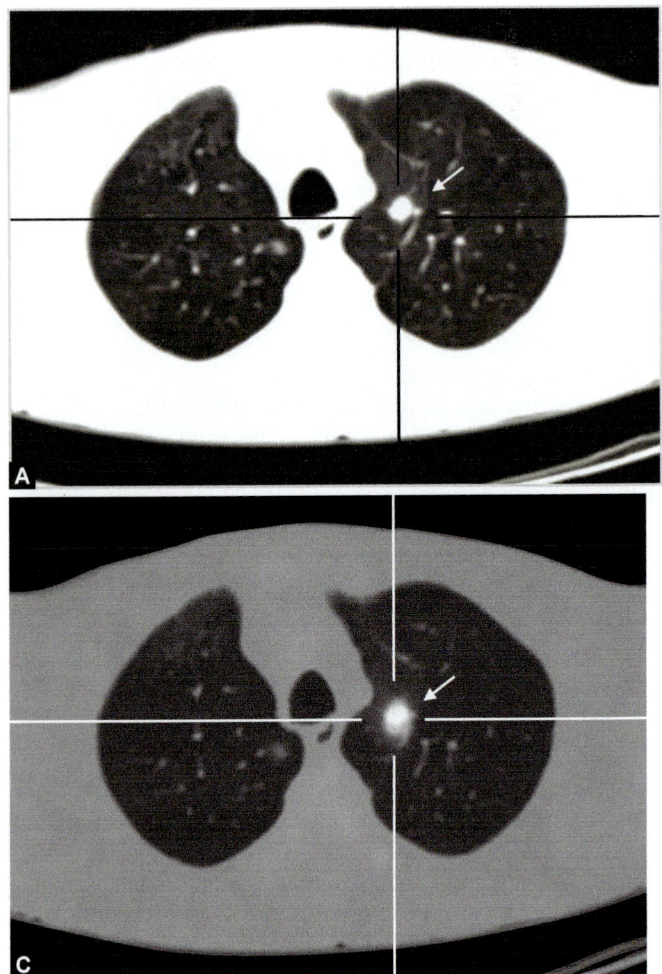

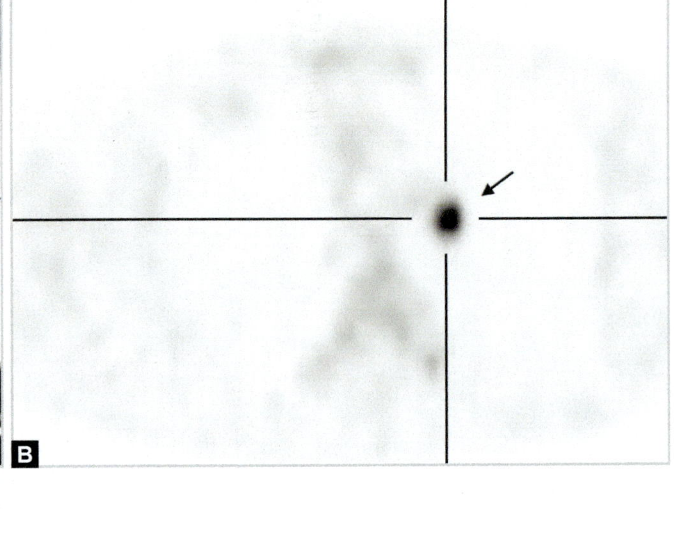

FIGS. 8A TO C: (A) CT of the chest (lung window); (B) ^{18}F-fluorodeoxyglucose positron emission tomography (FDG-PET) showing an SPN (arrow); and (C) positron emission tomography-computed tomography (PET-CT) image of the same patient showing increased uptake in the nodule (arrow).

Source: Dr TC Kalawat, Department of Nuclear Medicine, Sri Venkateswara Institute of Medical Sciences, Tirupati, Andhra Pradesh, India.

value (SUVmax) estimation is used as a semiquantitative method of evaluation of SPNs. In malignant SPNs, metabolism of glucose is typically increased and an SUVmax cutoff of 2.5 has been used to differentiate benign from malignant SPNs.[44] Currently, PET-CT is recommended only for nodules that are >8–10 mm in diameter.

For SPNs greater than 10 mm in size, FDG-PET has a sensitivity and specificity of 97% and 78%, respectively for characterizing it as malignant.[45-47] Malignant causes of an SPN, such as a well-differentiated adenocarcinoma of lung (especially with a bronchioloalveolar cell carcinoma) and a peripheral carcinoid tumor can produce false-negative PET-CT results. The PET-CT has a low sensitivity for lesions of <1 cm in diameter and the use of this technique in this setting is limited; but, if PET-CT results are positive, it would almost certainly prompt biopsy or resection. Common causes resulting in a false-positive PET result include active granulomatous inflammation, focal areas of organizing or resolving pneumonia, and rarely hamartomas.

Computer-aided Diagnosis

Computer-aided diagnosis (CAD) techniques have been developed as a method of assisting interpretation by means of computerized image analysis. There is a large body of published literature on the application of this technique in detection and characterization of SPNs. The CAD, acting as a second interpreter, facilitates assessment of nodule size, volume, attenuation, and enhancement characteristics by performing global analysis of high-resolution MDCT data of the entire nodule. Some reports suggest that CAD may be useful in identifying clinically significant nodules that have been missed by the radiologists.[48-50] Further refinements in CAD, such as integration of multifunctional CAD platforms into picture archiving and communication systems (PACS) that provide easy accessibility during reader interpretation may facilitate more widespread use of these techniques.[2] The salient imaging features that facilitate categorization of an SPN as benign are shown in **Table 2**.

TABLE 2: Radiologic features suggestive of benign and malignant solitary pulmonary nodules.

Radiologic feature	Benign	Malignant
Size of the lesion	Smaller the size of lesion, lesser the risk of malignancy	Larger the size of lesion, greater the risk of malignancy
Border	Smooth	Irregular or spiculated (*corona radiata*)
Density	Dense and solid	Nonsolid, ground-glass
Calcification	Concentric, central, popcorn-like, or homogeneous patterns are common	Usually, noncalcified or eccentric calcification
Satellite lesions	Common in granulomatous lesions	Rare
Wall thickness in a cavity	<5 mm	>15 mm
Doubling time	<1 month; >1 year	1 month–1 year

TISSUE SAMPLING TECHNIQUES

In spite of widespread use of various imaging techniques, characterization of some SPNs as benign or malignant is not possible and will warrant tissue sampling and histopathological or cytopathological diagnosis. Various methods, such as image-guided transthoracic fine needle aspiration cytology (FNAC), needle biopsy, bronchoscopic biopsy with or without electromagnetic navigation systems, video-assisted thoracoscopic surgery (VATS), electromagnetic navigation, radial endobronchial ultrasound (R EBUS), ultrathin bronchoscopes, and robotic-assisted bronchoscopy or open thoracotomy have been employed for procuring the tissue.[1-6]

Image-guided Procedures

Image-guided transthoracic needle FNAC biopsy is frequently used for confirming the etiological diagnosis in patients with SPN in whom the pretest probability of a malignant lesion is high. The test is performed under CT guidance or ultrasonography guidance (peripherally located or pleura-based lesions). This technique is highly accurate in ascertaining the etiological diagnosis of malignant SPNs (sensitivity >90% for lesions >5 mm in size). Contraindications for transthoracic FNAC and biopsy include an uncooperative patient, presence of bleeding diathesis, severe bullous emphysema, and prior pneumonectomy. Important complications of transthoracic needle biopsy include pneumothorax (seen in 20% of patients) and bleeding, which is usually minor and self-limiting.[1-6]

Video-assisted Thoracoscopic Surgery

The VATS technique facilitates procurement of tissue for frozen section examination to assist in decision about whether to proceed with a full lobectomy, especially from peripherally located SPNs and some centrally located SPNs in the lower lobe. Presently, VATS offers a lower morbidity and a shorter hospital stay compared to conventional thoracotomy.[1,51]

Fiberoptic Bronchoscopy

The sensitivity of fiberoptic bronchoscopy (FOB) for detecting a malignant SPN ranges from 10% for SPNs that are <1.5 cm diameter to 40–60% for SPNs that are 2–3 cm in diameter. Other factors that influence diagnostic yield of FOB include its proximity to bronchial tree and the prevalence of cancer in the given area.[1-6] Several newer bronchoscopic modalities have emerged for evaluation of SPN in the recent years.

Radial-probe Endobronchial Ultrasound

The R-EBUS utilizes ultrasound to visualize structures within and adjacent to the airway wall. R-EBUS permits visualization of internal structure of peripheral pulmonary nodules (PPNs); this information may be helpful in predicting the histology of the lesion. Advances in R-EBUS technology have permitted visualization and performance of transbronchial biopsies of PPNs without exposure to radiation. R-EBUS has an overall diagnostic yield ranging from 34 to 84%; even for nodules <30 mm, the diagnostic yield of R-EBUS and transbronchial biopsy approaches close to 80%.[52] Combining R-EBUS with other modalities has been shown to increase the diagnostic yield.[1-6,52]

Electromagnetic Navigation

Electromagnetic navigational bronchoscopy (ENB) is a novel image-guided localization technique based on the principles of electromagnetism that facilitates placing endobronchial accessories in the target areas of lung. In evaluating PPNs, the diagnostic yield of ENB has been found to be 59–85%; combining ENB and R-EBUS has been found to increase the diagnostic yield close to 90%.[53]

Ultrathin Bronchoscopy

The size of conventional bronchoscope prevents it from being advanced beyond a segmental or subsegmental bronchus level. Ultrathin bronchoscope by virtue of its smaller diameter (2.8–3.5 mm) has the advantage of facilitating insertion beyond the sixth-generation bronchi. For small peripheral lesions (<30 mm), this technique has a diagnostic yield ranging from 57 to 81%. CT fluoroscopy with ultrathin bronchoscopy has also been found to be useful for evaluation of SPNs.[54]

Virtual Bronchoscopic Navigation

Virtual bronchoscopy (VB) facilitates simulation of actual bronchoscopy by application of 3-dimensional (3D) display techniques to the airways. VB navigation (VBN) refers to use of virtual bronchoscopic images of bronchial path as a guide to navigate the bronchoscope. VBN coupled with ultrathin bronchoscopy, X-ray fluoroscopy, and EBUS has been found to be useful in evaluation of SPNs.[55]

MANAGEMENT

The management depends on several factors, including the degree of surgical risk, the presence or absence of comorbid conditions, the patient's preferences, radiological and surgical capability, and expertise available at the center where the patient is being evaluated.[49,50] The eventual goal is to ascertain the etiological diagnosis so that appropriate therapy can be instituted.

There are no consensus guidelines for evaluation and management of an incidentally-detected SPN. Evidence-based recommendations for follow-up and management of incidentally-detected SPNs based on the current American College of Chest Physicians guidelines[9] and the Fleischner Society guidelines[10] are shown in **Tables 3 and 4**. These are likely to evolve further as more information becomes available.

TABLE 3: Guidelines for the management of solitary pulmonary nodules.

Nodule diameter	American College of Chest Physicians[9]	Fleischner Society[10]
<6 mm	*≤4 mm:* • *Low-risk:* Patient discussion and follow-up optional • *High-risk:* Follow-up CT at 12 months (if stable, no further follow-up) *>4–6 mm:* • *Low-risk:* Follow-up CT at 12 months (if stable, no further follow-up) • *High-risk:* Follow-up CT at 6-12 months (if stable, follow-up at 18–24 months)	*<6 mm (<100 mm^3):* • *Low-risk:* No follow-up • *High-risk:* Optional follow-up CT in 12 months
6–8 mm	*>6–<8 mm:* • *Low-risk:* Follow-up CT at 6–12 months (if stable, follow-up at 18–24 months) • *High-risk:* Follow-up CT at 3–6 months (if stable, then 9–12 months and 24 months)	*6–8 mm (100–250 mm^3):* • *Low-risk:* Follow-up CT in 6–12 months, then consider follow-up CT at 18–24 months • *High-risk:* Follow-up CT in 6–12 months, then repeat CT in 18–24 months
≥8 mm	• *Pretest probability of malignancy <5%:* Surveillance CT in 3 months • *Pretest probability of malignancy is 5–65%:* PET-CT to determine continued surveillance, nonsurgical biopsy, or surgical biopsy/resection • *Pretest probability malignancy >65%:* Referral for surgical biopsy or resection after appropriate staging work-up	*>8 mm (>250 mm^3):* • *Low-risk:* Consider follow-up CT at 3 months, PET-CT, or tissue sampling • *High-risk:* Consider follow-up CT at 3 months, PET-CT, or tissue sampling

(CT: computed tomography; PET-CT: positron emission tomography-computed tomography)

TABLE 4: Guidelines for the management of subsolid solitary pulmonary nodules.

American College of Chest Physicians[9]	Fleischner Society[10]
≤5 mm: No follow-up	*<6 mm (<100 mm^3):* • *Ground-glass nodule:* No routine follow-up • *Part-solid:* No routine follow-up

>5 mm:
• *Ground-glass nodule:* Follow-up CT at 12 months then annual through 3 years
• *Part-solid nodule:*
  ○ *≤8 mm solid component:* Follow-up CT scan at 3, 12, and 24 months then annual until 5 years
  ○ *>8 mm solid component:* Follow-up CT at 3 months, further evaluation with PET-CT, nonsurgical biopsy, and/or resection if persists
	≥6 mm (>100 mm^3):
	• *Ground-glass nodule:* Follow-up CT 6–12 months, then every 2–5 years
	• *Part-solid nodule:* Follow-up CT 3–6 months then annually for 5 years

(CT: computed tomography; PET-CT: positron emission tomography-computed tomography)

SUMMARY

The goal of evaluating a patient presenting with an SPN is to correctly differentiate malignant SPNs from benign lesions so that appropriate therapy is instituted. The approach to a patient is based on the pretest probability of cancer determined according to the size of the nodule, the presence or absence of risk factors for lung cancer, such as history of tobacco smoking, patient's age, and imaging features of the SPN. When the pretest probability of cancer is low, the nodule should be monitored with serial high-resolution CT. When the probability of cancer is high, diagnostic work-up should be directed to establish the histopathological or cytopathological tissue diagnosis.

REFERENCES

1. Mazzone PJ, Lam L. Evaluating the patient with a pulmonary nodule: A review. JAMA. 2022;327(3):264-73.
2. Mohan A, Vijayalakshmi Devi B, Chandra A. Solitary pulmonary nodule. In: Jindal SK (Ed). Textbook of pulmonary and critical care medicine. New Delhi: Jaypee Brothers Medical Publishers (P) Ltd; 2011. pp. 1470-81.
3. Mohan A, Vijayalakshmi Devi B, Kumar PD, et al. Solitary pulmonary nodule: Approach to diagnosis. In: Thakur BB (Ed). Postgraduate Medicine. Mumbai: Indian College of Physicians, Academic wing of the Association of Physicians of India; 2012. pp. 467-79.
4. Mohan A, Vijayalakshmi Devi B, Chandra A. Solitary pulmonary nodule. In: Jindal SK (Ed). Textbook of pulmonary and critical care medicine, 2nd edition. New Delhi: Jaypee Brothers Medical Publishers (P) Ltd; 2017. pp. 1345-56.
5. Mohan A, Vijalakshmi Devi B, Chandra A. Clinical evaluation and management of a solitary pulmonary nodule in 2017. In: Raju YS (Ed). Clinical Medicine Update 2017. Kolkata: Indian Association of Clinical Medicine; 2017. pp. 32-8.
6. Chandra A, Mohan A, Rao MH, et al. Solitary pulmonary nodule: Experience at a tertiary care teaching hospital. Indian J Thorac Cardiovasc Surg. 2006;22:88.
7. Cruickshank A, Stieler G, Ameer F. Evaluation of the solitary pulmonary nodule. Intern Med J. 2019;49:306-15.
8. Sim YT, Poon FW. Imaging of solitary pulmonary nodule: a clinical review. Quant Imaging Med Surg. 2013;3(6):316-26.
9. Gould MK, Donington J, Lynch WR, et al. Evaluation of individuals with pulmonary nodules. When is it lung cancer? Diagnosis and management of lung cancer, 3rd edition: American College of Chest Physicians evidence-based clinical practice guidelines. Chest. 2013;143(5 Suppl):e93S-e120S.
10. MacMahon H, Naidich DP, Goo JM, et al. Guidelines for management of incidental pulmonary nodules detected on CT images: From the Fleischner Society 2017. Radiology. 2017; 284(1):228-43.
11. American College of Radiology. Committee on Lung-RADS. (2019). Lung-RADS Assessment Categories Version 1.1. [online] Available from https://www.acr.org/-/media/ACR/Files/RADS/Lung-RADS/LungRADSAssessmentCategoriesv1-1.pdf. [Last accessed September, 2024].
12. Ost D, Fein AM, Feinsilver SH. Clinical practice. The solitary pulmonary nodule. N Engl J Med. 2003;348(25):2535-42.
13. Erasmus JJ, Connolly JE, McAdams HP, et al. Solitary pulmonary nodules: Part I. Morphologic evaluation for differentiation of benign and malignant lesions. Radiographics. 2000;20(1):43-58.
14. Holin SM, Dwork RE, Glaser S, et al. Solitary pulmonary nodules found in a community-wide chest roentgenographic survey: A five-year follow-up study. Am Rev Tuberc. 1959;79(4):427-39.
15. de Koning HJ, van der Aalst CM, de Jong PA, et al. Reduced lung-cancer mortality with volume CT screening in a randomized trial. N Engl J Med. 2020;382(6):503-13.
16. Oken MM, Marcus PM, Hu P, et al.; PLCO Project Team. Baseline chest radiograph for lung cancer detection in the randomized prostate, lung, colorectal and ovarian cancer screening trial. J Natl Cancer Inst. 2005;97(24):1832-9.
17. Church TR, Black WC, Aberle DR, et al; National Lung Screening Trial Research Team. Results of initial low-dose computed tomographic screening for lung cancer. N Engl J Med. 2013; 368(21):1980-91.
18. Mohan A, Chandra A, Nagarajan A, et al. Clinical manifestations and treatment–outcome in patients with pulmonary tuberculomas. Am J Respir Crit Care Med. 2009;179:A3202.
19. Agarwal R, Srinivas R, Aggarwal AN. Parenchymal pseudotumoral tuberculosis: Case series and systematic review of literature. Respir Med. 2008;102(3):382-9.
20. Chandra A. Surgery for pleuropulmonary tuberculosis. In: Sharma SK, Mohan A (Eds). Tuberculosis, 3rd edition. New Delhi: Jaypee Brothers Medical Publishers (P) Ltd; 2020. pp. 644-53.
21. Swensen SJ, Silverstein MD, Ilstrup DM, et al. The probability of malignancy in solitary pulmonary nodules. Application to small radiologically indeterminate nodules. Arch Intern Med. 1997;157(8):849-55.
22. Gurney JW. Determining the likelihood of malignancy in solitary pulmonary nodules with Bayesian analysis. Part I. Theory. Radiology. 1993;186(2):405-13.
23. Herder GJ, van Tinteren H, Golding RP, et al. Clinical prediction model to characterize pulmonary nodules: Validation and added value of 18F-fluorodeoxyglucose positron emission tomography. Chest. 2005;128(4):2490-6.
24. Gould MK, Ananth L, Barnett PG; Veterans Affairs SNAP Cooperative Study Group. A clinical model to estimate the pretest probability of lung cancer in patients with solitary pulmonary nodules. Chest. 2007;131(2):383-8.
25. Cummings SR, Lillington GA, Richard RJ. Estimating the probability of malignancy in solitary pulmonary nodules. A Bayesian approach. Am Rev Respir Dis. 1986;134(3):449-52.
26. Matsuki Y, Nakamura K, Watanabe H, et al. Usefulness of an artificial neural network for differentiating benign from malignant pulmonary nodules on high-resolution CT: Evaluation with receiver operating characteristic analysis. AJR Am J Roentgenol. 2002;178(3):657-63.
27. Zhang R, Wei Y, Shi F, et al. The diagnostic and prognostic value of radiomics and deep learning technologies for patients with solid pulmonary nodules in chest CT images. BMC Cancer. 2022;22:1118.

28. McWilliams A, Tammemagi MC, Mayo JR, et al. Probability of cancer in pulmonary nodules detected on first screening CT. N Engl J Med. 2013;369(10):910-9.
29. Reid M, Choi HK, Han X, et al. Development of a risk prediction model to estimate the probability of malignancy in pulmonary nodules being considered for biopsy. Chest. 2019;156(2):367-75.
30. Arenas-Jiménez JJ, García-Garrigós E, Ureña Vacas A, et al. Organizing pneumonia. Radiologia (Engl Ed). 2022;64(Suppl 3): 240-9.
31. Woodring JH, Fried AM. Significance of wall thickness in solitary cavities of the lung: A follow-up study. AJR Am J Roentgenol. 1983;140(3):473-4.
32. Zwirewich CV, Vedal S, Miller RR, et al. Solitary pulmonary nodule: High-resolution CT and radiologic-pathologic correlation. Radiology. 1991;179(2):469-76.
33. Kuriyama K, Tateishi R, Doi O, et al. Prevalence of air bronchograms in small peripheral carcinomas of the lung on thin-section CT: Comparison with benign tumors. AJR Am J Roentgenol. 1991;156(5):921-4.
34. Suzuki K, Asamura H, Kusumoto M, et al. "Early" peripheral lung cancer: Prognostic significance of ground glass opacity on thin-section computed tomographic scan. Ann Thorac Surg. 2002;74:1635-9.
35. Swensen SJ, Viggiano RW, Midthun DE, et al. Lung nodule enhancement at CT: Multicenter study. Radiology. 2000;214: 73-80.
36. Swensen SJ, Brown LR, Colby TV, et al. Pulmonary nodules: CT evaluation of enhancement with iodinated contrast material. Radiology. 1995;194(2):393-8.
37. Yamashita K, Matsunobe S, Tsuda T, et al. Solitary pulmonary nodule: Preliminary study of evaluation with incremental dynamic CT. Radiology. 1995;194(2):399-405.
38. Nathan MH, Collins VP, Adams RA. Differentiation of benign and malignant pulmonary nodules by growth rate. Radiology. 1962; 79:221-32.
39. Weiss W. Tumor doubling time and survival of men with bronchogenic carcinoma. Chest. 1974;65(1):3-8.
40. Friberg S, Mattson S. On the growth rates of human malignant tumors: Implications for medical decision making. J Surg Oncol. 1997;65(4):284-97.
41. Schroeder T, Ruehm SG, Debatin JF, et al. Detection of pulmonary nodules using a 2D HASTE MR sequence: Comparison with MDCT. AJR Am J Roentgenol. 2005;185(4):979-84.
42. Vogt FM, Herborn CU, Hunold P, et al. HASTE MRI versus chest radiography in the detection of pulmonary nodules: Comparison with MDCT. AJR Am J Roentgenol. 2004;183(1):71-8.
43. Bruegel M, Gaa J, Woertler K, et al. MRI of the lung: Value of different turbo spin-echo, single-shot turbo spin-echo, and 3D gradient-echo pulse sequences for the detection of pulmonary metastases. J Magn Reson Imaging. 2007;25(1):73-81.
44. Lowe VJ, Hoffman JM, DeLong DM, et al. Semiquantitative and visual analysis of FDG-PET images in pulmonary abnormalities. J Nucl Med. 1994;35(11):1771-6.
45. Gould MK, Maclean CC, Kuschner WG, et al. Accuracy of positron emission tomography for diagnosis of pulmonary nodules and mass lesions: A meta-analysis. JAMA. 2001;285(7):914-24.
46. Mosmann MP, Borba MA, de Macedo FP, et al. Solitary pulmonary nodule and (18)F-FDG PET/CT. Part 1: Epidemiology, morphological evaluation and cancer probability. Radiol Bras. 2016;49(1):35-42.
47. Groheux D, Quere G, Blanc E, et al. FDG PET-CT for solitary pulmonary nodule and lung cancer: Literature review. Diagn Interv Imaging. 2016;97(10):1003-17.
48. Armato SG 3rd, Li F, Giger ML, et al. Lung cancer: Performance of automated lung nodule detection applied to cancers missed in a CT screening program. Radiology. 2002;225(3): 685-92.
49. Shiraishi J, Li F, Doi K. Computer-aided diagnosis for improved detection of lung nodules by use of posterior–anterior and lateral chest radiographs. Acad Radiol. 2007;14(1):28-37.
50. Marten K, Engelke C, Seyfarth T, et al. Computer-aided detection of pulmonary nodules: influence of nodule characteristics on detection performance. Clin Radiol. 2005;60(2):196-206.
51. Kumar A, Mohan A, Sharma SK, et al. Video assisted thoracoscopic surgery (VATS) in the diagnosis of intrathoracic pathology: initial experience. Indian J Chest Dis Allied Sci. 1999; 41(1):5-13.
52. Narula T, Machuzak MS, Mehta AC. Newer modalities in the work-up of peripheral pulmonary nodules. Clin Chest Med. 2013;34(3):395-415.
53. Folch EE, Pritchett MA, Nead MA, et al; NAVIGATE Study Investigators. Electromagnetic navigation bronchoscopy for peripheral pulmonary lesions: One-year results of the prospective, multicenter NAVIGATE study. J Thorac Oncol. 2019;14:445-58.
54. Oki M, Saka H, Asano F, et al. Use of an ultrathin vs thin bronchoscope for peripheral pulmonary lesions: A randomized trial. Chest. 2019;156(5):954-64.
55. Patel VK, Naik SK, Naidich DP, et al. A practical algorithmic approach to the diagnosis and management of solitary pulmonary nodules: Part 1: Radiologic characteristics and imaging modalities. Chest. 2013;143(3):825-39.

Hematopoietic and Lymphoid Neoplasm of Lungs

CHAPTER 155

Charanpreet Singh, Gaurav Prakash, Pankaj Malhotra

INTRODUCTION

Hematolymphoid neoplasms of the lungs can present either as primary lung neoplasms, where the tumor originates from the lung or tracheobronchial tree or as secondary lung involvement by a hematolymphoid neoplasm that originates elsewhere in the body.[1-4] Primary lung involvement by hematolymphoid neoplasms is rare, and the diagnosis is often not suspected initially. On the other hand, secondary lung involvement is more common. Differential diagnosis should consider more common infections rather than neoplastic lung involvement. Prognosis and treatment of these disorders can vary significantly, depending on several factors such as the patient's age, duration of symptoms, performance status, comorbidities, and stage of the disease.

The lungs can be affected not only by lymphoma but also by the side effects of systemic chemotherapy or radiotherapy used to treat lymphomas.[5-7] Lymphomas and leukemias may also affect the pulmonary vasculature and indirectly affect pulmonary function. This is predominantly in two ways—pulmonary thromboembolism (secondary to a thrombophilic state due to the malignancy) and leukostasis and hyperviscosity, which can be seen in patients with acute leukemia with very high counts at presentation as well as malignancies such as Waldenström macroglobulinemia if paraprotein levels at presentation are high. It is crucial to assess baseline lung function before initiating chemotherapy or radiotherapy, as certain antineoplastic drugs may require modifications in the presence of lung dysfunction.

LYMPHOMAS

Lymphomas are a diverse group of neoplastic disorders that originate from lymphoid tissue. In most cases, lymphoid tissue of nodal origin is involved. But, lymphomas can also develop in the extranodal lymphoid tissue present in various organs of normal individuals. In the case of the lungs, the main site of lymphoid tissue is the bronchial mucosa-associated lymphoid tissue (MALT), which is often involved in primary pulmonary lymphomas.

Lymphomas are generally classified into two main types based on histopathology and immunohistochemistry: Hodgkin lymphoma (HL) and non-Hodgkin lymphoma (NHL). NHL accounts for approximately 80–85% of all lymphomas. Primary pulmonary lymphoma, which affects the trachea, bronchus, and lung parenchyma, is rare and represents only 0.3% of all primary pulmonary neoplasms, less than 1% of all NHLs, and 3–4% of all extra nodal NHLs.[2,3] Mediastinal lymph node involvement is common in NHL but is not considered part of pulmonary neoplasms.

Lymphomas are typically systemic diseases, and the classification of primary and secondary involvement of a specific body site can sometimes be arbitrary. Secondary involvement of the lungs can occur through circulation or spread from neighboring sites.[8,9] Although the definition may seem arbitrary, classifying the involvement is important due to its implications for treatment and prognosis.

For the purpose of simplification, both HL and NHL are discussed separately, but there are some general considerations that apply to both. The diagnostic work-up for both HL and NHL is similar.

General Considerations

In lymphoma, the duration of symptoms can vary from weeks to months and sometimes even years, depending on the rate of disease progression. Generally, younger age is associated with more aggressive disease, while both low-grade and high-grade presentations of lymphomas are common as age advances. Systemic symptoms such as fever, weight loss, and night sweats, if present, indicate aggressive behavior and high tumor burden, classifying the patient as category B. The absence of these symptoms is denoted as category A. The involvement of lymphoma in extra nodal sites is categorized as E. Since the lung is a non-lymphoid tissue, any involvement of the lung is labeled as "E." If a patient has lymphoma elsewhere in the body and the lung is involved via hematogenous spread, it is labeled as stage IV E (IV due to metastatic involvement of the lung and E due to the lung being an extranodal organ). If the lung is the primary and the

BOX 1 Ann Arbor staging of lymphomas.

- *Stage I*: Involvement of a single lymph node or of a single extranodal organ or site (IE)
- *Stage II*: Involvement of two or more lymph node regions on the same side of the diaphragm, or localized involvement of an extranodal site or organ (IIE) and one or more lymph node regions on the same side of the diaphragm
- *Stage III*: Involvement of lymph node regions on both sides of the diaphragm, which may be accompanied by localized involvement of an extranodal organ or site (III E) or spleen (III S) or both (III SE)
- *Stage IV*: Diffuse or disseminated involvement of one or more distant extranodal organs with or without associated lymph node involvement
- *Fever >38°C, night sweats and weight loss >10% of body weight in the last 6 months of diagnosis are defined as systemic symptoms*
- *Spleen involvement is considered as nodal*

only site of lymphoma, it is stage IE. A tumor mass larger than 10 cm is labeled as X. Therefore, a patient with primary NHL of the lung with a size of 14 cm and no systemic symptoms would be labeled as "Primary pulmonary NHL, stage I AEX."

Diagnosis of lymphoma requires proper categorization based on the most recent WHO classification of hematopoietic and lymphoid neoplasms.[10] The World Health Organization (WHO) classification is based on lymphoma morphology, cell of origin (B, T, or NK-cell lineage), immunophenotyping, and chromosomal and molecular characteristics. Staging is necessary once the diagnosis of lymphoma is confirmed. Both HL and NHL are staged using the Ann Arbor staging system **(Box 1)**. Detailed investigations are required for a comprehensive workup **(Box 2)**. Staging helps in prognostication and making therapeutic decisions. In rare cases, surgery may be curative for localized lymphoma of the lung parenchyma if complete resection of the lesion is possible.

Prognosis of NHL is defined by the International Prognostic Index (IPI),[11] which takes into account age, disease stage, lactate dehydrogenase (LDH) levels, performance status, and extranodal site involvement. The higher the stage, the worse the prognosis. HL also has a similar prognostic score based on hemoglobin, white blood cell count, age, stage, serum albumin, and lymphocytopenia. During treatment, nonresponsiveness to one to two cycles of chemotherapy is considered an important adverse feature. Response criteria to systemic chemotherapy are now standardized.[12]

Primary Lung Involvement by Lymphomas

Involvement of the tracheobronchial tree and lung parenchyma by lymphomas without the involvement of adjacent lymph nodes or other structures is quite rare. The diagnosis requires the demonstration of clonal lymphoid proliferation in the lung parenchyma, trachea, or bronchi without detectable involvement of extrapulmonary sites at the time of diagnosis and during the following 3 months.[1-4]

BOX 2 Workup of a lymphoma patient.

- Lymph node biopsy (excisional or core) with immunohistochemistry
- FDG PET CT of whole body
- Complete blood counts, ESR and bone marrow examination (aspiration and trephine biopsy)
- Biochemical (urea, creatinine, uric acid, calcium, phosphorus, bilirubin, SGOT, SGPT, alkaline phosphatase, blood sugar)
- EKG, echocardiography or MUGA scan
- Urine examination
- Serum LDH, serum beta-2 microglobulin
- HbsAg, anti-HBc, anti-HCV, HIV
- PFT (Hodgkin lymphoma)

Work-up in resource constraints (depending upon resources):

- Clinical staging, chest X-ray, ultrasound abdomen, CECT chest/abdomen/pelvis

(anti-HBc: hepatitis B core antibody; anti-HCV: antibodies to the hepatitis C virus; CT: computed tomography; CECT: contrast-enhanced CT; EKG: electrocardiogram; ESR: erythrocyte sedimentation rate; FDG: fluorodeoxyglucose; HBsAg: hepatitis B surface antigen; LDH: lactate dehydrogenase; MUGA: multigated acquisition; PET: positron emission tomography; PFT: pulmonary function test; SGOT: serum glutamic-oxaloacetic transaminase; SGPT: serum glutamic pyruvic transaminase)

Epidemiology

Primary NHL and HL of lung account for <1% of all lymphoma and 3–4% of all extranodal lymphoma. Based on isolated case reports and series, it appears that most cases are reported in the middle and older age groups.[13-19] In some series, there is predominance of cases in the female population. Systemic symptoms (B symptoms) are more commonly observed at presentation. There are no known risk factors for the development of these lymphomas, except for low-grade primary NHL of the lung, specifically MALT lymphomas (discussed further).

Clinical Features

Patients commonly present with persistent cough, hemoptysis, dyspnea, wheezing, chest pain, discomfort, or stridor. They may also experience systemic symptoms such as fever, weight loss, and night sweats (B symptoms). The initial investigations usually involve a chest X-ray, which may reveal the presence of nodules, masses, atelectasis, cavitation, or other abnormalities.[20-23] The differential diagnosis includes infectious diseases (such as tuberculosis and histoplasmosis) as well as noninfectious conditions (such as lung carcinoma, bronchial carcinoid, sarcoidosis, and granulomatosis).[24,25] In some cases, both lymphoma and infection can coexist in the lung, necessitating a biopsy for accurate diagnosis.

Diagnosis

Sputum examination for malignant cytology can sometimes provide clues to the diagnosis. Obtaining an adequate tissue specimen with bronchoscopy, other interventional procedures or open lung biopsy is crucial in establishing the diagnosis.[26-29] Morphological examination, along with immunohistochemical stains and occasionally molecular analysis of the tissue specimen is essential for confirming the diagnosis. If obtaining sufficient tissue is not feasible, cytology with immunocytochemistry can suggest and help confirm the diagnosis. Flow cytometry run on a cytology sample often yields the diagnosis in a short period of time.

Treatment and Outcome

Patients presenting with obstructive endobronchial lesions typically require rigid bronchoscopy and stenting.[30,31] In some cases, laser therapy using Neodymium: Yttrium-Aluminum Garnet Laser (Nd:YAG) or photodynamic laser therapy (PDT) has been employed to treat these life-threatening obstructions. Previous case reports and case series have shown successful outcomes with surgery alone or surgery followed by radiotherapy.[32] However, in recent times, chemotherapy has been increasingly utilized in primary lymphomas of the lungs due to the adverse long-term effects associated with radiotherapy on lung parenchyma. The treatment approach varies based on the histology and staging of the lymphoma.[33]

SECONDARY LUNG INVOLVEMENT IN HODGKIN LYMPHOMA

Mediastinal lymph node involvement occurs in almost two thirds of patients with HL while lung parenchymal involvement occurs in 10% of patients, usually as an extension from the involved lymph nodes.[20,21] The most common histological type of HL is nodular sclerosis. If mediastinal lymphadenopathy is more than one third the size of the internal thoracic diameter or if the transverse diameter is >10 cm, it is defined as bulky disease, and these patients are candidates for mediastinal radiation after chemotherapy. The involved lymph nodes are typically found in the anterior mediastinum, paratracheal, hilar, subcarinal, peridiaphragmatic, paraesophageal, and internal mammary regions, in decreasing frequency.[21] Extension into the lung parenchyma manifests as interstitial linear infiltrates or small nodules. If this extension is in direct continuity with the involved lymph nodes, a separate procedure to confirm lung involvement by HL may not be necessary. In some cases, these lesions may be caused by an infectious process, and therefore, fine-needle aspiration, bronchial lavage, or, rarely, an open biopsy may be used for documentation. Isolated lung parenchymal involvement without involvement of the mediastinal lymph nodes is exceedingly rare.

Hodgkin lymphoma is considered a curable malignancy depending on the stage of the disease. Therefore, it is important to determine the stage of the disease before initiating chemotherapy. HL is also highly responsive to radiation therapy. Treatment approaches for HL have evolved from radiotherapy alone to chemotherapy alone or a combination of chemotherapy and radiotherapy. The most common chemotherapy protocol used to treat HL is ABVD (Adriamycin, Bleomycin, Vinblastine, Dacarbazine). In general, for stage I and II disease, two to four cycles of chemotherapy (ABVD) followed by radiotherapy are used. Stage III and IV HL are usually treated with chemotherapy alone. If bulky disease is present at any stage (defined as a tumor size > 10 cm), radiotherapy is always combined with chemotherapy. As a general rule, patients with early stage disease (Stages IA, IB, IIA) are generally given two to four cycles of ABVD protocol followed by radiation. Advanced HL (Stages IIB, III, IV) are treated with six cycles of ABVD protocol. Patients with a bulky disease, which has not achieved complete remission after six cycles of chemotherapy, may be considered as candidates for radiotherapy to the involved site.

Hodgkin lymphoma with secondary lung involvement is initially treated with chemotherapy to reduce tumor size. Bleomycin, included in the ABVD protocol, is also toxic to the lungs, so close monitoring with pulmonary function tests is necessary for these patients. Female patients who receive mediastinal radiation for the treatment of a mediastinal mass are at risk of developing secondary breast and thyroid cancer. These patients should be closely followed up for many years. In this subgroup, it is advisable to begin screening for breast cancer with mammography at least 5 years before the recommended age for breast cancer screening.[8]

Primary Lung Involvement in Non-Hodgkin Lymphoma

In NHL, lymph node involvement typically occurs in a noncontiguous manner, unlike the contiguous spread seen in HL. Lung involvement can occur in up to 40% of NHL patients. NHLs are generally classified into indolent and aggressive subtypes. The most common indolent lymphoma variety is MALT while aggressive lymphoma subtypes that have a predilection for the lungs include diffuse large B-cell lymphoma, lymphoblastic lymphoma, and anaplastic large-cell lymphoma. The treatment and prognosis differ between aggressive and indolent NHL.

Mucosa-associated Lymphoid Tissue Lymphoma

The most common type of primary pulmonary lymphoma is MALT lymphoma, which is characterized by clonal proliferation of lymphocytes in the bronchus-associated lymphoid tissue.[34-36] This type of lymphoma is classified as a low-grade B-cell NHL and originates from the lymphoid tissue in the bronchus or lung parenchyma, often due to prolonged antigenic stimulation. Similar to gastrointestinal

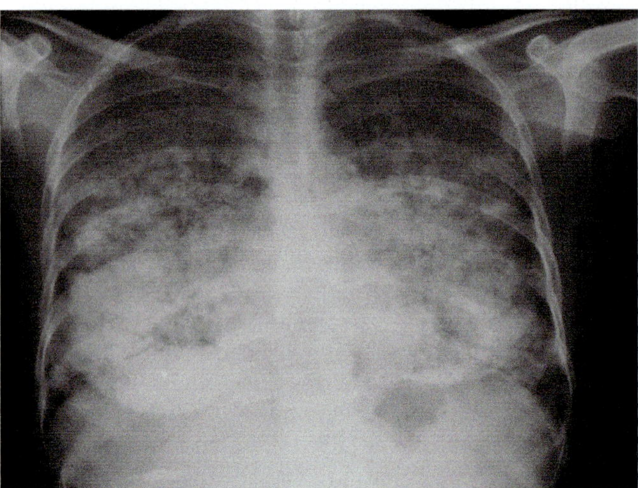

FIG. 1: Mucosa-associated lymphoid tissue lymphoma presentation in a 40-year-old lady.

MALT lymphomas, which are mainly associated with persistent antigenic stimulation from *Helicobacter pylori* infection, the cause of MALT lymphoma in the lung parenchyma is not attributed to a single organism, but rather to recurrent infections or autoimmune/rheumatological disorders of the body.[37-40]

Patients with MALT lymphoma may be asymptomatic, and the lesions are often detected incidentally on routine chest X-rays, or they may experience nonspecific chest symptoms that can be attributed to other causes **(Fig. 1)**.[40] Due to the rarity of these lymphomas, the diagnosis is primarily based on histology and immunohistochemistry of resected tissue. In approximately 25% of patients, MALT lymphoma may also present simultaneously at other sites, such as the orbit, salivary glands, or bone marrow. Differential diagnosis includes other lung conditions characterized by lymphocyte proliferation, such as follicular hyperplasia, lymphocytic interstitial pneumonia (typically bilateral), or hypersensitivity pneumonitis. Molecular techniques may sometimes be required for an accurate diagnosis of MALT lymphoma. In some cases, these lymphomas can transform into a higher-grade variety with systemic symptoms when present for an extended period.

As low-grade lymphomas are considered incurable, treatment is initiated when the disease becomes symptomatic or progressive. The choice of treatment depends on the disease stage, patient's age, and performance status. Rarely, surgery alone or in combination with radiotherapy may be considered. Although response to treatment are generally excellent, the disease tends to recur after some time.[39]

Secondary Involvement of Lungs by High-grade NHL

High-grade NHL generally presents with large mediastinal masses and can involve the lung parenchyma, with either contiguous or noncontiguous. The most common types are precursor T-cell lymphoblastic lymphoma/leukemia and primary mediastinal large B-cell lymphoma.

Primary Mediastinal Large B-cell Lymphoma

Primary mediastinal large B-cell lymphomas are recognized as a distinct entity in the WHO classification of lymphoma. They originate from the thymus and constitute approximately 2–3% of all NHL cases. These lymphomas show a slight female preponderance and typically occur in younger age groups.[41-43] The main presenting symptoms result from the rapid growth of a mediastinal mass, which compresses various structures in the mediastinum. The enlarging mass can also infiltrate the adjacent lung parenchyma, chest wall, pleura, and pericardium. The common symptoms include cough, hoarseness of voice, chest pain, and dyspnea. Systemic B symptoms are present in approximately one fifth of patients. The diagnostic workup for these patients is similar to that for other high-grade NHL cases, involving mediastinal lymph node core biopsy guided by ultrasound, endoscopy, or thoracoscopy for accurate classification.

The treatment approach for primary mediastinal large B-cell lymphoma is similar to that for other diffuse large B-cell lymphomas, typically involving the R-CHOP [cyclophosphamide, doxorubicin hydrochloride (hydroxydaunorubicin), vincristine sulfate (Oncovin), and prednisone] chemotherapy regimen, although some physicians may opt for third-generation chemotherapy regimens.[41] The recent data suggests that the use of infusional Dose-Adjusted EPOCH-R (DA-EPOCH-R) regimen may be preferred as radiotherapy to the mediastinum may be avoided in patients who achieve a complete response after chemotherapy. Response rates with DA-EPOCH-R are high and these patients have an excellent prognosis if treated early.

Precursor T-cell Leukemia/Lymphoma

In the WHO classification of lymphohematopoietic disorders, the distinction between lymphoma with lymphoblast-like cells and lymphoblastic leukemia has not been made because the treatment approaches for both conditions are similar.[11] T-cell lymphoma/leukemia typically presents as a large mediastinal mass in young males and is generally associated with a poor prognosis. The presenting symptoms arise due to the rapid enlargement of the mediastinal mass, causing compression on adjacent structures. In most cases, the disease is associated with human T-lymphotropic virus type 1 (HTLV-1) infection. The treatment involves intensive chemotherapy, during which a combination of various chemotherapeutic agents is administered over a few months as the intensive phase. This is followed by maintenance chemotherapy for a total duration of 2–3 years to prevent disease recurrence.

Diffuse Large B-cell Lymphoma Associated with Chronic Inflammation

This is a unique entity of diffuse large b-cell lymphoma (DLBCL), which occurs in the setting of chronic inflammation. The setting for chronic inflammation may be varied, such as a long-standing hydrocele, a metallic stent or a chronic infective focus. One of the most common examples is a chronic pyothorax such as seen in patients with tuberculosis, often referred to as a pyothorax-associated lymphoma. The median age of patients at the time of presentation is above 70 years, patients generally have other comorbidities. The presenting symptoms consist of pain in chest or back along with systemic symptoms such as fever and weight loss. Chest skiagram is usually the first investigation followed by either CT or MRI scans. The differential diagnosis includes other chest tumors such as mesothelioma and lung carcinoma. The diagnosis is achieved by performing a core biopsy of the mass and with immunohistochemistry.[44] Further, staging of lymphoma is done as mentioned earlier. Bone marrow involvement by lymphoma is rare. The treatment is given with chemotherapy as used for other large B-cell lymphoma. Sometimes, radiation is required if the tumor does not resolve completely after the chemotherapy. The prognosis is dismal in most cases because of the presence of comorbidities.[45]

Fluid Overload-associated B-cell Lymphoma

This is a new entity which has been included in the recent 2022 WHO classification of lymphoid neoplasms. It is commonly confused with its counterpart of primary effusion lymphoma (PEL) which is associated with human herpesvirus 8 (HHV-8) infection. Patients are usually elderly and have an underlying condition which predisposes them to fluid overload, such as cirrhosis or chronic kidney disease. Pathologically, the lymphoma is composed of large cells which are positive for B-cell such as CD19 and CD20. Lymphoma usually occurs in the body cavities, most commonly the pleural cavity. Epstein-Barr virus (EBV) may be detected in 13–30% of patients. Overall, these patients respond well to therapy and have a favorable prognosis.

Primary Effusion Lymphoma

Primary effusion lymphoma (PEL) is a distinct clinicopathological entity seen in patients who are elderly or immunocompromised. It is associated with infection by HHV8 virus, and a coinfection with EBV is also seen in the majority of patients. It can affect any of the body cavities, including the pericardium, peritoneum as well as the pleural space. The disease has an aggressive course and does not respond well to standard chemotherapeutic regimens such as CHOP and is associated with a poor prognosis.

Lymphomatoid Granulomatosis

Lymphomatoid granulomatosis (LYG) is a condition that can be mistaken for various malignant and nonmalignant lung disorders. The cause of this condition is unknown, but it is often found in patients with immunological abnormalities. The disease is characterized by the presence of lung nodules or masses, typically located in the lower lobes or periphery of the lung fields. A significant number of patients may also experience central nervous system (CNS) abnormalities, such as seizures or focal deficits, as well as dermatological involvement, including erythematous skin rashes, skin nodules, or ulcers. LYG has been described as resembling posttransplant lymphoproliferative disorder. It usually affects middle-to-elderly-aged individuals, and common symptoms include cough, hemoptysis, and dyspnea.

The diagnosis of LYG is typically made through surgical biopsy of the resected nodule or mass. Differential diagnoses to consider include Wegener's granulomatosis (WG) and T-cell lymphoma. Like WG, LYG involves granuloma formation, but the cells in LYG are atypical and immature, and most B-cells show infection with EBV. Similar to T-cell lymphoma, LYG granulomas are surrounded by reactive T-cells, but LYG does not typically present with cytopenias and paraproteinemias, which are often seen in T-cell lymphomas. Histologically, LYG is further graded into three types based on the number of cells infected with EBV. The aggressiveness of the disease increases as the histological grade progresses from one to three, and treatment strategies vary accordingly. Grade one and sometimes grade two LYG may be observed without treatment, whereas grade three LYG always requires treatment, usually similar to that for patients with diffuse large B-cell lymphoma.

SECONDARY INVOLVEMENT OF LUNG BY OTHER SYSTEMIC HEMATOPOIETIC AND LYMPHOID DISORDERS[46-48]

Castleman Disease[46]

Castleman disease (angiofollicular lymph node hyperplasia) was initially described in 1954 as a benign localized mass of lymph nodes in the mediastinum. Subsequently, additional types of this condition were identified, and it is now categorized into unicentric and multicentric forms, histologically classified as hyaline-vascular variant and plasma cell variant.

Unicentric CD presents as a single-mass lesion that can occur in the mediastinum, pleura, chest wall, and rarely in the lungs. It predominantly affects young adults and middle-aged individuals. Unless it compresses important nerves or vessels, the disease is mostly asymptomatic. Surgical resection of the mass can lead to a cure, while asymptomatic cases do not require treatment. The prevalence of the unicentric plasma cell variant is rarer compared to the multicentric plasma cell variant.

Multicentric CD typically manifests in middle-aged to elderly individuals and has become more common in the presence of HIV infection. The lesions can occur in the mediastinum, lungs, as well as various extrathoracic and retroperitoneal regions. Most patients experience systemic symptoms, such as fever, weight loss, and fatigue. In many cases, the disease has been associated with HHV-8 infection, which can be demonstrated in the resected tissue specimen. Treatment for patients with multicentric CD involves systemic chemotherapy. If the disease is associated with HIV infection, initiation of antiretroviral therapy is recommended promptly. Periodic flare-ups of the disease may occur.

PLASMA CELL DYSCRASIAS[47,48]

Plasma cell dyscrasias encompass various disorders, including multiple myeloma, solitary or multiple plasmacytomas, Waldenström macroglobulinemia, and primary amyloidosis. These disorders are characterized by the neoplastic proliferation of plasma cells that produce immunoglobulins. Lung involvement in these diseases is secondary. The most common thoracic manifestation of multiple myeloma is plasmacytoma of the ribs or adjacent vertebral column. Intraparenchymal nodules and interstitial infiltrates are less common but recognized manifestations. While the upper aerodigestive tract is a common, site for extramedullary plasmacytomas, primary pulmonary plasmacytoma is rare.

Due to the relative rarity of these lung disorders, their diagnosis often requires a biopsy or fine-needle aspiration cytology (FNAC) of the tissue. It is essential to conduct necessary investigations to detect systemic involvement in all cases of pulmonary plasma cell dyscrasia. These investigations may include serum and urine electrophoresis and bone marrow examination to identify clonal proliferation of plasma cells. Lung biopsy is often necessary to rule out infectious diseases as the cause of lung involvement. The treatment is primarily focused on addressing the systemic disease, and significant lung involvement is associated with a poor prognosis.

POSTTRANSPLANT LYMPHOPROLIFERATIVE DISORDERS

Lymphoproliferative disorders that develop after organ transplantation are considered a distinct entity, with a prevalence rate of up to 20% in different series. Their spectrum ranges from benign polyclonal lymphoproliferation to malignant lymphomas. Most disorders occur within the first year after transplantation. EBV infection acquired posttransplantation is one of the important risk factors, along with the degree of immunosuppression. The prevalence of posttransplant lymphoproliferative disorders (PTLDs) varies among different organ transplantations, with a higher risk observed in lung and heart transplantation due to increased immunosuppression.[49]

Intrathoracic presentation of PTLD occurs in up to 29% of patients.[50] The most common manifestations are lung nodules, patchy airspace disease, and mediastinal lymphadenopathy. The differential diagnosis includes infectious diseases that can occur in immunosuppressed patients. Therefore, a surgical biopsy of the lesion or an image-guided biopsy from the intrathoracic lymph node is necessary. More than 90% of lesions show positivity for EBV infection. Initial treatment involves reducing immunosuppression, which may only be effective in early-stage lesions. For advanced lesions, combination chemotherapy is the treatment of choice.[51] The prognosis depends on multiple factors, such as the stage and grade of the lesion, transplanted organ function, and performance status of the patient. Mortality rates are usually high, reaching up to 50% in some series.

CHEMOTHERAPEUTIC DRUGS LUNG TOXICITY[52-58]

The use of antineoplastic drugs can lead to lung toxicity, which can be challenging to differentiate from infectious diseases occurring in patients with hematological malignancies. Lung toxicity is a recognized complication of anticancer drugs. It can manifest as various lung disorders, including nonspecific interstitial pneumonitis, organizing pneumonia, desquamative interstitial pneumonia, eosinophilic pneumonia, granulomatous pneumonitis, diffuse alveolar hemorrhage, retinoic acid syndrome, noncardiogenic pulmonary edema, and acute respiratory distress syndrome. These symptoms have been associated with different classes of drugs, such as anthracyclines, purine analogs, antiangiogenesis drugs, monoclonal antibodies, proteasome inhibitors, alkylating agents, antibiotics, arsenic trioxide, and all-trans-retinoic acid. Respiratory symptoms typically appear 2–14 days after initiating the offending drug. Initially, most patients are treated for infectious complications, as infectious diseases are more common than drug toxicity. However, suspicion should remain high in patients who do not have identified infectious agents and whose symptoms correlate temporally with drug administration. Administration of corticosteroids in cases of drug-induced toxicity is generally associated with favorable outcomes.

MISCELLANEOUS MECHANISMS OF PULMONARY INVOLVEMENT

There are other ways in which hematolymphoid neoplasms can affect the pulmonary system, including involvement of the vasculature or the pleura.

Pulmonary Thromboembolism

Hematological malignancies, like other types of malignancies, are associated with a hypercoagulable state and an increased risk of deep venous thrombosis (DVT) and pulmonary thromboembolism (PTE). The risk of DVT and PTE is further elevated in these patients due to poor performance status at presentation and frequent immobility. Thrombosis is more commonly observed in patients with aggressive lymphomas compared to those with chronic lymphoproliferative disorders. Presentation can vary, with some patients having asymptomatic PTE detected during staging or response assessment scans, while others may experience symptoms due to a large PTE that may require thrombolysis. Treatment involves anticoagulation with low molecular weight heparin or non-vitamin K antagonist oral anticoagulants (NOACs) such as Apixaban or Rivaroxaban. Anticoagulation should continue for at least 3 months after the patient achieves remission.

Hyperviscosity and Leukostasis

Although hyperviscosity and leukostasis are distinct pathological conditions, they are being discussed together due to their similar presentations and mechanisms. In patients with leukemia, who have very high white blood cell counts at presentation, leukocytes can accumulate in the pulmonary capillaries, leading to pulmonary symptoms, profound dyspnea, and hypoxia. Similarly, patients with lymphomas, particularly Waldenstrom macroglobulinemia, may experience increased blood viscosity due to elevated immunoglobulin levels, resulting in impaired blood flow and stasis in the pulmonary vasculature. These patients may also exhibit significant CNS symptoms due to similar pathophysiological mechanisms occurring in the CNS vasculature. Treatment usually involves urgent leukapheresis or plasmapheresis to reduce the white blood cell count and immunoglobulin levels, respectively. Alongside apheresis, targeted therapy against the underlying neoplasm should be initiated as soon as possible since apheresis is only a temporary measure.

Nonmalignant Pleural Effusions

Patients with hematolymphoid malignancies may develop pleural effusions through mechanisms unrelated to neoplastic infiltration. For instance, patients with a large mediastinal mass may develop superior vena cava syndrome, leading to the development of a transudative pleural effusion. Peripheral pulmonary thromboembolism can also present with a pleural effusion. An important consideration for patients with a hematolymphoid malignancy and an effusion is chylous effusion, which occurs when the lymphomatous process disrupts the normal lymphatic channels. Chylous effusions can be seen in both NHL and HL **(Fig. 2)**.

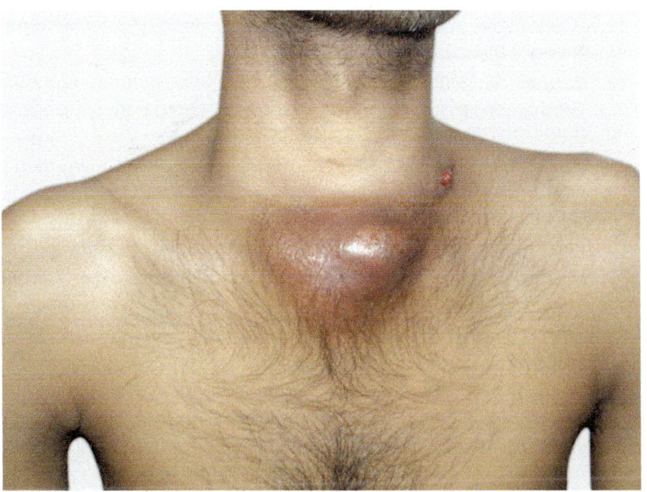

FIG. 2: Hodgkin lymphoma presenting as chest wall mass in a 22-year-old man.

SUMMARY

Lung involvement by hematolymphoid neoplasms is not uncommon and occurs in a variety of conditions. Primary lung involvement is, however, rare and generally missed. Many a type of these neoplasms are potentially treatable. It is, therefore, important to make an early diagnosis and differentiation from other common causes of lung involvement such as infections and nonlymphomatous tumors.

REFERENCES

1. Chilosi M, Zinzani PL, Poletti V. Lymphoproliferative lung disorders. Semin Respir Crit Care Med. 2005;26(5):490-501.
2. Vallisa D, Trabacchi E, Cavanna L. Primary lung lymphoma. Curr Drug Targets Inflamm Allergy. 2004;3(4):469-71.
3. Cadranel J, Wislez M, Antoine M. Primary pulmonary lymphoma. Eur Respir J. 2002;20(3):750-62.
4. Wannesson L, Ćavalli F, Zucca E. Primary pulmonary lymphoma: current status. Clin Lymphoma Myeloma. 2005;6(3):220-7.
5. Travis LB, Gospodarowicz M, Curtis RE, et al. Lung cancer following chemotherapy and radiotherapy for Hodgkin's disease. J Natl Cancer Inst. 2002;94(3):182-92.
6. Lorigan P, Radford J, Howell A, et al. Lung cancer after treatment for Hodgkin's lymphoma: a systematic review. Lancet Oncol. 2005;6(10):773-9.
7. Vahid B, Marik PE. Infiltrative lung diseases: complications of novel antineoplastic agents in patients with hematological malignancies. Can Respir J. 2008;15(4):211-6.
8. Chen YF, Li YC, Chen LM, et al. Primary cutaneous diffuse large B cell lymphoma relapsed solely as a huge lung tumor mimicking a primary pulmonary lymphoma. Int J Hematol. 2010;91(1):112-6.
9. Hsu PK, Hsu HS, Li AFY, et al. Non-Hodgkin's lymphoma presenting as a large chest wall mass. Ann Thorac Surg. 2006;81(4):1214-8.
10. Alaggio R, Amador C, Anagnostopoulos I, et al. The 5th edition of the World Health Organization Classification of Haematolymphoid Tumours: Lymphoid Neoplasms. Leukemia. 2022;36(7):1720-48.

11. A predictive model for aggressive non-Hodgkin's lymphoma. N Engl J Med. 1993;329(14):987-94.
12. Younes A, Hilden P, Coiffier B, et al. International Working Group consensus response evaluation criteria in lymphoma (RECIL 2017). Ann Oncol. 2017;28(7):1436.
13. Huang J, Lin T, Li ZM, et al. Primary pulmonary non-Hodgkin's lymphoma: a retrospective analysis of 29 cases in a Chinese population. Am J Hematol. 2010;85(7):523-5.
14. Kiani B, Magro CM, Ross P. Endobronchial presentation of Hodgkin lymphoma: A review of the literature. Ann Thorac Surg. 2003;76(3):967-72.
15. Kim JH, Lee SH, Park J, et al. Primary pulmonary non-Hodgkin's lymphoma. Jpn J Clin Oncol. 2004;34(9):510-4.
16. Solomonov A, Zuckerman T, Goralnik L, et al. Non-Hodgkin's lymphoma presenting as an endobronchial tumor: report of eight cases and literature review. Am J Hematol. 2008;83(5): 416-9.
17. Ferraro P, Trastek VF, Adlakha H, et al. Primary non-Hodgkin's lymphoma of the lung. Ann Thorac Surg. 2000;69(4):993-7.
18. Han SH, Maeng YH, Kim YS, et al. Primary anaplastic large cell lymphoma of the lung presenting with acute atelectasis. Thorac Cancer. 2014;5(1):78.
19. Cordier JF, Chailleux E, Lauque D, et al. Primary pulmonary lymphomas. A clinical study of 70 cases in nonimmunocompromised patients. Chest. 1993;103(1):201-8.
20. Bae YA, Lee KS. Cross-sectional evaluation of thoracic lymphoma. Thorac Surg Clin. 2010;20(1):175-86.
21. Sharma A, Fidias P, Hayman LA, et al. Patterns of lymphadenopathy in thoracic malignancies. Radiographics. 2004;24(2): 419-34.
22. Do KH, Jin SL, Joon BS, et al. Pulmonary parenchymal involvement of low-grade lymphoproliferative disorders. J Comput Assist Tomogr. 2005;29(6):825-30.
23. Chua SC, Rozalli FI, O'Connor SR. Imaging features of primary extranodal lymphomas. Clin Radiol. 2009;64(6):574-88.
24. Karakas Z, Agaoglu L, Taravari B, et al. Pulmonary tuberculosis in children with Hodgkin's lymphoma. Hematol J. 2003;4(1):78-81.
25. Codrich D, Monai M, Pelizzo G, et al. Primary pulmonary Hodgkin's disease and tuberculosis in an 11-year-old boy: case report and review of the literature. Pediatr Pulmonol. 2006; 41(7):694-8.
26. Takamura K, Nasuhara Y, Mishina T, et al. Intravascular lymphomatosis diagnosed by transbronchial lung biopsy. Eur Resp J. 1997;10(4):955-7.
27. Yamagata T, Okamoto Y, Ota K, et al. A case of pulmonary intravascular lymphomatosis diagnosed by thoracoscopic lung biopsy. Respiration. 2003;70(4):414-8.
28. Diehl LF, Hopper KD, Giguere J, et al. The pattern of intrathoracic Hodgkin's disease assessed by computed tomography. J Clin Oncol. 1991;9(3):438-43.
29. Bégueret H, Vergier B, Parrens M, et al. Primary Lung Small B-Cell Lymphoma versus Lymphoid Hyperplasia: Evaluation of Diagnostic Criteria in 26 Cases. Am J Surg Pathol. 2002;26(1): 76-81.
30. Huang IA, Hsia SH, Wu CT, et al. Combined chemotherapy and tracheobronchial stenting for life-threatening airway obstruction in a child with endobronchial non-Hodgkin lymphoma. Pediatr Hematol Oncol. 2004;21(8):725-9.
31. Ranu H, Madden BP. Endobronchial stenting in the management of large airway pathology. Postgrad Med J. 2009;85(1010): 682-7.
32. Vanden Eynden F, Fadel E, de Perrot M, et al. Role of surgery in the treatment of primary pulmonary B-cell lymphoma. Ann Thorac Surg. 2007;83(1):236-40.
33. Zinzani PL, Martelli M, Poletti V, et al. Practice guidelines for the management of extranodal non-Hodgkin's lymphomas of adult non-immunodeficient patients. Part I: primary lung and mediastinal lymphomas. A project of the Italian Society of Hematology, the Italian Society of Experimental Hematology and the Italian Group for Bone Marrow Transplantation. Haematologica. 2008;93(9):1364-71.
34. Ahmed S, Kussick SJ, Siddiqui AK, et al. Bronchial-associated lymphoid tissue lymphoma: A clinical study of a rare disease. Eur J Cancer. 2004;40(9):1320-6.
35. Arnaoutakis K, Oo TH. Bronchus-associated lymphoid tissue lymphomas. South Med J. 2009;102(12):1229-33.
36. Ahmed S, Siddiqui AK, Rai KR. Low-grade B-cell bronchial associated lymphoid tissue (BALT) lymphoma. Cancer Invest. 2002;20(7–8):1059-68.
37. Imai H, Sunaga N, Kaira K, et al. Clinicopathological features of patients with bronchial-associated lymphoid tissue lymphoma. Intern Med. 2009;48(5):301-6.
38. Klein T-O, Soll BA, Issel BF, et al. Bronchus-Associated Lymphoid Tissue Lymphoma and *Mycobacterium tuberculosis* Infection: An Unusual Case and a Review of the Literature. Respir Care. 2007;52(6).
39. Zinzani PL, Poletti V, Zompatori M, et al. Bronchus-associated lymphoid tissue lymphomas: an update of a rare extranodal maltoma. Clin Lymphoma Myeloma. 2007;7(9):566-72.
40. Zinzani PL, Tani M, Gabriele A, et al. Extranodal marginal zone B-cell lymphoma of MALT-type of the lung: single-center experience with 12 patients. Leuk Lymphoma. 2003;44(5):821-4.
41. Rodríguez J, Gutiérrez A, Piris M. Primary mediastinal B-cell lymphoma: treatment and therapeutic targets. Leuk Lymphoma. 2008;49(6):1050-61.
42. Martelli M, Ferreri A, Di Rocco A, Ansuinelli M, Johnson PWM. Primary mediastinal large B-cell lymphoma. Crit Rev Oncol Hematol. 2017;113:318-27.
43. Dunleavy K. Primary mediastinal B-cell lymphoma: biology and evolving therapeutic strategies. Hematology. 2017;2017(1): 298-303.
44. Petitjean B, Jardin F, Joly B, et al. Pyothorax-associated lymphoma: a peculiar clinicopathologic entity derived from B cells at late stage of differentiation and with occasional aberrant dual B- and T-cell phenotype. Am J Surg Pathol. 2002;26(6): 724-32.
45. Nakatsuka S ichi, Yao M, Hoshida Y, et al. Pyothorax-associated lymphoma: a review of 106 cases. J Clin Oncol. 2002;20(20): 4255-60.
46. Sharma OP. Paraproteinemias and the lungs. Curr Opin Pulm Med. 2005;11(5):408-11.
47. Kyrtsonis MC, Angelopoulou MK, Kontopidou FN, et al. Primary lung involvement in Waldenström's macroglobulinaemia: report of two cases and review of the literature. Acta Haematol. 2001;105(2):92-6.
48. Allam JS, Kennedy CC, Aksamit TR, Dispenzieri A. Pulmonary manifestations in patients with POEMS syndrome: a retrospective review of 137 patients. Chest. 2008;133(4):969-74.
49. Parker A, Bowles K, Bradley JA, et al. Diagnosis of post-transplant lymphoproliferative disorder in solid organ transplant recipients - BCSH and BTS Guidelines. Br J Haematol. 2010;149(5):675-92.

50. Halkos ME, Miller JI, Mann KP, et al. Thoracic presentations of posttransplant lymphoproliferative disorders. Chest. 2004; 126(6):2013-20.
51. Parker A, Bowles K, Bradley JA, et al. Management of post-transplant lymphoproliferative disorder in adult solid organ transplant recipients - BCSH and BTS Guidelines. Br J Haematol. 2010;149(5):693-705.
52. Kalkanis D, Stefanovic A, Paes F, et al. [18F]-fluorodeoxyglucose positron emission tomography combined with computed tomography detection of asymptomatic late pulmonary toxicity in patients with non-Hodgkin lymphoma treated with rituximab-containing chemotherapy. Leuk Lymphoma. 2009; 50(6):904-11.
53. Artinian V, Kvale PA. Cancer and interstitial lung disease. Curr Opin Pulm Med. 2004;10(5):425-34.
54. Lim KH, Yoon H II, Kang YA, et al. Severe pulmonary adverse effects in lymphoma patients treated with cyclophosphamide, doxorubicin, vincristine, and prednisone (CHOP) regimen plus rituximab. Korean J Intern Med. 2010;25(1):86-92.
55. Wagner SA, Mehta AC, Laber DA. Rituximab-induced interstitial lung disease. Am J Hematol. 2007;82(10):916-9.
56. Heresi GA, Farver CF, Stoller JK. Interstitial pneumonitis and alveolar hemorrhage complicating use of rituximab: case report and review of the literature. Respiration. 2008;76(4):449-53.
57. Liu X, Hong XN, Gu YJ, et al. Interstitial pneumonitis during rituximab-containing chemotherapy for non-Hodgkin lymphoma. Leuk Lymphoma. 2008;49(9):1778-83.
58. Herishanu Y, Polliack A, Leider-Trejo L, et al. Fatal interstitial pneumonitis related to rituximab-containing regimen. Clin Lymphoma Myeloma. 2006;6(5):407-9.

CHAPTER 156

Lung Cancer Screening

Mateus Fernandes, Viera Lakticova, Brett Bade, Suhail Raoof

INTRODUCTION

Lung cancer is the leading cause of death from cancer worldwide.[1] Compared to other common cancer types, lung cancer survival is shorter due to most cases being diagnosed in advanced stage disease.[2] Screening facilitates early diagnosis and curative treatments by identifying cancers before patients develop symptoms. Indeed, for many years, early diagnosis for breast, colon, and cervical cancers has been facilitated by screening efforts.[3] Unfortunately, despite the high mortality and lower survival rates associated with lung cancer, early screening efforts with chest X-ray and sputum cytology were ineffective.[4]

More recently, two large clinical trials in the United States and Europe have shown that annual screening with low-dose computed tomography (LDCT) can identify cancers at early stages, reducing lung cancer mortality by 20–24%.[5-7] Thus, to significantly improve lung cancer mortality and survival, physicians should incorporate screening into their practice. The shared decision-making insurance requirement for lung cancer screening in the United States emphasizes the importance of understanding the risks and benefits of screening. There are several important aspects of lung cancer screening that should guide patient discussions. In this chapter, we will review the topics that physicians should be most familiar with for shared decision-making, including (1) the benefits and evidence of lung cancer screening, (2) available guidelines recommending lung cancer screening, (3) tobacco cessation, (4) risks, (5) the shared decision-making process, and (6) how to manage screen-detected findings.

BENEFITS OF SCREENING

The primary goal of lung cancer screening is to detect lung cancer in an early stage, before any symptoms develop. Compared to patients with metastatic disease, treatment of early-stage lung cancers is more likely to result in cure or long-term survival.[8] As referenced above, early approaches to lung cancer screening included chest X-ray and sputum cytology.[4] These techniques identified some lung cancers, though there was no reduction in lung cancer mortality.[4]

More recent lung cancer screening studies have incorporated LDCT and included patients at high risk for lung cancer according to age and tobacco smoking history. Compared to chest X-ray, LDCT allows visualization of much smaller lung nodules.[9,10] Using LDCT, more recent clinical trials have shown promising results **(Table 1)**,[11-16] though most studies were unable to confirm reduction in lung cancer mortality due to small sample sizes. Only the National Lung Screening Trial (NLST) and the Nederlands-Leuvens Longkanker Screenings Onderzoek Study (NELSON) possessed the statistical power to confirm that lung cancer screening produces a statistically significant reduction in lung cancer mortality. The NLST performed three annual LDCTs and showed a lung cancer mortality reduction of 20%[6] The NELSON study performed four LDCTs (baseline, 1, 3, and 5.5 years) and identified a lung cancer mortality reduction of 24%. A pooled meta-analysis of eight trials found an overall mortality reduction of 19%.[17] In summary, using annual LDCT in patients at high risk for lung cancer has the potential to reduce lung cancer mortality by 20–24%.

Based on the results of NLST, US guidelines for lung cancer screening were formulated, and payer coverage for screening was provided in 2015 **(Table 2)**.[18] The United States Preventive Services Task Force (USPSTF) initially approved lung cancer screening in patients aged 55–80 years, with a ≥ 30 pack-year smoking history, and in patients who currently smoke or quit within the last 15 years.[19] More recently, the guidelines were updated to include younger patients with a less cigarette smoking history: Ages 50–80 years and a 20 pack-year smoking history.[18,19] The NELSON trial opened the door for lung cancer screening in Europe.[20] In 2019, the European Society for Medical Oncology (ESMO) convened a roundtable discussion, and an expert panel concluded that national health policy groups in Europe should start to implement CT screening for lung cancer.[20] Examples of individual health policy groups screening recommendations are outlined in **Table 2**.

TABLE 1: Summary of studies evaluating lung cancer screening.

Study (*n* = number of participants)	Participant characteristics	Lung cancer mortality reduction
NLST (*n* = 53, 454) National Lung Screening Trial 2013[6]	Age: 55–74 years >30 pack-years <15 years' cessation	20%*
NELSON (*n* = 15, 775) Nederlands–Leuvens Longkanker Screenings Onderzoek Study 2020[7]	Age: 50–75 years >15 cigarettes/day for >25 years or >10 cigarettes/day for >30 years <10 years' cessation	24% in men* 33% in women
DANTE (*n* = 2,472) Detection and Screening of Early Lung Cancer by Novel Imaging Technology and Molecular Essays Trial 2015[11]	Age: 60–74 years > 20 pack-years <10 years' cessation	No difference
DLCST (*n* = 4,104) Danish Lung Cancer Screening Trial 2016[12]	Age: 50–70 years >20 pack-years <10 years' cessation	No difference
ITALUNG (*n* = 3,206) Italian Lung Cancer Screening Trial 2017[13]	Age: 55–69 years >20 pack-years <10 years' cessation	30%
MILD trial (*n* = 4,099) Multi-centric Italian Lung Detection 2019[14]	Age: >49 years >20 pack-years <10 years' cessation	39%*
LUSI (*n* = 4,039) German Lung Cancer Screening Intervention Trial 2020[15]	Age: 50–69 years >15 cigarettes/day for >25 years or >10 cigarettes/day for >30 years <10 years' cessation	26%
UKLS (*n* = 4,055) United Kingdom Lung Screening Study 2016[16]	Age: 50–75 years Risk score† > 5%	Not reported

*Statistically significant ($p < 0.05$).

†Risk score refers to the score obtained on the Liverpool Lung Project lung cancer risk prediction algorithm version 2, which was a risk-based model used in the UKLS.

TABLE 2: Selected guidelines and eligibility recommendations for lung cancer screening.

Guideline	Screening recommendations or eligibility
United States Preventive Services Task Force (USPSTF)[10]	Recommend annual LDCT for adults aged 50–80 years who have ≥20 pack-year smoking history and currently smoke or have quit within the past 15 years
Centers for Medicare and Medicaid Services[21]	Recommend annual LDCT for adults aged 50–77 years who have ≥20 pack-year smoking history and currently smoke or have quit within the past 15 years
American College of Chest Physicians[17]	• Recommend annual LDCT for asymptomatic adults aged 55–77 years with 30 pack-years or more and either continue to smoke or have quit within the past 15 years • Suggest annual LDCT for asymptomatic individuals who do not meet the smoking and/or age criteria in recommendation 1, are age 50–80 years, have smoked 20 pack-years or more, and either continue to smoke or have quit within the past 15 years • Suggest annual LDCT for asymptomatic individuals who do not meet the smoking and/or age criteria in recommendations 1 and 2 but are projected to have a high net benefit from lung cancer screening based on the results of validated clinical risk prediction calculations and life expectancy estimates or based on life-year gained calculations
United Kingdom National Screening Committee[22]	Recommend targeted screening for lung cancer for people aged 55–74 identified as being at high risk of lung cancer
Canadian Task Force for Preventative Health[23]	Recommend annual LDCT in high-risk adults aged 55–74 years who are current or former smokers with a smoking history of at least 30 pack-years
European Commission A new EU approach to cancer screening (press release September 2022)[20]	Recommend screening for current and ex-smokers who have quit smoking within the previous 15 years, are aged 50–75 years, and have a smoking history of 30 pack-years

(LDCT: low-dose computed tomography)

Compared to established screening guidelines for other types of cancer, lung cancer screening is highly effective. In the NLST, the baseline risk of death from lung cancer was 1.7%, and the number needed to screen to prevent one death from lung cancer was 323 participants.[24] In other words, for every 1,000 individuals screened, 3 deaths from lung cancer were prevented.[24] Compared to screening for breast cancer, the numbers needed to screen with mammography to prevent one death from breast cancer range from 380 participants for high-risk individuals (60–69 years of age, with 0.9% baseline risk) to 1,900 participants for lower risk individuals (39–49 years of age, with 0.3% baseline risk).[25-27] Compared to prostate cancer screening with prostate-specific antigen (PSA), one study found that the number needed to screen was 1,400 to prevent one death from prostate cancer, in individuals with a 0.4% baseline risk.[28] This relatively high effectiveness of lung cancer screening may be due to more targeted screening of a high-risk population. For example, lung cancer screening incorporates both age and smoking histories, whereas breast and colon cancer screening primarily focus on age.

The updated USPSTF LCS guidelines in 2021 increased lung cancer screening eligibility by ~80%,[29] highlighting that many patients are at high risk for developing lung cancer but not included in the USPSTF guidelines. To more accurately identify patients at high risk of lung cancer, various risk prediction tools have been developed to more comprehensively estimate risk. These tools are discussed further below.

SCREENING CONSIDERATIONS AND ASSOCIATED RISKS

While lung cancer screening offers life-saving benefits, it is essential to consider the possible harms that may arise from both (1) the screening process itself and (2) the consequences of investigating abnormal test results.[30]

High False-positive Rate

With the increase in the use of LDCT for lung cancer screening, the identification of lung nodules that are not due to cancer (i.e., falsely positive LDCTs) is common. The rate of false positives varies significantly by definition of a positive screen. For example, nodule size criteria for a positive screen varies from 4 to 6 mm in most studies.[25] In the NLST, a positive screen was defined by the presence of a nodule ≥ 4 mm in size. Using this criterion, 24% of participants had a positive screen, and the false-positive rate was 96.4%.[5] United States veterans undergoing lung cancer screening (who are generally older and have the potential for occupational inhaled exposures) had positive screening in 50–60% of cases.[31] Due to high false-positive rates and patient anxiety related to lung nodule identification, shared decision-making should emphasize that identifying lung nodules is common in patients undergoing screening, and most lung nodules are not due to lung cancer. However, identified lung nodules must undergo sufficient follow-up, which is most commonly a repeat LDCT to ensure that there is no change in the nodule size.[17] Management of screen-detected pulmonary nodules is discussed below.

Psychological Consequences

One of the foremost risks and patient concerns is the psychological impact on individuals who have screen-detected lung nodules. The process of identifying and evaluating these nodules can be emotionally taxing and may lead to stress and anxiety. Studies indicate that individuals found to have a screen-detected lung nodule may experience temporary emotional and psychological distress.[32] However, distress does not appear to have a long-term adverse effect on anxiety levels or overall quality of life.[32] When performing shared decision-making, it is essential to ensure that patients understand what to expect from the process and weigh these short-term emotional effects against the potential benefits of early cancer detection and treatment.

Cumulative Radiation Exposure

Low-dose CT screening exposes individuals to cumulative radiation. Although the radiation dose from an individual LDCT scan is low, there is a concern that repeated LDCTs could potentially increase the risk of cancer over time. A single LDCT scan utilizes an effective radiation dose of 1.5 millisieverts (mSv), which is about 80% less radiation compared to a regular chest CT scan (7 mSv).[33]

For perspective, the average annual radiation exposure per person in the United States is about 6 mSv, of which about 48% is attributable to medical imaging **(Table 3)**.[34] The other major source of radiation exposure is background radiation, which occurs due to natural sources such as minerals undergoing radioactive decay (radon and thoron being the major contributors) or space/cosmic radiation. Notably, there have been no studies finding a causative association between cumulative background radiation and cancer risk.[35]

With perfect adherence to the NLST protocol, which entailed annual LDCT screening from age 55–77 years, the lifetime attributable risk of radiation-related lung cancer mortality is 0.07% for men and 0.14% for women.[36] This

TABLE 3: Estimated radiation dose from selected medical imaging, compared to other common exposures.[33,34]

Exposure	Radiation (mSv)
Air travel for 10 hours	0.04
Chest radiograph	0.1
Mammogram	0.4
Low-dose CT	1.5
Annual background radiation	2–4
Conventional CT	7

translates to one cancer death for every 2,500 persons screened. Remembering that one death is prevented for every 320 persons screened, this risk is relatively low.

Overdiagnosis and Competing Causes of Death

Overdiagnosis is a complex and important issue in lung cancer screening. Broadly speaking, overdiagnosis refers to the detection of indolent cancers that are either clinically insignificant or occur in individuals with competing comorbidities that would lead to death before the cancer becomes a significant health concern.[37] Though lung cancer is generally recognized as a more aggressive disease with shorter survival than other cancer types, there is a spectrum of growth patterns. Some lung cancers are slow to develop and grow. For example, adenocarcinoma-in-situ (previously known as bronchoalveolar carcinoma) tends to have slow growth. These lesions often radiographically appear as ground-glass nodules.[38] Several studies have shown heterogenicity in the growth rates of LDCT-detected lung cancer, which indicates that there is a reservoir of indolent cancers within the screening population.

Individuals eligible for lung cancer screening have significant tobacco smoking histories; thus, smoking-related comorbidities are common [e.g., coronary artery disease, chronic obstructive pulmonary disease (COPD)].[39] Since patients with slow-growing lung cancers may live for many years (or even their entire lifetime) without requiring intervention, decision-making for such nodules is often individualized.[40]

Estimates of overdiagnosis rates vary across studies. In the NLST, the overall overdiagnosis rate was 18.5% in the LDCT arm,[41] similar to the NELSON trial estimating 19.7% overdiagnosis at 4.5 years after the final screening round.[7]

Much like the identification of a lung nodule, there are psychological impacts on overdiagnosis. A diagnosis of cancer, even if it is ultimately determined to be slow growing, can cause significant anxiety, distress, and impairment of quality of life.[32] These challenges further highlight the need for shared decision-making for lung cancer screening, such that patients are prepared for the potential findings from undergoing a LDCT.[17,42]

Risk of Diagnostic Procedures

Patients must be aware that suspicious lesions found during screening may require invasive procedures. Potential procedures for screen-detected pulmonary nodules include bronchoscopy, CT-guided biopsy, or a surgical resection. The most common risks of these diagnostic procedures include bleeding and pneumothorax.[43] In NLST, for every 1,000 persons screened, false-positive results led to 17 invasive procedures (number needed to harm was 59) and fewer than 1 person having a major complication.[43] Importantly, the risk of major adverse effects during a diagnostic procedure is low, at 5 per 10,000 persons screened.[43] In the NLST, mortality was 0.8% in the procedure arm and 0.02% in the CT arm in those with benign nodules. Certain subgroups, such as individuals with COPD, may be at a higher risk for complications.[39] Thus, shared decision-making discussions are needed before LDCT, preparing patients for anticipated findings and weighing the risks and benefits of individual procedures, respectively.

Diagnostic procedures resulting from lung cancer screening are not limited to the lungs. In addition to recognizing lung nodules, LDCT of the chest often visualizes organs beyond the lungs: Heart, thyroid, thymus, kidneys, and adrenal glands. Therefore, other "incidental" findings in the thyroid, renal, and adrenal glands may need to be addressed. The rate of surgeries for benign diseases is a notable outcome of screening, and it varies across studies. In the NLST, about 25% of surgical procedures in LDCT arms were conducted for benign disease. For example, conditions such as coronary artery disease requiring surgery were detected during lung cancer screening. There is limited data to determine the impact of these interventions on overall mortality. Overall, the potential consequences of screening and subsequent interventions, including those unrelated to cancer, require careful consideration.[17]

Cost-effectiveness

Assessing the cost-effectiveness of LDCT screening is a crucial consideration. Current standards in the United States deem LDCT screening to be cost-effective when compared to other commonly screened cancers, as shown in **Table 4**.[44] However, cost-effectiveness can vary significantly depending on factors such as patient selection (e.g., comorbidities), the false-positive rate, and the rate of invasive procedures. Moreover, the cost associated with evaluating and managing findings unrelated to lung cancer on LDCT scans were not fully accounted for in cost-effectiveness analyses.[45] A recent cost-effectiveness analysis performed in Australia showed that applying the NELSON-based screening protocol may be more effective than the NLST screening algorithm.[46]

TABLE 4: Comparing the cost per life-year saved for commonly screened cancers.*

Type of cancer	Screening method	Cost per life-year saved (US dollars, year of original study)	Date of original study	Cost per life-year saved (US dollars, 2012 equivalent)
Cervical	Pap smear	33,000	2000	50,162–75,181
Colorectal	Colonoscopy	11,900	1999	18,705–28,958
Breast	Mammography	18,800	1997	31,309–51,274
Lung	LDCT	18,862	2012	18,862

*Data derived from an actuarial analysis assessing the cost-effectiveness of lung cancer screening.[45]

(LDCT: low-dose computed tomography)

INTEGRATING SMOKING CESSATION IN LUNG CANCER SCREENING

Screening for lung cancer offers a unique opportunity to engage individuals in discussions about smoking cessation. Tobacco smoking is the leading cause of preventable death in the United States, including heart disease, vascular disease, lung disease, and cancer. Studies find that individuals undergoing LDCT screening exhibit higher rates of smoking cessation when compared to those in usual care groups.[17] This suggests that LDCT screening may serve as a motivating factor for individuals to quit smoking, thereby potentially reducing their lung cancer risk. Individuals with screen-detected lung nodules are also more likely to quit smoking compared to those with negative screening results.[47] Prior work has shown that, in combination, tobacco smoking cessation and lung cancer screening provide additive benefit. As such, shared decision-making visits must address tobacco smoking cessation.[17]

ADHERENCE

The NLST and NELSON trials exhibited high adherence to screening and follow-up (>90%). Real-world studies show highly variable adherence rates.[48] A systematic review of lung cancer screening programs found an average adherence rate of 57–65%.[49] Patients with lower risk categories such as Lung-RADS 1 or 2 were less likely to be adherent.[49] Patients referred for screening by a specialist (such as a pulmonologist or a thoracic surgeon) were more likely to adhere. Other barriers to adherence include psychological, cognitive, social and environmental factors, which are consistent with other forms of cancer screening.[50] Finally, there is mounting evidence that markers of socioeconomic status affect lung cancer screening enrollment and adherence.[51,52] It is therefore essential to consider barriers and facilitators of adherence when enrolling a patient in lung cancer screening.

RISK ASSESSMENT TOOLS

When evaluating the efficacy and suitability of lung cancer screening, the use of clinical risk assessment tools should be considered to identify individuals at an elevated risk.[17] Indeed, the American College of Chest Physicians (ACCP) guidelines on lung cancer screening recommend that patients at high risk of lung cancer based on individualized risk assessment tools undergo lung cancer screening.[17] Compared to dichotomous criteria such as those from the NLST or the USPSTF, such an individualized approach can help to optimize the balance between screening benefits and potential harms.

Beyond age and smoking criteria used in current guidelines, additional data points can enhance risk prediction, improve screening efficiency, and reduce disparities in eligibility for screening among different racial, ethnic, and gender groups.[53]

There are two main types of prediction models used in risk assessment:

1. *Risk-based models*: These models predict the incidence of lung cancer or lung cancer-related deaths. They incorporate significant risk factors such as age, sex, race/ethnicity, the presence of comorbidities, and smoking history.[54] Risk models consider variables related to the presence of nodule, the risks associated with nodule evaluation, the risks of lung cancer treatment, survival after treatment, and overall survival. Risk models tend to select older individuals with more comorbidities detecting highest risk groups, thus possibly disrupting the balance of benefits and harms of screening.
2. *Benefit (i.e., life-gained) models*: Benefit models, such as the Life-Years From Screening with Computed Tomography (LYFS-CT) model, calculate the life-years gained through lung cancer screening. These models consider factors that influence life expectancy, which are similar to those used in risk models, but further expand to include educational status and body mass index (BMI), among others.[55]

The use of benefit models that consider life-years gained could help optimize screening outcomes when combined with risk models. Benefit models tend to select older but healthier individuals. Overall, individuals with limited life expectancy may be less likely to benefit from screening and more likely to experience harm.

Examples of commonly used risk and benefit models are outlined in **Table 5** below. Additional work is needed to determine which type of assessment tool is ideally suited to select patients for lung cancer screening eligibility.

TABLE 5: Risk and benefit models, and a comparison of factors used.

Type of model	Model	Factors
Risk	Bach[56]	Age, tobacco use, gender, asbestos exposure
	Brock University (PLCOm2014)[57]	Age, race/ethnicity, BMI, tobacco use, history of cancer, lung disease
	PLCOm2012[58]	Age, race/ethnicity, BMI, tobacco use, history of cancer, lung disease
	LCRAT[55]	Age, gender, race/ethnicity, education, BMI, tobacco use, history of cancer
Benefit	LYFS-CT[55]	Age, tobacco use, gender, race/ethnicity, comorbidities, education, BMI, history of cancer

(LCRAT: lung cancer risk assessment tool; LYFS-CT: Life-Years From Screening with Computed Tomography; PLCOm: lung cancer risk model developed from the Prostate, Lung, Colorectal and Ovarian Cancer Screening Trial)

SHARED DECISION-MAKING

Discussing the complexities associated with lung cancer screening is essential in making informed decisions about the benefits and risks of LDCT screening programs.[59] The benefits of early detection and reduced mortality must be carefully weighed against the potential drawbacks and uncertainties outlined above. Individuals at the highest risk for lung cancer (i.e., older patients with comorbidities such as COPD) are more likely to develop lung cancer and need diagnostic studies or procedures.[39] These individuals are also at a higher risk for complications from invasive procedures. Therefore, preparing patients for potential findings from the lung cancer screening process, possible diagnostic procedures for detected findings, and associated risk from procedures is an important and complex aspect of lung cancer screening.

In addition to addressing potential risks, lung cancer screening is generally considered to be preference-sensitive. Preference-sensitive screening is a type of screening where the benefits and harms of screening vary despite meeting eligibility requirements, involving significant tradeoffs affecting the patient's quality and/or length of life.[60] In the context of lung cancer screening, preference-sensitive screening refers to individuals who may or may not benefit from screening based on their personal values and priorities.[61] For example, in the United States Department of Veterans Affairs Lung Cancer Screening Demonstration Project, just 32% of veterans pursued lung cancer screening after engaging in shared decision-making.[62]

Preference-insensitive screening is a type of screening where the benefits and harms of screening are valued equally for all individuals.[60] In the context of lung cancer screening, preference-insensitive screening refers to individuals who are likely to benefit from screening regardless of their personal values and priorities.

Factors that should prompt a preference-sensitive decision include the following:[51,63]

- *Life expectancy*: Individuals with a limited life expectancy may be less likely to benefit from screening due to the lower likelihood of living long enough to experience the benefits of screening.
- *Competing mortality*: Individuals with high competing mortality from other causes may be less likely to benefit from screening due to the lower likelihood of dying from lung cancer.
- *Values and priorities*: Individuals who place a high value on avoiding false positives or overdiagnosis may be less likely to benefit from screening.

MANAGING SCREEN-DETECTED LUNG NODULES

In the context of LDCT screening, lung nodules are frequently identified. However, as outlined above, there is a high false-positive rate, and many of these nodules are benign. The decisions made regarding the management of screen-detected nodules have significant implications for the net benefit associated with screening.

When a nodule is detected, several factors such as size, rate of growth, and appearance are evaluated to determine the next step. In general, smaller nodules that do not change over time are more likely to be benign, and surveillance imaging is recommended.[64] Larger nodules that grow over time are more likely to be malignant, and guidelines recommend additional workup that may include functional imaging or biopsy[17,64] The ACCP guidelines recommend that lung cancer screening programs use a standardized reporting system for recommended follow-up of screen-detected findings.[17]

The American College of Radiology provides the Lung CT Screening Reporting and Data System (Lung-RADS) tool to standardize the approach to screen detected nodules, as outlined in **Tables 6 and 7**.[65]

Two scenarios deserve special mention and were updated in the most recent version of Lung-RADS.[65] Endotracheal or endobronchial abnormalities (outside the lung parenchyma) are also detected with lung cancer screening. Airway nodules that are segmental or more proximal are categorized as Lung-RADS 4A. However, the presence of air within these nodules suggests secretions rather than malignancy, and these are instead categorized as Lung-RADS 2.[65]

More distal nodules (subsegmental) are categorized as Lung-RADS 2. Since endobronchial abnormalities related to mucus often resolve at follow-up, persistent nodules in these areas after a 3-month follow-up raise suspicion for malignancy. Thus, these persistent endobronchial nodules warrant an upgrade to Lung-RADS 4B, with a recommended course of further clinical evaluation, typically involving bronchoscopy.[65]

Atypical pulmonary cysts are also identified during lung cancer screening. Whereas typical pulmonary cysts have thin walls and no internal complexity, atypical cysts may have one or both features.[66] To properly classify screen-detected cysts, it is important to determine what is the dominant feature of the cysts if there is a solid component, and if there is internal complexity.[66] Thin-walled, unilocular cysts (wall thickness <2 mm) are more likely to be benign and are not managed with the Lung-RADS classification system. Unilocular thick-walled cysts (walls thickness ≥2 mm) are managed as atypical pulmonary cysts. Multilocular cysts (thin or thick walled with internal septations) are also managed as atypical pulmonary cysts.[66]

Atypical pulmonary cysts should be distinguished from cavitary lung nodules. If there is a cavitary nodule with wall thickening being the dominant feature, this nodule should be classified as a solid or a part-solid nodule using total diameter and volumetric measurements as outlined above (rather than a pulmonary cyst). Cysts with an adjacent internal or external nodule should be classified based on the most concerning feature (solid, part-solid, or ground glass). Fluid-containing cysts more likely represent an infectious process and are not classified using Lung-RADS unless other concerning features are identified.[64] Finally, multiple cysts should prompt an alternative diagnosis and are not classified in Lung-RADS unless other concerning features are identified.[65,66]

TABLE 6: Approach to management of screen detected nodule according to Lung-RADS.*

	2 12-month LDCT	3 6-month LDCT	4A 3-month LDCT	4B Diagnostic chest CT
Solid	<6 mm (<113 mm^3) at baseline OR New <4 mm (<34 mm^3)	≥6 to <8 mm (≥113 to <268 mm^3) at baseline OR New 4 to <6 mm (34 to <113 mm^3)	≥8 to <15 mm (≥268 to <1,767 mm^3) at baseline OR Growing <8 mm (<268 mm^3) OR New 6 to <8 mm (113 to <268 mm^3)	≥15 mm (≥1767 mm^3) at baseline OR New or growing ≥8 mm (≥268 mm^3)
Part-solid	<6 mm total mean diameter (<113 mm^3) at baseline	≥6 mm total mean diameter (≥113 mm^3) with solid component < 6 mm (<113 mm^3) at baseline OR New <6 mm total mean diameter (<113 mm^3)	≥6 mm total mean diameter (≥113 mm^3) with solid component ≥6 mm to <8 mm (≥113 to <268 mm^3) at baseline OR New or growing <4 mm (<34 mm^3) solid component	Solid component ≥8 mm (≥268 mm^3) at baseline OR New or growing ≥4 mm (≥34 mm^3) solid component
Nonsolid (ground-glass opacity)	<30 mm (<14,137 mm^3) at baseline, new, or growing OR ≥30 mm (≥14,137 mm^3) stable or slowly growing	≥30 mm (≥14,137 mm^3) at baseline or new	–	–
Notes			PET/CT may be considered if there is a ≥8 mm (≥268 mm^3) solid nodule or solid component	PET/CT may be considered if there is a ≥8 mm (≥268 mm^3) solid nodule or solid component; tissue sampling; and/or referral for further clinical evaluation

(LDCT: low-dose computed tomography)

*Guidelines derived from the American College of Radiology Lung-RADS 2022 version.[65]

TABLE 7: Approach to management of screen-detected airway nodules and atypical pulmonary cysts according to Lung-RADS.*

	2 12-month screening LDCT	3 6-month LDCT	4A 3-month LDCT	4B Diagnostic chest CT
Airway nodule	Subsegmental at baseline, new, or stable	–	Segmental or more proximal at baseline	Segmental or more proximal; stable or growing
Atypical pulmonary cyst	–	Growing cystic component (mean diameter) of a thick-walled cyst	Thick-walled cyst OR Multilocular cyst at baseline OR Thin- or thick-walled cyst that becomes multilocular	Thick-walled cyst with growing wall thickness/ nodularity OR Growing multilocular cyst (mean diameter) OR Multilocular cyst with increased loculation or new/increased opacity (nodular, ground-glass, or consolidation)

(LDCT: low-dose computed tomography)

*Based on the American College of Radiology Lung-RADS 2022 version.[65]

SUMMARY

Lung cancer screening reduces cancer-associated mortality by 20–24%. Incorporating lung cancer screening into clinical practice requires an understanding of multiple topics, including risk, benefits, tobacco cessation, and individualized discussions of patient preferences.

There are several models available to further determine lung cancer risk based on clinical factors and nodule characteristics. Screening-detected nodules should be followed up according to risk category, and barriers and facilitators of screening adherence should be assessed.

REFERENCES

1. Ferlay J, Ervik M, Lam F, et al. Global Cancer Observatory: Cancer Today. Lyon, France: International Agency for Research on Cancer; 2024.
2. Schabath MB, Cote ML. Cancer Progress and Priorities: Lung Cancer. Cancer Epidemiol Biomarkers Prev. 2019;28(10):1563-79.
3. Smith RA, Andrews KS, Brooks D, et al. Cancer screening in the United States, 2019: A review of current American Cancer Society guidelines and current issues in cancer screening. CA Cancer J Clin. 2019;69(3):184-210.
4. Humphrey LL, Teutsch S, Johnson M; US Preventive Services Task Force. Lung cancer screening with sputum cytologic examination, chest radiography, and computed tomography: an update for the US Preventive Services Task Force. Ann Intern Med. 2004;140(9):740-53.
5. National Lung Screening Trial Research Team. Aberle DR, Adams AM, Berg CD, et al. Reduced lung-cancer mortality with low-dose computed tomographic screening. N Engl J Med. 2011;365(5):395-409.
6. National Lung Screening Trial Research Team. Church TR, Black WC, Aberle DR, et al. Results of initial low-dose computed tomographic screening for lung cancer. N Engl J Med. 2013;368(21):1980-91.
7. de Koning HJ, van der Aalst CM, de Jong PA, et al. Reduced Lung-Cancer Mortality with Volume CT Screening in a Randomized Trial. N Engl J Med. 2020;382(6):503-13.
8. Yang P. Epidemiology of lung cancer prognosis: quantity and quality of life. Methods Mol Biol. 2009;471:469-86.
9. Doria-Rose VP, Szabo E. Screening and prevention of lung cancer. In: Kernstine KH, Reckamp KL (Eds). Lung Cancer: A Multidisciplinary Approach to Diagnosis and Management. New York: Demos Medical Publishing; 2010. pp. 53-72.
10. Henschke CI, McCauley DI, Yankelevitz DF, et al. Early Lung Cancer Action Project: overall design and findings from baseline screening. Lancet. 1999;354:99-105.
11. Infante M, Cavuto S, Lutman FR, et al. Long-term Follow-up Results of the DANTE Trial, a Randomized Study of Lung Cancer Screening with Spiral Computed Tomography. Am J Respir Crit Care Med. 2015;191(10):1166-75.
12. Wille MM, Dirksen A, Ashraf H, et al. Results of the Randomized Danish Lung Cancer Screening Trial with Focus on High-risk Profiling. Am J Respir Crit Care Med. 2016;193(5):542-51.
13. Paci E, Puliti D, Lopes Pegna A, et al. Mortality, survival and incidence rates in the ITALUNG randomised lung cancer screening trial. Thorax. 2017;72(9):825-31.
14. Pastorino U, Rossi M, Rosato V, et al. Annual or biennial CT screening versus observation in heavy smokers: 5-year results of the MILD trial. Eur J Cancer Prev. 2012;21(3):308-15.
15. Becker N, Motsch E, Trotter A, et al. Lung cancer mortality reduction by LDCT screening-Results from the randomized German LUSI trial. Int J Cancer. 2020;146(6):1503-13.
16. Field JK, Duffy SW, Baldwin DR, et al. The UK Lung Cancer Screening Trial: a pilot randomised controlled trial of low-dose computed tomography screening for the early detection of lung cancer. Health Technol Assess. 2016;20(40):1-146.
17. Mazzone PJ, Silvestri GA, Souter LH, et al. Screening for Lung Cancer: CHEST Guideline and Expert Panel Report. Chest. 2021;160(5):e427-94.
18. Potter AL, Bajaj SS, Yang C-FJ. The 2021 USPSTF lung cancer screening guidelines: a new frontier. Lancet Respir Med. 2021;9(7):689-91.
19. Moyer VA; US Preventive Services Task Force. Screening for lung cancer: US Preventive Services Task Force recommendation statement. Ann Intern Med. 2014;160(5):330-8.
20. Official Journal of the European Union. (2022). Council Recommendation of 9 December 2022 on strengthening prevention through early detection: A new EU approach on cancer screening replacing Council Recommendation 2003/878/EC 2022/C 473/01. EUR-Lex. [online] Available from https://eur-lex.europa.eu/legal-content/EN/TXT/?uri=uriserv%3AOJ.C_.2022.473.01.0001.01.ENG [Last accessed September, 2024].
21. Centers for Medicare & Medicaid Services. (2022). Screening for lung cancer with low dose computed tomography (LDCT). [online] Available from https://www.cms.gov/medicare-coverage-database/view/ncacal-decision-memo.aspx?proposed=N&ncaid=304 [Last accessed September, 2024].
22. United Kingdom National Screening Committee. (2022). Targeted screening for lung cancer in individuals at increased risk. External review against programme appraisal criteria for the UK National Screening Committee. [online] Available from https://view-health-screening-recommendations.service.gov.uk/lung-cancer/ [Last accessed September, 2024].
23. Canadian Task Force on Preventive Health Care. Recommendations on screening for lung cancer. CMAJ. 2016;188(6):425-32.
24. Richardson A. Screening and the number needed to treat. J Med Screen. 2001;8(3):125-7.
25. Jonas DE, Reuland DS, Reddy SM, et al. Screening for Lung Cancer with Low-dose Computed Tomography: Updated Evidence Report and Systematic Review for the US Preventive Services Task Force. JAMA. 2021;325(10):971-87.
26. Nelson HD, Tyne K, Naik A, et al. Screening for breast cancer: an update for the US Preventive Services Task Force. Ann Intern Med. 2009;151(10):727-37, W237-42.
27. Andriole GL, Crawford ED, Grubb RL, et al. Prostate cancer screening in the randomized Prostate, Lung, Colorectal, and Ovarian Cancer Screening Trial: mortality results after 13 years of follow-up. J Natl Cancer Inst. 2012;104(2):125-32.
28. Schröder FH, Hugosson J, Roobol MJ, et al. Screening and prostate cancer mortality in a randomized European study. N Engl J Med. 2009;360(13):1320-8.
29. Landy R, Young CD, Skarzynski M, et al. Using Prediction Models to Reduce Persistent Racial and Ethnic Disparities in the Draft 2020 USPSTF Lung Cancer Screening Guidelines. J Natl Cancer Inst. 2021;113(11):1590-4.
30. Tanoue LT, Tanner NT, Gould MK, et al. Lung cancer screening. Am J Respir Crit Care Med. 2015;191(1):19-33.
31. Caverly TJ, Fagerlin A, Wiener RS, et al. Comparison of Observed Harms and Expected Mortality Benefit for Persons in the Veterans Health Affairs Lung Cancer Screening Demonstration Project. JAMA Intern Med. 2018;178(3):426-8.
32. Brain K, Lifford KJ, Carter B, et al. Long-term psychosocial outcomes of low-dose CT screening: results of the UK Lung Cancer Screening randomised controlled trial. Thorax. 2016;71(11):996-1005.

33. McCollough CH, Bushberg JT, Fletcher JG, et al. Answers to Common Questions About the Use and Safety of CT Scans. Mayo Clin Proc. 2015;90(10):1380-92.
34. The United States Environmental Protection Agency. (2016). Radiation doses and sources. [online] Available from https://www.epa.gov/radiation/radiation-sources-and-doses#averagedoses [Last accessed September, 2024].
35. David E, Wolfson M, Fraifeld VE. Background radiation impacts human longevity and cancer mortality: reconsidering the linear no-threshold paradigm. Biogerontology. 2021;22(2):189-95.
36. Frank L, Christodoulou E, Kazerooni EA. Radiation risk of lung cancer screening. Semin Respir Crit Care Med. 2013;34(6): 738-47.
37. Brodersen J, Schwartz LM, Heneghan C, et al. Overdiagnosis: what it is and what it isn't. BMJ Evid Based Med. 2018;23(1):1-3.
38. Lee SM, Goo JM, Park CM, et al. A new classification of adenocarcinoma: what the radiologists need to know. Diagn Interv Radiol. 2012;18(6):519-26.
39. Rivera MP, Tanner NT, Silvestri GA, et al.; American Thoracic Society Assembly on Thoracic Oncology. Incorporating Coexisting Chronic Illness into Decisions about Patient Selection for Lung Cancer Screening. An Official American Thoracic Society Research Statement. Am J Respir Crit Care Med. 2018;198(2):e3-e13.
40. Bleyer A, Welch HG. Effect of three decades of screening mammography on breast-cancer incidence. N Engl J Med. 2012;367(21):1998-2005.
41. Patz EF Jr, Pinsky P, Gatsonis C, et al; NLST Overdiagnosis Manuscript Writing Team. Overdiagnosis in low-dose computed tomography screening for lung cancer. JAMA Intern Med. 2014;174(2):269-74.
42. Brodersen J, Voss T, Martiny F, et al. Overdiagnosis of lung cancer with low-dose computed tomography screening: meta-analysis of the randomised clinical trials. Breathe (Sheff). 2020;16(1):200013.
43. Yang S, Shih YT, Huo J, et al. Procedural complications associated with invasive diagnostic procedures after lung cancer screening with low-dose computed tomography. Lung Cancer. 2022;165:141-4.
44. Jonas DE, Reuland DS, Reddy SM, et al. Screening for Lung Cancer with Low-dose Computed Tomography: Updated Evidence Report and Systematic Review for the US Preventive Services Task Force. JAMA. 2021;325(10):971-87.
45. Pyenson BS, Sander MS, Jiang Y, et al. An Actuarial Analysis Shows That Offering Lung Cancer Screening as an Insurance Benefit Would Save Lives at Relatively Low Cost. Health Affairs. 2012;31(4):770-9.
46. Behar Harpaz S, Weber MF, Wade S, et al. Updated cost-effectiveness analysis of lung cancer screening for Australia, capturing differences in the health economic impact of NELSON and NLST outcomes. Br J Cancer. 2023;128(1):91-101.
47. Slatore CG, Baumann C, Pappas M, et al. Smoking behaviors among patients receiving computed tomography for lung cancer screening. Systematic review in support of the US preventive services task force. Ann Am Thorac Soc. 2014;11(4):619-27.
48. Castro S, Sosa E, Lozano V, et al. The impact of income and education on lung cancer screening utilization, eligibility, and outcomes: a narrative review of socioeconomic disparities in lung cancer screening. J Thorac Dis. 2021;13(6):3745-57.
49. Lin Y, Liang L, Ding R, et al. Factors Associated with Nonadherence to Lung Cancer Screening Across Multiple Screening Time Points. JAMA Netw Open. 2023;6(5):e2315250.
50. Carter-Harris L, Davis LL, Rawl SM. Lung Cancer Screening Participation: Developing a Conceptual Model to Guide Research. Res Theory Nurs Pract. 2016;30(4):333-52.
51. Fernandes M, Milla C, Gubran A, et al. Assessing the impact of socioeconomic status on incidental lung nodules at an urban safety net hospital. BMC Pulm Med. 2023;23(1):469.
52. Bellinger C, Foley K, Genese F, et al. Factors Affecting Patient Adherence to Lung Cancer Screening. South Med J. 2020;113(11):564-7.
53. Pasquinelli MM, Tammemägi CM, Kovitz KL, et al. Risk Prediction Model versus United States Preventive Services Task Force Lung Cancer Screening Eligibility Criteria – Reducing Race Disparities. J Thorac Oncol. 2020;15(11):1738-47.
54. Katki HA, Kovalchik SA, Berg CD, et al. Development and Validation of Risk Models to Select Ever-Smokers for CT Lung Cancer Screening. JAMA. 2016;315(21):2300-11.
55. Cheung LC, Berg CD, Castle PE, et al. Life-Gained-Based versus Risk-Based Selection of Smokers for Lung Cancer Screening. Ann Intern Med. 2019;171(9):623-32.
56. Bach PB, Kattan MW, Thornquist MD, et al. Variations in lung cancer risk among smokers. J Natl Cancer Inst. 2003;95:470-8.
57. Tammemägi M, Church T, Hocking W, et al. Evaluation of the Lung Cancer Risks at which to Screen Ever- and Never-Smokers: Screening Rules Applied to the PLCO and NLST Cohorts. PLoS Med. 2014;11(12): e1001764.
58. Tammemagi MC, Katki HA, Hocking WG, et al. Selection Criteria for Lung-Cancer Screening. New Engl J Med. 2013;368(8):728-36.
59. Sferra SR, Cheng JS, Boynton Z, et al. Aiding shared decision making in lung cancer screening: two decision tools. J Public Health (Oxf). 2021;43(3):673-80.
60. Wennberg JE. Preference-Sensitive Care: A Dartmouth Atlas Project Topic Brief. Lebanon (NH): The Dartmouth Institute for Health Policy and Clinical Practice; 2007. [online] Available from https://www.ncbi.nlm.nih.gov/books/NBK586631/ [Last accessed September, 2024].
61. Caverly TJ, Cao P, Hayward RA, et al. Identifying Patients for Whom Lung Cancer Screening is Preference-Sensitive: A Microsimulation Study. Ann Intern Med. 2018;169(1):1-9.
62. Núñez ER, Caverly TJ, Zhang S, et al. Factors Associated with Declining Lung Cancer Screening after Discussion with a Physician in a Cohort of US Veterans. JAMA Netw Open. 2022;5(8):e2227126.
63. Gould MK. Precision Screening for Lung Cancer: Risk-Based but Not Always Preference-Sensitive? Ann Intern Med. 2018;169:52-3.
64. Mohamed Hoesein FA, de Jong PA, Mets OM. Optimizing lung cancer screening: nodule size, volume doubling time, morphology and evaluation of other diseases. Ann Transl Med. 2015;3(2):19.
65. Christensen J, Prosper AE, Wu CC, et al. ACR Lung-RADS v2022: Assessment Categories and Management Recommendations. J Am Coll Radiol. 2023:S1546-1440(23)00761-5.
66. Raoof S, Bondalapati P, Vydyula R, et al. Cystic Lung Diseases: Algorithmic Approach. Chest. 2016;150(4):945-65.

Lung Cancer Screening: An Indian Perspective

CHAPTER 157

Vikram Damaraju, Adimulam Ganga Ravindra

INTRODUCTION

Lung cancer is the leading cause of cancer-related mortality globally.[1] An estimated 238,000 new cases will be diagnosed, and 127,000 deaths will occur in the United States of America in 2023.[2] The 5-year survival rate for lung cancer is approximately 22%, as most patients are diagnosed at an advanced stage.[3] However, the 5-year survival rates for localized disease are approximately 56%. The effectiveness of screening programs for cervical, breast, and colon cancers has provided the thrust for developing an efficient lung cancer screening program.

SCREENING

Clinically, adult patients presenting with cough, hemoptysis, dyspnea, hoarseness of voice, and unintentional weight loss are suspected to have lung cancer. The incidence, morbidity, and mortality related to lung cancer are high enough and mandate screening. The goal of screening is to diagnose lung cancer at an early stage even before symptoms develop and when treatment results in a reduction of mortality rates. Screening should improve the quality of life and increase life expectancy. An ideal screening test should be effective, have a low false-positive rate (to prevent additional testing), have a low risk of complications (not to harm those without the disease; with an acceptable safety profile), and should be cost-effective (to decrease the healthcare burden).

RISK FACTORS FOR LUNG CANCER

Smoking tobacco is the most important risk factor; approximately two-thirds of lung cancers are caused by smoking. Cigarette smoking accounts for nearly 80% of lung cancer deaths and 30% of all cancer deaths.[4] Current smokers have a 20-fold higher risk of developing lung cancer, compared to never smokers.[5] Even individuals who quit smoking are at a higher risk of developing lung cancer compared to never smokers, with the risk decreasing every year since quitting. There are major age, gender, and geographic differences in the incidence of lung cancer, particularly in Asia, where 60–80% of women with lung cancer are never smokers. Never smokers with lung cancer were characteristically younger. Secondhand smoke exposure (passive smoking or environmental tobacco smoke) is also a common risk for adults who do not smoke. This exposure can begin at birth and extends across the life span.

Other occupational/environmental risk factors include asbestos, radon, indoor burning of biomass fuels (wood and coal), diesel exhaust, and air pollution. However, their contribution to lung cancer is relatively small compared to smoking tobacco. The risk increases if the survivors continue to smoke. Similarly, first-degree relatives of individuals with lung cancer are at risk of developing lung cancer. Other benign lung disorders like pulmonary fibrosis, chronic obstructive pulmonary disease, and alpha-1 anti-trypsin deficiency are associated with an increased risk of lung cancer. The risk for lung cancer is higher in individuals with pulmonary fibrosis, even after adjusting for age, gender, and smoking.[6] Some oncogenic viruses like human papillomavirus have a causal role in lung cancer.

MODES OF SCREENING: CHEST RADIOGRAPHY AND SPUTUM CYTOLOGY

Screening for lung cancer by chest radiography (and/or sputum cytology) has been extensively studied in at least seven trials (of which six were randomized trials). None of them has shown a mortality benefit by screening with chest radiography. Five studies compared less intense chest radiography screening (and/or sputum cytology) with more frequent chest radiography screening. There was significant heterogeneity in the pooled analysis with the risk ratio of death from lung cancer being 1.11. Two other studies compared annual chest radiography with annual chest radiography and sputum cytology (4 monthly). The pooled analysis showed a trend toward a reduction in mortality; however, this was not statistically significant. The diagnosis of lung cancer was delayed by more than a year when screened with chest radiography [than computed tomography (CT)] in a retrospective analysis.[7] The miss rate with chest radiography was 70% for lesions < 10 mm in size. The overall accuracy, sensitivity, and specificity of interpretation of lung cancer by chest radiography were 61%, 23%, and 96%, respectively, when compared to CT. The sensitivity and specificity of sputum cytology are <70% and 100%, respectively, for lung cancer detection. Hence, screening for lung cancer by chest radiography and sputum cytology is no longer recommended.

LOW-DOSE COMPUTED TOMOGRAPHY

Repeated scans with normal CT are impractical due to the large amount of radiation exposure (one CT chest = 750 chest radiographs) associated with it. The evolution of CT scan techniques has led to the development of low-dose computed tomography (LDCT) scans. LDCT is a noncontrast scan obtained by a multidetector helical CT scan with high-resolution image reconstruction. The effective dose of radiation exposure is 1.5 millisievert (mSv), compared to 0.013 and 10 mSv with a chest radiograph and CT chest, respectively.[8] The reduced radiation exposure is a result of reduced voltage and tube current–time product. The voltage and tube current–time product range from 80 to 140 kVp and 40 to 80 mAs, respectively, for the LDCT scan.

Evidence

Several observational studies have shown that LDCT is beneficial in lung cancer screening. The Japanese Anti-lung Cancer Action (ACLA) project and the US Early Lung Cancer Action Project (ELCAP) had shown that LDCT was superior to chest radiography in the detection of lung cancer in its early stage.[9,10] However, these studies did not measure the effect of LDCT screening on lung cancer mortality. Subsequently, several randomized controlled trials (RCTs) were conducted to assess the benefit of LDCT on cancer-related mortality.

The National Lung Screening Trial (NLST) was a multicenter RCT conducted in the USA.[11] Between 2002 and 2004, approximately 53,000 individuals were enrolled and underwent either LDCT or chest radiograph. Three scans (T0, T1, and T2) were performed at 1-year intervals. The individuals included were heavy smokers (with at least 30 pack years), aged between 55 and 74 years. A positive test was reported if there was adenopathy, effusion, and any noncalcified nodule measuring at least 4 mm in the chest radiography arm. The positive rate after the T2 screening round had decreased in both arms (16.8% vs. 5.0%). The overall lung cancer detection rate was 3.6% and the false-positive rate was 96.4% with the LDCT scan. The deaths from lung cancer were 356 (LDCT arm) and 443 (chest radiograph arm). There was a 20% reduction in the rate of death from lung cancer with the LDCT scan. The number needed to screen was 320 to prevent one death from lung cancer. The all-cause mortality was reduced by 6.7% with the LDCT scan after a median follow-up of 6.5 years.

The NELSON trial was a large-scale population-based trial conducted in the Netherlands and Belgium.[12] The participants included were aged between 50 and 75 years and with a smoking history of >15 cigarettes/day for 25 years or >10 cigarettes/day for 30 years. The individuals were randomized to either no screening or LDCT scan (at baseline, 1 year, 3 years, and 5.5 years). A positive result was noted if the volume of a solid nodule (SN) was >500 mm^3 or the volume was 50–500 mm^3 with a volume doubling time of <400 days. An indeterminate result was noted if the volume doubling time is between 400 and 600 days and the nodule volume is <50 mm^3. Individuals with indeterminate scans were asked to get a repeat scan after 6–12 weeks depending on the screening round. The lung cancer detection rate was 3.2% with a reduction in lung cancer-related deaths by 26% in men and 33% in women. But there was no significant difference in all-cause mortality between the two groups.

Other Studies from Tuberculosis-endemic Regions

Despite recommendations by several organizations, lung cancer screening has not been established as a routine public health practice in several developing countries because of several reasons. The majority of trials conducted in lung cancer screening was in areas where there is a low prevalence of tuberculosis (TB). In developing countries like India, the burden of TB is much higher than that in developed countries.[13] TB and other granulomatous diseases can result in false-positive results during LDCT screening due to lung nodules from active infection, fibrosis, or intrapulmonary lymph nodes.[14] This might result in higher rates of false-positive results resulting in unnecessary investigations, which might result in procedure-related complications and mental stress. However, available studies have yielded conflicting results. In a secondary analysis of the NLST trial **(Table 1)**, assessing factors (patient-specific and center-specific) associated with positive baseline LDCT results, patients enrolled from a histoplasmosis-endemic region were 30% more likely to have positive results at baseline [odds ratio (OR) 1.30; 95% confidence interval (CI) 1.21–1.40]. Follow-up scans were required to confirm the stability of these findings to ensure their benign nature.[14]

In a lung cancer screening trial from Brazil (BRELT1), a country with a high prevalence of TB, 790 subjects underwent LDCT screening. Among them, positive LDCT scans were reported in 312 (39.5%) subjects, compared to 27.3% in NLST. The lung cancer detection rate was 1.3%, similar to that reported by the NLST trial (1%).[15] The results of the BRELT1 study suggest that even though there were high numbers of positive scans on the first screen, the number of patients undergoing invasive procedures and the number of lung cancers detected were similar to other trials.

In a study to assess the effect of prior pulmonary TB on LDCT screening in North India, the screen-positive rate and

TABLE 1: Screen-positive rate with LDCT after the first round in countries with different incidences of tuberculosis.

Country	Study	Tuberculosis incidence rate per 100,000 population	Positivity criterion	LDCT-positivity rate after first round
USA	NLST[11]	3.0	Nodule size ≥ 4 mm	27%
Netherlands and Belgium	NELSON[12]	5.3 and 9.0	Nodule volume ≥ 50 mm^3*	22%*
Brazil	dos Santos 2016 (BRELT1)[15]	45.0	Nodule size ≥ 4 mm	39%
			Nodule size ≥ 6 mm	18.4%
China	Yang 2018[53]	61.0	Nodule size ≥ 4 mm	23%
South Korea	Kim 2020 (K-LUCAS)[54]	66	Nodule size ≥ 6 mm	16%
India	Damaraju V, 2023[16]	199	Nodule size ≥ 6 mm	32%

*Includes both indeterminate cases (nodule volume ≥ 50–500 mm^3; these subjects underwent another LDCT after 3 months) and positive cases (nodule volume > 500 mm^3).

(LDCT: low-dose computed tomography)

lung cancer detection rate were 32% and 1.6%, respectively.[16] In a multivariate analysis, only smoking (pack-years) predicted a positive LDCT scan. On exploratory analysis with ≥4 mm cutoff, the screen-positive rate was 45.1%. Both pack-years and prior TB were associated with positive LDCT with ≥4 mm cutoff. Regardless of the cutoff used, the screen-positive rates observed in this study from a TB-endemic region were higher than those reported rates from nonendemic regions. Prior TB was a predictor of positive scans when using the ≥4 mm cutoff. LDCT scans from TB-endemic areas should be interpreted with caution, especially when using smaller cutoffs for lung nodules.[16]

Lung Cancer Screening in Never Smokers

Lung cancer in never smokers has a high incidence in Asia with an approximate rate of 40% of lung cancers in China and South Korea, compared to 10% in North America and Europe.[17] The difference can be attributed to genetic mutations and environmental exposures. Women of Asian lineage living in America or European countries have a lower incidence of lung cancer, supporting an environmental cause. Up to 80% of women with lung cancers are never smokers in Asian countries.[18]

The majority of the lung cancer screening trials included heavy smokers. Only a small number of LDCT screening trials recruited never smokers. In a population-based screening study (individuals aged 50–74 years) in Japan, approximately 18,000 individuals underwent LDCT scans and 15,500 individuals underwent chest radiography in 8 years.[19] Never smokers comprised 54% and 66% in the LDCT arm and chest radiography arm, respectively. LDCT screening improved the lung cancer detection rate [hazard ratio (HR) = 1.79] and lung cancer mortality rate (HR = 0.41) among the never smokers. Similar studies from China and South Korea observed that LDCT scans could identify lung cancer in never smokers, although the cost-effectiveness and risk-benefit ratio were not evaluated. The TALENT study from Taiwan recruited never smokers, aged 55–75 years, with any of the following risks: Family history of lung cancer, secondhand smoking exposure, TB, cooking index > 110, and poor ventilation during cooking. Lung nodules were detected in 17% and the lung cancer detection rate was 2.6%.[20]

The current lung cancer screening guidelines of the United States recommend screening for high-risk individuals only (like heavy smokers) as evidenced by the very low incidence (0.35%) of lung cancer in the Prostate Lung Colorectal Ovarian Trial cohort of the white population and never smokers.[21,22] These recommendations do not necessarily apply to the Asian population.

Selection of Screening Population

Screening of high-risk individuals is essential to mitigate complications, false-positive results, and invasive procedures. Several approaches were attempted based on risk factors and risk prediction models. The NLST and NELSON trials recruited smokers according to their age, pack-years of smoking, and years since quitting (YSQ) smoking. Later on, several guidelines expanded the criteria to screen more individuals. The age range has been expanded to 50–80 years and pack-years of smoking reduced to 20. This allows more individuals, especially women, to be recruited for screening as they are at risk of lung cancer even with less smoking history.

Lung cancer screening based on personal risk prediction may improve screening efficacy. The majority of the models was developed based on a multivariable mathematical prediction of lung cancer diagnosis or lung cancer-related mortality. Some of the well-evaluated models are the Bach model, Lung Cancer Death Risk Assessment Tool (LCDRAT),

PLCOm2012 model, and Liverpool Lung Project (LLP) model. The PLCOm2012 model is the most validated prediction model till now. It includes age, education, body mass index, chronic obstructive pulmonary disease (COPD), personal history of cancer, ethnicity, family history of lung cancer, smoking status (current or former), pack-years smoked, and years since quitting in former smokers. At a 6-year risk threshold of 1.34%, the PLCOm2012 model had significantly higher sensitivity (83% vs. 71%) and positive predictive value (4% vs. 3.4%) than the NLST eligibility criteria.[23] The LLP risk model considers age, gender, smoking history, personal and family history of lung cancer, asbestos exposure, and history of pneumonia, bronchitis, emphysema, and TB. At a threshold of a 5-year risk of 5%, the lung cancer detection rate was 2.1% after a single LDCT scan in the United Kingdom Lung Screen (UKLS) trial.[24]

Recent models also include biomarker information in addition to the clinical profile, which further introduces complexity to decision-making. Risk-based screening usually recruits high-risk older, aged individuals with short life expectancy, minimizing the cost-effectiveness of a screening program. A risk prediction model which includes the personal risk of individuals and life expectancy may have the potential to improve all-cause mortality besides averting lung-cancer-related deaths.

Management of Abnormalities Found on Low-dose Computed Tomography Screening

Various findings can be observed on a baseline LDCT scan: Nodule, endobronchial growth, mass, lung collapse/atelectasis, significant mediastinal lymphadenopathy (>10 mm), significant unilateral pleural effusion, or pericardial effusion. Nodules with irregular, spiculated, or lobulated margins can be considered to be malignant. Well-defined and rounded nodules can be considered to be benign. The presence of notches in the nodules can be a sign of malignancy. Perifissural nodules may represent intrapulmonary lymph nodes. Lesions with diffuse, central, laminar, rim, or popcorn calcification can be benign. Other types of calcification (eccentric, stippled, amorphous, punctate, or reticular) can be considered to be due to a possibly malignant etiology. The presence of fat in a nodule is an indicator of benign etiology.

Nodule Density and Measurements

Some nonsolid nodules (NSN) which have slow growth or do not resolve in the interval scans have a high risk of malignancy, especially adenocarcinoma. SN and solid components of PSN have more chances of becoming invasive. The assessment of the size of the nodule can be measured as a mean of the shortest and longest diameters [rounded to the nearest whole number (mm)] or by calculating the volume of the nodule (semiautomated estimation after 3D reconstruction). The advantage of volume measurement is based on the notion that the nodule's size varies with respiration and is not always geometrically perfect. The National Comprehensive Cancer Network (NCCN) and the recent Lung-imaging Reporting and Data System (Lung-RADS) developed by American College of Radiology (ACR) also advocate using volume measurements as a more reproducible alternative to linear measurements.[25] Lung-RADS decreases the false-positive rate from greater than 1 in four individuals (in NLST) to approximately 1 in 10 individuals screened.[26,27]

Growth

Solid nodule and PSN are considered positive if they measure ≥6 mm. NSN are considered positive if they measure ≥2 cm and ≥3 cm according to the NCCN and Lung-RADS size criteria respectively.[25] Growth is defined as an increase in nodule size > 1.5 mm or an increase in the attenuation of the ground-glass component of the PSN or NSN. However, when the size increases but does not meet the growth criteria of 1.5 mm, the follow-up recommendations do not change. Corresponding volumetric thresholds have also been defined by the Lung-RADS. From an analysis of the NELSON trial, volumetric analysis and volume doubling time measurements had the highest specificity (95% vs. 90%) and positive predictive value (14% vs. 8%) than the linear measurements.[28]

Risk Prediction Model Based on Nodule

Several risk prediction models based on nodule characteristics were developed in the last two decades. The majority of these models (PanCan, Mayo Clinic, Peking, UKLS) include age, size, calcification, and density of the nodules. The PanCan model has the best predictive accuracy with an area under the curve (AUC) of 0.94 after external validation.[29] In the PanCan model female gender, large-sized nodules, upper lobe nodules, and spiculated nodules were associated with a diagnosis of cancer. The other models also included a family history of lung cancer, COPD, nodule count, and volume. Some deep learning models developed recently incorporated clinical, biological, and epidemiological factors to reduce the false-positive rate and overdiagnosis, which however require external validation.[30]

Frequency of Screening

The interval duration between two regular screening rounds has a crucial role in determining the benefit–harm ratio. Reducing the interval duration increases the cumulative radiation exposure and cost. Delaying the interval scan can reduce the cost and radiation exposure, however increasing the risk of interval cancers and the number of late-stage cancers. Most countries recommend annual screening based on the NLST data. The MILD trial recruited high-risk individuals and performed annual or biennial screening versus no screening and reported no difference in lung cancer mortality and overall mortality after 10 years of baseline scan. The biennial screening arm had 44% fewer follow-up scans without any increase in interval cancers or late-stage cancers. However, the MILD trial was underpowered to extrapolate these results.[31] Individuals with negative baseline LDCT had a lower 2-year probability of lung cancer compared to those with intermediate- or high-risk nodules. However, the number of interval cancers and late-stage cancers detected was higher after a 2.5-year interval scan, compared to 1 and 2-year intervals. This suggests that a screening interval > 2 years may not be justifiable.[12]

Incidental Findings

The frequency of incidental findings ranged from 28 to 94% depending on the site of imaging (community vs. tertiary care center).[32] Emphysema, bronchiectasis, thyroid nodule, emphysema, thoracic aortic aneurysm, interstitial lung disease, adrenal nodule, renal cyst or mass, hepatic lesion, and osteoporosis are the common incidental findings. Incidental findings can increase the risk of further radiation exposure (due to follow-up imaging), anxiety, complications of diagnostic procedures, and the cost required for additional testing. Appropriate management is required to mitigate the risks involved in further evaluation of incidental findings.

Drawbacks of Low-dose Computed Tomography

Benign intrapulmonary lymph nodes and noncalcified granulomas were the most common causes of false-positive results. Using Lung-RADS specifically for lung cancer developed by the ACR has improved the detection of lung cancer and decreased the false-positive results in NLST to approximately 10%.[27,33] In the NLST trial, there were 24% positive screens with LDCT, of which 96% were false positive. A further diagnostic evaluation was required in 75% of the subjects with positive screens. Invasive procedures were done in 7% of false-positive subjects; complications related to invasive procedures were noted in only 0.06%. Of the 4% of lung cancers detected, 18% of them were indolent.[11,34] Baseline CT scans found more indolent cancers; however, follow-up annual scans detected more rapidly growing cancers. The rate of false positivity with two annual screens was decreased to 33%.[11,35,36]

False Negatives

Missing lung cancer nodules in an LDCT scan may be a result of interpretation error or detection error. Subtle lesions appearing as ground-glass opacities or obscuration of nodules by vascular structures can lead to detection errors. Interpretation errors are commonly observed in those with underlying pulmonary disorders like TB, interstitial lung disease, or empyema. Computer-aided detection (CAD) method reduces the false-negative rate by automated lung nodule detection. However, these systems are not available widely.

Radiation Exposure

With the advances in reconstruction algorithms, the quality of the images has improved even with dose reduction. The radiation dose of conventional CT is an average of 7 mSv compared to 1.5 mSv of a low-dose CT scan. The cumulative risk of radiation exposure for an individual beginning at the age of 50 years raises the concern for radiation-induced cancer risk. In the MILD trial, the median cumulative effective dose after 10 years of annual screening was 9 and 13 mSv for men and women, respectively, with a 0.05% risk of radiation-induced cancers.[31] A study estimated an increase in lung cancer cases (radiation-related) by 2% if half of all eligible individuals were to undergo annual LDCT scans.[37] However, with the advent of ultra-low-dose CT (ULDCT), the risk of radiation exposure may decrease further.

Smoking Cessation and Lung Cancer Screening

Lung cancer screening provides an additional interaction between a smoker and the healthcare system. LDCT screening combined with smoking abstinence for >15 years resulted in a 38% reduction in lung cancer-specific mortality (HR 0.62).[38] In the NELSON trial, 17% of the trial population quit smoking.[39] This suggests that screening for lung cancer represents a teachable moment for smoking cessation, especially for those who have a positive result.[40]

Cost–benefit Analysis and Cost-effective Analysis

The estimated cost of an LDCT scan in the United States is about 332 USD.[41] If three fourths of approximately 6 million risk population undergo screening, an estimated 240,000 USD is required to prevent one lung cancer death.[42] Cost-benefit analysis gives dollar values for outcomes, while cost-effective analysis provides cost-per-life-year gained. Several analyses have noted a cost-effectiveness ratio of 100,000 USD or less per quality-adjusted life-years (QALY) gained by an effective screening program.[43] The high estimated number of false-positive scans and the cost per LDCT scan make it difficult to implement lung cancer screening programs in India.

Issues with the Implementation of Lung Cancer Screening Guidelines (Table 2)

Routine lung cancer screening has not been implemented in many countries. Government or insurance agency-funded lung cancer screening programs are established in countries like the USA, South Korea, Poland, and Croatia. Pilot projects or small-scale programs have started in many European countries.[44] Major challenges for implementing nationwide programs are the need for resources, team (dedicated and experienced), identification of high-risk individuals (especially in Asian countries), adequate participant recruitment, high-quality acquisition of low-dose CT (according to the protocol), appropriate interpretation and nodule risk stratification, safe and prompt intervention according to the LDCT results, and timely communication for follow-up. Strategies like lowering the cost of LDCT in low- and middle-income countries, educating the common man through awareness programs, risk prediction model-based recruitment of individuals, mobile LDCT scans, standardizing LDCT scan protocols, dedicated individuals for interpreting the results of LDCT, automated electronic reminders for follow-up, and screening coordinators to bridge the gap between participants and healthcare providers can address the challenges and maximize the benefit while minimizing the harm.[45]

Positron Emission Tomography

Positron emission tomography (PET) is frequently suggested in the diagnostic evaluation of nodules detected in LDCT. However, in regions with a high prevalence of TB, PET may be false positive.[46]

Ultra-low-dose Computed Tomography

Advances in technology have led to improved image quality and diagnostic accuracy even with radiation doses of <1 mSv (sub milliSievert dose). Dose reduction is achieved by lowering the tube current and/or voltage. Reducing the dose would lead to decreased image quality. Hence, these techniques are mostly combined with iterative reconstruction protocols. The diagnostic sensitivity for ULDCT in detecting lung nodules varied from 60 to 100%.[47] However, the studies included had heterogeneous populations, with varying outcome measures and poor precision estimates. In a recent observational study, the intrasubject agreement was excellent between LDCT and ULDCT (87–90%) with significant dose reduction.[48] Several other smaller studies noted comparable diagnostic ability of ULDCT with LDCT. Lung cancer screening by ULDCT seems to be a feasible approach; however, the lack of randomized trials restricts its wider use.

TABLE 2: Recommended eligibility criteria for lung cancer screening in different countries.

Country/Region	Year	Criteria for lung cancer screening
Japan[55]	2013	Age ≥ 50 years and ≥30 pack-year smoking
Korea[56]	2015	Age 55–74 years and ≥30 pack-year smoking history, who currently smoke or quit within the past 15 years
Canada[57]	2016	Age 55–74 years and ≥30 pack-year smoking history, who currently smoke or quit within the past 15 years
European Union[58]	2017	Should use a validated risk approach like PLCOm2012 or LLPv2
China[59]	2018	Age 50–74 years and ≥20 pack-year smoking history, who currently smoke or quit within the past 5 years
Poland[60]	2018	Age 55–74 years and ≥20 pack-year smoking history, who currently smoke or quit within the past 15 years OR Age 50–74 years if no additional risk factor
Singapore[61]	2019	Age 55–74 years and ≥30 pack-year smoking history, who currently smoke or quit within the past 15 years
Germany[62]	2019	Age 55–74 years and ≥30 pack-year smoking history, who currently smoke or quit within the past 15 years OR Age ≥ 50 years and ≥20 years of smoking and at least one of the following risk factors: History of lung cancer, family history of lung cancer, history of malignant ear, nose, or throat tumor or other malignant tumor associated with smoking, history of lymphoma, exposure to asbestos, COPD, or pulmonary fibrosis
Croatia[63]	2020	Age 50–70 years and ≥30 pack-year smoking history, who currently smoke or quit within the past 15 years
USA[64]	2021	Age 50–80 years and ≥20 pack-year smoking history, who currently smoke or quit within the past 15 years
Australia[65]	2022	Age 50–70 years and ≥30 pack-year smoking history, who currently smoke or quit within the past 10 years
UK[66]	2022	Age 55–74 years with a history of smoking and PLCOm2012 risk of >1.51% over 6 years or LLPv2 risk > 2.5% over 5 years

(LLP: Liverpool Lung Project; PLCO: Prostate, Lung, Colorectal, and Ovarian study model)

Blood-based Biomarkers

Blood-based biomarkers can help in managing indeterminate nodules, besides personalizing the frequency of follow-up scans. The false-positive rate reduced from 19 to 3.7% in the MILD trial, with the use of a microRNA signature. The combination of a blood-based biomarker and a positive LDCT can help in decision-making regarding the timing of follow-up scans and biopsies. Blood-based biomarkers can also help in selecting individuals for screening. The INTEGRAL consortium identified high-risk individuals using blood-based biomarkers and observed an AUC of 0.83 for lung cancer screening.[49] The blood-based biomarkers under evaluation are circulating tumor DNA, DNA methylation, single nucleotide polymorphisms, and complement fragments.[50]

Other Newer Modalities

Autofluorescence bronchoscopy (AFB), when used with conventional bronchoscopy, identifies areas of abnormal thickness and vascularity as abnormal fluorescence and aids in the diagnosis of dysplastic and intraepithelial neoplasms.[51] Owing to its poor specificity, autofluorescence imaging (AFI) has been developed to distinguish benign and preinvasive lesions by color. Electronic nose (EN) detects volatile organic compounds (alkanes and benzene derivatives) in the exhaled breath with sensitivity and specificity of 100% and 81%, respectively.[52] Though EN has been reported to diagnose lung cancer with fairly better accuracies, the lack of large-scale studies limits its broader implementation.

From different countries, there are different reports of screen-positive rates with LDCT after the first round **(Table 1)**.[11,12,15,16,53,54] Similarly, the recommended eligibility criteria for lung cancer screening also differ **(Table 2)**.[55-66]

SUMMARY

Lung cancer screening in high-risk individuals has been shown to reduce lung cancer-specific mortality. Screening using a risk prediction model which includes a personal risk of individuals and life expectancy may have the potential to improve all-cause mortality besides averting lung-cancer-related deaths. Screening for lung cancer represents a teachable moment for smoking cessation, especially for those who have a positive result. Implementing nationwide programs faces several challenges, including reducing LDCT costs in low- and middle-income countries, increasing public awareness, adopting risk prediction models for recruitment, utilizing mobile LDCT units, standardizing scan protocols, assigning dedicated interpreters, implementing automated follow-up reminders, and employing screening coordinators to improve communication between participants and healthcare providers. Addressing these challenges can help maximize benefits and minimize harm.

REFERENCES

1. Sung H, Ferlay J, Siegel RL, et al. Global Cancer Statistics 2020: GLOBOCAN Estimates of Incidence and Mortality Worldwide for 36 Cancers in 185 Countries. CA Cancer J Clin. 2021;71(3):209-49.
2. Siegel RL, Miller KD, Wagle NS, et al. Cancer statistics, 2023. CA Cancer J Clin. 2023;73(1):17-48.
3. SEER*Explorer: An interactive website for SEER cancer statistics [Internet]. Surveillance Research Program National Cancer Institute [online] Available from https://seer.cancer.gov/statistics-network/explorer/ [Last accessed September, 2024].
4. Jamal A, Phillips E, Gentzke AS, Homa DM, et al. Current Cigarette Smoking among Adults - United States, 2016. MMWR Morb Mortal Wkly Rep. 2018;67(2):53-9.
5. Office of the Surgeon G, Office on S, Health. Reports of the Surgeon General. The Health Consequences of Smoking: A Report of the Surgeon General. Atlanta (GA): Centers for Disease Control and Prevention (US); 2004.
6. Turner-Warwick M, Lebowitz M, Burrows B, et al. Cryptogenic fibrosing alveolitis and lung cancer. Thorax. 1980;35(7):496-9.
7. Quekel LG, Kessels AG, Goei R, et al. Miss rate of lung cancer on the chest radiograph in clinical practice. Chest. 1999;115(3):720-4.
8. Bach PB, Mirkin JN, Oliver TK, et al. Benefits and harms of CT screening for lung cancer: a systematic review. JAMA. 2012;307(22):2418-29.
9. Henschke CI, McCauley DI, Yankelevitz DF, et al. Early Lung Cancer Action Project: overall design and findings from baseline screening. Lancet. 1999;354(9173):99-105.
10. Kaneko M, Eguchi K, Ohmatsu H, et al. Peripheral lung cancer: screening and detection with low-dose spiral CT versus radiography. Radiology. 1996;201(3):798-802.
11. Aberle DR, Adams AM, Berg CD, et al. Reduced lung-cancer mortality with low-dose computed tomographic screening. N Engl J Med. 2011;365(5):395-409.
12. de Koning HJ, van der Aalst CM, de Jong PA, et al. Reduced Lung-Cancer Mortality with Volume CT Screening in a Randomized Trial. N Engl J Med. 2020;382(6):503-13.
13. Global tuberculosis Report 2022. Geneva: World Health Organization; 2022.
14. Balekian AA, Tanner NT, Fisher JM, et al. Factors Associated with a Positive Baseline Screening Exam Result in the National Lung Screening Trial. Ann Am Thorac Soc. 2016;13(9):1568-74.
15. dos Santos RS, Franceschini JP, Chate RC, et al. Do Current Lung Cancer Screening Guidelines Apply for Populations with High Prevalence of Granulomatous Disease? Results from the First Brazilian Lung Cancer Screening Trial (BRELT1). Ann Thorac Surg. 2016;101(2):481-6; discussion 7-8.
16. Damaraju V, Singh N, Garg M, et al. Effect of prior pulmonary TB on low-dose computed tomography during lung cancer screening. Int J Tuberc Lung Dis. 2023;27(3):223-5.

17. McCarthy WJ, Meza R, Jeon J, et al. Chapter 6: Lung cancer in never smokers: epidemiology and risk prediction models. Risk Anal. 2012;32 Suppl 1(Suppl 1):S69-84.
18. Barta JA, Powell CA, Wisnivesky JP. Global Epidemiology of Lung Cancer. Ann Glob Health. 2019;85(1):8.
19. Nawa T, Nakagawa T, Mizoue T, et al. A decrease in lung cancer mortality following the introduction of low-dose chest CT screening in Hitachi, Japan. Lung Cancer. 2012;78(3):225-8.
20. Yang P. PS01.02 National Lung Cancer Screening Program in Taiwan: The TALENT Study. J Thorac Oncol. 2021;16(3):S58.
21. Tammemägi MC, Church TR, Hocking WG, et al. Evaluation of the lung cancer risks at which to screen ever- and never-smokers: screening rules applied to the PLCO and NLST cohorts. PLoS Med. 2014;11(12):e1001764.
22. Ten Haaf K, de Koning HJ. Should Never-Smokers at Increased Risk for Lung Cancer be Screened? J Thorac Oncol. 2015;10(9):1285-91.
23. Tammemagi CM, Pinsky PF, Caporaso NE, et al. Lung cancer risk prediction: Prostate, Lung, Colorectal and Ovarian Cancer Screening Trial models and validation. J Natl Cancer Inst. 2011;103(13):1058-68.
24. Toumazis I, Bastani M, Han SS, et al. Risk-based lung cancer screening: A systematic review. Lung Cancer. 2020;147:154-86.
25. National Comprehensive Cancer Network. The NCCN Clinical Practice Guidelines in Oncology (NCCN Guidelines®): Lung Cancer Screening (version 2.2023). [online] Available from https://www.nccn.org/professionals/physician_gls/default.aspx. [Last accessed September, 2024].
26. Mazzone P, Powell CA, Arenberg D, et al. Components necessary for high-quality lung cancer screening: American College of Chest Physicians and American Thoracic Society Policy Statement. Chest. 2015;147(2):295-303.
27. McKee BJ, Regis SM, McKee AB, et al. Performance of ACR Lung-RADS in a clinical CT lung screening program. J Am Coll Radiol. 2015;12(3):273-6.
28. Horeweg N, van Rosmalen J, Heuvelmans MA, et al. Lung cancer probability in patients with CT-detected pulmonary nodules: a prespecified analysis of data from the NELSON trial of low-dose CT screening. Lancet Oncol. 2014;15(12):1332-41.
29. Callister ME, Baldwin DR, Akram AR, et al. British Thoracic Society guidelines for the investigation and management of pulmonary nodules. Thorax. 2015;70(Suppl 2):ii1-ii54.
30. Wu Z, Wang F, Cao W, et al. Lung cancer risk prediction models based on pulmonary nodules: A systematic review. Thorac Cancer. 2022;13(5):664-77.
31. Pastorino U, Sverzellati N, Sestini S, et al. Ten-year results of the Multicentric Italian Lung Detection trial demonstrate the safety and efficacy of biennial lung cancer screening. Eur J Cancer. 2019;118:142-8.
32. Janssen K, Schertz K, Rubin N, et al. Incidental Findings in a Decentralized Lung Cancer Screening Program. Ann Am Thorac Soc. 2019;16(9):1198-201.
33. Pinsky PF, Gierada DS, Black W, et al. Performance of Lung-RADS in the National Lung Screening Trial: a retrospective assessment. Ann Intern Med. 2015;162(7):485-91.
34. Patz EF Jr, Pinsky P, Gatsonis C, et al. Overdiagnosis in low-dose computed tomography screening for lung cancer. JAMA Intern Med. 2014;174(2):269-74.
35. Kramer BS, Berg CD, Aberle DR, et al. Lung cancer screening with low-dose helical CT: results from the National Lung Screening Trial (NLST). J Med Screen. 2011;18(3):109-11.
36. Walter JE, Heuvelmans MA, de Jong PA, et al. Occurrence and lung cancer probability of new solid nodules at incidence screening with low-dose CT: analysis of data from the randomised, controlled NELSON trial. Lancet Oncol. 2016;17(7):907-16.
37. Frank L, Christodoulou E, Kazerooni EA. Radiation risk of lung cancer screening. Semin Respir Crit Care Med. 2013;34(6):738-47.
38. Tanner NT, Kanodra NM, Gebregziabher M, et al. The Association between Smoking Abstinence and Mortality in the National Lung Screening Trial. Am J Respir Crit Care Med. 2016;193(5):534-41.
39. van der Aalst CM, van den Bergh KA, Willemsen MC, et al. Lung cancer screening and smoking abstinence: 2 year follow-up data from the Dutch-Belgian randomised controlled lung cancer screening trial. Thorax. 2010;65(7):600-5.
40. Brain K, Carter B, Lifford KJ, et al. Impact of low-dose CT screening on smoking cessation among high-risk participants in the UK Lung Cancer Screening Trial. Thorax. 2017;72(10):912-8.
41. Tailor TD, Bell S, Fendrick AM, et al. Total and Out-of-Pocket Costs of Procedures after Lung Cancer Screening in a National Commercially Insured Population: Estimating an Episode of Care. J Am Coll Radiol. 2022;19(1 Pt A):35-46.
42. Goulart BH, Ramsey SD. Moving beyond the national lung screening trial: discussing strategies for implementation of lung cancer screening programs. Oncologist. 2013;18(8):941-6.
43. Puggina A, Broumas A, Ricciardi W, et al. Cost-effectiveness of screening for lung cancer with low-dose computed tomography: a systematic literature review. Eur J Public Health. 2016;26(1):168-75.
44. van Meerbeeck JP, Franck C. Lung cancer screening in Europe: where are we in 2021? Transl Lung Cancer Res. 2021;10(5):2407-17.
45. Shankar A, Saini D, Dubey A, et al. Feasibility of lung cancer screening in developing countries: challenges, opportunities and way forward. Transl Lung Cancer Res. 2019;8(Suppl 1):S106-s21.
46. Purandare NC, Pramesh CS, Agarwal JP, et al. Solitary pulmonary nodule evaluation in regions endemic for infectious diseases: Do regional variations impact the effectiveness of fluorodeoxyglucose positron emission tomography/computed tomography. Indian J Cancer. 2017;54(1):271-5.
47. Tække M, Kristjánsdóttir B, Graumann O, et al. Diagnostic accuracy of low-dose and ultra-low-dose CT in detection of chest pathology: a systematic review. Clin Imaging. 2021;74:139-48.
48. Milanese G, Ledda RE, Sabia F, et al. Ultra-low dose computed tomography protocols using spectral shaping for lung cancer screening: Comparison with low-dose for volumetric LungRADS classification. Eur J Radiol. 2023;161:110760.
49. Guida F, Sun N, Bantis LE, et al. Assessment of Lung Cancer Risk on the Basis of a Biomarker Panel of Circulating Proteins. JAMA Oncol. 2018;4(10):e182078.
50. Horst C, Dickson JL, Tisi S, et al. Delivering low-dose CT screening for lung cancer: a pragmatic approach. Thorax. 2020;75(10):831-2.
51. Edell E, Lam S, Pass H, et al. Detection and localization of intraepithelial neoplasia and invasive carcinoma using fluorescence-reflectance bronchoscopy: an international, multicenter clinical trial. J Thorac Oncol. 2009;4(1):49-54.

52. Chapman EA, Thomas PS, Stone E, et al. A breath test for malignant mesothelioma using an electronic nose. Eur Respir J. 2012;40(2):448-54.
53. Yang W, Qian F, Teng J, et al. Community-based lung cancer screening with low-dose CT in China: Results of the baseline screening. Lung Cancer. 2018;117:20-6.
54. Kim H, Kim HY, Goo JM, et al. Lung Cancer CT Screening and Lung-RADS in a Tuberculosis-endemic Country: The Korean Lung Cancer Screening Project (K-LUCAS). Radiology. 2020;296(1):181-8.
55. Japan Radiological Society (JRS) and Japanese College of Radiology (JCR) . The Japanese Imaging Guideline. 2013. [online] Available from http://www.radiology.jp/content/files/diagnostic_imaging_guidelines_2013_e. pdf. [Last accessed September, 2024].
56. Jang SH, Sheen S, Kim HY, et al. The Korean guideline for lung cancer screening. J Kor Med Assoc. 2015;58(4):291-301.
57. Canadian Task Force on Preventive Health Care. Recommendations on screening for lung cancer. CMAJ. 2016;188(6):425-32.
58. Oudkerk M, Devaraj A, Vliegenthart R, et al. European position statement on lung cancer screening. Lancet Oncol. 2017;18(12):e754-e66.
59. Zhou Q, Fan Y, Wang Y, et al. China National Lung Cancer Screening Guideline with Low-dose Computed Tomography (2018 version). Zhongguo Fei Ai Za Zhi. 2018;21(2):67-75.
60. Rzyman W, Szurowska E, Adamek M. Implementation of lung cancer screening at the national level: Polish example. Transl Lung Cancer Res. 2019;8(Suppl 1):S95-s105.
61. Academy of Medicine Singapore. Report of the Screening Test Review Committee [Internet]. Singapore: Academy of Medicine; 2019 [last accessed 2024 Sep]. Available from: https://www.ams.edu.sg/view-pdf.aspx?file=media%5C4817_fi_59.pdf&ofile=STRC+Report+March+2019.pdf
62. Herth FJF, Reinmuth N, Wormanns D, et al. Joint Statement of the German Radiological Society and the German Respiratory Society on a Quality-Assured Early Detection Program for Lung Cancer with Low-dose CT. Pneumologie. 2019;73(10):573-7.
63. N1. (2020). Croatia first EU country to introduce early lung cancer screening nationwide. [online] Available from https://hr.n1info.com/english/news/a475221-croatia-first-eu-countryto-introduce-early-lung-cancer- screening-nationwide/ [Last accessed September, 2024].
64. Krist AH, Davidson KW, Mangione CM, et al. Screening for Lung Cancer: US Preventive Services Task Force Recommendation Statement. JAMA. 2021;325(10):962-70.
65. Australian Government Medical Services Advisory Committee. Application No. 1699 – National Lung Cancer Screening Program [Internet]. Canberra: Australian Government Department of Health; 2022 Jul [accessed September 2024]. Available from: http://www.msac.gov.au/internet/msac/publishing.nsf/Content/C77B956C49CD6841CA25876D000392DF $File/1699%20 Final%20PSD_Jul2022.pdf
66. UK National Screening Committee. Lung cancer. [online] Available from https://view-health-screening-recommendations.service.gov.uk/lung-cancer/ [Last accessed September, 2024].

SECTION

17

Respiratory Critical Care

SECTION OUTLINE

Clinical Approach to Hypoxia

CHAPTER 158

Aloke Gopal Ghoshal, Angira Dasgupta, Avik Ghoshal

INTRODUCTION

Hypoxia is a state of "insufficient oxygen", a medical emergency needing immediate attention. This is especially so since the human brain ceases to function if it remains without oxygen for a period as short as 10 minutes. Hypoxemia is often imprecisely equated to hypoxia.[1] Fundamentally, "hypoxemia" is a decrease in the oxygen content of the blood, whereas "hypoxia" denotes reduced oxygen at the tissue level.[2,3]

JOURNEY OF OXYGEN

The journey of oxygen in the human body starts with its inhalation from the ambient air **(Fig. 1)**. The ambient air at normal atmospheric pressure at a sea level of 760 mm Hg contains approximately 78% nitrogen, 21% oxygen, 1% argon, and traces of other gases, such as carbon dioxide, nitrogen dioxide, carbon monoxide, ammonia, neon, methane, helium, krypton, xenon, ozone, and few others.[4] The inhaled oxygen passes through the various generations of airways in the respiratory tract to reach that part of the lungs where it diffuses across the alveolocapillary barrier into the bloodstream until equilibrium is achieved **(Fig. 1)**. It is then transported to the tissues/organs in two main forms: (1) Major part (97–98%) binds to hemoglobin in the red blood cells (RBC) and (2) the remaining (2–3%) is dissolved in the blood. In the tissues, oxygen is utilized by the cellular mitochondria for adenosine triphosphate (ATP) or energy synthesis.[4-7]

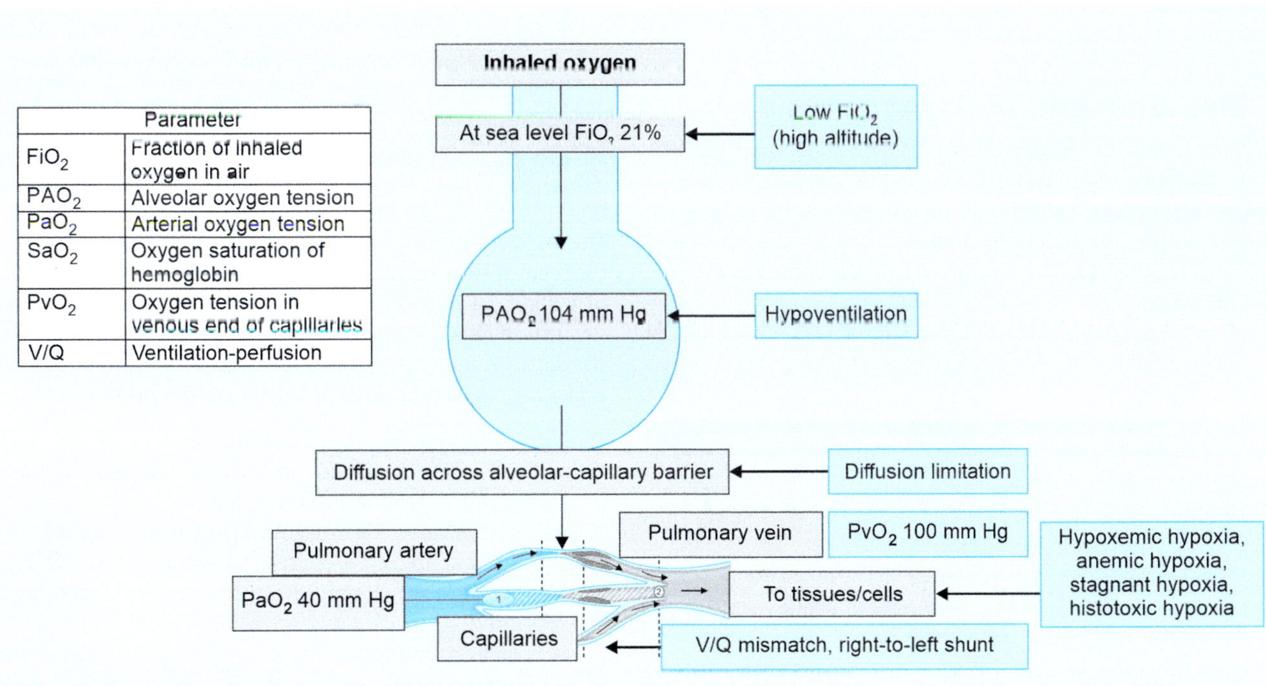

FIG. 1: Oxygen transport and types of hypoxemias and hypoxia. Thick arrows indicate mechanism of hypoxemia and hypoxia.

DEVELOPMENT OF HYPOXIA AND HYPOXEMIA

Mechanistically, hypoxia may develop due to one or more of the following conditions: (1) When the overall oxygen content of blood is low (hypoxemic hypoxia), (2) when there is a deficiency of hemoglobin which is the main carrier of oxygen (anemic hypoxia), (3) reduction in blood flow (stagnant hypoxia) as may occur in heart failure, or (4) issues with utilization of oxygen at the cellular level as in cyanide poisoning (histotoxic hypoxia). On the other hand, hypoxemia may occur due to problems in oxygen diffusion from air into the lungs and subsequent transport to the tissues. Depending on the stage of oxygen transport that is affected, hypoxemia may be classified as due to: (1) Low inspired PO_2, (2) hypoventilation, (3) diffusion limitation, (4) ventilation–perfusion (V/Q) mismatch, and (5) right-to-left shunt **(Fig. 1)**.

Interestingly, in the absence of any definitive threshold of oxygen below which tissue hypoxia occurs, it is seen that both hypoxemia and hypoxia can coexist or as standalone conditions.[1,2] There may be hypoxemia without hypoxia due to a compensatory increase in the hemoglobin level and cardiac output. On the other hand, there can be tissue hypoxia without hypoxemia as in cyanide poisoning where cells are unable to utilize oxygen despite having normal blood and tissue oxygen levels. Thus, a wide variety of diseases may cause hypoxemia and/or hypoxia. It remains a challenge for physicians to be able to tease out the particular reason for the lack of oxygen in a particular subject and to subsequently manage it.

In this chapter, we will discuss the various types of hypoxia and their mechanisms and finally relate them to case scenarios in order to propose a clinical approach.

Measurements of Oxygen Levels

Oxygen levels in the blood can be measured in various ways. Notably, some parameters can be measured directly while others are calculated parameters which help in understanding the pathophysiology of oxygen transport and utilization **(Box 1)**. The important measurements include the following:

- *Arterial oxygen saturation (SaO_2)*: SaO_2 is a measure of the proportion of hemoglobin bound to oxygen compared to the amount of unbound hemoglobin. This can be measured with the help of a pulse oximeter which is a noninvasive device to measure oxygen saturation (SpO_2) when placed over a person's finger. The principle used is to measure light wavelengths to determine the ratio of levels of oxygenated hemoglobin to that of deoxygenated hemoglobin. The use of pulse oximetry has become a standard of care in medicine.[5] Although a relatively crude measure, SaO_2 value below 90% indicates hypoxemia.
- *Partial pressure of oxygen or arterial oxygen tension (PaO_2)*: The arterial oxygen tension (PaO_2) is the amount of oxygen dissolved in the plasma, which can be estimated from arterial blood gas measurements.[4,5]
- *Alveolar to arterial (A–a) oxygen gradient [$P(A–a)O_2$]*: It is a common measure of oxygenation and helps to assess the integrity of the alveolar capillary unit. It is defined as the difference between the partial pressure of oxygen in the alveoli (PAO_2) and that of oxygen dissolved in the plasma (PaO_2), i.e., $PAO_2 - PaO_2$.

A natural gradient exists due to both physiological right-to-left shunt and a physiological V/Q mismatch caused by gravity-dependent differences between various lung zones. The A–a oxygen gradient indicates the effectiveness of gas exchange which depends on the surface area available for exchange, the integrity of the alveolocapillary membrane, and also the capillary transit time.[4,5] The A–a oxygen difference is <10 mm Hg in young healthy adults and increases with age. Clinically, the alveolar-arterial oxygen gradient P(A–a) O_2 is useful to differentiate between the mechanisms of hypoxemia. Intuitively, the causes of hypoxia with increased $P(A–a)O_2$ and those of preserved P(A–a) O_2 are different.

- *PaO_2/FiO_2 ratio*: It is the ratio of arterial oxygen partial pressure to the fraction of oxygen in inspired air. A normal PaO_2/FiO_2 ratio is 300–500, with values <300 indicating abnormal gas exchange and values <200 mm Hg indicating severe hypoxemia.

BOX 1 Normal values and calculations.

- The normal SaO_2 is >94–95%
- The normal value for the partial pressure of arterial oxygen (PaO_2) irrespective of age is greater than 80 mm Hg/10.6 kPa
- The normal PaO_2 for a given age can be predicted from PaO_2 = 104 mm Hg/13.8 kPa – 0.27 × age in years
- At sea level, the alveolar gas equation:
  - $PAO_2 = (760 - 47)\ 0.21 - 40/0.8 = 99.7$ mm Hg
  - $P(A–a)\ O_2 = 2.5 + 0.21 \times$ age in years

Oxygen–Hemoglobin Dissociation Curve (Fig. 2)

The oxygen–hemoglobin dissociation curve is a graphical representation of the relationship of the partial pressure of oxygen in blood (PO_2 along the *X*-axis) and the oxygen saturation (SaO_2 along the *Y*-axis). The curve is sigmoidal in shape, with a steep slope at low partial pressures of oxygen and a more gradual slope at higher partial pressures.

The curve characteristics are as follows:

- *p50*: It is the pressure at which hemoglobin is 50% saturated (27 mm Hg on the *X*-axis).
- *Arterial blood*: Hemoglobin is approximately 100% saturated at an oxygen partial pressure of 100 mm Hg.
- *Venous blood*: Hemoglobin is approximately 75% saturated.

In certain situations of hypoxia, where more oxygen needs to be delivered to the hypoxic tissues, the binding of O_2 with hemoglobin becomes "relaxed" or loose to enable easy release

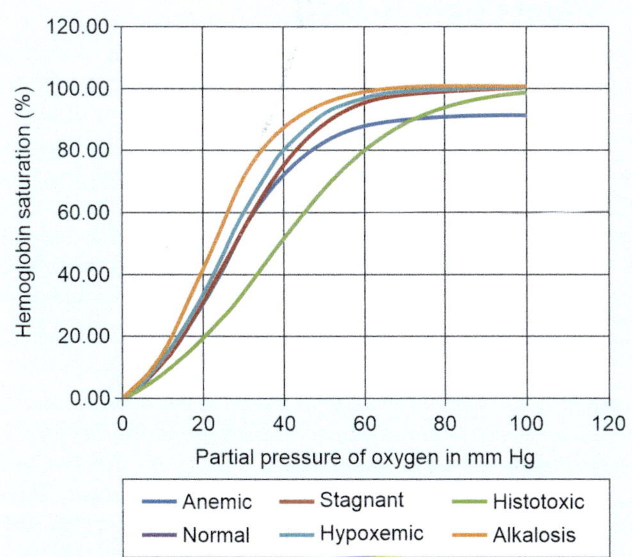

FIG. 2: Oxygen-hemoglobin dissociation curve with shift to right (as in hypoxemic, stagnant, and histotoxic hypoxia) and shift to left (in alkalosis) demonstrated with simulated data.

of the oxygen molecules. This shifts the curve to the right. Increases in carbon dioxide, hydrogen ion concentration (pH), temperature, and 2,3-diphosphoglycerate in blood are some of the causes when the curve shifts to the right. The reverse occurs when levels of any of the above factors fall.

CAUSES OF HYPOXIA

Depending upon one of the five major pathophysiologic mechanisms, hypoxia may be classified as one of the following types: Hypoxemic hypoxia, anemic hypoxia, stagnant hypoxia, and histotoxic hypoxia. Hypoxemia can be further classified on the basis of the underlying cause as (1) low inspired PO_2, (2) hypoventilation, (3) diffusion limitation, (4) V/Q mismatch, and (5) right-to-left shunt.[8,9]

Hypoxia due to Low FiO_2

Hypoxia due to low FiO_2 occurs when the barometric pressure falls such as with the increase in altitude. The concentration of oxygen in ambient air remains constant. But as the barometric pressure decreases, the partial pressure of oxygen decreases proportionately. This condition has been appropriately referred to as hypobaric hypoxia.[5]

Case 1: *A 53-year-old gentleman was holidaying and enjoying tea-tasting in a tea garden located at 2,850 m, when he suddenly started to feel breathless, exhausted, and dizzy with a headache. He was managed at a close-by healthcare facility with oxygen and intravenous fluids, without much relief. On examination, he was slightly drowsy with a pulse rate of 108 beats/min, blood pressure of 130/80 mm Hg, respiratory rate of 35 breaths/min, temperature of 101°F, and SpO_2 80% in room air. Systemic examination was unremarkable. His laboratory reports were normal except a raised total cell count of 12,000/cu mm. An arterial blood gas (ABG) analysis showed pH 7.40, PCO_2 in arterial blood ($PaCO_2$) 39 mm Hg, PaO_2 50 mm Hg, SaO_2 80%, and HCO_3 25 mEq/L. The ECG showed sinus tachycardia, whereas the chest X-ray revealed diffuse bilateral perihilar infiltrates. Echocardiography was within normal limits and the noncontrast CT head did not show anything remarkable.*

In case 1, the hypoxia is an example of acute mountain sickness (AMS) with high-altitude pulmonary edema (HAPE). High-altitude sickness comprises AMS, high-altitude cerebral edema (HACE), and HAPE. Its incidence is approximately 0.1–4%.[6]

A situation like this occurs when one climbs rapidly to high altitudes without adequate time for acclimatization or without prophylactic medications. At heights above 2,500–3,000 m, the atmospheric pressure becomes low and the subject becomes hypoxic, especially when the underlying lung is diseased. The peripheral chemoreceptors sense low arterial PaO_2 and stimulates an increase in ventilation through their input to the medullary respiratory center. The resulting hyperventilation typically reduces $PaCO_2$ while keeping the $P(A\text{–}a)O_2$ normal.[7-9]

Diffusion Limitation

Oxygen diffusion occurs at the end of inhalation. It is a passive process where oxygen diffuses from the alveoli to the adjacent blood capillaries. Diffusion continues until the oxygen in the alveoli (PAO_2) equilibrates with the end-capillary blood ($PeCO_2$), and this happens well before the blood leaves with oxygen. A similar process occurs with carbon dioxide, except that it passes from mixed venous blood to the alveoli until equilibrium is established.

Hypoxia due to diffusion limitation may be due to. (1) a decrease in lung surface area for diffusion (e.g., emphysema in which there is a loss of alveolar walls and capillaries), (2) inflammation and fibrosis of the alveolocapillary membrane [e.g., interstitial lung disease (ILD)], (3) low alveolar oxygen (e.g., high-altitude sickness), and (4) extremely short time capillary transit. A normal pulmonary capillary transit time is 0.75 seconds, and the time required to complete gas exchange is 0.25 seconds approximately.

Case 2: *A 54-year-old female presented with exertional shortness of breath. Her breathing was normal at rest but worsened with exertion. On clinical examination, she had bibasal velcro rales. Spirometry showed moderate restrictive pattern with a diffusion capacity of KCO of 67% predicted. Her saturation was 95% at rest in room air which dropped to 80% after 6 minutes of walking. High-resolution computed tomography (HRCT) thorax revealed bilateral basal peripheral honeycombing suggesting a diagnosis of ILD. ABGs at end-exercise are: pH 7.34, $PaCO_2$ 30 mm Hg, HCO_3 18 mEq/L, and PaO_2 81 mm Hg.*

In case 2, the patient has ILD and is hypoxic due to diffusion limitation. Patients with such diseases may have normal oxygen pressures at rest but develops hypoxemia with exercise. In fact, development or worsening of hypoxemia during exercise is regarded as an early sign of diffusion limitation. It is believed that patients with pulmonary fibrosis do not have adequate reserve to recruit additional capillaries and thus develops exercise-induced/exaggerated hypoxemia.[7,8]

The reasons for exercise desaturation are manifold. Exercise increases the amount of oxygen extracted from arterial blood in the systemic circulation, which tends to reduce the partial pressure of oxygen in the mixed venous blood. Therefore, more oxygen has to be taken up in the lungs in order to reach the normal oxygenation levels of arterial blood. Exercise also increases the pulmonary blood flow which reduces the transit time for gas transfer from the alveoli to the blood and vice versa. Further, the capillary transit time is shortened due to rise in cardiac output and increased oxygen extraction by the tissues.[9,10]

Ventilation–Perfusion Mismatch

This is the most common cause of hypoxemia and is associated with an increased $P(A\text{-}a)O_2$ due to an anatomical and/or physiological imbalance between V and Q. Both are higher at the base and lower at the apex of the lungs. However, the V/Q ratio is higher at the apex and lower at the base. This is due to the fact that the rise from the base to apex in perfusion is much more than the rise in ventilation. The normal V/Q level is 0.8.

Clinical examples of V/Q mismatch beyond the physiological range include airway diseases (asthma, COPD, bronchiectasis, cystic fibrosis), ILDs, pulmonary hypertension, pulmonary vasculitis, and thromboembolic disease.

Case 3: *A 35-year-old female with a history of moderate-to-severe COVID-19 came for follow-up in the rehabilitation services. Her HRCT scan of thorax revealed bilateral ground-glass opacities (GGOs), lung fibrosis interspersed with areas of consolidation and bronchiectasis (CORAD score 3/5). Functional assessment was done with spirometry [forced expiratory volume in 1 second (FEV_1) 65% predicted, forced vital capacity (FVC) 60% predicted with a ratio of 89], and a SpO_2 of 87% at rest. The 6-minute walk test showed significant desaturation (>4%). ABGs at the end of 6-minute walk showed pH 7.35, $PaCO_2$ 35 mm Hg, HCO_3 19, and PaO_2 61 mm Hg in room air.*

In case 3, the young lady has low oxygen levels even at rest. However, the $P(A\text{-}a)O_2$ is increased. Another common clinical scenario which may cause worsening of existing hypoxemia is while treating acute severe asthma with only bronchodilator nebulization. Hypoxemias due to V/Q mismatch can be corrected with supplemental oxygen and the increase in PaO_2 has a steep response when sufficient supplemental oxygen is administered.[9-11]

Shunt (Right to Left)

A shunt is said to exist when blood from the right side of the heart enters the left side without taking part in any gas exchange. In health, a small percentage of shunt of about 2–3% of cardiac output normally exists. This is attributed to the flow of blood through bronchial veins draining into pulmonary veins or a few of the coronary veins (called thebesian veins) draining directly into the left ventricle. A shunt may be imagined as the extreme degree of V/Q mismatch where there is no ventilation. The feature that differentiates a shunt from other causes of hypoxemia is its poor response to supplemental oxygen therapy.

Case 4: *A 32-year-old male who works in train maintenance develops severe acute respiratory distress syndrome (ARDS) secondary to bacterial pneumonia and septic shock. Chest X-ray reveals bilateral pneumonia with bronchiectasis. There was no growth in the culture of respiratory secretions. An ABG on mechanical ventilation with a FiO_2 of 0.80 reveals pH 7.28, PaO_2 67 mm Hg, and $PaCO_2$ 61 mm Hg.*

In case 4, where the disease state results from filling of the alveolar spaces with fluid or collapse, a part of the cardiac output goes through the pulmonary vasculature without coming into contact with alveolar air. Other examples of shunts include pneumonia, pulmonary edema, alveolar collapse, pulmonary arteriovenous communication, and ARDS. In congenital cyanotic heart diseases, deoxygenated right heart blood flows straight to the left side bypassing the lungs.

In hypoxemia from shunts, the $P(A\text{-}a)O_2$ is elevated with a normal $PaCO_2$. In fact, hypercapnia is uncommon until the shunt fraction reaches near 50%. This is due to stimulation of the respiratory center by a chemoreceptor as the $PaCO_2$ in the arterial blood leaving the shunt unit is high. Arterial PaO_2 does not rise to the normal level even if the patient is given 100% oxygen to breathe.

PaO_2/FiO_2 is a rough estimate of shunt fraction. If PaO_2/FiO_2 is <200, shunt fraction is > 20%, whereas a PaO_2/FiO_2 of >200 indicates a shunt fraction of <20%.[8,9]

Hypoventilation

Hypoventilation refers to conditions in which alveolar ventilation is abnormally low in relation to oxygen uptake or carbon dioxide output. The alveolar PAO_2 which is the nondead-space ventilation reaches a lower level than normal. The alveolar $PACO_2$ and therefore arterial $PaCO_2$ are raised (hypercapnia) with a normal $P(A\text{-}a)O_2$.

Hypoxia occurs if the balance between O_2 delivery (V) and O_2 removal (blood flow, Q) gets altered. In the above example, there is hypoventilation with a normal blood flow which results in a low V/Q ratio (less delivery and unchanged removal of O_2), which lowers PAO_2 and consequently $PeCO_2$. Increasing the FiO_2 can alleviate the hypoxemia. However, correction of hypercapnia is only possible by elimination of CO_2 through increased assisted ventilation with the help of noninvasive or invasive mechanical ventilators.

Case 5: *An 82-year-old female presented with persistent cough and chest wall pain with a history of stage 4 breast cancer. Her physician prescribed an opioid-containing antitussive to reduce the cough and chest wall pain. On examination, the respiratory rate was 14 per minute with normal chest findings. Chest X-ray was clear. The SaO_2 was 90% in room air at rest. An ABG analysis reveals pH 7.17, PaO_2 55 mm Hg, and $PaCO_2$ 67 mm Hg.*

In case 5, the patient with breast cancer was put on opioids for persistent cough. Opioids are known to suppress the respiratory center leading to a fall in the respiratory rate which in turn causes hypoventilation as evidenced in ABG analysis by a raised $PaCO_2$. Other common causes of hypoventilation include airway obstructive diseases, extreme obesity, neuromuscular diseases, lack of stimulus from the respiratory center to the brainstem, spinal cord, myoneural junction (myasthenia gravis), and drug-induced (morphine derivatives, barbiturates) depression of the respiratory center.[8]

APPROACH TO HYPOXIA (FLOWCHART 1)

The approach to a subject with hypoxia depends on an in-depth understanding of the mechanisms of hypoxia. The first step is to record a thorough history. The history should be such that the underlying mechanism of hypoxia is somewhat clear. For example, there may be a history of climbing heights indicating AMS as a probable cause for hypoxia. Investigations to rule out other diseases with similar presentations are also important.

The next step is to calculate the $P(A-a)O_2$ gradient, check for the levels of $PaCO_2$, and assess if the low levels of oxygen get easily corrected with additional oxygen therapy.

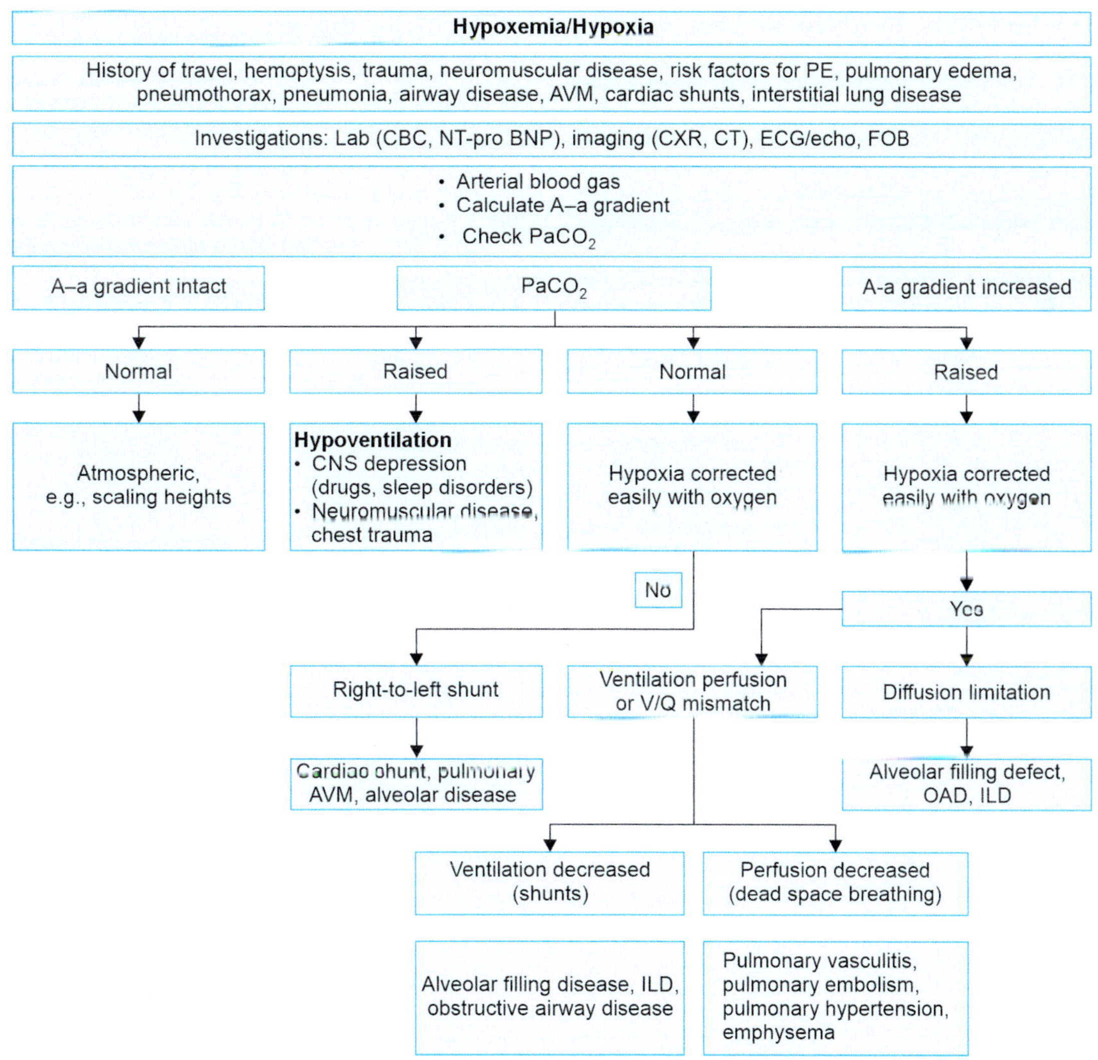

FLOWCHART 1: An approach to hypoxemia and hypoxia.

(AVM: arteriovenous malformation; CBC: complete blood count; CNS: central nervous system; CXR: chest X-ray; FOB: fiberoptic bronchoscopy; ILD: interstitial disease; PE: pulmonary embolism; NT-pro-BNP: N-terminal prohormone of brain natriuretic peptide)

An algorithm for a clinical approach to hypoxia is suggested **(Flowchart 1)**.

SUMMARY

While the causes of hypoxia are many, treating such patients with hypoxia depends on an in-depth understanding of the mechanisms of hypoxia. The first step is to record a thorough history. The history, if taken well, should be able to identify the underlying mechanism of hypoxia somewhat clearly. The next step is to perform an arterial blood gas analysis and calculate the P(A–a) O_2 gradient, check for the levels of $PaCO_2$, and assess if the low levels of oxygen get easily corrected with additional oxygen therapy. If corrected, the possible reasons are some forms of diffusion defect or something which causes a ventilation or perfusion defect. If hypoxia is not corrected by oxygen, the etiology is related to the presence of a right to left shunt. This chapter describes the approach to hypoxia with the help of clinical cases using the concepts of the pathophysiology of hypoxia.

REFERENCES

1. Rodríguez-Roisin R, Roca J. Mechanisms of hypoxemia. Intensive Care Med. 2005;31:1017-9.
2. Bhutta BS, Alghoula F, Berim I. Hypoxia [Updated 2022 Aug 9]. In: StatPearls [Internet]. Treasure Island (FL): StatPearls Publishing; 2023 Jan. [online] Available from https://www.ncbi.nlm.nih.gov/books/NBK482316/ [Last accessed September, 2024].
3. Greene KE, Peters JI. Pathophysiology of acute respiratory failure. Clin Chest Med. 1994;15(1):1-12.
4. Sharma S, Hashmi MF. Partial Pressure of Oxygen [Updated 2022 Dec 22]. In: StatPearls [Internet]. Treasure Island (FL): StatPearls Publishing; 2023 Jan. [online] Available from https://www.ncbi.nlm.nih.gov/books/NBK493219/ [Last accessed September, 2024].
5. Hafen BB, Sharma S. Oxygen saturation [Updated 2022 Nov 23]. In: StatPearls [Internet]. Treasure Island (FL): StatPearls Publishing; 2023 Jan. [online] Available from https://www.ncbi.nlm.nih.gov/books/NBK525974/ [Last accessed September, 2024].
6. Pittman RN. Oxygen transport in normal and pathological situations: Defects and compensations. Regulation of Tissue Oxygenation. San Rafael, CA: Morgan & Claypool Life Sciences; 2011. (Chapter 7) [online] Available from https://www.ncbi.nlm.nih.gov/books/NBK54113/ [Last accessed September, 2024].
7. Bonora M, Patergnani S, Rimessi A, et al. ATP synthesis and storage. Purinergic Signal. 2012;8(3):343-57.
8. Petersson J, Glenny RW. Gas exchange and ventilation-perfusion relationships in the lung. Eur Respir J. 2014;44(4):1023-41.
9. Grocott M, Montgomery H, Vercueil A. High-altitude physiology and pathophysiology: implications and relevance for intensive care medicine. Crit Care. 2007;11(1):203.
10. Sarkar M, Niranjan N, Banyal PK. Mechanisms of hypoxemia. Lung India. 2017;34(1):47-60. [Erratum in: Lung India;34(2):220]. [Last accessed September, 2024].
11. Brinkman JE, Toro F, Sharma S. Physiology, Respiratory Drive [Updated 2022 Jun 8]. In: StatPearls [Internet]. Treasure Island (FL): StatPearls Publishing; 2023 Jan. [online] Available from https://www.ncbi.nlm.nih.gov/books/NBK482414/

CHAPTER 159

High-flow Nasal Cannula Oxygen

Amit Mandal

INTRODUCTION

The high-flow nasal cannula (HFNC) is a medical device that delivers a high flow of heated and humidified oxygen to patients in need of respiratory support. It has gained popularity in recent years as an alternative to traditional oxygen therapy and noninvasive ventilation (NIV) methods.[1,2] The newer systems which are designed to deliver warm and humidified oxygen at high flows have lead to the increased use of HFNC in adults, particularly during the COVID-19 pandemic.[3] HFNC now is a standard method of oxygen administration in both pediatric and adult patients with milder forms of respiratory failure and deoxygentation.[4] It was more commonly used for pediatric population but has now gained popularity in adults. HFNC comprises an air-oxygen blender, an active humidifier, a single heated circuit, and a nasal cannula. Herein we deliberate on the physiological basis, indications, and current evidence on the use of HFNC in adults.

MECHANISM OF ACTION AND PHYSIOLOGICAL EFFECTS

The HFNC system includes the nasal cannula with a wide-bore interface. The gas blender mixes oxygen and air to achieve the desired oxygen concentration, while the heated humidifier warms and humidifies the gas to improve the patient comfort.[5,6] The high flow rates provided by the device may range from 20 to 60 L/min, exceeding the patient's peak inspiratory flow rate.

The high flow of gas delivered through the nasal cannula creates positive end-expiratory pressure (PEEP), reduces airway resistance, washes out nasopharyngeal dead space, and flushes out carbon dioxide.[7] The combination of these effects improves oxygenation and reduces work of breathing.

Heated and humidified oxygen at high flow has the following physiological effects:[7-9]

- Removal of carbon dioxide from the anatomical dead space without an increase in the tidal volume. It may also reduce work of breathing and improve thoracoabdominal synchrony. There is also a reduction in respiratory rate and minute ventilation without causing an increase in the $PaCO_2$.
- HFNC provides a PEEP of up to 3 cm H_2O with the closed mouth. This is not likely with the open mouth which most patients with acute respiratory failure (ARF) breathe through. HFNC at a higher flow rate has multiple beneficial effects such as:
  - Improved end-expiratory lung volumes,
  - Improvement of dynamic lung compliance,
  - Improved oxygenation,
  - Homogenization of ventilation distribution, and
  - Decrease in respiratory rate.
- HFNC assures a constant FiO_2. During ARF, there are significant variations in the inspiratory flow and the tidal volume. With HFNC, the delivered FiO_2 is closer to the depicted FiO_2, especially at high flow.
- The gas delivered through HFNC is heated and humidified as is used with critical care ventilators.

CLINICAL INDICATIONS

High flow nasal cannula is commonly used in various clinical settings and patient populations with hypoxia and deoxygenation. Some of the clinical indications for HFNC include the following:

- *Acute respiratory failure*: There are potential benefits of HFNC in different settings of ARF management. HFNC can be used as a first-line treatment or as a step-up therapy in patients with ARF, including hypoxemic respiratory failure and hypercapnic respiratory failure.[10-13] HFNC when compared to standard oxygen therapy leads to less treatment failure but probably makes no difference to treatment failure when compared to NIV.[14-16]
- *Postextubation support*: HFNC has been proposed to reduce the rate of reintubation in patients at high risk of extubation failure, such as those with a history of chronic obstructive pulmonary disease (COPD), congestive heart failure (CHF), or high Acute Physiology and Chronic

Health Evaluation (APACHE) scores.[17-19] In a systemic review and meta-analysis of the available literature to assess the efficacy of HFNC versus NIV in patients at high risk of extubation failure, it was concluded that HFNC reduced the incidence of adverse events but did not affect reintubation and mortality.[17] Similarly, the efficacy of HFNC versus NIV for AECOPD (acute exacerbation of chronic obstructive pulmonary disease) patients after extubation was analyzed using a systemic review and meta-analysis of the available randomized controlled trials.[18] It was reported that HFNC could be used as an alternative to NIV after extubation in AECOPD patients with hypercapnia but found to be less effective in normocapnic patients.[18]

- *Bronchiolitis*: HFNC has emerged as an effective treatment modality for infants with bronchiolitis, providing improved oxygenation, reduced respiratory distress, and decreased treatment failure rates compared to traditional oxygen therapy.[20]
- *Preoxygenation and apnea oxygenation*: HFNC can be used during intubation procedures to provide preoxygenation and apnea oxygenation, maintaining oxygen saturation levels and reducing the risk of hypoxemia.[21,22] There is lack of evidence in the use of HFNC during intubation in high-risk groups such as obese patients, those with a PaO_2:FiO_2 ratio of <150 mm Hg, and those who are difficult-to-intubate patients.
- *Postoperative patients*: HFNC significantly reduced the reintubation rate and escalation of respiratory support in the immediate postoperative period in patients undergoing cardiac or thoracic surgeries. There was no change in mortality, hospital and intensive care unit stay, or incidence of postoperative hypoxia.[23]
- *Palliative therapy and do-not-intubate patients*: HFNC can be effectively used in setting where intubation is being refused and it has been shown to have better tolerance than NIV.[24-26] HFNC is associated with less patient discomfort and less frequent complications which are otherwise common with NIV (such as claustrophobia, pressure ulcers, and inability to communicate, eat, or expectorate).
- *Bronchoscopy*: HFNC performs well to prevent oxygen saturation falling below 90% during bronchoscopy. It allows insertion of bronchoscope and improves oxygenation during the procedure.[27-29] HFNC performs better than NIV which is associated with mask intolerance. Moreover, it is difficult to manipulate the bronchoscope through the NIV mask.

BENEFITS OF HIGH-FLOW NASAL CANNULA

The use of HFNC offers several benefits over conventional oxygen therapy and NIV methods:[2,8,10,30-32]

- *Improved patient comfort*: The heated and humidified gas delivered by HFNC enhances patient comfort, reducing nasal dryness, congestion, and discomfort associated with traditional oxygen masks.
- *Reduced work of breathing*: HFNC reduces respiratory effort by providing a high flow of gas that helps to flush out carbon dioxide, improving gas exchange and reducing the work of breathing.
- *Enhanced oxygenation*: HFNC can achieve higher oxygen concentrations compared to conventional oxygen therapy, ensuring optimal oxygenation in patients with hypoxemia.
- *PEEP effect*: HFNC provides a mild positive end-expiratory pressure (PEEP) effect, which helps to recruit collapsed alveoli and improve oxygenation.
- *Decreased airway resistance*: The high flow rates delivered by HFNC reduce airway resistance, improving respiratory mechanics and facilitating easier breathing.
- Ability to deliver constant FiO_2.
- Decrease in anatomical dead space.

INSTITUTION OF HIGH-FLOW NASAL CANNULA

An algorithm generally follows the ROX index, i.e., ratio of oxygen saturation (measured by pulse oximetry) divided by FiO_2 to respiratory rate ratio **(Flowchart 1)**.

- *Initiation*: The first step is assembling the unit and the patient interface using the correct size nasal canula. It is important to properly set the temperature and oxygen flow. An initial flow of 30–40 L/m can be used. The oxygen flow may be adjusted to achieve the desired level of oxygen saturation.

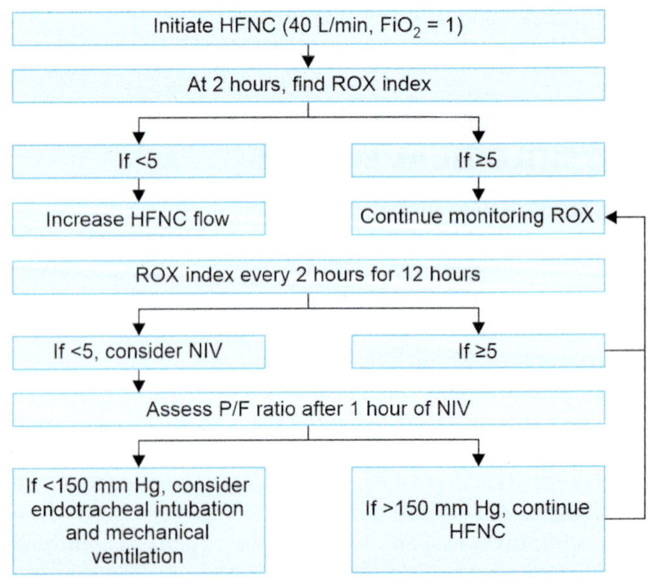

FLOWCHART 1: Algorithm regarding the use of HFNC for the management of hypoxia in acute respiratory failure (ROX = Oxygen saturation by pulse oximetry divided by FiO_2 to respiratory rate ratio).

(HFNC: high-flow nasal cannula; NIV: noninvasive ventilation)

- *Evaluating the efficacy of therapy*: An important concern during the HFNC therapy is early identification of the patient who is not showing signs of improvement and is likely to need intubation. The ROX index (ratio of oxygen saturation as measured by pulse oximetry/FiO_2 to respiratory rate) is considered a valuable tool for such determination.[10] An ROX index ≥4.88 measured at 2, 6, or 1 hours is a determinant of HFNC success. An ROX index <2.85, <3.47, and <3.85 at 2, 6 and 12 hours of HFNC initiation, respectively, were predictive of HFNC failure.[33]
- *Weaning from HFNC*: The first step is to reduce the FiO_2 until an acceptable oxygenation can be achieved. Once the FiO_2 required is less than 50%, the flows may be gradually reduced. The patient can be weaned off HFNC once the patient is stable on flows < 20 L/m and FiO_2 < 50%.

COMPLICATIONS

While HFNC is generally considered safe, it is important to be aware of potential complications:

- *Nasal discomfort and epistaxis*: Prolonged or high-flow use of HFNC may cause nasal discomfort, dryness, or epistaxis. Appropriate humidification and regular nasal care can help minimize these complications.
- *Gastric distension*: In patients with compromised lower esophageal sphincter function or gastrointestinal obstruction, high flow rates of HFNC may lead to gastric distension. Monitoring and adjustment of flow rates can mitigate this risk.
- *Delayed recognition of clinical deterioration*: Continuous monitoring of patients on HFNC is crucial to identify signs of clinical deterioration promptly. Careful assessment of respiratory parameters and clinical status is necessary to ensure timely intervention if needed.[34]

EVIDENCE AND RESEARCH

Numerous studies have evaluated the efficacy and safety of HFNC in different clinical scenarios. The evidence suggests that HFNC can improve oxygenation, decrease respiratory distress, and reduce the need for invasive ventilation. The FLORALI trial, published in 2015, demonstrated the effectiveness of HFNC in a well-defined subset of patients, demonstrating a significant improvement in 90-day mortality compared to either NIV or standard oxygen therapy (12% vs. 28% vs. 23%).[35] The FLORALI-2, another multicenter, open-label randomized controlled trial evaluated the efficacy of preoxygenation with NIV as compared to HFNC in reducing the risk of severe hypoxemia during intubation. The results of the trial did not demonstrate a change in the risk of severe hypoxemia with either of the modalities.[36] The SOHO-COVID randomized clinical trial evaluated the benefit of HFNC in patients with respiratory failure due to COVID-19. The use of HFNC was not associated with significant reduction in mortality at day 28 compared to standard oxygen therapy.[36,37] However, further research is still needed to establish optimal flow rates, patient selection criteria, and long-term outcomes associated with HFNC use.

SUMMARY

High-flow nasal cannula therapy is a valuable tool in respiratory support, providing improved oxygenation, reduced work of breathing, and enhanced patient comfort. It has found utility in various clinical indications, including ARF, postextubation support, bronchiolitis, and preoxygenation during intubation. Although generally safe, close monitoring of patients and awareness of potential complications are essential. Ongoing research is essential to further define the optimal application and benefits of HFNC in different patient populations.

REFERENCES

1. Helviz Y, Einav S. A Systematic Review of the High-flow Nasal Cannula for Adult Patients. Crit Care. 2018;22(1):71.
2. Rochwerg B, Einav S, Chaudhuri D, et al. The role for high flow nasal cannula as a respiratory support strategy in adults: a clinical practice guideline. Intensive Care Med. 2020;46(12):2226-37.
3. Crimi C, Pierucci P, Renda T, et al. High-Flow Nasal Cannula and COVID-19: A Clinical Review. Respir Care. 2022;67(2):227-40.
4. Kwon JW. High-flow nasal cannula oxygen therapy in children: a clinical review. Clin Exp Pediatr. 2020;63(1):3-7.
5. Ritchie JE, Williams AB, Gerard C, et al. Evaluation of a humidified nasal high-flow oxygen system, using oxygraphy, capnography and measurement of upper airway pressures. Anaesth Intensive Care. 2011;39(6):1103-10.
6. Chanques G, Riboulet F, Molinari N, et al. Comparison of three high flow oxygen therapy delivery devices: a clinical physiological cross-over study. Minerva Anestesiol. 2013;79(12):1344-55.
7. Vargas F, Saint-Leger M, Boyer A, et al. Physiologic Effects of High-Flow Nasal Cannula Oxygen in Critical Care Subjects. Respir Care. 2015;60(10):1369-76.
8. Sztrymf B, Messika J, Bertrand F, et al. Beneficial effects of humidified high flow nasal oxygen in critical care patients: a prospective pilot study. Intensive Care Med. 2011;37(11):1780-6.
9. Wettstein RB, Shelledy DC, Peters JI. Delivered oxygen concentrations using low-flow and high-flow nasal cannulas. Respir Care. 2005;50(5):604-9.
10. Sehgal IS, Dhooria S, Agarwal R. High-Flow Nasal Cannula Oxygen in Respiratory Failure. N Engl J Med. 2015;373(14):1374.
11. Mauri T, Alban L, Turrini C, et al. Optimum support by high-flow nasal cannula in acute hypoxemic respiratory failure: effects of increasing flow rates. Intensive Care Med. 2017;43(10):1453-63.

12. Bräunlich J, Dellweg D, Bastian A, et al. Nasal high-flow versus noninvasive ventilation in patients with chronic hypercapnic COPD. Int J Chron Obstruct Pulmon Dis. 2019;14:1411-21.
13. Ricard JD, Roca O, Lemiale V, et al. Use of nasal high flow oxygen during acute respiratory failure. Intensive Care Med. 2020;46(12):2238-47.
14. Lewis SR, Baker PE, Parker R, et al. High-flow nasal cannulae for respiratory support in adult intensive care patients. Cochrane Database Syst Rev. 20213(3):CD010172.
15. Rochwerg B, Granton D, Wang DX, et al. High flow nasal cannula compared with conventional oxygen therapy for acute hypoxemic respiratory failure: a systematic review and meta-analysis. Intensive Care Med. 2019;45(5):563-72.
16. Messika J, Ben Ahmed K, Gaudry S, et al. Use of High-Flow Nasal Cannula Oxygen Therapy in Subjects with ARDS: A 1-year Observational Study. Respir Care. 2015;60(2):162-9.
17. Wang Q, Peng Y, Xu S, et al. The efficacy of high-flow nasal cannula (HFNC) versus non-invasive ventilation (NIV) in patients at high risk of extubation failure: a systematic review and meta-analysis. Eur J Med Res. 2023;28(1):120
18. Feng Z, Zhang L, Yu H, et al. High-Flow Nasal Cannula Oxygen Therapy versus Noninvasive Ventilation for AECOPD Patients After Extubation: A Systematic Review and Meta-analysis of Randomized Controlled Trials. Int J Chron Obstruct Pulmon Dis. 2022;17:1987-99.
19. Hernández G, Vaquero C, González P, et al. Effect of Postextubation High-Flow Nasal Cannula vs Conventional Oxygen Therapy on Reintubation in Low-Risk Patients: A Randomized Clinical Trial. JAMA. 2016;315(13):1354-61.
20. Fainardi V, Abelli L, Muscarà M, et al. Update on the Role of High-Flow Nasal Cannula in Infants with Bronchiolitis. Children (Basel). 2021;8(2):66.
21. Meunier J, Guitton C. Place de l'oxygénothérapie haut débit dans la pré-oxygénation pour l'intubation et la pratique des gestes invasifs [The role of HFNC oxygen in pre-oxygenation prior to intubation and the practice of invasive procedures]. Rev Mal Respir. 2023;40(1):47-60.
22. Chaudhuri D, Granton D, Wang DX, et al. Moderate Certainty Evidence Suggests the Use of High-Flow Nasal Cannula Does Not Decrease Hypoxia When Compared with Conventional Oxygen Therapy in the Peri-Intubation Period: Results of a Systematic Review and Meta-analysis. Crit Care Med. 2020;48(4):571-8.
23. Chaudhuri D, Granton D, Wang DX, et al. High-Flow Nasal Cannula in the Immediate Postoperative Period: A Systematic Review and Meta-analysis. Chest. 2020;158(5):1934-46.
24. Wilson ME, Mittal A, Dobler CC, et al. High-Flow Nasal Cannula Oxygen in Patients with Acute Respiratory Failure and Do-Not-Intubate or Do-Not-Resuscitate Orders: A Systematic Review. J Hosp Med. 2020;15(2):101-6.
25. Koyauchi T, Hasegawa H, Kanata K, et al. Efficacy and Tolerability of High-Flow Nasal Cannula Oxygen Therapy for Hypoxemic Respiratory Failure in Patients with Interstitial Lung Disease with Do-Not-Intubate Orders: A Retrospective Single-Center Study. Respiration. 2018;96(4):323-9.
26. Peters SG, Holets SR, Gay PC. High-flow nasal cannula therapy in do-not-intubate patients with hypoxemic respiratory distress. Respir Care. 2013;58(4):597-600.
27. Lucangelo U, Vassallo FG, Marras E, et al. High-flow nasal interface improves oxygenation in patients undergoing bronchoscopy. Crit Care Res Pract. 2012;2012:506382.
28. Simon M, Braune S, Frings D, et al. High-flow nasal cannula oxygen versus non-invasive ventilation in patients with acute hypoxaemic respiratory failure undergoing flexible bronchoscopy—a prospective randomised trial. Crit Care. 2014; 18(6):712.
29. La Combe B, Messika J, Labbé V, et al. High-flow nasal oxygen for bronchoalveolar lavage in acute respiratory failure patients. Eur Respir J. 2016;47(4):1283-6.
30. Bräunlich J, Köhler M, Wirtz H. Nasal highflow improves ventilation in patients with COPD. Int J Chron Obstruct Pulmon Dis. 2016;11:1077-85.
31. Fraser JF, Spooner AJ, Dunster KR, et al. Nasal high flow oxygen therapy in patients with COPD reduces respiratory rate and tissue carbon dioxide while increasing tidal and end-expiratory lung volumes: a randomised crossover trial. Thorax. 2016;71(8):759-61.
32. Pilcher J, Richards M, Eastlake L, et al. High flow or titrated oxygen for obese medical inpatients: a randomised crossover trial. Med J Aust. 2017;207(10):430-4.
33. Roca O, Caralt B, Messika J, et al. An Index Combining Respiratory Rate and Oxygenation to Predict Outcome of Nasal High-Flow Therapy. Am J Respir Crit Care Med. 2019;199(11):1368-76.
34. Kang BJ, Koh Y, Lim CM, et al. Failure of high-flow nasal cannula therapy may delay intubation and increase mortality. Intensive Care Med. 2015;41(4):623-32.
35. Frat JP, Thille AW, Mercat A, et al. FLORALI Study Group; REVA Network. High-flow oxygen through nasal cannula in acute hypoxemic respiratory failure. N Engl J Med. 2015;372(23): 2185-96.
36. Frat JP, Ricard JD, Quenot JP, et al. FLORALI-2 study group; REVA network. Non-invasive ventilation versus high-flow nasal cannula oxygen therapy with apnoeic oxygenation for preoxygenation before intubation of patients with acute hypoxaemic respiratory failure: a randomised, multicentre, open-label trial. Lancet Respir Med. 2019;7(4):303-12.
37. Frat JP, Quenot JP, Badie J, et al.; SOHO-COVID Study Group and the REVA Network. Effect of High-Flow Nasal Cannula Oxygen vs Standard Oxygen Therapy on Mortality in Patients with Respiratory Failure due to COVID-19: The SOHO-COVID Randomized Clinical Trial. JAMA. 2022;328(12):1212-22.

Noninvasive Ventilation

CHAPTER 160

GC Khilnani, Vijay Hadda

INTRODUCTION

Assisted ventilation is an integral part of critical care that has significantly improved the outcome of these patients. Conventional mechanical ventilation is associated with several complications, a large proportion of these are related to endotracheal intubation. Noninvasive ventilation (NIV) refers to technique of augmenting alveolar ventilation without an endotracheal airway, thereby avoiding many of these complications. Since its first use in 1980s in patients with neuromuscular respiratory failure, NIV is considered as one of the most important additions in the field of mechanical ventilation and critical care armamentarium. Over the last two decades, it has gained widespread acceptance as a mode of assisted ventilation for the management of acute, as well as chronic respiratory failure in different settings including in emergency departments, intensive Care Units (ICUs), wards, and at home.[1-5]

Technically, NIV refers to the provision of inspiratory pressure support plus positive end-expiratory pressure (PEEP) via a nasal or face mask. Although continuous positive airway pressure (CPAP) does not actively assist inspiration and is not a ventilatory support mode, it is considered a form of NIV, when used as a therapy for respiratory failure. The use of NIV therapy in selected patients with acute respiratory failure (ARF) is associated with significantly reduced need for endotracheal intubation and conventional ventilation. The available evidence suggests that the benefits of this therapy are not limited to hypercapnic (ARF) but extend to hypoxemic ARF as well. The successful application of NIV requires training and collaboration of an experienced ICU team, including intensivists, nurses, and respiratory physiotherapists. An expanded awareness of NIV devices and techniques promises to increase the therapeutic options for patients with severe respiratory insufficiency.

TECHNICAL ASPECT OF NONINVASIVE VENTILATION

Types of Noninvasive Ventilation

Noninvasive mechanical ventilation support can be either negative pressure ventilation or positive pressure ventilation.

Negative Pressure Ventilation

The negative pressure ventilators were widely used during polio epidemics, the classical example was the "iron lung". The principle of negative pressure ventilation involves the application of external subatmospheric pressure to the chest wall, resulting in its expansion during inspiration, expiration occurs as the pressure around the chest wall is allowed to return to atmospheric level. During negative pressure ventilation, tidal volume is related to peak inspiratory negative pressure (more the negative pressure, more the tidal volume) and the pressure waveform (a square wave produces a greater tidal volume than a half sine wave) generated by the ventilator pump. This type of ventilation has been used in patients with respiratory failure due to chest wall deformity, neuromuscular diseases, or central hypoventilation.[6,7] Negative pressure ventilation has been shown to be associated with a higher partial pressure of oxygen (PaO_2), a lower partial pressure of carbon dioxide ($PaCO_2$) (despite identical minute ventilation), and less lung injury in an animal study.[8] It may motivate the researchers for similar trials in human subjects. However, the use of negative pressure ventilation is limited by their propensity of causing upper airway obstruction leading to oxygen desaturation and poor acceptance by patients due to the awkward size of devices.[7] The positive pressure ventilation administered by nasal mask, overcame some of these shortcomings, especially ameliorating the nocturnal oxygen desaturation.

Noninvasive Positive Pressure Ventilation

For several decades, positive pressure ventilation has been delivered by endotracheal intubation as standard of care for patients with various forms of respiratory failure. Noninvasive Positive Pressure Ventilation (NIPPV) refers to the positive pressure ventilation provided without the use of endotracheal intubation. The technique requires a mechanical ventilator, connected by tubing to an interface (nasal, orofacial, and other types of mask). The ventilator delivers continuous or intermittent positive airway pressure through the upper airway and actively assists the ventilation. NIPPV is used in selected patients with various forms of respiratory failure.[1,9-12]

The Equipment of NIPPV Ventilator Device

The primary requirement for NIPPV is a device to deliver positive pressure ventilation (ventilator) and an appropriate patient-ventilator interface (orofacial or nasal mask). The choice of ventilators available to provide noninvasive ventilatory support has continued to expand. Noninvasive ventilatory support may be provided either by using large bedside critical care volume ventilators or a specialty ventilator devoted to NIV. A dedicated NIPPV ventilator is a small, compact, portable machine connected to the interface (nasal, orofacial, or other types of masks) via tubing **(Fig. 1)**. Many critical care ventilators currently in use also have a NIPPV option, either as part of the original device or available as an upgrade option. While the critical care ventilators have options of several modes and better oxygen blending, they are also less tolerant of leaks. The specialty ventilators have fewer options and range but are more leak tolerant. The ideal device is dependent on a number of factors, including the familiarity of the staff and the availability of options. The differences between the bedside critical care ventilator and specialty noninvasive ventilator continue to diminish as the differences related to ventilator options, range of support, and leak tolerance are corrected in both devices. The size is an important consideration. Therefore, specialty ventilators which are small in size **(Fig. 1)** are used both in hospitals and in homes.

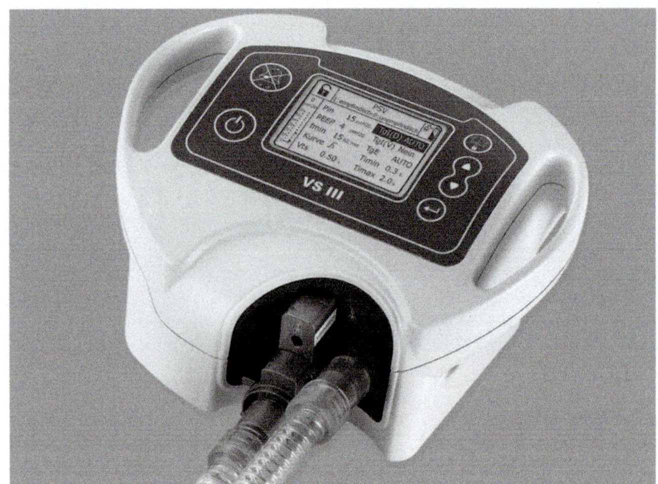

FIG. 1: Noninvasive ventilation machine.

Interfaces

The interface between the machine and the patient is a tight-fitting mask that is made of silicon **(Figs. 2A and B)**. Nasal masks and orofacial masks were the earliest interfaces, with subsequent development and use of full-face masks, mouthpieces, nasal pillows, and helmets.[5] This advancement gives liberty to the care provider to select interface as per indication and tolerance of the patient. Nasal masks and orofacial masks are still the most commonly used interfaces. Both nasal and a full-face mask are held in place by cloth straps or Velcro **(Fig. 3)**. These masks are available in various sizes. The choice of mask depends upon the comfort and compliance of the patient, as well as on the operator's choice.

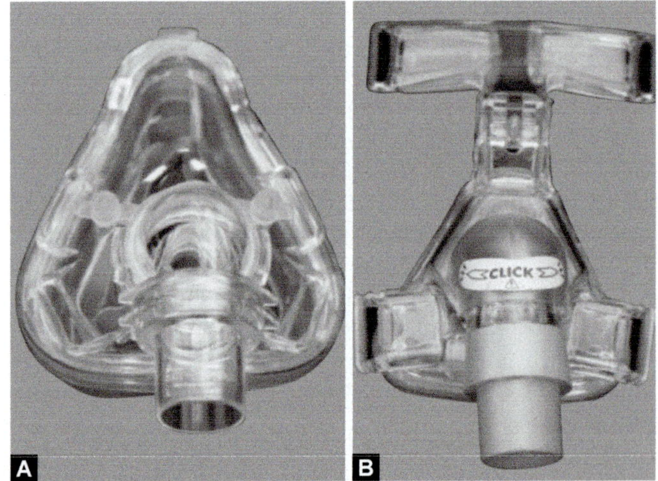

FIGS. 2A AND B: Silicone mask interfaces. (A) Orofacial and (B) Nasal mask.

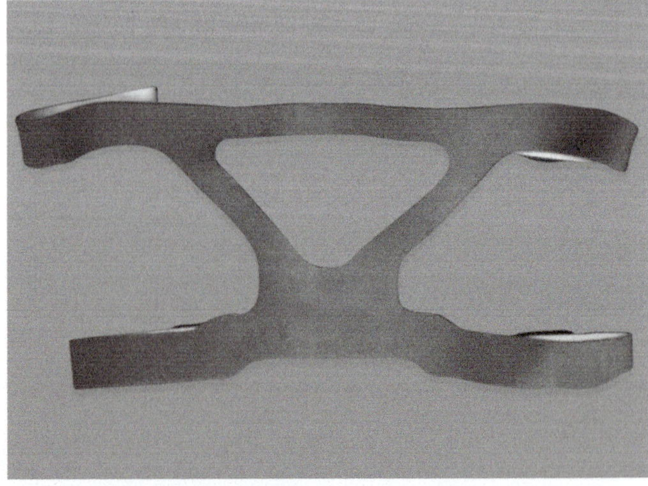

FIG. 3: A typical headgear to hold the interface.

Orofacial masks are the most frequently used interface for management of acute respiratory failure. Use of these masks compared to nasal masks leads to faster correction of blood gases. Orofacial masks are preferred in patients who are less cooperative, have a higher severity of illness, are mouth-breathers or pursed lips breathers, edentulous, and those requiring more effective ventilation. However, these masks are associated with claustrophobia, hindrance in speaking and coughing, and carry a small risk of aspiration with emesis. Nasal masks are best suited for more cooperative patients with a lesser severity of illness. These are not claustrophobic, allow speaking, drinking, coughing, secretion clearance, and carry lesser risk of aspiration and emesis. However, these are associated with more air leaks (e.g., mouth-breathing or edentulous patients) and effectiveness is limited in patients with nasal deformities or blockade. Importantly, mask should be the proper sized, so that it snugly fits and there is no air leak. Indeed, selection of appropriate mask and its proper application is of paramount importance for success of this form of ventilation; air leak leads to ineffective ventilation. Leaks are the bane of all of the interfaces, but excess pressure applied with the straps is discomforting to the patients, increases the risk of pressure necrosis, and skin breakdown. Some amount of air leak at times is inevitable; however, most of the machines have facility for leak compensation. Therefore, one should be careful to minimize excess pressure on the face or nose. Straps should be tight enough to prevent significant leaks but with enough slack to allow passage of 1 or 2 fingers between the face and the straps.[1,5]

Various Modes of Ventilation

The NIPPV usually provides a form of assisted ventilation, where every breath is supported by the ventilator. Two types of breaths can be used, either volume-targeted or pressure-targeted.

Volume-targeted Noninvasive Positive Pressure Ventilation

During volume-targeted breaths, a predetermined tidal volume is delivered, usually with a set peak-flow rate and a controlled flow wave shape, over a fixed inspiratory time. It is frequently recommended to set tidal volume higher than usual, to compensate for possible leaks (12–14 mL/kg). In "invasively" ventilated patients, much attention has been paid to the importance of the peak-flow setting for relieving the patient's dyspnea and reducing effort.[13] Surprisingly, little attention is paid to the importance of this peak-flow setting, while providing volume-controlled ventilation with NIPPV. The usual peak-flow rate of 45–60 L/min is essential to decrease patient's inspiratory effort. Excessive peak-flow rates, however, also have adverse effects, as they can increase the sense of dyspnea (the patient receives "too much air").[13,14] Unfortunately, some of the "old" generation ventilators cannot be used for volume-targeted NIPPV. Modern ventilators have been designed to deliver volume-targeted NIPPV; however, in the case of leaks, the delivered volume is reduced, with no adaptation by the ventilator.

Pressure-targeted Noninvasive Positive Pressure Ventilation

In case of pressure-targeted NIPPV, the ventilator maintains a constant preset pressure after the breath has been triggered by the patient and stops when the flow indicates the end of the patient's effort, or after a fixed, preset inspiratory time (assist pressure control). The potential advantages of a pressure-targeted NIPPV include:

- The preset pressure is maintained in case of leaks, which facilitates achieving an appropriate delivered volume
- The likelihood of leaks and its side effects is reduced because the pressure is limited in the mask
- Synchrony between the patient and the ventilator is usually good since these modes have been primarily designed to facilitate the patient's effort to breathe
- The combination of pressure-support ventilation (PSV) and PEEP has been shown to be very efficient in reducing the work of breathing.[15]

Choosing the initial mode of ventilation is based in parts on the underlying disease, the ventilator available, and the past experience. Pressure-targeted ventilation with CPAP is the most basic level of support and is not considered as a mode of NIPPV in true sense. CPAP is most frequently used for management of cardiogenic pulmonary edema and obstructive sleep apnea.

Most patients on NIPPV require pressure support mode of ventilation with PEEP [popularly called bilevel positive airway pressure (BiPAP)]. During BiPAP mode, patient receives ventilatory support during both phases of respiration, as preset inspiratory positive airway pressure (IPAP) and expiratory positive airway pressure (EPAP). The difference between IPAP and EPAP is a reflection of the amount of PSV provided to the patient and EPAP is synonymous with PEEP. Some noninvasive ventilators have facilities of proportional-assist ventilation (PAV), which provides flow and volume assistance with each breath. While volume ventilators can be used to provide noninvasive ventilatory support, pressure-targeted modes are preferred because they provide better patient comfort and synchrony and are more tolerant of the leaks that accompany all noninvasive ventilatory interfaces.

Mechanism of Action of Noninvasive Positive Pressure Ventilation

Intermittent positive pressure is transmitted through upper airway to the alveoli, increasing transpulmonary pressure, inflating the lungs, and assisting alveolar ventilation, as in the case with positive pressure ventilation through an artificial airway. It has been stated that NIPPV improves daytime ventilatory muscle function by reducing chronic respiratory muscle fatigue, improving respiratory system compliance through reversal of micro atelectasis of lung, and preventing nocturnal hypoventilation by resetting the respiratory center's sensitivity to carbon dioxide.

STEPS TO SUCCESSFUL PROVISION OF NONINVASIVE POSITIVE PRESSURE VENTILATION

Several considerations can enhance the likelihood of successful NIPPV, such as proper selection of patient, settings (ICU/ward/home), the type of interface used, underlying disease, and patient's cooperation. In addition to these factors, the experience and expertise of healthcare providers, including the nurses and the respiratory physiotherapist, are important for the success of NIPPV.

Choosing the Patients

It is most essential to choose the right patient for initiating NIPPV. A poor selection of patient leads to higher rate of failure of NIPPV. It is important to ensure that patient is able to understand the instructions. Although altered level of consciousness is a relative contraindication, patients with chronic obstructive pulmonary disease (COPD) with impaired consciousness may be given a trial of NIPPV for 30–60 minutes; quite often, there is improvement in the level of consciousness. Other contraindications to its use include hemodynamic instability, presence of copious respiratory secretions, impaired swallowing reflex, active upper gastrointestinal bleeding, and orofacial trauma.

Hemodynamic parameters are important considerations; presence of hemodynamic instability or associated organ failure in a patient with respiratory failure carries a risk of failure of NIPPV. Recent facial surgery, trauma, or deformity are obvious contraindications. Patients should be carefully assessed for contraindications before the decision to initiate NIPPV is taken **(Box 1)**.

Location of Noninvasive Positive Pressure Ventilation Application

Initially, it was recommended that NIPPV should be initiated only in the ICU since some proportion of patients would require endotracheal intubation. It has now been recognized that this modality can be used in general wards.[4,16] Many other trials have demonstrated its therapeutic use outside ICUs in the emergency room, general wards, and high-dependency units (HDUs) subjected to the availability of trained and experienced nursing staff and respiratory therapists.[2,3,16] With years of experience, we are able to manage many patients on NIPPV in our ward. The location of NIPPV therapy is largely determined by the severity of the illness. For example, patients with ARF due to exacerbation of COPD with pH <7.25 are best managed in ICU.

BOX 1 **Contraindications to use of noninvasive positive pressure ventilation (NIPPV).**

- Uncooperative/obtunded patient
- Agitated patient
- Hemodynamic instability or presence of organ failure
- Severe comorbidity
- Recent facial/upper airway trauma
- Recent upper gastrointestinal tract surgery
- Intestinal obstruction
- Excessive secretions in the airways
- Undrained pneumothorax

Explanation and Evaluation

Physician should explain to the patient about the breathing support being provided to him and its benefits. Patients should also be provided a feel of the interface. It can be done by holding the mask with hands, without applying straps. It is useful to inform the patient that some discomfort might occur in the beginning due to tight-fitting mask and the repeated gush of air with each inspiration. This helps the patient in understanding the working of the device, which leads to a reduction in the anxiety and better cooperation.

Initial Ventilator Settings and Adjustments

The primary goals of NIPPV are adequate ventilation and oxygenation, correction of respiratory failure, and adequate patient tolerance and comfort.[17] The ventilatory settings and adjustments are made to achieve these endpoints. Initial settings focus on achieving adequate tidal volumes, usually in the range of 5–7 mL/kg. Additional support is provided to reduce the respiratory rate to <25 breaths/minute. Oxygen is adjusted to achieve adequate oxygenation, so as to achieve hemoglobin oxygen saturation of >90%. Serial arterial blood gas (ABG) measurements are essential to monitor the response to therapy and to guide further adjustments in the ventilator settings.

All patients should be initiated on a pressure support that is lower than the target level. To start with, an IPAP of 6 cm of water with EPAP of 2 cm of water is a reasonable setting. A pressure difference of 4 cm of water between IPAP and EPAP is desirable. Pressure may be augmented every few minutes by 2 cm of water, to reach a target level necessary to achieve the therapeutic endpoints. The maximum recommended level of IPAP is 24 cm of water, whereas that of EPAP is 16 cm of water. If any patient requires IPAP/EPAP of more than that, one should strongly consider endotracheal intubation. Oxygen should be supplemented through a port provided in the mask or in the NIPPV machine at a flow rate so as to maintain oxygen saturation above 90%.

Monitoring of Patients on Noninvasive Positive Pressure Ventilation

Patient should be monitored for patient-ventilator asynchrony, deterioration of sensorium, gastric distention,

TABLE 1: Indications of discontinuation of noninvasive positive pressure ventilation (NIPPV).

Major criteria (One of these)	Minor criteria (Two of these)
• Respiratory arrest • Loss of consciousness • Gasping for air • Psychomotor agitation requiring sedation • Heart rate <50 beats/minute with loss of alertness • Hemodynamic instability	• Respiratory rate > 35 breaths/minute • pH < 7.30 and decreased from onset • Partial pressure of oxygen (PaO_2) < 45 mm Hg despite oxygen • Increase in encephalopathy and decreased level of consciousness

and development of air leaks as patient changes posture or speaks. Pulse rate, blood pressure, respiratory rate, signs of respiratory distress, and oxygen saturation should be monitored during the 1st hour. ABG must be repeated within the 1st hour and monitored as and when necessary. A rising $PaCO_2$ with fall in pH should be taken as a sign of failure of NIPPV; discontinuation of NIPPV and administration of invasive ventilation should be considered **(Table 1)**. It must be remembered that a delay in decision regarding initiation of invasive ventilation is far worse than not considering NIPPV at all.

Predictors of Response to Noninvasive Positive Pressure Ventilation

It is important to recognize that certain parameters may predict success or failure of NIPPV, so that patients are not subjected to unduly prolonged treatment with NIPPV, when optimal treatment requires endotracheal intubation and conventional mechanical ventilation. These parameters should be observed during a trial of NIV **(Box 2)**. These parameters, in turn, are a reflection of the patient's ability to cooperate with NIV, patient-ventilatory synchrony, and efficacy of NIV for the clinical situation. Trials of NIPPV are usually of ~2-hour duration and are useful to determine if a patient can be managed by this modality. Extended trials without significant improvement are not recommended; this only delays intubation and mechanical ventilation (unless patients have "do-not-intubate" status). Trials may be as short as of a few minutes in patients with immediate failure and probably should not exceed 2 hours if patients fail to improve.

Objective criteria for discontinuation are important to limit trials in patients in whom NIV ultimately fails **(Table 1)**. The patients who are fulfilling these criteria are best managed by invasive mechanical ventilation, hence also referred as intubation criteria. These criteria, although carry a subjective element, have been defined in investigational studies. All these criteria are subject to some degree of interpretation in the context of the patient's clinical status. However, most patients who meet these criteria are candidates for intubation.

BOX 2 Predictors of response to noninvasive positive pressure ventilation (NIPPV).

- *Predictors of successful response to trial of NIPPV (1–2 hours):*
  - Improvement in $PaCO_2$ (a decrease of greater than 8 mm Hg)
  - Improvement in pH (> 0.06)
  - Correction of respiratory acidosis
- *Predictors of failure:*
  - Severity of illness:
    - Acidosis (pH < 7.25)
    - Hypercapnia (>80 and pH < 7.25)
    - Acute Physiology and Chronic Health Evaluation II (APACHE II) score higher than 20
  - Level of consciousness:
    - Neurologic score (>4 = stuporous, arousal only after vigorous stimulation; inconsistently follows commands)
    - Encephalopathy score (>3 = major confusion, daytime sleepiness, or agitation)
    - Glasgow Coma Scale score lower than 8
  - Failure of improvement with 12–24 hours of noninvasive ventilation
- *Late failures (>48 hours after initiation of NIPPV):*
  - Admission predictors of failure:
    - Lower functional status (Activity score < 2 = dyspnea on light activity)
    - Initial acidosis (pH < 7.22)
    - Hospital complications (pneumonia, shock, and coma)

($PaCO_2$: partial pressure of carbon dioxide)

CLINICAL USES OF NONINVASIVE POSITIVE PRESSURE VENTILATION: EVIDENCE AND RECOMMENDATIONS

Hypercapnic Respiratory Failure

Chronic Obstructive Pulmonary Disease

After several randomized controlled trials, a general consensus has been reached that NIPPV has an important role in the management of selected patients with ARF due to exacerbation of COPD.[5,18-20] This therapeutic modality has also been used in chronic stable phase of COPD and for facilitation of extubation in patients who required intubation.

- *NIPPV in acute exacerbation of COPD:* Use of NIPPV for management of ARF secondary to acute exacerbation of COPD is now the standard of care. NIPPV acts primarily by reducing patients' effort and work of breathing in patients with COPD presenting with acute exacerbation.[18,19] Several randomized trials have documented reduction in requirement of endotracheal intubation, ICU and hospital stay, and mortality.[21-23] There have been several randomized trials that have documented benefit of this modality in patients with ARF secondary to COPD.[24,25] NIPPV also leads to reduced rate of nosocomial pneumonia and other complications related to endotracheal intubation. Therefore, all the patients with ARF secondary to COPD should receive benefit of NIPPV, unless there are contraindications. Patients with type II respiratory failure secondary to COPD with altered level of consciousness improve within 30–60 minutes with NIPPV. Therefore, such patients should get the therapy under close monitoring.

- *NIPPV in chronic stable COPD:* The possibility that NIPPV might aid patients with severe COPD has intrigued clinicians for decades. Earlier investigators thought that the intermittent use of NIPPV might give rest to the mechanically disadvantaged respiratory muscles, relieving chronic fatigue and enhancing ventilatory and overall functions. NIPPV led to improvement in ABGs, unloading of respiratory muscles when pressures were set according to patients' comfort, and improvement in ABGs in COPD patients with chronic hypercapnia.[26] Use of nocturnal NIPPV in chronic stable COPD patients with CO_2 retention leads to significant improvement in day time blood gases and sleep quality, compared to those receiving oxygen therapy alone.[26] The principal mechanisms for improved gas exchange in patients with COPD following NIPPV include decreased gas trapping and increased ventilatory sensitivity to $PaCO_2$.[27] Changes in some volitional muscle strength measures may reflect improved patient effort.

The NIPPV is also shown to significantly reduce ICU admissions, and improve alveolar ventilation, exercise capacity, quality of life.[28,29] Not all the studies have shown benefit of NIPPV in chronic COPD. Some investigators have failed to show additional benefits from NIPPV over oxygen therapy and comprehensive rehabilitation programs. In some studies, the long-term use of NIPPV is discouraged in severe stable COPD patients without significant hypercapnia.[30] Nocturnal NIPPV provides significant physiological and clinical benefits to stable patients with severe COPD with significant hypercapnia. NIPPV may be more effective in selected patients with hypercapnia and hypoxemia.[5,18] The use of NIPPV among patients with stable COPD and hypercapnia was also shown to be associated with significantly lower death rate as compared to standard treatment.[31]

Clearly, the data on mortality benefit of NIPPV use in long-term management of severe COPD is not robust enough to justify the routine use of NIPPV for home ventilation. However, given the positive impact of nocturnal use of NIPPV on physiological parameters, as well as subjective symptoms, there is significant benefit in terms of reduction of morbidity and possibly mortality. In fact, a selected group of patients may well benefit from domiciliary mechanical ventilation, we need to identify who they are. Moreover, NIPPV can be a new strategy to improve exercise tolerance in COPD patients. Larger studies designed to determine the impact of NIPPV on long-term mortality in these patients are required and a routine use of NIPPV must await such data.[5,32]

Facilitating Extubation in Chronic Obstructive Pulmonary Disease

Based on success of NIPPV in managing patients with ARF, there have been efforts to try the same in patients on conventional mechanical ventilation, in order to facilitate weaning and prevent reintubation in patients with COPD. In these patients, NIPPV can be used in three ways:

1. Using NIPPV after early extubation, in order to reduce duration of invasive mechanical ventilation
2. Using NIPPV as a prophylactic measure to avoid respiratory failure and reintubation
3. Using NIPPV as a therapeutic option in patients who develop respiratory distress after extubation, in order to avert endotracheal intubation.

The evidence suggests that NIPPV weaning was significantly associated with reduced mortality; fewer ventilator-associated pneumonia; lesser length of ICU stay and hospitalization; reduced total duration of ventilation and duration of invasive ventilation; and need for tracheostomy.[33,34] Benefits in mortality and weaning failures were significantly greater in trials that exclusively enrolled patients with COPD versus mixed populations.[34] Based on these findings, patients intubated for hypercapnic respiratory failure due to COPD who fail spontaneous breathing trials should be considered for a trial of extubation to NIPPV. This approach should be reserved for patients who are good candidates for NIPPV in other respects and who are able to tolerate levels of pressure support easily administered via mask (i.e., 15 cmH_2O). In addition, there should not have been a difficult intubation.

Bronchial Asthma

Asthma exacerbations are similar to COPD exacerbations. There is increased airway obstruction, dynamic hyperinflation, and impaired ventilatory effort, leading to respiratory muscle fatigue. However, there is a paucity of randomized controlled trials on the use of NIPPV in asthma. Initial positive results have been reported in a limited number of case reports, case series, or uncontrolled studies with both CPAP and BiPAP.[35-38] NIPPV in asthma patients with ARF has been associated with improved gas exchange and avoidance of intubation in an uncontrolled study. A prospective randomized controlled study including 53 patients with acute severe asthma showed that addition of NIPPV to standard therapy was associated with trends toward accelerated lung functions and decrease in dose of bronchodilators and duration of stay in hospital and ICU.[39]

A trial of NIPPV before intubation and mechanical ventilation should be considered in selected patients with acute asthma and respiratory failure (evidence category B). These would include patients who can tolerate and cooperate with this therapy. In view of lack of strong data, NIPPV should only be used under close observation of the experienced respiratory therapists, nurses, and physicians and in an area with facility for immediate intubation, if needed.[40]

Hypoxemic Respiratory Failure

Cardiogenic Pulmonary Edema

The NIPPV has been used in patients with cardiogenic pulmonary edema for quite a long time; both CPAP and BiPAP have been used for the same. The favorable effects on lung mechanics include improvements in alveolar recruitment and functional residual capacity and reduction in anatomic shunting. It also reduces the work of breathing by decreasing the preload and afterload. There is suggestion that the patients with cardiogenic pulmonary edema secondary to acute myocardial infarction get maximum benefits from this therapy.[41] There is always a concern of recurrence of myocardial infarction in these patients; however, there is enough evidence that use of NIPPV does not add to the risk of myocardial infarction and should not be considered a contraindication to this therapy.[42] It may be avoided in patients who require emergency life-saving procedure, such as percutaneous coronary intervention.

The NIPPV use has been shown to be associated with reductions in intubation and mortality rates.[43-45] A large trial has challenged these findings in which no mortality benefit of NIPPV was observed in patients with acute cardiogenic pulmonary edema, although it showed a more rapid improvement in respiratory distress and metabolic disturbances than the standard oxygen therapy.[42] NIPPV should be used to treat acute cardiogenic pulmonary edema with expectations of success in terms of rapid improvement in symptoms and metabolic disturbances and probably reduced mortality and intubation rate (level A).[13]

Pneumonia

Noninvasive positive pressure ventilation has been used in patients with pneumonia and ARF with variable results.[46-48] The benefits of NIPPV include reduced intubation rates, ICU length of stay, and mortality rates. Among these, the patients with underlying COPD respond better than those without the same. However, there is no strong evidence to support the routine use of NIPPV in patients with ARF due to pneumonia. NIPPV has been extensively employed in the recent coronavirus disease-2019 (COVID-19) pandemic in patients with severe COVID pneumonia with benefit.[49,50]

Acute Lung Injury/Acute Respiratory Distress Syndrome

Patients with acute lung injury (ALI)/acute respiratory distress syndrome (ARDS) require conventional mechanical ventilation using various strategies. NIPPV has been tried in patients with ALI/ARDS in an effort to avoid endotracheal intubation.[51-55] Benefits of this modality are not well documented in these trials. Therefore, NIPPV should be used in these patients with caution; endotracheal intubation should not be delayed.

Respiratory Failure in Immunocompromised Patients

Immunocompromised patients who require endotracheal intubation have higher rate of ventilator-associated pneumonia. The use of NIPPV in such patients leads to reduced rate of nosocomial infection, which results in reduced mortality and ICU stay.[56] Therefore, the current recommendations strongly favor (level A) the use of NIPPV in immunocompromised patients with ARF.[57,58]

Postoperative Respiratory Failure

The NIPPV is widely used during postoperative period in patients with abdominal and thoracic surgery.[59-61] It is believed that it provides better patient comfort and oxygenation after extubation. The current evidence shows only some usefulness of this modality, it does not strongly support the routine use of CPAP or NIPPV in postoperative patients, either prophylactically in high-risk patients or as an early therapy of respiratory insufficiency. Although data is sparse to support NIPPV, it can be safely used for respiratory distress in these patients.

Weaning or Postextubation Respiratory Failure

Noninvasive positive pressure ventilation (NIPPV) during weaning or postextubation period has been used in three ways:

1. A *facilitation technique* for early extubation in patients who fail to meet standard extubation criteria[33,62]
2. A *rescue or curative technique* for avoiding reintubation in patients who fail extubation[63,64]
3. A *preventive or prophylactic technique* for preventing extubation failure[65-67]

The NIPPV has been suggested as a means to avoid reintubation and improve outcomes in patients with failed weaning. The first report to assess the role of NIPPV for weaning dates back to 1992, when it was successfully used in assisting the return of spontaneous breathing in a small group of patients with chronic respiratory insufficiency and weaning difficulties.[68] There have been conflicting results from various trials in patients with extubation failure. NIPPV reduced the need for reintubation, ventilator-associated pneumonia, need for tracheostomy, and ICU mortality.[65,67] Notably, patients with hypercapnic respiratory failure (mainly COPD) benefitted the most. Currently available data suggest that the potential effectiveness of NIPPV for facilitating ventilator weaning and early extubation varies across patient population and that the benefit seems greatest for COPD patients. However, early indiscriminate use in all patients with risk factors is discouraged. Patients with extubation failure treated with NIPPV should be closely monitored and delays in needed intubation be avoided. Further studies are required to better identify those subcategories of patients with non-COPD respiratory failure who are most likely to benefit from NIPPV.

Palliative Care and Do-not-intubate Status

Noninvasive ventilation may be particularly useful in patients reporting to the emergency room for ARF, with a do-not-intubate (DNI) status, due to advanced age or other critical conditions. There are very few studies that have addressed this issue.[69,70] The current evidence suggests that if the patient and/or family desire prolonged survival, the NIPPV use should be reserved primarily for COPD and congestive heart failure patients.[17] On the other hand, if the goal is to palliate, relieve dyspnea, or to delay death, then NIPPV can be used for other diagnoses as well.[17] However, it should be reassessed frequently and stopped if the goal of palliation is not being met.

Other Intensive Care Unit Applications of Noninvasive Positive Pressure Ventilation

Preoxygenation before Intubation

Preoxygenation by face mask is standard of care for improving the oxygen status of the patients requiring endotracheal intubation. NIPPV has been tried by few intensive care providers considering the fact that it has the potential to improve oxygenation more effectively than oxygen by face mask.[71] It was also noticed that NIPPV might be a useful preoxygenation technique in the hypoxemic critically ill patient. However, the current evidence is insufficient to suggest the routine use of NIPPV for this purpose and further studies are required before reaching any conclusion.

Before Fiberoptic Bronchoscopy

Fiberoptic bronchoscopy (FOB) is an important tool for determining the etiological diagnosis of pneumonia. Arterial oxygen tension routinely decreases by 10–20 mm Hg in patients after they undergo uncomplicated FOB, this may complicate hypoxemia in patients with already compromised oxygen status, which puts them on high risk for developing respiratory failure or serious cardiac arrhythmias. NIPPV seems a logical approach in such situations. There is some data to suggest that its use is associated with improved oxygenation and reduces postprocedure respiratory failure in patients with severe hypoxemia undergoing bronchoscopy.[72,73] However, the ICU team must be prepared for the possibility of emergent intubation.

Chronic Ventilation Failure

Chronic ventilation failure is observed in many conditions, including the chest wall diseases, neuromuscular disease, sleep apneas, and obesity-hypoventilation syndrome.[74-76] Mechanical ventilatory support in the form of NIPPV, especially at night, may be helpful in improving ventilation in these conditions. The benefits of this modality include a reduction in need for hospitalization for respiratory illness, improvement in daytime ABGs and respiratory muscle strength, and improvement in activities of daily living.[74] Data also suggest a good long-term survival benefit of home ventilation with NIPPV.[77] For sleep apnea syndrome, NIPPV is the standard modality of therapy.

HIGH-FLOW NASAL CANNULA VERSUS NONINVASIVE VENTILATION

High-flow nasal canula (HFNC) is relatively newer mode of respiratory therapy that is capable of delivering humidified and heated oxygen with an fraction of inspired oxygen (FiO_2) ranging from 0.21 to 1.0 and a flow that can be up to 60–70 L/min. HFNC also generates a positive pharyngeal pressure of 3–6 cmH_2O that may act as a PEEP.[78] During use of HFNC, patient can eat, drink, and vocalize. Thus, HFNC allows the treating physician more control over delivery of FiO_2 (with some PEEP) with better patient comfort and compliance to the therapy. Studies comparing HFNC with NIV have shown that HFNC is not inferior to NIV in treatment of hypoxemic respiratory failure.[78] Therefore, HFNC and NIV are used interchangeably for many patients. We suggest that for patients with increased work of breathing (as evidenced by the use of accessory muscles of respiration) NIV may be preferred over HFNC.

SUMMARY

The role of NIPPV in the management of ARF has been further clarified in the recent years **(Table 2)**. Evidence is strong to support its use in the initial management of ARF in patients with COPD exacerbations, acute cardiogenic pulmonary edema, immunocompromised state, and to facilitate extubation in patients with COPD with failed spontaneous breathing trials. A trial of NIPPV is justified in patients with asthma exacerbations, postoperative respiratory failure, extubation failure or a "do-not-resuscitate" status. Supporting evidence for these indications is not strong; they should be carefully selected according to available guidelines and clinical judgment. The response to NIPPV after the 1–2 hours is the best predictor of eventual outcome, if the patient does not have a favorable initial response to NIPPV, the clinician should consider intubation.

TABLE 2: Noninvasive positive pressure ventilation (NIPPV) for various types of acute respiratory failure (ARF): Evidence for efficacy and strength of recommendation.

Type of ARF	Level of evidence[a]	Strength of recommendation[b]
Hypercapnic respiratory failure: COPD exacerbation	A	Recommended
Asthma Facilitation of extubation (COPD)	C A	Option Guideline
Hypoxemic respiratory failure: Cardiogenic pulmonary edema	A	Recommended
Pneumonia ALI/ARDS Immunocompromised Postoperative respiratory failure Extubation failure Do-not-intubate status Preintubation oxygenation	C C A B C C B	Option Option Recommended Guideline Guideline Guideline Option
Facilitation of bronchoscopy	B	Guideline

Note:

a:

A: Supported by multiple randomized controlled trials and meta-analyses;

B: Supported by more than one randomized controlled trial or case control series or cohort studies;

C: Case series or experts' consensus/opinion.

b:

Recommended: First choice for ventilatory support in selected patients Guideline: Can be used in appropriate patients with careful monitoring.

Option: Suitable for a very carefully selected minority of patients under close monitoring.

(ALI: acute lung injury; ARDS: acute respiratory distress syndrome; COPD: chronic obstructive pulmonary disease)

REFERENCES

1. Mehta S, Hill NS. Noninvasive ventilation. Am J Respir Crit Care Med. 2001;163(2):540-77.
2. Conti G, Antonelli M, Navalesi P, et al. Noninvasive vs. conventional mechanical ventilation in patients with chronic obstructive pulmonary disease after failure of medical treatment in the ward: A randomized trial. Intensive Care Med. 2002;28(12):1701-7.
3. Wood KA, Lewis L, Von Harz B, et al. The use of noninvasive positive pressure ventilation in the emergency department: Results of a randomized clinical trial. Chest. 1998;113(5):1339-46.
4. Plant PK, Owen JL, Elliott MW. Early use of non-invasive ventilation for acute exacerbations of chronic obstructive pulmonary disease on general respiratory wards: A multicentre randomised controlled trial. Lancet. 2000;355(9219):1931-5.
5. Khilnani GC, Banga A. Noninvasive ventilation in patients with chronic obstructive airway disease. Int J Chron Obstruct Pulmon Dis. 2008;3(3):351-7.
6. Unterborn JN, Hill NS. Options for mechanical ventilation in neuromuscular diseases. Clin Chest Med. 1994;15(4):765-81.
7. Goldstein RS, Molotiu N, Skrastins R, et al. Reversal of sleep-induced hypoventilation and chronic respiratory failure by nocturnal negative pressure ventilation in patients with restrictive ventilatory impairment. Am Rev Respir Dis. 1987;135(5):1049-55.
8. Grasso F, Engelberts D, Helm E, et al. Negative-pressure ventilation: Better oxygenation and less lung injury. Am J Respir Crit Care Med. 2008;177(4):412-8.
9. Ambrosino N, Vagheggini G. Non-invasive ventilation in exacerbations of COPD. Int J Chron Obstruct Pulmon Dis. 2007;2(4):471-6.
10. Mehta S, Al-Hashim AH, Keenan SP. Noninvasive ventilation in patients with acute cardiogenic pulmonary edema. Respir Care. 2009;54(2):186-95; discussion 95-7.
11. Ram FS, Wellington S, Rowe BH, et al. Non-invasive positive pressure ventilation for treatment of respiratory failure due to severe acute exacerbations of asthma. Cochrane Database Syst Rev. 2005(1):CD004360.
12. Schönhofer B, Kuhlen R, Neumann P, et al. Clinical practice guideline: Non-invasive mechanical ventilation as treatment of acute respiratory failure. Dtsch Arztebl Int. 2008;105(24):424-33.
13. Cinnella G, Conti G, Lofaso F, et al. Effects of assisted ventilation on the work of breathing: Volume-controlled versus pressure-controlled ventilation. Am J Respir Crit Care Med. 1996;153(3):1025-33.
14. Manning HL, Molinary EJ, Leiter JC. Effect of inspiratory flow rate on respiratory sensation and pattern of breathing. Am J Respir Crit Care Med. 1995;151(3 Pt 1):751-7.
15. Bunburaphong T, Imanaka H, Nishimura M, et al. Performance characteristics of bilevel pressure ventilators: A lung model study. Chest. 1997;111(4):1050-60.
16. Khalid I, Sherbini N, Qushmaq I, et al. Outcomes of patients treated with noninvasive ventilation by a medical emergency team on the wards. Respir Care. 2014;59(2):186-92.

17. Curtis JR, Cook DJ, Sinuff T, et al. Noninvasive positive pressure ventilation in critical and palliative care settings: Understanding the goals of therapy. Crit Care Med. 2007;35(3):932-9.
18. Davidson AC, Banham S, Elliott M, et al. "BTS/ICS guideline for the ventilatory management of acute hypercapnic respiratory failure in adults". Thorax. 2017; 71(Suppl 2): ii1–i35.
19. Rochwerg B, Brochard L, Elliott MW, et al. Official ERS/ATS clinical practice guidelines: Noninvasive ventilation for acute respiratory failure. Eur Respir J. 2017; 50(2):1602426.
20. Raveling T, Vonk J, Struik FM, et al. Chronic non-invasive ventilation for chronic obstructive pulmonary disease. Cochrane Database Syst Rev. 2021(8): CD002878.
21. Collaborative Research Group of Noninvasive Mechanical Ventilation for Chronic Obstructive Pulmonary Disease. Early use of non-invasive positive pressure ventilation for acute exacerbations of chronic obstructive pulmonary disease: A multicentre randomized controlled trial. Chin Med J (Engl). 2005;118(24):2034-40.
22. Lightowler JV, Wedzicha JA, Elliott MW, et al. Non-invasive positive pressure ventilation to treat respiratory failure resulting from exacerbations of chronic obstructive pulmonary disease: Cochrane systematic review and meta-analysis. BMJ. 2003;326(7382):185.
23. Khilnani GC, Saikia N, Banga A, et al. Non-invasive ventilation for acute exacerbation of COPD with very high $PaCO_2$: A randomized controlled trial. Lung India. 2010;27(3):125-30.
24. Brochard L, Isabey D, Piquet J, et al. Reversal of acute exacerbations of chronic obstructive lung disease by inspiratory assistance with a face mask. N Engl J Med. 1990;323(22):1523-30.
25. Kramer N, Meyer TJ, Meharg J, et al. Randomized, prospective trial of noninvasive positive pressure ventilation in acute respiratory failure. Am J Respir Crit Care Med. 1995;151(6):1799-806.
26. Vitacca M, Nava S, Confalonieri M, et al. The appropriate setting of noninvasive pressure support ventilation in stable COPD patients. Chest. 2000;118(5):1286-93.
27. Meecham Jones DJ, Paul EA, Jones PW, et al. Nasal pressure support ventilation plus oxygen compared with oxygen therapy alone in hypercapnic COPD. Am J Respir Crit Care Med. 1995;152(2):538-44.
28. Clini E, Sturani C, Porta R, et al. Outcome of COPD patients performing nocturnal non-invasive mechanical ventilation. Respir Med. 1998;92(10):1215-22.
29. Perrin C, El Far Y, Vandenbos F, et al. Domiciliary nasal intermittent positive pressure ventilation in severe COPD: Effects on lung function and quality of life. Eur Respir J. 1997;10(12):2835-9.
30. Shapiro SH, Ernst P, Gray-Donald K, et al. Effect of negative pressure ventilation in severe chronic obstructive pulmonary disease. Lancet. 1992;340(8833):1425-9.
31. Köhnlein T, Windisch W, Köhler D, et al. Non-invasive positive pressure ventilation for the treatment of severe stable chronic obstructive pulmonary disease: A prospective, multicentre, randomised, controlled clinical trial. Lancet Respir Med. 2014;2(9):698-705.
32. Díaz-Lobato S, Alises SM, Rodriguez EP. Current status of noninvasive ventilation in stable COPD patients. Int J Chron Obstruct Pulmon Dis. 2006;1(2):129-35.
33. Ferrer M, Esquinas A, Arancibia F, et al. Noninvasive ventilation during persistent weaning failure: A randomized controlled trial. Am J Respir Crit Care Med. 2003;168(1):70-6.
34. Burns KE, Meade MO, Premji A, et al. Noninvasive positive-pressure ventilation as a weaning strategy for intubated adults with respiratory failure. Cochrane Database Syst Rev. 2013;12:CD004127.
35. Shivaram U, Miro AM, Cash ME, et al. Cardiopulmonary responses to continuous positive airway pressure in acute asthma. J Crit Care. 1993;8(2):87-92.
36. Meduri GU, Turner RE, Abou-Shala N, et al. Noninvasive positive pressure ventilation via face mask. First-line intervention in patients with acute hypercapnic and hypoxemic respiratory failure. Chest. 1996;109(1):179-93.
37. Beers SL, Abramo TJ, Bracken A, et al. Bilevel positive airway pressure in the treatment of status asthmaticus in pediatrics. Am J Emerg Med. 2007;25(1):6-9.
38. Gupta D, Nath A, Agarwal R, et al. A prospective randomized controlled trial on the efficacy of noninvasive ventilation in severe acute asthma. Respir Care. 2010;55(5):536-43.
39. Soroksky A, Stav D, Shpirer I. A pilot prospective, randomized, placebo-controlled trial of bilevel positive airway pressure in acute asthmatic attack. Chest. 2003;123(4):1018-25.
40. Lim WJ, Mohammed Akram R, Carson KV, et al. Non-invasive positive pressure ventilation for treatment of respiratory failure due to severe acute exacerbations of asthma. Cochrane Database Syst Rev. 2012;12:CD004360.
41. Weng CL, Zhao YT, Liu QH, et al. Meta-analysis: Noninvasive ventilation in acute cardiogenic pulmonary edema. Ann Intern Med. 2010;152(9):590-600.
42. Gray A, Goodacre S, Newby DE, et al. Noninvasive ventilation in acute cardiogenic pulmonary edema. N Engl J Med. 2008;359(2):142-51.
43. Masip J, Roque M, Sanchez B, et al. Noninvasive ventilation in acute cardiogenic pulmonary edema: Systematic review and meta-analysis. JAMA. 2005;294(24):3124-30.
44. Winck JC, Azevedo LF, Costa-Pereira A, et al. Efficacy and safety of non-invasive ventilation in the treatment of acute cardiogenic pulmonary edema—a systematic review and meta-analysis. Crit Care. 2006;10(2):R69.
45. Berbenetz N, Wang Y, Brown J, et al. Non-invasive positive pressure ventilation (CPAP or bilevel NPPV) for cardiogenic pulmonary oedema. Cochrane Database Syst Rev. 2019;(4): CD005351.
46. Honrubia T, García López FJ, Franco N, et al. Noninvasive vs conventional mechanical ventilation in acute respiratory failure: a multicenter, randomized controlled trial. Chest. 2005;128(6):3916-24.
47. Nicolini A, Ferraioli G, Ferrari-Bravo M, et al. Early non-invasive ventilation treatment for respiratory failure due to severe community-acquired pneumonia. Clin Respir J. 2016;10(1): 98-103.
48. Carrillo A, Gonzalez-Diaz G, Ferrer M, et al. Non-invasive ventilation in community-acquired pneumonia and severe acute respiratory failure. Intensive Care Med. 2012;38(3):458-66.
49. Forrest IS, Jaladanki SK, Paranjpe I, et al. Non-invasive ventilation versus mechanical ventilation in hypoxemic patients with COVID-19. Infection. 2021;49(5):989-97.
50. Murthy S, Gomersall CD, Fowler RA. Care for critically ill patients with COVID-19. JAMA. 2020;323(15):1499-500.
51. Yoshida Y, Takeda S, Akada S, et al. Factors predicting successful noninvasive ventilation in acute lung injury. J Anesth. 2008;22(3):201-6.
52. Antonelli M, Conti G, Esquinas A, et al. A multiple-center survey on the use in clinical practice of noninvasive ventilation as a first-line intervention for acute respiratory distress syndrome. Crit Care Med. 2007;35(1):18-25.

53. Thille AW, Contou D, Fragnoli C, et al. Non-invasive ventilation for acute hypoxemic respiratory failure: intubation rate and risk factors. Crit Care. 2013;17(6):R269.
54. Pierson DJ. History and epidemiology of noninvasive ventilation in the acute-care setting. Respiratory Care. 2009;54(1):40-52.
55. Rittayamai N, Grieco DL, Brochard, L. Noninvasive respiratory support in intensive care medicine. Intensive Care Med. 2022;48(9):1211-14.
56. Confalonieri M, Calderini E, Terraciano S, et al. Noninvasive ventilation for treating acute respiratory failure in AIDS patients with *Pneumocystis carinii* pneumonia. Intensive Care Med. 2002;28(9):1233-8.
57. Keenan SP, Sinuff T, Burns KE, et al. Clinical practice guidelines for the use of noninvasive positive-pressure ventilation and noninvasive continuous positive airway pressure in the acute care setting. CMAJ. 2011;183(3):E195-214.
58. Schönhofer B, Kuhlen R, Neumann P, et al. Non-invasive ventilation as treatment for acute respiratory insufficiency. Essentials from the new S3 guidelines. Anaesthesist. 2008;57(11):1091-102.
59. Squadrone V, Coha M, Cerutti E, et al. Continuous positive airway pressure for treatment of postoperative hypoxemia: A randomized controlled trial. JAMA. 2005;293(5):589-95.
60. Wallet F, Schoeffler M, Reynaud M, et al. Factors associated with noninvasive ventilation failure in postoperative acute respiratory insufficiency: An observational study. Eur J Anaesthesiol. 2010;27(3):270-4.
61. Kilger E, Möhnle P, Nassau K, et al. Noninvasive mechanical ventilation in patients with acute respiratory failure after cardiac surgery. Heart Surg Forum. 2010;13(2):E91-5.
62. Kilger E, Briegel J, Haller M, et al. Effects of noninvasive positive pressure ventilatory support in non-COPD patients with acute respiratory insufficiency after early extubation. Intensive Care Med. 1999;25(12):1374-80.
63. Keenan SP, Powers C, McCormack DG, et al. Noninvasive positive-pressure ventilation for postextubation respiratory distress: A randomized controlled trial. JAMA. 2002;287(24):3238-44.
64. Esteban A, Frutos-Vivar F, Ferguson ND, et al. Noninvasive positive-pressure ventilation for respiratory failure after extubation. N Engl J Med. 2004;350(24):2452-60.
65. Nava S, Gregoretti C, Fanfulla F, et al. Noninvasive ventilation to prevent respiratory failure after extubation in high-risk patients. Crit Care Med. 2005;33(11):2465-70.
66. Ferrer M, Valencia M, Nicolas JM, et al. Early noninvasive ventilation averts extubation failure in patients at risk: A randomized trial. Am J Respir Crit Care Med. 2006;173(2):164-70.
67. Khilnani GC, Galle AD, Hadda V, et al. Non-invasive ventilation after extubation in patients with chronic obstructive airways disease: A randomised controlled trial. Anaesth Intensive Care. 2011;39(2):217-23.
68. Udwadia ZF, Santis GK, Steven MH, et al. Nasal ventilation to facilitate weaning in patients with chronic respiratory insufficiency. Thorax. 1992;47(9):715-8.
69. Levy M, Tanios MA, Nelson D, et al. Outcomes of patients with do-not-intubate orders treated with noninvasive ventilation. Crit Care Med. 2004;32(10):2002-7.
70. Scarpazza P, Incorvaia C, di Franco G, et al. Effect of noninvasive mechanical ventilation in elderly patients with hypercapnic acute-on-chronic respiratory failure and a do-not-intubate order. Int J Chron Obstruct Pulmon Dis. 2008;3(4):797-801.
71. Baillard C, Fosse JP, Sebbane M, et al. Noninvasive ventilation improves preoxygenation before intubation of hypoxic patients. Am J Respir Crit Care Med. 2006;174(2):171-7.
72. Antonelli M, Conti G, Rocco M, et al. Noninvasive positive-pressure ventilation vs. conventional oxygen supplementation in hypoxemic patients undergoing diagnostic bronchoscopy. Chest. 2002;121(4):1149-54.
73. Heunks LM, de Bruin CJ, van der Hoeven JG, et al. Non-invasive mechanical ventilation for diagnostic bronchoscopy using a new face mask: An observational feasibility study. Intensive Care Med. 2010;36(1):143-7.
74. Baumann HJ, Klose H, Simon M, et al. Fiber optic bronchoscopy in patients with acute hypoxemic respiratory failure requiring noninvasive ventilation—a feasibility study. Crit Care. 2011;15(4):R179.
75. Simonds AK. Nocturnal ventilation in neuromuscular disease--when and how? Monaldi Arch Chest Dis. 2002;57(5-6):273-6.
76. Mokhlesi B, Masa JF, Brozek JL, et al. Evaluation and management of obesity hypoventilation syndrome. An official American thoracic society clinical practice guideline. Am J Respir Crit Care Med. 2019;200(3):e6–e24.
77. Simonds AK. Home ventilation. Eur Respir J Suppl. 2003,47.38s-46s.
78. Oczkowski S, Ergan B, Bos L, et al. ERS clinical practice guidelines: High flow nasal cannula in acute respiratory failure. Eur Respir J. 2022;59(4):2101574.

Mechanical Ventilation: General Principles and Modes

CHAPTER 161

GC Khilnani, Vijay Hadda

INTRODUCTION

Mechanical ventilation is an important method to save the life of critically ill patients. In both forms, invasive and noninvasive, positive-pressure ventilation is widely used worldwide. About one-third of adult intensive care unit (ICU) patients receive mechanical ventilation.[1,2] Conceptually, mechanical ventilation is a process to provide O_2 and CO_2 transport between the environment and the alveolar pulmonary capillary interface, with the help of a device with the objectives to maintain appropriate PaO_2 and $PaCO_2$ in arterial blood and reduction in work of breathing. Originally, a mechanical ventilator (MV) consisted of a simple, manually driven pump device, which over the period has developed into an advanced positive-pressure ventilator for continuous support of patients in respiratory failure. The earlier MVs delivered fixed volumes or pressures with fixed rates and breath durations; however, later advancements allow the patient to trigger the ventilator with their own effort, which can then be cycled off on time criteria or when certain flow criteria are met.[3] Latest MVs provide many variables, which may be controlled to provide the ventilatory support depending on the underlying disease in an intermittent fashion, mimicking natural breathing. With these advancements, the survival rate in patients requiring mechanical ventilation has significantly improved.[4] The basic principles and application of different ventilators are broadly similar.

INDICATIONS OF MECHANICAL VENTILATION

Mechanical ventilation is often used to manage ventilatory or oxygenation failure or an impending failure. Failure to ventilate or oxygenate adequately may be caused by several pulmonary or extrapulmonary conditions, belonging to three distinct groups:

1. *Depressed respiratory drive*: This group includes drug overdose (narcotic, sedative, alcohol, etc.), acute spinal cord injury, head trauma, neurologic disorders (coma, stroke, etc.), sleep disorders (e.g., sleep apnea), and metabolic alkalosis.
2. *Excessive ventilatory workload*: This group includes acute airflow obstruction, e.g., chronic obstructive pulmonary disease (COPD), asthma or epiglottitis, dead-space ventilation (pulmonary embolism and emphysema), acute lung injury (ALI), e.g., acute respiratory distress syndrome (ARDS), cardiovascular decompensation [decreased cardiac output, ventilation/perfusion (V/Q) mismatch], shock, increased metabolic rate (fever), drugs, and decreased compliance (atelectasis, pneumothorax, and obesity).
3. *Ventilatory pump failure*: This includes chest trauma (flail chest, tension pneumothorax), premature birth (idiopathic respiratory distress syndrome), electrolyte imbalance (hyperkalemia or hypokalemia), and geriatric patients (muscle fatigue).

BASIC ASPECTS OF MECHANICAL VENTILATION

Phase Variables

The actual factors that provide the four components of a ventilator-delivered breath are called the phase variables. These factors or variables are responsible for changing of one phase of the respiratory cycle into the next and for controlling what occurs during that portion of the breath. The four phases of a breath consists of:

1. Inspiratory phase
2. Change from inspiration to expiration
3. Expiratory phase
4. Change from expiration to inspiration

In each of these four phases, a certain variable (time, pressure, volume, or flow) is measured and used to initiate, maintain, and end the phase.

Triggering of Breath

Triggering is the term applied to the variable that changes from expiration to inspiration.

When a variable, such as time, pressure, volume, or flow, reaches a preset value and causes the ventilator to change from expiration to inspiration, the ventilator is said to be triggered by that parameter. The ventilator is said to be time-triggered, where inspiration begins when a certain time has elapsed. This occurs independent from a patient's spontaneous effort. In pressure triggering, the ventilator senses the patient's inspiratory effort sufficient to cause a drop in the baseline airway pressure by preset value and initiates inspiration. The breath occurs regardless of the set rate. It is essential to find the individual patient's need and set sensitivity accordingly; otherwise, either the patient has to work hard or there will be autotriggering. A ventilator is said to be flow-triggered, when the baseline flow variable drops below a preset flow and initiate inspiration. Ventilators can also be manually triggered in most cases. This is accomplished by activating the "manual breath" control.

Limiting a Breath

Limiting is a term used to describe the variables that have a limiting value during inspiration or expiration, which could be time, flow, or pressure. The length of inspiration is the time from the beginning of inspiratory flow to the start of expiratory flow. During the inspiratory phase, the ventilator can control pressure, volume, or flow as described previously in this section. In addition, the ventilator can also limit these variables. Limiting in simple words means that the variable can reach the preset value but never goes higher than it.

Cycling of Breath

Cycling is defined by the preset variable, causing the ventilator to end the inspiration and switch it to expiration. During this process, a preset variable (time, pressure, volume, or flow) is actually measured by the ventilator; this information is used by the ventilator to determine when to end the inspiratory flow.

Time-cycled ventilation: This is one of the common cycling mechanisms used in clinical practice; time-cycling terminates the inspiratory gas flow and changes to the expiratory phase, when a preselected time interval has elapsed after the start of inspiration. At the designated time, the exhalation valve opens and the delivered tidal volume (VT) is vented to the ambient atmosphere. At a constant gas flow and controlled time interval, VT can be predicted according to the following relationship:

$$\text{Volume} = \text{Flow (volume/unit time)} \times \text{Time}$$

Pressure-cycled ventilation: In this cycling, ventilation terminates the inspiratory phase, when a preselected airway pressure is achieved. The exhalation valve then opens, initiating the expiratory phase. VT and the time of active flow delivery will vary in pressure-cycled ventilation, depending on the airway resistance, chest wall, and lung compliance and the integrity of the ventilator circuit. As the volume delivery is unpredictable with pressure cycling, this mode is uncommonly used in intensive care settings. They are used predominately for intermittent positive-pressure breathing, ventilator support at home, and while using inverse ratio ventilation (IRV).

Volume-cycled ventilation: In volume-cycled ventilation, the inspiration is terminated when a preselected volume of gas has been delivered. There is fear of development of excessive airway pressure, in case of airway obstruction; therefore, volume-cycled ventilators have pressure-limiting valves that prevent excessive pressure within the system. Without this pressure-limiting valve, excessive pressure may lead to barotrauma. There has been a belief that volume-cycled ventilation maintains constant VT delivery to the patient, regardless of changes in resistance and compliance. This characteristic is largely responsible for the popularity of these devices in critical care settings. But the volume of gas received by the patient may vary considerably with volume-cycled ventilation. The variability occurs, since the gas flows into the circuit and the patient. When the ventilator triggers, a larger proportion of the volume is lost within the circuit due to expansion of the tubing and compression of the inspiratory gas within the humidifier or nebulizer, water traps, bellows, or cylinder and connectors. Conversely, if the patient's compliance improves, less inspiratory gas is retained within the circuit.

Flow-cycled ventilation: The inspiration ends when a preset flow is achieved. Flow-cycled ventilation is independent of airway pressure, VT, or duration of inspiration. Flow-cycled mode is most commonly used during pressure-support (PS) ventilation, in which it is common for the ventilator to cycle into exhalation when the flow during inspiration has dropped to 25% of the peak inspiratory flow.

Patient–ventilator Interactions

Most of the modern MVs utilize piston or bellow systems of high-pressure gas source to drive the gas flow. The newer MVs provide "interactive" modes in that the patient can interact with ventilator and affect its functions. These interactions can range from simple triggering of mechanical breaths to more complex processes, which can affect various aspects of tidal breath, such as the flow pattern and breath timing. The patient interacts with the ventilator based on three physiological variables:[5]

1. Ventilatory drive when inspiration starts
2. Ventilatory requirement, i.e., how much flow and volume are required to satisfy the metabolic demand
3. Timing of the integrated circuits generating the respiratory rhythm, as measured by the duration and ratio of inspiratory time (TI) to total breath cycle duration

Similarly, a ventilator interacts with the patient based on three technologic variables:

1. The inspiratory trigger or when the ventilator starts to deliver flow, volume, and pressure
2. The delivery of the gas, i.e., the algorithm used by the ventilator to assist ventilation through delivery of flow, volume, or pressure

3. Cycling or when the ventilator stops assisting the inspiratory effort and lets the patient exhale spontaneously

Interactive modes allow for muscle activity, which when done at nonfatiguing or physiologic levels may prevent muscle atrophy and facilitate fatigue recovery.[6,7] In addition, permitting spontaneous patient ventilator activity and using comfortable interactive modes may reduce the need for sedation and/or of neuromuscular blockers, which are often required to prevent patients from "fighting" controlled ventilation.[8] For the ventilation to be effective, these interactions should be synchronous during different phases of interactive breathe delivery, i.e., breathe triggering, ventilator flow delivery, and breathe cycling.

Synchronous interactions imply that the ventilator is sensitive to the initiation, modulation, and termination of a patient's ventilatory effort. The importance of these variables is described as follows.

Interactions during breath triggering: During the interactive mode of ventilation, MVs need to sense a spontaneous effort (a drop in airway pressure or flow change), in order to trigger a mechanical response. Even with modern advanced sensors, there is some unavoidable dyssynchrony in the triggering process due to the artifacts triggering the ventilator (i.e., autocycling) or a certain inherent delay (system responsiveness) in opening of demand valve. Both of these factors can result in a significant work of breathing during the triggering process. In the setting of air trapping and auto-positive end expiratory pressure (PEEP), the elevated alveolar pressure at end expiration can serve as a significant triggering threshold load on the ventilatory muscles. In these circumstances, appropriate use of external PEEP can equilibrate expiratory pressure throughout the lungs and ventilator circuit to reduce this triggering load.[9]

Interaction during ventilator-delivered flow: During an interactive breath, ventilatory muscles contract.[10] At this point, the ventilator flow delivery should be adequate to meet one of three goals:

1. Fully unload the contracting ventilatory muscles in patients with severely overloaded and fatigued muscles.
2. Partially unload the contracting ventilatory muscles in patients recovering from muscle fatigue.
3. Add no imposed loads on muscles in patients during spontaneous breathing trials, i.e., continuous positive airway pressure (CPAP).

Synchronous flow interactions are required to achieve these goals. There is evidence that suggests that pressure-targeting breathe, by providing a variable flow, tends to synchronize better with patient effort than the fixed flow pattern of the flow-targeted breath.[11] Moreover, a single, consistent assisted or supported breath pattern more readily synchronizes with breath types. Thus, when partial support is desired, pressure-support/-assist (PS or PA) approach alone appears preferable to synchronized intermittent mandatory ventilation (SIMV). Although SIMV offers the advantage of a guaranteed ventilator rate during partial support, the PA control mode can similarly provide both interactive pressure-targeted assisted breaths and backup pressure-targeted controlled breaths.

Interaction during breath-cycling: Cycling dyssynchrony can occur in one of two ways: (1) If the breath lasts beyond patient effort, an inadequate expiratory time (TE) may develop (along with air trapping) and/or patient expiratory efforts may be required to terminate the breath, and (2) if the breath terminates before the patient's effort ends, the patient may be left demanding additional flow without any tidal breathe being delivered by the machine, which significantly imposes loading and/or double-breath triggering may result. Cycle dyssynchrony can be addressed by adjusting the VT or TI in flow/volume-targeted ventilation, by adjusting the TI in PA-control ventilation, or by adjusting the cycle criteria in PS mode of ventilation.

In recent years, certain innovations have been introduced to improve patient–ventilator synchrony during interactive modes of ventilation, such as automatic tube compensation, inspiratory pressure slope, and proportional-assist ventilation (PAV). These have significantly reduced the problem of patient–ventilator dyssynchrony.

MODES OF MECHANICAL VENTILATION

Technological advances have provided a number of different modes, by which a patient can be mechanically ventilated. However, the primary targets are to improve gas exchange, provide patient comfort, and speed up weaning from mechanical ventilation. All the ventilators are equipped to deliver either volume-set or pressure-set ventilation. In volume-set ventilation, a preset VT is delivered at whatever pressure it is required. On the other hand, in pressure-set modes, a fixed inspiratory pressure (P_{insp}) is applied to the respiratory system. Whatever the resulting VT, both usually achieve the same level of ventilation in fully paralyzed patients. In these patients, plateau pressure (P_{plat}) is determined by VT and static respiratory system compliance (C_{rs}):

$$P_{plat} = VT/C_{rs} + PEEP \text{ (including auto-PEEP)}$$

Further, VT is predictable (in paralyzed patients), if C_{rs} is known:

$$VT = (P_{insp} - PEEP) \times C_{rs}$$

Though the physician's comfort level with volume-set and pressure-set modes may vary, both modes are similarly tied to each other through the patient's C_{rs}. The potential advantage of pressure-set ventilation is probably greater physician control over the peak airway pressure (P_{rw}) and the peak alveolar pressure (P_{alv}), hence reduction of ventilator-induced lung injury (VILI). However, it could be also attainable with low VT (typically 5–8 mL/kg) in volume-set ventilation. Other advantages of pressure-set modes are greater control over inspiratory flow rate and therefore potentially increased comfort. The disadvantage of pressure-set modes is the increased airflow resistance or lung stiffness, which decreases the minute ventilation. Volume-set modes provide ventilation but require pressure alarms to detect new abnormalities in respiratory mechanics.

Controlled Mechanical Ventilation

The term controlled mechanical ventilation (CMV) has been used to describe a volume or pressure-controlled and time-triggered form of ventilation. The operator sets the desired VT (volume controlled) or peak airway pressure (pressure controlled), respiratory rate/frequency (*f*), TI, and I:E ratio. The patient's ventilation is totally controlled by ventilator and the patient cannot trigger the ventilator **(Fig. 1)**. However, the controlled ventilation does not guarantee that the patient will not attempt to initiate spontaneous ventilation. In such situations, the ventilator will not respond if it is used strictly in a control mode implying that the ventilator sensitivity is kept "off". This may result in patient-ventilator asynchrony; that is, the patient attempts to take more breaths than what the ventilator can provide. It adds to significant patient apprehension, results in CO_2 retention, and increased work of breathing. To overcome the problem, the patients need heavy sedation and/or neuromuscular blockade. The complications observed with use of CMV include excessive ventilation, use of sedatives and muscle relaxants, and muscle atrophy resulting from disuse.[7,12,13] Further, use of heavy sedation/neuromuscular blockade imposes a great risk of apnea/hypoxia in case of accidental ventilator disconnection.

Volume-controlled (Targeted) Ventilation

Volume-controlled (targeted) mode requires that the operator set a desired VT. Usually, the operator also sets the rate or TI and gas flow, including flow pattern. During this mode of ventilation, the peak pressure varies from breath to breath depending on several factors, primarily a patient's lung compliance. However, volume delivered is usually constant.

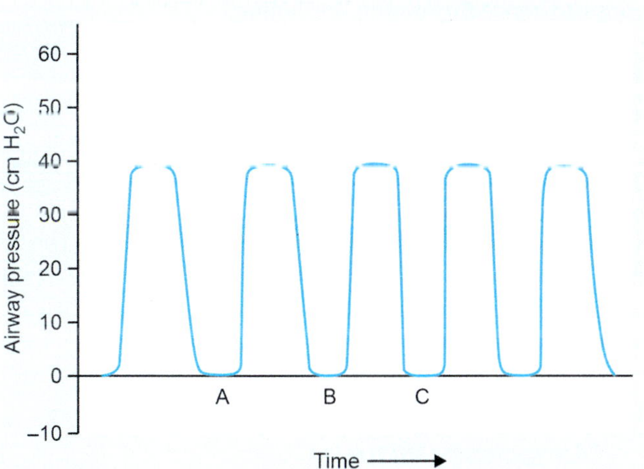

FIG. 1: A graphical presentation of controlled mechanical ventilation (CMV).

Pressure-controlled (Targeted) Ventilation

Pressure-controlled ventilation (PCV), unlike volume targeted modes, is pressure and time cycled and generates VTs that vary with the impedance of the respiratory system. The ventilation is determined by *f*, the inspiratory pressure increment (P_{insp} – PEEP), and I:E ratio. A working understanding of the factors that determine volume delivery is necessary for proper implementation of this mode of ventilation.

During the inspiratory phase of PCV, gas flows briskly into the ventilator circuit to pressurize the system to a specified target. Once the target pressure has been reached, flow is adjusted to maintain a flat or "square wave" pressure profile over the remainder of the set TI.[14] This is achieved by measuring airway pressure approximately every 2 ms to provide critical feedback to flow controller mechanisms within the ventilator. By tracking the rate of change in pressure during inspiration, appropriate deceleration can occur as the pressure ceiling is approached. Flow is brisk, if the gradient between the circuit pressure and the pressure target is large. As in patients without severe obstruction, given a sufficiently long TI, there is equilibrium between the ventilator-determined P_{insp} and P_{alv} and inspiratory flow ceases. In such cases, VT can be predicted based on P_{insp} (=P_{alv}) and the mechanical properties of the respiratory system (C_{rs}). As the gradient between the recorded pressure and preset target narrows, flow decelerates to prevent overshoot. In situations of severe airflow obstruction or if TI is too short to allow equilibration between ventilator and alveoli, VT will fall below the predicted, based on P_{insp} and C_{rs}.

Advantages of Pressure-controlled Ventilation

Pressure-controlled ventilation facilitates ventilation with a lung-protective strategy. When one of the goals of ventilator management is to limit alveolar overdistention, PCV ensures that P_{alv} never exceeds the prefixed threshold value (usually 30–35 cm H_2O). Pressure limits and decelerating flow profiles are thought to produce more uniform distribution of forces within the lung, possibly reducing the risk of barotrauma. PCV leads to improved oxygenation and higher static and dynamic compliance along with improved measures of work of breathing. PCV is increasingly used in patients with ARDS to deliver inspiratory reserve volume (IRV), in which the TI exceeds the TE.

Disadvantage of Pressure-controlled Ventilation

Pressure-controlled ventilation, especially when done as IRV, generally requires sedation and sometimes leads to paralysis, which may have adverse effects on weaning.

Assist-control Mode of Ventilation

Assist-control mode of ventilation (ACMV) is the most commonly used mode of ventilation all over the world. It delivers controlled breaths as well as assists patient-triggered breaths. During ACMV, the operator can set the inspiratory flow rate (V•), frequency (*f*), and VT. In some ventilators, one must set the total minute ventilation and rate, thereby determining VT and indirectly determining V•. In fully paralyzed or sedated patients, ACMV behaves like CMV delivering tidal breaths per minute at an operator set rate. VT and V• determine the TI, TE, and I:E ratio. In turn, P_{plat} depends on VT and C_{rs}. A patient who has their own adequate respiratory effort can trigger the ventilator **(Fig. 2)**. During such a breath, the ventilator assists the patient and delivers the set VT at the patient's respiratory rate. This ability to trigger extra breaths may change TI, TE, and I:E ratio and may create or increase auto-PEEP. This can be overcome by setting controlled ventilator frequency, a few breaths per minute below the patient's rate, so the control rate serves as an adequate support should the patient stop initiating breaths. If high inspiratory effort continues during the ventilator-delivered breath (few patients may trigger a second or third superimposed/stacked breath), it will lead to breath stacking.

On the ACMV mode, patients continue to perform inspiratory work even on a ventilator.[6] This may not be easily appreciated, despite careful examination of the patient, unless intrathoracic pressures (esophageal pressure or central venous pressure) are measured. Since effort at the end of the breath will affect the peak pressure (P_{pk}) and P_{plat}, determination of respiratory system mechanics may be unreliable. Clues to patient effort are also often available from the airway pressure tracing **(Fig. 2)**. If a patient assists every breath, the work of breathing can be increased, by either increasing the magnitude of the trigger or by lowering VT. Lowering of "*f*" at the same VT generally has no effect on work of breathing.

Indications of Assist-control Mode of Ventilation

The ACMV mode is most often used to provide full ventilatory support in the first place. Typically, these patients have stable respiratory drive (an adequate inspiratory effort of at least 10–12 breaths/min) and therefore can trigger the ventilator into inspiration. The time-triggering control rate (backup rate) is generally considered as safety net, to provide adequate ventilation in case the patient stops triggering the ventilator. In general, the accepted minimum control rate for

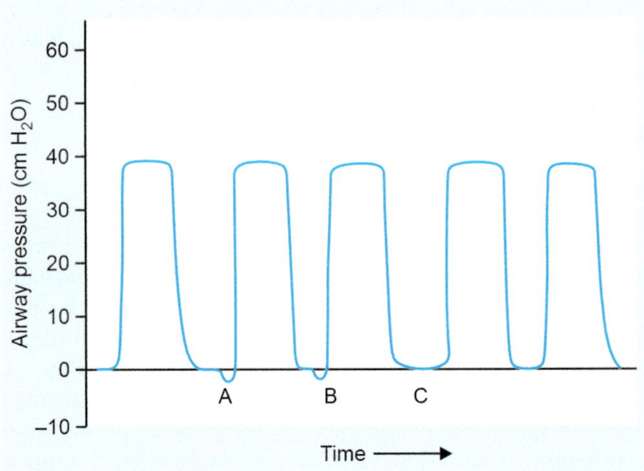

FIG. 2: A graphical presentation of assist controlled mechanical ventilation (ACMV). Each assisted as well as controlled breath triggers a mechanical ventilator to deliver tidal volume. The assisted breath is characterized by a negative deflection at the beginning of inspiration (breaths A and B) while in controlled breathing, there is no negative deflection at the onset of inspiration (breath C).

the ACMV mode is 2–4 breaths/min, lower than the patient's assist rate or a minimum control rate of 12–15 breaths/min.

Advantages of Assist-control Mode of Ventilation

There are two advantages of ACMV mode. First, the work of breathing which is required is minimal when trigger sensitivity is set appropriately and when the ventilator supplies adequate flow that meets or exceeds a patient's inspiratory demand. Second, if the patient has an appropriate ventilatory drive, this mode allows the patient to control the respiratory rate and hence the minute ventilation.

Complications of Assist-control Mode of Ventilation

Alveolar hyperventilation or respiratory alkalosis is the most important complication associated with the ACMV mode. Patients on ACMV had higher pH and lower $PaCO_2$, when compared to intermittent mandatory ventilation (IMV).[15] This is an important consideration in patients having inappropriately high respiratory drive/rate due to disease/injury to the respiratory center.

Synchronized Intermittent Mandatory Ventilation

Synchronized intermittent mandatory ventilation works as CMV in fully paralyzed patients, where ventilation is determined by the mandatory *f*, VT, and V. In SIMV, if the patient has breathing effort, he or she may perform respiratory

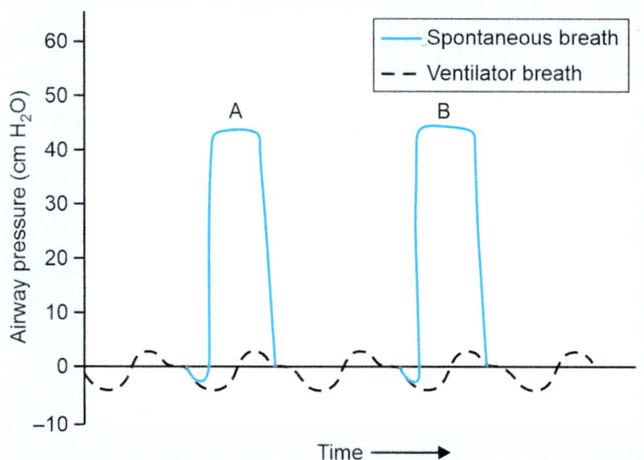

FIG. 3: A graphical presentation of synchronized intermittent mandatory ventilation (SIMV). Tracing is showing two mandatory breaths (A and B) and five triggered breaths. In SIMV, the mandatory breaths may be delivered slightly sooner or later (during a small window period) than the preset time, so that the anticipated breath during this is converted into mechanical breath.

work during the mandatory breaths also. Moreover, the patient can trigger additional breaths, by lowering airway opening pressure (P_{ao}) below the trigger threshold **(Fig. 3)**. If this triggering effort comes in a brief, defined interval (synchronization window) before the next mandatory breath is due, the ventilator will deliver the mandatory breath ahead of the scheduled breath, in order to synchronize with the patient's inspiratory effort. If a breath is initiated outside the synchronization window VT, V and I:E ratio are determined by a patient's effort and respiratory mechanics, not by ventilator settings. These spontaneous breaths tend to be small and variable from breath to breath. In the absence of breathing effort by the patient, the ventilator will deliver a tidal breath with preset VT and rate. The SIMV mode is often used to gradually augment the patient's work of breathing for weaning. This can be achieved by lowering either the mandatory breath or the VT. This approach prolongs the process of weaning.[16]

Indications for Synchronized Intermittent Mandatory Ventilation mode

The primary indication of SIMV is to provide partial ventilatory support, so the patient is actively involved in providing part of minute volume. For practical purposes, full ventilatory support is provided usually for the first 24 hours. After this initial period of full ventilator support, the usual practice of partial ventilatory support, such as SIMV, is tried. SIMV have been used for weaning by gradually reducing the rate, but it prolongs weaning, as compared to that with PS or spontaneous breathing trial. SIMV promotes spontaneous breathing and use of respiratory muscles to provide the following beneficial acts:

- Maintenance of respiratory muscle strength and avoidance of muscle atrophy
- Reduced ventilation-perfusion mismatch
- Decreased mean airway pressure
- Help in weaning

Synchronized intermittent mandatory ventilation has an inherent property to provide a spontaneous breathing workload that gradually increases a patient's muscle strength and endurance. The primary disadvantage is breath wasting, which may occur when the patient breathes outside the synchronization window. Although SIMV is commonly used for weaning, this approach prolongs the process of weaning.

Pressure-support Ventilation

Pressure-support ventilation is delivered to the mechanically ventilated patient during spontaneous breathing. It is a triggered mode, with changes in airway pressure or flow used as the trigger signal. Ventilation is determined by P_{insp}, patient-determined *f*, and patient effort. Following detection of spontaneous patient effort, the ventilator delivers a breath, i.e., flow cycled but time limited. Once a breath is triggered, the ventilator attempts to maintain P_{ao} at the preset P_{insp} using whatever flow is necessary. Eventually, flow begins to fall due to cessation of the patient's inspiratory effort or due to increasing elastic recoil of the respiratory system as VT rises. The termination point is determined by the algorithm within the ventilator; it is usually a function of the delivered VT. At the termination point, inspiratory flow ceases and the breath cycles directly into expiration.

Pressure-support ventilation, although is commonly used for weaning purpose, has a potential for providing full ventilatory support. A potential advantage of PS ventilation is improved patient comfort.[17] When a patient is well maintained [on clinical and arterial blood gas (ABG) parameters] at a PS of 5–7 cm H_2O, it indicates that the patient can be extubated. The patient's own effort is essential for PSV. PSV can account for a large fraction of total minute ventilation, even when set at rather low levels in patients with normal respiratory system mechanics. Old ventilators do not have a back support with PSV; therefore, there is a risk of apnea/hypoxia. PS ventilation is commonly used for weaning.

Positive End Expiratory Pressure

Positive end expiratory pressure increases the end expiratory or baseline airway pressure to a value greater than atmospheric pressure **(Fig. 4)**. PEEP is not a standalone mode; it is rather applied in conjunction with other ventilatory modes. It is used mainly to recruit or stabilize lung units and improve oxygenation in patients with hypoxemic respiratory failure.

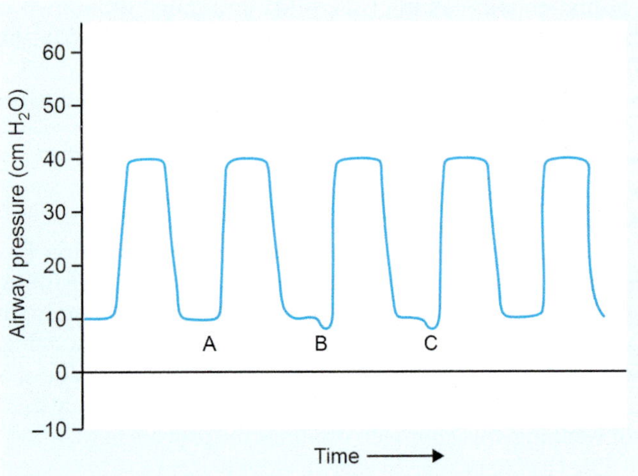

FIG. 4: A graphical presentation of positive end-expiratory pressure (PEEP). It is a pressure tracing of assist-controlled mode of mechanical ventilation with a PEEP of 10 cm H_2O. "A" is controlled breath, while "B" and "C" are assisted breaths with PEEP.

Advantages of Positive End Expiratory Pressure

Use of PEEP has positive effects on both the gas exchange and lung mechanics with the following advantages:[18,19]

- *Gas exchange*:
  - Redistributes fluid within the alveoli and reduces intrapulmonary shunting
  - Improves arterial oxygenation (PaO_2)
  - Reduces FiO_2 requirement and risk of oxygen toxicity
- *Lung mechanics*:
  - Helps in preventing alveolar collapse
  - Stabilizes and recruits lung units
  - Increases functional residual capacity (FRC)
  - Improves lung compliance
  - Shifts tidal deflections to the right along the inspiratory pressure–volume curve, minimizing potential for VILI, by preventing repetitive collapse of lung units at end expiration followed by reopening during inspiration.
  - May decrease the inspiratory work of breathing due to auto-PEEP in patients with obstructive airway disease.

Indications of Positive End Expiratory Pressure

Indications of PEEP include the respiratory failure either due to intrapulmonary shunting or due to decreased FRC, e.g., ALI and ARDS, cardiogenic pulmonary edema, diffuse pneumonia requiring mechanical ventilation, atelectasis associated with severe hypoxemia, and other forms of severe hypoxemic respiratory failure. PEEP is also used in patients with COPD, where there is significant intrinsic PEEP. External PEEP is given approximately at the level of 80% of the intrinsic PEEP. It helps in the easy triggering of breath by counteracting intrinsic PEEP.

Complications of Positive End Expiratory Pressure

The hazards associated with the use of PEEP include the following:

- Decreased venous return and cardiac output leading to hypotension
- Barotrauma
- Increased intracranial pressure
- Alteration in renal function and water metabolism

Continuous Positive Airway Pressure

Conceptually, CPAP is not a mode of ventilation but rather a means of raising FRC while the patient is breathing spontaneously. In this mode, ventilatory support is pressure-limited and pressure- or flow-triggered; i.e., the spontaneous breath has a pressure limit that remains nearly the same (within few centimeters of water) during both inspiration and expiration **(Fig. 5)**. The patient's inspiratory effort causes the ventilator to increase the flow to the patient to maintain the same pressure during inspiration. During expiration, the flow out of the exhalation valve maintains the expiratory pressure fairly uniform. No mechanical positive pressure breaths are given.

Indications of Continuous Positive Airway Pressure

Continuous positive airway pressure is frequently used to assess the patient's ability to breathe without ventilatory support. The advantages of CPAP for weaning over T-piece breathing are:

- Improved oxygenation
- Detection of low minute ventilation and apnea (as ventilator alarms remain in place)
- The patient's spontaneous VT and rate can be easily read
- The work of breathing is reduced, if auto-PEEP is present.[20,21]

Bi-leveled Positive Airway Pressure

Conceptually, bi-leveled positive airway pressure (Bi-PAP) is a mode which combines PEEP with PS and is used more in context of noninvasive ventilation (NIV) using a nasal or oronasal mask. In this mode, both expiratory positive airway pressure (EPAP) and inspiratory positive airway pressure (IPAP) are adjustable. IPAP helps in improving alveolar ventilation, normalization of $PaCO_2$, and reduction in work of breathing, whereas EPAP improves oxygenation by reducing intrapulmonary shunting. Previously, Bi-PAP could be given by dedicated NIV machines. Majority

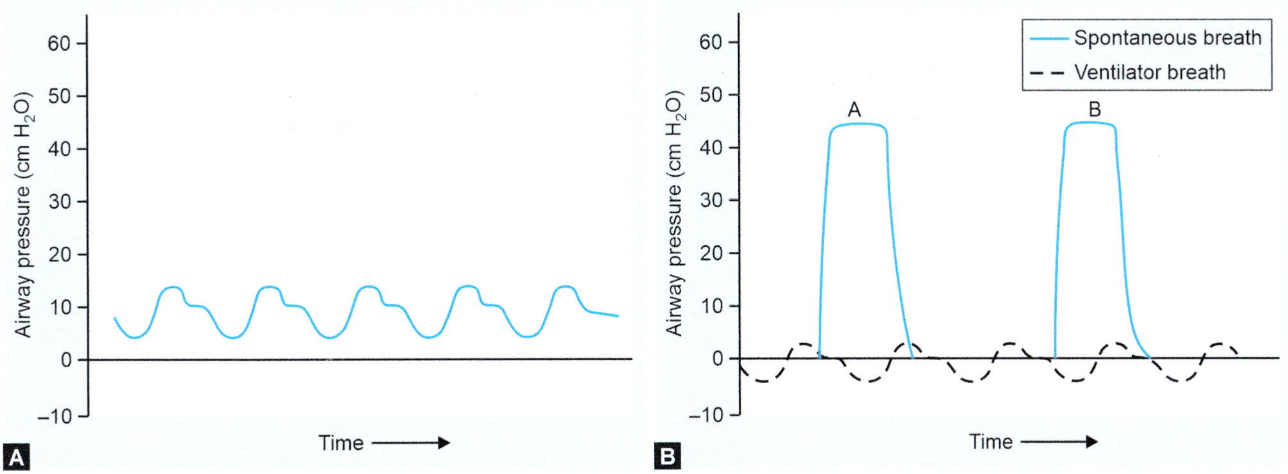

FIGS. 5A AND B: Graphical presentation of continuous positive airway pressure (CPAP) of 14 cm H_2O.

of the newer ventilators have this facility with an inbuilt pressure-controlling valve to maintain desired EPAP and IPAP levels. Inspiration is triggered at the inspiratory flow of >40 mL/sec for more than 30 ms. Expiratory flow is detected when the inspiratory flow decreases below a manufacturer determined threshold level (flow cycled) or when IPAP is longer than 3 seconds (time cycled). Usual initial setting of EPAP and IPAP are 4 cm H_2O and 8 cm H_2O, respectively. Further adjustments are done based on the cardiopulmonary response. If the response is positive, the IPAP may be increased with increment of 2 cm H_2O to improve alveolar ventilation. Similarly, EPAP may also be increased to improve oxygenation. When EPAP and IPAP are equal, it behaves like CPAP.

Indications of Bi-leveled Positive Airway Pressure

Bi-leveled positive airway pressure is useful in preventing endotracheal intubation in several conditions leading to respiratory failure, such as COPD, pulmonary edema, pneumonia, ALI, and ARDS. It also helps in weaning and avoiding intubation in patients with respiratory failure during the postextubation period.

NEWER MODES OF MECHANICAL VENTILATION

Inverse Ratio Ventilation

Inverse ratio ventilation is not a different mode of ventilation; instead, it is a maneuver to improve oxygenation in cases with severe hypoxic respiratory failure. During IRV, TI is kept equal to/more than TE resulting in an I:E ratio > 1. There are two general ways to apply IRV:

1. Pressure-controlled IRV (PC-IRV), in which a preset airway pressure is delivered for a fixed period of time
2. Volume-controlled IRV (VC-IRV), in which a VT is delivered at a slow (decelerating) inspiratory flow rate, keeping I:E ratio > 1.

For PC-IRV, variables controlled by the physician must specify the inspiratory airway pressure, *f*, and I:E ratio, while VT and flow profile are determined by respiratory system impedance as discussed for PCV. The commonly used initial settings for PC-IRV are:

P_{insp} = 20–40 cm H_2O (or 10–30 cm H_2O above the PEEP), *f* = 20/min, and I:E = 2:1–4:1. For VC-IRV, the operator selects a VT, *f*, *V* (a low value), flow profile, and possibly an end inspiratory pause. The chosen values result in an I:E ratio > 1:1 and as high as 5:1. As there a risk of auto-PEEP, the PC-IRV is preferred over VC-IRV. Compared with conventional modes of ventilation, lung oxygen exchange is often improved on IRV. The mechanisms involved are increased mean alveolar pressure and volume and creation of auto-PEEP, which reduces shunt by redistributing alveolar edema into the pulmonary interstitium.[22] A major disadvantage of IRC (both PC-IRV and VC-IRV) is requirement of heavy sedation with or without muscle paralysis, which may have an adverse effect on the outcome.

High-frequency Ventilation

High-frequency ventilation (HFV) attempts to achieve adequate gas exchange, by using asymmetrical velocity profiles when combining very high respiratory rates with VT smaller than the volume of anatomic dead space **(Fig. 6)**. These modes include high-frequency oscillatory ventilation (HFOV) and high-frequency jet ventilation (HFJV). It is used more commonly in neonates and infants with neonatal respiratory failure. There has been a renewed interest in using HFV in adult patients with ALI/ARDS, with the rationale that the small VT may cause less ventilator-associated lung injury. Theoretical benefits of HFV include a lower risk of barotrauma due to smaller tidal excursions, improved gas exchange

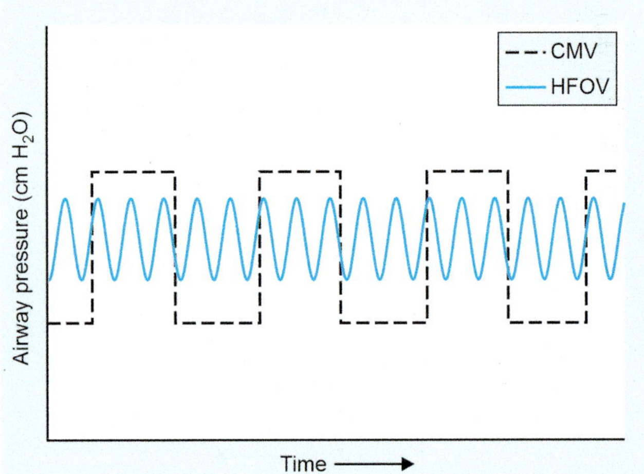

FIG. 6: A graphical presentation of high-frequency ventilation (solid line), comparing the controlled ventilation (dotted line).

(CMV: controlled mechanical ventilation; HFOV: high-frequency oscillatory ventilation)

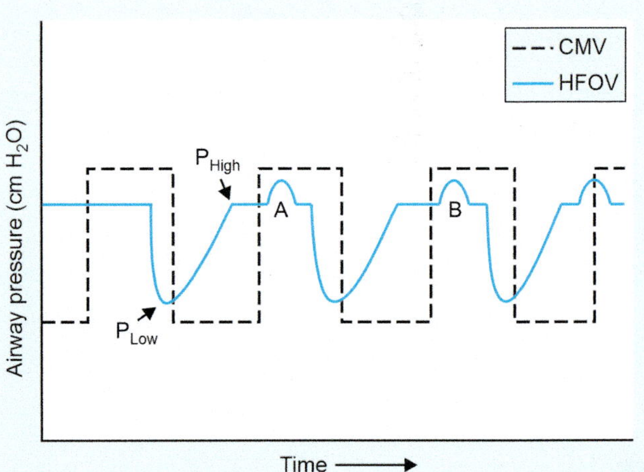

FIG. 7: A graphical presentation of airway pressure release ventilation (solid line), as compared to controlled ventilation (dotted line). This pressure–time tracing is showing two spontaneous breaths (A and B) at P_{High}.

(CMV: controlled mechanical ventilation; HFOV: high-frequency oscillatory ventilation)

through a more uniform distribution of ventilation, and improved healing of bronchopleural fistulas.[23] A substantial risk is that dynamic hyperinflation is the rule. However, more trials are necessary to determine whether HFV can improve mortality outcomes in these patients.

Airway Pressure Release Ventilation

Airway pressure release ventilation (APRV) is similar to CPAP in that the patient is allowed to breathe spontaneously without restriction. During APRV, the clinician sets a "pressure high", "pressure low" and a time at each level (time high and time low) **(Fig. 7)**. Ventilation occurs during the release from pressure high to pressure low. The "time low" is typically 0.2–0.8 seconds in restrictive lung disease and 0.8–1.5 seconds in obstructive lung disease. It is probably most prudent to start at 0.8 and titrate to meet individual patient requirements. The time low is also referred to as the release phase.[24] During spontaneous exhalation, the PEEP is dropped (released) to a lower level; this action simulates the process of exhalation. A common occurrence in this mode is setting the "time low" too long. This essentially mimics a pressure-targeted SIMV strategy. The patient typically spends 4–6 seconds in "time high". In the paralyzed patient, the APRV/Bi-level is identical to pressure-targeted IRV. For these reasons, some have described this mode as IRV. However, a major difference between APRV/Bi-level and IRV is that IRV typically requires chemical paralysis or heavy sedation. APRV/Bi-level allows for spontaneous breathing throughout both pressure levels, making it relatively more comfortable and typically does not require heavy sedation or paralysis. APRV/Bi-level has gained popularity in patients with hypoxemic respiratory failure because it improves oxygenation by optimizing alveolar recruitment and V/Q matching.[25]

Proportional-assist Ventilation

Proportional-assist ventilation is a form of partial ventilatory support developed to avoid some of the adverse effects of CMV, such as excessive ventilation, use of sedative/paralytic agents, and muscle disuse atrophy. PAV is based on the principle that during partial support, the pressure applied to the respiratory system (PRS) is contributed by the pressure produced by the respiratory muscles (PMUS) and the ventilator (PAW), the latter of which represents the amount of assistance delivered:

$$PRS = PMUS + PAW$$

The load imposed on the respiratory muscles during assisted ventilation can be described by the equation of motion as follows:

$$PMUS = R \times V\bullet + E \times VT + PEEPi - PAW$$

where V is flow, VT indicates volume displacement, R is respiratory system resistance, E is respiratory system elastance, and PEEPi is the end-expiratory elastic recoil pressure, which the respiratory muscles must overcome at the onset of inspiration to trigger the ventilator. During PAV, the ventilator instantaneously delivers positive pressure throughout inspiration, in proportion to patient-generated flow (flow assist, units cm $H_2O/L/s$) and volume (volume assist, units cm H_2O/L). The pressure applied by the ventilator (PAW) therefore is:

$$PAW = FA \times V\bullet + VA \times VT$$

During PAV, the ventilatory support depends on a patient's efforts; the more the demand, the greater will apply a set pressure, flow, or volume. Instead, it boosts the sensed patient's effort according to a proportion set by the clinician. This contrasts with volume-assist ventilation, where flow and volume may be "pulled down" by the effort. PAV also contrasts with PA/PS, in which flow and volume are affected by the effort but pressure is not.

Advantages of Proportional-assist Ventilation

Proportional-assist ventilation has been shown to be effective in unloading the respiratory muscles, without imposing a fixed breathing pattern, in enhancing patient comfort and patient-ventilator interaction.[21,26-28] Two recent, randomized clinical trials have demonstrated improved patient comfort during NIV with PAV compared with PSV.[29,30]

Complications of Proportional-assist Ventilation

Despite these positive results, PAV still seems to be more of an intellectually satisfying research tool than a ventilatory treatment in the clinical setting. There are a number of practical limitations which hinder the use of PAV.[31] The most important limitation is that proper adjustments of PAV settings require knowledge of the mechanical characteristics of the respiratory system; this information is not easy to obtain in patients receiving partial support.[32-34] Furthermore, the PAV algorithm is based on the equation of motion, which assumes resistance and elastance to be linear within the tidal breathing range. This assumption may not always be valid in ICU patients. Moreover, neuromechanical coupling, the transformation of respiratory muscle activation into mechanical output (PMUS), is important for tidal breaths. There are several factors which can lead to neuromechanical uncoupling in an ICU setting, such as fatigue, electrolyte, acid-base disorders, and shock contributing to decreased PMUS.[35,36] Other problems which may be observed during PAV include ventilator-patient asynchrony and the presence of air leaks.[30]

Proportional-assist Ventilation Plus and Proportional Pressure Support

Proportional-assist ventilation plus (PAV+) and proportional pressure support (PPS) are forms of synchronized ventilatory assistance, where the ventilator generates pressure in proportion to the patient's effort; i.e., the greater the effort, the more the pressure the ventilator generates. Therefore, the clinician determines the level of resistive and elastic unloading, irrespective of volume or flow requirements.

Neurally Adjusted Ventilatory Assist

Neurally adjusted ventilatory assist (NAVA) was developed in an attempt to overcome the limitations of PAV while maintaining all of its potential advantages. During this mode of ventilation, the electrical activity of the inspiratory muscles is used as an index of the inspiratory neural drive. The neural drive is measured as crural diaphragm electrical activity (EA_{di}), detected by means of esophageal bipolar electrodes, as it expresses global diaphragm activation.[37,38] Further, esophageal electrodes are not affected by the activity of postural and expiratory muscles (cross-talk) or by the subcutaneous tissues, which can be a problem with skin surface electrodes. The array of bipolar electrodes can be mounted on a nasogastric tube, which is introduced in almost all critically ill patients. The signal obtained by these electrodes is then transferred to the ventilator to regulate the ventilation support, which is therefore instantaneously applied in relation to EA_{di}. Thus, cycling and the intrabreath assist profile are determined directly by the EA_{di}, whereas the amount of assistance for a given EA_{di} depends on a user-controlled gain factor. As the ventilator is triggered directly by EA_{di} with NAVA, the synchrony between neural and mechanical TI is guaranteed both at the onset and at the end of inspiration, regardless of PEEPi, air leaks, and respiratory mechanics.

Advantages of Neurally Adjusted Ventilatory Assist

In the absence of any significant disease of the respiratory centers, phrenic nerves and neuromuscular junctions and drugs suppressing the ventilatory drive, the ventilator support provided corresponds to the ventilatory demand of the patient, irrespective of variations in muscle length or contractility. The use of neural control of mechanical ventilation has the capability to dramatically enhance the coordination between mechanical ventilation and respiratory muscle activity, thereby improving patient comfort.

Limitations of Neurally Adjusted Ventilatory Assist

Although NAVA may be considered as a major advance in the care of the critically ill, it is not currently available for clinical use and serves only as a research tool. It has been used primarily in healthy subjects for short-term studies, by only a few investigators. The effects of this mode on breathing pattern and gas exchange have yet to be evaluated and it remains to determine whether NAVA can maintain adequate levels of support in different kinds of respiratory failure from admission to weaning.

Biologically Variable Ventilation

Biologically variable ventilation (BVV) is a new mode, which was designed to improve the management of ARDS. CMV is often required for the treatment of ARDS; however, the loss of physiological variability of breathing pattern may contribute to deterioration in respiratory mechanics and gas exchange.[39] BVV mimics spontaneous breath-to-breath variability, incorporating natural variable noise into volume-targeted CMV, which may overcome this limitation. The ventilator has a program to modulate respiratory rate and VT while maintaining a fixed minute ventilation based on a previously generated data file.[39] It is important to recollect that recruitment is a continuous and progressive phenomenon that depends not only on PEEP, but also on the inflation volume.[40,41] The rationale behind BVV is based on the concept that the alveolar recruitment achieved by high volumes exceeds the derecruitment caused by small volumes, resulting in improvement in lung compliance and oxygenation without an increase in mean airway pressure.[42]

Advantages of Biologically Variable Ventilation

Biologically variable ventilation has been compared with conventional controlled ventilation in a series of animal studies. BVV significantly improved oxygenation in healthy animals during general anesthesia.[43] It has been shown to be useful after re-expansion of a collapsed lung and in ARDS, with and without PEEP.[39,44] BVV variability results in periodic deep inflations and the mere application of periodic sighs has also been shown to provide beneficial effects.[40,45] Comparing these two strategies, BVV is found to be more effective than periodic sighs of the same magnitude and frequency as the higher BVV VT.[44]

Limitations of Biologically Variable Ventilation

Although there are impressive results with BVV use in animal studies, no human study has been conducted yet. There are dissimilarities between different animal species; therefore, the effects observed in animals should be carefully extrapolated to humans. Indeed, others have failed to reproduce the benefits of BVV in a canine model of oleic acid-induced ARDS.[46] Further, its effects on conditions of different severity or diverse origins are also not clear.[42]

Hybrid or Mixed Modes

Some ventilators allow combinations of modes, most commonly SIMV plus PSV. There is a little reason to use such a hybrid mode, although some physicians use the SIMV mode as a means to add sighs to PSV, an option not otherwise generally available. It is advantageous in that SIMV plus PSV guarantees some backup minute ventilation (which PSV does not). It is many times used for difficult-to-wean patients.

INITIATING MECHANICAL VENTILATION

Initial Ventilator Settings

Initial ventilator settings depend on the goals of ventilation, i.e., full respiratory muscle rest versus partial exercise, the patient's respiratory system mechanics, and the needed minute ventilation. Each critically ill patient presents unique challenges. Some common clinical scenarios are described in the following text.

Patients with Normal Lung Mechanics and Gas Exchange[47]

These patients may require mechanical ventilation because of:

- Loss of central drive to breathe (drug overdose or structural injury to the brainstem)
- Due to neuromuscular weakness (high cervical myelopathy, myasthenia gravis)
- Treatment of shock (as adjuvant therapy)
- To achieve hyperventilation (treatment of raised intracranial pressure)

Following are the acceptable initial setting after intubation:

FiO_2 of 0.5–1.0

VT 8–12 mL/kg, *f* of 8–12/min

Inspiratory flow rate of 40–60 L/min

In patients with preserved respiratory drive and without profound weakness, PSV can be used. The PS is adjusted (usually 10–20 cm H_2O above PEEP), to bring the respiratory rate down into the low twenties, usually corresponding to VT of about 500 cc. It should be noted that PSV is entirely spontaneous, with no machine backup. Therefore, hypoventilation may occur despite the use of PSV, if there is further deterioration of muscle strength or blunting of respiratory drive. Once stabilized, effort should be made to bring down $FiO_2 < 0.6$. For hyperventilation, the initial respiratory rate should be increased to the range of 16–20 breaths/min. If the patient complains of air hunger, the inspiratory flow rate can be increased, but 40–50 L/min is often sufficient; flow > 60 L/min is rarely required.

Airway pressure and flow waveforms should be inspected for evidence of patient-ventilator dyssynchrony or undesired patient effort. To provide full rest, the patient's drive can be suppressed by increasing the inspiratory flow rate, frequency, or VT.[48] If such adjustments are ineffective, then sedation may be necessary. If sedatives also do not abolish inspiratory efforts and full rest is essential (as in shock), muscle paralysis should be considered. Preventive measures for atelectasis should include sighs (6–12/h at 1.5–2 times the VT) or small amounts of PEEP (5–7.5 cm H_2O). This is specially required in patients with neuromuscular diseases. Three point turning and chest physiotherapy are desirable in all patients, unless other conditions preclude their use. Rotating beds are effective in some patients in preventing atelectasis and pneumonia.[49]

Patients with Severe Airflow Obstruction

The common conditions included in this category are bronchial asthma and COPD.

Bronchial Asthma

Patients with acute severe asthma requiring mechanical ventilation are usually extremely anxious and distressed. Deep sedation should be routinely provided; a few patients may require therapeutic paralysis, although paralytic drugs occasionally cause long-lasting weakness.[50] These interventions help to reduce oxygen consumption (and hence carbon dioxide production), to lower airway pressures, and to reduce the risk of self-extubation. The gas exchange abnormalities of airflow obstruction are largely due to ventilation-perfusion mismatch. Ventilation should be initiated using the assist/control (A/C) mode (or SIMV), the VT should be small (5–7 mL/kg), and the respiratory rate should be 12–15 breaths/min. A peak flow of 60 L/min is recommended; higher flow rates do not increase expiratory rate significantly. An FiO_2 of 0.5 suffices in the vast majority of patients.[51]

Requirements for a higher FiO_2 should prompt a search for an alveolar filling problem or for lobar atelectasis. Finally, if the patient is triggering the ventilator, some PEEP should be added to reduce the work of triggering, although this may occasionally compound the dynamic hyperinflation, potentially compromising the cardiac output. Usually, auto-PEEP increases little as long as PEEP is not set higher than about 85% of the auto-PEEP.[52] The targets should be to minimize alveolar overdistention ($P_{plat} < 30$) and dynamic hyperinflation (auto-PEEP below 10 cm H_2O or end-inspiratory lung volume < 20 mL/kg), a strategy that largely prevents barotrauma.[53] Reducing minute ventilation to achieve these goals generally causes the PCO_2 to rise above 40 mm Hg (permissive hypercapnia), often to 70 mm Hg or higher. This requires sedation, such that permissive hypercapnia is quite well tolerated. Careful attention should be paid to the inspiratory flow and flow profile. The flow changes, which have little effect in a normal individual without airflow obstruction, can have a dramatic impact in obstructed patients. Specifically, reduction in the inspiratory flow or switching to a decelerating flow profile reduces the airway pressures and the amount of ventilator alarming. But the same actually worsens auto-PEEP, by prolonging inspiration. Therefore, a close watch should be kept on auto-PEEP and expiratory flow profile.

Chronic Obstructive Pulmonary Disease

Unlike patients with status asthmaticus, patients with COPD have expiratory flow limitation, arising largely from loss of elastic recoil. As a consequence, in a patient with COPD, the peak airway pressures on the ventilator tends not to be extraordinarily high; still auto-PEEP and its consequences are common.[54] The majority of patients with COPD will appear exhausted at the time when mechanical support is instituted and will sleep with minimal sedation. To the extent that muscle fatigue has played a role in a patient's functional decline, rest and sleep are desirable. Also, such a patient has underlying compensated respiratory acidosis. Hyperventilation carries the risk of severe respiratory alkalosis and bicarbonate wasting by the kidney. The initial ventilator settings of a VT of 5–7 mL/kg and a respiratory rate of 24–28 breaths/min, with either an SIMV or an A/C mode, set on minimal sensitivity can achieve the goal of rest and relative hypoventilation. Usually, good oxygenation can be achieved with an FiO_2 of 0.4. Inspiratory flow rates may be adjusted for patient comfort, but usually in the range of 60 L/min. PEEP should be used, when the patient is triggering the ventilator, but is not required in a sedated patient. Usually, 2–3 days of rest restore biochemical and functional changes associated with muscle fatigue, but 24 hours is probably not sufficient.[35] A few patients on the ventilator are difficult to rest and continue to demonstrate a high work of breathing. Airway pressure and flow waveforms may be used to identify these patients and strategies for improving the ventilator settings. Auto-PEEP may be responsible for this problem, when addition of extrinsic PEEP to nearly counterbalance the auto-PEEP may dramatically improve the patient's comfort.

Another approach is to increase minute ventilation, although this worsens auto-PEEP and bicarbonate loss. A careful search should be made for problems that might drive the patient to a respiratory rate higher than what is desirable, e.g., hypoperfusion, pleural effusion, or pain. If the patient continues to make significant inspiratory efforts after correction, judicious sedation is advised. Once the patient improves and the respiratory muscles are adequately rested, the patient should assume some of the work of breathing and be evaluated for weaning. During this phase, some extrinsic PEEP is typically useful to reduce the work of triggering.[54]

Patients with Acute Lung Injury or Adult Respiratory Distress Syndrome

Acute lung injury and ARDS are inflammatory conditions, resulting from a broad spectrum of lung injury leading to mild respiratory abnormality to severe respiratory derangement. Respiratory dysfunction often develops during the early phase of (within 48 hours) of the physiologic insult and may take weeks to months to resolve.[55] Regardless of the cause, the pulmonary physiology and the mechanics are altered, leading to hypoxemic respiratory failure. The use of positive-pressure ventilation itself may cause lung injury (VILI), which may amplify preexisting injury, delay lung recovery, and result in adverse outcomes. In ARDS, the FRC is reduced due to alveolar flooding and collapse, leaving fewer alveoli to accept the VT. This results in stiff lung; the work of breathing is increased dramatically.

The ARDS lung should be viewed as a small lung (baby lung), rather than a stiff lung. In line with this current conception of ARDS, ventilatory strategies have evolved markedly in the past decade. The goals of ventilation are to reduce shunt, avoid toxic concentrations of oxygen, and choose ventilator settings that do not amplify lung damage. The initial FiO_2 should be 1.0, in view of the typically extreme hypoxemia. PEEP should be instituted immediately, beginning with 15 cm H_2O, rapidly adjusted thereafter either to produce an arterial saturation of 90% on an FiO, <0.6 "least PEEP approach", or a PEEP of 2 cm H_2O higher than the lower inflection point of the inflation pressure-volume curve "open-lung approach".[56] The VT should be 5-7 mL/kg on A/C or SIMV, since higher VT usually overdistend the lung at end inspiration, as judged by the upper inflection point of the respiratory pressure-volume curve, which may even contribute to systemic inflammation.[57] Alternatively, PCV can be used with an inspiratory pressure (PEEP plus the pressure increment) of 30-35 cm H_2O. This will generally drive VT of 350-550 mL/kg. In both modes, the respiratory rate of 24-28 breaths/min is acceptable as long as there is no auto-PEEP. The combination of high levels of PEEP (especially when the open-lung approach is used) and low end-inspiratory pressures, leaving only a small range for tidal ventilation, is called lung protective ventilatory (LPV) strategy. A common consequence of LPV is hypercapnia ("permissive hypercapnia"). The ventilatory settings, which are followed most widely, are based on ARDSnet trial.[58] The same protocol is summarized below:

A. Target a VT of 6 mL/kg predicted body weight (PBW), with a goal of plateau pressures of 30 cm H_2O or lower and adjust VT according to ARDSNet guidelines. For patients who develop ALI, while receiving VT in excess of 6 mL/kg, stepwise reductions in VT of 1 mL/kg every 15 minutes, with concomitant increases in respiratory rate to maintain constant minute ventilation, are advised to ease the transition.
   1. *Choose a mode of ventilation*: Although any mode may be used, the sentinel ARDSNet trial results were based on the use of continuous mandatory ventilation (assist/control) mode with volume-controlled ventilation setting. Importantly, plateau pressure may not reflect trans-pulmonary pressure in pressure-limited modes (PCV and PS ventilation). If the patient is making active inspiratory efforts that lower the pleural pressure, in this situation, delivered VT and transpulmonary pressures may approximate those in the control arm (12 mL/kg) of the ARDSNet trial.
   2. *Calculate PBW*:
      - Males: PBW (kg) = 50 + 2.3 [height (inches) 60]
      - Females: PBW (kg) = 45.5 + 2.3 [height (inches) 60]
   3. Choose VT goal of 6 mL/kg PBW.
   4. Set PEEP to 5 cm H_2O or higher.
   5. Measure and record plateau pressure, at least every 4 hours and after any changes in VT and PEEP:
      a. If plateau pressure > 30 cm H_2O, reduce VT to 5 mL/kg and then to 4 mL/kg PBW, if necessary and to decrease plateau pressure to 30 cm H_2O or lower.
      b. If VT < 6 mL/kg PBW and plateau pressure < 25 cm H_2O, increase VT by 1 mL/kg PBW to a maximum of 6 mL/kg.
   6. *Adjust respiratory rate or VT according to pH goals*:
      a. If pH < 7.30, consider increasing the respiratory rate to as high as 35/min, while monitoring for development of auto-PEEP.
      b. If pH < 7.15 and respiratory rate > 35/min, consider increasing VT and suspending the plateau pressure limit, depending on patient's tolerance of the acidemia.
   7. If severe dyspnea (less than three double-triggered breaths per minute or if airway pressure remains at or below PEEP level during inspiration), increase VT to 7-8 mL/kg PBW, if plateau pressure remains <30 cm H_2O. If plateau pressure > 30 cm H_2O on 7 or 8 mL/kg PBW, revert to lower VT, consider ventilator adjustments to improve patient synchrony, and consider more sedation.
   8. Set PEEP or FiO_2, to achieve an oxygenation target of PaO_2 55-80 mm Hg or SpO_2 of 88-95%, using the PEEP and FiO_2 combinations.
      a. Increase FiO_2 or PEEP within 5 minutes of consistent measurements below the oxygenation target range.
      b. Reduce FiO_2 or PEEP within 30 minutes of consistent measurements above the oxygenation target range.
      c. Assess lung recruitability for patients with PaO_2/FiO_2 lower than 150 (with PEEP = 5 cm H_2O), consider using the higher PEEP/lower FiO_2 to set PEEP and FiO_2, if either or both of the following occur when PEEP is increased:
         i. Increase in respiratory system compliance (when PEEP is increased from 5 to 15 cm H_2O)
         ii. Reduced dead-space fraction (or decrease in $PaCO_2$ at constant minute ventilation and VT), when PEEP is increased from 5 to 15 cm H_2O.

B. Select PEEP and FiO_2, according to oxygenation criteria, using PEEP-FiO_2 combinations within the two ranges tested in the alveoli trial. In patients with high FiO_2 requirements (PaO_2/FiO_2 < 150 with PEEP 5 cm H_2O), who demonstrate a reduction in dead-space fraction (or a fall in $PaCO_2$ at constant minute ventilation and VT) or an improvement in respiratory system compliance, when PEEP is increased from 5 to 15 cm H_2O, the authors advise use of the higher PEEP/lower FiO_2 table. For patients who experience a fall in respiratory compliance or a rise in dead-space fraction, when PEEP is increased to 15 cm H_2O (indicating overdistension) or who have active barotrauma or adverse PEEP-induced cardiovascular changes, the authors advise use of the lower PEEP/higher FiO_2 table. The two approaches produce similar clinical outcomes, when applied to patients who have ALI/ARDS, regardless of lung recruitability. This stratification aims at targeting higher PEEP, to the recruitable subset of patients; although such an approach is logical, it remains to be shown, whether such an approach improves outcomes.

C. Minimize contributors to patient–ventilator dyssynchrony (e.g., adequate sedation, trigger sensitivity, flow, and other factors).

COMPLICATIONS OF MECHANICAL VENTILATION

Mechanical ventilation is associated with multiple complications **(Box 1)**; some of them may be related temporally and not caused by ventilatory support per se, but many are a direct result of positive-pressure ventilation. A successful outcome of mechanical ventilation depends upon the avoidance and presentation of complications. Comprehensive intensive care of patient can therefore be considered as an essential component of mechanical ventilation.

BOX 1 Common complications associated with MV.

Endotracheal intubation complications

- *During intubation trauma to teeth and soft tissue:*
    - Esophageal intubation
    - Vomiting and aspiration
    - Hypoxia
    - Arrhythmia
    - Bradycardia
- *While intubated obstruction:*
    - Pneumonia and atelectasis
    - Aspiration
    - Kinking of endotracheal (ET) tube
    - Mucosal injury
    - Improper position
    - Accidental extubation
- *Postextubation aspiration:*
    - Laryngospasm
    - Hoarseness
    - Laryngeal or subglottic edema
    - Laryngeal stenosis
    - Tracheal stenosis

Positive-pressure ventilation

- *Pulmonary:*
    - Barotrauma
    - Ventilator-associated pneumonia
    - Deconditioning of respiratory muscles
    - Oxygen toxicity
- *Extrapulmonary:*
    - Raised intracranial tension
    - Hypotension
    - Stress ulcer and cholestasis
    - Renal dysfunction

SUMMARY

Mechanical ventilation is a life-saving intervention for patients with respiratory failure admitted in the intensive care unit. During mechanical ventilation a positive pressure is delivered to the lungs to improve oxygenation and ventilation, either alone or in combination. There are various modes which can be selected to deliver breath using the positive pressure during mechanical ventilation. Latest mechanical ventilators provide many variables, which may be controlled to provide the ventilatory support depending on the underlying disease in an intermittent fashion, mimicking natural breathing. Appropriate selection of modes and variables such as tidal volume, respiratory rate, inspiratory time, pressure support, fraction of oxygen, etc. are crucial to get maximum benefits and minimize the adverse effects of mechanical ventilation. Therefore, an in-depth knowledge of various modes of mechanical ventilation, their advantages and disadvantages, indications and contraindication is a must before using this life saving intervention. This chapter provides an over view of general principles and various modes of mechanical ventilation.

REFERENCES

1. Esteban A, Anzueto A, Alia I, et al. How is mechanical ventilation employed in the intensive care unit? An international utilization review. Am J Respir Crit Care Med. 2000;161(5):1450-8.
2. Esteban A, Anzueto A, Frutos F, et al. Characteristics and outcomes in adult patients receiving mechanical ventilation: a 28-day international study. JAMA. 2002; 287(3):345-55.
3. Slutsky AS. History of Mechanical Ventilation. From Vesalius to Ventilator-induced Lung Injury. Am J Respir Crit Care Med. 2915;191(10):1106-15.
4. Mauri T, Pivi S, Bigatello LM. Prolonged mechanical ventilation after critical illness. Minerva Anestesiol. 2008;74(6):297-301.
5. Jolliet P, Tassaux D. Clinical review: patient-ventilator interaction in chronic obstructive pulmonary disease. Crit Care. 2006;10(6):236.
6. Marini JJ, Rodriguez RM, Lamb V. The inspiratory workload of patient-initiated mechanical ventilation. Am Rev Respir Dis. 1986;134(5):902-9.
7. Goligher EC, Dres M, Fan E, et al. Mechanical Ventilation-induced Diaphragm Atrophy Strongly Impacts Clinical Outcomes. Am J Respir Crit Care Med. 2018;197(2):204-13.
8. Hansen-Flaschen JH, Brazinsky S, Basile C, et al. Use of sedating drugs and neuromuscular blocking agents in patients requiring

mechanical ventilation for respiratory failure. A national survey. JAMA. 1991;266(20):2870-5.

9. O'Donoghue FJ, Catcheside PG, Jordan AS, et al. Effect of CPAP on intrinsic PEEP, inspiratory effort, and lung volume in severe stable COPD. Thorax. 2002;57(6):533-9.
10. Flick GR, Bellamy PE, Simmons DH. Diaphragmatic contraction during assisted mechanical ventilation. Chest. 1989;96(1):130-5.
11. Yang LY, Huang YC, Macintyre NR. Patient-ventilator synchrony during pressure-targeted versus flow-targeted small tidal volume assisted ventilation. J Crit Care. 2007;22(3):252-7.
12. Kilburn KH. Shock, seizures, and coma with alkalosis during mechanical ventilation. Ann Intern Med. 1966;65(5):977-84.
13. Powers SK, Kavazis AN, Levine S. Prolonged mechanical ventilation alters diaphragmatic structure and function. Crit Care Med. 2009;37(10 Suppl):S347-53.
14. McKibben AW, Ravenscraft SA. Pressure-controlled and volume-cycled mechanical ventilation. Clin Chest Med. 1996;17(3):395-410.
15. Hooper RG, Browning M. Acid-base changes and ventilator mode during maintenance ventilation. Crit Care Med. 1985;13(1):44-5.
16. Esteban A, Frutos F, Tobin MJ, et al. A comparison of four methods of weaning patients from mechanical ventilation. Spanish Lung Failure Collaborative Group. N Engl J Med. 1995;332(6):345-50.
17. MacIntyre NR. Respiratory function during pressure support ventilation. Chest. 1986;89(5):677-83.
18. Maggiore SM, Jonson B, Richard JC, et al. Alveolar derecruitment at decremental positive end expiratory pressure levels in acute lung injury: comparison with the lower inflection point, oxygenation, and compliance. Am J Respir Crit Care Med. 2001;164(5):795-801.
19. Richard JC, Brochard L, Vandelet P, et al. Respective effects of end-expiratory and end-inspiratory pressures on alveolar recruitment in acute lung injury. Crit Care Med. 2003;31(1):89- 92.
20. Shivaram U, Miro AM, Cash ME, et al. Cardiopulmonary responses to continuous positive airway pressure in acute asthma. J Crit Care. 1993;8(2):87-92.
21. Appendini L, Purro A, Patessio A, et al. Partitioning of inspiratory muscle workload and pressure assistance in ventilator-dependent COPD patients. Am J Respir Crit Care Med. 1996;154(5):1301-9.
22. Duncan SR, Rizk NW, Raffin TA. Inverse ratio ventilation. PEEP in disguise? Chest. 1987;92(3):390-2.
23. Turnbull AD, Carlon G, Howland WS, et al. High-frequency jet ventilation in major airway or pulmonary disruption. Ann Thorac Surg. 1981;32(5):468-74.
24. Habashi NM. Other approaches to open-lung ventilation: airway pressure release ventilation. Crit Care Med. 2005; 33(3 Suppl):S228-40.
25. Putensen C, Rasanen J, Lopez FA. Ventilation-perfusion distributions during mechanical ventilation with superimposed spontaneous breathing in canine lung injury. Am J Respir Crit Care Med. 1994;150(1):101-8.
26. Navalesi P, Costa R. New modes of mechanical ventilation: proportional assist ventilation, neurally adjusted ventilatory assist, and fractal ventilation. Curr Opin Crit Care. 2003;9(1):51-8.
27. Vitacca M, Clini E, Pagani M, et al. Physiologic effects of early administered mask proportional assist ventilation in patients with chronic obstructive pulmonary disease and acute respiratory failure. Crit Care Med. 2000;28(6):1791-7.
28. Grasso S, Puntillo F, Mascia L, et al. Compensation for increase in respiratory workload during mechanical ventilation. Pressure support versus proportional-assist ventilation. Am J Respir Crit Care Med. 2000;161(3 Pt 1):819-26.
29. Gay PC, Hess DR, Hill NS. Noninvasive proportional assist ventilation for acute respiratory insufficiency. Comparison with pressure support ventilation. Am J Respir Crit Care Med. 2001;164(9):1606-11.
30. Wysocki M, Richard JC, Meshaka P. Noninvasive proportional assist ventilation compared with noninvasive pressure support ventilation in hypercapnic acute respiratory failure. Crit Care Med. 2002;30(2):323-9.
31. Grasso S, Ranieri VM. Proportional assist ventilation. Respir Care Clin N Am. 2001;7(3):465-73, ix-x.
32. Navalesi P, Pollini A. Acute respiratory failure in patients with severe community-acquired pneumonia: a prospective randomized evaluation of noninvasive ventilation. Am J Respir Crit Care Med. 2000;162(2 Pt 1):761-2.
33. Younes M, Webster K, Kun J, et al. A method for measuring passive elastance during proportional assist ventilation. Am J Respir Crit Care Med. 2001;164(1):50-60.
34. Farre R, Mancini M, Rotger M, et al. Oscillatory resistance measured during noninvasive proportional assist ventilation. Am J Respir Crit Care Med. 2001;164(5):790-4.
35. Laghi F, D'Alfonso N, Tobin MJ. Pattern of recovery from diaphragmatic fatigue over 24 hours. J Appl Physiol. 1995;79(2):539-46.
36. Nava S, Bellemare F. Cardiovascular failure and apnea in shock. J Appl Physiol. 1989;66(1):184-9.
37. Sinderby C, Beck J, Spahija J, et al. Voluntary activation of the human diaphragm in health and disease. J Appl Physiol. 1998;85(6):2146-58.
38. Beck J, Gottfried SB, Navalesi P, et al. Electrical activity of the diaphragm during pressure support ventilation in acute respiratory failure. Am J Respir Crit Care Med. 2001;164(3):419-24.
39 Lefevre GR, Kowalski SE, Girling LG, et al. Improved arterial oxygenation after oleic acid lung injury in the pig using a computer-controlled mechanical ventilator. Am J Respir Crit Care Med. 1996;154(5):1567-72.
40. Polese G, Vitacca M, Bianchi L, et al. Nasal proportional assist ventilation unloads the inspiratory muscles of stable patients with hypercapnia due to COPD. Eur Respir J. 2000;16(3):491-8.
41. Jonson B, Richard JC, Straus C, et al. Pressure-volume curves and compliance in acute lung injury: evidence of recruitment above the lower inflection point. Am J Respir Crit Care Med. 1999;159(4 Pt 1):1172-8.
42. Suki B, Barabasi AL, Hantos Z, et al. Avalanches and power law behaviour in lung inflation. Nature. 1994;368(6472):615-8.
43. Mutch WA, Eschun GM, Kowalski SE, et al. Biologically variable ventilation prevents deterioration of gas exchange during prolonged anaesthesia. Br J Anaesth. 2000;84(2):197-203.
44. Mutch WA, Harms S, Ruth Graham M, et al. Biologically variable or naturally noisy mechanical ventilation recruits atelectatic lung. Am J Respir Crit Care Med. 2000;162(1):319-23.
45. Patroniti N, Foti G, Cortinovis B, et al. Sigh improves gas exchange and lung volume in patients with acute respiratory distress syndrome undergoing pressure support ventilation. Anesthesiology. 2002;96(4):788-94.
46. Nam AJ, Brower RG, Fessler HE, et al. Biologic variability in mechanical ventilation rate and tidal volume does not improve

oxygenation or lung mechanics in canine oleic acid lung injury. Am J Respir Crit Care Med. 2000;161(6):1797-804.

47. Arold SP, Mora R, Lutchen KR, et al. Variable tidal volume ventilation improves lung mechanics and gas exchange in a rodent model of acute lung injury. Am J Respir Crit Care Med. 2002;165(3):366-71.
48. Tobert DG, Simon PM, Stroetz RW, et al. The determinants of respiratory rate during mechanical ventilation. Am J Respir Crit Care Med. 1997;155(2):485-92.
49. Nelson LD, Choi SC. Kinetic therapy in critically ill trauma patients. Clin Intensive Care. 1992;3(6):248-52.
50. Leatherman JW, Fluegel WL, David WS, et al. Muscle weakness in mechanically ventilated patients with severe asthma. Am J Respir Crit Care Med. 1996;153(5):1686-90.
51. Rodriguez-Roisin R, Ballester E, Roca J, et al. Mechanisms of hypoxemia in patients with status asthmaticus requiring mechanical ventilation. Am Rev Respir Dis. 1989;139(3):732-9.
52. Tobin MJ, Lodato RF. PEEP, auto-PEEP, and waterfalls. Chest. 1989;96(3):449-51.
53. Tuxen DV, Williams TJ, Scheinkestel CD, et al. Use of a measurement of pulmonary hyperinflation to control the level of mechanical ventilation in patients with acute severe asthma. Am Rev Respir Dis. 1992;146(5 Pt 1):1136-42.
54. Ranieri VM, Giuliani R, Cinnella G, et al. Physiologic effects of positive end-expiratory pressure in patients with chronic obstructive pulmonary disease during acute ventilatory failure and controlled mechanical ventilation. Am Rev Respir Dis. 1993;147(1):5-13.
55. Ware LB, Matthay MA. The acute respiratory distress syndrome. N Engl J Med. 2000;342(18):1334-49.
56. Amato MB, Barbas CS, Medeiros DM, et al. Beneficial effects of the "open lung approach" with low distending pressures in acute respiratory distress syndrome. A prospective randomized study on mechanical ventilation. Am J Respir Crit Care Med. 1995;152(6 Pt 1):1835-46.
57. Roupie E, Dambrosio M, Servillo G, et al. Titration of tidal volume and induced hypercapnia in acute respiratory distress syndrome. Am J Respir Crit Care Med. 1995;152(1):121-8.
58. Ventilation with lower tidal volumes as compared with traditional tidal volumes for acute lung injury and the acute respiratory distress syndrome. The Acute Respiratory Distress Syndrome Network. N Engl J Med. 2000;342(18):1301-8.

CHAPTER

162

Respiratory Failure

Abinash Sherindar Singh Paul, Ritesh Agarwal

INTRODUCTION

Respiratory failure can be defined as a syndrome in which the respiratory system fails to meet one or both of its gas exchange functions: Oxygenation and carbon dioxide (CO_2) elimination.[1] In practice, respiratory failure is said to be present if the partial pressure of oxygen in alveoli (PaO_2) values are <60 mm Hg while breathing room air. It is further classified into type I (or hypoxemic respiratory failure) if the partial pressure of carbon dioxide ($PaCO_2$) levels are <45 mm Hg or type II (or hypercapnic respiratory failure) if the $PaCO_2$ levels are ≥45 mm Hg.[2] Some authors also classify it further into type III (perioperative respiratory failure), and type IV (shock-related respiratory failure). However, there is no real advantage of doing so.

At sea level, the normal value of PaO_2 in healthy adults is 80–100 mm Hg.[3] The PaO_2 falls progressively after the age of 10 years at approximately 5 mm Hg/decade. The 70–70 rule is a good way of remembering the normal decline with age. At 70 years of age, the PaO_2 drops to 70 mm Hg and this declines further to 60 mm Hg at 80 years, and then to 50 mm Hg at 90 years of age. The health status of seniors varies widely, and normal values are difficult to establish in the later decades of life.

CLASSIFICATION

The respiratory system serves to remove CO_2 from the blood entering the pulmonary circulation. It provides oxygen (O_2) to it before it leaves the pulmonary circulation.

For this to happen, all links in the supply chain must function. There must be fresh air in the alveoli (ventilation), adequate circulation of blood through the pulmonary vessels (perfusion), movement of gas between the alveoli and the pulmonary capillaries (diffusion), and a good match between alveolar gas and pulmonary capillary blood [ventilation–perfusion (V/Q) matching].

Respiratory failure is also classified as acute or chronic depending on how fast it develops **(Table 1)**. Acute respiratory failure (ARF) refers to disorders of recent onset (hours to days). ARF is characterized by the absence of physiologic compensation. On the other hand, chronic respiratory failure (CRF) develops over months to years, allowing compensatory mechanisms to improve oxygen transport and to buffer respiratory acidosis.[4-6] ARF can also be superimposed on CRF, as in acute exacerbations of chronic obstructive pulmonary disease (COPD). ARF is characterized by life-threatening derangements in arterial blood gases and acid–base status while the manifestations of CRF are less dramatic and may not be as readily apparent.[7] Acute type 1 respiratory failure is usually seen in diseases of lung parenchyma, cardiovascular system, and lower airways. Most causes lead to a V/Q mismatch but other mechanisms such as low inspired concentration of oxygen, impairment of diffusion, intrapulmonary shunting, and low mixed venous oxygen content can all contribute **(Table 1)**.

The coronavirus disease 2019 (COVID-19) pandemic brought respiratory failure to every neighborhood and

TABLE 1: Causes of respiratory failure.

Acute	Chronic
Type 1	
• Acute pulmonary edema • Pneumonia • Acute lung injury/acute respiratory distress syndrome • Pneumothorax • Severe acute asthma	• *Interstitial lung diseases*: Idiopathic pulmonary fibrosis, sarcoidosis, and others • Lymphangitis carcinomatosis • Chronic pulmonary embolism • Chronic heart failure
Type 2	
• Acute exacerbations of chronic obstructive pulmonary disease • Tension pneumothorax • Guillain–Barré syndrome • Myasthenia gravis • Laryngeal edema • Inhaled foreign body	• Chronic obstructive pulmonary disease • Obesity hypoventilation syndrome • Motor neuron disease and other neuromuscular disorders

small hospital. Communities tried to deal with the flood of patients needing oxygen supplementation in unorthodox ways like organizing concentrators and oxygen plants in community centers and places of worship. Governmental agencies set up large camp-like treatment centers with facilities for supplementation and ventilation. The use of awake proning was a powerful lesson learned during this time. It is an example of a simple, cost-free maneuver, which proved effective in a significant number of cases during the epidemic. The theoretical basis for its effectiveness makes interesting reading. It may or may not apply to other causes of respiratory failure.[8]

MECHANISMS OF RESPIRATORY FAILURE

Hypoxemic (Type 1) Respiratory Failure

A low PaO_2 and a normal or low $PaCO_2$ characterizes hypoxemic respiratory failure (also called type 1 or nonventilatory or normocapnic respiratory failure).[9,10] Although there are four pathophysiological mechanisms that can cause hypoxemia, namely, low fraction of inspired oxygen (FiO_2), diffusion impairment, right-to-left shunt, and V/Q mismatch, the underlying physiologic aberration causing hypoxemia is predominantly V/Q mismatch. The classic example of acute hypoxemic respiratory failure is the acute lung injury (ALI)/ acute respiratory distress syndrome (ARDS). To put it simply, the injured alveoli are full of leaked fluid, and therefore cannot fill with air, even if oxygen is given or mechanical ventilation is attempted.

Both O_2 and CO_2 diffuse readily, down their concentration gradients, through the alveolar wall and pulmonary capillary endothelium.[11] Under normal circumstances, equilibration of both gases is complete within one-third of the transit time of erythrocytes through the pulmonary capillary bed. Thus, even in disease states in which diffusion of gases is impaired, the impairment is unlikely to be severe enough to prevent equilibration of CO_2 and O_2. In patients with interstitial lung diseases, a diffusion abnormality only rarely results in arterial hypoxemia at rest.[12] However, if the transit time in the pulmonary circulation is shortened, as occurs with exercise, and diffusion is impaired, then diffusion limitation may contribute to hypoxemia. Exercise testing can often demonstrate such physiologically significant abnormalities due to impaired diffusion. The ratio of pulmonary ventilation to pulmonary blood flow for the whole lung at rest is about 0.8–1 (4–6 liters of minute ventilation divided by 5–6 liters of blood flow every minute). It is this matching of distribution of ventilation and perfusion that is the most important determinant of gas exchange.[13]

The V/Q mismatch is the final common pathway to hypoxemia in most pulmonary diseases **(Fig. 1)**. An area of lung that is well-perfused but not ventilated acts as a right-to-left shunt (physiological shunt) whereas an area that is well-ventilated but not perfused acts like a dead space (physiological dead space). The spectrum of V/Q ratios in a healthy lung varies between zero (perfused but not ventilated) to infinity (ventilated but not perfused). The ideal V/Q ratio of one indicates perfectly matched ventilation and perfusion. Although V/Q mismatch encompasses both physiologic shunt and physiologic dead space but in clinical parlance, the term generally denotes physiologic shunt mechanism. Physiologic dead space is rarely, if ever, the cause of hypoxemia. In an alveolar-capillary unit with a V/Q ratio of zero (physiologic shunt), the blood leaving the unit has the composition of mixed venous blood entering the pulmonary capillaries, i.e., partial pressure of oxygen (PO_2) of 40 mm Hg and PCO_2 of 46 mm Hg whereas in an alveolar-capillary unit with a high V/Q ratio (physiologic dead space) the small amount of blood leaving the unit has a PaO_2 of 150 mm Hg and $PaCO_2$ of 0 mm Hg (approaching the composition of inspired gas).[12,13]

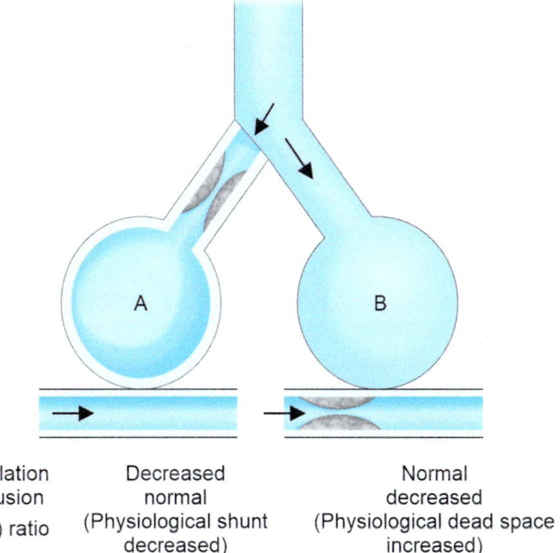

FIG. 1: Primary mechanism of hypoxemic respiratory failure—shunt physiology.

The efficiency of gas exchange can be evaluated clinically by measuring the PaO_2, $PaCO_2$, and the alveolar-arterial (A-a) global oxygen delivery (DO_2) gradient.[14] Thus, patients with hypoxemia may be divided into those with a normal gradient and those with an increased gradient **(Flowchart 1)**. The alveolar PO_2 (PAO_2) can be calculated from the alveolar air equation: $PAO_2 = (P_B - P_{H2O})\ FiO_2 - (PaCO_2/R)$, where, P_B is barometric pressure (760 mm Hg at sea level), P_{H2O} is the water vapor pressure (47 mm Hg at sea level) and R is the respiratory exchange ratio (assumed to be 0.8).

The alveolar-arterial gradient is then derived by subtracting PaO_2 from PAO_2. In a healthy individual, the (A-a) DO_2 is normally <15 mm Hg at room air; this value increases by 3 mm Hg every decade and can be as high as 30 mm Hg in elderly patients. Hypoxemic respiratory failure most often occurs due to conditions that increase the (A-a) DO_2.[15]

SECTION 17: RESPIRATORY CRITICAL CARE

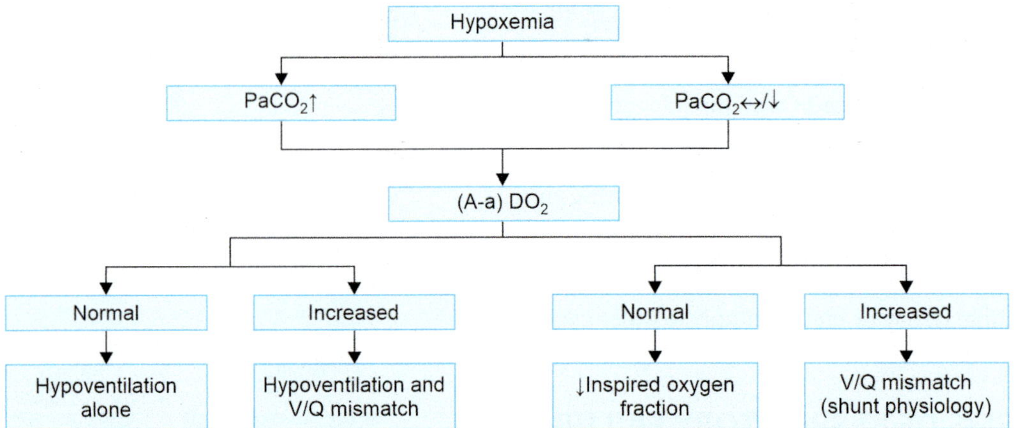

FLOWCHART 1: Importance of calculating alveolar–arterial gradient in patients with acute respiratory failure.
(A-a: alveolar–arterial; DO_2: global oxygen delivery; $PaCO_2$: partial pressure of carbon dioxide; V/Q: ventilation–perfusion)

Hypercapnic (Type 2) Respiratory Failure

The normal respiratory rate is about 12–16 breaths per minute with a tidal volume of around 500 mL. About 30% of the air inspired with each breath remains in the conducting airways of the lung and does not reach the alveoli. This component of the breath, that is not available for gas exchange, is called the anatomic dead space component. The remaining 70% reaches the alveolar zone and can participate in gas exchange. If the total ventilation each minute is 7 L, then 2 L/min is the dead space ventilation and 5 L/min is the alveolar ventilation. In diseases where some alveoli are ventilated but not perfused, the component dead space increases.[12,13] If total dead space ventilation increases but total minute ventilation remains unchanged, then alveolar ventilation (V_A) falls. Gas exchange is critically dependent on (V_A) rather than total minute ventilation. The $PaCO_2$ is directly proportional to the amount of CO_2 produced per minute and inversely proportional to V_A; according to the relationship: $PaCO_2 = 0.863 \times VCO_2/V_A$, where CO_2 is expressed in mL/min, V_A in L/min, and $PaCO_2$ in mm Hg. VCO_2 is the volume of carbon dioxide produced in mL per minute.

At fixed CO_2, when V_A increases, $PaCO_2$ falls, and when V_A decreases, $PaCO_2$ rises. Maintaining a normal level of O_2 in the alveoli (and consequently in arterial blood) also depends on provision of adequate alveolar ventilation to replenish alveolar O_2. Thus, hypercapnic respiratory failure results from any cause that leads to decrease in V_A.[4-6,11,14] Multiple mechanisms operate to cause hypercapnia in COPD, the most common cause of type 2 respiratory failure. The mechanisms can be easily remembered by the mnemonic COPD.

- *C*: Central hypoventilation
- *O*: Obstructive physiology with air trapping
- *P*: Peripheral inspiratory muscle weakness due to inflammatory cytokines
- *D*: Diaphragmatic dysfunction

CLINICAL MANIFESTATIONS OF RESPIRATORY FAILURE

A combination of arterial hypoxemia and tissue hypoxia leads to the typical manifestations of hypoxemic failure. Hypoxemia causes hyperventilation due to stimulation of carotid body chemoreceptors with resultant tachypnea. There may be cyanosis; the degree of which depends on the concentration of the hemoglobin and the patient's perfusion. Hypoxia stimulates anaerobic metabolism with generation of lactic acid that further stimulates ventilation. Mild hypoxia may also lead to impaired mental performance. With progression of hypoxia, alteration in the sensorium, somnolence, coma, and seizures can occur leading to permanent brain damage. Hypoxemia causes stimulation of the sympathetic nervous system resulting in tachycardia, diaphoresis, and systemic vasoconstriction. Severe hypoxia can lead to bradycardia, vasodilation, hypotension, myocardial ischemia, infarction, arrhythmias, and cardiac failure. Symptoms and signs also reflect not just acute hypoxemia but also the underlying cause of respiratory failure. Patients with acute hypercapnic respiratory failure largely present with central nervous system (CNS) disturbances. Hypercapnia causes CNS depression leading to lethargy, somnolence, coma, asterixis, restlessness, tremors, slurred speech, headache, and papilledema. Symptoms of hypercapnia may overlap those of hypoxemia.

DIAGNOSIS

Arterial Blood Gas Analysis

Respiratory failure may be associated with a variety of clinical manifestations. As these are nonspecific and respiratory failure may be present without dramatic signs or symptoms, this emphasizes the importance of measuring arterial blood gases in all patients in whom respiratory failure is suspected.

The arterial blood gas analysis measures pH, PaO_2, $PaCO_2$, and bicarbonate (HCO_3). The partial pressure is the driving pressure for the gas in blood and not a measure of the quantity of gas in the blood. Thus, the actual O_2 content in the blood depends on the solubility of O_2 in plasma and the quantity of hemoglobin. The PaO_2 determines what percentage of hemoglobin is saturated with O_2, based on the position on the oxyhemoglobin dissociation curve. Oxygen content in blood can be determined by adding the amount of O_2 dissolved in plasma to the amount bound to hemoglobin; According to the equation: O_2 content = 1.34 × (hemoglobin) × O_2 saturation + 0.0031 × PaO_2.

In arterial blood, the amount of O_2 transported dissolved in plasma (approximately 0.3 mL O_2 per deciliter of blood) is trivial compared to the amount bound to hemoglobin (approximately 20 mL O_2 per deciliter of blood). In arterial blood gas analysis, PaO_2 is the measurement used to assess the effect of respiratory disease on the oxygenation status. The PaO_2 gives an assessment of the hypoxemia whereas the oxygen content denotes the level of hypoxia.[15]

Pulse Oximetry

Pulse oximetry is a noninvasive assessment of the oxygenation status as measurement of PaO_2 requires arterial puncture. The pulse oximeter calculates oxygen saturation (rather than PaO_2) based on measurements of absorption of two wavelengths of light by hemoglobin in pulsatile, cutaneous arterial blood. Because of differential absorption of the two wavelengths of light by oxygenated and nonoxygenated hemoglobin, the percentage of hemoglobin that is saturated with oxygen, i.e., the SaO_2 can be calculated and displayed instantaneously. Because the oxyhemoglobin dissociation curve becomes relatively flat above PaO_2 of 60 mm Hg (corresponding to SaO_2 of 90%), the oximeter is relatively insensitive to changes in PaO_2 above this level. In conditions where cutaneous perfusion is decreased such as hypotension, the signal from the oximeter may be less reliable or even unobtainable. Other forms of hemoglobin, such as carboxyhemoglobin and methemoglobin, are not distinguishable from oxyhemoglobin when only two wavelengths of light are used. The SaO_2 values are not reliable in the presence of significant amounts of either of these forms of hemoglobin. Finally, the pulse oximeter does not indicate anything about CO_2 elimination.[15]

Chest Radiograph

Chest radiography is essential because it frequently reveals the cause of respiratory failure. However, distinguishing between cardiogenic and noncardiogenic pulmonary edema often is difficult, and may require clinical judgment and echocardiography.

Pulmonary Function Tests

Generally, pulmonary function tests (PFTs) should not be performed in patients with ARF. However, PFTs are valuable in the evaluation of CRF.

A decrease in FEV_1/FVC ratio indicates airflow obstruction, whereas a reduction in both the volume of air exhaled in the first second of a forced exhalation (FEV_1) and forced vital capacity of the lungs (FVC) and maintenance of the FEV_1/FVC ratio suggest restrictive lung disease. Respiratory failure is uncommon in obstructive diseases when the FEV_1 is greater than 1 L and in restrictive diseases when the FVC is more than 1 L.

TREATMENT

The principles of managing respiratory failure are outlined below:

- As most patients are critically ill, management should take place in a high-dependency unit/intensive care unit (ICU) setting.
- Alleviation of hypoxia is the immediate aim of treatment.
- Treatment of the basic underlying conditions such as pneumonia, pulmonary edema, etc., should be done.
- Support with mechanical ventilation either noninvasive or invasive. This is to "buy" time for specific therapies such as antibiotics to act.
- Immune status of the patient should be ascertained as it often changes the list of differential diagnoses while treating ARF.[16]

Oxygen Therapy

Hypoxemia is the major immediate threat to organ function. Therefore, the first objective is to reverse and/or prevent tissue hypoxia.[12] Oxygen therapy is started immediately on admission after an arterial blood sample is obtained for assessment of blood gas tensions. The goal of supplemental oxygen is to maintain a PaO_2 of 55–60 mm Hg corresponding to SpO_2 of 89–92%.[17] A common mistake committed by physicians, nursing staff, and occasionally the patient's attendants is to increase the flow of oxygen to improve oxygen saturation. However, one should not forget that oxygen is a "drug" and should be carefully administered since excessive oxygen has undesirable effects. In a patient with COPD who has chronic type II respiratory failure and hypercapnia, the ventilatory stimulus for hypercapnia is blunted and the ventilatory drive is maintained primarily by hypoxemia. Theoretically, excess amounts of oxygen can blunt this "hypoxic drive" with resultant hypercapnia and worsening respiratory acidosis. Excessive oxygen therapy has been shown to prolong hospital stay, probably, because it can lead to generation of harmful reactive oxygen species, which can exacerbate tissue injury. Excessive oxygen supplementation can also lead to hypercapnia by increasing V/Q disturbances, the Haldane effect (in the presence of increased O_2, the affinity of hemoglobin for CO_2 decreases), and by causing numerous areas of absorption atelectasis. Another reason why PaO_2 should not be increased beyond 60 mm Hg is because it corresponds to an oxygen saturation (SaO_2) of around 90%; from the oxygen content equation, we can conclude that there is no benefit in increasing PaO_2 above 60 mm Hg except in situations of hyperbaric oxygen delivery. In arterial blood, the amount of O_2 transported dissolved in plasma (approximately 0.3 mL O_2 per deciliter of blood) is trivial compared to the amount bound to hemoglobin (approximately 20 mL O_2 per deciliter of blood). Because of the sigmoid shape of the oxyhemoglobin dissociation curve, it is important to differentiate between the partial pressure and the content of oxygen in the blood. The partial pressure is a measure of the driving pressure for the gas in blood and not a measure of the quantity of gas in the blood. Thus, the actual O_2 content in the blood depends on the solubility of O_2 in plasma and the quantity of hemoglobin. The PaO_2 determines what percentage of hemoglobin is saturated with O_2, based on the position on the oxyhemoglobin dissociation curve. Hemoglobin is almost fully (>90%) saturated at a PaO_2 of 60 mm Hg, and little additional O_2 is carried by hemoglobin even with a substantial elevation of PaO_2 above 60 mm Hg. On the other hand, significant O_2 desaturation of hemoglobin occurs once PaO_2 falls below 60 mm Hg and onto the steep descending limb of the curve.

Choosing the most appropriate type of oxygen delivery device is important. Low-flow oxygen delivery systems provide oxygen at flow rates that are lower than patient's inspiratory demands; thus when the total ventilation exceeds the capacity of the oxygen reservoir, room air is entrained.[18-20] The final concentration of oxygen delivered depends on the ventilatory demands of the patient, the size of the oxygen reservoir, and the rate at which the reservoir is filled. At a constant flow, the larger the tidal volume, the lower the FiO_2 and vice versa.[12] In contrast, the high-flow systems provide a constant FiO_2 by delivering the gas at flow rates that exceed the patient's peak inspiratory flow and by using devices that entrain a fixed proportion of room air. In acute situations, it is always better to use high-flow devices as one can, to a reasonable extent, guarantee the oxygen delivered. On the other hand, with the use of a low-flow device, oxygen delivery would be dependent on the patient's minute ventilation. Once the patient has been stabilized, one can shift to nasal prongs as these are more comfortable for the patient.

The appropriate FiO_2 is selected with the help of alveolar gas equation.[12] We also know that the ratio of PaO_2 to PAO_2 is independent of FiO_2. For example, a patient with COPD has PaO_2 of 35 mm Hg and $PaCO_2$ of 58 mm Hg on room air; the FiO_2 requirement to bring PaO_2 to 60 mm Hg is calculated as follows:

$$PAO_2 = [FiO_2 (P_{ATM} - P_{H2O})] - (PaCO_2/R)$$

$$= [0.21 (760 - 47)] - (58/0.8) = 77.3$$

$$PaO_2/PAO_2 = 35/77 = 0.45$$

To get the desired PaO_2 of 60 mm Hg, the PAO_2 must increase for the same PaO_2/PAO_2 ratio, i.e.,

$$35/77 = 60/\ PAO_2\ (x) = 0.45$$

$$PAO_2\ (x) = 77 \times 60/35$$

$$PAO_2 = 133.3$$

The desired FiO_2 (for PaO_2 of 60 mm Hg) can be determined again from the alveolar gas equation as above, i.e.,

$$133 = FiO_2 \times 713 - (58/0.8)$$

$$FiO_2 = 28.8$$

High-flow Nasal Cannula

A relatively new oxygen delivery device namely the high-flow nasal cannula (HFNC) has been used in adults with respiratory failure. It was extensively used during the pandemic as an alternative to noninvasive ventilation (NIV). Like NIV, it is ideally applied in a closely monitored setting. It delivers high-flow heated humidified oxygen through wide-bore nasal prongs and supplies much higher flow rates (up to 60 L/min) than the traditional nasal cannula. It is of benefit for short-term use in patients with severe hypoxemia.[21] It is often preferred by patients as the nasal prongs are small and relatively comfortable to wear. The unit ensures that the oxygen is warmed to body temperature and humidified. The high flow rate can create a mild positive end-expiratory pressure (PEEP) effect, which has been documented in several studies. This is a mild effect and has been quantified as an increase of 0.7 cmH_2O for every 10 L/min increase in flow (if the mouth is closed). Unlike low-flow systems where entrainment of ambient air can significantly lower the concentration of the O_2 being supplied, an HFNC does not allow this to happen. The flow rate and the FiO_2can be set. Flows from 5 to 60 L/min are possible, and one can start mid-range and titrate as required. The FiO_2 is set to target a desired oxygen saturation. It is preferred to use increased flows rather than use oxygen fractions above 60%. A nebulizer chamber cannot be placed in the HFNC circuit, and it must be used separately through a mouthpiece. HFNC is not a substitute for NIV in cases of type II respiratory failure.[22]

Noninvasive Ventilation

Noninvasive ventilation refers to the provision of inspiratory pressure support plus continuous positive airway pressure (CPAP) via a nasal or facemask, i.e., without an endotracheal airway.[23-28] It has been used for diverse forms of respiratory failure and has revolutionized the management of respiratory failure.[29-35] Although CPAP does not actively assist inspiration and is not traditionally a ventilatory mode, it is considered a form of NIV when used as a therapy for respiratory failure. The key to the successful application of NIV is good patient selection. Patients who clearly require immediate intubation should be excluded. Careful assessment of the patient determines whether the patient requires and is likely to respond to NIV.[24] This requires clinical evaluation and may also involve a NIV trial. NIV is an effective tool in improving the clinical outcomes of patients with ARF. Etiologies likely to respond best include-acute exacerbations of COPD,[36] cardiogenic pulmonary edema,[23,24] weaning patients with CRF especially COPD,[37] and management of ARF in immunocompromised patients.[38,39] It not only avoids the need for endotracheal intubation but also reduces other complications such as occurrence of nosocomial infections, duration of ICU stay, and the overall cost of hospitalization.[40]

Important determinants of NIV success include a comfortable, properly fitting interface and appropriate ventilator settings.[24,35] Masks are firmly secured with elastic straps to the face in order to avoid air leaks and consequent malfunction. The nasal mask is usually well tolerated because it causes less claustrophobia and discomfort.[41] It allows eating, drinking, and expectorating. A full-face mask is preferable in severe respiratory failure. Dyspneic patients mouth-breathe in order to bypass resistance of the nasal passages. Mouth opening during nasal mask ventilation results in air leakage and decreased effectiveness.[42] Full-face masks are used for ARF whereas nasal masks are preferred in the chronic setting. Optimal ventilator settings are determined by the ability to reduce the work of breathing (assessed clinically by reduction in respiratory rate to <30–35 breaths per minute) by providing an adequate level of pressure support (usually >8–10 cmH_2O) without causing discomfort from high pressures **(Box 1)**.

The NIV should be applied only in an area where staff trained in the use of NIV is constantly present.[43] To assure the success of NIV, close monitoring is necessary, especially during the first few hours. Patients need to be monitored with close clinical observation, continuous pulse oximetry, and on-demand arterial blood gas measurements. Favorable subjective responses such as tolerance of the mask and NIV pressures and reduction of respiratory distress predict good results. Although the optimal duration of an NIV trial remains uncertain, a response within 1–4 hours of initiation is a reasonable expectation.[44] Finally, patients who are failing an NIV trial should be promptly intubated and mechanically ventilated as delays in endotracheal intubation in patients being managed with NIV have been shown to be associated with decreased survival.[45]

BOX 1 Protocol for application of noninvasive ventilation in acute respiratory failure.

- Full-face masks are better tolerated in acute settings
- Start with an inspiratory pressure support of 6–8 cmH_2O and CPAP of 3–4 cmH_2O
- *Adjustments*:
  - Increase inspiratory pressure and CPAP by 2 and 1 cmH_2O, respectively
  - Titrate to tidal volume (5–7 mL/kg), respiratory rate (<35 breaths/min), according to blood gases
  - Maximum inspiratory pressure and CPAP generally used is 15–16 cmH_2O and 7–8 cmH_2O, respectively
- Air leaks should be minimized
- CPAP is rarely used in acute respiratory failure

(CPAP: continuous positive airway pressure)

We have significant experience with the use of NIV.[46] In a study involving 63 patients, NIV failures were higher in ARF associated with other causes (15/39, 38.4%) compared to ARF associated with COPD (3/24, 12.5%). Only the etiology of ARF (ARF due to other causes) was associated with NIV failure in a multivariate analysis.[26] In another study involving 40 patients with hypoxemic ARF, NIV failures were higher in ARDS group (12/21, 57.1%) than in hypoxemic ARF due to other causes (7/12, 36.8%). The only factor associated with NIV failure was the baseline PaO_2–FiO_2 ratio on a univariate analysis.[27] In a recently conducted randomized controlled trial, we randomized patients with acute asthma to the standard medical therapy (SMT) arm ($n = 28$) or NIV plus SMT arm ($n = 25$). The improvement in respiratory rate, FEV_1, and PaO_2–FiO_2 were seen equally in both groups. However, increment in FEV_1 by 50% at 4 hours was greater in the NIV arm. Not only the mean dose of bronchodilators required was lesser in the NIV group, but the ICU and hospital length of stay was significantly shorter in NIV group. There were four instances of SMT failure, and all these patients improved with the application of NIV. Two patients failed NIV and required endotracheal intubation.[47]

With the remarkable success of NIV in COPD, it has been tempting to try and use this in the setting of asthma, which seems similar. However, most trials do not show unequivocal benefits in asthma. NIV must be used cautiously, if at all in asthma. The mask should not be allowed to delay or interfere with inhaled therapy in any case.[48] There are constant efforts to try and expand the role of NIV beyond the currently accepted four settings mentioned earlier. In these, benefit has been proven beyond doubt.

Endotracheal Intubation and Invasive Ventilation

Patients who are in severe respiratory distress and those who fail treatment with oxygen and NIV generally require endotracheal intubation and invasive ventilation. Another indication for intubation is airway protection in patients with altered mental status. The aim of invasive ventilation is to correct hypoxemia and maintain alveolar ventilation appropriate to patient's metabolic requirements. It has been recognized since 1970 that mechanical ventilation if not applied properly could cause harm.[49] However, only recently has this concept been applied in day to day practice. A new era of ventilatory management began in 1990 when it was showed that minimizing pulmonary overdistension and allowing permissive hypercapnia decreased mortality in patients with ARDS.[50] The clinical importance of ventilator-associated lung injury was aptly highlighted by the ARDS Network study.[51] Although patients without ALI were, till recently, ventilated with large tidal volumes, recent studies have shown that use of higher tidal volumes can cause ventilator-associated lung injury even in patients with normal lungs.[52-60] Recognition of this fact has led to a paradigm shift in the ventilatory management with use of lower tidal volumes even in patients with normal lungs. The current ventilatory strategy aims at minimizing complications of mechanical ventilation. The principles are to prevent initiation of additional alveolar injury and facilitate healing of the underlying condition. The ventilation is thus pressure-targeted employing lower tidal volumes. The aim is to have adequate blood gases and normalization of physiological parameters is not considered important **(Table 2)**.

An important consideration is the ventilator that should be used for mechanically ventilating these patients. No ventilator is clearly better than any other. The machine is selected based on the spectrum of patients, the financial resources of the ICU, and the available expertise in handling the equipment. Clearly, the people operating the ventilator are more important than the machine. Other important issue is the mode to be used for mechanical ventilation. No mode is clearly superior. The choice of a particular mode is often guided by institutional policy or personal preference. One controversial area is the choice of a volume-controlled or pressure-controlled strategy. There is no strong evidence base for the pressure-controlled ventilation although logically it is likely to be equivalent to the volume-controlled mode because it is the settings rather than the mode that is the important issue. It is best to initiate ventilation with a volume assist controlled mode, and once the patient improves, shift the patient to pressure-support ventilation. As a protocol, we rarely, if ever, use synchronized intermittent mandatory ventilation for either initial ventilation or later weaning. Newer modes of ventilation are increasingly being promoted to decrease the hazards of conventional ventilation and improve patient–ventilator interactions. However, none of the newer modes of ventilation has been shown superior to conventional modes. Also, the indications, efficacy, and safety are still clinically uncertain and are not being widely utilized. Much controversy has been witnessed over lung-protective ventilation with all the adjunctive maneuvers versus high-frequency ventilation and finally extracorporeal membrane oxygenation (ECMO).[61]

Extracorporeal Membrane Oxygenation

The use of ECMO for severe ARF in adults has grown rapidly, especially during the pandemic. ECMO is a complex, high-risk, and costly modality. It should be utilized only in centers with the expertise to ensure it is used safely. An international consensus opinion on ECMO was published a decade ago, with the aim of providing physicians, ECMO centers, and policymakers a description of the optimal approach to organizing ECMO programs for ARF in adult patients. It helped to ensure that ECMO was delivered safely and proficiently, and facilitated clinical trials under homogeneous and optimal conditions.[62] This modality is beginning to be more frequently used in Indian centers at present. It is the most useful intervention in ARDS not responding to other measures.[63] Significant benefit was seen in the better quality studies of venovenous ECMO and the subgroup with H1N1.[64] More recently the COVID-19 pandemic has allowed much experience to be gained with the modality.[65] The indications for ECMO in COVID-19-related ARDS are similar to any viral pneumonia.[22,66,67] The venovenous modality suffices for patients with pulmonary involvement refractory to other

TABLE 2: Parameters and goals for invasive mechanical ventilation in different categories of respiratory failure.

	Restricted lung	Obstructed lung	Normal lung
Prototype	ARDS	Acute asthma	Neuromuscular respiratory failure
Mode	V-ACMV	V-ACMV	V-ACMV
Initial tidal volumes	4–6 mL/kg	4–6 mL/kg	6–8 mL/kg
Respiratory rate	18–35 breaths/min	8–12 breaths/min	14–18 breaths/min
PEEP	$FiO_2 \times 20$	5–8 cmH_2O	Up to 5 cmH_2O
I: E	1:1–1:2	1:3–1:6	1:2–1:3
Flow waveform	Descending ramp	Square waveform	–
Plateau pressure	30 cmH_2O	30 cmH_2O	–
PaO_2	~ 55–60 mm Hg	~ 55–60 mm Hg	~ 60–80 mm Hg
pH	7.2–7.4	7.2–7.4	–

(ARDS: acute respiratory distress syndrome; FiO_2: fraction of inspired oxygen; I:E: inspiration:expiration ratio; PaO_2: partial pressure of oxygen; PEEP: positive end-expiratory pressure; V-ACMV: volume-assist controlled mechanical ventilation)

modalities. The venoarterial mode provides both pulmonary and cardiac support and is useful in patients with severe cardiac dysfunction in addition to ARDS. Benefits in reversing hypoxemia may not necessarily translate into mortality benefit.[68,69] Even with conditions usually associated with a high chance of death, almost 50% of patients receiving ECMO survive up to discharge. Complications are frequent and most often comprise renal failure, pneumonia or sepsis, and bleeding.[70] The experience gained with the modality during the pandemic is likely to see it being used far more frequently than before.

SUMMARY

The management of respiratory failure hinges on two basic principles, i.e., alleviation of hypoxemia, and aggressive treatment of the underlying basic disease. Oxygen should be administered through high-flow (Venturi mask) system. NIV should be judiciously used in ARF as inappropriate use of NIV may lead to delayed intubation in some patients. Eventually, mechanical ventilation is required in patients who fail NIV or develop respiratory arrest. ECMO is useful in patients who remain hypoxemic despite 100% oxygen.

REFERENCES

1. Wood LDH, Naureckas ET. The pathophysiology and differential diagnosis of acute respiratory failure. In: Hall JB, Schmidt GA, Wood LDH (Eds). Principles of Critical Care. New Delhi: McGraw-Hill; 2005. pp. 417-26.
2. Ceriana P, Nava S. Hypoxic and hypercapnic respiratory failure. Eur Respir Mon. 2006;36:1-15.
3. Campbell EJ. Respiratory Failure. BMJ. 1965;1(5448):1451-60.
4. Campbell EJ. Respiratory failure. Definition, mechanisms and recent developments. Bull Eur Physiopathol Respir. 1979;15 Suppl:1-13.
5. Duncan SR, Raffin TA. Mechanisms and management of respiratory failure. Compr Ther. 1986;12(7):55-63.
6. Froelich R. Mechanisms underlying respiratory failure. J Contin Educ Nurs. 1979;10(4):31-9.
7. Adrogué HJ, Tobin MJ. Respiratory Failure. Massachussets: Blackwell Science; 1997.
8. Sodhi K, Chanchalani G. Awake proning: Current evidence and practical considerations. Indian J Crit Care Med. 2020;24(12):1236-41.
9. Esan A, Hess DR, Raoof S, et al. Severe hypoxemic respiratory failure: Part 1–ventilatory strategies. Chest. 2010;137(5):1203-16.
10. Raoof S, Goulet K, Esan A, et al. Severe hypoxemic respiratory failure: Part 2–nonventilatory strategies. Chest. 2010;137(6):1437-48.
11. Conference report: Mechanisms of acute respiratory failure. Am Rev Respir Dis. 1977;115(6):1071-8.
12. Jindal SK, Agarwal R. Oxygen Therapy, 2nd edition. New Delhi: Jaypee Brothers Medical Publishers (P) Ltd; 2008.
13. Lumb AB, Nunn JF. Nunn's Applied Respiratory Physiology. Oxford, UK: Butterworth Heinemann; 2000.
14. D'Alonzo GE, Dantzker DR. Respiratory failure, mechanisms of abnormal gas exchange, and oxygen delivery. Med Clin North Am. 1983;67(3):557-71.
15. Dakin J, Griffiths M. The pulmonary physician in critical care 1: Pulmonary investigations for acute respiratory failure. Thorax. 2002;57(1):79-85.
16. Sarkar P, Rasheed HF. Clinical review: Respiratory failure in HIV-infected patients–a changing picture. Crit Care. 2013;17(3):228.
17. Jindal SK, Agarwal R. Long-term oxygen therapy. Expert Rev Respir Med. 2012;6(6):639-49.
18. Agarwal R, Gupta D. What are high-flow and low-flow oxygen delivery systems? Stroke. 2005;36(10):2066-7; author reply 2067.
19. Agarwal R. Supplemental oxygen and risk of surgical wound infection. JAMA. 2006;295(14):1641.
20. Agarwal R. The low-flow or high-flow oxygen delivery system and a low-flow or high-flow nonrebreather mask. Am J Respir Crit Care Med. 2006;174(9):1055.
21. Sotello D, Rivas M, Mulkey Z, et al. High-flow nasal cannula oxygen in adult patients: A narrative review. Am J Med Sci. 2015; 349(2):179-85.
22. Anand S, Baishya M, Singh A, et al. Effect of awake prone positioning in COVID-19 patients-A systematic review. Tren Anaesth Crit Care. 2021;36:17-22.
23. Agarwal R, Aggarwal AN, Gupta D. Is noninvasive pressure support ventilation as effective and safe as continuous positive airway pressure in cardiogenic pulmonary oedema? Singapore Med J. 2009;50(6):595-603.
24. Agarwal R, Aggarwal AN, Gupta D, et al. Non-invasive ventilation in acute cardiogenic pulmonary oedema. Postgrad Med J. 2005;81(960):637-43.
25. Agarwal R, Aggarwal AN, Gupta D, et al. Role of noninvasive positive-pressure ventilation in postextubation respiratory failure: A meta-analysis. Respir Care. 2007;52(11):1472-9.
26. Agarwal R, Gupta R, Aggarwal AN, et al. Noninvasive positive pressure ventilation in acute respiratory failure due to COPD vs other causes: Effectiveness and predictors of failure in a respiratory ICU in North India. Int J Chron Obstruct Pulmon Dis. 2008;3(4):737-43.
27. Agarwal R, Handa A, Aggarwal AN, et al. Outcomes of noninvasive ventilation in acute hypoxemic respiratory failure in a respiratory intensive care unit in North India. Respir Care. 2009;54(12):1679-87.
28. Agarwal R, Reddy C, Aggarwal AN, et al. Is there a role for noninvasive ventilation in acute respiratory distress syndrome? A meta-analysis. Respir Med. 2006;100(12):2235-8.
29. Brochard L. Noninvasive pressure support ventilation in acute respiratory failure. Monaldi Arch Chest Dis. 1998;53(4):486-7.
30. Organized jointly by the American Thoracic Society, the European Respiratory Society, the European Society of Intensive Care Medicine, and the Société de Réanimation de Langue Française, and approved by ATS Board of Directors. International Consensus Conferences in Intensive Care Medicine: Noninvasive positive pressure ventilation in acute respiratory failure. Am J Respir Crit Care Med. 2001;163(1):283-91.
31. Brochard L. Noninvasive ventilation for acute respiratory failure. JAMA. 2002;288(8):932-5.
32. Hamel DS, Klonin H. The role of noninvasive ventilation for acute respiratory failure. Respir Care Clin N Am. 2006;12(3):421-35.
33. Hill NS, Brennan J, Garpestad E, et al. Noninvasive ventilation in acute respiratory failure. Crit Care Med. 2007;35(10):2402-7.

34. Miletin MS, Detsky AS, Lapinsky SE, et al. Non-invasive ventilation in acute hypoxemic respiratory failure. Intensive Care Med. 2000;26(2):242-5.
35. Nava S, Hill N. Non-invasive ventilation in acute respiratory failure. Lancet. 2009;374(9685):250-9.
36. Ram FSF, Picot J, Lightowler J, et al. Non-invasive positive pressure ventilation for treatment of respiratory failure due to exacerbations of chronic obstructive pulmonary disease. Cochrane Database Syst Review. 2004;3(CD004104).
37. Ferrer M, Sellarés J, Valencia M, et al. Non-invasive ventilation after extubation in hypercapnic patients with chronic respiratory disorders: randomised controlled trial. Lancet. 2009; 374(9695):1082-8.
38. Hilbert G, Gruson D, Vargas F, et al. Noninvasive continuous positive airway pressure in neutropenic patients with acute respiratory failure requiring intensive care unit admission. Crit Care Med. 2000;28(9):3185-90.
39. Hilbert G, Gruson D, Vargas F, et al. Noninvasive ventilation in immunosuppressed patients with pulmonary infiltrates, fever, and acute respiratory failure. N Engl J Med. 2001;344(7):481-7.
40. Brochard L, Mancebo J, Elliott MW. Noninvasive ventilation for acute respiratory failure. Eur Respir J. 2002;19(4):712-21.
41. Navalesi P, Fanfulla F, Frigerio P, et al. Physiologic evaluation of noninvasive mechanical ventilation delivered with three types of masks in patients with chronic hypercapnic respiratory failure. Crit Care Med. 2000;28(6):1785-90.
42. Kwok H, McCormack J, Cece R, et al. Controlled trial of oronasal versus nasal mask ventilation in the treatment of acute respiratory failure. Crit Care Med. 2003;31(2):468-73.
43. Carlucci A, Delmastro M, Rubini F, et al. Changes in the practice of non-invasive ventilation in treating COPD patients over 8 years. Intensive Care Med. 2003;29(3):419-25.
44. Agarwal R. Noninvasive ventilation in acute lung injury/acute respiratory distress syndrome. In: Esquinas AM (Ed). Noninvasive Mechanical Ventilation: Theory, Equipment, and Clinical Applications, 1st edition. Berlin, Germany: Springer; 2010.
45. Nava S, Ceriana P. Causes of failure of noninvasive mechanical ventilation. Respir Care. 2004;49(3):295-303.
46. Sharma S, Agarwal R, Aggarwal AN, et al. A survey of noninvasive ventilation practices in a respiratory ICU of North India. Respir Care. 2012;57(7):1145-53.
47. Gupta D, Nath A, Agarwal R, et al. A prospective randomized controlled trial on the efficacy of noninvasive ventilation in severe acute asthma. Respir Care. 2010;55(5):536-43.
48. Lim WJ, Mohammed Akram R, Carson KV, et al. Non-invasive positive pressure ventilation for treatment of respiratory failure due to severe acute exacerbations of asthma. Cochrane Database Systematic Rev. 2012;12:CD004360.
49. Mead J, Takishima T, Leith D. Stress distribution in lungs: A model of pulmonary elasticity. J Appl Physiol. 1970;28(5):596-608.
50. Hickling KG, Henderson SJ, Jackson R. Low mortality associated with low volume pressure limited ventilation with permissive hypercapnia in severe adult respiratory distress syndrome. Intensive Care Med. 1990;16(6):372-7.
51. Acute Respiratory Distress Syndrome Network; Brower RG, Matthay MA, Morris A, et al. Ventilation with lower tidal volumes as compared with traditional tidal volumes for acute lung injury and the acute respiratory distress syndrome. The Acute Respiratory Distress Syndrome Network. N Engl J Med. 2000;342(18):1301-8.
52. Gama de Abreu M, Heintz M, Heller A, et al. One-lung ventilation with high tidal volumes and zero positive end-expiratory pressure is injurious in the isolated rabbit lung model. Anesth Analg. 2003;96(1):220-8.
53. Choi G, Wolthuis EK, Bresser P, et al. Mechanical ventilation with lower tidal volumes and positive end-expiratory pressure prevents alveolar coagulation in patients without lung injury. Anesthesiology. 2006;105(4):689-5.
54. Mascia L, Zavala E, Bosma K, et al. High tidal volume is associated with the development of acute lung injury after severe brain injury: An international observational study. Crit Care Med. 2007;35(8):1815-20.
55. Yilmaz M, Keegan MT, Iscimen R, et al. Toward the prevention of acute lung injury: Protocol-guided limitation of large tidal volume ventilation and inappropriate transfusion. Crit Care Med. 2007;35(7):1660-6; quiz 1667.
56. Meier T, Lange A, Papenberg H, et al. Pulmonary cytokine responses during mechanical ventilation of noninjured lungs with and without end-expiratory pressure. Anesth Analg. 2008; 107(4):1265-75.
57. Wolthuis EK, Choi G, Dessing MC, et al. Mechanical ventilation with lower tidal volumes and positive end-expiratory pressure prevents pulmonary inflammation in patients without preexisting lung injury. Anesthesiology. 2008;108(1):46-54.
58. Determann RM, Royakkers A, Wolthuis EK, et al. Ventilation with lower tidal volumes as compared with conventional tidal volumes for patients without acute lung injury: A preventive randomized controlled trial. Critical Care. 2010;14(1):R1.
59. Hong CM, Xu DZ, Lu Q, et al. Low tidal volume and high positive end-expiratory pressure mechanical ventilation results in increased inflammation and ventilator-associated lung injury in normal lungs. Anesth Analg. 2010;110(6):1652-60.
60. Weingarten TN, Whalen FX, Warner DO, et al. Comparison of two ventilatory strategies in elderly patients undergoing major abdominal surgery. Br J Anaesth. 2010;104(1):16-22.
61. Shekar K, Davies AR, Mullany DV, et al. To ventilate, oscillate, or cannulate? J Critical Care. 2013;28(5):655-62.
62. Combes A, Brodie D, Bartlett R, et al. Position paper for the organization of extracorporeal membrane oxygenation programs for acute respiratory failure in adult patients. Am J Respir Crit Care Med. 2014;190(5):488-96.
63. MacLaren G, Brain MJ, Butt WW. ECMO in acute and chronic adult respiratory failure: Recent trends and future directions. Minerva Anestesiol. 2013;79(9):1059-65.
64. Munshi L, Telesnicki T, Walkey A, et al. Extracorporeal life support for acute respiratory failure. A systematic review and metaanalysis. Ann Am Thorac Soc. 2014;11(5):802-10.
65. Combes A, Peek GJ, Hajage D, et al. ECMO for severe ARDS: Systematic review and individual patient data meta-analysis. Intensive Care Med. 2020;46(11):2048-57.
66. Bertini P, Guarracino F, Falcone M, et al. ECMO in COVID-19 patients: A systematic review and meta-analysis. J Cardiothorac VascAnesth. 2022;36(8):2700-6.
67. Ramanathan K, Shekar K, Ling RR, et al. Extracorporeal membrane oxygenation for COVID-19: A systematic review and meta-analysis. Crit Care. 2021;25(1):1-11.
68. Pierrakos C, Karanikolas M, Scolletta S, et al. Acute respiratory distress syndrome: Pathophysiology and therapeutic options. J Clin Med Res. 2012;4(1):7-16.
69. Zampieri FG, Mendes PV, Ranzani OT, et al. Extracorporeal membrane oxygenation for severe respiratory failure in adult patients: A systematic review and meta-analysis of current evidence. J Crit Care. 2013;28(6):998-1005.
70. Zangrillo A, Landoni G, Biondi-Zoccai G, et al. A meta-analysis of complications and mortality of extracorporeal membrane oxygenation. Crit Care Resusc.2013;15(3):172-8.

Acute Respiratory Distress Syndrome: Epidemiology, Etiology, Pathophysiology, Definition, and Subphenotypes

CHAPTER 163

Valliappan Muthu, Kuruswamy Thurai Prasad, Ritesh Agarwal

INTRODUCTION

Acute respiratory distress syndrome (ARDS) is a clinical syndrome consequent to various etiologies.[1] The condition was first described in 1967 in a series of 12 patients with tachypnea, hypoxemia, and diffuse lung infiltrates following various causes (most commonly trauma). The authors considered a possible link to surface active agents of the lung since the clinical and pathological features in ARDS resembled the respiratory distress encountered in infants with surfactant deficiency. A beneficial role of positive end-expiratory pressure (PEEP) and inconsistent benefit with systemic corticosteroids (in a subset of patients) were few other pertinent observations in this landmark study, which have stood the test of time.[2]

Despite several decades of research, ARDS continues to remain an enigmatic entity with a high mortality rate. The complexity of ARDS is partly due to the heterogeneity of etiology, which may have differing courses and responses to various therapies.[3] In this chapter, we will review the epidemiology, definition, etiology, pathophysiology, and subphenotypes of ARDS.

EPIDEMIOLOGY OF ACUTE RESPIRATORY DISTRESS SYNDROME

Population-based studies from the United States and Iceland have estimated the annual incidence rate of ARDS from 3.6 to 82.4 per 100,000 person-years.[4,5] The prevalence of ARDS in intensive care units (ICUs) was 10.4% in a large observational study enrolling 29,144 patients in 459 ICUs across 50 countries.[6] In another study, the prevalence of ARDS from an Indian ICU was 12.4% of all ICU admissions over 16 years.[7] There is substantial underrecognition and undertreatment of ARDS. The Large Observational Study to Understand the Global Impact of Severe Acute Respiratory Failure (LUNG SAFE) study noted that ARDS was clinically suspected in only 51% of the mild and 78% of the severe ARDS cases. The ICU (35%) and in-hospital (40%) mortality associated with ARDS was also high.[6] In the latter study, the in-hospital mortality rates for mild, moderate, and severe ARDS were 34.9%, 40.3%, and 46.1%, respectively. The incidence and outcome of ARDS are likely to vary depending on the case mix, age, sex, severity of illness at admission, race, and possibly genetic and other modifiable risk factors such as alcohol use disorder.[7-10]

The trend of ARDS and its etiology over time is unclear. A longitudinal study over several years observed a reduction in the incidence of ARDS, possibly due to adopting a hospital-wide ARDS-prevention strategy (such as lung protective ventilation, protection against aspiration, and others).[5] On the contrary, another study suggested an increase in the incidence of ARDS over time.[4,11] The data on mortality trends is also conflicting, with a few studies suggesting an improvement in survival over the years,[11] while others note that the mortality has remained unchanged.[12]

DEFINITION OF ACUTE RESPIRATORY DISTRESS SYNDROME

Acute respiratory distress syndrome is not a disease entity; instead, it is a clinical pattern, and attempts to find the cause of respiratory failure is crucial.[13] The original description by Ashbaugh et al. is sufficient to identify ARDS at the bedside, and a few experts have criticized the need for newer definitions.[3,14] Nevertheless, a uniform definition is required for timely recognition and enrolling patients in clinical trials evaluating the management strategies for ARDS.

The first formal attempt at defining ARDS was published by Murray et al. in 1988, where they used oxygenation, PEEP, chest radiograph, and respiratory system compliance (when available) to assign a lung injury score (LIS).[15] The LIS appears to have limited utility and prognostic advantage over the various criteria developed later [the Berlin definition and the American-European Consensus Conference (AECC) consensus criteria].[16] The AECC definition of ARDS, published in 1994, was the first widely accepted and used definition, framed after several rounds of discussions and conferences from 1992. The AECC definition categorized patients as having acute lung injury (ALI) or ARDS based on the oxygenation criteria **(Table 1)**. However, along with a few other limitations, the AECC definition lacked a clear cutoff to define "acute onset". Also, nearly 50% of patients diagnosed with ARDS (using the AECC definition) lacked histological evidence of DAD. Subsequent studies also found that pulmonary artery catheterization-guided management of ALI did not improve clinical outcomes and was associated with a higher complication rate than the standard of care.[17] In 2005, a modified definition was proposed (based on a Delphi consensus)[18] which also compared with the LIS score and AECC definitions.[19] Although the Delphi consensus criteria

TABLE 1: Definitions of ARDS.

	American-European Consensus Conference definition on ARDS (1994)[82]	Berlin consensus definition (2012)[20]	New global definition of ARDS (2023)[28]
Criteria	Acute lung injury (ALI) • Acute onset • *Oxygenation*: $PaO_2/FiO_2 \leq 300$ mm Hg (regardless of PEEP) • Bilateral infiltrates on chest radiograph • Pulmonary arterial wedge pressure ≤ 18 mm Hg or no clinical evidence of left atrial hypertension *ARDS*: Same as ALI, except oxygenation criteria $PaO_2/FiO_2 \leq 200$ mm Hg	*Timing*: Respiratory failure within 1 week of clinical insult or new/worsening respiratory symptoms *Chest radiograph*: Bilateral opacities not fully explained by pleural effusion, lung collapse or nodules *Origin of lung edema*: Not fully explainable by cardiac failure or fluid overload An objective assessment (e.g., echocardiography) suggested to exclude cardiogenic edema if no risk factors present *Oxygenation criteria on a PEEP of ≥5 cmH_2O*: PaO_2/FiO_2 ratio of >200 to ≤300 mm Hg (mild) PaO_2/FiO_2 of >100 to ≤200 mm Hg (moderate) $PaO_2/FiO_2 \leq 100$ mm Hg (severe)	*Risk factors*: Respiratory failure precipitated by an acute predisposing risk factor such as pneumonia, aspiration, nonpulmonary infection, trauma, transfusion, or shock Pulmonary edema not attributable (exclusively or primarily) to cardiogenic causes or fluid overload. ARDS may be considered in the setting of cardiogenic pulmonary edema if predisposing risk factors are present *Timing*: Respiratory failure within 1 week of clinical insult or new/worsening respiratory symptoms *Chest imaging*: bilateral opacities on chest radiograph, computed tomography, or bilateral B-lines or consolidations on ultrasonography, not explained by atelectasis, effusions, or nodules *Oxygenation criteria*: For three different categories: 1. *Nonintubated ARDS*: $PaO_2/FiO_2 \leq 300$ mm Hg or $SpO_2/FiO_2 \leq 315$ (if $SpO_2 \leq 97\%$) on HFNO with a flow of ≥30 L/min or NIV/CPAP (at least 5 cmH_2O PEEP) 2. *Intubated ARDS:* • Mild: PaO_2/FIO_2 ratio of >200 to ≤300 or SpO_2/FiO_2 >235 to ≤315 (if $SpO_2 \leq 97\%$) • Moderate: PaO_2/FIO_2 of >100 to ≤200 or SpO_2/FiO_2 > 148 to ≤ 235 (if $SpO_2 \leq 97\%$) • Severe: $PaO_2/FiO_2 \leq 100$ or $SpO_2/FiO_2 \leq 148$ (if $SpO_2 \leq 97\%$) 3. *Modified definition for resource-variable settings*: $SpO_2/FiO_2 \leq 315$ (if $SpO_2 \leq 97\%$). PEEP or a minimum oxygen flow is not required in these settings
Strengths	• Easy to apply • Several trials have been conducted using the above criteria	• The time frame was defined • More refined radiological criteria with illustrative examples • The three categories of ARDS had distinct mortality rates, and the definition had a better predictive value for ARDS mortality than the AECC definition	• Simpler to use • Inclusion of HFNO in the definition • Enables identification of ARDS even in low-income countries • Obviates the need for PEEP to diagnose ARDS

Continued

Continued

	American-European Consensus Conference definition on ARDS (1994)[82]	Berlin consensus definition (2012)[20]	New global definition of ARDS (2023)[28]
Limitations	• No clear definition for the "acute" onset • Does not account for PEEP while stratifying and diagnosing ARDS based on the oxygenation criteria • Interobserver variability in interpreting the chest radiograph • The need for pulmonary artery catheterization • Several trials have been conducted using the above criteria	• Heterogeneity of ARDS not addressed • Recent advances such as HFNO need to be considered in defining ARDS • May overestimate ARDS • In resource-limited settings, ARDS may be missed	• Quality assurance of pulse oximetry devices and difficulty using them in dark-skinned patients or those with circulatory failure • Operator dependence of ultrasonography • Likely to dilute the definition and overestimate ARDS • Likely to increase the heterogeneity, making it difficult to interpret the trials

(ALI: acute lung injury; ARDS: acute respiratory distress syndrome; CPAP: continuous positive airway pressure; FiO_2: fraction of inspired oxygen; HFNO: high-flow nasal oxygen; NIV: noninvasive ventilation; PaO_2: partial pressure of arterial oxygen; PEEP: positive end-expiratory pressure; SpO_2: peripheral oxygen saturation measured by pulse oximeter)

were not widely followed, the underrecognition of ARDS and the poor specificity of the AECC definition were important observations.[19] The poor specificity and underrecognition led to the proposal of the refined Berlin criteria of ARDS.

The Berlin definition of ARDS defined the time frame for diagnosing ARDS, eliminated the need for pulmonary artery catheterization, and provided illustrative examples to improve the chest radiograph interpretation.[20] Unlike the AECC definition, the Berlin criteria were validated. The three categories (mild, moderate, and severe) of ARDS identified by the Berlin definition were found to be different in terms of severity (median ventilator-free days, mortality) than the AECC classification.[21] The Berlin definition was subsequently used for several trials and in clinical practice. Nevertheless, the underrecognition of ARDS continued, and a few studies also showed that the predictive ability of 28-day mortality with the Berlin definition [area under the receiver operating characteristic (AURoC) curve of 0.5664] was not different from the AECC definition (AURoC of 0.5625).[22] While the Berlin criteria was sensitive (89%), it lacked specificity (63%), when compared against the histopathological finding of diffuse alveolar damage (DAD).[23] The histological correlation was better in patients with moderate or severe ARDS and those who had a longer duration of illness (>72 hours). Later studies suggest that the use of a higher PEEP (≥10 cmH_2O) and FiO_2 (≥0.5) after 24 hours of standard ventilatory and supportive care could improve risk stratification and may be used for the inclusion of participants in trials.[24,25]

The global applicability of the ARDS definitions has been questioned, and challenges in resource-constrained settings, such as the scarcity of mechanical ventilators and facilities for chest radiographs or arterial blood gas analyzers, led to the Kigali Modification of the Berlin definition.[26] The modifications included the use of $SpO_2/FiO_2 < 315$ (instead of PaO_2/FiO_2 ratio), eliminating the need for PEEP in the criteria, and allowing the use of either chest radiograph or thoracic ultrasound to document lung infiltrates. A study conducted in Rwanda showed that the standard Berlin definition would have missed all cases of ARDS, compared to the Kigali modification (detected 4% ARDS).[26] The validity of Kigali modification in mechanically ventilated patients remains to be seen, and a recent study from the Netherlands suggested a high false positivity in this population, primarily due to the inclusion of ultrasonography to diagnose lung infiltrates.[27]

Global Consensus Definition of ARDS (2023)

A new definition was recently proposed to address the Berlin definition's limitation and improve its applicability even in resource-limited settings.[28] The fundamental changes from the earlier definition include the following:

- *New categories of ARDS*: (1) Nonintubated ARDS—high-flow nasal oxygen (HFNO, threshold of oxygen delivery of at least 30 L/min) and noninvasive ventilation (NIV); (2) intubated ARDS, and (3) ARDS diagnosed in resource-limited settings (formal adoption of the Kigali modification of Berlin definition)
- SpO_2/FiO_2 as an alternative to the PaO_2/FiO_2 ratio when arterial blood gas estimation is unavailable. Pulse oximetry should be performed after ensuring adequate waveform, oximeter placement, and is considered valid only when SpO_2 is ≤97%.
- Thoracic ultrasound (performed by trained operators) for detecting bilateral lung infiltrates as an alternative when chest radiographs or computed tomography are unavailable.

The new consensus criteria are more liberal and overcome one of the major drawbacks of the existing definitions, i.e., underdiagnosis of ARDS.[6] However, the newer definition is fraught with the risk of overdiagnosis, especially with an operator-dependent investigation (ultrasonography) to identify non-aerated lung parenchyma, unexplained by collapse, effusion or nodules. While the consensus definition emphasizes, the need for ultrasound training and more robust protocols for using lung ultrasound (LUS),[29] the impact of this modification needs to be prospectively studied. Moreover, LUS has been evaluated in ARDS patients versus healthy volunteers,[30] and their performance in the critical care unit with other respiratory illnesses, nonpulmonary causes of ARDS, obesity, or underlying chronic respiratory diseases would be a significant challenge.[31] The impact of such a watered-down definition of ARDS at the bedside and in clinical trials must be prospectively evaluated.

PRECIPITATING CAUSES OF ACUTE RESPIRATORY DISTRESS SYNDROME

Acute respiratory distress syndrome may be triggered by infectious or noninfectious illness, directly affecting the lung due to local inflammation or indirectly through inflammatory mediators from a systemic illness **(Fig. 1)**. Pneumonia (59%), extrapulmonary sepsis (16%), and aspiration (14%) were the leading causes of ARDS in a large multinational study.[6] Data from India also suggest a similar trend.[32,33] Of the infectious causes of ARDS, pneumonia (bacterial or viral) is the most common, followed by a systemic source of infection and sepsis. Pancreatitis, trauma, obesity, and transfusions are a few important noninfectious contributors to ARDS.[32,34-36] It is vital to recognize that patients admitted with various other illnesses may develop ARDS during hospitalization (hospital-acquired ARDS).[37] A population-based case-control study identified several factors for hospital-acquired ARDS, including excessive fluid administration, transfusions (especially plasma-containing products), aspiration of gastric contents, mechanical ventilation (MV) with a tidal volume > 8 mL/kg body weight, and others.[38] Thoracic (more than abdominal) surgeries, cardiopulmonary bypass, and organ transplantation are a few other known factors for ARDS.[39-41]

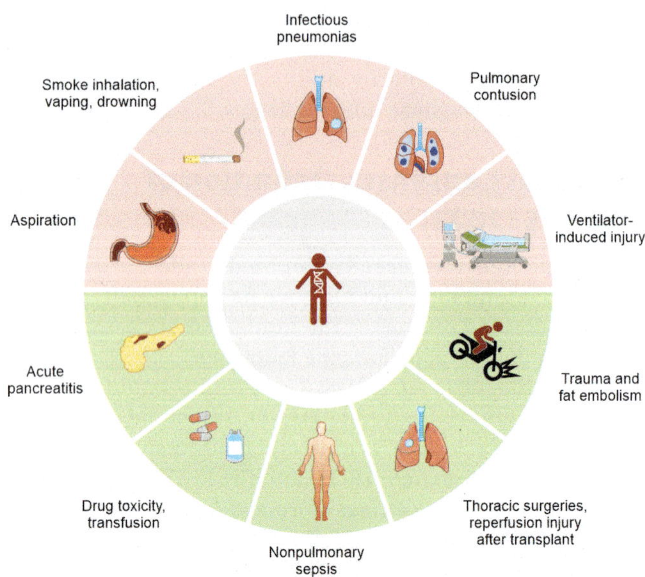

FIG. 1: Precipitating causes of ARDS. The upper half of the figure (highlighted in red) mentions the pulmonary causes (direct lung injury) of ARDS. In contrast, the lower half (green) shows few extrapulmonary causes (indirect lung injury). Underlying genetic factors may contribute to the development of ARDS (purple, center).

(ARDS: acute respiratory distress syndrome)

Genetic factors may underlie the development and severity of ARDS in some individuals. However, there are no single-gene disorders or simple Mendelian inheritance to explain ARDS. Possible association of ARDS has been noted with *surfactant protein B* gene, *angiotensin-converting enzyme* gene, *selectin P ligand* gene, and others.[42] Environmental and modifiable risk factors that can augment the risk of ARDS include cigarette smoking,[39] particulate matter < 2.5 μm ($PM_{2.5}$), and ozone.[43]

The epidemiology and etiology of ARDS may vary depending on the setting (ward or ICU, medical or surgical ICU, and others), and the population where the study is conducted (developed vs. developing nations).[32,33,44-48] Causes unique to tropical and developing nations, especially scrub typhus,[49] malaria, enteric fever, and other zoonotic diseases (dengue, chikungunya, and others) should also be considered and evaluated as many of them have specific and effective treatment.[33,46,50-53] In one study, among subjects admitted in ICU with active pulmonary tuberculosis, nearly one-third had ARDS.[7,54,55] However, tuberculosis is an uncommon cause (3.8%) of ARDS even in India. Drugs and toxins are other underrecognized causes of ARDS, and the clinician should be aware of the regional/geographical differences in etiology. For instance, paraquat poisoning is not an uncommon cause of ARDS in India and nearly 50% of the fatal cases may have DAD, a hallmark of ARDS.[32,56,57]

PATHOPHYSIOLOGY OF ACUTE RESPIRATORY DISTRESS SYNDROME

Our understanding of the pathophysiology of ARDS has improved over time, yet it is incomplete. The complexity of ARDS and the challenges in studying critically ill subjects are major hurdles. The alveolar-capillary barrier comprises a layer of alveolar epithelium separated from the capillary endothelium by a thin basement membrane **(Fig. 2)**. Based on the histopathological examination of lung tissue, Bachofen et al. described three phases of ARDS with pathophysiological implications: (1) exudative phase—interstitial edema and

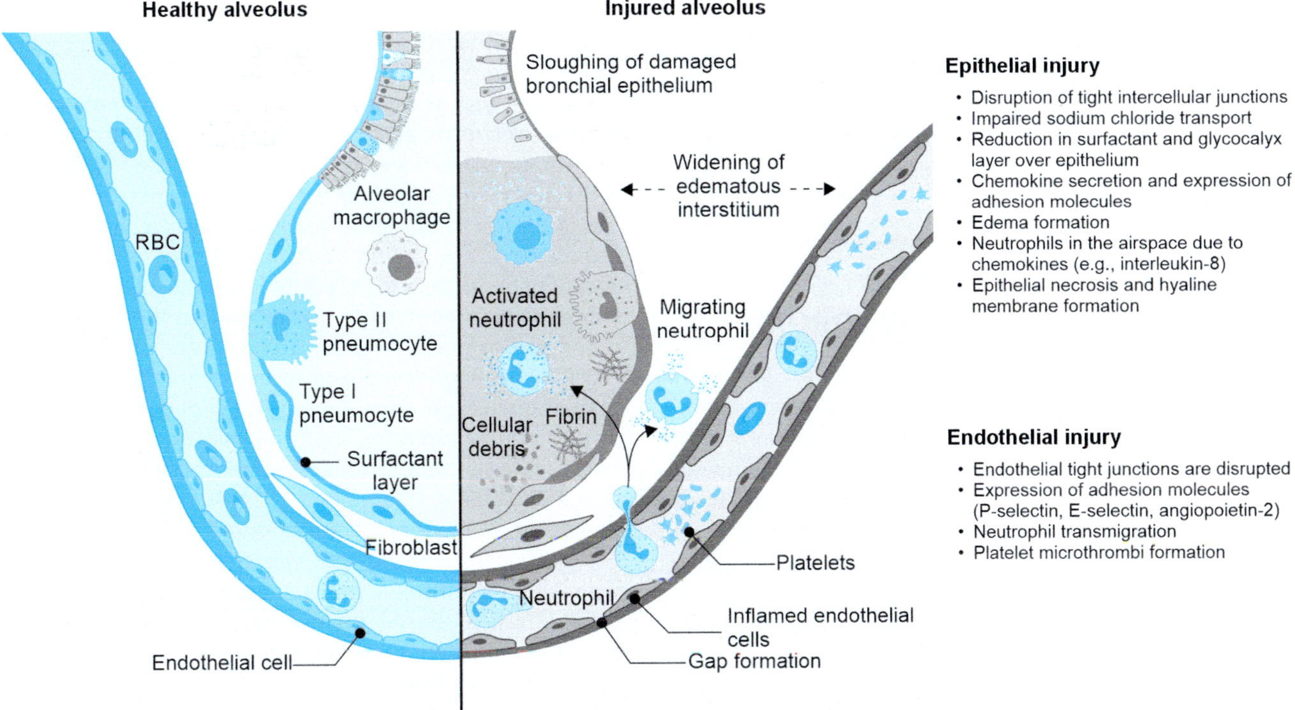

FIG. 2: Representative diagram showing the injury to the capillary endothelium and alveolar epithelium in ARDS. Depicted on the left side of the diagram is an intact, tight epithelial cell layer composed primarily of type I pneumocytes with a few interspersed type II pneumocytes and occasional macrophages. The alveoli are maintained dry in health due to the tight cellular junctions and the intact transport mechanism of sodium and chloride. On the contrary, a direct insult to the alveolar epithelium (usually pulmonary causes of ARDS) or capillary endothelium (more prominent in extrapulmonary ARDS) would result in disruption of the cellular junction and membrane transport of sodium, leading to varying degrees of edema. The injury to the glycocalyx layer of epithelium, along with several proinflammatory proteins in the alveoli, releases chemokines, tissue factor, and activation of the coagulation pathway, resulting in intraalveolar fibrin formation.

(ARDS: acute respiratory distress syndrome)

alveolar flooding, (2) proliferative phase—alveolar type II cell infiltration and fibroblast proliferation, and (3) fibrotic phase—macrophage infiltration, collagen deposition, and resolution.[58] Exudative changes are prominent in the first week of ARDS, while proliferative changes and fibrosis dominate after 3 weeks. However, a considerable overlap is now known between these phases of ARDS.[59] Injury to the endothelial and epithelial barriers of the lung are central to the physiological (hypoxemia and decreased lung compliance) and pathological changes (DAD) that are encountered in ARDS.[1,60]

Epithelial Injury

Alveolar epithelium is a thin but tightly arranged sheet of predominantly type I epithelial cells interspersed with type II alveolar epithelial cells (that secretes surfactants) covered by a glycocalyx layer. Mechanical disruption of the tight epithelial barrier leads to fluid extravasation into the alveolar space. In contrast, the injury to the type II cells may alter surfactant production, and the injury to the glycocalyx exposes and activates an inflammatory cascade. The net alveolar fluid clearance is thus reduced, and there is resultant edema in the lungs.[61] The clinical severity of ARDS and its outcome depends on the extent of the epithelial injury, which can range from mild disruption of the barrier to frank necrosis and cell death. Activated epithelial cells secrete chemokines and adhesion molecules, resulting in neutrophil migration into alveoli. The neutrophils release proteases and reactive oxygen species and promote further epithelial-endothelial injury from the formation of neutrophil extracellular traps.

Endothelial Injury

The usually intact endothelium has tight intercellular junctions and does not express adhesion molecules. However, following an insult (e.g., pathogens and their circulating products, cell-free hemoglobin, and others), vascular endothelial cadherins are inhibited, and the resultant disruption of tight junctions. Injury to endothelium leads to the shedding of anticoagulant molecules on the cell surface (such as thrombomodulin, protein-C receptor) and upregulation of procoagulant factors, prompting the formation of microvascular thrombi.[62] The microvascular thrombi may be responsible for severe impairment in gas exchange and acute right ventricular dysfunction seen in some patients, both of which are poor prognostic markers in ARDS.[63,64]

SUBPHENOTYPES OF ACUTE RESPIRATORY DISTRESS SYNDROME

Interaction of environmental exposures and genotypes results in clinically observable traits called phenotypes.[65] ARDS in itself is a phenotype where several possible etiologies can culminate into a common pathophysiology of alveoli-capillary damage resulting in non-inflammatory edema and a similar clinical presentation (with diffuse infiltrates and hypoxemia). Based on any arbitrary cutoff, ARDS patients may be classified into "subgroups" (e.g., PaO_2:FiO_2 ratio-based cutoffs).[66,67] However, such subgroups are arbitrary, and patients may often switch between categories over time. In contrast, subgroups that can be reliably and accurately differentiated from one another qualify for a subphenotype.[68] Subphenotypes, attributable to a distinct pathobiological basis, constitute endotypes. The unselected phenotypes of ARDS were ideal for evaluating several strategies, such as low tidal volume ventilation and others, which are effective against the common pathophysiologic pathways. Recruitable and nonrecruitable subphenotypes of ARDS have also been described based on the response to recruitment maneuvers and MV.[69] Nevertheless, several therapies with a biological basis (such as anti-inflammatory agents) have failed to show any benefit due to the heterogeneous nature of ARDS.[70] Several subphenotypes are described in ARDS based on a clinical, radiological, or biological basis.[69,71,72] The ultimate aim of such classification is the identification of treatable traits.

Radiological subphenotypes (focal and nonfocal) have been identified in chest CT, with potential clinical implications.[73] Nonfocal pattern is characterized by diffuse and patchy loss of aeration on imaging and responds well to alveolar recruitment. Focal patterns (predominant dorsal-inferior consolidations) respond well to prone ventilation.[74] A randomized controlled trial evaluated personalized MV based on the radiological pattern; however, no significant improvement in the 90-day survival was noted. Notably, 21% of patients were misclassified, and the mortality in these subjects was significantly higher than in the appropriately managed subjects.[73] Thus, an accurate classification is required before personalized strategies are tried. Further, CT may not be readily available in ARDS patients, and relying on chest radiographs to classify patients is prone to errors. In many of these studies, subphenotype classification is usually based on static data obtained at 24–48 hours of intubation, and dynamic changes are not captured.

Biological subphenotypes were first described in subjects with ARDS adopting a statistical modeling strategy (latent class analysis) based on plasma biomarkers data from two trials.[75] Calfee et al. identified two distinct biological subphenotypes **(Table 2)**—hyperinflammatory and hypo-inflammatory. The subphenotypes have been confirmed in several other studies and have been observed to be stable over time.[1,68,71,76-78] The prevalence of hyperinflammatory subphenotype in ARDS has been found to range from 26% to 40% across various studies, whereas the hypoinflammatory accounts for 48–74%.[68] Notably, COVID-19 ARDS, widely discussed as having "cytokine storm" had much lesser levels of these inflammatory cytokines (compared to non-COVID-19 ARDS), and most cases belonged to the hypoinflammatory subphenotype.[79] Apart from the prognostic implication of the two biological subphenotypes **(Table 2)**, a differential response to treatment strategy has been observed.[80] A better response to higher PEEP, benefit from simvastatin treatment, and a worse outcome with liberal fluid strategy have been noted in the hyperinflammatory ARDS, based on the reanalysis of data from multiple RCTs.[68,71,80,81]

TABLE 2: Features of hyperinflammatory subphenotype (compared to hypoinflammatory) of acute respiratory distress syndrome.

Characteristics	• Higher plasma concentration of interleukins (IL)-6, IL-8. Tumor necrosis factor receptor • Lower concentration of bicarbonate and protein-C
Clinical features	• A higher proportion of severe shock • Higher risk of metabolic acidosis • More frequently had extrapulmonary causes of sepsis
Impact on outcomes	• Longer intensive care unit (ICU) stay • Fewer ventilator-free days • Higher 90-day mortality
Response to treatment	• A higher PEEP strategy was more effective • Improved survival with simvastatin (but not rosuvastatin) in hyperinflammatory ARDS • Higher mortality with liberal fluid strategy

SUMMARY

Acute respiratory distress syndrome is a clinical syndrome, rather than a single disease, occurring secondary to various systemic diseases (e.g., sepsis, pancreatitis) or local insults to the lung (e.g., pneumonia). Injury to the alveolar epithelium and capillary endothelium leads to pathological changes that present as diffuse lung infiltrates (non-cardiogenic pulmonary edema), and hypoxemia. While identifying ARDS as a pattern may have advantages for conducting trials and evaluating supportive care strategies (such as fluid and ventilatory management), categorizing them into biological subphenotypes would be required to identify specific pharmacotherapies for ARDS.

ACKNOWLEDGMENT

We thank Dr Akshit Tuli, Internal Medicine, PGIMER, for his valuable inputs.

The figures have been Created with Biorender.com and we have obtained the required license to publish.

REFERENCES

1. Bos LDJ, Ware LB. Acute respiratory distress syndrome: Causes, pathophysiology, and phenotypes. Lancet. 2022;400(10358): 1145-56.
2. Ashbaugh DG, Bigelow DB, Petty TL, et al. Acute respiratory distress in adults. Lancet. 1967;2(7511):319-23.
3. Vincent JL, Santacruz C. Do we need ARDS? Intensive Care Med. 2016;42(2):282-3.
4. Pham T, Rubenfeld GD. Fifty years of research in ARDS. The epidemiology of acute respiratory distress syndrome. A 50th birthday review. Am J Respir Crit Care Med. 2017;195(7):860-70.
5. Li G, Malinchoc M, Cartin-Ceba R, et al. Eight-year trend of acute respiratory distress syndrome: A population-based study in olmsted county, minnesota. Am J Respir Crit Care Med. 2011;183(1):59-66.
6. Bellani G, Laffey JG, Pham T, et al. Epidemiology, patterns of care, and mortality for patients with acute respiratory distress syndrome in intensive care units in 50 countries. JAMA. 2016; 315(8):788-800.
7. Muthu V, Dhooria S, Aggarwal AN, et al. Acute respiratory distress syndrome due to tuberculosis in a respiratory ICU over a 16-year period. Crit Care Med. 2017;45(10):E1087-90.
8. Muthu V, Agarwal R, Dhooria S, et al. Epidemiology, lung mechanics and outcomes of ARDS: A comparison between pregnant and non-pregnant subjects. J Crit Care. 2019;50:207-12.
9. Erickson SE, Shlipak MG, Martin GS, et al. Racial and ethnic disparities in mortality from acute lung injury. Crit Care Med. 2009;37(1):1-6.
10. Moss M, Parsons PE, Steinberg KP, et al Chronic alcohol abuse is associated with an increased incidence of acute respiratory distress syndrome and severity of multiple organ dysfunction in patients with septic shock. Crit Care Med. 2003;31(3):869-77.
11. Sigurdsson MI, Sigvaldason K, et al. Acute respiratory distress syndrome: Nationwide changes in incidence, treatment and mortality over 23 years. Acta Anaesthesiol Scand. 2013;57(1): 37-45.
12. Phua J, Badia JR, Adhikari NK, et al. Has mortality from acute respiratory distress syndrome decreased over time?: a systematic review. Am J Respir Crit Care Med. 2009;179(3):220-7.
13. Tobin MJ. ARDS: Hidden perils of an overburdened diagnosis. Crit Care. 2022;26(1):392.
14. Tobin MJ. Defining acute respiratory distress syndrome (again): A plea for honesty. Am J Respir Crit Care Med. 2023;207(5):625.
15. Murray JF, Matthay MA, Luce JM, et al. An expanded definition of the adult respiratory distress syndrome. Am Rev Respir Dis. 1988;138(3):720-3.
16. Kangelaris KN, Calfee CS, May AK, et al. Is there still a role for the lung injury score in the era of the Berlin definition ARDS? Ann Intensive Care. 2014;4(1):4.
17. Wheeler AP, Bernard GR, Thompson BT, et al. Pulmonary-artery versus central venous catheter to guide treatment of acute lung injury. N Engl J Med. 2006;354(21):2213-24.
18. Ferguson ND, Davis AM, Slutsky AS, et al. Development of a clinical definition for acute respiratory distress syndrome using the Delphi technique. J Crit Care. 2005;20(2):147-54.
19. Ferguson ND, Frutos-Vivar F, Esteban A, et al. Acute respiratory distress syndrome: Underrecognition by clinicians and diagnostic accuracy of three clinical definitions. Crit Care Med. 2005;33(10):2228-34.
20. Ranieri VM, Rubenfeld GD, Thompson BT, et al Acute respiratory distress syndrome: The Berlin definition. JAMA. 2012;307(23):2526-33.
21. Ferguson ND, Fan E, Camporota L, et al. The Berlin definition Of ARDS: An expanded rationale, justification, and supplementary material. Intensive Care Med. 2012;38(10):1573-82.
22. Caser EB, Zandonade E, Pereira E, et al. Impact of distinct definitions of acute lung injury on its incidence and outcomes in Brazilian icus: Prospective evaluation of 7,133 patients. Crit Care Med. 2014;42(3):574-82.
23. Thille AW, Esteban A, Fernández-Segoviano P, et al. Comparison of the Berlin definition for acute respiratory distress syndrome with autopsy. Am J Respir Crit Care Med. 2013;187(7):761-7.
24. Villar J, Pérez-Méndez L, Blanco J, et al. A universal definition of ARDS: the pao2/fio2 ratio under a standard ventilatory setting--A prospective, multicenter validation study. Intensive Care Med. 2013;39(4):583-92.
25. Villar J, Fernández RL, Ambrós A, et al. A Clinical classification of the acute respiratory distress syndrome for predicting outcome and guiding medical therapy. Crit Care Med. 2015;43(2):346-53.
26. Riviello ED, Kiviri W, Twagirumugabe T, et al. Hospital incidence and outcomes of the acute respiratory distress syndrome using the Kigali modification of the Berlin definition. Am J Respir Crit Care Med. 2016;193(1):52-9.
27. Vercesi V, Pisani L, Van Tongeren PSI, et al. External confirmation and exploration of the Kigali modification for diagnosing moderate or severe ARDS. Intensive Care Med. 2018;44(4): 523-4.
28. Smit MR, Brower RG, Parsons PE, et al. The global definition of acute respiratory distress syndrome: ready for prime time? Am J Respir Crit Care Med. 2024;209(1):14-16.

29. Smit MR, Hagens LA, Heijnen NFL, et al. Lung ultrasound prediction model for acute respiratory distress syndrome: A multicenter prospective observational study. Am J Respir Crit Care Med. 2023;207(12):1591-601.
30. Lichtenstein D, Goldstein I, Mourgeon E, et al. Comparative diagnostic performances of auscultation, chest radiography, and lung ultrasonography in acute respiratory distress syndrome. Anesthesiology. 2004;100(1):9-15.
31. Ware LB. Improving acute respiratory distress syndrome diagnosis: Is lung ultrasound the answer? Am J Respir Crit Care Med. 2023;207(12):1548-9.
32. Agarwal R, Aggarwal AN, Gupta D, et al. Etiology and outcomes of pulmonary and extrapulmonary acute lung injury/ards in a respiratory ICU in north India. Chest. 2006;130(3):724-9.
33. Sharma SK, Gupta A, Biswas A, et al. Aetiology, Outcomes & predictors of mortality in acute respiratory distress syndrome from a tertiary care centre in north India. Indian J Med Res. 2016;143(6):782-92.
34. Gong MN, Bajwa EK, Thompson BT, et al. Body mass index is associated with the development of acute respiratory distress syndrome. Thorax. 2010;65(1):44-50.
35. Bux J, Sachs UJ. The pathogenesis of transfusion-related acute lung injury (TRALI). Br J Haematol. 2007;136(6):788-99.
36. Khan H, Belsher J, Yilmaz M, et al. Fresh-frozen plasma and platelet transfusions are associated with development of acute lung injury in critically ill medical patients. Chest. 2007;131(5):1308-14.
37. Yadav H, Thompson BT, Gajic O. Fifty years of research in ARDS. Is acute respiratory distress syndrome a preventable disease? Am J Respir Crit Care Med. 2017;195(6):725-36.
38. Ahmed AH, Litell JM, Malinchoc M, et al. The role of potentially preventable hospital exposures in the development of acute respiratory distress syndrome: A population-based study. Crit Care Med. 2014;42(1):31-9.
39. Kotloff RM, Ahya VN, Crawford SW. Pulmonary complications of solid organ and hematopoietic stem cell transplantation. Am J Respir Crit Care Med. 2004;170(1):22-48.
40. Messent M, Sullivan K, Keogh BF, et al. Adult Respiratory distress syndrome following cardiopulmonary bypass: Incidence and prediction. Anaesthesia. 1992;47(3):267-8.
41. Serpa Neto A, Hemmes SN, Barbas CS, et al. Incidence of mortality and morbidity related to postoperative lung injury in patients who have undergone abdominal or thoracic surgery: A systematic review and meta-analysis. Lancet Respir Med. 2014;2(12):1007-15.
42. Gong MN. Genetic epidemiology of acute respiratory distress syndrome: implications for future prevention and treatment. Clin Chest Med. 2006;27(4):705-24; Abstract X.
43. Rhee J, Dominici F, Zanobetti A, et al. Impact of long-term exposures to ambient pm(2.5) and ozone on ARDS risk for older adults in the United States. Chest. 2019;156(1):71-9.
44. Jindal SK, Aggarwal AN, Gupta D. Adult respiratory distress syndrome in the tropics. Clin Chest Med. 2002;23(2):445-55.
45. Kumar SS, Selvarajan Chettiar KP, Nambiar R. Etiology and outcomes of ARDS in a resource limited urban tropical setting. J Natl Med Assoc. 2018;110(4):352-7.
46. Balakrishnan N, Thabah MM, Dineshbabu S, et al. Aetiology And short-term outcome of acute respiratory distress syndrome: A real-world experience from a medical intensive care unit in southern India. J R Coll Physicians Edinb. 2020;50(1):12-8.
47. Gupta D, Ramanathan RP, Aggarwal AN, et al. Assessment of factors predicting outcome of acute respiratory distress syndrome in North India. Respirology. 2001;6(2):125-30.
48. Hendrickson KW, Peltan ID, Brown SM. The epidemiology of acute respiratory distress syndrome before and after Coronavirus disease 2019. Crit Care Clin. 2021;37(4):703-16.
49. George T, Viswanathan S, Karnam AH, et al. Etiology And Outcomes Of ARDS in a rural-urban fringe hospital of South India. Crit Care Res Pract. 2014;2014:181593.
50. Agrawal PN, Ramanathan RM, Gupta D, et al. Acute respiratory distress syndrome complicating typhoid fever. Indian J Chest Dis Allied Sci. 1999;41(4):225-9.
51. Atam V, Singh AS, Yathish BE, et al. Acute pancreatitis and acute respiratory distress syndrome complicating Plasmodium Vivax Malaria. J Vector Borne Dis. 2013;50(2):151-4.
52. Singh A. Acute respiratory distress syndrome: An Unusual presentation of chikungunya fever viral infection. J Glob Infect Dis. 2017;9(1):33-4.
53. Agarwal R, Nath A, Gupta D. Noninvasive ventilation in Plasmodium vivax related ALI/ARDS. Intern Med. 2007;46(24): 2007-11.
54. Muthu V, Dhooria S, Agarwal R, et al. Profile of patients with active tuberculosis admitted to a respiratory intensive care unit in a tertiary care center of North India. Indian J Crit Care Med. 2018;22(2):63-6.
55. Agarwal R, Gupta D, Aggarwal AN, et al. Experience with ARDS caused by tuberculosis in a respiratory intensive care unit. Intensive Care Med. 2005;31(9):1284-7.
56. Kumar S, Gupta S, Bansal YS, et al. Pulmonary histopathology in fatal paraquat poisoning. Autops Case Rep. 2021;11:E2021342.
57. Sharma DS, Prajapati AM, Shah DM. Review of a case of paraquat poisoning in a tertiary care rural-based ICU. Indian J Crit Care Med. 2019;23(6):284-6.
58. Bachofen M, Weibel ER. Alterations of the gas exchange apparatus in adult respiratory insufficiency associated with septicemia. Am Rev Respir Dis. 1977;116(4):589-615.
59. Thille AW, Esteban A, Fernández-Segoviano P, et al. Chronology of histological lesions in acute respiratory distress syndrome with diffuse alveolar damage: A prospective cohort study of clinical autopsies. Lancet Respir Med. 2013;1(5):395-401.
60. Matthay MA, Zemans RL, Zimmerman GA, et al. acute respiratory distress syndrome. Nat Rev Dis Primers. 2019;5(1):18.
61. Ware LB, Matthay MA. Alveolar fluid clearance is impaired in the majority of patients with acute lung injury and the acute respiratory distress syndrome. Am J Respir Crit Care Med. 2001;163(6):1376-83.
62. Livingstone SA, Wildi KS, Dalton HJ,et al. Coagulation dysfunction in acute respiratory distress syndrome and its potential impact in inflammatory subphenotypes. Front Med (Lausanne). 2021;8:723217.
63. Petit M, Jullien E, Vieillard-Baron A. Right ventricular function in acute respiratory distress syndrome: Impact on outcome, respiratory strategy and use of veno-venous extracorporeal membrane oxygenation. Front Physiol. 2021;12:797252.
64. Osman D, Monnet X, Castelain V, et al. Incidence and prognostic value of right ventricular failure in acute respiratory distress syndrome. Intensive Care Med. 2009;35(1):69-76.
65. Agache I, Akdis CA. Precision medicine and phenotypes, endotypes, genotypes, regiotypes, and theratypes of allergic diseases. J Clin Invest. 2019;129(4):1493-503.

66. Sehgal IS, Agarwal R, Dhooria S, et al. Risk stratification of acute respiratory distress syndrome using a PaO_2: FiO_2 threshold of 150 mm Hg: A retrospective analysis from an Indian intensive care unit. Lung India. 2020;37(6):473-8.
67. Sehgal IS, Dhooria S, Behera D, et al. Acute respiratory distress syndrome: Pulmonary and extrapulmonary not so similar. Indian J Crit Care Med. 2016;20(3):194-7.
68. Reilly JP, Calfee CS, Christie JD. Acute respiratory distress syndrome phenotypes. Semin Respir Crit Care Med. 2019;40(1): 19-30.
69. Wendel Garcia PD, Caccioppola A, et al. Latent class analysis to predict intensive care outcomes in acute respiratory distress syndrome: A proposal of two pulmonary phenotypes. Crit Care. 2021;25(1):154.
70. Mcauley DF, Laffey JG, O'Kane CM, et al. Simvastatin In the acute respiratory distress syndrome. N Engl J Med. 2014;371(18):1695-703.
71. Heijnen NFL, Hagens LA, Smit MR,et al. Biological subphenotypes of acute respiratory distress syndrome show prognostic enrichment in mechanically ventilated patients without acute respiratory distress syndrome. Am J Respir Crit Care Med. 2021;203(12):1503-11.
72. Heijnen NFL, Hagens LA, Smit MR, et al. Biological subphenotypes of acute respiratory distress syndrome may not reflect differences in alveolar inflammation. Physiol Rep. 2021;9(3): E14693.
73. Constantin JM, Jabaudon M, Lefrant JY, et al. Personalised mechanical ventilation tailored to lung morphology versus low positive end-expiratory pressure for patients with acute respiratory distress syndrome in France (The LIVE Study): A multicentre, single-blind, randomised controlled trial. Lancet Respir Med. 2019;7(10):870-80.
74. Constantin JM, Grasso S, Chanques G, et al. Lung morphology predicts response to recruitment maneuver in patients with acute respiratory distress syndrome. Crit Care Med. 2010;38(4): 1108-17.
75. Calfee CS, Delucchi K, Parsons PE, et al Subphenotypes in acute respiratory distress syndrome: Latent class analysis of data from two randomised controlled trials. Lancet Respir Med. 2014;2(8):611-20.
76. Bos LDJ, Sjoding M, Sinha P, et al. Longitudinal respiratory subphenotypes in patients with covid-19-related acute respiratory distress syndrome: Results from three observational cohorts. Lancet Respir Med. 2021;9(12):1377-86.
77. Alipanah N, Calfee CS. Phenotyping in acute respiratory distress syndrome: State of the art and clinical implications. Curr Opin Crit Care. 2022;28(1):1-8.
78. Delucchi K, Famous KR, Ware LB, et al. Stability of ARDS subphenotypes over time in two randomised controlled trials. Thorax. 2018;73(5):439-45.
79. Leisman DE, Ronner L, Pinotti R, et al. Cytokine elevation in severe and critical COVID-19: A rapid systematic review, meta-analysis, and comparison with other inflammatory syndromes. Lancet Respir Med. 2020;8(12):1233-44.
80. Calfee CS, Delucchi KL, Sinha P, et al. Acute respiratory distress syndrome subphenotypes and differential response to simvastatin: secondary analysis of a randomised controlled trial. Lancet Respir Med. 2018;6(9):691-8.
81. Famous KR, Delucchi K, Ware LB, et al. Acute respiratory distress syndrome subphenotypes respond differently to randomized fluid management strategy. Am J Respir Crit Care Med. 2017; 195(3):331-8.
82. Bernard GR, Artigas A, Brigham KL, e al. Report of the American-European Consensus Conference on ARDS: Definitions, Mechanisms, relevant outcomes and clinical trial coordination. The Consensus Committee. Intensive Care Med. 1994;20(3): 225-32.

Acute Respiratory Distress Syndrome: Respiratory Mechanics, Management, and Long-term Outcomes

CHAPTER

164

Valliappan Muthu, Inderpaul Singh Sehgal, Ritesh Agarwal

INTRODUCTION

Managing acute respiratory distress syndrome (ARDS) centers around optimizing mechanical ventilation (MV), conservative fluid strategy, and supportive care. Apart from the treatment of specific etiologic triggers, no disease-modifying therapy has been consistently shown to be effective for ARDS. Knowledge of respiratory mechanics is essential in ARDS to minimize lung injury and improve intensive care unit (ICU) morbidity and mortality. Understanding the complexities and advances in personalized ventilation strategies are areas of research that might further improve outcomes. In this chapter, we will discuss respiratory mechanics and their implications for ventilatory management of ARDS. We will also discuss nonventilatory management and advances in the field. The management of coronavirus disease 2019 (COVID-19)-associated ARDS also follows the same principles outlined in this chapter and should be like any other cause of ARDS (except for the use of specific pharmacotherapeutic agents, such as glucocorticoids, tocilizumab, and others).

APPLIED RESPIRATORY MECHANICS

Acute respiratory distress syndrome lungs were initially regarded as uniformly stiff (with low compliance); however, computed tomography (CT) studies have shown regional abnormalities composed of a mix of consolidation, atelectasis, and normal (or near-normal) aerated lung parenchyma.[1,2] The loss of aerated lung parenchyma accounts for reduced functional residual capacity (FRC). Notably, the aerated lung parenchyma had normal compliance (instead of uniformly "stiff" lung). The latter concept was widely discussed as the "baby lung", wherein the functioning aerated lung parenchyma equated to that seen in a healthy child of around 5 years of age (small functioning lungs instead of diffusely stiff lungs).[3] Although the lungs may be uniformly affected by the disease process and edema is diffuse, the heavy edematous portions of the nondependent lung parenchyma force the air out of the dependent portions. Thus, due to the physiological heterogeneity of ARDS, some alveoli may be normally distended while others may be over or under-distended, even with the same tidal volume (Vt).

Positive End-expiratory Pressure

In ARDS, the lack of surfactant and several other factors result in collapse and derecruitment of variable portions of the lungs. Positive end-expiratory pressure (PEEP) (external PEEP or applied PEEP) is the pressure maintained in the alveoli at the end of expiration. It prevents the collapse of the alveoli and distal airway during each expiration. An intrinsic PEEP or auto-PEEP is the alveolar pressure accumulating secondary to incomplete expiration. The beneficial effect of PEEP on ARDS has been recognized since the initial description of ARDS.[4] However, increasing PEEP beyond a certain threshold can have hemodynamic consequences due to increased intrathoracic pressure and right atrial pressure, which in turn compromises venous return and cardiac output. PEEP can also increase the after-load of the right heart by increasing pulmonary vascular resistance.[5] Excessive PEEP can increase lung stress and strain, leading to ventilator-induced lung injury (VILI). "Stress" is the distribution of internal forces per unit area induced by external force applied to a material (e.g., lung tissue in the current context), and the consequent change in the dimension of that material is called "strain".[6] Currently used surrogates for stress and strain are the plateau pressure and Vt (Vt/FRC better represents strain). However, they are inadequate and fail to account for the inhomogeneity of the ARDS lungs. More robust estimation methods are required to avoid the harmful effects of excessive PEEP. The various methods to set the PEEP during MV are discussed in later sections of this chapter.

Mechanisms and Strategies to Mitigate Ventilator-induced Lung Injury

Mechanical ventilation has revolutionized the management of ARDS and the outcomes have improved over the past few decades. Nevertheless, significant intra and interindividual variations in ARDS are increasingly recognized. The use of positive pressure ventilation may lead to or accentuate the pre-existing lung injury due to several reasons, resulting in VILI.[7] VILI may occur at low or high lung volumes. The earlier practice of using a high Vt (12 mL/kg or even higher)[8] was challenged by several small studies, and finally, the landmark ARDS network trial established the superiority of lower Vt, i.e., 6 mL/kg of predicted body weight (PBW) over 12 mL/kg.[9] A high lung volume would result in alveolar overdistension and subsequent injury ("*volutrauma*"). A study conducted two decades ago suggested a 1.3 odd increase in the risk of acute lung injury for every mL/kg increment in Vt above 6 mL/kg of PBW.[10] A larger Vt also increases end-inspiratory transpulmonary pressure (TPP), which is the pressure difference between the alveoli and intrapleural pressure and may lead to complications (*barotrauma*) such as pneumothorax, pneumomediastinum, and subcutaneous emphysema. The incidence of barotrauma has considerably decreased after the widespread adoption of lung protective ventilatory strategy by modulating the PEEP along with a low Vt to maintain a plateau pressure (Pplat) target of <30 cmH_2O.[11,12]

Transpulmonary Pressure

The pleural space between the elastic lungs and the noncollapsible chest wall has a slight negative pressure (around -5 cmH_2O). During inspiration, the intrapleural pressure becomes more negative and allows air entry into the lungs. The pressure holding the lung open is called TPP and is measured as the difference between the airway and pleural pressures. While airway pressure can be easily measured in ventilated patients, pleural pressure measurement is difficult. Esophageal pressure measured by placing a pressure transducer at the lower end of the esophagus has been successfully used in trials as a surrogate for pleural pressure.[13] TPP >25 cmH_2O at the end of inspiration is a marker of overdistension and can result in VILI, whereas TPP <0 at the end of expiration can cause closure of alveoli and derecruitment. VILI occurring at low lung volumes due to repeated opening and closure of the alveoli and distal small airways is known as "atelectotrauma" and can be counteracted by applying PEEP. Atelectotrauma is possibly due to the sudden and transient swings in end-inspiratory TPP, and a TPP monitoring strategy can help titrate optimal PEEP. Mechanical injury to the alveoli by volutrauma or atelectotrauma subsequently leads to *biotrauma*, mediated by pulmonary and systemic inflammatory mediators [tumor necrosis factor-α, interleukin-6 (IL-6), IL-8, matrix metalloproteinases, and others].[10,14]

Driving Pressure

Driving pressure (Δp) is another proposed parameter for monitoring ventilation strategies.[15,16] At the bedside, ΔP can be easily calculated as the difference between Pplat and PEEP (in a passively ventilated patient, ΔP = Pplat – PEEP), and multiple studies have shown baseline driving pressure to be independent predictors of mortality.[15,17-19] ΔP equals Vt/compliance of the respiratory system, and the compliance is directly proportional to the FRC. ΔP, thus, represents the relationship between the Vt and the amount of functional lung tissue available to receive the breath.[7] In an individual patient data analysis from nine randomized control trials (RCTs) of ARDS, ΔP was independently associated with survival in ARDS, and increasing ΔP was associated with a higher risk of death even in those on lung protective ventilation (Vt ≤7 mL/kg/PBW and Pplat ≤30 cmH_2O).[19] ΔP (target <15 cmH_2O)-guided ventilation is feasible,[20] and needs further evaluation prospective trials.

The application of low Vt (6 mL/kg of PBW) and high PEEP, together called "lung protective ventilation", are thus crucial in mitigating the adverse effects of MV. Optimizing PEEP and Vt has improved ARDS outcomes over the past few decades.

PRACTICAL ASPECTS OF MECHANICAL VENTILATION

Noninvasive Versus Invasive Ventilation

Hypoxemia is the central feature of ARDS, and oxygenation targets can be achieved with standard oxygen therapy, high-flow nasal oxygen (HFNO), and noninvasive and invasive MV. Noninvasive ventilation (NIV) can improve oxygenation, decrease the work of breathing, and may avoid endotracheal intubation and its complications. However, the use of NIV in ARDS may result in the delivery of a large Vt. Higher inspiratory demand and large TPP during NIV can worsen the underlying lung injury and should preferably be avoided.[21] Also, delaying intubation in ARDS has been shown to have poor outcomes.[22] HFNO is another recently introduced noninvasive oxygenation mode and was widely used during the COVID-19 pandemic. Although a few studies suggest NIV (with helmet) and HFNO to help avoid endotracheal intubation, the evidence is equivocal. Multicenter RCTs conducted before and during the COVID-19 pandemic failed to demonstrate a decreased intubation rate with NIV or HFNO compared to standard oxygen therapy.[23,24] Further, the large LUNG-SAFE study reporting observational data from 50 countries showed that NIV use was independently associated with ICU mortality in patients with severe ARDS [partial pressure of oxygen (PaO_2)/ fraction of inspired oxygen (FiO_2) ratio <150 mm Hg].[25] Thus, invasive MV should be the preferred strategy in most patients; NIV may be initially used under close supervision in an occasional patient with less severe ARDS, who is hemodynamically stable, and has no immediate indication for intubation.

Initial Mechanical Ventilation Settings

Mode of ventilation: Both volume- or pressure-control modes of ventilation are suitable for managing patients with ARDS, and there is insufficient evidence to recommend one over the other. We suggest volume-limited ventilation mode for the initial management of ARDS as most physicians are familiar with it, and importantly, volume-limited modes ensure delivery of desired Vt. However, the patient tolerance of volume-limited modes is poor, and there is a risk of increased airway pressure. A better patient tolerance in pressure-limited ventilation is offset by the inconsistency in Vt and minute ventilation. A systematic review of three RCTs failed to show any clinically important differences in hospital mortality, duration of hospital stays, barotrauma, or the development of organ dysfunction between volume and pressure-limited modes.[26] Irrespective of the volume- or pressure-limited modes, an assist-control mode should be preferred over partially supported modes such as synchronized intermittent mandatory ventilation. High-frequency oscillatory ventilation (HFOV) is not recommended for adults with ARDS.[27]

Selection of Vt and respiratory rate (RR): The current standard of management for ARDS should be like the landmark ARDS network trial, and initial Vt could be set at 6 mL/kg of PBW with an RR appropriate to meet the patient's minute ventilation (RR should, however, be ≤35 breaths/min). The calculation of PBW for men and women is described in **Table 1**. Alveolar hypoventilation consequential to low-tidal-volume ventilation (LTVV) can result in hypercapnic respiratory acidosis [partial pressure of carbon dioxide ($PaCO_2$) >45 mm Hg and pH <7.35], which is usually well-tolerated. The higher RR used to compensate for the hypoventilation may result in incomplete expiration and auto-PEEP. LTVV is unconventional and requires increased sedation to avoid patient-ventilator dyssynchrony. Nevertheless, the benefit outweighs these potential adverse events, and LTVV should be the standard of care for ARDS.

PEEP and oxygenation: Initially, a PEEP of at least 5 cmH_2O is set along with the FiO_2 of 1 (tapered over the next 1 hour), targeting a peripheral oxygen saturation (SpO_2) of 90–94%. Further, titration of PEEP and FiO_2 is performed per the settings **(Table 1)** used in the ARDS network trial.[9] While a systematic review of 25 RCTs among critically ill subjects (including sepsis, stroke, and others) suggested increased 30-day mortality with liberal oxygenation target (median baseline SpO_2 of 96%),[28] a recent RCT conducted in 205 ARDS subjects did not find a better survival at 28 days with

TABLE 1: The initial ventilator settings for managing patients with ARDS and the PEEP/FiO_2 table for titrating PEEP to achieve oxygenation targets.

Initial ventilator settings								
Calculation of predicted body weight (PBW)								
Male	50 + 2.3 [height (in inches) – 60] or							
	50 + 0.91 [height (in cm) – 152.4]							
Female	45.5 + 2.3 [height (in inches) – 60] or							
	45.5 + 0.91 [height (in cm) – 152.4]							
Mode: Volume assist-control								
Set initial Vt to 6 mL/kg PBW								
Set initial respiratory rate to ≤35 breaths/minute to match baseline minute ventilation								
Subsequent Vt adjustment								
Ensure Pplat ≤30 cmH_2O								
Check inspiratory Pplat with 0.5 second inspiratory pause at least every 4 hours and after each change in PEEP or tidal volume								
If Pplat >30 cmH_2O, decrease Vt in 1 mL/kg PBW steps to 5, or if necessary to 4 mL/kg PBW								
If Pplat <25 cmH_2O and Vt <6 mL/kg, increase Vt by 1 mL/kg PBW until Pplat >25 cmH_2O or Vt is 6 mL/kg								
If breath stacking (autoPEEP) or severe dyspnea occurs, Vt may be increased to 7 or 8 mL/kg PBW provided Pplat remains ≤30 cmH_2O								
Arterial oxygenation and PEEP								
Oxygenation target: PaO_2 = 55–80 mm Hg or SpO_2 = 90–94%.								
FiO_2/PEEP combinations to achieve oxygenation goal								
FiO_2	0.3	0.4	0.5	0.6	0.7	0.8	0.9	1.0
PEEP, cmH_2O	5	5–8	8–10	10	10–14	14	14–18	18–24
PEEP should be applied starting with the minimum value for a given FiO_2.								
Note: The above table has been adapted from the acute respiratory distress syndrome (ARDS) network trial on low-tidal-volume ventilation (LTVV).								
(FiO_2: fraction of inspired oxygen; PaO_2: arterial oxygen tension; PEEP: positive end-expiratory pressure; Pplat: plateau pressure; SpO_2: oxyhemoglobin saturation; Vt: tidal volume)								

conservative oxygenation (target PaO_2 of 55–70 mmHg; SpO_2 of 88–92%) strategy.[29] On the contrary, increased 90-day mortality and mesenteric ischemia were noted in the conservative oxygenation group than in the more liberal oxygenation group (target of 90–105 mmHg; $SpO_2 \geq 96\%$).[29]

As discussed earlier, PEEP serves to improve and maintain alveolar recruitment in ARDS. The selection of initial PEEP is usually per the standard PEEP: FiO_2 table. Alternatively, a pressure-volume (PV) curve may be used for selecting the optimal PEEP. The pressure (x-axis) to volume (y-axis) relation is readily available for monitoring in ventilators. The usual PV curve in ARDS is S-shaped, with a flat curve during the initial portion (low lung compliance), followed by a steep rise (higher compliance) and flattening of the curve beyond a particular volume (represents overdistension).[30] The transition point from low to high compliance in the PV curve denotes the lower inflection point (LIP), and selecting a PEEP value above this LIP (initial PEEP) is likely to provide maximal improvement. The requirement of neuromuscular blockade (NMB) or deep sedation to construct a PV curve is a significant limitation. Further, a PV curve with an S-shape and a clear LIP may not be seen in several patients.

Recruitment maneuvers (RM): RMs involve strategies to transiently increase TPP and airway pressures to aerate previously gasless lungs (i.e., recruitment). Application of a high PEEP for a brief duration (e.g., 35 cmH_2O for less than 40 seconds) is one of the most common RM and can improve oxygenation. However, the role of RM in ARDS is controversial as the existing evidence does not suggest an improvement in survival, hospital length of stay, and others.[31-33] Although oxygenation may improve following RMs, they may be potentially harmful (barotrauma, pneumothorax, and others).[33,34] RMs may be used independently or with LTVV and high PEEP (collectively called "open lung ventilation"). Based on the existing evidence, the routine use of RM is not recommended.[33] The use of RM may be limited to scenarios where circuit disconnection (suctioning, patient positioning, bronchoscopy, and others) leads to derecruitment. Frequent (>1 per day) or prolonged (>40 seconds) RM and RM after seven days of ARDS (usually the fibroproliferative phase) are likely harmful and should be avoided.[33]

Monitoring and Positive End-expiratory Pressure Titration

Patients being mechanically ventilated for ARDS should be monitored using clinical parameters, gas exchange, and ventilatory parameters. The Vt, RR, and PEEP are modified based on the pH, PaO_2, or SpO_2 levels. A pH of 7.25–7.35 on low Vt ventilation (with Pplat < 30 cmH_2O) can be safely continued. For patients unable to achieve adequate oxygenation, PEEP titration is attempted within the safe limits of Pplat and ΔP. The optimal strategy to titrate PEEP is unclear and several methods have been described, although there is no convincing evidence to recommend them over the standard PEEP/FiO_2 table targeting oxygenation.[32]

- The PEEP/FiO_2 **(Table 1)** is the most widely used method to titrate PEEP, targeting the desired oxygenation levels.
- *Esophageal pressure monitoring and TPP:* A catheter is inserted via the nasogastric or orogastric route (and used for enteral feeding), ensuring the catheter's transducer is at the lower end of the esophagus. Constant TPP monitoring to ensure end-expiratory TPP above 0 cmH_2O (and <10 cmH_2O) avoids alveolar derecruitment, and end-inspiratory TPP ≤25 cmH_2O avoids alveolar overdistension. In an RCT of 200 patients, the esophageal pressure-guided PEEP titration reduced the need for rescue therapies in ARDS [prone ventilation and extracorporeal membrane oxygenation (ECMO), and others] than the high PEEP-FiO_2 strategy. However, there was no difference in the primary trial outcomes of mortality or ventilation-free days.[35] Esophageal pressure-guided PEEP titration may be helpful in specific scenarios where the airway pressures do not accurately reflect the pressures across the lung (e.g., obesity, chest wall deformities, and others). However, considering the cost, expertise, and availability, routine use is not suggested.
- *Stress index (SI):* SI is another helpful bedside observation that could assist in titrating PEEP or Vt. Using a constant inspiratory flow, observing the pressure–time graph may provide information regarding recruitment success. The convex shape of the pressure–time graph indicates SI < 1 and PEEP can be increased. A straight slope of the pressure–time graph is consistent with an SI of 1 and successful recruitment, while a concave shape suggests SI > 1 and overdistension. Although not a perfect tool for monitoring, it is simple to use and dynamic.[36]
- *Imaging:* Assessment of lung aeration by chest CT can guide the titration of PEEP. However, it is cumbersome, often impractical, and has been used in research settings. More recently, electrical impedance tomography and bedside ultrasound to assess lung recruitment and individualized PEEP titration have been suggested.[37,38] Rigorous studies are required to assess the superiority of image-guided PEEP titration over the current standard of care.

In patients who improve with the above strategy, gradual weaning may be attempted. In those who continue to have refractory hypoxemia, further escalation of care should be considered, and the options include prone ventilation, ECMO, and rarely lung transplantation (LT).

MANAGEMENT OF REFRACTORY HYPOXEMIA

Prone Ventilation

Ventilation of patients in the prone position favorably alters the respiratory mechanics (decreasing the ventral-to-dorsal TPP, reducing compression of the lung by the heart, and improving lung perfusion) and usually results in improved oxygenation. Prone ventilation is strongly recommended in patients with severe hypoxemia (PaO_2:FiO_2 < 150 mm Hg on PEEP at least 5 cmH_2O, and FiO_2 ≥ 0.6 while on LTVV).[32] Prone ventilation improves hypoxemia[39] and reduces mortality, especially when initiated early (12–24 hours of intubation) and continued for at least 16 hours every session.[40] Prone ventilation may be discontinued if there is an improvement in oxygenation (PaO_2:FiO_2 ≥150 mm Hg, PEEP of ≤10 cm H_2O, and a FiO_2 of ≤0.6) when assessed after 4 hours of supine positioning, or if it is ineffective, i.e., a decrease in PaO_2:FiO_2 ratio by 20% of that in the supine position. Immediate termination of the prone session would also be required with the development of complications such as tube dislodgement, cardiac arrest, and others.[40] Notably, in the landmark PROSEVA trial, the incidence of complications was not significantly different with prone (experimental arm) and supine ventilation (control arm).[40]

Extracorporeal Life Support

Extracorporeal life support (ECLS) is an advanced life support system that facilitates gas exchange or provides circulatory support. Analogous to dialysis, ECLS involves blood circulation through a "membrane" that performs gas exchange. ECLS includes ECMO and extracorporeal carbon dioxide removal ($ECCO_2R$). The major components of an ECLS circuit are the drainage and reinfusion cannulae, circulatory pump, membrane lung, connecting tubings, oxygen, and heat source. Depending on the drainage and reinfusion circuits, ECMO can be venovenous (VV) (blood drained from a central vein or venous chamber and infused back into a venous chamber or vein) or venoarterial (VA) [drainage from a venous chamber and reinfusion into an artery (usually femoral)]. VV ECMO is primarily used in respiratory failure to provide gas exchange and oxygenation, whereas VA ECMO is used when circulatory support is needed (cardiac failure). An additional reinfusion cannula may be added to a preexisting circuit, for example, arterial reinfusion cannula in an ARDS patient on VV-ECMO when cardiac support is required (hybrid ECMO). In ARDS, ECMO may be used in refractory cases for gas exchange or as a bridge to LT if there are no contraindications, such as uncontrolled bleeding or the underlying disease is likely irreversible with little chance of recovery (e.g., irreversible hypoxemic insult to the brain). Currently, there is low-to-moderate evidence to support improvement in survival with the use of ECMO in patients with severe ARDS (PaO_2:FiO_2 <50 mm Hg for 3 hours, PaO_2:FiO_2 < 80 mm Hg for 6 hours, or arterial pH <7.25 with a $PaCO_2$ >60 mm Hg for at least 6 hours).[41] ECMO has an increased risk of serious bleeding (requiring blood transfusions) and severe thrombocytopenia.[42-44] ECMO should be offered at centers with expertise after ensuring lung protective ventilation, prone ventilation, and others.[44,45]

The $ECCO_2R$ helps remove carbon dioxide and can support ultra-low Vt (≤3 mL/kg of PBW). In a pragmatic RCT of 412 patients randomized to $ECCO_2R$-facilitated ultra LTVV versus the standard of care, 90-day mortality was not significantly different. A high complication rate (including intracranial hemorrhage, bleeding at other sites, and infections) was noted in the above trial.[46] Currently, $ECCO_2R$ is not recommended in clinical practice (only to be used in clinical trials).[32]

Lung Transplantation

Lung transplantation is an established treatment option for patients with chronic respiratory failure due to end-stage lung diseases. However, there is limited data on LT for ARDS. LT may be considered in high-volume transplant centers in patients aged <65 years, lacking any significant comorbidities and organ failure limited only to the lungs, provided the following basic requirements are met: (1) No radiological or clinical improvement for at least 4 weeks after the onset of illness; (2) persisting hypoxemia, poor lung compliance, and ECMO requirement; (3) no evidence of systemic illness, sepsis or shock; and[4] willingness for transplantation, post-transplant social support, and physiotherapy.[47] In appropriately selected patients, a few case series suggest a 1-year survival rate between 70–80%.[48-50] The reported 5-year survival was 54% in a 13-patient multicenter European study (the median age of the patients was 29 years).[51]

Supportive Care

Conservative Fluid Strategy

The increased capillary permeability in ARDS places them at a higher risk of pulmonary edema, and thus a positive fluid balance should be avoided. In a multicenter RCT, a conservative fluid strategy (central venous pressure <4 mm Hg or, when available, pulmonary artery occlusion pressure < 8 mm Hg) was found to improve oxygenation and ventilator-free days significantly than a more liberal strategy (although no mortality benefit).[44] The conservative strategy can be achieved either by judicious fluid restriction or intravenous diuretics, ensuring that the mean arterial pressure is ≥60 mm Hg (without inotropes) and there is no evidence of hypoperfusion (including urine output of at least 0.5 mL/kg of body weight per hour).

Neuromuscular Blockade

NMB in MV patients is used to reduce ventilator–patient dyssynchrony and reduce the work of breathing. However, NMB usage would require higher doses of sedation, can prolong ICU stay, and increase the risk of ICU-acquired weakness. Two major trials evaluated NMBs in ARDS, and currently, the routine use of NMB is not recommended in patients with moderate-to-severe ARDS.[43] In the first multicenter (ACURASYS) trial on NMBs, enrolling 340 moderate-to-severe ARDS patients managed on LTVV, the use of cisatracurium infusion for 48 hours improved 90-day survival as compared to placebo infusion, and the incidence of neuromuscular weakness was not significantly different.[52] The second major trial conducted in 2019 compared cisatracurium for 48 hours with light sedation (targeting Richmond Agitation–Sedation Scale of 0 or -1) along with the standard of care management for ARDS (LTVV, prone ventilation, and others). There was no significant difference in hospital mortality, ventilator-free days, or ICU-acquired weakness.[53] Although the mean PEEP and FiO_2 were lower with cisatracurium, the incidence of barotrauma was not significantly lower with NMB. The use of NMB may be considered in the early phase of ARDS in individuals at risk for pneumothorax[32] and to facilitate MV (if not achieved by sedation).[54-56]

Others

Sedation (light sedation), nutritional support, glycemic control (random blood glucose of 140–180 mg/dL), venous thromboembolism, and stress ulcer prophylaxis should be used in ARDS patients like other critically ill subjects. Standard ICU practices to prevent hospital-acquired infections (particularly ventilator-associated pneumonia) must be implemented in these patients.[57]

Pharmacotherapy

Acute respiratory distress syndrome is an inflammatory condition with noncardiogenic pulmonary edema, and several immunomodulators and anti-inflammatory agents have been tried with little success.[58] Activated protein C, aspirin, interferon-β, mucolytics (N-acetylcysteine), surfactants, antioxidants, vitamin D, statins, and others have been evaluated and are not recommended for use.[59-66] The heterogeneity in ARDS could be a prime factor for the lack of benefit with several of these agents. While inhaled pulmonary vasodilators such as nitric oxide transiently improve oxygenation, there is insufficient evidence to recommend its use in ARDS.[67] There is a suggestion that subphenotyping of ARDS patients may identify potential subgroups who might benefit from a therapy,[68-70] and clinical trials in enriched populations should be conducted in future.[32] The effectiveness of several specific therapies for ARDS in COVID-19 exemplifies the need for subphenotyping in the future clinical trials. Dexamethasone (6 mg/day for up to 10 days in hypoxemic COVID-19) and adjunctive tocilizumab (single intravenous dose of 8 mg/kg) or baricitinib for patients with persisting oxygen requirement are currently the standard of care for improving survival in COVID-19 ARDS.[71-73]

LONG-TERM OUTCOME OF ACUTE RESPIRATORY DISTRESS SYNDROME

The ARDS and ICU survivors have significant morbidity and even mortality on follow-up.[74] Among ARDS survivors, cognitive, psychological, and physical morbidities are well known. Psychiatric illnesses can occur in more than half of the ARDS survivors and include depression, post-traumatic stress disorder, anxiety, and others.[75,76] Poor quality of life, decreased exercise tolerance, and muscle weakness are also common among ARDS survivors.[77] Pre-existing illnesses, duration of ICU stay, delirium, use of sedation, and NMB are associated with morbidity during follow-up. Overall, morbidity affects the patient's ability to return to work and has a significant economic impact.[78] In a 5-year follow-up study, nearly 77% could return to work,[77] whereas in another study, 44% of survivors could not resume work by 1 year.[78]

SUMMARY

ARDS has considerable morbidity and morbidity. Management of ARDS includes primarily invasive MV, conservative fluid management, and supportive care. LTVV, high applied PEEP, and prone ventilation are essential to improve survival in patients with moderate-to-severe ARDS. There are no specific pharmacologic therapies for ARDS, except for a few conditions such as COVID-19-associated ARDS. Long-term follow-up to assess for morbidities and psychosocial support to manage them are essential in ARDS survivors.

REFERENCES

1. Gattinoni L, Caironi P, Valenza F, et al. The role of CT-scan studies for the diagnosis and therapy of acute respiratory distress syndrome. Clin Chest Med. 2006;27(4):559-70; abstract vii.
2. Puybasset L, Gusman P, Muller JC, et al. Regional distribution of gas and tissue in acute respiratory distress syndrome. III. Consequences for the effects of positive end-expiratory pressure. CT Scan ARDS Study Group. Adult Respiratory Distress Syndrome. Intensive Care Med. 2000;26(9):1215-27.
3. Gattinoni L, Pesenti A. The concept of "baby lung". Intensive Care Med. 2005;31(6):776-84.
4. Ashbaugh DG, Bigelow DB, Petty TL, et al. Acute respiratory distress in adults. Lancet. 1967;2(7511):319-23.
5. Sahetya SK, Goligher EC, Brower RG. Fifty Years of Research in ARDS. Setting Positive End-Expiratory Pressure in Acute Respiratory Distress Syndrome. Am J Respir Crit Care Med. 2017;195(11):1429-38.

6. Gattinoni L, Carlesso E, Caironi P. Stress and strain within the lung. Curr Opin Crit Care. 2012;18(1):42-7.
7. Henderson WR, Chen L, Amato MBP, et al. Fifty Years of Research in ARDS. Respiratory Mechanics in Acute Respiratory Distress Syndrome. Am J Respir Crit Care Med. 2017;196(7): 822-33.
8. Pontoppidan H, Geffin B, Lowenstein E. Acute respiratory failure in the adult. 3. N Engl J Med. 1972;287(16):799-806.
9. Acute Respiratory Distress Syndrome Network; Brower RG, Matthay MA, Morris A, et al. Ventilation with lower tidal volumes as compared with traditional tidal volumes for acute lung injury and the acute respiratory distress syndrome. N Engl J Med. 2000;342(18):1301-8.
10. Gajic O, Dara SI, Mendez JL, et al. Ventilator-associated lung injury in patients without acute lung injury at the onset of mechanical ventilation. Crit Care Med. 2004;32(9):1817-24.
11. Anzueto A, Frutos-Vivar F, Esteban A, et al. Incidence, risk factors and outcome of barotrauma in mechanically ventilated patients. Intensive Care Med. 2004;30(4):612-9.
12. Boussarsar M, Thierry G, Jaber S, et al. Relationship between ventilatory settings and barotrauma in the acute respiratory distress syndrome. Intensive Care Med. 2002;28(4):406-13.
13. Talmor D, Sarge T, Malhotra A, et al. Mechanical ventilation guided by esophageal pressure in acute lung injury. N Engl J Med. 2008;359(20):2095-104.
14. Pugin J, Dunn I, Jolliet P, et al. Activation of human macrophages by mechanical ventilation in vitro. Am J Physiol. 1998;275(6): L1040-50.
15. Toufen Junior C, De Santis Santiago RR, Hirota AS, et al. Driving pressure and long-term outcomes in moderate/severe acute respiratory distress syndrome. Ann Intensive Care. 2018;8(1):119.
16. Neto AS, Hemmes SN, Barbas CS, et al. Association between driving pressure and development of postoperative pulmonary complications in patients undergoing mechanical ventilation for general anaesthesia: A meta-analysis of individual patient data. Lancet Respir Med. 2016;4(4):272-80.
17. Muthu V, Agarwal R, Dhooria S, et al. Epidemiology, lung mechanics and outcomes of ARDS: A comparison between pregnant and non-pregnant subjects. J Crit Care. 2019;50:207-12.
18. Muthu V, Dhooria S, Aggarwal AN, et al. Acute respiratory distress syndrome due to tuberculosis in a respiratory ICU over a 16-year period. Crit Care Med. 2017;45(10):e1087-e90.
19. Amato MB, Meade MO, Slutsky AS, et al. Driving pressure and survival in the acute respiratory distress syndrome. N Engl J Med. 2015;372(8):747-55.
20. Pereira Romano ML, Maia IS, Laranjeira LN, et al. Driving pressure-limited strategy for patients with acute respiratory distress syndrome. A pilot randomized clinical trial. Ann Am Thorac Soc. 2020;17(5):596-604.
21. Agarwal R, Reddy C, Aggarwal AN, et al. Is there a role for noninvasive ventilation in acute respiratory distress syndrome? A meta-analysis. Respir Med. 2006;100(12):2235-8.
22. Kangelaris KN, Ware LB, Wang CY, et al. Timing of intubation and clinical outcomes in adults with acute respiratory distress syndrome. Crit Care Med. 2016;44(1):120-9.
23. Frat JP, Thille AW, Mercat A, et al. High-flow oxygen through nasal cannula in acute hypoxemic respiratory failure. N Engl J Med. 2015;372(23):2185-96.
24. Monro-Somerville T, Sim M, Ruddy J, et al. The effect of high-flow nasal cannula oxygen therapy on mortality and intubation rate in acute respiratory failure: A systematic review and meta-analysis. Crit Care Med. 2017;45(4):e449-e56.
25. Bellani G, Laffey JG, Pham T, et al. Noninvasive ventilation of patients with acute respiratory distress syndrome. Insights from the LUNG SAFE study. Am J Respir Crit Care Med. 2017;195(1): 67-77.
26. Chacko B, Peter JV, Tharyan P, et al. Pressure-controlled versus volume-controlled ventilation for acute respiratory failure due to acute lung injury (ALI) or acute respiratory distress syndrome (ARDS). Cochrane Database Syst Rev. 2015;1(1):CD008807.
27. Young D, Lamb SE, Shah S, et al. High-frequency oscillation for acute respiratory distress syndrome. N Engl J Med. 2013;368(9): 806-13.
28. Chu DK, Kim LH, Young PJ, et al. Mortality and morbidity in acutely ill adults treated with liberal versus conservative oxygen therapy (IOTA): A systematic review and meta-analysis. Lancet. 2018;391(10131):1693-705.
29. Barrot L, Asfar P, Mauny F, et al. Liberal or conservative oxygen therapy for acute respiratory distress syndrome. N Engl J Med. 2020;382(11):999-1008.
30. Muscedere JG, Mullen JB, Gan K, et al. Tidal ventilation at low airway pressures can augment lung injury. Am J Respir Crit Care Med. 1994;149(5):1327-34.
31. Hodgson C, Keating JL, Holland AE, et al. Recruitment manoeuvres for adults with acute lung injury receiving mechanical ventilation. Cochrane Database Syst Rev. 2009;(2): CD006667.
32. Grasselli G, Calfee CS, Camporota L, et al. ESICM guidelines on acute respiratory distress syndrome: Definition, phenotyping and respiratory support strategies. Intensive Care Med. 2023; 49(7):727-59.
33. Writing Group for the Alveolar Recruitment for Acute Respiratory Distress Syndrome Trial (ART) Investigators; Cavalcanti AB, Suzumura ÉA, Laranjeira LN, et al. Effect of lung recruitment and titrated positive end-expiratory pressure (PEEP) vs low PEEP on mortality in patients with acute respiratory distress syndrome: A randomized clinical trial. JAMA. 2017;318(14):1335-45.
34. Hess DR. Recruitment maneuvers and PEEP titration. Respir Care. 2015;60(11):1688-704.
35. Beitler JR, Sarge T, Banner-Goodspeed VM, et al. Effect of titrating positive end-expiratory pressure (PEEP) with an esophageal pressure-guided strategy vs an empirical high PEEP-FiO2 strategy on death and days free from mechanical ventilation among patients with acute respiratory distress syndrome: A randomized clinical trial. JAMA. 2019;321(9):846-57.
36. Terragni PP, Filippini C, Slutsky AS, et al. Accuracy of plateau pressure and stress index to identify injurious ventilation in patients with acute respiratory distress syndrome. Anesthesiology. 2013;119(4):880-9.
37. van der Zee P, Somhorst P, Endeman H, et al. Electrical impedance tomography for positive end-expiratory pressure titration in COVID-19-related acute respiratory distress syndrome. Am J Respir Crit Care Med. 2020;202(2):280-4.
38. Ball L, Robba C, Maiello L, et al. Computed tomography assessment of PEEP-induced alveolar recruitment in patients with severe COVID-19 pneumonia. Crit Care. 2021;25(1):81.

39. Bloomfield R, Noble DW, Sudlow A. Prone position for acute respiratory failure in adults. Cochrane Database Syst Rev. 2015;2015(11):CD008095.
40. Guérin C, Reignier J, Richard JC, et al. Prone positioning in severe acute respiratory distress syndrome. N Engl J Med. 2013;368(23): 2159-68.
41. Burrell A, Kim J, Alliegro P, et al. Extracorporeal membrane oxygenation for critically ill adults. Cochrane Database Syst Rev. 2023;9(9):CD010381.
42. Friedrichson B, Mutlak H, Zacharowski K, et al. Insight into ECMO, mortality and ARDS: A nationwide analysis of 45,647 ECMO runs. Crit Care. 2021;25(1):38.
43. Combes A, Peek GJ, Hajage D, et al. ECMO for severe ARDS: Systematic review and individual patient data meta-analysis. Intensive Care Med. 2020;46(11):2048-57.
44. Combes A, Hajage D, Capellier G, et al. Extracorporeal Membrane Oxygenation for Severe Acute Respiratory Distress Syndrome. N Engl J Med. 2018;378(21):1965-75.
45. Peek GJ, Mugford M, Tiruvoipati R, et al. Efficacy and economic assessment of conventional ventilatory support versus extracorporeal membrane oxygenation for severe adult respiratory failure (CESAR): A multicentre randomised controlled trial. Lancet. 2009;374(9698):1351-63.
46. McNamee JJ, Gillies MA, Barrett NA, et al. Effect of lower tidal volume ventilation facilitated by extracorporeal carbon dioxide removal vs standard care ventilation on 90-day mortality in patients with acute hypoxemic respiratory failure: The REST randomized clinical trial. JAMA. 2021;326(11):1013-23.
47. Hoetzenecker K, Schwarz S, Keshavjee S, et al. Lung transplantation for acute respiratory distress syndrome. J Thorac Cardiovasc Surg. 2023;165(4):1596-601.
48. Harano T, Ryan JP, Chan EG, et al. Lung transplantation for the treatment of irreversible acute respiratory distress syndrome. Clin Transplant. 2021;35(2):e14182.
49. Frick AE, Gan CT, Vos R, et al. Lung transplantation for acute respiratory distress syndrome: A multicenter experience. Am J Transplant. 2022;22(1):144-53.
50. Chang Y, Lee SO, Shim TS, et al. Lung Transplantation as a therapeutic option in acute respiratory distress syndrome. Transplantation. 2018;102(5):829-37.
51. Bharat A, Machuca TN, Querrey M, et al. Early outcomes after lung transplantation for severe COVID-19: A series of the first consecutive cases from four countries. Lancet Respir Med. 2021;9(5):487-97.
52. Papazian L, Forel JM, Gacouin A, et al. Neuromuscular blockers in early acute respiratory distress syndrome. N Engl J Med. 2010;363(12):1107-16.
53. National Heart, Lung, and Blood Institute PETAL Clinical Trials Network; Moss M, Huang DT, Brower RG, et al. Early neuromuscular blockade in the acute respiratory distress syndrome. N Engl J Med. 2019;380(21):1997-2008.
54. Bourenne J, Hraiech S, Roch A, et al. Sedation and neuromuscular blocking agents in acute respiratory distress syndrome. Ann Transl Med. 2017;5(14):291.
55. Forel JM, Roch A, Marin V, al. Neuromuscular blocking agents decrease inflammatory response in patients presenting with acute respiratory distress syndrome. Crit Care Med. 2006;34(11): 2749-57.
56. Guervilly C, Bisbal M, Forel JM, et al. Effects of neuromuscular blockers on transpulmonary pressures in moderate to severe acute respiratory distress syndrome. Intensive Care Med. 2017;43(3):408-18.
57. Torres A, Niederman MS, Chastre J, et al. International ERS/ESICM/ESCMID/ALAT guidelines for the management of hospital-acquired pneumonia and ventilator-associated pneumonia: Guidelines for the management of hospital-acquired pneumonia (HAP)/ventilator-associated pneumonia (VAP) of the European Respiratory Society (ERS), European Society of Intensive Care Medicine (ESICM), European Society of Clinical Microbiology and Infectious Diseases (ESCMID) and Asociación Latinoamericana del Tórax (ALAT). Eur Respir J. 2017;50(3):1700582.
58. Gorman EA, O'Kane CM, McAuley DF. Acute respiratory distress syndrome in adults: Diagnosis, outcomes, long-term sequelae, and management. Lancet. 2022;400(10358):1157-70.
59. Li C, Bo L, Liu W, et al. Enteral immunomodulatory diet (omega-3 fatty acid, γ-linolenic acid and antioxidant supplementation) for acute lung injury and acute respiratory distress syndrome: An updated systematic review and meta-analysis. Nutrients. 2015;7(7):5572-85.
60. Liu KD, Levitt J, Zhuo H, et al. Randomized clinical trial of activated protein C for the treatment of acute lung injury. Am J Respir Crit Care Med. 2008;178(6):618-23.
61. Kor DJ, Carter RE, Park PK, et al. Effect of aspirin on development of ARDS in at-risk patients presenting to the emergency department: The LIPS-A randomized clinical trial. JAMA. 2016; 315(22):2406-14.
62. Gao Smith F, Perkins GD, Gates S, et al. Effect of intravenous β-2 agonist treatment on clinical outcomes in acute respiratory distress syndrome (BALTI-2): A multicentre, randomised controlled trial. Lancet. 2012;379(9812):229-35.
63. Ranieri VM, Pettilä V, Karvonen MK, et al. Effect of intravenous interferon β-1a on death and days free from mechanical ventilation among patients with moderate to severe acute respiratory distress syndrome: A randomized clinical trial. JAMA. 2020;323(8):725-33.
64. Randomized, placebo-controlled trial of lisofylline for early treatment of acute lung injury and acute respiratory distress syndrome. Crit Care Med. 2002;30(1):1-6.
65. Bo L, Jin F, Ma Z, et al. Redox signaling and antioxidant therapies in acute respiratory distress syndrome: A systematic review and meta-analysis. Expert Rev Respir Med. 2021;15(10):1355-65.
66. McAuley DF, Laffey JG, O'Kane CM, et al. Simvastatin in the acute respiratory distress syndrome. N Engl J Med. 2014;371(18): 1695-703.
67. Gebistorf F, Karam O, Wetterslev J, et al. Inhaled nitric oxide for acute respiratory distress syndrome (ARDS) in children and adults. Cochrane Database Syst Rev. 2016;2016(6):CD002787.
68. Boyle AJ, Ferris P, Bradbury I, et al. Baseline plasma IL-18 may predict simvastatin treatment response in patients with ARDS: A secondary analysis of the HARP-2 randomised clinical trial. Crit Care. 2022;26(1):164.
69. Torbic H, Bulgarelli L, Deliberato RO, et al. Potential impact of subphenotyping in pharmacologic management of acute respiratory distress syndrome. J Pharm Pract. 2024;37(4): 955-66.

70. Sinha P, Calfee CS, Cherian S, et al. Prevalence of phenotypes of acute respiratory distress syndrome in critically ill patients with COVID-19: A prospective observational study. Lancet Respir Med. 2020;8(12):1209-18.
71. RECOVERY Collaborative Group; Horby P, Lim WS, Emberson JR, et al. Dexamethasone in hospitalized patients with Covid-19. N Engl J Med. 2021;384(8):693-704.
72. RECOVERY Collaborative Group; Tocilizumab in patients admitted to hospital with COVID-19 (RECOVERY): A randomised, controlled, open-label, platform trial. Lancet. 2021;397(10285): 1637-45.
73. Baricitinib in patients admitted to hospital with COVID-19 (RECOVERY): a randomised, controlled, open-label, platform trial and updated meta-analysis. Lancet. 2022;400(10349):359-68.
74. Kodati R, Muthu V, Agarwal R, et al. Long-term survival and quality of life among survivors discharged from a respiratory ICU in North India: A prospective study. Indian J Crit Care Med. 2022;26(10):1078-85.
75. Bienvenu OJ, Colantuoni E, Mendez-Tellez PA, et al. Depressive symptoms and impaired physical function after acute lung injury: A 2-year longitudinal study. Am J Respir Crit Care Med. 2012;185(5):517-24.
76. Huang M, Parker AM, Bienvenu OJ, et al. Psychiatric symptoms in acute respiratory distress syndrome survivors: A 1-Year National Multicenter Study. Crit Care Med. 2016;44(5):954-65.
77. Herridge MS, Tansey CM, Matté A, et al. Functional disability 5 years after acute respiratory distress syndrome. N Engl J Med. 2011;364(14):1293-304.
78. Kamdar BB, Huang M, Dinglas VD, et al. Joblessness and lost earnings after acute respiratory distress syndrome in a 1-year national multicenter study. Am J Respir Crit Care Med. 2017;196(8):1012-20.

Sepsis and Septic Shock

CHAPTER 165

Dhruva Chaudhry, Lokesh Kumar Lalwani

INTRODUCTION

Sepsis is not a definite illness but a syndrome associated with still uncertain pathobiology. It can be recognized by the combination of clinical signs and symptoms in a patient with suspicion of infection.[1] The prevalence of sepsis patients has been rising in recent years because of the population's increasing age and rising comorbidities like chronic organ failure, immunosuppressive diseases, and cancer. This rising trend of sepsis is associated with higher mortality, morbidity, and healthcare utilization. The estimated cost for treating sepsis is around \$55 per patient in India[2] to \$129,632 per patient in the United States,[3] despite the fact, mortality rate is as high as 33% and 66% in sepsis and septic shock, respectively.[4] Early and prompt identification of sepsis and appropriate management in the early hours after developing sepsis are crucial and improve outcomes.

DEFINITION

Sepsis is defined as a "life-threatening organ dysfunction caused by a dysregulated host response to infection". Organ dysfunction associated with sepsis can be picked out as a change in total sequential organ failure assessment (SOFA) score ≥2 points along with suspicion of infection.[5] The parameters required to calculate SOFA score are cumbersome and need laboratory values that are not readily available. Multiple tools were used for screening of sepsis, such as systemic inflammatory response syndrome (SIRS) criteria, quick SOFA(qSOFA), or modified early warning score (MEWS) **(Table 1)**.[6,7] MEWS is validated in medical-surgical patients and identify risk of clinical deterioration and mortality when score is ≥5. It comprises five physiologic variables: Systolic blood pressure, heart rate, respiratory rate, temperature, and mental status.[8] In comparison with

TABLE 1: Screening criteria of sepsis. Systemic inflammatory response syndrome (SIRS) criteria; quick sequential organ failure score (qSOFA); and modified early warning score (MEWS).

SIRS (≥2 points)	• Body temperature ≥38°C, or ≤36°C • Heart rate of ≥90 beats/min • Respiratory rate of ≥ 20 breaths/min • White blood cell count of ≥12,000/mm³ or ≤4,000/mm³ or >10% bands						
qSOFA (≥2 points)	• Respiratory rate ≥ 22 breaths/min • Systolic blood pressure < 100 mm Hg • Altered mental status						
MEWS (≥ 5 points)	Score						
	3	2	1	0	1	2	3
Respiratory rate (min^{-1})		≤8		9–14	15–20	21–29	>29
Heart rate (min^{-1})		≤40	41–50	51–100	101–110	111–129	>129
Systolic BP (mm Hg)	≤70	71–80	81–100	101–199		≥200	
Urine output (mL/kg/h)	Nil	<0.5					
Temperature (°C)		≤35	35.1–36	36.1–38	38.1–38.5	≥38.6	
Neurological				Alert	Reacting to voice	Reacting to pain	Unresponsive

SIRS, qSOFA score is found to be more specific but less sensitive for early identification of sepsis in the emergency department.[9] More complex MEWS has not performed better for screening of sepsis.[6]

Septic shock is defined as a "subset of sepsis in which fundamental circulatory, cellular, and metabolic abnormalities are extreme enough to increase mortality substantially".[5] Septic shock may be identified with a clinical history consistent with sepsis along with continuous hypotension and needs vasopressor support to maintain mean arterial pressure (MAP) ≥65 mm Hg and having serum lactate level >2 mmol/L (18 mg/dL) despite adequate volume resuscitation. In presence of shock, mortality rate rises by 40% in sepsis.[5]

PHENOTYPES OF SEPSIS

Four phenotypes named α, β, γ, and δ were identified as subgroups of sepsis.[10] The α phenotype is associated with lesser abnormal laboratory values and less organ dysfunction. Patients with β phenotype were identified as older, had a higher chronic illness, and most presented with renal dysfunction. Those who present with γ phenotype had a higher temperature and lower albumin levels and were more likely to have raised inflammatory markers such as white blood cell count, premature neutrophil count, erythrocyte sedimentation rate, or C-reactive protein. A group of patients with δ phenotype of sepsis have elevated serum lactate levels, higher values of transaminases, and hypotension.[11]

RISK FACTORS AND ETIOLOGY OF SEPSIS

Several risk factors and etiologies of sepsis have been identified. Older age and male gender were associated with a greater incidence of sepsis.[12] Pre-existing comorbidities such as chronic obstructive pulmonary disease (COPD), alcohol dependence, immunosuppressive disorders, diabetes, malignancy, and hemodialysis have also been identified as risk factors.[13] A positive association was found between sepsis and invasive interventions in the intensive care unit (ICU) including urinary catheterization, central venous catheters, and nasogastric tube insertion for parenteral nutrition.[14] Abdominal surgery and laparotomy are also recognized as independent risk factors for developing sepsis. Increased levels of biomarkers, namely soluble platelet selectin (sP-selectin), SE-selectin, and Gc-globulin have been found to be associated with sepsis.[15] In addition to these risk factors, infection is identified as the most common etiology of sepsis. Not only the bacteria but other microorganisms including viruses, fungi, and parasites can cause sepsis **(Fig. 1)**.[16,17] The most frequent site of infection was identified as respiratory system (44%), followed by the abdomen (31%) and urinary tract (8%). A total 4% of patients had multiple sites of entry for microorganisms.[18] *Pseudomonas aeruginosa* and *Klebsiella pneumoniae* are the most common gram-negative bacteria causing sepsis.[19] In modern intensive care settings, incidence of sepsis and septic shock associated with gram-positive bacteria, e.g., *Staphylococcus aureus* or *Streptococcus pneumoniae* is rising and accounts for up

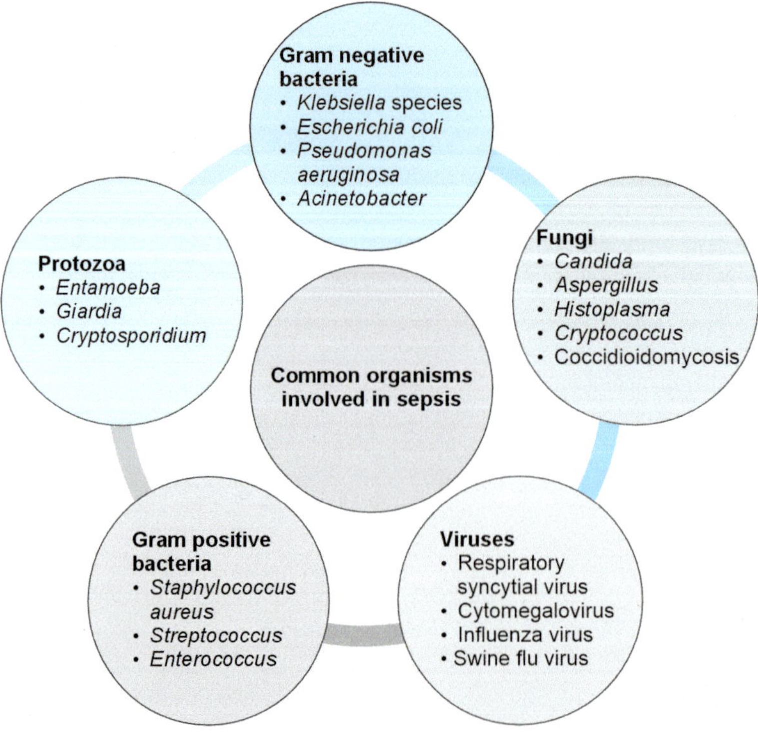

FIG. 1: Common organisms involved in sepsis.

to 50%.[20] Most common parasite associated with sepsis is falciparum malaria and it leads to life-threatening organ dysfunction.[21] *Burkholderia pseudomallei* and Rickettsial infections are also associated with sepsis.[22] Sepsis due to fungal infection is rising rapidly and causes up to 15% of total sepsis cases.[23]

PATHOGENESIS OF SEPSIS

There are heterogeneous pathophysiologic processes involved in the pathogenesis of sepsis **(Fig. 2)**. Interlinkage of microbiological products with a host, which is prone because of its genetic and other factors including immune modulatory mediators, leads to cellular and organ dysfunction.[5] The severity of sepsis is affected by an activation cascade that will further progress to an auto-amplifying cytokine production termed *"cytokine storm"* which is mostly responsible for the diverse, local, and remote signals related to infection.[24] The most common pathways responsible for sepsis are described below:

- *Innate immunity and inflammatory mediators:* At the beginning of the cascade, activation of the innate immune system against pathogens is initiated, which is composed of mainly macrophages, neutrophils, monocytes, and natural killer cells.[25] It happens by attaching pathogen-associated molecular patterns (PAMPs), like bacterial endotoxin and fungal β-glucans, to specific recognition receptors on these inflammatory cells. This reaction can also happen by damage-associated molecular patterns (DAMPs) that can be

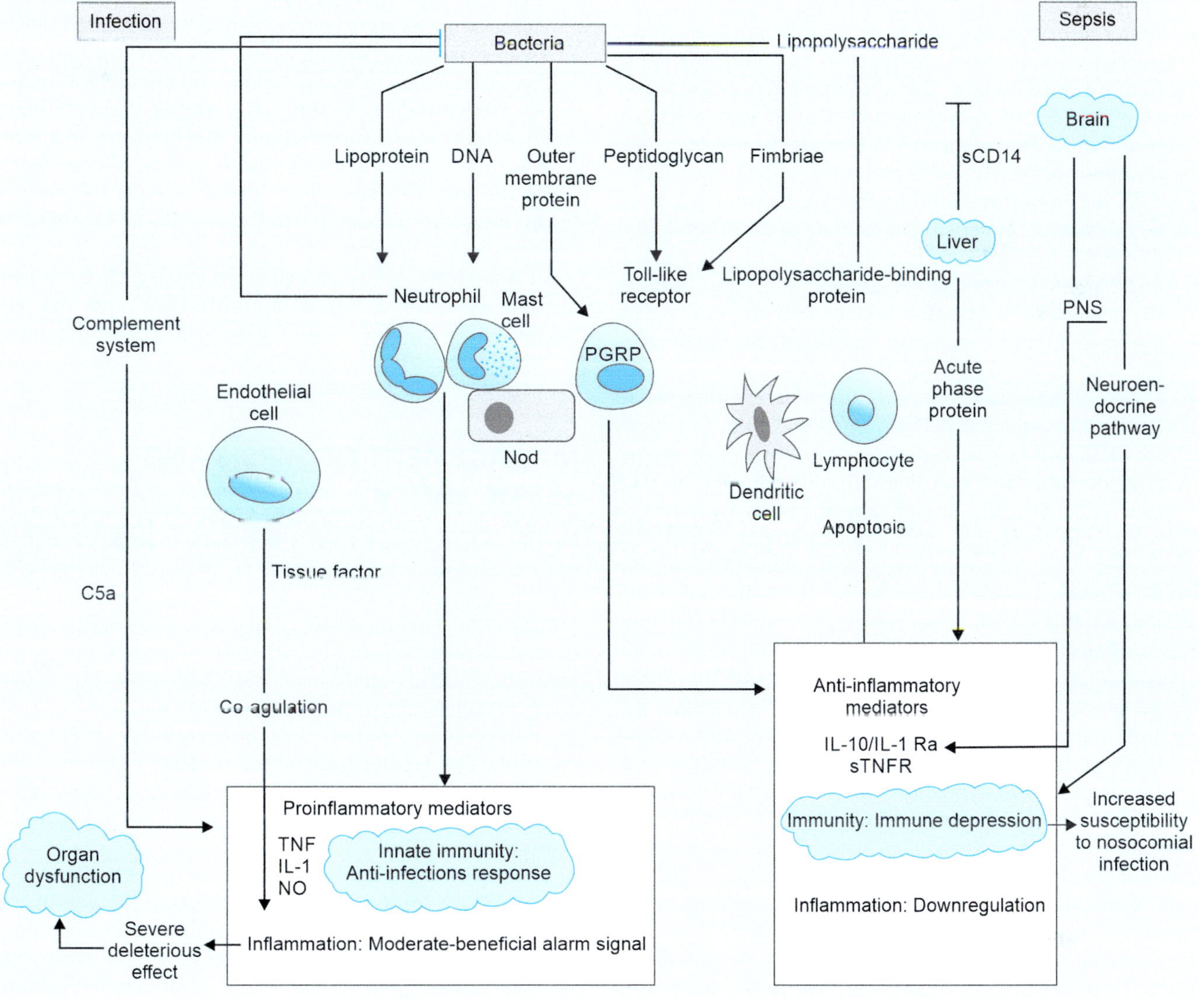

FIG. 2: Complex pathogenesis of sepsis.

(CD: cluster of differentiation; C5a: complement 5a; DNA: deoxyribonucleic acid; IL: interleukin; NO: nitric oxide; NOD: nucleotide-binding oligomerization domain; PNS: peripheral nervous system; PGRP: peptidoglycan recognition protein; sTNFR: soluble tumor necrosis factor receptor; TNF: tumor necrosis factor)

molecules extracted from dead or damaged host cells, such as adenosine triphosphate (ATP) and mitochondrial deoxyribonucleic acid (DNA).

- *Dysregulation of hemostasis:* Sepsis leads to the interaction of inflammatory and hemostatic pathways with the activation of the inflammatory and coagulation cascade. This interaction can vary from mild thrombocytopenia to severe disseminated intravascular coagulation (DIC). The dysregulation of coagulation can be multifactorial in sepsis. Hypercoagulability in sepsis results from the liberation of tissue factors from disrupted endothelial cells.[26] Bacteriemia and endotoxin accelerate the blockade of tissue factors and inhibit inflammation-induced thrombin production.[27] Tissue factors further cause the activation of platelets and the development of platelet-fibrin clots. This microthrombi can lead to perfusion defects and result in tissue hypoxia and organ dysfunction.
- *Immunosuppression:* The early proinflammatory phase of sepsis mainly takes the place of an enlarged state of immune suppression. The number of T cells decreases as a product of apoptosis and a decreased response to inflammatory cytokines.[28] Studies have shown that inhibition of cluster of differentiation 4 (CD4+) and CD8+ cells is commonly found in the lymphoid organ, such as the spleen. In sepsis, the activity of neutrophils has diminished chemotaxis response to interleukin 8 (IL-8) and expresses fewer chemokine receptors. These findings express that the immune system fails to generate an adequate immune response against infective pathogens like bacteria, virus, or fungi.[29]
- *Cellular, tissue, and organ dysfunction:* Hypoperfusion leads to diminished delivery and utilization of oxygen by cells and is the underlying mechanism of sepsis. Hypoperfusion is the result of cardiovascular dysfunction that is evident in sepsis.[30] Septic cardiomyopathy is acute and reversible. It is associated with circulatory cytokines like tumor necrosis factor alpha (TNF-α) and IL-1β, which leads to depression of cardiac myocytes and hampers the functioning of mitochondria. Further, it will decrease the left ventricular ejection fraction and is associated with low or average left ventricular filling pressure with raised left ventricular compliance.[31] Inflammatory mediators lead to arterial and venous dilation and, subsequently, decreased venous return, causing a state of hypotension and distributive shock.

Disturbance in barrier function of endothelium leads to increased leucocyte adhesion and vasodilation, and development of a procoagulant state. This results in the accumulation of edema fluid in the interstitial spaces, subcutaneous tissue, and body cavities. In the lungs, collection of protein-rich fluid in the interstitial pulmonary spaces and alveoli leads to a ventilation-perfusion mismatch, decreased lung compliance, hypoxia, and acute respiratory distress syndrome (ARDS).

In the renal system, disruption in microvasculature and tubules produces a combination of reduced renal perfusion, acute tubular necrosis, and a varying degree of acute kidney injury. In the liver, difficulty in bilirubin clearance leads to cholestasis. In the gastrointestinal tract, raised permeability of the mucosal lining results in autodigestion of the bowel by luminal enzymes and bacterial translocation across the bowel wall. Septic encephalopathy includes oxidative stress, neurotransmitter disruption, changes of cerebral edema, and white matter damage in its clinical spectrum and varies from mild confusion to profound delirium and coma. Significant muscular breakdown happens in sepsis to produce amino acids that provide a source of power to the immune cells. Additionally, raised insulin resistance produces a state of hyperglycemia. The effect of sepsis on different organ systems is shown in **Figure 3**.

- *Mitochondrial and microcirculatory distress syndrome (MMDS):* It can be a part of SIRS. It is defined as cytopathic tissue hypoxia, which is not corrected by oxygen transport optimization. It is also attached to an acquired defect in using oxygen and energy production in mitochondria, leading to multiple organ failures. Dysfunction of auto-regulatory mechanisms, including microcirculatory dysfunction, is a determining factor in the pathophysiology of sepsis. It leads to decrease in microcirculatory partial pressure of O_2 (pO_2) in comparison to venous pO_2 and is termed as "pO_2 gap". It is the primary reason behind microcirculatory distress and systemic hemodynamic-derived and oxygen-derived variables cannot diagnose it. Heterogenous inducible nitric oxide synthase (iNOS) expression leads to pathological flow shunting.

MANAGEMENT OF SEPSIS AND SEPTIC SHOCK

In 2001, a benchmark study showed the mortality benefit of early goal-directed therapy (EGDT) and used an algorithm including blood transfusion, fluid resuscitation, and use of inotropes and vasopressors to maintain the targeted MAP, central venous pressure (CVP), and mixed venous oxygen saturation.[32] This trial was conducted when pulmonary artery catheters were routinely placed in most sepsis patients to monitor these parameters. Subsequently, there were contradictory results from other studies.[33] However, the principles of fluid resuscitation and hemodynamic goals are still the same and considered in the Surviving Sepsis Campaign guidelines.[34]

- *Screening and diagnosis:* Initial management should not be delayed for further diagnostic tests in the presence of a strong suspicion of sepsis based on screening criteria (qSOFA or SIRS) and measures of sepsis-induced organ dysfunction **(Flowchart 1)**. A blood culture should be taken before antibiotic administration, along with a urine culture, if there is suspicion of urinary tract

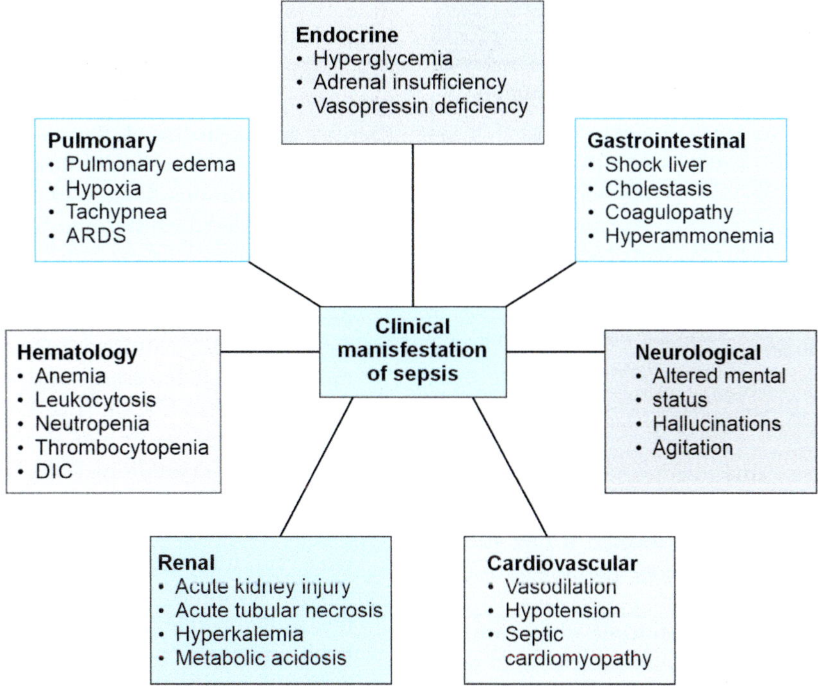

FIG. 3: Clinical manifestation of sepsis on different organ systems.
(DIC: disseminated intravascular coagulation)

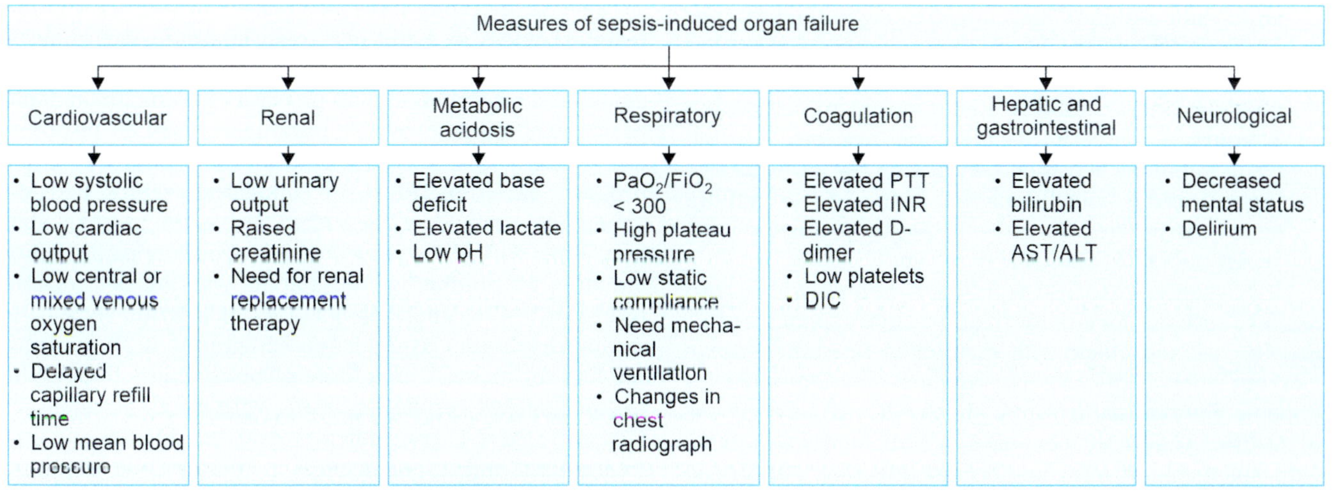

FLOWCHART 1: Measures of sepsis-induced organ failure.
(ALT: alanine aminotransferase; AST: aspartate aminotransferase; DIC: disseminated intravascular coagulation; FiO_2: fraction of oxygen; INR: international normalized ratio; PaO_2: partial pressure of oxygen; PTT: partial thromboplastin time)

infection. A chest X-ray is to be done as a routine to rule out pneumonia. Further imaging, like a computed tomography (CT) scan of the abdomen is to be done if there is suspicion of intra-abdominal infection, e.g., abscess or diverticulitis.

- *Biomarkers of sepsis:* Early recognition of the infectious etiology helps initiate targeted treatment, improves the outcome, and decreases mortality. Presepsin (sCD-14ST) is a potential biomarker, whose level increases in response to microbial infection in the host. The serum level of presepsin to discriminate between sepsis and noninfectious organ failure is 582 pg/mL while 1,285 pg/mL is the cutoff value for differentiating between sepsis and septic shock. Patients with presepsin levels of <821 pg/mL have shown a mortality rate of 18.4%, and mortality of 33.3% is associated with higher presepsin levels (≥ 821 pg/mL).[35]

TABLE 2: Initial resuscitation bundles for sepsis and septic shock.	
3-hour resuscitation bundle	**6-hour septic shock bundle**
Measure initial lactate level	Apply vasopressor (for hypotension after initial fluid resuscitation) to maintain MAP ≥65 mm Hg
Obtain blood culture before antibiotic administration	
Administer broad-spectrum antibiotics	In the event of persistent hypotension, despite fluid resuscitation or lactate ≥4 mmol/L, measure central venous pressure and superior vena cava oxygen saturation
Administer 30 mL/Kg crystalloids for hypotension or lactate ≥4 mmol/L	
(MAP: mean arterial pressure)	

Serum procalcitonin levels are not recommended to decide when to start antibiotics though it has shown effectiveness in the cessation of antibiotic therapy to reduce cumulative exposure.[36]

- *Antibiotics and source control:* Multiple observational studies have suggested that early administration of antibiotics is associated with favorable outcomes. If sepsis is definite or probable, antimicrobials should be administered immediately, ideally within 1 hour of recognition, regardless of shock. However, if sepsis is possible, administer antimicrobials immediately in the presence of shock. If shock is absent, then rapid assessment has to be done for infectious versus noninfectious causes of acute illness, and administer antimicrobials within 3 hours if concern for infection persists.[34] Initial resuscitation for sepsis and septic shock was categorized into a 3-and 6-hour bundle but both of these bundles were incorporated in a 1-hour bundle of the surviving sepsis guideline **(Table 2)**.[37]

It is suggested to use combined therapy with gram-negative coverage for empiric treatment over monotherapy.[38] Empiric antimicrobials with methicillin-resistant *Staphylococcus aureus* (MRSA) coverage are recommended for patients with sepsis or septic shock who are at high risk of MRSA. Anaerobic coverage is indicated in patients with suspicion of intra-abdominal infection. Antifungal and antiviral therapy may be considered for patients with immune deficiencies or immune suppression. INTEREST trial concluded that combination therapy with intravenous doxycycline and azithromycin was a better therapeutic option for treatment of severe scrub typhus than monotherapy with either drug alone.[39]

Prolonged infusion of antimicrobials especially β-lactam antibiotics for maintenance over conventional bolus of antibiotics is recommended for sepsis management and organ-specific infections **(Flowchart 2)**.

Inappropriate use of antimicrobial agents has been shown to contribute to the occurrence of multidrug-resistant (MDR) organisms. To deal with MDR organisms with the aim of battling drug resistance, improving patient outcomes, and decreasing the health care cost, a novel strategy of antimicrobial stewardship program (AMS) looks to be effective and is strongly recommended in ICUs.[40] The primary concern of AMS is to provide the best empirical therapy related to the patient's clinical condition, source of infection, local antimicrobial resistance pattern, and previous antibiotics history to avoid repeating the same antibiotic and, on the other side, to halt antibiotics in patients without infection.[41]

- *Fluid resuscitation:* Reduced duration of hypotension in sepsis is associated with decreased mortality in septic shock.[42] Fluid resuscitation is important to maintain cardiac output and MAP in the presence of pathologic vasodilation. The Surviving Sepsis Campaign recommended an initial fluid bolus of 30 mL/kg of intravenous crystalloid fluid. This amount of fluid is adequate for most of the patients but causes concern when this amount of fluid is excessive for some patients. Observational studies have demonstrated that excess volume administration is associated with higher mortality, probably due to adjunct pulmonary edema needing prolonged mechanical ventilation and worsened kidney injury.[43] Crystalloid solution is the first choice for initial fluid resuscitation of sepsis and septic shock patients. Starches and gelatin are not recommended for resuscitation.

Several methods have been used to predict volume responsiveness to avoid over-resuscitation. According to Surviving Sepsis Guidelines, dynamic measures are better to guide fluid resuscitation than physical examination or static parameters alone. Dynamic parameters include response to a passive leg raise, stroke volume variation (SVV), pulse pressure variation (PPV), or echocardiography. Bedside echocardiography has been identified as the most reliable tool, along with an increase in the carbon monoxide before and after a "minibus" of 100–250 mL working as a reliable indicator.[44] Checking collapsibility of inferior vena cava during inspiration using echocardiography is an accurate method for analysis of volume responsiveness in patients on mechanical ventilation along with paralytic agents.[45] However, there is contradictory evidence for this method to examine fluid responsiveness in spontaneous breathing patients.[46] Doppler measurements of dynamic carotid artery parameters such as carotid blood flow (CBF) and carotid flow time (CFT) are being studied as potential indicators of fluid responsiveness. A cutoff of 10% increase in CBF was considered positive response to fluid bolus. There was a significant change in CBF after fluid bolus, but CFT has shown no difference. These facts demonstrate no correlation between CBF and CFT, and CFT did not predict fluid responsiveness.[47]

- *Target blood pressure:* Various retrospective data suggest that a higher mortality risk and renal injury are associated with MAP <85 mm Hg.[48] When comparing lower MAP target (65–70) with a higher MAP target (80–85), there is no mortality benefit of one over other.[49] However,

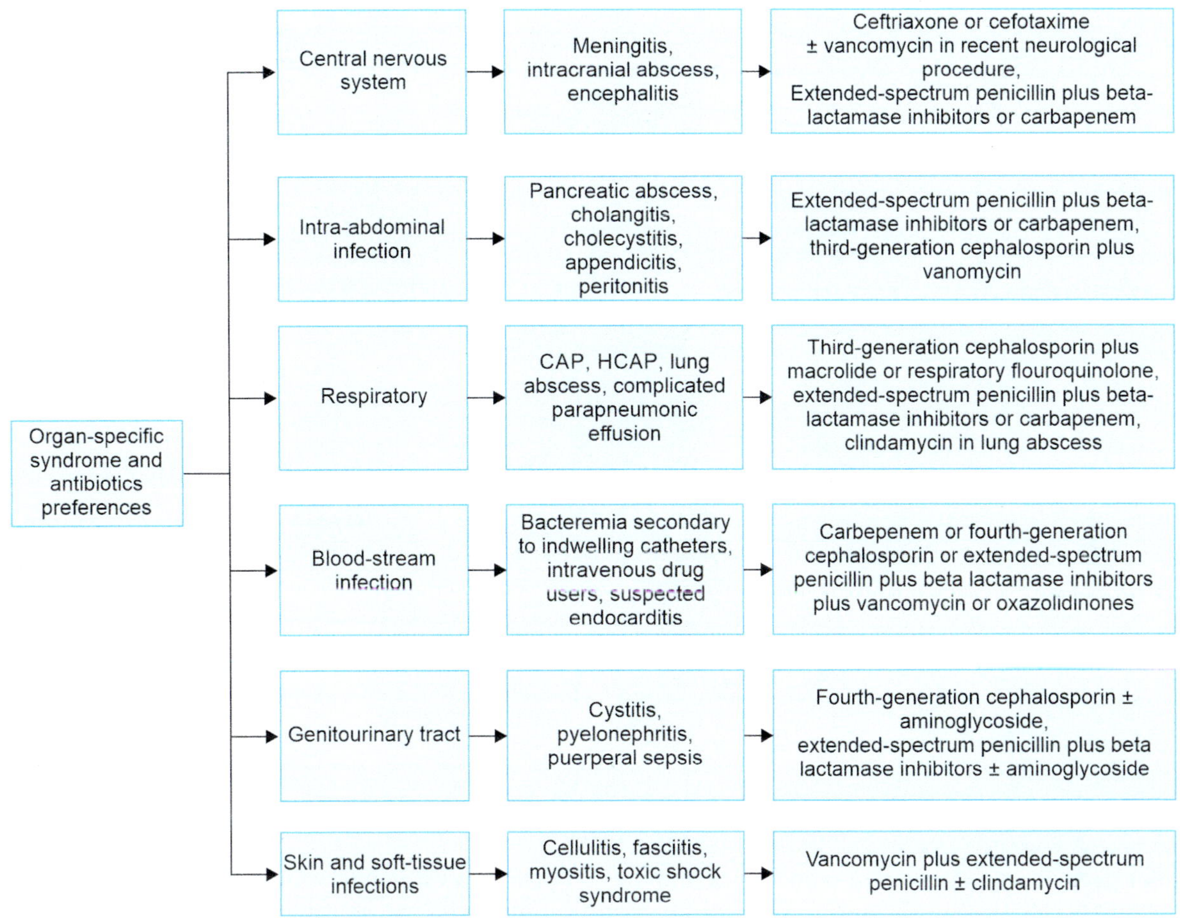

FLOWCHART 2: Organ-specific syndrome and antibiotics preferences.
(CAP: community-acquired pneumonia; HCAP: healthcare-associated pneumonia)

the Surviving Sepsis Guidelines recommend a target MAP of at least 65 mm Hg for titration of vasopressor support.[34]

- *Vasopressor choice:* Vasopressors are the next choice during and after fluid resuscitation for maintaining blood pressure in patients with septic shock. Randomized controlled trials that evaluated the safety of dopamine in comparison with norepinephrine as an initial choice for shock have demonstrated higher incidences of tachyarrhythmia and worsened mortality with dopamine.[50] Hence, norepinephrine is recommended as a first-line agent according to Surviving Sepsis Campaign.[34] Epinephrine was also compared with norepinephrine as the initial drug of choice in septic shock patients but it did not show a mortality benefit.[51] Epinephrine may be added for inotropic benefit to maintain perfusion in cases where septic patients with hypotension also have decreased cardiac output. Vasopressin is a noncatecholamine substance that directly acts on V1 and V2 receptors and, compared to norepinephrine, shows no mortality advantage.[52] Angiotensin II is a product of the renin-angiotensin-aldosterone system. Addition of human angiotensin II to catecholamine and vasopressin therapy increased MAP in patients with vasodilatory shock, allowing reductions in the dose of catecholamines.[53] Oral midodrine administered at total 3 doses of 10 mg every 8 hourly [in addition to the usual sepsis care, including subsequent initiation of intravenous vasopressors (IVPs)] demonstrated a decreased median duration of IVPs, decreased total IVP requirement in the first 24 hours of ICU stay, and shorter ICU length of stay; but these results were not significant.[54]
- *Adjunct therapies:* Several adjunct therapies have been evaluated in sepsis patients to fight against dysregulated inflammatory response. Systemic steroids have been investigated in multiple randomized trials, but the results of these trials have not demonstrated mortality benefits. The latest ADRENAL trial evaluated continuous infusion of hydrocortisone in patients of septic shock and found nil benefit compared to placebo.[55] The APROCCHSS trial evaluated the use of bolus hydrocortisone every 6 hours and a single daily dose of fludrocortisone and demonstrated a modest mortality benefit.[56] Possibly,

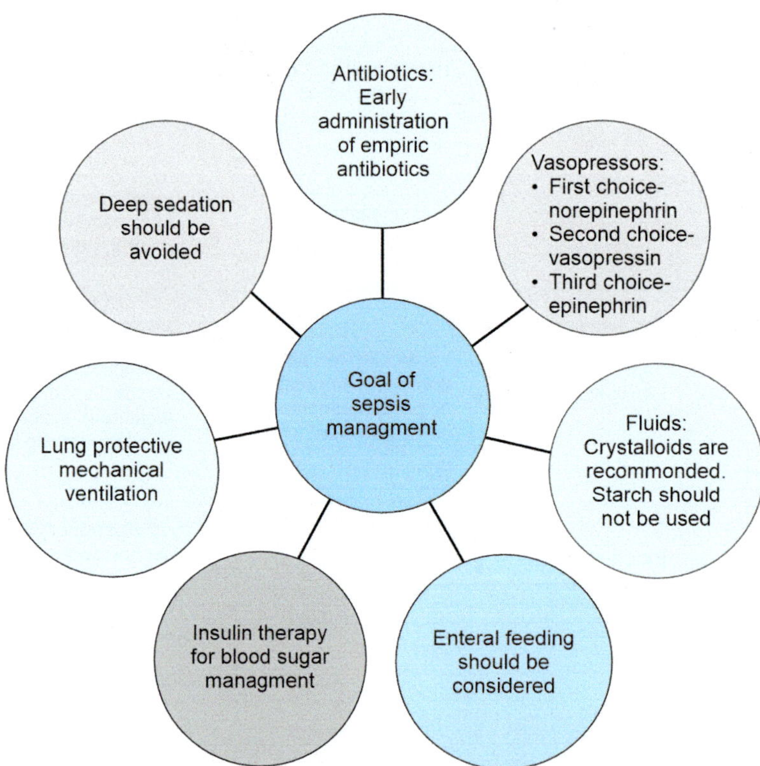

FIG. 4: Various strategies used in sepsis and septic shock management.

steroids decrease the duration of septic shock and the time spent on life support therapy in ICUs but the use of steroids did not lead to lesser deaths when overall compared with the group not receiving steroids.[55]

Ascorbic acid (Vitamin C) is recognized as an antioxidant that may decrease the dysregulated response to sepsis. In small studies, the use of cocktail therapy, including ascorbic acid, thiamine, and hydrocortisone, was evaluated and found promising results.[57] The CITRIS-ALI trial examined ascorbic acid's role on organ dysfunction scores in septic patients and ARDS and found no significant difference.[58] Surviving Sepsis Campaign 2021 suggests against using intravenous vitamin C for adults with sepsis or septic shock.[34]

- *Ventilation:* Different strategies are used in management of sepsis **(Fig. 4)**. There is inadequate evidence to recommend oxygen targets in adults with sepsis-induced hypoxemic respiratory failure. Only moderate progress has been achieved in patients with sepsis and respiratory insufficiency in the field of mechanical ventilation as a supportive measure. The primary goal of mechanical ventilation is to improve gaseous exchange, reduce the work of breathing, along with preventing high airway pressures and iatrogenic damage to lung tissue. Guidelines recommend high-flow oxygen therapy over noninvasive ventilation in sepsis-induced hypoxemic respiratory failure patients. In sepsis-inspired ARDS, the recommendation for a protective lung ventilation strategy with a tidal volume of 6 mL/Kg ideal body weight with a higher limit for plateau pressure of 30 cmH_2O is still valid.[59] Prone positioning in ARDS is strongly recommended as associated with lower mortality. Despite having only minor complications and being better at reducing driving pressure, it has been shown in an observational study that prone positioning is only used for 32.9% of severe ARDS patients.[60]

POST-SEPSIS SYNDROME

Post-sepsis syndrome is a cumulative term used for long-term physical and psychological symptoms observed in roughly 50% of sepsis survivors.[61] Common symptoms include cognitive decline, fatigue, shortness of breath, weakness, new onset of anxiety or depression, post-traumatic stress disorder, and sleep disturbances. In some cases of post-sepsis syndrome, people may develop more severe health issues, including organ damage to the heart, lungs, and kidneys. Long-term effects of the post-sepsis syndrome consist of persistent immune, cognitive, neuropsychiatric, and cardiovascular dysfunctions, resulting in frequent rehospitalization, increased mortality, and decreased quality of life compared to survivors of other acute medical conditions. Understanding the pathophysiology of these issues is crucial to developing new therapeutic opportunities to improve the survival rate and quality of life of sepsis survivors. These novel strategies include modulating the immune system and addressing mitochondrial dysfunction.[62]

SUMMARY

Sepsis and septic shock are the most common causes of inpatient mortality. Sepsis is recently appreciated as life-threatening organ dysfunction caused by the dysregulated host response to infective etiology. Septic shock is defined as persistent hypotension and elevated lactate levels and is associated with increased mortality compared to sepsis alone. Multiple etiologies and risk factors are identified in the pathogenesis of sepsis. The SIRS and qSOFA scores are helpful in the early screening of sepsis suspects, but SIRS is associated with lower specificity, and the qSOFA score is left behind in sensitivity. Early therapy against sepsis includes broad-spectrum antimicrobial therapy directed against the most likely pathogen, along with fluid resuscitation guided by dynamic methods of fluid responsiveness and vasopressors. The first choice of vasopressor agent is norepinephrine. However, multiple vasopressor agents of different classes are required in severe hypotension to avoid the deleterious adverse effects of increasing one vasopressor alone. Adjunct therapies are under evaluation for their benefit in sepsis, including corticosteroids and vitamin supplementation.

REFERENCES

1. Taeb AM, Hooper MH, Marik PE. Sepsis: Current definition, pathophysiology, diagnosis, and management. Nutr Clin Pract. 2017;32(3):296-308.
2. Garg P, Krishak R, Shukla DK. NICU in a community level hospital. Indian J Pediatr. 2005;72(1):27-30.
3. Balamuth F, Weiss SL, Neuman MI, et al. Pediatric severe sepsis in U.S. children's hospitals. Pediatr Crit Care Med. 2014;15(9):798-805.
4. Rudd KE, Kissoon N, Limmathurotsakul D, et al. The global burden of sepsis: Barriers and potential solutions. Crit Care. 2018;22(1):232.
5. Singer M, Deutschman CS, Seymour CW, et al. The Third International Consensus definitions for sepsis and septic shock (sepsis-3). JAMA. 2016;315(8):801-10.
6. Brunetti E, Isaia G, Rinaldi G, et al. Comparison of diagnostic accuracies of qSOFA, NEWS, and MEWS to identify sepsis in older inpatients with suspected infection. J Am Med Dir Assoc. 2022;23(5):865-71.e2.
7. Usman OA, Usman AA, Ward MA. Comparison of SIRS, qSOFA, and NEWS for the early identification of sepsis in the emergency department. Am J Emerg Med. 2019;37(8):1490-7.
8. Subbe CP, Kruger M, Rutherford P, et al. Validation of a modified early warning score in medical admissions. QJM. 2001;94(10):521-6.
9. Herwanto V, Shetty A, Nalos M, et al. Accuracy of quick sequential organ failure assessment score to predict sepsis mortality in 121 studies including 1,716,017 individuals: A systematic review and meta-analysis. Crit Care Explor. 2019;1(9):e0043.
10. Knaus WA, Marks RD. New phenotypes for sepsis: The promise and problem of applying machine learning and artificial intelligence in clinical research. JAMA. 2019;321(20):1981-2.
11. Seymour CW, Kennedy JN, Wang S, et al. Derivation, validation, and potential treatment implications of novel clinical phenotypes for sepsis. JAMA. 2019;321(20):2003-17.
12. Moromizato T, Litonjua AA, Braun AB, et al.Association of low serum 25-hydroxyvitamin D levels and sepsis in the critically ill. Crit Care Med. 2014;42(1):97-107.
13. Fathi M, Markazi-Moghaddam N, Ramezankhani A. A systematic review on risk factors associated with sepsis in patients admitted to intensive care units. Aust Crit Care. 2019;32(2):155-64.
14. Elias AC, Matsuo T, Grion CM, et al. Incidence and risk factors for sepsis in surgical patients: A cohort study. J Crit Care. 2012;27(2):159-66.
15. Geppert A, Zorn G, Karth GD, et al. Soluble selectins and the systemic inflammatory response syndrome after successful cardiopulmonary resuscitation. Crit Care Med. 2000;28(7):2360-5.
16. Lin GL, McGinley JP, Drysdale SB, et al. Epidemiology and immune pathogenesis of viral sepsis. Front Immunol. 2018;9:2147.
17. Delaloye J, Calandra T. Invasive candidiasis as a cause of sepsis in the critically ill patient. Virulence. 2014;5(1):161-9.
18. Rosolem MM, Rabello LS, Lisboa T, et al. Critically ill patients with cancer and sepsis: Clinical course and prognostic factors. J Crit Care. 2012;27(3):301-7.
19. Torres V, Azevedo LC, Silva U, et al. Sepsis-associated outcomes in critically ill patients with malignancies. Ann Am Thorac Soc. 2015;12(8):1185-92.
20. Sriskandan S, Cohen J. Gram-positive SEPSIS: Mechanisms and differences from gram-negative sepsis. Infect Dis Clin North Am. 1999;13(2):397-412.
21. Schultz MJ, Dunser MW, Dondorp AM, et al. Current challenges in the management of sepsis in ICUs in resource-poor settings and suggestions for the future. Intensive Care Med. 2017;43(5):612-24.
22. Cheng AC, West TE, Limmathurotsakul D, et al. Strategies to reduce mortality from bacterial sepsis in adults in developing countries. PLoS Med. 2008;5(8):e175.
23. Dolin HH, Papadimos TJ, Chen X, et al. Characterization of pathogenic sepsis etiologies and patient profiles. A novel approach to triage and treatment. Microbiol Insights. 2019;12:1178636118825081.
24. Chousterman BG, Swirski FK, Weber GF. Cytokine storm and sepsis disease pathogenesis. Semin Immunopathol. 2017;39(5):517-28.
25. Vincent JL, Moreno R, Takala J, et al. The SOFA (Sepsis-related Organ Failure Assessment) score to describe organ dysfunction/failure. On behalf of the Working Group on Sepsis-Related Problems of the European Society of Intensive Care Medicine. Intensive Care Med. 1996;22(7):707-10.
26. Remick DG. Pathophysiology of sepsis. Am J Pathol. 2007;170(5):1435-44.

27. van der Poll T, Opal SM. Host-pathogen interactions in sepsis. Lancet Infect Dis. 2008;8(1):32-43.
28. Eckle I, Seitz R, Egbring R, et al. Protein C degradation in vitro by neutrophil elastase. Biol Chem Hoppe Seyler. 1991;372(11): 1007-13.
29. Heagy W, Hansen C, Nieman K, et al. Impaired ex vivo lipopolysaccharide-stimulated whole blood tumor necrosis factor production may identify "septic" intensive care unit patients. Shock. 2000;14(3):271-6; discussion 276-7.
30. Jones AE, Puskarich MA. Sepsis-induced tissue hypoperfusion. Crit Care Nurs Clin North Am. 2011;23(1):115-25.
31. Boissier F, Aissaoui N. Septic cardiomyopathy: Diagnosis and management. J Intensive Med. 2021;2(1):8-16.
32. Rivers E, Nguyen B, Havstad S, et al. Early goal-directed therapy in the treatment of severe sepsis and septic shock. N Engl J Med. 2001;345(19):1368-77.
33. ProCESS Investigators; Yealy DM, Kellum JA, Huang DT, et al. A randomized trial of protocol-based care for early septic shock. N Engl J Med. 2014;370(18):1683-93.
34. Evans L, Rhodes A, Alhazzani W, et al. Surviving sepsis campaign: International guidelines for management of sepsis and septic shock 2021. Intensive Care Med. 2021;47(11):1181-247.
35. Lee S, Song J, Park DW, et al. Diagnostic and prognostic value of presepsin and procalcitonin in non-infectious organ failure, sepsis, and septic shock: A prospective observational study according to the Sepsis-3 definitions. BMC Infect Dis. 2022; 22(1):8.
36. Gregoriano C, Heilmann E, Molitor A, et al. Role of procalcitonin use in the management of sepsis. J Thorac Dis. 2020;12 (Suppl 1):S5-s15.
37. Levy MM, Evans LE, Rhodes A. The surviving sepsis campaign bundle: 2018 update. Intensive Care Med. 2018;44(6):925-8.
38. Luyt CE, Bréchot N, Trouillet JL, et al. Antibiotic stewardship in the intensive care unit. Crit Care. 2014;18(5):480.
39. Varghese GM, Dayanand D, Gunasekaran K, et al. Intravenous doxycycline, azithromycin, or both for severe scrub typhus. N Engl J Med. 2023;388(9):792-803.
40. Kollef MH, Bassetti M, Francois B, et al. The intensive care medicine research agenda on multidrug-resistant bacteria, antibiotics, and stewardship. Intensive Care Med. 2017;43(9): 1187-97.
41. Trouillet JL, Vuagnat A, Combes A, et al. Pseudomonas aeruginosa ventilator-associated pneumonia: Comparison of episodes due to piperacillin-resistant versus piperacillin-susceptible organisms. Clin Infect Dis. 2002;34(8):1047-54.
42. Kumar A, Roberts D, Wood KE, et al. Duration of hypotension before initiation of effective antimicrobial therapy is the critical determinant of survival in human septic shock. Crit Care Med. 2006;34(6):1589-96.
43. Acheampong A, Vincent JL. A positive fluid balance is an independent prognostic factor in patients with sepsis. Crit Care. 2015;19(1):251.
44. Muller L, Toumi M, Bousquet PJ, et al. An increase in aortic blood flow after an infusion of 100 ml colloid over 1 minute can predict fluid responsiveness: The mini-fluid challenge study. Anesthesiology. 2011;115(3):541-7.
45. Muller L, Bobbia X, Toumi M, et al. Respiratory variations of inferior vena cava diameter to predict fluid responsiveness in spontaneously breathing patients with acute circulatory failure: Need for a cautious use. Crit Care. 2012;16(5):R188.
46. Marik PE, Cavallazzi R, Vasu T, et al. Dynamic changes in arterial waveform derived variables and fluid responsiveness in mechanically ventilated patients: A systematic review of the literature. Crit Care Med. 2009;37(9):2642-7.
47. Judson PI, Abhilash KPP, Pichamuthu K, et al. Evaluation of carotid flow time to assess fluid responsiveness in the emergency department. J Med Ultrasound. 2021;29(2):99-104.
48. Maheshwari K, Nathanson BH, Munson SH, et al. The relationship between ICU hypotension and in-hospital mortality and morbidity in septic patients. Intensive Care Med. 2018;44(6): 857-67.
49. Asfar P, Meziani F, Hamel JF, et al. High versus low blood-pressure target in patients with septic shock. N Engl J Med. 2014;370(17):1583-93.
50. De Backer D, Biston P, Devriendt J, et al. Comparison of dopamine and norepinephrine in the treatment of shock. N Engl J Med. 2010;362(9):779-89.
51. Myburgh JA, Higgins A, Jovanovska A, et al. A comparison of epinephrine and norepinephrine in critically ill patients. Intensive Care Med. 2008;34(12):2226-34.
52. Russell JA, Walley KR, Singer J, et al. Vasopressin versus norepinephrine infusion in patients with septic shock. N Engl J Med. 2008;358(9):877-87.
53. Khanna A, English SW, Wang XS, et al. Angiotensin II for the treatment of vasodilatory shock. N Eng J Med. 2017;377(5): 419-30.
54. Lal A, Trivedi V, Rizvi MS, et al. Oral midodrine administration during the first 24 hours of sepsis to reduce the need of vasoactive agents: Placebo-controlled feasibility clinical trial. Crit Care Explor. 2021;3(5):e0382.
55. Venkatesh B, Finfer S, Cohen J, et al. Adjunctive Glucocorticoid Therapy in Patients with Septic Shock. N Engl J Med. 2018; 378(9):797-808.
56. Annane D, Renault A, Brun-Buisson C, et al. Hydrocortisone plus fludrocortisone for adults with septic shock. N Engl J Med. 2018;378(9):809-18.
57. Marik PE, Khangoora V, Rivera R, et al. Hydrocortisone, vitamin C, and thiamine for the treatment of severe sepsis and septic shock: A retrospective before-after study. Chest. 2017;151(6): 1229-38.
58. Fowler AA 3rd, Truwit JD, Hite RD, et al. Effect of vitamin C infusion on organ failure and biomarkers of inflammation and vascular injury in patients with sepsis and severe acute respiratory failure: The CITRIS-ALI randomized clinical trial. JAMA. 2019;322(13):1261-70.
59. Sklar MC, Patel BK, Beitler JR, et al. Optimal ventilator strategies in acute respiratory distress syndrome. Semin Respir Crit Care Med. 2019;40(1):81-93.
60. Guérin C, Reignier J, Richard JC, et al. Prone positioning in severe acute respiratory distress syndrome. N Engl J Med. 2013;368(23):2159-68.
61. van der Slikke EC, An AY, Hancock REW, et al. Exploring the pathophysiology of post-sepsis syndrome to identify therapeutic opportunities. EBioMedicine. 2020;61:103044.
62. Mostel Z, Perl A, Marck M, et al. Post-sepsis syndrome–an evolving entity that afflicts survivors of sepsis. Mol Med. 2019;26(1):6.

Nonpulmonary Critical Care I

CHAPTER 166

Liziamma George, Ivan Wong

INTRODUCTION

Patients are admitted to critical care units with several disease processes other than respiratory failure. In addition, patients admitted with respiratory failure often develop further organ dysfunctions that require aggressive management. It is important for a pulmonary intensivist to diagnose and manage both pulmonary and nonpulmonary problems effectively. We will discuss some of the common nonpulmonary critical care diagnoses and their corresponding management.

GASTROINTESTINAL AND HEPATIC PROBLEMS IN CRITICAL CARE

Gastrointestinal Bleeding

Gastrointestinal (GI) bleeding may be a medical emergency necessitating admission to the critical care unit **(Boxes 1 and 2)**. It is common in male and elderly patients. Upper GI bleed is defined as bleeding above the level of the ligament of Treitz, while lower GI bleed is bleeding below the level of the ligament of Treitz. Upper GI bleed tends to occur more commonly than its lower GI counterpart and has a mortality that ranges from 6 to 12% as opposed to 5% in lower GI bleed.[1,2] Recurrent acute or chronic bleeding from the digestive tract without an obvious etiology after a normal esophagogastroduodenoscopy (EGD) and colonoscopy is known as an obscure GI bleed.[3]

BOX 1 Common causes of upper gastrointestinal bleeding.

- Peptic ulcer disease—MCC worldwide (duodenal ulcers, gastric ulcers, stomal ulcers)
- Erosive gastritis, esophagitis, and duodenitis (alcohol, aspirin, and NSAIDs)
- Esophageal and gastric varices (caused by portal hypertension)
- Mallory–Weiss syndrome
- Stress ulcers
- AVM
- Malignancy
- Aortoenteric fistula
- Dieulafoy lesion

(AVM: arteriovenous malformation; MCC: most common cause; NSAIDs: nonsteroidal anti-inflammatory drugs)

Upper Gastrointestinal Bleeding

Clinical Features

Clinical manifestations depend on the rate and amount of bleeding. These patients should be promptly assessed for hemodynamic status. A pulse ≥100 beats/min, systolic blood pressure <100 mm Hg, postural changes, an increase in the pulse of ≥20 beats/min, or a drop in systolic blood pressure of ≥20 mm Hg on standing are significant for hypovolemic shock. Airway protection is needed for patients with altered mental status or massive hematemesis. History of alcohol abuse, nonsteroidal anti-inflammatory drug (NSAID) usage, liver disease, family history of GI or other malignancies, recent retching, prior surgery, and other medication usage may aid in identifying the etiology of GI bleeding. Elderly patients, who potentially have an age-related compromised cardiac reserve, may present with symptoms of chest pain and shortness of breath rather than GI bleed, suggestive of myocardial ischemia. Other symptoms such as fatigue and dyspnea tend to occur with chronic blood loss. Signs specific

BOX 2 Common causes of lower gastrointestinal bleeding.

- Diverticulosis
- Hemorrhoids
- AVM/Angiodysplasia/Aortoenteric fistula
- Neoplasia
- Polyps
- Benign anorectal disease (fissures and ulcers)
- Upper GI source
- Small bowel source

(AVM: arteriovenous malformation; GI: gastrointestinal)

for upper GI bleed include hematemesis, bloody gastric lavage, melena, and hematochezia. Bright red bleeding through the rectum is usually indicative of lower GI bleed; however, a brisk upper GI bleed can cause fresh blood to pass through the rectum. Because of the possible contributing factors and associated complications, patients should also be examined for signs of liver and cardiac disease.

Diagnosis

Nasogastric lavage is a method of sampling contents from the stomach. Once a nasogastric tube is properly inserted, a minimum of 100–200 mL of room temperature water or normal saline is inserted through the tube and into the stomach and then aspirated. While a coffee-ground aspirate or fresh blood is diagnostic of upper GI bleed, its absence will not rule out upper GI bleed in up to 20% of patients. The presence of blood in the stomach is an indication of an urgent EGD for either diagnostic and/or therapeutic purposes. Despite its advantages as a diagnostic tool, the routine use of nasogastric lavage in suspected GI bleed failed to demonstrate a benefit with respect to clinical outcomes such as mortality, hospital length of stay, or need for blood transfusions.[4] The use of cold or iced saline lavages has also not been shown to improve outcomes.

Essential laboratory tests should be performed to assess the severity of GI bleeding as well as to evaluate for any contributing etiological factors. Blood samples should also be sent for typing and crossmatching. It is important to note that the hematocrit may be normal in recent massive GI bleed and can therefore result in an underestimation of the severity.

Management

Irrespective of the bleeding site, management of acute GI bleeding should include hemodynamic stabilization, localization of the bleeding site, and specific therapeutic intervention.[5] Supplemental oxygen should be provided to ensure adequate tissue oxygenation and all patients should also be placed on cardiac monitors.

Intravascular volume repletion with crystalloid infusion through two large bores (16- or 18-gauge) intravenous (IV) lines should begin immediately. Patients with unstable vital signs even after initial stabilization should be transfused with packed red cells as per guidelines for hemodynamic assessment and transfusion requirement **(Table 1)**.[6]

In cases with exsanguinating blood loss, attempts at localization, and control of bleeding through endoscopic or surgical procedures should be done simultaneously. The threshold for transfusion must be individualized. Most hemodynamically stable patients do not require a transfusion for a hemoglobin (Hb) level > 7 g/dL, while hypotensive and actively bleeding patients will require more aggressive transfusions.[7]

The Blatchford and Rockall scoring systems are used for risk stratification of upper GI bleeding **(Tables 2 and 3)**.[8,9] Higher scores are indicative of rebleeding and death, while lower scores identify patients who do not need urgent

TABLE 1: Signs, symptoms, and fluid replacement strategies in patients with hypovolemic (hemorrhagic) shock.

Blood loss (mL)	<750	750–1,500	1,500–2,000	>2,000
Blood loss (% BV)	<15%	15–30%	30–40%	<40%
Pulse rate	<100	>100	>120	>140
Blood pressure	Normal	Normal	Decreased	Decreased
Pulse pressure (mm Hg)	Normal or increased	Decreased	Decreased	Decreased
Respiratory rate (breaths/min)	14–20	20–30	30–40	>35
Urine output (mL/h)	>30	20–30	5–15	Insignificant
Mental status	Slightly anxious	Mildly anxious	Anxious and confused	Confused and lethargic
Fluid replacement	Crystalloid	Crystalloid	Crystalloid and blood	Crystalloid and blood

(BV: blood volume)

TABLE 2: Blatchford bleeding score which predicts the need for treatment in patients with upper gastrointestinal bleeding. A higher score (≥6) is associated with an increased risk of rebleeding, while a lower score (<6) is associated with a decreased rebleeding risk.

At presentation	Points
Systolic blood pressure (mm Hg)	
100–109	1
90–99	2
<90	3
Blood urea nitrogen	
6.5–7.9 mmol/L	2
8.0–9.9 mmol/L	3
10–24.9 mmol/L	4
≥25 mmol/L	6
Hemoglobin for men	
12.0–12.9 g/dL	1
10.0–11.9 g/dL	3
<10.0 g/dL	6
Hemoglobin for women	
10.0–11.9 g/dL	1
<10.0 g/dL	6
Other variables at presentation	
Pulse ≥ 100	1
Melena	1
Syncope	2
Hepatic disease	2
Cardiac failure	2

TABLE 3: Rockall scoring system which is used to identify patients at risk for developing unfavorable outcomes following acute upper gastrointestinal bleeding. A complete Rockall score of ≤2, i.e., following endoscopy is associated with a good prognosis, i.e., low risk for rebleeding and death.

Variable	Points		
Age (years)			
<60	0	Clinical Rockall score (0–7)	Complete Rockall score (0–11)
60–79	1		
>80	2		
Hemodynamic status			
Shock absent: SBP > 100 mm Hg and HR <100 beats/min	0		
Shock absent: SBP > 100 mm Hg and HR > 100 beats/min	1		
Shock present: SBP < 100 mm Hg and HR > 100 beats/min	2		
Coexisting illness			
Ischemic heart disease, congestive heart failure, other major illness	2		
Renal failure, hepatic failure, metastatic cancer	3		
Endoscopic diagnosis			
No lesion observed, Mallory–Weiss tear	0		
Peptic ulcer, erosive disease, esophagitis	1		
Cancer of upper GI tract	2		
Endoscopic stigmata of recent hemorrhage			
Clean-based ulcer, flat pigmented spot	0		
Blood in upper GI tract, active bleeding, visible vessel, clot	2		
(GI: gastrointestinal; HR: heart rate; SBP: systolic blood pressure)			

intervention.[10] Localization of the bleeding site is the cornerstone in the management of upper GI bleed. Endoscopy should be performed within 24 hours of patient presentation. The administration of IV erythromycin as a single dose is recommended before endoscopy in patients with clinically severe or ongoing active upper GI bleeding. Pre endoscopy erythromycin infusion has been shown to improve gastric mucosa visualization and reduce length of stay; in addition, it is generally safe and well tolerated.[11] The risk of rebleeding based on endoscopic findings can be assessed using Forrest classification **(Table 4)**.[12] Patients with grades 2C and 3 are considered low risk for rebleeding, while patients with high-risk lesions should undergo endoscopic hemostasis to prevent recurrent bleeding. A second-look endoscopy is not routinely recommended. In patients with coagulation abnormalities, endoscopy should not be delayed and the risk/benefit ratio should be assessed carefully.

Medical therapy should be used as an adjunct to endoscopic therapy. Pre-endoscopic continuous infusion of proton pump inhibitors (PPIs) decreases the need for endoscopic intervention.[13] Administration of a PPI has also been shown to decrease rebleeding, surgical intervention, and mortality.[14] Continuous PPI infusion is given for 72 hours for acute GI bleed. In addition, it is reported that in patients with recurrent bleeding, repeat endoscopy is preferred to surgical intervention.

TABLE 4: Endoscopic appearance and associated rebleeding risk in patients with upper gastrointestinal bleeding.

Class	Appearance	Risk of rebleeding
1A	Spurting blood	Very high → Early surgical intervention
1B	Oozing blood	Very high
2A	Nonbleeding visible vessel	High
2B	Adhering clot	High
2C	Flat lesions and pigmented spot	Low
3	Clean-based ulcer	Low

For patients taking antithrombotic agents presenting with an acute upper GI bleed, aspirin if taken as monotherapy or as dual antiplatelet therapy for secondary cardiovascular prophylaxis, aspirin should not be interrupted, and the second antiplatelet agent should be held, preferably to be restarted within 5 days. In patients who are taking vitamin K antagonists with clinical instability, low-dose vitamin K supplemented with IV prothrombin complex concentrate (PCC) or fresh frozen plasma (FFP) (if PCC is unavailable) should be administered. In patients taking direct oral anticoagulants (DOACs), the anticoagulant should be held and the use of reversal agents or IV PCC should be considered.[11] Idarucizumab is used for reversal of the direct thrombin inhibitor dabigatran and andexanet alfa is for the reversal of direct factor Xa inhibitors such as apixaban and rivaroxaban **(Table 5)**. However, the administration of these reversal agents should not delay endoscopy.[15]

Angiography with embolization is recommended for patients in whom acute bleeding is not controlled by endoscopic treatment. Successful angiographic identification of the bleeding site requires a bleeding rate of 0.5–1 mL/min.[16] The complications of this procedure include bowel ischemia, infarction, and contrast-induced renal failure.

The surgical team should be involved early in the management of these patients to augment prompt response when all have failed in ensuring hemostasis. Early endoscopy (within 24 hours) and an algorithm approach constitute the cornerstone for management **(Flowchart 1)**.[16]

Lower Gastrointestinal Bleeding

Clinical Features

Lower GI bleeding is defined as bleeding distal to the ligament of Treitz which happens due to multiple etiologies **(Box 2)**. These patients tend to present with hematochezia or maroon-colored stools. Rarely, patients can also present with melena with bleeding from the cecum or right colon. About 15% of patients with presumed lower GI bleed are ultimately found to have an upper GI bleed.[17]

Diagnosis

The initial stabilization of lower GI bleed is not different from that of upper GI bleed. However, in patients with hematochezia associated with hemodynamic instability, an upper endoscopy should be performed to rule out a brisk upper GI bleed. A nasogastric lavage in this case would also be useful to assess for possible upper GI source of bleeding.[17] Localization of bleeding is done by colonoscopy, which identifies the bleeding in 60–80% of cases. Once the patient is hemodynamically stable, colonoscopy should be performed within 24 hours of the patient presentation after adequate colon cleansing. A nasogastric tube can be used to facilitate colon preparation in patients who are intolerant to oral intake and at low risk of aspiration.[17]

Other imaging modalities utilized for localization of the bleeding include nuclear scanning using technetium-99 m-labeled red blood cell (Tc99m RBC) scan, computed tomography (CT) angiography, and arteriography. Radionuclide scanning is more sensitive but less specific as it may not localize the lesion and no therapeutic intervention can done and requires at least 0.1–0.5 mL of bleeding per minute. Barium studies have no role in the evaluation of lower GI bleed. A multidetector CT scan was used to localize massive GI bleeding in some reports.[18] Arteriography of both superior and inferior mesenteric arteries can be used to identify the source of bleeding. Some studies recommend radionuclide scanning before angiography to decrease the incidence of negative tests.

Management

An algorithm approach should be followed for the management of lower GI bleed **(Flowchart 2)**.[19] In patients on antithrombotic agents with acute lower GI bleed, a multidisciplinary approach with the cardiology, hematology, neurology, and vascular and gastroenterology physicians should be held in deciding the discontinuation, use of reversal

TABLE 5: Reversal of antithrombotics due to life-threatening bleeding.

Medication	Mechanism of action	Treatment
Warfarin	Vitamin K antagonist	Vitamin K 10 mg intravenous piggyback and • *For INR > 2*: 4-factor prothrombin complex concentrate • If PCC is unavailable, give fresh frozen plasma 10–15 mL/kg
Dabigatran	Direct thrombin inhibitor	• Idarucizumab 2.5 g × 2 doses • Activated charcoal (25 g) if ingestion was within 2 hours
Rivaroxaban and apixaban	Factor Xa inhibitor	*Andexanet alfa low dose*: 400 mg IV bolus at 30 mg/min, followed by 4 mg/min up to 120 minutes if rivaroxaban dose ≤ 10 mg or apixaban dose ≤ 5 mg, or *High dose*: 800 mg IV at 30 mg/min, followed by 8 mg/min up to 120 minutes if rivaroxaban dose > 10 mg or dose unknown or apixaban dose > 5 mg or dose unknown
Unfractionated heparin	Potentiates the action of antithrombin III	Protamine sulfate 1 mg per 100 units of heparin received in the previous 2.5 hours
Low-molecular-weight heparin	Inhibits factor Xa and thrombin	Protamine sulfate although does not completely neutralize antifactor Xa activity, it is therefore controversial

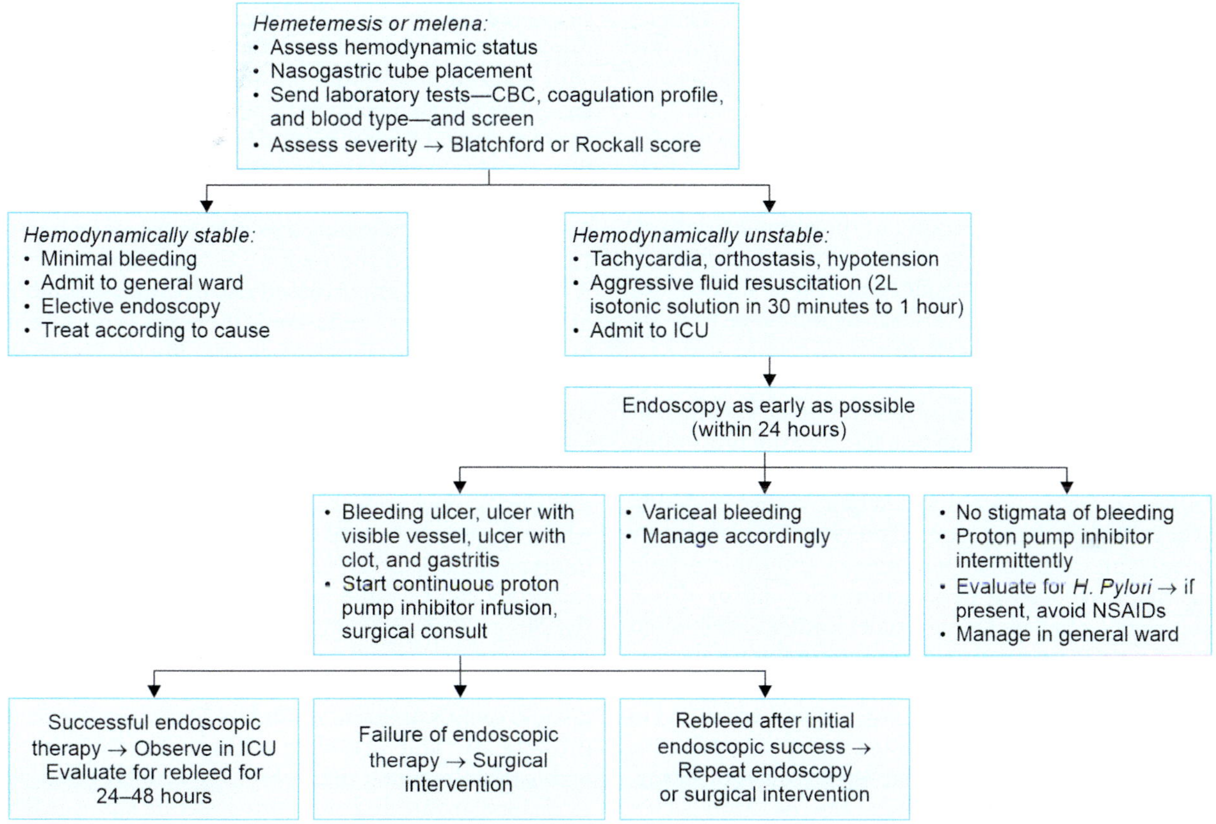

FLOWCHART 1: Management of upper gastrointestinal bleeding, which is focused around hemodynamic stabilization and localization of the bleeding site.

(CBC: complete blood count; ICU: intensive care unit; *H. pylori*: *Helicobacter pylori*; NSAID: nonsteroidal anti-inflammatory drug)

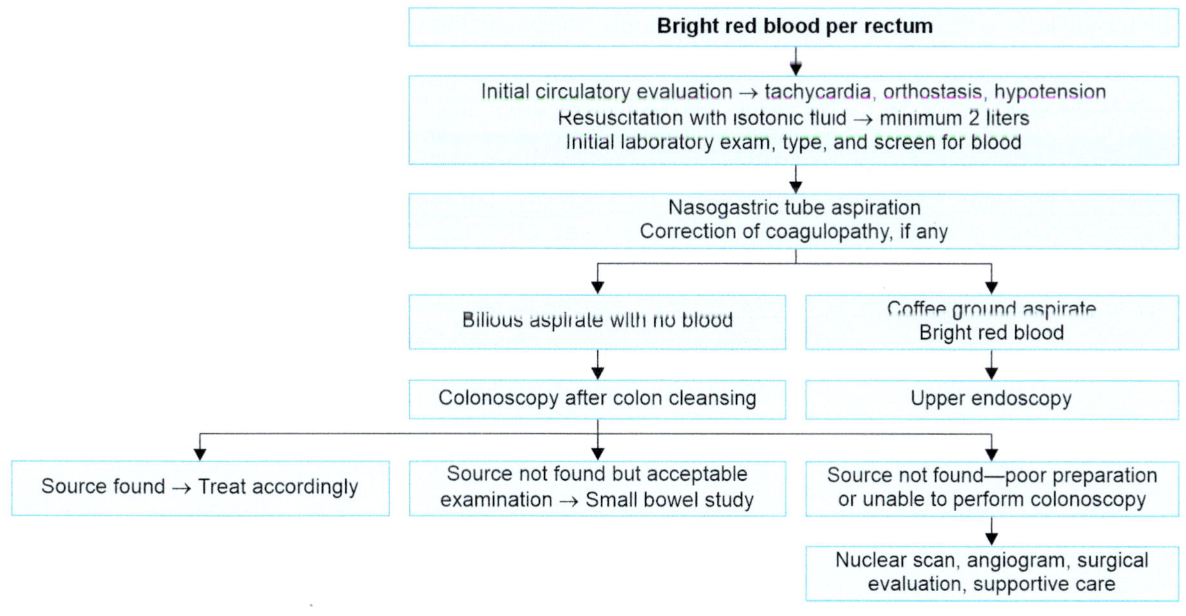

FLOWCHART 2: An algorithmic approach to the management of lower gastrointestinal bleeding.

agents, and resumption of antithrombotic agents.[17] Platelet and FFP transfusions should be considered for patients receiving massive RBC transfusions (defined as three or more units of packed RBC) given within 1 hour.[17]

Acute Variceal Hemorrhage

Acute variceal hemorrhage is one of the complications of portal hypertension requiring critical care unit admission. Patients with Child–Pugh classification of B or C **(Table 6)** have a higher incidence of variceal hemorrhage and are associated with a mortality of 15–20%.

The specific treatment strategies include the use of medications, endoscopy, surgical interventions, transjugular intrahepatic shunt, balloon tamponade, and the prevention of recurrent bleeding. After initial stabilization of the patient, medications directed toward splanchnic vasoconstriction should be utilized to decrease portal pressure. The commonly used agents are vasopressin, terlipressin, and somatostatin analogs such as octreotide. Vasopressin causes direct vasoconstriction of splanchnic arterioles leading to decreased portal pressure. The major side effects include systemic vasoconstriction, particularly to the coronary vessels. The use of nitrates in addition to vasopressin is recommended to decrease these side effects with added therapeutic benefits. Notably, vasopressin has minimal effects on rebleeding. Terlipressin, a vasopressin analog, can be used as an alternative to vasopressin, which has fewer side effects than vasopressin. Somatostatin, an indirect vasoconstrictor of splanchnic circulation, rapidly decreases the portal pressure with minimal side effects. It is superior to vasopressin in patients with variceal hemorrhage. The infusion is continued for 2–5 days and has no significant effect on mortality. Antibiotic prophylaxis with IV ceftriaxone for a maximum of 7 days should be given as early as variceal bleeding is suspected to prevent spontaneous bacterial peritonitis (SBP). Administration of antibiotic prophylaxis has been associated with reduced rebleeding rate and lower mortality.[20,21] PPIs should be initiated because peptic ulcers are a very common cause of upper GI bleeding and are discontinued once portal hypertensive bleeding is confirmed.

Endoscopic variceal ligation is the definitive treatment for acute variceal bleeding and should be performed within 12 hours.[20] Delayed endoscopy, >15 hours after presentation, is correlated with an increased risk of death. A combination of both medical and endoscopic therapies is most beneficial to control bleeding. Endoscopic sclerotherapy is considered only when endoscopic ligation is unavailable. Endoscopic therapies are associated with complications such as ulceration, mediastinitis, and esophageal perforation as well as sepsis. Balloon tamponade is considered when medical and endoscopic approaches fail to achieve hemostasis or when there is a lack of expertise to perform endoscopic interventions. This is a temporary measure until definitive treatment can be undertaken. The common tubes used are the Sengstaken–Blakemore tube or the Minnesota tube. Rebleeding is a significant problem that is associated with high risk of death. Predictive risk factors include Child class C, hepatic venous pressure gradient > 20 mm Hg, portal venous thrombosis, and presence of hemodynamic instability with a systolic blood pressure < 100 mm Hg at admission. Transjugular intrahepatic portosystemic shunt (TIPS) can be used to reduce the portal venous pressure by creating a shunt between the hepatic and portal veins. Rescue TIPS is indicated in patients with persistent bleeding or early rebleeding despite optimal treatment with vasoconstrictors and endoscopic variceal ligation.

In decompensated liver cirrhosis, prolongation of prothrombin time does not reflect bleeding tendency; therefore, correction of the international normalized ratio (INR) with

TABLE 6: Modified Child–Pugh classification of the severity of liver disease with the associated risk of mortality.

Parameters	Points assigned		
	1	2	3
Ascites	Absent	Slight	Moderate
Bilirubin	<2 mg/dL (<34.2 µmol/L)	2–3 mg/dL (34.2 to –51.3 µmol/L)	>3 mg/dL (>51.3 µmol/L)
Albumin	>3.5 g/dL (35 g/L)	2.8–3.5 g/dL (28–35 g/L)	<2.8 g/dL (<28 g/L)
Prothrombin time (seconds over normal)	<4	4–6	>6
INR	1.7	1.7–2.3	>2.3
Encephalopathy	None	Grade 1–2 (lethargy, apathy)	Grade 3–4 (somnolence and coma)
Grades	**A (well compensated)**	**B (functional compromise)**	**C (decompensated)**
Total points	5–6	7–9	10–15
Mortality % (1–2 years)	0–15	20–40	55–65

(INR: international normalized ratio)

FFP should not be performed. Administration of recombinant factor VIIa or desmopressin has not been shown to have any benefit in controlling variceal bleeding in clinical trials.[22,23]

Other disorders associated with liver disease necessitating intensive care unit (ICU) admission include lung disorders associated with liver failure. The major conditions are hepatopulmonary syndrome (HPS), hepatic hydrothorax, and portopulmonary hypertension.

The HPS is a pulmonary vascular disorder characterized by pulmonary vascular dilatation and intrapulmonary arteriovenous shunting, leading to ventilation-perfusion mismatch in the setting of liver disease. It has no association with the severity of liver disease.[24,25] Patients usually present with shortness of breath associated with platypnea and orthodeoxia (dyspnea and desaturation when the position changed to sitting from recumbent position). The chest X-ray is usually normal or may show increased vascular markings; arterial blood gas shows hypoxemia partial pressure of oxygen (PaO_2) < 80 mm Hg with increased alveolar-arterial gradient (>15 mm Hg). Contrast echocardiography (microbubbles in left atrium three to six cardiac cycles) or perfusion lung scanning using technetium labeled macroaggregates of albumin (presence of isotope in brain and kidney) can be performed to confirm the presence of intrapulmonary vasodilatation. Perfusion lung scanning however would not be able to distinguish between intrapulmonary and intracardiac shunts.[24] Liver transplantation is the treatment of choice.[26]

Portopulmonary hypertension occurs in patients with portal hypertension and is managed similarly to other diseases that fall under class 1 pulmonary arterial hypertension.

Hepatic hydrothorax presents as massive pleural effusion mostly involving the right hemithorax.[27] The first step in management is therapy with low sodium diet (70–90 mEq/day) and diuretics **(Flowchart 3)**. If there is no response to diuretics, therapeutic thoracentesis of approximately 2 liters can be attempted followed by diuretics at lower doses if possible. If patients do not respond to diuretics or develop complications, they should be considered for a TIPS placement. This measure may help as a bridge to liver transplantation. TIPS placement is best considered in patients younger than 60 years of age, without hepatic encephalopathy and/or those with Child class A or B cirrhosis. For patients who cannot undergo TIPS placement, pleurodesis or diaphragmatic repair by thoracoscopy should be considered. Chest tube placement should be avoided as it is associated with severe complications.[28]

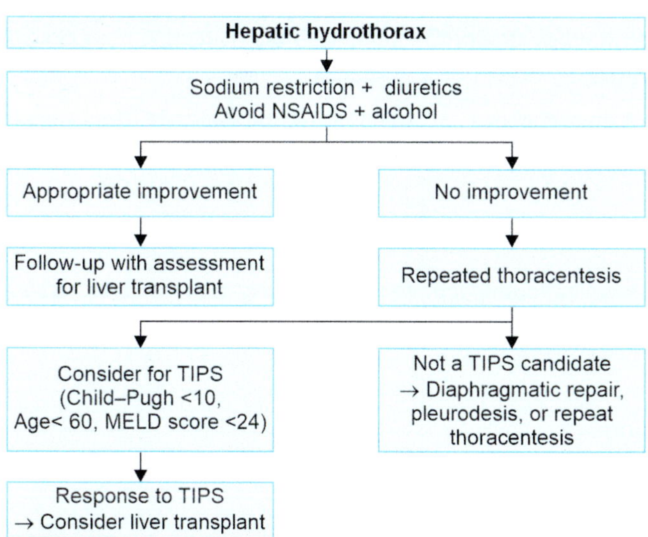

FLOWCHART 3: An algorithm outlining the management of patients presenting with hepatic hydrothorax.

(MELD: model for end-stage liver disease; NSAID: nonsteroidal anti-inflammatory drug; TIPS: transesophageal portosystemic shunt)

Acute Liver Failure

Acute liver failure is an uncommon but severe disease that is defined as acute liver injury in a patient without pre-existing liver disease, presenting with acute hepatic encephalopathy and coagulopathy (INR > 1.5) within 28 weeks of symptom onset.[29] Patients should be managed in a critical care unit at the onset of encephalopathy.[30]

While acetaminophen toxicity is the major cause of liver failure in the western world, infections are the predominant etiology in developing countries. The most common causes of hepatic failure in India include hepatitis E virus (44%), hepatitis B virus (15%), hepatitis A virus (2%), and unknown (31%).[31] The treatment of liver failure depends on the specific etiology **(Table 7)**. N-acetylcysteine (NAC) should also be administered to patients presenting with acute liver failure regardless of the underlying etiology. In nonacetaminophen-related acute liver failure, NAC has been shown to significantly improve overall survival, post-transplant survival, and transplant free survival.[32]

Management of Complications

Hepatic encephalopathy is a reversible neurological dysfunction, occurring in patients with liver failure. Neurotoxins such as ammonia, oxidative stress, production of false neurotransmitters, and alteration of the blood-brain barrier are implicated in its development. In addition to correction of precipitating factors, ammonia production in the gut is reduced with the use of lactulose and nonabsorbable antibiotics such as neomycin and rifaximin.[33] Infections contribute significantly to the mortality of these patients and should be treated aggressively. For patients developing hypotension intravascular volume repletion if they are hypovolemic, vasopressors and inotropic support for vasodilatation and low cardiac state should be instituted.

Psychomotor agitation seen in patients with hepatic encephalopathy may be worsened by benzodiazepines and propofol through gamma-aminobutyric acid pathways. Flumazenil, a benzodiazepine antagonist, is reported to have short-term benefits in patients with hepatic encephalopathy. For analgesia, fentanyl is used in these patients.[34] The

TABLE 7: Etiology, treatment, and transplant criteria for acute liver failure.

Etiology	Treatment	Criteria for transplant
Acetaminophen	NAC Oral: 140 mg load, then 70 mg/kg every 4 hours NAC IV: 150 mg/kg load, then 12.5 mg/kg hourly × 4 hours, then 6.25 mg/kg hourly	Arterial pH 7.3 or all of the following: • PT > 100 seconds (INR > 6.5) • Creatinine > 3.4 mg/dL • Grade III or IV encephalopathy MELD > 33, APACHE > 15
Amanita (mushroom)	Penicillin G: 1 g/kg daily IV and NAC as above	
HSV	Acyclovir 30 mg/kg daily IV	PT > 100 seconds (INR > 6.5) or any three of the following: 1. NANB/drug/halothane etiology 2. Jaundice to encephalopathy > 7 days
AIH	Methylprednisolone 60 mg/day IV	3. Age < 10 or >40 years 4. PT > 50 seconds (INR > 3.5)
HBV	Lamivudine 100–150 mg/daily orally	5. Bilirubin > 17.4 mg/dL
AFLP/HELLP	Delivery of fetus	6. Hepatocyte necrosis > 70%

(AFLP: acute fatty liver of pregnancy; AIH: autoimmune hepatitis; APACHE: acute physiology and chronic health evaluation; Cr: creatinine; HBV: hepatitis B virus, HELLP: hemolysis, elevated liver enzymes, low platelets; HSV: herpes simplex virus; INR: international normalized ratio; IV: intravenous; MELD: model for end-stage liver disease; NAC: N-acetylcysteine; NANB: non-A, non-B hepatitis; PT: prothrombin time)

occurrence of upper GI bleeding is prevented using either H2 blockers or PPIs. Parenteral vitamin K is recommended for all patients with acute liver failure; however, routine FFP administration is not recommended, and cryoprecipitate is given when fibrinogen levels are <100 mg/dL. Recombinant factor VIIa is recommended if there is volume overload and FFP fails to correct coagulopathy or before invasive procedures with a high risk of bleeding.[35] Further studies are needed to define the exact role of this agent. Nevertheless, factor VIIa should not be given to patients with acute myocardial infarction, stroke, or other thromboembolic disorders. Nutritional supplementation through the enteral route is preferred to parenteral nutrition in these patients.[36] Also, patients with hypoglycemia should receive IV dextrose infusion.

Nonconvulsive seizures can also occur in these patients; however, routine seizure prophylaxis is not recommended. Electroencephalography monitoring is suggested for patients with grade III or IV encephalopathy, sudden deterioration of mental status, or myoclonus.

Acute liver failure patients who develop hypotension should be treated aggressively, initially with fluids to correct volume status and subsequently with vasopressors if fluid administration alone does not correct the hypotension.

Cerebral edema and raised intracranial pressure (ICP) due to hyperammonemia increase the morbidity and mortality for these patients. CT of brain is recommended for patients with advanced hepatic encephalopathy. The placement of ICP monitoring devices for these patients is controversial at this time but should be considered for liver transplant candidates. The management of a patient with intracranial hypertension includes keeping the head of bed at 30° in a neutral position and maintenance of euthermia; however, prophylactic hyperventilation is not recommended. Conversely, acute hyperventilation can be given to patients with brain herniation. Specific therapies such as mannitol are utilized when ICP is >25 mm Hg for >10 minutes. The dose ranges from 0.25 to 1.0 g/kg over 30 minutes. The dose can be repeated if serum osmolality is <320 mOsm/L or ICP > 25 mm Hg. Other treatment modalities include hypertonic saline, induction of moderate hypothermia, barbiturate coma, and indomethacin infusion. Patients with acute liver failure are candidates for orthotopic liver transplantation **(Table 7)**.[37]

Renal failure occurs in 40–80% of patients with acute liver failure and is associated with poor prognosis. Renal replacement therapy (RRT) has clinically been shown to significantly clear serum ammonia levels and is directly correlated to the ultrafiltration rate.[38] Therefore, patients with persistent hyperammonemia, hyponatremia, metabolic acidosis, or progressive hepatic encephalopathy should be initiated on RRT early. Continuous RRT is preferred to intermittent dialysis to avoid the metabolic and hemodynamic fluctuations that may increase ICP during intermittent dialysis.[39]

Extracorporeal albumin liver dialysis (ECAD) has been used as a rescue therapy or a bridge to transplantation. Albumin dialysis facilitates the removal of albumin-bound toxins, along with proinflammatory cytokines.[40] High-volume plasma exchange for 3 days compared to standard medical treatment demonstrated improvement in overall survival.[41] Standard-volume plasma exchange in patients with ALF has been shown to be safe and effective and improves transplant-free survival.[42]

Acute-on-chronic Liver Failure

Acute-on-chronic liver failure is a syndrome associated with a high risk of short-term death within 28 days. This term applies to patients with acutely decompensated cirrhosis who present with an intense inflammatory state, due to a precipitating event and is associated with at least a single or multiorgan failure. Organ failures can be defined by shock, grade 3 or 4 hepatic encephalopathy, or the need for dialysis or mechanical ventilation.[43]

Clinical Features

Patients with acute-on-chronic liver failure typically present simultaneously with or very early after acute decompensation. Among patients with alcoholic cirrhosis, 60% of patients have a known precipitating condition, such as alcoholic hepatitis or infection. A hepatitis B infection flare is a common precipitating factor for acute-on-chronic liver failure in Asia and is associated with high rates of complications due to bacterial or fungal infections, hepatorenal syndrome, and GI bleeding.

Management

The mainstay treatment of this syndrome is to identify and treat the precipitating event and provide supportive care. Trials with extracorporeal liver support did not improve survival in patients with acute-on-chronic liver failure compared to standard medical therapy.

Liver transplantation has demonstrated 80% 1-year posttransplant survival compared to 20% in those who did not receive liver transplantation.[43]

Spontaneous Bacterial Peritonitis

Spontaneous bacterial peritonitis is an infection of ascitic fluid in the absence of an intra-abdominal source of infection.[44,45] It is a common and life-threatening complication of cirrhosis. SBP occurrence is rare in noncirrhotic patients as opposed to cirrhotic ones. Bacterial translocation into ascitic fluid is commonly believed to be a causative factor for the development of SBP; however, current research shows that SBP is the result of the interplay of several factors such as prolonged bacteremia resulting from defective local and humoral immunity, intrahepatic shunting of blood, defective bactericidal action of ascitic fluid, and transabdominal introduction of infection. The microorganisms responsible for SBP are isolated in 60–70% of cases and colonic bacteria are cultured in 65% of cases, with *Escherichia coli* and *Klebsiella* species being the common organisms isolated.

Clinical Features

Spontaneous bacterial peritonitis should be suspected in all cirrhotic patients with ascites, as the clinical manifestations can be very subtle as well as nonspecific, with a broad range of clinical expression. Ascitic fluid analysis should be performed in all patients with ascites who are admitted to the hospital, especially in those presenting with abdominal pain, fever, and encephalopathy.

Diagnosis and Management

Spontaneous bacterial peritonitis is identified when an ascitic fluid analysis demonstrates a polymorphonuclear (PMN) cell count > 250 cells/mm^3. A positive culture of ascitic fluid is noted in only 30% of cases and is usually not required for diagnosis. First-line antibiotics, with third-generation cephalosporins, should be started immediately after a positive ascitic fluid tap.[46] Given the growing number of multidrug-resistant organisms, cephalosporins may become less effective. Therefore, initial antibiotic therapy with carbapenems should be initiated in those with nosocomial infection or recent hospitalization and critically ill patients admitted to the ICU. A diagnostic paracentesis should also be repeated 48 hours after initiation of antibiotics to assess response to therapy. A negative response is defined by a decrease in PMN < 25% from baseline and should lead to broadening the antibiotic coverage.[47]

Renal dysfunction can also occur in patients with SBP because of large-volume paracentesis. IV albumin administration has been shown to reduce the risk of renal impairment taking place.[48] However, albumin has been proposed to be used in patients with serum creatinine >1 mg/dl, blood urea nitrogen >30 mg/dL, and total bilirubin >4 mg/dL.[49] Following a single episode of SBP, patients should receive long-term prophylaxis with either norfloxacin, ciprofloxacin, or trimethoprim-sulfamethoxazole.

Severe Acute Pancreatitis

Acute pancreatitis is an inflammatory condition of the pancreas resulting in abdominal pain and elevation of the serum levels of the pancreatic enzymes. It is a self-limited disease in most cases. About 20% of patients develop acute necrotizing pancreatitis, which increases the risk of multiorgan failure and death. The common etiologies include gallstones, alcohol consumption, hypertriglyceridemia (HTG), smoking, hypercalcemia, drugs, trauma, pancreatic divisum, and infections.

Clinical Features

Pancreatic enzymes are activated within the acini, causing damage to the pancreatic tissues and vasculature. In necrotizing pancreatitis, the inflammation extends into the adjacent tissues. Patients present to the ICU with fever, tachycardia, shock, and multiorgan dysfunction.

Diagnosis

A CT scan of the abdomen and magnetic resonance pancreaticoduodenography [magnetic resonance cholangiopancreatography (MRCP)] are the best radiological tests for the diagnosis and staging of acute pancreatitis, however, MRCP gives a better image of the pancreatic and biliary duct system.[50] A number of scoring systems have been developed to assess the severity of pancreatitis such as Ranson's criteria

TABLE 8: Ranson's criteria for predicting the severity of acute pancreatitis. Each parameter is assigned a score of 1 if present. A higher score is associated with higher mortality (score: <3 → <3% mortality; 3–6 → 15% mortality; >6 → 40% mortality).

0 hour	
Age	>55
White blood cell count	>16,000/mm^3
Blood glucose	>200 mg/dL (11.1 mmol/L)
LDH	>350 U/L
AST	>250 U/L
48 hours	
Hematocrit	Fall by ≥10%
Blood urea nitrogen	Increase by ≥5 mg/dL (1.8 mmol/L) despite fluids
Serum calcium	<8 mg/dL (2 mmol/L)
PO_2	<60 mm Hg
Base deficit	>4 mEq/L
Fluid sequestation	>6,000 mL

(AST: aspartate aminotransferase; LDH: lactate dehydrogenase; PO_2: partial pressure of oxygen)

TABLE 9: Bedside index for severity in acute pancreatitis (BISAP) composite score ≥ 3 is associated with 5–20% mortality.

*B*UN	BUN > 25 mg/dL (1 point)
*I*mpaired mental status	Impaired mental status, GCS < 15 (1 point)
*S*IRS	Evidence of ≥2 SIRS criteria (1 point)
*A*ge	Age > 60 years (1 point)
*P*leural effusion	Evidence of a pleural effusion on imaging (1 point)

(BUN: blood urea nitrogen; GCS: Glasgow Coma Scale; SIRS: systemic inflammatory response syndrome)

(Table 8), APACHE II scores (≥8 is considered significant), bedside index for severity in acute pancreatitis (BISAP) scores (≥ 3), and CT scan grading are accurate means to risk stratify patients with acute pancreatitis. The benefit of utilizing the BISAP score is that its components are clinically relevant and easy to obtain **(Table 9)**.[51]

Management (Flowchart 4)

A contrast-enhanced abdominal CT scan should be performed for patients with acute pancreatitis who require admission to the ICU. Fluid resuscitation is the hallmark in the treatment of acute pancreatitis. Moderate fluid resuscitation with 10 mL/kg followed by 1.5 mL/kg/h infusion is recommended over aggressive fluid resuscitation at 20 mL/kg followed by

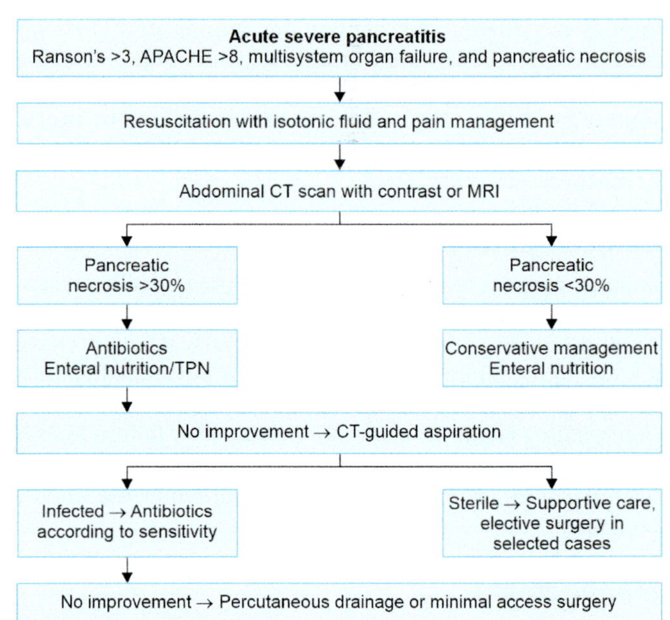

FLOWCHART 4: An algorithmic approach to the management of acute pancreatitis.

(APACHE: acute physiology and chronic health evaluation; CT: computed tomography; MRI: magnetic resonance imaging; TPN: total parental nutrition)

3 mL/kg/h due to the increased incidence of fluid overload.[52] There is evidence that demonstrates that lactated ringer's solution is associated with reduced C-reactive protein levels compared to normal saline.[53] Additionally, in a systematic review and meta-analysis, administration of lactated ringer's solution is associated with a significant reduction of ICU admission and development of local complications.[54]

In addition to the vital signs, monitoring hematocrit for hemoconcentration can guide the adequacy of fluid resuscitation. Pain is managed with meperidine, morphine, or fentanyl. About 20% of patients with acute pancreatitis will have necrotizing pancreatitis. The higher degree of necrosis portends a higher mortality. Patients with infected necrotizing pancreatitis require immediate antibiotic therapy to cover for aerobic and anaerobic gram-negative and gram-positive microorganisms. First-line antibiotics are carbapenems with fluoroquinolones being second-line.[55] Prophylactic antibiotics are not recommended for these patients, due to increased incidence of invasive candidiasis of the pancreas that is associated with increased mortality.[56,57] There are no studies that support the routine use of prophylactic antifungals in severe acute pancreatitis. CT-guided aspiration and drainage of collections should be performed in patients in whom infection is suspected. Open necrosectomy is not favored.[58] Early oral feeding or enteral feeding via a nasojejunostomy or nasogastric tube is associated with decreased infectious complications and early recovery compared to parenteral nutrition.[57,59] In patients with gallstone pancreatitis, urgent (within 24 hours of admission) endoscopic retrograde cholangiopancreatography (ERCP) is recommended in those with acute cholangitis. Early ERCP (within 72 hours of admission) is recommended if suspicion of persistent bile duct stones remains high.[60] A large cohort study demonstrated that urgent ERCP in patients with acute biliary pancreatitis without cholangitis did not have significant mortality benefit or length of stay.[61]

Although uncommon, HTG is a well-established etiology of acute pancreatitis with a reported incidence of 2–4%. HTG-induced pancreatitis should be managed no differently than what has already been discussed with the addition of treatment specific to HTG. Insulin and heparin infusion can be used to lower triglyceride levels. However, due to concern for rebound HTG and hemorrhage into the pancreas, insulin is favored over heparin. Plasmapheresis can rapidly remove triglycerides as well as proinflammatory markers and cytokines in HTG-induced pancreatitis. However, there is no mortality benefit compared to conservative therapy. There is also no mortality benefit in the initiation of plasmapheresis early (within 36 hours of admission) versus late (after 36 hours).[62]

SUMMARY

This section focuses on managing nonpulmonary critical care issues, particularly gastrointestinal and hepatic complications in critically ill patients. It highlights the diagnosis and treatment of acute gastrointestinal bleeding, including both upper and lower GI bleeds, as well as variceal hemorrhage linked to portal hypertension. Key interventions discussed include endoscopy, transfusion strategies, and pharmacological treatments. Additionally, the section addresses acute liver failure, acute-on-chronic liver failure, and complications such as spontaneous bacterial peritonitis, emphasizing the importance of timely intervention and multidisciplinary care to improve outcomes in the ICU.

REFERENCES

1. Strate LL, Ayanian JZ, Kotler G, et al. Risk factors for mortality in lower intestinal bleeding. Clin Gastroenterol Hepatol. 2008;6: 1004-10.
2. Sostres C, Lanas A. Epidemiology and demographics of upper gastrointesinal bleeding: prevalence, incidence and mortality. Gastrointest Endosc Clin N Am. 2011;21:567-81.
3. Westerhof J, Weersma RK, Koornstra JJ. Investigating obscure gastrointestinal bleeding: capsule endoscopy or double balloon enteroscopy? Neth J Med. 2009;67:260-5.
4. Huang ES, Karsan S, Kanwal F, et al. Impact of nasogastric lavage on outcomes in acute GI bleeding. Gastrointest Endosc. 2011;74:971-80.
5. Khamaysi I, Gralnek IM. Acute upper gastrointestinal bleeding (UGIB) - initial evaluation and management. Best Pract Res Clin Gastroenterol. 2013;27:633-8.
6. Grenvik A, Ayres SM, Holbrook PR, et al. Textbook of Critical Care, 4th edition. Philadelphia: WB Saunders Company; 2000.
7. Villanueva C, Colomo A, Bosch A, et al. Transfusion strategies for acute upper gastrointestinal bleeding. N Engl J Med. 2013; 368:11-21.
8. Blatchford O, Murray WR, Blatchford M. A risk score to predict need for treatment for upper-gastrointestinal haemorrhage. Lancet. 2000;356:1318-21.
9. Tham TC, James C, Kelly M. Predicting outcome of acute non-variceal upper gastrointestinal haemorrhage without endoscopy using the clinical Rockall Score. Postgrad Med J. 2006;82:757-9.
10. Masaoka T, Suzuki H, Hori S, et al. Blatchford scoring system is a useful scoring system for detecting patients with upper gastrointestinal bleeding who do not need endoscopic intervention. J Gastroenterol Hepatol. 2007;22:1404-8.
11. Gralnek IM, Stanley AJ, Morris AJ, et al. Endoscopic diagnosis and management of nonvariceal upper gastrointestinal hemorrhage (NVUGIH): European Society of Gastrointestinal Endoscopy (ESGE) Guideline - Update 2021. Endoscopy. 2021; 53(3):300-32.
12. Hadzibulic E, Govedarica S. Significance of Forrest classification, Rockall's and Blatchford's risk scoring system in prediction of rebleeding in peptic ulcer disease. Acta Medica Medianae. 2007; 46:38-43.
13. Lau JY, Leung WK, Wu JC, et al. Omeprazole before endoscopy in patients with gastrointestinal bleeding. N Engl J Med. 2007; 356:1631-40.
14. Leontiadis GI, Sharma VK, Howden CW. Systematic review and meta-analysis: enhanced efficacy of proton-pump inhibitor therapy for peptic ulcer bleeding in Asia–a post hoc analysis from the Cochrane Collaboration. Aliment Pharmacol Ther. 2005;21:1055-61.
15. White K, Faruqi U, Cohen AAT. New agents for DOAC reversal: a practical management review. Br J Cardiol. 2022;29(1):1.
16. Palmer KR. Non-variceal upper gastrointestinal haemorrhage: guidelines. Gut. 2002;51:iv1-6.
17. Strate LL, Gralnek IM. ACG Clinical Guideline: Management of Patients With Acute Lower Gastrointestinal Bleeding. Am J Gastroenterol. 2016;111(4):459-74.
18. Yoon W, Jeong YY, Shin SS, et al. Acute massive gastrointestinal bleeding: detection and localization with arterial phase multi-detector row helical CT. Radiology. 2006;239:160-7.
19. Barnert J, Messmann H. Diagnosis and management of lower gastrointestinal bleeding. Nat Rev Gastroenterol Hepatol. 2009; 6:637-46.
20. Garcia-Tsao G, Sanyal A, Grace N, et al. AASLD Practice Guidelines: Prevention and management of gastroesophageal varices and variceal hemorrhage in cirrhosis. Hepatology. 2007; 46:922-38.
21. Soares-Weiser K, Brezis M, Tur-Kaspa R, et al. Antibiotic prophylaxis for cirrhotic patients with gastrointestinal bleeding. Cochrane Database Syst Rev. 2002:CD002907.
22. Lisman T, Caldwell SH, Burroughs AK, et al. Hemostasis and thrombosis in patients with liver disease: the ups and downs. J Hepatol. 2010;53(2):362-71.

23. Bosch J, Thabut D, Albillos A, et al. Recombinant factor VIIa for variceal bleeding in patients with advanced cirrhosis: A randomized, controlled trial. Hepatology. 2008;47(5):1604-14.
24. Rodriguez-Roisin R, Krowka MJ. Hepatopulmonary syndrome–a liver-induced lung vascular disorder. N Engl J Med. 2008;358: 2378-7.
25. Gandhi KD, Taweesedt PT, Sharma M, et al. Hepatopulmonary syndrome: An update. World J Hepatol. 2021;13(11):1699-706.
26. Rodriguez-Roisin R, Krowka MJ, Herve P, et al. Pulmonary-Hepatic vascular Disorders (PHD). Eur Respir J. 2004;24:861-80.
27. Garcia N Jr, Mihas AA. Hepatic hydrothorax: pathophysiology, diagnosis, and management. J Clin Gastroenterol. 2004;38:52-8.
28. Xiol X, Guardiola J. Hepatic hydrothorax. Curr Opin Pulm Med. 1998;4:239-42.
29. Escorsell À, Castellote J, Sánchez-Delgado J, et al. Management of acute liver failure. Clinical guideline from the Catalan Society of Digestology. Gastroenterol Hepatol. 2019;42(1):51-64.
30. Stravitz RT, Kramer AH, Davern T, et al. Intensive care of patients with acute liver failure: recommendations of the U.S. Acute Liver Failure Study Group. Crit Care Med. 2007;35:2498-508.
31. Bernal W, Wendon J. Acute liver failure. N Engl J Med. 2013;369: 2525-34.
32. Walayat S, Shoaib H, Asghar M, et al. Role of N-acetylcysteine in non-acetaminophen-related acute liver failure: an updated meta-analysis and systematic review. Ann Gastroenterol. 2021; 34(2):235-40.
33. Bass NM, Mullen KD, Sangal A, et al. Rifaximin treatment in hepatic encephalopathy. N Engl J Med. 2010;362:1071-81.
34. Jacobi J, Fraser GL, Coursin DB, et al. Clinical practice guidelines for the sustained use of sedatives and analgesics in the critically ill adult. Crit Care Med. 2002;30:119141.
35. Jeffers L, Chalasani N, Balart L, et al. Safety and efficacy of recombinant factor VIIa in patients with liver disease undergoing laparoscopic liver biopsy. Gastroenterology. 2002;123:118-26.
36. Plauth M, Riggoo O, Assis-Camilo M, et al. ESPEN guidelines on enteral nutrition: liver disease. Clin Nut. 2006;25:285-94.
37. Takahashi Y, Kumada H, Shimizu M, et al. A multicenter study on the prognosis of fulminant viral hepatitis: early prediction for liver transplantation. Hepatology. 1994;19:1065-71.
38. Slack AJ, Auzinger G, Willars C, et al. Ammonia clearance with haemofiltration in adults with liver disease. Liver Int. 2014;34(1): 42-8.
39. European Association for the Study of the Liver; Clinical practice guidelines panel; Wendon J; Cordoba J, Dhawan A, Larsen FS, et al.; EASL Governing Board representative; Bernardi M. EASL Clinical Practical Guidelines on the management of acute (fulminant) liver failure. J Hepatol. 2017;66(5):1047-81.
40. Saliba F, Bañares R, Larsen FS, et al. Artificial liver support in patients with liver failure: a modified DELPHI consensus of international experts. Intensive Care Med. 2022;48(10):1352-67.
41. Larsen FS, Schmidt LE, Bernsmeier C, et al. High-volume plasma exchange in patients with acute liver failure: An open randomised controlled trial. J Hepatol. 2016;64(1):69-78.
42. Maiwall R, Bajpai M, Singh A, et al. Standard-Volume Plasma Exchange Improves Outcomes in Patients With Acute Liver Failure: A Randomized Controlled Trial. Clin Gastroenterol Hepatol. 2022;20(4):e831-54.
43. Arroyo V, Moreau R, Jalan R. Acute-on-Chronic Liver Failure. N Engl J Med. 2020;382(22):2137-45.
44. Lata J, Stiburek O, Kopacova M. Spontaneous bacterial peritonitis: a severe complication of liver cirrhosis. World J Gastroenterol. 2009;15:5505-10.
45. Rimola A, Garcia-Tsao G, Navasa M, et al. Diagnosis, treatment and prophylaxis of spontaneous bacterial peritonitis: a consensus document. International Ascites Club. J Hepatol. 2000;32:142-53.
46. Moore KP, Wong F, Gines P, et al. The management of ascites in cirrhosis: report on the consensus conference of the International Ascites Club. Hepatology. 2003;38:258-66.
47. Biggins SW, Angeli P, Garcia-Tsao G, et al. Diagnosis, Evaluation, and Management of Ascites, Spontaneous Bacterial Peritonitis and Hepatorenal Syndrome: 2021 Practice Guidance by the American Association for the Study of Liver Diseases. Hepatology. 2021;74(2):1014-48.
48. Bass NM. Intravenous albumin for spontaneous bacterial peritonitis in patients with cirrhosis. N Engl J Med. 1999;341: 443-4.
49. Sigal SH, Stanca CM, Fernandez J, et al. Restricted use of albumin for spontaneous bacterial peritonitis. Gut. 2007;56:597-9.
50. Balthazar EJ, Freeny PC, van Sonnenberg E. Imaging and intervention in acute pancreatitis. Radiology. 1994;193:297-306.
51. Wu BU, Johannes RS, Sun X, et al. The early prediction of mortality in acute pancreatitis: a large population-based study. Gut. 2008;57(12):1698-703.
52. de-Madaria E, Buxbaum JL, Maisonneuve P, et al.; ERICA Consortium. Aggressive or Moderate Fluid Resuscitation in Acute Pancreatitis. N Engl J Med. 2022;387(11):989-1000.
53. de-Madaria E, Herrera-Marante I, González-Camacho V, et al. Fluid resuscitation with lactated Ringer's solution vs normal saline in acute pancreatitis: A triple-blind, randomized, controlled trial. United European Gastroenterol J. 2018;6(1):63-72.
54. Kow CS, Burud IAS, Hasan SS. Fluid Resuscitation With Lactated Ringer's Solution Versus Normal Saline in Acute Pancreatitis: A Systematic Review and Meta-Analysis of Randomized Trials. Pancreas. 2022;51(7):752-5.
55. Purschke B, Bolm L, Meyer MN, et al. Interventional strategies in infected necrotizing pancreatitis: Indications, timing, and outcomes. World J Gastroenterol. 2022;28(27):3383-97.
56. Leonard-Murali S, Lezotte J, Kalu R, et al. Necrotizing pancreatitis: A review for the acute care surgeon. Am J Surg. 2021;221(5):927-34.
57. Tenner S, Baillie J, DeWitt J, et al. American College of Gastroenterology Guideline: Management of acute pancreatitis. Am J Gastroenterol. 2013;108:14001415.
58. Besselink MG, Verwer TJ, Schoenmaeckers EJ, et al. Timing of surgical intervention in necrotizing pancreatitis. Arch Surg. 2007;142:1194-201.
59. Szatmary P, Grammatikopoulos T, Cai W, et al. Acute Pancreatitis: Diagnosis and Treatment. Drugs. 2022;82(12):1251-76.
60. Fogel EL, Sherman S. ERCP for gallstone pancreatitis. N Engl J Med. 2014;370(2):150-7.
61. Kabaria S, Mutneja H, Makar M, et al. Timing of endoscopic retrograde cholangiopancreatography in acute biliary pancreatitis without cholangitis: a nationwide inpatient cohort study. Ann Gastroenterol. 2021;34(4):575-81.
62. Garg R, Rustagi T. Management of Hypertriglyceridemia Induced Acute Pancreatitis. Biomed Res Int. 2018;2018:4721357.

Nonpulmonary Critical Care II (Hematological and Renal Problems)

CHAPTER 167

Liziamma George, Ivan Wong

INTRODUCTION

Hematological and renal disorders are prevalent in critically ill patients and play a pivotal role in the complexity of intensive care management. These conditions, whether occurring independently or as part of broader systemic dysfunctions, contribute significantly to morbidity and mortality in the ICU. Anemia, thrombocytopenia, and coagulopathies are common hematological challenges, often exacerbated by the inflammatory state of critical illness. Simultaneously, acute kidney injury (AKI) frequently develops, complicating fluid and electrolyte balance, and further straining the body's ability to recover. Understanding the intricate interplay between these systems and applying targeted therapeutic interventions are essential for optimizing patient outcomes. This chapter explores the mechanisms, diagnosis, and management strategies for both hematological and renal disorders in the critical care setting.

HEMATOLOGY IN CRITICAL CARE

ANEMIA

Anemia, acute or chronic, is a frequent problem in critically ill patients admitted into intensive care units (ICUs) and can result from several causes **(Table 1)**.[1,2] The proinflammatory state seen in critically ill patients results in a blunted erythropoietic response to anemia in addition to abnormalities in iron metabolism, further complicating the clinical course.[3-5] In normal and anemic patients, cardiac output is regulated to maintain oxygen delivery (DO_2) at five times the oxygen consumption (VO_2) (DO_2:VO_2 = 5:1). Changes to VO_2 will trigger a compensatory response in DO_2, however, not the other way around. Therefore, if cardiac output is impaired, the decrease in DO_2 is compensated by increased oxygen extraction by tissues from the capillary blood to meet the oxygen demands, resulting in a decrease in venous oxygen content and saturation (mixed venous oxygen saturation).

Anaerobic metabolism and lactic acidosis occur when DO_2 is inadequate to meet oxygen demands at DO_2:VO_2 < 2:1. The decision to transfuse packed red blood cells (PRBCs) to increase the oxygen content and therefore, DO_2 should be based on the patient's individual physiologic status and not an arbitrary level of hemoglobin (Hb) or hematocrit.[6] It has been reported that 63% and 29% of critically ill patients admitted into the ICU have an admitting Hb concentration of <12.0 and 10.0 g/dL, respectively, with Hb concentrations on average decreasing by approximately 0.5 g/dL/day in nonseptic patients (without active bleeding or hemolysis) during the first 3 days of ICU stay.[7] The Hb concentration remains stable thereafter in these patients. Conversely in septic patients, Hb concentrations, on average, decrease

TABLE 1: Different etiologies of anemia in the intensive care unit.

Mechanism	Etiology
Blood loss	• Phlebotomy • Gastrointestinal bleeding • Other sources of bleeding • Surgery and other invasive procedures
Diminished erythropoiesis	• Decreased erythropoietin synthesis • Erythropoietin resistance • Iron deficiency • Nutritional deficiencies • Myelosuppressive drugs or toxins • Bone marrow disorders • Endocrine disorders
Pre-existing chronic anemia	Anemia of chronic disease
Increased erythrocyte destruction	• Defective production of Hb subunits • Hemolysis • Autoimmune diseases • Drugs
Hemodilution	Aggressive fluid resuscitation

(Hb: hemoglobin)

by 0.8 g/dL/day during the first 3 days in the ICU and subsequently by 0.3 g/dL/day. Historically, the lower limits of normal Hb concentration in adults have been suggested to range from 12.7 to 13.7 g/dL in men and 11.5–12.2 g/dL in women. Maintaining Hb concentration of 7.0–9.0 g/dL has been sufficient and red cell transfusion is considered when Hb concentration is <7.0–8 g/dL.[8,9] Clinicians must weigh the potential benefits against the possible risks, including an increased incidence of infection as well as other complications of red cell transfusions.[10]

Clinical Features

The clinical consequences of anemia will depend on the degree of anemia, the rate at which it has developed, and the oxygen demands of the patient which tend to be high in the critically ill, as well as the ability of the patient to compensate for these changes. High-risk groups in which anemia is less tolerated and more vulnerable to adverse outcomes include the elderly, critically ill patients, and patients with chronic respiratory, coronary, or cerebrovascular disease. The symptoms and signs are nonspecific.

Diagnosis

Detailed clinical history and physical examination supplemented with laboratory evaluations will give some clues about the etiology of anemia. Laboratory tests include a complete blood count (CBC) including red blood cell (RBC) indices and white blood cell (WBC) differentials. It is important to compare these results with prior CBCs to determine the onset of anemia, as well as identify trends and progression of the disease. Other laboratory tests that can be performed as indicated to determine the etiology of anemia include peripheral blood smear; iron profile studies and folate and vitamin B12 levels to evaluate nutritional deficiencies; bilirubin level, lactate dehydrogenase (LDH) levels, haptoglobin levels, and Coombs test to evaluate degree and type of hemolysis; Hb electrophoresis; thyroid function tests; blood urea nitrogen (BUN) and creatinine levels; and bone marrow examinations.[11]

Management

Anemia of acute onset, such as gastrointestinal bleeding, is typically treated with the administration of physiologic crystalloids, colloidal fluids, or red cell transfusions.[2] However, in patients with a more chronic evolution of anemia, treatment will depend on the underlying etiology. Iatrogenic causes such as phlebotomy are common in the ICU and range from 40 to 70 mL/day.[2,5] Blood conservation techniques such as the use of small-volume phlebotomy tubes and point-of-care analysis and closed, no-waste sampling systems may contribute to the reduction in anemia.[7]

Approximately 70% of critically ill patients are transfused and receive their initial transfusion within the first 48 hours in the ICU.[5] For those patients staying greater than a week in the ICU, about 73–85% of them will receive red cell transfusions.[1,5] The benefits of red cell transfusions must be weighed against such risks as immunosuppression, allergic reactions, and infectious transmissions.[5] Higher transfusion rates have been reported to be associated with increased hospital-acquired infections, increased ICU length of stay, higher rates of coagulation abnormalities, and more severe organ failure, as well as increased mortality rates.[5,8,10] In light of these risks, alternative treatment strategies have been explored in critically ill patients such as the administration of exogenous human recombinant erythropoietin which has not been reported to result in a decrease in red cell transfusion. Erythropoietin is associated with more thrombotic events.[12,13] There are no widely accepted treatment guidelines for managing anemia in critically ill patients and practice varies between centers. Further research and understanding of anemia, in addition to innovative treatment strategies, may promote improved clinical outcomes for critically ill patients.

Indications for Red Blood Cell Transfusion in the Intensive Care Unit

In patients with hemorrhagic shock, initial resuscitation should begin with crystalloids. If the shock is not corrected after 2 liters of crystalloids, PRBC transfusion is indicated to improve DO_2 to the tissues and should be guided by hemodynamic parameters rather than Hb measurement. Aggressive measures to control bleeding should accompany resuscitation. Blood lactate levels can be used to guide the adequacy of resuscitation.[14] In patients with hemodynamically stable anemia, transfusion is considered if the Hb level drops below 7 g/dL and should be guided by the patient's condition rather than the absolute number. Transfusion to improve Hb > 9 g/dL is not indicated in mechanically ventilated patients, patients with stable coronary disease, and stable trauma patients. Patients with acute coronary symptoms may benefit from higher levels of Hb.[15] Whenever possible, transfusion should be given in single units.[16]

Massive transfusions are necessary for patients with hemorrhagic shock; however, such transfusions are associated with hypothermia, metabolic acidosis, and coagulopathy. Hypothermia occurs due to transfusion of stored cold blood and impairment of metabolism leading to delayed clearing of toxins and cytokines. Dilutional coagulopathy along with consumption coagulopathy occurs in these patients and this is further exacerbated by hypothermia that can occur with massive transfusions. A transfusion ratio of 1:1:1 [RBC, fresh frozen plasma (FFP), and platelets] or whole blood has been recommended in case of massive transfusions but remains controversial.[17] Massive transfusions are also associated with hyperkalemia, hypocalcemia, hypomagnesemia, metabolic alkalosis, and acidosis.[17] Transfusion-associated acute lung injury (TRALI) occurs within 6 hours of transfusion with signs and symptoms of acute respiratory failure. The proposed mechanisms are the reaction of donor antibodies against the recipient WBCs and pulmonary vascular endothelial activation, leading to WBC sequestration and endothelial damage. Transfusion-associated circulatory overload (TACO) is the second most common transfusion-associated mortality. It is defined as the presence of acute respiratory distress—dyspnea, orthopnea, cough, elevated brain natriuretic peptide, central venous pressure, presence of left heart failure, positive fluid balance, and radiographic evidence of pulmonary edema within 6 hours of transfusion. The incidence of TACO is prevented by careful evaluation of the fluid status of the patients and administration of diuretics in high-risk patients along with supportive care.

THROMBOCYTOPENIA

Thrombocytopenia occurs frequently in critically ill patients and is the most common coagulation problem in this group of patients.[18,19] Approximately 50% of critically ill patients may not present with thrombocytopenia at the time of admission into ICU; however, whether present on admission or developing during the ICU course, thrombocytopenia in critically ill patients suggests poor prognosis.[18,19] Depending on the cutoff level utilized to define thrombocytopenia (i.e., <150 × 10^9/L vs. <100 × 10^9/L), the type of population being assessed (e.g., medical vs. surgical/trauma) and the period of the ICU course (e.g., <4 days vs. ≥4 days) being studied, the incidence of thrombocytopenia has been reported to range from 15 to 60%.[20] The decreased risk of bleeding with platelet counts between 100 and 150 × 10^9/L has resulted in a cutoff level of <100 × 10^9/L being proposed as the definition of thrombocytopenia in the critically ill.[19] In addition to increased bleeding risks and consequent necessity for transfusions, thrombocytopenia has also been associated with an increased length of ICU and hospital stay, as well as an increased mortality.[19,20] Not only has the severity of thrombocytopenia been independently associated with a poorer outcome, but the degree of decline in platelet count (i.e., 30–50%) over time has also been associated with a higher mortality, even if it remains within the normal range.[20-22] The relationship between a low or declining platelet count and mortality is doubtful to be causal but rather influenced by the disease or factors contributing to the development of thrombocytopenia. These etiological factors include but are not limited to sepsis, organ failure, drugs, disseminated intravascular coagulation (DIC), thrombotic thrombocytopenic purpura (TTP), atypical hemolytic uremic syndrome (aHUS), hemophagocytic lymphohistiocytosis (HLH), catastrophic antiphospholipid syndrome, nutritional deficiencies, and transfusion.[19,22]

The mechanisms which may elucidate the development of thrombocytopenia are sometimes spurious (e.g., laboratory error) or the disorders of distribution (e.g., splenomegaly), dilution (e.g., massive transfusions), increased platelet destruction (e.g., DIC), and decreased platelet production (e.g., drugs).[19,23] Correction of the underlying cause may contribute to improving platelet counts and consequently prevent delays in required invasive procedures as well as limit the use of platelet transfusions. Heparin-induced thrombocytopenia (HIT), an antibody-mediated reaction against platelet factor 4 occurs approximately 4 days after initiation of treatment and is associated with thrombotic rather than bleeding risk. Diagnosis is suspected when the platelet count decreases by 50% from the initial value. Treatment is with thrombin inhibitors—argatroban, hirudin, or danaparoid—until platelet count reaches >150 × 10^9/L.[21,23]

TABLE 2: The degree of thrombocytopenia and associated bleeding risk.

Platelet count (cells × 10^9/L)	Risk
<100	10-fold increased bleeding risk compared to platelet counts 100–150
<50	Invasive procedures commonly avoided (surgical bleeding uncommon if platelet counts > 50)
<20	Risk of spontaneous bleeding
<10	Risk of severe, life-threatening bleeding

Clinical Features

The signs and symptoms of thrombocytopenia tend to take place rapidly as platelets have a relatively short 10-day half-life. The type of bleeding may be comparatively mild as in mucosal or cutaneous bleeding, e.g., epistaxis, gingival bleeding, petechiae, or more severe as in spontaneous intracerebral hemorrhage. The risk of bleeding depends on the degree of thrombocytopenia **(Table 2)**.

Diagnosis

The evaluation of a patient with thrombocytopenia involves a complete history and physical examination, assessing for what may be contributing to or causing the patient's low platelets such as splenomegaly, recent infections, comorbidities, or medications the patient may be taking or recently have taken. A peripheral blood smear can be essential in determining the etiology of the patient's thrombocytopenia **(Table 3)**.

Management

Platelet concentrates are made by centrifugation of either whole blood or plasma and by apheresis of blood. Simply transfusing patients with platelets to raise levels may be unwarranted, ineffective, and even contraindicated in some critically ill thrombocytopenic patients. It is essential to determine the typically multifactorial etiology of thrombocytopenia in these patients and subsequently correct the underlying cause **(Table 4)**. This usually

TABLE 3: Possible peripheral blood smear findings and their corresponding etiology and initial diagnostic step.

Smear	Possible etiology	Diagnostic step
Normal	• Hypersplenism • Immune-mediated (drugs) • Idiopathic thrombocytopenic purpura (ITP)	• Physical exam; imaging test • Review medications • Diagnosis of exclusion
• Platelet clumping • Platelet satellitism	Pseudothrombocytopenia	Redraw specimen in heparin or citrate tube; repeat manual or automated count
Fragmented red blood cells (schistocytes, helmet cells)	Microangiopathic hemolytic anemia*	Further evaluation based on suspected etiology
Atypical lymphocytes	Viral infection	Viral studies ± further evaluation based on suspected etiology
• Oval macrocytes • Hyperpigmented polymorphonuclear cells	Vitamin B12 deficiency Folate deficiency	Check vitamin B12 and folate levels
Leukoerythroblastosis	Myelophthisis	Bone marrow biopsy
Blasts	• Leukemia • Myelodysplastic syndrome	Bone marrow biopsy
• Dyserythropoiesis • Dysgranulopoiesis • Dysmegakaryopoiesis	Myelodysplastic syndrome	Bone marrow biopsy
White blood cell left shift	Sepsis	Septic workup

*Microangiopathic hemolytic anemia—thrombotic thrombocytopenic purpura (TTP), hemolytic uremic syndrome (HUS), disseminated intravascular coagulation (DIC), malignant hypertension, preeclampsia/eclampsia, HELLP syndrome (hemolysis, elevated liver enzymes, and low platelets), disseminated carcinoma, malfunctioning prosthetic heart valve, vasculitis, and scleroderma renal crisis.

TABLE 4: The different causes, mechanisms, and treatment of thrombocytopenia.

Mechanism	Pathophysiology	Etiology	Treatment
Spurious	Clumping of platelets in specimen tube	Laboratory order	Specimen redrawn in heparin or citrate tube
Decreased platelet production	Bone marrow suppression	Nutritional deficiency	Replete deficiencies
		Drugs, toxins	Stop offending agent
		Viral infections	Supportive care
		Metastases	Chemotherapy, radiation therapy
Increased platelet destruction	Nonimmune mediated	DIC	Treat underlying etiology, anticoagulation
		TTP	Plasma exchange
		HELLP	Delivery of infant
	Immune mediated	Drugs	Stop offending drug
		Type 2 HIT	Stop heparin administration; start direct thrombin inhibitor
		ITP	Steroids, IV Ig, splenectomy
Dilutional	Infusion of massive amounts of blood products and intravenous fluids	Transfusion for massive blood loss	Platelet transfusion, supportive care
Distributional	Increased platelet sequestration	Splenomegaly, portal hypertension	Supportive care, splenectomy

(DIC: disseminated intravascular coagulation; HELLP: hemolysis, elevated liver enzymes, low platelets; HIT: heparin-induced thrombocytopenia; ITP: idiopathic thrombocytopenic purpura; IVIg: intravenous immunoglobulin; TTP: thrombotic thrombocytopenic purpura) results in an increase in platelet counts and possibly limits exposure to the risks of platelet transfusions as well as prevents delays in the requirement for invasive procedures. Prophylactic platelet transfusion is given to patients who are actively bleeding with thrombocytopenia or when platelet counts fall below 10 × 10^9/L.[24,25] The dose for prophylactic transfusion of platelets is controversial. The choice of low-, medium-, or high-dose platelet transfusion does not affect the incidence of bleeding. Therapeutic transfusion is given to patients with thrombocytopenia associated with gross hemorrhage. Usually, this bleeding is multifactorial and may not be corrected with platelet transfusion alone. In patients who require interventions, a platelet count > 50 × 10^9/L for trauma and general surgery and >100 × 10^9/L for neurological interventions is required. Each platelet concentrate should produce an increase in platelet count of approximately 5–10 × 10^9/L in an average 70 kg adult. Refractoriness to platelet transfusion may be due to alloimmunization or nonimmune factors. Alloimmunization can be prevented by giving ABO-matched platelets and HLA-compatible donors. In patients with life-threatening bleeding and platelet refractoriness, giving frequent small transfusions, intravenous immunoglobulin G (IgG) administration, plasma exchange, rituximab, use of antifibrinolytic agents, and transfusion of factor VIIa may be helpful.[26]

THROMBOTIC THROMBOCYTOPENIC PURPURA

Thrombotic thrombocytopenic purpura is a thrombotic microangiopathic disease that is caused by a deficiency in ADAMTS13, commonly due to antibodies that inhibit ADAMTS13. Due to prompt recognition and treatment, mortality rates have improved from 80% to 10–20%. Although a low ADAMTS13 < 10% is diagnostic, it may take days to obtain results. Therefore, the classic clinical features such as altered mental status, fever, acute kidney injury (AKI), thrombocytopenia, and hemolytic anemia should allude to the diagnosis of TTP. A PLASMIC score **(Table 5)** of 5 or higher has high sensitivity and negative predictive value in the diagnosis of TTP.[27] Once TTP is suspected, emergent hematology consultation and initiation of therapeutic plasma exchange are needed to remove autoantibodies and replace ADAMTS13. If plasma exchange is not available, transfusion of FFP to transiently replace ADAMTS13 until definitive treatment can be arranged. Corticosteroids should also be given early, and sometimes at pulse doses for 3 days, if there is severe disease or neurological involvement.[27]

TABLE 5: A PLASMIC score of 5 or higher has a high sensitivity and negative predictive value in the diagnosis of TTP.

*P*latelet count < 30 × 10^9/L	1 point
Hemo*L*ysis variables	1 point
No *A*ctive cancer	1 point
No history of *S*olid-organ or stem-cell transplant	1 point
*M*CV < 90 fL	1 point
*I*NR < 1.5	1 point
*C*reatinine < 2.0 mg/dL	1 point

(INR: international normalized ratio; MCV: mean corpuscular volume; TTP: thrombotic thrombocytopenic purpura)

Hemophagocytic lymphohistiocytosis is defined as an extreme form of the inflammatory process, with a failure in feedback between pro- and anti-inflammatory pathways in response to a trigger, leading to uncontrolled macrophage and lymphocyte activation and proliferation. HLH in the ICU, regardless of etiology, is associated with a 57% mortality rate. Diagnosis of HLH in the ICU is difficult. Diagnostic criteria include clinical and biological parameters (fever, adenopathy, splenomegaly, hepatomegaly, cytopenia, hyperferritinemia, hypertriglyceridemia, and hypofibrinogenemia). Treatment usually involves supportive care, corticosteroids, and etoposide. Emapalumab is an anti-interferon-gamma immunoglobulin that is approved for familial, refractory, and recurrent HLH.[28]

RISKS OF TRANSFUSION

The administration of blood products is not without risk. These risks could be infectious or immune-mediated in nature **(Table 6)**, but the greatest risk results from human error.[29,30] Although the incidence of infectious and immune-mediated events such as ABO incompatibility has been on the decrease, in recent times, the transfusion of blood products has been associated with organ dysfunction, immune suppression, hospital-acquired infections, increased ICU stay, and decreased survival. Significant progress has been made in diminishing the risks, particularly infectious risks, associated with the transfusion of blood products. Early recognition of adverse events associated with transfusion is vital for patient safety.

COAGULOPATHY IN THE INTENSIVE CARE UNIT

Coagulopathy occurs in critically ill patients due to the underlying illness or medications. There is no recommendation to transfuse patients with coagulopathy if they are not actively bleeding. FFP is indicated for the replacement of single coagulation factor deficiency and multiple factor deficiencies, for patients with DIC associated with bleeding, during plasma exchange in patients with TTP, and for severe bleeding associated with warfarin-induced coagulopathy. Prothrombin complex concentrates can be used as an alternative to FFP for the reversal of anticoagulation due to warfarin. They achieve more rapid reversal with significantly less fluid administration.[31] Cryoprecipitate is given

TABLE 6: Infectious and noninfectious complications of blood transfusion.

Infectious	HIV	**Noninfectious**	Febrile reactions
	Hepatitis A, B, and C virus		*Allergic*: • Urticarial/Cutaneous reaction • Anaphylaxis
	Bacterial: • *Yersinia enterocolitica* • *Staphylococcus aureus* • *Klebsiella pneumonia* • *Serratia marcescens* • *Staphylococcus epidermidis*		*Hemolytic reaction*: • Acute • Delayed
	Parasites: • Plasmodium • Babesia • Trypanosoma		Circulatory overload
	Other viruses: • HTLV types I and II • CMV • EBV		*Alloimmunization*: • Red blood cell mediated • Human leukocyte antigen mediated
	Emerging infections: • Creutzfeldt–Jakob disease • West Nile virus • B19 Parvovirus		• TRALI • GVHD • Transfusion-related iron overload • Transfusion-related immunomodulation

(CMV: cytomegalovirus; EBV: Epstein–Barr virus; GVHD: graft-versus-host disease; HIV: human immunodeficiency virus; HTLV: human T-cell lymphotropic virus; TRALI: transfusion-associated lung injury)

to patients when plasma fibrinogen levels are <1.5–2.0 g/L. Tranexamic acid, an inhibitor of fibrinolysis, should be considered for trauma patients at risk for significant bleeding in whom it is demonstrated to improve survival and decrease the need for transfusions.[32] Recombinant factor VIIa is used in patients with hemophilia and factor VIII and factor IX inhibitors. Both prothrombin complex concentrates and recombinant VIIA have been used to reverse the new oral anticoagulants, thrombin, and Xa inhibitors but are not proven therapies in this setting.[33] They have also been utilized in the setting of massive and refractory hemorrhage.[34] The use of recombinant human soluble thrombomodulin has been studied in patients with sepsis-induced DIC and was not shown to reduce all-cause mortality.[35]

RENAL DISEASE IN CRITICAL CARE

ACUTE KIDNEY INJURY

A normally functioning kidney eliminates urea and other nitrogenous waste products, in addition to regulating fluid, electrolyte, and acid–base equilibrium. Conversely, renal dysfunction results in the buildup of uremic toxins and nitrogenous waste products (azotemia), as well as an imbalance in the fluid, electrolyte, and acid–base equilibrium because of a reduction in the glomerular filtration rate (GFR).[36] AKI, formerly referred to as acute renal failure, is said to occur when renal dysfunction takes place suddenly and/or rapidly.[37,38]

Various definitions for AKI have been reported in the literature, resulting in wide-ranging incidence and mortality rates of 1–25% and 15–90%, respectively, in ICUs.[39-42] The need for a consensus definition for AKI resulted in the development of the RIFLE classification **(Table 7)** by the Acute Dialysis Quality Initiative (ADQI) group.[40,43,44]

The definition was later modified and validated in many studies by the Acute Kidney Injury Network (AKIN). The AKIN definition comprised smaller increases in serum creatinine, the introduction of a time frame (48 hours) to the diagnosis of AKI, and the elimination of loss and end-stage renal disease as categories **(Table 6)**.[45,46] Both classifications are associated with increased mortality with worsening degrees of AKI. The change in nomenclature to AKI now encompasses a broader spectrum of diseases with different levels of severity, ranging from minor renal dysfunction to total organ failure necessitating renal replacement therapy (RRT).[47,48] The etiology of AKI has typically been separated into three categories, namely prerenal, intrinsic renal, and postrenal azotemia **(Table 8)**,[38] thereby guiding the mode of therapeutic intervention. However, in ICU patients, the etiology of AKI is usually a result of multiple factors which could easily fall into any, or more commonly, a combination

TABLE 7: The RIFLE and AKIN classification of acute kidney injury.

	GFR criteria	Urine output criteria
RIFLE category		
Risk	Increased serum creatinine × 1.5 or GFR decrease > 25%	UO < 0.5 mL/kg/h × 6 hours
Injury	Increased serum creatinine × 2 or GFR decrease > 50%	UO < 0.5 mL/kg/h × 12 hours
Failure	Increased serum creatinine × 3 or GFR decrease > 75% or serum creatinine ≥ 4 mg/dL (with acute rise ≥ 0.5 mg/dL)	UO < 0.3 mL/kg/h × 24 hours or anuria × 12 hours
Loss	Persistent ARF → complete loss of renal function > 4 weeks	
ESRD	ESRD → complete loss of renal function > 3 months	
AKIN stage		
1	Increased serum creatinine ≥ 0.3mg/dL (≥ 26.4 μmol/L) or increase ≥ 150% to 200% (1.5- to 2-fold) from baseline	UO < 0.5 mL/kg/h for >6 hours
2	Increased serum creatinine > 200% to 300% (> 2- to 3-fold) from baseline	UO < 0.5 mL/kg/h for >12 hours
3	Increased serum creatinine > 300% (3-fold) from baseline or serum creatinine ≥ 4.0 mg/dL with an acute increase of at least 0.5 mg/dL	UO < 0.3 mL/kg/h for >24 hours or anuria for 12 hours

(AKIN: acute kidney injury network; ARF: acute renal failure; ESRD: end-stage renal disease; GFR: glomerular filtration rate; UO: urine output)

TABLE 8: Various causes of acute kidney failure in intensive care unit.

Prerenal		Intrinsic		Postrenal
Sepsis*	Acute tubular necrosis	Glomerulonephritis	Interstitial nephritis	Bladder neck obstruction (prostate disease)
	Hypotension/Shock	Postinfectious GN	Medications (NSAID, antibiotics, diuretics)	
Low cardiac output state	Sepsis*	Vasculitis (Wegener's granulomatosis, lupus nephritis)	Infections	Ureteric obstruction (pelvic malignancy, renal calculi)
Medications (diuretics, NSAID)	Rhabdomyolysis	Goodpasture syndrome	Immunologic causes	
Burns	Medications (antibiotics, antivirals, antifungals, radiocontrast dye)	Rapidly progressive GN		Neurogenic bladder
Surgery (cardiac, vascular)	Burns	Medications (NSAID, biphosphonates)		
• Shock (anaphylactic, hemorrhagic, hypovolemic) • Hepatorenal syndrome • Abdominal compartment syndrome	• Transfusion reactions Hemolysis • Tumor lysis syndrome			

* Sepsis is the most common cause of acute kidney injury in the intensive care unit in up to 50% of cases.

(GN: glomerulonephritis; NSAID: nonsteroidal anti-inflammatory drug)

of the categories, thus complicating the way such patients can be treated successfully.[38]

Clinical Presentation

Acute kidney injury can affect multiple organ systems. The reduction in GFR and urine output can result in fluid overload, which may further progress into congestive heart failure and hypotension, raised intra-abdominal pressure from retroperitoneal tissue edema and ascites, and hypertension from intravascular volume overload, as well as pulmonary compromise from congestion and pleural effusions. Electrolyte abnormalities such as metabolic acidosis and hyperkalemia commonly occur predisposing to cardiac arrhythmias. Critically ill patients with AKI can also develop a compromised inflammatory and immune response which increases the risk of infection, pneumonia, shock, or other multiorgan failure. The uremic state in these patients can contribute to the development of anorexia, vomiting, encephalopathy, pericarditis, bleeding diathesis, polyneuropathy, and anemia from increased erythrocyte destruction, which can be further complicated by weakness and easy fatiguability. These multiple adverse effects contribute to the increased mortality in critically ill patients with AKI.[49]

Diagnosis

The diagnosis of AKI involves taking a detailed clinical history, physical examination, and the performance of relevant tests which may aid in determining the etiology, such as BUN, serum creatinine, urine microscopy, urine chemistry, and renal ultrasound.[38,49] Serum creatinine is a commonly used tool in diagnosing AKI; however, it is important to note that like all approximations of GFR, it is not an accurate reflection of the latter in ICU patients who tend to be in a nonsteady state. In such patients, it tends to underestimate the degree of renal dysfunction such that large changes in GFR are mirrored by only small changes in the serum creatinine.[38,41] Nonetheless, it is the change in serum creatinine that provides clinical benefit in diagnosing AKI. Urine chemistries such as the fractional excretion of sodium and urea **(Box 1)** may help in distinguishing prerenal from renal causes of AKI **(Table 9)**, although in ICU patients, these tend to coexist.[38,50] Finally, due to limitations of the aforementioned diagnostic tools, AKI biomarkers, which indicate different aspects of kidney injury such as cysteine-rich protein 61, neutrophil gelatinase-associated lipocalin, kidney injury molecule-1, cystatin C, and urine interleukin-18, are actively being investigated as alternatives for the earlier detection of AKI prior to functional deterioration.[51] So far, there is no clear evidence for using biomarkers for the prediction of kidney injury.

BOX 1 Calculation formulas for the fractional excretions of sodium and urea.

Fractional excretion of sodium

$$FE_{Na} = \{(U_{Na}/P_{Na}) \div (U_{Cr}/P_{Cr})\} \times 100$$

*Fractional excretion of urea**

$$FE_{Ur} = \{(U_{Ur}/P_{Ur}) \div (U_{Cr}/P_{Cr})\} \times 100$$

*Provides information similar to the fractional excretion of sodium, but in contrast, it can be used in patients on diuretic therapy

[FE_{Na}: fractional excretion of sodium; FE_{Ur}: fractional excretion of urea; P_{Cr}: plasma creatinine concentration (mg/dL); P_{Na}: plasma sodium concentration (mEq/L); P_{Ur}: plasma urea concentration (mg/dL); U_{Cr}: urine creatinine concentration (mg/dL); U_{Na}: urine sodium concentration (mEq/L); U_{ur}: urine urea concentration (mg/dL)]

TABLE 9: Delineating laboratory features for differentiating prerenal and renal causes of acute kidney injury.

Urinary diagnostic indices	Prerenal	Renal
BUN:Cr ratio	>20:1	< 20:1
Urine sodium (mEq/L)	<20	>40
FE_{Na} (%)	<1	>2
FE_{Ur} (%)	<35	>50
Urine osmolality (mOsm/L)	>500	<350
Urine microscopy	Normal (except for occasional hyaline casts)	Abnormal

(BUN: blood urea nitrogen; Cr: creatinine; FENa: fractional excretion of sodium; FEUr: fractional excretion of urea)

Management

The treatment of ICU patients with AKI can be challenging as many of these patients develop AKI from multiple precipitating factors and commonly have coexisting multiorgan failure. Nonetheless, treatment strategies are initially targeted at correcting the suspected underlying cause. Such treatment may include but is not limited to fluid resuscitation with or without inotropic or vasopressor support to maintain hemodynamic stability and renal perfusion, correction of metabolic abnormalities, discontinuation of nephrotoxic agents, or dosage adjustments of medications eliminated through the kidney, as well as the provision of adequate nutrition.

With regards to fluid resuscitation, there is no difference in survival when comparing crystalloids with colloids (albumin).[52] In patients with head trauma, colloid resuscitation has been found to increase mortality.[53] In addition, synthetic colloids, in particular hydroxyethyl starch with high molecular weights, are associated with an increased incidence of kidney injury.[54]

Furthermore, though fluid resuscitation can be crucial in these patients, a positive fluid balance is also associated with increased mortality.[55] However, AKI secondary to rhabdomyolysis should get adequate fluid resuscitation. The role of diuretic agents in the treatment of AKI remains controversial.[38,56] Diuretics did not improve overall mortality, need for RRT, or shorten the duration of AKI.[56]

At present, there is no evidence supporting the routine use of diuretics in patients with AKI or to convert oliguric renal failure to nonoliguric renal failure. In addition, there is no consensus regarding the most appropriate time to start RRT for AKI and should be individualized. However, severe hyperkalemia, severe metabolic acidosis, and uremic complications such as encephalopathy, pericarditis, pleuritis or bleeding diathesis, and volume overload are generally considered to be absolute indications for RRT, which could either be continuous or intermittent.[57] The choice of modality depends on the local expertise. Continuous RRT as a first modality in patients with severe AKI has not been shown to improve survival or renal recovery compared to intermittent hemodialysis.[58]

Similarly, there is also no consensus regarding the dose of hemofiltration or the renal replacement modality, i.e., continuous versus intermittent. A detailed description of modes of RRT is beyond the scope of this chapter.

PREVENTION OF ACUTE KIDNEY INJURY

Early recognition of underlying risk factors and prevention of additional injuries in high-risk patients are particularly important. Maintaining adequate renal perfusion, prevention of hyperglycemia, and avoidance of nephrotoxins are some of the strategies used for this purpose.

Radioiodine contrast-induced nephropathy can be prevented by using a low-volume nonionic low-osmolar or iso-osmolar agent in a well-hydrated patient. There is no significant advantage in using sodium bicarbonate over sodium chloride solution.[59] Prophylactic administration of N-acetylcysteine to prevent renal failure is also controversial.[60] In patients who must undergo radiological studies utilizing contrast, adequate hydration, use of prophylactic N-acetyl cysteine, avoidance of other nephrotoxic agents, and use of low-volume nonionic low or iso-osmolar agents are recommended.

Acute kidney injury is common in patients with hepatic failure admitted to ICUs. In cirrhotic patients requiring large-volume paracentesis and in patients with spontaneous bacterial peritonitis, the administration of intravenous albumin decreases the incidence of AKI.[38] In patients with hepatorenal syndrome, the use of terlipressin with albumin has been shown to improve kidney function.[61] Noradrenaline has also been reported to be as effective as terlipressin in decreasing serum creatinine.[62] Similarly, other agents such as octreotide and midodrine have been found useful in this condition.[63] Nonetheless, the definitive treatment for hepatorenal syndrome is liver transplantation.

SUMMARY

Acute kidney failure is common in critically ill patients and is associated with a significant increase in mortality. Prevention of renal injury is important. Most of the treatment modalities are controversial and need further studies.

REFERENCES

1. Hebert PC, Tinmouth A, Corwin H. Anemia and red cell transfusion in critically ill patients. Crit Care Med. 2003;31:S672-7.
2. DeBellis RJ. Anemia in critical care patients: incidence, etiology, impact, management, and use of treatment guidelines and protocols. Am J Health Syst Pharm. 2007;64:S14-21.
3. Corwin HL. Anemia and blood transfusion in the critically ill patient: role of erythropoietin. Crit Care. 2004;8(Suppl 2):S42-4.
4. Fink MP. Pathophysiology of intensive care unit-acquired anemia. Crit Care. 2004;8(Suppl 2):S9-10.
5. Shander A. Anemia in the critically ill. Crit Care Clin. 2004;20: 159-70.
6. Spinelli E, Bartlett RH. Anemia and Transfusion in Critical Care: Physiology and Management. J Intensive Care Med. 2016;31(5): 295-306.
7. Fowler RA, Rizoli SB, Levin PD, et al. Blood conservation for critically ill patients. Crit Care Clin. 2004;20:313-24.
8. Carson J, Carless P. Hebert P. Outcomes using lower vs higher hemoglobin threshold for red blood cell transfusion. JAMA. 2013;309(1):83-4.
9. Hebert PC, Wells G, Blajchman MA, et al. A multicenter, randomized, controlled clinical trial of transfusion requirements in critical care. Transfusion Requirements in Critical Care Investigators, Canadian Critical Care Trials Group. N Engl J Med. 1999; 340:409-17.
10. Rhode J, Dimcheff D, Blumberg N, et al. Health care-associated infection after red blood cell transfusion; a systematic review and meta-analysis. JAMA. 2014;311:1317-26.
11. Bain BJ. Diagnosis from the blood smear. N Engl J Med. 2005; 353:498-507.
12. Corwin HL, Gettinger A, Pearl RG, et al. Efficacy of recombinant human erythropoietin in critically ill patients: a randomized controlled trial. JAMA. 2002;288:2827-35.
13. Corwin HL, Gettinger A, Fabian TC, et al. Efficacy and safety of epoetin alfa in critically ill patients. N Engl J Med. 2007;357: 965-76.
14. Spahn DR, Cerny V, Coats TJ, et al. Management of bleeding following major trauma: a European guideline. Crit Care. 2007; 11:R17.
15. Carson JL, Broos MM, Abbott J, et al. Liberal versus restrictive transfusion threshold for patients with symptomatic coronary artery disease. Am Heart J. 2013;165:964-71.
16. Napolitano LM, Kurek S, Luchette FA, et al. Clinical practice guideline. red blood cell transfusion in adult trauma and critical care. Crit Care Med. 2009;37:3124-57.
17. Pham Hp, Shaz BH. Update on massive transfusion. Br J Anaesth. 2013;111 Suppl 1:i72-82.
18. Vanderschueren S, De Weerdt A, Malbrain M, et al. Thrombocytopenia and prognosis in intensive care. Crit Care Med. 2000;28:1871-6.
19. Rice TW, Wheeler AP. Coagulopathy in critically ill patients: part 1: platelet disorders. Chest. 2009;136:1622-30.
20. Moreau D, Timsit JF, Vesin A, et al. Platelet count decline: an early prognostic marker in critically ill patients with prolonged ICU stays. Chest. 2007;131:1735-41.
21. Mercer KW, Gail Macik B, Williams ME. Hematologic disorders in critically ill patients. Semin Respir Crit Care Med. 2006;27: 286-96.
22. Strauss R, Wehler M, Mehler K, et al. Thrombocytopenia in patients in the medical intensive care unit: bleeding prevalence, transfusion requirements, and outcome. Crit Care Med. 2002; 30:1765-71.
23. Aster RH, Bougie DW. Drug-induced immune thrombocytopenia. N Engl J Med. 2007;357:580-7.

24. Stanworth S, Estcourt L, Powter G, et al. A no-prophylaxis platelet-transfusion strategy for hematologic cancers. N Engl J Med. 2013;368:1771-80.
25. Slichter SJ, Kaufman RM, Assmann SF, et al. Dose of prophylactic platelet transfusions and prevention of hemorrhage. N Engl J Med. 2010;362:600-13.
26. Vassallo R. Management of the platelet-transfusion-refractory patient. In: Sweeney JD, Lozano M (Eds). Platelet Transfusion Therapy, 1st edition. Bethesda: AABB Press; 2013. pp. 321-58.
27. Spring J, Munshi L. Hematology Emergencies in Critically Ill Adults: Benign Hematology. Chest. 2022;161(5):1285-96.
28. Bichon A, Bourenne J, Allardet-Servent J, et al. High Mortality of HLH in ICU Regardless Etiology or Treatment. Front Med (Lausanne). 2021;8:735796.
29. Hajjar LA, Auler Junior J, Santos L, et al. Blood transfusion in critically ill patients: state of the art. Clinics (Sao Paulo). 2007; 62:507-24.
30. Klein HG, Spahn DR, Carson JL. Red blood cell transfusion in clinical practice. Lancet. 2007;370:415-26.
31. Rodgers GM. Prothrombin complex concentrates in emergency bleeding disorders. Am J Hematol. 2012;87:898-902.
32. Shakur H, Roberts I, Bautista R, et al. Effects of tranexamic acid on death, vascular occlusive events, and blood transfusion in trauma patients with significant haemorrhage (CRASH-2); a randomized controlled trial. Lancet. 2011;377:10961101.
33. Majeed A, Schulman S. Bleeding and antidotes in new oral anticoagulants. Best Pract Clin Haematol. 2013;26:191-202.
34. Goodnough LT. A reappraisal of plasma, prothrombin complex concentrates, and recombinant factor VIIa in patient blood management. Crit Care Clin. 2012;28:413426.
35. Vincent JL, Francois B, Zabolotskikh I, et al.; SCARLET Trial Group. Effect of a Recombinant Human Soluble Thrombomodulin on Mortality in Patients With Sepsis-Associated Coagulopathy: The SCARLET Randomized Clinical Trial. JAMA. 2019;321(20):1993-2002.
36. Kellum JA. Acute kidney injury. Crit Care Med. 2008;36:S141-5.
37. Venkataraman R, Kellum JA. Prevention of acute renal failure. Chest. 2007;131:300308.
38. Abuelo JG. Normotensive ischemic acute renal failure. N Engl J Med. 2007;357:797805.
39. Dennen P, Douglas IS, Anderson R. Acute kidney injury in the intensive care unit: an update and primer for the intensivist. Crit Care Med. 2010;38:261-75.
40. Kellum JA, Levin N, Bouman C, et al. Developing a consensus classification system for acute renal failure. Curr Opin Crit Care. 2002;8:509-14.
41. Uchino S, Kellum JA, Bellomo R, et al. Acute renal failure in critically ill patients: a multinational, multicenter study. JAMA. 2005;294:813-8.
42. Nisula S, Kaukonen KM, Vaara ST, et al.; FINNAKI Study Group. Incidence, risk factors and 90-day mortality of patients with acute kidney injury in Finnish intensive care units: The FINNAKI study. Intensive Care Med. 2013;39:420-8.
43. Mehta RL, Chertow GM. Acute renal failure definitions and classification: time for change? J Am Soc Nephrol. 2003;14: 2178-87.
44. Bellomo R. Defining, quantifying, and classifying acute renal failure. Crit Care Clin. 2005;21:223-37.
45. Bellomo R, Ronco C, Kellum JA, et al. Acute renal failure - definition, outcome measures, animal models, fluid therapy and information technology needs: the Second International Consensus Conference of the Acute Dialysis Quality Initiative (ADQI) Group. Crit Care. 2004;8:R204-12.
46. Mehta RL, Kellum JA, Shah SV, et al. Acute Kidney Injury Network: report of an initiative to improve outcomes in acute kidney injury. Crit Care. 2007;11:R31.
47. Crowley S, Peixoto A. Acute kidney injury in the intensive care unit. Clin Chest Med. 2009;30:29-43.
48. Case J, Khan S, Khan A. Epidemiology of acute kidney injury in the intensive care unit. Crit Care Res Pract. 2013;2013:449730.
49. Hoste EA, De Waele JJ. Physiologic consequences of acute renal failure on the critically ill. Crit Care Clin. 2005;21:251-60.
50. Himmelfarb J, Joannidis M, Molitoris B, et al. Evaluation and initial management of acute kidney injury. Clin J Am Soc Nephrol. 2008;3:962-7.
51. DeGeus HRN, Betjes MG, Bakker J. Biomarkers for the prediction of acute kidney injury: a narrative review on current status and future challenges. Clin Kidney J. 2012;5(2):102-8.
52. Finfer S, Bellomo R, Boyce N, et al. A comparison of albumin and saline for fluid resuscitation in the intensive care unit. N Engl J Med. 2004;350:2247-56.
53. Myburgh J, Cooper DJ, Finfer S, et al. Saline or albumin for fluid resuscitation in patients with traumatic brain injury. N Engl J Med. 2007;357:874-84.
54. Wiedermann CJ. Systematic review of randomized clinical trials on the use of hydroxyethyl starch for fluid management in sepsis. BMC Emerg Med. 2008;8:1.
55. Payen D, de Pont AC, Sakr Y, et al. A positive fluid balance is associated with a worse outcome in patients with acute renal failure. Crit Care. 2008;12:R74.
56. Nadeau-Fredette AC, Bouchard J. Fluid management and the use of diuretics in acute kidney injury. Adv Chronic Kidney Dis. 2013;20:45-55.
57. KDIGO Workgroup. Dialysis Interventions for treatment of AKI. Kidney Int Suppl. 2012;2:89-115.
58. Gaudry S, Grolleau F, Barbar S, et al. Continuous renal replacement therapy versus intermittent hemodialysis as first modality for renal replacement therapy in severe acute kidney injury: a secondary analysis of AKIKI and IDEAL-ICU studies. Crit Care. 2022;26(1):93.
59. Brar SS, Shen AY, Jorgensen MB, et al. Sodium bicarbonate vs sodium chloride for the prevention of contrast medium-induced nephropathy in patients undergoing coronary angiography: a randomized trial. JAMA. 2008;300:1038-46.
60. Gonzales DA, Norsworthy KJ, Kern SJ, et al. A meta-analysis of N-acetylcysteine in contrast-induced nephrotoxicity: unsupervised clustering to resolve heterogeneity. BMC Med. 2007;5:32.
61. Wong F, Pappas SC, Curry MP, et al.; CONFIRM Study Investigators. Terlipressin plus Albumin for the Treatment of Type 1 Hepatorenal Syndrome. N Engl J Med. 2021;384(9):818-28.
62. Sharma P, Kumar A, Shrama BC, et al. An open label, pilot, randomized controlled trial of noradrenaline versus terlipressin in the treatment of type 1 hepatorenal syndrome and predictors of response. Am J Gastroenterol. 2008;103:1689-97.
63. Skagen C, Einstein M, Lucey MR, et al. Combination treatment with octreotide, midodrine, and albumin improves survival in patients with type 1 and type 2 hepatorenal syndrome. J Clin Gastroenterol. 2009;43:680-5.

Nonpulmonary Critical Care III (Endocrinal and Neurological Problems)

Liziamma George, Ivan Wong

CHAPTER 168

INTRODUCTION

Patients with endocrine emergencies are commonly admitted to critical care units. The accurate and early diagnosis of these entities is important for better outcomes in these patients. In this section, we discuss the clinical presentation, diagnosis, and management of common endocrine emergencies.

THYROID STORM

Hyperthyroid patients present with palpitations, unexplained weight loss, diarrhea, intolerance to heat, and muscle weakness. A thyroid storm is an endocrine emergency that is characterized by multiple organ failure due to thyrotoxicosis and is associated with 8–25% mortality.[1,2] The common causes are Graves' disease, chronic and subacute thyroiditis, toxic thyroid adenoma, postpartum thyroiditis, and excessive iodine intake. It can also be precipitated by stress, surgery, sepsis, or cardiovascular events in a preexisting hyperthyroid patient.

Clinical and Diagnostic Features

Patients can present with cardiac arrhythmias, widened pulse pressure, congestive heart failure, systemic inflammatory response syndrome, hypotension, psychosis, delirium, and coma. A scoring system based on the signs and symptoms seen in thyroid storm is commonly used **(Table 1)**.[3] The laboratory findings specific to the thyroid gland include a low or undetectable thyroid-stimulating hormone (TSH) level and a high thyroxine (T4) level.

TABLE 1: The scoring system for the clinical evaluation of a thyroid storm.

Thermoregulatory dysfunction		**Cardiovascular dysfunction**	
Temperature		Tachycardia	
99–99.9	5	99–109	5
100–100.9	10	110–119	10
101–101.9	15	120–129	15
102–102.9	20	130–139	20
103–103.9	25	≥140	25
≥104.0	30	**Congestive heart failure**	
Central nervous system effects		*Mild*	5
Mild	10	Pedal edema	
Agitation		*Moderate*	10
Moderate	20	Bibasilar rales	
Delirium, psychosis		*Severe*	15
Extreme lethargy		Pulmonary edema	
Severe	30	Atrial fibrillation	10
Seizure		**Precipitant history**	
Coma		Negative	0
Gastrointestinal (GI)/hepatic dysfunction		Positive	10
Moderate	10	**Total score**	**Diagnosis**
Diarrhea, abdominal pain		≥45	More likely
Nausea/vomiting		25–44	Suggestive
Severe	20	≤25	Less likely
Unexplained jaundice			

Management

The key is to start treatment as soon as the thyroid storm is clinically suspected. The therapeutic regimen involves the use of various agents. Patients should be stabilized with fluids if hypotensive or with diuretics in case of congestive heart failure. Adequate oxygenation should be maintained and often these patients may need mechanical ventilatory support. Fever should be controlled by cooling and the use of acetaminophen. After initial stabilization, therapy directed to decreasing adrenergic tone with beta-blockers should be given, with propranolol being the drug of choice. Propranolol is typically given 40–80 mg every 4–6 hours.

Specific treatment is given to reduce thyroid hormone synthesis by using thionamides. Either propylthiouracil or methimazole can be used. Propylthiouracil has the advantage of decreasing peripheral conversion of T4 to triiodothyronine (T3). Propylthiouracil is given at a dose of 200 mg every 4 hours and methimazole is given at a dose of 30 mg every 6 hours. Unlike propylthiouracil, methimazole cannot be given in pregnancy. The serious side effects of thionamides are agranulocytosis (dose dependent), antineutrophil cytoplasmic antibody- (ANCA)-positive vasculitis, and hepatic failure.

To prevent the release of synthesized thyroid hormone from the thyroid gland, Lugol's iodine (10 drops three times daily) or saturated solutions of potassium iodide [SSKI (five drops every 6 hours)] is given. It is important to give iodine only after giving thionamide agents to prevent the increase in thyroid hormone synthesis. Lithium carbonate also decreases the release of thyroid hormone but is rarely used due to its toxicity. Bile acid sequestrants such as cholestyramine (4 g given four times daily) are given in severe cases to reduce gut recycling of thyroid hormone. In patients who respond poorly to the abovementioned management, plasmapheresis and thyroidectomy have been used to treat thyroid storm.[1]

MYXEDEMA COMA

Myxedema coma is a rare but life-threatening complication that results from severe untreated hypothyroidism or long-standing hypothyroidism. It can be precipitated by trauma, surgery, severe infection, and cold stress, especially with the usage of sedative, hypnotic, and narcotic medications.[4]

Clinical and Diagnostic Features

Myxedema is characterized by distinct clinical features rather than by laboratory findings suggestive of hypothyroidism **(Table 2)**. The role of laboratory findings is to confirm the diagnosis and delineate coexisting or precipitating conditions. Low TSH levels along with low total and free serum T4 and T3 levels are noted in primary hypothyroidism. High TSH levels with below-normal levels of T3 are seen in secondary hypothyroidism. Low sodium levels with elevated levels of lactate dehydrogenase (LDH) and creatinine are also seen.

TABLE 2: The clinical features of myxedema coma based on the organ system involved.

System	Clinical features
Neurological	Mental obtundation, delayed relaxation phase of reflexes
Cardiovascular	Bradycardia, hypotension, electrocardiogram (EKG) changes, pericardial effusions
Endocrine	Hypoglycemia, hyponatremia, hypothermia
Respiratory	Hypoventilation, pleural effusions
Gastrointestinal	Paralytic ileus, ascites
Genitourinary	Atonic bladder, urinary retention
Integumentary	Alopecia, coarse dry skin, myxedema facies

Management

Because of the high mortality associated with this condition, patients should be monitored in the intensive care unit (ICU).[5] Supportive care, treatment of hypothermia, and monitoring of the neurological and respiratory status should be emphasized along with the supplementation of thyroid hormones **(Table 3)**.[6] The type of thyroid hormone replacement whether to use T4 alone, T3 alone, or both in combination is controversial. The concern with giving T4 alone in critically ill patients in myxedema coma is the potential reduced deiodination and conversion of T4 to T3, resulting in a delay in recovery. Although T3 is more active, when given high doses in patients with underlying cardiac disease, higher mortality rates have been reported.[7] Both thyroid storm and myxedema coma are associated with significant mortality and early recognition and treatment are important for a favorable outcome.

ACUTE ADRENAL INSUFFICIENCY

Acute adrenal insufficiency is seen in patients with bilateral adrenal hemorrhage, undiagnosed adrenal insufficiency with stress, trauma, surgery, drugs, especially etomidate and previous steroid therapy, and pituitary apoplexy.[8,9] Diagnosis is made on the basis of the clinical and laboratory features associated with acute adrenal insufficiency or adrenal crisis

TABLE 3: The management of myxedema coma in a critical care setting

Supportive care	• Invasive mechanical ventilation to bypass mechanical obstruction caused by large tongue • Fluid and vasopressor administration for hypotension • Passive rewarming for hypothermia • Stress-dose corticosteroids for possible coexisting adrenal insufficiency • Monitoring and correction of electrolyte abnormalities
Replacement of thyroid hormone	• Both T4 and T3 given intravenously • Bolus of 300–500 µg followed by 50–100 µg daily • Use caution in elderly patients and patients with myocardial injury • Pregnant patients may need higher doses
Management of coexisting conditions	Panculture and initiation of broad-spectrum antibiotics

(Box 1). Diagnosis is difficult due to the diurnal variation of cortisol secretion. Cortisol levels are higher in the morning and lower in the evening. A random morning cortisol level of <3 µg/dL is strongly suggestive of adrenal insufficiency.[10] The adrenocorticotropic hormone (ACTH) stimulation test or cosyntropin test is used to establish a definitive diagnosis of primary but not secondary adrenal insufficiency.[11] In cases of suspected adrenal crisis, treatment with hydrocortisone or dexamethasone should be started immediately and not delayed by confirmatory tests. The supportive measures include volume administration with isotonic fluids with glucose in case of hypoglycemia. Precipitating causes must be sought and treated. Management of adrenal insufficiency in patients with septic shock will be described elsewhere.

BOX 1 The clinical and laboratory findings seen in patients with adrenal crisis.

- Dehydration, hypotension, or shock out of proportion to severity of current illness
- Nausea and vomiting with a history of weight loss and anorexia
- Abdominal pain (acute abdomen)
- Unexplained hypoglycemia
- Unexplained fever
- Hyponatremia, hyperkalemia, azotemia, hypercalcemia, or eosinophilia
- Hyperpigmentation or vitiligo
- Other autoimmune endocrine deficiencies, such as hypothyroidism or gonadal failure

DIABETIC KETOACIDOSIS AND HYPEROSMOLAR HYPERGLYCEMIC STATE

Diabetic ketoacidosis (DKA), hyperosmolar hyperglycemic state (HHS), and drug-induced hypoglycemia are the major complications of diabetes mellitus. Both DKA and HHS are due to insulin deficiency and excessive counterregulatory hormones. A detailed description is beyond the scope of this chapter; however, a brief synopsis of pathogenesis, precipitating factors contributing to the development of DKA and HHS will help **(Flowchart 1 and Table 4)**.[12,13]

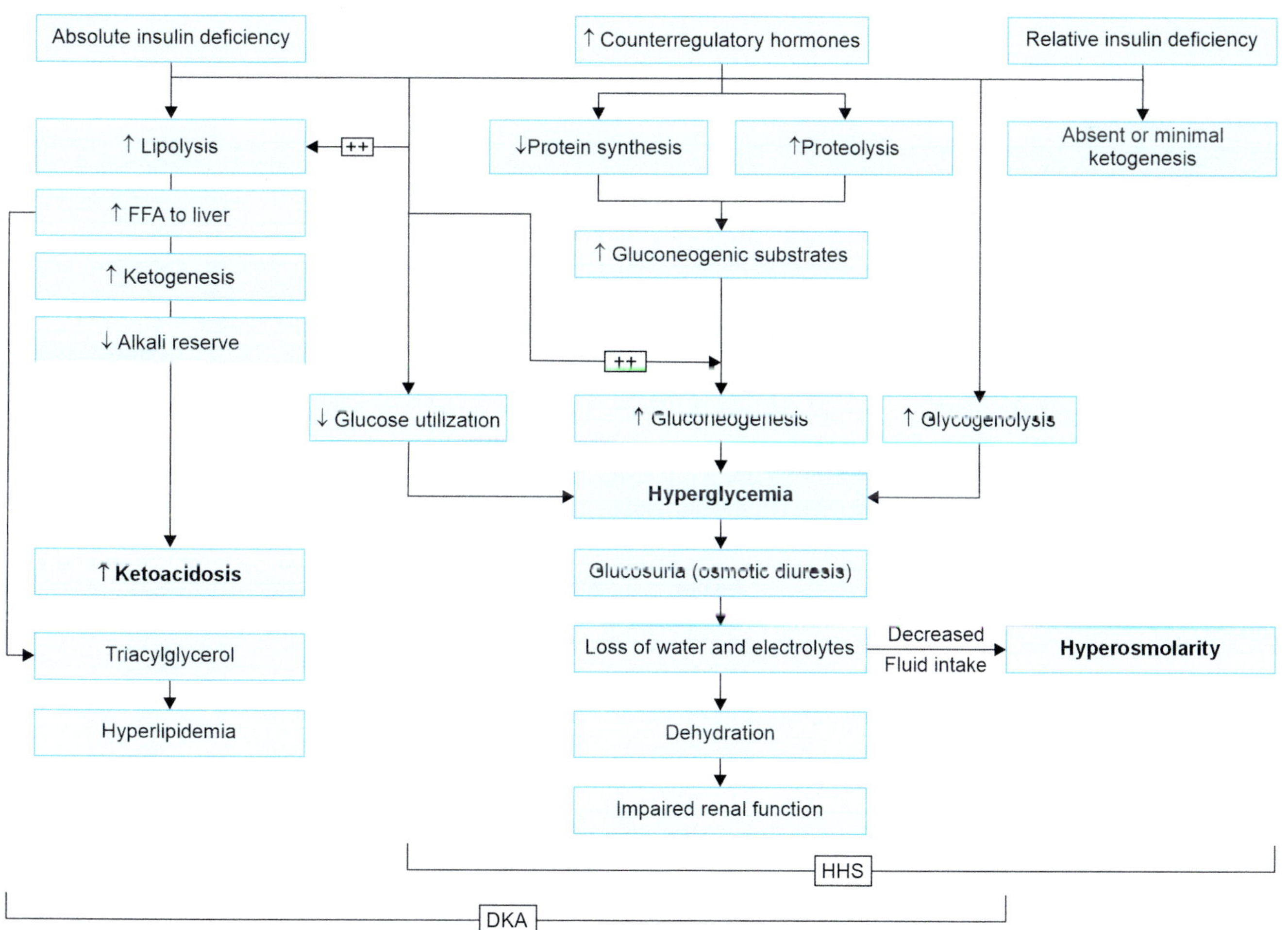

FLOWCHART 1: Pathophysiology of DKA and HHS.
(DKA: diabetic ketoacidosis; FFA: free fatty acid; HHS: hyperosmolar hyperglycemic syndrome)

Clinical and Diagnostic Features

Diabetic ketoacidosis and HHS patients usually present with nausea, vomiting, abdominal pain, shortness of breath, polyuria, and polydipsia. As the condition worsens, they develop neurological symptoms which may progress to coma. The initial evaluation should assess hemodynamic status and airways. The investigations to be performed include white blood cell (WBC) count, complete metabolic panel, plasma osmolality, urine analysis, serum and urine ketones, arterial blood gases, electrocardiogram (ECG), and chest X-ray (CXR) **(Table 5)**.[13] Metabolic acidosis is the hallmark of DKA **(Table 6)**.

Management

Patients should be managed in the ICU following a management algorithm **(Flowchart 2)**. If potassium is <3 mEq/L, replenish potassium to above 3.3 mEq/L before initiating insulin. Sodium bicarbonate is given only when the arterial pH is <7. The insulin infusion is typically continued until ketoacidosis is resolved. Blood glucose should

TABLE 4: Some precipitating factors that can contribute to the development of hyperosmolar hyperglycemic nonketotic syndrome and DKA.

Precipitating factors for HHS	
Inadequate insulin treatment or noncompliance	21–41%
Acute illness	32–60%
Infection	Pneumonia, urinary tract infection, sepsis
Neurological	CVA
Endocrine	Acromegaly, thyrotoxicosis, Cushing syndrome
Gastrointestinal	Peritoneal dialysis, mesenteric thrombosis, acute pancreatitis
Cardiopulmonary	Acute PE, MI
Other	Heat stroke, hypothermia, severe burns
Predisposing factors for DKA	
Inadequate insulin treatment or noncompliance	Most common cause
New-onset diabetes	20–25%
Acute illness	Infection (30–40%), CVA, MI, acute pancreatitis
Drugs	Infection (30–40%), CVA, MI, acute pancreatitis

(CVA: cerebrovascular accident; DKA: diabetic ketoacidosis; HHS: hyperosmolar hyperglycemic state; MI: myocardial infarction; PE: pulmonary embolus)

TABLE 5: The criteria utilized in diagnosing diabetic ketoacidosis (DKA) and hyperosmolar hyperglycemic syndrome (HHS).

	DKA			
Parameter	**Mild**	**Moderate**	**Severe**	**HHS**
Plasma glucose (mg/dL)	>250	>250	>250	>600
Arterial pH	7.25–7.30	7.00–7.24	<7.00	>7.30
Serum bicarbonate (mEq/L)	15–18	10 to <15	<10	>18
Urine ketones	Positive	Positive	Positive	Small
Serum ketones	Positive	Positive	Positive	Small
Effective serum osmolality (mOsm/kg)	Variable	Variable	Variable	>320
Anion gap	>10	>12	>12	Variable
Alteration in sensoria or mental obtundation	Alert	Alert/drowsy	Stupor/coma	Stupor/coma

TABLE 6: The laboratory evaluation of the metabolic causes of acidosis and coma.

	Starvation or high fat intake	DKA	Lactic acidosis	Uremic acidosis	Alcoholic ketosis (starvation)	Salicylate intoxication	Methanol or ethylene glycol intoxication	Hyperosmolar coma	Hypoglycemic coma	Rhabdomyolysis
pH	Normal	↓	↓	Mild ↓	↓↑	↓↑	↓	Normal	Normal	Mild ↓ may be ↓↓
Plasma glucose	Normal	↑	Normal	Normal	↓ or normal	Normal or ↓	Normal	↑↑ >500 mg/dL	↓↓ <30 mg/dL	Normal
Glycosuria	Negative	++	Negative	Negative	Negative	Negative•	Negative	++	Negative	Negative
Total plasma ketones Δ	Slight ↑	↑↑	Normal	Normal	Slight to moderate ↑	Normal	Normal	Normal or slight ↑	Normal or slight ↑	Normal
Anion gap	Slight ↑	↑	↑	Slight ↑	↑	↑	↑	Normal	Normal or slight ↑	↑↑
Osmolality	Normal	↑	Normal	↑	Normal	Normal	↑↑	↑↑ >330 mOsm/kg	Normal	Normal or slight ↑
Uric acid	Mild (starvation)	↑	Normal	Normal	↑	Normal	Normal	Normal	Normal	↑
Miscellaneous		May give false positive for ethylene glycol	Serum lactate > 7 mmol/L	BUN > 200 mg/dL		Serum salicylate positive	Serum levels positive			Myoglobinuria, hemoglobinuria

- Acetest and Ketostix measure acetoacetic acid only—values obtained may be misleading and low because the majority of ketone bodies are β-hydroxybutyrate; + Positive
- Respiratory alkalosis/metabolic acidosis; Δ may get false-positive or false-negative urinary glucose caused by the presence of salicylate or its metabolites.

(BUN: blood urea nitrogen; DKA: diabetes ketoacidosis)

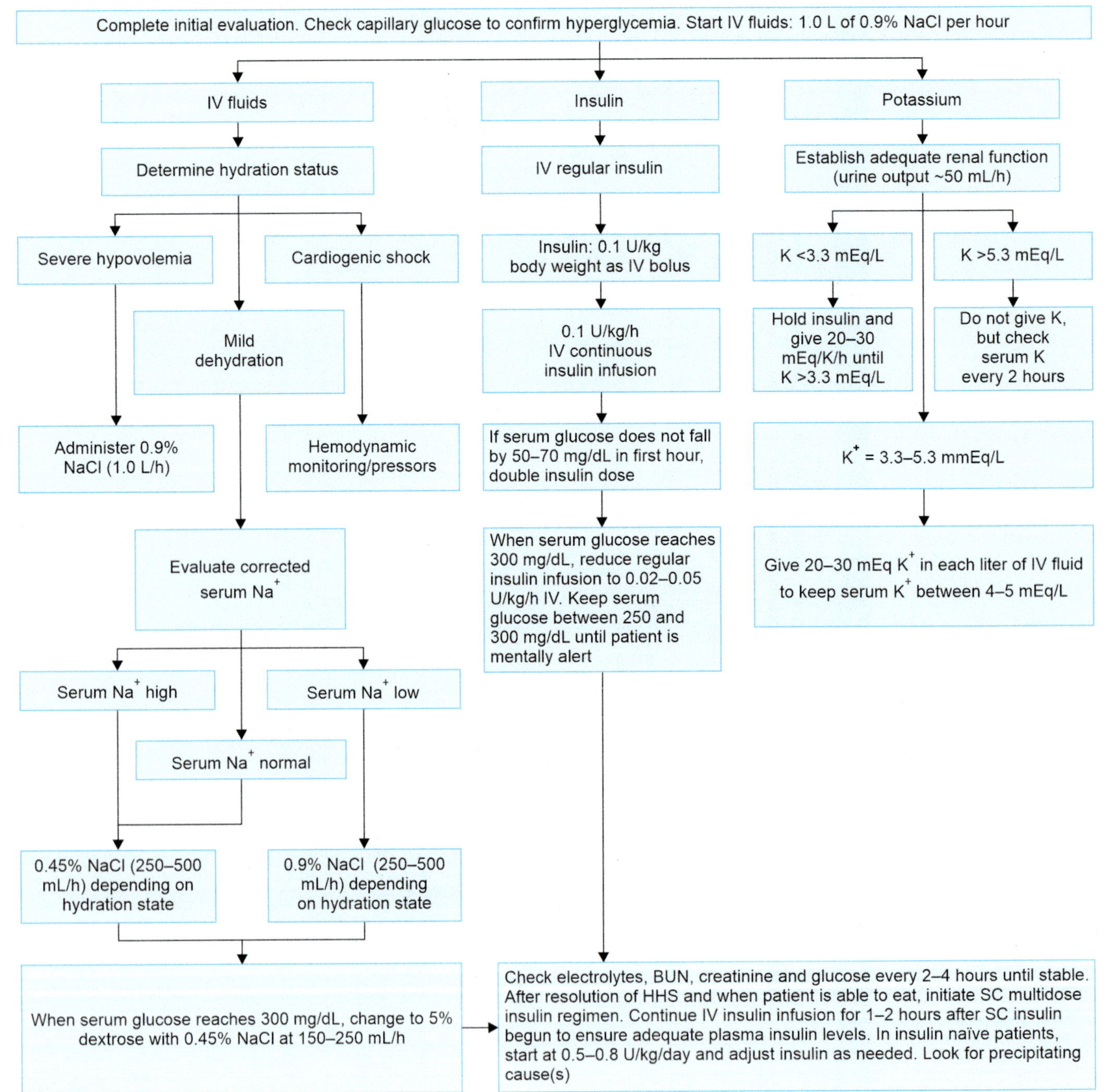

FLOWCHART 2: Algorithm on the management of patients with hyperosmolar hyperglycemic nonketotic syndrome and diabetic ketoacidosis.

(BUN: blood urea nitrogen; HHS: hyperosmolar hyperglycemic; IV: intravenous; SC: subcutaneous)

be monitored every hour while on an insulin infusion, while other laboratory tests, i.e., basic metabolic profile are monitored every 3–4 hours. The complications of untreated DKA and HHS are cerebral edema, particularly in children, and noncardiogenic pulmonary edema.[14] Patients must be monitored for hypoglycemia and hypokalemia. Almost all patients with DKA develop a nonanion gap metabolic acidosis with treatment and phosphate repletion is not recommended for patients with DKA.

Hypoglycemia in diabetic patients occurs either due to insulin excess or because of failure of the counterregulatory hormones. Symptoms and signs are usually nonspecific.

Severe hypoglycemia causes seizure and coma and should be treated with glucagon 0.5–1 mg subcutaneously or intramuscularly, as well as intravenous (IV) glucose (dextrose).

NEUROLOGICAL DISORDERS IN CRITICAL CARE

ACUTE ISCHEMIC STROKE

A stroke is a focal neurological deficit that is typically of acute onset and results from a disruption of the cerebral blood flow. It usually occurs suddenly but occasionally progresses in a more gradual fashion. Many stroke presentations result from cerebral ischemia, while hemorrhage (intracerebral or subarachnoid) causes the rest.[15] Acute ischemic stroke is being discussed here while intracerebral and subarachnoid hemorrhages (SAH) are discussed in subsequent chapters. The mechanisms causing ischemic strokes could be grouped into atherothrombotic, cardioembolic, lacunar, and cryptogenic types **(Table 7)**. Strokes may result in permanent disability and prognosis tends to be poorer in older patients, as well as patients with underlying comorbidities such as diabetes or heart disease.[15] Time is of the essence in the management of these patients. The advent and widespread utilization of thrombolytic therapy within 4.5 hours of developing ischemic stroke has revolutionized the management of what was once considered a condition with few treatment choices.[16-19] Despite this, up to 69% of stroke patients are ineligible to receive thrombolytic therapy due to delayed hospital presentation.[16] Endovascular therapy (EVT) has therefore further revolutionized the management of acute ischemic stroke.

Clinical Features

Thrombotic strokes tend to present with clinical features that evolve over hours to days, whereas embolic strokes have a sudden or rapid onset at maximum severity at the time of presentation. The pattern of neurological impairment will depend on the vascular territory involved **(Table 8)**.

Diagnosis

It is essential to obtain a comprehensive history, particularly determining the time of symptom onset, any recent events such as trauma, surgery, myocardial infarction, prior stroke, medication use such as anticoagulants, insulin, or antihypertensives, and evaluation of other comorbidities.[15] A complete physical examination with emphasis on the neurological system should also be performed when a

TABLE 7: The different pathophysiological mechanisms contributing to the development of ischemic stroke.

Pathophysiology	Frequency of ischemic stroke
Atherosclerotic cerebrovascular disease • Hypoperfusion • Arteriogenic emboli	20%
Lacunar (small penetrating artery disease) • Arterial thrombosis 2°atheroma formation or lip hyalinosis	25%
Cardiogenic embolism • Atrial fibrillation • Valvular heart disease • Atrial or ventricular thrombi • Atrial myxoma • Bacterial endocarditis	20%
Cryptogenic	30%
Other • Prothrombotic states • Dissections • Arteritis • Migraines/vasospasms • Drug abuse	5%

TABLE 8: The clinical presentation of acute ischemic stroke in relation to the vascular region involved.

Vascular territory	Neurological deficit
Anterior cerebral artery	Contralateral hemiparesis and hemisensory deficit (leg > arm), urinary incontinence, abulia, confusion, primitive reflexes (sucking, grasp), apraxia
Middle cerebral artery	Contralateral hemiparesis and hemisensory deficit (face and arm > leg and foot), homonymous hemianopsia, ipsilateral gaze preference, aphasia (Broca's and Wernicke) with dominant (left-sided) hemisphere lesion, neglect with no-dominant (right-sided) hemisphere lesion
Posterior cerebral artery	Contralateral hemiparesis and hemisensory deficit, altered mental status, ophthalmoplegia from third cranial nerve palsy, macular-sparing homonymous hemianopsia, visual agnosia, visual hallucinations, alexia without agraphia, disorders of color perception, amnesia
Vertebrobasilar	Deficits involve the medulla (medial or lateral medullary syndrome), pons (locked-in syndrome), midbrain, and cerebellum and consist of dysphagia, dysarthria, diplopia, dizziness, vertigo, nausea, vomiting, Horner's syndrome, cranial nerve palsies, limb and gait ataxia, and motor and sensory deficits involving both parts of the body
Lacunar	Pure hemiparesis, pure hemisensory deficit, ataxic hemiparesis, dysarthria–clumsy hand

patient presents with a neurological deficit suggestive of an ischemic event. Certain conditions that are known to mimic the clinical features of ischemic strokes include but are not limited to intracranial bleeds, seizures with postictal paresis, syncope, systemic infection, brain tumors, complicated migraines, conversion disorders, and hypertensive encephalopathy.[15] It is important to distinguish these mimics from ischemic strokes to treat the patients appropriately. The National Institute of Health Stroke Scale (NIHSS) is a 42-point scale based on neurological deficits elicited by physical examination **(Table 9)**. It is commonly utilized to quantify the severity of the neurological deficit. Initial general

TABLE 9: The National Institute of Health Stroke Scale (NIHSS). A score of ≥16 is associated with a high likelihood of severe disability or death, while a score of ≤6 is associated with a good prognosis.

Entity	Score
1a. *Level of consciousness*: A 3 is scored only if the patient makes no movement (other than reflexive posturing) in response to noxious stimulation.	• 0 = Alert; keenly responsive • 1 = Not alert; but arousable by minor stimulation to obey, answer, or respond. • 2 = Not alert; requires repeated stimulation to attend, or is obtunded and requires strong or painful stimulation to make movements (not stereotyped) • 3 = Responds only with reflex motor or autonomic effects or totally unresponsive, flaccid, and areflexic
1b. *LOC questions*: The patient is asked the month and his/her age. The answer must be correct—there is no partial credit for being close.	• 0 = Answers both questions correctly • 1 = Answers one question correctly • 2 = Answers neither question correctly
1c. *LOC commands*: The patient is asked to open and close the eyes and then to grip and release the nonparetic hand. Substitute another one-step command if the hands cannot be used.	• 0 = Performs both tasks correctly • 1 = Performs one task correctly • 2 = Performs neither task correctly
2. *Best gaze*: Only horizontal eye movements will be tested. Voluntary or reflexive (oculocephalic) eye movements will be scored, but caloric testing is not done.	• 0 = Normal. • 1 = Partial gaze palsy; gaze is abnormal in one or both eyes, but forced deviation or total gaze paresis is not present • 2 = Forced deviation, or total gaze paresis not overcome by the oculocephalic maneuver
3. *Visual*: Visual fields (upper and lower quadrants) are tested by confrontation, using finger counting or visual threat, as appropriate. Patients may be encouraged, but if they look at the side of the moving fingers appropriately, this can be scored as normal. If there is unilateral blindness or enucleation, visual fields in the remaining eye are scored.	• 0 = No visual loss • 1 = Partial hemianopia • 2 = Complete hemianopia • 3 = Bilateral hemianopia (blind including cortical blindness)
4. *Facial palsy*: Ask—or use pantomime to encourage—the patient to show teeth or raise eyebrows and close eyes. Score symmetry of grimace in response to noxious stimuli in the poorly responsive or noncomprehending patient.	• 0 = Normal symmetrical movements • 1 = Minor paralysis (flattened nasolabial fold, asymmetry on smiling) • 2 = Partial paralysis (total or near-total paralysis of lower face) • 3 = Complete paralysis of one or both sides (absence of facial movement in the upper and lower face)
5. *Motor arm*: The limb is placed in the appropriate position: Extend the arms (palms down) 90°(if sitting) or 45°(if supine). Drift is scored if the arm falls before 10 seconds. The aphasic patient is encouraged using urgency in the voice and pantomime but not noxious stimulation. Each limb is tested in turn, beginning with the nonparetic arm. Only in the case of amputation or joint fusion at the shoulder, the examiner should record the score as untestable (UN) and clearly write the explanation for this choice.	• 0 = No drift; limb holds 90 (or 45) degrees for full 10 seconds • 1 = Drift; limb holds 90 (or 45) degrees but drifts down before full 10 seconds; does not hit bed or other support • 2 = Some effort against gravity; limb cannot get to or maintain (if cued) 90 (or 45) degrees, drifts down to bed but has some effort against gravity • 3 = No effort against gravity; limb falls • 4 = No movement • UN = Amputation or joint fusion • 5a. Left arm • 5b. Right arm

Continued

Continued

Entity	Score
6. *Motor leg*: The limb is placed in the appropriate position—hold the leg at 30°(always tested supine). Drift is scored if the leg falls before 5 seconds. The aphasic patient is encouraged to use urgency in the voice and pantomime but not noxious stimulation.	• 0 = No drift; leg holds 30°position for full 5 seconds • 1 = Drift; leg falls by the end of the 5-second period but does not hit bed • 2 = Some effort against gravity; leg falls to bed by 5 seconds but has some effort against gravity • 3 = No effort against gravity; leg falls to bed immediately • 4 = No movement • UN = Amputation or joint fusion • 6a. Left leg • 6b. Right leg
7. *Limb ataxia*: This item is aimed at finding evidence of a unilateral cerebellar lesion. Test with eyes open. In case of visual defect, ensure testing is done in an intact visual field.	• 0 = Absent • 1 = Present in one limb • 2 = Present in two limbs • UN = Amputation or joint fusion
8. *Sensory*: Sensation or grimace to pinprick when tested, or withdrawal from noxious stimulus in the obtunded or aphasic patient. Only sensory loss attributed to stroke is scored as abnormal and the examiner should test as many body areas [arms (not hands), legs, trunk, face] as needed to accurately check for hemisensory loss.	• 0 = Normal; no sensory loss • 1 = Mild-to-moderate sensory loss; patient feels pinprick is less sharp or is dull on the affected side; or there is a loss of superficial pain with pinprick, but patient is aware of being touched • 2 = Severe to total sensory loss; patient is not aware of being touched in the face, arm, and leg
9. *Best language*: A great deal of information about comprehension will be obtained during the preceding sections of the examination. For this scale item, the patient is asked to describe what is happening in the attached picture, name the items on the attached naming sheet, and to read from the attached list of sentences.	• 0 = No aphasia; normal • 1 = Mild-to-moderate aphasia; some obvious loss of fluency or facility of comprehension, without significant limitation on ideas expressed or form of expression. Reduction of speech and/or comprehension, however, makes conversation about provided materials difficult or impossible. For example, in conversation about provided materials, examiner can identify picture or naming card content from patient's response • 2 = Severe aphasia; all communication is through fragmentary expression; great need for inference, questioning, and guessing by the listener. Range of information that can be exchanged is limited; listener carries burden of communication. Examiner cannot identify materials provided from patient response • 3 = Mute, global aphasia; no usable speech or auditory comprehension
10. *Dysarthria*: If patient is thought to be normal, an adequate sample of speech must be obtained by asking patient to read or repeat words from the attached list.	• 0 = Normal • 1 = Mild-to-moderate dysarthria; patient slurs at least some words and, at worst, can be understood with some difficulty • 2 = Severe dysarthria; patient's speech is so slurred as to be unintelligible in the absence of or out of proportion to any dysphasia, or is mute/anarthric UN = Intubated or other physical barrier
11. *Extinction and inattention (formerly neglect)*: Sufficient information to identify neglect may be obtained during the prior testing.	• 0 = No abnormality • 1 = Visual, tactile, auditory, spatial, or personal inattention or extinction to bilateral simultaneous stimulation in one of the sensory modalities • 2 = Profound hemi-inattention or extinction to more than one modality; does not recognize own hand or orients to only one side of space

tests to be performed include complete blood count (CBC), coagulation profile, serum electrolytes, serum glucose, renal function, electrocardiography, and chest radiography. Specific tests that are to be performed promptly are computed tomography (CT) scan or magnetic resonance imaging (MRI) of the brain to distinguish the etiology and nature of the stroke, and later once the diagnosis is established, carotid duplex ultrasonography and transthoracic echocardiography with or without bubble contrast.[15]

Management

The initial management at the time of presentation involves stabilizing the patient and performing a prompt clinical evaluation, as well as laboratory and imaging studies, thereby assessing the need for resuscitation, oxygen supplementation or intubation, fever, blood sugar, or blood pressure control, and thrombolysis. Fever, hyperglycemia, and hypotension following an ischemic stroke have been associated with poorer outcomes and should be treated. Immediate treatment of hypertension is controversial and currently recommended for patients with systolic pressures > 220 mm Hg not undergoing fibrinolysis. The National Institute of Neurological Disorders and Stroke Recombinant Tissue Plasminogen Activator (NINDS rt-PA) stroke trial demonstrated that ischemic stroke patients treated with thrombolysis using IV recombinant tissue plasminogen activator (rt-PA), i.e., alteplase within 3 hours after the onset of symptoms were 31–50% more likely to have a better clinical outcome at 3 months in contrast to the 20–38% in those who received placebo, although there was no difference in mortality.[20,21] Despite being the only available treatment during its time, of all patients with acute ischemic stroke, only up to 5.2% of patients received IV thrombolytic therapy. The main reason for this is that the limited time window excluded many potential candidates. Therefore, the American Stroke Association extended the r-tPA window from 3 to 4.5 hours in 2009, which increased the utilization of tPA to 20% of acute ischemic stroke patients.[16] In patients who wake up with stroke symptoms with an unclear time of symptom onset, diffusion-weighted MRI can be useful to identify potential IV r-tPA candidates if they are within 4.5 hours of stroke symptom recognition.[16,18] There is an associated risk of intracranial hemorrhage associated with thrombolysis. Prevention of this complication is of the utmost importance; therefore, only carefully selected patients who fulfill certain criteria **(Box 2)** can receive thrombolysis.

Patients need to be monitored closely either in an ICU or stroke unit following thrombolysis, with vital sign checks every 15 minutes for 2 hours, then every 30 minutes for 6 hours, and then every hour for 16 hours. Additionally, arterial punctures need to be avoided and all antiplatelet or anticoagulation therapy should be withheld for the first 24 hours following r-tPA administration because of the increased risk of bleeding. EVT, in addition to standard medical care, has improved overall outcomes in patients with acute ischemic stroke. Patients who are eligible for IV thrombolysis should receive IV alteplase even if EVT is being considered as it has also been shown to improve outcomes in this subset of patients as well.[16,18,22] Studies have also shown that the time window for EVT may be extended to 24 hours post symptom onset in patients with a mismatch between clinical deficit and the infarct size or perfusion mismatch.[16] In patients with large ischemic strokes complicated by massive swelling, hemicraniectomy has emerged as an option and may benefit a select group of patients.[23-25]

Stroke patients develop significant morbidity either because of the disease itself, for example, impaired swallowing, seizures, cerebral edema, infections such as pneumonia or urinary tract infection, or because of complications following treatment, for example, hemorrhagic transformation. The early recognition and appropriate treatment of these conditions, where possible, is essential in improving clinical outcome.

BOX 2 The indications and contraindications for thrombolytic therapy in patients with acute ischemic stroke.

Indications

- Ischemic stroke with symptom onset < 3 hours
- Measurable neurological deficit
  - Signs should not be clearing spontaneously
  - Signs should not be minor and isolated
  - Ideal candidates have NIHSS scores of 4–20 (estimation of risk/benefit ratio required)
  - Caution in patients with major deficits
- Patient and/or patient's designee/family comprehend potential risks and benefits of thrombolysis

Contraindications

- CT or MRI of brain demonstrates:
  - Intracranial hemorrhage
  - Hypodensity of more than one third of cerebral hemisphere
- Head trauma or stroke in the preceding 3 months
- Myocardial infarction in the preceding 3 months
- Gastrointestinal and urinary tract hemorrhage in last 21 days
- Arterial puncture at a noncompressible site in the last 7 days
- Major surgery in the last 14 days
- Systolic blood pressure ≥ 185 mm Hg or diastolic blood pressure ≥ 110 mm Hg
- History of prior intracranial hemorrhage
- Evidence of active bleeding or acute trauma on physical examination
- Use of oral anticoagulation with INR > 1.7
- Use of heparin in the last 48 hours with a prolonged aPTT level
- Platelet count ≥ 100 x 10^9/L
- Blood glucose level < 50 mg/dL
- Seizure with postictal residual neurological deficit

(aPTT: activated partial thromboplastin time; CT: computed tomography; INR: international normalized ratio; MRI: magnetic resonance imaging; NIHSS: National Institute of Health Stroke Scale)

SUBARACHNOID HEMORRHAGE

Subarachnoid hemorrhage accounts for 10% of cerebrovascular accidents (CVAs) and is associated with significant morbidity and mortality (50%). SAH may be spontaneous or traumatic **(Table 10)**.[26] The risk factors for SAH include cigarette smoking, heavy alcohol consumption, uncontrolled hypertension, use of sympathomimetic drugs, cocaine abuse, estrogen deficiency, and some hereditary conditions such as polycystic kidney and Ehlers-Danlos syndrome.[27]

Clinical Features

Patients present with unusual or severe sudden-onset headaches. Warning bleeds and sentinel headaches are relatively uncommon. Clinical features and physical examination may provide some indication of the diagnosis and location of the bleeding **(Table 11)**.

TABLE 10: The common and uncommon causes of spontaneous subarachnoid hemorrhage.

Common	• Cerebral aneurysms • Arteriovenous malformation (AVM)
Uncommon	• Neoplasms • Dural AVM • Venous angiomas • Infectious aneurysms

TABLE 11: The clinical symptoms and physical examination findings in subarachnoid hemorrhage (SAH).

Clinical history	
Onset of headache: Abrupt, maximal at onset, "thunderclap"	
Severity: Very severe or worst of life	
Associated signs and symptoms: Loss of consciousness, diplopia, seizure, and focal neurological signs	
Physical findings	
Finding	*Likely location of aneurysm*
Diminished consciousness	Any
Nuchal rigidity	Any
Papilledema	Any
Retinal and subhyaloid hemorrhage	Any
Third nerve palsy	Posterior communicating artery
Sixth nerve palsy	Posterior fossa
B/I weakness in legs or abulia	Anterior communicating artery
Nystagmus or ataxia	Posterior fossa
Aphasia, hemiparesis, left-sided visual neglect	Middle cerebral artery

Diagnosis

The initial screening test to confirm the diagnosis is a non-contrast CT scan of the brain; however, the diagnostic yield depends on the time that has elapsed between symptom onset to performance of the CT scan (sensitivity 98% in first 12 hours and 54% at 5 days). Other conditions such as intracerebral hemorrhage (ICH), mass effect, and hydrocephalus, which may present in a similar manner, can also be differentiated with the initial CT scan. A false-negative CT scan can result from severe anemia or small-volume hemorrhage. A lumbar puncture should be performed after an initial negative CT scan, and SAH patients will display high opening pressure, red blood cells in the cerebrospinal fluid (CSF) that do not clear, and xanthochromia which may persist for up to 2 weeks. A definitive diagnosis is made by angiography, which can identify the source of bleeding. Other tests which can be used are digital subtraction angiography or magnetic resonance angiography. The amount, location, and extent of bleed correlates with prognosis. Several grading systems are used in practice to standardize the clinical classification of patients with SAH based on the initial neurologic examination and the appearance of blood on the initial head CT. They include the Glasgow Coma Scale (GCS) system, the Hunt and Hess grading system, and The World Federation of Neurological Surgeons' System **(Tables 12 and 13)**.

TABLE 12: The Glasgow Coma Scale (GCS) which is scored between 3 and 15—3 being the worst and 15 the best. It is composed of three parameters—best eye response, best verbal response, and best motor response. A score of 13 or higher is associated with mild brain injury, a score of 9 to 12 is associated with moderate injury, and a score of 8 or less represents severe brain injury.

Eye opening	
Spontaneous	4
Response to verbal command	3
Response to pain	2
No eye opening	1
Best verbal response	
Oriented	5
Confused	4
Inappropriate words	3
Incomprehensible sounds	2
No verbal response	1
Best motor response	
Obeys commands	6
Localizing response to pain	5
Withdrawal response to pain	4
Flexion to pain	3
Extension to pain	2
No motor response	1

TABLE 13: The Hunt and Hess grading system for assessing the severity of subarachnoid hemorrhage. Mortality is minimum with grade 1 but maximum with grade 5.

Grade	Presentation
1	Asymptomatic or mild headache and slight nuchal rigidity
2	Moderate-to-severe headache, stiff neck, no neurologic deficit except cranial nerve palsy
3	Drowsy or confused, mild focal neurologic deficit
4	Stupor, moderate or severe hemiparesis
5	Deep coma, decerebrate posturing

Management

The management of SAH is centered on three aspects **(Box 3)**, namely general management, definitive treatment (identifying and treating the causative lesion and preventing rebleeding), and treatment of complications.[28-33]

General management involves ICU monitoring, discontinuation of all antithrombotic medications, and correction of any coagulopathy if present. Blood pressure control is essential if elevated in these patients and may also be guided by monitoring of the patient's level of consciousness or intracranial pressure (ICP). The calcium channel blocker, nimodipine, has been shown to improve outcomes in SAH patients; however, the exact mechanism of this improvement is unknown and has been attributed to the prevention of vasospasm. The use of antiepileptic medication in SAH is controversial; therefore, the routine use of antiepileptics is discouraged due to the poor neurologic outcome that has been reported with its use. In addition, antifibrinolytic agents such as tranexamic acid and epsilon aminocaproic acid have been shown to decrease rebleed in SAH patients, but this is also without a significant effect on the general outcome of these patients. This has been attributed to the development of generalized cerebral ischemia; hence, these agents are not used routinely in SAH patients. The administration of glucocorticoids has also not been shown to be beneficial in these patients. The systemic factors contributing to the increased mortality include hypoxemia, metabolic acidosis, hyperglycemia, and cardiovascular instability. Definitive treatment involves either surgical clipping or endovascular coiling. There is a decreased mortality and a nonsignificant increase in rebleeding in patients treated with endovascular coiling as opposed to surgical clipping. The timing of intervention should be as early as feasible.

Complications of SAH **(Table 14)** and rebleeding manifest with worsening neurological status and carry significant morbidity and mortality. The definitive therapy involves treatment of aneurysms. Vasospasm starts approximately 3 days after the initial bleed and peaks after 7–8 days. It is associated with cerebral ischemia and neurological deficits, and the extent of vasospasm can be monitored using transcranial Dopplers. Irrigation of the cistern magna with urokinase following surgical or endovascular intervention has been shown to prevent vasospasm but is associated with significant complications. In addition, statins may prevent vasospasm, though the data has been inconsistent.

BOX 3 The steps involved in the management of subarachnoid hemorrhage.

General management

- Admission to an intensive care unit
- Oxygen supplementation and mechanical ventilation, if indicated
- Stool softeners, bed rest, and analgesia to diminish hemodynamic fluctuations
- Correction of coagulopathy, if any
- Control blood pressure
- Deep venous thrombosis (DVT) prophylaxis with pneumatic compression stockings; subcutaneous unfractionated heparin 5,000 units three times daily can be added for prophylaxis once the aneurysm is treated
- Monitor and treat elevated intracranial pressure
- Seizure prophylaxis

Identifying and treating the causative lesion and preventing rebleeding

- Team of experienced surgeons and endovascular practitioners
- To consider the neurologic grade and clinical status of the patient, the availability of expertise in surgical and endovascular techniques, the anatomic characteristics of the aneurysm, including the location and the size of the aneurysm and its neck
- Timing of surgery is controversial although early surgery is preferred
- Neurosurgical clipping preferable over endovascular coiling

Treatment of complications

- *Treating hydrocephalus*
  - Ventricular drain placement for deteriorating level of consciousness and no improvement in hydrocephalus within 24 hours
- *Treating and preventing vasospasm*
  - Inflammatory reaction in the blood vessel wall
  - Develops between days 4 and 12 after subarachnoid hemorrhage
  - Transcranial Doppler ultrasonography is performed either daily or every other day
  - Treated with hypervolemia and induced hypertension
  - May require treatment with temporary external ventricular drainage or the placement of a permanent shunt
- *Rebleeding*
  - Manifests as worsening neurological state
  - Treat underlying cause

Maintenance of euvolemia is recommended to prevent vasospasm. Induced hypertension should be considered for patients with delayed cerebral ischemia due to vasospasm. Balloon angioplasty and the administration of intra-arterial vasodilators are indicated in patients with vasospasm that

TABLE 14: The complications of subarachnoid hemorrhage.

Complication	Features
Hydrocephalus	May develop in 24 hours due to obstruction to CSF flow by clotted blood
Seizures	Prophylaxis with antiseizure medications
Raised intracranial pressure	Monitor closely
Rebleeding	20% in 2 weeks with peak incidence on day 1 (4%) and 1.5% per day for 2 weeks
Vasospasm	Arterial smooth muscle contraction
Neurological deficits	Cerebral ischemia
Hypothalamic dysfunction	Sympathetic stimulation leading to myocardial ischemia and labile blood pressure
Hyponatremia	SIADH
Pulmonary edema	Neurogenic and non-neurogenic causes
Complications from ICU stay	Identify and treat appropriately

(CSF: cerebrospinal fluid; ICU: intensive care unit; SIADH: syndrome of inappropriate antidiuretic hormone)

is refractory to medical therapy. Hydrocephalus is common in elderly patients with intraventricular bleed, posterior circulation aneurysms, and treatment with antifibrinolytic agents. Spontaneous resolution occurs in about 50% of cases. Hyponatremia can develop secondary to the syndrome of inappropriate antidiuretic hormone (SIADH) or with cerebral salt wasting. Clear distinction between these two entities is important for proper management: SIADH patients are euvolemic, while cerebral salt-wasting patients are hypovolemic.

INTRACEREBRAL HEMORRHAGE

Intracerebral hemorrhage occurs within the brain parenchyma or surrounding meningeal spaces. Brain hemorrhage can occur from defects in the vessel wall, such as aneurysms, arteriovenous malformations (AVMs), small vessel microaneurysms, coagulopathy, increased blood pressure, or trauma. ICH accounts for 10–30% of all stroke hospital admissions and is associated with high mortality. ICH can be classified into primary or secondary depending on the underlying cause of bleeding **(Table 15 and Box 4)**. ICH commonly occurs in the cerebral lobes, cerebellum, basal ganglia, thalamus, and brainstem, with extension into ventricles with large hematomas. Cerebral edema and neuronal damage in the surrounding parenchyma also occur. There are several mechanisms of brain injury in ICH:[34]

- Primary direct mechanical injury to brain parenchyma by the expanding clot
- Increased ICP
- Herniation secondary to mass effect

TABLE 15: The classification of intracerebral hemorrhage based on the cause of the bleed.

Primary intracerebral hemorrhage	• Accounts for majority of cases • Caused by spontaneous rupture of small vessels damaged by chronic hypertension or amyloid angiopathy
Secondary intracerebral hemorrhage	• Occurs in minority of patients • Secondary to vascular abnormalities, tumors, and impaired coagulation

BOX 4 **The various etiologies of intracerebral hemorrhage with hypertension being the most common.**

- Hypertension
- Amyloid angiopathy
- Arteriovenous malformation
- Intracranial aneurysm
- Cavernous hemangioma
- Venous angioma
- Coagulopathy
- Vasculitis
- Intracranial neoplasm
- Hemorrhagic ischemic stroke
- Cocaine or alcohol usage

Clinical Features

The neurologic symptoms usually increase gradually over minutes to a few hours. Patients present with decreased level of consciousness because of increased ICP and direct compression of thalamic and brain stem reticular activating system (RAS). Most patients are hypertensive at the time of presentation. Other symptoms include headache, seizures, and vomiting which are more common with ICH than ischemic stroke. Stupor or coma in ICH is a warning sign except for patients with thalamic hemorrhage, in whom involvement of the RAS is the cause of stupor rather than diffuse brain injury. These patients often recover after reabsorption of blood. Neurological signs vary depending on the location of hemorrhage. In cases of severe intracerebral bleeding, herniation can take place **(Table 16)**.

Diagnosis

Intracerebral hemorrhage is a neurologic and medical emergency as it is related with a high risk of ongoing bleeding, progressive neurologic deterioration, permanent disability, and death. Although rapid onset of abnormalities and decreased level of consciousness suggest the diagnosis, imaging with CT scan of brain is needed to confirm the diagnosis.[35] CT scan of the brain is the initial diagnostic test and a cerebral angiography should be performed in patients who are younger than 70 years of age with lobar ICH, less than 45 years of age with deep or posterior fossa ICH, and

TABLE 16: The herniation syndromes that can be seen with intracerebral bleeding.

Type	Causes	Clinical hallmark
Lateral transtentorial (uncal)	Temporal lobe mass lesion	• Ipsilateral third cranial nerve (CN 3) palsy • Contralateral or bilateral motor posturing
Central transtentorial	• Diffuse cerebral edema • Hydrocephalus	• Progression from bilateral decorticate to decerebrate posturing • Rostral-caudal loss of brainstem reflexes
Subfalcine	Frontal or parietal mass lesion	• Asymmetric motor posturing (contralateral > ipsilateral) • Preserved oculocephalic reflex

45-70 year-old patients with no history of hypertension.[36] In addition to the CT scan, patients should get CBC, coagulation profile, and comprehensive metabolic panel. MRI can be useful in identifying large AVMs and may be used in selected patients.

Management

All patients with ICH should be monitored closely in the ICU.[37-44] Initial management includes evaluation of the airways, breathing, and circulation **(Box 5)**. Mechanical ventilatory support is usually recommended for patients with GCS of less than 8 but should be guided by the clinical presentation. The secondary effects of ICH include expansion of the hematoma, increased ICP, perihematomal edema, intraventricular hemorrhage, and hydrocephalus. Treatment involves a combination of both medical and surgical interventions. Elevated blood pressure is common in patients with ICH and is feared to contribute to the expansion of hematoma. The management of hypertension and hypotension **(Table 17)** and lowering blood pressure to <140 mm Hg systolic did not decrease hematoma volume or mortality but may in a subset of patients improve functional outcomes. Raised ICP contributes to the mortality of these patients and should be managed expediently. It is defined as a pressure > 20 mm Hg for >5 minutes. As soon as raised ICP is suspected, the head of the bed should be raised to 30° keeping the head at midline. Hypovolemia should be treated expediently to prevent postural hypotension.

Osmotic therapy with mannitol decreases the swelling of an edematous brain, decreases the viscosity of blood, and increases cardiac preload, thus increasing the cerebral perfusion pressure (CPP). The target osmolality is 310-320 osmols. Mannitol is given in a dose of 0.25-1 g/kg every 4-6 hours. Side effects include volume overload and osmotic renal failure. The effect of mannitol is seen within 30 minutes to 1 hour and is guided by clinical improvement. Hypertonic saline, either as 3% saline 150 mL bolus every 6 hours or as a continuous infusion of 0.5 mL to 1 mL/kg/h, can also be utilized for the treatment of raised ICP. Frequent serum sodium monitoring is required with hypertonic saline administration. Alternatively, 7.5% saline as a 250 mL bolus or 23.4% saline in doses of 30-60 mL over 20 minutes can be used when other modalities are unsuccessful. Sudden increases in sodium can contribute to the development of coma and seizures. Steroids are not recommended for cerebral edema secondary to CVA.

Hyperventilation has an immediate and transient effect on cerebral circulation. It lowers CPP by cerebral vasoconstriction and may be associated with exacerbations of ischemia in local regions of the brain. It is recommended to lower the $PaCO_2$ to 30-35 mm Hg in situations of an intractable rise in CPP.[40] Hyperthermia worsens neurological damage by increasing the metabolism in ischemic brain tissues. Therapeutic cooling to control temperature of 36°C and gradual rewarming may improve outcomes. The role of ventriculostomy and CSF drainage has not been studied prospectively, but it is an effective method of decreasing ICP, especially in the phase of hydrocephalus.[41] Interventricular

BOX 5 The steps involved in the management of intracerebral hemorrhage.

- *General management*
  - Reversal of anticoagulation
  - Treatment of fever source
  - Prevent and address hyperglycemia and hypoglycemia
  - Adequate treatment of pain
  - Seizure prophylaxis and treatment
  - DVT prophylaxis
  - Supplemental oxygen or intubation as indicated
- *ICP*
  - Elevate head of bed
  - Hypovolemia should be treated
  - Ventriculostomy and CSF drainage for hydrocephalus
  - Osmotic therapy with mannitol, hypertonic saline
  - Sedation and paralysis as needed
  - Maintain ICP 5-20 (aggressive measures to decrease ICP)
  - Maintain cerebral perfusion pressure > 70 mm Hg
- *Maintenance of optimum blood pressure*
  - MAP < 110 (some suggested medications are shown in **Table 17**)
- *Address metabolic and nutritional needs*
  - Early administration of TPN worsens ICH
  - Start TPN after 2-3 days with a high concentration of calories from lipids

(CSF: cerebrospinal fluid; DVT: deep vein thrombosis; ICH: intracerebral hemorrhage; ICP: intracranial pressure monitoring; MAP: mean arterial pressure; TPN: total parenteral nutrition)

TABLE 17: The management of hypotension and hypertension in acute intracerebral hemorrhage.

High blood pressure	
If SBP is >200 mm Hg, or MAP > 150 mm Hg on two readings 20 minutes apart	Start intravenous labetalol, esmolol, enalapril, or other smaller doses of easily titratable intravenous medications such as diltiazem, lisinopril, or verapamil
If SBP is >180 mm Hg and MAP < 130 mm Hg with elevated ICP	Start intravenous antihypertensives (agents shown below)
If SBP is >180 mm Hg and MAP < 130 mm Hg with no elevation of ICP	• Intermittent or continuous antihypertensives can be used. • The goal is to keep SBP < 160 mm Hg and MAP ≈ 110 mm Hg
Labetalol	5–100 mg/h by intermittent bolus doses of 10–40 mg or continuous drip (2–8 mg/min)
Esmolol	500 µg/kg as a load; maintenance → 50–200 µg/kg/min
Nitroprusside	0.5–10 µg/kg/min
Hydralazine	10–20 mg every 4–6 hours
Enalapril	0.625–1.2 mg every 6 hours as needed
Low blood pressure	
Volume replenishment is the first line of approach. If hypotension persists after correction of volume deficit, continuous infusions of pressors should be considered, particularly for low systolic blood pressure such as <90 mm Hg	
Phenylephrine	2–10 µg/kg/min
Dopamine	2–20 µg/kg/min
Norepinephrine	Titrate from 0.05–0.2 µg/kg/min
(ICP: intracranial pressure; MAP: mean arterial pressure; SBP: systolic blood pressure)	

hemorrhage and infection are notable complications of this procedure.

In addition to these specific treatments, patients should be treated adequately for pain. Sedation and neuromuscular blockade may be needed for patients who are intubated. Also, blood glucose should be lowered to >150 mg/dL, but hypoglycemia should be avoided. Since most of the seizures are nonconvulsive in nature, prophylactic seizure medications must be used initially.

Patients with ICH have a high incidence of venous thromboembolism and should receive prophylaxis initially with pneumatic compression stockings and later subcutaneous heparin 5,000 units every 8 hours after day 4 of ICH onset.[42] Patients who developed venous thromboembolism should be treated with an inferior vena caval (IVC) filter. Warfarin treatment increases the incidence of ICH, and the risk is proportional to the degree of anticoagulation and the presence of amyloid vasculopathy. The anticoagulant effect can be reversed using vitamin K 10 mg intravenously, fresh frozen plasma (FFP), or prothrombin complex concentrate. In patients taking vitamin K antagonists with an elevated international normalized ratio (INR), and prothrombin complex concentrate was found to be superior to FFP in reducing INR and reducing the incidence of hematoma expansion.[36] The reinstitution of warfarin therapy should be carefully assessed on an individual basis. ICH associated with antifibrinolytic therapy carries a worse prognosis than warfarin-associated ICH and is treated with platelets and cryoprecipitate.

Surgical treatment is not beneficial except in certain selected conditions.[44] Recommendations for surgery are as follows: (1) cerebellar hematoma with neurological deterioration, brainstem compression, or hydrocephalus should be removed as soon as possible; (2) patient with large lobar clots within 1 cm of the surface of the brain, evacuation of supratentorial ICH by standard craniotomy may be considered; and (3) the usefulness of urokinase infusion into the clot or minimally invasive evacuation of the clot or routine decompressive craniotomy is currently unknown.

Prognosis

A simple six-point clinical grading scale called the ICH score had been devised to predict mortality after ICH. This scale incorporates several clinical components that may be independent predictors of outcome. The ICH score is determined by adding the score from each component **(Table 18)**.

STATUS EPILEPTICUS

Seizures are a common condition seen in 3.3–34% of ICU patients.[45] They can result from either a primary neurological pathology, such as a stroke, brain tumor, or central nervous system (CNS) infection, or develop as a neurological complication of critical illness as in patients with metabolic abnormalities, drug/substance toxicity or withdrawal, or hypoxemia.[45,46] Status epilepticus is said to occur when

TABLE 18: The six-point ICH scoring used to predict mortality after the development of ICH. A cumulative ICH score is obtained by adding the points from each component.

Scale	Points
Glasgow Coma Scale (GCS) score	
3–4	2
5–12	1
13–15	0
Intracerebral hemorrhage (ICH) volume	
≥30 cm^3	1
≤30 cm^3	0
Intraventricular extension of hemorrhage	
Present	1
Absent	0
Infratentorial origin	
Yes	1
No	0
Age	
≥80 years	1
≤80 years	0

seizures are recurrent or refractory lasting >5 minutes or repetitive in nature without regaining consciousness in between episodes **(Box 6)**.[46] It is a life-threatening emergency that necessitates urgent diagnosis and treatment and is classified as either being convulsive or nonconvulsive. The convulsive form tends to be the more severe and common type and is characterized by repeated seizure episodes associated with a postictal state, while the nonconvulsive form is characterized typically by an altered mental status and a lack of obvious physical manifestations.

BOX 6 The different etiologies associated with the development of status epilepticus.

- Antiepileptic drug noncompliance
- Alcohol related
- Cerebrovascular accidents
- Vascular malformations
- Drug toxicity (cephalosporins, penicillin, ciprofloxacin, tacrolimus, cyclosporin, theophylline, and cocaine)
- Central nervous system (CNS) infections (meningitis, encephalitis, abscess)
- CNS tumors (primary or secondary)
- Metabolic disturbances (electrolyte abnormalities, sepsis, and uremia)
- Head trauma
- Surgery
- Cerebral anoxia/hypoxia
- Hypoglycemia or hyperglycemia
- Vasculitis

Clinical Features and Diagnosis

Patients with convulsive status epilepticus are easy to recognize as they present with classic motor manifestations. Conversely, patients with nonconvulsive status epilepticus often go unrecognized because of the lack of obvious signs. The use of electroencephalography (EEG) is therefore an essential tool in the diagnosis of the nonconvulsive type. The basic diagnostic workup also includes a rapid assessment of glucose levels, CBC, electrolytes, liver function, arterial blood gas analysis, and toxicology screen, in addition to imaging studies such as CT scan or MRI of the brain. A lumbar puncture may also be performed in selected patients to evaluate the CSF for possible secondary causes of the seizure episodes. The prompt diagnosis and treatment of status epilepticus is essential as prolonged or recurrent seizure episodes are associated with worsening neurological injury, and systemic complications such as lactic acidosis, hyperthermia, arrhythmias, aspiration, rhabdomyolysis, renal failure, and trauma.[45]

Management

The EEG not only serves as a diagnostic tool but also aids in monitoring response to treatment, as patients may still be actively seizing even though motor signs have subsided. Treatment involves eliminating seizure activity as well as preventing the development of further episodes. The general and pharmacological strategies employed in the management of status epilepticus **(Flowchart 3)** include an initial step in evaluating the respiratory and cardiovascular status of the patient. Patients are frequently intubated to preserve the airway and enhance oxygenation. A rapid blood glucose test is usually performed at bedside and treated for levels < 60 mg/dL, and at the same time blood is sent off for blood tests as listed earlier. Benzodiazepines are the initial drug of choice. IV lorazepam 1–2 mg, midazolam 2–5 mg, or diazepam 10–20 mg can be given at first, but these doses can be increased up to 5–10 mg, 5–20 mg, or 20–40 mg over 5 minutes in cases of recurrent or refractory seizures.[47,48] Intramuscular midazolam is an effective alternative if IV access is not available.[49] In patients not responding to the increased doses of benzodiazepines, second-line agents that have been used include phenytoin (loading dose 20 mg/kg at 50 mg/min) or fosphenytoin (20 mg/min at 150 mg/min). Other alternative second-line agents that can be used include IV medications such as levetiracetam and valproic acid.[48,50] In patients who still continue to have seizure episodes (>60 minutes), induction of a pharmacological coma may be necessary with infusions of phenobarbital, propofol, or midazolam. Continuous EEG monitoring is also preferred, particularly in patients with nonconvulsive status

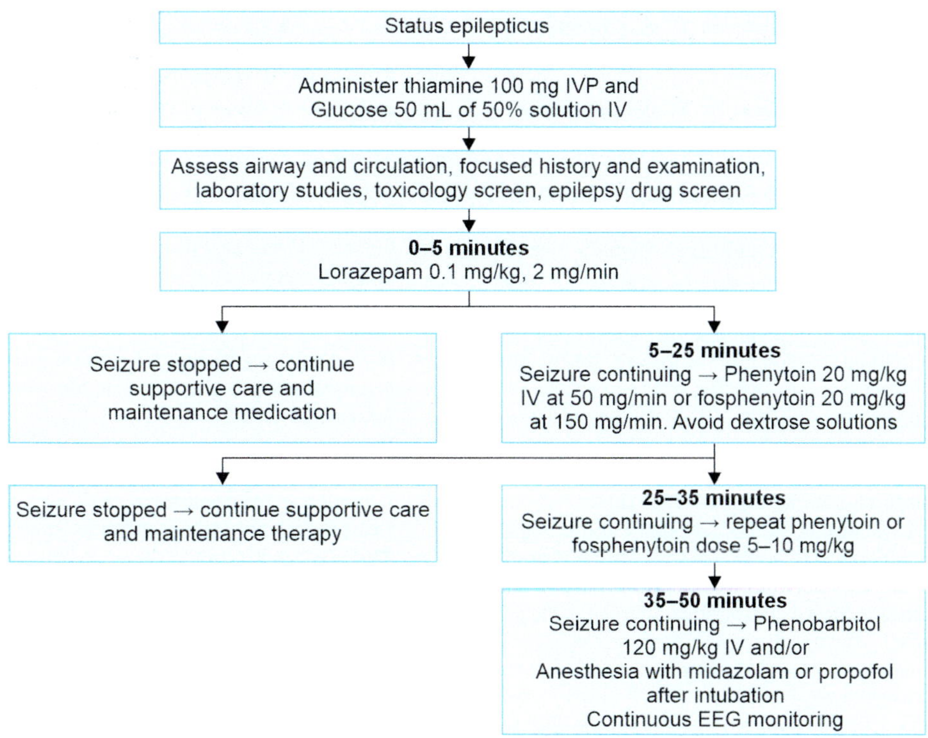

FLOWCHART 3: An algorithmic approach to the management of status epilepticus.
(EEG: electroencephalogram; IV: intravenous; IVP: intravenous push)

epilepticus.[48,51,52] Status epilepticus is a serious condition in critically ill patients and is associated with a mortality of approximately 20%.[53] Early recognition and treatment are necessary to prevent potentially severe neurological consequences.

SUMMARY

Endocrinal and neurological emergencies can develop in patients with pre-existing diseases or in patients admitted in critical care units with other disorders. Early diagnosis is important for management in these patients. Diabetic, thyroid and adrenal emergencies are most common endocrinal problems requiring critical care. On the other hand, stroke, convulsive and hemorrhagic disorders are common neurological conditions requiring critical care. Status epilepticus is a serious neurological condition in critically ill patients which is usually associated with a high mortality. Early recognition and treatment are necessary to prevent potentially severe consequences.

REFERENCES

1. Ross DS, Burch HB, Cooper DS, et al. 2016 American Thyroid Association Guidelines for Diagnosis and Management of Hyperthyroidism and Other Causes of Thyrotoxicosis. Thyroid. 2016;26(10):1343-421.
2. Satoh T, Isozaki O, Suzuki A, et al. 2016 Guidelines for the management of thyroid storm from The Japan Thyroid Association and Japan Endocrine Society (First edition). Endocr J. 2016;63(12):1025-64.
3. Burch HB, Wartofsky L. Life-threatening thyrotoxicosis. Thyroid storm. Endocrinol Metab Clin North Am. 1993;22:263-77.
4. Wartofsky L. Myxedema coma. Endocrinol Metab Clin North Am. 2006;35:687-98, vii-viii.
5. Beynon J, Akhtar S, Kearney T. Predictors of outcome in myxoedema coma. Crit Care. 2008;12:111.
6. Wall CR. Myxedema coma: diagnosis and treatment. Am Fam Physician. 2000;62:2485-90.
7. Ylli D, Klubo-Gwiezdzinska J, Wartofsky L. Thyroid emergencies. Pol Arch Intern Med. 2019;129(7-8):526-34.
8. Rolih CA, Ober KP. Pituitary apoplexy. Endocrinol Metab Clin North Am. 1993;22:291-302.
9. Cuthbertson BH, Sprung CL, Annane D, et al. The effects of etomidate on adrenal responsiveness and mortality in patients with septic shock. Intensive Care Med. 2009;35:1868-76.
10. Charmandari E, Nicolaides N, Chrousos GP. Adrenal insufficiency. Lancet. 2014;383:2152-67.
11. Bancos I, Hahner S, Tomlinson J, et al. Diagnosis and management of adrenal insufficiency. Lancet Diabetes Endocrinol. 2015;3(3):216-26.
12. Kitabchi AE, Umpierrez GE, Murphy MB, et al. Management of hyperglycemic crises in patients with diabetes. Diabetes Care. 2001;24:131-53.

13. Kitabchi AE, Umpierrez GE, Miles JM, et al. Hyperglycemic crises in adult patients with diabetes. Diabetes Care. 2009;32: 1335-43.
14. Umpierrez GE, Murphy MB, Kitabchi AE. Diabetic Ketoacidosis and Hyperglycemic Hyperosmolar Syndrome. Diabetes Spectrum. 2002;15:28-36.
15. van der Worp HB, van Gijn J. Clinical practice. Acute ischemic stroke. N Engl J Med. 2007;357:572-9.
16. Herpich F, Rincon F. Management of Acute Ischemic Stroke. Crit Care Med. 2020;48(11):1654-63.
17. Saver JL, Goyal M, van der Lugt A, et al. HERMES Collaborators. Time to Treatment With Endovascular Thrombectomy and Outcomes From Ischemic Stroke: A Meta-analysis. JAMA. 2016; 316(12):1279-88.
18. Warner JJ, Harrington RA, Sacco RL, et al. Guidelines for the Early Management of Patients With Acute Ischemic Stroke: 2019 Update to the 2018 Guidelines for the Early Management of Acute Ischemic Stroke. Stroke. 2019;50(12):3331-2.
19. Jauch E, Saver J, Adams H, et al. Guidelines for the early management of patients with acute ischemic stroke: A guideline for health care professionals from the American Heart Association/American Stroke Association. Stroke. 2013;44: 870-947.
20. Al Mahdy H. Management of acute ischaemic stroke. Br J Hosp Med (Lond). 2009;70:572-7.
21. Lansburg M, O'Donnell M, Khatri P, et al. Antithrombotic and thrombolytic therapy for ischemic stroke. Antithrombotic therapy and prevention of thrombosis 9th ed: American College of Chest Physicians evidence-based clinical practice guidelines. Chest. 2012;141(2 Suppl):e601S-36S.
22. Ciccine E, Valsassori L, Nichelatti M, et al. Endovascular treatment for acute stroke. N Engl J Med. 2013;368:904-13.
23. Chimowitz M. Endovascular treatment for acute ischemic stroke—still unproven. N Engl J Med. 2013;368:952-5.
24. Wijdicks E, Sheth K, Carter B, et al. Recommendations for the management of cerebral and cerebellar infarction with swelling. A statement for healthcare professionals from the American Heart Association/American Stroke Association. Stroke. 2014;45:1222-38.
25. Juttler E, Unterberg A, Woitzik J, et al. Hemicraniectomy in older patients with extensive middle cerebral artery syndrome. N Engl J Med. 2014;370:1091-100.
26. van Gijn J, Rinkel GJ. Subarachnoid haemorrhage: diagnosis, causes and management. Brain. 2001;124:249-78.
27. Rinkel GJ, Djibuti M, Algra A, et al. Prevalence and risk of rupture of intracranial aneurysms: a systematic review. Stroke. 1998;29:251-6.
28. Connolly E, Rabinstein E, Carhuapoma R, et al. Guidelines for the management of aneurysmal subarachnoid hemorrhage: a guideline for healthcare professionals from statement for healthcare professionals from, American Heart Association/ American Stroke Association. Stroke. 2012;44:1711-37.
29. Bardach NS, Olson SJ, Elkins JS, et al. Regionalization of treatment for subarachnoid hemorrhage: a cost-utility analysis. Circulation. 2004;109:2207-12.
30. Naidech AM, Kreiter KT, Janjua N, et al. Phenytoin exposure is associated with functional and cognitive disability after subarachnoid hemorrhage. Stroke. 2005;36:583-7.
31. Roos YB, Rinkel GJ, Vermeulen M, et al. Antifibrinolytic therapy for aneurysmal subarachnoid haemorrhage. Cochrane Database Syst Rev. 2003;2:CD001245.
32. Bauer A, Ramussen P. Treatment of intracranial vasospam following subarachnoid hemorrhage. Front Neuro. 2014;5:1-7.
33. Sillberg VA, Wells GA, Perry JJ. Do statins improve outcomes and reduce the incidence of vasospasm after aneurysmal subarachnoid hemorrhage: a metaanalysis. Stroke. 2008;39: 2622-6.
34. Gebel JM, Broderick JP. Intracerebral hemorrhage. Neurol Clin. 2000;18:419-38.
35. Rincon F, Mayer SA. Intracerebral hemorrhage: getting ready for effective treatments. Curr Opin Neurol. 2010;23:59-64.
36. Sheth KN. Spontaneous Intracerebral Hemorrhage. N Engl J Med. 2022;387(17):1589-96.
37. Hemphill JC 3rd, Bonovich DC, Besmertis L, et al. The ICH score: a simple, reliable grading scale for intracerebral hemorrhage. Stroke. 2001;32:891-7.
38. Morgenstern L, Hemphill C, Anderson C, et al. Guidelines for the management of spontaneous intracerebral hemorrhage: A guideline for healthcare professionals from the American Heart Association/American Stroke Association. Stroke. 2010;41: 2108-29.
39. Anderson C, Heeley Huang Y, Wang J, et al. Rapid blood pressure lowering in patients with acute intracerebral hemorrhage. N Engl J Med. 2013;368:2355-61.
40. Marshall S, Kalanuria A, Markandaya M, et al. Management of intracerebral pressure in the neurosciences critical care unit. Neurosurg Clin N Am. 2013;24:361373.
41. Belur P, Chang J, He S, et al. Emerging experimental therapies for intracerebral hemorrhage: targeting mechanism of secondary brain injury. Neurosurg Focus. 2013;34:E9.
42. Vespa PM, O'Phelan K, Shah M, et al. Acute seizures after intracerebral hemorrhage: a factor in progressive midline shift and outcome. Neurology. 2003;60:1441-6.
43. Lacut K, Bressollette L, Le Gal G, et al. Prevention of venous thrombosis in patients with acute intracerebral hemorrhage. Neurology. 2005;65:865-9.
44. Medenlow D, Gregson B, Rowan E, et al. Early surgery versus initial conservative treatment in patients with spontaneous supratentorial lobar intracerebral hematomas (STICH II) a randomized trial. Lancet. 2013;382:397-408.
45. Varelas PN, Spanaki M. Management of seizures in the critically ill. Neurologist. 2006;12:127-39.
46. Mirski MA, Varelas PN. Seizures and status epilepticus in the critically ill. Crit Care Clin. 2008;24:115-47, ix.
47. Lowenstein DH, Alldredge BK. Status epilepticus. N Engl J Med. 1998;338:970-6.
48. Talati R, White CM, Coleman CI. Status epilepticus: a review of current pharmacologic treatments. Conn Med. 2009;73:525-8.
49. Brophy G, Bell R, Claassen J, et al. Guidelines for the evaluation and management of status epilepticus. Neurocrit Care. 2012;17: 13-23.
50. Silbergleit R, Durkalski V, Lowenstein D, et al. Intramuscular versus intravenous therapy for prehospital status epilepticus. N Engl J Med. 2012;366:591-600.
51. Moddel G, Bunten S, Dobis C, et al. Intravenous levetiracetam: a new treatment alternative for refractory status epilepticus. J Neurol Neurosurg Psychiatry. 2009;80:689-92.
52. Wheless JW, Vazquez BR, Kanner AM, et al. Rapid infusion with valproate sodium is well tolerated in patients with epilepsy. Neurology. 2004;63:1507-8.
53. Kumar A, Bleck TP. Intravenous midazolam for the treatment of refractory status epilepticus. Crit Care Med. 1992;20:483-8.

CHAPTER 169

Toxic Inhalations

Clayton T Cowl

INTRODUCTION

Environmental exposures to inhaled toxic substances may occur in occupational settings, at home, or in any of a variety of situations—from accidental mass casualty events to individual exposures. This chapter will focus on acute inhalational toxicity, defined by the adverse effects of a substance that result either from a single exposure or from multiple exposures in a short period of time (usually less than 24 hours).[1] These compounds make up an array of irritant and nonirritant gases, vapors, fumes, and airborne particles that may affect the upper or lower respiratory tract resulting in airway or parenchymal injury and/or result in systemic disease. Examples of respirable toxicants include inhalation of combustible materials from fires (structural or forest fires), industrial accidents, inappropriate home use, and direct intentional releases of compounds during military conflicts or from terroristic actions.[2] Between 1981 and 1983, the United States National Institute for Occupational Safety and Health (NIOSH) conducted its National Occupational Exposure Survey (NOES) and determined that at that time, based upon on-site visits to 4,490 establishments in 522 industry types that employed approximately 1,800,000 workers in 377 occupational categories, nearly 13,000 different potential exposure agents and more than 100,000 unique tradename products were observed during those on-site visits.[3] Although the database has not been updated since 1990 due to resource limitations, it has been calculated that thousands of workers have been victims of acute toxic inhalation exposures over the past three and a half decades. Inhaled toxicants have been classified in a standard fashion into what has been termed "the Purple Book." This "Globally Harmonized System of Classification and Labelling of Chemicals" or GHS is a system developed by the United Nations for standardizing and harmonizing the classification and labeling of chemicals globally and is regularly updated.[4] However, in a clinical environment, many cases with exposure acutely to toxic gases, including inhalations of breakdown products of combustible materials and explosions, involve simultaneous exposure to multiple compounds at varying concentrations.[5]

Because of direct contact from the ambient air with the conducting systems of the respiratory tract, including the nasal passages, oropharynx, and trachea as well as proximal and distal airways, acute toxic inhalations are primarily a respiratory system issue with other organs less commonly affected.[6] There are a variety of factors that play a role in the severity of injury, including concentration of the substance in the offending environment, the pre-existing status of the victim (e.g., prior smoking history, pre-existing airway conditions), the presence or absence of ventilation or surrounding air flow, and the physical nature of the toxicant. Initial onset of symptoms may occur instantaneously to the exposure or up to several days or longer. Downstream clinical effects may occur grossly with mucosal involvement of the airway as well as at the cellular level and can result in immediate respiratory distress or death, systemic illness experienced over weeks or months, or development of a chronic respiratory disease. Injury may also involve contact of the offending agent with the conjunctivae and skin or involve inadvertent aspiration or ingestion of a toxicant. Smoke, gases, and vapors are the most common forms of inhaled toxic substances, but liquids and solids may also be inhaled as dusts, aerosols, or fine mists.[1] Often, the precise substance is unknown or can be described only in terms of its physical properties or the nature of the symptoms experienced.

Despite the many thousands of potential individual chemicals that may cause inhaled injury to victims, the most common form of toxic inhalation encountered is that from breathing air contaminated with breakdown products of combustion. Classic "smoke inhalation" associated with structural fires and/or from close proximity to wildfires (note that airborne pollution is covered elsewhere in this textbook) is the most common form of acute toxic inhalation and complicates burns in 10–20% of patients with exposure to fires with acute smoke inhalation, increasing morbidity and mortality significantly.[1,7] The primary determinants of injury to the airways hinge on concentration of particulates, duration of smoke exposure, and smoke composition. Among victims of fires, increased exposure results in high prevalence of lung injury and morbidity/mortality regardless of geography. Smoke inhalation victims sustain injuries from three main sources including heat injury, chemical irritation throughout the respiratory tract, and systemic toxicity that may occur with inhalation of carbon monoxide, cyanide, or other compounds. A combination of these injuries may also occur.[8] As a general observation, thermal injuries are typically seen in the supraglottic structures and chemical injuries are noted in the lower airways. Individuals with smoke inhalation are typically plagued with respiratory tract edema, and as the mucosal lining of the airway is injured by superheated moisture within the airway and chemical breakdown products with toxicants, bronchoconstriction occurs. More distally, a release of proteolytic elastases is usually noted, in turn leading to release of inflammatory mediators, fluid shifts, and development of pulmonary edema and atelectasis. Decreased levels of surfactant and immunomodulators such as interleukins and tumor necrosis factor-α further propagate the injury.[9] The effects of acute toxicity from smoke inhalation result from asphyxiation (physical or chemical), systemic toxicity from cyanide-based compounds or carbon monoxide, chlorine-based metabolites from combustion of polyvinyl chloride (PVC) found in plastics, or direct injury to the respiratory mucosa.[10]

PHYSICAL PROPERTIES OF GASES AS A DIAGNOSTIC TOOL

It is not uncommon to encounter patients with acute symptoms of a toxic inhalation from unknown or undefined exposures. A chemical spill may contain several compounds or result in toxic metabolites if certain substances react with water or other chemicals. For example, a train derailment may result in varying concentrations of exposures depending on the nature of the volume of release of the substances, the proximity to the spill of the victim, and the volatility of various spilled compounds that may mix or become reactive if they come in contact with moisture from the environment or by leaks into natural waterways, or combust and result in inhalation of multiple heated particulates. Another example could involve a domestic mishap such as mixing ammonia and bleach in a bathtub or enclosed shower, resulting in chloramine compounds that directly irritate the respiratory mucosa. The mixture is heavier than air and therefore sinks to the lowest level of the room or enclosure, magnifying the concentration of the gaseous inhalation for an individual bending over to clean the area. Even when the precise identity of an inhaled toxicant remains unknown, the physical properties of a gas may help to estimate or anticipate the nature of the pathologic effects of the toxic inhalation.

Among the variables to consider during initial assessment of an acute toxic inhalation are the size of inhaled particles and the water solubility of the inhaled substance.[5,6,10] Larger particles (>10 μm) tend to affect the nasopharynx and upper airway where the mucociliary lining will bind and stabilize particles; however, this protective mechanism is often overwhelmed when an individual is involved in an environment in which there is a very high concentration of the offending agent (e.g., inside a tank, rooms without exhaust ventilation, or other confined spaces). This concentrated exposure may also be affected by the total time an individual is exposed such as when a victim is unable to evacuate the source of the untoward inhalation or who becomes incapacitated at the time of the exposure. Smaller particles (5–10 μm or less) are often inhaled into the distal airways resulting in a cascade of intracellular mechanisms that may result in acute and chronic inflammation, fluid shifts, free radical production, or direct cellular destruction.

Water solubility of a compound not only provides critical clues for identification of the inhaled toxicant, but also helps to anticipate potential respiratory system effects and prognosis. A more water-soluble compound (e.g., ammonia) tends to affect the moist surfaces of the upper respiratory tract rapidly such as the conjunctivae, nasopharyngeal and oropharyngeal mucosa, and upper tracheal mucosa. Less water-soluble compounds such as oxides of nitrogen, or phosgene, do not affect the upper airways immediately and often have delayed effects that may allow for longer exposures associated with more pulmonary parenchymal damage. Other factors to consider in acute toxic inhalations include the concentration of the inhalant in the ambient air, the total duration of exposure, the density of the substance (i.e., heavier gases will tend to sink toward the ground), the color of the gas (e.g., elemental chlorine will tend to appear yellow-green when exposed to ambient air), its smell (e.g. the smell of sulfur-based compounds in rotten eggs or the irritating pungent odor of chlorine gas or sulfur dioxide), the presence or absence of ventilation, whether the patient utilized any form of personal respiratory protection such as a respirator, whether coworkers or other individuals at the scene were affected, and a variety of other host factors such as age, smoking status, comorbid diseases (e.g., concurrent heart disease or preexisting pulmonary conditions), and genetic susceptibility.[5] **Box 1** outlines some of the more common physical properties to consider when evaluating a patient suspected of an inhaled toxic exposure.

PATHOPHYSIOLOGY OF ACUTE TOXIC INHALATION INJURY

There have been a variety of major pathophysiological changes identified during and subsequent to an acute toxic inhalation injury. Although heat and steam can directly injure the tracheobronchial tree in smoke inhalation from a combustion source,[11] other known respiratory irritants are produced by combustion products. These include compounds such as halogen acids, unsaturated aldehydes such as acrolein, and formaldehyde.[11,12] The presence of

BOX 1 **Physical characteristics of gases causing acute toxic inhalations.**

Characteristics of inhaled gas:
- Size of particle
- Water-solubility
- Color
- Density (i.e., Is the gas heavier than air and sink toward the ground?)
- Concentration of gas
- Odor/Smell

Individual host factors:
- Presence/Absence of ventilation
- Loss of consciousness
- Presence/Absence of personal respiratory protection
- Age
- Smoking status
- Medical comorbidities
- Genetic factors

these substances triggers a host inflammatory response, often resulting in sloughing of the tracheobronchial mucosa, and is frequently accompanied by direct toxic effects to the airway at a cellular level. Airway injury leads to production of neuropeptides from sensory and vasomotor nerve endings such as substance P and calcitonin gene-related peptide.[11,13] Furthermore, these neuropeptides have been associated with inducing bronchoconstriction and stimulating nitric oxide synthetase that, in turn, produces reactive oxygen species that cause toxic effects on cells. The neuropeptides have also been described as functioning like tachykinins to create increased vascular permeability and lymphatic flow and result in pulmonary edema.[14] Decreased levels of surfactant and immunomodulators such as interleukins and tumor necrosis factor-α accentuate the injury.[9] Once this cascade ensues, additional local cellular injury occurs with loss of hypoxic pulmonary vasoconstriction. This, in turn, causes bronchial blood flow to increase dramatically within just 20 minutes of the inhalational injury. In animal models, once reactive oxygen species cause mitochondrial dysfunction and cellular apoptosis, the injured respiratory epithelial cells and alveolar macrophages trigger the extrinsic coagulation cascade which then impairs the homeostatic balance of coagulation at the level of the inducing plasminogen activator-I, thereby creating a hypercoagulable state.[15] Additional bronchial blood flow seems to accumulate polymorphonuclear lymphocytes and cytokines in the interstitium, potentiating the inflammatory response.[16] Shifts of plasma proteins into the airways with cast and exudate formation cause alveolar collapse or complete occlusion of the distal airways. When animal experiments were conducted to intentionally decrease bronchial blood flow, it revealed that airway obstruction was reduced and intraparenchymal fluid was limited, with oxygenation being consequently improved.[17,18] Additional studies have shown that antagonists to calcitonin gene-related peptide and substance P slowed the fluid shifts and inflammation in a sheep model.[13] Neutrophilic movement into the airway with production of reactive oxygen species and peroxynitrite ($ONOO^-$) during acute toxic inhalations has been targeted for anti-inflammatory therapies. Peroxynitrite decomposition catalysts have been demonstrated to be cytoprotective in animal models studying smoke inhalation injury.[19,20]

ESTIMATING CLINICAL SEVERITY IN ACUTE TOXIC LUNG INJURY

Initial clinical manifestations of smoke inhalation usually result from a large airway epithelial injury. They consist of mucosal hyperemia, edema and ulceration, cast formation, and, in severe cases, bronchial obstruction. Although visualizing the airway via flexible bronchoscopy is considered the standard technique to assess the severity of inhalation injury, other modalities such as CT imaging of the thorax, sequential carboxyhemoglobin measurements, and spirometry all continue to be available as adjuncts depending on the severity and nature of the toxic inhalation.[21] There have been efforts to predict mortality in order to gauge the level of resuscitation that will be required by utilizing the calculation of PaO_2/FiO_2 after resuscitation[22,23] and by use of CT imaging of the thorax in animal models.[24] Approximately one-third of patients with inhalation injury develop acute lung injury (ALI) over the first 3 days after smoke exposure.[25] This pulmonary response to smoke inhalation is characterized by an inflammatory process and manifests clinically with decreased Pao_2/FiO_2, decreased respiratory compliance, and requirement for mechanical ventilation.

RESPIRATORY SYSTEM EFFECTS FROM SPECIFIC INHALED TOXICANTS

Although smoke inhalation from combustible materials is the most prevalent form of acute toxic inhalation and involves inhalation of a variety of respiratory irritants, a variety of specific toxic gas inhalations are encountered in practice from industrial leaks and spills, agricultural uses, or household sources. Several of the most common gases that result in acute toxic inhalations and their main characteristics are outlined in **Table 1**.

Chlorine and Its Derivatives

Chlorine gas reacts with water to form hydrochloric acid (HCl) and hypochlorous acid (HOCl), each being a strong caustic irritant to the respiratory mucosa. Unlike chlorine gas alone that is neither strongly water-soluble nor lipophilic, it may affect both the upper and lower respiratory tracts, causing direct cellular damage through use of oxygen-free

TABLE 1: Physical characteristics of several common gases causing respiratory injury.

Gas	Color	Density (i.e., heavier than air)	Water solubility	Anatomic region of impact	Other characteristics
Ammonia	Colorless	No	High	Conjunctivae, nasopharynx	Pungent odor, alkali burns
Chlorine	Yellow-green	Yes	Intermediate	Pharynx	Acid burns, reactive oxygen species, reactive nitrogen species
Sulfur dioxide	Colorless	Yes	High	Larynx	Pungent "rotten eggs" odor
Nitrogen dioxide	Red-orange	Yes	Low	Bronchioles	Inhaled in "silo filler's disease"
Phosgene	White to pale yellow	Yes	Low	Alveoli	At low concentrations, smells like newly mown hay
Ozone	Colorless	Yes	Low	Toxicity via oxidation of membrane lipids	Forms reactive nitrogen species. Plastics manufacturing, fabric bleach, water disinfectant
Sulfur dioxide	Colorless	Yes	High	Conjunctivae, nasopharynx	"Rotten eggs" odor
Hydrogen sulfide	Colorless, flammable	Yes	Intermediate	Asphyxiant olfactory nerves for low concentration, airways for high concentration exposures	Foul-smelling breakdown product of manure gas and if exposed in confined spaces can be lethal
Zinc chloride	White	Yes	Intermediate to high	Nasopharynx and upper airway	Used for smoke bombs

radical formation. Its derivatives are highly water-soluble and react with moisture in the conjunctiva as well as the oropharyngeal mucosa and upper tracheal regions resulting in severe cough, chest tightness, burning and tearing of the eyes, and dysphonia.[26] Lower respiratory tract involvement is less common but may occur with high-intensity exposures associated with events in which an individual was unable to escape or was incapacitated in the environment where the exposure existed.

Although historically used as a chemical warfare agent, these products are common to industrial, environmental, and domestic settings today. Its uses are ubiquitous in textile and paper industries as a bleaching agent, in water purification processes, in sewage treatment, and as a cleaning disinfectant.[27] Common clinical presentations also may come from domestic use of chlorine derivatives mixed with other chemicals such as with household cleaning agents. For example, chloramine gas is formed when chloride or hypochlorous gas is mixed with ammonia.[28-30] When combined with water, which is typically used while performing household cleaning, a variety of highly water-soluble irritant gases are formed resulting in acute primarily upper respiratory tract irritation. Similar clinical presentations have been reported in situations in which chlorine used for water purification can react with natural organic matter introduced into the water by swimmers, forming potentially harmful chlorination by-products.[31] Many of these cases have been associated with excessive use of chlorine in a pool or hot tub water beyond the manufacturer's dosing recommendations.

Ammonia

Ammonia is among the most widely produced chemicals within the world, a majority of which is used for chemical fertilizers or as various animal feeds, but also utilized in the manufacture of cyanides, synthetic fibers, plastics, and explosives manufacturing.[32] Other common uses include that of serving as a cooling agent within refrigeration systems, as a cleaning agent, and in petroleum refining. Exposures most commonly occur through gas leaks within the process of producing the gas, storing it, or transporting it. Because of its high nitrogen content, it is utilized as a fertilizer within the soil and its off-gassing after application into the ground may affect agricultural workers. Industrial and household cleaning agents may also include significant concentrations of ammonia within its dissolved form, and since it is also released from manure, it can affect farmers who work in animal confinement buildings.[33]

As a highly water-soluble chemical, ammonia gas or vapors result in immediate irritation to the conjunctiva, skin, oral nasopharynx, larynx, and trachea. Its rapid interaction with water results in the formation of ammonium hydroxide that is converted into hydroxyl ions, producing not only a strongly alkaline reaction, but also an exothermic reaction that may contribute to thermal burns of the eyes, skin, and upper airway. Alkali burns can be deeply penetrating into the tissues resulting in tissue liquefaction. Cutaneous burns, which maybe disfiguring, tend to be most prominent in areas where moisture or water is of the highest concentration. Contact with the eyes may result in permanent visual acuity loss including direct damage to the corneal endothelium, stroma, lens, and iris. Inhalation of ammonia may result in mucosal edema, hemorrhage, and sloughing of tissue, resulting in fatal upper airway obstruction in the most severe cases.[34] The severity of injury is highly dependent on the concentration and length of exposure to the caustic irritant. Given a high-volume exposure, not only is the upper airway affected, but the lower respiratory tract can also be injured including reported episodes of acute pneumonitis, development of airway obstruction associated with respiratory failure, and episodes of infectious pneumonitis with bacterial organisms. Later stages may include development of bronchiectasis and/or focal bronchiolitis obliterans. There have been prior reports of pneumothoraces and pulmonary fibrosis as well.[35,36]

Treatment hinges on rapid removal from the initial exposure followed by immediate irrigation of all body surfaces exposed to the gas, notably the eyes and skin with water flushes. Importantly, the upper airway should be secured with a low threshold for intubation, even if in early stages postexposure the patient seems relatively clinically stable (but there is a well-documented history of a recent high-volume ammonia exposure). Although corticosteroids and empiric antibiotics have been used previously, there is lack of compelling data to demonstrate their long-term clinical benefit.[37]

Sulfur Dioxide

Sulfur dioxide (SO_2) is one of the "criteria air pollutants" monitored by regulatory agencies across the world, and population-based effects from ambient air pollution are discussed elsewhere in this textbook. In terms of acute exposure, various meta-analyses have identified increased mortality associated with short-term exposure to this toxic inhalant.[38,39] SO_2 is a colorless heavier-than-air gas frequently utilized in a number of industrial processes and also encountered in bleaching of wood pulp and wool, certain forms for olfactory (smell) testing, mining, and sugar refinery operations and may be encountered environmentally from volcanic exposure.[40,41]

Since this gas is highly water-soluble and reacts with water to form sulfuric acid, it is highly reactive to the upper airway. In addition to respiratory injury that may include both the upper and lower respiratory tracts, acute exposures can result in dose-dependent conjunctival and corneal burns and ulcerations. Severe airflow obstruction has been reported in individuals surviving the initial exposure but later developing bronchiolitis obliterans or being diagnosed with reactive airways dysfunction syndrome (RADS).[42,43] High concentration exposures may lead to lethal consequences within just minutes secondary to severe alveolar hemorrhage and edema leading to respiratory failure. In addition, there are also asphyxiant effects with high concentrations.[44]

Treatment of acute toxic exposure from sulfur dioxide centers on supportive care such as providing adequate hydration, supplemental oxygenation, maintaining an adequate upper airway, and use of short-acting bronchodilators as needed for symptomatic relief. Intravenous or oral corticosteroids have been utilized without clearly documented long-term benefits, but anecdotal benefits have also been reported.

Oxides of Nitrogen

Another "criteria air pollutant," nitrogen dioxide, and similar compounds are present within ambient air pollution but may also be involved in acute individual high-intensity exposures that have been noted in mining operations, agricultural activities such as those encountered with silo gas due to breakdown of organic matter (often referred to a "silo filler's disease"), present in the explosives industry, and acetylene welding operations.[45]

Since oxides of nitrogen (NO_x) are lower in water-solubility, acute symptoms are not always present and the lower respiratory tract seems to be more affected. NO_x react with water to form nitric acid and therefore higher volume exposures can result in pulmonary parenchymal injury, including pulmonary edema and airflow obstruction involving the lower airways with less intense exposures sometimes reaching complete resolution without further sequelae. It is not uncommon for late-onset symptoms, even hours after the initial exposure, making recognition of the specific type of toxic inhalation critical since acute respiratory distress syndrome (ARDS) may occur with late onset and cases have been reported in which individuals have presented for medical assessment and have been sent home, only to have subsequent severe untoward outcomes.[46] Even weeks after the initial exposure, development of bronchiolitis obliterans has been reported and therefore, the patient should be followed closely after the acute exposure symptoms have been addressed.

Phosgene

Phosgene, a colorless gas with the smell of freshly cut grass or hay at low concentrations and irritating pungent odors at higher exposure concentrations, was responsible for 85% or more of chemical weapon-related fatalities during the First World War.[47] A compound of low water solubility, phosgene is utilized in the production of various pharmaceuticals, pesticides, and as an industrial chemical reaction catalyst. These reactions include production of polyurethane residence, toluene diisocyanate, and certain dyes.[48] With its lower water solubility, most of its effects are associated with lower respiratory tract injury including the pulmonary parenchyma. Phosgene interacts with water to produce HCl, resulting in direct cellular toxicity and epithelial necrosis. This also results in increased alveolar permeability with the development of pulmonary edema and ARDS. There seems to be a direct correlation between concentration and length of exposure with severity of ultimate respiratory disease. As with many toxic inhaled exposures, supportive care is the mainstay of therapy. However, various immunomodulating agents and anti-inflammatory drugs such as N-acetyl cysteine, ibuprofen, aminophylline, and isoproterenol have been studied in animal models with emphasis placed on reducing free radical species responsible for lipid peroxidation, correcting the imbalance in the glutathione redox state, and preventing the release of biological mediators such as leukotrienes that account for the increased permeability at the cellular level.[49]

Hydrogen Sulfide

Hydrogen sulfide (H_2S) is also known as hydrosulfuric acid, sewer gas, or stink damp and has a characteristic smell of rotten eggs. The gas is slightly heavier than air and is corrosive, flammable, and may be explosive. The compound is slightly water soluble and, subsequent to combustion, may result in the formation of sulfur dioxide. Common locations for toxic exposures include wherever breakdown of organic matter occurs coupled with anaerobic conditions. This accounts for why most reported clinically relevant exposures occur around animal feeding operations, manure pits, sewer drains, undersea vents, sulfur springs, and stagnant bodies of water without ventilation. The compound is used in the production of various pesticides, dyes, and pharmaceuticals as well as within the nuclear energy sector in large quantities as part of "heavy water" separation containing the hydrogen isotope deuterium from that of regular water.[50] Sadly, there have been reports of this compound being used for suicides (dubbed "detergent suicides"). The reported cases involved mixing HCI (found in commercial pool and toilet bowl cleaners) with either lime sulfur (found in common pesticides) or bath sulfur (available in Japan) in an enclosed space to generate toxic levels of H_2S gas.[51]

Hydrogen sulfide odor can be detected by the olfactory system at concentrations as low as 0.0005 ppm, but the sense of smell is lost after 2–15 minutes at just 100 ppm, making use of the physical property of smell for H_2S unreliable and potentially dangerous as a proactive warning to significant inhaled toxic exposure. Where environmental scenarios involving highly concentrated ambient levels of the gas exist, a process known as "knockdown" may occur in which an exposed individual simply passes out.[52] Not only are survival rates extremely low in this situation if the individual is not removed from the exposure, particularly if the exposure occurs in a confined space, but also the incapacitation of the victim will often prompt emergency responders to enter the area rapidly, resulting in additional victims. Where there are environments involving very high concentrations of >500 ppm of H_2S, immediate syncope and death may result. This is thought to be, in part, due to cardiopulmonary paralysis or asphyxiation.[53]

Ozone

Generated as a secondary pollutant from various breakdown reactions occurring from nitrogen oxides, ozone is considered an ambient air pollutant associated with upper and lower respiratory tract bronchial inflammation and airway hyperresponsiveness from oxidative injury and cellular inflammation.[54] Although ozone is known to be a naturally occurring gas involving the upper troposphere that protects the earth from ultraviolet radiation, it is also a primary component of environmental smog.[34] Long-term effects of increased ambient ozone prevalence remain unclear, but longitudinal studies seem to suggest increased declines in lung function and progression of emphysema and those with these parenchymal changes. Treatment is generally supportive.

Cadmium

Exposure to this highly corrosive-resistant metal is present in a variety of occupational settings, and most toxic exposures are associated with cadmium vapors encountered within confined spaces or poorly ventilated rooms. Cadmium is used in soldering and brazing as well as in battery and bearing manufacturing and in electroplating or galvanizing metal surfaces of all types.[55,56] Clinical presentation involves development of generalized myalgias, fevers, and chills several hours after exposure followed by cough, chest tightness, shortness of breath, as well as radiographic changes consistent with bilateral infiltrates involving the pulmonary parenchyma.[56] Spirometry can often reveal airflow restriction, and reduction in diffusing capacity is also noted. Exposure to high concentrations of cadmium vapor may result in a pneumonitis with rapid progression to ARDS and subsequent respiratory failure.[57] As with many other inhaled toxicants, treatment generally centers on supportive care, particularly as it pertains to ALI due to cadmium fume inhalation. Corticosteroids have been utilized to help improve outcomes but again, efficacy has not been well established. Although serum and urine cadmium levels may establish prior exposure, it does not produce specific threshold levels that help gauge prognosis. Urine levels actually better measure total body cadmium burden. Occasionally, clinicians will be asked to comment on elevated cadmium levels obtained in the blood or urine of individuals without known industrial exposures; these often are associated with significant smoking history.[58]

Mercury

Toxic inhalation of mercury vapor is often associated with little or no upper airway symptoms, making it more likely that an individual could be exposed to these toxicants for an extended period of time without acute symptoms. The symptoms typically include cough, shortness of breath, or dysphonia that can occur within 24 hours after exposure.

There may be systemic effects such as fever, gastrointestinal symptoms including nausea or diarrhea, and dysgeusia associated with metallic taste. Unlike other toxic inhalations causing systemic effects, mercury inhalation may have persistent progression involving pneumonitis associated with progressive respiratory failure, and in several cases pneumothoraces have been reported prior to eventual death.[59] Mercury vapor has direct irritant effects of the distal airways including both alveolar and bronchiolar level cellular destruction. Chelating agents [e.g., succimer, dimercaprol (BAL) or unithiol, penicillamine, and dimercaprol] have not been shown to be effective in modifying long-term outcomes for patients with ALI from mercury inhalation.[60]

SUMMARY

Assessment and therapy for acute toxic inhalations are challenging, particularly when the inhaled compound is unknown or there are multiple substances that have been inhaled concurrently as a result of explosions, leaks, or fire. Recognizing the physical properties of a specific inhaled toxic gas as well as some basic characteristics of gases seen more commonly in clinical practice can be helpful in targeting therapy. Maintaining and supporting the airway is a critical component of treatment, and having a low threshold for intubation to protect the airway is important, particularly for exposure to high concentration of specific toxicants.

REFERENCES

1. Gorguner M, Akgun A. Acute inhalation injury. Eurasian J Med. 2010;42(1):28-35.
2. Chen TM, Malli H, Maslove DM, et al. Toxic inhalational exposures. J Intensive Care Med. 2013;28(6):323-33.
3. National Occupational Exposure Survey. National Institute for Occupational Safety and Health. Centers for Disease Control and Prevention. [online] Available from https://web.archive.org/web/20110716084755/http:/www.cdc.gov/noes/ [Last accessed September, 2024].
4. United Nations Globally Harmonized System of Classification and Labelling of Chemicals (GHS), 10th revised edition. New York: United Nations; 2023. [online] Available from http://www.unece.org/trans/danger/publi/ghs/ghs_rev00/00files_e.html [Last accessed September, 2024].
5. Cowl CT. Assessment and treatment of acute toxic inhalations. Curr Opin Pulm Med. 2019;25(2):211-6.
6. Jing J, Schwartz DA. Acute and chronic responses to toxic inhalations. In: Grippi MA, Elias JA, Fishman JA, et al. (Eds). Fishman's Pulmonary Diseases and Disorders, 5th edition. New York: McGraw-Hill; 2015.
7. Dries DJ, Endorf FW. Inhalation injury: epidemiology, pathology, treatment strategies. Scand J Trauma Resusc Emerg Med. 2013;21:31.
8. Deutsch CJ, Tan A, Smailes S, et al. The diagnosis and management of inhalation injury: An evidence based approach. Burns. 2018;44(5):1040-51.
9. Gupta K, Mehrotra M, Kumar P, et al. Smoke Inhalation Injury: Etiopathogenesis, Diagnosis, and Management. Indian J Crit Care Med. 2018;22(3):180-8.
10. Rehberg S, Maybauer MO, Enkhbaatar P, et al. Pathophysiology, management and treatment of smoke inhalation injury. Expert Rev Respir Med. 2009;3(3):283-97.
11. Albright JM, Davis CS, Bird MD. et al. The acute pulmonary inflammatory response to the graded severity of smoke inhalation injury. Crit Care Med. 2012;40(4):1113-21.
12. Fontán JJ, Cortright DN, Krause JE, et al. Substance P and neurokinin-1 receptor expression by intrinsic airway neurons in the rat. Am J Physiol Lung Cell Mol Physiol. 2000;278(2): L344-55.
13. Lange M, Enkhbaatar P, Traber DL, et al. Role of calcitonin gene-related peptide (CGRP) in ovine burn and smoke inhalation injury. J Appl Physiol (1985). 2009;107(1):176-84.
14. Kraneveld AD, Nijkamp FP. Tachykinins and neuro-immune interactions in asthma. Int Immunopharmacol. 2001;1(9-10): 1629-50.
15. Walker PF, Buehner MF, Wood LA, et al. Diagnosis and management of inhalation injury: an updated review. Crit Care. 2015;19:351.
16. Murakami K, Traber DL. Pathophysiological basis of smoke inhalation injury. News Physiol Sci. 2003;18:125-9.
17. Morita N, Enkhbaatar P, Maybauer DM, et al. Impact of bronchial circulation on bronchial exudates following combined burn and smoke inhalation injury in sheep. Burns, 2011;37(3):465-73.
18. Enkhbaatar P, Pruitt Jr BA, Suman O, et al. Pathophysiology, research challenges, and clinical management of smoke inhalation injury. Lancet. 2016;388(10052):1437-46.
19. Lange M, Szabo C, Enkhbaatar P, et al. Beneficial pulmonary effects of a metalloporphyrinic peroxynitrite decomposition catalyst in burn and smoke inhalation injury. Am J Physiol Lung Cell Mol Physiol. 2011;300(2):L167-75.
20. Hamahata A, Enkhbaatar P, Lange M, et al. Administration of a peroxynitrite decomposition catalyst into the bronchial artery attenuates pulmonary dysfunction after smoke inhalation and burn injury in sheep. Shock. 2012,38(5).543-8.
21. Hassan Z, Wong JK, Bush J, et al. Assessing the severity of inhalation injuries in adults. Burns. 2010;36(2):212-6.
22. Ryan CM, Fagan SP, Goverman J, et al. Grading inhalation injury by admission bronchoscopy. Crit Care Med. 2012;40(4):1345-6.
23. Cancio LC, Galvez Jr E, Turner CE, et al. Base deficit and alveolar-arterial gradient during resuscitation contribute independently but modestly to the prediction of mortality after burn injury. J Burn Care Res. 2006;27(3):289-96; discussion 296-7.
24. Park MS, Cancio LC, Batchinsky AI, et al. Assessment of severity of ovine smoke inhalation injury by analysis of computed tomographic scans. J Trauma. 2003;55(3): 417-27; discussion 427-9.
25. Mosier MJ, et al.Pham TN, Park DR, et al. Predictive value of bronchoscopy in assessing the severity of inhalation injury. J Burn Care Res. 2012;33(1):65-73.
26. Evans RB. Chlorine: state of the art. Lung. 2005;183(3):151-67.
27. Winder C. The toxicology of chlorine. Environ Res. 2001;85(2): 105-14.
28. Reisz GE, Gammon RS. Toxic pneumonitis from mixing household cleaners. Chest. 1986;89(1):49-52.

SECTION 17: RESPIRATORY CRITICAL CARE

29. Lin GD, Wu JY, Peng XB, et al. Chlorine poisoning caused by improper mixing of household disinfectants during the COVID-19 pandemic: Case series. World J Clin Cases. 2022;10(25): 8872-9.
30. Mrvos R, Dean BS, Krenzelok EP. Home exposures to chlorine/chloramine gas: review of 216 cases. South Med J. 1993;86(6): 654-7.
31. Couto M, Bernard A, Delgado L, et al. Health effects of exposure to chlorination by-products in swimming pools. Allergy. 2021;76(11):3257-5.
32. Ballal SG, Ali BA, Albar AA, et al. Bronchial asthma in two chemical fertilizer producing factories in eastern Saudi Arabia. Int J Tuberc Lung Dis. 1998;2(4):330-5.
33. Choudat D, Goehen M, Korobaeff M, et al. Respiratory symptoms and bronchial reactivity among pig and dairy farmers. Scand J Work Environ Health. 1994;20(1):48-54.
34. Jolly AJ, Schwartz DA. Acute and chronic responses to toxic inhalations. In: Grippi MA, Antin-Ozerkis DE, Dela-Cruz CS (Eds). Fishman's Pulmonary Diseases and Disorders, 6th edition. New York: McGraw-Hill Education; 2023.
35. Pangeni RP, Timilsina B, Oli PR, et al. A multidisciplinary approach to accidental inhalational ammonia injury: A case report. Ann Med Surg (Lond). 2022;82:104741.
36. Brautbar N, Wu MP, Richter ED. Chronic ammonia inhalation and interstitial pulmonary fibrosis: a case report and review of the literature. Arch Environ Health. 2003;58(9):592-6.
37. de Lange DW, Meulenbelt J. Do corticosteroids have a role in preventing or reducing acute toxic lung injury caused by inhalation of chemical agents? Clin Toxicol (Phila). 2011;49(2): 61-71.
38. Orellano P, Reynoso J, Quaranta N. Short-term exposure to sulphur dioxide (SO2) and all-cause and respiratory mortality: A systematic review and meta-analysis. Environ. Int. 2021;150: 106434.
39. Yorifuji T, Kashima S, Suryadhi MAH, et al. Acute exposure to sulfur dioxide and mortality: Historical data from Yokkaichi, Japan. Arch Environ Occup Health. 2019;74(5):271-8.
40. Carlsen HK, Valdimarsdóttir U, Briem H, et al. Severe volcanic SO(2) exposure and respiratory morbidity in the Icelandic population - a register study. Environ Health. 2021;20(1):23.
41. Sprowl GM. Hazards of Hawai'i Volcanoes National Park. Hawaii J Med Public Health. 2014;73(11 Suppl 2):17-20.
42. Woodford DM, Coutu RE, Gaensler EA. Obstructive lung disease from acute sulfur dioxide exposure. Respiration. 1979;38(4): 238-45.
43. Bardana EJ Jr. Reactive airways dysfunction syndrome (RADS): guidelines for diagnosis and treatment and insight into likely prognosis. Ann Allergy Asthma Immunol. 1999;83(6 Pt 2):583-6.
44. Charan NB, Myers CG, Lakshminarayan S, et al. Pulmonary injuries associated with acute sulfur dioxide inhalation. Am Rev Respir Dis. 1979;119(4):555-60.
45. Amaducci A, Downs JW. Nitrogen Dioxide Toxicity. In: StatPearls [Internet]. Treasure Island (FL): StatPearls Publishing; 2024 Jan.
46. Aggarwal AN, Ramanathan RM, Jindal SK. Acute respiratory distress syndrome following nitrogen dioxide exposure. Indian J Chest Dis Allied Sci. 1998;40(4):275-9.
47. Fitzgerald GJ. Chemical warfare and medical response during World War I. Am J Public Health. 2008;98(4):611-25.
48. Cao CL, Zhang L, Shen J. Phosgene-Induced acute lung injury: Approaches for mechanism-based treatment strategies. Front Immunol. 2022;13:917395.
49. Sciuto AM, Hurt HH. Therapeutic treatments of phosgene-induced lung injury. Inhal Toxicol. 2004;16(8):565-80.
50. Rayner-Canham G, Overton T. Descriptive Inorganic Chemistry. The Group 16 Elements The Chalcogens. New York: W.H. Freeman and Company; 2009.
51. Morii D, Miyagatani Y, Nakamae N, et al. Japanese experience of hydrogen sulfide: the suicide craze in 2008. J Occup Med Toxicol. 2010;5:28.
52. Chou SO, Pohl JM, Hana R. (2016). Toxicological profile for hydrogen sulfide and carbonyl sulfide. [online] Available from https://stacks.cdc.gov/view/cdc/43468 [Last accessed September, 2024].
53. Xiao Q, Ying J, Zhang C. The biologic effect of hydrogen sulfide and its function in various diseases. Medicine (Baltimore). 2018;97(44):e13065.
54. Kim SY, Kim E, Kim WJ. Health Effects of Ozone on Respiratory Diseases. Tuberc Respir Dis (Seoul). 2020;83(Suppl 1):S6-11.
55. Rafati Rahimzadeh M, Rafati Rahimzadeh M, Kazemi S, et al. Cadmium toxicity and treatment: An update. Caspian J Intern Med. 2017;8(3):135-45.
56. Charkiewicz AE, Omeljaniuk WJ, Nowak K, et al. Cadmium Toxicity and Health Effects: A Brief Summary. Molecules. 2023; 28(18):6620.
57. Leduc D, de Francquen P, Jacobovitz D, et al. Association of cadmium exposure with rapidly progressive emphysema in a smoker. Thorax. 1993;48(5):570-1.
58. Brockhaus A, Freier I, Ewers U, et al. Levels of cadmium and lead in blood in relation to smoking, sex, occupation, and other factors in an adult population of the FRG. Int Arch Occup Environ Health. 1983;52(2):167-75.
59. Oz SG, Tozlu M, Yalcin SS, et al. Mercury vapor inhalation and poisoning of a family. Inhal Toxicol. 2012;24(10): 652-8.
60. Clarkson TW, Magos L, Myers GJ. The toxicology of mercury--current exposures and clinical manifestations. N Engl J Med. 2003;349(18):1731-7.

Pulmonary Arterial Hypertension in the Intensive Care Unit

CHAPTER **170**

Himanshu Deshwal, Linda Benes, Roxana Sulica

INTRODUCTION

Pulmonary arterial hypertension (PAH) is characterized by pulmonary vascular remodeling, which ultimately leads to right ventricular failure (RVF) and death. Hemodynamic definition of pulmonary hypertension (PH) has undergone several modifications; latest European Society of Cardiology (ESC) and European Respiratory Society (ERS) 2022 guidelines define PH as mean pulmonary artery pressure (mPAP) > 20 mm Hg with different phenotypes classified based on pulmonary artery wedge pressure (PAWP) and pulmonary vascular resistance (PVR), i.e., PAWP ≤ 15 mm Hg, and PVR ≥ 2 Wood units (WU) **(Table 1)**[1]. The major modification was the reduction in PVR from 3 to 2 WU as it reflects the upper limit of normal, captures more patients with precapillary disease early, and is associated with progression to RVF and mortality.[2,3]

Pulmonary hypertension is classified into five broad categories based on the etiology and hemodynamic presentation, and the therapeutic approach depends on this classification **(Table 2)**.[1] While most of the therapeutic focus lies on Group I PAH, improved understanding of the underlying pathophysiology, emerging therapeutic targets, and early recognition of the disease have expanded the therapeutic horizon to individualized, evidence-based care.

Pulmonary hypertension with RVF in the critical care setting is associated with significant morbidity and mortality and warrants early recognition, close monitoring, and aggressive therapeutic management. RVF, respiratory failure, infection, missed medications, infections, arrhythmias, and bleeding are the most common causes of hospitalization, with the majority (66.9%) requiring intensive care unit (ICU) admission.[4] RVF alone contributes to 16–18% of ICU hospitalization.[5,6] Patients admitted to ICU have higher mortality ranging from 27.1% to 52%.[5-8] Several prognostic indicators for in-hospital mortality have been described. Hyponatremia, acute kidney injury (AKI), systemic hypotension, need for mechanical ventilation, brain natriuretic peptide, higher inotropic dose, and higher SOFA and APACHE II scores are significant predictors of in-hospital mortality in various studies.[6-9]

In this chapter, we highlight the underlying pathophysiology of RVF and suggest an approach to diagnosing, treating, and managing complications such as triggering factors.

PATHOPHYSIOLOGY OF RIGHT HEART FAILURE IN PULMONARY HYPERTENSION

Normal Right Ventricular Physiology

The right ventricle is a low-pressure and high-compliance chamber with the ability to accommodate large variations in the venous return without altering the end-diastolic

TABLE 1: New hemodynamic definitions of pulmonary hypertension based on the ERS/ESC 2022 guidelines.

Pulmonary hypertension phenotype	Hemodynamic definition
Pulmonary hypertension	mPAP > 20 mm Hg
Precapillary pulmonary hypertension	mPAP > 20 mm Hg, PAWP ≤ 15 mm Hg and PVR > 2 WU
Postcapillary pulmonary hypertension • Isolated postcapillary PH (IpcPH) • Combined pre- and postcapillary PH (CpcPH)	mPAP > 20 mm Hg and PAWP > 15 mm Hg • mPAP > 20 mm Hg, PAWP > 15 mm Hg and PVR ≤ 2 WU • mPAP > 20 mm Hg, PAWP > 15 mm Hg and PVR > 2 WU
Exercise Pulmonary Hypertension	mPAP/CO slope > 3 mm Hg/L/min
Unclassified Pulmonary Hypertension	mPAP > 20 mm Hg, PAWP ≤ 15 mm Hg and PVR ≤ 2 WU

(mPAP: mean pulmonary artery pressure; PAWP: pulmonary artery wedge pressure; PVR: pulmonary vascular resistance; CO: cardiac output; WU: Wood units; ERS/ESC: European Respiratory Society/European Society of Cardiology)

TABLE 2: Clinical classification of pulmonary hypertension based on etiology and pathophysiology.

Clinical classification of pulmonary hypertension	
Group I	Pulmonary arterial hypertension
Group II	Pulmonary hypertension associated with left heart disease
Group III	Pulmonary hypertension associated with lung diseases/hypoxia
Group IV	Pulmonary hypertension associated with pulmonary artery obstruction
Group V	Pulmonary hypertension due to unclear or multifactorial mechanisms

pressure. The muscular conformation of the right ventricle is based on the Torrent-Guasp Helical model, suggesting two interconnected myofibril loops (basal and apical).[10] The longitudinally oriented muscle fibers contribute to the stroke volume more than the radial/obliquely arranged muscle fibers.[10] The muscular arrangement of the RV and left ventricle (LV) are interconnected, and thus, the LV contraction contributes significantly to the RV stroke volume via the interventricular septum.[11] In disease states, the flattening or paradoxical septal motion may suggest significant RV dysfunction and loss of LV contribution.[12]

The RV contraction defers from the LV such that it is more peristaltic/sequential than pulsatile. Due to high compliance of the pulmonary vasculature, the RV generates less than one fifth of the systolic pressures generated by the LV. Hence, the RV has increased sensitivity to augmented afterload.[13] The load-independent measure of RV contractility is the end-systolic elastance (measured using pressure-volume loops as a ratio of end-systolic pressure and stroke volume) which is coupled with the RV afterload, effectively described as the pulmonary vascular elastance.[14] The pulmonary vascular elastance is a better RV afterload marker than PVR as it includes both pulsatile and resistive components of the pulmonary vasculature.[15] This RV-to-PA coupling is maintained in general health to provide adequate stroke volume and LV preload. The primary determinants of RV function are similar to the LV and include preload, afterload, inotropy, and lusitropy (active relaxation).[15]

Right Ventricular Response to Increased Afterload

The response of the right ventricular function is different in acute vs. chronic loading conditions as several pathophysiologic changes occur in the right ventricular morphology to maintain RV-PA coupling and stroke volume. In states of acute increase in RV afterload, such as acute pulmonary embolism, acute respiratory distress syndrome, and hypoxia, the RV does not have sufficient time to adapt to the stress, which results in dilation of the right heart chambers. This leads to RV wall stress, increased myocardial oxygen demand, and ischemia, further deterioration of RV function, with reduced stroke volume and cardiogenic shock.[16] Therefore, it is essential to treat the etiology of the increased afterload (oxygen supplementation, lung protective mechanical ventilation, anticoagulation/thrombolysis, or suction thrombectomy).

In chronic loading conditions such as PAH, the RV myocardium undergoes hypertrophy to maintain contractility, RV–PA coupling, and stroke volume. As the disease state progresses and RV contraction is insufficient, the right heart chambers dilate to accommodate a larger volume of blood to maintain adequate stroke volume. At this stage, the RV end-systolic elastance changes, and RV–PA uncoupling starts to occur. A loss of lusitropy leads to increased RV filling pressures as measured by right atrial or central venous pressures.[15] A subsequent increase in RV wall stress results in myocardial ischemia, neurohumoral activation, and myocardial fibrosis resulting in further RV dysfunction. Subsequently, there is a loss of septal contribution of the LV contraction resulting in RV–PA uncoupling and a reduction in stroke volume.[15] This vicious cycle results in a clinically volume-overloaded state, cardiogenic shock, and increased risk for supraventricular tachycardia, myocardial edema, pericardial effusion, and death.

PULMONARY HYPERTENSION IN THE CRITICALLY ILL PATIENT

Evaluation and Monitoring

Close monitoring and evaluation are required for patients with PAH admitted to ICU. In addition to clinical examination, noninvasive and invasive methods may be utilized to assess and monitor the severity of illness, prognosis, and response to therapy (**Table 3**).

Biomarkers/Laboratory Testing

While biomarkers have been used to prognosticate in the ambulatory setting, their utility in critical care setting is less well studied. Elevation of serum troponin I levels as a marker of RV myocyte injury and troponin levels to risk-stratify the severity of pulmonary embolism and assist in therapeutic decision-making have been used. Serum brain natriuretic peptide (BNP) or N-terminal BNP are easily reproducible and relatively inexpensive biomarkers often used to assess the severity of heart failure. Although not specific to right heart failure, in the context of PAH, it has significant prognostic value and is a part of several risk stratification tools.[11,17] In ambulatory settings, BNP is inversely correlated to a 6-minute walk distance and VO_2max in patients with idiopathic PAH.[18]

TABLE 3: Clinical evaluation and monitoring of pulmonary hypertension patient in intensive care unit.

Evaluation and monitoring for pulmonary hypertension in the intensive care unit		
Clinical evaluation	**Test modality**	**Parameters**
Heart rate and rhythm	Continuous cardiac monitor	Tachyarrhythmia, bradycardia, heart blocks
Respiratory Status	• Pulse oximetry • Arterial blood gas • Hemoglobin	• Goal O_2 saturation > 90% • Goal PaO_2 > 60 mm Hg • Goal hemoglobin >8–10 mm Hg
Systemic Perfusion	• Blood pressure • Urine output and renal function • Serum lactate	• Arterial line if unstable • Strict input and output, Sodium level, blood urea nitrogen and creatinine levels • Serum lactate < 2 mmol/L
Pulmonary hypertension, right ventricular dysfunction, and fluid status	• Pulmonary artery catheterization • Echocardiography • Biomarkers • Urine Output	• CVP, mPAP, PAWP, CO/CI, PVR, PAPi, CVP:PAWP ratio, PAO_2 saturation • RA/RV morphology and function, pericardial effusion, IVC dilation • Brain natriuretic peptide, serum troponin • Negative fluid balance

(CVP: central venous pressure; mPAP: mean pulmonary artery pressure; PAWP: pulmonary artery wedge pressure; PVR: pulmonary vascular resistance; CO: cardiac output; WU: Wood units, PAPi: pulmonary artery pulsatility index; IVC: inferior vena cava)

More recent studies have identified BNP as a predictor of mortality in PAH patients admitted to ICU.[5,6]

Patients admitted to ICU may have several metabolic derangements, including renal dysfunction and electrolyte imbalance. Elevated blood urea nitrogen, serum creatinine, and hyponatremia are independent predictors of mortality in PAH patients admitted to ICU.[6,19] Cardiorenal AKI can be seen in a volume overload state and is associated with worse outcomes.[20] Hepatic derangement may be seen in congestive hepatopathy or as a result of adverse medication effects, requiring thorough evaluation.[6]

Echocardiography

Echocardiography is an essential noninvasive, portable, and easy to use tool used to screen for PH and assess right ventricular structure and function in the ICU. In patients with an established diagnosis of PAH, an echocardiogram can be the first-line modality to assess the interval progression of the disease and changes in the RV function and morphology.[1] It can be easily used for point-of-care testing and frequently repeated to guide management. While the complex anatomy of RV makes accurate functional assessment difficult, several echocardiographic markers can be utilized to screen for PH, assess the severity of RV dysfunction, and for prognostic purposes.[21]

Enlargement of the right atrium and ventricle, along with paradoxical septal motion in systole and diastole, may suggest RV pressure and volume overload and is an important marker of increased RV afterload (**Figs. 1A to D**).[12,21] In addition, pericardial effusion and right atrial enlargement are often markers of an advanced disease state and are associated with poor outcomes.[22] The longitudinal motion of the tricuspid annulus assessed using tricuspid annular planar systolic excursion (TAPSE) or tissue Doppler (s') correlates with RV ejection fraction and can provide insight into the RV function.[1,21] Continuous Doppler assessment of the tricuspid regurgitant (TR) jet is utilized to assess the maximum TR velocity, which can help estimate right ventricular systolic pressures (RVSP) using Bernoulli's equation (**Figs. 2A to D**). A TR velocity > 2.8 m/s is often utilized as a screening tool for elevated PAPs.[23] Both overestimation and underestimation of PAP occur frequently. Accuracy of an echocardiogram to estimate the PAP is dependent on multiple factors, including the quality of echocardiographic windows, the severity of tricuspid regurgitation, body habitus, presence of mechanical valve, etc.[21,23]

Dilated inferior vena cava with minimal respiratory variation may suggest elevated right atrial pressures. In the parasternal short-axis view, assessing the right ventricular outflow tract (RVOT) and pulmonary valve with pulsed wave Doppler can also be utilized to evaluate for increased RV afterload. Reduced pulmonary acceleration time and mid-to-late systolic notching of the RVOT waveform are highly suggestive of increased RV afterload either due to pulmonary embolism or pulmonary vasculopathy/hypertension.[24]

Patient size, difficulty in positioning a critically ill patient, and the technician's experience level can result in a poor-quality study. A transesophageal echocardiogram yields a higher sensitivity and specificity for patients who can tolerate the procedure. It is frequently reserved for patients with poor transthoracic windows, suspected valvular disease, endocarditis, or pulmonary embolism.[25]

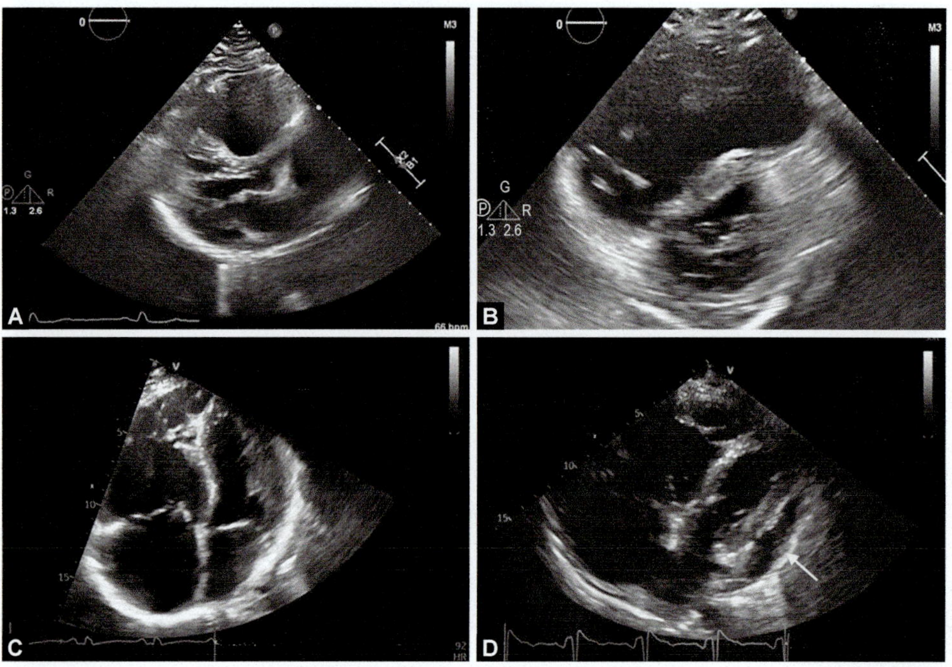

FIGS. 1A TO D: Echocardiographic assessment of RV function and PH. (A) Parasternal long-axis view demonstrating severely dilated right ventricle with bulging of the interventricular septum into the left ventricle. (B) Parasternal short-axis view demonstrating severely dilated right ventricle with flattening of the interventricular septum into the left ventricle during systole and diastole suggesting RV pressure and volume overload. (C) Four-chamber view demonstrating enlargement of right atrium and ventricle with RV forming the apex. (D) Four-chamber view demonstrating severely dilated right atrium and ventricle along with moderate pericardial effusion (arrow) along the left ventricular border.

(PH: pulmonary hypertension; RV: right ventricle)

Swan-Ganz Catheterization/Right Heart Catheterization

Right heart catheterization is the gold standard for diagnosing PH.[1] This is accomplished in the ICU setting by using a pulmonary artery (PA) catheter that is inserted through either the right internal jugular (RIJ) vein, the left subclavian vein, or the femoral veins (right preferred). The RIJ is the preferred route of access as the PA catheter may be left in place for continuous monitoring of cardiac pressures.

Values measured include right atrial pressure/central venous pressure, PA systolic, diastolic, and mean pressures, PAWP, and PVR. A PAWP ≥ 15 mm Hg suggests left-sided disease, while a PAWP ≤ 15 mm Hg is consistent with pulmonary arterial hypertension/precapillary PH. Cardiac output (CO) and cardiac index can be measured by thermodilution or the Fick method. Fick's principle relies on knowing the uptake of oxygen by an organ and the concentration of oxygen in the arterial and venous circulations. Due to the cumbersome nature of calculating oxygen consumption, the indirect Fick's determination uses a fixed value for oxygen consumption, allowing one to calculate the CO more easily. However, the thermodilution CO method is recommended as indirect Fick's CO may be inaccurate or unreliable due to assumed O_2 consumption, which can be significantly different in each individual and disease state. An important calculation during right heart catheterization is PVR expressed in WU. Measurement of the oxygen saturation in the PA is an important marker of the adequacy of systemic oxygen delivery, and it is a useful parameter to guide the use of inotropes in the ICU patient with PH.[26] Several other markers of RV function can be calculated using the obtained hemodynamic variables with clinical and prognostic implications (**Table 4**).

Even though the use of pulmonary artery catheterization in the ICU has declined over the past years due to the lack of impact on the outcome and potential complications, none of the investigations leading to those conclusions have included patients with PH and RVF. As such, in certain cases of critically ill patients with PH, PA catheterization may be indicated for monitoring and treatment guidance.[27] The risks of PA catheterization in critically ill PH patients are also unknown. Still, in the outpatient setting and with experienced providers, the mortality risk from the procedure is 0.055%, with PA rupture as the most important cause of death.[28] It is likely that, particularly in the critical care setting, the risk of complications may decrease by floating the catheter with fluoroscopic guidance and reducing the number of manipulations in the PA.

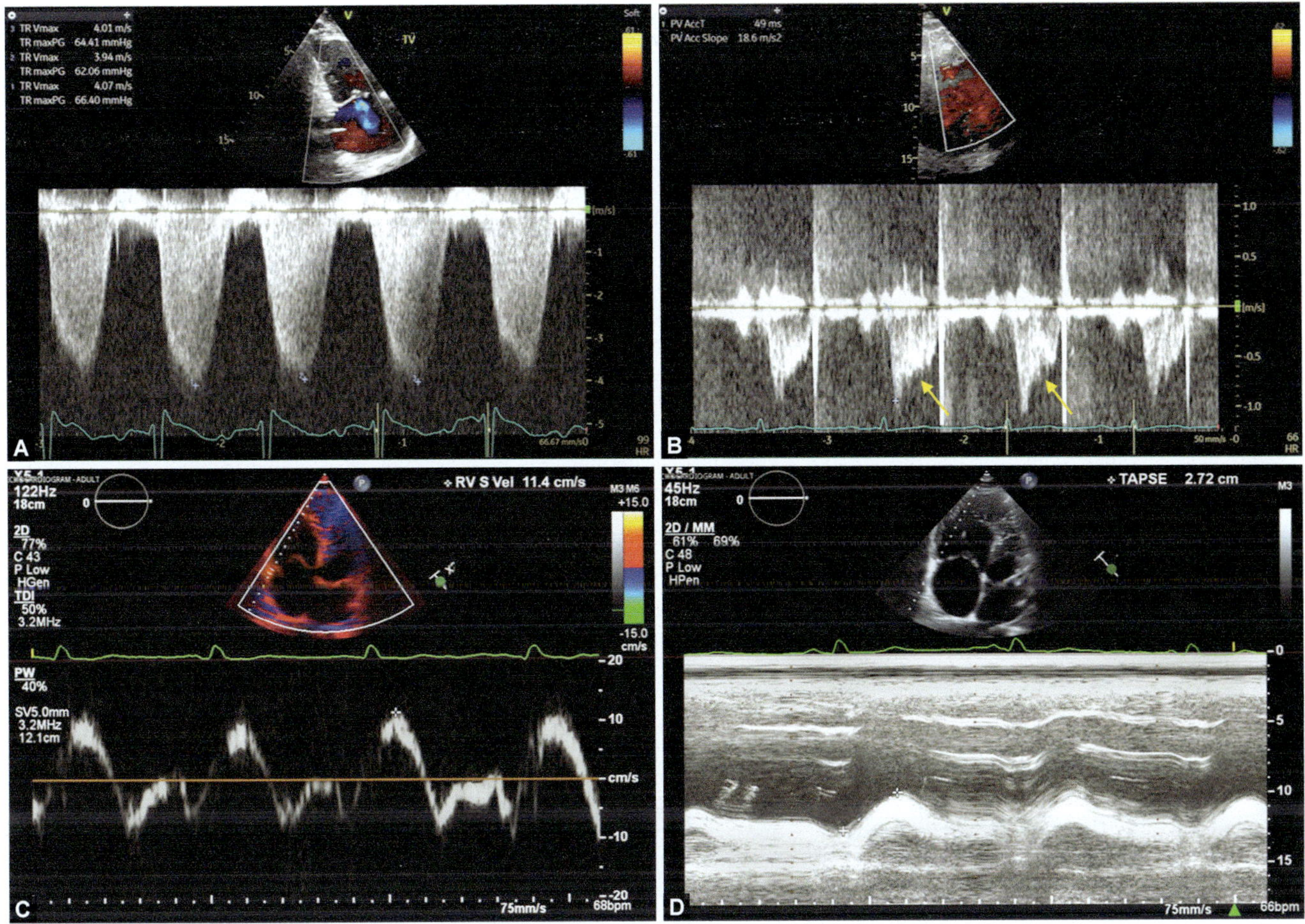

FIGS. 2A TO D: Doppler assessment in PH and RV failure. (A) Continuous-wave Doppler in four chamber view assessing the tricuspid regurgitant velocity that can be used to assess the right ventricular systolic pressure. (B) Pulsed-wave Doppler across the right ventricular outflow tract in parasternal short axis view demonstrating a reduced pulmonary acceleration time and mid-systolic notching (arrows), suggesting increased RV afterload and PA pressures. (C) Tissue Doppler across the lateral tricuspid annulus assessing the longitudinal right ventricular function (TDI s') which is closely correlated to RV ejection fraction. (D) M-mode demonstrating tricuspid annular planar systolic excursion (TAPSE) which is also an indirect marker of RV ejection fraction and function.

(PH: pulmonary hypertension; RV: right ventricle)

MANAGEMENT

General principles for patients with PAH in RVF are identifying and treating triggering factors, improving RV function by optimizing RV preload, reducing RV afterload, increasing cardiac contractility, and maintaining adequate tissue perfusion (**Fig. 3**).

Identify and Treat the Triggering Factors

Supraventricular Tachycardia

Advanced disease state and morphologic remodeling of the right atrium may commonly precipitate supraventricular tachycardia in PAH. The estimated prevalence is 11–35% and is poorly tolerated in right ventricular failure due to loss of atrioventricular (AV) synchrony.[29] In a compensated state, the right atrial kick contributes to maintaining RV stroke volume in PAH. The loss of AV synchrony can precipitate clinical decompensation in PAH patients; therefore, restoring the sinus rhythm is paramount. The AV nodal blocking agents, such as calcium channel blockers or beta-blockers, are poorly tolerated due to negative inotropic and chronotropic effects. Antiarrhythmic medications such as amiodarone can be used in PAH. However, amiodarone inhibits the cytochrome P450 pathway, and cautious medication reconciliation is required to prevent drug interaction with medications such as endothelin receptor antagonists. Electrical cardioversion can be utilized in acutely decompensated patients with hemodynamic instability. Radiofrequency ablation is generally required as a definitive treatment in atrial flutter or reentrant arrhythmias to prevent recurrence.[30]

TABLE 4: Calculated variables obtained from pulmonary artery catheterization.

Parameter	Calculation
Diastolic pulmonary gradient (mm Hg)	dPAP – PAWP
Transpulmonary gradient (mm Hg)	mPAP – PAWP
Cardiac output (CO) by Fick's principle	$\frac{VO_2 \text{ (}O_2\text{ Consumption)}}{\text{(Arterial }O_2\text{ Content – Venous }O_2\text{ Content)}}$
Pulmonary vascular resistance (PVR) (Wood units)	$\frac{\text{mPAP – PAWP}}{\text{CO}}$
Systemic vascular resistance (SVR) (dyne/s/cm^{-5})	$\frac{\text{MAP – CVP} \times 80}{\text{CO}}$
Pulmonary artery compliance (mL/mm Hg)	$\frac{\text{Stroke volume}}{\text{sPAP – dPAP}}$
Pulmonary artery pulsatility index (PAPi)	$\frac{\text{sPAP – dPAP}}{\text{CVP}}$
Cardiac power output (Watts)	$\frac{\text{MAP} \times \text{CO}}{451}$

sPAP: systolic pulmonary artery pressure; dPAP: diastolic pulmonary artery pressure; mPAP: mean pulmonary artery pressure; PAWP: pulmonary artery venous pressure; MAP: mean arterial pressure, CVP: central venous pressure/mean right atrial pressure.

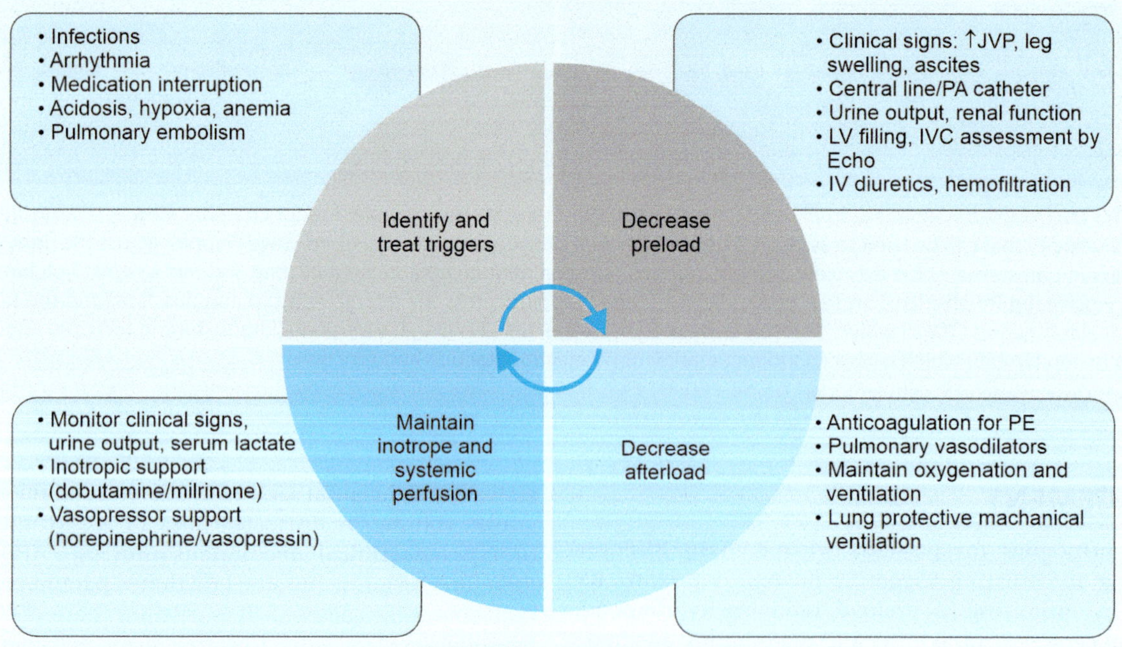

FIG. 3: Management of pulmonary hypertension patient with decompensated right ventricular failure in the intensive care unit. (LV: left ventricular; IVC: inferior vena cava; IV: intravenous; JVP: jugular venous pressure; PA: pulmonary artery)

Pericardial Effusion

Pericardial effusion is a poor prognostic indicator in PAH and poses a therapeutic challenge. Draining a pericardial effusion, if needed, has to be done with utmost caution, due to the risk of a sudden increase in RV preload, interventricular interdependence, and reduction in LV stroke volume, leading to cardiac arrest.[31] In addition, due to RV remodeling, classic echocardiographic features of tamponade physiology may be absent in PAH.[22] Left atrial collapse, >25% variation in mitral inflow with respiration, and diastolic flow reversal in hepatic veins during expiration are reliable markers of tamponade physiology in PAH.[22] While smaller effusions may eventually improve with medical therapy, large pericardial effusion with tamponade physiology requires a multidisciplinary approach to deciding whether to drain. Pericardiocentesis with gradual fluid removal not exceeding 50–100 cc/day and central venous pressure monitoring has been suggested in some case series.[32]

Infection

Infections contribute to 16% of hospitalization in PAH patients and are associated with significant morbidity and mortality.[7] While most common cause of infection is pneumonia, in patients with indwelling catheters prostacyclin administration, a low index of suspicion is required for prompt diagnosis and treatment. Blood cultures must be obtained, and the infected catheter should be removed immediately. Broad-spectrum antibiotics should be initiated and adjusted to narrow spectrum based on culture sensitivity. In sepsis, close monitoring and cautious resuscitation are required to prevent volume overload and RV decompensation.

Optimizing Various Facets of Right Ventricular Failure

Improving Right Ventricular Preload

Optimizing the RV preload is a key pillar in managing RVF. Physiology of RVF in PAH is RV afterload dependent and has a distinct response to fluid loading compared to RV myocardial ischemia. The failing RV in PAH is functioning on the descending segment of the Frank-Starling curve, and further volume loading may lead to a decline in stroke volume. In addition, an overdistended RV may impair left ventricular preload and stroke volume by means of septal shift into the left ventricle leading to ventricular interdependence or reverse Bernheim effect. Increased venous congestion may subsequently lead to cardiorenal AKI, an important prognostic factor in hospitalized PAH patients.[20] Reducing the stressed intravascular volume employing diuresis or extracorporeal fluid removal is essential in improving RV function and stroke volume.[33] Fluid restriction and intravenous loop diuretics are the first-line treatment for optimizing RV preload. In patients not responding to loop diuretics, the addition of thiazide (chlorthalidone) may improve diuresis via diuretic synergy.[34] If medical therapy is insufficient, continuous renal replacement therapy may be warranted in reducing the volume overload state. Close monitoring and replacement of electrolytes are essential to avoid precipitating arrhythmias. Documentation and review of baseline dry weight prior to hospitalization is important and can be utilized to target diuretic therapy.[34,35]

Improving Right Ventricular Afterload

Pulmonary vasodilator therapies are the cornerstone of the management of PAH with RVF in the ICU. Care must be taken to exclude left ventricular dysfunction or elevated left ventricular end-diastolic pressure (elevated PAWP), as injudicious use of pulmonary vasodilators may precipitate pulmonary edema.

In patients with an established diagnosis of PAH on appropriate therapy, the PH medications should not be discontinued or dose adjusted. This is particularly important with continuous prostacyclin therapy as acute withdrawal may precipitate RVF leading to cardiovascular collapse.[36] The PH medications should be reinitiated under the guidance of the PH expert if the reason for hospitalization was RVF secondary to missed medications.[36]

Inhaled pulmonary vasodilators can be considered in patients with hemodynamic instability and respiratory failure. Inhaled nitric oxide (NO) has been studied extensively in acute respiratory distress syndrome with improvement in oxygenation, although no significant effect on overall mortality.[37] Inhaled NO can be utilized in acutely unstable PAH patients as it has been shown to reduce PVR and improve CO without significant systemic hypotension due to rapid inactivation in the pulmonary capillaries. In addition, inhaled NO has the advantage of selective pulmonary vasodilation in well-ventilated areas leading to improved ventilation-perfusion matching. The main concerns with inhaled NO include the need for continuous administration and potential toxicity leading to methemoglobinemia.[38] Inhaled prostacyclin analogs in the ICU are studied mainly in the postoperative cardiothoracic surgical settings but can be utilized if parenteral formulations are unavailable.[27]

Intravenous prostacyclin analogs such as epoprostenol and treprostinil are potent pulmonary vasodilators and are the drug of choice for PAH with RVF in the ICU.[6,39] A dedicated central venous catheter with an air-filter is often required to administer continuous prostacyclin analog infusions and must be considered under the guidance of a PH expert. Systemic hypotension due to direct systemic vasodilation is common with parenteral prostacyclin therapies.[39]

In patients with acute RVF precipitated by pulmonary embolism, prompt initiation of anticoagulation is important. In addition, several institutions have developed a pulmonary embolism response team (PERT) to offer multidisciplinary decision-making involving the cardiothoracic surgeon, intensivist, PH specialist, and interventional radiologist.[40] A decision to perform catheter-based thrombolysis or suction thrombectomy vs. surgical thromboembolectomy may be considered depending on the severity of hemodynamic compromise.[41]

Improving Inotropy

Inotropic support is required in patients with evidence of cardiogenic shock and evidence of decreased tissue oxygen delivery. While most inotropic agents overcome their systemic vasodilatory effects by increasing CO, concurrent vasopressor support is often required.[42] Several inotropic agents with different mechanisms of action are available; however, it is paramount to review their advantages and disadvantages (**Table 5**). Dobutamine has a

TABLE 5: Inotropic and vasopressor agents of choice in pulmonary hypertension and right ventricular failure in intensive care unit.

Inotropic and vasopressor agents in pulmonary hypertension in intensive care unit			
	Site of receptor activity	**Mechanism of action**	**Adverse effects/limitation**
Inotropic agents (Maintenance of RV contractility and stroke volume)			
Dobutamine	β_1, β_2	↑ Cardiac output/inotrope ↓ PVR, ↓SVR, ↑ RV: PA coupling	Tachycardia Hypotension
Milrinone	PDE-3 inhibitor	↑ Cardiac output/inotrope ↓ PVR, ↓SVR, ↑ RV: PA coupling	Tachycardia Hypotension
Epinephrine	α_1, α_2, β_1, β_2	↑ Cardiac output/inotrope ↑ PVR (RV afterload), ↑SVR ↑ MAP (systemic perfusion)	Tachycardia Lactate elevation Increased RV afterload
Levosimendan	Troponin C Ca^{2+} sensitization	↑ Cardiac output/inotrope ↓ PVR, ↓SVR, ↑ RV: PA coupling	Tachycardia Hypotension
Vasopressor agents (Maintenance of systemic perfusion)			
Norepinephrine	α_1, β_1	↑ Cardiac output (↑) PVR, ↑SVR ↑ MAP (systemic perfusion) ↑ RV:PA coupling	Lactate elevation
Vasopressin (low-dose)	V_1	(↑↓) PVR, ↑↑SVR ↑ MAP (systemic perfusion) ↑ RV:PA coupling	ADH activity
Phenylephrine	α_1	↑↑ PVR (RV afterload), ↑↑SVR ↑ MAP (systemic perfusion)	Increased RV afterload

(PVR: pulmonary vascular resistance; SVR: systemic vascular resistance; RV: right ventricle; PA: pulmonary artery; MAP: mean arterial pressure; ADH: anti-diuretic hormone)

dose-dependent decrease in PVR and increased RV contractility and CO, leading to improved RV-to-PA coupling efficiency. However, tachycardia is often a limiting factor and a dose of maximum 5–10 µg/kg/min dose is usually recommended to avoid side effects.[42] Milrinone also significantly lowers RV afterload and improves RV contractility; however, it has more systemic vasodilation leading to hypotension, often requiring vasopressor support. In addition, milrinone is renally cleared, leading to drug accumulation in patients with AKI.[43] Epinephrine is a potent inotropic agent; however, it also significantly increases PVR, increases the risk of tachyarrhythmias, and is generally avoided.

Improving Systemic Perfusion

In systemic hypotension, the CO may be insufficient to meet the body's metabolic demands leading to decreased perfusion of the vital organs (kidney, liver, coronaries, and brain), and vasopressor support is often required in RV failure (**Table 5**). However, vasopressors should be used judiciously as cardiogenic shock is associated with concurrent sympathetic overdrive, significantly impacting peripheral and pulmonary vascular resistance. Higher doses of available vasopressors may further increase RV afterload and worsen RV failure.

Norepinephrine is the drug of choice in PAH with systemic hypotension. It has been shown to improve RV-to-PA coupling at lower doses via direct inotropic effect, albeit to a smaller degree than dobutamine. Norepinephrine increases systemic blood pressure through α1-mediated peripheral vasoconstriction and β1-mediated inotropic effect.[44]

Vasopressin at lower doses is a potent peripheral vasoconstrictor and can be used with inotropic agents. Animal studies have demonstrated nitric oxide-mediated pulmonary vasodilation at lower doses; however, its effect on pulmonary circulation in humans has been inconsistent. In addition, higher doses may induce a negative inotropic effect along with increased PVR.

Phenylephrine is a potent peripheral vasoconstrictor with sole α1- mediated activity. It is generally avoided in chronic PH patients due to a significant increase in RV afterload.[45]

MANAGEMENT OF RESPIRATORY FAILURE IN PAH IN ICU

Respiratory failure is common in decompensated PH patients and can be challenging to manage. Hypoxia worsens PH and can occur due to several reasons, including pneumonia, atelectasis, right-to-left shunting, or progression of underlying coexisting lung disease. Hypercapnia may further increase pulmonary vasoconstriction leading to increase PVR and mean PA pressures.[46]

Early recognition of clinical worsening and appropriate strategies to treat hypoxemia and hypercapnia is often required as invasive mechanical ventilation (IMV) is often associated with significant mortality.[7,47] The goal of early respiratory support in the ICU is to improve oxygenation and ventilation and avoid the need for IMV.[42,48]

For hypoxic respiratory failure, initial management includes oxygen supplementation with a nasal cannula or high-flow nasal cannula (HFNC). The advantages of HFNC include delivery of higher flow rates to match the patient's flow demands, oxygenation of dead space, decreased sympathetic drive, and provision of minimal positive end-expiratory pressure to allow recruitment of atelectatic airways without the risk of barotrauma.[49] HFNC is well tolerated in PH patients as it does not impact hemodynamics while improving ventilation-perfusion matching and may overcome coexisting hypoxic vasoconstriction. In decompensated PH patients, inhaled pulmonary vasodilators can be delivered through HFNC to improve RV afterload further and V/Q matching in directly ventilated areas.

Positive-pressure ventilation (PPV) may be required for patients with acute hypercapnic respiratory failure or those in respiratory distress; however, it must be approached carefully due to its direct effect on reducing venous return (RV preload) and increasing RV afterload leading to hemodynamic decompensation. Non-invasive positive-pressure ventilation (NIPV) can be utilized at lower settings to improve respiratory distress or hypercapnia if it offsets the need for IMV. Bilevel NIPV or automated volume-assured positive-pressure support (AVAPS) may be utilized in hypercapnic patients with close monitoring.

Multidisciplinary planning is often required in advance if intubation and IMV are anticipated in a PH patient, as there is a significant risk of cardiovascular collapse and mortality during the peri-intubation phase.[47] A thorough preintubation preparation is required to minimize the risk of intubation.

Volume status and systemic perfusion should be optimized using appropriate diuretics and vasopressor support with norepinephrine or vasopressin. Parenteral or inhaled pulmonary vasodilators should be continued through the periintubation phase to optimize RV afterload. Carefully assessing the airway and anticipating the difficulty of intubation may guide physicians in deciding on the modality of induction and intubation.

Induction agents such as propofol are associated with negative inotrope and hypotension and should be avoided.[50] Etomidate is generally considered safe for rapid sequence induction; however, the possibility of an acute adrenal crisis must be entertained in chronically ill patients.[51] The decision to use neuromuscular blockade must also be weighed carefully as patients may be maintaining their hemodynamics on their sympathetic drive, which can be blunted during paralysis with the potential for decompensation.

Delayed sequence induction using ketamine infusion followed by benzodiazepines and opioids for analgesia (fentanyl) are often utilized, given their minimal impact on the airway reflexes, respiratory drive, and hemodynamics.[52,53] Applying local anesthetics such as lidocaine in the upper airway and trachea may prevent vagal reflex and reduce pain periintubation. The most experienced provider must attempt endotracheal intubation to minimize complications and improve the chances of a successful first pass. Direct laryngoscopy or fiberoptic video laryngoscopy can be utilized depending on the provider's comfort of use. Awake intubation using fiberoptic bronchoscopy has been utilized safely in critically ill PH patients using nasally delivered NIPV or HFNC for continuous respiratory support.[54]

Similarly to lung-protective ventilation strategies, RV-protective mechanical ventilation has been recommended for patients with PAH.[55] RV-protective IMV must be utilized to reduce the impact of PPV on PH physiology and RV failure. The goal of RV-protective IMV includes optimizing oxygenation and ventilation to minimize hypoxic vasoconstriction, reducing lung stress and barotrauma by limiting driving pressure, and minimizing the impact of PPV on PH physiology and RVF.[56] Pulmonary vascular resistance follows a U-shaped relationship with lung volumes with the lowest PVR at functional residual capacity. Ventilator settings should be adjusted to deliver tidal volumes in the range of 4–8 mL/kg per ideal body weight as long as the plateau pressures remain below 27 cm H_2O and driving pressures below 17 cm H_2O to minimize barotrauma and lung stress. A low positive end-expiratory pressure (PEEP) strategy can be applied to overcome hyperinflation if oxygen saturation is maintained above 94%. Daily assessment for spontaneous breathing trials and readiness for extubation should be considered for early liberation from IMV.

Mechanical Circulatory Support

Extracorporeal mechanical circulatory support (EMCS) may be considered in decompensated PH with RVF refractory to maximal medical management. When considering EMCS, a multidisciplinary team consisting of a PH specialist, cardiothoracic surgeon, intensivist, and anesthesiologist should be utilized in decision-making.[57] The goal of using EMCS must be either a bridge to the recovery of RV failure, a bridge to pulmonary thromboendarterectomy [in chronic thromboembolic pulmonary hypertension (CTEPH)], or a bridge to lung transplantation.[58] In patients with end-stage PAH listed for lung transplantation, utilizing EMCS can significantly reduce waiting list mortality, albeit at the cost of prolonged hospitalization and ICU stay.[58]

Several factors, such as the identifiable etiology of acute RV decompensation (infection, pulmonary embolism, and tachyarrhythmias) versus chronic RVF due to progressive pulmonary arterial hypertension, may help decide the goal of utilizing EMCS. A thorough evaluation of indication and contraindications should be utilized in this complex decision-making, and EMCS should be avoided if no identifiable destination therapy is identified (recovery or transplantation). In addition, multiorgan failure, active malignancy with poor life expectancy, coagulopathy, or active systemic infections may preclude the use of MCS.[59,60] If the goal is to bridge to lung transplantation, central VA-ECMO is preferred as it allows for physical rehabilitation and conditioning in preparation for the transplantation; however, it requires general anesthesia and sternotomy.[57] Peripheral cannulation may be considered in acutely decompensating patients. An alternate approach includes peripheral upper limb cannulation that may allow ambulation.[57]

SUMMARY

The management of PH patients in the ICU requires a thorough understanding of the pathophysiology of the disease and RVF. Close monitoring using non-invasive and invasive tools may be necessary to obtain useful information and guide management. Targeting the triggering factor and optimizing various determinants of RV function (preload, afterload, inotropy, and lusitropy) is the primary goal of treatment to improve outcomes. In patients with respiratory failure, a trial of non-invasive ventilation should take precedence with careful consideration of invasive mechanical ventilation. Right ventricle-protective mechanical ventilation is recommended to reduce the impact of PPV on the hemodynamics and the RV afterload. Extracorporeal mechanical circulatory support may be required as a bridge to recovery when a triggering factor is identified or as a bridge to lung transplantation.

REFERENCES

1. Humbert M, Kovacs G, Hoeper MM, et al. 2022 ESC/ERS Guidelines for the diagnosis and treatment of pulmonary hypertension: Developed by the task force for the diagnosis and treatment of pulmonary hypertension of the European Society of Cardiology (ESC) and the European Respiratory Society (ERS). Endorsed by the International Society for Heart and Lung Transplantation (ISHLT) and the European Reference Network on rare respiratory diseases (ERN-LUNG). Eur Heart J. 2022;43(38):3618-731.
2. Maron BA, Brittain EL, Hess E, et al. Pulmonary vascular resistance and clinical outcomes in patients with pulmonary hypertension: a retrospective cohort study. Lancet Resp Med. 2020;8(9):873-84.
3. Kovacs G, Berghold A, Scheidl S, et al. Pulmonary arterial pressure during rest and exercise in healthy subjects: a systematic review. Eur Respir J. 2009;34(4):888-94.
4. Bauchmuller K, Condliffe R, Southern J, et al. Critical care outcomes in patients with pre-existing pulmonary hypertension: insights from the ASPIRE registry. ERJ Open Research. 2021;7(2):00046-2021.
5. Sztrymf B, Souza R, Bertoletti L, et al. Prognostic factors of acute heart failure in patients with pulmonary arterial hypertension. Eur Respir J. 2010;35(6):1286-93.
6. Naranjo M, Mercurio V, Hassan H, et al. Causes and outcomes of ICU hospitalisations in patients with pulmonary arterial hypertension. ERJ open research. 2022;8(2):00002-2022.
7. Campo A, Mathai SC, Le Pavec J, et al. Outcomes of hospitalisation for right heart failure in pulmonary arterial hypertension. Eur Resp J. 2011;38(2):359.
8. Garcia MVF, Souza R, Costa ELV, et al. Outcomes and prognostic factors of decompensated pulmonary hypertension in the intensive care unit. Resp Med. 2021;190:106685.
9. Huynh TN, Weigt SS, Sugar CA, et al. Prognostic factors and outcomes of patients with pulmonary hypertension admitted to the intensive care unit. J Crit Care. 2012;27(6):739.e7-13.
10. Torrent-Guasp F, Buckberg GD, Clemente C, et al. The structure and function of the helical heart and its buttress wrapping. I. The normal macroscopic structure of the heart. Semin Thorac Cardiovasc Surg. 2001;13(4):301-19.
11. Benza RL, Gomberg-Maitland M, Elliott CG, et al. Predicting survival in patients with pulmonary arterial hypertension: The REVEAL risk score calculator 2.0 and comparison with esc/ers-based risk assessment strategies. Chest. 2019;156(2):323-37.
12. Clancy DJ, McLean A, Slama M, et al. Paradoxical septal motion: A diagnostic approach and clinical relevance. Australasian J Ultrasound Med. 2018;21(2):79-86.
13. Vandenheuvel MA, Bouchez S, Wouters PF, et al. A pathophysiological approach towards right ventricular function and failure. Eur J Anaesthesiol. 2013;30(7):386-94.
14. Vonk Noordegraaf A, Chin KM, Haddad F, et al. Pathophysiology of the right ventricle and of the pulmonary circulation in pulmonary hypertension: an update. Eur Resp J. 2019;53(1):1801900.
15. Houston BA, Brittain EL, Tedford RJ. Right ventricular failure. N Engl J Med. 2023;388(12):1111-25.
16. Lualdi JC, Goldhaber SZ. Right ventricular dysfunction after acute pulmonary embolism: pathophysiologic factors, detection, and therapeutic implications. Am Heart J. 1995;130(6):1276-82.
17. Chin KM, Rubin LJ, Channick R, et al. Association of n-terminal pro brain natriuretic peptide and long-term outcome in patients with pulmonary arterial hypertension. Circulation. 2019;139(21):2440-50.
18. Leuchte HH, Holzapfel M, Baumgartner RA, et al. Clinical significance of brain natriuretic peptide in primary pulmonary hypertension. J Am Coll Cardio. 2004;43(5):764-70.

19. Campo A, Mathai SC, Pavec JL, et al. Outcomes of hospitalisation for right heart failure in pulmonary arterial hypertension. Eur Resp J. 2011;38(2):359.
20. Haddad F, Fuh E, Peterson T, et al. Incidence, correlates, and consequences of acute kidney injury in patients with pulmonary arterial hypertension hospitalized with acute right-side heart failure. Journal of Cardiac Failure. 2011;17(7):533-9.
21. Augustine DX, Coates-Bradshaw LD, Willis J, et al. Echocardiographic assessment of pulmonary hypertension: A guideline protocol from the British Society of Echocardiography. Echo Res Pract. 2018;5(3):G11-g24.
22. Sahay S, Tonelli AR. Pericardial effusion in pulmonary arterial hypertension. Pulm Circ. 2013;3(3):467-77.
23. Schneider M, Pistritto AM, Gerges C, et al. Multi-view approach for the diagnosis of pulmonary hypertension using transthoracic echocardiography. Int J Cardiovasc Imaging. 2018;34(5):695-700.
24. Parker MW, Gottbrecht MF, Aurigemma GP. Midsystolic notch and pulmonary hypertension: pathophysiologic mechanism and technical considerations. journal of the american society of echocardiography: Official publication of the American Society of Echocardiography. J Am Soc Echocardiogr. 2021;34(6):693-5.
25. Ashes C, Roscoe A. Transesophageal echocardiography in thoracic anesthesia: pulmonary hypertension and right ventricular function. Curr Opin Anaesthesiol. 2015;28(1):38-44.
26. Adie SK, Abdul-Aziz AA, Ketcham SW, et al. Considerations for inotrope and vasopressor use in critically ill patients with pulmonary arterial hypertension. J Cardiovasc Pharmacol. 2022;79(1):e11-7.
27. Price LC, Wort SJ, Finney SJ, et al. Pulmonary vascular and right ventricular dysfunction in adult critical care: Current and emerging options for management: a systematic literature review. Crit Care (London, England). 2010;14(5):R169.
28. Stephan R, Ioana RP. Right heart catheterisation: best practice and pitfalls in pulmonary hypertension. Eur Resp Rev. 2015;24(138):642.
29. Fingrova Z, Ambroz D, Jansa P,et al. The prevalence and clinical outcome of supraventricular tachycardia in different etiologies of pulmonary hypertension. PloS one. 2021;16(1):e0245752.
30. Wanamaker B, Cascino T, McLaughlin V, et al. Atrial Arrhythmias in pulmonary hypertension: Pathogenesis, prognosis and management. Arrhythm Electrophysiol Rev. 2018;7(1):43-8.
31. Stewart RH, Cox CS, Allen SJ, et al. Myocardial edema provides a link between pulmonary arterial hypertension and pericardial effusion. Circulation. 2022;145(11):793-5.
32. Case BC, Yang M, Kagan CM, et al. Safety and feasibility of performing pericardiocentesis on patients with significant pulmonary hypertension. Cardiovasc Revasc Med. 2019;20(12): 1090-5.
33. Spiegel R. Stressed vs. unstressed volume and its relevance to critical care practitioners. Clin Exp Emerg Med. 2016;3(1):52-4.
34. Hansen L, Burks M, Kingman M, et al. Volume management in pulmonary arterial hypertension patients: an expert pulmonary hypertension clinician perspective. Pulm Ther. 2018;4(1):13-27.
35. Sinha AD, Agarwal R. Setting the dry weight and its cardiovascular implications. Seminars in Dialysis. 2017;30(6):481-8.
36. Narechania S, Torbic H, Tonelli AR. Treatment discontinuation or interruption in pulmonary arterial hypertension. J Cardiovas Pharmacol Ther. 2019;25(2).131-41.
37. Taylor RW, Zimmerman JL, Dellinger RP, et al. Low-dose inhaled nitric oxide in patients with acute lung injury: A randomized controlled trial. JAMA. 2004;291(13):1603-9.
38. Weinberger B, Laskin DL, Heck DE, et al. The toxicology of inhaled nitric oxide. Toxicol Sci 2001;59(1):5-16.
39. Harrison WF, Wendy G-S. Practical considerations for therapies targeting the prostacyclin pathway. European Resp Rev. 2016;25(142):418.
40. Derlis Fleitas S, Andrew LL, Huaqing Z, et al. Impact of pulmonary embolism response teams on acute pulmonary embolism: a systematic review and meta-analysis. Eur Resp Rev. 2022;31(165):220023.
41. Tu T, Toma C, Tapson VF, et al. A prospective, single-arm, multicenter trial of catheter-directed mechanical thrombectomy for intermediate-risk acute pulmonary embolism: The FLARE Study. JACC Cardiovasc Interv. 2019;12(9):859-69.
42. Olsson KM, Halank M, Egenlauf B, et al. Decompensated right heart failure, intensive care and perioperative management in patients with pulmonary hypertension: Updated recommendations from the Cologne Consensus Conference 2018. Int J Cardiol. 2018;272s:46-52.
43. Chong LYZ, Satya K, Kim B, et al. Milrinone dosing and a culture of caution in clinical practice. Cardiol Rev. 2018;26(1):35-42.
44. Overgaard CB, Dzavík V. Inotropes and vasopressors: Review of physiology and clinical use in cardiovascular disease. Circulation. 2008;118(10):1047-56.
45. Adie SK, Abdul-Aziz AA, Ketcham SW, et al. Considerations for inotrope and vasopressor use in critically ill patients with pulmonary arterial hypertension. J Cardiovasc Pharmacol. 2022;79(1).
46. Viitanen A, Salmenperä M, Heinonen J. Right ventricular response to hypercarbia after cardiac surgery. Anesthesiology. 1990;73(3):393-400.
47. Marcos VFG, Rogerio S, Pedro C. Predictors of invasive mechanical ventilation use in patients with acute decompensated pulmonary hypertension admitted to the intensive care unit. ERJ Open Res. 2023;9(2):00598-2022.
48. Marius MH, Raymond LB, Paul C, et al. Intensive care, right ventricular support and lung transplantation in patients with pulmonary hypertension. Eur Resp J. 2019;53(1):1801906.
49. Spiesshoefer J, Bannwitz B, Mohr M, et al. Effects of nasal high flow on sympathovagal balance, sleep, and sleep-related breathing in patients with precapillary pulmonary hypertension. Sleep Breath. 2021;25(2):705-17.
50. Hoeper MM, Granton J. Intensive care unit management of patients with severe pulmonary hypertension and right heart failure. Am J Respir Crit Care Med. 2011;184(10):1114-24.
51. Chan CM, Mitchell AL, Shorr AF. Etomidate is associated with mortality and adrenal insufficiency in sepsis: A meta-analysis. Crit Care Med. 2012;40(11):2945-53.
52. Matchett G, Gasanova I, Riccio CA, et al. Etomidate versus ketamine for emergency endotracheal intubation: A randomized clinical trial. Intensive Care Med. 2022;48(1):78-91.
53. Weingart SD, Trueger NS, Wong N, et al. Delayed sequence intubation: A prospective observational study. Ann Emerg Med. 2015;65(4):349-55.
54. Johannes J, Berlin DA, Patel P, et al. A technique of awake bronchoscopic endotracheal intubation for respiratory failure in patients with right heart failure and pulmonary hypertension. Crit Care Med. 2017;45(9).

55. Alexis P, Xavier R, Antoine V-B. Rationale and description of right ventricle-protective ventilation in ARDS. Resp Care. 2016;61(10):1391.
56. Vieillard-Baron A, Price LC, Matthay MA. Acute cor pulmonale in ARDS. Intensive Care Med. 2013;39(10):1836-8.
57. Machuca TN, de Perrot M. Mechanical support for the failing right ventricle in patients with precapillary pulmonary hypertension. Circulation. 2015;132(6):526-36.
58. de Perrot M, Granton JT, McRae K, et al. Impact of extracorporeal life support on outcome in patients with idiopathic pulmonary arterial hypertension awaiting lung transplantation. J Heart Lung Transplant. 2011;30(9):997-1002.
59. Cypel M, Keshavjee S. Extracorporeal life support as a bridge to lung transplantation. Clin Chest Med. 2011;32(2):245-51.
60. Tsuneyoshi H, Rao V. The role of extracorporeal membrane oxygenation (ECMO) therapy in acute heart failure. Int Anesthesiol Clin. 2012;50(3):114-22.

Hemodynamic Monitoring in Intensive Care Unit

CHAPTER 171

Rajkalyan Chakrabarti, Purvesh R Patel, Pralay K Sarkar

INTRODUCTION

Hemodynamic monitoring is one of the major pillars on which management of critically ill patients stands. Hemodynamic instability is a common reason for admission to critical care units. Failure to timely optimize hemodynamic parameters, organ perfusion, and tissue oxygen delivery leads to progressive end-organ damage that alters the clinical course and adds to morbidity and mortality. In this chapter, we will focus on conceptual understanding of some commonly available monitoring tools. It is useful to remember that in hemodynamic monitoring, interpretation of waveform displays is as important as the digitally displayed values. Recognizing trends of hemodynamic variables is more important than a single data point. The importance of interpreting hemodynamic data in context of good history and physical examination cannot be overemphasized.

CONCEPTUAL FRAMEWORK OF HEMODYNAMIC MONITORING AND MANAGEMENT

Human organ function is critically dependent on tissue oxygen delivery. The ultimate function of cardiovascular system is delivery of adequate amount of oxygen to every organ. An ideal tool of hemodynamic monitoring could be the measurement of tissue partial pressure of oxygen in an organ. However, in current state of medical technology development, such tools are limited in availability and application. Adequacy of tissue oxygen delivery in turn depends on adequacy of blood flow to any organ. Regional blood flow measurement can then be the next ideal goal of hemodynamic monitoring. However, there is no easily applicable tool for monitoring regional perfusion, for example, blood flow to brain and kidneys. Regional blood flow is also controlled by local autoregulation, which cannot be manipulated for therapeutic purposes. The most pragmatic goal of hemodynamic optimization, therefore, remains to ensure adequate cardiac output (CO) and adequate blood pressure (BP). An inherent assumption remains that if CO and BP are optimized, regional blood flow and oxygen delivery will be maintained. CO is, therefore, a reasonable proxy for oxygen delivery. Maintaining adequate BP remains another major goal of hemodynamic management. This conceptual framework is shown schematically in **Figure 1**.

CLINICAL AND LABORATORY MEASURES OF TISSUE PERFUSION

Assessment of simple clinical parameters usually first indicates that a circulatory problem exists, which then necessitates deployment of monitoring tools. A deteriorating trend in vital signs is often missed as the absolute value in early stages can still be within normal range. Tachycardia,

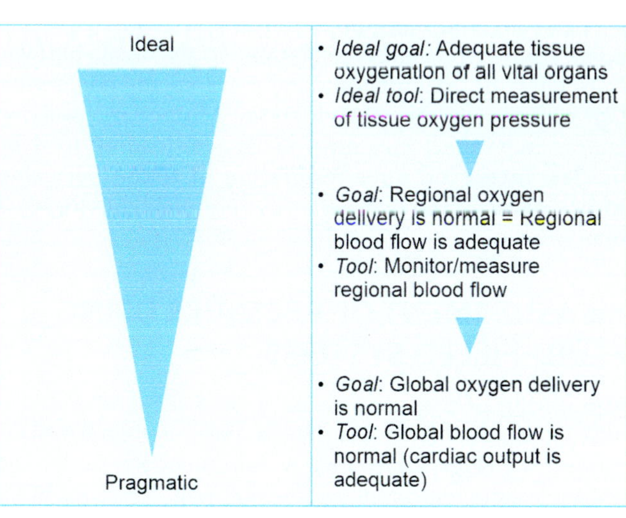

FIG. 1: A conceptual framework of hemodynamic monitoring.

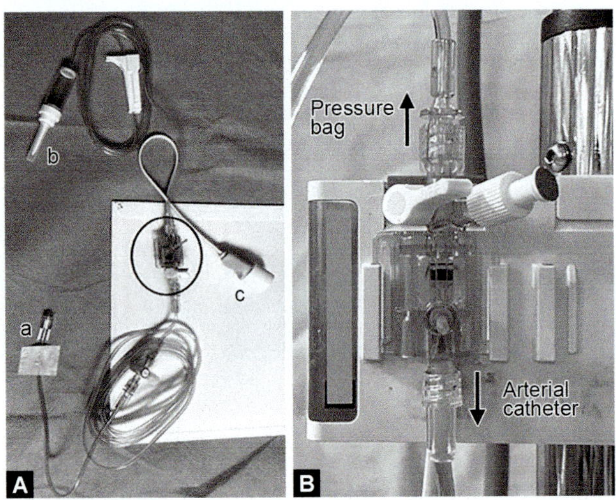

FIGS. 2A AND B: Disposable transducer and monitoring set-up. (A) The connection to the patient (a), the connection to the high-pressure bag (b), and the electronic monitoring cable (c) are shown. The pressure bag is maintained at 300 mm Hg and used for flushing the line. (B) The red stopper indicates a side port that can be opened for zero referencing. By pulling on the blue elastic chord, pressure flush can be activated.

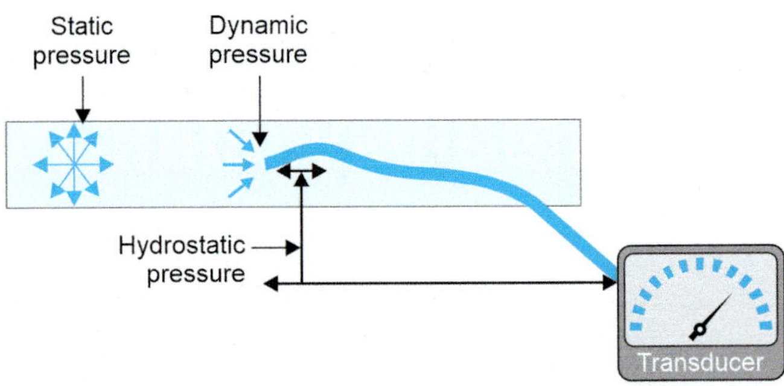

FIG. 3: Different constituents affecting pressure measurement. The goal is to measure the static pressure and eliminate the hydrostatic pressure component, which is a source of error. Dynamic pressure component is unavoidable, especially when high pressure is being measured in high flow areas.

tachypnea, confusion, or agitation can come early. As the circulatory dysfunction progresses, signs of low perfusion, for example, cold and clammy skin, decreased urine output, and encephalopathy become apparent. On examination, comparison of central and peripheral temperature and checking capillary filling time are important. Both skin mottling and capillary refill time have been shown to be predictors of morbidity and mortality in sepsis and indicators of decreased visceral perfusion in critically ill patients.[1-3] Blood lactate is a key marker of global tissue hypoperfusion and measured commonly both to diagnose shock states and monitor response to therapy. However, apart from hypoxemia, activation of glycolytic pathway from effect of inflammation and elevated catecholamines can cause elevation of lactate. Moreover, multiple factors may affect clearance of lactate, leading to delay in clearance even after restoration of tissue perfusion. Measurement of lactate is part of current guidelines for sepsis management.[4]

MEASUREMENT OF PRESSURE USING FLUID-FILLED SYSTEMS

Monitoring of pressures using a fluid-filled system and small transducers is ubiquitous part of hemodynamic monitoring **(Figs. 2A and B)**. A transducer is a device that senses a particular biophysical event (e.g., pressure in the context of hemodynamic monitoring) and converts it into a useful electrical signal that can be calibrated and measured.

A pressure transducer used in cardiovascular monitoring is a form of mechanical or displacement transducer. It has a mechanical component that is displaced or deformed by the intravascular pressure.

The value of intravascular pressure measured through a fluid-filled column has three components **(Fig. 3)**:[5]

1. *Residual or static pressure:* This is the pressure component that we aim to measure.
2. *Dynamic pressure:* Component contributed by the kinetic energy of the moving blood.
3. *Hydrostatic pressure head:* This comes from the weight of the fluid within the connecting system and is proportional to the vertical height of fluid column between the catheter and the reference port. The reference port is that port of the transducer that is exposed to air (air–fluid interface) to establish a "zero reference" point.

Hydrostatic pressure component is the most consistent source of errors in pressure monitoring in day-to-day clinical practice. To eliminate the error related to this component, the tip of the intravascular catheter and the air-reference port of the transducer need to be at the same vertical level. As the exact position of the tip of an intravascular catheter cannot be judged, a common convention is to place the transducer's air-reference port at the same level as mid-chest point (mid-way mark on lateral chest from anterior and posterior chest). Alternatively, closely approximating the previous level, the phlebostatic axis can be used; it is the junction of the fourth intercostal space and mid-axillary line. It is assumed that in a supine patient, the catheter tip will closely approximate the mid-chest level. After adjusting the position of the patient and/or transducer, zeroing of the system is next done by opening the air-reference port to atmosphere. After zeroing is performed, accuracy of pressure reading will be maintained as long as the air-reference port remains at the same horizontal level as the mid-chest or with an equivalent point of mid-sternum in lateral position **(Figs. 4A and B)**. The system needs to be re-zeroed after each

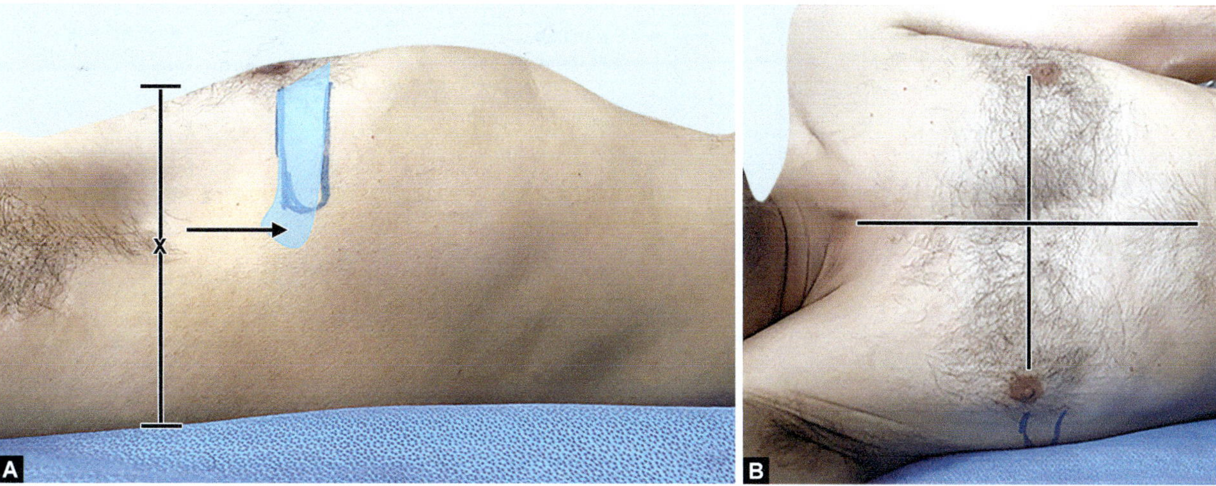

FIGS. 4A AND B: Reference level for pressure measurement, in supine and lateral positions. (A) In supine position, the reference point is either the midway (marked "X") between anterior and posterior chest or the phlebostatic axis, which is the junction between fourth intercostal space (shaded in blue) and the mid-axillary line (arrow). (B) In lateral position, the reference point is the junction of the nipple line and the mid-sternal line or lateral sternal border.

change in relative vertical positions of the air-reference port and the patient. Alternatively, the zero-reference port and the mid-chest need to be brought back at the same level to maintain the accuracy of the measured value.

The use of a fluid-filled system between the catheter tip and the transducer inherently imposes the risks associated with distortion and dampening of the pressure signals by the inertia of the fluid and the physical characteristics of the tubing system. Two characteristics of the connecting system (including catheter, tubing, and stopcocks) are important in altering pressure signals: (1) Resonant frequency of the system, i.e., how rapidly the fluid-filled system oscillates and how close that frequency of oscillation is to the pressure wave itself; (2) damping coefficient of the system, indicating how quickly the natural oscillation can come to rest. Natural resonant frequency and damping coefficient act in opposite directions and by their interactions decide the dynamic response of the system. Important pressure signal distortions due to unfavorable natural resonant frequency and/or damping coefficient come from tubing length, diameter, stiffness, and presence of air bubbles or blood clots. Standard steps should be taken to avoid errors in pressure measurement related to the monitoring system **(Box 1)**. Dynamic response of the system can be easily tested at bedside by the fast flush (square wave) test.[6] By activating the fast flush valve, the transducer is exposed to 300 mm Hg pressure in the pressurized saline bag. This produces a square waveform that rises sharply, forms a plateau, and drops off sharply when the flush valve is released. After the fast flush ends, the transducer returns to baseline after a brief period of oscillation. By inspection of the nature of the oscillation, it can be deduced whether the system is underdamped, overdamped, or optimally damped **(Figs. 5A to C)**.

BOX 1 Optimizing against errors in invasive hemodynamic pressure monitoring.

- *Keep catheter and tubing length minimum (< 3–4 feet):* Increased tubing length accentuates the pressure signal
- *Use stiff noncompliant tubing:* Compliant tubing is compressible by the transmitted vascular pressure and leads to attenuation of pressure signal
- *Use large diameter catheter:*
    - Small catheter leads to frictional loss of transmitted pressure
    - Use 7-FR or larger catheter in adults
    - Balance risk of vessel thrombus formation in selecting catheter
- *Eliminate all air bubbles from the system:* Air bubbles are compressible and lead to loss of energy of transmitted pressure waves (attenuation)
- *Prevent blood clot formation within the system:*
    - Same effect as air bubbles
    - Continuous low-volume infusion reduces the risk of clot formation
- *Reduce number of stopcocks within the system:*
    - Changes in lumen diameter at each stopcock site distort signal
    - Each stopcock site is a convenient place for air bubbles or clots to lodge

SYSTEMIC BLOOD PRESSURE MEASUREMENT

Physiology of Arterial Blood Pressure

With each contraction of left ventricle (LV), a volume of blood equivalent to stroke volume (SV) is ejected to proximal aorta and stretches the aorta. The pressure generated by

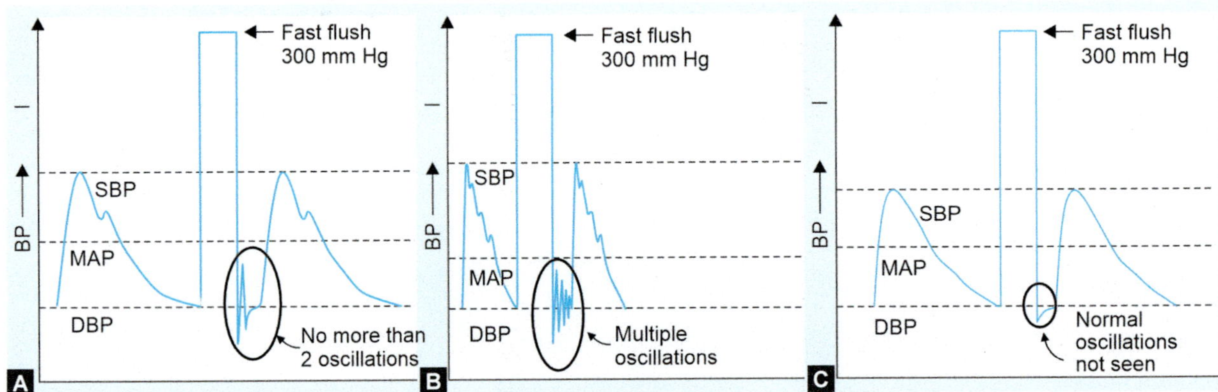

FIGS. 5A TO C: Dynamic response testing by rapid flush test. (A) In a monitoring system with optimal dynamic response, there is no more than two oscillations; the amplitude of the second oscillation is usually no more than one-third of the first oscillation. The time interval between the oscillations reflects the natural frequency of the monitoring system and should be <30 ms. Also, note that a distinct dicrotic notch indicates that the system is not overdamped. (B) In an underdamped system, multiple oscillations take place after the fast flush. Also note artefacts seen on pressure waveform. SBP is overestimated and DBP is underestimated in an underdamped system. MAP remains more accurate. (C) In an overdamped system, the pressure tracing fails to oscillate normally after the fast flush. Also, note the rounded contour of the waveform and loss of dicrotic notch. SBP is underestimated and DBP is overestimated in an overdamped system. MAP is less affected.

(BP: blood pressure; DBP: diastolic blood pressure; MAP: mean arterial pressure; SBP: systolic blood pressure)

this process is dependent on the volume of blood and the resistance to ejection. The stretching of aorta creates a pressure wave that transmits along contiguous segments in the vascular tree and is felt as pulse in any distal artery. The speed at which the pressure wave propagates depends on the compliance of the arterial wall.

Location of Measurement and Difference in Blood Pressure

Arterial blood pressure (BP) measured in more distal locations is higher than BP measured in proximal locations. It appears counterintuitive at first glance. This is due to summation of reflected waves on the primary systolic wave. Pressure measured in radial or femoral artery is higher than brachial or aortic pressure. Systolic blood pressure (SBP) measured in femoral artery can be higher by 25–50 mm Hg than in brachial or radial artery; diastolic and mean BP values are closer across different sites.

Arterial Pulse Waveform

Arterial pressure waveform has *three* clearly defined components **(Fig. 6)**. With ejection of blood from LV, the pressure rises rapidly to reach a peak, and it is defined as systolic blood pressure. With continuous blood runoff from proximal aorta to distal arterial bed, the pressure starts to fall. As and when aortic pressure becomes higher than the LV pressure that is now in diastole, the aortic valve closes, marking the end of systole. This is seen on arterial pressure curve as a short sharp rise followed by continued fall. This creates a notch in the pressure tracing known as *incisura* when recorded in central aorta and as *dicrotic notch* when recorded in peripheral arteries. The systolic peak on arterial tracing occurs after the QRS complex on electrocardiograph (ECG), the interval varies depending on the site of monitoring. Diastolic (more correctly, end-diastolic) pressure is measured just before the

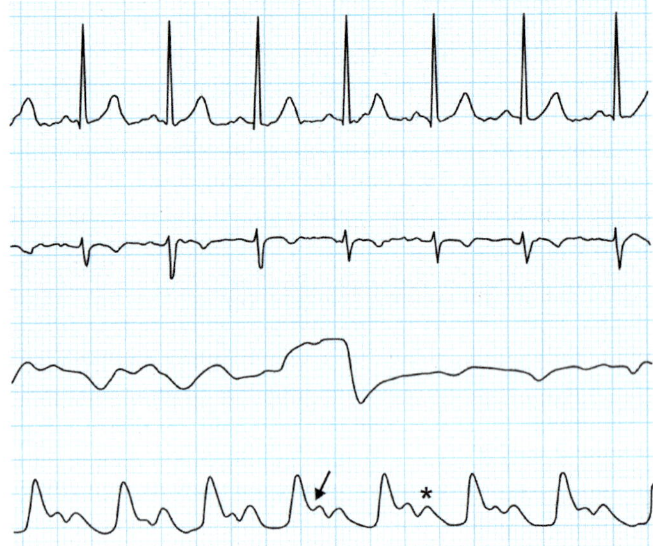

FIG. 6: Arterial waveform. The systolic peak occurs immediately after QRS complex. Diastole is measured just before the next upstroke. The dicrotic notch (arrow) occurs after T wave of electrocardiograph (ECG). A secondary diastolic wave is also seen(*).

next upstroke. The dicrotic notch comes after the T wave of ECG. Mean arterial pressure (MAP) is the BP average over time. More specifically, MAP is equal to the area under curve of the arterial pressure waveform divided by the beat period.

Secondary wave or reflected wave also explains the difference in contour of the arterial waveforms seen in different arteries. Starting from aorta, more distal the location is, sharper and later in the waveform is the peak and less prominent is the dicrotic notch. Secondary waves can be distinctly visible in arterial waveform during systole or diastole **(Fig. 6)**. The arterial waveform also changes with aging due to arterial stiffening with increased pulse wave velocity. In an older person, the arterial waveform shows a late systolic peak and a smooth diastolic pressure drop without secondary diastolic wave.

Methods of Blood Pressure Measurement

Methods of blood pressure measurement can be divided into invasive (direct) blood pressure measurement (ABP) and noninvasive (indirect) blood pressure measurement (NIBP). A summary and comparison are given in **Table 1**.

TABLE 1: Comparison of methods of blood pressure measurement in an intensive care unit (ICU).

	Invasive (direct) blood pressure monitoring	Noninvasive (indirect) blood pressure monitoring
Principle	Measures intra-arterial pressure directly by connecting the blood through a noncompressible column of fluid to a pressure transducer.	Employs a known external counterpressure through a pneumatic cuff to occlude blood flow distal to the point of compression. Blood pressure is calculated indirectly by detecting various changes in distal flow as external pressure is altered.
Common technologies		• Oscillometric method • Auscultatory method
Advantage	• Accuracy • Continuous monitoring • Diagnostic clues from arterial pressure waveform[40] • Frequent blood sampling	• Widely available • Equipment is durable, reusable, and does not need calibration • Does not need invasive procedure • Needs minimal training
Disadvantage	• Needs invasive procedure • Needs special kit and electronic monitoring equipment • Needs frequent calibration to ensure reliability • Adequate staff training is required	• Continuous monitoring not possible • Frequent monitoring for extensive periods is labor-intensive • Patient discomfort from frequent inflation of cuff • *Complications*: Venostasis, limb edema, neuropathy, and soft-tissue damage • Unreliable record at extreme ranges of blood pressure
Sources of errors	• Transducer position relative to heart • Transducer calibration • Dampening of signal by clot or air bubble in the system • Compression by surgical retractor at a site proximal to the arterial line	*Technical:* • Wrong cuff size relative to size of arm or inability to find a right size cuff in very large or very small size patients: ○ The cuff should be 20% wider than the diameter of the part of the limb being used (or cover two thirds its length) • Manometer error • Rapid deflation of the cuff (> 3 mm Hg/sec) • External pressure against the cuff • Movement of limb during measurement and shivering • Leak in the cuff, hoses, or connections *Physiological:* • *Cardiac dysrhythmias:* Atrial fibrillation, frequent ectopic beats, and severe bradycardia • *Peripheral vascular disease:* Noncompliant vessels, for example, calcified artery will alter measured blood pressure • Large cyclic or beat-to-beat variation in pulse volume/blood pressure from spontaneous or assisted ventilation, hypovolemia, seizure, and straining[9]

Understanding the physical principles behind noninvasive and invasive BP measurement is important for sound judgment about reliability of measured value in frequently encountered clinical scenarios when a discrepancy is noted between BP measured by invasive and noninvasive methods.

Invasive (Direct) Blood Pressure Measurement

Direct intraarterial measurement of blood pressure, i.e., ABP is a commonly used monitoring tool in any critical care unit. It is more accurate than NIBP under certain circumstances. It has the advantage of providing beat-to-beat information, and therefore, it is very useful in circumstances where a short-term fluctuation of blood pressure can be harmful (e.g., hypertensive emergency and intracranial bleeding) or rapid titration of medications for hypotension or hypertension is needed (e.g., shock states and hypertensive emergencies). Examination of arterial waveform and fluctuation of BP with respiratory cycle can provide important diagnostic information.

Intra-arterial Pressure Monitoring

Intra-arterial pressure monitoring is obtained by connecting an intra-arterial catheter placed in a peripheral artery with fluid-filled pressure transduction system. The basic principle is to provide an uninterrupted column of liquid connecting arterial blood to a pressure transducer (hydraulic coupling).[7] The real-time record shows SBP, diastolic blood pressure (DBP), and MAP. Careful attention to the waveform and dynamic response of the system should be ensured to get accurate reading (see above and **Box 1**). Indications of ABP monitoring are presented in **Box 2**.

Noninvasive Blood Pressure Measurement

Principle of Counterpressure

French Physiologist Étienne-Jules Marey, in 1876, developed the concept of applying counterpressure to measure BP noninvasively in humans.[8] The measurement of oscillations in pressure in the outside cuff is the basis of oscillometric method described here. By recording and characterizing the sounds, as generated by the changing flow in the underlying artery, BP is measured by auscultatory method.

BOX 2 Indications for invasive blood pressure monitoring.

- Labile blood pressure
- Frequent blood pressure recording is needed
- Rapid titration of medications is needed, for example, in hypertensive emergency and shock
- Major blood pressure instability is expected, for example, major surgery with possibility of substantial blood loss
- *Inaccuracy of NIBP suspected/possible:* Peripheral vascular disease, inability to find well-fitted blood pressure cuff, obesity, and cardiac arrhythmias
- NIBP data does not correlate with rest of clinical examination

(NIBP: noninvasive blood pressure)

Oscillometric method: Oscillometric method is the underlying technology of most automated NIBP devices used in clinical practice.[9] In this method, a cuff is inflated around a limb, and the pressure within the cuff is monitored by a solid-state transducer. This cuff pressure is the counterpressure applied against the arterial pressure. With each arterial pulse, there is a rise followed by fall in the volume of the limb under the cuff. This change in volume causes a pulsatile change in pressure within the surrounding cuff. As the cuff is inflated above the level of SBP, all flow stops in the artery and no oscillation in pressure is detected. After inflating the cuff to a higher pressure for another 1–2 seconds, the machine starts to gradually lower the pressure in a stepwise fashion following an algorithm **(Fig. 7)**. When the cuff pressure falls to the level of peak arterial pressure, a small pressure wave is detected. The amplitude of these pressure waves increases in size, with the increasing pressure difference between the limb and cuff, reaching a peak. With further lowering of pressure, the amplitude of these fluctuations falls and eventually stops. The cuff pressure for maximum amplitude corresponds to MAP. Systolic pressure corresponds to the point where the *rate of increase in the size of oscillation* is maximal; diastolic pressure is represented by the *maximal rate of decrease* in size of oscillation.[9,10]

Auscultatory method: First described in 1905 by Nicolai Korotkoff, a Russian army sergeant, auscultatory method is based on detecting different phases of sound created when blood flow restarts after being occluded by an external cuff. Five phases of sounds are described. The BP at which the first phase ("snapping tone") appears is taken as the SBP. The pressure at which the sound disappears (fifth phase) is taken as the DBP, which normally corresponds to the lowest pressure within the arteries before the next pulse arrives.[10] If sound continues to be audible on complete deflation of the cuff, the fourth phase ("muffled tone") is taken as DBP.[11] When the disappearance point is ≥10 mm Hg lower than the point of muffling, the disappearance point is falsely low and the muffling point is taken as DBP. This situation happens in hyperkinetic circulatory states. If the difference is >10 mm Hg, it is a good practice to record both the pressures corresponding to muffling and disappearance of sound, for example, BP 140/70–40.

Direct versus Indirect Blood Pressure Measurements

In general, ABP shows slightly higher systolic pressure and slightly lower diastolic pressure (5–10 mm Hg) than NIBP measurements. A common dilemma in intensive care unit (ICU) practice is the discrepancies noted between ABP

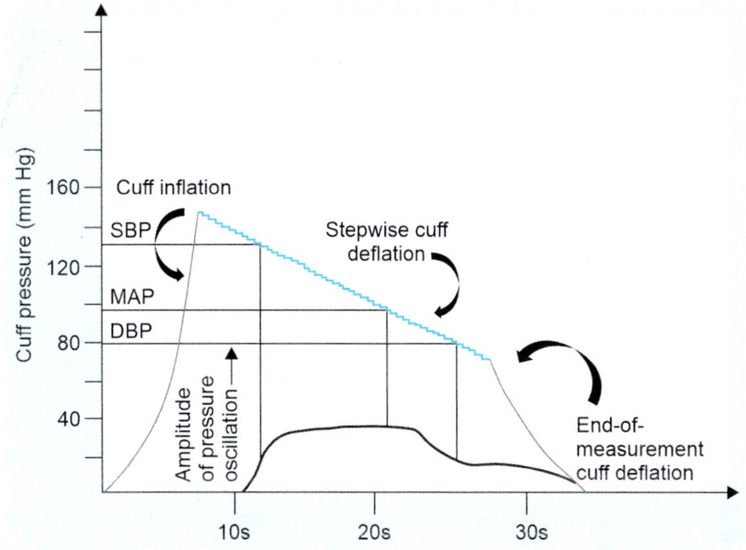

FIG. 7: NIBP measurement by principle of counterpressure. As the external cuff pressure is lowered, the amplitude of oscillation in the cuff pressure becomes higher and reaches a maximal value; the corresponding cuff pressure is MAP.
(DBP: diastolic blood pressure; MAP: mean arterial pressure; NIBP: noninvasive blood pressure; SBP: systolic blood pressure)

and NIBP in a given patient. There are several potential reasons:

- *These techniques measure different parameters:* ABP measures pressure at the monitoring site and NIBP measures flow (in auscultatory method) or consequence of flow (e.g., external pressure fluctuation from flow as in oscillometric method), beneath or beyond the occluding cuff.
- There are gradients within the arterial circulation, for example, normal peripheral pulse pressure widening, severe vasoconstriction, and shock.
- *In any given patient, it is rarely possible to measure ABP and NIBP at the same site at repeated intervals:* Common site for ABP is radial artery and for NIBP it is the brachial artery.
- Sources of technical errors in either invasive or non-invasive or both techniques in pressure measurement in the same patient at one point in time or over the period of monitoring **(Table 1)**.

Studies vary in results in the degree of correlation between ABP and NIBP. Some studies show within-patient variability, between-patient variability, and variability with changes in clinical condition over time in the same patient.[12] Given this uncertainty, some general principles can be adapted for routine clinical practice:

- In normotensive patients, SBP measured by noninvasive methods gives similar or slightly lower value compared to ABP.
- In hypertensive patients, NIBP underestimates SBP.
- In hypotensive patients, SBP is overestimated by NIBP.
- Majority of data indicate that indirect measurements of MAP give equal value or slightly overestimate direct MAP values.
- Most useful information about acute changes in circulation in ICUs comes from SBP and MAP, and DBP adds little extra value.
- DBP measured by indirect methods slightly overestimates directly measured values.
- NIBP is less reliable whenever there are rapid pressure changes and dysrhythmias.
- Whenever significant discrepancy is noted, careful review should be made to rule out technical sources of errors in ABP and/or NIBP measurements.

CENTRAL VENOUS PRESSURE AND RIGHT ATRIAL PRESSURE MONITORING

Central venous lines (CVLs) are frequently placed in critically ill patients for secured access to administration of vasopressors and other medications. If internal jugular or subclavian vein is used for placement of CVLs, central venous pressure (CVP) can readily be measured. CVP is a reflection of right atrial pressure (RAP) and has similar waveforms. Though CVP is no longer thought to be a reliable measure of volume status and volume responsiveness, it provides useful measure of preload of right side of heart in patients with right heart disease, for example, in pulmonary hypertension patients. The CVP and RAP pressure waveforms are identical; the waveform and the physiological explanation are described below and shown in **Figure 8**. The waveform

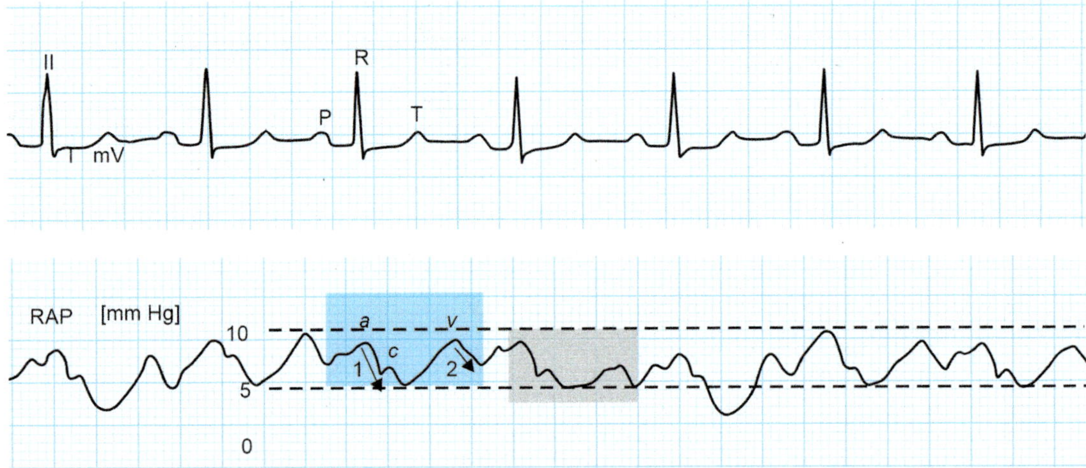

FIG. 8: Right atrial waveform and the physiological events. Note the relationship of the waves with ECG. The a wave is seen after P wave of ECG or at some point within the PR interval. The descent that immediately follows a wave is termed *x* descent (arrow 1). The *c* wave is seen on the downward slope of *x* descent. The *v* wave is seen near the end of T wave or anytime during TP interval of ECG. The *y* descent (arrow 2) follows the *v* wave. This tracing is from a spontaneously breathing patient. The waveform complex just before inspiratory drop in RAP has been chosen for measurements. The blue box shows end-expiratory measurement and the gray box represents the pressure drop in inspiration.

(ECG: electrocardiograph; RAP: right atrial pressure)

consists of two major positive waves, *a* and *v*, and one minor one, *c*. Atrial contraction produces *a* wave. It is generally seen 80–100 ms after P wave of ECG or at some point within the PR interval. The descent that immediately follows *a* wave is caused by atrial relaxation and is termed *x* descent. As the right ventricle (RV) starts contracting, the RV pressure rises and causes closure of the tricuspid valve. This event creates a minor positive wave, called *c* wave, usually on the downward slope of *x* descent. Sometimes, *c* wave appears as a notch on *a* wave. The *c* wave corresponds to the RST junction of ECG and timing of this wave depends on the PR interval. As the RV systole continues, the pressure in RA increases due to venous return against a closed tricuspid valve, resulting in *v* wave. The *v* wave is seen near the end of T wave or anytime during TP interval of ECG. The *y* descent follows the *v* wave and is produced by opening of tricuspid valve and rapid emptying of right atrium.

Measurement of Mean Right Atrial Pressure

Atrial pressure rises during atrial systole (*a* wave) and diastole (*v* wave) are usually within 3-4 mm Hg of each other. In this scenario, the midpoint of these pressure waves can be taken as mean right atrial pressure (RAPm). However, if either of these waves is much more elevated than the other, the RAPm is calculated only from *a* wave. Exaggerated *v* wave is commonly seen in clinical practice, for example, in case of tricuspid regurgitation. The electronic monitoring system usually includes the *v* wave in reporting the RAPm and reports a higher value though it would not represent the actual filling pressure of the right heart. In such a situation, the RAPm can be calculated from the waveform by locating the peak and trough of *a* wave and taking the midpoint. If a *c* wave is clearly visible, corresponding pressure can be used as RAPm as *c* wave indicates end of (ventricular) diastole.

RIGHT HEART/PULMONARY ARTERY CATHETERIZATION

Pulmonary artery catheterization (PAC) is considered the most invasive compared to other commonly employed monitoring techniques. Its advantage lies in the fact that in addition to CO, it also provides pulmonary artery (PA) pressure, right and left-sided filling pressure [RAP and pulmonary artery wedge pressure (PAWP) respectively], and mixed venous oxygen saturation (SVO_2). Though cardiac catheterization was developed many decades ago, the use of PAC outside catheterization laboratories only started after development of balloon-flotation catheters in early 1970s. As happens with any new technique, PAC was overused and abused and at the same time, it made invaluable contribution to understanding hemodynamic changes in critically ill patients and correlation with echocardiographic findings.[13] During the peak use years of bedside PAC, it has been used in medical and surgical ICUs for determining cause of hypotension and for differentiating between cardiogenic and noncardiogenic pulmonary edema. It has also been used to calculate tissue oxygen delivery in order to optimize it or to achieve supranormal tissue oxygen delivery. Use of diuretics and inotropes was guided by PAC data for many years in medical and surgical ICUs. Carefully conducted randomized controlled trials in the high-risk patients in ICUs, patients with acute respiratory distress syndrome (ARDS), and high-risk surgical patients did not show any benefits.[14-17] In light of current evidence and considering availability of other monitoring tools, PAC remains useful in the following situations in ICU practice:

- In several publications, PAC has been reported to improve outcomes in patients with acute cardiogenic shock. In this group of patients, a more accurate categorization of clinical phenotypes helps to guide therapy.[18,19] This group includes patients with cardiogenic shock after left and/or right ventricular infarction following reperfusion therapy and cardiogenic shock in patients without acute myocardial infarction (AMI).
- Decompensated chronic heart failure where expected improvement is not seen after initial management.
- Decompensated chronic heart failure where mechanical circulatory support is being planned.
- Perioperative monitoring of patients with pulmonary hypertension who are high-risk and/or undergoing high-risk surgery.[20]
- Perioperative management of patients undergoing heart, lung, or heart-lung transplantation.

A detailed description of procedural steps for placement of PAC is beyond the scope of this chapter. Technical details for accurate measurement of PAC data are well described in pulmonary hypertension literature and are equally applicable when PAC is used in ICU setting.[21,22] Like all hemodynamic pressures, PAC-derived pressures are also measured in end-expiration in both ventilated and nonventilated patients. The measurement of RAP has been described in the previous section. PA and RV waveforms obtained during right heart catheterization (RHC) are shown in **Figures 9A and B**. The measurement of RV and PA pressure is usually straightforward. The terms PAWP and pulmonary artery occlusion pressure (PAOP) are usually used interchangeably (PAWP will be used here). When the catheter with inflated balloon is advanced to a small branch of pulmonary artery, it occludes the forward flow in that segment of pulmonary artery and creates a "static" column of blood between the catheter tip and left atrium (LA); the pressure shown reflects the events in left atrial pressure. It is an intrinsically difficult measurement and most prone to errors. PAWP measurement is also most subject to controversy in pulmonary hypertension and heart failure literature.[23-25] Few important points will be noted here:

- With the PA catheter in the wedge position, the inflated balloon stops all forward blood flow. Post-balloon static column of blood reflects the pulmonary venous and ultimately left atrial pressure due to pressure equalization. However, if the surrounding alveolar pressure (P_A) exceeds the pressure within small vessels, then the monitored pressure essentially reflects the P_A **(Fig. 10A)**. To accurately reflect downstream pressure, the pulmonary arterial (P_a) and venous (P_v) pressures need to exceed P_A, a condition fulfilled in West zone 3.[26,27]
- In chest X-ray (CXR), a proper zone 3 positioning of PA catheter can be checked by the following criteria: (a) The tip should appear 3–5 cm from the midline and within 2 cm from the hilum and (b) the tip of the catheter should be inferior to the LA position **(Fig. 10B)**.
- As PAWP reflects left atrial physiological events **(Fig. 11)**, the waveform reflects the same pattern as in RAP and

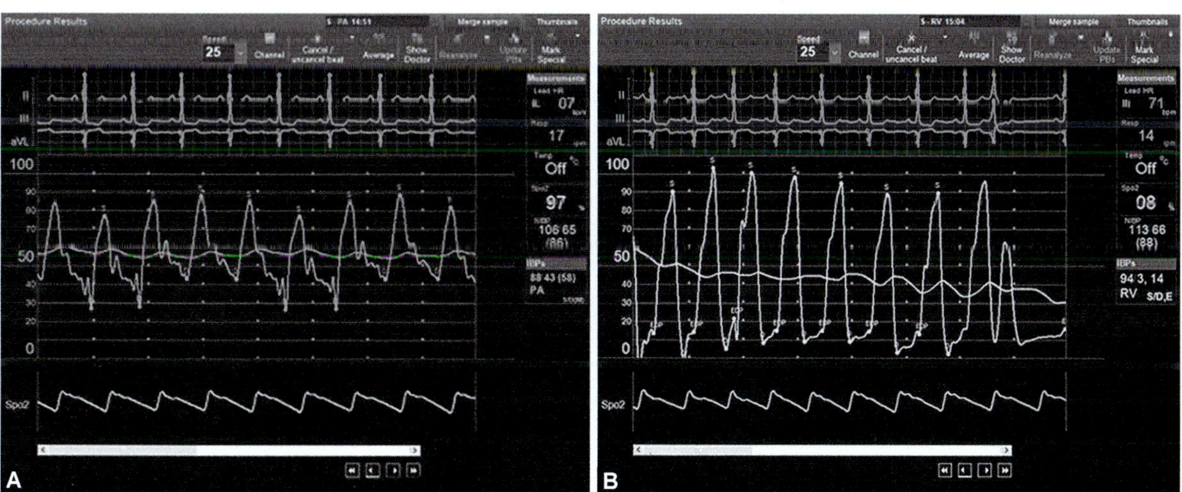

FIGS. 9A AND B: PA and RV waveform in a patient with severe pulmonary hypertension admitted with RV failure. (A) In the PA waveform, note the high pressure. (B) In the RV waveform, note the high end-diastolic pressure (EDP), indicating the decompensated state of the RV.

(PA: pulmonary artery; RV: right ventricle)

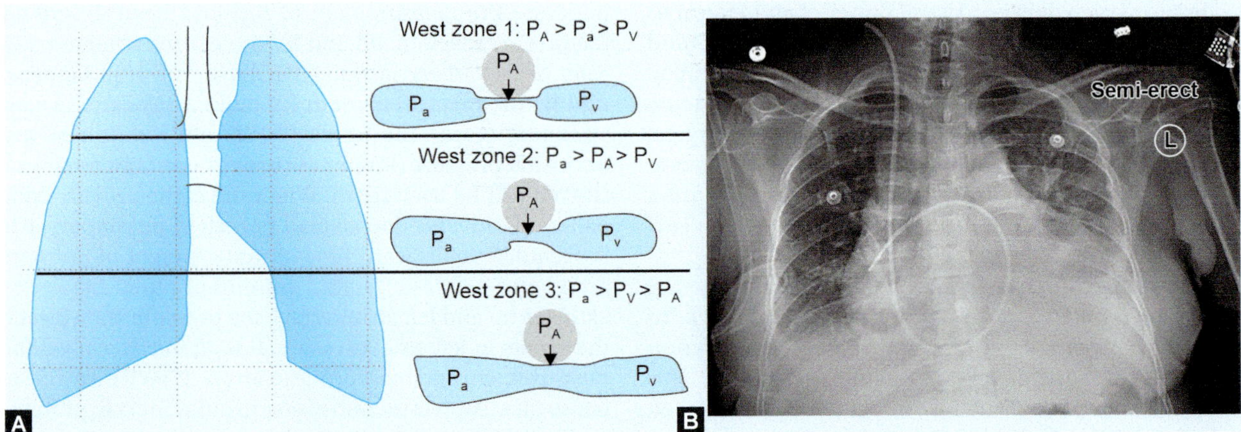

FIGS. 10A AND B: (A) PA catheter placement in relation to West zones influences PAWP measurement. Within the lung, the relative magnitudes of arterial, venous, and alveolar pressures differ, with difference in regional blood flow. In zone 3, venous pressure exceeds alveolar pressure and continuous blood flow is achieved. In zone 3, PA occlusion pressure reflects downstream pressure. (B) CXR showing tip of PA catheter in right lower lung zone.

(CXR: chest X-ray; P_A: alveolar pressure; P_a: arterial pressure; P_v: venous pressure; PA: pulmonary artery; PAWP: pulmonary artery wedge pressure)

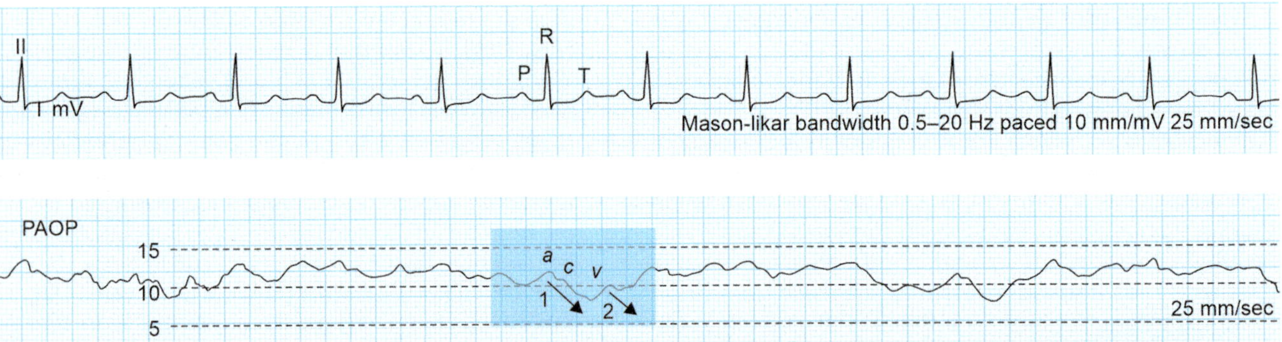

FIG. 11: Normal PAWP tracing. PAWP tracing in a patient with normal wedge pressure. The explanation of different parts of the waveform is the same as in RAP waveform (see Fig. 8). Both *a* and *v* waves are close to each other in values and <12 mm Hg, indicating normal wedge pressure.

(PAWP: pulmonary artery wedge pressure; PAOP: pulmonary artery occlusion pressure; RAP: right atrial pressure)

has similar explanation for different components. A greater time delay is noted between the electrical event and corresponding pressure wave, compared to RAP waveform, as the pressure wave has to travel longer to be recorded at PA catheter tip.

- There is a phase delay of 130– 200 ms between PAWP and ECG.
- The *c* wave (caused by closure of mitral valve) is often lost in retrograde transmission and not seen.
- The *a* and *v* waves are normally close to each other and the mean of the 2 waves represents mean PAWP.
- In automated monitoring systems used for pressure monitoring, the digital pressure displayed in the system is the average over the duration of cardiac cycle; the reported pressure may then be reported at higher level if either *a* or *v* wave is abnormally high. This displayed pressure reflects better the sum total of passive pressure to which the pulmonary vasculature is exposed.[23]
- If either *a* or *v* wave is higher than the other and dominant, the mean of *a* wave should be reported as mean pressure, as a measure of LV end-diastolic pressure or LV filling pressure. The height of the *v* wave should also be noted and reported **(Fig. 12)**.
- In pulmonary hypertension literature, different pressure values (e.g., mean pressure calculated as described earlier and PAWP at the onset of QRS complex) are used for the calculation of diastolic pressure gradient (DPG) and transpulmonary gradient (TPG), and for accurate classification of precapillary versus postcapillary pulmonary hypertension.[23,25] However, this is less relevant from ICU perspective and PAWP mean remains the most important pressure.

Serious complications may arise from PAC placement and monitoring and are listed in **Table 2**.

In summary, PAC is a useful tool when used properly. PAC is a diagnostic tool, and correct interpretation of the data and its incorporation in patient management need good knowledge of cardiorespiratory physiology. Interpretation of waveforms needs skills and experience. Incorporation of PAC-derived numbers alone into any rigid algorithm of patient management, without careful integration of all relevant and available clinical data, is likely to result in adverse outcomes. A major criticism of the studies that showed no benefits and/or detrimental effects of PAC is that they included patients where prolonged catheterization was frequently performed with no known reversible therapy.[13]

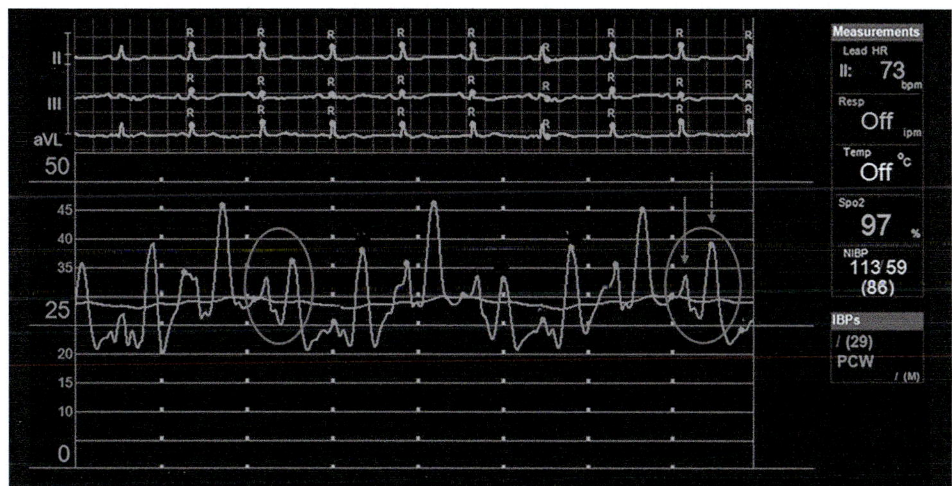

FIG. 12: PAWP tracing with markedly elevated wedge pressure. Note that both *a* (arrow) and *v* (dashed arrow) waves are >20 mm Hg and *v* wave is significantly higher than *a* wave. Here, the midpoint of *a* wave should be used to report mean PAWP. Height of *a* and *v* waves should also be noted. The circles correspond to heart beats at end-expiration and chosen for pressure measurement.
(PAWP: pulmonary artery wedge pressure)

TABLE 2: Complications of PAC.*

Complication	Cause	Prevention	Management
Arrhythmia: • Often transient • PVCs and nonsustained VT most common • Shock, myocardial ischemia, and electrolyte abnormalities increase risk	Myocardial irritation by the catheter	• To cross RV as quickly as feasible • Minimal catheter manipulation in RA or RV	• None, if transient • Usual management, if sustained along with consideration for deferring or terminating the procedure
Heart block: RBBB; complete heart block if patient has previous LBBB		Least manipulation of catheter in RV	• To use a PAC with pacing capability • To prepare for transvenous pacing
Infection: • Catheter-related blood-stream infection • Septic endocarditis of right-sided heart valve	• Lack of adequate aseptic technique • Prolonged catheterization	• Aseptic technique in placement of catheter • Scrupulous cleaning while accessing ports • Limiting duration of PAC monitoring to <3 days when feasible • Use of nonglucose IV solutions	• Blood culture and appropriate antibiotics • Removal of catheter

Continued

Continued

Complication	Cause	Prevention	Management
Pulmonary infarction	• Embolization from the catheter • Prolonged wedging as a result of forward migration of the catheter • Balloon left inflated inadvertently	• Monitoring of position in CXR • Monitoring display of pressure waveform from distal lumen to look for loss of PA waveform • Brief and infrequent wedging • Using PAEDP as surrogate for PAOP	• To monitor for hemoptysis and pleuritic chest pain • Removal of catheter
Thrombosis: Low CO states, DIC, and congestive heart failure are risk factors	Thrombogenic effect of catheter	• Infusion of heparinized solution through side arm of introducing sheath • Aspiration of the catheter before flushing	
Pulmonary artery rupture: • Severe and fatal complication • Suspected when patient develops hemoptysis	• Advancing catheter without balloon inflation • Balloon inflation in over-wedged position • Overdistension of balloon	• Balloon inflated slowly and waveform was continuously monitored during PAOP measurement • Distal lumen waveform and CXR should be monitored for distal migration of catheter • Catheter should not be flushed unless balloon deflated • PAEDP can be monitored if there is close agreement with PAOP	• Patient monitored in lateral position with catheter side in dependent position • Airway management for massive hemoptysis • Surgical intervention though many of these patients are too sick for operative intervention
Cardiac tamponade	Perforation of cardiac wall by catheter tip	Catheter should not be advanced within heart unless the balloon is inflated	Emergent pericardiocentesis
Catheter coiling	• Dilated RA or RV • Excessive length of catheter insertion	• If no pressure change while advancing 15 cm from RA to RV and then RV to PA, the catheter should be withdrawn and readvanced • Use of fluoroscopy if either patient or machine can be mobilized	

*Complications related to vascular access are not listed.

(CXR: chest X-ray; DIC: disseminated intravascular coagulation; LBBB: left bundle branch block; PAC: pulmonary artery catheterization; PVC: premature ventricular contraction; PAOP: pulmonary artery occlusion pressure; PAEDP: PA end-diastolic pressure; RA: right atrium; RV: right ventricle; RBBB: right bundle branch block; VT: ventricular tachycardia)

ADVANCED CRITICAL CARE ECHOCARDIOGRAPHY IN HEMODYNAMIC MONITORING

Advanced critical care echocardiography (ACCE) differs from basic critical care echocardiography in extent of data obtained for hemodynamic management. With comprehensive use of Doppler, a wide range of hemodynamic data can be obtained by an intensivist and can be rapidly integrated into care of a patient. It is critical that ACCE is performed by the intensivist who has proficiency in other aspects of critical care ultrasonography and has adequate training in both critical care medicine and ACCE to reap the maximum benefits of ACCE. As a hemodynamic monitoring tool, echocardiography has the unique advantage of being able to provide data about both structure and function of cardiovascular system at the same time. The extent of an examination can be tailored to the need of a particular case, for example, calculation of SV and CO in a shock state or measurement of right ventricular systolic pressure in suspected right ventricular dysfunction or acute cor pulmonale. The rise of ACCE as a hemodynamic monitoring tool in ICU has been timely, especially with the waning use of PAC since the beginning of new millennium. Though individual aspects of the data provided by ACCE can be obtained from other monitoring equipment/tools, ACCE remains unique in its speed, ease of use, and reliability. Repeated use to monitor evolution of disease and response to treatment are also major advantages.

Concept of Doppler

Use of Doppler remains the fundamental basis of ACCE. Doppler phenomenon, discovered by Austrian physicist Christian Doppler in 1842, describes the apparent shift in frequency of sound when either the source of sound or observer is moving in relation to each other. By noting the

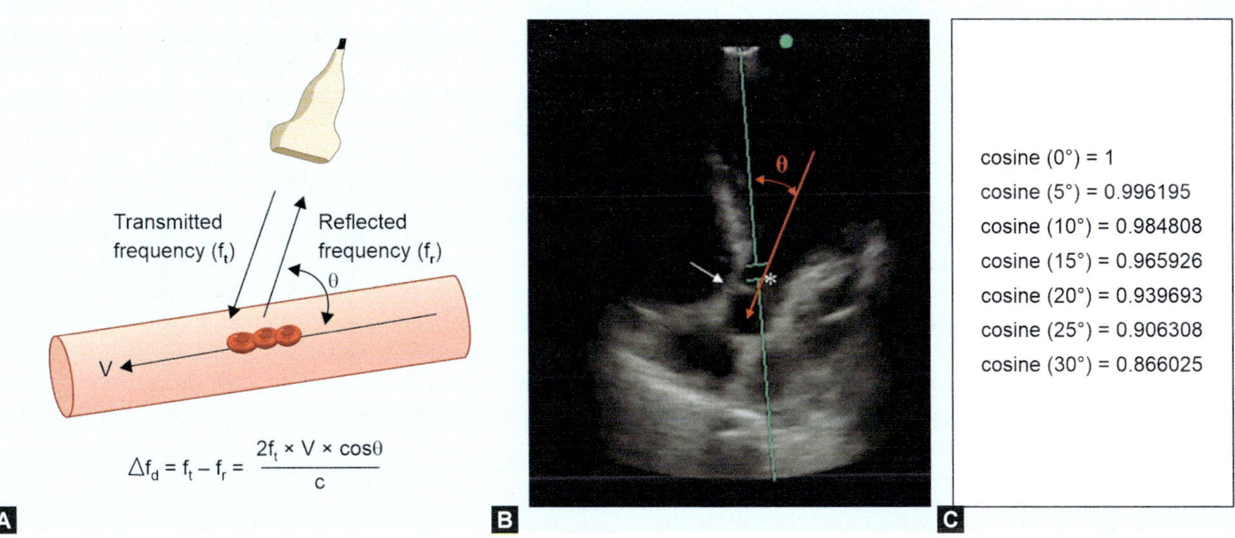

FIGS. 13A TO C: (A) Doppler equation. Note that the measured velocity is directly proportional to the frequency shift. (B) Measurement of blood flow velocity at LVOT (*). The light green line is the line of Doppler interrogation and the red line is the direction of blood flow. Note the angle between the 2 lines (θ). The white arrow points to aortic valve. (C) cos θ value at different angles.
(LVOT: left ventricular outflow tract)

shift in frequency, the speed of the moving object can be determined as per the Doppler equation **(Figs. 13A to C)**:

Thus, the Doppler frequency shift

$$= \Delta f_d = f_t - f_r = \frac{2f_t \times v \times \cos\theta}{c}$$

where,

c = The speed of sound in tissue

cos = Cosine

v = Flow velocity

θ = Angle between the direction of blood flow and the axis of the ultrasound beam

f_t = Transmitted frequency

f_r = Received frequency

Therefore, the change in Doppler frequency shift is proportional to the flow velocity. Most important technical factor is the alignment of the line of Doppler interrogation with the direction of blood flow. For any angle above 0°, there is an underestimation of velocity. As will be clear from cosine angle chart shown in **Figures 13A to C**, the degree of underestimation is significant when the angle exceeds 20°.

In echocardiography, the moving objects inside the heart include blood and cardiac tissue (e.g., valve annulus and myocardial tissue). The echocardiography probe with Doppler capability emits sound of known frequency and receives and measures the frequency of the reflected sound. As the probe remains stationary at any particular window of examination, by detecting the frequency shift, velocity of moving blood or tissue within the heart can be measured. The precise location of measurements is guided by 2D images. All modern echocardiography machines, including the ones designed for ICU use, have full Doppler capability including presets that let an examiner to switch easily between measuring blood flow velocity and cardiac tissue velocity.

Modes of Doppler Examination

Spectral Doppler

Spectral Doppler represents the graphical presentation of velocity spectrum against time. *Instantaneous* Doppler-measured velocity is plotted along *y*-axis and time is plotted along *x*-axis **(Fig. 14A)**. Results from both pulse-wave (PW) and continuous-wave (CW) Doppler examinations are essentially spectral representations of instantaneous velocity against time.

Pulse-wave Doppler

In PW Doppler examination, velocity of blood or tissue is measured at a precise location and plotted against time. Examples include measurement of blood flow velocity at left ventricular outflow tract (LVOT) during systole **(Fig. 14A)**, measurement of blood flow velocity at mitral valve tip during diastole, and measurement of velocity of mitral annulus during diastole. In PW examination, the same transducer element that sends the sound receives the echo from the moving target. An important limitation is inability to measure correctly high velocities, for example, from *any* valvular regurgitation.

Continuous-wave Doppler (Fig. 14B)

In CW Doppler, separate transducer elements within the same probe housing emit sounds and receive reflected sounds. During the period of examination, these elements continuously do their respective functions. CW Doppler is useful in measuring any high velocity along the path of interrogation though is unable to precisely locate the area of the high velocity. This limitation is known as range ambiguity. In practice, from the knowledge of the path of interrogation from 2D image, the user can determine the source of abnormal high velocity. High velocities within the cardiac chambers arise from *any* valvular regurgitant lesions or septal defects between a high-pressure and a low-pressure chamber, for example, ventricular septal defect (VSD).

Tissue Doppler (Fig. 14C)

Tissue Doppler (TD) is an application of PW Doppler where the moving velocity of a specific part of a structure/tissue (e.g., annulus velocity of mitral or tricuspid valve during echocardiography) is being measured. Tissue-movement velocity is typically lower than the blood-flow velocity though the strength of the echo (i.e., intensity) generated from moving tissue is higher than the strength of echo generated by the moving blood. When TD mode is chosen in machine settings (readily available in all portable ICU-ready machines in current generation), the machine automatically adjusts filters to suppress the echoes generated from the moving blood and plots the velocity spectrum of the moving tissue against time.

Color Doppler (Fig. 14D)

Color Doppler is a form of PW Doppler examination. During the examination, within the color box, at multiple points, the velocity of blood flow is measured. The machine converts the velocities as per a color code and superimposes the color-coded flow velocity pattern on the 2D image. By convention, any blood flow toward the probe is coded in red and any blood flow away from the probe is displayed in blue.

The velocity scale is also displayed.

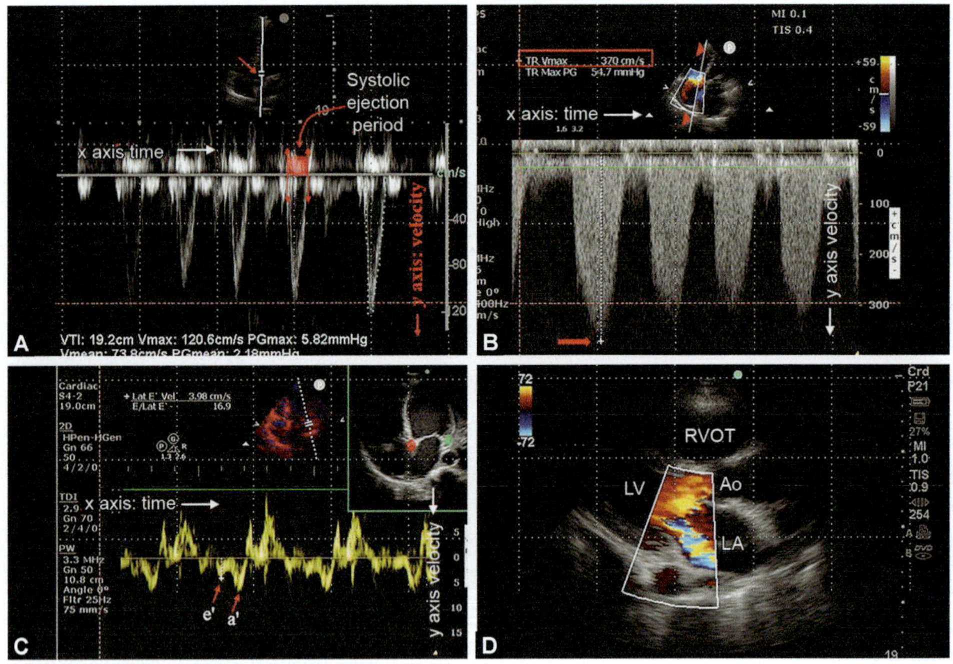

FIGS. 14A TO D: Modes of Doppler examination. (A) Pulse wave Doppler. Velocity is measured at LVOT (indicated by red arrow). Spectrum of instantaneous velocity is displayed along *y*-axis against time along *x*-axis. The period of systolic ejection period through LVOT is shown on the time axis. By common convention, the velocity is plotted above baseline if the blood is flowing toward the probe and below baseline if the blood is flowing away from the probe. (B) Continuous wave (CW) Doppler. Velocity is measured along the line and displayed against time. From the knowledge of cardiac anatomy, the location of maximum velocity can be known. In this patient with tricuspid regurgitation (TR), the line of CW Doppler interrogation (red arrowheads) runs along RV and RA through the tricuspid valve (and through the regurgitant jet shown in color Doppler). The maximum velocity represents the velocity of TR jet at tricuspid valve level (red arrow, measured at 3.7 m/sec). The highest velocities come from the narrowest point in the path of examination, which is the leaking valve or in the case of VSD, the site of the septal defect. (C) Tissue Doppler. Measurement of mitral valve lateral annulus relaxation velocity during diastole is shown from apical four-chamber (A4C) view. During diastole, as the LV relaxes, the annulus moves away from the probe that is placed as cardiac apex; the velocities are therefore depicted below the baseline on *y*-axis of the spectral presentation. The velocity corresponding to early rapid ventricular relaxation phase is termed e'; the velocity corresponding to the late part and coinciding with atrial contraction is termed a' (red arrows). The early relaxation velocity e' reduces with myocardial disease and progression of left ventricular diastolic dysfunction and provides important hemodynamic measurement. (D) Color Doppler. Examination of the mitral valve, showing mitral regurgitation. In this systolic frame, blood flow from LV to aorta is depicted in red; regurgitant jet from LV to LA is shown in multicolored hues as expected for a turbulent flow associated with regurgitation.

(LVOT: left ventricular outflow tract; LA: left atrium; LV: left ventricle; RA: right atrium; RV: right ventricle; RVOT: right ventricular outflow tract; VSD: ventricular septal defect)

Fundamental Mechanisms of Use of Doppler

Velocity–time Integral: Measurement of Flow

Velocity–time integral (VTI) is a key concept in quantitative Doppler echocardiography for hemodynamic monitoring. It is used to measure volume of blood shift or flow between two areas within heart during a specified period of time, for example, systolic ejection period. Most common application is measurement of SV at LVOT. If it is conceptualized that any volume shift during a cardiac cycle completely fills an empty cylinder, measuring the volume of the cylinder will calculate the shifted volume. For example, in left ventricular SV measurement, it is conceptualized that a cylinder is placed just above the aortic valve and the blood moving through the LVOT and aortic valve during LV systole fills up this imaginary cylinder. The volume of the cylinder will, therefore, represent LVSV. To measure the volume of a cylinder, the diameter and length of the cylinder need to be determined.

Volume (cylinder) = $\pi r^2 l$, where r is the radius of the cylinder and l is the length of the cylinder.

The VTI is used to calculate the length of the imaginary cylinder **(Figs. 15A and B)**. This is a use of PW Doppler, by which velocity is measured over the time of a flow period.

A detailed description of the SV and CO measurement is given in the CO section of this chapter.

Measurement of Pressure Gradient from Flow Velocity

Within the cardiac chambers, flow of blood across valves is along pressure gradients (measured in mm Hg). The velocity of the flow is dependent on the pressure gradient. As Doppler allows measurement of velocity of blood flow across cardiac valves, it can be used to measure the pressure gradient between two cardiac chambers. Presence of a regurgitant or stenotic lesion makes the gradient calculation possible. Modified Bernoulli's equation is used to measure the pressure gradient:

$\Delta P = P2 - P1 = 4V^2$

where,

ΔP = Pressure gradient

P1 = Pressure in the receiving chamber

P2 = Pressure in the upstream chamber

V = Maximum instantaneous velocity of flow between two chambers

Therefore, if two of the three parameters (P1, P2, and V) are known, the third parameter can be calculated using the Bernoulli's equation.

This concept of Doppler use is demonstrated in **Figures 16A and B** and summarized in **Table 3**.

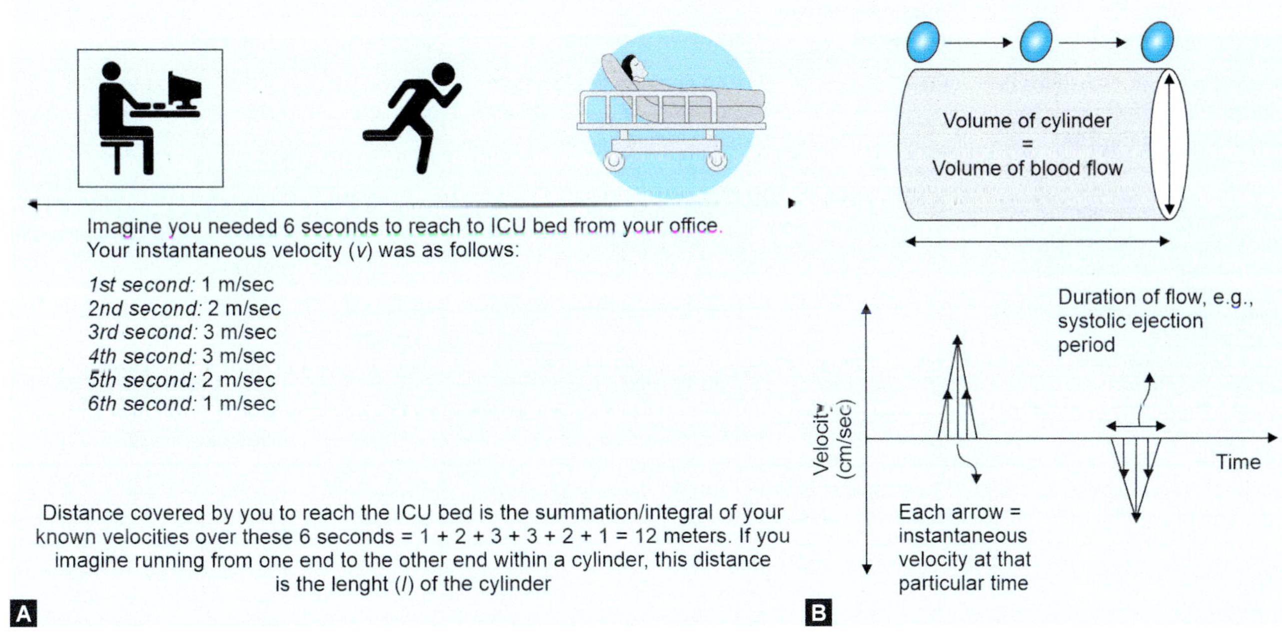

FIGS. 15A AND B: Concept of VTI. (A) Cartoon illustration of the concept. By summing up the instantaneous velocities over any given period of time, the distance covered during that time period can be calculated. (B) Blood (a group of RBCs) has traveled from one end of the cylinder to another end during the period of flow, i.e., systolic ejection period. If the instantaneous velocities obtained by PW Doppler are summed up, the distance covered can be calculated and it represents the length of the cylinder. The diameter of the cylinder is calculated at the respective site as discussed under CO measurement.

(CO: cardiac output; PW: pulse wave; RBCs: red blood cells; VTI: velocity–time integral)

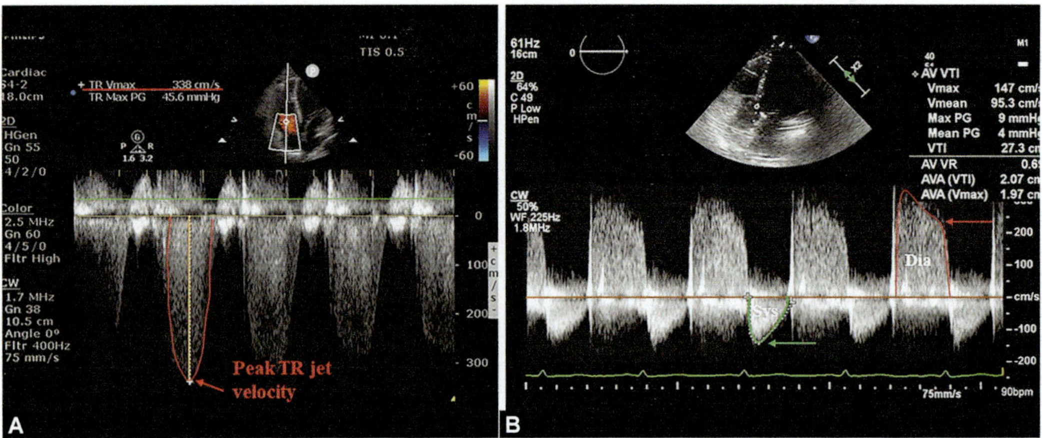

FIGS. 16A AND B: Measurement of pressure gradient from Doppler. (A) Measurement of RV systolic pressure from tricuspid regurgitation (TR) jet velocity. The peak jet velocity is 3.38 m/sec. The peak pressure gradient between RV and RA (mm Hg) is $4 \times (3.38)^2 = 45.6$ mm Hg. If the right atrial pressure is known, then RV systolic pressure can be calculated from the gradient. TR velocity profile is outlined by red envelope and the maximum instantaneous velocity measurement is also marked (orange line, red arrow). (B) Measurement of LV end-diastolic pressure (LVEDP) from aortic regurgitation (AR) velocity. The end-diastolic velocity (red arrow) of the regurgitant jet (red envelope) is 2.4 m/sec. At the time of the echocardiogram, patient's BP was 104/40 mm Hg. By applying modified Bernoulli's equation, the pressure gradient between aortic diastolic pressure and LVEDP (DBP – LVEDP) would be $4 \times (2.4)^2 = 23$ mm Hg. LVEDP, therefore can be calculated as 17 mm Hg. Also, note the systolic velocity profile (green envelope) across the aortic valve. The peak velocity is 1.47 m/sec (green arrow). The calculated systolic gradient, $4 \times (1.47)^2$ is 9 mm Hg, showing that there is no significant aortic valve stenosis.

(BP: blood pressure; DBP: diastolic blood pressure; LA: left atrium; LV: left ventricle; RA: right atrium; RV: right ventricle)

TABLE 3: Measurement of important pressure gradients using Doppler.

Velocity measured	Pressure gradient measured	Known pressure	Derived pressure	Comments
Tricuspid regurgitation (maximal) velocity (CW Doppler across tricuspid valve) **(Fig. 16A)**	RV–RA	RA pressure (known from central line or IVC size and respiratory variation)	RV systolic pressure	If there is no pulmonic valve stenosis, RV systolic pressure represents PA systolic pressure
Peak velocity across aortic valve **(Fig. 16B)** (CW Doppler along a line through LVOT and AV)	LV–Aorta	Peak aortic pressure (systolic blood pressure)	LV Peak pressure	In presence of aortic stenosis, gradient will be high
Mitral valve regurgitation (peak) velocity	LV–LA	LV pressure (same as SBP)	(Peak) LA pressure	
Aortic regurgitation velocity at the end of regurgitation period **(Fig. 16B)**	Aortic diastolic pressure–LVEDP	Aortic diastolic pressure	LVEDP	More peripherally measured DBP is taken as aortic diastolic pressure
Pulmonary regurgitation velocity at the end of regurgitation period	PA diastolic pressure–RV diastolic pressure	RV end-diastolic pressure	PA diastolic pressure	RV end-diastolic pressure is most closely represented by RAPmean, which can be calculated from central venous line tracing

(AV: atrioventricular; CW: continuous wave; DBP: diastolic blood pressure; IVC: inferior vena cava; LA: left atrium; LV: left ventricle; LVEDP: left ventricular end-diastolic pressure; LVOT: left ventricular outflow tract; PA: pulmonary artery; RV: right ventricle; SBP: systolic blood pressure)

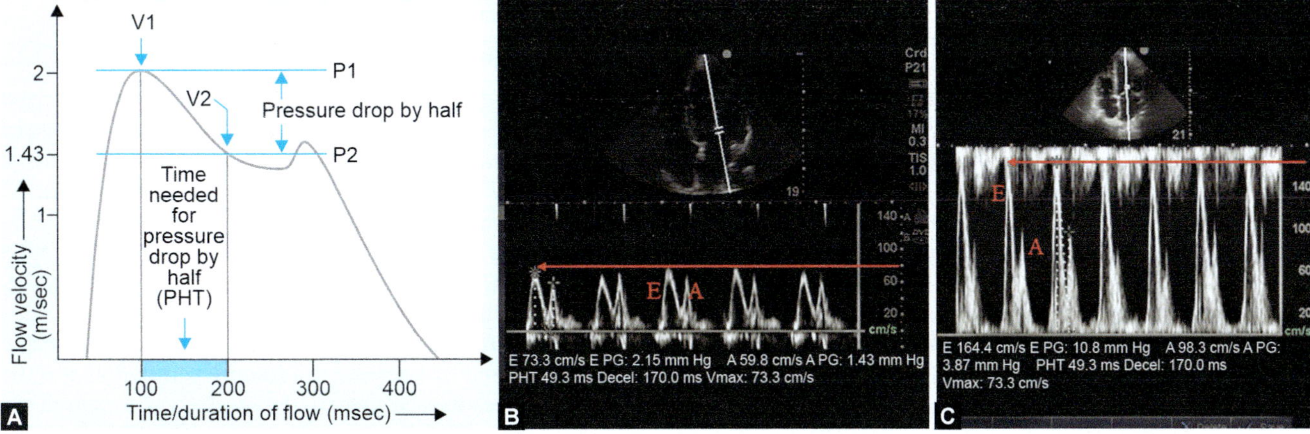

FIGS. 17A TO C: Concept of pressure half-time. (A) Illustration of the concept. By measuring change in flow velocity over time, we can measure change in pressure gradient over the same time period. At any given instant during the period of blood flow, the instantaneous velocity depends on the pressure gradient between the upstream and downstream chambers. When the flow velocity is maximum (V1, 2 m/sec in the example), the pressure gradient is highest (P1). At a velocity V2 (1.43 m/sec in the example), the pressure gradient is exactly half of highest-pressure gradient (P2). The time interval that is needed for the velocity to change this much is called pressure half-time (P1/2t, PHT), which is 100 ms in this example. (B) Measurement of diastolic flow velocity at tip of mitral valve by PW Doppler. The early peak velocity (E, red arrow) represents the pressure gradient between left atrium and left ventricle during early rapid filling phase of ventricular diastole. It is an important parameter for volume overload, left atrial pressure, cardiac function, and hemodynamic management. The E velocity is normal in this example. By tracing the slope of the declining flow velocity, pressure half-time (PHT) is calculated by the machine software. A represents the velocity of flow during late diastolic phase as a result of atrial contraction. (C) Mitral valve inflow velocity in a patient with volume overload. Note the high E velocity, denoting high pressure gradient between LA and LV at the beginning of diastole. Use of this parameter in hemodynamic management is discussed later in this chapter. In absence of mitral valve disease, high E wave velocity will indicate high left atrial pressure and high pulmonary artery wedge pressure.

(LA: left atrium; LV: left ventricle; PW: pulse wave)

Measurement of Pressure Half-time

Blood flow velocity across a valve depends on the pressure gradient. Therefore, by measuring the change in flow velocity over the duration of blood flow, the rate of change in pressure gradient can be calculated. This concept has most immediate application in measuring mitral stenosis severity: More severe the stenosis, the longer it takes the pressure gradient to fall across mitral valve **(Figs. 17A to C)**. Direct application of this concept in daily critical care practice is less. However, the blood flow velocities from LA to LV during diastole are used to measure diastolic dysfunction and left ventricular filling pressures. Measurement of left-sided filling pressures from mitral valve blood flow velocity has immense application in hemodynamic diagnosis and management in ICU **(Figs. 17A to C)**.

BOX 3 **Determinants of cardiac output.**

Cardiac output (CO) = Heart rate (HR) × Stroke volume (SV)

- *HR:*
  - HR response rapidly adjusts cardiac output
  - *Most effective method of changing CO:* 2–3 times increase can be done in CO in a healthy person by change in HR alone
  - With increase in HR, a slight increase in ventricular contractility occurs (Bowditch's law)
  - *Decrease in HR:* CO may not fall as an increase in diastolic filling time increases SV
- *SV depends on:*
  - Ventricular end-diastolic volume (preload)
  - Myocardial contractility
  - Ventricular afterload

MEASUREMENT OF CARDIAC OUTPUT

Cardiac output monitoring should be a routine component of management of hemodynamically unstable patients in ICU. CO measurement, in conjunction with other commonly measured hemodynamic parameters, helps to derive calculated indices to categorize shock state and optimize management strategy. No clinical (e.g., blood pressure) or laboratory parameter (e.g., serum lactate level) correlate well with CO on a consistent basis and each of those parameters can have other confounders. Therefore, direct measurement of CO is stressed. Determinants of CO are listed in **Box 3**.

Important milestones in development of principles and techniques of CO monitoring are presented in **Box 4** *with important references for an interested reader to find additional literature.* Based on these principles, a wide array of CO monitoring tools are available commercially, though an ideal technology remains elusive. Desirable traits of an ideal CO monitoring system are presented in **Box 5**. Lack of high-quality data from head-to-head trials of different systems makes it difficult to choose one above the other. A comparison of major methods/systems used in clinical practice is presented in **Table 4**. It is notable that not all technologies have traveled widely beyond their country/continent of origin to find worldwide use. Many technologies have not been successful commercially and had their demise with time. Details of important CO monitoring principles, methods, and related systems are presented here.

BOX 4 Important milestones in development of cardiac output (CO) monitoring.

- *1870:* Adolf Fick described computation of CO from arterial and venous blood oxygen measurements[41]
- *1897:* Stewart's indicator dilution method[42]
- *1928–1932:* Development of Stewart-Hamilton equation[43-45]
- *1954:* Development of thermodilution method[46]
- *1963:* Measurement of CO in human using thermodilution[47]
- *1966:* Bioimpedance-based measurement of CO in clinical practice[48]
- *1970:* Development of flow-directed balloon-tipped pulmonary artery (PA) catheter[49]
- *1971:* Thermodilution measurement in human using PA catheter[50]
- *1980:* Gas rebreathing[33]
- *1993,* 1998: Continuous thermodilution monitoring through PA catheter[51,52]
- *1993:* Description of lithium dilution technique for CO measurement[53]
- *1994:* Description of transcardiopulmonary indicator dilution technique[54]

BOX 5 Desirable features of an ideal cardiac output (CO)-monitoring technology.

- Noninvasive/minimally invasive
- Widely applicable in all patient groups (awake/sedated/anesthetized/critically ill)
- Real-time beat-to-beat result
- Accurate and repeatable results
- Short learning curve for implementation and analysis
- Operator independent
- Cost-effective
- Minimal risk of complications

Fick's Principle of Cardiac Output Measurement

First developed in 1870, Fick's principle has been summarized as, *"the total uptake of (or release of) a substance by the peripheral tissues is equal to the product of the blood flow to the peripheral tissues and the arterial-venous concentration difference (gradient) of the substance".*

While this principle is widely applicable, it can most easily be explained in terms of oxygen consumption **(Fig. 18)**, which is explained as follows:

- The amount of oxygen consumed per minute of time can be measured by knowing the minute ventilation and the partial pressure of oxygen in the inspired and expired air.
- This amount of oxygen is the difference between the amount of oxygen delivered to tissues via arterial blood each minute and the amount of oxygen left in blood returning to heart, for example, mixed venous blood.
- By knowing the hemoglobin (Hb, g/L), arterial blood oxygen saturation (SaO_2), partial pressure of oxygen (PaO_2), and the oxygen content per unit of arterial blood (CaO_2) can be calculated:
$$CaO_2\,(mL/L) = [SaO_2 \times Hb\,(g/L) \times 1.34] + [PaO_2\,(mm\,Hg) \times 0.003]$$
- Similarly, oxygen content of venous blood (CvO_2) can be calculated from oxygen saturation (SvO_2) and partial pressure of oxygen (PvO_2) of mixed venous blood.
$$CvO_2\,(mL/L) = [SvO_2 \times Hb\,(g/L) \times 1.34] + [PvO_2\,(mm\,Hg) \times 0.003]$$
- If the total amount of oxygen consumption per minute is known and the oxygen content difference between per unit of arterial and venous blood is known, then the number of units of blood required to deliver the amount of oxygen per minute can be calculated and represents cardiac output (CO).

$$VO_2 = (CO \times CaO_2) - (CO \times CvO_2)$$

where:
VO_2 is the total oxygen consumption, as a volume per unit time (e.g., L/min)
CO is the cardiac output, also as volume per unit time (L/min)
CaO_2 and CvO_2 are the arterial and venous oxygen content (e.g., mL/L)
To rearrange things,

$$CO = VO_2/(CaO_2 - CvO_2)$$

Measurement of CO in ICU by direct Fick's method is impractical as accurate measurement of oxygen consumption is cumbersome and mixed venous O_2 sampling requires placement of a PA catheter. Moreover, CO measurement by this method cannot be repeated easily.

In *indirect Fick method,* one or more of the variables from the Fick equation are estimated rather than measured. Most commonly, oxygen consumption is calculated from

TABLE 4: Comparison of different cardiac output (CO) measurement techniques.

Method of CO measurement	Invasiveness	Equipment required	Proprietary system required	Advantages	Limitations
Direct Fick principle	+++	• Arterial sampling and PA catheter • Direct measurement of oxygen consumption	No	Sound physiological principles	Accurate and repeated calculation of oxygen consumption impractical in ICU patients
Indirect Fick method	+++	Depends on which variables estimated	No		Relies on estimation of one or more variables used in Fick equation
PAC—intermittent thermodilution (TD)	+++	• Central venous access • Thermodilution-capable PAC	No	Additional hemodynamic data through PAC	Not continuous
PAC—continuous TD	+++	• Central venous access • Specialized PAC	No	• Additional hemodynamic data through PAC • Continuous CO	Time lag in reflecting change in CO
PiCCO	++	• Thermistor-tipped arteria line in a central vessel • Requires intermittent calibration • Central venous access	Yes	• Being a calibrated system, more reliable in patients with vasodilatation, for example, sepsis and liver failure • Continuous estimation of real-time CO	
LiDCO	++	Arterial line, central venous line/peripheral vein	Yes	Combines beat-to-beat CO through pulse wave analysis and advantage of calibration	Cannot be used in patients who are on lithium therapy
FloTrac/Vigileo	+	Arterial line	Yes	• Minimally invasive • Continuous estimation of real-time CO	• More reliable in monitoring trends than measuring absolute value • Less accurate than calibrated PWA systems • Less reliable with significant aortic regurgitation, arrhythmia, and intra-aortic balloon pump
Esophageal Doppler	+	Transesophageal Doppler probe	Yes	Minimally invasive	• Poorly tolerated unless tracheal tube present • Relies on assumed proportion of blood flow through descending aorta
USCOM	(–)	Transthoracic Doppler probe	Yes	Noninvasive	• Uses nomogram for valve area estimation • Not accurate with significant valve stenosis
Gas rebreathing	++	Rebreathing circuit	Yes	Real-time beat-to-beat CO monitoring	Requires tracheal intubation and stable tidal volume during measurement
Thoracic bioimpedance	(–)	Cutaneous electrodes	Yes	Noninvasive	Accuracy with hemodynamic instability not well-tested

(ICU: intensive care unit; LiDCO: lithium dilution cardiac output; PA: pulmonary artery; PAC: pulmonary artery catheterization; PiCCO: pulse index continuous cardiac output)

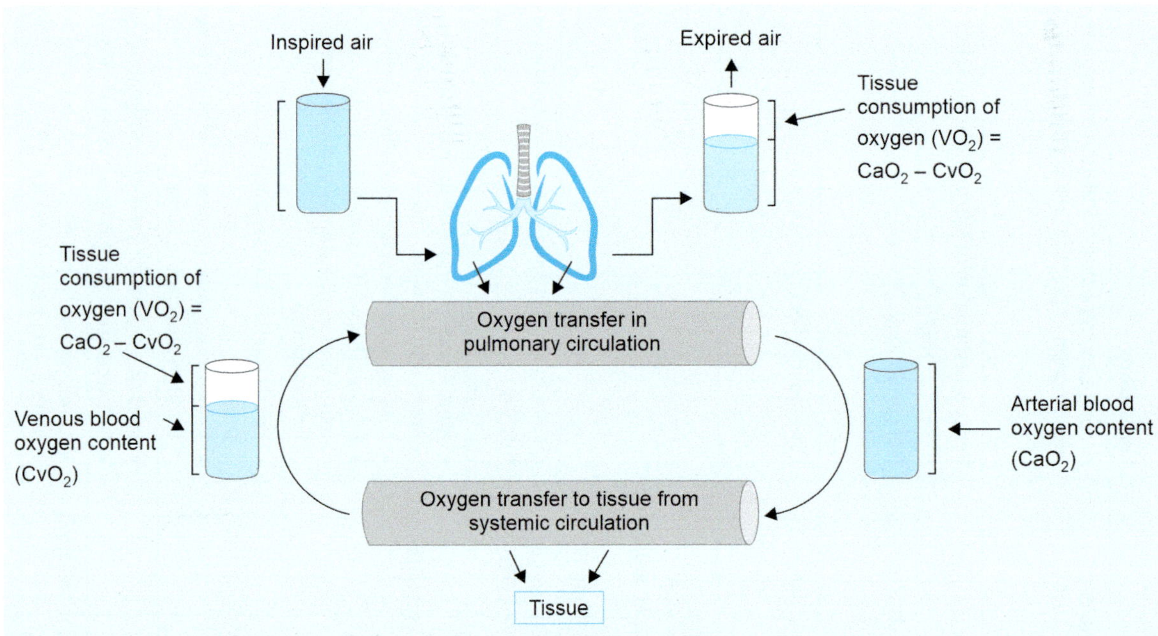

FIG. 18: Fick principle. The difference in oxygen content between inspired and expired air is the amount of oxygen consumed during any period of time. If the oxygen content per unit of arterial and mixed venous blood is known, then it can be calculated how many units of blood have flown through the tissues to deliver the same amount of oxygen to tissues.

nomograms. A variation of indirect Fick method is applied in calculation of CO by partial gas rebreathing techniques.

Indicator Dilution Principle

Any CO measurement using indicator dilution technique involves injecting a known volume and concentration of an indicator upstream of heart, for example, in a central or peripheral vein. The indicator is mixed with blood and is carried downstream by the moving blood flow. The concentration of the indicator is measured downstream (post right or LV). As measured at the downstream point, the indicator concentration rises and then falls, and a time concentration curve can be constructed. Stewart developed the original formulation in 1897. In 1928, Hamilton modified the formula used for CO calculation, incorporating the fact that the concentration of the indicator rises and falls in a nonstepwise fashion **(Fig. 19)**. The final formulation, still used today, has come to be known as Stewart-Hamilton equation. It would suffice to remember that CO = amount of indicator injected/area under the time-concentration curve.

Thermodilution

Thermodilution method of CO measurement is an adaptation of indicator dilution principle. Here, a known volume of fluid with a known/measured temperature is injected proximal to heart. The bolus of "cold" or "negative heat" is therefore the indicator. As the fluid/saline colder than blood gets mixed with flowing blood, the temperature of the blood at the distal measuring point changes and is measured with a thermistor. Just like the concentration of a chemical indicator, the temperature change at the measuring point can be plotted against time to provide an indicator dilution curve.

There are two important assumptions in any indicator dilution technique using Stewart-Hamilton equation:

i. Complete mixing of blood and indicator (dye or cold fluid) is happening with no loss of indicator.
ii. Blood flow remains constant during the measurement.

Limitations of indicator dilution techniques are presented in **Box 6**, in context of the most widely practiced technique, for example, intermittent bolus thermodilution through PAC.

Pulmonary Artery Catheter and Intermittent Bolus Thermodilution (IB-PATD)

Pulmonary artery catheter remains the gold standard amongst all "bedside techniques" since it was introduced in 1970.

Either iced or room air saline or 5% dextrose is injected through a proximal port and in-built thermistor measures the temperature in the PA. Several studies show equivalent results of using 10-mL room temperature and 10-mL iced injectates over a wide range of COs, though some reports also show significant differences, particularly in low- and high-flow states. The highest reproducibility of CO measurements in critically ill patients was demonstrated with 10-mL iced injectate. Since its introduction, its use became widespread

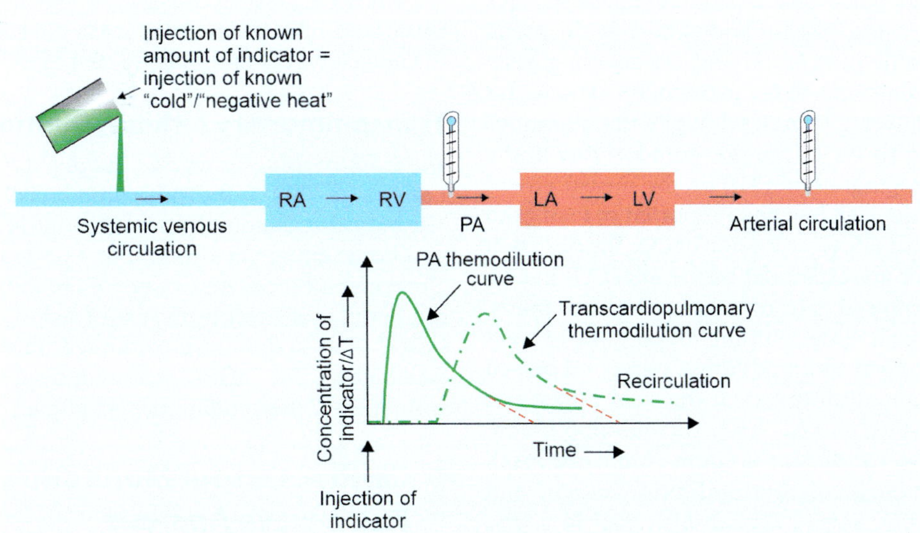

FIG. 19: CO monitoring by indicator dilution technique. Thermodilution is used as an example of the principle. Indicator is injected upstream of right heart, i.e., in systemic venous circulation, either through a peripheral vein or central vein, depending on the method. Indicator concentration (temperature change in thermodilution techniques, ΔT) is measured post right heart or post left heart. The long tail of the curve is due to recirculation of the indicator. Computer algorithm for calculation of CO extrapolates the curve to baseline (as shown as red part of the concentration–time curve) after a set time to calculate the area under curve.

(CO: cardiac output; LA: left atrium; LV: left ventricle; PA: pulmonary artery; RA: right atrium; RV: right: ventricle)

BOX 6 Limitations and sources of errors in indicator dilution techniques.

- *Loss of indicator before injection [any loss of indicator overestimates cardiac output (CO)]:*
  - Loss of injectate (from leak)
  - Erroneously lower volume of injectate
- *Loss of indicator during injection:*
  - Occult warming of the injectate before it enters bloodstream:
    - From mixing of injectate with fluid already within catheter
    - Transfer of heat from blood surrounding the catheter (catheter volume and rate of injection affect this loss)
- *Loss of indicator after injection:*
  - Conductive rewarming of indicator by surrounding tissue:
    - Pronounced in low-flow states
    - When the indicator travels longer distances en route to the measuring thermistor, for example, the more the distance traveled by the indicator, more is the loss in TCPTD compared with the IB-PATD
  - *Diversion of cold indicator:* Right-to-left shunt and venovenous extracorporeal lung assist
  - Tricuspid regurgitation (TR) by increasing transit time and allowing more time for gain of heat and smaller effective cold bolus
- *Recirculation of indicator—underestimates cardiac output:*
  - Left-to-right shunt
  - *Significant TR: By increasing circulation time:*
- *Fluctuation in baseline temperature:*
  - Active cooling or rewarming of the patient
  - Concurrent IV infusions
  - Fluctuation of PA temperature from cardiac and respiratory oscillations
- *Fluctuation in CO:*
  - Significant change in CO with respiratory cycle under certain conditions
  - Arrhythmias
- Truncation and extrapolation algorithms of thermodilution curve

(IB-PATD: pulmonary artery catheter and intermittent bolus thermodilution; IV: intravenous; PA: pulmonary artery; TCPTD: transcardiopulmonary thermodilution)

till early 21st century when several studies showed its lack of benefit in improving patient outcomes. Widespread availability of portable ultrasound and echocardiography also was timely to contribute to fall in use of PA catheter for hemodynamic monitoring in general. While the numerous sources of errors in IB-PATD are presented in **Box 6**, the effect of tricuspid regurgitation (TR) on the measurement needs special mention. TR has been reported to lead both to overestimation and underestimation of CO. The direction and amount of error are explained by the effect TR has on transit time and scope of gain of heat by the cold bolus. An increase in transit time without much gain of heat will lead to a prolonged thermodilution curve, increased AUC, and underestimation of CO. If the cold bolus part of TR volume gains much heat from surrounding blood, it amounts to a lower indicator amount (indicator loss), lower area under curve of thermodilution curve, and overestimation of CO. Severe TR can also lead to a true decrease in forward flow, and therefore measured CO. The effect of TR on thermodilution-derived CO remains an unsolved question.[28-30]

Continuous Pulmonary Artery Thermodilution—Cardiac Output

In *continuous PA thermodilution CO (CPATD-CO)*, blood flowing through the superior vena cava is heated intermittently by an electric filament attached to the PAC approximately 15–25 cm before its tip and blood temperature is measured more distally. Use of this method will depend on the availability of a commercially available system and suitable catheter. CO measured by CPATD correlates well with intermittent bolus thermodilution as well as other methods of comparison, for example, electromagnetometry and ultrasound using aortic flow probes. Though IB-PATD and CPATD correlate well in general, a notable exception is patients recovering from hypothermia, for example, patient recovering from cardiopulmonary bypass, where IB-PATD is less affected by thermal noise. Also, in times of rapid hemodynamic change, CPATD is less reliable given inherent time delay in reflecting the change.

Transcardiopulmonary Thermodilution

The pulse index continuous cardiac output (PiCCO) (Pulsion Medical Systems, Munich, Germany) is the main commercial system available using transcardiopulmonary thermodilution (TCPTD). In this method, "cold injectate" is given in a central vein. The cold indicator gets mixed with blood and travels through the right heart, pulmonary circulation, and left heart. Resulting thermal changes are measured typically by a transistor-tipped femoral artery catheter and a thermodilution curve is plotted. In addition to TCPTD, PiCCO system provides beat-to-beat CO monitoring by pulse contour analysis.

The PiCCO device has been extensively studied and compared with pulmonary artery thermodilution-derived CO measurement and generally correlates well.

Transpulmonary Lithium Dilution

The lithium dilution cardiac output [LiDCO-Plus (LiDCO, Cambridge, UK)] is the only commercially available system. The indicator, isotonic lithium chloride (150 mM), is injected as a bolus either via a central or a peripheral venous route. The concentration-time curve of the indicator is generated in a peripheral artery by the use of an ion-selective electrode. LiDCO-Plus system also combined pulse contour analysis (see below). The LiDCO system derived CO correlates well with the PAC thermodilution technique.

Cardiac Output Monitoring using Pulse-wave Analysis

The concept of CO measurement by pulse wave analysis (PWA) was first suggested by Otto Frank in 1899 and later described by Erlanger and Hooker in 1904. Any PW-based method aims to measure blood flow changes by analysis of BP waveform. With each contraction, an amount of blood equivalent to the SV enters aorta and starts an arterial waveform. The waveform depends on the amount of SV but is obviously affected by the impedance and compliance of the aorta and peripheral vascular resistance. Scientific models and algorithms differ from one system to another system of BP wave-based SV measurement and a detailed discussion of various principles of waveform analysis (e.g., Windkessel models, long time interval analysis technique, and pulse power analysis) is beyond the scope of this chapter. It is obvious that vascular tree characteristics are important part of any algorithm that uses any principle based on pressure waveform analysis. CO monitoring systems based on PWA may be invasive, minimally-invasive, and noninvasive. They are most effectively classified according to the method a system uses to calibrate estimated CO values in externally calibrated systems, internally calibrated systems, and uncalibrated systems. We will briefly discuss the commonly available systems.

Invasive and minimally-invasive PWA technologies all need an arterial catheter. Externally calibrated PWA systems estimate CO from the invasively measured arterial pressure waveform. A reference method is used to calibrate the CO measurements from PWA.

- *PiCCO system*: This system uses the area under the systolic part of the arterial pressure wave curve, averaged over 30 seconds period, to continuously estimate CO. Calibration is done by intermittent TCPTD. Therefore, a central venous catheter (used for the injection of the cold indicator solution) and a dedicated thermistor-tipped arterial catheter are needed. The arterial catheter needs to be placed in a central artery (femoral, brachial, or axillary artery). Any intervention or clinical event that might change vascular tone, for example, change in vasoactive agents and fluid administration would need recalibration by thermodilution to maintain reliability of the PWA CO measurement.

- *The LiDCO-plus system (LiDCO, Cambridge, UK)*: This system uses a proprietary algorithm (Pulse CO) to estimate CO using pulse power analysis principle. The system is calibrated by intermittent transcardiopulmonary lithium dilution (described earlier). In patients on lithium therapy, lithium dilution-derived CO will be overestimated. In addition, use of some neuromuscular blocking agents containing quaternary ammonium residues may be detected by the lithium sensor, making CO calibration inaccurate.
- *FloTrac/Vigileo system (Edwards Lifesciences, Irvine, California, USA):* It is a less invasive system. CVP line is not needed as there is no role of intermittent external calibration. Lack of calibration is a potential source of error. It utilizes a blood flow sensor attached to a standard arterial catheter. CO is calculated every 20 seconds using an algorithm that has been updated multiple times by the manufacturer during the lifecycle of system. Multiplication of arterial pulsatility (standard deviation of pressure wave over 20 seconds) and a constant (K) derived from the patient's specific vascular compliance results in SV, which is then multiplied by heart rate to calculate CO. The specific vascular compliance is updated every minute and is based on age, height, gender, and weight and waveform characteristic. The performance of the FloTrac/Vigileo system has also been researched in a range of clinical situations, in comparison with both PACs and PiCCO devices, with conflicting results. It has been suggested that the FloTrac/Vigileo may be more useful for measuring trends than absolute values.

Cardiac output monitoring utilizing PWA is one of the most extensively studied of all the minimally-invasive monitoring system. In general, they show good agreement with CO measurements made using a PAC. Despite this, the user should be aware of several sources of potential error, which may be more pronounced in some clinical settings. All pulse contour analysis monitors rely on an optimal arterial signal. Over or underdamped traces may lead to inaccurate CO measurement. Arrhythmias, aortic regurgitation, and the use of an intra-aortic balloon pump affect the pulse contour and have been shown to affect accuracy. Changes in systemic vascular resistance (SVR) may also lead to inaccuracies in CO measurement.

Doppler-based Flow Measurement by Velocity Summation Method

General principle of measurement of flow, for example, CO by summation of flow velocities has been covered under advanced echocardiography section.

Transthoracic Echocardiography with Doppler to Measure Stroke Volume at Left Ventricular Outflow Tract or Right Ventricular Outflow Tract

This method will be described in detail as it is noninvasive and most easily applied, using portable bedside ultrasound machines commonly used in ICUs.

Measurement of SV at LVOT is shown in **Figures 20A to D** and can be broken down into the following steps:[31]

1. Measurement of SV is quantitative estimation of the volume of blood that passes through LVOT during each systole. It can be thought of as measuring the volume of a cylinder that is completely filled, with the blood ejected during each systole. The cross-sectional area of this imaginary cylinder is equal to the cross-sectional area of LVOT **(Fig. 20A)**.
2. The diameter of LVOT can be measured on parasternal long-axis view **(Fig. 20A)**. LVOT diameter is used to calculate the cross-sectional area of LVOT (LVOT is assumed as a circle, the area, therefore, is calculated by the formula πr^2, where r = radius of LVOT; d/2).
3. From an apical window, an apical five-chamber view is obtained that includes the LVOT **(Fig. 20B)**. A pulsed-wave Doppler interrogation box is placed at the center of LVOT. A velocity-time plot/velocity envelope is obtained.
4. VTI is calculated **(Fig. 20C)** and represents the length of this imaginary cylinder.
5. SV is calculated as follows **(Fig. 20D)**:
   SV (mL) = LVOT cross-sectional area (cm^2) × VTI (cm)

Aortic Doppler

The USCOM device (Ultrasonic Cardiac Output Monitors, Sydney, Australia) is truly noninvasive and uses a CW Doppler probe placed suprasternally to measure flow through the ascending aorta or on the left chest to measure main PA flow. Just like transthoracic measurement at LVOT, VTI is calculated from the area under the velocity-time curve and used as stroke distance (i.e., the length of cylinder, as shown in **Figs. 15A and B**). An estimate of aortic cross-section area (CSA) is taken either from a nomogram (height, weight, and age) or from utilizing M-mode ultrasound. Estimation of CSA may be an important source of error for this method of CO measurement. The use of nomogram may introduce measurement error, especially as CSA will change with change in vascular tone and volume status, more than the change in cross sectional area of LVOT. USCOM devices have shown variable results, especially in low and high CO states.

The Esophageal Doppler

Esophageal Doppler (EDM) uses technology to insert specialized probes, either orally or nasally, to measure blood

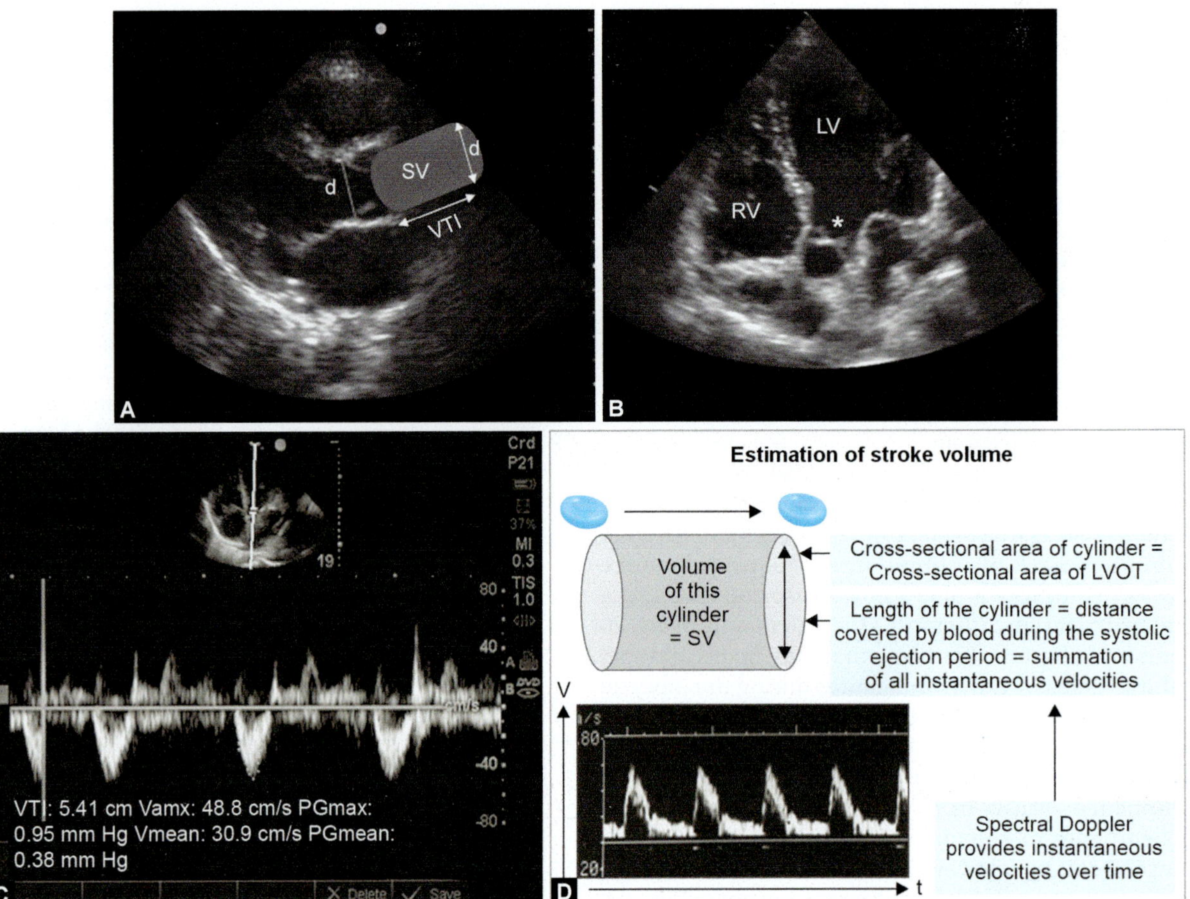

FIGS. 20A TO D: Measurement of stroke volume (SV) by echocardiography. (A) SV can be imagined as a cylindrical volume of blood ejected during each systole. Left ventricular outflow tract (LVOT) diameter (d) is measured in systole at the level of aortic annulus from a parasternal long-axis view. The distance is measured between the point where the anterior aortic cusp meets the ventricular septum and the point where the posterior aortic cusp meets the anterior mitral leaflet. The line should be perpendicular to the anterior aortic wall. (B) An apical five-chamber view visualizes the LVOT; a pulse Doppler interrogation box is placed at the center of LVOT (*). (C) Doppler measurement of flow velocity and VTI at LVOT. (D) Schematic representation of the principle of SV measurement.

(LV: left ventricle; RV: right: ventricle; VTI: velocity–time integral)

Source: Reproduced with permission from Sarkar et al. (2020).

flow in descending thoracic aorta. The probes are generally only tolerated in anesthetized or sedated patients, and there is a steep learning curve for optimal use. Optimal probe position is crucial in reducing measurement error for both blood flow measurement and aortic CSA measurement. Like any Doppler-based measurement, Doppler equation assumes that laminar flow and any turbulent flow in aorta will reduce measurement accuracy. Systems using EDM derive aortic area calculation either from M-mode measurement of diameter or from standard nomograms based on height, weight, age, and sex. The method also assumes fixed ratio of blood supply between upper and lower body (30% cephalic), though in reality, it is variable. A correction factor must be used as measurement utilizes the descending aorta assuming 70% of CO passes through the vessel.

Thoracic Bioimpedance and Bioreactance

The techniques of thoracic electrical bioimpedance (TEB) and thoracic electrical bioreactance (TEBR) both depend on measurement of change in electrical current during transmission across the thoracic cavity. Theoretical premise behind these technologies is that the thoracic cavity is a cylinder perfused with fluid (blood and tissue fluid). All other tissue remaining the same, the amount of fluid/blood determines the electrical conduction properties. The amount of blood in thoracic cavity and impedance changes during the cardiac cycle. Changes in CO will change the amount of aortic blood and will be reflected in a change in TEB. In TEB method, a known voltage of very low-intensity current is applied through voltage-delivering electrode pads, and voltage is measured through sensor electrodes placed elsewhere on the patient. With cardiac cycle, as the impedance (opposite of conductivity) changes, numeric value of impedance can be plotted as a waveform, and cardiac cycle events (e.g., opening and closing of aortic valve) can be identified in correlation with ECG. SV is calculated by a formula using patient-specific parameters (gender, height, and weight), ECG R-R interval, and parameters measured from TEB data.

TEB offers advantage of continuous CO monitoring in a noninvasive way. The system is very sensitive to movement, and thus less reliable in awake patients in critical care than in intraoperative patients. Arrhythmias may also lead to inaccuracy due to irregular R-R interval. Further evidence is still needed to determine the accuracy of TEB devices in hemodynamically unstable patients.

Compared to TEB, TEBR measures phase shift of electrical current applied across thorax. From technical point of view, TEBR is more reliable, has better signal fidelity, better noise filtering capacity, and is not affected by the distance between electrodes. It is also not affected by changes in other thoracic cavity fluids (chest wall edema, effusions, pulmonary edema, pulmonary and venous circulation).

Gas Rebreathing

Rebreathing techniques for CO monitoring have used both inert gases and CO_2. These techniques depend on application of Fick principle in some form as explained below.

The Fick equation written for CO_2 as the indicator gas is as follows:

$$CO = VCO_2/(CvCO_2 - CaCO_2)$$

where, VCO_2 is CO_2 excreted by the lungs, and $CaCO_2$ and $CvCO_2$ are the arterial and mixed venous CO_2 contents, respectively. It can be stated that at steady state, the amount of CO_2 entering the lungs via the pulmonary artery ($CvCO_2$) is proportional to the CO and equal to the sum of the amount exiting the lung via expiration (VCO_2) and via pulmonary veins (i.e., remaining in arterial blood exiting lungs, $CaCO_2$).

To apply the Fick method directly, both the CO_2 excretion by lungs and direct/invasive sampling of arterial and mixed venous blood will be required. Rebreathing techniques *estimate* arterial and mixed venous CO_2 contents from measurements of end-tidal CO_2 partial pressure ($P_{ET}CO_2$) generated in the mouth during normal breathing and rebreathing maneuvers, making it a noninvasive way to measure CO.[32] In cooperative patients, VCO_2 can be measured with acceptable accuracy using commercially available metabolic gas monitors. During normal breathing, $P_{ET}CO_2$ reflects the partial pressure of CO_2 in blood exiting the lungs and $CaCO_2$ can be calculated. During a period of total rebreathing, all CO_2 excretion is eliminated. Therefore, the $P_{ET}CO_2$ will progressively rise till it equalizes the CO_2 level in mixed venous blood entering lungs and $CvCO_2$ can be calculated. This "total rebreathing" method cannot be applied to an intubated critically ill patients due to technical limitations and a partial rebreathing method has been developed. Partial rebreathing technique uses the ratio of the change in the numerator and denominator of the Fick equation (differential form of Fick equation) to measure CO. Changes in CO_2 elimination (ΔVCO_2) and $\Delta P_{ET}CO_2$, in response to a brief change in effective ventilation are used to measure cardiac output.[33] Two sets of measurements are obtained either by changing minute ventilation or by adding dead space by using a commercial system [NICO system (Novametrix Medical Systems, Wallingford, Connecticut, USA) was such a commercially available system]. Lack of current availability of any commercial system and paucity of new clinical publications about this method show that this method did not reach mainstream. Based on the theme of differential CO_2 Fick method, in recent years, capnotracking and capnodynamics have been developed as ways to measure pulmonary blood flow, in effect reflecting CO.[34,35] Both of these methods involve automated change in ventilation to generate the data for differential Fick equation. However, they are yet to reach a level of clinical validity enough to be accepted widely.

APPLICATION OF HEMODYNAMIC DATA

Noninvasive Cardiac Catheterization

Cardiac catheterization, right and left heart, provides precise cardiac chamber pressures and opportunity to measure CO. Using most commonly used noninvasive or minimally-invasive hemodynamic monitoring tools, data can be gathered to reflect the cardiac chamber pressures and CO. These data in turn can be used to obtain derived indices that help to categorize shock states as well as tissue blood flow and oxygen delivery. This concept is presented in **Table 5** and **Box 7**.

Categorization of Shock State

An important function of day-to-day ICU practice is early recognition of shock and correct categorization of shock. Following a simple checklist including clinical data (history and physical examination findings) and laboratory data (e.g., renal function, serum lactate, and measured and derived hemodynamic indices), correct categorization of shock can be made. A simple framework for approaching shock is shown in **(Box 8)**. It is stressed that all relevant data should be collected first before reaching a conclusion about the etiology of hemodynamic failure. Omission of collecting important data and premature conclusions about etiology of shock can lead to misclassification of shock and disastrous consequences.[31] Similarly, suboptimal management of

TABLE 5: Noninvasive/minimally-invasive cardiac catheterization.

Hemodynamic parameter measured by cardiac catheterization	Alternative (Noninvasive/minimally invasive)	Limitation	Comments
RA pressure	From ultrasound, IVC size and size variation with sniff maneuver by the patient	• Inadequate view • Increased IAP, a source of error • No widely accepted formulation in non-ventilated patients	Semi-quantitative measurement (low/normal/elevated) (see **Box 7**)
Central venous pressure (CVP)/RA pressure	Central venous line (CVL) waveform/CVP	Needs CVL	• RAPmean best estimate of right ventricular filling pressure • Almost identical to RAP, measured through PAC if CVL positioning is satisfactory
RV systolic pressure (RVSP)	From TR jet velocity measured by Doppler echocardiography	TR jet may be insufficient even when RV pressure is significantly elevated	
RV diastolic pressure	RAPmean/a wave closest approximation of end-diastolic pressure	CVL needed	
PA systolic pressure	≈ RVSP	Lack of adequate TR jet	In absence of pulmonic valve stenosis, RV systolic pressure matches PA systolic pressure
PA diastolic pressure	Calculated from PR jet velocity and RAP **(Box 2)**	Measurable PR jet may not be present	PA diastolic pressure can be used as a proxy for PAOP
Left atrial pressure/PAWP (mean) (see **Box 7**)	• Early diastolic mitral inflow velocity (E) and early relaxation velocity of mitral annular tissue (e') and quotient (E/e' ratio) of these 2 values a widely studied parameter • Normal E/e' does not rule out high LAP • E/e' > 15 (calculated using lateral mitral annular velocity) has high specificity in identifying a high LAP[55-57] • Lateral E/e' of < 8 has shown good diagnostic accuracy to predict PAWP < 18 mm Hg[58]	Cannot be used with mitral annular calcification or mitral valve stenosis	• Semi-quantitative measurement (normal/indeterminate/elevated) • In critically ill patients with hypoxic respiratory failure and RV dysfunction, the cumulative hemodynamic load of RV is best represented by mean LAP • In any hemodynamic measurement, use of a single parameter should be avoided • E/e' should be used along with other data[59,60]
LV systolic pressure	From ABP		In absence of aortic stenosis, LV systolic pressure closely approximates SBP
CO	• VTI at LVOT/RVOT by transthoracic echocardiography • PWA-based techniques	• Not adequate view and/or good Doppler alignment in all patients • Needs arterial line and good arterial waveform	Relative merits and demerits discussed under CO section
Mixed venous oxygen saturation (SVO_2)	Central venous catheter-derived oxygen saturation ($ScVO_2$)	Not identical as venous return from lower body not accounted for	In shock states, SVO_2 is lower than $ScVO_2$ as higher desaturation occurs in splanchnic circulation
CI	CO/BSA		
PVR	(MPAP – LAP)/CO	All data may not be available in each patient to calculate PVR	• Expressed in Wood units • To express in dynes/sec/cm^{-5}, Wood unit value is multiplied by 80

Continued

Continued

Hemodynamic parameter measured by cardiac catheterization	Alternative (Noninvasive/minimally invasive)	Limitation	Comments
SVR	(MAP – RAP)/CO		To express in dynes/sec/cm^{-5}, Wood unit value is multiplied by 80
Tissue oxygen delivery (DO_2)	CO × CaO_2		CaO_2 (mL/L) = [SaO_2 × Hb (g/L) × 1.37] + [PaO_2 (mm Hg) × 0.003]

(ABP: invasive blood pressure; BSA: body surface area; CI: cardiac index; CO: cardiac output; CaO_2: oxygen content of arterial blood; IAP: intra-abdominal pressure; IVC: inferior vena cava; LV: left ventricle; LAP: left atrial pressure; LVOT: left ventricular outflow tract; MPAP: mean pulmonary arterial pressure; PA; pulmonary artery; PR: pulmonary resistance; PAC: pulmonary artery catheter; PVR: pulmonary vascular resistance; PWA: pulse wave analysis; PAOP: pulmonary artery occlusion pressure; PAWP: pulmonary artery wedge pressure; RA: right atrium; RAP: right atrial pressure; RV: right ventricle; RVOT: right ventricular outflow tract; RVSP: right ventricular systolic pressure; SBP: systolic blood pressure; SVR: systemic vascular resistance; TR: tricuspid regurgitation; VTI: velocity–time integral)

BOX 7 Calculation and right atrial and left atrial pressure from echocardiography.[61]

- *Right atrial pressure (RAP):*
  - IVC size ≤ 2.1 cm; collapses >50% during sniff = RAP 0–5 mm Hg
  - IVC size > 2.1 cm; collapses >50% during sniff = RAP 5–10 mm Hg
  - IVC size > 2.1; collapses < 50% during sniff = RAP 10–20 mm Hg
- *Left atrial pressure (LAP):*
  - Normal E/e′ does not rule out high LAP
  - Lateral E/e′ >15 has high specificity in identifying a high LAP[55-57]
  - Lateral E/e′ of <8 has shown good diagnostic accuracy to predict PAOP <18 mm Hg[58]

(E/e′: early diastolic mitral inflow velocity/early relaxation velocity of mitral annular tissue; IVC: inferior vena cava; PAOP: pulmonary artery occlusion pressure)

shock can lead to very poor outcomes **(Figs. 21A and B)**. Two illustrative cases show the subtlety and thoroughness that are needed for diagnosis of etiology of shock **(Case Studies 1 and 2)**.

Preload Assessment/Assessment of Volume Responsiveness

Preload assessment is an issue that intensivists encounter every day and there is no parameter that performs well in all patient groups and under all circumstances. When there is a question of judging preload sensitivity, an intensivist is left with three potential approaches:

1. Blind fluid challenge to see whether hemodynamic parameters improve or not.
2. *To use traditional pressure-based approach*: CVP-, PAWP-, PAC-derived indices.

BOX 8 A conceptual framework for diagnosis and management of shock.

- *Shock is due to:*
  - Inadequate cardiac output
  - Maldistribution of cardiac output [~abnormal systemic vascular resistance (SVR)]
- *Major categories of shock:[62]*
  - Hypovolemic
  - Cardiogenic:
    - Myocardial failure
    - Valvular pathology
  - Obstructive:
    - Cardiac tamponade
    - Tension pneumothorax
    - Pulmonary embolism
    - Aortic stenosis
    - Distributive
    - Sepsis
    - Neurogenic
    - Anaphylaxis
  - Others:
    - Adrenal crisis
- *In physiological terms, any hemodynamic assessment should lead to three simple questions:*
  - i. Is it a preload problem?
  - ii. Is it a problem of cardiac contractility?
  - iii. Is it a problem of afterload?
- *Any hemodynamic assessment should lead to few simple alternatives:*
  - i. Whether to give fluid therapy
  - ii. Whether to give inotropic agents
  - iii. Whether to give vasopressors
  - iv. Any combination of the above choices
- *Etiology of shock:*
  - Hemodynamic data, interpreted in light of other clinical and laboratory investigations, often will provide a rapid diagnosis.

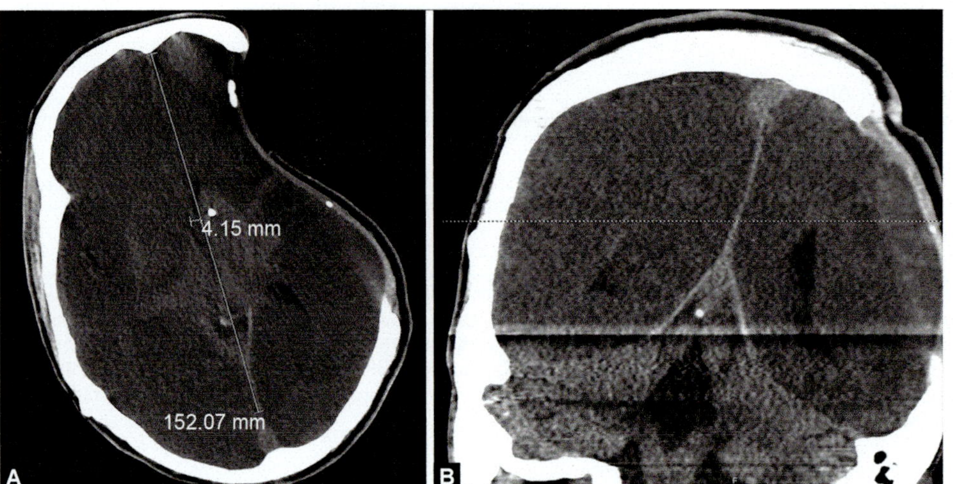

FIGS. 21A AND B: Consequence of shock. This middle-aged patient was independent and functional in his daily life in spite of previous hemicraniectomy. He was admitted with urinary tract infection, septic shock, and metabolic encephalopathy. Management during early hours included empiric use of multiple vasopressors without any assessment of volume status or cardiac output. His mental status deteriorated in first 24 hours, and he developed deep unresponsiveness, in spite of no sedation. CT head on day 3 of hospitalization showed global infarction from low-flow state.

CASES

CASE STUDY 1

A 61-year-old man presented with 2-day history of fatigue and dizziness. He had known history of diffuse large B-cell lymphoma and received a cycle of chemotherapy 3 weeks prior to presentation. He had previous episodes of acute pulmonary embolism and was on apixaban. He also had history of systolic heart failure with LV ejection fraction of 45% on echocardiography 3 months prior to this admission. Apart from fatigue, he reported experiencing fevers and chills at home. He had decreased oral intake for 2 days prior to presentation, and had nausea, 2 episodes of vomiting without hematemesis, and 2 episodes of dark maroon/black stools over 24 hours. There was no history of chest pain, dyspnea, and any localized symptoms of infection. At admission, he was found to have hypotension and elevated lactate. Additional workup showed severe anemia (hemoglobin 4 gm% at admission, 8.4 gm% 1 week ago) and severe thrombocytopenia (platelet count <10,000/mL, 128,000/mL 1 week ago). Serum troponin I was 1.09 ng/mL (normal <0.04 ng/mL). Ultrasound showed IVC diameter of 2.4 cm and a drop in LV systolic function by visual assessment and a drop in CO, as measured by Doppler echocardiography, compared to the previous echo. A diagnosis of cardiogenic shock was therefore made. It was thought that severe anemia developed over a short period of time caused diffuse ischemic injury to the heart leading to a drop in LV contractility and CO. He showed rapid clinical improvement with blood transfusion with careful monitoring to avoid volume overload and decompensation of heart failure. This case shows the importance of complete initial data gathering and correct categorization of shock. Instead of strong evidence of gastrointestinal (GI) bleeding, the patient had cardiogenic shock and not hypovolemic shock.

CASE STUDY 2

A 61-year-old woman with known end-stage renal disease (ESRD) was admitted with acute cholecystitis, sepsis, and septic shock. Along with initial volume resuscitation and antibiotics, she required vasopressor support for initial stabilization of her BP. Given hemodynamic instability and sepsis, she was started on continuous renal replacement therapy (CRRT). On day 3, an increasing vasopressor requirement was noted over few hours. A worsening of sepsis was suspected and a complete shock assessment was undertaken. Her ABP was 127/47 (MAP was 75) and heart rate was 80 beats/minute during echocardiographic examination. Her height was 162 cm, weight 56 kg, and body surface area (BSA) was 1.6 kg/m.^{2}

Bedside ECG showed: Left ventricular hypertrophy with small LV cavity, diastolic dysfunction with normal left-sided filling pressure, and small IVC. Quantitative measurements were as follows:

- Mitral valve (MV) inflow velocity (cm/sec): E 60, A 93
- MV lateral annulus e' (cm/sec): 6.38

- MV medial annulus e′ (cm/sec): 6.38
- LVOT VTI (cm): 23.7
- SV = 50 mL
- CO = 4 L/minute
- Estimated RAP 0–5 mm Hg
- Calculated SVR = 1,400 dynes/s/cm^5

(e′ = early relaxation velocity of mitral annular tissue)

The parameters indicated clear evidence of hypovolemia with low-to-normal filling pressure on both sides of heart. Low CO and high normal SVR also supported a diagnosis of hypovolemia. Persistent unrecognized hypovolemia was thought more likely as the cause for worsening vasopressor requirement than vasodilatory shock. Additional volume resuscitation was given as small aliquots of fluid boluses. CRRT fluid balance goal was also adjusted. Vasopressors could be weaned off over next several hours.

3. To determine which patients are preload sensitive and give volume to them.
   - Nonultrasound-based methods, e.g., SV by PWA
   - Ultrasound/echocardiography-based methods

If a blind fluid challenge is given, it is important to judge the margin of safety, i.e., to assess the potential of serious harm if the clinical judgment about the requirement of volume is wrong. As an example, a fluid challenge of 1L may be safe in a patient with documented normal right heart function who is on ventilator with low fraction of inspired oxygen (FIO_2) requirement, while the same volume challenge may be detrimental with a patient with known pulmonary hypertension and RV dysfunction. Both echocardiography and lung ultrasound, along with routine physiological data can be used to judge this margin of safety. The goal is to rule out with reasonable certainty, RV dysfunction, elevation of LV filling pressure, and identification of pulmonary edema.

Various parameters used in judging volume responsiveness can be divided into static and dynamic parameters and summarized in **Table 6**. Dynamic parameters in turn fall under two broad categories, those using passive leg raising (PLR), thereby proving an internal and reversible fluid challenge of ~300 mL, and the parameters using cardiorespiratory interactions during mechanical ventilation. It is imperative for an intensivist to be familiar with the parameters and understand the limitation(s) of these parameters. Few general points should be noted:

- Many studies have been done on small number of patients. Definition and method of testing of volume responsiveness have not always been uniform either. For example, while volume loading and measurement for increase in CO has been used in large number of studies, a large study, comparing respiratory variations of different parameters [e.g., inferior vena cava (IVC) size variation, superior vena cava (SVC) size variation, and peak aortic velocity variation] used PLR-induced change in Vpeak as measure of volume responsiveness.[36]
- A large study of comparison of different echocardiographic parameters has shown lower diagnostic accuracies than pioneer studies of different parameters.[36]
- Various cutoff values mentioned in different studies should not be interpreted as dichotomous decision points in patient management. Cutoff points quoted in **Table 6** are from initial/early reports of the corresponding technique.
- PLR can be applied in a wide range of patients with or without spontaneous breathing and even in presence of cardiac arrhythmias. However, its implementation at bedside is not always easy from a practical standpoint.
- All clinical and ancillary data should be woven into the decision.
- Early, frequent, and repeated assessment is necessary.
- Realistically, not every parameter is obtainable in every patient.

Dynamic indices should play a greater role in uncertain clinical scenarios. If one wants to train his/her team in a handful of dynamic parameters, variation in aortic VTI or Vpeak with PLR or with respiratory cycle are suggested as suitable ones **(Figs. 22A and B)**. These parameters have strong performance characteristics, supported by multiple studies, systemic review and meta-analysis of multiple studies.[37,38] A step-by-step guide to performing PLR is described by Monnet et al.[39] and shown in **Figure 23.** A pragmatic approach to assessment of volume responsiveness is shown in **Flowchart 1**.

When the volume status cannot be assessed with reasonable certainty from available data, the authors suggest that any intervention or manipulation of intravascular volumes should be in small increments with close clinical monitoring of the effects on end-organ function and adverse effects.

TABLE 6: Static and dynamic indices of intravenous fluid/volume responsiveness/preload sensitivity.[a,b,c]

Parameter	Significant change	Advantage	Limitation	Other comments	References
Postural drop in blood pressure	Decrease in SBP of >20 mm Hg or decrease in DBP >10 mm Hg when moving from recumbency to standing	Simple bedside test of significant hypovolemia	Patient may be too sick to properly change posture	Straightforward application in acute bleeding	
CVP	No cutoff value reliably predicts volume responsiveness	Widely available	Poor correlation with volume responsiveness	Selective role in heart-failure management	63
PAWP	PAWP <12 mm Hg does not have enough predictive power for fluid responsiveness		Available and applicable only in selected patients during heart-failure management	• Trend may be more important than single reading • Not for use in general ICU patients for shock management	64
End-systolic LV cavity obliteration (hyperdynamic LV)		Easy to learn and reliable			
Inferior vena cava (IVC) size	• <1 cm = Fluid responsive • >2.5 = No role of volume loading	Noninvasive and easy to learn	Multiple sources of technical error	A wide "grey zone" where IVC size alone is not helpful	
IVC size changes with respiration (Two methods described)	• IVC diameter (DIVC) variation (ΔD_{ivc}) of ≥ 12% • ΔD_{ivc} calculated as the difference between the maximum and the minimum DIVC value, expressed as a percentage of the two values • IVC "distensibility index (dIVC)" of ≥18% [IVC diameter (D) measured at end-expiration (Dmin) and at end-inspiration (Dmax) (dIVC) was calculated as the ratio of (Dmax – Dmin)/Dmin, and was expressed as a percentage	Easily obtained in most patients	• Requires patient intubated and passive with ventilator • Result dependent on TV/PEEP • Invalidated by any process that influences IVC dynamics (elevated IAP, adjacent compression, and preexisting right heart disease) • Subject to translational artifact, off-axis artifact, and interobserver and intraobserver variability	• False negatives in case of low TV, low lung compliance • Small number of patients in initial studies	65,66
SVC collapsibility (Calculated as maximum diameter on expiration – minimum diameter on inspiration)/maximum diameter on expiration	SVC collapsibility of ≥ 36%		• Needs TEE • Needs patients passive on ventilator with stable cardiac rhythm • Needs relatively high TV		67
Change in Doppler indices of CO: SV, VTI, and peak aortic flow velocity (Vpeak) *with respiratory cycle*	Respiratory variation of Vpeak of ≥12% (Calculated as the difference between maximum and minimum of Vpeak values during respiratory cycle, divided by the mean of the two values, expressed as a percentage)	Noninvasive	• Requires passive ventilator interaction • Regular rhythm • TV, PEEP, and vasopressor-sensitive • Severe RV failure may invalidate result • Cardiac translation of Doppler angle may induce error		36,68,69

Continued

Continued

Parameter	Significant change	Advantage	Limitation	Other comments	References
Pulse pressure (PP) variation *with respiratory cycle*	Respiratory changes in pulse pressure (ΔPP) calculated as the difference between maximum and minimum PP divided by the mean of the two values and expressed as a percentage. ΔPP >13% allowed discrimination between responders and nonresponders	Simple to obtain through an arterial line tracing	Same limitations as with Doppler indices measured during respiratory cycle TV dependent		70,71
Change in Doppler indices of CO: SV, VTI, and peak aortic flow velocity (Vpeak) with *passive leg raising (PLR)*	• SV or any parameter linearly changing with SV (e.g., VTI and Vpeak) can be studied • Increase of CO or SV ≥12% • Vpeak change of ≥10%	• Can be used regardless of breathing activity, cardiac rhythm, TV, and lung compliance • *Intuitively attractive:* Give volume and observe the effect on SV directly • Excellent performance characteristics	• Takes time • Needs efficient team effort • *Drawbacks of Doppler:* Angle dependence and translational artifact	• Effect of intra-abdominal pressure should be <16 mm Hg • Effect of PLR peaks in the minute after starting the test • Real-time measurement is best	36,37, 72-76
Pulse pressure variation *with PLR*	≥12% increase in PP		Change in PP imperfectly reflects change in CO	Less reliable than direct measurement of CO	38,74
End-tidal CO_2 monitoring *with PLR*	≥5%	Easy to apply	Only in intubated patients who are passive on ventilator		76,77
Lung ultrasonography	A-line pattern associated with normal PAWP	Easy to learn and perform	B-line pattern does not automatically indicate high PAWP	Helps to judge margin of safety for volume challenge when assessment of volume responsiveness is inconclusive	78,79
Perfusion index calculated from pulse oximetry plethysmography signals *with respiratory cycle and PLR*	• >14% with respiration and • ≥9% with PLR	Noninvasive and widely available		More data needed	80,81

[a] List of tests for preload sensitivity is neither complete nor exhaustive. Included are the tests most practical and familiar.
[b] Cutoff values mentioned are from original/pioneering studies. Later studies and meta-analyses reported some differences.
[c] No cutoff value should be used as dichotomous decision-making point and all clinical and laboratory data should be taken into consideration.

(CO: cardiac output; CVP: central venous pressure; DBP: diastolic blood pressure; ICU: intensive care unit; IV: intravenous; IAP: intra-abdominal pressure; LV: left ventricle; PAWP: pulmonary artery wedge pressure; SBP: systolic blood pressure; SVC: superior vena cava; SV: stroke volume; TEE: transesophageal echocardiography; TV: tidal volume; PEEP: positive end-expiratory pressure; VTI: velocity–time integral)

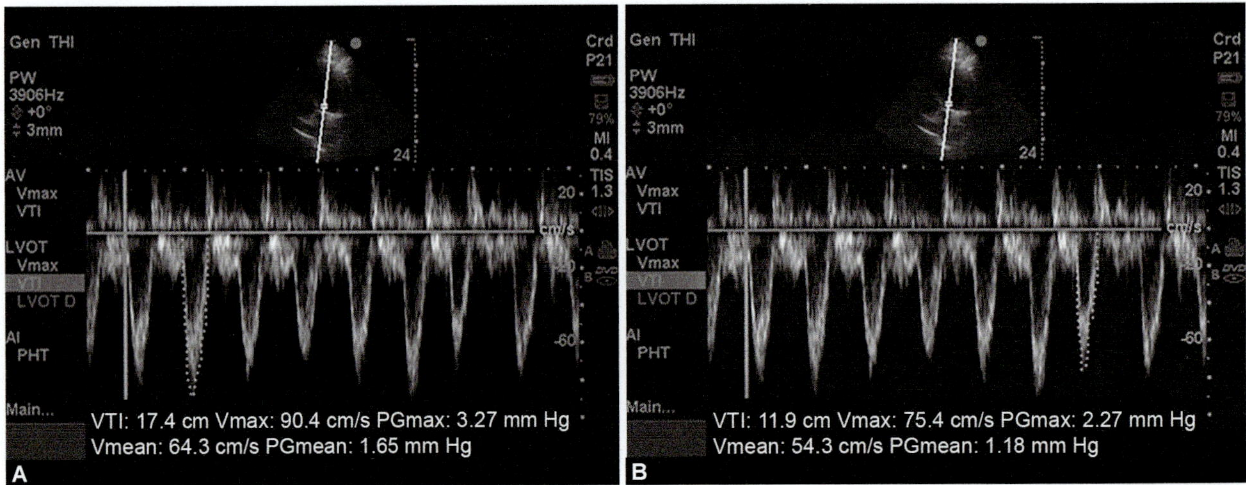

FIGS. 22A AND B: Respiratory variation of velocity–time integral (VTI) and Vpeak. (A) VTI is 17.4 cm and Vpeak is 90.4 cm/sec. (B) VTI is 11.9 cm and Vpeak is 75.4 cm/sec. VTI and Vpeak show >30% and 15% change, respectively with respiration, suggesting strong volume responsiveness. Careful volume administration in this somnolent stroke patient led to improvement in hemodynamic parameters and level of consciousness.

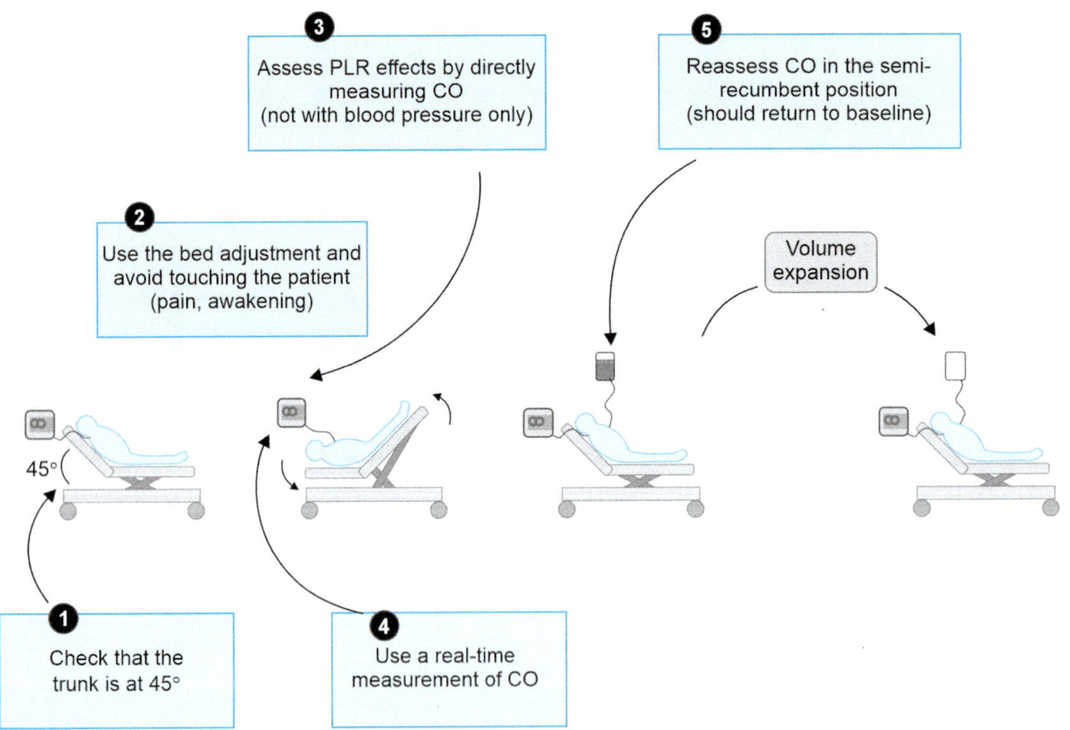

FIG. 23: Correct way of performing passive leg raising (PLR).

(CO: cardiac output)

Source: Reproduced from Monnet et al. (2015).

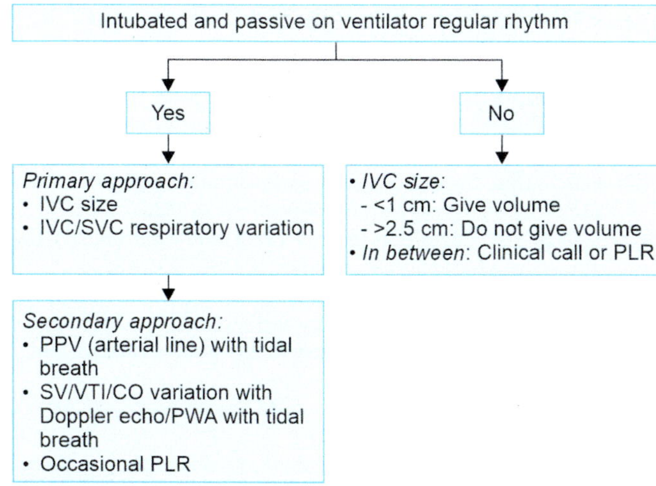

FLOWCHART 1: A suggested approach to assessment of volume responsiveness.

(CO: cardiac output; IVC: inferior vena cava; PLR: passive leg raising; PPV: pulse pressure variation; PWA: pulse wave analysis; SV: stroke volume; SVC: superior vena cava; VTI: velocity–time integral)

SUMMARY

Availability of myriad of tools for hemodynamic monitoring makes this a difficult area to master. A sound understanding of cardiorespiratory physiology and cardiopulmonary interaction during mechanical ventilation is an essential element of good clinical practice in this area. Given rapid change in technology, proprietary nature, and limited geographic spread of many technologies, especially for CO monitoring, decisions about adoption of any particular technology in an ICU should be made cautiously. In this chapter, we have stressed on elements that help in understanding physiologic principles and have wide applicability. An emphasis on bedside hemodynamic pressure monitoring and echocardiography is deliberate given their wide availability, nondependence on proprietary expensive technology, easy implementation, and/or noninvasive nature.

REFERENCES

1. Ait-Oufella H, Lemoinne S, Boelle PY, et al. Mottling score predicts survival in septic shock. Intensive Care Med. 2011;37(5):801-7.
2. Ait-Oufella H, Bige N, Boelle PY, et al. Capillary refill time exploration during septic shock. Intensive Care Medicine. 2014;40(7):958-64.
3. Brunauer A, Koköfer A, Bataar O, et al. Changes in peripheral perfusion relate to visceral organ perfusion in early septic shock: A pilot study. J Crit Care. 2016;35:105-9.
4. Evans L, Rhodes A, Alhazzani W, et al. Surviving sepsis campaign: International guidelines for management of sepsis and septic shock 2021. Intensive Care Medi. 2021;47(11):1181-247.
5. Principles and Hazards of Monitoring Equipments. In: Daily EK, Schroeder JS (Eds). Techniques in Bedside Hemodynamic Monitoring. Missouri: United States: CV Mosby Company; 1985.
6. Kleinman B, Powell S, Kumar P, et al. The fast flush test measures the dynamic response of the entire blood pressure monitoring system. Anesthesiology. 1992;77(6):1215-20.
7. Ward M, Langton JA. Blood pressure measurement. BJA Educ. 2007;7(4):122-6.
8. Geddes LA. Counterpressure: The concept that made the indirect measurement of blood pressure possible. IEEE Eng Med Biol Mag. 1998;17(6):85-7.
9. Ramsey M 3rd. Blood pressure monitoring: Automated oscillometric devices. J Clin Monit. 1991;7(1):56-67.
10. Lewis PS; British and Irish Hypertension Society's Blood Pressure Measurement Working Party. Oscillometric measurement of blood pressure: A simplified explanation. A technical note on behalf of the British and Irish Hypertension Society. J Hum Hypertens. 2019;33(5):349-51.
11. Pickering TG, Hall JE, Appel LJ, et al. Recommendations for blood pressure measurement in humans and experimental animals: Part 1: Blood pressure measurement in humans: A statement for professionals from the Subcommittee of Professional and Public Education of the American Heart Association Council on High Blood Pressure Research. Circulation. 2005;111(5):697-716.
12. Gravlee GP, Brockschmidt JK. Accuracy of four indirect methods of blood pressure measurement, with hemodynamic correlations. J Clin Monit. 1990;6(4):284-98.
13. Chatterjee K. The Swan-Ganz catheters: Past, present, and future. A viewpoint. Circulation. 2009;119(1):147-52.
14. Harvey S, Harrison DA, Singer M, et al. Assessment of the clinical effectiveness of pulmonary artery catheters in management of patients in intensive care (PAC-Man): A randomised controlled trial. Lancet. 2005;366(9484):472-7.
15. Sandham JD, Hull RD, Brant RF, et al. A randomized, controlled trial of the use of pulmonary-artery catheters in high-risk surgical patients. N Engl J Med. 2003;348(1):5-14.
16. National Heart, Lung, and Blood Institute Acute Respiratory Distress Syndrome (ARDS) Clinical Trials Network; Wheeler AP, Bernard GR, Thompson BT, et al. Pulmonary-artery versus central venous catheter to guide treatment of acute lung injury. N Eng J Med. 2006;354(21):2213-24.
17. National Heart, Lung, and Blood Institute Acute Respiratory Distress Syndrome (ARDS) Clinical Trials Network; Wiedemann HP, Wheeler AP, Bernard GR, et al. Comparison of two fluid-management strategies in acute lung injury. N Eng J Med. 2006;354(24):2564-75.
18. Garan AR, Kanwar M, Thayer KL, et al. Complete hemodynamic profiling with pulmonary artery catheters in cardiogenic shock is associated with lower in-hospital mortality. JACC Heart Fail. 2020;8(11):903-13.
19. Ranka S, Mastoris I, Kapur NK, et al. Right heart catheterization in cardiogenic shock is associated with improved outcomes: Insights from the nationwide readmissions database. J Am Heart Assoc. 2021;10(17):e019843.
20. McGlothlin DP, Granton J, Klepetko W, et al. ISHLT consensus statement: Perioperative management of patients with

pulmonary hypertension and right heart failure undergoing surgery. J Heart Lung Transplant. 2022;41(9):1135-94.
21. Soto FJ, Kleczka JF. Cardiopulmonary hemodynamics in pulmonary hypertension: Pressure tracings, waveforms, and more. Advances in Pulmonary Hypertension. 2008;7(4):386-93.
22. Rosenkranz S, Preston IR. Right heart catheterisation: Best practice and pitfalls in pulmonary hypertension. Eur Respir Rev. 2015;24(138):642-52.
23. Houston BA, Tedford RJ. What we talk about when we talk about the wedge pressure. Circ Heart Fail. 2017;10(9):e004450.
24. Tampakakis E, Tedford RJ. Balancing the positives and negatives of the diastolic pulmonary gradient. Eur J Heart Fail. 2017;19(1):98-100.
25. Wright SP, Moayedi Y, Foroutan F, et al. Diastolic pressure difference to classify pulmonary hypertension in the assessment of heart transplant candidates. Circ Heart Fail. 2017;10(9): e004077.
26. Bootsma IT, Boerma EC, de Lange F, et al. The contemporary pulmonary artery catheter. Part 1: Placement and waveform analysis. J Clinical Monit Comput. 2022;36(1):5-15.
27. West JB, Dollery CT, Naimark A. Distribution of blood flow in isolated lung; relation to vascular and alveolar pressures. J Appl Physiol. 1964;19:713-24.
28. Boerboom LE, Kinney TE, Olinger GN, et al. Validity of cardiac output measurement by the thermodilution method in the presence of acute tricuspid regurgitation. J Thorac Cardiovasc Surg. 1993;106(4):636-42.
29. Reuter DA, Huang C, Edrich T, et al. Cardiac output monitoring using indicator-dilution techniques: Basics, limits, and perspectives. Anesth Analg. 2010;110(3):799-811.
30. Heerdt PM, Blessios GA, Beach ML, et al. Flow dependency of error in thermodilution measurement of cardiac output during acute tricuspid regurgitation. J Cardiothorac Vasc Anesth. 2001;15(2):183-7.
31. Sarkar PK, Patel PR. A 53-year-old Man with Acute Liver Failure. Chest. 2020;157(2):e53-7.
32. Haryadi DG, Orr JA, Kuck K, et al. Partial CO_2 rebreathing indirect Fick technique for non-invasive measurement of cardiac output. J Clin Monit Comput. 2000;16(5-6):361-74.
33. Gedeon A, Forslund L, Hedenstierna G, et al. A new method for noninvasive bedside determination of pulmonary blood flow. Med Biol Eng Comput. 1980;18(4):411-8.
34. Sigmundsson TS, Öhman T, Hallbäck M, et al. Performance of a capnodynamic method estimating effective pulmonary blood flow during transient and sustained hypercapnia. J Clin Monit Comput. 2018;32(2):311-9.
35. Karlsson J, Winberg P, Scarr B, et al. Validation of capnodynamic determination of cardiac output by measuring effective pulmonary blood flow: A study in anaesthetised children and piglets. Br J Anaesth. 2018;121(3):550-8.
36. Vignon P, Repessé X, Bégot E, et al. Comparison of echocardiographic indices used to predict fluid responsiveness in ventilated patients. Am J Respir Crit Care Med. 2017;195(8): 1022-32.
37. Cherpanath TG, Hirsch A, Geerts BF, et al. Predicting fluid responsiveness by passive leg raising: A systematic review and meta-analysis of 23 clinical trials. Crit Care Med. 2016;44(5): 981-91.
38. Monnet X, Marik P, Teboul JL. Passive leg raising for predicting fluid responsiveness: A systematic review and meta-analysis. Intensive Care Med. 2016;42(12):1935-47.
39. Monnet X, Teboul JL. Passive leg raising: Five rules, not a drop of fluid! Crit Care. 2015;19(1):18.
40. Eather KF, Peterson LH, Dripps RD. Studies of the circulation of anesthetized patients by a new method for recording arterial pressure and pressure pulse contours. Anesthesiology. 1949;10(2):125-32.
41. Fick A. Uber die messung des Blutquantums in den Hertzvent rikeln. Sitzber Physik Med Ges Wurzburg. 1870:36.
42. Stewart GN. Researches on the circulation time and on the influences which affect it. J Physiol. 1897;22(3):159-83.
43. Hamilton WF, Moore JW, Kinsman JM, et al. Simultaneous determination of the pulmonary and systemic circulation times in man and of a figure related to the cardiac output. Am J Physiol. 1928;84(2):338-44.
44. Hamilton WF, Moore JW, Kinsman JM. Studies on the circulation. Am J Physiol. 1932;99(3):534-51.
45. Kinsman JM, Moore JW, Hamilton WF. Studies on the circulation. Am J Physiol. 1929;89(2):322-330.
46. Fegler G. Measurement of cardiac output in anaesthetized animals by a thermodilution method. Q J Exp Physiol Cogn Med Sci. 1954;39(3):153-164.
47. Khalil HH. Determination of cardiac output in man by a new method based on thermodilution. Lancet. 1963;1(7295):1352-4.
48. Kubicek WG, Karnegis JN, Patterson RP, et al. Development and evaluation of an impedance cardiac output system. Aerospace Med. 1966;37(12):1208-12.
49. Swan HJ, Ganz W, Forrester J, et al. Catheterization of the heart in man with use of a flow-directed balloon-tipped catheter. New Engl J Med. 1970;283(9):447-51.
50. Ganz W, Donoso R, Marcus HS. A new technique for measurement of cardiac output by thermodilution in man. Am J Cardiol. 1971;27(4):392-6.
51. Yelderman M. Continuous measurement of cardiac output with the use of stochastic system identification techniques. J Clin Monit. 1990;6(4):322-32.
52. Mihm FG, Gettinger A, Hanson CW 3rd, et al. A multicenter evaluation of a new continuous cardiac output pulmonary artery catheter system. Critical Care Med. 1998;26(8):1346-50.
53. Linton RA, Band DM, Haire KM. A new method of measuring cardiac output in man using lithium dilution. Br J Anaesth. 1993;71(2):262-6.
54. Weyland A, Buhre W, Hoeft A, et al. Application of a transpulmonary double indicator dilution method for postoperative assessment of cardiac index, pulmonary vascular resistance index, and extravascular lung water in children undergoing total cavopulmonary anastomosis: Preliminary results in six patients. J Cardiothorac Vasc Anesth. 1994;8(6):636-41.
55. Lancellotti P, Galderisi M, Edvardsen T, et al. Echo-Doppler estimation of left ventricular filling pressure: Results of the multicentre EACVI Euro-Filling study. Eur Heart J Cardiovasc Imaging. 2017;18(9):961-8.
56. Nagueh SF, Smiseth OA, Appleton CP, et al. Recommendations for the evaluation of left ventricular diastolic function by echocardiography: An update from the American Society of Echocardiography and the European Association of Cardiovascular Imaging. J Am Soc Echocardiogr. 2016;29(4): 277-314.
57. Obokata M, Borlaug BA. The strengths and limitations of E/e′ in heart failure with preserved ejection fraction. Eur J Heart Fail. 2018;20(9):1312-4.

58. Vignon P, AitHssain A, Francois B, et al. Echocardiographic assessment of pulmonary artery occlusion pressure in ventilated patients: A transoesophageal study. Crit Care. 2008;12(1):R18.
59. Bowcock EM, McLean A. Bedside assessment of left atrial pressure in critical care: A multifaceted gem. Crit Care. 2022; 26(1):247.
60. Nauta JF, Hummel YM, van der Meer P, et al. Correlation with invasive left ventricular filling pressures and prognostic relevance of the echocardiographic diastolic parameters used in the 2016 ESC heart failure guidelines and in the 2016 ASE/EACVI recommendations: A systematic review in patients with heart failure with preserved ejection fraction. Eur J Heart Fail. 2018;20(9):1303-11.
61. Porter TR, Shillcutt SK, Adams MS, et al. Guidelines for the use of echocardiography as a monitor for therapeutic intervention in adults: A report from the American Society of Echocardiography. J Am Soc Echocardiogr. 2015;28(1):40-56.
62. Weil MH, Shubin H. Proposed reclassification of shock states with special reference to distributive defects. In: Hinshaw LB, Cox BG (Eds). The Fundamental Mechanisms of Shock: Proceedings of a Symposium Held in Oklahoma City, Oklahoma, October 1–2, 1971. Boston, MA: Springer US; 1972. pp. 13-23.
63. Marik PE, Cavallazzi R. Does the central venous pressure predict fluid responsiveness? An updated meta-analysis and a plea for some common sense. Critical Care Med. 2013;41(7):1774-81.
64. Osman D, Ridel C, Ray P, et al. Cardiac filling pressures are not appropriate to predict hemodynamic response to volume challenge. Critical Care Med. 2007;35(1):64-8.
65. Barbier C, Loubières Y, Schmit C, et al. Respiratory changes in inferior vena cava diameter are helpful in predicting fluid responsiveness in ventilated septic patients. Intensive Care Med. 2004;30(9):1740-6.
66. Feissel M, Michard F, Faller JP, et al. The respiratory variation in inferior vena cava diameter as a guide to fluid therapy. Intensive Care Med. 2004;30(9):1834-7.
67. Vieillard-Baron A, Chergui K, Rabiller A, et al. Superior vena caval collapsibility as a gauge of volume status in ventilated septic patients. Intensive Care Med. 2004;30(9):1734-9.
68. Slama M, Masson H, Teboul JL, et al. Respiratory variations of aortic VTI: A new index of hypovolemia and fluid responsiveness. Am J Physiol Heart Circ Physiol. 2002;283(4):H1729-33.
69. Feissel M, Michard F, Mangin I, et al. Respiratory changes in aortic blood velocity as an indicator of fluid responsiveness in ventilated patients with septic shock. Chest. 2001;119(3): 867-73.
70. Michard F, Boussat S, Chemla D, et al. Relation between respiratory changes in arterial pulse pressure and fluid responsiveness in septic patients with acute circulatory failure. Am J Respir Crit Care Med. 2000;162(1):134-8.
71. De Backer D, Heenen S, Piagnerelli M, et al. Pulse pressure variations to predict fluid responsiveness: Influence of tidal volume. Intensive Care Med. 2005;31(4):517-23.
72. Maizel J, Airapetian N, Lorne E, et al. Diagnosis of central hypovolemia by using passive leg raising. Intensive Care Med. 2007;33(7):1133-8.
73. Lamia B, Ochagavia A, Monnet X, et al. Echocardiographic prediction of volume responsiveness in critically ill patients with spontaneously breathing activity. Intensive Care Med. 2007;33(7):1125-32.
74. Monnet X, Rienzo M, Osman D, et al. Passive leg raising predicts fluid responsiveness in the critically ill. Critical Care Med. 2006;34(5):1402-7.
75. Cavallaro F, Sandroni C, Marano C, et al. Diagnostic accuracy of passive leg raising for prediction of fluid responsiveness in adults: Systematic review and meta-analysis of clinical studies. Intensive Care Med. 2010;36(9):1475-83.
76. Monge García MI, Gil Cano A, Gracia Romero M, et al. Non-invasive assessment of fluid responsiveness by changes in partial end-tidal CO_2 pressure during a passive leg-raising maneuver. Ann Intensive Care. 2012;2:9.
77. Monnet X, Bataille A, Magalhaes E, et al. End-tidal carbon dioxide is better than arterial pressure for predicting volume responsiveness by the passive leg raising test. Intensive Care Med. 2013;39(1):93-100.
78. Lichtenstein DA, Mezière GA, Lagoueyte JF, et al. A-lines and B-lines: Lung ultrasound as a bedside tool for predicting pulmonary artery occlusion pressure in the critically ill. Chest. 2009;136(4):1014-20.
79. Volpicelli G, Skurzak S, Boero E, et al. Lung ultrasound predicts well extravascular lung water but is of limited usefulness in the prediction of wedge pressure. Anesthesiology. 2014;121(2): 320-7.
80. Cannesson M, Desebbe O, Rosamel P, et al. Pleth variability index to monitor the respiratory variations in the pulse oximeter plethysmographic waveform amplitude and predict fluid responsiveness in the operating theatre. Br J Anaesth. 2008; 101(2):200-6.
81. Beurton A, Teboul JL, Gavelli F, et al. The effects of passive leg raising may be detected by the plethysmographic oxygen saturation signal in critically ill patients. Crit Care. 2019;23(1):19.

CHAPTER 172

Right Heart Catheterization

Parmeet Saini, Vishal K Patel, Albina Guri, Anthony Saleh

INTRODUCTION

Warner Forssmann in 1929 introduced a catheter into his own heart and demonstrated that right heart catheterization is feasible in humans, although the catheter was advanced only into the right atrium. In 1956, Drs Cournand and Richards enhanced this catheter, which could be further advanced into the pulmonary arteries. Forssmann, Cournand, and Richards were honored with the Nobel Prize in Medicine for this invention.[1] After various improvements, Scheinman, Abbott, and Rapaport developed a flow-directed right heart catheter to measure right-sided cardiac pressures.[2] A year later in 1970, Swan and William Ganz enhanced the previous flow-directed catheter by adding a balloon flotation feature, giving rise to the currently known "Swan–Ganz catheters".[3] Further modification of these catheters enabled them to measure cardiac output by the thermodilution technique, to pace the right atrium and right ventricle, and to measure right-sided pressures including pulmonary capillary occlusion pressure.[4]

Initially used for hemodynamic monitoring in patients with acute myocardial infarction, pulmonary artery catheterization (PAC) rapidly grew in popularity and was used extensively in the management of critically ill patients with shock, further extended to peri- and postoperative hemodynamic monitoring in surgical and nonsurgical patients. Since then, PAC use has been the topic of controversial debate and focus of many trials in attempts to distinguish and refine appropriate clinical uses **(Box 1)**. It is now well established that while the catheter certainly offers significant theoretical advantages in the management of critically ill patients, there is no mortality benefit from this relatively invasive procedure. For this reason, routine use of PAC in critically ill patients is not recommended. There is a general consensus among different societies that PAC monitoring can provide valuable information in patients with pulmonary hypertension, cardiogenic shock (CS), patients on mechanical circulatory devices [ventricular assist devices (VADs), Impella, intra-aortic balloon pump, extracorporeal membrane oxygenation (ECMO)], and peri- and postoperative monitoring in heart, lung, and liver transplant patients. The catheter remains the gold standard for diagnosis and management of pulmonary hypertension.

BOX 1 Indications and contraindications of PAC.[5]

Indications

- *Diagnostic*:
  - Diagnosis of circulatory shock states
  - Differentiation of high versus low pressure pulmonary edema
  - Diagnosis of pulmonary hypertension
  - Diagnosis of valvular disease, intracardiac shunts, cardiac tamponade, constrictive pericarditis, and pulmonary embolus
  - Monitoring and management of complicated acute myocardial infarction
  - Assessing hemodynamic response to therapies
  - Management of multiorgan system failure and/or severe burns
  - Perioperative hemodynamic monitoring in cardiac surgery
  - Assessment of response to treatment in patients with pulmonary arterial hypertension
  - Preoperative assessment in heart or lung transplantation
  - Mechanical circulatory support devices
  - Preimplantation assessment of left ventricular assist devices
  - Postimplantation optimization after left ventricular assist device placement
- *Therapeutic*:
  - Aspiration of air emboli

Contraindications

- Tricuspid or pulmonary valve mechanical prosthesis
- Tricuspid or pulmonary valve endocarditis
- Right-sided intracardiac mass (thrombus and/or tumor)
- Preexisting left bundle branch block
- Coagulopathy
- Uncooperative patients
- Ongoing malignant arrhythmias

(PAC: pulmonary artery catheter)

SETUP

The pulmonary artery (PA) catheter is a multilumen (usually four to five lumens) catheter of 110 cm in length demarcated in 10 cm intervals **(Figs. 1A and B)**. It is constructed from polyvinylchloride and is pliable. The external diameters range from 5 to 8 Fr (1 Fr = 0.0335 mm). All catheters have a distal port, typically yellow, that connects to the catheter tip. Most catheters also have a proximal port, typically blue, that connects to a lumen 30 cm from the tip for central venous pressure monitoring, fluids, or drug administration. Larger catheters usually have an accessory infusion port, typically clear or white, that also terminates approximately 30 cm from the tip. The distal port or PA port has a balloon just proximal to it. When inflated, it guides the catheter from the right heart chambers into the PA and also protrudes beyond the catheter tip minimizing the chances of endocardial damage or arrhythmia.

Typically, the balloon is inflated with 1.5 cc of air; however, if a right-to-left intracardiac shunt or a pulmonary arteriovenous fistula is suspected, then the balloon should be inflated with filtered carbon dioxide to avoid rupture.[6] If carbon dioxide is used, periodic deflation and inflation are required as carbon dioxide diffuses through the latex balloon at a rate of 0.5 mL/min. Liquids should not be used for balloon inflation.

Approximately, 4 cm proximal to the balloon is the thermistor that is used to measure temperature changes utilized for the calculation of cardiac output. In the most commonly used quadruple-lumen catheter, additional ports are present at 19 and 30 cm from the tip. Also available, a five-lumen catheter has an additional port at 40 cm from the tip, which can be used for fluid or medication infusion. Some catheters are coated with heparin and others have connections for temporary ventricular pacing.

Pressure transducer: The conversion of intravascular pressures into an electrical signal is done by a catheter-tubing-transducer system. Transmission of pressures from the catheter to the display system is achieved via connecting it to a semirigid, noncompliant tubing filled with isotonic saline. This is then connected to a fluid-filled pressure transducer. This system accurately transmits intracardiac pressures to the transducer, causing small amounts of movement in the transducer membrane. This movement generates a proportional electric current that is amplified and transmitted to the monitor.

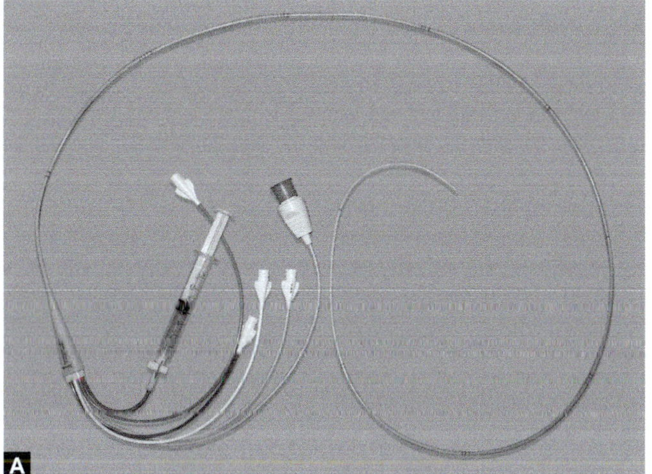

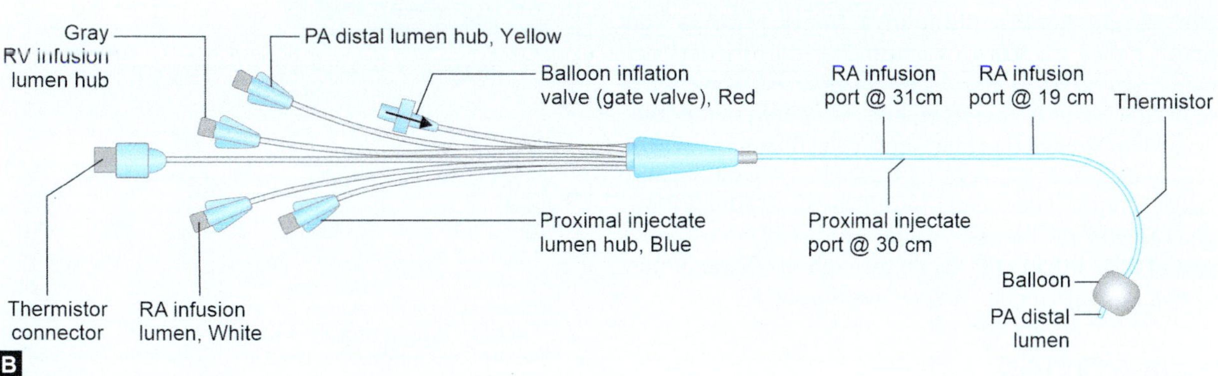

FIGS. 1A AND B: Pulmonary artery catheter.[7]

(PA: pulmonary artery; RA: right atrial; RV: right ventricular)

Courtesy: Reproduced with permission from Edwards Lifesciences.

INSERTION

The PA catheter is usually inserted percutaneously into the internal jugular, subclavian, or femoral veins. The right internal jugular approach has the shortest and straightest path to the heart and the left subclavian approach does not necessitate the PAC turning at an acute angle, thus making them the preferred approaches over other sites. The femoral vein approach may make it difficult to pass a PAC into the heart given the distance from the heart and often requires fluoroscopic guidance; this is particularly true if the right-sided heart chambers are enlarged.

Venous access using an introducer is performed under sterile fashion in the Trendelenburg position under ultrasound guidance, while the insertion of the PAC can be done in a flat or slightly upright position. Before insertion, it is important to check the PAC for kinks and balloon integrity. Connect all the lumens to stopcocks and flush them all with isotonic saline to eliminate air bubbles. Flick the PAC tip to check the response on the monitor after connecting it to the transducer. Finally, the PAC is passed through a sterile sleeve before insertion to ensure sterility.

The existing curve of the PAC is adjusted before insertion to facilitate entry into the PA. Once the catheter displays the right atrial (RA) pressure waveforms (at approximately the 10–20 cm mark), the balloon is slowly inflated with air. The catheter is passed downstream to obtain RV, PA, and PA occlusion pressures (PAOP). Inflation of the balloon facilitates the advancement of the catheter and prevents endocardial trauma.[8] The catheter is always withdrawn with the balloon deflated to avoid valvular rupture or pulmonary endothelial injury. Usually, the right atrium is entered at 15–20 cm, the right ventricle at 25–30 cm, and the PAOP can be identified at 40–50 cm when using the internal jugular or the subclavian approach. It is essential to monitor the electrocardiogram during the insertion of the PA catheter in the RV because of the propensity to cause arrhythmias.

Special considerations: Patients should have normal coagulation parameters before a central venous access is attempted; however, critically ill patients in the intensive care unit (ICU) frequently require anticoagulation. Intravenous heparin should be discontinued 4 hours prior to the procedure. If the patient is on warfarin, then the international normalized ratio (INR) should be normalized using fresh frozen plasma prior to the procedure. In certain conditions such as severe right atrial or right ventricular dilatation, severe pulmonary hypertension, severe tricuspid regurgitation, and low cardiac output states, it may be difficult to position a flow-directed catheter and this may warrant the use of fluoroscopy. Infusion of 5–10 mL of cold saline through the distal lumen may stiffen the catheter and help in positioning it.

INTERPRETATION

Once the PA catheter has been inserted, it becomes imperative to appropriately interpret the available data. PA catheterization allows measurement of RA, right ventricular (RV), PA, and PAO pressures along with cardiac output, mixed venous oxygen saturation, and oxygen saturation in the right-sided chambers to detect intracardiac shunting.

The normal resting RA pressure is 0–8 mm Hg. Two major positive RA waves are usually recorded: A wave and V wave. The A wave is produced by atrial contraction and follows the electrocardiographic P wave.[9] The A-wave peak generally follows the electrocardiographic P-wave peak by 80 msec.[10] The V wave is produced by venous filling of the right atrium while the tricuspid valve is closed. The peak of the V wave occurs at the end of ventricular systole when the atrium is maximally filled. This follows the electrocardiographic T wave. A third wave, known as the C wave, is a minor positive wave due to sudden motion of the tricuspid valve ring toward the right atrium and can be seen in cases of electrocardiographic P–R prolongation. The X descent follows the A wave and is due to atrial relaxation. The Y descent follows the V wave and is due to rapid emptying of the right atrium **(Fig. 2)**.

The normal resting RV pressure is 20–25/0–8 mm Hg. The RV systolic pressure equals the PA systolic pressure except in cases of pulmonic stenosis or RV outflow tract obstruction. The RV diastolic pressure equals the mean RA pressure during diastole when the valve is open. The RV waveform is identified by a sudden upstroke (and downstroke) representing ventricular systole in the tracing during catheter advancement. Particular attention must be paid to exit the right ventricle as quickly as possible as the presence of the catheter is arrhythmogenic.

The PA waveform is distinguished from the RV waveform by a progressive decrease rather than an increase in pressure

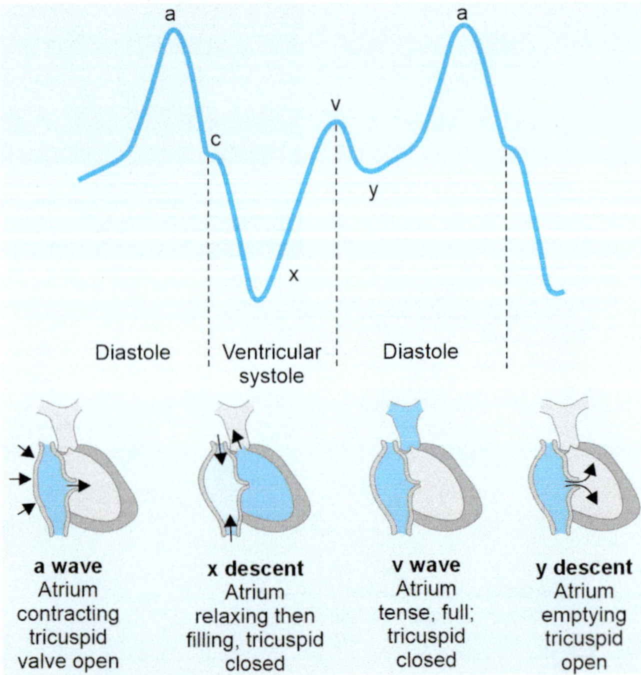

FIG. 2: Right atrial waveforms.[11]

Courtesy: Reproduced with permission from Oxford University Press.

during diastole, an overall increase in diastolic pressure, and a dicrotic notch due to the closure of the pulmonic valve. The PA diastolic pressure is usually 1–3 mm Hg higher than the PAOP **(Fig. 3)**. So the PA diastolic pressure can be used as an index of left ventricular filling pressure in patients whom an occlusion pressure may be unobtainable.

The normal PAOP is 2–15 mm Hg. The PAOP waveform is similar to the RA waveform except that the V waves on a PAOP tracing are larger than the A waves. Once the PAOP is obtained, the balloon should be deflated to reproduce PA waveforms and help confirm accurate positioning. If the PA waveform does not reappear, the catheter should be withdrawn until it does. Wedge position can be further confirmed by withdrawing a blood specimen from the distal lumen and measuring its oxygen saturation. If the measured oxygen saturation is higher than 95%, it confirms the wedge position. A chest radiograph should also be obtained to verify appropriate location and lung zone.

Pulmonary artery occlusion pressure should always be measured at the end of exhalation. This provides an optimal reference point because pleural pressures return to baseline and are closest to the atmospheric pressure. Pleural pressures can be higher with active expiratory muscle contraction or with the use of positive end-expiratory pressure (PEEP).[13] The effect is typically negligible when the positive end-expiratory pressure is <10 cm of water. With PEEP > 10, the pulmonary vasculature is compressed due to the increased alveolar and hence intrathoracic pressure. In such cases, half the applied PEEP (converted from cm of water to mm Hg) must be subtracted from the measured PAOP.[14] The respiratory variation differences in the PAOP tracing between a patient spontaneously breathing and that on positive-pressure ventilation are shown in **Figures 4A and B**. PAOP should ideally correlate with left ventricular end-diastolic pressure (LVEDP), provided the patient has a normal mitral valve and normal left ventricular function. PAOP most accurately estimates pulmonary venous pressure and, therefore, left atrial pressure if the catheter tip is in zone 3 of the lungs. In zone 3, pulmonary arterial and venous pressures are greater than alveolar pressures, providing an uninterrupted column of blood between the catheter tip and the pulmonary veins.[15] A catheter wedged in either zone 1 or 2 shows marked respiratory variations and irregular waveforms which may be misinterpreted as higher pressures **(Fig. 5)**.

It is important to note that PA catheters give data on pressures opposed to volume. Conceptually, PAOP should be indicative of LVEDP. Nevertheless, the assumption that PAOP reflects pulmonary venous pressure in agreement with LVEDP is not always correct in critically ill patients. There are certain conditions in which a discrepancy between PAOP and LVEDP may exist **(Table 1; Fig. 6)**. PAOP is useful when there is a linear relationship between pressure and volume at the end of ventricular diastole. However, as evidenced by the Frank–Starling law, this relationship is often curvilinear. A physician must always acknowledge that underlying anatomic abnormalities, decreased left ventricular compliance, mitral valve disorders, and pulmonary disease may falsely increase or decrease the PAOP. Furthermore, PAOP does not take into account pulmonary capillary permeability, interstitial pressure, or pulmonary capillary resistance.

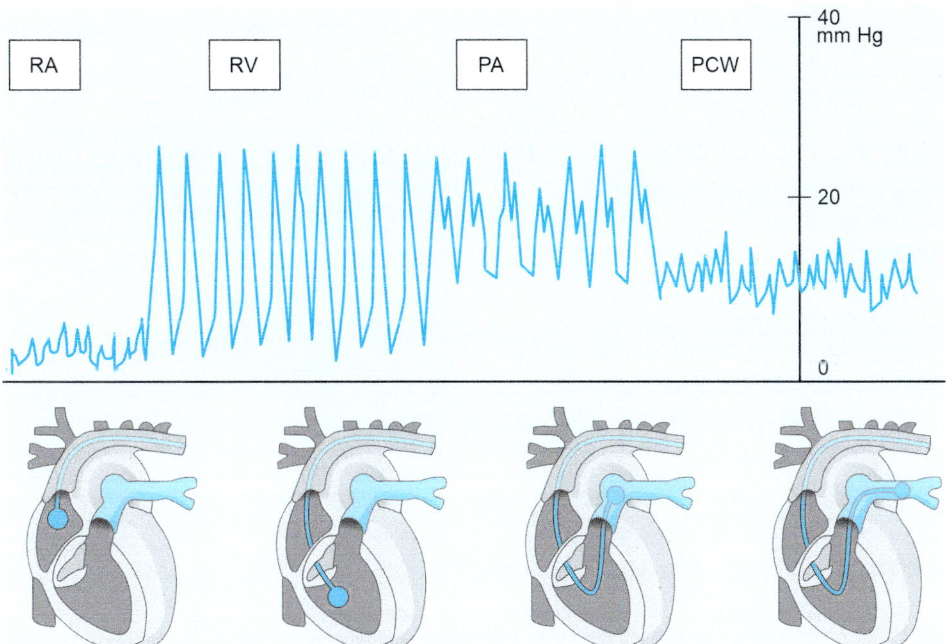

FIG. 3: Typical waveform progression as the PAC floats through the cardiac chambers.[12]
(PA: pulmonary artery; PCW: pulmonary capillary wedge; RA: right atrial; RV: right ventricular)
Courtesy: Reproduced with permission from The Internet Journal of Anesthesiology.

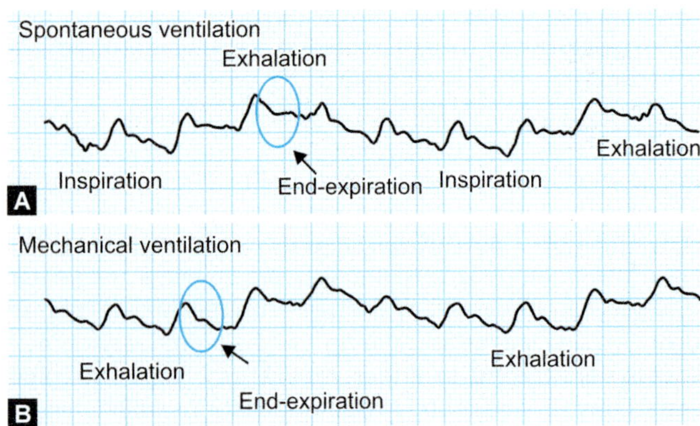

FIGS. 4A AND B: PAOP waveforms during spontaneous versus mechanical ventilation.

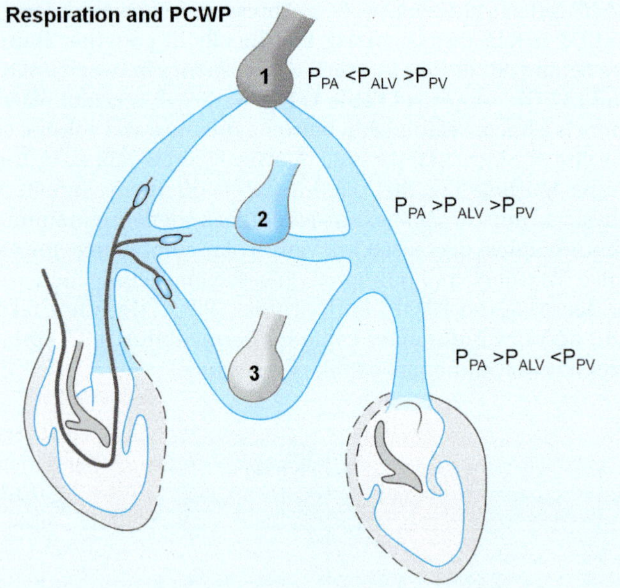

FIG. 5: Physiologic lung zones in an upright patient.[16]
(PCWP: pulmonary capillary wedge pressure)
Courtesy: Reproduced with permission from McGraw Hill.

After obtaining measurements from each chamber, the cardiac output can be recorded by connecting the thermistor to the monitor and then injecting a cold saline bolus through the proximal port into the right atrium (thermodilution technique). On a plot of temperature against time, the area under the curve is inversely proportional to the cardiac output **(Figs. 7A to D)**. The measurement is repeated until at least three consistent results have been obtained, and then the average of the results is calculated as final.[18]

Once the catheter has been inserted and the position is confirmed, the critical job of interpreting the data accurately and making the necessary interventions is left up to the clinician. Using the measured pressures (RA, RV, PA, and PAO pressures), the remaining hemodynamic parameters can be calculated **(Table 2)**. Cardiac output can be either measured using the thermodilution technique or calculated using Fick's method.

TABLE 1: Conditions causing discrepant PAOP and LVEDP readings.[17]

PAOP < LVEDP	PAOP > LVEDP
Aortic insufficiency	Increased intrathoracic pressure
Pneumonectomy	• Positive pressure ventilation
Pulmonary embolism	• PEEP
Decreased LV compliance	Tachycardia
• Increased LV mass	Mitral valve disease
• Increased LV stiffness	• Insufficiency
○ Scar from prior ischemia	• Stenosis
○ Sepsis	• Thrombosis
○ Diabetes mellitus	COPD
○ Aging	Pulmonary venous disease
○ Infiltrative disorders (sarcoidosis, amyloidosis)	

(COPD: chronic obstructive pulmonary disease; LV: left ventricular; LVEDP: left ventricular end-diastolic pressure; PAOP: pulmonary artery occlusion pressure; PEEP: positive end-expiratory pressure)

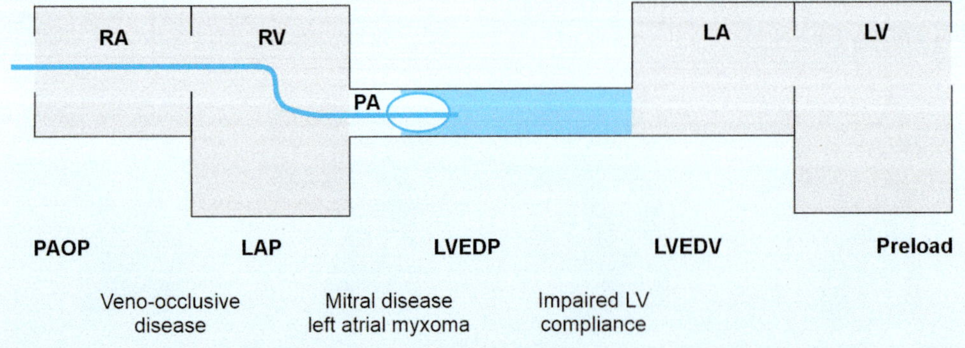

FIG. 6: PAOP as a reflection of LVEDP and conditions causing discrepancies.
(PAOP: pulmonary artery occlusion pressure; LAP: left atrial pressure; LVEDP: left ventricular end-diastolic pressure; LVEDV: left ventricular end-diastolic volume; RA: right atrial; RV: right ventricular; LA: left atrial; LV: left ventricular; PA: pulmonary artery;)

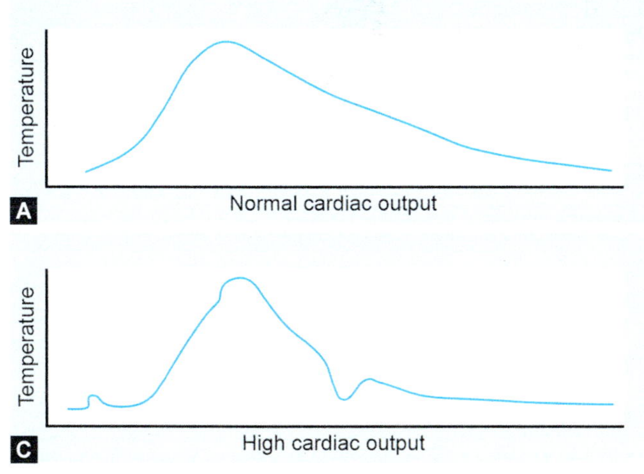

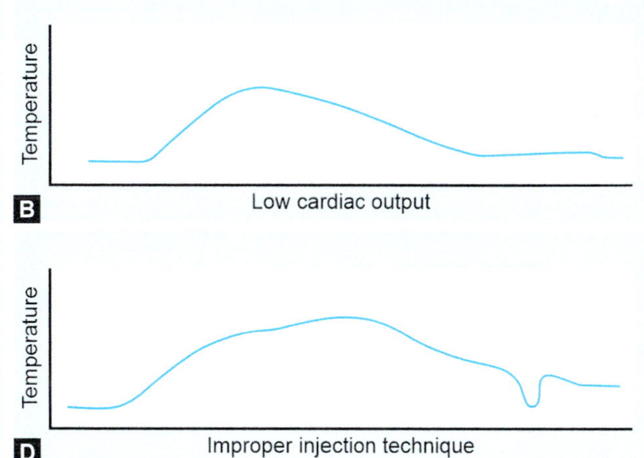

FIGS. 7A TO D: Thermodilution curves.[18]
Courtesy: Reproduced with permission from Elsevier Saunders.

There are a variety of conditions, which can be either definitely diagnosed (VSD, pulmonary hypertension) or highly suggested due to their trends (cardiogenic pulmonary edema, cardiac tamponade) via PA catheterization. Additionally, certain conditions such as septic shock, hypovolemic shock, and pulmonary embolism can be entertained with PA catheterization as well **(Tables 3 and 4)**.

COMPLICATIONS

Pulmonary artery catheterization is associated with a variety of complications. These can be divided into those related to central venous access and those specific to the PA catheter insertion **(Box 2)**.

Pulmonary infarction is a potentially preventable complication of PA catheterization caused by distal migration of the PA catheter tip into the smaller branches of the PA causing persistent wedging.[20] It is, therefore, important to recognize when the catheter is overwedged. This is identified when the balloon is inflated and a blunted upward trend is seen on the tracing **(Fig. 8)**. In such cases, the balloon must be immediately deflated, and the catheter withdrawn to visualize an accurate PA waveform. Pulmonary infarction may also be seen if the balloon is left inflated in the wedge position for an extended period of the time.[21] Wedging should not be performed for more than 15 minutes at a time. Another potentially fatal and feared complication of PA catheterization is rupture of the PA. It has been reported in 0.1–0.2% of patients with a mortality of 45–65%.[22,23] It can occur during insertion or a few days after insertion.[24] It can also occur as a result of overwedging or if air is inflated too rapidly while attempting to obtain a PAOP. It presents typically with massive hemoptysis, hypoxemia, and shock. Emergency management includes immediate angiography with embolization, selective intubation of the unaffected lung, and cardiothoracic surgery referral.

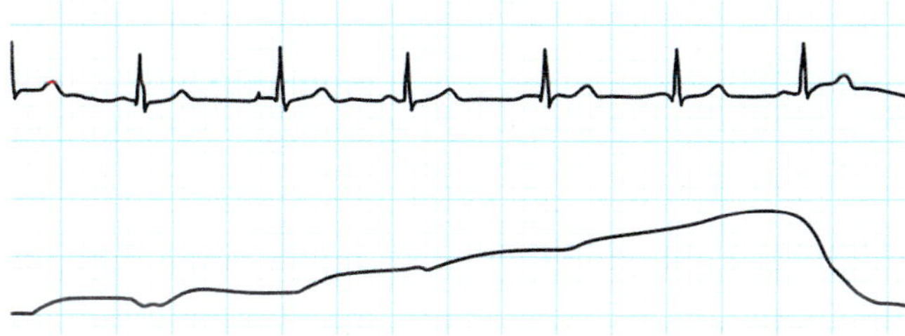

FIG. 8: Overwedged PAOP tracing.

The PA catheter, being a foreign body in a vascular system, can damage the endothelium and cause thrombosis. These thrombi can encase the tip of the catheter or form anywhere in the venous system acting as pulmonary emboli. A changing relationship between the PA diastolic pressure and PAOP over a period of time should increase suspicion for thrombosis at the catheter tip. Knotting of the catheter results when the catheter forms a loop in the cardiac chamber and the catheter is repeatedly withdrawn and advanced.[25] Knotting is avoided by not advancing the catheter beyond the anticipated distance. Knotted catheters can be removed transvenously or surgically. Knotting of the PA catheter around intracardiac structures, other intravascular catheters, and intracardiac sutures has been reported.[26-28]

Balloon rupture is associated with air emboli gaining intravascular entry and/or balloon fragments embolizing into the distal pulmonary circulation. If the rupture occurs during catheter insertion, the loss of the balloon's protective function can cause endocardial damage and/or arrhythmia. Atrial and ventricular arrhythmias are common during the insertion of a PA catheter. Most arrhythmias are self-limited and do not necessitate treatment; however, up to 3% of sustained arrhythmias warrant treatment.[29,30] Transient right bundle branch blocks can be seen during catheter insertion and patients with preexisting left bundle branch blocks can

TABLE 2: Calculation of cardiac output and vascular resistance using Fick's method.[17]

Value	Equation	Normal values
Cardiac output (L/min)	$CO = \frac{VO_2}{C_a - C_v}$ which can be simplified to $CO = \frac{VO_2}{1.36 \times Hgb \times (SaO_2 - SVO_2) \times 10}$	4.8–73 for an average adult
Cardiac index (L/min/m²)	$CI = \frac{CO}{BSA}$	2.8–4.2
Systemic vascular resistance (dyn/sec/cm^{-5})	$SVR = \frac{MAP - RA}{CO} \times 80$	700–1,600
Pulmonary vascular resistance (dyn/sec/cm^{-5})	$PVR = \frac{PA - PCWP}{CO} \times 80$	20–130

[1.36: oxygen-carrying capacity of hemoglobin (mL/g); 10 = conversion factor; BSA: body surface area; C_a: oxygen content of arterial blood; C_v: oxygen content of the venous blood; SaO_2: arterial oxygen saturation; SvO_2: mixed venous oxygen saturation; VO_2: oxygen consumption (mL/min) ~ 125 mL/min/m²]

Courtesy: Reproduced with permission from The New England Journal of Medicine.

TABLE 3: Summary of PA catheter findings in selected clinical situations.

	RA	RV	PA	PAOP	BP	CI	SVR	PVR
Normal	0–8	25/0–8	25/8–15	8–15	120/80	>2.5	~1,500	<250
Hypovolemic shock	0–2	15–20/0–2	15–20/2–6	2–6	<90/60	<2.0	>1,500	<250
Early septic shock	0–2	20–25/0–2	20–25/0–6	0–6	<90/60	>2.5	<1,500	<250
Late septic shock	0–4	25/4–10	25/4–10	4–10	<90/60	<2.0	>1,500	>250
Cardiogenic shock	>8	50/>8	50/35 (>15)	35 (>15)	<90/60	<2.0	>1500	<250
Cardiac tamponade	12–18	25/12–18	25/12–18	12–18	<90/60	<2.0	>1,500	>450
Acute MI with LVF	0–8	30–40/0–8	30–40/18–25	>15	>120/80	>2.0	>1,500	>250
Acute MI without LVF	0–8	25/0–8	25/12–18	<15	>120/80	<2.5	~1,500	<250
Acute ventricular septal rupture	6	60/6–8	60/35	30	<90/60	<2.0	>1,500	>250
Biventricular failure	>6	50–60/>6	50–60/25	18–25	120/80	~2.0	>1,500	>250
RV failure	12–20	30/12–20	30/12	<15	<90/60	<2.0	>1,500	>250
Acute massive PE	8–12	>30/12	>30/12–15	<15	<90/60	<2.0	>1,500	>450
Cor pulmonale	>6	>50 (80) />6	>50 (80) />15	<15	120/80	~2.0	>1,500	>400
Pulmonary hypertension	0–6	>50 (80–100)/40	>50 (80–100)/>15	<15	<120/80	<2.0	>1,500	>500

(BP: blood pressure; CI: cardiac index; PA: pulmonary artery; PAOP: pulmonary artery occlusion pressure; PVR: pulmonary vascular resistance; RA: right atrium; RV: right ventricle; SVR: systemic vascular resistance;)

be at risk of complete heart block due to transient right heart block during catheter insertion.

Damage to the right atrium, right ventricle, pulmonic valve, tricuspid valve, and supporting chordae can occur during insertion or withdrawal of the catheter. It is most commonly seen while withdrawing a catheter with the balloon inflated.

CLINICAL CONTROVERSY

In 2003, the American Society of Anesthesiologists Task Force published practice guidelines for the use of PAC. PAC monitoring was deemed appropriate in two groups of patients: Surgical patients undergoing procedures associated with a high risk of complications from hemodynamic changes and

TABLE 4: General trends in certain clinical conditions.[7]

Condition	HR	MAP	CO/ CI	CVP/RAP	PAP/PAOP	Notes
Left ventricular failure	↑	↓	↓	↑	↑	
Pulmonary edema (cardiogenic)	↑	N,↓	↓	↑	↑ PAOP > 25 mm Hg	
Massive pulmonary embolism	↑	↓	↓	↑,N	↑PAD > PAOP by >5 mm Hg	↑ PVR
Acute ventricular septal defect	↑	↓	↓	↑	↑ Giant "v" waves on PAOP tracing	O_2 step-up noted in SvO_2
Acute mitral valve regurgitation	↑	↓	↓	↑	↑ Giant "v" waves on PAOP tracing	No O_2 step-up noted in SvO_2
Cardiac tamponade	↑	↓	↓	↑	↑ CVP, PAD, and PAOP equalized	↓RVEDV1
Right ventricular failure	↑,V	↓,V	↓	↑	PAP ↑, PAOPN/↓	↑RVEDVI
Hypovolemic shock	↑	↓	↓	↓	↓	↑ Oxygen extraction ↑SVR
Cardiogenic shock	↑	↓	↓	N,↑	↑	↑ Oxygen extraction ↑SVR
Septic shock	↑	↓	↓	↓,N	↓,N	SVR changes. ↓ Oxygen extraction ↓SVR

(CO: cardiac output; CVP: central venous pressure; HR: heart rate; MAP: mean arterial pressure; PAD: pulmonary artery diastolic; PAP: pulmonary artery pressure; PAOP: pulmonary artery occlusion pressure; RAP: right atrial pressure; RVEDV: right ventricular end-diastolic volume; SVR: systemic vascular resistance)

Courtesy: Reproduced with permission from Edwards Lifesciences.

BOX 2 Complications.

Central venous access puncture:
- Bleeding
- Local hematomas
- Injury to thoracic duct
- Injury to the carotid artery
- Pseudoaneurysm formation
- Pneumothorax
- Hemothorax
- Infection
- Air embolism

PA catheterization
- Atrial or ventricular tachyarrhythmias
- Bradyarrhythmias—complete heart block
- Pulmonary infarction
- PA rupture
- Myocardial perforation
- Thrombus formation
- Knotting of the catheter
- Valvular injury
- Infection
- Air embolism

Systemic hypotension related to vasoreactivity testing for pulmonary hypertension

(PA: pulmonary artery)

surgical patients with advanced cardiopulmonary disease who would be at an increased risk for adverse perioperative events.[31] Similar guidelines published in 2004 by the American College of Cardiology/American Heart Association (AHA) suggested PAC use in progressive hypotensive patients unresponsive to fluid resuscitation as well as mechanical complications of acute myocardial infarction as Class I indications. Class IIA indications addressed PAC utility in CS and severe congestive heart failure to guide inotropic therapy.[19]

Since then, a number of randomized controlled studies have not shown a mortality benefit in patients who underwent placement of a PAC compared to those who did not, specifically in septic shock, acute respiratory distress syndrome, acute decompensated heart failure, or those patients undergoing high-risk surgery. A clinical controversy ensued from these studies as critics claimed that the acutely ill patients in the ICU are more likely to undergo PAC placement. There are several landmark studies that have recently changed the perception and utility of right heart catheterization.[32-40]

It goes without question that the use of a PAC has declined over time with the advent of the stated trials. A time-trend analysis on national estimates of PAC use in the United States from 1993 to 2004, using data from the Nationwide Inpatient Sample, found a 65% and 63% decrease in PAC use in all medical and surgical patients, respectively,[41] during that period; the most prominent decline, by 81%, was in use of PACs for myocardial infarction.[41] Because of the paucity of evidence, there is significant variability in PAC catheter use among physicians and institutions, mainly seen in large academic centers and those with advanced heart failure programs. For the same reason, there are a few strong recommendations by society guidelines regarding the use of PAC.

At this time, there are two groups of patients in whom PAC use is strongly recommended by society guidelines: (1) PAC use in diagnosing, classifying, and guiding treatment decisions in patients with pulmonary hypertension (Class 1, Level B recommendation in 2022 ECS/ERS Guidelines)[42] and (2) PAC use in all adult candidates in preparation for listing for cardiac transplantation and periodically until transplantation [Class 1, Level C recommendation in 2016 International Society for Heart Lung Transplantation (ISHLT) Guidelines].[43]

In the most recent AHA guidelines in 2022, AHA does not recommend routine invasive hemodynamic monitoring PAC, but it does have a Class IIA recommendation of PAC monitoring to guide management in decompensated heart failure patients who fail to improve with treatment, require inotropic support, and have uncertain hemodynamics and worsening renal failure (Class IIA recommendation in 2022 AHA guidelines).[44]

There is limited data on PAC monitoring in patients with CS with or without mechanical support devices. The approach to hemodynamic monitoring in these patients is adopted from data on heart failure patients; however, it is important to note that the landmark trial showing no benefit of PAC in decompensated heart failure (ESCAPE trial) excluded patients in CS. The ISHLT recommend PAC hemodynamic monitoring in decompensated heart failure patients requiring mechanical assist devices (Class IIA) and serial hemodynamic measurements 3–6 months after LVAD implantation to assess for reversibility of pulmonary hypertension (Class IIA, Level C).[43] In a single-center prospective registry from 2005 to 2009, use of PAC monitoring in patients with CS without acute coronary syndrome (ACS) was associated with lower short-term and long-term mortality rates.[45] Recent data from a large multicenter registry suggest that complete hemodynamic profiling with PAC in CS is associated with lower in-hospital mortality.[46] Unfortunately, these lack empiric evidence at present.

SUMMARY

The PA catheter remains a powerful tool in assessment and monitoring of cardiovascular physiology. Following its introduction, a large number of retrospective, prospective uncontrolled and observational studies have questioned the utility and safety of PAC use. To date, the literature does not show improved patient outcomes in routine PAC use without specific interventions. There were no differences in the number of deaths during hospital stay, days spent in general ICUs, and days spent in the hospital between patients who did and did not have a PAC inserted.[47] It should be noted that the patient groups studied in the early studies are the ones with little gain from PAC use, and a number of studies did not use a predefined treatment protocol.

Strong indications for ongoing PAC use still exist, particularly in cases of high output states ("pseudosepsis states"), severe congestive heart failure requiring inotropic and vasodilator agents, acute CS, and preoperative workup for solid organ transplantation.[48] Additionally, recent retrospective studies have suggested mortality benefits associated with PAC hemodynamic profiling in CS patients. Unfortunately, these lack empiric evidence at present. Future studies must shift the focus on identifying the subgroup of patients PAC is most useful rather than *if* it is useful.

As the pendulum on PAC use continues to shift among health professionals, there is a consensus among the societies that routine use of PAC monitoring in critical care settings does not benefit patient outcomes; however, PAC remains an important diagnostic and hemodynamic monitoring tool to be utilized only in selected patients by well-trained physicians but not a therapeutic intervention.

REFERENCES

1. Cournand A. Cardiac catheterization: development of the technique, its contributions to experimental medicine, and its initial application in man. Acta Med Scand Suppl. 1975;579:3-32.
2. Scheinman M, Abbott J, Rapaport E. Clinical uses of a flow-directed right heart catheter. Arch Intern Med. 1969;124(1): 19-24.
3. Swan HJC, Ganz W, Forrester J, et al. Catheterization of the heart in man with use of a flow-directed balloon-tipped catheter. N Engl J Med. 1970;283(9):447-51.
4. Chatterjee K, Swan HJ, Ganz W, et al. Use of a balloon-tipped flotation electrode catheter for cardiac mounting. Am J Cardiol. 1975;36(1):56-61.
5. Mueller HS, Chatterjee K, Davis KB, et al. ACC expert consensus document. Present use of bedside right heart catheterization in patients with cardiac disease. J Am Coll Cardiol. 1998;32(3):840-64.
6. Irwin RS, Rippe JM, Curley FJ, et al. (Eds). Procedures and Techniques in Intensive Care Medicine. Boston: Little, Brown and Company; 2003.
7. McGee W, Headley J. Frazler J. Quick Guide to Cardiopulmonary Care. California: Edwards Lifesciences; 2009. pp. 162-3.
8. Ginosar Y. Bone's Atlas of Pulmonary and Critical Care Medicine. Philadelphia: Lippincott Williams & Wilkins; 1999. pp. 1-17.
9. Barry WA, Braunwald E. Heart Disease: Textbook of Cardiovascular Medicine, Vol. 1, Philadelphia: W.B. Saunders; 1988. p. 287.
10. Sharkey SW. Beyond the wedge: Clinical physiology and the Swan-Ganz catheter. Am J Med. 1987;83:111.
11. Longmore JM, et al. The Oxford Handbook of Clinical Medicine, 5th edition. Oxford: Oxford University Press; p. 79.
12. Mathews L. Paradigm Shift in Hemodynamic Monitoring. Internet J Anesthesiol. 2007;11(2).

13. Wiedemann HP, Matthay MA, Matthay RA. Cardiovascular-pulmonary monitoring in the intensive care unit. Chest. 1984;85(5):656-68.
14. Marini J. Estimation of transmural cardiac pressure during ventilation with PEEP. J Appl Physiol. 1982;53:384-91.
15. West JB, Dollery CT, Naimark A. Distribution of blood flow in isolated lung; relation to vascular and alveolar pressures. J Appl Physiol. 1964;19:713-24.
16. Raoof S, George L, Saleh A. ACP Manual of Critical Care. New York: McGraw Hill Professional Publishing; 2008. p. 26.
17. Brandsetter R. Swan-Ganz catheter: Misconceptions, pitfalls, and incomplete user knowledge-an unidentified trilogy in need of correction. Heart Lung. 1998;27:218-22.
18. Christopher K. Pulmonary-Artery Catheterization. N Engl J Med. 2013;369:e35.
19. Libby P, Braunwald E. Braunwald's Heart Disease. Philadelphia: Elsevier Saunders; 2007.
20. Foote GA, Schabel SI, Hodges M. Pulmonary complications of the flow-directed balloon-tipped catheter. N Engl J Med. 1974;290(17):927-31.
21. Wechsler RJ, Steiner RM, Kinori I. Monitoring the monitors: the radiology of thoracic catheters, wires, and tubes. Semin Roentgenol. 1988;23(1):61-84.
22. McDaniel DD, Stone JG, Faltas AN, et al. Catheter-induced pulmonary artery hemorrhage. Diagnosis and management in cardiac operations. J Thorac Cardiovasc Surg. 1981;82(1):1-4.
23. Shah KB, Rao TL, Laughlin S, et al. A review of pulmonary artery catheterization in 6,245 patients. Anesthesiology. 1984;61(3):271-5.
24. Carlson TA, Goldenberg IF, Murray PD, et al. Catheter-induced delayed recurrent pulmonary artery hemorrhage. Intervention with therapeutic embolism of the pulmonary artery. JAMA. 1989;261(13):1943-5.
25. Lipp H, O'Donoghue K, Resnekov L. Intracardiac knotting of a flow-directed balloon catheter. N Engl J Med. 1971;284(4):220.
26. Meister SG, Furr CM, Engel TR, et al. Knotting of a flow-directed catheter about a cardiac structure. Cathet Cardiovasc Diagn. 1977;3(2):171-5.
27. Swaroop S. Knotting of two central venous monitoring catheters. Am J Med. 1972;53(3):386-8.
28. Lazzam C, Sanborn TA, Christian F Jr. Ventricular entrapment of a Swan-Ganz catheter: a technique for nonsurgical removal. J Am Coll Cardiol. 1989;13(6):1422-4.
29. Sprung CL, Pozen RG, Rozanski JJ, et al. Advanced ventricular arrhythmias during bedside pulmonary artery catheterization. Am J Med. 1982;72(2):203-8.
30. Iberti TJ, Benjamin E, Gruppi L, et al. Ventricular arrhythmias during pulmonary artery catheterization in the intensive care unit. Prospective study. Am J Med. 1985;78(3):451-4.
31. American Society of Anesthesiologists. Practice Guidelines for Pulmonary Artery Catheterization. Anesthesiology. 2003;99: 988-1014.
32. Rhodes A, Cusack RJ, Newman PJ, et al. A randomized, controlled trial of the pulmonary artery catheter in critically ill patients. Intensive Care Med. 2002;28(3):256-64.
33. Sandham JD, Hull RD, Brant RF, et al. A randomized, controlled trial of the use of pulmonary-artery catheters in high-risk surgical patients. N Engl J Med. 2003;348(1):5-14.
34. Richard C, Warszawski J, Anguel N, et al. Early use of the pulmonary artery catheter and outcomes in patients with shock and acute respiratory distress syndrome: a randomized controlled trial. JAMA. 2003;290(20):2713-20.
35. Harvey S, Harrison DA, Singer M, et al. Assessment of the clinical effectiveness of pulmonary artery catheters in management of patients in intensive care (PAC-Man): a randomised controlled trial. Lancet. 2005; 366(9484): 472-7.
36. Binanay C, Califf RM, Hasselblad V, et al.; ESCAPE Investigators and ESCAPE study coordinators. Evaluation study of congestive heart failure and pulmonary artery catheterization effectiveness: the ESCAPE trial. JAMA. 2005;294(13):1625-33.
37. Shah MR, Hasselblad V, Stevenson LW, et al. Impact of the pulmonary artery catheter in critically ill patients: meta-analysis of randomized clinical trials. JAMA. 2005;294(13):1664-70.
38. Wheeler AP, Bernard GR, Thompson BT, et al. Pulmonary-artery versus central venous catheter to guide treatment of acute lung injury. N Engl J Med. 2006;354(21):2213-24.
39. Djaiani G, Karski J, Yudin M, et al. Clinical outcomes in patients undergoing elective coronary artery bypass graft surgery with and without utilization of pulmonary artery catheter-generated data. J Cardiothorac Vasc Anesth. 2006;20(3):307-10.
40. Clermont G, Kong L, Weissfeld LA, et al. The effect of pulmonary artery catheter use on costs and long-term outcomes of acute lung injury. PLoS One. 2011;6(7):e22512.
41. Wiener RS, Welch HG. Trends in the use of the pulmonary artery catheter in the United States, 1993-2004. JAMA. 2007;298(4):423-9.
42. Humbert M, Kovacs G, Hoeper MM, et al. 2022 ESC/ERS Guidelines for the diagnosis and treatment of pulmonary hypertension. Eur Heart J. 2022;43(38):3618-731.
43. Mehra MR, Canter CE, Hannan MM, et al. The 2016 international society for heart lung transplantation listing criteria for Heart Transplantation: A 10-year update. J Heart Lung Transpl. 2016;35(1):1-23.
44. Heidenreich PA, Bozkurt B, Aguilar D, et al. 2022 ACC/AHA/HFSA guideline for the management of heart failure. J Cardiac Fail. 2022;28(5). https://doi.org/10.1161/CIR.0000000000001063.
45. Rossello X, Vila M, Rivas-Lasarte M, et al. Impact of pulmonary artery catheter use on short- and long-term mortality in patients with cardiogenic shock. Cardiology. 2016;136(1):61-9.
46. Garan AR, Kanwar M, Thayer KL, et al. Complete hemodynamic profiling with pulmonary artery catheters in cardiogenic shock is associated with lower in-hospital mortality. JACC Heart Fail. 2020;8(11):903-13.
47. Rajaram SS, Desai NK, Kalra A, et al. Pulmonary artery catheters for adult patients in intensive care. Cochrane Database Syst Rev. 2013;2018(12):CD003408.
48. Chatterjee K. The Swan-Ganz catheters: Past, present, and future. Circulation. 2009;119(1):147-52.

Role of Ultrasonography in Critical Care Medicine

CHAPTER 173

Pralay K Sarkar, Seth J Koenig, Paul H Mayo

INTRODUCTION

For more than the last two decades, ultrasonography has found major application in the practice of critical care medicine. Efficiently and thoroughly utilized, ultrasonography can have a major impact in advancing the quality of care in critically ill patients. The advantages of critical care ultrasonography (CCUS) are evident: The intensivist personally performs the ultrasonography examination so they are in a position to immediately interpret the results in order to answer the clinical question under consideration. Thus, ultrasonography allows rapid diagnosis and therapeutic interventions at the bedside. Standard radiology or cardiology department-based ultrasonography service inevitably introduces a time delay between the need for the examination, which is immediate, and the performance of the examination, which is delayed, often by many hours. In addition, radiologists or cardiologists have minimal knowledge of the clinical situation. The time delay and clinical dissociation of the offline reader prevent their results from being integrated into the clinical plan quickly and efficiently as can be done by the intensivists. Performance of ultrasonography by intensivists also avoids the risk associated with transportation of critically ill patients out of the intensive care unit (ICU) for imaging studies.

By definition, the intensivist performs all aspects of the CCUS examination at bedside: Image acquisition, image interpretation, and clinical application. The field of CCUS has therefore been developed by critical care physicians and is separate conceptually from the ultrasonography as practiced by the radiology and cardiology community. For this reason, the risks associated with the inexperienced intensivist ultrasonographer misinterpreting ultrasound results, misdiagnosing, and mistreating their patients cannot be overstated.[1] Therein lies the importance of fellowship training programs incorporating a formal ultrasonography curriculum for their fellows, including supervised, hands-on training.[1] Incorporation of ultrasonography into routine frontline critical care practice requires that professional societies develop high-quality educational programs in order to ensure that attending/faculty-level intensivists are fully trained in the discipline and many professional societies have done the same.[2-5]

Healthcare quality has been usefully defined around six fundamental domains.[6] The usefulness and limitations of ultrasonography in improving care of critically ill patients can be described in reference to these quality care domains as summarized in **Table 1**.[7]

This chapter will review important applications of ultrasonography in critical care medicine. For a more comprehensive review of the field, the reader is referred to standard texts. **(See Further Readings.)**

TABLE 1: Benefits and limitations of ultrasound (US) in impacting quality of care in critical care medicine.

Quality of care domain	Definition	Advantages of US	Limitations of US
Safety	Reducing/eliminating errors that happen during healthcare experience	• Safe, noninvasive • Available 24/7 at bedside with immediate interpretations • Eliminates risks associated with moving patients off ICU monitoring for diagnostic tests • Improves safety for procedures	• Expertise variable • Inaccurate interpretation by an inexperienced operator may lead to serious errors • Potential of excess use because of easy availability, often at expense of meticulous physical examination • May fail to use, more difficult to obtain, but better diagnostic tests

Continued

Continued

Quality of Care Domain	Definition	Advantages of US	Limitations of US
Effectiveness	Using well-established, evidence-based principles, provides experience, and patient values in achieving the desired care	Guidelines for clear indications of ultrasound use in critical care are emerging	• Requires adequate operator training/ experience • Requires adequate acoustic window/ imaging condition for satisfactory data gathering
Efficiency	Using finite resources in the best possible way to optimize the value of resources	Being performed by the ICU physicians themselves, focused evaluation in a given clinical context can lead to efficient care without delay	Enough operator experience should be there for efficient data gathering and utilization of data in the care of the patient being operated and interpreted by the clinician, lack of objectivity and confirmatory bias remain
Equity	Equal access to healthcare resources by all patients	Ultrasound is cheaper than many other imaging modalities and	Costs of initial investment for equipment and personnel training mean that it will remain inaccessible in many ICUs in near future
Timeliness	Providing diagnostic and therapeutic services to patients in a timely fashion when they need them	CCUS is largely performed by intensivists themselves, being available readily if intensivists are trained to perform CCUS	Intensivists proficient in using CCUS may not be available 24/7
Patient centeredness	Providing care and services to patients where they need it in a way that lead to a satisfactory healthcare experience	• Use of a safe, fast modality reduces the burden on the related to unnecessary transport and pain • Immediate information can be communicated to the patient and family • Immediate implementation of actions based on results can improve patient satisfaction	Not available in all ICUs round the clock

(CCUS: critical care ultrasonography; ICU: intensive care unit)

TRAINING IN CRITICAL CARE ULTRASONOGRAPHY

The intensivist who seeks to develop competence in CCUS follows an organized approach to training. A key question that needs to be answered is what constitutes the subject matter of the field. With knowledge of this, the learner has a roadmap to follow. The American College of Chest Physicians (ACCP), in partnership with La Société de Réanimation de Langue Française (SRLF), developed the first consensus statement that defined competence in CCUS **(Box 1)**.[4] This statement outlined in a simple format the elements of the field that define competence. Other professional societies have also developed similar guidelines.[2,8-10]

Training in CCUS requires mastery of the cognitive elements of the field; this is available in the standard textbooks and medical literature and in many well-designed e-learning formats. Image acquisition is the second mandatory component of competence and can only be learned by repeated practice, initially with normal subjects followed by practice on patients. Image acquisition is a key element of competence because the intensivist personally performs the ultrasonography examination at the bedside. Mastery of image acquisition requires knowledge of machine control, transducer manipulation, and scanning protocol, requiring that the learner be trained by a knowledgeable supervisor. There is also a major autodidactic component to acquiring skill at image acquisition, so the trainee should devote many hours of hands-on practice. The third component of training in image interpretation requires a review of both normal and abnormal images, not only for purposes of identification of disease, but also for integrating the knowledge into clinical management. Like image acquisition, image interpretation requires many hours of review of relevant images. It is not clear at the present time how many scans must be performed or images reviewed to achieve competence. An international expert statement on training standards for CCUS has been published.[11] This statement used ACCP-SRLF statement as the foundation. The expert panel reached the agreement that a formal certification is not required. However, there is a general consensus that competence-based training in basic critical care echocardiography (CCE) and general CCUS should be included in the curriculum of any intensivist. A Systematic Review of International Training Competencies and Program published in 2019 concluded that the majority of countries lacked a formal training program, with variability in training standards and definition of competence even in countries with formal training programs.[9]

BOX 1 ACCP expert consensus statement on competence in critical care ultrasound.[4]

Basic principles

- Understanding of fundamental principles of ultrasound physics
- Knowledge of machine and transducer controls
- Knowledge of normal and abnormal ultrasound anatomy
- Knowledge of and the pathophysiologic consequence of the imaged abnormality
- Knowledge of image interpretation, clinical applications, and specific limitations of ultrasonography
- Ability to understand the goal-directed nature of ultrasound examination in a critical care setting, in search of a specific clinical question

Pleural ultrasonography

- Identification of the presence of pleural effusion as a relatively hypoechoic or echo-free space surrounded by typical anatomic boundaries: Diaphragm, chest wall, ribs, normal/abnormal lung
- Identification of other important structures in the neighborhood: Liver, spleen, kidney, heart, pericardium, spinal column, aorta, inferior vena cava
- Identification of characteristic dynamic findings of pleural fluid
- Characterization of fluid
- Identification of miscellaneous findings, such as pleural-based masses or thickening
- Performance of semiquantitative assessment of fluid volume
- Recognition of specific limitations of ultrasonography to identify pleural fluid due to inadequate image acquisition conditions or nature of pleural fluid/other pleural pathology

Lung ultrasonography

- Identification and characterization of the normal aeration pattern
- Identification and characterization of consolidated lung with or without air bronchograms
- Identification and characterization of alveolar interstitial pattern
- Identification and characterization of air artifacts to rule out pneumothorax
- Identification and characterization of findings that rule in pneumothorax presence of lung point (both by 2D imaging and M mode)

Abdominal ultrasonography

- Identification and characterization of intraperitoneal fluid by static and dynamic image characteristics. Qualitative assessment of intraperitoneal fluid volume
- Identification of all the relevant abdominal structures: Abdominal wall, diaphragm, liver, gallbladder, spleen, kidney, bladder, bowel, uterus, spinal column, aorta, inferior vena cava
- Assessment of the urinary tract: Identification of bladder, identification of urinary catheter, identification of abnormal bladder contents; differentiation of distended bladder from ascites
- Identification of both kidneys, presence or absence of hydronephrosis, measurement of kidney in longitudinal axis
- Identification of abdominal aorta, assessment of the aorta, identification of abdominal aortic aneurysm

Vascular ultrasonography: guidance of vascular access

- Identification of relevant central and peripheral veins and arteries: Internal jugular/carotid, subclavian vein/artery, axillary vein/artery, brachial vein/artery, radial artery, femoral vein/artery vein, peripheral veins such as basilic, cephalic, external jugular
- Differentiation of vein from artery based on anatomic position, compressibility, phasic changes during respiration
- Identification of adjacent nonvenous structures such as muscle, mass, lymph node
- Identification of normal anatomic variability in structure and position
- Identification of vascular thrombosis

Vascular ultrasonography: Diagnosis of venous thrombosis

- Identification of relevant veins and their associated artery: Internal jugular, subclavian, axillary, brachial, basilic, common femoral, proximal saphenous, superficial femoral, popliteal
- Identification of venous thrombosis by visualization of endoluminal thrombus
- Knowledge of correct performance of compression study with identification of normal and abnormal results
- Identification of adjacent structures, e.g., lymph node, mass, hematoma, ruptured Baker cyst

TECHNICAL CONSIDERATIONS

In CCUS, the intensivist is responsible for all aspects of image acquisition. This requires a knowledge of basic ultrasound physics, an understanding of common artifacts of ultrasound imaging, and knowledge of machine function.

Physics of Ultrasound

Sound is created when a moving/vibrating object creates alternate pressure or density changes in sequential layers of surrounding media. The media can be conceptualized to be comprised of columns/layers; within each layer, the matter undergoes alternate compression and rarefaction or alternate high and low points of pressure change **(Fig. 1)**. One layer, during the pressure change, transmits some energy to the next layer and thereby the sound propagates.

Several parameters are used to describe the properties of sound **(Fig. 1)**:

Cycle and period: A *cycle* is one complete vibration of the medium with a change of pressure/density of the medium from baseline to a high point through a low point back to the resting position. The time necessary for the sound wave to complete one cycle is known as its *period (T)*. Period is measured in units of time, usually µsec.

Wavelength: The length of a single cycle measured in units of length is called a *wavelength (λ)*. The wavelength of sound in a particular medium is inversely proportional to the frequency of the sound and is defined by the formula:

Wavelength = Speed of the sound in the medium/ Frequency

The wavelength of diagnostic ultrasound is 0.1–0.6 mm.

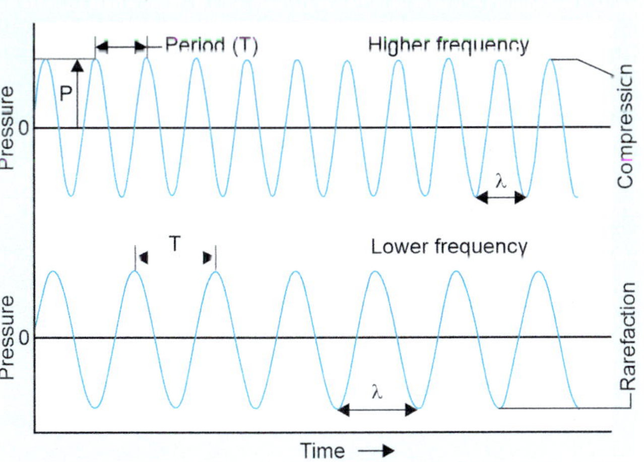

FIG. 1: Characteristics of sound. Sound propagation can be represented in a sinusoidal waveform. As sound propagates, each layer of medium undergoes compression and rarefaction and pressure changes. Note the inverse relationship between frequency and wavelength of sound.

Courtesy: Reproduced with permission from www.usra.ca.

Frequency (f): The number of cycles completed in 1 second is known as *frequency*. A standard measure of frequency is Hertz (Hz): 1 Hertz is one cycle per second (cps) (1 Hz = 1 cps). Ultrasound, by definition, is sound with a frequency of >20 kHz (1 kHz = 1,000 Hz). Typical frequencies used in diagnostic ultrasound range from 2 to 10 MHz (1 MHz = 1 million Hz). Most emitted and reflected sounds contain a lowest frequency, known as the *fundamental frequency*, and multiples of the fundamental frequency, known as *harmonic frequencies* or simply *harmonics*.

Amplitude: With propagation of sound, the particles in the medium move from their resting position leading to change in pressure and density. The particles come back to their resting positions and pressure and density also return to the baseline. The difference between the peak and resting values of any of these parameters, pressure and density, is called the *amplitude (P)* of the sound. Amplitude is a reflection of the "loudness" and the energy of the sound. The amplitude of the sound is described on a logarithmic scale; the units of this scale are Bells. A decibel (dB) is 0.1 of Bells.

Power: The amount of energy delivered per second is defined as *power*. Power = $k \times (\text{amplitude})^2$ (k is the coefficient). The unit of power is Watts.

Intensity: This is the amount of energy delivered per second to the surface of the medium and is defined as power per unit area (expressed in the unit watts/cm^2). It is directly proportional to power (amplitude) and inversely proportional to the area. Intensity of ultrasound determines the biological effects of ultrasound such as tissue heating. Diagnostic ultrasound typically uses an intensity of 0.001–100 watts/cm^2.

Speed: Propagation speed of sound in a particular medium is determined by the density of the medium. The speed of sound is 1,540 m/s in soft tissue; 1,450 m/s in fat; 300–1,200 m/s in lungs; and 2,000–4,000 m/s in bone.

Generation of Ultrasound and the Ultrasound Image

Generation of ultrasound is based on the principle of piezoelectricity. Piezoelectricity is the ability of some natural and artificially made materials to generate an electrical potential when a mechanical stress is applied to them. The induction of a voltage across the material on application of mechanical stress is known as *direct piezoelectric effect*. The same materials also exhibit the *reverse piezoelectric effect:* Production of stress and/or strain when an electric field is applied. The piezoelectric material used in the ultrasound transducer is usually lead zirconate titanate (PZT) crystals.

An ultrasound probe contains multiple elements of a piezoelectric material. These elements act as acoustic transducers. Under an electric voltage, these elements undergo mechanical distortion. When the applied voltage is turned off, the crystals come back to their original shape.

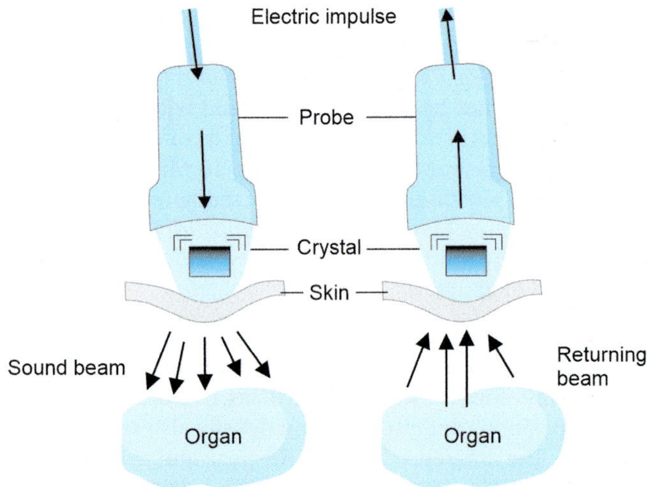

FIG. 2: Generation of ultrasound. Application of a voltage to PZT crystals leads to their mechanical distortion and generation of ultrasound waves. Reflected ultrasound waves deform the crystals leading to the generation of electrical impulse. (PZT: lead zirconate titanate)

Courtesy: Reproduced with permission from www.usra.ca.

During this change of shape, some of the mechanical energy is converted into sound energy which is emitted by the transducer toward the target organ. Whenever the ultrasound waves encounter a surface or an interface with a different density, part of the sound wave is reflected back to the probe and is detected as an echo (see below). The energy of the reflected sound wave deforms the crystals. This generates an electrical current that the machine processes and displays as a pixel **(Fig. 2)**. The stronger the reflection, the greater is the strength of the returning echo and the greater is the strength of the electrical current it generates. An ultrasound beam contains multiple wavelets, each one after reflection contributing a pixel in the image. Thus, multiple wavelets within an ultrasound beam, after reflection from multiple adjacent points within a target organ, create a collection of pixels: Image of the organ. Ultrasonography machines perform all the time calculations assuming that the speed of travel of ultrasound waves in human tissues is 1,540 m/sec. The distance from the transducer of the object causing the echo is calculated from the time delay between generation of the ultrasound from the transducer and reception of the reflected sound. The longer the delay, the deeper the structure will be represented within the image.

Interaction of Ultrasound with the Medium and at Interfaces

As ultrasound travels from its source through a medium (tissue), it undergoes progressive loss of energy (i.e., reduction in amplitude), known as *attenuation*. Ultrasound is absorbed by the medium causing attenuation and in the process generates heat. Attenuation depends on the frequency of ultrasound and the nature of the medium. In any given medium, the higher the frequency of the ultrasound (i.e., shorter wavelength), the greater will be attenuation.

At the interface between two mediums (or two different tissue layers), part of the ultrasound beam undergoes reflection and part is transmitted forward **(Fig. 3A)**. The reflected part of the ultrasound (echo) forms the basis of all diagnostic imaging. The amount of reflection at any interface depends on the difference in the acoustic impedance of the two media and the wavelength of the ultrasound. Most soft tissues have similar impedance; typically, at the boundary of two soft tissues (i.e., kidney/fat), only 1% of the ultrasound is reflected. On the other hand, ultrasound is intensely reflected at the surface of bones; as no ultrasound can penetrate the bone, no structure can be seen beyond a bony structure. Ultrasound also undergoes scattering (i.e., intense multidirectional reflection) in air **(Fig. 3B)**. If air is interposed between the ultrasound beam and the target object, the energy in the ultrasound beam is lost by scattering; the returned echo is minimal and a satisfactory image cannot be obtained.

Reflection is also determined by the wavelength of the ultrasound. The smaller the wavelength, the smaller will be the size of object capable of reflecting it. If the boundary between two media is imagined as made up of multiple small reflectors, it follows that the finer details of the boundary can be seen if the wavelength of the ultrasound is smaller than the size of those small components of the boundary. In other words, resolution (i.e., ability to see two close-by objects separately) improves. Similarly, if two components of the boundary or two objects are separated by a distance greater than the wavelength of the emitted ultrasound, they are clearly seen as separate objects.

The intensivist ultrasonographer needs to have a clear understanding of the relationship between penetration, resolution, and the frequency of ultrasound. Ultrasound waves of higher frequency (i.e., shorter wavelength) are reflected easily by smaller objects, thereby improving resolution. However, as more energy is reflected by superficial structures and through attenuation, the ability of

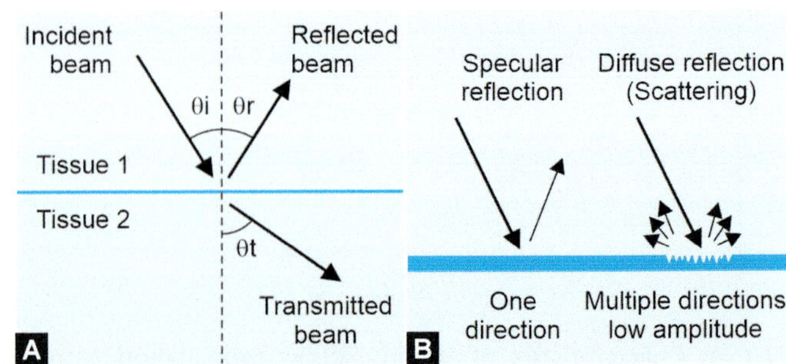

FIGS. 3A AND B: Interaction of ultrasound with the medium and at interfaces. (A) Refraction and reflection of ultrasound at the interface between two media; (B) Specular reflection and scattering.

Courtesy: Reproduced with permission from www.usra.ca.

higher frequency ultrasound to penetrate deeper structures is limited. Higher frequency ultrasound images superficial structures in greater detail but cannot penetrate to image deeper structures. Higher frequency ultrasound is therefore used for vascular studies and studies of superficial structures. Conversely, lower frequency ultrasound is used to image deeper structures although with a predictable loss of resolution (e.g., in abdominal ultrasonography).

Important Terminologies Related to Ultrasound

Attenuation: The progressive decline in amplitude or strength of ultrasound as it passes deeper through the tissues is known as attenuation. While attenuation is the result of absorption of sound energy as it passes through the tissue, reflection of ultrasound at each level also weakens the strength of the beam that penetrates further.

Echogenicity: The term echogenicity refers to the brightness of an element in an ultrasound image. Echogenicity depends on the strength (amplitude) of the reflected ultrasound. A hypoechoic structure appears less echogenic than the surrounding anatomical structures. A hyperechoic structure appears more echogenic than the surrounding anatomical structures. An isoechoic structure has the same echogenicity as the surrounding anatomical structures. An anechoic structure has absent echogenicity and it appears black. Fluid-filled structures are often anechoic. Some ultrasonographers use the liver as the reference standard to judge echogenicity for other structures.

Resolution: Resolution, specifically spatial resolution, refers to the ability of the machine to show two closely spaced objects as separate entities with a distinct outline. Resolution determines the details of a structure. *Axial resolution* refers to the minimum distance between two objects placed along the axis of the beam, where the two structures are identified as separate. Axial resolution depends on the frequency of the ultrasound **(Figs. 4A and B)**. Lateral resolution is defined as the minimum distance between two objects placed along a line perpendicular to beam axis, where the two structures are identified as separate. Lateral resolution is largely dependent on the width of the ultrasound beam and may be improved to some extent by altering the focal zone of the transducer **(Figs. 5A to C)**. Line density contributes to lateral resolution, a factor that can be modified by a machine with sophisticated controls.

Artifacts: These are features of the image that do not originate from the object being imaged.[12] The intensivist ultrasonographer needs to be able to identify different types of artifacts in order to avoid errors related to their misinterpretation. Artifacts may arise because of equipment problems, patient-related factors (e.g., obesity), unsatisfactory operator technique (e.g., due to inappropriate gain setting),

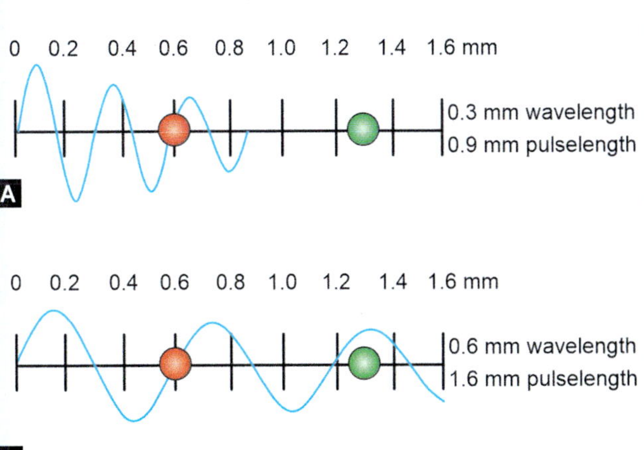

FIGS. 4A AND B: Axial resolution depends on pulse length. An ultrasound pulse commonly consists of two or three sound cycles of the same frequency. A higher frequency ultrasound has a shorter cycle length and therefore provides better axial resolution. (A) Axial resolution is sufficient to distinguish the two target objects as separate because the incident wave hits target 1 (brown) before hitting target 2 (green). (B) Both targets 1 (brown) and 2 (green) are hit by the same wave and both target objects are seen as one.

Courtesy: Reproduced with permission from www.usra.ca.

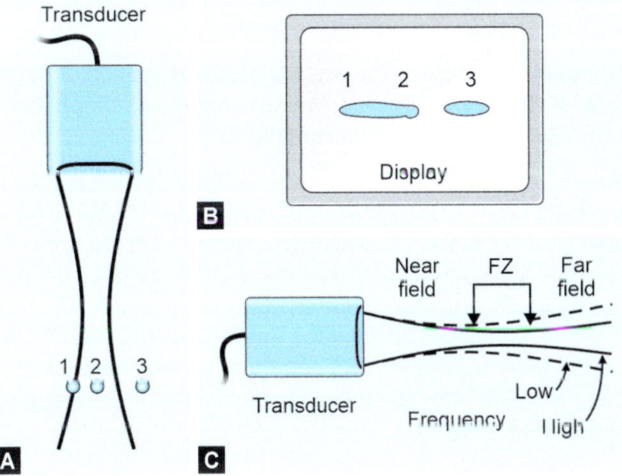

FIGS. 5A TO C: Lateral resolution depends on the ultrasound beam width, which in turn is inversely related to the ultrasound frequency. Lateral resolution is poor when the two structures lie at the same depth within the same beam width. Because the returning echoes overlap with each other side by side, the two structures (1 and 2 in figure) will appear as one on the display (A and B). Lateral resolution is best at the focal zone where the width of the beam is also narrowest (C). Keeping the target object at the focal zone helps to obtain the best resolution.

Courtesy: Reproduced with permission from www.usra.ca.

movement of the target organ (e.g., due to translational respiratory artifacts) or because of sound-tissue interactions. This last category of artifacts (sound-tissue artifacts) results from the physical characteristics of ultrasound and the way it reacts with tissue. Common types of sound-tissue artifacts are discussed below.

Acoustic shadow artifact: This artifact occurs when a structure near total reflects the incident ultrasound beam and the ultrasound beam penetration is severely impeded. No structure beyond the reflector is visible, as the deep structures are shadowed by the reflector. Examples of acoustic shadow artifact include a gallbladder stone with a shadowing deep to it **(Fig. 6A)** or rib shadows.

Reverberation artifact: This artifact occurs when the ultrasound beam is reflected back and forth between two surfaces. The depth of an image is calculated by the ultrasound machine by the time delay between sending the ultrasound beam and receiving the reflected echo. With each reflection in the closed space between two surfaces, part of the reflected beam escapes and reaches the transducer after a delay that is an exact multiplicative of the time that the first reflection needed to reach the transducer. To the machine, each such reflection is exactly the same as the first reflection but arriving at a different time. Each reflection is therefore interpreted by the machine as an object that resembles the original reflective surface, at a depth that is multiplicative of the distance between the two reflective surfaces **(Fig. 6B)**. Some of the important findings in lung ultrasound are based on the principle of reverberation artifacts.

Mirror image artifact: This artifact occurs if a reflector in the path of the beam has a curved structure (e.g., diaphragm) and reflects sound like a mirror **(Fig. 6C)**.

Posterior acoustic enhancement artifact: This artifact is typically seen as a hyperechoic area deep to a fluid-filled (anechoic) structure. The beam passes through the area of a very low attenuation coefficient and enters an area deep to the structure with more energy than the ultrasound beam that has not passed through the fluid-filled structure. As the beam enters an area of higher attenuation with more energy, there is much stronger reflection, making that area appear hyperechoic **(Fig. 6D)**.

Different Ultrasound Modalities

- *Two-dimensional (2D) imaging:* Most CCUS is performed with the 2D imaging technique, also known as B-mode ultrasonography. The most common transducer is either a phased array or a linear array design. The ultrasound beam is rapidly cycled across the transducer head, typically at 30 or more times per second. At this frame rate, the operator observes an uninterrupted pattern of organ motion on the 2D image.
- *M mode (motion mode):* An M-mode image displays the movement of all structures against time along a single beam line **(Fig. 7)**. The single beam line is displayed against a time axis. Each reflecting structure in the path of the beam is represented by a line; the undulation of the line along the *y* axis of the image reflects the movement

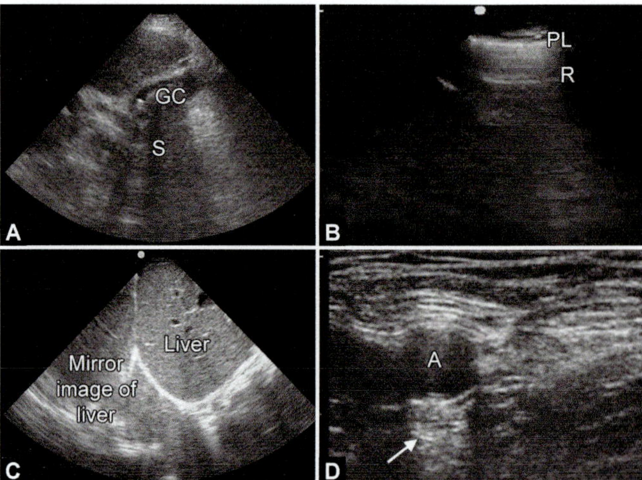

FIGS. 6A TO D: Common ultrasound imaging artifacts. (A) Gallbladder stone (GC) with acoustic shadow artifact (S). (B) Reverberation artifact (R) from reverberation of ultrasound from pleural line (PL). In lung ultrasonography, these artifacts are known as A lines. (C) Mirror image artifact. Strong reflection of ultrasound from a specular reflector-like diaphragm creates a mirror image of liver. (D) Posterior acoustic enhancement artifact, appearing as a hyperechoic region (arrow) deep to a fluid-filled structure (e.g., a vessel, A = artery).

Courtesy: (D) Reproduced with permission from www.usra.ca.

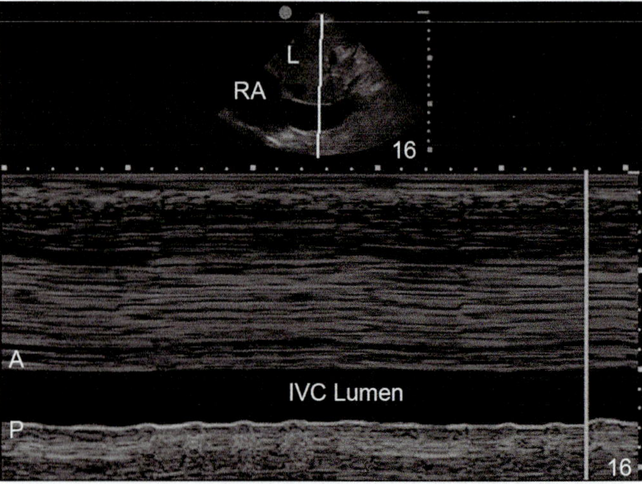

FIG. 7: M-mode examination of IVC. The upper panel of the figure shows the level (longitudinal section at the right paramedian location) where the M-mode examination was performed. A represents the anterior wall of IVC and P represents the posterior wall of IVC. In this case, minimal respiratory variation of IVC lumen size is indicated by minimal undulation of the lines A and P.

(L: liver; RA: right atrium)

of the structure while time is represented along the *x* axis. If a structure in the path of the beam has no movement over time, it will be reflected as a straight line. M-mode is useful for measuring rapidly moving cardiac structures as the sampling frequency is much higher than the 2D imaging, on the order of approximately 2,000 sampling cycles per second.

- *Doppler imaging:* Doppler is particularly useful for the measurement of blood flow velocity. It has extensive utility in advanced CCE but is seldom used in other aspects of CCUS. The physics and imaging strategy of Doppler ultrasonography are beyond the scope of this text. The reader is referred to definitive resources.[13]

Machine controls: The intensivist ultrasonographer is responsible for all aspects of image acquisition. This requires knowledge of machine controls **(Fig. 8)**. Machines of different manufactures have control surfaces of radically different designs. It is not possible to describe here the details of the machine controls that are specific to a wide variety of machines. Some full capability ultrasonography machines have very complex controls that require a sophisticated ultrasonography technician for their proper operation. In general, portable machines are designed for the ease of operation and the control surfaces are relatively simple. A well-designed portable machine with straightforward controls can be mastered easily by the intensivist. In a generic sense, the operator must be able to locate and learn to manipulate the following basic controls:

Depth: All modern ultrasonography machines of use in ICU allow for depth control. The operator can choose to examine superficial or deep structures by altering the depth of penetration of the ultrasound beam. As a general rule, the depth is set so that the target structure is located at the middle of the screen.

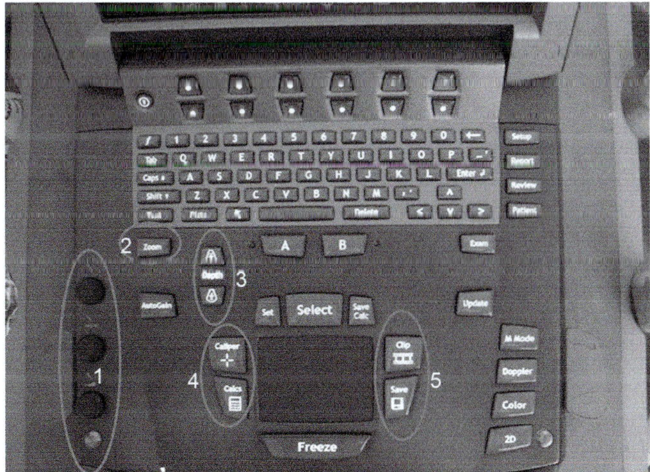

FIG. 8: User interface showing common control buttons in a portable ultrasonography machine. 1. Gain; 2. Zoom; 3. Depth; 4. Caliper and calculation function; 5. Memory functions for saving still and video clips. (See the text for description.)

(The authors do not intend to endorse use of any particular brand of ultrasound machine.)

Projection indicator: All machines have an indicator on the screen that is referenced to a marker on the transducer. In any given ultrasound image, the structures which are on the side of the transducer marker are projected to the indicator side of the screen image. By international convention, abdominal, thoracic and vascular ultrasonography is performed with the screen image indicator set to the left of the screen, whereas echocardiography is performed with the screen indicator on the right of the screen.

Gain: All modern ultrasound machines have a gain control. The gain control is adjusted to optimize the brightness of the image. The gain is a feature of image processing that amplifies the returned echo. The effect of increasing gain is to increase the brightness of the image. The strength of the echo returning from deeper structures is often weak. Increasing the gain may improve image quality, and the structures will be better seen on the screen. If the gain is set too high, nonspecific brightness will be seen throughout the image. Image quality will be degraded with details and discriminations among different structures being lost. Brightness of different parts/depths of the image can be adjusted individually to obtain an optimum image quality. This allows the ultrasonographer to adjust the gain individually for different objects at different depths from the surface. Echoes from the objects from near field are stronger and can be reduced in amplitude (gain reduced); the echoes from objects in far field (farther from the transducer) are weaker and can be increased in amplitude.

Zoom: Most machines allow the operator to magnify a specific part of the image for more detailed analysis.

Focus: Some machines have a focus control. This allows the operator to alter the width of the ultrasound beam at a specific point in the image, thereby improving lateral resolution in the area of interest. Other machines have automated this function such that the optimal focus point is at the center of the ultrasound image without need for machine adjustment.

Doppler control: Control of Doppler ultrasound function requires knowledge of Doppler physics and is beyond the scope of this chapter.

Calipers and freeze function: Most ultrasound machines allow the operator to freeze the image, to replay the image in slow motion for review, and to make accurate measurements of distance and area from the frozen image.

Memory function: Most modern ultrasound machines are designed with the ability to store both frozen images and video clips. Image and video capture is an essential component of good ultrasonography practice as it permits documentation, offline analysis, education, and quality review. Commercially available enterprise software solutions are available for remote storage of images and integration with picture archiving and communication system (PACS) and electronic medical records.

THORACIC ULTRASONOGRAPHY

Thoracic ultrasonography, which includes examination of lung and pleura, is a key skill for the intensivist. It is easy to learn and has useful applications at the bedside in day-to-day practice of critical care medicine. For example, it has utility for rapid diagnosis of patients with respiratory failure or for evaluation of acute dyspnea. Standard supine chest radiographs frequently are difficult to interpret due to a nonspecific opacification pattern, whereas thoracic ultrasonography allows for accurate identification of pleural effusion, consolidation, atelectatic lung, alveolar interstitial syndrome, and pneumothorax.[14] Ultrasonography has the potential to reduce the need for chest radiographs and chest computerized tomography with its high radiation exposure.[15,16]

Dr Daniel Lichtenstein is responsible for the development of lung ultrasonography. His original work in the 1990s defined the field and has been validated by many other groups. The basic principles of thoracic ultrasonography have been defined by Lichtenstein:[17]

- In the thorax, air and fluid have opposite gravitational dynamics; so by inference, in the supine patient, pleural effusion will be seen posteriorly and pneumothorax will be seen anteriorly.
- The lung is the most voluminous organ.
- All lung signs arise at the level of the pleural line.
- Lung ultrasonography is based on the analysis of artifacts.
- Lung patterns are dynamic: Serial examinations are valuable.
- Most acute lung disorders abut the lung surface.

Equipment: Any ultrasound machine that is capable of abdominal or cardiac imaging can be used for thoracic ultrasonography. Most general ultrasonography is performed with transducers with a frequency of 3.5–5 MHz. A probe of this frequency and of convex sector design can be conveniently used for longitudinal scanning through the intercostal spaces. Transducers of the 3.5–5.0 MHz frequency range do not have sufficient resolution for a detailed analysis of pleural surface pathology. However, they offer better penetration so that deeper structures can be visualized. High-frequency probes (7.5–10 MHz), designed for vascular examination, can be used for detailed pleural examination. These transducers allow excellent resolution of the pleural surface but at the expense of limited penetration and visibility of deeper structures. Most standard ultrasound machines are adequate for thoracic ultrasonography. However, some modern handheld units may lack adequate near-field resolution. When there is a pleural effusion, the inside of the chest wall may not be clearly visualized; this might lead to error in estimating the depth of needle penetration when performing thoracentesis. Some recent-generation ultrasonography machines use extensive image processing for image smoothing. This may mask standard lung ultrasound findings such as lung sliding.

Examination protocol: Lung ultrasonography in the critically ill is generally performed with the patient in supine position. It is useful to follow an organized protocol. During the SARS-CoV-2 (COVID-19) pandemic, various protocols of lung ultrasonography were proposed, differing in number of lung zones or anatomical points examined. However, a 12-zone scanning protocol, including the superior and inferior areas of the anterior, lateral, and posterior regions/zones of the chest **(Fig. 9C)**, is easy for consistent practice and remain equally useful compared to more extensive protocols.[18] The anterior zone (zone 1) is the area between the sternum and the anterior axillary line, and the lateral zone (zone 2) is defined as the area between the anterior and posterior axillary lines. With the transducer held perpendicular to the skin surface in a longitudinal scanning axis **(Fig. 9A)**, the clinician examines the underlying pleural surface and lung through the rib interspaces. By moving the transducer over adjacent interspaces, the examiner can lay down a series of scan lines and develop a three-dimensional model of the thorax by using a multiple tomographic plane approach. The posterior zone, which lies between the posterior axillary line and the spine, cannot be imaged with the patient in the supine position. If there is a requirement to examine the posterior compartment, the patient can be rolled into a lateral decubitus position; alternatively, the transducer can be pressed into the mattress and angled toward the central body mass to obtain a partial view of the posterior structures **(Fig. 9B)**. The probe should always be orientated so that the marker on the probe points cephalad **(Figs. 9A to C)**; the machine should be set to project the screen marker to the left. Maintaining this rule in probe position and machine setup helps the operator to remain orientated to the anatomic axis of scanning, as the cephalad structures of the image are always projected to the left of the screen.[19] The gain and depth setting should be optimized to achieve adequate magnification, resolution, and brightness of the structures being examined. For example, for examining the pleural surface, the depth setting should be reduced for near-field examination. For examining the underlying lung, a deeper depth setting should be used. As lung ultrasonography is often performed to address a specific question, complete scanning of all lung zones may not always be required. Supine examination of the anterior and lateral chest wall can answer many clinically important questions. Examination of the anterior chest wall rapidly rules out pneumothorax and interstitial syndrome. Examination of the lateral chest wall is useful for identification of free-flowing pleural effusions and alveolar consolidations. Small pleural effusions and posterior consolidation can be detected by examining the posterior compartment.[19]

As a standard protocol, the clinician should routinely visualize both hemidiaphragms. In a longitudinal scanning

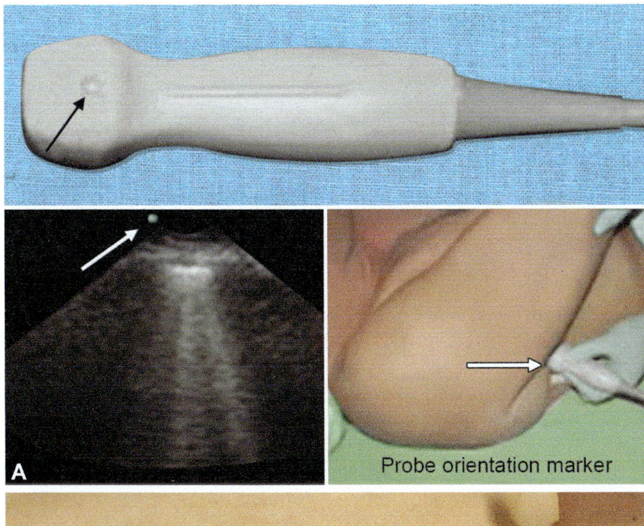

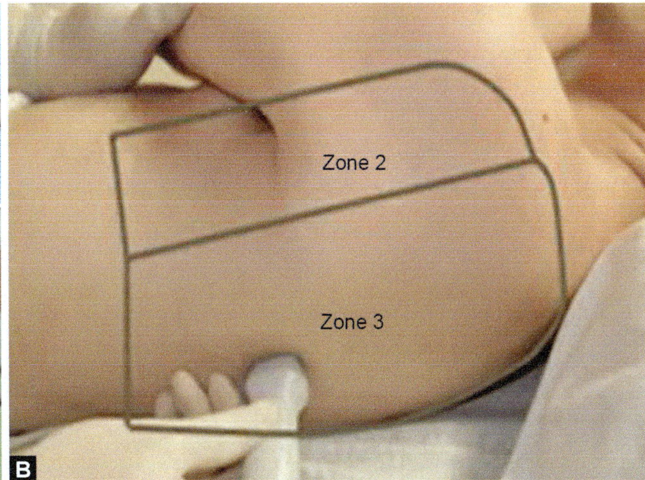

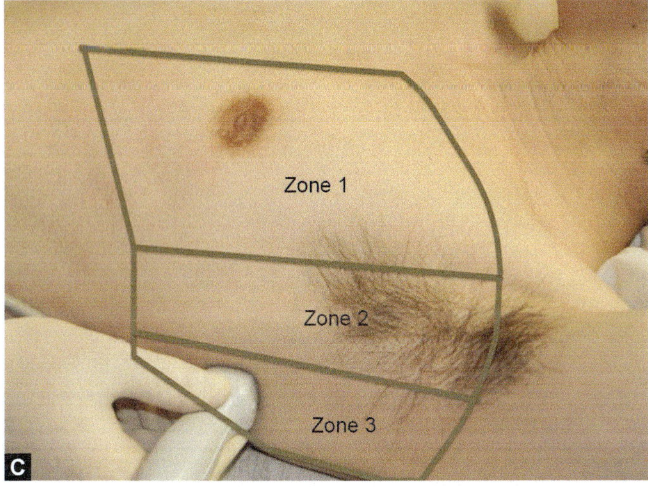

FIGS. 9A TO C: Technique of thoracic ultrasonography. (A) Probe is placed longitudinally across the intercostals space with the orientation mark pointing upward; (B) Probe placement in a supine patient to look for posterior effusion; (C) The lung can be divided into compartments for imaging.

Courtesy: Dr Pierre Kory, Pulmonologist and Intensivist, USA.

axis, the diaphragm appears as a bright curvilinear structure **(Fig. 10)** that moves in synchrony with respiration.

As an organizing principle, the large difference in acoustic impedance of ultrasound between air and tissue leads to intense reflection at any air-tissue interface. When parenchymal air is replaced by fluid or an infiltrative process, depending on the ratio of air to fluid, ultrasound findings progress from a normal aeration pattern to alveolar/interstitial edema pattern to tissue density pattern **(Figs. 11 to 13)**.

Normal findings: In a longitudinal scan through an intercostal space, the rib shadows are seen on both sides of the image and serve as a basic landmark **(Fig. 11A)**. Related to the major difference in the acoustic impedance between the chest wall and underlying air-filled lung tissue, the ultrasound beam is strongly reflected from the surface of the lung. This point of reflection of ultrasound from the lung surface corresponds to the pleural surface. It appears as a bright, highly echogenic line between two adjacent ribs, ~0.5 cm below the periosteal origin of the rib shadow **(Figs. 11A and B)**. The normal pleura is 0.2–0.4 mm thick.[20] A 3.5–5.0 MHz probe does not allow

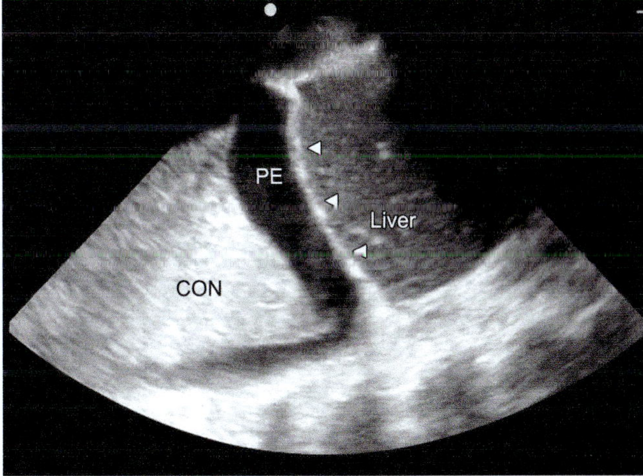

FIG. 10: In the longitudinal scanning axis, the diaphragm appears as a bright curvilinear structure (arrowheads). Also seen in the image are liver, consolidated lung (CON), and a small amount of pleural effusion (PE). The dense area of airless consolidated lung appears to have the same echodensity as liver, known as sonographic hepatization (see text).

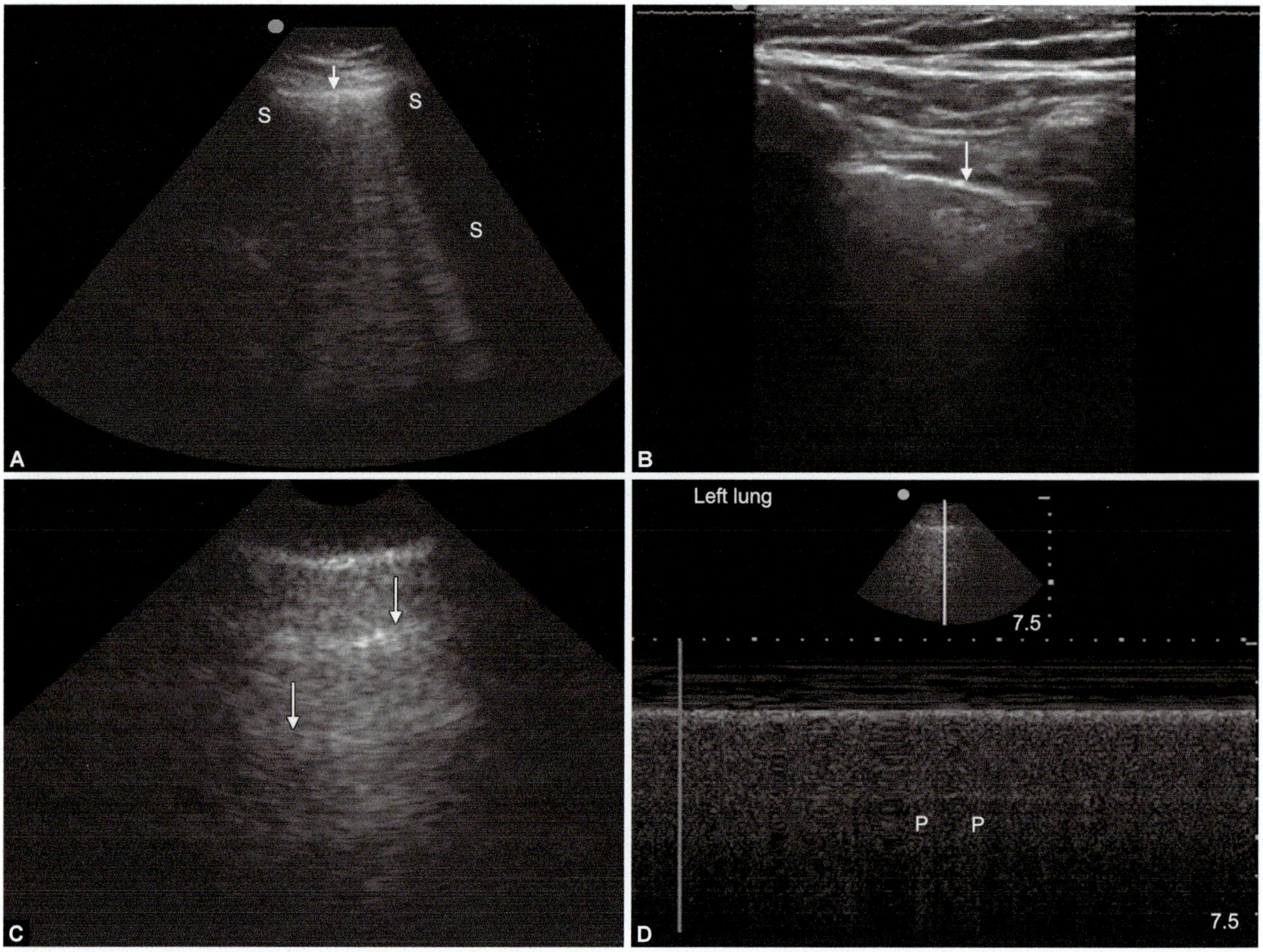

FIGS. 11A TO D: Normal findings in lung ultrasonography. (A) In longitudinal scanning through an intercostals space, the rib shadows (S) serve as the basic landmark. Pleura is seen as a bright echogenic line (arrow). (B) A high-frequency probe (7.5 MHz in this image) shows the pleural line (arrow) in greater resolution. (C) A lines (arrows) are generated by reverberation of ultrasound, a normal finding. (D) M-mode record lung sliding generates "sea-shore" pattern. Lung pulse (P) is also shown in the image.

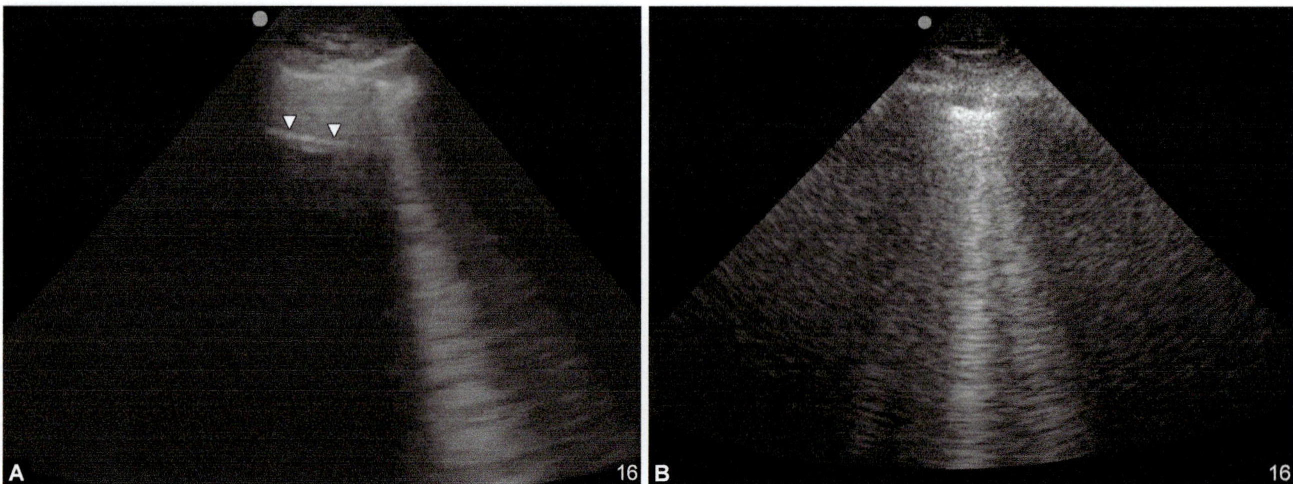

FIGS. 12A TO D: *Continued*

Continued

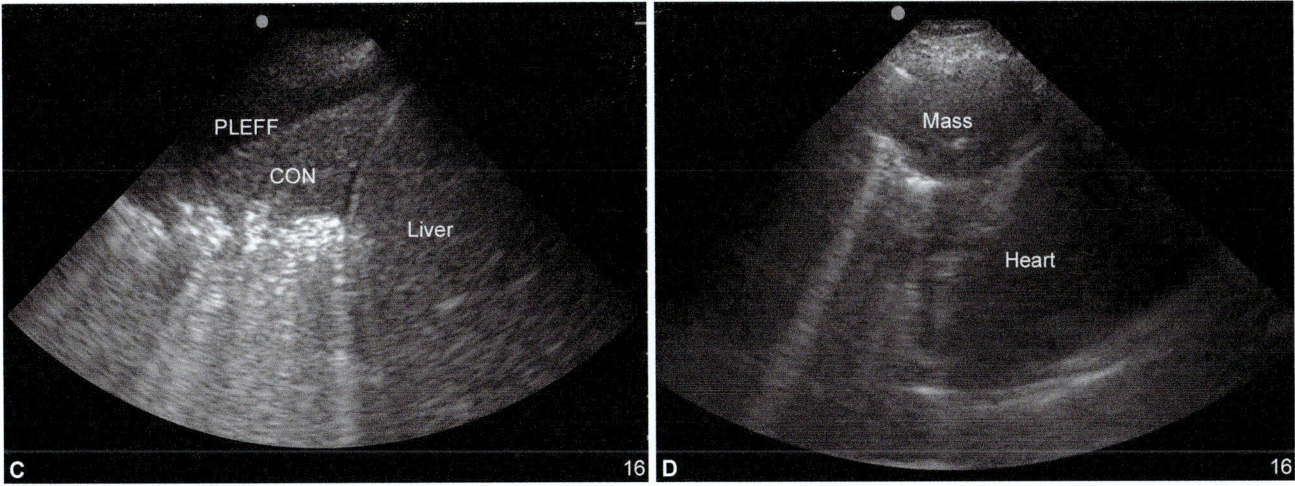

FIGS. 12A TO D: B line(s) arises from the pleural line (A) and effaces A line (arrowheads) at the intersection. Three or more B lines in a single longitudinal scan plane are considered pathological (B). (C) Multiple B lines (lung rocket) arising from the margin of an area of consolidation (CON). A small pleural effusion (PLEFF) is also seen. (D) A single B line arising from the margin of subpleural lung mass. Of note, the lung mass provided an acoustic window to visualize the heart in this scan plane. Consolidated lung can also provide a suitable acoustic window to visualize a deeper intrathoracic structure.

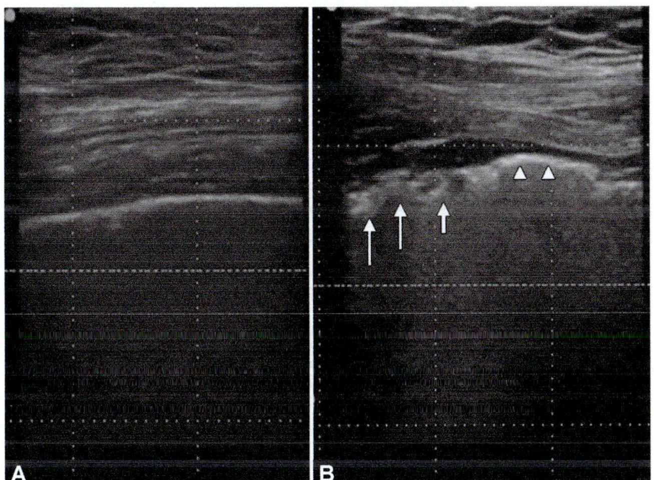

FIGS. 13A AND B: Normal and abnormal pleural morphology. (A) Normal pleural line imaged with a high-frequency probe. It is thin, smooth, and regular. (B) Pleural line in a patient with bilateral pneumonia. The pleural line is irregular and thickened at places (thin arrows). A small subpleural consolidation is also seen (thick arrow). An adjacent area of normal pleura is indicated also (arrowheads).

sufficient resolution to visualize the parietal and visceral pleural surfaces separately so that the pleural line represents a single summation interface. Aerated lung is not seen as an anatomically distinct entity because of strong reflection of the ultrasound beam at the pleural interface. However, aerated lung has a distinctive ultrasound pattern that results from reverberation artifact. Aerated lung is characterized by the presence of *A* lines which are horizontally orientated curvilinear hyperechoic lines observed deeper and parallel to the pleural line **(Fig. 11C)**. *A* lines may occur in single or multiple numbers and result from the reverberation of the ultrasound beam between the pleural surface and skin. If there is more than one *A* line in the ultrasound image, the distance between *A* lines will be a multiplicative of the distance between the pleural surface and the skin. Several *A* lines are often visible. The actual number of *A* lines has no significance as long as there is at least one.[21] *A* lines are strongly correlated with a normal aeration pattern on the chest CT scan at the site of the transducer application to the chest wall.[14] Examination of the pleural interface is characterized by two dynamic findings:

1. *Lung sliding*. This occurs due to the movement of the visceral pleura against parietal pleura in phase with respiration. Lung sliding appears as a "twinkling" at the level of the pleural line, in rhythm with respiration.[21] An M-mode examination of the pleural line reveals a pattern known as the "*sea shore*" pattern and allows the examiner to document the presence of lung sliding with a single, frozen image that can be easily printed out for documentation **(Fig. 11D)**. Lung sliding is minimal at the apex and maximal at the lung bases. The presence of lung sliding indicates apposition of parietal and visceral pleural surfaces at the site of transducer placement. The presence of lung sliding rules out pneumothorax at the site of transducer placement on the chest wall. The examiner may quickly examine multiple interspaces over the anterior lung zones, thereby excluding pneumothorax with a high level of certainty.
2. *Lung pulse*: This occurs due to the movement of the visceral pleura against parietal pleura in phase with

cardiac contractions.[22] Lung pulse is best seen at pleural surfaces adjacent to the heart, but may be observed over the right chest as well. Lung pulse can be recorded with M mode for purpose of easy documentation **(Fig. 11D)**. The presence of lung pulse indicates apposition of the parietal and the visceral pleural surfaces at the site of transducer placement. The presence of lung pulse rules out the presence of pneumothorax at the site of transducer placement on the chest wall. The examiner may quickly examine multiple interspaces over the anterior lung zones, thereby excluding pneumothorax with a high level of certainty.

Abnormal Findings in Thoracic Ultrasound

B line(s): These is an important finding of lung ultrasonography and often reflects the presence of pulmonary pathology. They have characteristic features which are as follows[21] **(Fig. 12A)**:

- They are vertical in orientation.
- They rise from the pleural line and move with the movement of the pleural line (in synchrony with lung sliding and lung pulse).
- They spread to the bottom edge of the image.
- They efface A lines at the point of intersection.
- They are narrow at their point of origin at the pleural surface and spread out as they approach the edge of the image.

It is very important that the clinician ensures these criteria are fulfilled for definitive identification of B lines. B lines may reflect significant lung abnormality and can be mistaken for mimickers (Z line and I line).[21] The location, distribution, and number of B lines determine their significance. A few B lines are often found in the lower lateral intercostal spaces in normal subjects.[23-25] Multiple B lines in the nondependent areas of lung are usually of pathological significance, particularly if they appear as multiple comet-tail artifacts. Multiple B lines evoke a pattern similar to a rocket at lift-off, and the term "lung rockets" has been used to describe the pattern **(Fig. 12B)**. A pattern that is definitively pathologic occurs when at least three B lines are detected in a single scanning position over the anterior chest **(Fig. 12B)**.[24,25]

B lines or comet-tail artifacts result from successive reverberation at the interface between air and pathologically thickened interlobular septa, at the lung visceral pleural interface.[24] This occurs most frequently when interlobular septae are distended with fluid or other infiltrative or inflammatory processes. These include interstitial lung disease, e.g., idiopathic pulmonary fibrosis or sarcoidosis,[26] acute cardiogenic pulmonary edema, lung contusion, acute lung injury, acute respiratory distress syndrome (ARDS), lymphangitic carcinomatosis, and early/resolving lung consolidation.[23,24,27,28] B lines, when focal in location, suggest a localized process such as pneumonia. The presence of diffuse B lines suggests a generalized process such as cardiogenic pulmonary edema. Comet-tail artifacts have been associated with alveolar-interstitial shadows seen on a chest radiograph and they can be considered equivalent to Kerley B lines seen on a plain radiograph. Lichtenstein et al. demonstrated tomodensitometric correlations of the thickened subpleural interlobular septa, as well as ground-glass areas, two lesions present in acute pulmonary edema, with the presence of the comet-tail artifact.[24] They compared chest CT findings with ultrasound findings and found 95% accuracy of ultrasonography in the diagnosis of alveolar-interstitial syndrome in comparison to CT scan.[14]

Acute cardiogenic pulmonary edema results in B lines. An elevation of left-sided cardiac pressures causes distension of interlobular septa in the nondependent lung zones. This distension of interlobular septa causes multiple B lines or comet-tail artifacts in the nondependent lung zones. The finding of multiple B lines is therefore a sensitive but nonspecific means of detecting cardiogenic, i.e., hydrostatic, edema. The presence of A lines in the nondependent lung zones is strong evidence that left-sided cardiac pressures are not elevated. Lichtenstein et al. have demonstrated that the presence of A lines in the anterior lung zones with the patient in the supine position indicates that the pulmonary artery occlusion pressure (PAOP) is always ≤18 mm Hg and usually ≤13 mm Hg.[29] The presence of A lines therefore excludes cardiogenic pulmonary edema as the cause for respiratory dysfunction. This fact has important clinical application as will be discussed later.

Close examination of pleural line can give a clue to the etiology of B lines. A diffuse B-line pattern due to cardiogenic pulmonary edema is associated with a smooth pleural line. If B lines result from an underlying inflammatory pathology (e.g., ARDS, interstitial lung disease, or pneumonia), the pleural surface is often irregular and additional small subpleural areas of lung consolidation may be seen **(Figs. 13A and B)**.[30]

Alveolar Consolidation

Alveolar consolidation can be diagnosed by thoracic ultrasonography. Consolidated lung has tissue density without change in dimension with respiration. It has similar echodensity to liver; hence, the term sonographic hepatization of lung has been used for descriptive purposes **(Figs. 14A to F)**. The border between the tissue density of alveolar consolidation and aerated lung may be irregular and may exhibit B lines or comet-tail artifact **(Fig. 14A)**. Punctate echogenic foci may be visible within an area of alveolar consolidation. These represent air-filled bronchi and are termed "sonographic air bronchogram".[31] Depending on the plane of scanning, they may appear as nonpulsatile, linear echoes converging toward the root of the lung or scattered echoes of variable lengths **(Fig. 14A)**. Posterior reverberation artifacts or acoustic shadowing may also be produced by echoes related to large proximal bronchi.[32] The sonographic

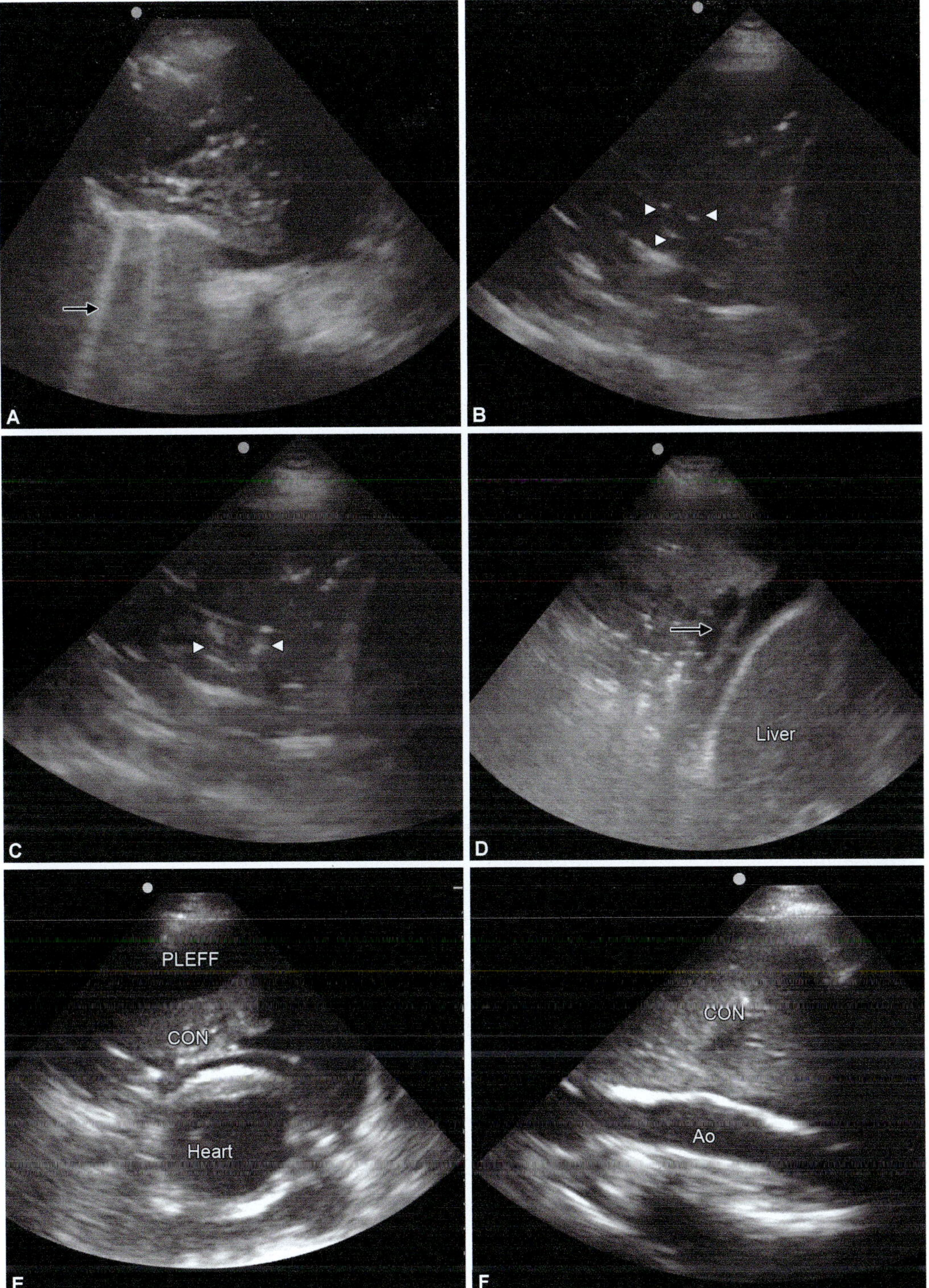

FIGS. 14A TO F: Alveolar consolidation. (A) An area of consolidation with sonographic air bronchogram (bright echogenic spots within the area of consolidation). Also seen are B lines (arrow) arising from the margin of the consolidation. (B) Dynamic air bronchogram. During expiration, within the area of consolidation, air bronchogram appears as punctuate bright spots (arrowheads). (C) During inspiration, the echogenic spots expand centrifugally toward the pleural surface into branching, echogenic structures (arrowheads) and represent air movement in the bronchi within the area of consolidation. (D) Microabscesses within an area of consolidation (arrow) in a case of necrotizing pneumonia. (E) Pleural effusion (PLEFF) providing a good window to visualize an underlying area of consolidation (CON) and the heart. (F) An area of consolidation (CON) proving a view to the underlying descending aorta (Ao); scanning done in a sagittal plane from the left infra-axillary area.

air bronchogram may be mobile and may exhibit movement that is independent of the surrounding movement of the lung related to respiratory cycle **(Figs. 14B and C)**. The mobile air bronchogram (also known as dynamic air bronchogram) indicates that the bronchus supplying that area of alveolar consolidation is patent and not blocked by endobronchial pathology. In some cases, multiple, branching, nonpulsatile, anechoic, tubular structures can be seen within the area of consolidation representing fluid-filled bronchi. These are known as sonographic "fluid bronchogram".[33] Alternatively, they may represent pulmonary vascular structures; the distinction between the two may be made by color Doppler. Sonographic alveolar consolidation can be observed only if the process abuts the pleura allowing ultrasound to penetrate through the abnormality. If the area of consolidation is deep within the lung, it cannot be visualized as aerated lung tissue between pleura and the area of consolidation will block the ultrasound. In the majority of cases, alveolar consolidation abuts the pleura, making it easily accessible to ultrasound analysis.[34] Where a pleural effusion is present, it provides an acoustic window to visualize the underlying consolidation **(Fig. 14E)**. Likewise, the presence of consolidation provides an acoustic window to visualize underlying structures that will not normally be visible, such as heart or great vessels **(Fig. 14F)**.

The finding of sonographic alveolar consolidation pattern is descriptive and does not imply a specific diagnosis such as pneumonia. Similar to plain radiography and CT scan, a sonographic consolidation pattern may result from a wide variety of pathological processes. Any disease process that results in airless alveolar structures can give rise to a sonographic consolidation pattern: Atelectasis, infiltrative processes (tumor, purulent material as in pneumonia), severe pulmonary edema with flooding of alveoli, etc.

Alveolar consolidation can be accurately diagnosed by ultrasonography. In a study of critically ill patients, ultrasonography was found to have a sensitivity of 90% and specificity of 98% with high interobserver concordance for the diagnosis of alveolar consolidation using CT scan as the gold standard.[34] Alveolar consolidation may be localized to any part of lung and its identification requires clinical correlation. In a patient presenting with fever, cough, purulent sputum, and dyspnea, demonstration of an area of consolidation suggests a diagnosis of pneumonia. In patients with necrotizing pneumonia, ultrasound is sensitive in detecting microabscesses **(Fig. 14D)**; in complicated cases, it can be used for needle aspiration guidance in order to obtain etiologic diagnosis with minor and infrequent complications.[31] Ultrasonography has been used to follow response to treatment of both community-acquired pneumonia (CAP) and ventilator-associated pneumonia (VAP). A decrease in size/number or disappearance of lesions indicates improvement in CAP.[35] In a study on VAP, gradual reaeration of consolidated areas in response to antibiotic treatment was reflected by a continuum of changing ultrasound patterns. Significant correlations between CT and ultrasonography with higher accuracy than chest radiography have been shown in predicting lung reaeration in this study.[28]

Areas of sonographic alveolar consolidation may be observed in cases of pulmonary embolism (PE). In patients with clinical suspicion of PE, the diagnosis is supported by the sonographic finding of one or more triangular/rounded/wedge-shaped areas of consolidation (consistent with pulmonary infarcts) with or without localized/basal pleural effusion.[36-38] The area of consolidation may show a central hyperechoic reflex corresponding to a bronchiole within the area of consolidation. Fresh reperfusion infarcts are homogeneous and hypoechoic; older infarcts are less homogeneous and well demarcated. Two or more triangular or rounded pleural-based sonographic ultrasound consolidations have been shown to have high specificity for the diagnosis of PE in patients with high pretest probability.[39]

The presence of dynamic air bronchogram is useful in differentiating pneumonia from postobstructive resorptive atelectasis. A pleural effusion commonly causes compressive atelectasis of the adjacent lung that has a sonographic alveolar consolidation pattern. In the case of compressive atelectasis, the bright echoes, representing air bronchogram, appear crowded toward the root of the lung.[32] Dynamic air bronchogram has been described as a helpful feature in differentiating pneumonia from postobstructive (resorptive) atelectasis **(Figs. 14B and C)**.[40] When present, they are considered evidence against resorptive atelectasis and favor the diagnosis of pneumonia. Lung sliding also suggests absence of resorptive atelectasis.[22]

Pleural Effusion

Ultrasonography is useful in the identification of pleural effusion. When the ultrasound detection of pleural effusion has been compared to chest CT scan or clinical confirmation by aspiration of fluid, its sensitivity and specificity of >90% has been recorded.[14,41] Ultrasonography is the imaging modality of choice in diagnosing pleural effusion in a supine critically ill patient.

The three cardinal features of ultrasonographic identification of pleural effusion are as follows:[19]

1. Presence of a relatively echo-free space
2. Typical anatomic boundaries that surround this space: Chest wall, diaphragm, and visceral pleural surface of the lung **(Fig. 15A)**
3. Typical dynamic findings: Movement of compressed lung during respiration.

Pleural fluid, depending on its composition, may be anechoic or hypoechoic. A simple transudate may appear black **(Fig. 15B)**, whereas a complicated pleural effusion may be more echoic **(Figs. 16A to D)**.

The typical anatomic boundaries are the inside of chest wall, the diaphragm, and the visceral pleural surface of the lung. The inside of the chest wall may be difficult to visualize if there is near-field clutter artifact. Its identification is important in order to estimate the depth of needle penetration

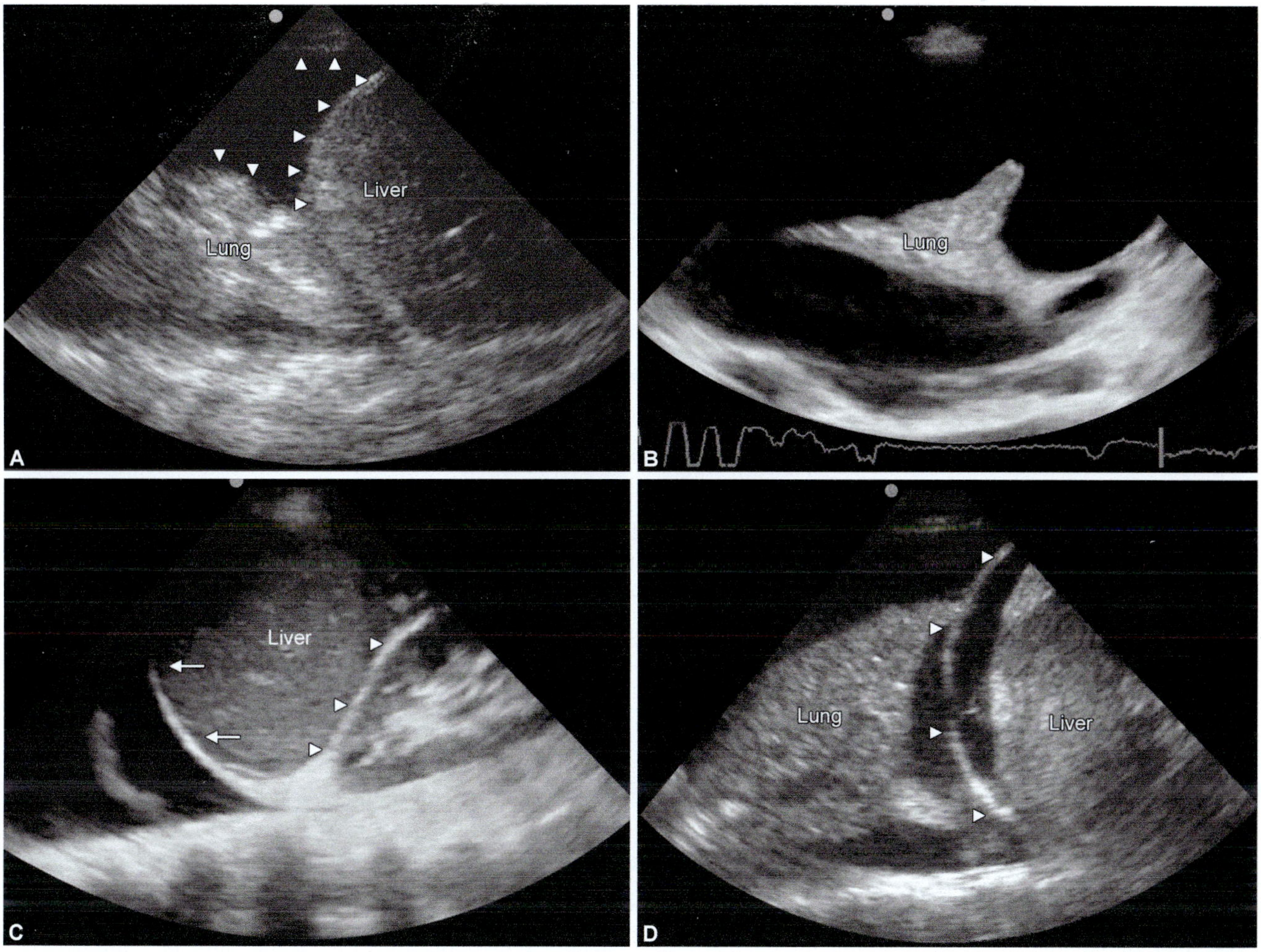

FIGS. 15A TO D: Pleural effusion. (A) Pleural effusion is identified by the typical anatomical boundaries (arrows): Chest wall (above), diaphragm (right), and visceral pleural surface (left). (B) Large pleural effusion. A typical transudative effusion is completely anechoic. (C) Identifying the diaphragm (arrows) and liver/spleen below the diaphragm is critically important. The hepatorenal recess (arrowheads) may be erroneously identified as diaphragm and the liver as a complex pleural effusion, by an inexperienced operator. An attempted thoracentesis, in such a case, will lead to liver injury. (D) Small pleural effusion. The patient also has ascites, seen as a hypoechoic area below the diaphragm (arrowheads). Compressed lung shows an alveolar consolidation pattern.

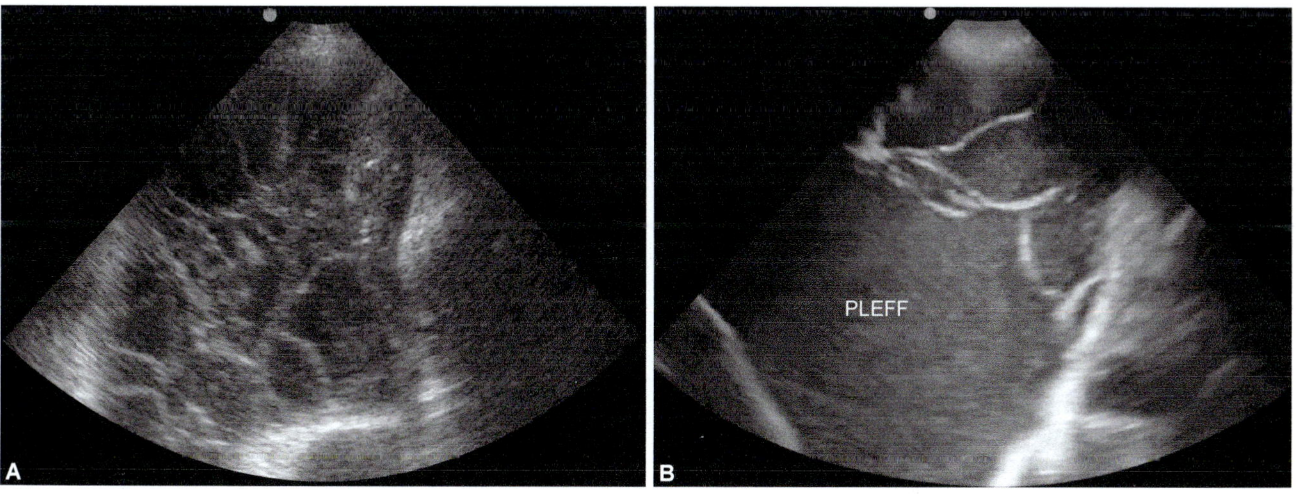

FIGS. 16A TO D: *Continued*

Continued

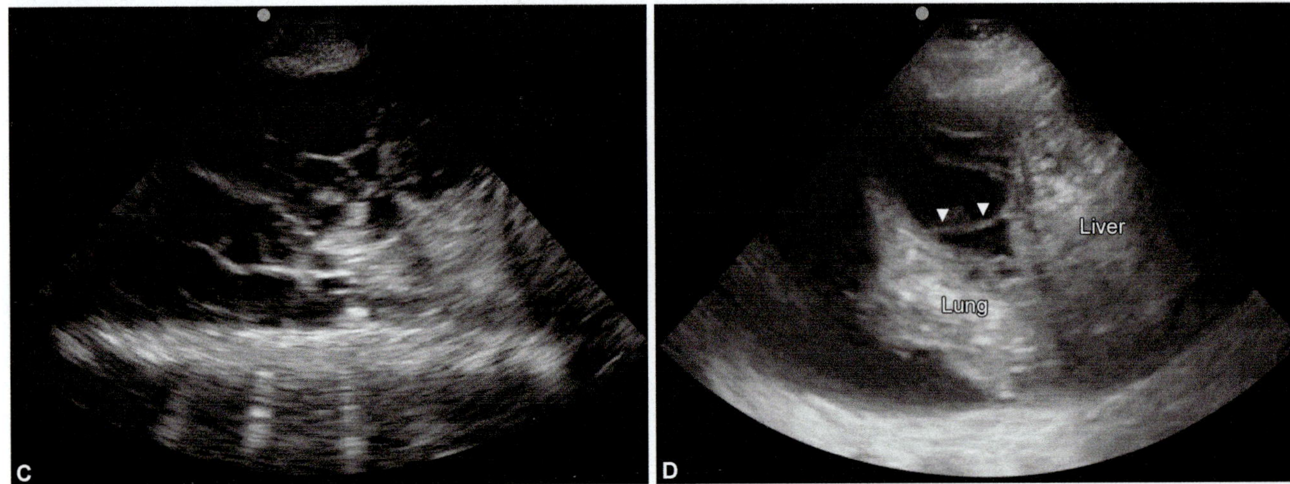

FIGS. 16A TO D: Complex pleural effusion. (A) Echogenicity within the pleural fluid indicates complex pleural effusion. Also note the developing septations and loculations. (B) Echogenic pleural fluid (PLEFF) in a case of hemothorax. (C) Complex pleural effusion with multiple loculi. (D) Septations (arrowheads) within a pleural fluid collection.

needed to enter the pleural space. The diaphragm is identified as a curvilinear hyperechoic structure that moves with the respiratory cycle. The liver or spleen is identified below the diaphragm **(Fig. 15C)**. The visceral pleural surface of the lung demarcates the lung adjacent to the pleural effusion. The lung that is adjacent to a pleural effusion will have features of an ultrasonographic alveolar consolidation pattern due to compressive atelectasis **(Fig. 15D)**.

The dynamic findings characteristic of pleural effusion **(Figs. 17A to C)** include *lung flapping* or *jellyfish sign* **(Fig. 17B)** which is the undulating movement of compressed lung within the pleural effusion. A *curtain sign* occurs when the aerated lung enters the scanning field during the respiratory cycle and obscures visualization of the effusion. Cellular components within an effusion may have respirophasic or cardiophasic movement known as *plankton sign* **(Fig. 17A)**. Complex effusion may have undulating septations or fronds **(Fig. 16D)**. M-mode ultrasound examination of the visceral pleural surface at the interface of the effusion often shows a *sinusoidal pattern*, reflecting movement of the pleural surface within the fluid-filled space **(Fig. 18)**.

Free-flowing fluid within the pleural cavity assumes a dependent position within the thorax due to gravitational forces. A loculated pleural effusion may be located in non-dependent areas of the thorax. In supine patients, a moderate-to-large pleural effusion can generally be identified by scanning in the mid or posterior axillary line. Small pleural effusion may be difficult to identify due to a posterior location. The operator may need to press the transducer on the mattress and angle the ultrasound beam toward the central body mass **(Fig. 9C)**. Alternatively, the patient needs to be placed in lateral decubitus position to scan the posterior areas.

Estimation of pleural fluid volume (PEV): Several methods have been described for accurate estimation of pleural fluid volume based on ultrasonography findings.[42,43] Remérand et al. described a multiplanar approach to measure PEV.[44] In their study, contiguous paravertebral intercostal spaces were scanned to detect the upper and the lower limits of the effusion. They showed good correlation of ultrasound PEV with either the volume of the drained pleural effusion or CT-based estimation of PEV.[44] The advantage of very accurate estimation of PEV remains to be established. In frontline critical care practice, it may suffice to identify the volume in qualitative terms: Small, moderate, or large, to guide the intensivist in the management of the effusion.

Characterization of pleural fluid: Pleural fluid echogenicity, in combination with a patient's clinical history, gives important clues regarding its etiology. Transudates are generally anechoic. Exudative effusions have a variable amount of echogenicity. However, exudative effusions may occasionally be anechoic. Exudative effusions may demonstrate the *plankton sign* (see above) or swirling echoes and strands that give them a heterogeneously echogenic appearance. Highly cellular exudates like empyema or hemothorax can have a homogeneously echogenic appearance **(Fig. 16B)**. Such richly cellular effusions can form a bilayer effect where the cellular components sediment in a dependent area within the effusion under gravitational effect (*hematocrit sign*; **Fig. 17C**). A complex parapneumonic effusion or empyema can be suspected by finding septations, loculations, or stranding within the effusion **(Figs. 16A to D)**. Pleural ultrasonography is superior in identifying septations within pleural fluid compared to CT scan.[45]

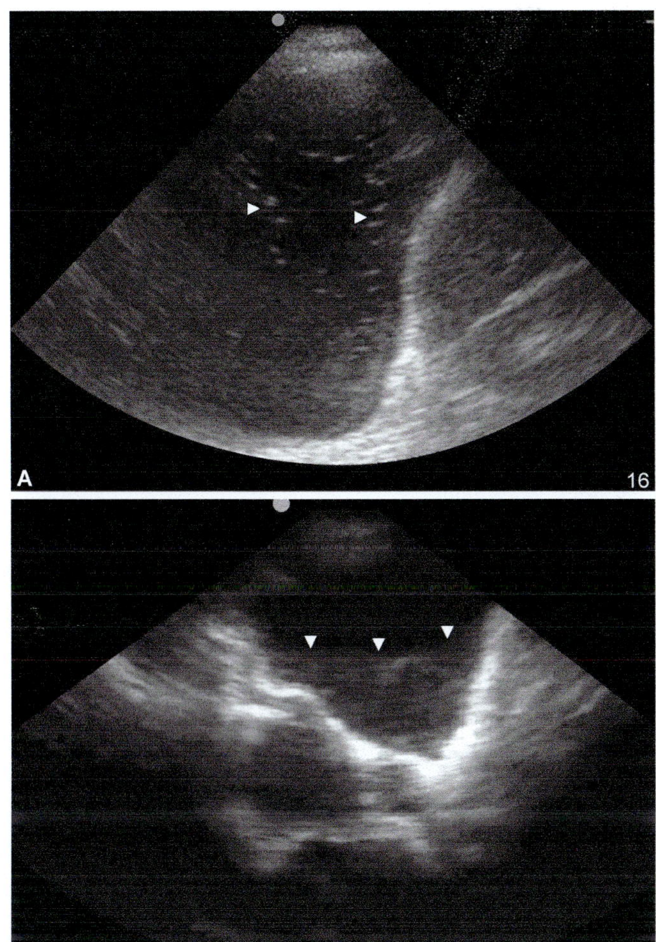

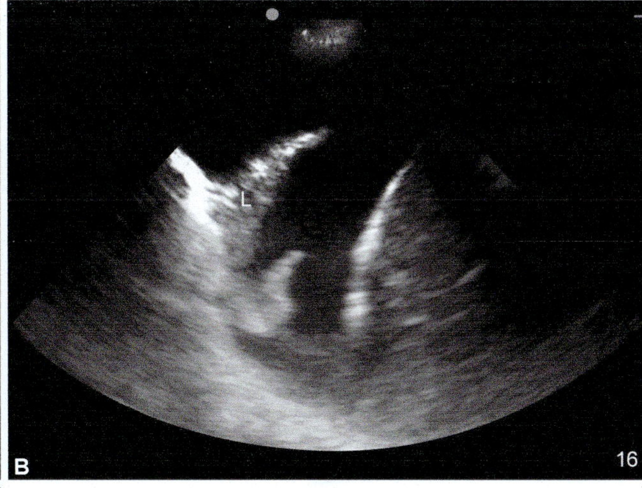

FIGS. 17A TO C: Other signs in pleural effusion. (A) Complex pleural effusion with multiple echogenic foci (arrowheads). In real-time scanning, slow swirling motion of this echogenic material is known as "plankton sign". (B) In real-time scanning, the compressed lung shows an undulating movement, known as lung flapping or jellyfish sign. (C) Hematocrit sign: In a richly cellular effusion, the cellular components can sediment forming a bilayer effect (arrowheads).

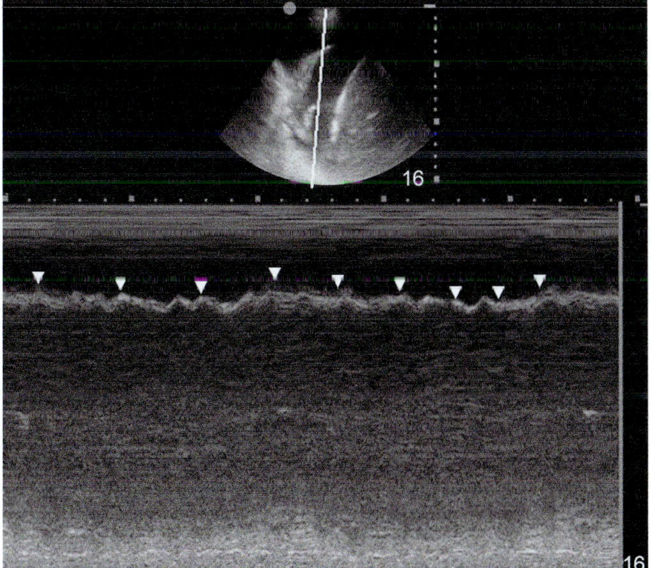

FIG. 18: Sinusoid sign. M-mode examination of the visceral pleural surface shows a sinusoidal pattern (arrowheads) reflecting movement of the visceral pleural surface within the effusion.

Important Clinical Applications of Thoracic Ultrasonography

The knowledge of thoracic ultrasonography gives the intensivist the ability to immediately assess the critically ill patient at point of care. The clinician can immediately and repeatedly gather information or identify major problems more rapidly and accurately than can be obtained by the standard supine chest radiography. The reader is strongly encouraged to develop skill in thoracic ultrasonography and become proficient in its clinical application in the bedside management of their ICU patient.

Evaluation for Pneumothorax

Pneumothorax may occur following procedures, may be an underlying cause for cardiopulmonary failure, and, when it occurs in a patient on mechanical ventilatory support, it may be immediately life-threatening due to tension physiology. Standard chest radiography is unreliable in diagnosing pneumothorax.[46,47-49] Thoracic ultrasonography is a reliable method to exclude pneumothorax with diagnostic performance that is comparable to the reference standard and CT scan[49,50] and superior to chest radiography. It may decrease the need for CT.[51] The presence of sliding lung rules out pneumothorax at the site of examination with 100% negative predictive value.[52] The presence of lung pulse[22] or B lines rules out pneumothorax as the generation of these ultrasound signs depends on apposition of the two pleural surfaces.[17,24] In the supine patient, free air in a pneumothorax space accumulates anteriorly (with the rare exception of loculated pneumothorax)[53] so that rapid scanning at several points over the anterior lung zones rules out pneumothorax if lung sliding is present.

While the *presence* of lung sliding rules out pneumothorax in an absolute sense, its *absence* does not rule in pneumothorax. The absence of lung sliding or lung pulse is only suggestive of a pneumothorax. A pneumothorax interposes air between the visceral and the parietal pleura so that lung sliding and lung pulse are lost. However, there are other causes of loss of lung sliding:

- Pleural symphysis
- Inadequate respirophasic expansion of lung: Dense consolidation, severe ARDS, advanced fibrosis, and atelectasis from endobronchial occlusion, may all cause loss of lung sliding due to the fact that the underlying disease process restricts air entry during respiration. Lung pulse and B lines may still be present in these cases which is helpful. Apnea will result in loss of lung sliding although lung pulse continues until cardiac arrest supervenes.

When the intensivist checks for lung sliding immediately before central venous access or thoracentesis, the finding of loss of lung sliding immediately following the procedure is strong evidence of procedure-related pneumothorax.[54,55] The absence of lung sliding can easily be documented on an M-mode examination of lung **(Fig. 19A)**.

While the absence of lung sliding can only suggest the presence of pneumothorax, thoracic ultrasonography may be used to diagnose pneumothorax if the intensivist can identify a *"lung point"*. In a pneumothorax space, the partially collapsed lung will still be apposed to the inside of the chest wall. If the ultrasound transducer is placed at the border of apposition, the partially collapsed lung will enter the scanning plane on an intermittent basis coincident with respiratory cycle. The operator will observe intermittent lung sliding or B lines as the partially collapsed lung enters the scanning plane during the respiratory activity.[56] This sign is demonstrable at the border of the pneumothorax. This can be shown and documented by M-mode examination at the margin of pneumothorax **(Fig. 19B)**. The lung point can identify a small pneumothorax and can diagnose pneumothorax when a chest radiograph is nondiagnostic. The more lateral the lung point, the larger the volume of the pneumothorax.[51] Lung point may be absent in a large pneumothorax with complete collapse of the lung. Identification of the lung point requires advanced scanning skills as it is a subtle finding, making it a specific but not a sensitive finding.

A pneumothorax space is air filled and therefore has an exclusive *A*-line pattern. The combination of absence of lung sliding with an exclusive *A*-line pattern has a high specificity for diagnosis of pneumothorax.[56,57]

Guidance for Thoracentesis

A major application of ultrasonography is for guidance of safe thoracentesis (see Procedure section).

Clarification of Supine Chest Radiograph

Standard supine chest radiographs in the ICU are often difficult to interpret. The image is a two-dimensional representation of a complex three-dimensional structure.

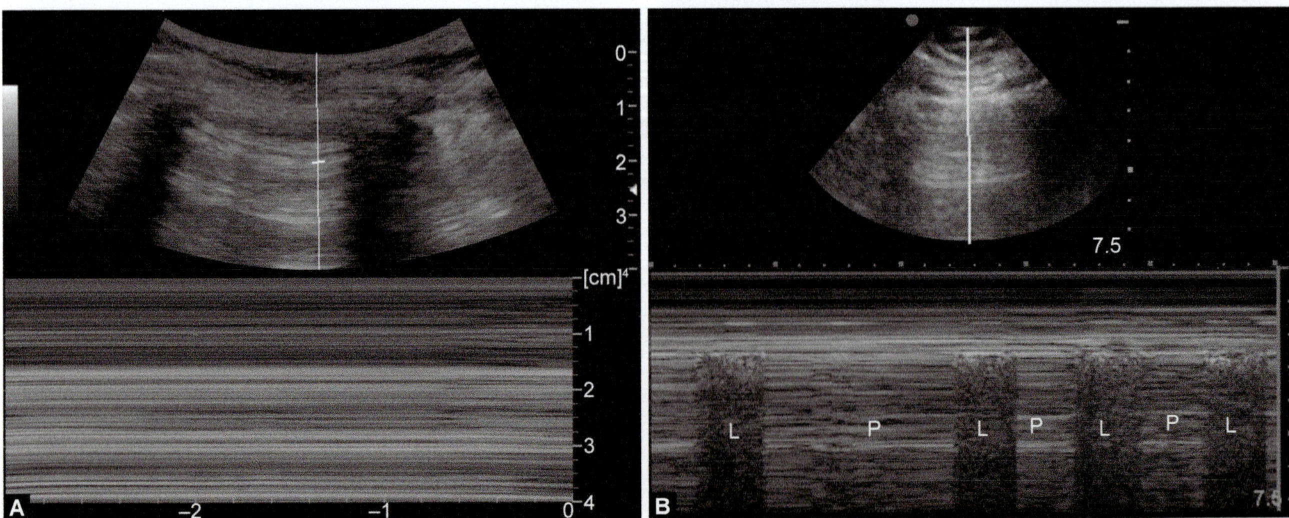

FIGS. 19A AND B: (A) M-mode examination of the lung in a case of pneumothorax. The absence of lung sliding is reflected by a straight pleural line. Also note the exclusive A-line pattern in the upper panel image. (B) Demonstration of lung point by M mode. M-mode examination at the margin of the pneumothorax shows intermittent/alternating normal lung pattern (L) and pneumothorax (P) pattern.

Combined with problems related to penetration and rotation artifacts, the resultant image results in a nonspecific summation radiodensity of the lung fields. Using ultrasonography, the examiner can rapidly and repeatedly develop a three-dimensional construct of the thoracic compartment that is superior to that derived from a supine chest radiograph. By using an organized scan line protocol, thoracic ultrasonography can diagnose pneumothorax, normal aeration pattern, alveolar interstitial pattern, consolidation pattern, and/or pleural effusion.

Ultrasound Assessment of Respiratory Decompensation

Acute respiratory failure is a common problem in the ICU. It may present in a patient who is breathing spontaneously or who is decompensating while already on mechanical ventilatory support. In either case, thoracic ultrasonography, when combined with basic goal-directed echocardiography (GDE) and lower extremity venous examination, helps the clinician to reach a diagnosis and decide upon an immediate management strategy. Lichtenstein et al. have demonstrated the excellent performance of thoracic ultrasonography for assessment of acute respiratory failure.[58] The authors proposed an algorithm for evaluation of patients with acute respiratory distress termed *bedside lung ultrasound in emergency* or the BLUE protocol. Studying a cohort of 260 patients, thoracic ultrasound alone yielded correct diagnoses in 90.5% of cases. Integration of ultrasonography data with clinical assessment is likely to yield even better results.

Thoracic ultrasonography permits the intensivist to rapidly categorize the cause of acute respiratory failure. Pneumothorax, normal aeration pattern, alveolar–interstitial pattern, consolidation, and/or pleural effusion are readily identified at the bedside of the decompensated patient. A very specific application of thoracic ultrasonography is in the management of the acutely dyspneic patient who may have respiratory failure due to cardiogenic pulmonary edema. Cardiogenic pulmonary edema results from elevation of hydrostatic pressure within the pulmonary capillary system due to elevation of left heart filling pressures. Lichtenstein et al. have demonstrated that presence of anterior *A* lines indicates that PAOP is ≤18 mm Hg and usually ≤13 mm Hg. Therefore, in an acutely dyspneic patient, presence of *A* lines rules out cardiogenic pulmonary edema in an absolute sense. In an acutely dyspneic patient, anterior *A* line suggests airway disease, metabolic dysfunction, PE, or neurological causes for the dyspnea. However, the presence of multiple anterior B lines is a nonspecific finding. Multiple anterior B lines may result from hydrostatic pulmonary edema but may have many other potential causes.

Miscellaneous Applications

Lung ultrasonography can be integrated in the hemodynamic evaluation of acute circulatory failure. After ruling out an obstructive cause of shock, e.g., PE, empirical fluid challenge can be considered if lung ultrasonography shows an A-line pattern.[59] Similarly, lung ultrasonography can be used to determine the end-point of fluid resuscitation as development of new B lines will indicate an increase in extravascular lung water.[60] During mechanical ventilation, lung ultrasound can be a useful tool in titration of positive end expiratory pressure (PEEP) for lung recruitment.[61] Ultrasound changes in lung aeration during a spontaneous breathing trial have been reported to predict postextubation respiratory distress.[62]

Limitations of Thoracic Ultrasonography

Thoracic ultrasonography has some specific limitations:[19]

- Obesity, edema, subcutaneous emphysema, chest wall dressings, wounds, and body position all may prevent adequate image acquisition.
- Some modern machines with extensive postacquisition image processing have near-field clutter which degrades image quality.
- Difficulty may arise in differentiating a complex pleural effusion from a consolidation. A hemothorax or empyema may be hyperechoic and lack dynamic findings. Air within a pleural effusion may further confuse the interpretation. With this complexity, chest CT may be required in this type of difficult cases. An air or fluid bronchogram supports a diagnosis of consolidation whereas a sinusoidal pattern on M-mode examination is typical of pleural effusion.[34]
- Thoracic ultrasonography requires that the clinician is adequately trained in the field. For example, in identifying B lines, the examiner must have knowledge of their mimics: I and Z lines.[21] Sliding lung and lung point may be subtle findings.
- Identification of a pleural effusion is straightforward if it is a large anechoic collection. On the other hand, an empyema or hemothorax may have a dense homogeneous echogenic pattern, similar to liver and spleen, without any visible septation. They may lack dynamic changes due to their density.
- Application of lung ultrasonography results requires that the intensivist be able to integrate the findings into their overall analysis of pathophysiology and clinical circumstances.

CRITICAL CARE ECHOCARDIOGRAPHY

Introduction

Hemodynamic failure is a common feature of critical illness as is respiratory failure that derives from cardiac dysfunction. Echocardiographic assessment of hemodynamics is a key component of assessment and management of the critically ill. Mastery of CCE is therefore an important component of CCUS. CCE has become an essential branch of CCUS and has gained general acceptance.[63]

Basic Critical Care Echocardiography Versus Advanced Critical Care Echocardiography

Critical care echocardiography may be divided into two levels of competence: Basic and advanced. Basic CCE is a skill that can be acquired with a short period of training and should be considered as a standard part of competence in CCUS. Competence in advanced CCE requires a long period of training similar in scope to that required for cardiology echocardiographers.[64] For the purpose of frontline critical care applications, most intensivists do not need advanced-level competence in echocardiography, as important clinical problems may be identified and managed by the intensivist with the basic-level training.

Basic CCE uses rapid, real-time, visual two-dimensional assessment of cardiac structure and function with specific focused objectives.[65,66] It includes assessment of cardiac anatomy, global wall motion, biventricular function, gross valvular pathology, pericardium, and IVC size **(Box 2)**.[4]

Advanced CCE includes all elements of the basic examination with the comprehensive assessment of segmental wall function, valvular function, and all elements of standard cardiology-type Doppler examination (color and spectral). Advanced CCE also includes assessment of preload sensitivity and hemodynamic function, applications specific to critical care practice. Consensus competency guidelines for intensivists in advanced CCE have been published.[4,64]

Both basic and advanced CCE are performed within the context of the clinician being competent in the other aspects of CCUS. The value of the cardiac evaluation is amplified if the intensivist uses a whole-body approach to CCUS.

Equipment

Both basic and advanced CCE require an ultrasonography machine capable of cardiac imaging, with a phased array transducer with the frequency range of 3.5–5.0 MHz. Phased array transducers used for cardiac ultrasonography have a small footprint so that they can scan between rib interspaces. Transducers used for cardiac ultrasonography are capable of performing other aspects of CCUS. Full Doppler capability is essential for performing advanced CCE. Basic CCE may be performed without Doppler capability.

BOX 2 Competence in basic critical care echocardiography.[4]

- Ability to recognize common echocardiographic patterns
- Ability to assess LV size and global systolic function
- Ability to recognize homogeneous and heterogeneous LV contraction pattern
- Ability to assess global RV size and contraction
- Assessment for pericardial fluid and diagnosis of tamponade
- IVC size and respiratory variation
- Basic color Doppler assessment for (severe) valvular regurgitation

(IVC: inferior vena cava; LV: left ventricular; RV: right ventricular)

Basic CCE

Image Acquisition

Basic CCE relies on five views that are used to answer a limited number of clinical questions.

1. *Parasternal longitudinal-axis view (PSL):* The transducer is placed in the left parasternal area, in the fourth intercostal space, with the index marker oriented toward the right shoulder. By adjustment of probe angle and position, the examiner seeks a tomographic plane such that the image includes right ventricular outflow tract (RVOT), interventricular septum, left atrium (LA), left ventricular outflow tract (LVOT), aortic valve (AV), and mitral valve (MV) **(Fig. 20A)**. An adequate PSL view bisects the aortic and mitral valves and includes the LV cavity in its longest axis. The PSL view allows evaluation of left ventricular (LV) size and function, RVOT, septal kinetics, valvular morphology, and pericardial effusion.
2. *Parasternal short-axis view (PSS)*: Once an adequate PSL has been obtained, the transducer is rotated 90° clockwise without any angulation or tilting. This yields the PSS view. By movement and angulation of the transducer, the examiner seeks to establish a cross-sectional view of LV at the papillary muscle level, RV, and interventricular septum **(Fig. 20B)**. An adequate view positions the LV cavity at the center of the screen. The PSS view allows evaluation for pericardial effusion, global and segmental LV function, and septal kinetics.
3. *Apical four-chamber view (A4C):* The transducer is placed at the LV apex with the index marker oriented toward the left shoulder. By movement and angulation of the transducer, the examiner seeks to establish a view from the apex of the RV, the LV, the right atrium (RA), and the LA that bisects the mitral orifice. In this view, both ventricles, atria, interatrial and interventricular septa, mitral valve and the tricuspid valve (TV), and pericardium can be visualized **(Fig. 20C)**. The A4C view allows evaluation of RV/LV size and function, septal kinetics, and pericardial effusion. This view has major utility in advanced CCE for Doppler-based examination of mitral and TVs and segmental analysis. These are not within the scope of basic CCE.
4. *Subcostal view*: The transducer is placed below the xiphoid process with the index marker oriented toward the left flank. The transducer is held on its top surface in near horizontal position with the bottom surface contacting the patient. The subcostal view allows evaluation for RV/LV size and function, interatrial septal anatomy and function, and pericardial effusion **(Fig. 20D)**.
5. *Inferior vena cava (IVC) view:* The transducer is placed in the right paramedian subcostal position in order to scan the IVC in a longitudinal axis. If air within the transverse

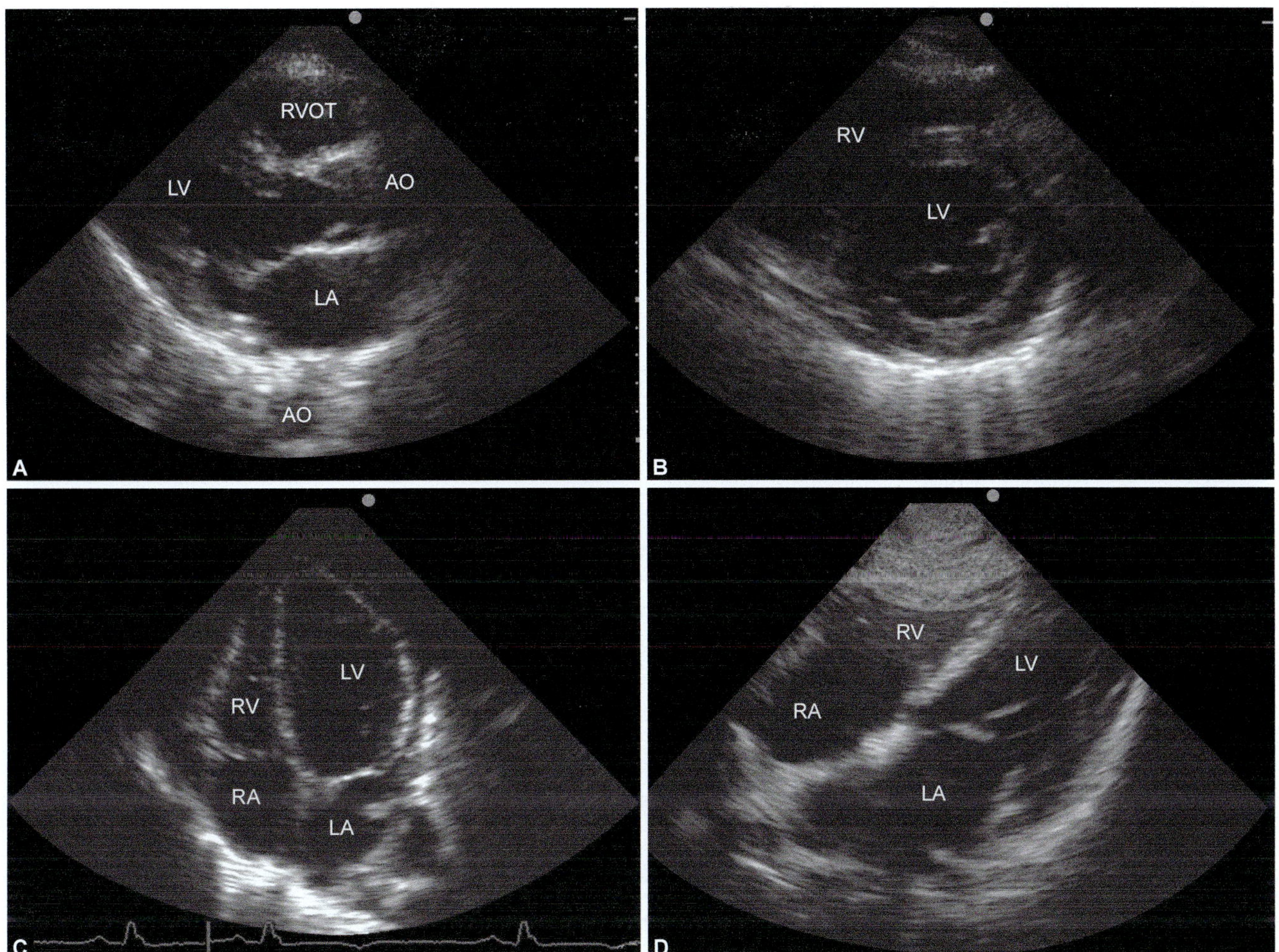

FIGS. 20A TO D: Standard view in basic CCE. (A) Parasternal long-axis view; (B) Parasternal short-axis view; (C) Apical four-chamber view; (D) Subcostal (four-chamber) view.
(CCE: critical care echocardiography)

colon blocks this view, the examiner may attempt a transcostal right paramedian longitudinal axis view or a right lower midaxillary longitudinal axis view. This view visualizes the IVC in the longitudinal axis and is useful in assessing preload sensitivity.

Competence in basic CCE may include qualitative assessment of valve function using color Doppler to assess for severe valvular regurgitation. Comprehensive assessment of valvular function is beyond the scope of basic CCE.

Challenges in image acquisition: Compared to other aspects of CCUS, image acquisition for CCE is more difficult. Ribs block transmission of ultrasound and so represent a barrier to easy examination. The air-filled lung blocks adequate examination and is often interposed between the transducer and the heart. Hyperinflation due to COPD or PEEP may block all image acquisition from anterior chest and the examiner may have to rely on the subcostal image alone. In patients with obesity, heavy musculature, wounds, or chest dressings, adequate examination may be blocked. Positioning the patient in lateral decubitus frequently improves image quality but may be a major challenge in the ICU. Translational artifacts happen when the heart moves with respiratory movement. Patients who are dyspneic and are on mechanical ventilation have considerable movement of the heart during examination. The examiner may interpret changes as deriving from intrinsic cardiac contraction when they may represent movement of heart across tomographic planes related to respiratory translation. The position of the heart in the chest may result in suboptimal image acquisition. For instance, diaphragmatic elevation shifts the heart to a more vertically oriented position in the supine patient. Adequate PSL and PSS views are not possible in these circumstances.

In addition to the physical impediments, poor technique may yield factitious information. For example, in an off-axis image of the LV in a PSL view, the small size of the LV cavity may cause the examiner to conclude that the patient has a hyperdynamic LV with end-systolic effacement suggesting severe hypovolemia. In the AP4, the size of the RV may appear to be very small if the transducer is rotated too far in the counterclockwise position.

Clinical Applications

Basic CCE, performed as a part of whole-body ultrasound approach, is used for rapid assessment of cardiopulmonary failure.[67] In approaching a patient in shock, the intensivist seeks to categorize the cause of the shock and to develop an initial management strategy. The frontline intensivist uses a simple differential diagnosis for the shock state: Obstructive, cardiogenic, hypovolemic, or distributive, with the understanding that these causes may frequently coexist. Basic CCE allows the intensivist to identify the primary cause of shock. The examination may be repeated to track the effect of the intervention. A few examples will highlight the use of basic CCE in assessment of shock. Obstructive shock may be caused by pericardial tamponade or acute cor pulmonale due to massive PE. In the former, the examiner identifies a pericardial effusion of consequential size **(Fig. 21A)**. There may be accompanying signs of tamponade effect: RV diastolic collapse or RA systolic collapse **(Fig. 21B)**. In the right clinical context, the pericardial tamponade is identified and lifesaving pericardiocentesis may proceed forthwith. In case of a patient with shock and a large hypocontractile RV **(Figs. 21C and D),** massive PE is a major consideration. Lung ultrasonography with predominant A lines and presence of a deep vein thrombosis (DVT) may confirm the diagnosis and lead to immediate intervention. Within the category of cardiogenic shock, severely impaired LV function will be identified **(Fig. 21E)**. Occasionally, marked mechanical disruption of valve function and gross valvular regurgitation will be identified by the basic echocardiographer in a patient with cardiogenic shock **(Figs. 21G and H)**. Severe hypovolemic shock results in hyperdynamic LV with end-systolic effacement of cavity **(Fig. 21F)** and/or IVC that is very small in diameter (see the following text for a detailed discussion of preload sensitivity). Distributive shock may present with relatively normal echocardiographic findings. It is obvious that echocardiographic findings must always be interpreted within the overall clinical situation. Chronic cardiac dysfunction may result in major abnormality on

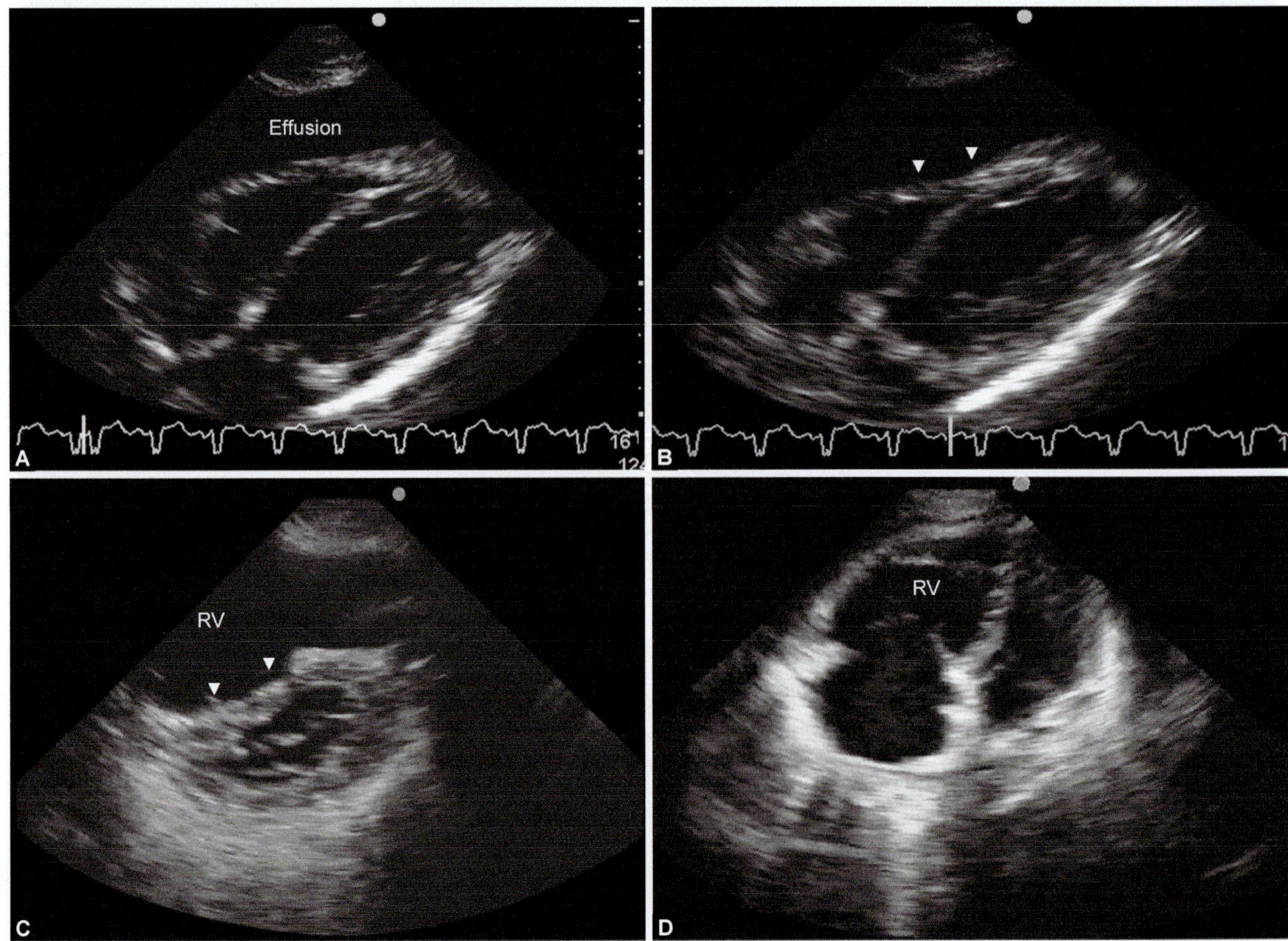

FIGS. 21A TO H: *Continued*

Continued

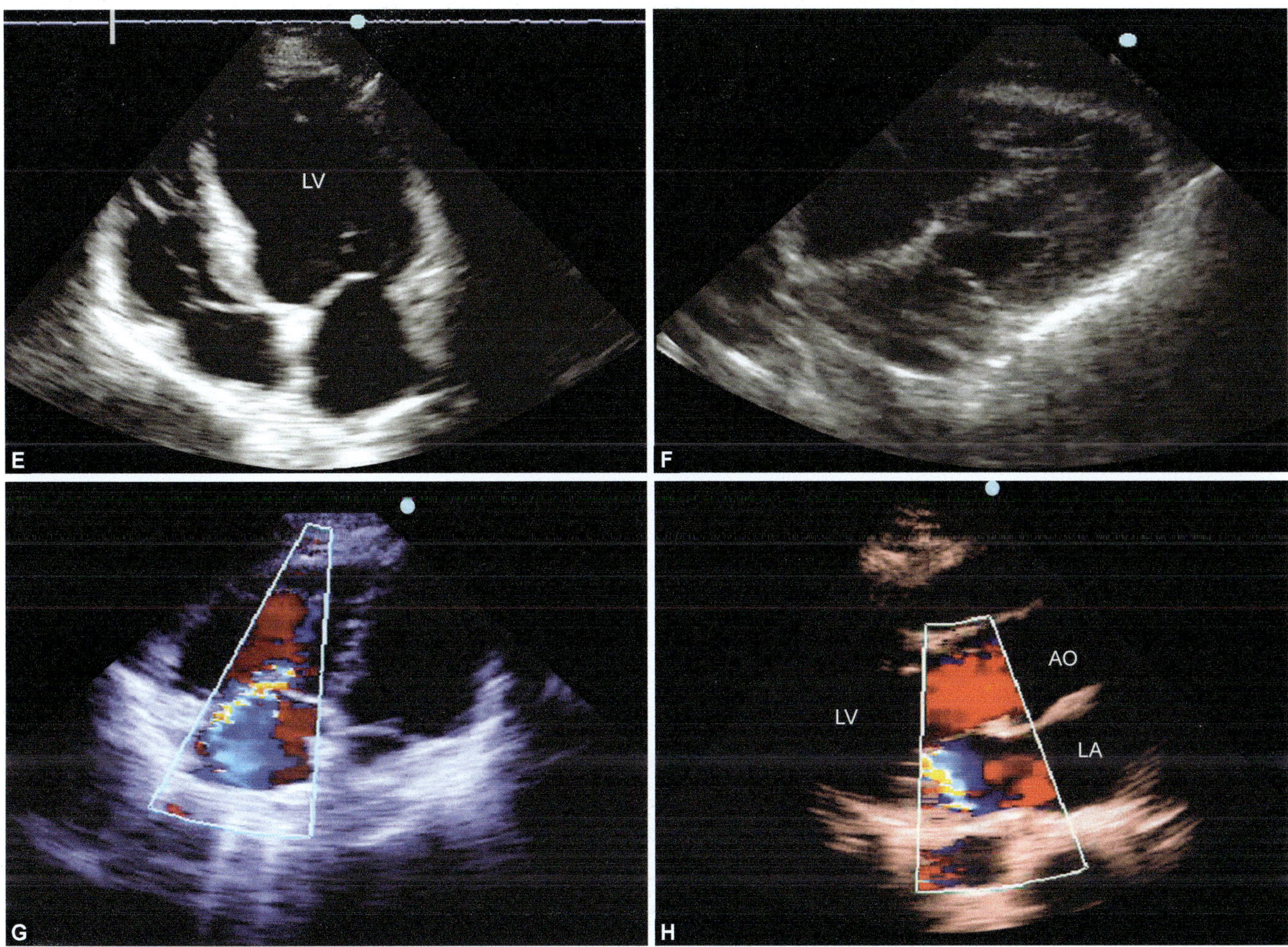

FIGS. 21A TO H: Basic CCE in the differential diagnosis of shock. (A) Large pericardial effusion. (B) RV diastolic collapse in subcostal view (arrowheads). The ECG tracing and open position of the mitral valve show that the ventricles are in diastole. (C) Large RV in parasternal short-axis view. Note the leftward displacement of interventricular septum (arrowhead), giving the LV a "D"-shaped appearance and indicating RV pressure overload. (D) Apical four-chamber view showing RV dilatation. In this view, a normal RV is usually smaller than the LV. (E) Large LV in a patient with poor LV function and hypotension. (F) Small hypercontractile LV in a patient with hypovolemic shock. Note the complete effacement of LV cavity in systole in this parasternal short-axis view (LV cavity marked by the solid white circle). (G) Color Doppler examination of tricuspid valve showing massive TR (A4C view). (H) Color Doppler interrogation of mitral valve showing MR (PSL view).

(CCE: critical care echocardiography; LV: left ventricular; RV: right ventricular; MR: mitral regurgitation; PSL: parasternal longitudinal-axis view)

screening examination, but it may not be the primary cause of the shock state. Often, there may be more than one primary cause of hemodynamic failure. The integration of image acquisition, image interpretation, and cognitive elements of CCUS is required for full application of echocardiographic findings at the bedside. An intensivist who becomes competent in basic CCE will be able to identify different clinical syndromes as listed in **Box 3**.[4]

Advanced CCE

Advanced CCE allows for comprehensive assessment of cardiac structure and function. The intensivist with competence in advanced CCE has the same level of capability in image acquisition and interpretation as a cardiologist who is fully trained in echocardiography, with the exception of comprehensive assessment of prosthetic valve function, complex congenital heart disease, cardiac source of systemic embolism, and stress echocardiography.[4] Beyond sophisticated image interpretation and interpretation skills, the practice of advanced CCE requires that the intensivist has a broad-based knowledge of the pathophysiology of cardiopulmonary failure in order to integrate the findings into the care of the patient. The cognitive aspects of competence in advanced CCE and the key questions that can be addressed

BOX 3 Competence in basic CCE: Required cognitive skills in recognition of clinical syndromes.

Severe hypovolemia
- Small, hyperdynamic ventricles with end systolic cavity obliteration
- Small (virtual) IVC, IVC with marked respiratory variation in caliber

LV pump failure
- Global hypocontractility of LV suggests pump failure
- Segmental hypocontractility suggests myocardial ischemia
- LV cavity dilatation indicates chronic cardiac disease

RV failure
- Acute cor pulmonale is manifested by RV dilatation and paradoxical septal motion
- Isolated RV dilatation suggests RV infarct
- Dilated, noncollapsible IVC is a corroborative finding

Cardiac tamponade
- Pericardial effusion (size inconsequential if tamponade is clinically suspected)
- RA/RV diastolic collapse
- Dilated, noncollapsible IVC supports the diagnosis

Acute massive left-sided valvular regurgitation
- Normal LV cavity size (LV has no time to dilate)
- Normal/hyperdynamic LV systolic function (LV volume overload)
- Massive color Doppler regurgitant flow

Cardiac arrest: Clue to etiology (see text for details)
- Tamponade
- Acute cor pulmonale
- Global LV systolic dysfunction
- Heterogeneous contractility pattern

(CCE: critical care echocardiography; IVC: inferior vena cava; LV: left ventricular; RA: right atrial; RV: right ventricular)

with advanced CCE have been defined in the ACCP-SRLF competence statement and subsequently in an international consensus statement.[4,64]

Transesophageal echocardiography (TEE) is an important component of competence in advanced CCE. In some countries, TEE is used on a routine basis by intensivists with both basic and advanced skill levels. While this is a desirable practice pattern, we recognize that many ICUs do not have availability of TEE, particularly in North America and Asia. There are certain situations where TEE is superior to TTE. Patients with inadequate TTE image quality may require TEE for definitive evaluation of cardiac function. Obesity, edema, high PEEP levels, and thoracic wounds or dressings may prohibit adequate TTE imaging. Especially problematic are patients who have thoracic trauma or have undergone post-open heart surgery. Older studies report that TTE in the ICU leads to a successful examination in 50% of attempts[68,69] in comparison to TEE with success in 90% of attempts.[70] However, evolution of TTE technology in the form of high-quality portable machines has greatly improved the yield of TTE in the critically ill. In our opinion, most patients in the medical ICU can be imaged adequately with the TTE technique. The other indication of TEE is to examine cardiac structure and function that is not well imaged with TTE by virtue of its anatomic position. TEE is particularly suited for the detailed analysis of posterior cardiac structures such as the LA and the pulmonary veins with Doppler analysis. The superior vena cava is also better visualized with TEE.

Advanced CCE differs from basic CCE in that it focuses on quantitative analysis of cardiac function and structure, whereas basic CCE gives the intensivist a qualitative assessment. Advanced CCE necessarily includes use of both color and spectral Doppler, whereas basic CCE does not. The use of Doppler requires that the intensivist has full knowledge of the physics of the technique as well as the limitations and pitfalls. Detailed discussion of the physics, limitations, and pitfalls of Doppler is beyond the scope of discussion of a Pulmonary and Critical Care Medicine textbook. A focused discussion of Doppler principle and use has been included in "Hemodynamic Monitoring in Intensive Care Unit" chapter. Competence in advanced CCE requires many hundred hours of training and image interpretation under direct supervision of an experienced echocardiographer and supervisor.

Specific Components

- *Assessment of LV structure and function*:
  - *LV volume:* End-diastolic LV area may be measured in multiple axes and used for the identification of hypovolemia. The end-diastolic area of the LV at the papillary muscle level in the PSS view is a parameter that can be used to identify preload sensitivity (see below).[71] The measurement of LV end-diastolic and end-systolic areas may be used to measure stroke volume (SV) using Simpson's method.
  - *LV contraction:* A global subjective assessment of LV function can be made and graded as hyperdynamic, normal, mildly reduced, moderately reduced, or severely reduced. Visual estimate of ejection fraction (EF) may be made very accurately when compared to quantitative measurement of EF. Assessment of LV contractile function includes observation of LV segmental function based on a standard 17-segment model defined by the American Heart Association (AHA).[72,73] The visual analysis of segmental wall function is based on thickening of the wall segments and the endocardial excursion of the wall segment.
  - M-mode analysis of cardiac function is part of advanced CCE. It is useful for a detailed analysis of high-frequency cardiac functions such as valve fluttering, premature coaptation of valve leaflets, systolic anterior motion of mitral valve, mitral valve prolapse, septal kinetics, and pulmonary valve function. The utility of M-mode examination of

ventricular function has major limitations; assessment of fractional shortening and EF by M-mode examination is prone to inaccuracy related to the complex three-dimensional structure of the heart and the possibility of asymmetric segmental wall function.

- Stroke volume may be measured with both TTE and TEE. Typically, it is measured in the LVOT but may be measured at other valve orifices, if the examiner seeks to measure quantitative valve regurgitation/stenosis or for shunt physiology. Once SV is measured, cardiac output (CO) is known and multiple hemodynamic indices can be derived using standard formula, such as systemic vascular resistance, pulmonary vascular resistance, and indices of ventricular work.

  Principles and steps in SV measurement have been discussed in "Hemodynamic Monitoring in Intensive Care Unit" chapter of this textbook.
- Other measures of LV systolic function may be derived from Doppler assessment. In the presence of mitral regurgitation (MR), continuous wave Doppler examination of the MR jet permits calculation of the rate of pressure increase (dP/dt) within the LV during isovolumetric contraction. This dP/dt is sensitive to changes in contractility and is independent of preload or afterload.[74] Systolic mitral annular descent measured by tissue Doppler gives an estimate of global LV function.[75]
- Assessment of LV diastolic function is based on Doppler assessment of transmitral filling, pulmonary venous flow pattern, and lateral mitral annular velocity. These values may be used for quantitative assessment of PAWP. Use of TEE is particularly suited for detailed analysis of pulmonary vein inflow, the results of which may be used to estimate PAWP.

- *Assessment of RV structure and function*:

Right ventricular diastolic overload/volume overload is manifested as RV dilatation. It can impair LV diastolic function, can contribute to hemodynamic failure, and has implications when assessing a patient for fluid therapy. A visual comparison of LV and RV size and RV cavity shape gives qualitative information about RV diastolic overload. A normal RV is smaller than the LV and crescentic in shape from the PSS view **(Fig. 20B)**. Both ventricular areas can be measured at end-diastole from an A4C view. Other authors have used the subcostal view.[76] The normal RVEDA:LVEDA ratio is between 0.36 and 0.6 (0.48 ± 0.12).[77] Moderate dilatation is defined as a ratio of 0.7–0.9 and severe dilatation as ratio > 1 **(Fig. 22A)**. Some authors have shown that visual analysis of RV dilatation by a trained echocardiographer correlates well with quantitative measurement.[78] RV diastolic overload results in a characteristic diastolic septal dyskinesia pattern measured with M mode and that is identified as septal paradox by 2D echocardiography.

Assessment of RV systolic function is based on a qualitative visual analysis of RV free wall and interventricular septum contraction. The contractile function can be graded as normal, mild, moderate, or severely reduced. In a patient with abnormal RV systolic function, evidence of RV systolic overload may also be present. Septal dyskinesia is the hallmark of RV systolic overload. It results when an increase in RV afterload leads to a prolongation in RV contraction beyond the end of LV ejection. This leads to a transient increase in RV pressure over LV pressure when RV is still contracting though LV has started to relax. This leads to a posterior movement of the interventricular septum.[79] This paradoxical septal motion can be observed visually and can be more precisely recorded by M mode at the mid-ventricular level from a PSL view **(Fig. 22B)**. Septal dyskinesia can also be diagnosed by measuring systolic eccentricity index (EI). From a PSS view of the LV at the papillary muscle level, measurements are taken at end-systole. D1 is measured as a diameter that bisects the papillary muscles and D2 as an orthogonal diameter to D1. D2/D1 is taken as the EI. A normal systolic EI is 1; EI > 1 indicates septal dyskinesia **(Fig. 22C)**.[80]

Right ventricular free wall thickness is assessed at end-diastole on the subcostal view. The normal thickness is 3.3 ± 0.6 mm. In the presence of features of RV systolic overload, significant thickening of RV free wall helps to differentiate between acute and subacute/chronic cor pulmonale.

- *Assessment of valve function*: Advanced CCE permits comprehensive assessment of valve function. This may be an important component of assessment of a patient with cardiopulmonary failure. In the ICU, major valve failure may be the cause of the problem. Alternatively, presence of significant valve dysfunction may contribute to compromise of hemodynamics in the patient who has another life-threatening disorder. The comprehensive assessment of valvular function requires competence in detailed 2D assessment of the anatomy of the valve apparatus. This includes identification of valve vegetations and their mimics as well as subtle findings such as valve thickening and disruption of paravalvular structures. Complete evaluation of prosthetic valve anatomy and function requires a highly competent echocardiographer who has specific training in the subject. The intensivist with competence in advanced CCE may provide screening service but may wish to call for consultation in this situation. Generally speaking, TEE is required for full evaluation of prosthetic valve function.

The evaluation of valve function starts with 2D assessment and color Doppler analysis. If significant valvular dysfunction is suspected, spectral Doppler analysis allows for quantification of both stenotic and regurgitation dysfunction. Color Doppler is frequently used in a qualitative fashion to grade the degree of

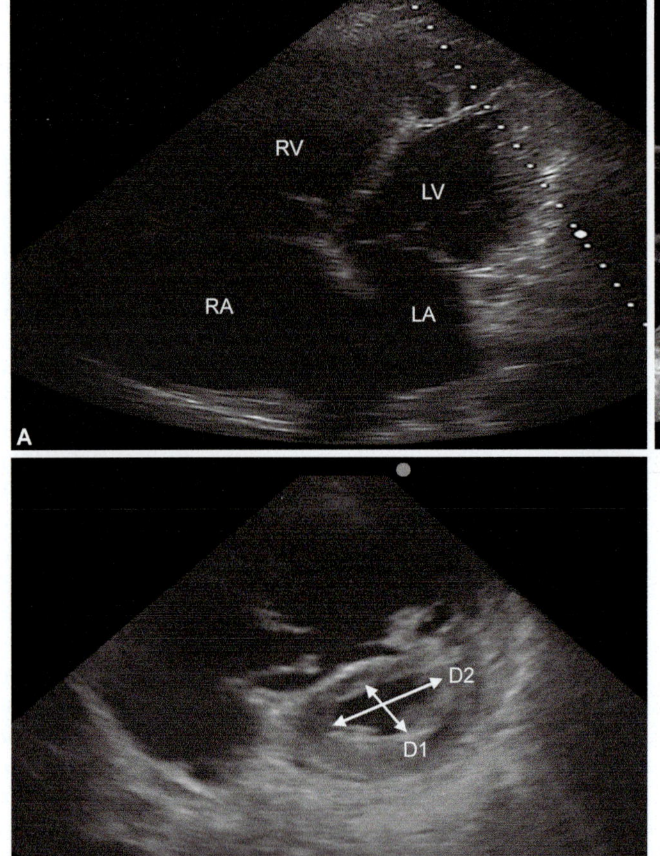

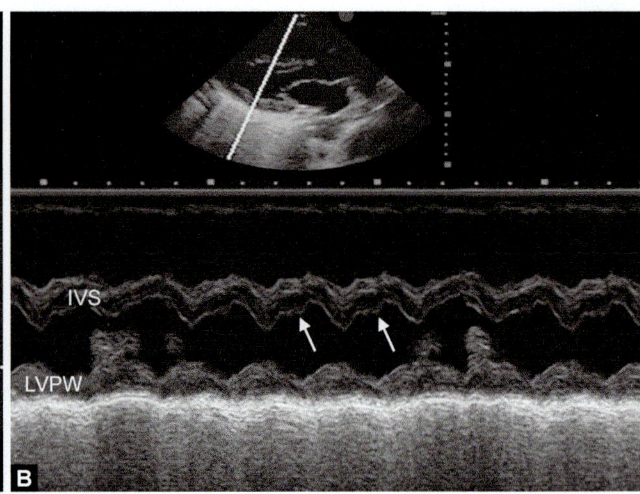

FIGS. 22A TO C: Assessment of RV function. (A) A4C view showing marked dilatation of RV. Note that the apex of heart is being formed by RV. (B) M-mode examination from PSL at the mid-cavity level. The early diastolic dip in septum (indicated by arrows) toward the LV cavity indicates prolonged RV ejection period and pressure overload. LV posterior wall (LVPW) and interventricular septum (IVS) are shown. In systole, they come toward each other; in diastole, they move away from each other. (C) Eccentricity index (D2/D1) of >1 in a patient with marked RV pressure overload. D1 is measured as a diameter that bisects the papillary muscles and D2 as an orthogonal diameter to D1.

valve regurgitation. Methods of quantitative assessment include use of the continuity equation method, the proximal isovelocity surface area method, and/or the measurement of vena contracta. Identification of significant stenosis or regurgitation includes determination of the possible etiology such as endocarditis, rheumatic heart disease, subvalvular stenosis, congenital lesion, and chordae/papillary muscle dysfunction.

- *Examination of cardiac pressures*: Advanced CCE has in common with standard cardiology echo the measurement of a wide variety of intracardiac pressures. Using spectral Doppler, the intensivist can accurately measure pressures such as pulmonary artery systolic pressure, pulmonary artery diastolic pressure, left atrial pressure (LAP), and left ventricular end-diastolic pressure. Generally, measurement of intracardiac pressures with Doppler requires that there will be some degree of valvular regurgitation or stenosis. A more detailed discussion can be found in "Hemodynamic Monitoring in Intensive Care Unit" chapter.
- *Examination of pericardial space*: The identification of pericardial effusion and qualitative identification of RV and/or RA collapse is part of the skill set for basic CCE. Advanced CCE allows the intensivist to examine other features to identify more precisely findings that favor the presence of cardiac tamponade physiology. The use of M mode permits accurate timing of wall movement of the RV and RA free wall in the PSS, subcostal, and A4C views. Tamponade physiology is suggested by diastolic collapse of the RV free wall and/or systolic collapse of RA free wall. It causes increased variation in MV and TV inflow velocities during respiratory cycling. Neither chamber compression nor variation of diastolic inflow is highly specific or sensitive for the presence of tamponade, and multiple confounders may be present in any given patient. The diagnosis of cardiac tamponade cannot be made by echo alone but rather is based on the clinical context.

Clinical Applications

It is beyond the scope of this discussion to review all aspects of advanced CCE that are relevant to critical care practice. What follows is a review of an important component of advanced CCE that is of particular interest to the intensivist but is not often included in the echocardiography performed by a cardiologist: Identification of preload sensitivity.

When managing a patient with shock, a key question is whether an infusion of volume will result in improved CO/SV, in other words, whether the patient is volume responsive (preload sensitive) or not. This is a key question for the clinician, as volume resuscitation may be of great benefit to a patient in shock but dangerous if given in the wrong circumstance. Inappropriate volume resuscitation has been associated with poor outcome.[81] There are several approaches to identifying whether the patient in shock is volume responsive. From a physiological point of view, the clinician seeks to determine whether the ventricles are on the steep portion of the Frank–Starling curve (where there will be SV augmentation with volume resuscitation) or whether they are on the flat portion (where volume infusion will not increase SV). In some clinical situations, the need for volume is clear from the history (e.g., history of blood loss, vomiting, diarrhea) and physical examination (e.g., poor skin turgor); in such cases, volume replacement is clearly warranted and can be undertaken without any further study.

A traditional approach, based on static measurement of pressures e.g. CVP and PAWP, are now known to be poor predictors of volume responsiveness with the exception of the occasional patient who has very low cardiac filling pressures.[82,83] The end-diastolic LV diameter and area are criteria that can be used for identification of volume responsiveness; an end-diastolic LV diameter of <25 mm and LV end-diastolic area of <55 cm^2 are criteria used for the diagnosis of hypovolemia.[71] End-systolic cavity obliteration is also a sensitive sign of hypovolemia and low preload.[84]

Advanced CCE permits the intensivist to make a variety of dynamic measurements that predict volume-responsive shock with a high level of accuracy. Michard and Teboul showed that significant variations in pulse pressure (PP) in patients on mechanical ventilatory support identify preload responsiveness.[85] The patients had to be passive on mechanical ventilatory support and in sinus rhythm. An arterial PP variation between inhalation and exhalation of >13% is strongly predictive of preload sensitivity and far superior to common static pressure measurements. PP in this situation is directly proportional to SV, so that the observation of significant PP variation actually represents a significant variation of SV. Using this physiological insight, the advanced echocardiographer may examine directly the variation of SV in reference to cyclical variation of intrathoracic pressure in a patient on mechanical ventilation provided the patient is passive and in regular cardiac rhythm. The ventilator, by increasing intrathoracic pressure during inspiration, alters the preload of ventricles. Elevation of intrathoracic pressure during inspiration has the effect of reducing the preload of the RV and augmenting the preload of the LV; during exhalation, the effect is reversed. Therefore, during mechanical ventilation, if SV that is measured by real-time echo varies to a significant extent, there is a high probability that the patient will have augmentation of SV following volume infusion. If there is a lack of change in SV, the patient will not have augmentation of SV following volume infusion and therefore should not receive it. As a surrogate of SV, Feissel et al. have used the velocity time integral (VTI) or flow velocity measured in the descending aorta.[86] This technique requires a transesophageal Doppler transducer and is less practical than measuring SV directly at LVOT by TTE. A variation of >12% in SV, VTI, or the flow velocity in this position indicates that the patient in shock will have improvement in SV and therefore CO following volume resuscitation.

The method of measuring SV variation with respiration has been shown to be useful only in patients who are passive on ventilatory support in normal rhythm and therefore has limited application. An alternative technique, which has been shown to be effective in spontaneously breathing patients, uses passive leg raising (PLR). Raising both legs in the supine patient to 45° results in rapid augmentation of venous return to the heart. With this simple maneuver, about 300 mL blood is delivered to the intrathoracic compartment constituting a major volume challenge which is completely reversible when legs are lowered. In performing the PLR maneuver, the intensivist measures the LVOT VTI, before and 1 minute after the maneuver. A PLR-induced increase in SV of >12% has been shown to be predictive of central hypovolemia; the same also predicted an increase in stroke volume of >15% in response to volume expansion.[87,88]

Measurement of SV variation during ventilator cycling or with PLR requires advanced CCE skills. It may be limited by poor image quality and takes time. These limitations have encouraged investigators to look for a simpler noninvasive surrogate of aortic VTI and LV stroke volume. Brachial artery peak velocity ($Vpeak_{brach}$) is one such parameter that can be measured using Doppler. Monge Garcia et al. have studied respiratory variation of brachial artery peak velocity ($\Delta Vpeak_{brach}$) to predict fluid responsiveness in mechanically ventilated patients.[89] A $\Delta Vpeak_{brach}$ value > 10% predicted fluid responsiveness, defined as ≥15% increase in SV index, after volume expansion with a sensitivity of 74% and a specificity of 95% **(Fig. 23)**. Préau et al. have shown that PLR combined with measurement of change in femoral artery flow velocity is useful in identifying preload sensitivity in spontaneously breathing patients.[90] Conceptually, variation in brachial artery or femoral artery flow is similar to measurement of PP variation with an arterial catheter and has the major advantage that it can be performed easily by clinicians with minimal training in ultrasonography.[91]

Lung ultrasonography has a role in guiding volume resuscitation in critically ill patients with shock. If such a patient has *A*-line predominance in anterior lung zone, Lichtenstein et al. have demonstrated that PAOP is ≤18 mm Hg and in high proportion of cases ≤13 mm Hg.[29] The presence of *A*-line predominance does not indicate the need of volume resuscitation but indicates that volume resuscitation can be

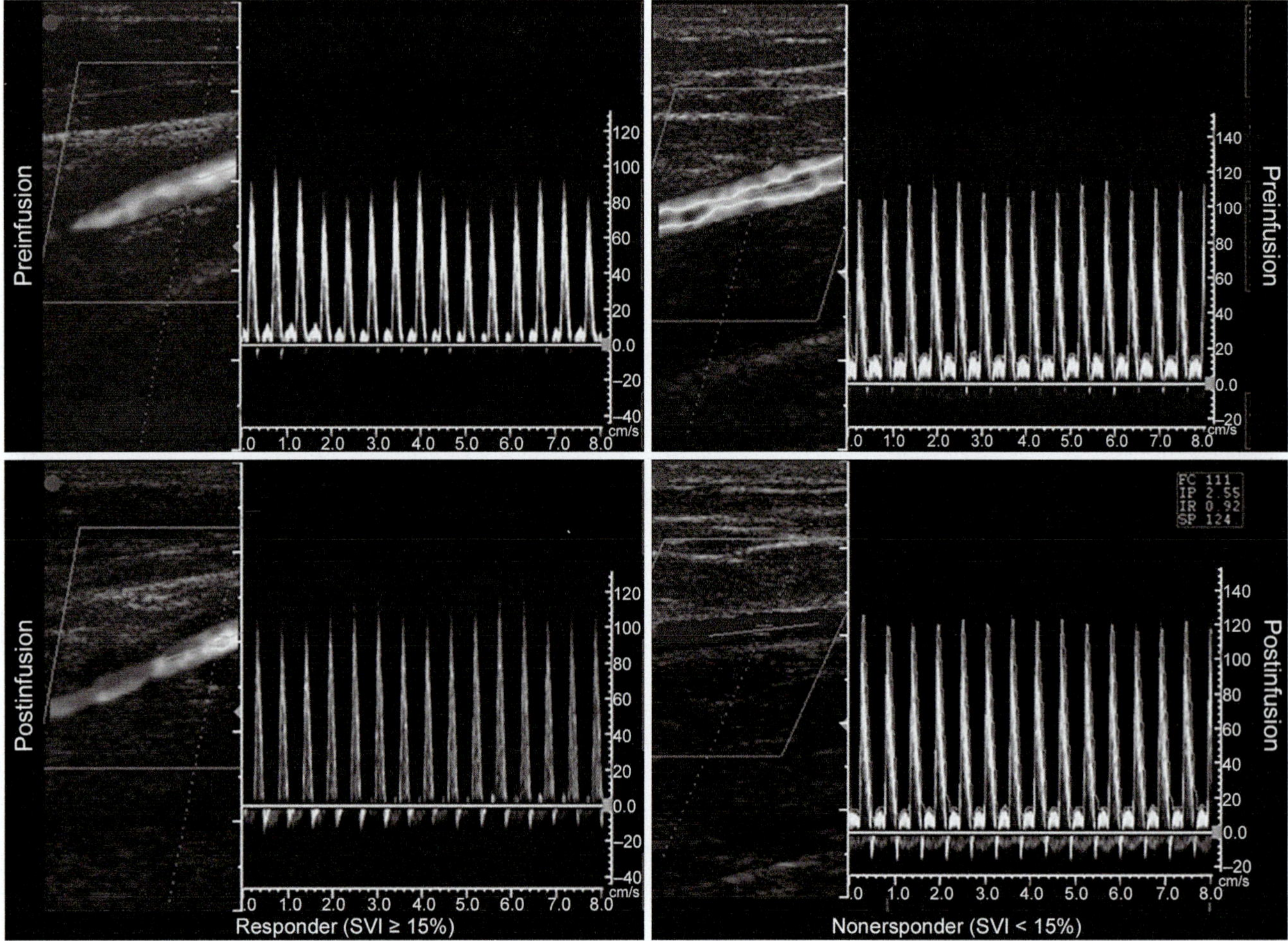

FIG. 23: Illustrative example of Doppler evaluation of brachial artery peak velocity variation in a responder and nonresponder. In the responder (left), volume expansion (VE) induced a decrease of brachial artery peak velocity variation ($\Delta Vpeak_{brach}$) by 15% (from 23% at baseline to 8% after VE). Response to volume challenge was evident in 27% increase in stroke volume index in this patient (not shown in the figure). In the nonresponder (right), volume expansion did not induce any significant change in $\Delta Vpeak_{brach}$ (from 9% to 9% after VE). Stroke volume index increased only 8% after VE in this patient.

Source: Reproduced from Monge Garcia MI, Gil Cano A, Diaz Monrove JC. Brachial artery peak velocity variation to predict fluid responsiveness in mechanically ventilated patients. Crit Care 2009;13:R142. Original publisher: BioMed Central Ltd. Image reproduced within the scope of open access policy of BioMed Central.

safely given to the patient, as the presence of *A* lines indicates that the LAP is not elevated (*vide supra*). On the other hand, appearance of *B* lines or interstitial syndrome after fluid resuscitation will suggest an end-point to fluid resuscitation.[92] Combining clinical data, basic bedside echocardiography, and lung ultrasonography, a rapid differential diagnosis of acute circulatory failure is possible.

Assessment of IVC size and its variation with respiration have been used to predict fluid responsiveness **(Figs. 24A to F)**. The exact location used for measurement of IVC diameter varies in different reports.[93,94-96,97-100] IVC diameter can be measured 2–3 cm from the RA in a longitudinal view. For accurate measurements, an M-mode tracing, perpendicular to the IVC, is used **(Fig. 24B)**. An IVC diameter of <10 mm may predict a positive response to fluid infusion.[99] Cutoff values for the difference in IVC diameter between inspiration and expiration of 12% (using max-min/mean) and 18% (using max-min/min) for IVC have been reported to accurately separate responders from nonresponders.[96,99] The above measures have been validated only in patients who are passive on mechanical ventilation, are in regular rhythm, and have normal RV function.

Variation of superior vena cava size coincident with ventilator cycling may also be used to predict preload sensitivity.[101] This requires use of TEE. A complementary and extended discussion of testing for volume responsiveness has been included in "Hemodynamic Monitoring in Intensive Care Unit" chapter.

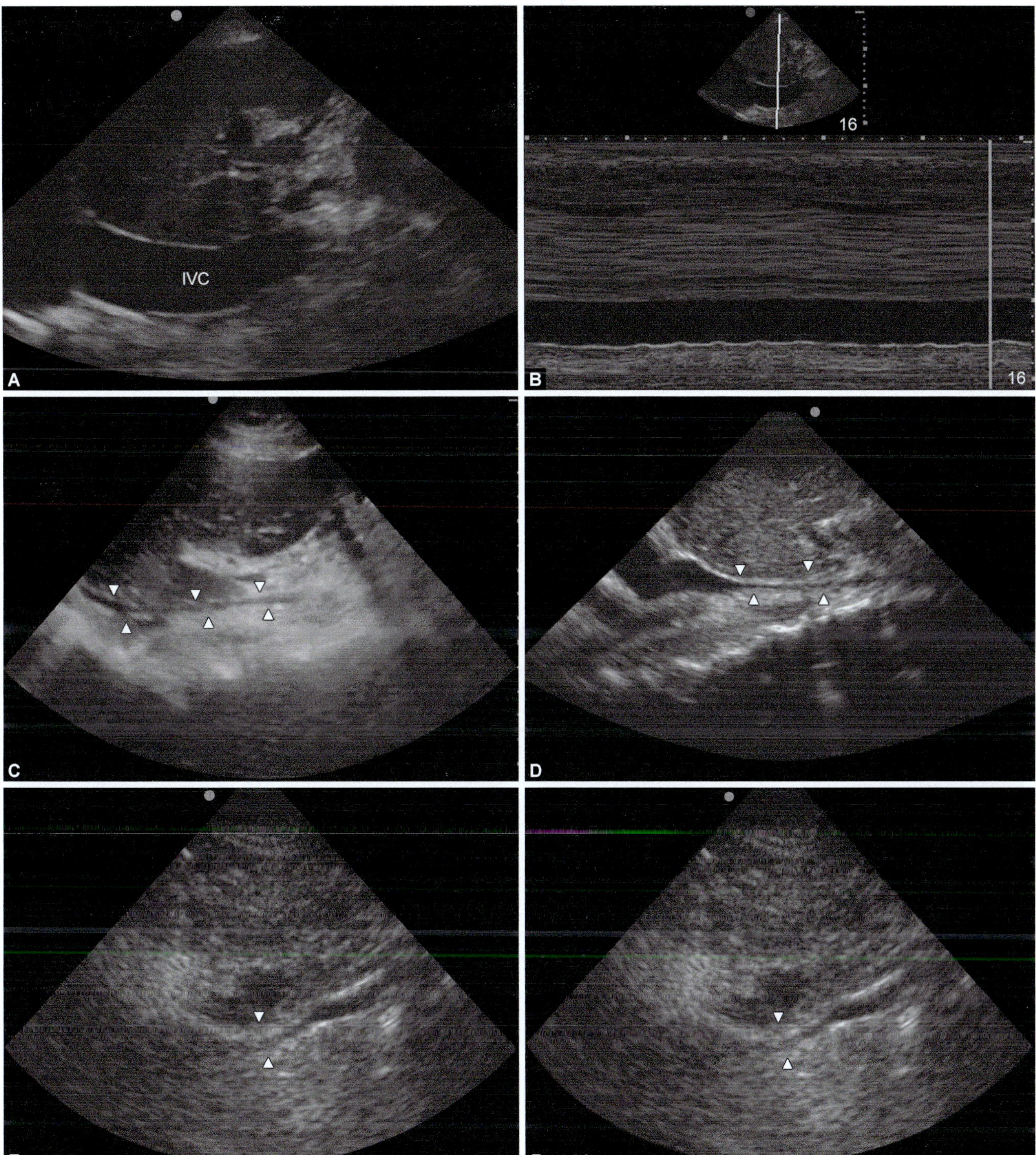

FIGS. 24A TO F: IVC diameter and its variation help to predict fluid responsiveness. (A) Large dilated IVC; (B) M-mode examination of the IVC shows little respiratory variation of diameter; (C and D) Very small or "virtual" IVC (arrowheads) in a volume-depleted patient; (E and F) Significant respiratory variation of IVC diameter during mechanical ventilation in a volume-depleted patient. E shows IVC diameter in inspiration and F shows IVC diameter in expiration.

(IVC: inferior vena cava)

ABDOMINAL ULTRASOUND: SCOPE IN INTENSIVE CARE UNIT

For the intensivist, abdominal ultrasonography has important but limited applications in the ICU. It is neither necessary nor realistic for the intensivist to become fully trained in all aspects of abdominal ultrasonography. Abdominal ultrasonography is used to answer important specific questions, so the modality is best deployed as a screening tool. As the intensivist uses ultrasonography for screening purposes, they must understand when to refer the patient for more complete study by a fully trained ultrasonographer. Abdominal ultrasonography has specific technical limitations, and abdominal CT may be required for definitive imaging. However, abdominal CT requires transport of the unstable patient, has considerable radiation dose, and cannot be performed repeatedly. Ultrasonography is performed quickly at the bedside and answers certain clinical questions with a high level of accuracy. Schacherer et al. reported the experience of 400 ultrasonography examinations in the ICU.[102] New pathological findings were detected in one third of cases with confirmation of known pathology in another third. In 80% of cases, no other imaging test had to be performed. We will review the aspects of abdominal ultrasonography that are relevant to the intensivist.

Equipment: Modern portable machines have full capability for abdominal ultrasonography. Doppler is not required for applications typical to the ICU. A curved array transducer that is specifically designed for abdominal ultrasonography is desirable but adds significant cost to the purchase price of the ICU machine. A phased array cardiac transducer provides acceptable image quality while reducing acquisition cost.

Clinical Applications

Identification of intra-abdominal fluid (ascites): A focused abdominal ultrasound examination performed by non-radiologists originated from the concept of focused assessment with sonography for trauma (FAST).[103,104] The FAST is a limited abdominal examination performed by emergency department physicians or trauma surgeons specifically to determine whether the patient has intra-abdominal fluid collection. Ultrasonography can detect as little as 100 cc of free fluid in the peritoneal cavity.[105] The FAST protocol was developed to detect blood in patients with blunt abdominal trauma. It consists of three abdominal views: Examination of the hepatorenal recess, the splenorenal recess, and the rectovesical/rectovaginal region. A variation of the FAST examination includes a subxiphoid window for pericardial fluid and examination of the aorta. The FAST examination has reduced the need of diagnostic peritoneal lavage in trauma patients.[106]

The FAST exam has utility in the ICU, as the presence of ascites has implications for diagnosis and management. Identification of ascites requires the operator to perform the standard components of FAST exam **(Figs. 25A and B)**. In addition, the intensivist should examine the paracolic gutter and subphrenic regions for a more comprehensive evaluation. Ascites is hypoechoic, subtended by typical anatomic boundaries (intra-abdominal organs), and has typical dynamic findings. Unlike pleural fluid, it undergoes shape change with force application by the transducer on the abdominal wall. Mimickers of ascites include fluid-filled intestine, distended bladder, and distended gallbladder. Anechoic ascites **(Fig. 25B)** is generally transudative. While exudative ascites is often hyperechoic. Ultrasound cannot differentiate between fresh blood and ascitic fluid as both are usually anechoic. The presence of fluid with echogenicity or internal loculations/septations usually indicates an exudate and suggests the need for further investigation **(Fig. 25C)**. Identification of ascites is an important ultrasound finding in itself but always has to be interpreted within the clinical context. A patient with cirrhosis and a large amount of anechoic fluid may not require further diagnostic evaluation. Intra-abdominal fluid with increased echogenicity and loculations, combined with signs of sepsis or findings of acute abdominal presentation, suggests peritonitis with hollow viscus perforation or a neglected hemoperitoneum. The identification of ascites mandates a decision whether to perform paracentesis as part of a diagnostic or therapeutic response.

Evaluation of kidneys: Both kidneys can be readily imaged at the bedside in the ICU. The optimal position for kidney imaging is with the patient in lateral decubitus position. This is usually not feasible in the critically ill because of hemodynamic and respiratory instability. The examination starts with the longitudinal axis view of the kidneys followed by transverse axis imaging. A single tomographic plane is not sufficient, and the intensivist should scan through the organs in multiple tomographic planes in order to develop a three-dimensional construct of the kidneys. The longitudinal length, parenchymal thickness, parenchymal echogenicity, and corticomedullary differentiation are determined. Normal longitudinal length is 9–12 cm; normal cortical thickness is between 1.5 and 1.8 cm. Normal renal cortex is hypoechoic or isoechoic compared to the liver or spleen. A visible distinction between the cortex and the medulla is normal. Renal parenchyma surrounds the renal sinus which contains the pelvis, the calyces, and major branches of renal vasculature. It appears hyperechoic because of the presence of fatty tissue.

Ultrasonography is the preferred imaging modality for patients with acute renal failure in the ICU. A primary objective of the examination is to rule out obstructive uropathy as the cause of renal failure. A dilated pelvicalyceal system indicates obstructive uropathy and can be diagnosed with a high level of sensitivity **(Fig. 25E)**. The severity of the obstruction may be classified and its chronicity can be estimated by the morphologic characteristics of the dilatation. Stones within the collecting system may be observed with an accompanying acoustic shadow artifact. There may be pitfalls in the examination for hydronephrosis. A patient with significant coexistent intrinsic renal parenchymal disease, who also has a urinary obstruction, may not develop hydronephrosis due to lack of urine production. Rarely, infiltrative diseases of the kidney may restrict pelvicalyceal dilatation in the obstructed kidney. Acute obstruction will not result in discernible hydronephrosis immediately, and the finding may be delayed for many hours.

Acute kidney injury with renal failure results in normal or enlarged kidney size. Chronic renal disease causes increased cortical echogenicity and reduction in cortical thickness **(Fig. 25D)**.

A problem facing intensivists in performing renal ultrasonography is the discovery of an abnormality that is beyond their level of competence. Renal cysts, both simple and complicated, unusual variants of normal anatomy, or malignancy, may present as ambiguous findings on ultrasound examination when the intensivists' primary concern is to rule out obstruction. In this case, the screening ultrasonographer has an obligation to call for a definitive examination by a fully trained ultrasonographer or by other diagnostic modalities like CT scan.

Evaluation of the urinary bladder: The urinary bladder is readily imaged using a transverse and longitudinal axis approach at the suprapubic area. The distended bladder appears as a large anechoic space in the appropriate anatomic location **(Fig. 25F)**.

A primary indication for bladder ultrasonography is in the evaluation of anuria. This often results from blockage or misplacement of a urinary catheter. In the case of a blocked urinary catheter, the fluid-filled catheter balloon is readily visualized in the distended bladder **(Fig. 25F)**. Flushing or manipulating the catheter will result in renewed urine flow in these cases. The examination of the urinary bladder should always be performed in conjunction with the kidneys. In imaging the urinary bladder, the intensivist must be prepared for the possibility of ambiguous ultrasonography findings, such as bladder tumor. Just as is the case with the kidneys, this requires definitive imaging by a fully trained ultrasonographer.

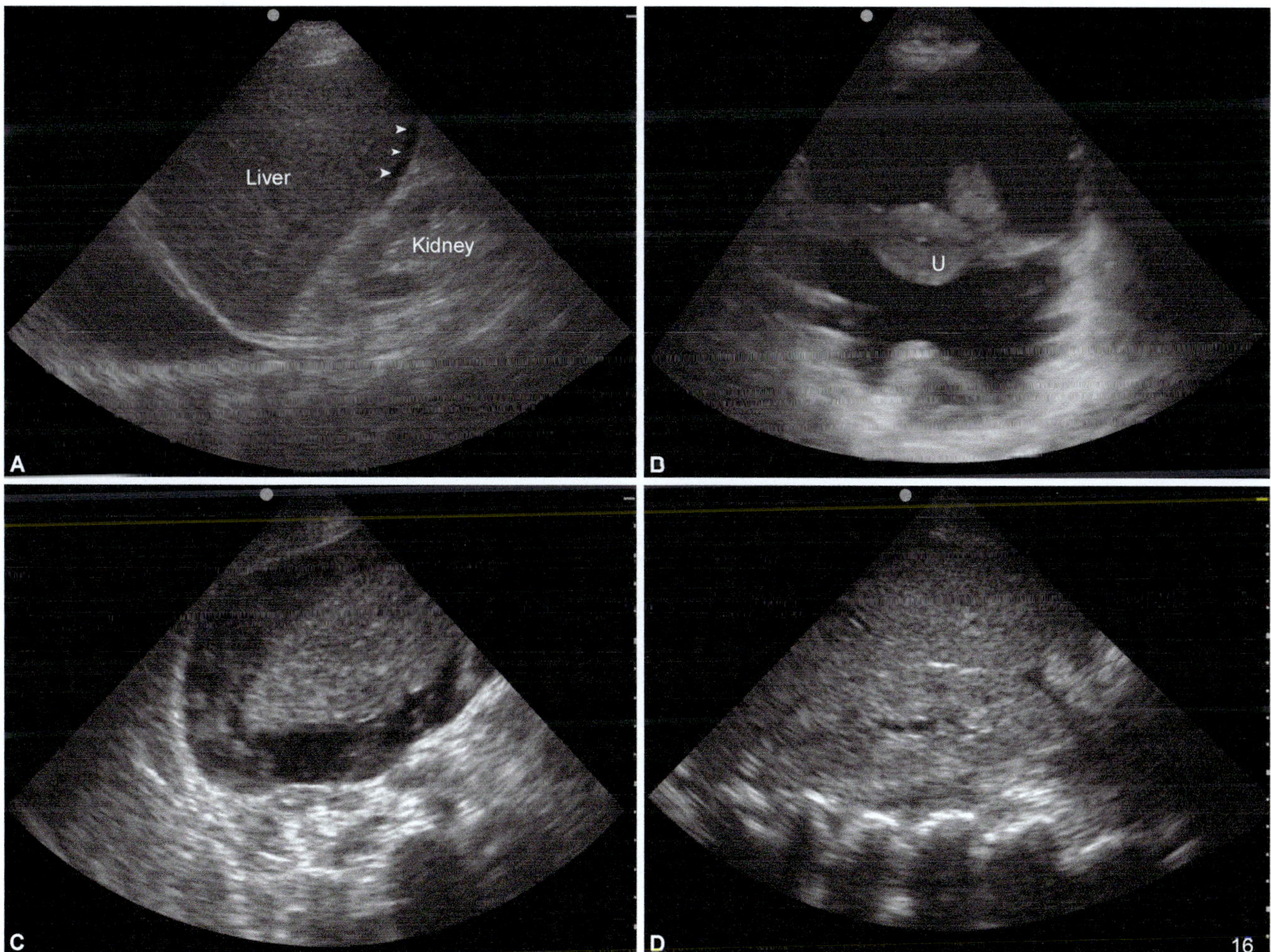

FIGS. 25A TO F: *Continued*

Continued

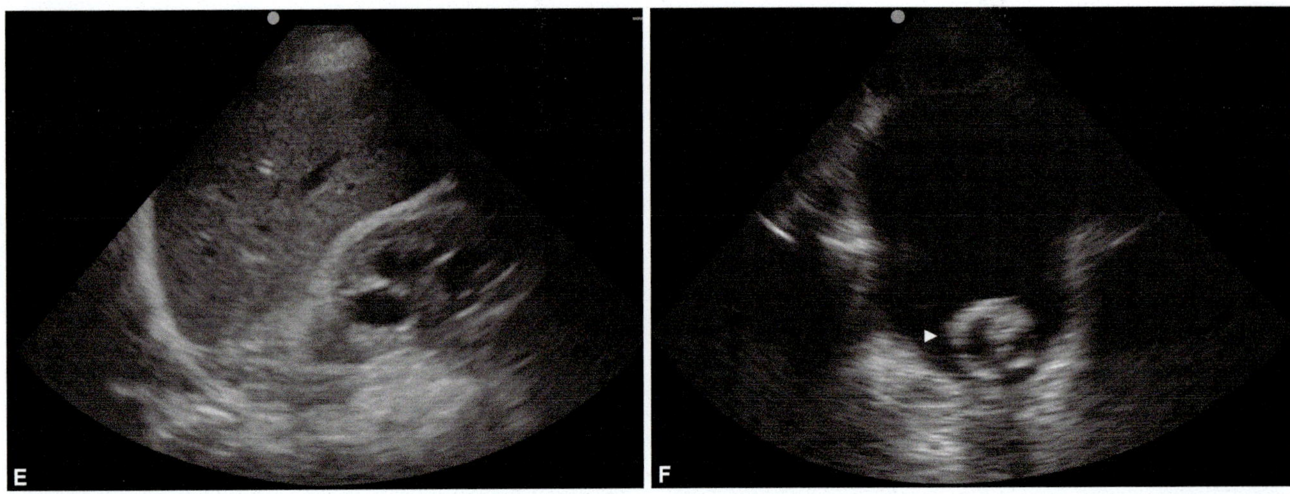

FIGS. 25A TO F: Common applications of abdominal ultrasound in critical care unit. (A) Minimal ascites in the hepatorenal recess (arrowheads). In a patient with blunt abdominal trauma, such findings are highly significant. (B) Pelvic scan showing a large amount of anechoic ascites (uterus is indicated by U). (C) Complex ascites. Echogenic ascitic fluid may indicate exudative and often infected ascitic fluid. (D) Small kidney with loss of corticomedullary differentiation in a patient with chronic renal failure. (E) Hydronephrosis of right kidney. (F) Distended urinary bladder in a patient with blocked Foley's catheter. The balloon of the catheter can be seen inside the distended bladder (arrowhead).

Evaluation for pneumoperitoneum: Ultrasonography has been described as a more sensitive modality than plain radiography for the diagnosis of pneumoperitoneum with a high sensitivity, specificity, and positive predictive value.[107,108] To detect pneumoperitoneum, the epigastric area and right upper quadrant are scanned in the supine patient. Sonographically, air will appear as echogenic areas with posterior reverberation artifacts **(Fig. 26A)**.[109,110] Pneumoperitoneum also causes enhancement of the peritoneal stripe.[111] Presence of air bubbles within ascitic fluid will also point to a diagnosis of pneumoperitoneum **(Fig. 26B)**.[110] A lack of peritoneal sliding also indicates the possibility of pneumoperitoneum. Massive pneumoperitoneum may make it impossible to visualize any abdominal organ, indirectly suggesting the diagnosis **(Fig. 26C)**.

Evaluation of abdominal aorta: The abdominal aorta may be imaged in both longitudinal and transverse axes in order to determine whether an aortic aneurysm or other major pathology exists **(Figs. 27A and B)**. An enlarged aorta (>3 cm, measured from outside wall to outside wall) with luminal thrombus and irregularity suggests an aortic aneurysm.

Evaluation of other abdominal organ systems: Ultrasonography may be used to assess all organ systems within the abdomen. However, the intensivist needs to be aware that developing comprehensive skill in all aspects of abdominal ultrasonography requires dedicated and time-consuming training. The authors suggest that this is not necessary for routine critical care function. The intensivists may appropriately limit abdominal ultrasonography to a specific targeted screening approach.

The liver is imaged in longitudinal and transverse planes. If sepsis is suspected, assessment of liver can give valuable clues: Presence of single or multiple hypoechoic lesions may be indicative of abscesses. For suspected biliary disease, ultrasonography is the initial investigation of choice. Intrahepatic biliary ductal dilatation is the hallmark of obstructive biliary pathology **(Fig. 27C)**. In patients with jaundice, abnormal liver function tests, sepsis of unknown etiology, or new fever, biliary ductal dilatation assumes importance. The gallbladder should be imaged in multiple tomographic planes to look for stone and biliary sludge **(Fig. 27D)**. Features of acute cholecystitis include gallbladder wall thickening, pericholecystic fluid, and sonographic elicitation of Murphy's sign. In the absence of stone, the above signs along with an enlarged gallbladder indicate a possible diagnosis of acalculous cholecystitis **(Figs. 27E and F)**.[112] Evidence of gallbladder stone, sludge, and biliary obstruction has important implications in a patient admitted with pancreatitis.

Ultrasonography is useful for evaluation of the gastrointestinal tract. For example, typical findings of enteritis include thickened bowel wall (>4 mm) and echoic bowel content. Toxic megacolon may be identified by imaging fluid-filled ascending colon > 10 cm in diameter **(Fig. 27G)**. The presence of bowel peristalsis by ultrasonography rules out ischemic bowel or peritonitis with a high level of certainty.

The pancreas is frequently difficult to image with ultrasonography in the poorly prepared critically ill patient. Identification of retroperitoneal pathology such as retroperitoneal lymph node (LN) or hematoma is also challenging to anyone other than a fully trained ultrasonographer. The spleen may be readily imaged for such abnormalities as abscess, but much splenic pathology is not readily visible to a screening ultrasonographer; for example, splenic hematoma may be isoechoic to adjacent normal splenic parenchyma.

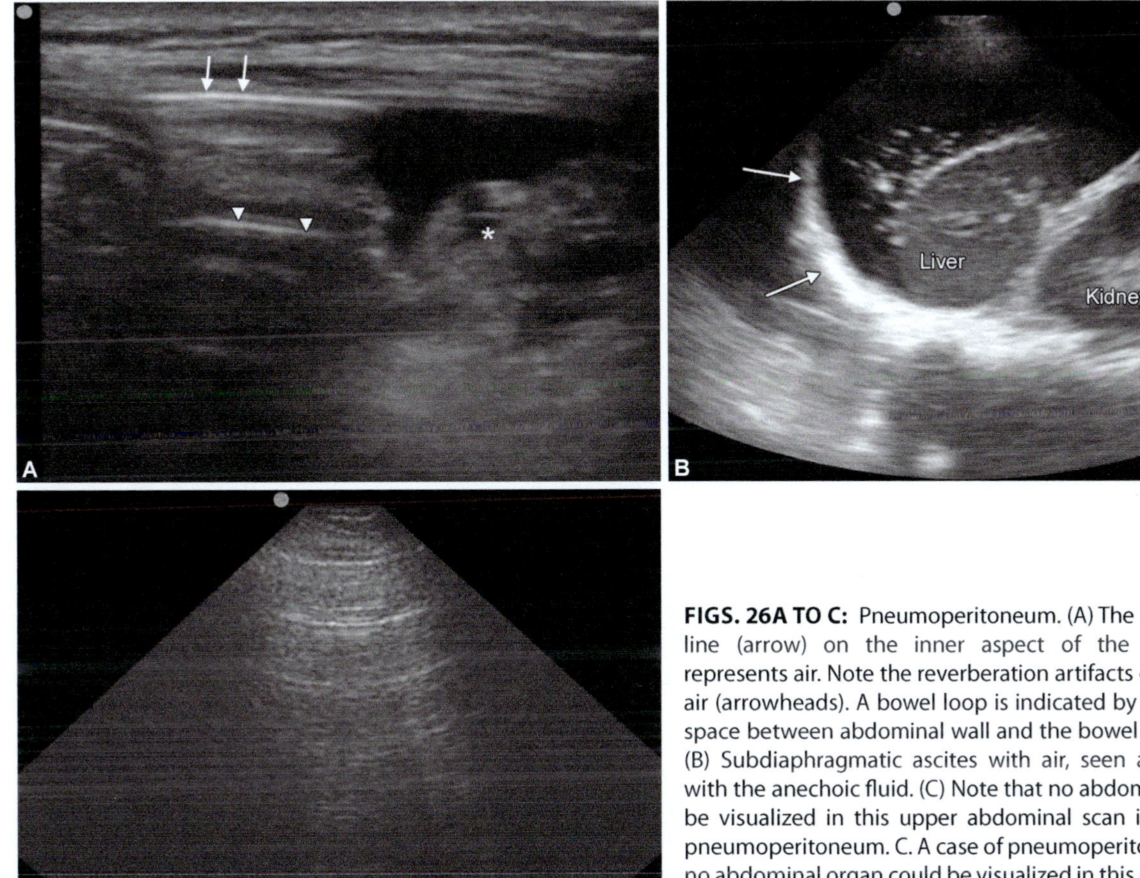

FIGS. 26A TO C: Pneumoperitoneum. (A) The bright echogenic line (arrow) on the inner aspect of the abdominal wall represents air. Note the reverberation artifacts generated by the air (arrowheads). A bowel loop is indicated by (*) and the black space between abdominal wall and the bowel loop is free fluid. (B) Subdiaphragmatic ascites with air, seen as bright echoes with the anechoic fluid. (C) Note that no abdominal organ could be visualized in this upper abdominal scan in a patient with pneumoperitoneum. C. A case of pneumoperitoneum. Note that no abdominal organ could be visualized in this upper abdominal scan. Exclusive air pattern, as seen in this photo, can raise the suspicion of pneumoperitoneum In the right clinical scenario; The scan mimics A-line pattern seen in normal lung ultrasound.

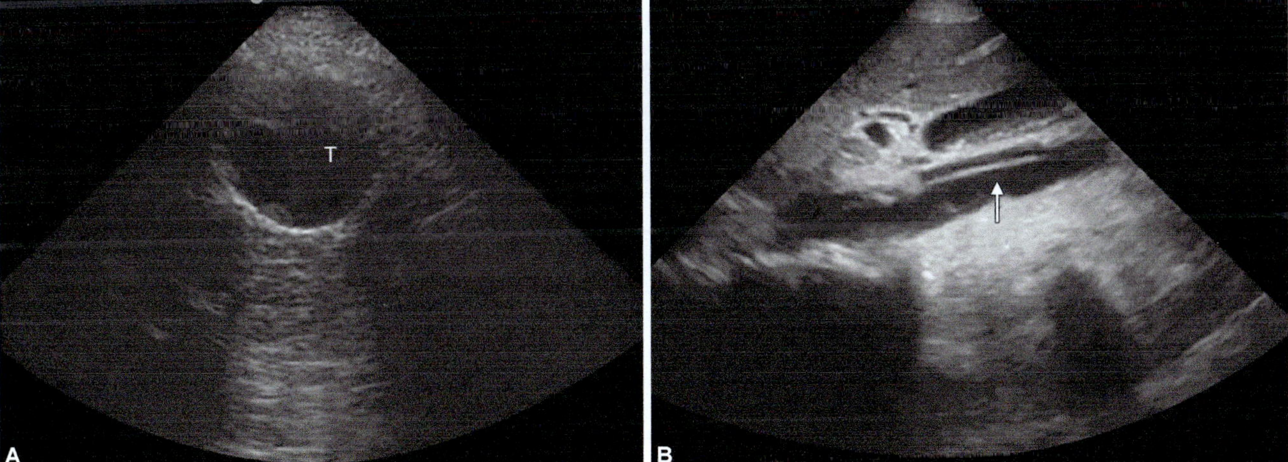

FIGS. 27A TO H: *Continued*

Continued

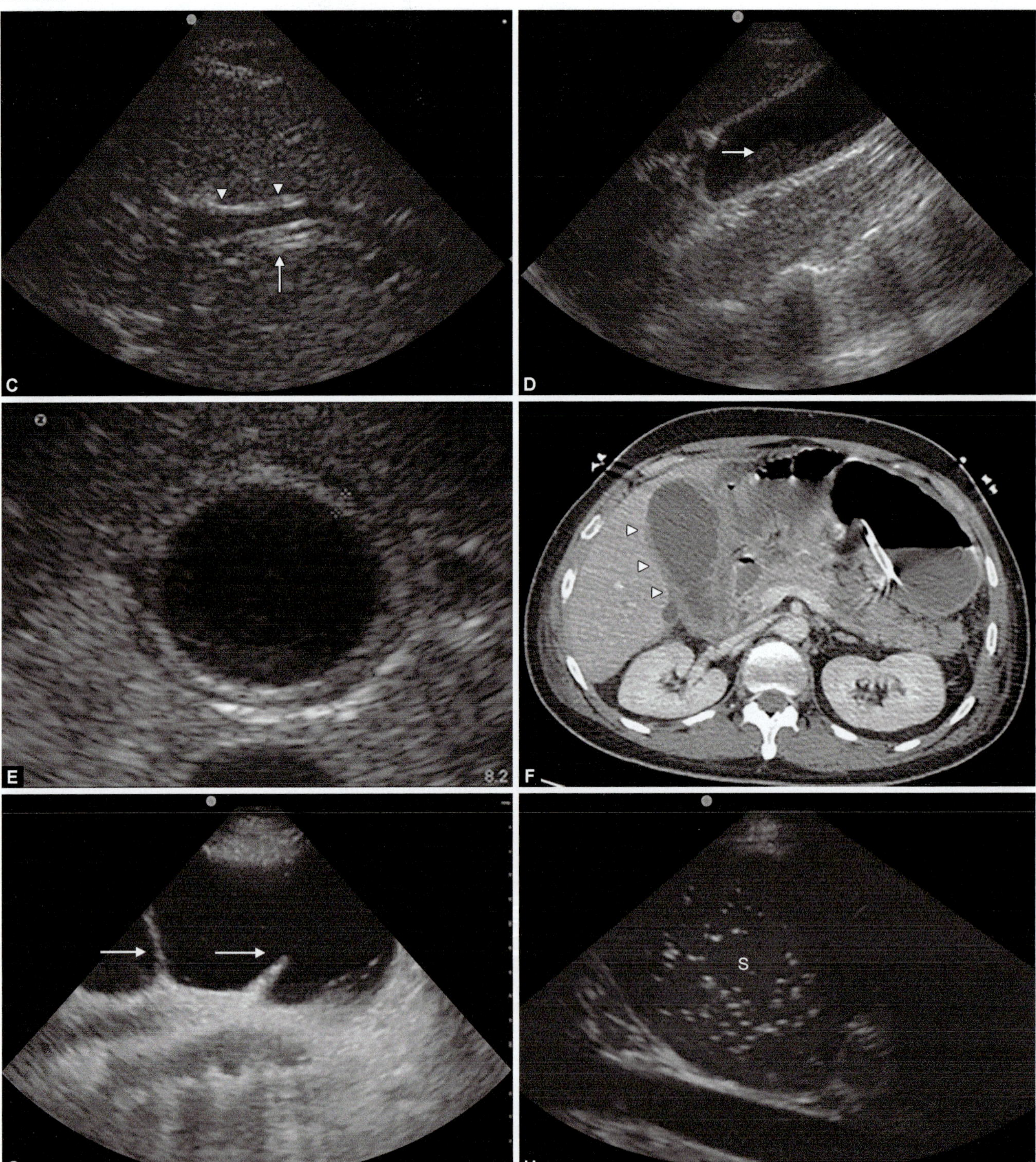

FIGS. 27A TO H: Other applications of abdominal ultrasound. (A) Abdominal aortic aneurysm with partial thrombosis of the lumen (T). (B) Aortic dissection, the intimal flap can be seen in this longitudinal view of the aorta (arrow). (C) Dilated intrahepatic biliary duct in a case of obstructive jaundice (arrowheads). Note the accompanying normal-looking portal vein branch (arrow). (D) Gallbladder sludge (arrow). (E) Dilated gallbladder with thickened wall in a case of acalculous cholecystitis. (F) Abdominal CT scan of the patient in (E) shows large dilated gallbladder (arrowheads). (G) Dilated loop of colon. Note the colonic haustra (arrow). (H) Dilated fluid-filled stomach seen in a preintubation scan (S).

ULTRASOUND ASSESSMENT OF VENOUS THROMBOEMBOLISM

There are several circumstances in which an intensivist may wish to search for DVT. These include physical examination findings that suggest DVT or an acute deterioration of respiratory or circulatory status where DVT is sought as a surrogate marker for PE. DVT may be observed as an incidental finding while examining veins for cannulation. When the intensivist decides to obtain a study for DVT, they have two choices: Either they may call for a study being performed by a vascular technician/radiologist or they may choose to perform the study themselves at point of care. Waiting for a radiologist-performed study introduces a dangerous delay in the process of diagnosis and management of DVT. Intensivists and other nonradiologists may perform DVT study with the same level of accuracy as radiology department-based services.[113,114] The study technique is easy to learn and has immediate bedside application. The intensivist who is skilled at DVT study can obtain immediate diagnosis very rapidly at bedside.

Equipment: Modern portable bedside ultrasound machines, equipped with a high-frequency linear vascular transducer, are suitable to detect DVT. Doppler capability, while desirable, is not a requirement in order to perform an accurate study: DVT can be diagnosed using two-dimensional compression ultrasonography alone.[115,116]

Examination protocol: For lower extremity examination, the patient should be placed in reverse Trendelenburg position, in order to promote distension of the leg veins, with the leg externally rotated and the knee slightly flexed. The examination should be bilateral and comparative. The examination starts at the level of the inguinal ligament (femoral crease) where the external iliac vein becomes the common femoral veins. Careful consideration should be given to the area where the great saphenous vein drains into the common femoral vein. The common femoral vein is scanned at multiple points up to its bifurcation into the superficial femoral vein and the deep femoral veins. The superficial vein is examined at multiple points until it enters the adductor canal. The popliteal vein is assessed where it runs behind the knee joint, in the popliteal fossa. The different levels of lower extremity deep venous system where a DVT should be looked for are shown in **Figures 28A to F**. In the upper extremity and neck vein examination, the veins are imaged at regular intervals in transverse plane along their course to avoid missing a clot.[117,118]

At each level of examination, in transverse scanning plane, the vein and the companion artery are identified. Before compression, the vein is examined for a visible clot. Visible clot appears as echogenic material that can be mobile and/or adherent to the vessel wall. It is diagnostic of DVT and does not need compression. Thrombi may be seen in the internal jugular, subclavian, or axillary veins. While compressions on transverse scan are used for internal jugular, axillary, and brachial veins, the subclavian vein cannot be compressed effectively so Doppler study may be necessary. After obtaining a satisfactory picture on a transverse scan, the transducer can be rotated 90° to get a longitudinal image of the vessel, suitable for rapid survey of veins and assessment of extent and nature of a thrombus when seen.

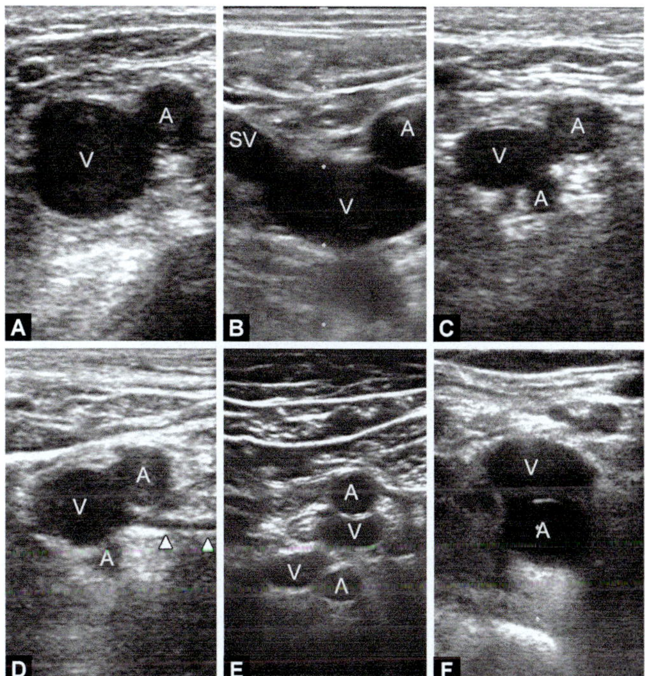

FIGS. 28A TO F: Lower limb DVT study in a critical care setting. It is important to be familiar with different anatomical levels that should be identified for adequate compression ultrasonography. (A) Below the inguinal ligament where the common femoral artery (A) and common femoral vein (V) are seen; (B) At the level where saphenous vein (SV) enters the common femoral vein (V) from the medial side; (C) Bifurcation of common femoral artery into superficial femoral artery and arteria profunda femoris; (D) A lateral perforator vein (arrowhead) joining the common femoral vein (V); (E) Image at a level after bifurcation of both common femoral artery and common femoral vein; (F) Popliteal artery (A) and popliteal vein (V). (A: artery; DVT: deep vein thrombosis; V: vein)

At each site of examination, if no clot is visible, the vein is identified by its location, by the company of an artery and on occasions by visualizing valve movement within the vein. A thrombus may be visible as a distinct echogenic structure within the vein **(Fig. 29 lower panel)**; no compression maneuver is required in this circumstance. If no clot is visualized, the examiner applies sufficient pressure to deform the vein. A normal vein is compressible with mild pressure (0.5–1.0 kg/cm^2). Complete compressibility is defined as apposition of walls with effacement of lumen **(Fig. 29, upper panel.)**. Complete compressibility excludes DVT at the site of examination. Incomplete compressibility of vein indicates presence of DVT and is the only validated diagnostic criterion for DVT. Abnormal compression ultrasonography **(Fig. 29, middle panel)** has high sensitivity and specificity for diagnosis of femoropopliteal DVT.[119,120]

Clinical Issues

DVT as a surrogate marker for PE: Compression ultrasonography shows a DVT in 30–50% of patients with PE. Finding a proximal DVT in patients suspected of PE is sufficient to start anticoagulation without further testing.[121,122] Additionally, multiorgan ultrasonography involving basic CCE, lung ultrasonography, and DVT study, when used in conjunction with clinical probability scores, safely reduces the need for CT pulmonary angiograms in patients with suspected PE.[123] Similarly, another study showed that a screening, point-of-care ultrasonography protocol may reduce the number of CTPAs either by documenting DVT or by finding an alternative diagnosis.[124]

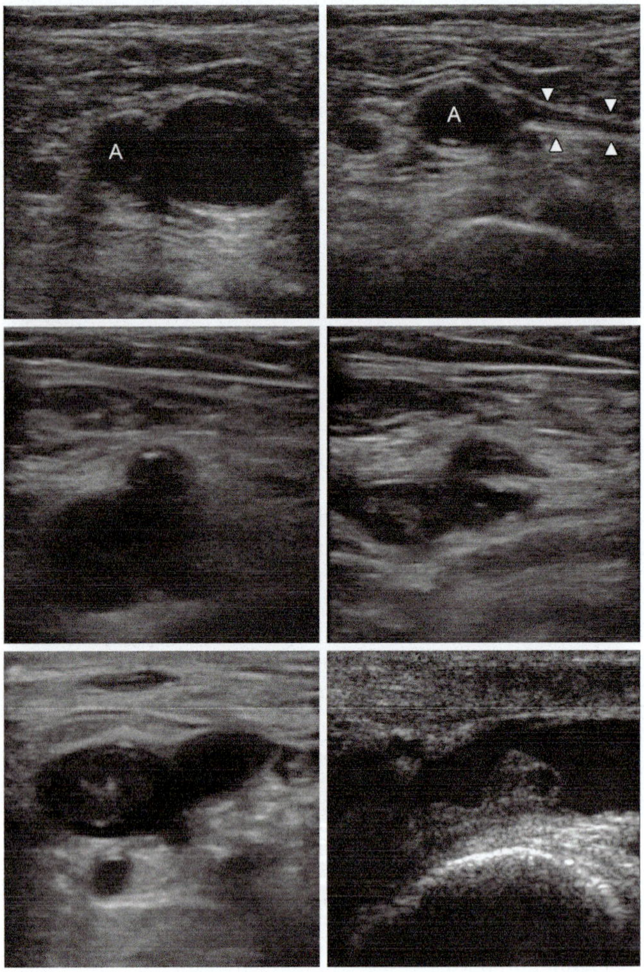

FIG. 29: Ultrasonography in the diagnosis of DVT. *Upper panel, left:* A normal common femoral vein before compression (A: arterial lumen). *Upper panel, right:* A normal common femoral vein after compression. Note the complete obliteration of venous lumen on application of compression (arrowheads). *Middle panel, left:* Common femoral vein DVT before compression. *Middle panel, right:* Common femoral vein DVT after compression. Note that the lumen cannot be obliterated. The thrombus is also visible as echogenic material within the venous lumen after compression. *Lower panel, left:* Common femoral vein thrombosis. The thrombus is visible within the venous lumen. Compression should not be applied if the thrombus is already visible. *Lower panel, right:* A longitudinal view of the common femoral vein shows the clot.
(DVT: deep vein thrombosis)

Importance/Frequency of upper extremity DVT: About 10% of all cases of upper extremity DVT have been reported to result in PE.[125] Certain groups of patients are more prone to developing upper extremity DVT: Cancer patients with central venous port systems,[126] patients with peripherally inserted central venous catheters,[127] and patients with central venous catheters (both internal jugular and axillary/subclavian).[128,129] Few studies have examined ultrasonography for the diagnosis of upper extremity DVT. These studies are of inferior methodology. In the absence of a good alternative test in ICU patients, compression ultrasonography remains a practical choice for the diagnosis of upper extremity DVT.[130]

Importance of studying calf veins: Ultrasound study of calf veins for DVT requires operator experience, significant additional time, and difficulties in positioning the patient. The accuracy of ultrasonography in the diagnosis of calf DVT has been reported to be lower than in the diagnosis of proximal DVT.[131] Our opinion is that it is not realistic for intensivists to develop this skill level. One strategy is for the intensivist to repeat the DVT study of the popliteal and femoral veins serially at 24–48-hour intervals in those patients who are at very high risk for DVT.

DVT proximal to femoral veins: In nontrauma patients, isolated iliac vein or IVC thrombosis is very uncommon but is always a concern, especially in cases of previous femoral vein cannulation.[132] These veins may not readily be imaged with ultrasonography except in patients with slender body habitus. In trauma patients, as well as in patients with pelvic disorders and obstetric patients, isolated pelvic vein thrombosis may need to be explored with the use of Doppler or other imaging modalities.

Limitations

- The examiner must have adequate training and familiarity with the venous anatomy.
- Patients who are obese, are edematous, or have wounds or dressings may have inadequate image quality.
- The identification of a thrombus does not indicate its age. There are criteria that can be used to identify recent or old (presumably) inactive thrombi. However, these are not completely reliable.
- The subclavian vein may not be compressible, particularly in obese or muscular individuals. Unless an echogenic clot is visualized within the subclavian vein,

lack of compressibility does not necessarily indicate the presence of an isoechoic clot within the SV.

ULTRASOUND GUIDANCE FOR PROCEDURES

Ultrasound-guided Vascular Access

Ultrasonography may be used to guide vascular access in the ICU. Several studies and two meta-analyses have shown the benefits of ultrasound guidance in central venous catheter placement:[133-136] Ultrasound guidance for central venous access is recommended by national quality organizations in the United States and the United Kingdom.[137,138] It improves success and reduces complication rate for central venous access and can be used for arterial and peripheral vascular access. In a recently published international evidence-based recommendation, ultrasound guidance has been suggested as the method of choice for any kind of vascular cannulation considering its high safety and efficacy.[139] In this section, we will discuss the general principles for performing vascular access under ultrasound guidance. This discussion assumes that the reader has full knowledge of the mechanical aspects of vascular access such as site preparation and physical manipulation of needle, dilator, and cannula. For detailed site-specific discussion, the reader is referred to comprehensive review articles.[140-142]

Advantages of using ultrasound to guide vascular access

- *Localization of vessels*: Following identification of the anatomical landmarks, prepuncture ultrasound examination of the proposed site helps in the identification of the target vessel and its relationship with the surrounding structures [e.g., carotid artery, thyroid gland, and trachea in case of internal jugular vein (IJV) cannulation]. The ultrasound images are used to identify anatomical variations and to fine-tune the selection of the puncture site **(Figs. 30A and B)**.
- *Assessment of suitability for vascular cannulation*: Examination of the target vessel allows for determination that the vessel is suitable for line placement. Ultrasonography permits visualization of features that prohibit vascular access which cannot be identified by simple visual examination. There may be marked difference in vessel caliber **(Fig. 30C)**[143,144] and variability of vessel position relative to the adjacent artery in ~5% of the general population.[141,145] A partial or complete thrombosis of the vessel, a vascular stenosis, or a perivascular hematoma can only be identified with ultrasonography **(Fig. 30D)**. Hypovolemia may reduce the size of target vessel, and marked respiratory efforts may cause variability of vascular size **(Fig. 30C)**, making it impossible to cannulate the IJV and subclavian vein. These cannot be identified without ultrasonography. Use of ultrasound, therefore, reduces the chances of failure associated with blind technique.
- *Reduction of procedure time*: Ultrasound guidance of central venous access reduces the number of attempts required and improves first-pass success rate, improving the safety and comfort of the patient.
- *Use in arterial puncture and peripheral venous access*: Ultrasonography is useful in guiding all forms of arterial access and is particularly useful in patients who are hypovolemic or hypotensive or who develop vasospasm secondary to multiple cannulation attempts.[146,147] The diameter of the radial artery, a common site for arterial line placement, is only ~3 mm[148] so that blind line insertion at this site may be challenging. Ultrasound guidance improves the success rate of peripheral venous access.[149,150]
- *Evaluation of potential complication*: Ultrasonography may be used to immediately identify procedural complications of vascular access such as hematoma or pneumothorax. It may be used to confirm guidewire placement prior to dilatation. This is useful to avoid inadvertent arterial injury during central venous access. The correct placement of guidewire **(Fig. 31B** and catheter **(Figs. 31C and D)** can be checked immediately at bedside.

Equipment requirement

- Vascular access is generally performed by using a high-frequency (7–10 MHz) linear transducer. The higher frequency provides excellent resolution with the tradeoff that penetration is limited. Fortunately, barring massive obesity, vessels commonly accessed for cannulation are superficial.
- In performing real-time ultrasound guidance of vascular access, the use of a purpose designed sterile probe cover is mandatory. An attempt to jerry-rig a sterile transducer cover using a glove is inappropriate and violates the basic principles of central line sterile precautions.

General principles of ultrasound guidance of vascular access

- In addition to full mastery of machine control and transducer manipulation, the operator must place the machine in such a way that the screen is easily visible without much movement on the part of the operator. This might require rearrangement of equipment and bed position in a crowded work environment. The operator should avoid a situation where the screen is not easily visible.
- The operator must have knowledge of local anatomy. With understanding of the anatomy, a key objective of using ultrasonography is to unequivocally identify the target and to differentiate veins from arteries. A vein is identified initially by its typical location and relationship with the surrounding structures. Once identified, the operator must confirm that the vascular structure is in fact a vein. The vein is easily compressible, whereas the adjacent artery is not. The vein has respirophasic change of caliber and may have mobile venous valves that are visible with ultrasonography. Performance of Valsalva

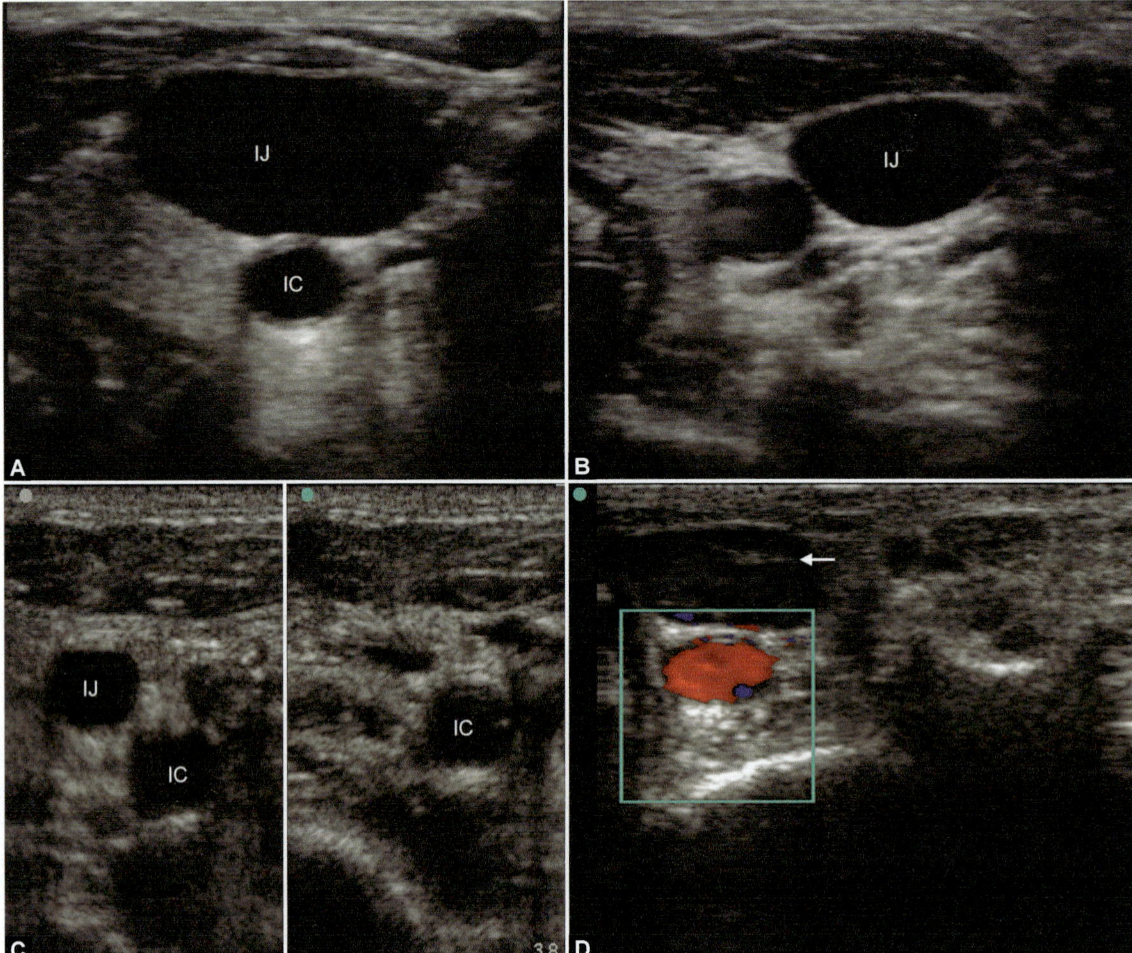

FIGS. 30A TO D: Ultrasonography helps in selection of a suitable vessel for cannulation. (A) Internal jugular vein (IJ) is located directly in front of the internal carotid artery (IC). Attempted cannulation at this site will carry a high risk of inadvertent puncture of the carotid artery. (B) As the internal jugular vein is imaged at different points along its course in the neck, at this location the vein lies outside the carotid artery. Attempted venous puncture will not have much risk of accidental carotid artery puncture. (C) Small left IJ with near-complete obliteration of the lumen during spontaneous breathing. Cannulation of this vessel will be very difficult. (D) IJ thrombus (arrow). Note that the thrombosed IJ does not show any color flow signal while the carotid artery does.

maneuver increases the caliber of the vein but has no effect on the caliber of the artery. The artery is pulsatile. In general, Doppler analysis is not required to differentiate veins from arteries with the exception of subclavian position. In the subclavian position, particularly in muscular or obese individuals, compression of the subclavian vein may be difficult; venous valve and respirophasic change may also be difficult to recognize. Doppler ultrasound may be used to identify subclavian vein.

- Before performing subclavian or internal jugular venous access, the contralateral vein should be examined in order to identify the best site in terms of vessel position, size, and condition. In addition, the operator should document the presence of sliding lung bilaterally before starting the procedure in order to rule out pneumothorax.
- Following insertion of the guidewire and before dilatation of the vessel, the operator should always document that the guidewire is in the vein **(Fig. 31B)**. Inadvertent placement of a guidewire into the adjacent artery is of no clinical consequence as the vessel defect is small. The wire may be removed with local vascular compression to follow. However, inadvertent dilatation of the artery due to unrecognized wire insertion leaves a much larger defect and constitutes a major complication.
- Following the procedure, the operator should document sliding lung. Its presence rules out procedural pneumothorax. Loss of lung sliding following internal jugular or subclavian venous access, where it was known to be present before the procedure, is a strong evidence of procedure-related pneumothorax.

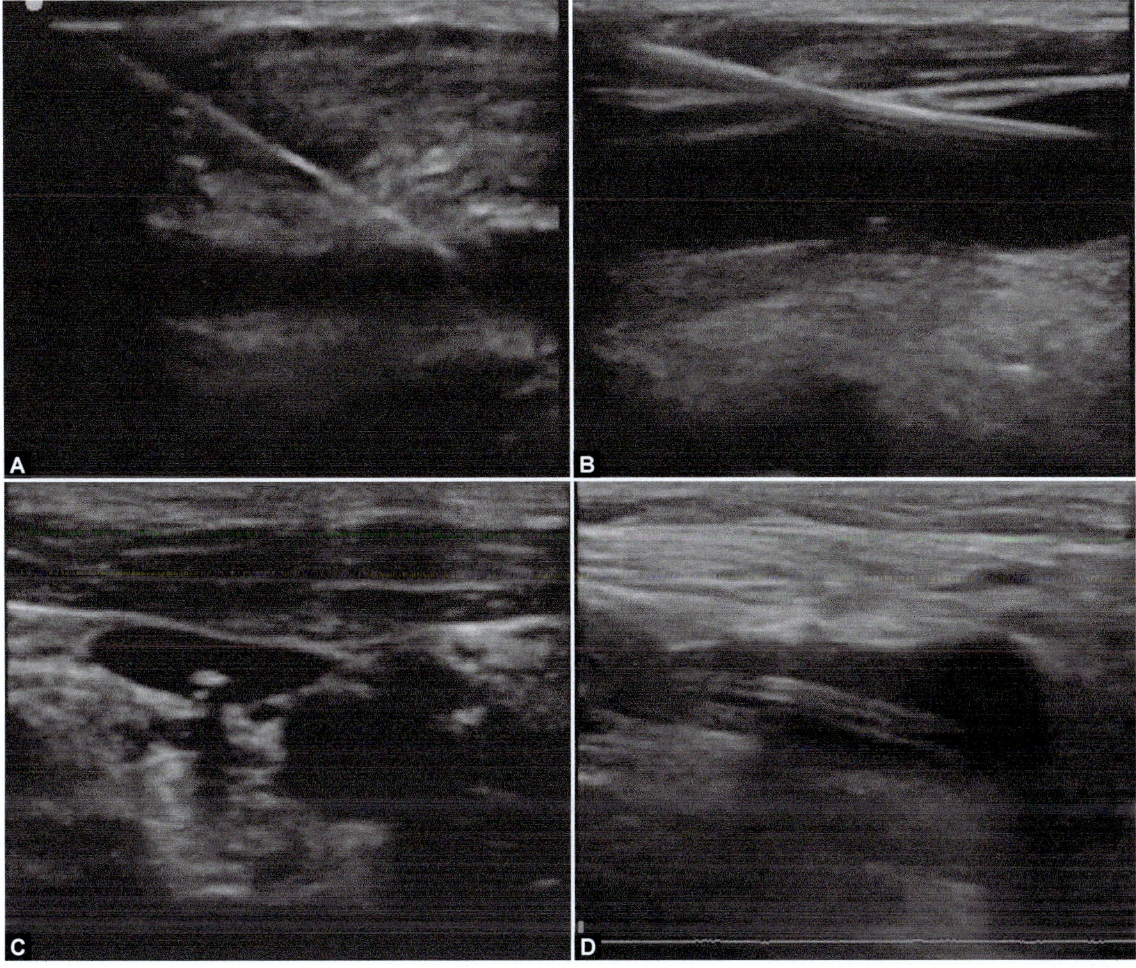

FIGS. 31A TO D: Vascular cannulation under ultrasound guidance. (A) Subclavian vein is punctured under ultrasound guidance. The vein is visualized in the long axis and the needle trajectory is under direct visual control. (B) Correct placement of guidewire is confirmed before dilatation. (C) Correct placement of catheter can easily be confirmed using ultrasound. A cross-sectional view of IJ shows the catheter inside the vascular lumen. (D) The catheter can also be visualized inside the vein in longitudinal view.

Technique for vascular cannulation

There are two general approaches to ultrasound guidance for vascular access: Short-axis and long-axis approaches.

Using the short axis approach, the transducer is oriented such that the image shows a cross-sectional view of the vessel. The needle is inserted at a point away from the transducer and angled toward the center of the image. Some operators track the needle tip as it moves forward by moving the transducer along with the needle in synchrony, thereby guiding the needle tip real time in the vessel. The alternative is to hold the transducer in a stable position and estimate the angle and depth in which the needle should be inserted in order that the needle tip intersects the scanning plane in the lumen (center) of the target vessel. Neither method is conclusively known to be superior to the other and should be used according to operator preference.

Using the long-axis approach, the transducer is oriented such that the image shows a longitudinal image of the vessel. The needle is introduced at the side of the transducer and advanced so that the entire needle is visualized throughout the insertion process **(Fig. 31A)**.

At internal jugular and femoral insertion sites, both short-axis and long-axis approaches are effective. In the authors' experience, scanning the vessel in transverse axis is the preferred method for accessing femoral vein and IJV. Most operators prefer to use this approach. The final choice should be predicated to operator experience.

Specific issues related to access site

Internal jugular vein: In the authors' experience, most operators image the jugular vein in its transverse axis, although some prefer a longitudinal approach.[151] In using ultrasound for guidance of IJV access, it becomes clear that the landmark-based blind posterior approach places the carotid artery deep to the IJ vein. This risks inadvertent puncture of the carotid artery as the needle can easily pass through the IJV. The anterior approach is favored when using ultrasound guidance as a point of puncture can be chosen so that the vein is positioned lateral to the artery. This underlines one major advantage of using ultrasound for vascular access; the angle of needle insertion is determined by the image rather than relying on the blind landmark method.

Subclavian vein: A traditional landmark-based technique requires the operator to use the clavicle as the definitive landmark for the procedure. When using the ultrasound for subclavian vein access, the operator should choose a much more lateral position for insertion than is used for the blind technique.[152] Using ultrasound, the vein may be punctured near the point where the axillary vein becomes the subclavian vein (before it crosses the outer border of the first rib). The vein in this location is more caudal and superficial. Several advantages of this ultrasound-guided (more lateral) axillary vein puncture over traditional blind subclavian puncture have been suggested: (1) There is a reduction of accidental arterial punctures; (2) there is less discomfort, as there is no contact of the needle with the periosteum of the clavicle; (3) the catheter enters the vein well before the vein passes the narrow space between the first rib and the clavicle, so there is less risk of pinching and transection of the catheter;[153] (4) with ultrasound guidance, the vein can be entered close to the clavicle; here we have the attachment of the vein to the clavicle preventing the anterior wall from collapsing during puncture;[141] and (5) after the guidewire is placed, the distal internal jugular vein can be examined; if the wire is seen into IJV, it can be repositioned under ultrasound guidance.[154]

Subclavian venous access under ultrasound guidance is best performed with the vessel imaged in the longitudinal axis **(Fig. 31A)**. In this way, the needle can be visualized in its entirety throughout the insertion. This level of needle control is important as the pleural surface is close to the posterior vessel wall.

Femoral vein: The femoral vein is usually accessed using transverse imaging axis. If the image plane is below the inguinal ligament, the vein will be positioned deep to the artery. This is inappropriate position for access, as there is a high risk for arterial injury. The transducer position should be adjusted such that the common femoral vein is imaged medial to the artery. Slight external rotation of the leg helps to bring the vessels side by side.

Arterial catheterization: Ultrasound-guided radial artery cannulation has been shown to have a higher success rate than the blind technique.[147] Radial artery cannulation may be difficult at the standard wrist site due to vasospasm, hematoma formation, or intimal dissection after repeated attempts. In these cases, successful cannulation of the radial artery at a more proximal (mid forearm) location, deep to the brachioradialis muscle, has been reported using real-time ultrasonography.[155] Femoral artery cannulation is similar to central venous line placement at this site in terms of ultrasound technique.[156] Ultrasound may identify significant atheromata at the femoral artery precluding that site.

Peripheral venous cannulation ***(Figs. 32A to C):*** For those patients who have difficult peripheral venous access, ultrasound improves the success rate, reduces the number of unsuccessful attempts, requires less time, and improves patient satisfaction.[149,150] In patients with difficult peripheral venous access, placement of an ultrasound-guided peripheral venous line can reduce the number of central line use in ICUs or help in earlier discontinuation of central venous line. Safety of administration of vasoactive medications through the peripheral vein has been well demonstrated[157] and a well-placed peripheral IV line obviates the need of central line placement for vasopressor administration.

Ultrasound Guidance of Thoracentesis

Ultrasonography may be used to guide thoracentesis with improved success and reduced pneumothorax rate.[158] Ultrasound guidance for thoracentesis is important in the ICU as standard supine chest radiographs have severe limitations in the identification of a safe site for needle insertion. In the patient on mechanical ventilatory support, a

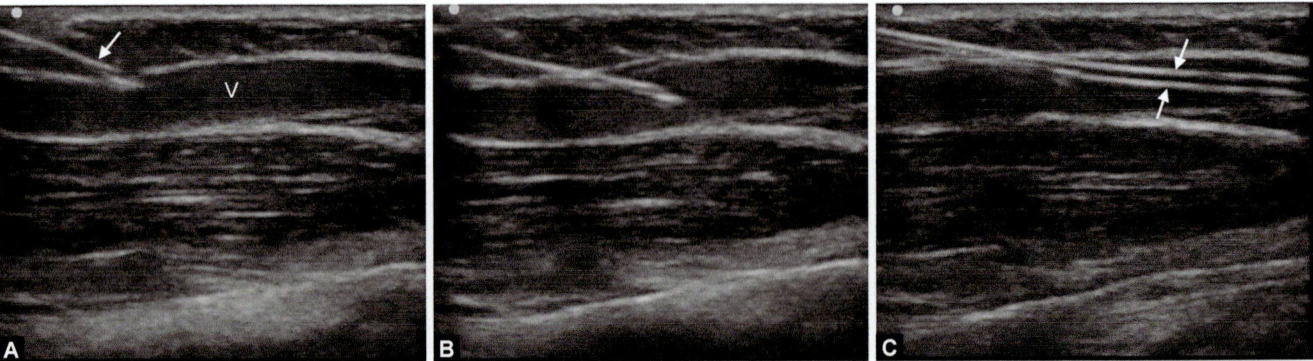

FIGS. 32A TO C: Peripheral IV insertion under ultrasound guidance. (A) The vein (V) is visualized in longitudinal plane. The needle with catheter (arrow) is seen puncturing the vein. (B) The catheter and needle are inside the vein. (C) The catheter is advanced over the needle and seen within the vein (arrows).

pneumothorax resulting from a thoracentesis effort may have catastrophic complications. Several studies have addressed the safety of ultrasound for guidance of thoracentesis in mechanically ventilated patients and have shown that the procedure may be performed with a low complication rate.[41,159]

The purpose of ultrasonography for procedural guidance of thoracentesis is to identity a safe site, angle, and depth for needle penetration that avoids injury to lung, subdiaphragmatic organs, and the heart. The critically ill patient is often supine, so by gravitational effect the pleural fluid takes a dependent posterior position in the thorax (unless loculated). The scanning plane should be in the longitudinal axis in the posterior to mid-axillary line. The transducer is angled and/or moved to find an anechoic space that is subtended by typical anatomical boundaries and that has typical dynamic findings, consistent with a pleural effusion. Before any consideration of needle insertion, the examiner must make unequivocal identification of the diaphragm. The neophyte ultrasonographer may misidentify the hepatorenal or splenorenal space, which is curvilinear, as the diaphragm. This is a serious error, as this could lead to laceration of these organs. There should be at least 10 mm of space between the inside of chest wall and the visceral pleural surface.[41,159] Once a suitable site is identified and marked, the depth of the penetration is measured from a frozen ultrasound image. Thoracentesis should be performed promptly after ultrasound marking without any patient movement to avoid shifting of fluid from the intended aspiration site. The syringe and the needle assembly should be introduced in the same angle in which the transducer was held while determining the best access site. This is best accomplished when the operator performs the procedure immediately following the examination. Following the procedure, the operator should check for pneumothorax by examining for lung sliding.[160] Ultrasound guidance of needle insertion may be used for simple thoracentesis or for insertion of pleural drainage system of any size.

An important pitfall is that firm pressure by the probe on the skin, particularly in an edematous patient, may indent the skin at the site of examination. This leads to the underestimation of the depth at which fluid will be reached when aspiration is attempted. The operator should be able to recognize this problem and needs to insert the needle more than the measured distance.

A rare but dreaded complication of any pleural procedure is intercostal artery injury. Some operators routinely look for the presence of an aberrantly positioned intercostal artery in the intercostal space **(Fig. 33)** to avoid any potential injury.

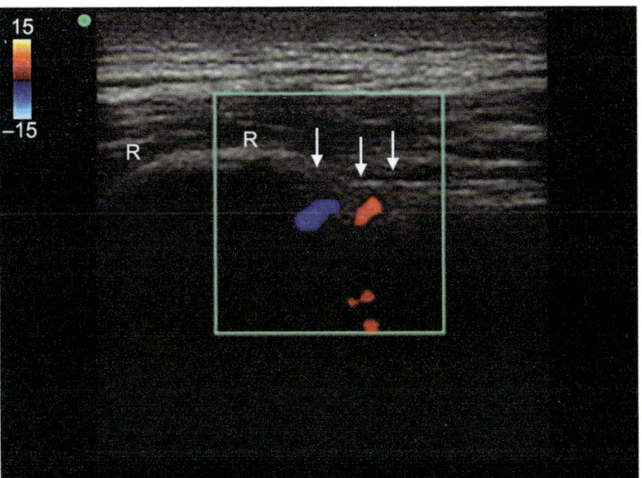

FIG. 33: Longitudinal scan through an intercostal space with a high frequency (vascular) probe shows the intercostal vessels (seen on color Doppler) sagging into the intercostal space (arrows). R = upper rib.

Ultrasound Guidance of Pericardiocentesis

Echocardiography-guided pericardiocentesis is the current standard of care for drainage of pericardial effusion. The traditional subxiphoid approach to pericardiocentesis, with or without fluoroscopic guidance, should be replaced in favor of ultrasound-guided pericardiocentesis.[161] In a report of 1,127 consecutive echocardiography-guided pericardiocenteses, success was achieved in 97% cases, including 89% cases where fluid could be obtained with a single needle pass. Major complications (chamber laceration or injury to an intercostal vessel necessitating surgery, pneumothoraces requiring chest tube placement, ventricular tachycardia, and bacteremia) were reported in 1.2% cases with death of one patient.[162] A similar success rate has been reported in another large series.[163]

To perform pericardiocentesis under ultrasound guidance, the examiner scans using multiple windows in order to determine a safe site, angle, and depth of needle penetration **(Figs. 34A and B)**. The ideal entry site is the point where the largest collection of fluid can be reached by the shortest distance from the skin following a straight trajectory and avoiding any vital structure.[161] Under ultrasound guidance, the left anterior chest wall is the entry site of the needle in the majority of the cases. The subxiphoid approach is often not indicated as the effusion is not of sufficient size or the liver blocks safe needle insertion. The patient's body position may be shifted in order to redistribute the pericardial fluid for better access. At least 10 mm of fluid depth is required to perform safe pericardiocentesis. The heart may exhibit marked movement both in swinging form and between systole and diastole, so the safe depth of needle penetration needs to be measured within the context of cardiac movement. Once the clinician marks the site for access, the patient should not move until the procedure is performed, out of concern that patient movement will cause redistribution of fluid within the pericardium. The site is prepared with sterile technique, and all equipment is prepared. A sterile transducer cover should be included in the setup. After the preparation and before needle insertion, the intensivist performs a confirmatory scan to document the best site, angle, and depth for needle insertion. Real-time guidance of needle insertion is not required for pericardiocentesis (similar to thoracentesis) provided the operator performs the scan immediately before the needle insertion. The needle and syringe assembly are held in the angle in which the transducer was held. Skin compression artifact may be problematic. This occurs when the transducer is applied firmly to the skin of the patient so that the measured depth underestimates the depth required to access fluid. The operator must take care to avoid asymmetric force application to the skin mark, as this may cause an inaccurate site of insertion. Placing a depth guard on the needle and introducing the needle in a straight line without any lateral movement ensure further safety of needle advancement. Once the needle has penetrated the pericardial fluid space, a wire and/or catheter may be introduced with prompt removal of the needle. The final catheter type is up to the discretion of the operator. The catheter position may be confirmed either by directly identifying the catheter within the pericardial space **(Fig. 34C)** or by injecting agitated saline through the catheter and visualizing the same in the pericardial space **(Fig. 34D)**.

Ultrasound Guidance of Paracentesis

Diagnostic and therapeutic paracentesis are common procedures performed in ICUs. Often, paracentesis is performed by a blind technique with reliance on physical examination to identify a suitable site. The safety and success of paracentesis can be improved by the use of ultrasonography.[164] Ultrasound guidance of paracentesis is preferable under certain circumstances: Advanced pregnancy, significant bowel distension, and extensive/multiple previous abdominal surgeries. The blind paracentesis is relatively contraindicated if any of these conditions is present.[165]

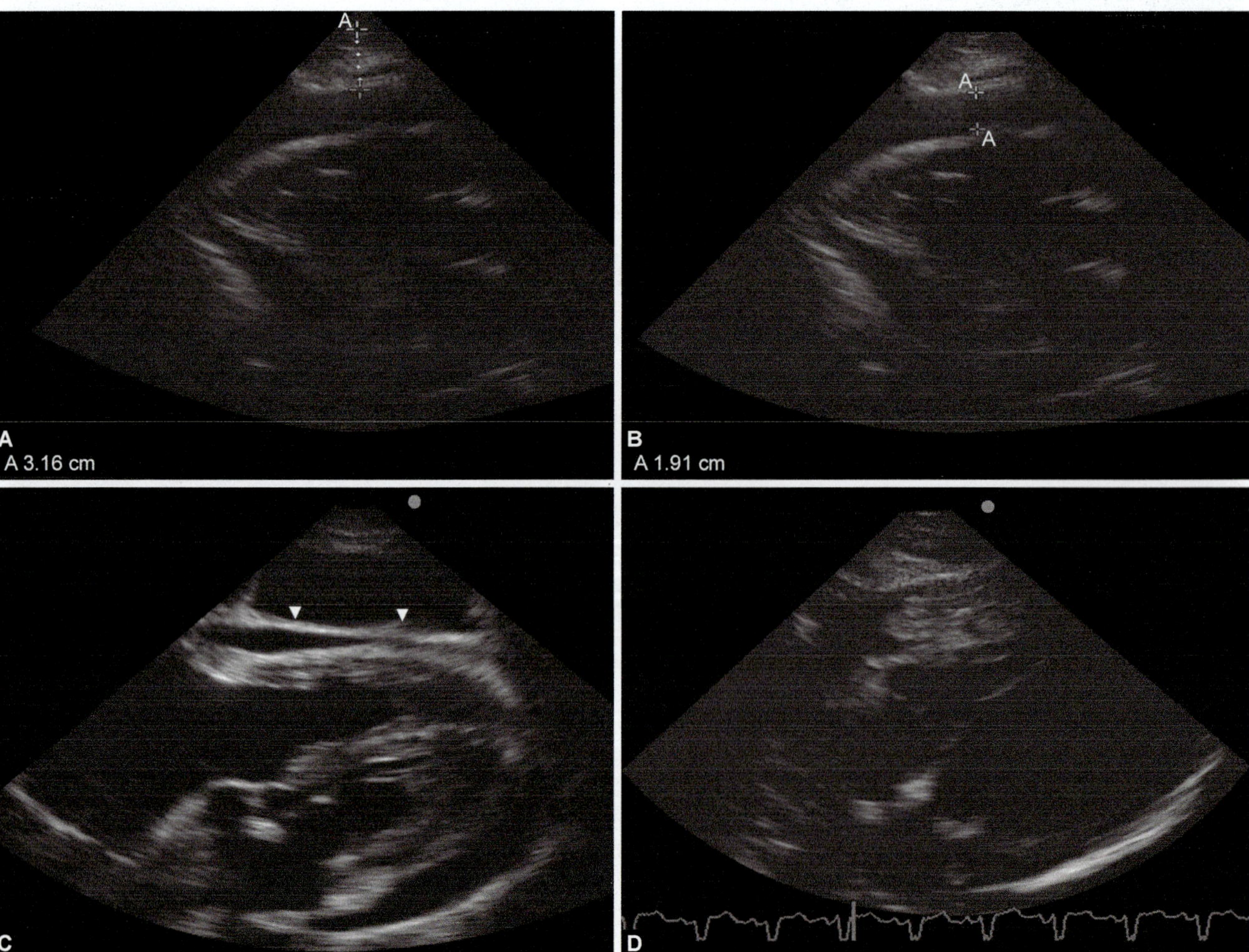

FIGS. 34A TO D: Pericardiocentesis under ultrasound guidance. (A and B) Large pericardial effusion. In PSL view, anterior effusion of 1.91 cm thickness was seen at a depth of 3.16 cm from the skin. Pericardiocentesis was performed from a left parasternal access. (C) The drainage catheter in the pericardial space (arrowheads) shown in the subcostal view. (D) Injection of agitated saline through the catheter helped to confirm the position of the catheter by opacification of the pericardial space.

In patients who have peritoneal adhesions from previous surgeries or peritonitis, the fluid may not be located at typical abdominal sites where blind paracentesis is attempted. The chance of success with blind paracentesis depends on the amount of fluid present. In patients who have a small amount of fluid, ultrasonography helps to confirm the presence of fluid and locate the best site for performing the procedure. In some patients thought to have ascites by clinical examination, ultrasonography may negate the presence of the same or may show too little fluid for safe paracentesis. Ultrasonography reduces unsuccessful blind attempts.[166]

Ultrasound-guided paracentesis uses the same skillset required to perform thoracentesis and pericardiocentesis. The operator scans the lower lateral abdomen and suprapubic area in order to identify the best site, angle, and depth for needle entry. The inferior epigastric artery **(Fig. 35A)** runs in the lateral rectus sheath and is generally sufficiently medial in position that it is not at risk for inadvertent needle injury. For maximal safety, the operator may examine the proposed insertion trajectory using a linear vascular probe for aberrant vascular structures **(Fig. 35B)** or other abnormalities **(Fig. 35C)** that might increase the risk of bleeding. Identification of linea alba provides an avascular plane for performing paracentesis in patients with coagulopathy **(Fig. 35D)**. Ascites has its mimics; a distended bladder or fluid-filled intestinal structures may be mistaken for ascites. They have anatomic patterns that allow the operator to differentiate from intra-abdominal fluid. Ascites changes in shape when the transducer is pushed into the abdominal wall. Like thoracentesis and pericardiocentesis, paracentesis need not be performed with real-time guidance provided the operator performs the procedure immediately following site identification without any interval patient

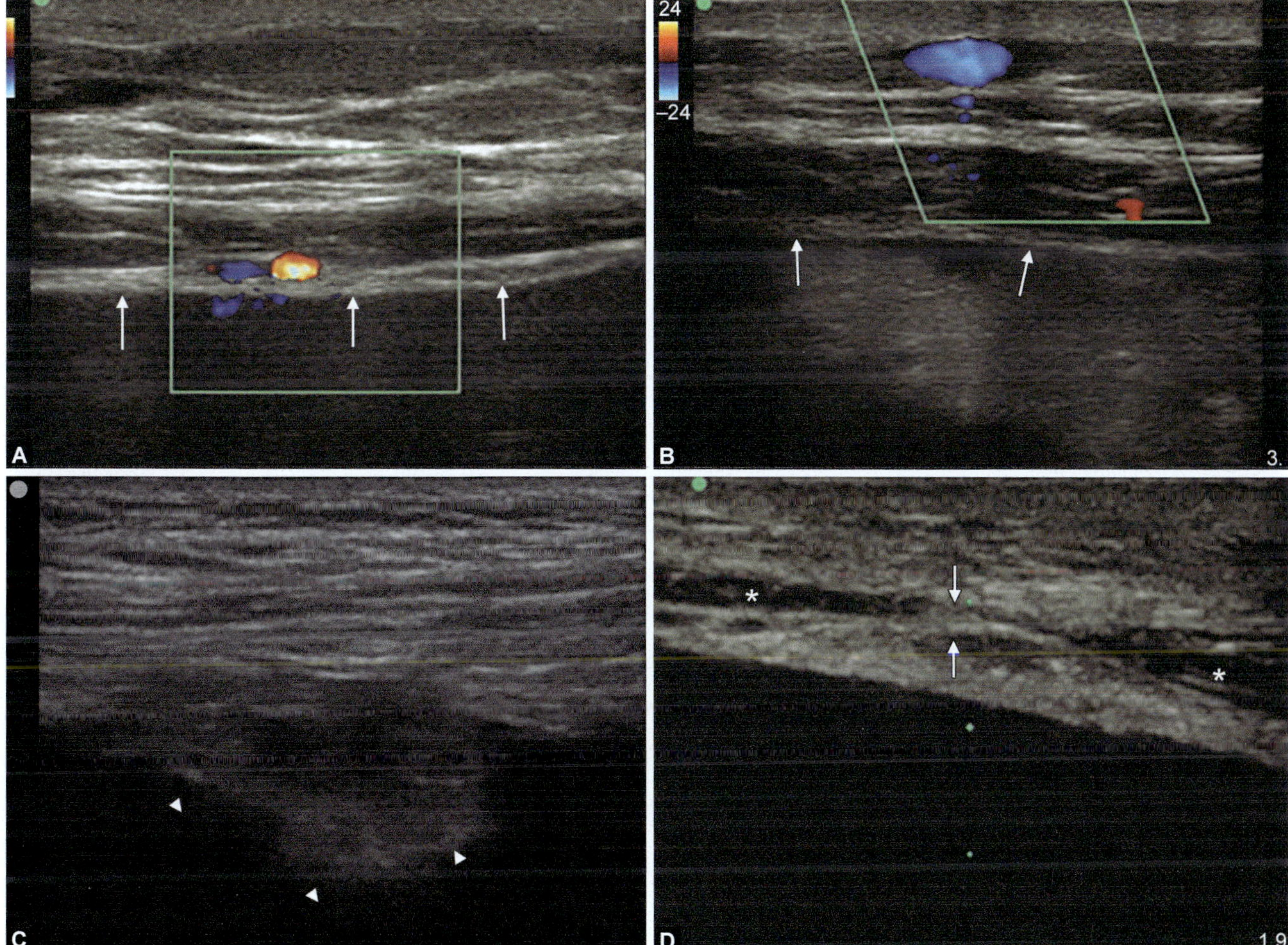

FIGS. 35A TO D: Paracentesis can be made safer with the use of ultrasound. (A) Epigastric vessels can easily be identified and avoided (arrows mark peritoneal lining). (B) Other aberrant vessels can be identified and avoided. In this patient with portal hypertension, the initially identified spot for paracentesis had a large dilated vein in the abdominal wall when checked with a high-frequency vascular probe (arrows mark peritoneal lining). (C) Peritoneal metastasis identified with ultrasound (arrowheads) in a patient who needed paracentesis. Traversing this spot for paracentesis would risk serious intraperitoneal hemorrhage. (D) Linea alba (arrow) can be identified with ultrasound in obese patients and offers a safe path for paracentesis. Rectus abdominis muscles shown (marked *).

movement. For ultrasound guidance of paracentesis, a suitable site is one where a collection of fluid is seen and a straight path of approach to the fluid from the skin surface avoids bowel loops and other organs.

Ultrasound for Airway Management

Ultrasonography can be helpful in airway management of critically ill patients.[167] It has been studied for preintubation measurement of anterior neck softtissue thickness, particularly in obese patients, showing positive correlation with difficulty in laryngoscopy.[168]

Ultrasonography can be used to confirm endotracheal intubation in two ways. By obtaining a midline longitudinal section of the trachea at the level of the cricoid cartilage, the endotracheal tube (ETT) can be visualized as an echogenic line below the anterior tracheal wall, provided there is no air artifact between tracheal wall and ETT. Whereas the endotracheal position of the tube can be confirmed, it is not possible to determine where the tip of the ETT is located. As an alternative, the presence of bilateral lung sliding and diaphragmatic movement with ventilation confirm ETT position. Ultrasonography may also be used to identify inadvertent mainstem bronchial intubation. In this case, if the ETT has been advanced to right mainstem bronchus with the inflated cuff blocking air entry to left, the patient will exhibit lung sliding with ventilation on the right side but will lack the same on the left side as no air entry occurs. The patient will have lung pulse on the left.[22] Very soon after the mainstem intubation, the left lung will develop resorptive atelectasis, particularly if the patient is on high FiO_2; the left lung will develop a consolidation pattern on ultrasonography. Drawing back of the ETT may be guided by lung ultrasonography.

Ultrasonography has been studied to predict extubation outcome. The degree of diaphragmatic movement during spontaneous breathing trial, measured as displacement of liver/spleen, has been reported to have more accuracy in predicting successful extubation than traditional weaning parameters.[169]

Ultrasonography has been used to guide percutaneous dilatational tracheostomy.[170-172] Ultrasound study of the thyroid and cricoid cartilages, tracheal rings, paratracheal soft tissues, thyroid gland, and vascular structures allows the intensivist to select the optimal puncture site of the trachea. The identification of a large aberrant midline vein or an innominate artery that is unusually high in position allows the intensivist to avoid catastrophic complication of major vessel injury **(Figs. 36A to C)**. With the help of ultrasonography, patients who have unfavorable anatomy for percutaneous dilatational tracheostomy can be identified and referred for surgical tracheostomy.[173]

During emergency endotracheal intubation, unrecognized gastric fluid collection may result in a life-threatening aspiration event. Ultrasonography can be used to rapidly identify a significant gastric fluid collection during the setup of emergency ETT **(Fig. 27H)**. This allows the team to empty the stomach with the insertion of a gastric tube, thereby avoiding the risk of a dangerous aspiration event.[174] If the patient is too unstable for gastric tube insertion, the team may take specific measures to prevent aspiration of gastric contents with the fore knowledge of the risk.

Ultrasound for Confirmation of Gastric Tube Placement

Ultrasonography can be used to confirm the proper location of a gastric tube. By scanning the left upper quadrant, the gastric tube may be seen as a discrete structure. Injection of air or fluid yields a characteristic pattern of air bubbles within the stomach. Bedside ultrasonography has been used to guide placement of nasoenteric feeding tubes[175,176]

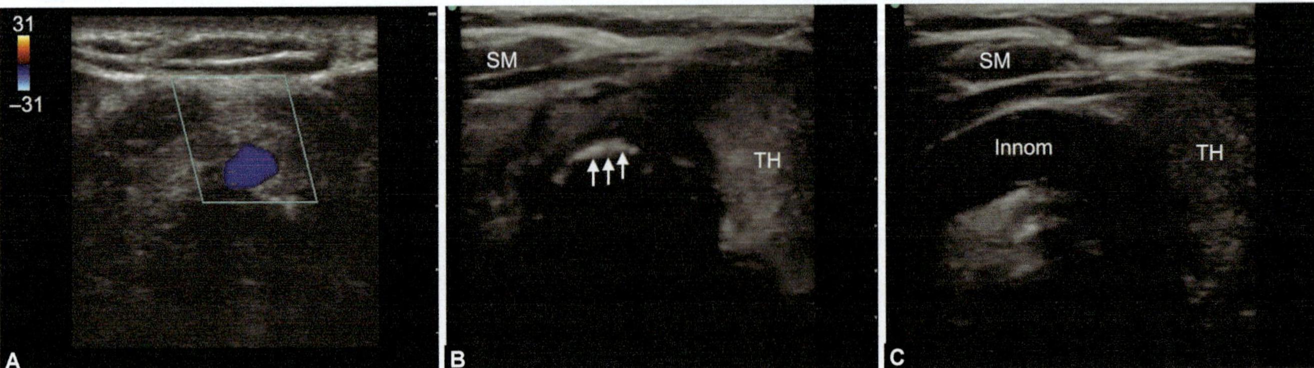

FIGS. 36A TO C: Role of ultrasonography in selection of case for percutaneous dilatational tracheostomy. (A) Prominent anterior thyroid vein close to the midline makes the case unsuitable for percutaneous tracheostomy. (B) Transverse scan over trachea to identify a suitable site. At this level, the airway could be identified, the bright line (arrows) indicating the tracheal mucosal interface. (SM= strap muscle; TH = thyroid gland) (C) Transverse scan over the lower part of cervical trachea, ~2 cm below the level shown in (B). Note the innominate artery (INNOM) arching over the right side of trachea, bringing a high risk of arterial injury if percutaneous tracheostomy is tried.

and to replace dislodged gastrostomy tubes.[177] The tip of the tube is visualized with ultrasonography; visualization can be improved by injecting air through the tube as air acts as a contrast for ultrasound imaging.[176]

Lumbar Puncture

Use of ultrasonography to facilitate spinal puncture has been reported in obstetric anesthesia literature. Using an initial paramedian longitudinal scan plane approach, the level of vertebral interspaces such as L_5–S_1 and L_4–L_5 are identified and marked. A transverse scan of each individual space is then performed. The processes flanking each vertebral interspace are identified as small hyperechoic signals. When the plane of transverse scanning passes exactly through an interspace, a hyperechoic band-like shadow of the ligamentum flavum and the dorsal dura is visualized. The best site, angle, and depth of puncture can be accurately judged. Use of ultrasound decreases procedure time and improves patient comfort.[178]

Other Procedures

Ultrasonography allows for accurate placement of needle, wire, or a drainage device into a wide variety of clinically important targets. For example, abscesses, LNs, lung masses, mediastinal masses, and fluid collections of all types may be accessed under ultrasound control. The principles of ultrasound guidance remain the same regardless of the procedure. The operator identifies the target and adjacent anatomic structures that must be avoided during the needle insertion. The best site, angle, and depth are determined. In many cases, real-time control is not necessary. For small targets, the operator must be proficient with real-time guidance. In the authors' experience, this is best done with the needle being scanned in its entirety along its long axis throughout insertion. The entry of needle into the target allows for simple aspiration or biopsy or may be followed by the drainage device of the operator's choice.

SUMMARY

Ultrasonography has major utility in critical care medicine. High-quality portable machines are widely available and permit point-of-care scanning by the frontline intensivist. Ultrasound imaging of the lung, pleura, vascular structures, heart, and abdominal organs allows rapid diagnosis and guides management at the bedside of the critically ill. Ultrasonography increases the safety and success rate of many common ICU procedures. We hope that this chapter serves to inform and motivate the intensivists to develop competence in the field of CCUS as defined in the ACCP-SRLF statement on competence in the field.

REFERENCES

1. Schmidt GA. ICU ultrasound. The coming boom. Chest. 2009;135(6):1407-8.
2. Frankel HL, Kirkpatrick AW, Elbarbary M, et al. Guidelines for the Appropriate Use of Bedside General and Cardiac Ultrasonography in the Evaluation of Critically Ill Patients—Part I: General Ultrasonography. Crit Care Med. 2015;43(11):2479-502.
3. Demi L, Wolfram F, Klersy C, et al. New International Guidelines and Consensus on the Use of Lung Ultrasound. J Ultrasound Med. 2023;42(2):309-44.
4. Mayo PH, Beaulieu Y, Doelken P, et al. American College of Chest Physicians/La SociÃ©tÃ© de RÃ©animation de Langue FranÃ§aise Statement on Competence in Critical Care Ultrasonography. Chest. 2009;135(4):1050-60.
5. Greenstein YY, Littauer R, Narasimhan M, et al. Effectiveness of a Critical Care Ultrasonography Course. Chest. 2017;151(1):34-40.
6. Institute of Medicine (US) Committee on Quality of Health Care in America. Crossing the Quality Chasm: A New Health System for the 21st Century. Washington, DC: National Academies Press; 2001.
7. Slonim A. The Use of Ultrasound in the ICU: Potential Impact on Care. In: Levitov A MP, Slonim AD (Eds). Critical Care Ultrasonography. New York: McGraw Hill Medical; 2009. pp. 3-10.
8. Levitov A, Frankel HL, Blaivas M, et al. Guidelines for the Appropriate Use of Bedside General and Cardiac Ultrasonography in the Evaluation of Critically Ill Patients-Part II: Cardiac Ultrasonography. Crit Care Med. 2016;44(6):1206-27.
9. Wong A, Galarza L, Duska F. Critical Care Ultrasound: A Systematic Review of International Training Competencies and Program. Crit Care Med. 2019;47(3):e256-62.
10. Robba C, Wong A, Poole D, et al. Basic ultrasound head-to-toe skills for intensivists in the general and neuro intensive care unit population: consensus and expert recommendations of the European Society of Intensive Care Medicine. Intensive Care Med. 2021;47(12):1347-67.
11. International expert statement on training standards for critical care ultrasonography. Intensive Care Med. 2011;37(7):1077-83.
12. Hagen-Ansert SL. Foundations of sonography. In: Hagen-Ansert SL (Ed). Textbook of Diagnostic Ultrasonography. Vol. 1. Berlin: Mosby Elsevier; 2006. pp. 3-32.
13. Doppler echocardiography and color flow imaging. Comprehensive noninvasive hemodynamic assessment. In: Oh JK SJ, Tajik AJ (Eds). The Echo Manual. Gurugram: Wolters Kluwer India; 2006. pp. 59-79.
14. Lichtenstein D, Goldstein I, Mourgeon E, et al. Comparative diagnostic performances of auscultation, chest radiography, and lung ultrasonography in acute respiratory distress syndrome. Anesthesiology. 2004;100(1):9-15.
15. Hendrikse KA, Gratama JW, Hove W, et al. Low value of routine chest radiographs in a mixed medical-surgical ICU. Chest. 2007;132(3):823-8.
16. Brenner DJ, Hall EJ. Computed tomography--an increasing source of radiation exposure. N Engl J Med. 2007;357(22):2277-84.

17. Lichtenstein DA. Ultrasound examination of the lungs in the intensive care unit. Pediatr Crit Care Med. 2009;10(6):693-8.
18. Tung-Chen Y, Ossaba-Velez S, Acosta Velasquez KS, et al. The Impact of Different Lung Ultrasound Protocols in the Assessment of Lung Lesions in COVID-19 Patients: Is There an Ideal Lung Ultrasound Protocol? J Ultrasound. 2022;25(3): 483-91.
19. Mayo PH, Doelken P. Pleural ultrasonography. Clin Chest Med. 2006;27(2):215-27.
20. Reuss J. The pleura. In: Mathis G, Lessnau KD (Eds). Atlas of Chest Sonography. Berlin: Springer-Verlag; 2003. pp. 17-35.
21. Lichtenstein DA. Pneumothorax and introduction to ultrasound signs in the lung. In: General Ultrasound in the Critically Ill. Berlin: Springer-Verlag; 2005. pp. 105-15.
22. Lichtenstein DA, Lascols N, Prin S, et al. The "lung pulse": an early ultrasound sign of complete atelectasis. Intensive Care Med. 2003;29(12):2187-92.
23. Soldati G, Testa A, Silva FR, et al. Chest ultrasonography in lung contusion. Chest. 2006;130(2):533-8.
24. Lichtenstein D, Meziere G, Biderman P, et al. The comet-tail artifact. An ultrasound sign of alveolar-interstitial syndrome. Am J Respir Crit Care Med. 1997;156(5):1640-6.
25. Volpicelli G, Mussa A, Garofalo G, et al. Bedside lung ultrasound in the assessment of alveolar-interstitial syndrome. Am J Emerg Med. 2006;24(6):689-96.
26. Targhetta R, Chavagneux R, Balmes P, et al. Sonographic lung surface evaluation in pulmonary sarcoidosis: preliminary results. J Ultrasound Med. 1994;13(5):381-8.
27. Reissig A, Kroegel C. Transthoracic sonography of diffuse parenchymal lung disease: the role of comet tail artifacts. J Ultrasound Med. 2003;22(2):173-80.
28. Bouhemad B, Liu ZH, Arbelot C, et al. Ultrasound assessment of antibiotic-induced pulmonary reaeration in ventilator-associated pneumonia. Crit Care Med. 2010;38(1):84-92.
29. Lichtenstein DA, Meziere GA, Lagoueyte JF, et al. A-lines and B-lines: lung ultrasound as a bedside tool for predicting pulmonary artery occlusion pressure in the critically ill. Chest. 2009;136(4):1014-20.
30. Volpicelli G, Elbarbary M, Blaivas M, et al. International evidence-based recommendations for point-of-care lung ultrasound. Intensive Care Med. 2012;38(4):577-91.
31. Yang PC, Luh KT, Chang DB, et al. Ultrasonographic evaluation of pulmonary consolidation. Am Rev Respir Dis. 1992;146(3): 757-62.
32. Weinberg B, Diakoumakis EE, Kass EG, et al. The air bronchogram: sonographic demonstration. AJR Am J Roentgenol. 1986;147(3):593-5.
33. Dorne HL. Differentiation of pulmonary parenchymal consolidation from pleural disease using the sonographic fluid bronchogram. Radiology. 1986;158(1):41-2.
34. Lichtenstein DA, Lascols N, Meziere G, et al. Ultrasound diagnosis of alveolar consolidation in the critically ill. Intensive Care Med. 2004;30(2):276-81.
35. Reissig A, Kroegel C. Sonographic diagnosis and follow-up of pneumonia: a prospective study. Respiration. 2007;74(5):537-47.
36. Mathis G, Bitschnau R, Gehmacher O, et al. Chest ultrasound in diagnosis of pulmonary embolism in comparison to helical CT. Ultraschall Med. 1999;20(2):54-9.
37. Pfeil A, Reissig A, Heyne JP, et al. Transthoracic sonography in comparison to multislice computed tomography in detection of peripheral pulmonary embolism. Lung. 188(1):43-50.
38. Reissig A, Heyne JP, Kroegel C. Sonography of lung and pleura in pulmonary embolism: sonomorphologic characterization and comparison with spiral CT scanning. Chest. 2001;120(6): 1977-83.
39. Mathis G, Blank W, Reissig A, et al. Thoracic ultrasound for diagnosing pulmonary embolism: a prospective multicenter study of 352 patients. Chest. 2005;128(3):1531-8.
40. Lichtenstein D, Meziere G, Seitz J. The dynamic air bronchogram. A lung ultrasound sign of alveolar consolidation ruling out atelectasis. Chest. 2009;135(6):1421-5.
41. Lichtenstein D, Hulot JS, Rabiller A, et al. Feasibility and safety of ultrasound-aided thoracentesis in mechanically ventilated patients. Intensive Care Med. 1999;25(9):955-8.
42. Vignon P, Chastagner C, Berkane V, et al. Quantitative assessment of pleural effusion in critically ill patients by means of ultrasonography. Crit Care Med. 2005;33(8):1757-63.
43. Balik M, Plasil P, Waldauf P, et al. Ultrasound estimation of volume of pleural fluid in mechanically ventilated patients. Intensive Care Med. 2006;32(2):318-21.
44. Remérand F, Dellamonica J, Mao Z, et al. Multiplane ultrasound approach to quantify pleural effusion at the bedside. Intensive Care Med. 2010;36(4):656-64.
45. McLoud TC, Flower CD. Imaging the pleura: sonography, CT, and MR imaging. AJR Am J Roentgenol. 1991;156(6):1145-53.
46. Tocino IM, Miller MH, Fairfax WR. Distribution of pneumothorax in the supine and semirecumbent critically ill adult. AJR Am J Roentgenol. 1985;144(5):901-5.
47. Lamb AD, Qadan M, Gray AJ. Detection of occult pneumothoraces in the significantly injured adult with blunt trauma. Eur J Emerg Med. 2007;14(2):65-7.
48. Trupka A, Waydhas C, Hallfeldt KK, et al. Value of thoracic computed tomography in the first assessment of severely injured patients with blunt chest trauma: results of a prospective study. J Trauma. 1997;43(3):405-11; discussion 411-402.
49. Soldati G, Testa A, Sher S, et al. Occult traumatic pneumothorax: diagnostic accuracy of lung ultrasonography in the emergency department. Chest. 2008;133(1):204-11.
50. Soldati G, Testa A, Pignataro G, et al. The ultrasonographic deep sulcus sign in traumatic pneumothorax. Ultrasound Med Biol. 2006;32(8):1157-63.
51. Lichtenstein DA, Meziere G, Lascols N, et al. Ultrasound diagnosis of occult pneumothorax. Crit Care Med. 2005;33(6):1231-8.
52. Lichtenstein DA, Menu Y. A bedside ultrasound sign ruling out pneumothorax in the critically ill. Lung sliding. Chest. 1995;108(5):1345-8.
53. Chiles C, Ravin CE. Radiographic recognition of pneumothorax in the intensive care unit. Crit Care Med. 1986;14(8):677-80.
54. Sartori S, Tombesi P, Trevisani L, et al. Accuracy of transthoracic sonography in detection of pneumothorax after sonographically guided lung biopsy: prospective comparison with chest radiography. AJR Am J Roentgenol. 2007;188(1):37-41.
55. Reissig A, Kroegel C. Accuracy of transthoracic sonography in excluding post-interventional pneumothorax and hydropneumothorax. Comparison to chest radiography. Eur J Radiol. 2005;53(3):463-70.

56. Lichtenstein D, Meziere G, Biderman P, et al. The "lung point": an ultrasound sign specific to pneumothorax. Intensive Care Med. 2000;26(10):1434-40.
57. Lichtenstein D, Meziere G, Biderman P, et al. The comet-tail artifact: an ultrasound sign ruling out pneumothorax. Intensive Care Med. 1999;25(4):383-8.
58. Lichtenstein DA, Meziere GA. Relevance of lung ultrasound in the diagnosis of acute respiratory failure: the BLUE protocol. Chest. 2008;134(1):117-25.
59. Lichtenstein D, Karakitsos D. Integrating lung ultrasound in the hemodynamic evaluation of acute circulatory failure (the fluid administration limited by lung sonography protocol). J Crit Care. 2012;533.e11-9.
60. Theerawit P, Touman N, Sutherasan Y, et al. Transthoracic ultrasound assessment of B-lines for identifying the increment of extravascular lung water in shock patients requiring fluid resuscitation. Indian J Crit Care Med. 2014;18(4):195-9.
61. Stefanidis K, Dimopoulos S, Tripodaki ES, et al. Lung sonography and recruitment in patients with early acute respiratory distress syndrome - a pilot study. Crit Care. 2011;15(4):R185.
62. Soummer A, Perbet S, Brisson H, et al. Ultrasound assessment of lung aeration loss during a successful weaning trial predicts postextubation distress. Crit Care Med. 2012;40(7):2064-72.
63. Vieillard-Baron A, Millington SJ, Sanfilippo F, et al. A decade of progress in critical care echocardiography: a narrative review. Intensive Care Med. 2019;45(6):770-88.
64. Expert Round Table on Echocardiography in ICU. International consensus statement on training standards for advanced critical care echocardiography. Intensive Care Med. 2014;40(5):654-66.
65. Oropello JM MA, Goldman M. Goal-directed echocardiography in the ICU. In: Levitov AB, Mayo PH, Slonim AD (Eds). Critical Care Ultrasonography. New York: McGraw Hill Medical; 2009. pp. 67-78.
66. Manasia AR, Nagaraj HM, Kodali RB, et al. Feasibility and potential clinical utility of goal-directed transthoracic echocardiography performed by noncardiologist intensivists using a small hand-carried device (SonoHeart) in critically ill patients. J Cardiothorac Vasc Anesth. 2005;19(2):155-9.
67. Volpicelli G, Lamorte A, Tullio M, et al. Point-of-care multiorgan ultrasonography for the evaluation of undifferentiated hypotension in the emergency department. Intensive Care Med. 2013;39(7):1290-8.
68. Pearson AC. Noninvasive evaluation of the hemodynamically unstable patient: the advantages of seeing clearly. Mayo Clin Proc. 1995;70(10):1012-4.
69. Cook CH, Praba AC, Beery PR, et al. Transthoracic echocardiography is not cost-effective in critically ill surgical patients. J Trauma. 2002;52(2):280-4.
70. Pearson AC, Castello R, Labovitz AJ. Safety and utility of transesophageal echocardiography in the critically ill patient. Am Heart J. 1990;119(5):1083-9.
71. McLean AS. Transoesophageal echocardiography in the intensive care unit. Anaesth Intensive Care. 1998;26(1):22-5.
72. Cerqueira MD, Weissman NJ, Dilsizian V, et al. Standardized myocardial segmentation and nomenclature for tomographic imaging of the heart: a statement for healthcare professionals from the Cardiac Imaging Committee of the Council on Clinical Cardiology of the American Heart Association. Circulation. 2002;105(4):539-42.
73. Mitchell C, Rahko PS, Blauwet LA, et al. Guidelines for Performing a Comprehensive Transthoracic Echocardiographic Examination in Adults: Recommendations from the American Society of Echocardiography. J Am Soc Echocardiogr. 2019;32(1):1-64.
74. Bargiggia GS, Bertucci C, Recusani F, et al. A new method for estimating left ventricular dP/dt by continuous wave Doppler-echocardiography. Validation studies at cardiac catheterization. Circulation. 1989;80(5):1287-92.
75. Gulati VK, Katz WE, Follansbee WP, et al. Mitral annular descent velocity by tissue Doppler echocardiography as an index of global left ventricular function. Am J Cardiol. 1996;77(11):979-84.
76. Fremont B, Pacouret G, Jacobi D, et al. Prognostic value of echocardiographic right/left ventricular end-diastolic diameter ratio in patients with acute pulmonary embolism: results from a monocenter registry of 1,416 patients. Chest. 2008;133(2):358-62.
77. Jardin F, Dubourg O, Bourdarias JP. Echocardiographic pattern of acute cor pulmonale. Chest. 1997;111(1):209-17.
78. Vieillard-Baron A, Charron C, Chergui K, et al. Bedside echocardiographic evaluation of hemodynamics in sepsis: is a qualitative evaluation sufficient? Intensive Care Med. 2006;32(10):1547-52.
79. Elzinga G, Piene H, de Jong JP. Left and right ventricular pump function and consequences of having two pumps in one heart. A study on the isolated cat heart. Circ Res. 1980;46(4):564-74.
80. Ryan T, Petrovic O, Dillon JC, et al. An echocardiographic index for separation of right ventricular volume and pressure overload. J Am Coll Cardiol. 1985;5(4):918-27.
81. Durairaj L, Schmidt GA. Fluid therapy in resuscitated sepsis: less is more. Chest. 2008;133(1):252-63.
82. Michard F, Teboul JL. Predicting fluid responsiveness in ICU patients: a critical analysis of the evidence. Chest. 2002;121(6):2000-8.
83. Marik PE, Baram M, Vahid B. Does central venous pressure predict fluid responsiveness? A systematic review of the literature and the tale of seven mares. Chest. 2008;134(1):172-8.
84. Leung JM, Levine EH. Left ventricular end-systolic cavity obliteration as an estimate of intraoperative hypovolemia. Anesthesiology. 1994;81(5):1102-9.
85. Michard F, Boussat S, Chemla D, et al. Relation between respiratory changes in arterial pulse pressure and fluid responsiveness in septic patients with acute circulatory failure. Am J Respir Crit Care Med. 2000;162(1):134-8.
86. Feissel M, Michard F, Mangin I, et al. Respiratory changes in aortic blood velocity as an indicator of fluid responsiveness in ventilated patients with septic shock. Chest. 2001;119(3):867-73.
87. Lamia B, Ochagavia A, Monnet X, et al. Echocardiographic prediction of volume responsiveness in critically ill patients with spontaneously breathing activity. Intensive Care Med. 2007;33(7):1125-32.
88. Maizel J, Airapetian N, Lorne E, et al. Diagnosis of central hypovolemia by using passive leg raising. Intensive Care Med. 2007;33(7):1133-8.
89. Monge Garcia MI, Gil Cano A, Diaz Monrove JC. Brachial artery peak velocity variation to predict fluid responsiveness in mechanically ventilated patients. Crit Care. 2009;13(5):R142.
90. Preau S, Saulnier F, Dewavrin F, et al. Passive leg raising is predictive of fluid responsiveness in spontaneously breathing patients with severe sepsis or acute pancreatitis. Crit Care Med. 2009;38(3):819-25.

91. Brennan JM, Blair JE, Hampole C, et al. Radial artery pulse pressure variation correlates with brachial artery peak velocity variation in ventilated subjects when measured by internal medicine residents using hand-carried ultrasound devices. Chest. 2007;131(5):1301-7.
92. Lichtenstein D. FALLS-protocol: lung ultrasound in hemodynamic assessment of shock. Heart Lung Vessel. 2013;5(3):142-7.
93. Wallace DJ, Allison M, Stone MB. Inferior vena cava percentage collapse during respiration is affected by the sampling location: an ultrasound study in healthy volunteers. Acad Emerg Med. 2010;17(1):96-9.
94. Sakurai T, Ando Y, Masunaga Y, et al. Diameter of the inferior vena cava as an index of dry weight in patients undergoing CAPD. Perit Dial Int. 1996;16(2):183-5.
95. Lyon M, Blaivas M, Brannam L. Sonographic measurement of the inferior vena cava as a marker of blood loss. Am J Emerg Med. 2005;23(1):45-50.
96. Barbier C, Loubieres Y, Schmit C, et al. Respiratory changes in inferior vena cava diameter are helpful in predicting fluid responsiveness in ventilated septic patients. Intensive Care Med. 2004;30(9):1740-6.
97. Kircher BJ, Himelman RB, Schiller NB. Noninvasive estimation of right atrial pressure from the inspiratory collapse of the inferior vena cava. Am J Cardiol. 1990;66(4):493-6.
98. Brennan JM, Ronan A, Goonewardena S, et al. Handcarried ultrasound measurement of the inferior vena cava for assessment of intravascular volume status in the outpatient hemodialysis clinic. Clin J Am Soc Nephrol. 2006;1(4):749-53.
99. Feissel M, Michard F, Faller JP, et al. The respiratory variation in inferior vena cava diameter as a guide to fluid therapy. Intensive Care Med. 2004;30(9):1834-7.
100. Lichtenstein DA. Inferior vena cava. In: General Ultrasound in the Critically Ill. Berlin: Springer-Verlag; 2005. pp. 82-6.
101. Vieillard-Baron A, Chergui K, Rabiller A, et al. Superior vena caval collapsibility as a gauge of volume status in ventilated septic patients. Intensive Care Med. 2004;30(9):1734-9.
102. Schacherer D, Klebl F, Goetz D, et al. Abdominal ultrasound in the intensive care unit: a 3-year survey on 400 patients. Intensive Care Med. 2007;33(5):841-4.
103. Tso P, Rodriguez A, Cooper C, et al. Sonography in blunt abdominal trauma: a preliminary progress report. J Trauma. 1992;33(1):39-43; discussion 43-34.
104. Rozycki GS, Ochsner MG, Schmidt JA, et al. A prospective study of surgeon-performed ultrasound as the primary adjuvant modality for injured patient assessment. J Trauma. 1995;39(3):492-8; discussion 498-500.
105. Goldberg BB, Clearfield HR, Goodman GA, Morales JO. Ultrasonic determination of ascites. Arch Intern Med. 1973;131(2):217-20.
106. Ollerton JE, Sugrue M, Balogh Z, et al. Prospective study to evaluate the influence of FAST on trauma patient management. J Trauma. 2006;60(4):785-91.
107. Chen SC, Wang HP, Chen WJ, et al. Selective use of ultrasonography for the detection of pneumoperitoneum. Acad Emerg Med. 2002;9(6):643-5.
108. Moriwaki Y, Sugiyama M, Toyoda H, et al. Ultrasonography for the diagnosis of intraperitoneal free air in chest-abdominal-pelvic blunt trauma and critical acute abdominal pain. Arch Surg. 2009;144(2):137-41; discussion 142.
109. Jones R. Recognition of pneumoperitoneum using bedside ultrasound in critically ill patients presenting with acute abdominal pain. Am J Emerg Med. 2007;25(7):838-41.
110. Lee DH, Lim JH, Ko YT, et al. Sonographic detection of pneumoperitoneum in patients with acute abdomen. AJR Am J Roentgenol. 1990;154(1):107-9.
111. Muradali D, Wilson S, Burns PN, et al. A specific sign of pneumoperitoneum on sonography: enhancement of the peritoneal stripe. AJR Am J Roentgenol. 1999;173(5):1257-62.
112. Mirvis SE, Vainright JR, Nelson AW, et al. The diagnosis of acute acalculous cholecystitis: a comparison of sonography, scintigraphy, and CT. AJR Am J Roentgenol. 1986;147(6):1171-5.
113. Shiver SA, Lyon M, Blaivas M, et al. Prospective comparison of emergency physician-performed venous ultrasound and CT venography for deep venous thrombosis. Am J Emerg Med. 2010;28(3):354-8.
114. Reissig A, Kroegel C. Diagnosis of pulmonary embolism and pneumonia using transthoracic sonography. In: Bolliger CT, Herth FJF, Mayo FJF, et al. (Eds). Clinical Chest Ultrasound: From the ICU to the Bronchoscopy Suite. Vol. 37. Basel: Karger; 2009. pp. 43-50.
115. Lensing AW, Prandoni P, Brandjes D, et al. Detection of deep-vein thrombosis by real-time B-mode ultrasonography. N Engl J Med. 1989;320(6):342-5.
116. Lichtenstein DA. Lower extremity veins. In: General Ultrasound in the Critically Ill. Berlin: Springer-Verlag; 2005. pp. 87-95.
117. Maki DD, Kumar N, Nguyen B, et al. Distribution of thrombi in acute lower extremity deep venous thrombosis: implications for sonography and CT and MR venography. AJR Am J Roentgenol. 2000;175(5):1299-301.
118. Badgett DK, Comerota MC, Khan MN, et al. Duplex venous imaging: role for a comprehensive lower extremity examination. Ann Vasc Surg. 2000;14(1):73-6.
119. Vogel P, Laing FC, Jeffrey RB, Jr., et al. Deep venous thrombosis of the lower extremity: US evaluation. Radiology. 1987;163(3):747-51.
120. Labropoulos N, Bekelis K, Leon LR, Jr. Thrombosis in unusual sites of the lower extremity veins. J Vasc Surg. 2008;47(5):1022-7.
121. Le Gal G, Righini M, Sanchez O, et al. A positive compression ultrasonography of the lower limb veins is highly predictive of pulmonary embolism on computed tomography in suspected patients. Thromb Haemost. 2006;95(6):963-6.
122. Torbicki A, Perrier A, Konstantinides S, et al. Guidelines on the diagnosis and management of acute pulmonary embolism: the Task Force for the Diagnosis and Management of Acute Pulmonary Embolism of the European Society of Cardiology (ESC). Eur Heart J. 2008;29(18):2276-315.
123. Nazerian P, Vanni S, Volpicelli G, et al. Accuracy of point-of-care multiorgan ultrasonography for the diagnosis of pulmonary embolism. Chest. 2014;145(5):950-7.
124. Koenig S, Chandra S, Alaverdian A, et al. Ultrasound assessment of pulmonary embolism in patients receiving CT pulmonary angiography. Chest. 2014;145(4):818-23.
125. Becker DM, Philbrick JT, Walker FB 4th. Axillary and subclavian venous thrombosis. Prognosis and treatment. Arch Intern Med. 1991;151(10):1934-43.
126. Yukisawa S, Fujiwara Y, Yamamoto Y, et al. Upper-extremity deep vein thrombosis related to central venous port systems implanted in cancer patients. Br J Radiol. 2010;83(994):850-3.
127. Lobo BL, Vaidean G, Broyles J, et al. Risk of venous thromboembolism in hospitalized patients with peripherally inserted central catheters. J Hosp Med. 2009;4(7):417-22.

128. Verso M, Agnelli G, Kamphuisen PW, et al. Risk factors for upper limb deep vein thrombosis associated with the use of central vein catheter in cancer patients. Intern Emerg Med. 2008;3(2):117-22.
129. Martin C, Viviand X, Saux P, et al. Upper-extremity deep vein thrombosis after central venous catheterization via the axillary vein. Crit Care Med. 1999;27(12):2626-9.
130. Di Nisio M, van Sluis GL, Bossuyt PM, et al. Accuracy of diagnostic tests for clinically suspected upper extremity deep vein thrombosis: a systematic review. J Thromb Haemost. 2010;8(4):684-92.
131. Kearon C, Julian JA, Newman TE, et al. Noninvasive diagnosis of deep venous thrombosis. McMaster Diagnostic Imaging Practice Guidelines Initiative. Ann Intern Med. 1998;128(8):663-77.
132. Durbec O, Viviand X, Potie F, et al. A prospective evaluation of the use of femoral venous catheters in critically ill adults. Crit Care Med. 1997;25(12):1986-9.
133. Milling TJ, Jr, Rose J, Briggs WM, et al. Randomized, controlled clinical trial of point-of-care limited ultrasonography assistance of central venous cannulation: the Third Sonography Outcomes Assessment Program (SOAP-3) Trial. Crit Care Med. 2005;33(8):1764-9.
134. Karakitsos D, Labropoulos N, De Groot E, et al. Real-time ultrasound-guided catheterisation of the internal jugular vein: a prospective comparison with the landmark technique in critical care patients. Crit Care. 2006;10(6):R162.
135. Randolph AG, Cook DJ, Gonzales CA, et al. Ultrasound guidance for placement of central venous catheters: a meta-analysis of the literature. Crit Care Med. 1996;24(12):2053-8.
136. Hind D, Calvert N, McWilliams R, et al. Ultrasonic locating devices for central venous cannulation: meta-analysis. BMJ. 2003; 327(7411):361.
137. Rothschild JM. (2001). Ultrasound guidance of central vein catheterization. [online] Available from http://www.ahrq.gov/clinic/ptsafety/chap21.htm [Last accessed September, 2024].
138. Cecchini S, Schena E, Saccomandi P, et al. Cardiac output estimation in mechanically ventilated patients: a comparison between prolonged expiration method and thermodilution. Conf Proc IEEE Eng Med Biol Soc. 2012;2012:2708-11.
139. Lamperti M, Bodenham AR, Pittiruti M, et al. International evidence-based recommendations on ultrasound-guided vascular access. Intensive Care Med. 2012;38(7):1105-17.
140. Feller-Kopman D. Ultrasound-guided internal jugular access: a proposed standardized approach and implications for training and practice. Chest. 2007;132(1):302-9.
141. Pirotte T. Ultrasound-guided vascular access in adults and children: beyond the internal jugular vein puncture. Acta Anaesthesiol Belg. 2008;59(3):157-66.
142. Maecken T, Grau T. Ultrasound imaging in vascular access. Crit Care Med. 2007;35(5 Suppl):S178-85.
143. Lichtenstein D, Saifi R, Augarde R, et al. The Internal jugular veins are asymmetric. Usefulness of ultrasound before catheterization. Intensive Care Med. 2001;27(1):301-5.
144. Samy Modeliar S, Sevestre MA, de Cagny B, et al. Ultrasound evaluation of central veinsin the intensive care unit:effects of dynamic manoeuvres. Intensive Care Med. 2008;34(2):333-8.
145. Denys BG, Uretsky BF. Anatomical variations of internal jugular vein location: impact on central venous access. Crit Care Med. 1991;19(12):1516-9.
146. Shiver S, Blaivas M, Lyon M. A prospective comparison of ultrasound-guided and blindly placed radial arterial catheters. Acad Emerg Med. 2006;13(12):1275-9.
147. Levin PD, Sheinin O, Gozal Y. Use of ultrasound guidance in the insertion of radial artery catheters. Crit Care Med. 2003;31(2): 481-4.
148. Loh YJ, Nakao M, Tan WD, Lim CH, Tan YS, Chua YL. Factors influencing radial artery size. Asian Cardiovasc Thorac Ann. 2007;15(4):324-6.
149. Blaivas M, Lyon M. The effect of ultrasound guidance on the perceived difficulty of emergency nurse-obtained peripheral IV access. J Emerg Med. 2006;31(4):407-10.
150. Costantino TG, Parikh AK, Satz WA, et al. Ultrasonography-guided peripheral intravenous access versus traditional approaches in patients with difficult intravenous access. Ann Emerg Med. 2005;46(5):456-61.
151. Stone MB, Moon C, Sutijono D, et al. Needle tip visualization during ultrasound-guided vascular access: short-axis vs long-axis approach. Am J Emerg Med. 2010;28(3):343-7.
152. Orihashi K, Imai K, Sato K, et al. Extrathoracic subclavian venipuncture under ultrasound guidance. Circ J. 2005;69(9): 1111-5.
153. de Graaff JC, Bras LJ, Vos JA. Early transection of a central venous catheter in a sedated ICU patient. Br J Anaesth. 2006;97(6):832-4.
154. Howes B, Dell R. Ultrasound to detect incorrect guidewire positioning during subclavian line insertion. Anaesthesia. 2006; 61(6):615.
155. Sandhu NS, Patel B. Use of ultrasonography as a rescue technique for failed radial artery cannulation. J Clin Anesth. 2006;18(2):138-41.
156. Shiloh AL, Eisen LA. Ultrasound-guided arterial catheterization: a narrative review. Intensive Care Med. 2010;36(2):214-21.
157. Cardenas-Garcia J, Schaub KF, Belchikov YG, et al. Safety of peripheral intravenous administration of vasoactive medication. J Hosp Med. 2015;10(9):581-5.
158. Gordon CE, Feller-Kopman D, Balk EM, et al. Pneumothorax following thoracentesis: a systematic review and meta-analysis. Arch Intern Med. 170(4):332-9.
159. Mayo PH, Goltz HR, Tafreshi M, et al. Safety of ultrasound-guided thoracentesis in patients receiving mechanical ventilation. Chest. 2004;125(3):1059-62.
160. Saucier S, Motyka C, Killu K. Ultrasonography versus chest radiography after chest tube removal for the detection of pneumothorax. AACN Adv Crit Care. 21(1):34-8.
161. Tsang TS, Freeman WK, Sinak LJ, et al. Echocardiographically guided pericardiocentesis: evolution and state-of-the-art technique. Mayo Clin Proc. 1998;73(7):647-52.
162. Tsang TS, Enriquez-Sarano M, Freeman WK, et al. Consecutive 1127 therapeutic echocardiographically guided pericardiocenteses: clinical profile, practice patterns, and outcomes spanning 21 years. Mayo Clin Proc. 2002;77(5):429-36.
163. Cho BC, Kang SM, Kim DH, et al. Clinical and echocardiographic characteristics of pericardial effusion in patients who underwent echocardiographically guided pericardiocentesis: Yonsei Cardiovascular Center experience, 1993-2003. Yonsei Med J. 2004;45(3):462-8.
164. Bard C, Lafortune M, Breton G. Ascites: ultrasound guidance or blind paracentesis? CMAJ. 1986;135(3):209-10.
165. McGibbon A, Chen GI, Peltekian KM, et al. An evidence-based manual for abdominal paracentesis. Dig Dis Sci. 2007;52(12):3307-15.
166. Nazeer SR, Dewbre H, Miller AH. Ultrasound-assisted paracentesis performed by emergency physicians vs the traditional technique: a prospective, randomized study. Am J Emerg Med. 2005;23(3):363-7.

167. Åustic A. Role of ultrasound in the airway management of critically ill patients. Crit Care Med. 2007;35(5):S173-7.
168. Ezri T, Gewurtz G, Sessler DI, et al. Prediction of difficult laryngoscopy in obese patients by ultrasound quantification of anterior neck soft tissue. Anaesthesia. 2003;58(11):1111-4.
169. Jiang J-R, Tsai T-H, Jerng J-S, Yu C-J, et al Ultrasonographic Evaluation of Liver/Spleen Movements and Extubation Outcome. Chest. 2004;126(1):179-85.
170. Muhammad JK, Patton DW, Evans RM, et al. Percutaneous dilatational tracheostomy under ultrasound guidance. Br J Oral Maxillofac Surg. 1999;37(4):309-11.
171. Sustic A, Zupan Z, Krstulovic B. Ultrasonography and percutaneous dilatational tracheostomy. Acta Anaesthesiol Scand. 1999;43(10):1086-8.
172. Sustic A, Kovac D, Zgaljardic Z, et al. Ultrasound-guided percutaneous dilatational tracheostomy: a safe method to avoid cranial misplacement of the tracheostomy tube. Intensive Care Med. 2000;26(9):1379-81.
173. Muhammad JK, Major E, Patton DW. Evaluating the neck for percutaneous dilatational tracheostomy. J Craniomaxillofac Surg. 2000;28(6):336-42.
174. Koenig SJ, Lakticova V, Mayo PH. Utility of ultrasonography for detection of gastric fluid during urgent endotracheal intubation. Intensive Care Med. 2011;37(4):627-31.
175. Hernandez-Socorro CR, Marin J, Ruiz-Santana S, et al. Bedside sonographic-guided versus blind nasoenteric feeding tube placement in critically ill patients. Crit Care Med. 1996;24(10):1690-4.
176. Gubler C, Bauerfeind P, Vavricka SR, et al. Bedside sonographic control for positioning enteral feeding tubes: a controlled study in intensive care unit patients. Endoscopy. 2006;38(12):1256-60.
177. Wu TS, Leech SJ, Rosenberg M, et al. Ultrasound can accurately guide gastrostomy tube replacement and confirm proper tube placement at the bedside. J Emerg Med. 2009;36(3):280-4.
178. Carvalho JC. Ultrasound-facilitated epidurals and spinals in obstetrics. Anesthesiol Clin. 2008;26(1):145-58, vii-viii.

FURTHER READINGS

1. Levitov A, Mayo PH, Slonim AD (Eds). Critical Care Ultrasonography, 2nd edition. New York: McGraw Hill Medical; 2014.
2. Lichtenstein DA. Whole Body Ultrasonography in the Critically Ill, 1st edition. Berlin: Springer; 2010.

Sedation, Analgesia, and Delirium in the Intensive Care Unit

CHAPTER 174

Karan Madan, Ayush Goel, Ritesh Agarwal

INTRODUCTION

Critical care is full of potential stressors. Up to 70% of critically ill patients experience agitation, pain, anxiety, and confusion during their intensive care unit (ICU) stay. Common stressors include pain, sleeplessness, mechanical ventilation, presence of tracheal tubes, invasive procedures, intravenous lines, catheters, noise, thoughts of death, and uncertainty regarding recovery from illness. How much sedation is given, and for how long, is important in determining patient outcomes as both over and undersedation can have deleterious consequences. Undersedation can cause increased sympathetic response, accidental extubations, and physical and psychological stress whereas oversedation can lead to increased duration of invasive mechanical ventilation and prolonged duration of stay in the ICU. Sedation is the depression of a patients' awareness to its environment and reduction of their responsiveness to external stimulation. Depth of sedation is a continuum (**Table 1**).

ASSESSMENT OF PAIN, SEDATION, AND AGITATION IN THE INTENSIVE CARE UNIT

Assessment of level of consciousness, pain, agitation, and cognition is central to patient management. The use of validated assessment methods like pain and sedation scales provides homogeneity of assessment among different caregivers, means for objective measurement, and better communication. The use of scales permits medication titration to desired levels, thereby minimizing the risk of oversedation and providing provision of adequate analgesia.

Assessment of Pain

Various validated tools are available to detect and quantify pain, thus guiding the dose of analgesia.

Patients Who can Communicate

The gold standard for pain assessment is the patients' self-report. Common self-reported scales include numeric rating scale (NRS), visual analogical scale (VAS), and the verbal descriptor scale (VDS). The NRS rates pain on a 0–10 scale with 0 indicating no pain and 10 being the worst pain experienced.[1] It is the most feasible scale with studies showing that up to 90% of the patients with ability to follow simple commands are able to correctly use it. Having a tracheal tube should not restrict the physicians or nursing staff from using this scale.[2] The VDS includes five descriptors "no pain", "mild pain", "moderate pain", "severe pain", and "extreme pain". The patients' cultural and language differences must be kept in mind and appropriate changes should be made during assessment.

Patients Who cannot Communicate

In situations where the patients are not able to self-report pain, observation of the patient's pain behavior is used

TABLE 1: Depths of sedation.

	Minimal sedation (anxiolysis)	Moderate sedation (conscious sedation)	Deep sedation	General anesthesia
Responsiveness	Normal response to verbal stimuli	Purposeful response to verbal/tactile stimuli	Purposeful response following repeated or painful stimuli	Unarousable even with painful stimulus
Airway	Unaffected	Able to protect	Intervention may be required	Intervention often required
Spontaneous ventilation	Unaffected	Adequate	May be inadequate	Frequently inadequate
Cardiovascular function	Unaffected	Maintained	Maintained	May be impaired

to assess pain. The two most widely available scales with studies showing robust psychometric performance are the critical care pain observational tool (CPOT) and the behavior pain scale (BPS). These scales help standardize the observation of behaviors indicative of pain (facial expression, body movements/tonus, and vocalization/ventilator compliance).[3]

Behavioral pain scale is based on three variables as highlighted in **Table 2**. Each of these variables are thought to signify pain and are scored from 1 to 4. The score ranges from 3 (no pain), 4–5 (mild pain), and 6–12 (unacceptable amount of pain).[4]

TABLE 2: Behavioral pain scale (BPS).

Item	Description	Score
Facial expression	• Relaxed • Partially tightened (e.g., brow lowering) • Fully tightened (e.g., eyelid closure) • Grimacing	1 2 3 4
Upper limbs	• No movement • Partially bent • Fully bent with finger flexion • Permanently retracted	1 2 3 4
Compliance with ventilation	• Tolerating ventilation • Coughing but tolerating ventilation most of the time • Fighting ventilator but ventilation possible at times • Unable to control ventilation	1 2 3 4

Critical care pain observational tool uses four domains with assessment of muscle tension in addition to the ones included in BPS. Each variable is scored from 0 to 2 with total score ranging from 0 (no pain) to 8 (maximal pain)[5] **(Table 3)**. Both BPS and CPOT scales have been shown to have discriminant validity for the presence of pain and also possess fair inter-rater reliability.[6]

Patients Who cannot Communicate nor Express Pain Behaviors

Some patients in the ICU require deep sedation with or without neuromuscular blocking agents in view of severe neurological or respiratory conditions. Behavioral scales cannot be used in these settings due to decreased responsiveness. Newer electrophysiological devices based on measurement of multiple physiological markers related to sympathetic–parasympathetic responses to pain (heart rate variability, pupillary dilatation, temperature, skin conductance, body plethysmography, etc.), have been developed to assess pain in such situations.[7] The nociception level index (NOL) is an artificial intelligence-based technology that acquires physiological signals through four sensors, analyses pain-related patterns and finally displays result on a monitor from a scale of 0 (no pain) to 100 (maximal pain).[8] Pilot studies have shown that these methods can help discriminate pain and reduce analgesia use; however, larger studies are needed before their widespread application.[9]

Sedation Assessment Scales

Sedation scoring is a valuable tool for ICU teams to assess the depth of sedation in patients. This assessment allows for the

TABLE 3: Critical pain and observation tool (CPOT).

Indicator	Descriptor	Score	
Facial expression	• No muscle tension observed • Presence of frowning, brow lowering, orbit tightening, and levator contraction • All of the above movements plus eyelid tightly closed	Relaxed neutral Tense Grimacing	0 1 2
Body movements	• Does not move at all • Slow cautious movements like touching/rubbing pain site • Pulling tube, attempting to sit up, moving/thrashing limbs, and striking at staff	Absence of movements Protection Restlessness	0 1 2
Muscle tension (evaluate by passive flexion and extension of extremities)	• No resistance to passive movements • Resistance to passive movements • Strong resistance and inability to complete movement	Relaxed Tense and rigid Very tense or rigid	0 1 2
Compliance with the ventilator (intubated patients)	• Alarms not activated, easy ventilation • Alarms stop spontaneously • Asynchrony blocking ventilation with alarms frequently being activated	Tolerating ventilator Coughing but tolerating Fighting ventilator	0 1 2
Vocalization (extubated patient)	• Talking in normal tone or no sound • Sighing or moaning • Crying out or sobbing		0 1 2

TABLE 4: Various sedation assessment scales.

Scale	Consciousness	Agitation	Pain	Ventilator synchrony	Comprehension
Ramsay sedation scale (RSS)	+	+			
Sedation agitation scale (SAS)	+	+			
Motor activity assessment scale (MAAS)	+	+			
Richmond agitation sedation scale (RASS)	+	+		+	
Adaptation to intensive care environment (ATICE)	+	+	+	+	+

TABLE 5: Ramsay sedation scale (RSS).

Description	Score
Patient anxious and agitated or restless or both	1
Patient cooperative, orientated, and tranquil	2
Patient responds to commands only	3
Brisk response to a light glabellar tap or loud auditory stimulus	4
Sluggish response to a light glabellar tap or loud auditory stimulus	5
No response to a light glabellar tap or loud auditory stimulus	6

TABLE 6: Richmond agitation sedation scale (RASS).

Term	Description	Score
Combative	Overtly violent and immediate danger to staff	+4
Very agitated	Pulls on tubes/catheters or exhibits aggressive behavior toward staff	+3
Agitated	Patient–ventilator asynchrony or frequent nonpurposeful movement	+2
Restless	Anxious or apprehensive but movements are not aggressive	+2
Alert and calm		0
Drowsy	Not fully alert but sustained awakening (>10 s) with eye contact to voice	–1
Light sedation	Briefly (<10 s) awakens with eye contact to voice	–2
Moderate sedation	Any movement to voice without eye contact	–3
Deep sedation	No response to voice but responds to physical stimulation	–4
Unarousable	No response to physical stimulation	–5

targeting of patient-specific goals by adjusting analgesic and sedative therapies to achieve an optimal level of sedation.[10] It is crucial for sedation scoring to be objective, as guessing the level of sedation is unreliable and inconsistent. It is strongly recommended to utilize sedation scoring systems in the ICU, which involve evaluating a patient's response to verbal and physical stimuli. The patient's response determines a numerical score, indicating the level of sedation. Regular reassessment enables the titration of sedation for each patient, aiming to achieve an optimal level of sedation.[11] The ideal sedation assessment scale should be able to correctly identify the level of consciousness, agitation, pain, and comprehension while being simple and user-friendly with high interobserver reliability.[12] The Ramsay sedation scale was introduced almost half a century ago and since then a large number of scales have been developed **(Table 4)**.[13]

All of these scales assess the levels of patient sedation based on a common principle of observing response to increasing levels of stimulation. An initial observation is made to see whether the patient is awake. If not, the response to auditory and subsequently more intense (physical) stimulation is noted. The responses indicate a progressively deeper level of sedation.

The Ramsay scale **(Table 5)** is straightforward and provides three levels of awake states (score 1–3) and three levels of asleep states (score 4–6).[14] The Society of Critical Care Medicine (SCCM) guidelines suggest using the sedation agitation scale (SAS) or Richmond agitation sedation scale (RASS) as they have shown to have the highest psychometric scores. Both scales have demonstrated high degree of inter-rater reliability and have shown to be able to discriminate among different sedation levels.[15]

The RASS **(Table 6)** scores patients on a 10 point scale ranging from +4 (combative) to –5 (unarousable). RASS score of –2 to +1 corresponds to light sedation whereas a score of –3 to –5 denotes deep sedation.[16]

Sedation scoring is usually performed by the nursing staff and should be done every 4 hourly and more frequently if the patient is unstable or if their sedation medication needs frequent adjustment.

Objective Methods of Assessing Sedation

Measuring brain activity can be done using cerebral function monitors. The various available systems are the bispectral index (BIS),[13] patient state index (PSI),[17] narcotrend index,[18] and the cerebral state index (CSI).[19] Of these, the BIS is the most widely studied tool. It is a specialized electrocardiograph (EEG) monitor which provides a quantitative assessment of the patient's level of consciousness. The value ranges from 0 (indicating isoelectric line) to 100 (completely awake state).[13] It is best suited for sedative titration during deep sedation or neuromuscular blockade. BIS monitoring has good correlation with subjective sedation scales like RASS. A study reported that a score of 70 differentiated adequate from inadequate sedation with 85% sensitivity and 80% specificity.[20] Few small-size studies comparing BIS monitoring with a subjective tool have shown reduction in total sedative use and faster awakening time.[21]

Choosing the Optimum Depth of Sedation

Intensive care unit sedation practices have evolved dramatically over the years. Historically, patients were often deeply sedated, and controlled modes of mechanical ventilation were used. Such practice has consistently been shown to be strongly associated with poor outcomes. The current guidelines recommend to use minimum sedation and allow spontaneous awakening trials (SATs) daily while ensuring patient comfort.[15]

A trial done by Kress et al. in 2020 introduced and validated the concept of protocolized sedation. They showed that using ICU sedation protocols to target Ramsay score of 3–4 with daily interruption of sedation as opposed to local practices was associated with a significantly shorter duration of mechanical ventilation (4.9 vs. 7.3, $p = 0.004$). There was also a significant reduction in the amount of sedative (midazolam) and analgesic used (morphine).[22]

Numerous studies over the years have compared light sedation (Ramsay score 1–2) with deep sedation (Ramsay score 3–4). A randomized controlled trial done by Treggiari et al. among 137 patients showed that the mean duration of mechanical ventilation (2.9 vs. 5.5 days, $p = 0.02$) and ICU length of stay (4.0 vs. 5.5, $p = 0.03$) were all significantly shorter in the intervention arm (target sedation range Ramsay 1–2) as compared to the control arm (Ramsay 3–4). The post-traumatic stress disorder (PTSD) scores assessed at 4 weeks after discharge were also lower in the intervention arm.[23] The SPICE study also showed that early deep sedation (assessed at 48 hours) was associated with increased time to extubation and higher ICU/hospital mortality, thus advocating the upfront use of light sedation.[24]

The current SCCM guidelines recommend daily interruption of sedation followed by SAT and spontaneous breathing trial (SBT) for all patients. Every SAT should begin with a safety screen to identify patients where withdrawal of sedation can be harmful (active seizures, alcohol withdrawal, agitation, active myocardial ischemia, or raised intracranial pressure). For patients who pass the SAT screen, all sedation and analgesia should be withheld. The SAT continues until the trial fails [anxiety, agitation, respiratory rate (RR) >35 breaths/min, oxygen saturation (SpO_2) <88%, respiratory distress, or cardiac arrhythmia] or succeeds (patient opens his or her eyes to verbal commands and tolerates sedation interruption for >4 hours). Patients who pass the SAT should be subjected to SBT safety screen and SBT. For patient who fail the SAT, sedation should be restarted at 50% of the dose and gradually titrated upward to achieve the targeted level of sedation.[25]

Given the improved outcomes with light sedation and interruption of sedation, few trials have also looked into the concept of nonsedation wherein only analgesia is administered to the patients with use of sedative agents restricted to rescue therapy. The non-sedation (NON-SEDA) trial compared analgesia only (nonsedation group) to light sedation (RASS -2 to -3 using propofol/midazolam) among 700 patients. The all-cause mortality at 90 days was similar among the two groups [42.4% vs. 37%, 5.4% (-2.2 to 12.2)]. Patients in the nonsedation group had a lower risk of a major thromboembolic event [0.3% vs. 2.8%, -2.5% (-4.8 to -0.7)] with no difference in the days free from intermittent mandatory ventilation (IMV). Up to 27% patients in the nonsedation group needed rescue sedation and 8.9% patients had self-extubation warranting re-intubation.[26]

The optimum strategy lies somewhere between nonsedation and light sedation with greater emphasis on an analgesia-first approach. Continuous assessment and an individualized approach should be used to improve outcomes.

THE IDEAL SEDATIVE AGENT

The ideal sedation ceases to exist but should contain the following properties:

- *Pharmaceutics:*
  - Ease of administration
  - Easily prepared and long shelf life
- *Pharmacodynamics:*
  - Predictable dose-dependent effects, thus allowing for dose titration to target various levels of sedation
  - Provides sedation, anxiolysis, amnesia, and analgesia
  - No tolerance or withdrawal symptoms
  - Allows ventilator synchrony and provides procedural sedation
- *Pharmacokinetics:*
  - Short-acting, allowing patient assessment and rapid recovery following discontinuation, thus helping to perform SAT/SBT
  - Minimal metabolism, thus allowing use in patients with hepatic/renal impairment
  - Minimal or no side-effects

OPIOID ANALGESICS

Mechanism of Action of Opioids

Opioids exert their effects by stimulating opioid receptors. Among the opioid receptors, the μ receptor is the primary opioid receptor and can be further classified into μ1 and μ2 subtypes. The μ1 receptors are responsible for mediating analgesia while binding to μ2 receptors leads to constipation, nausea, and respiratory depression. Binding to κ receptors mediates spinal analgesia, pupillary constriction, and the sedative effects of opioids.[27]

It is worth noting that although the administration of opioids may result in a mild-to-moderate anxiolytic effect, they do not induce amnesia. Opioids also exhibit excellent action in suppressing cough. Furthermore, they provide significant relief in the subjective feeling of dyspnea. Due to the combination of these two effects, opioids can be particularly beneficial for mechanically ventilated patients.[28]

Morphine, fentanyl, and hydromorphone are the most commonly utilized opioid analgesic agents in the ICU. Some opioid analgesic agents are described as follows:

- *Morphine:* It acts as an agonist on μ receptors and exhibits weak agonistic activity on κ and δ receptors. Due to its poor lipid solubility, it has a relatively slow onset of action, typically taking 5–10 minutes. Both morphine and its active metabolites are excreted through the kidneys. Therefore, caution should be exercised when administering morphine to patients with renal insufficiency, as it can accumulate and prolong the drug's effects.[29]
- *Fentanyl:* It is a μ receptor agonist, which has high lipid solubility, and therefore has a rapid onset of action (<1 min). Fentanyl is preferred in patients with renal insufficiency. Cautious use should be done in patients with end-stage renal disease, as fentanyl itself may accumulate at high doses. Owing to its high lipophilicity, repeated dosing or infusion can lead to a prolonged duration of effect, as the drug re-enters the plasma after discontinuation. In acutely distressed patients, fentanyl is the preferred agent for rapid onset of analgesia.[28]
- *Hydromorphone:* It is a μ receptor agonist with a duration of action and half-life nearly similar to morphine. However, its hepatic metabolism (by glucuronidation) leads to inactive metabolites (hydromorphone-3 glucuronide) making hydromorphone the opioid of choice in patients with end stage renal disease.[30]
- *Remifentanil:* Remifentanil, an ultrashort-acting selective μ receptor agonist is emerging as a promising opioid analgesic for use in critically ill patients. The drug has unique pharmacokinetics, in that it undergoes rapid metabolism by nonspecific blood and tissue esterases to an inactive metabolite remifentanil acid. The drug is intensely lipophilic (onset of action <1 min) and approximately 250 times more potent than morphine. The terminal half-life of the drug is approximately 10–20 minutes.[30] Due to its short duration of action, remifentanil may be preferable for analgesia in patients requiring frequent neurological assessments. Although the ultrashort action is beneficial in avoidance of prolonged drug effects, pain may rapidly emerge after drug discontinuation and longer-acting agents may need to be administered to patients with ongoing pain.
- *Other agents:* Meperidine with an onset of action and half-life similar to morphine should not be routinely used for analgesia in the ICU. It has an active metabolite, normeperidine, a central nervous system (CNS) stimulant, which can cause neuroexcitation that manifests as tremors and seizures.[31]

Side Effects of Opioids

The side effects of opioids are as follows:

- *Respiratory depression:* Opioids lead to dose-dependent, centrally-mediated respiratory depression. At lower doses, the RR is decreased with preserved tidal volumes. As the dosage increases, tidal volume is also reduced and ventilatory response to hypoxia is obtunded.[28]
- *Hypotension:* Opioid-induced hypotension is of particular concern in hypovolemic and hemodynamically unstable patients and can occur in euvolemic patients also. By blunting the sympathetic tone, vagally-mediated bradycardia, histamine release, and increase in systemic venous capacitance, opioids can cause a precipitous fall in blood pressure.[32]
- *Gastric retention and ileus:* Routine use of stool softeners and stimulant laxatives may minimize opioid-induced constipation but they are often ineffective.
- *Other side effects:* Muscle rigidity, urinary retention, nausea, and pruritus

SEDATIVE MEDICATIONS

Benzodiazepines

Benzodiazepines act by potentiating the gamma-aminobutyric acid (GABA) receptors. Benzodiazepines possess anxiolytic and anticonvulsant properties. They are potent inducers of anterograde amnesia but do not cause retrograde amnesia. The pharmacological effect of benzodiazepines depends on the extent of GABA-receptor binding. Anxiolysis is associated with approximately 20% binding, sedation with 30–50% binding, and hypnosis with 60% binding.[33]

Benzodiazepines can cause respiratory depression, especially when coadministered with opioids, and the extent of this effect is dose-dependent. They may also result in hypotension, particularly in hypovolemic patients. Additionally, they can modulate the anticipatory pain response, leading to a reduction in the required dose of opioids (opioid sparing effect).[34]

Midazolam

Midazolam is a rapidly acting, water-soluble benzodiazepine (onset of action within 5 minutes) that has a short duration of action. It is oxidized by the cytochrome P450 (CYP3A4) enzyme system in the liver leading to the production of water-soluble hydroxylated metabolites. The primary metabolite is 1-hydroxymidazolam glucuronide, a CNS depressant that can cause prolonged sedation especially if kidney failure is present, as it is renally excreted. Obese patients and patients with hypoalbuminemia can also have prolonged sedation after midazolam administration.[35]

Because of unpredictable awakening and time to extubation when midazolam infusions continue longer than 48–72 hours, it is recommended for short-term use only. Midazolam is a preferred agent for rapid sedation of acutely agitated patients.

Lorazepam

Lorazepam has an onset of action within 5–20 minutes and the effect lasts for up to 6–8 hours. Unlike midazolam, hepatic metabolism of lorazepam leads to production of inactive metabolites, which are excreted by the kidney.[28] An important concern with lorazepam administration is propylene glycol toxicity. Propylene glycol is used as a solubility enhancer for the drug in intravenous preparations. The toxicity may manifest as hyperosmolar states, worsening metabolic acidosis, and acute tubular necrosis.[33] Monitoring of serum osmolal gap should be done in patients receiving 50 mg per day and greater or >1 mg/kg of lorazepam per day. An osmolal gap greater than 10–15 indicates significant accumulation of propylene glycol.[36] Treatment involves discontinuation of lorazepam infusion. In severe cases, hemodialysis provides effective removal of propylene glycol.

Propofol

Propofol (2,6 diisopropylphenol) is a widely used ICU sedative. Like the benzodiazepines, it possesses sedative and hypnotic properties and provides amnesia.[37] However, its site of binding on the GABA receptor is different from that of the benzodiazepines. It lacks analgesic properties, therefore patients may require a greater dose of opioids for pain relief if receiving propofol rather than benzodiazepines.[38]

It is profoundly lipophilic, therefore crosses the blood-brain barrier, and rapid redistribution after infusion discontinuation leads to quick emergence times.[28] SCCM guidelines recommend propofol as the preferred sedative agent when rapid awakening is important like in neurological assessment. Propofol reduces CNS metabolism, cerebral blood flow, and decreases intracranial pressure.

Although propofol is metabolized in the liver by conjugation to metabolically inactive metabolites, clearance apparently is not significantly altered by hepatic or renal disease. Propofol causes profound respiratory depression, and can also cause hypotension, especially in hypovolemic patients. Airway should be secured, or intubation should be on standby whenever administering propofol.[28]

Propofol is a caloric source, providing 1.1 kcal/mL primarily from its fat content.[39] Prolonged infusions may be associated with hypertriglyceridemia and also pancreatitis, therefore serum triglyceride levels should be monitored.[40] It is recommended to monitor triglyceride concentrations after 2 days of propofol infusion and also to include the total caloric intake from lipids in the nutrition-support prescription.

Propofol infusion syndrome (PRIS): It is a rare complication seen with infusion of propofol.[41] It is characterized by acute refractory bradycardia leading to asystole in the presence of one or more of the following: Metabolic acidosis (base deficit >10 mmol/L), rhabdomyolysis, hyperlipidemia, and enlarged or fatty liver. This potentially fatal condition is typically associated with propofol infusions at doses higher than 4 mg/kg/h for greater than 48 hours duration. This is likely to occur from mitochondrial respiratory chain inhibition or impaired mitochondrial fatty acid metabolism mediated by propofol. Treatment involves immediate discontinuation of propofol and supportive treatment with hemodialysis or hemoperfusion, as the clinical setting dictates.[41]

Dexmedetomidine

Dexmedetomidine is the dextro enantiomer of medetomidine, which is the methylated derivative of etomidine. It is a highly specific alpha-2 receptor agonist. The drug possesses anxiolytic, sedative, and analgesic properties. The mechanism of action is multipronged with sedation and anxiolysis via receptors within the locus coeruleus and analgesia via receptors in the spinal cord. The drug does not produce any significant respiratory depression. There is also mounting evidence that dexmedetomidine has protective effects against ischemic and hypoxic injury.[30]

The onset of action occurs after approximately 15 minutes of intravenous (IV) injection. The drug distribution occurs rapidly from the brain, leading to a short terminal half-life. Hepatic metabolism by glucuronidation leads to production of inactive metabolites. Dose reductions are required in the presence of both renal and liver diseases.[30] Dexmedetomidine can provide excellent sedation without respiratory depression during fiberoptic intubation or other difficult airway procedures. In these settings, it has added benefits of decreasing saliva production and airway secretions.[42]

Volatile Anesthetic Sedation

Volatile agents have been used to provide general anesthesia for more than a century. Expansion of their role as sedative agents in the ICU has gained popularity over the last few decades. They offer the advantage of having a quick onset and offset, being easy to titrate, having a pulmonary route of elimination (no impact of renal/hepatic impairment), and having a bronchodilator and anti-convulsant action. Isoflurane, desflurane, and sevoflurane are the most commonly used drugs.[43]

The major obstacles to the use of volatile anesthetics for ICU sedation are cost, concerns for environmental pollution, and the need for anesthetic expertise. Specialized volatile delivery systems such as AnaConDa ("anesthesia conserving device") and MIRUS allow the infusion of liquid volatile anesthetic through the breathing circuit of a standard ICU ventilator. Addition of these devices increases the dead space by around 100 mL and the minimum recommended tidal volume is 300–350 mL. Drug delivery may become a problem in patients with excessive bronchial secretions and having a genetic predisposition to malignant hyperthermia.

The use of volatile anesthetic sedation has demonstrated shorter emergence times (isoflurane vs. midazolam or propofol), shorter times to extubation (sevoflurane vs. propofol), better cognitive functions after emergence (desflurane vs. propofol), and a trend toward lesser propensity to develop delirium (isoflurane vs. midazolam).[44-47] Volatile anesthetic sedation provides an attractive alternative to routine use of IV sedative agents in the ICU, but further research to ensure patient safety with focus on long-term outcomes like mortality, delirium, cognitive impairment, and hospital length of stay is needed before adopting their widespread use.

Peripherally Acting μ-opioid Receptor Antagonists

Opioid use in the ICU is associated with a number of gastrointestinal side effects like constipation, ileus, and delayed gastric emptying. Peripherally acting μ-opioid receptor antagonists (PAMORAs) are a novel class of drugs that do not cross the blood–brain barrier to antagonize the central effects of opioids, thereby preserving the analgesic effects. They antagonize the peripheral side effects of opioids, importantly constipation and ileus.[48]

Methylnaltrexone and alvimopan are currently the Food and Drug Administration (FDA) approved PAMORAs. Subcutaneous methylnaltrexone is approved for the relief of opioid-induced constipation and oral alvimopan, to facilitate the return of gut dysfunction after anastomotic bowel surgery. This class of drugs may prove to be of great therapeutic potential in the management of patients in the ICU particularly in those requiring frequent and prolonged administration of opioids.

Tables 7 and 8 summarize the effects and dosage ranges of the commonly used agents.

CHOOSING THE APPROPRIATE SEDATIVE AGENT

The current sedation strategies focus on the analgesia-first approach or analgosedation. The most common reason for agitation in the ICU is pain. Lack of appropriate analgesia can lead to overuse of sedatives to control this agitation. Use of opioid and nonopioid analgesics to control pain remains the first step of all ICU pain-sedation protocols.[39] Analgesia alone can provide light levels of sedation in some patients as shown in the NON-SEDA trial.[26]

The most commonly used sedative agents include benzodiazepines (midazolam/lorazepam), dexmedetomidine, and propofol. The PADIS (prevention and management of pain, agitation/sedation, delirium, immobility, and sleep disruption in adult patients in the ICU) guidelines recommend using nonbenzodiazepine agents because of improved short-term outcomes such as ICU length of stay, duration of IMV, and incidence of delirium.[15] When comparing propofol to benzodiazepines, multiple trials reported shorter time to extubation [mean difference (MD) –11.6 hours; 95% confidence interval (CI) –15.6 to –7.6 hours] with no difference in delirium rates. The SEDCOM study compared dexmedetomidine with midazolam and showed reduction in duration of IMV (MD –1.9 days; 95% CI –2.32 to –1.48 days) and risk of delirium [RR (relative risk) 0.71; 95% CI 0.61–0.83].[49] The MENDS2 trial compared dexmedetomidine with propofol among 422 patients. The trial showed no difference in the primary endpoint of days alive without delirium at 14 days and secondary endpoint of ventilator-free days or overall mortality. Cognitive impairment at day 90 was also similar.[50]

The choice of agent is also influenced by the patient characteristics, side effect profile, and the desirable effect. Dexmedetomidine does not reduce the respiratory drive, and thus fails to provide deep sedation, which may be required among patients with acute respiratory distress syndrome to facilitate lung-protective ventilation.[51] Ketamine at full dissociative doses is reserved for use among patients with profound hypotension or status asthmaticus due to its vasoconstrictive and bronchodilator properties.[52] Propofol reduces the intracranial pressure and is the preferred agent in patients with traumatic brain injuries. Its short half-life also allows rapid recovery needed for frequent GCS monitoring in these patients. Dexmedetomidine is associated with bradycardia and hypotension, thus restricting its use in patients with heart blocks.[51]

Flowchart 1 provides a simplified approach to help select the appropriate sedative agent in the ICU.

DELIRIUM

The Diagnostic and Statistical Manual of Mental Disorders, Fifth Edition (DSM-V) lists four domains of delirium: Disturbance in attention and awareness, disturbance in

TABLE 7: Commonly used sedatives/analgesics in the intensive care unit.

Agent	Time to onset (minutes)	Time to offset	Analgesic effect	Provides deep sedation	Reduces respiratory drive	Risk for delirium	Risk for withdrawal
Opioid: Fentanyl	1–2	1–4 hours	+++	No	Yes	+	++
Dexmedetomidine	15–20	60–90 minutes	+	No	No	–	++
Midazolam	2–5	1–72 hours	–	Yes	Yes	+++	++
Propofol	0.5–1	5–10 minutes	–	Yes	Yes	+	–

TABLE 8: Dosage range of the commonly used sedatives/analgesics in the ICU.

Agent	Ampoule/Vial available	Commonly used dilution	Dosage range
Opioid: Fentanyl	500 µg/10 mL	*1,000 µg/50 mL:* 20 µg/mL	0.7–10 µg/kg/h 3–10 mL/h
Dexme-detomidine	500 µg/5 mL	*400 µg/50 mL:* 8 µg/mL	0.2–1.5 µg/kg/h 1.5–10 mL/h
Midazolam	5 mg/5 mL	*Undiluted:* 1 mg/mL	1–10 mg/h 1–10 mL/h
Propofol	200 mg/20 mL	*Undiluted:* 10 mg/mL	10–250 mg/h 1–10 mL/h

cognition (memory, language, or perception), development over a short period of time, and fluctuation. Other symptoms commonly associated with delirium include sleep disturbances, abnormal psychomotor activity, and emotional disturbances.[48] Patients may be agitated (hyperactive delirium), calm or lethargic (hypoactive delirium), or may fluctuate between the two. Hyperactive delirium can be associated with hallucinations or delusions, while hypoactive delirium is characterized by confusion and sedation, thus often being underdiagnosed in the ICU.[53]

Epidemiology and Risk Factors

Studies have shown that up to 80% of patients admitted to the ICU suffer from delirium. Hyperactive delirium is the most common subtype followed by mixed and hypoactive.[54] Patients with dementia, CNS disease, alcohol abuse, old age, and patients on IMV are predisposed. Common risk factors include electrolyte abnormalities (hypo/hypernatremia, hyperglycemia, and hypercalcemia), fever, sepsis, vasopressor requirement, use of certain medications (benzodiazepines, opioids, and anticholinergics), shock, anemia, and hypertension.[55]

Outcomes

Delirium among critically ill patients is strongly associated with cognitive impairment after hospital discharge.[56] It can prolong duration of IMV by hindering extubation, increase hospital length of stay, and maybe associated with increased mortality.[57]

Assessment of Delirium

Routine assessment of delirium is recommended in all critically ill patients.[15] This leads to early and timely identification so that appropriate measures can be taken, thus improving outcomes. Studies have shown that without validated screening tools, physicians and bedside nurses fail to identify delirium. The two most commonly used tools are the confusion assessment method for the ICU (CAM-ICU) and intensive care delirium screening checklist (ICDSC) tools, both of which can be administered within 2–5 minutes. The ICDSC also offers an advantage of detection of "subsyndromal" delirium, which over the course of time may progress to overt delirium. A score ≥4 is considered positive for delirium.[58] The components of CAM-ICU are mentioned in **Flowchart 2**.[59]

Treatment and Prevention of Delirium

Multicomponent nonpharmacological interventions aimed at reducing modifiable risk factors (avoiding excessive use of opiates and benzodiazepines, and correcting electrolytes), improving cognition by frequent reorientation and use of clocks, improving sleep (minimizing light and noise), reducing immobility,[60] and reducing visual or hearing impairment (by help of aids) have shown to reduce the risk as well as duration of delirium.[61] Currently, use of pharmacological agents is not recommended for prevention of delirium. In the REDUCE study, prophylactic use of haloperidol among high-risk critically ill patients did not improve survival or risk of delirium (33.3% vs. 33%).[62]

Treatment of delirium is also primarily focused on treating underlying disease and correcting the modifiable risk factors. Nonpharmacological interventions like increasing family time, daylight exposure, ambient temperature optimization, sleep promotion, and physical and occupational therapy are to be employed first. The SCCM guidelines do not recommend the routine use of typical or atypical antipsychotics for treating delirium.[15] Large-scaled trials have failed to show any benefit of haloperidol in improving survival or reducing the duration of delirium [days alive without delirium or coma at 90 days: 57.7 vs. 52.6; MD 5.1 (-1.2 to 11.3)].[63] However, patients who experience significant distress (anxiety, fear, and hallucinations), who are agitated and physically harmful to themselves or others may benefit from short-term use of antipsychotics. Haloperidol, olanzapine, and quetiapine are the commonly used agents. Haloperidol is usually administered by intermittent IV injections. Initially, a starting dose of 2 mg IV can be administered followed by repeated doses (doubling the previous dose) every 15–20 minutes. The loading dose is administered till the control of acute agitation. After the control of acute agitation, scheduled intermittent doses (25% of the loading dose) may be administered 6 hourly and then gradually tapered off.[64] Monitoring should be done for electrocardiographic changes (QT interval prolongation and arrhythmias) when receiving haloperidol.[1] Development of extrapyramidal syndrome (EPS) is another known complication of administration of neuroleptic agents. If EPS develops, haloperidol should be stopped and a trial of diphenhydramine or benztropine should be given.[65] Quetiapine is usually started at 25 mg bedtime and the dose is gradually up-titrated based on response and tolerability.

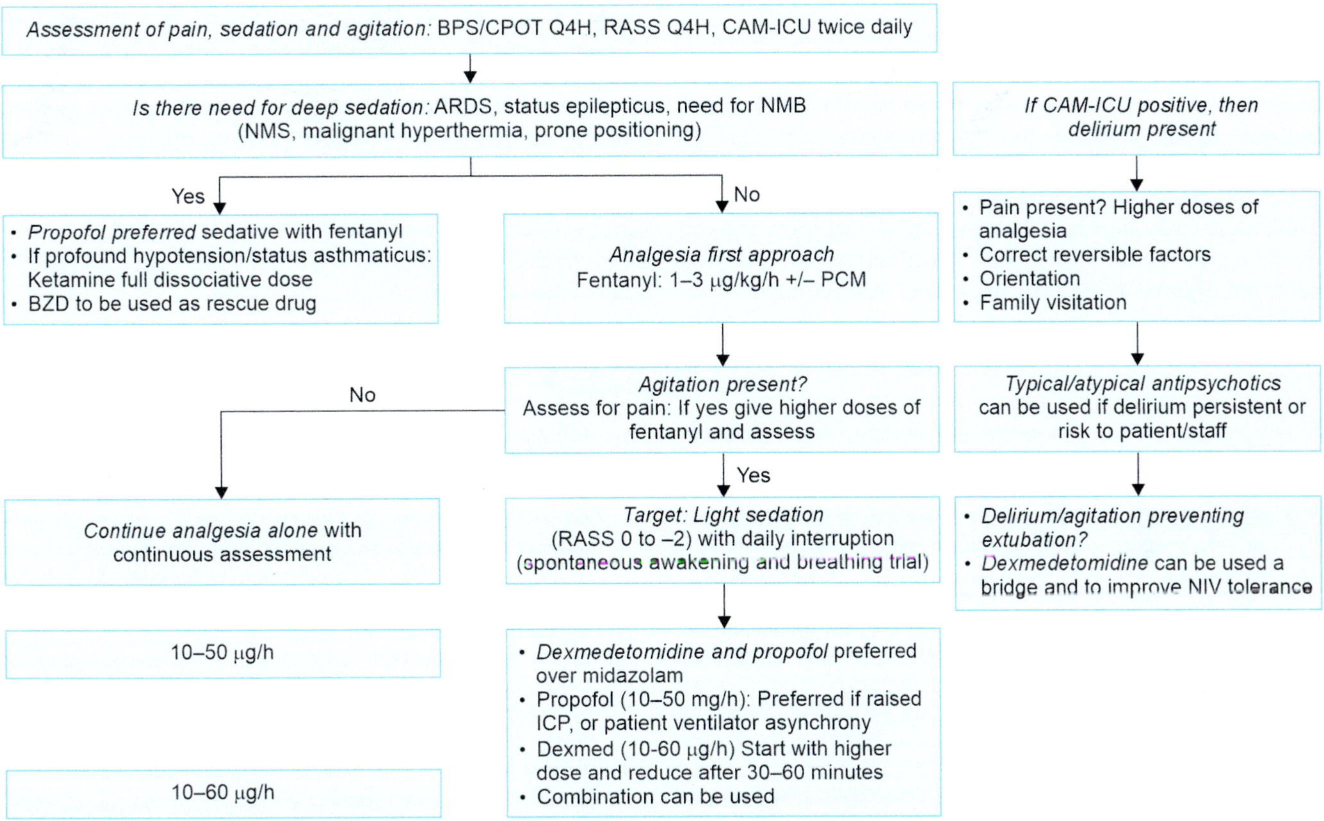

Assessment of pain, sedation and agitation: BPS/CPOT Q4H, RASS Q4H, CAM-ICU twice daily
Is there need for deep sedation: ARDS, status epilepticus, need for NMB (NMS, malignant hyperthermia, prone positioning)
If CAM-ICU positive, then delirium present
Yes
No
• Propofol preferred sedative with fentanyl
• If profound hypotension/status asthmaticus: Ketamine full dissociative dose
• BZD to be used as rescue drug
Analgesia first approach
Fentanyl: 1–3 µg/kg/h +/– PCM
• Pain present? Higher doses of analgesia
• Correct reversible factors
• Orientation
• Family visitation
No
Agitation present?
Assess for pain: If yes give higher doses of fentanyl and assess
Typical/atypical antipsychotics can be used if delirium persistent or risk to patient/staff
Yes
Continue analgesia alone with continuous assessment
Target: Light sedation
(RASS 0 to –2) with daily interruption (spontaneous awakening and breathing trial)
• Delirium/agitation preventing extubation?
• Dexmedetomidine can be used a bridge and to improve NIV tolerance
10–50 µg/h
• Dexmedetomidine and propofol preferred over midazolam
• Propofol (10–50 mg/h): Preferred if raised ICP, or patient ventilator asynchrony
• Dexmed (10-60 µg/h) Start with higher dose and reduce after 30–60 minutes
• Combination can be used
10–60 µg/h

FLOWCHART 1: A simplified approach to sedation and analgesia in critically ill patients.

(ARDS: acute respiratory distress syndrome; BPS: behavior pain scale; BZD: benzodiazepines; CAM-ICU: confusion assessment method for the ICU; CPOT: critical care pain observational tool; ICP: intracranial pressure; NIV: noninvasive ventilation; NMB: neuromuscular blockade; NMS: neuroleptic malignant syndrome; PCM: paracetamol; Q4H: every 4 hours; RAAS: Richmond agitation sedation scale)

Acute mental status change
Change from baseline OR fluctuations in past 24 hours?
No
CAM-ICU Negative no delirium
Yes
Inattention
• Squeeze hand whenever letter "A" is listed SAVEHAART
• Error: No squeeze on "A" AND/OR squeeze on letter other than "A"
0–2 errors
>2 error
Altered level of consciousness
RASS other than zero
Current RASS Level
RASS = Zero
Disorganized thinking
>1 error
CAM-ICU Positive for delirium
Ask the following:
• Will a stone float on water?
• Are there fish in the sea?
• Does 1 pound weigh more than 2?
• Can a hammer be used to pound a nail?
Commands:
• Hold up this many fingers
• Do the same thing with the other hand?
0–1 error
CAM-ICU negative no delirium

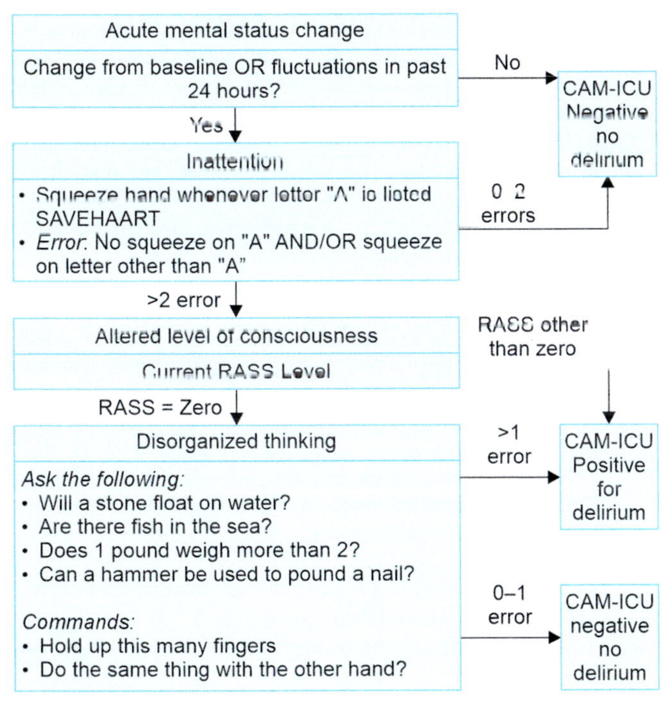

FLOWCHART 2: CAM-ICU algorithm.

(CAM-ICU: confusion assessment method for the ICU; RAAS: Richmond agitation sedation scale)

THE ABCDEF BUNDLE APPROACH

The ICU liberation bundle encompasses an advanced approach and methodology that aims to enhance patient care through the alleviation of pain, minimizing oversedation, mitigating delirium, reducing dependence on mechanical ventilation, promoting mobility, decreasing isolation, addressing sleep disruptions, and preventing ICU-associated weakness. Additionally, it strives to mitigate postdischarge consequences that can significantly impact patients' lives.[66]

It consists of the following individual elements:

A : Assess, prevent, and manage pain
B : SAT and SBT
C : Choice of analgesia and sedation
D : Delirium—assess, prevent and manage
E : Early mobility and exercise
F : Family engagement and empowerment

Implementation of this holistic approach has shown to reduce delirium and coma days by 25–50%, reduce the use of physical restraint by 60%, decrease the likelihood of hospital death, and reduce ICU readmissions.[67]

SUMMARY

Sedation is an often overlooked but an integral part of critical care medicine. Assessment of pain, depth of sedation, and delirium should be conducted using objective tools such as BPS, RAAS, and CAM-ICU. Protocolized practices targeting a light level of sedation have been shown to improve outcomes. Daily interruption of sedation and spontaneous awakening trials should be implemented. Various sedative agents, including propofol, dexmedetomidine, midazolam, and opioids, are available. The appropriate choice depends on the clinical scenario; however, an analgesia-first approach should be followed, with propofol or dexmedetomidine preferred over midazolam, as they reduce the risk of delirium.The treatment of delirium is primarily non-pharmacological and includes increasing family time and reorienting patients to their surroundings. Antipsychotics have not been shown to prevent or reduce the duration of delirium, so their use should be limited to controlling agitation.

REFERENCES

1. Puntillo KA, White C, Morris AB, et al. Patients' perceptions and responses to procedural pain: Results from Thunder Project II. Am J Crit Care. 2001;10(4):238-51.
2. Ahlers SJ, van Gulik L, van der Veen AM, et al. Comparison of different pain scoring systems in critically ill patients in a general ICU. Crit Care. 2008;12(1):R15.
3. Gélinas C, Joffe AM, Szumita PM, et al. A psychometric analysis update of behavioral pain assessment tools for noncommunicative, critically ill adults. AACN Adv Crit Care. 2019;30(4): 365-87.
4. Payen JF, Bru O, Bosson JL, et al. Assessing pain in critically ill sedated patients by using a behavioral pain scale. Crit Care Med. 2001;29(12):2258-63.
5. Gélinas C, Fillion L, Puntillo KA, et al. Validation of the critical-care pain observation tool in adult patients. Am J Crit Care. 2006;15(4):420-7.
6. Aïssaoui Y, Zeggwagh AA, Zekraoui A, et al. Validation of a behavioral pain scale in critically ill, sedated, and mechanically ventilated patients. Anesth Analg. 2005;101(5):1470-6.
7. Ledowski T. Objective monitoring of nociception: A review of current commercial solutions. Br J Anaesth. 2019;123(2): e312-21.
8. Gélinas C, Shahiri TS, Richard-Lalonde M, et al. Exploration of a multi-parameter technology for pain assessment in postoperative patients after cardiac surgery in the intensive care unit: The Nociception Level Index (NOL)™. J Pain Res. 2021;14:3723-31.
9. Shahiri TS, Richard-Lalonde M, Richebé P, et al. Exploration of the nociception level (NOL™) index for pain assessment during endotracheal suctioning in mechanically ventilated patients in the intensive care unit: An observational and feasibility study. Pain Manag Nurs. 2020;21(5):428-34.
10. Ramsay MAE. Intensive care: Problems of over- and under-sedation. Best Pract Res Clin Anaesthesiol. 2000;14(2):419-32.
11. Jacobi J, Fraser GL, Coursin DB, et al. Clinical practice guidelines for the sustained use of sedatives and analgesics in the critically ill adult. Crit Care Med. 2002;30(1):119-41.
12. De Jonghe B, Cook D, Appere-De-Vecchi C, et al. Using and understanding sedation scoring systems: A systematic review. Intensive Care Med. 2000;26(3):275-85.
13. LeBlanc JM, Dasta JF, Kane-Gill SL. Role of the bispectral index in sedation monitoring in the ICU. Ann Pharmacother. 2006;40(3):490-500.
14. Ramsay MA, Savege TM, Simpson BR, et al. Controlled sedation with alphaxalone-alphadolone. Br Med J. 1974;2(5920):656-9.
15. Devlin JW, Skrobik Y, Gélinas C, et al. Clinical Practice Guidelines for the Prevention and Management of Pain, Agitation/Sedation, Delirium, Immobility, and Sleep Disruption in Adult Patients in the ICU. Crit Care Med. 2018;46(9):e825-73.
16. Sessler CN, Gosnell MS, Grap MJ, et al. The richmond agitation-sedation scale: Validity and reliability in adult intensive care unit patients. Am J Respir Crit Care Med. 2002;166(10):1338-44.
17. Schneider G, Heglmeier S, Schneider J, et al. Patient State Index (PSI) measures depth of sedation in intensive care patients. Intensive Care Med. 2004;30(2):213-6.
18. Kreuer S, Wilhelm W, Grundmann U, et al. Narcotrend index versus bispectral index as electroencephalogram measures of anesthetic drug effect during propofol anesthesia. Anesth Analg. 2004;98(3):692–7, table of contents.
19. Cortínez LI, Delfino AE, Fuentes R, et al. Performance of the cerebral state index during increasing levels of propofol anesthesia: A comparison with the bispectral index. Anesth Analg. 2007;104(3):605-10.
20. Karamchandani K, Rewari V, Trikha A, et al. Bispectral index correlates well with Richmond agitation sedation scale in mechanically ventilated critically ill patients. J Anesth. 2010; 24(3):394-8.
21. Yang KS, Habib AS, Lu M, et al. A prospective evaluation of the incidence of adverse events in nurse-administered moderate sedation guided by sedation scores or Bispectral Index. Anesth Analg. 2014;119(1):43-8.
22. Kress JP, Pohlman AS, O'Connor MF, et al. Daily interruption of sedative infusions in critically ill patients undergoing mechanical ventilation. N Engl J Med. 2000;342(20):1471-7.
23. Treggiari MM, Romand JA, Yanez ND, et al. Randomized trial of light versus deep sedation on mental health after critical illness. Crit Care Med. 2009;37(9):2527-34.
24. Shehabi Y, Chan L, Kadiman S, et al. Sedation depth and long-term mortality in mechanically ventilated critically ill adults: A prospective longitudinal multicentre cohort study. Intensive Care Med. 2013;39(5):910-8.
25. Girard TD, Kress JP, Fuchs BD, et al. Efficacy and safety of a paired sedation and ventilator weaning protocol for mechanically ventilated patients in intensive care (Awakening and Breathing Controlled trial): A randomised controlled trial. Lancet. 2008;371(9607):126-34.
26. Olsen HT, Nedergaard HK, Strøm T, et al. Nonsedation or light sedation in critically ill, mechanically ventilated patients. N Engl J Med. 2020;382(12):1103-11.
27. Trescot AM, Datta S, Lee M, et al. Opioid pharmacology. Pain Physician. 2008;11(2 Suppl):S133-53.
28. Brush DR, Kress JP. Sedation and analgesia for the mechanically ventilated patient. Clin Chest Med. 2009;30(1):131-41, ix.

29. Pasternak GW, Bodnar RJ, Clark JA, et al. Morphine-6-glucuronide, a potent mu agonist. Life Sci. 1987;41(26):2845-9.
30. Panzer O, Moitra V, Sladen RN. Pharmacology of sedative-analgesic agents: Dexmedetomidine, remifentanil, ketamine, volatile anesthetics, and the role of peripheral mu antagonists. Crit Care Clin. 2009;25(3):451-69, vii.
31. Goetting MG, Thirman MJ. Neurotoxicity of meperidine. Ann Emerg Med. 1985;14(10):1007-9.
32. McArdle P. Intravenous analgesia. Crit Care Clin. 1999;15(1): 89-104.
33. Devlin JW, Roberts RJ. Pharmacology of commonly used analgesics and sedatives in the ICU: Benzodiazepines, propofol, and opioids. Crit Care Clin. 2009;25(3):431-49, vii.
34. Ghoneim MM, Mewaldt SP. Benzodiazepines and human memory: A review. Anesthesiology. 1990;72(5):926-38.
35. Spina SP, Ensom MHH. Clinical pharmacokinetic monitoring of midazolam in critically ill patients. Pharmacotherapy. 2007; 27(3):389-98.
36. Barnes BJ, Gerst C, Smith JR, et al. Osmol gap as a surrogate marker for serum propylene glycol concentrations in patients receiving lorazepam for sedation. Pharmacotherapy. 2006; 26(1):23-33.
37. McKeage K, Perry CM. Propofol: A review of its use in intensive care sedation of adults. CNS Drugs. 2003;17(4):235-72.
38. Kress JP, O'Connor MF, Pohlman AS, et al. Sedation of critically ill patients during mechanical ventilation. A comparison of propofol and midazolam. Am J Respir Crit Care Med. 1996; 153(3):1012-8.
39. Kress JP, Pohlman AS, Hall JB. Sedation and analgesia in the intensive care unit. Am J Respir Crit Care Med. 2002;166(8): 1024-8.
40. Devlin JW, Lau AK, Tanios MA. Propofol-associated hypertri-glyceridemia and pancreatitis in the intensive care unit: An analysis of frequency and risk factors. Pharmacotherapy. 2005; 25(10):1348-52.
41. Kam PC, Cardone D. Propofol infusion syndrome. Anaesthesia. 2007;62(7):690-701.
42. Bergese SD, Khabiri B, Roberts WD, et al. Dexmedetomidine for conscious sedation in difficult awake fiberoptic intubation cases. J Clin Anesth. 2007;19(2):141-4.
43. Jerath A, Parotto M, Wasowicz M, et al. Volatile anesthetics. Is a new player emerging in critical care sedation? Am J Respir Crit Care Med. 2016;193(11):1202-12.
44. Kong KL, Willatts SM, Prys-Roberts C. Isoflurane compared with midazolam for sedation in the intensive care unit. BMJ. 1989; 298(6683):1277-80.
45. Meiser A, Sirtl C, Bellgardt M, et al. Desflurane compared with propofol for postoperative sedation in the intensive care unit. Br J Anaesth. 2003;90(3):273-80.
46. Sackey PV, Martling CR, Carlswärd C, et al. Short- and long-term follow-up of intensive care unit patients after sedation with isoflurane and midazolam–a pilot study. Crit Care Med. 2008;36(3):801-6.
47. Röhm K, Wolf M, Boldt J, et al. Short-term sevoflurane sedation using the anaesthetic conserving device AnaConDa® after cardiac surgery: Feasibility, recovery and clinical issues. Crit Care. 2008;12(Suppl 2):P270.
48. European Delirium Association; American Delirium Society. The DSM-5 criteria, level of arousal and delirium diagnosis: Inclusiveness is safer. BMC Med. 2014;12:141.
49. Riker RR, Shehabi Y, Bokesch PM, et al. Dexmedetomidine vs midazolam for sedation of critically ill patients: A randomized trial. JAMA. 2009;301(5):489-99.
50. Hughes CG, Mailloux PT, Devlin JW, et al; MENDS2 Study Investigators. Dexmedetomidine or Propofol for Sedation in Mechanically Ventilated Adults with Sepsis. N Engl J Med. 2021; 384(15):1424-36.
51. Gertler R, Brown HC, Mitchell DH, et al. Dexmedetomidine: A novel sedative-analgesic agent. Proc (Bayl Univ Med Cent). 2001;14(1):13-21.
52. Kurdi MS, Theerth KA, Deva RS. Ketamine: Current applications in anesthesia, pain, and critical care. Anesth Essays Res. 2014; 8(3):283-90.
53. Kumar A, Bakhla AK, Gupta S, et al. Etiologic and cognitive differences in hyperactive and hypoactive delirium. Prim Care Companion CNS Disord. 2015;17(6).
54. Krewulak KD, Stelfox HT, Leigh JP, et al. Incidence and prevalence of delirium subtypes in an adult ICU: A systematic review and meta-analysis. Crit Care Med. 2018;46(12):2029-35.
55. Zaal IJ, Devlin JW, Peelen LM, et al. A systematic review of risk factors for delirium in the ICU. Crit Care Med. 2015;43(1):40-7.
56. Ely EW, Shintani A, Truman B, et al. Delirium as a predictor of mortality in mechanically ventilated patients in the intensive care unit. JAMA. 2004;291(14):1753-62.
57. Wolters AE, van Dijk D, Pasma W, et al. Long-term outcome of delirium during intensive care unit stay in survivors of critical illness: A prospective cohort study. Crit Care. 2014;18(3):R125.
58. Bergeron N, Dubois MJ, Dumont M, et al. Intensive care delirium screening checklist: Evaluation of a new screening tool. Intensive Care Med. 2001;27(5):859-64.
59. Ely EW, Inouye SK, Bernard GR, et al. Delirium in mechanically ventilated patients: Validity and reliability of the confusion assessment method for the intensive care unit. JAMA. 2001; 286(21):2703-10.
60. Hoyer EH, Friedman M, Lavezza A, et al. Promoting mobility and reducing length of stay in hospitalized general medicine patients: A quality-improvement project. J Hosp Med. 2016;11(5):341-7.
61. Balas MC, Vasilevskis EE, Olsen KM, et al. Effectiveness and safety of the awakening and breathing coordination, delirium monitoring/management, and early exercise/mobility bundle. Crit Care Med. 2014;42(5):1024-36.
62. van den Boogaard M, Slooter AJC, Brüggemann RJM, et al. Effect of haloperidol on survival among critically ill adults with a high risk of delirium: The REDUCE randomized clinical trial. JAMA. 2018;319(7):680-90.
63. Andersen-Ranberg NC, Poulsen LM, Perner A, et al. Haloperidol for the treatment of delirium in ICU patients. N Engl J Med. 2022;387(26):2425-35.
64. Wang EHZ, Mabasa VH, Loh GW et al. Haloperidol dosing strategies in the treatment of delirium in the critically-ill. Neurocritical Care. 2012;16(1):170-83.
65. Beach SR, Gross AF, Hartney KE, et al. Intravenous haloperidol: A systematic review of side effects and recommendations for clinical use. Gen Hosp Psychiatry. 2020;67:42-50.
66. Marra A, Ely EW, Pandharipande PP, et al. The ABCDEF bundle in critical care. Crit Care Clin. 2017;33(2):225-43.
67. Pun BT, Balas MC, Barnes-Daly MA, et al. Caring for critically ill patients with the ABCDEF bundle: Results of the ICU liberation collaborative in over 15,000 adults. Crit Care Med. 2019;47(1): 3-14.

Weaning from Mechanical Ventilation

CHAPTER 175

Ajmal Khan

INTRODUCTION

Apart from its ability to save lives, mechanical ventilation (MV) has several undesirable consequences and patient discomfort. Any intervention that promotes timely and swift transition from complete ventilatory support to spontaneous breathing improves the outcome. Thus, liberation from the ventilator should be initiated when the root cause that led to the MV has sufficiently improved and an unassisted spontaneous breathing is sustainable. Weaning is a process of abrupt or gradual transition from full ventilatory support to spontaneous breathing and/or removal of artificial airway.

The basis for rational decision in the weaning process is the balance between aggressiveness to wean and patient safety. A premature weaning attempt carries the risk of compromised gas exchange and airway protection, muscle fatigue, difficulty re-establishing the airway, and a 6- to 12-fold increased risk of mortality.[1] Similarly, any delay in the weaning process is associated with complications such as nosocomial pneumonia and iatrogenic lung injury, along with an increased cost of intensive care unit (ICU) care.

TYPES OF WEANING

The time spent on weaning, which can be up to 40–50% of the total duration of MV, provides an insight into the difficulties and complexities of the weaning process.

This process starts as early as the patient's intubation and usually ends with successful extubation **(Fig. 1)**. In approximately 70–75% of patients, MV can be abruptly

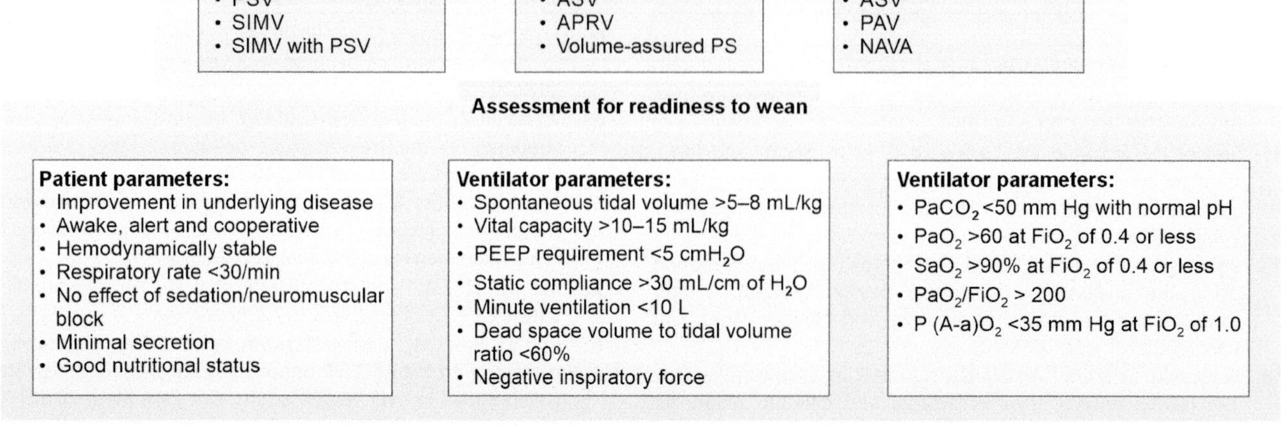

Extubation

Removal of endotracheal tube

Spontaneous breathing trials (SBTs)

Conventional method:
- SBT with T-piece
- PSV
- SIMV
- SIMV with PSV

Newer modes:
- ATC
- ASV
- APRV
- Volume-assured PS

Closed loop ventilation:
- SmartCare
- ASV
- PAV
- NAVA

Assessment for readiness to wean

Patient parameters:
- Improvement in underlying disease
- Awake, alert and cooperative
- Hemodynamically stable
- Respiratory rate <30/min
- No effect of sedation/neuromuscular block
- Minimal secretion
- Good nutritional status

Ventilator parameters:
- Spontaneous tidal volume >5–8 mL/kg
- Vital capacity >10–15 mL/kg
- PEEP requirement <5 cmH_2O
- Static compliance >30 mL/cm of H_2O
- Minute ventilation <10 L
- Dead space volume to tidal volume ratio <60%
- Negative inspiratory force

Ventilator parameters:
- $PaCO_2$ <50 mm Hg with normal pH
- PaO_2 >60 at FiO_2 of 0.4 or less
- SaO_2 >90% at FiO_2 of 0.4 or less
- PaO_2/FiO_2 > 200
- P $(A\text{-}a)O_2$ <35 mm Hg at FiO_2 of 1.0

FIG. 1: Methods and parameters employed for weaning and extubation.

(APRV: airway pressure release ventilation; ASV: adaptive support ventilation; ATC: automated tube compensation; NAVA: neurally adjusted ventilatory assist; PS: pressure support; PSV: pressure support ventilation; SIMV: synchronized intermittent mandatory ventilation; PAV: proportional assist ventilation)

discontinued as soon as the condition that caused respiratory failure has resolved. A gradual transition is required in some patents before they develop adequate respiratory muscle strength to maintain spontaneous breathing and adequate gas exchange.[2]

An international consensus conference classifies weaning based on number, timing, and results of spontaneous breathing trials (SBTs):[3]

- *Simple weaning*: Initiation of weaning to successful extubation on the first attempt without difficulty is simple weaning. It carries a better prognosis with an ICU and in-hospital mortality of approximately 5% and 12%, respectively.[4]
- *Difficult weaning*: Failure to tolerate initial SBT; successful weaning requiring up to three SBTs or up to 7 days from first SBT
- *Prolonged weaning*: Failure of at least three SBT or takes >7 days after the first SBT is prolonged weaning

Both difficult and prolonged weaning increase duration of hospitalization and consequently carry an ICU mortality of approximately 25%. During the 28-day study period in 349 ICUs, there were 2,174 successful weaning out of 4,559 mechanically ventilated patients; among those patients, 55% underwent simple weaning, 39% underwent difficult weaning, and 6% underwent prolonged weaning.[5,6] Patients who are directly extubated without SBT cannot be categorized by this classification, which is its major limitation. In addition, it cannot clarify the effect of these categories on morbidity and mortality.

The duration of ventilation from the first separation attempt of weaning was used to introduce the WIND (Weaning according to a New Definition) classification recently.[7] This was defined as an SBT or direct extubation for intubated patients, and 24 hours without ventilatory assistance for tracheostomized patients. Using these criteria, four mutually exclusive groups having a direct and immediate impact on morbidity and mortality, with differing prolongation of weaning were established. The initial attempt at separation as a critical milestone, and each extra day without a successful weaning corresponds to a higher crude mortality, were established.[7]

PATHOPHYSIOLOGY OF WEANING

A complex interplay of respiratory controllers, lung and chest wall mechanics, respiratory muscles, gas exchange characteristics, and cardiovascular hemodynamics determines the method and timing of weaning from MV. Disturbance at any level has the potential to prolong the weaning or weaning failure.

Altered Control of Breathing

Structural, functional, or metabolic abnormalities within the nervous system, including drugs affecting the brain and peripheral nerves, will alter afferent or efferent output, respiratory drive, and attenuate airway protective reflexes.[8,9] Each of these factors, alone or in combination, can contribute to weaning difficulty.

Altered Respiratory Mechanics

The force generated by the inspiratory muscle overcomes the elastic and resistive loads of the respiratory system during normal respiration. This entails signal synthesis in the brainstem's respiratory centers, anatomic and functional integrity of nerves that transmit the signal, uninterrupted neuromuscular transmission, and adequate muscle strength. Physiological variables such as dynamic hyperinflation, resistance, and elastance are most commonly altered during the weaning process. Four factors account for the increase in resistance—increase in ventilatory volume, a decrease in lung volume, accumulation of secretions, and bronchoconstriction.[10] Low respiratory system compliance occurs due to stiff chest wall, stiff lungs, and flooded or atelectatic alveoli. Dynamic hyperinflation not only increases an elastic load, but it also places the diaphragm in a mechanically disadvantageous position, which reduces its capacity to generate adequate transdiaphragmatic pressure. The dynamic hyperinflation causing intrinsic positive end expiratory pressure (auto-PEEP) increases the pressure gradient needed to inspire.[11] This increase in inspiratory threshold raises the work of breathing and leads to weaning failure.

Respiratory Muscle Dysfunction

Respiratory muscle weakness occurs commonly in the ICUs because of:

- Atrophy and remodeling from inactivity[12]
- Critical illness neuropathy and myopathy[13]
- Drugs (neuromuscular blockers, aminoglycoside, and corticosteroids)[14,15]
- Metabolic factors such as nutrition, electrolytes, and hormones
- Imbalance between respiratory muscle capacity and the load[16,17]

Electrolyte imbalance, particularly deficiency of phosphate and magnesium, impairs ventilatory muscle function.[18-20] Severe hypothyroidism and myxedema directly impair diaphragmatic function and blunt ventilatory responses to hypercapnia and hypoxia.[21] Besides thyroid hormone, insulin/glucagon and adrenal corticosteroids are also important for optimal muscle function. Deficiency of them may cause respiratory muscle dysfunction.

Cardiovascular Performance

Ventilatory work of respiratory muscles depends on efficient transport of oxygen by the cardiovascular system. Transition from mechanical ventilation to spontaneous breathing during weaning reverses the prior unloading of respiratory muscles, which can induce ischemia or heart failure in susceptible individuals with limited cardiac reserve.[22,23] Cardiovascular dysfunction during this shift occurs due to increased metabolic and circulatory demands, displacement of blood from the abdomen to thorax by contracting diaphragm and increase in left ventricular afterload imposed by negative pleural pressure swings.

Rapid changes in intrathoracic pressure from positive to negative during weaning and postextubation impact cardiorespiratory physiological functioning. This rapid swing toward more negative intrathoracic pressure increases right ventricular preload because of an increase in systemic venous return and decreases afterload by distending the pulmonary vasculature.[24] The increase in blood volume from the right heart amplifies preload and left ventricular transmural pressure, which augments its afterload. All these factors contribute to precipitate cardiac ischemia and failure and pulmonary edema, further increasing the work of breathing and weaning failure.[25,26]

PROCESS OF WEANING

Weaning encompasses a cumulative process that involves an assessment of readiness to wean from MV, the process of ventilatory support withdrawal, and finally the removal of an artificial airway. The main policy choice to minimize the duration of ventilation is to recognize preparedness for SBTs earlier and to discontinue MV more quickly. Ideally, weaning starts as early as the patient's intubation, but in routine clinical practice, it starts when the condition that led to has sufficiently improved in the presence of intact airway reflexes, afebrile status, and cardiovascular stability.

Assessment of Readiness to Wean

The most crucial step in the transition from full MV support to spontaneous breathing is the decision to assess the readiness to SBT. There is no defined optimal time to evaluate the patient for the assessment of the weaning, and both early and late decisions are associated with poor and challenging outcomes. Therefore, implementing a daily evaluation of the preparedness for a trial of unassisted breathing is a logical and reasoned strategy. To identify a patient's preparedness for weaning, it is possible to use either subjective or an objective criteria often known as protocol-driven criteria. The subjective criteria and clinical assessment alone often lead to an underestimation of the patient's ability to breathe spontaneously.[27-30] It is imperative to establish a rational justification for utilizing objective predictors in clinical decision-making when determining the readiness for successful weaning from MV.

In order to streamline the assessment process, a range of objective criteria have been devised. However, it is important to note that the objective criteria should primarily serve as a support for the physician's clinical judgment, and it is possible for patients to be weaned off even if they do not meet these criteria **(Fig. 1)**. These objective criteria are based on studies showing weaning success when used within the framework of weaning protocol.[31,32] The results of a multicenter observational research of weaning methods encompassing 1,868 patients from six geographic regions throughout the world reveal that there are considerable variations in practice.[33] Thus, a weaning protocol should be adapted to the patient demographic and ICU where they will be used because they may not be helpful in all settings.

There are some indices that are used to predict the results of the weaning trial even before implementing SBT. However, a lot of them need complicated testing and have limited predictive value.

- Simplified weaning index (SWI)[34]

$$\text{SWI} = \text{Fv} \times (\text{IP} - \text{PEEP})/\text{NIP} \times \text{PaCO}_2/40$$

Fv = Ventilaory frequency

IP = Inspiratory pressure

PEEP = Positive end-expiratory pressure

NIP = Maximum negative inspiratory pressure

$PaCO_2$ = Partial pressure of Carbon dioxide

A SWI < 9/min is 93% predictive of successful weaning, whereas a SWI > 11/min is 95% predictive of weaning failure.

- *CROP index (compliance, rate, oxygenation, pressure)*: This index is an integrative index incorporating dynamic respiratory system compliance (C_{rs}), spontaneous breathing frequency (*f*), PAO_2, alveolar partial pressure of oxygen (mm Hg), PaO_2, partial pressure of arterial oxygen (mm Hg), and PI_{max} in the following relationship:

$$\text{CROP index} = [\text{Cdyn} \times \text{MIP}] \times [\text{PaO}_2/\text{PAO}_2]/\text{f}$$

The link between the demands placed on the respiratory system and the respiratory muscles' capacity to withstand them is assessed by the CROP index. Weaning success is predicted by a CROP index > 13 mL/breath/min.[35]

- *Muscle load indices*: These require more sophisticated measurements, such as pleural pressure (estimated from esophageal pressure) to calculate the pressure time product (PTP) and pressure time index (PTI).[36] PTI can be a useful predictor of fatigue when it is >0.1.
- *Rapid shallow breathing index (RSBI)*: The RSBI is the ratio of respiratory frequency to tidal volume (f/V_T). The tidal volume can be calculated by dividing minute ventilation (i.e., total volume inspired and expired in 1 minute) by the frequency. Both handheld spirometer and ventilator can estimate minute ventilation. A negative RSBI of ≥105 breaths/min/L is better at identifying a weaning failure than a positive value of <105 breaths/min/L in successful weaning prediction.[37,38] It has a sensitivity, specificity, positive predictive value, and negative predictive value of 97%, 64%, 78%, and 95%, respectively.[35] The RSBI summarizes extubation outcome during the weaning trial; however, it may not reveal the underlying cause of its failure. Compared to other classic and frequently used parameters, the ratio of frequency to tidal volume (RSBI),

measured during the first minute of a T-piece trial at a threshold value of 105 breaths/min/L, was a considerably better predictor of weaning outcome.[35]

Small endotracheal tube, female gender, sepsis, supine position, anxiety, and restrictive lung diseases, all increase the RSBI and require caution while interpreting the results.[39] Another significant disadvantage of RSBI is that its threshold is affected by ventilatory support settings, experimental conditions, and the patient population.[40] In a meta-analysis of 48 studies focused on extubation outcome, RSBI had a pooled sensitivity and specificity of 83% and 58%, respectively, in predicting successful extubation. The findings of the study suggest that RSBI has a moderate predictive capacity to expect weaning failure and does not sufficiently predict successful extubation.

- *Diaphragmatic dysfunction*: The diaphragm as the principal respiratory muscle carries out the major part of the work of breathing. Diaphragmatic dysfunction is the inability to partially or completely generate pressure within its muscle fibers. It occurs when inflammatory or metabolic disorders, neuromyopathies, mechanical ventilation, or lung hyperinflation affect its mechanical coupling, neural, or contractile functions.[41] Disuse atrophy, critical illness polyneuropathy, myopathy, use of paralyzing agents, undernutrition, and metabolic abnormalities such as hypocalcemia, hypokalemia, or hypomagnesemia play a part in diaphragmatic dysfunction leading to a protracted course of MV.[42,43] Although diaphragmatic dysfunction is under recognized entity, its estimated prevalence in critically ill patients requiring MV is over 60% conferring a correlation with difficult weaning.[44]

Methods to evaluate diaphragmatic dysfunction:

- *Measurement of transdiaphragmatic pressure (P_{di})*: Uses dedicated catheter with esophageal and gastric balloon to measure its pressures. Thus, $P_{di} - P_{es} = P_{ab}$. Diaphragmatic dysfunction occurs when P_{di} is <11 cm H_2O.
- *Electrical activity of the diaphragm (EA_{di}) test*: Uses dedicated esophageal catheter with four electrode couples at the distal tip.
- *Ultrasound assessment of the diaphragm*: Uses ultrasound to detect diaphragmatic dysfunction and classify it into usual, reduced, or loss of function. Successful weaning predictors on ultrasound are:
  - Diaphragmatic excursion (DE): Maximum diaphragmatic displacement during breathing
  - Diaphragmatic thickness fraction (DTF, %): Difference between the end-inspiratory (Te-Insp) and end-expiratory (Te-Exp) thickness of the diaphragm divided by the end expiratory thickness.

Various studies done to evaluate these parameters alone or in combination to predict weaning success have mixed results because of a difference in study population and design.[45-47] A systematic review of 20 observational studies involving 875 patients shows diaphragm ultrasound is a feasible and reproducible tool to detect diphragmatic dysfunction in critically ill patients; it can predict extubation success or failure during weaning and SBTs.[47] Optical cutoffs for diphragmatic excursion and thickening fraction range from 10 to 14 mm and 30% to 36%, respectively.[47] Another systematic review of 19 cohort studies involving 1,114 patients shows superior diagnostic accuracy of the diaphragm thickening fraction (DTF) in comparison to other methods like diaphragm excursion (DE) and the RSBI for prediction of weaning outcome.[48] Randomized studies are needed to ascertain the clinical applicability and generalization of this simple and noninvasive technique in the future.

Diaphragm ultrasound is an important tool to assess morphology and function of the diaphragm. Its impact on clinical outcome is yet to be defined and validated. A comprehensive ultrasonographic evaluation of heart, lung, and diaphragm during the weaning can provide more valuable information than each on its own.

Spontaneous Breathing Trials

After a satisfactory assessment of readiness to wean, prompt removal of the artificial airway is a feasible option. However, given the high rates of postextubation distress and reintubation rates of approximately 40%, a formal weaning trial is required before extubation. Weaning trials increase the likelihood of tolerating extubation by reconditioning the respiratory muscles more effectively. A SBT is a traditional test to determine readiness for artificial airway removal by simulating the physiological state following extubation. It evaluates the patient's ability to maintain spontaneous respiration following extubation. Using a T-piece and continuous positive airway pressure of 0 cm H_2O more effectively simulates the physiologic parameters after extubation.[49] Several ventilatory modalities are available to support the gradual withdrawal of MV after a successful or failed SBT, but their respective effects on outcome vary between the modalities. The choice of which modality to use will primarily depend on physician preference and local protocols following a "Do Not Exhaust" policy.

Weaning from the ventilator and placing directly on T-piece with supplemental oxygen is the most traditional weaning approach to SBT. Low level of continuous positive airway pressure (CPAP) or pressure support ventilation (PSV) are an alternative method of providing SBT without ventilator removal, with an added advantage of quick reinstitution of ventilatory support in the face of SBT failure. Initial SBT is well tolerated in approximately 50–75% for successful extubation.[2,50] Daily SBTs, other weaning strategies, or an extubation with immediate noninvasive ventilatory (NIV) support are an option for those who fail initial SBT.

In a meta-analysis of 17 studies, protocolized weaning with daily SBTs resulted in a 26% reduction in the duration of mechanical ventilation. Similarly, protocolized weaning reduced weaning duration (8 studies) and ICU length of stay (9 studies) by 70% and 11%, respectively. Protocolized weaning had no significant effect on mortality or reintubation rates.[51] Because of nonuniformity in results across the ICUs, caution is required in generalizing these finding. Use of PSV-SBT as compared to T-piece is consistently superior, as evident from randomized trials and meta-analysis.[52-54]

Optimal SBT duration depends upon the duration of ventilation or the underlying cause for respiratory failure. Studies on optimal SBT duration suggest that 30 minutes is equivalent to 120 minutes with either T-piece or PSV.[55] A potential concern about the SBT is its safety. Unnecessary prolongation of a failing SBT may precipitate muscle fatigue, hemodynamic instability, and a worsening in gas exchange. Recognizing the failure of SBT early and terminating it does not contribute to an adverse outcome.[56,57] Thus, close monitoring during the initial few minutes of SBT avoids the detrimental effects of ventilatory muscle overload during failing SBT, which often occurs early.[58] To ensure maximum sensitivity and safety, it is advisable to continue SBT for at least 30 minutes, but not over 120 minutes.

Failure of SBT is defined by tachypnea, tachycardia, arrhythmia, hypertension, hypotension, hypoxemia, or the subjective evidence of agitation or distress, depressed mental status, and diaphoresis.[4] Failed SBTs are often because of persistent mechanical abnormalities of the respiratory system (especially the muscle fatigue) that are unlikely to reverse rapidly.[58] There is no benefit in conducting SBTs twice a day as compared to a single SBT, so the next SBT should be given only after 24 hours. The application of computer-driven assessments and clinician feedback tools for the assessment to perform SBTs and sedation optimization strategy can augment weaning.[31,59,60]

Methods of SBTs during weaning are:

- *Conventional methods*:
  - SBT with T-piece
  - PSV
  - Synchronized intermittent mandatory ventilation (SIMV)
  - SIMV with PSV
- *Newer modes*:
  - Automatic tube compensation
  - Adaptive support ventilation
  - Airway pressure-release ventilation
  - Volume assured pressure support
- *Closed-loop ventilation*:
  - SmartCare
  - Adaptive support ventilation
  - Proportional assist ventilation (PAV)
  - Neurally adjusted ventilatory assist (NAVA)

Pressure Support Ventilation

During the weaning process, a gradual reduction of PS is used as the sole mode of MV in 21% of patients.[5] It is a pressure-limited ventilation that recognizes the patient's inspiratory effort, ensures appropriate delivery at the time of inspiration, and cycles to the expiratory phase with no active patient exhalation. During PSV, breath is flow cycled to the expiratory phase when the flow decelerates to 5 L/min or 25% of the peak inspiratory flow. PSV is useful for counteracting the extra work imposed by breathing through an endotracheal tube.

TABLE 1: Comparative characteristics of three modes for weaning.

T-piece	T-Piece	SIMV	PSV
Work quantity	All or none	Adjusted by number of mandatory breaths	Adjusted by level of given pressure
Tidal volume	Determined by patient	Set by clinician	Patient interact with applied pressure
Minimum minute ventilation	Not assured	Assured	Not assured
Synchrony	Regular periods of irregular load	Regular load	Constant
Patient comfort	Least	Intermediate	Most
Equipment complexity	Simple	Intermediate	Maximum

Continuous Positive Airway Pressure

The CPAP by itself is not a mode, as it does not provide any inspiratory support. CPAP, when applied during spontaneous breathing in patients with acute respiratory insufficiency, reduces mean intrathoracic pressure, has beneficial effects on right and left ventricular performance, improves oxygenation, and reduces the work of breathing **(Table 1)**.[53,54]

Automated Weaning

Closed-loop weaning systems are automatic systems that use physiological feedback signals to adjust the weaning process. It identifies the ability to breathe spontaneously earlier than other modes to facilitate weaning through real-time monitoring and intervention. At present, several feedback systems are available, which decreases the amount of applied pressure in pressure-support breaths. These systems are useful for patients who are recovering from respiratory failure.[59,61] These algorithms include simple tidal volume targets, tidal volume targets with rate and inspiratory-expiratory time considerations, and tidal volume targets with rate and end-tidal CO_2 considerations. A meta-analysis of 39 randomized studies found PAV as an effective ventilatory mode for weaning success and lower reintubation and mortality rates than other modes. Small number of studies, variation in patient population and ventilatory setting prior to weaning are the major limitations of this study.[60]

Role of Noninvasive Ventilation in Weaning

Approximately 13–19% of patients require reintubation for respiratory failure following a gradual weaning process.[62] Reintubation is a marker of increased severity of illness and an independent predictor of mortality.[63] One of the strategy to prevent postextubation respiratory failure is the application of NIV for weaning as a bridge to spontaneous breathing. In hypercapnic respiratory failure, NIV reduces duration of MV, ICU, and hospital stays and improves survival both in the ICU and at 90 days.[64] NIV can facilitate weaning in mechanically ventilated patients, especially in the subgroup of patients with COPD.[65] However, NIV cannot avoid reintubation in postextubation hypoxemic respiratory failure.[65,66] The delay in reintubation correlates with worse survival rates in patients who received NIV for established post-extubation respiratory failure in these studies. NIV is definitely useful in facilitating weaning in hypercapnic respiratory failure and in prevention of post-extubation respiratory failure in high-risk patients **(Box 1)**.[67]

BOX 1 Criteria to prevent postextubation respiratory failure with NIV.

- Elderly patient (age > 65 years)
- More than one consecutive failure of weaning trial
- Chronic heart failure
- 4. $PaCO_2$ > 45 mm Hg after extubation
- More than one medical/surgical comorbid condition
- Poor cough reflex
- Upper airway stridor at extubation that does not require immediate re-intubation
- APACHE II score > 12 on the day of extubation

Weaning Failure

Although there is some variation in the definition of successful weaning, a consensus definition is the ability to maintain spontaneous breathing for at least 48 hours after extubation. In patients requiring mechanical ventilation, weaning failure is relatively common, with an estimated prevalence of 31% and a range 26–42%.[2] Failures are often because of persistent mechanical alterations in the respiratory system that are unlikely to reverse within a short time.[68] A failed trial can precipitate respiratory muscle fatigue and studies in healthy subjects suggest that complete recovery from fatigue can take longer than 24 hours.[58] Pressure support or assist-control ventilation modes are alternatives to failing initial trial.

SUMMARY

The weaning process is a critical component of ICU care. Both disease and management factors may lead to difficult weaning that require an assessment for the readiness of weaning. The SBTs in those patients passing the screen are the "gold standard" for ventilator withdrawal. Decision to extubate in successful SBT requires further assessment of patient's ability to protect the airway. In selected patient population especially with hypercapnic respiratory failure, NIV trial to facilitate weaning is warranted.

REFERENCES

1. Esteban A, Alia I, Gordo F, et al. Extubation outcome after spontaneous breathing trials with T-tube or pressure support ventilation. The Spanish Lung Failure Collaborative Group. Am J Respir Crit Care Med. 1997;156(2 Pt 1):459-65.
2. Brochard L, Rauss A, Benito S, et al. Comparison of three methods of gradual withdrawal from ventilatory support during weaning from mechanical ventilation. Am J Respir Crit Care Med. 1994;150(4):896-903.
3. Boles JM, Bion J, Connors A, et al. Weaning from mechanical ventilation. Eur Respir J. 2007;29(5):1033-56.
4. Vallverdu I, Calaf N, Subirana M, et al. Clinical characteristics, respiratory functional parameters, and outcome of a two-hour T-piece trial in patients weaning from mechanical ventilation. Am J Respir Crit Care Med. 1998;158(6):1855-62.
5. Esteban A, Anzueto A, Frutos F, et al. Characteristics and outcomes in adult patients receiving mechanical ventilation: a 28-day international study. JAMA. 2002;287(3):345-55.
6. Penuelas O, Frutos-Vivar F, Fernandez C, et al. Characteristics and outcomes of ventilated patients according to time to liberation from mechanical ventilation. Am J Respir Crit Care Med. 2011;184(4):430-7.
7. Beduneau G, Pham T, Schortgen F, et al. Epidemiology of Weaning Outcome according to a New Definition. The WIND Study. Am J Respir Crit Care Med. 2017;195(6):772 83.
8. Barrientos-Vega R, Mar Sanchez-Soria M, Morales-Garcia C, et al. Prolonged sedation of critically ill patients with midazolam or propofol: impact on weaning and costs. Crit Care Med. 1997;25(1):33-40.
9. Wheeler AP. Sedation, analgesia, and paralysis in the intensive care unit. Chest. 1993;104(2):566-77.
10. Straus C, Louis B, Isabey D, et al. Contribution of the endotracheal tube and the upper airway to breathing workload. Am J Respir Crit Care Med. 1998;157(1):23-30.
11. Vallverdu I, Mancebo J. Approach to patients who fail initial weaning trials. Respir Care Clin N Am. 2000;6(3):365-384;v.
12. Le Bourdelles G, Viires N, Boczkowski J, et al. Effects of mechanical ventilation on diaphragmatic contractile properties in rats. Am J Respir Crit Care Med. 1994;149(6):1539-44.
13. Bolton CF, Breuer AC. Critical illness polyneuropathy. Muscle Nerve. 1999;22(3):419-24.
14. Segredo V, Caldwell JE, Matthay MA, et al. Persistent paralysis in critically ill patients after long-term administration of vecuronium. N Engl J Med. 1992;327(8):524-8.

15. Decramer M, Lacquet LM, Fagard R, et al. Corticosteroids contribute to muscle weakness in chronic airflow obstruction. Am J Respir Crit Care Med. 1994;150(1):11-6.
16. Jubran A, Tobin MJ. Passive mechanics of lung and chest wall in patients who failed or succeeded in trials of weaning. Am J Respir Crit Care Med. 1997;155(3):916-21.
17. Tobin MJ, Laghi F, Jubran A. Respiratory muscle dysfunction in mechanically-ventilated patients. Mol Cell Biochem. 1998;179(1-2):87-98.
18. Aubier M, Murciano D, Lecocguic Y, et al. Effect of hypophosphatemia on diaphragmatic contractility in patients with acute respiratory failure. N Engl J Med. 1985;313(7):420-4.
19. Aubier M, Viires N, Piquet J, et al. Effects of hypocalcemia on diaphragmatic strength generation. J Appl Physiol (1985). 1985;58(6):2054-61.
20. Dhingra S, Solven F, Wilson A, McCarthy DS. Hypomagnesemia and respiratory muscle power. Am Rev Respir Dis. 1984;129(3):497-8.
21. Siafakas NM, Salesiotou V, Filaditaki V, et al. Respiratory muscle strength in hypothyroidism. Chest. 1992;102(1):189-94.
22. Chatila W, Ani S, Guaglianone D, et al. Cardiac ischemia during weaning from mechanical ventilation. Chest. 1996;109(6):1577-83.
23. Jubran A, Mathru M, Dries D, et al. Continuous recordings of mixed venous oxygen saturation during weaning from mechanical ventilation and the ramifications thereof. Am J Respir Crit Care Med. 1998;158(6):1763-9.
24. Haaksma ME, Tuinman PR, Heunks L. Weaning the patient: between protocols and physiology. Curr Opin Crit Care. 2021;27(1):29-36.
25. Teboul JL. Weaning-induced cardiac dysfunction: where are we today? Intensive Care Med. 2014;40(8):1069-79.
26. Bedet A, Tomberli F, Prat G, et al. Myocardial ischemia during ventilator weaning: a prospective multicenter cohort study. Crit Care. 2019;23(1):321.
27. Afessa B, Hogans L, Murphy R. Predicting 3-day and 7-day outcomes of weaning from mechanical ventilation. Chest. 1999;116(2):456-61.
28. Ely EW, Baker AM, Evans GW, et al. The prognostic significance of passing a daily screen of weaning parameters. Intensive Care Med. 1999;25(6):581-7.
29. Epstein SK, Nevins ML, Chung J. Effect of unplanned extubation on outcome of mechanical ventilation. Am J Respir Crit Care Med. 2000;161(6):1912-6.
30. Jordan J, Rose L, Dainty KN, et al. Factors that impact on the use of mechanical ventilation weaning protocols in critically ill adults and children: A qualitative evidence-synthesis. Cochrane Database Syst Rev. 2016;10(10):Cd011812.
31. Girard TD, Kress JP, Fuchs BD, et al. Efficacy and safety of a paired sedation and ventilator weaning protocol for mechanically ventilated patients in intensive care (Awakening and Breathing Controlled trial): A randomised controlled trial. Lancet. 2008;371(9607):126-34.
32. Tanios MA, Nevins ML, Hendra KP, et al. A randomized, controlled trial of the role of weaning predictors in clinical decision making. Crit Care Med. 2006;34(10):2530-5.
33. Burns KEA, Rizvi L, Cook DJ, et al. Ventilator Weaning and Discontinuation Practices for Critically Ill Patients. Jama. 2021;325(12):1173-84.
34. Jabour ER, Rabil DM, Truwit JD, et al. Evaluation of a new weaning index based on ventilatory endurance and the efficiency of gas exchange. Am Rev Respir Dis. 1991;144(3 Pt 1): 531-7.
35. Yang KL, Tobin MJ. A prospective study of indexes predicting the outcome of trials of weaning from mechanical ventilation. N Engl J Med. 1991;324(21):1445-50.
36. MacIntyre NR, Leatherman NE. Mechanical loads on the ventilatory muscles. A theoretical analysis. Am Rev Respir Dis. 1989;139(4):968-73.
37. Meade M, Guyatt G, Cook D, et al. Predicting success in weaning from mechanical ventilation. Chest. 2001;120(6 Suppl):400S-24S.
38. Tobin MJ, Jubran A. Variable performance of weaning-predictor tests: role of Bayes' theorem and spectrum and test-referral bias. Intensive Care Med. 2006;32(12):2002-12.
39. Seymour CW, Cross BJ, Cooke CR, et al. Physiologic impact of closed-system endotracheal suctioning in spontaneously breathing patients receiving mechanical ventilation. Respir Care. 2009;54(3):367-74.
40. El-Khatib MF, Zeineldine SM, Jamaleddine GW. Effect of pressure support ventilation and positive end expiratory pressure on the rapid shallow breathing index in intensive care unit patients. Intensive Care Med. 2008;34(3):505-10.
41. McCool FD, Tzelepis GE. Dysfunction of the diaphragm. N Engl J Med. 2012;366(10):932-42.
42. Chawla J, Gruener G. Management of critical illness polyneuropathy and myopathy. Neurol Clin. 2010;28(4):961-77.
43. Jaber S, Petrof BJ, Jung B, et al. Rapidly progressive diaphragmatic weakness and injury during mechanical ventilation in humans. Am J Respir Crit Care Med. 2011;183(3):364-71.
44. Vetrugno L, Guadagnin GM, Barbariol F, et al. Ultrasound imaging for diaphragm dysfunction: A narrative literature review. J Cardiothorac Vasc Anesth. 2019;33(9):2525.
45. Palkar A, Narasimhan M, Greenberg H, et al. Diaphragm excursion-time index: A new parameter using ultrasonography to predict extubation outcome. Chest. 2018;153(5):1213-20.
46. Carrie C, Gisbert-Mora C, Bonnardel E, et al. Ultrasonographic diaphragmatic excursion is inaccurate and not better than the MRC score for predicting weaning-failure in mechanically ventilated patients. Anaesth Crit Care Pain Med. 2017;36(1):9-14.
47. Zambon M, Greco M, Bocchino S, et al. Assessment of diaphragmatic dysfunction in the critically ill patient with ultrasound: A systematic review. Intensive Care Med. 2017;43(1):29-38.
48. Mahmoodpoor A, Fouladi S, Ramouz A, et al. Diaphragm ultrasound to predict weaning outcome: systematic review and meta-analysis. Anaesthesiol Intensive Ther. 2022;54(2):164-74.
49. Sklar MC, Burns K, Rittayamai N, et al. Effort to Breathe with Various Spontaneous Breathing Trial Techniques. A Physiologic Meta-analysis. Am J Respir Crit Care Med. 2017;195(11):1477-85.
50. Perkins GD, Mistry D, Gates S, et al. Effect of protocolized weaning with early extubation to noninvasive ventilation vs invasive weaning on time to liberation from mechanical ventilation among patients with respiratory failure: The breathe randomized clinical trial. JAMA. 2018;320(18):1881-8.
51. Blackwood B, Burns KE, Cardwell CR, et al. Protocolized versus non-protocolized weaning for reducing the duration of mechanical ventilation in critically ill adult patients. Cochrane Database Syst Rev. 2014;2014(11):Cd006904.
52. Ouellette DR, Patel S, Girard TD, et al. Liberation from mechanical ventilation in critically ill adults: An official American College of Chest Physicians/American Thoracic Society Clinical Practice Guideline: Inspiratory pressure augmentation during spontaneous breathing trials, protocols minimizing sedation, and noninvasive ventilation immediately after extubation. Chest. 2017;151(1):166-80.

53. Thille AW, Coudroy R, Nay MA, et al. Pressure-Support Ventilation vs T-Piece During Spontaneous Breathing Trials Before Extubation Among Patients at High Risk of Extubation Failure: A Post-Hoc Analysis of a Clinical Trial. Chest. 2020;158(4): 1446-55.
54. Thille AW, Gacouin A, Coudroy R, et al. Spontaneous-Breathing Trials with Pressure-Support Ventilation or a T-Piece. N Engl J Med. 2022;387(20):1843-54.
55. Perren A, Domenighetti G, Mauri S, et al. Protocol-directed weaning from mechanical ventilation: clinical outcome in patients randomized for a 30-min or 120-min trial with pressure support ventilation. Intensive Care Med. 2002;28(8):1058-63.
56. Capdevila X, Perrigault PF, Ramonatxo M, et al. Changes in breathing pattern and respiratory muscle performance parameters during difficult weaning. Crit Care Med. 1998;26(1): 79-87.
57. Dojat M, Harf A, Touchard D, et al. Evaluation of a knowledge-based system providing ventilatory management and decision for extubation. Am J Respir Crit Care Med. 1996;153(3):997-1004.
58. Vassilakopoulos T, Zakynthinos S, Roussos C. The tension-time index and the frequency/tidal volume ratio are the major pathophysiologic determinants of weaning failure and success. Am J Respir Crit Care Med. 1998;158(2):378-85.
59. Rose L, Presneill JJ, Johnston L, et al. A randomised, controlled trial of conventional versus automated weaning from mechanical ventilation using SmartCare/PS. Intensive Care Med. 2008;34(10):1788-95.
60. Jhou HJ, Chen PH, Ou-Yang LJ, et al. Methods of Weaning From Mechanical Ventilation in Adult: A Network Meta-Analysis. Front Med. 2021;8.
61. Lellouche F, Mancebo J, Jolliet P, et al. A multicenter randomized trial of computer-driven protocolized weaning from mechanical ventilation. Am J Respir Crit Care Med. 2006;174(8):894-900.
62. Chatila WM, Criner GJ. Complications of long-term mechanical ventilation. Respir Care Clin N Am. 2002;8(4):631-47.
63. Epstein SK, Ciubotaru RL. Independent effects of etiology of failure and time to reintubation on outcome for patients failing extubation. Am J Respir Crit Care Med. 1998;158(2):489-93.
64. Ferrer M, Esquinas A, Arancibia F, et al. Noninvasive ventilation during persistent weaning failure: a randomized controlled trial. Am J Respir Crit Care Med. 2003;168(1):70-6.
65. Burns KE, Adhikari NK, Meade MO. A meta-analysis of noninvasive weaning to facilitate liberation from mechanical ventilation. Can J Anaesth. 2006;53(3):305-15.
66. Esteban A, Frutos-Vivar F, Ferguson ND, et al. Noninvasive positive-pressure ventilation for respiratory failure after extubation. N Engl J Med. 2004;350(24):2452-60.
67. Keenan SP, Powers C, McCormack DG, Block G. Noninvasive positive-pressure ventilation for postextubation respiratory distress: A randomized controlled trial. JAMA. 2002;287(24): 3238-44.
68. Jubran A, Tobin MJ. Pathophysiologic basis of acute respiratory distress in patients who fail a trial of weaning from mechanical ventilation. Am J Respir Crit Care Med. 1997;155(3):906-15.

Hyperbaric Oxygen Therapy

CHAPTER 176

PS Tampi

INTRODUCTION

Hyperbaric oxygen therapy (HBOT) is the administration of oxygen at a pressure greater than that at sea level, which is 1 atmosphere. Hyperbaric medicine owes its origin to the problems encountered by deep-sea divers, exposed to high-pressure diving sports and commercial or military expeditions at depths of 10 m or more. In clinical medicine, this is simulated by exposing a patient to hyperbaric atmosphere in a closed monoplace or multiplace chamber. In either case, the partial pressure of oxygen (PaO_2) will approach 1,500 mm Hg at a pressure equivalent to 33 fsw (feet of seawater). A century of research in oxygen administration has established that the effects are dose related, and the hyperbaric environment merely provides the opportunity to give higher doses than can be achieved at sea level.

The history of HBOT factually begins from 1662 when the British physician Henshaw used compressed air for medical purposes in an airtight room called a "domicilium" in which variable climatic and pressure conditions could be produced, with pressure provided by a large pair of bellows. Several subsequent developments thereafter demonstrated the potential benefits of using oxygen under pressure for the treatment of decompression sickness and several other medical and surgical conditions.[1,2] Drager, in 1917, devised a hyperbaric system for treating diving accidents. In 1937, Behnke and Shaw actually used hyperbaric oxygen (HBO_2) signifying the arrival of the era of HBO_2 therapy. It was in this very year that Cunningham's "air chamber" hotel—the largest hyperbaric chamber at that time—was demolished in USA.

RATIONALE OF HYPERBARIC OXYGEN[3-6]

An increased atmospheric pressure increases the partial pressure of O_2 in the alveolar air and arterial blood, provided the fractional concentrations of oxygen remain the same. This is easily derived from the alveolar air equation. Since the oxygen dissolved in the plasma depends upon PaO_2, the dissolved O_2 content of blood is also increased. This is independent of Hb levels of the blood. Therefore, under hyperbaric conditions, the total oxygen-carrying capacity of the blood is significantly more **(Table 1)**. At 1 atmosphere (sea level), with a person breathing 100% O_2, the PaO_2 is about 670 mm Hg and the total oxygen content is 18.7 mL/dL. Increasing the pressure to 3 atmospheres, the PaO_2 increases to about 1,700–1,800 mm Hg and the total O_2 content to 22 mL/dL. Of this, about 25% (i.e., 5.5 mL/dL) is dissolved in plasma. This in fact is equivalent to the total oxygen content of blood under normal conditions, at a much lower Hb level of 4 g%. Therefore, under hyperbaric conditions, it is possible to maintain adequate oxygen content of blood as well as delivery to the tissues with a very low or no hemoglobin at all. However, it should be remembered that the whole of the tissue oxygen requirements can be met by dissolved oxygen, only if PaO_2 is around 2,025 mm Hg.

TABLE 1: Different components of oxygen content of the blood at different atmospheric pressures at a constant plasma hemoglobin of 14 g/dL, when breathing 100% O_2.

Pressure (atmospheres)	PaO_2 (mm Hg)	Dissolved O_2 (%)	Total O_2 content (mL/dL)
1	670	11	18.7
2	1,200–1,300	18	20
3	1,700–1,800	25	22

OTHER PHYSIOLOGICAL EFFECTS OF HYPERBARIC OXYGENATION

Effect on $PaCO_2$: An increased hemoglobin saturation of venous blood reduces its ability to carry CO_2, and results in carbon dioxide accumulation (Haldane effect).

Vasoconstriction: It occurs due to increase in PaO_2 and has a therapeutic value.

Angiogenesis: The mechanism by which this occurs is not known but occurs only when oxygen is administered at more than 1 atmospheres absolute (ATA) and does not occur with 100% oxygen at 1 ATA.

BENEFICIAL EFFECTS OF HYPERBARIC OXYGEN

Hyperbaric oxygen administration achieves two principal objectives:

1. It increases PaO_2 and tissue PO_2 to levels higher than those obtained at 1 atmosphere. This has several potential therapeutic benefits. The oxygen delivery to the tissues is increased, which may promote healing; the phagocytosis and antibiotic action on the microorganisms are augmented. Hyperoxia induces vasoconstriction, which reduces tissue edema. Finally, the oxygen dissolved in the plasma is available to the tissues, without any increase required in the hemoglobin level. This is not associated with any increase by blood transfusions. Problems of increased blood viscosity are therefore avoided.
2. There is an increase in the ambient pressure which increases interstitial tissue pressures as well. This is used to treat decompression sickness, which may occur in divers. Similarly, presence of air or gas in the blood either injected accidentally during some procedure or due to embolization can be absorbed with HBO_2 therapy.

MECHANISM OF ACTION OF HYPERBARIC OXYGEN

- HBO_2 increases dissolved oxygen in the plasma, which readily diffuses into the hypoxic tissues.
- Increased oxygenation results in vasoconstriction at the site, resulting in reduced transudation, reduction in capillary pressure, and thereby reducing the tissue edema.
- The reduction in tissue edema reduces compression of the cells, thereby enhancing the reabsorption of fluid.
- With edema being less, barriers of diffusion are reduced and oxygen diffusion to the tissues improves, resulting in improvement in tissue functions.
- Improved vascularization due to neovascularization results in speedy recovery of tissues and gives way to tissue regeneration.
- Oxide, hydroperoxide, and superoxide radicals of oxygen are toxic and interfere with the cell metabolism of bacteria and thereby destroy the bacteria.
- HBO_2 modulates the immune system and helps in the faster elimination of viruses.
- Bacterial killing effect of leukocytes is impaired in the hypoxic state. Increased oxygenation will enhance the killing power of leukocytes.

INDICATIONS

Enthusiasm with the use of HBO_2 now is almost similar to what was seen with the use of normobaric oxygen in the 19th century, when its therapeutic applications were first discovered. But this enthusiasm has helped to discover its beneficial role as an adjunct in the treatment of diverse clinical conditions.[5-8] Indications may vary in different countries in different settings. Some of the more definite indications are the decompression sickness, air embolism, gas gangrene, and carbon monoxide poisoning. The indications apprised by the Undersea and Hyperbaric Medical Society are rather limited and rely on the proof of efficacy of controlled studies.

Decompression Sickness[5,9-14]

Decompression sickness (DCS) occurs when the ambient air pressure is allowed to lower rapidly after a prolonged exposure to a higher pressure. This is commonly seen in the deep sea/scuba divers, after emerging from a diving juggernaut, and occasionally in the aviators or astronauts on reaching the outer atmosphere or space. Due to a sudden lowering of pressure, the inert gases dissolved in body fluids bubble out in both intravascular and extravascular compartments resulting in multiple symptoms. The common clinical manifestations can be classified into three types:

- *Type I*: It includes musculoskeletal pains, skin and lymphatic tissue, and often fatigue.
- *Type II*: It includes neurological symptoms (either central or peripheral such as paresthesias and sensorimotor deficits), cardiorespiratory (such as substernal pain, cough, dyspnea), audiovestibular (such as nausea, vomiting, nystagmus, tinnitus, hoarseness of voice), and shock.
- *Type III*: It is a syndrome with severe symptoms of DCS and arterial gas embolism (AGE) and can even be refractory to recompression and result in death. The bubbles in DCS can also injure the vascular endothelium which leads to platelet aggregation, denatured lipoproteins, and activation of leukocytes causing capillary leaks and proinflammatory events.

Hyperbaric oxygen is used to decrease the size of the bubbles, both by increasing the pressure and by using an oxygen gradient.

Hyperbaric oxygen and recompression in DCS type I to about 60 fsw for 2–20-minute periods, with a slow decompression to 30 fsw for another 20 minutes, constitute the mainstay of therapy. For DCS types II and III, patients are placed at 60 fsw (2.8 ATA) for at least three 20-minute intervals and are then slowly decompressed to 30 fsw. The duration a patient is kept at 60 or 30 fsw is dependent on the patient's response to therapy. Both steps help in the reduction and resolution of the bubbles and maintenance of tissue oxygenation. Increased occurrence of oxygen toxicity under higher pressure conditions limits the duration of use of HBO_2. Relapse may occur after discontinuation of therapy. Short-term observation, especially in patients with neurological symptoms for at least 6 hours, is generally recommended. Some people advocate the provision of observation units for about 4 hours after hyperbaric therapy.

Air Embolism[5,15-17]

Air bubbles may form in the venous circulation, due to sudden decompression (e.g. decompression sickness), or more commonly get introduced during central venous instrumentation, invasive medical and surgical procedures, hemodialysis, chest trauma, or positive-pressure ventilation, employing high levels of positive end expiratory pressures (PEEPs). These air bubbles finally end up in the lungs, causing obstruction of pulmonary circulation, and presenting a picture of pulmonary air embolism. It may occasionally be fatal if a large pulmonary vessel gets blocked. Bubbles may also form in the arterial circulation but are rare because of the higher hydrostatic pressure in the larger vessels. Arterial gas emboli due to pulmonary barotrauma causes symptoms within seconds to minutes of the event and can include loss of consciousness, confusion, neurological deficits, cardiac arrhythmias, or cardiac arrest. Cerebral air embolism is uncommon but more serious in nature.

Treatment of air embolism employs resuscitative and restorative measures for pulmonary circulation through removal and/or absorption of air from the pulmonary vessels. Attempts to remove the air bubbles include the direct needle aspiration, Trendelenburg position, or removal through a central venous catheter. Administration of 100% oxygen helps reabsorption of air. HBO_2 administration rapidly reduces the bubble size. Generally, 50% O_2 at a pressure of 165 feet is administered initially for a few minutes followed by intermittent periods of 100% oxygen at a lower pressure of 65 feet. A recent report on the use of US Navy Treatment suggests this use of oxygen-filled monoplace hyperbaric chamber as better tolerated and safer from oxygen toxicity point of view than a multiplace chamber, for the treatment of both decompression sickness and air embolism.

Gas Gangrene and Other Necrotizing Infections[18-21]

There is an increased evidence to suggest a major role of HBO_2 in inflammatory cytokines and mediators. It is shown to cause cytokine downregulation and growth factor upregulation. HBO_2, therefore, is likely to promote wound healing by suppressing inflammation and facilitating repair. It also augments the antibacterial action of leukocytes, which gets otherwise inhibited under hypoxic conditions and thereby improves the efficacy of antibiotics. These effects have been shown in a few clinical trials and clinical experience, when used as an adjunct treatment for gas gangrene, nonhealing wounds (e.g., diabetic foot), osteomyelitis, and necrotizing fasciitis. It is also shown to shorten the treatment with antibiotics for soft-tissue infections. Angiogenesis occurs in response to high oxygen concentration through fibroblast proliferation and collagen synthesis. HBO_2 also likely stimulates growth factors and has direct and indirect antimicrobial activity, thereby increasing intracellular leukocyte killing.

Hyperoxygenation in particular is valuable in gas gangrene, since it inhibits the growth of the causative anerobic microorganisms, i.e., *Clostridia*, and prevents formation of toxins responsible for necrotizing myositis and myonecrosis. Reports on the useful role of HBO_2 are available for treatment of all kinds of clostridial infections including necrotizing fasciitis of upper extremities, orbital gas gangrene, and recurrent crepitant cellulitis with extensive subcutaneous emphysema. It has also been used in patients with refractory mycoses, leprosy, and other intractable infections.

Carbon Monoxide Poisoning[11,22-25]

Carbon monoxide (CO), a by-product of incomplete combustion of coal, is a colorless and odorless poisonous gas. It is a common cause of death in miners and other personnel working with coal furnaces in foundries and factories. CO poisoning in India occurs in people burning indoor coal for heating and cooking during winter months in ill-ventilated houses. Deaths in this scenario are commonly reported in individuals sleeping in closed rooms. Malfunctioning air conditioning systems in cabins have been occasionally blamed for CO poisoning.

Carbon monoxide poisoning is generally insidious. Neurological complications are most frequent. Some of the common symptoms include headache, confusion, dizziness, nausea, and vomiting. In more serious forms, syncope, seizures and coma may precede death. Cardiac arrhythmias and pulmonary edema may also occur. CO has an affinity for hemoglobin, almost 300 times that of oxygen. CO also shifts the oxygen dissociation curve to the left (the Haldane effect), which decreases oxygen delivery to tissues. CO can also bind cytochrome oxidase aa3/C and myoglobin. Reperfusion injury can occur when free radicals and lipid peroxidation are produced.

Exposure to CO therefore quickly results in displacement of oxygen and formation of carboxyhemoglobin (HbCO). Treatment of CO poisoning needs to be prompt and aggressive. A great degree of evidence supports that hypoxia occurs late in CO poisoning. But the treatment of both, the actually poisoned persons and the environmental exposures, is based on a hypoxic theory of toxicity. Oxygen therapy is the mainstay of therapy besides other supportive care. Oxygen accelerates the dissociation of CO from hemoglobin and other heme proteins. Oxygen with an FiO_2 of 100% is administered with a high flow and the response is quick, provided the treatment is started in time before any organ damage has occurred. While breathing room air, this process takes about 300 minutes. With 100% oxygen nonbreather mask, this time is reduced to 90 minutes; with HBO_2, the time is further shortened to 32 minutes. HBO_2 restores cytochrome oxidase aa3/C and helps to prevent lipid peroxidation. HbCO level usually does not correlate well with symptoms or outcome and many patients with HbCO of 25–30% are treated.

Hyperbaric oxygen has been used in a few trials. It rapidly decreases blood HbCO concentration by the oxygen competitively displacing CO from hemoglobin. It may also delay the occurrence of delayed brain injury. HBO_2 is administered at 2.5 ATA for periods of 60–100 minutes for one to five sessions depending on severity and response. Multiple studies describe controversial methods and conclusions about the use of HBO_2 for CO poisoning.

Adjunct to Treatment of Cancers[26-30]

Hyperbaric oxygen may improve the treatment of malignant tumors by increasing the tumor sensitization to radiotherapy. A significant improvement is reported with HBO_2 followed by radiotherapy for local tumor control, mortality for cancers of the head and neck, and local tumor recurrences in cancers of head, neck, and uterine cavity. It also improves the response to photodynamic and chemotherapy, possibly by raising intratumoral oxygen tension. It was also shown to improve survival in locally advanced breast cancer undergoing neoadjuvant chemotherapy. It may also promote new vessel growth into areas with reduced oxygen tension, thereby promoting healing of radiation-induced tissue injury. There is a concern among clinicians and patients that HBO_2 may cause recurrence of malignancy or promote the growth of an existing tumor due to its known angiogenic effect. Feldmeier has reviewed this subject extensively and found that malignant angiogenesis follows a different pathway than angiogenesis related to wound healing.

Miscellaneous Conditions[31-42]

- *Plastic and reconstructive surgery*: For nonhealing wounds, including radiation wounds and venous leg ulcers, as an aid to the survival of skin flaps with marginal circulation, as an aid to reimplantation surgery, as an adjunct to the treatment of burns
- *Trauma, osteomyelitis, and other orthopedic indications*: Crush injury, compartment syndrome, soft-tissue sports injuries; nonunion of fractures, bone grafts, osteoradionecrosis
- *Neurological*: Stroke, multiple sclerosis, migraine, cerebral edema, multi-infarct dementia, spinal cord injury and vascular diseases of the spinal cord, brain abscess, peripheral neuropathy, cluster headaches and migraine, vegetative coma
- *Ophthalmology*: Occlusion of the central artery of retina
- *Peripheral vascular diseases*: Shock, myocardial ischemia, aid to cardiac surgery
- Chronic pain from fibromyalgia syndrome, myofascial pain syndrome, migraine, and cluster headache
- *Hematology*: Sickle cell crises, severe blood loss anemia
- *Gastrointestinal*: Gastric ulcer, necrotizing enterocolitis, and paralytic ileus, pneumatoides, cystoides intestinalis, hepatitis
- *Otorhinolaryngology*: Sudden idiopathic sensorineural deafness, acute acoustic trauma, labyrinthitis, Ménière's disease, malignant otitis externa (chronic infection)
- *Lung diseases*: Lung abscess, pulmonary embolism (adjunct to surgery)
- *Endocrine*: Diabetes
- *Obstetrics*: Complicated pregnancy, diabetes, eclampsia, heart disease, placental hypoxia, fetal hypoxia, congenital heart disease of the neonate
- *Asphyxiation*: Drowning, near-hanging, smoke inhalation
- *Aid to rehabilitation*: Spastic hemiplegia of stroke, paraplegia, chronic myocardial insufficiency, peripheral vascular disease

CONTRAINDICATIONS

Contraindications for HBO_2 therapy can be divided into absolute contraindications, which include untreated tension pneumothorax, and relative contraindications, which include upper respiratory infections, bronchial asthma, emphysema with CO_2 retention, symptomatic pulmonary lesions seen on chest X-ray, history of thoracic or ear surgery, Eustachian tube disorders, congenital spherocytosis, pacemakers, epidural pain pump, uncontrolled high fever, pregnancy, claustrophobia, seizure disorders, and malignant diseases.

COMPLICATIONS[43-48]

The complications in the use of HBO_2 are related to pressure changes and the toxic effects of oxygen. They include barotrauma to ear, sinuses, or lungs. Trauma to ears or sinuses may be averted with slow compression, the use of decongestants, patient education, and rarely myringotomy. Pulmonary barotrauma is very rare, perhaps occurring in 1 in 50,000 treatments. It can be prevented by careful pretreatment screening for pulmonary blebs, air trapping caused by bronchospasm or secretions, pre-existing pneumothorax, central lines, and ventilatory support. Oxygen toxicity with occurrence of grand mal seizures is noticed beyond a depth of 3 ATA (66 feet or 20 m of seawater). Damage of lung tissue, manifested by decrement in vital capacity and irritation to large airways, may occur due to oxygen toxicity following HBO_2. Increased pressure causes increased gas density and airway resistance. This produces an altered voice called the "Donald Duck voice" and an increased awareness of breathing.

Hypoventilation may result, especially in a patient with an underlying obstructive lung disease. Increased partial pressure of nitrogen at a pressure of 2.5 atmosphere causes symptoms of mild euphoria progressing to frank intoxication and decreased performance at over 4 atmospheres. Accumulation of O_2 may occur in the event of an exposure for several days. Hyperpnea and occasionally respiratory acidosis may result. Other toxic substances or pollutants, which may continue to accumulate in a closed chamber and reach toxic pressures, include alcohol (from disinfectant solution), sulfur dioxide, hydrocarbons, carbon monoxide, volatile substances, and mercury vapors. A regular monitoring is required for their concentrations. The nursing and medical personnel looking after the patient in a hyperbaric chamber may suffer from decompression sickness due to tissue bubble formation. The risk is rather low because the chamber is kept warm; exposure is short and decompression rate slow. The risk of an accidental fire is greater in hyperbaric conditions. All inflammable materials should therefore be kept away. Refractive changes and cataract in the lens of the eye may occur as a complication of prolonged HBOT.

Claustrophobia may be a problem in up to 10% of patients, especially in the monoplace chamber.

HYPERBARIC OXYGEN IN PEDIATRIC AGE GROUP

Since the proportion of surface area to body mass is much greater in children than in adults, and as the temperature within the chamber can fluctuate, the child needs to be kept warm without causing hyperthermia. Tympanostomy tube placements may be considered to prevent middle ear trauma.

POTENTIAL NEW INDICATIONS

Bisphosphonates-associated Osteonecrosis

Bisphosphonates are used in the treatment of bone metastases, osteoporosis, Paget's disease, and acute hypercalcemia. However, their use may lead to osteonecrosis in these patients. The pathophysiology leading to osteonecrosis is unknown. No reliable treatment for this condition is available at present. A pilot study using HBO_2 to treat bisphosphonate-associated osteonecrosis showed favorable results, and a randomized controlled trial (RCT) is currently underway.

HYPERBARIC CHAMBERS[49,50]

The main facility required for hyperbaric medicine is of course the hyperbaric chamber itself. This is essentially a chamber constructed to withstand pressurization so that oxygen can be administered inside at a pressure greater than at sea level. The size, shape, and pressure capabilities of the design chambers vary considerably. The technical details of each model, now available, are provided by the manufacturers.

TYPES OF HYPERBARIC CHAMBERS

- Monoplace chamber **(Fig. 1)**
- Multiplace or "walk-in" chambers **(Fig. 2)**
- Mobile or portable

Monoplace: Transportable by air, sea, or land. This is a unique, portable hyperbaric chamber used for the treatment of acute mountain sickness (AMS). By increasing air pressure around the patient to 1.5–1.7 ATA, the bag simulates descent of as much as 7,000 feet, thus relieving AMS symptoms. The bag is constructed of durable nylon and reinforced with circular nylon straps. A lengthwise zipper permits easy access and egress for the patient, and four clear windows allow visual contact. The bag is pressurized with ambient air to 2 pounds per square inch by use of a foot pump. Everything fits into a red pack with carrying handle, shoulder strap, and backpack straps. They are only approved by the Food and Drug Administration (FDA) for the treatment of high-altitude illness.

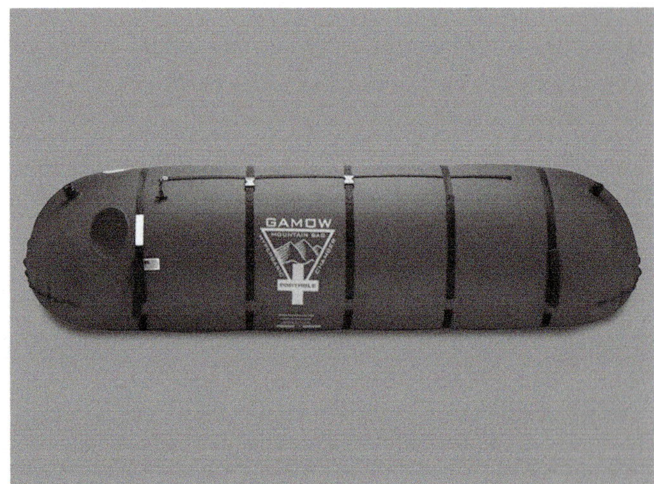

FIG. 1: Monoplace chamber—portable.

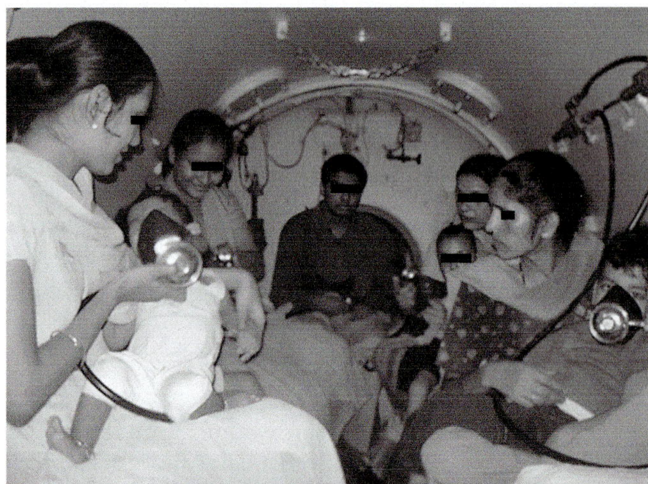

FIG. 2: Multiplace or "walk-in" chambers.

Multiplace: A chamber can be driven from place to place.
- Chambers for testing and training divers
- Small hyperbaric chambers
- For neonates
- For animal experiments
- Newer duoplace chambers can hold two patients at a time. Their operation is similar to that of a monoplace chamber.

OTHER CHAMBERS

Topical oxygen or Topox is administered through a small chamber that is placed over an extremity and pressurized with oxygen. The patient does not breathe the oxygen nor is the remainder of the body pressurized. The patient does not benefit from the systemic effects of HBO_2. Topox is based on the concept that oxygen diffuses through tissue at a depth of 30–50 µm.

TECHNIQUES OF HYPERBARIC OXYGENATION

The hyperbaric technician follows the prescribed instructions for the hyperbaric physician about pressure, duration, and frequency of treatment. Most of the treatments are given at pressures between 1.5 and 2.5 ATA, and the usual duration of a hyperbaric session is 60 minutes. Of this, 10 minutes are required for compression and 5 minutes for decompression if a pressure of 1.5 ATA is used. Thus, the maximal oxygen saturation is maintained for about 50 minutes. In the case of infections, the treatment duration is doubled. The treatment sessions for most chronic conditions are given daily, including on weekends.

WORLD DISTRIBUTION OF HYPERBARIC CHAMBERS

The largest number of chambers is located in China (around 1,800), followed by Russia (over 1,300). South Korea has the largest number per million inhabitants (4.9 compared with 3.6 in Russia). Europe has about 475 hyperbaric chambers. Within Europe, excluding Russia, Italy has the largest number of installations (34.1% of the European total) and also the largest number per million inhabitants (1.75). The number of hyperbaric chambers per million inhabitants has risen progressively since 1968 in all countries except Germany, where the number has actually declined. The fastest rise has been in China and Japan. The number of chambers does not necessarily correlate with the number of treatments given. There is no separation of multiplace and monoplace chambers in the statistics.

HYPERBARIC CHAMBERS IN INDIA

With the increasing awareness of medical professionals regarding the benefits of HBO_2 treatment, the availability of such facilities is continuing to increase in India. The Defence Research and Development Organisation (DRDO) has developed a hyperbaric chamber for the Indian Navy. This recompression chamber provides safe, reliable, and controlled atmospheric pressure, temperature, and quality of breathing air for treating and training deep-sea divers. This facility has been developed and commissioned in the Indian Naval Hospital-INHS Asvini, at Mumbai. Of the 22 hyperbaric chambers in India, 9 chambers are available with defense services and 13 chambers are with civil hospitals in metropolitan cities. Of course, the hyperbaric chambers available with the defense services are also being utilized by the civil population.

Of late, several corporate hospitals located in metropolitan cities have procured and offer monoplace hyperbaric chambers for HBOT. But considering the magnitude of hyperbaric chamber requirements in India, for over a billion population, the availability of chambers is grossly inadequate.

SUMMARY

Hyperbaric oxygen therapy involves breathing pure oxygen in a pressurized chamber to enhance the body's natural healing processes. This modality of treatment has been around since its first discovery in the 1600s. Since then the use of HBOT for medicinal purposes has been in and out of favour, but now is a firmly established modality of therapy worldwide for approved indications. HBOT increases oxygen levels in the body promoting wound healing and reducing inflammation. It also improves immune function and is used to treat several medical conditions such as decompression sickness, arterial gas embolism, carbon monoxide poisoning and many others. Patients can be treated in a closed "monoplace or a "multiplace hyperbaric chamber". HBOT is a noninvasive, relatively safe and evidence-based treatment.

REFERENCES

1. Moon RE, Camporesi EM. Hyperbaric oxygen therapy: From the nineteenth to the twenty-first century. Respir Care Clin N Am. 1999;5:1-5.
2. Edwards ML. Hyperbaric oxygen therapy. Part 1: History and principles. J Vet Emerg Crit Care. 2010;20:284-8.
3. Leach RM, Rees PJ, Wilmshurst P. ABC of oxygen: Hyperbaric oxygen therapy. Br Med J. 1998;317:1140-3.
4. Kirby JP, Snyder J, Schuerer DJE, et al. Essentials of hyperbaric oxygen therapy: 2019 review. Mol Med. 2019;116:176-9.
5. Ortega MA, Fraile-Martinez O, García-Montero C, et al. A general overview on the hyperbaric oxygen therapy: Applications, mechanisms and translational opportunities. Medicina (Kaunas). 2021;57(9):864.
6. Camporesi EM, Mascia MF, Thom SR. Physiological principles of hyperbaric oxygenation. In: Oriani G, Marroni A, Wattel F (Eds). Handbook on Hyperbaric Medicine. Milan: Springer; 1996. pp. 35-58.
7. Chen W, Liang X, Nong Z, et al. The multiple applications and possible mechanisms of the hyperbaric oxygenation therapy. Med Chem. 2019;15:459-71.
8. Choudhury R. Hypoxia and hyperbaric oxygen therapy: A review. Int J Gen Med. 2018;11:431-42.

9. Strauss RH. Diving medicine. Am Rev Respir Dis. 1979;119(6): 1001-23.
10. Tetzlaff K, Shank ES, Muth CM. Evaluation and management of decompression illness – an intensivist's perspective. Intensive Care Med. 2003;29(12):2128-36.
11. Mathieu D, Marroni A, Kot J. Tenth European Consensus Conference on Hyperbaric Medicine: Recommendations for Accepted and Non-Accepted Clinical Indications and Practice of Hyperbaric Oxygen Treatment. Diving Hyperb Med. 2017; 47(1):24-32.
12. Kirby JP. hyperbaric oxygen therapy emergencies. Mol Med. 2019;116:180-3.
13. Pollock NW, Buteau D. Updates in decompression illness. Emerg Med Clin N Am. 2017;35:301-19.
14. Vann RD, Butler FK, Mitchell SJ, et al. Decompression illness. Lancet. 2011;377:153-64.
15. Malik N, Claus PL, Illman JE, et al. Air embolism: Diagnosis and management. Future Cardiol. 2017;13:365-78.
16. Moon RE. Hyperbaric treatment of air or gas embolism: Current recommendations. Undersea Hyperb Med. 2019;46:673-83.
17. Yesilaras M, Atılla OD, Aksay E, et al. Retrograde cerebral air embolism. Am J Emerg Med. 2014;32:1562.e1-2.e2.
18. Shaw JJ, Psoinos CM, Emhoff TA, et al. Not just full of hot air: Hyperbaric oxygen therapy increases survival in cases of necrotizing soft tissue infections. Surg Infect. 2014;15:328-35.
19. Sanford NE, Wilkinson JE, Nguyen H, et al. Efficacy of hyperbaric oxygen therapy in bacterial biofilm eradication. J Wound Care. 2018;27:S20-8.
20. Halbach JL, Prieto JM, Wang AW, et al. Early hyperbaric oxygen therapy improves survival in a model of severe sepsis. Am J Physiol Regul Integr Comp Physiol. 2019;317:R160-8.
21. Perry BN, Floyd WE. Gas gangrene and necrotizing fasciitis in the upper extremity. J Surg Orthop Adv. 2004;13:57-68.
22. Prockop LD, Chichkova RI. Carbon monoxide intoxication: An updated review. J Neurol Sci. 2007;262(1-2):122-30.
23. Rhine DJ, Best T. Hyperbaric oxygen therapy in carbon monoxide poisoning: Effects on neurological sequelae. CJEM. 2000;2(1):22-4.
24. Stoller KP. Hyperbaric oxygen and carbon monoxide poisoning: a critical review. Neurol Res. 2007;29(2):146-55.
25. Casillas S, Galindo A, Camarillo-Reyes LA, et al. Effectiveness of hyperbaric oxygenation versus normobaric oxygenation therapy in carbon monoxide poisoning: A systematic review. Cureus. 2019;11:e5916.
26. Al-Waili NS, Butler GJ, Beale J, et al. Hyperbaric oxygen and malignancies: a potential role in radiotherapy, chemotherapy, tumor surgery and phototherapy. Med Sci Monit. 2005;11(9): RA279-89.
27. Bennett M, Feldmeier J, Smee R, et al. Hyperbaric oxygenation for tumor sensitization to radiotherapy. Cochrane Database Syst Rev. 2005;19:CD005007.
28. Kim SW, Kim IK, Lee SH. Role of hyperoxic treatment in cancer. Exp Biol Med. 2020;245:851-60.
29. Moen I, Stuhr LEB. Hyperbaric oxygen therapy and cancer—a review. Target Oncol. 2012;7:233-42.
30. Stępień K, Ostrowski RP, Matyja E. Hyperbaric oxygen as an adjunctive therapy in treatment of malignancies, including brain tumours. Med Oncol. 2016;33:101.
31. Bhutani S, Vishwanath G. Hyperbaric oxygen and wound healing. Indian J Plast Surg. 2012;45:316-24.
32. Sharma R, Sharma SK, Mudgal SK, et al. Efficacy of hyperbaric oxygen therapy for diabetic foot ulcer, a systematic review and meta-analysis of controlled clinical trials. Sci Rep. 2021;11:2189.
33. Brouwer RJ, Lalieu R, Hoencamp R, et al. A systematic review and meta-analysis of hyperbaric oxygen therapy for diabetic foot ulcers with arterial insufficiency. J Vasc Surg. 2020;71: 682-92.
34. Longobardi P, Hoxha K, Bennett MH. Is there a role for hyperbaric oxygen therapy in the treatment of refractory wounds of rare etiology? Diving Hyperb Med. 2019;49:216-24.
35. Rose D. Hyperbaric oxygen therapy for chronic refractory osteomyelitis. Am Fam Physician. 2012;86:888-93.
36. Savvidou OD, Kaspiris A, Bolia IK, et al. Effectiveness of hyperbaric oxygen therapy for the management of chronic osteomyelitis: A systematic review of the literature. Orthopedics. 2018;41: 193-9.
37. Nakamura H, Makiguchi T, Atomura D, et al. Changes in skin perfusion pressure after hyperbaric oxygen therapy following revascularization in patients with critical limb ischemia: a preliminary study. Int J Low Extrem Wounds. 2020;19:57-62.
38. Bennett MH, French C, Schnabel A, et al. Normobaric and hyperbaric oxygen therapy for the treatment and prevention of migraine and cluster headache. Cochrane Database Syst Rev. 2015;2015:CD005219.
39. Lin C-H, Su W-H, Chen Y-C, et al. Treatment with normobaric or hyperbaric oxygen and its effect on neuropsychometric dysfunction after carbon monoxide poisoning. Medicine. 2018; 97:e12456.
40. Sharma SN, Sapre GK, Kulkarni J, et al. Hyperbaric oxygen therapy in multiple sclerosis. J Assoc Physicians India. 1986; 34(3):221-4.
41. Olson EA, Lentz K. Central retinal artery occlusion: A literature review and the rationale for hyperbaric oxygen therapy. Mol Med. 2016;113:53-7.
42. Kim SH, Cha YS, Lee Y, et al. Successful treatment of central retinal artery occlusion using hyperbaric oxygen therapy. Clin Exp Emerg Med. 2018;5:278-81.
43. Van Meter KW. The effect of hyperbaric oxygen on severe anemia. Undersea Hyperb Med. 2012;39:937-42.
44. Rhee TM, Hwang D, Lee JS, et al. Addition of hyperbaric oxygen therapy vs. medical therapy alone for idiopathic sudden sensorineural hearing loss: A systematic review and meta-analysis. JAMA Otolaryngol Head Neck Surg. 2018;144:1153-61.
45. Cooper JS, Phuyal P, Shah N. Oxygen Toxicity. Treasure Island, FL: StatPearls Publishing; 2021. [online]. Available from https://www.ncbi.nlm.nih.gov/books/NBK430743/ [Last accessed September, 2024].
46. Nakane M. Biological effects of the oxygen molecule in critically ill patients. J Intensive Care. 2020;8:95.
47. Hadanny A, Zubari T, Tamir-Adler L, et al. Hyperbaric oxygen therapy effects on pulmonary functions: A prospective cohort study. BMC Pulm Med. 2019;19:148.
48. Arslan A. Hyperbaric oxygen therapy in carbon monoxide poisoning in pregnancy: Maternal and fetal outcome. Am J Emerg Med. 2021;43:41-5.
49. Lind F. A pro/con review comparing the use of mono- and multiplace hyperbaric chambers for critical care. Diving Hyperb Med. 2015;45:56-60.
50. Weaver LK. Monoplace hyperbaric chamber use of U.S. Navy Table 6: A 20-year experience. Undersea Hyperb Med. 2006;33(2):85-8.

SECTION

18

Surgical Aspects

SECTION OUTLINE

Surgical Management of Pneumonia

CHAPTER 177

Avantika Nathani, Pratibha G Gogia, Dean Schraufnagel, Atul C Mehta

INTRODUCTION

Pneumonias are a common cause of hospitalizations, morbidity, and mortality, especially among children, the elderly, and immunocompromised individuals. In 2021, the Centers for Disease Control estimated the mortality rate from pneumonia to be 12.4 per 100,000 population.[1] This number is higher within populations at extremes of age and in lower-income countries with 22% of deaths in children aged 1–5 years being attributed to pneumonia.[2] Prior to the advent of antibiotics, complications like empyema and abscesses were common and hence surgical drainage and radical surgery were the mainstays of therapy, although with a high mortality rate **(Fig. 1)**.[3-5] Over the last few decades, however, antibiotics have become the cornerstone of the management of pneumonia. This has significantly reduced the need for surgical management. In this chapter, we identify present-day indications for surgery for pneumonias as well as discuss appropriate perioperative care **(Table 1)**.

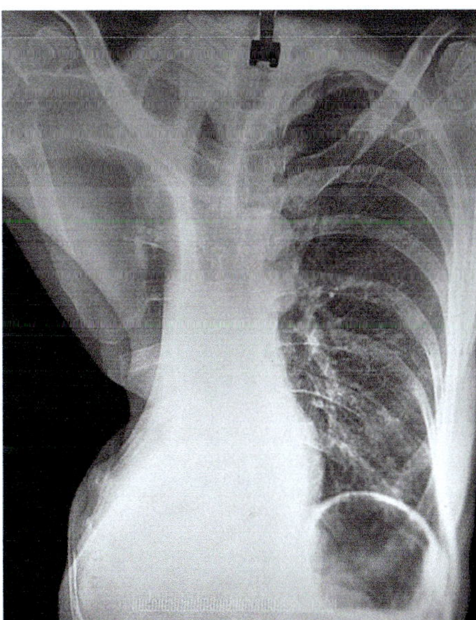

FIG. 1: Note remote right pneumonectomy and thoracoplasty for multidrug-resistant tuberculosis.

Courtesy: Dr R Singla, National Institute of Tuberculosis and Chest Diseases, New Delhi.

MODERN INDICATIONS

Failure of Medical Treatment

Treatment failure refers to "lack of clinical improvement within 72 hours of initiation of antibiotics".[6] Various host and organism factors contribute toward the treatment failure. The initial step is to reassess the presence of infection. Flexible bronchoscopy (FB) with bronchoalveolar lavage (BAL) sampling can help identify predominant offending microorganisms for appropriate therapy. If there is a lack of response to the appropriate drug, dose, and duration of therapy occasionally surgical resection of the affected area may be considered. Resection is generally indicated in infections with organisms pan-resistant to antibiotics that require source control. This includes segmentectomy, lobectomy, or, in some extreme cases, even pneumonectomy.

TABLE 1: Modern indications for surgery for Pneumonia

Indication	Examples
Failure of medical treatment	Progressive nonresolving pneumonia
Medical therapy is inappropriate	Pneumonias with complications • Abscess • Empyema • Fistula
Difficult-to-treat pneumonias	• Fungal pneumonia • Mycobacterial pneumonia
Special circumstances	• Postobstructive pneumonia • Lady Windermere syndrome • Right middle lobe syndrome • Broncholithiasis • Congenital abnormalities • Cystic fibrosis

Complications of pneumonia as detailed in the following sections are the frequent indications for the surgery.

Complications of Pneumonias

Long-standing pneumonias or those caused by highly virulent or anaerobic organisms can lead to complications such as lung abscesses, empyema, or a bronchopleural fistula.

Lung Abscess

A lung abscess is defined as a collection of suppurative necrosis of the lung parenchyma often surrounded by a cavity **(Figs. 2A and B)**. Antibiotics, including anaerobic coverage, remain the first line of treatment for lung abscesses. About 80–90% of lung abscesses resolve with medical treatment alone;[7] however, abscesses larger than 6 cm in diameter or the presence of symptoms for greater than 12 weeks' duration require additional measures. In these cases, conservative drainage of the abscess, either bronchoscopic or transthoracic, is recommended for the source control.[7] The abscess can be punctured bronchoscopically with a laser to evacuate abscess contents. Transthoracic drainage can be in the form of a surgical chest tube (using a trocar) or Seldinger's technique. Bear in mind that this approach could lead to a broncho-pleural-cutaneous fistula. Failure of conservative drainage techniques may necessitate surgical resection of the affected area.[8] Surgery may also be indicated in the event of persistent hemoptysis or if there is a spontaneous rupture of the abscess.[9]

Empyema

Empyema refers to the presence of pus in the pleural cavity. Positive pleural fluid Gram stain as well as cultures also fall in the definition of empyema. This commonly occurs due to infection of a parapneumonic effusion. In India, tuberculosis (TB) remains the most common cause of empyema.[10] The treatment of empyema depends on the stage of presentation. In acute empyema, antibiotics and in-dwelling pleural drains are considered as the first line of treatment. The goal is to completely evacuate the pleural space resulting in full expansion of the underlying lung. Surgical management of the acute phase involves entering the pleural space via an open thoracotomy or video-assisted thoracic surgery (VATS) to clear the pleural space of fibrinous bands, pus, and adhesions **(Fig. 3)**.[11]

Chronic or long-standing empyema pose a different challenge as they often present with an organized rind around the lung, calcified pleura, rib crowding, or even rib destruction **(Figs. 4A to C)**. Surgery is the gold standard for the treatment of chronic empyema. Surgical management consists of decortication either via VATS or an open thoracotomy **(Figs. 5A and B)**, thoracoplasty, and rib resection. Patients with TB often need a window or drainage procedure for source control. An Eloesser flap, its modified form, lets the infected pleural fluid drain passively and involves the creation of a one-way valve using autologous tissue to allow the egress of fluid from the chest cavity without the return of air.[12] A modified version of this is Clagette window which is a larger opening designed to be used as a temporary measure to drain infected pleural fluid and allow decontamination with subsequent closure **(Figs. 6A to C)**.[13]

Bronchopulmonary Fistula

A bronchopleural fistula is a sinus tract that is formed between the bronchial tree and the pleural space.[14] Suppurative necrotizing pneumonias, especially TB or *Pseudomonas*, can create fistulas due to the destruction of the bronchial wall and lung parenchyma resulting in this pathological communication. The first step in the management includes antibiotics to cover the underlying infection as well as pleural drainage to evacuate the air

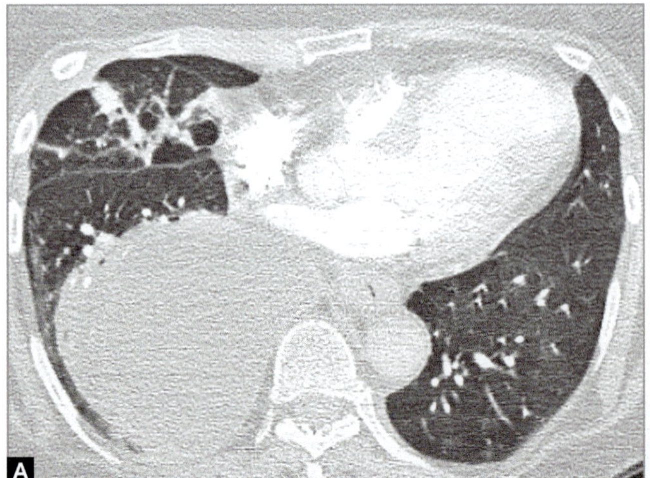

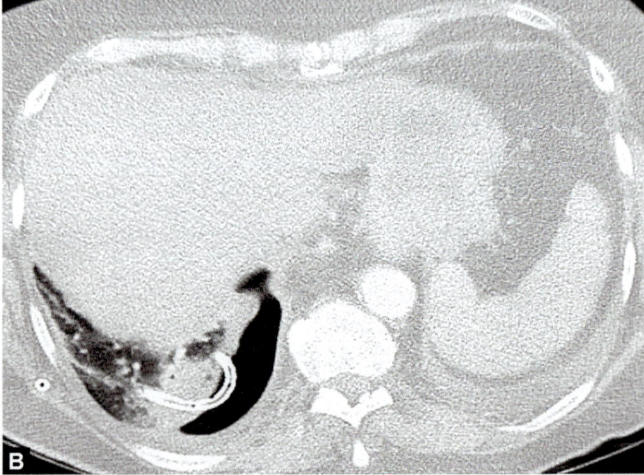

FIGS. 2A AND B: Lung abscess in right lower lobe managed by percutaneous drainage leading to a bronchopleural fistula.

and fluid in the pleural space. If the fistula does not resolve spontaneously, a surgical intervention is indicated. This can be performed bronchoscopically with the use of a bronchial blocker or one-way valves. Surgical management includes VATS or open thoracotomy for the identification and excision or closure of the fistulous defect.

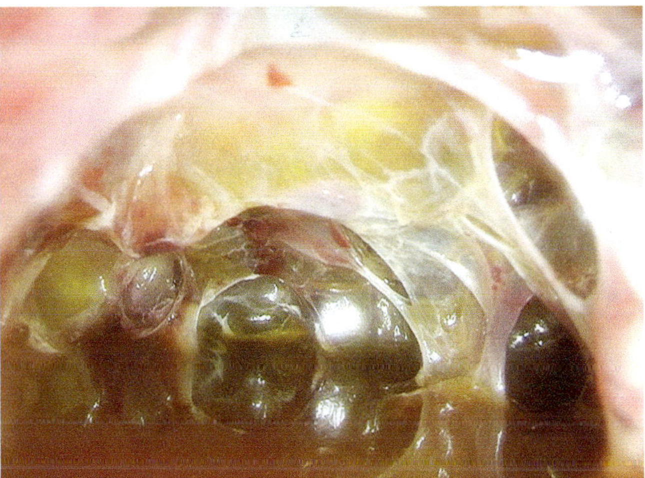

FIG. 3: Video-assisted thoracoscopic surgery (VATS) view of empyema with multiple fibrinous bands.

Bronchiectasis

Recurrent pneumonias can often lead to bronchiectasis. If localized, this can be managed with surgery (vide infra).

Difficult-to-treat Pneumonias

Surgical management is sometimes indicated for difficult-to-treat pneumonias, particularly those pneumonia caused by fungal organisms or TB.

Fungal Pneumonia

Fungal infections, particularly pneumonia, are common in immunocompromised individuals as well as in those who live in endemic areas. Surgery is indicated as a salvage therapy if antifungals fail or there are complications.

Pulmonary aspergilloma occurs due to colonization of aspergillus in a preexisting lesion like tuberculous or sarcoid cavities or an emphysematous bleb **(Fig. 7)**.

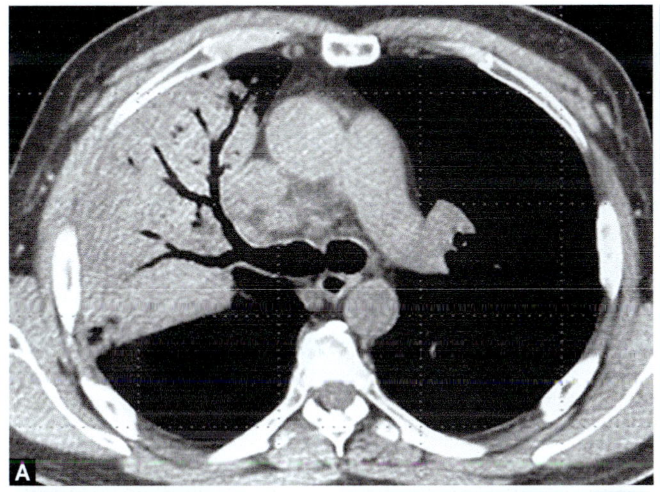

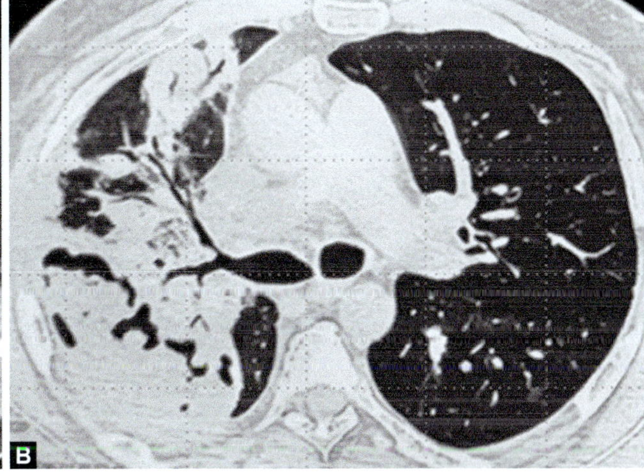

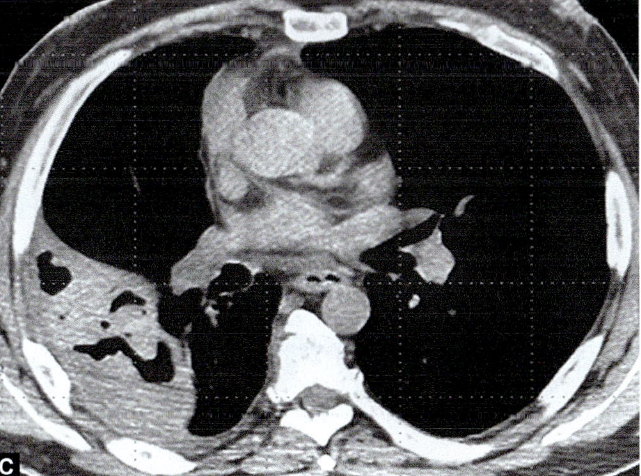

FIGS. 4A TO C: (A) Right upper lobe in *Klebsiella pneumoniae* (bulging fissure sign), turning into a lung abscess (B) and developing empyema (C) requiring surgical intervention in a patient with common variable immune deficiency.
Courtesy: Dr Avadesh Bansal, Apollo Hospital, New Delhi.

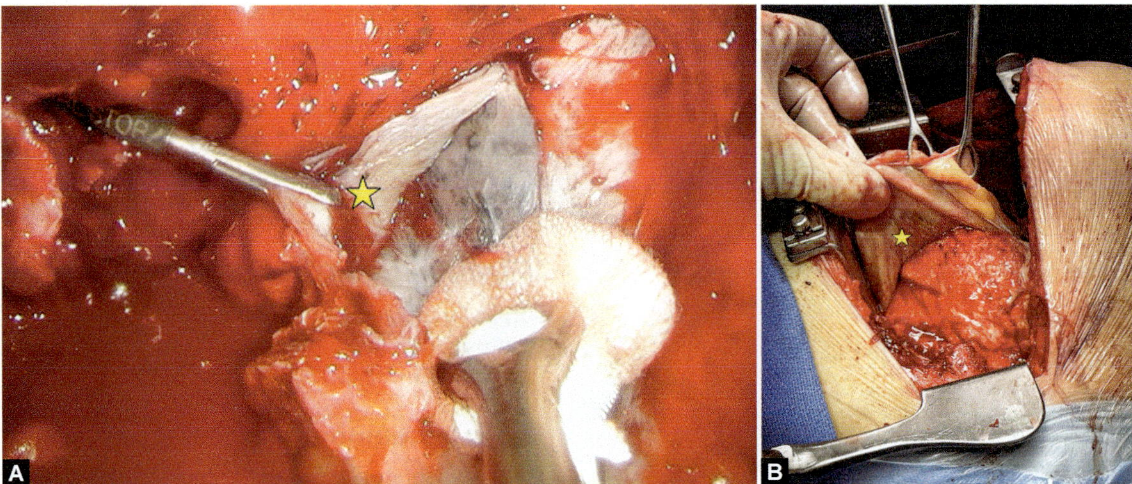

FIGS. 5A AND B: (A) Video-assisted thoracotomy (VATS) decortication of rind (yellow star) around an early empyema; (B) Open thoracotomy decortication of chronic empyema with thick rind (yellow star).

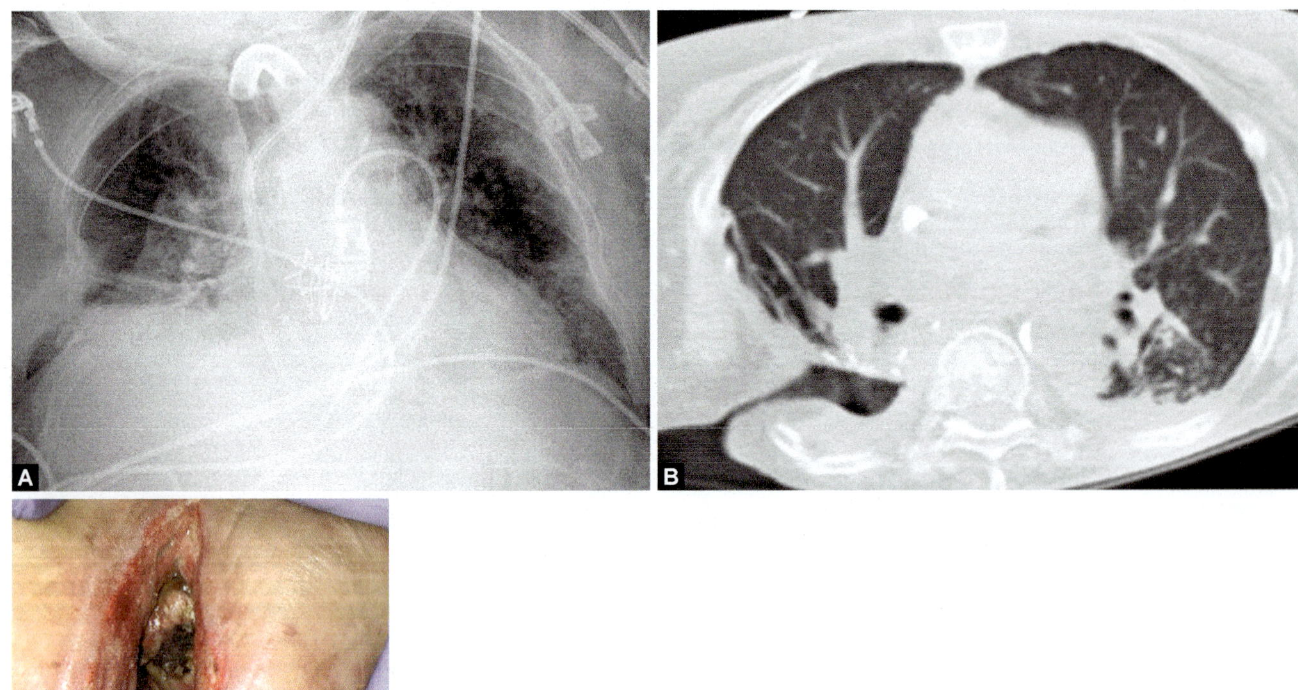

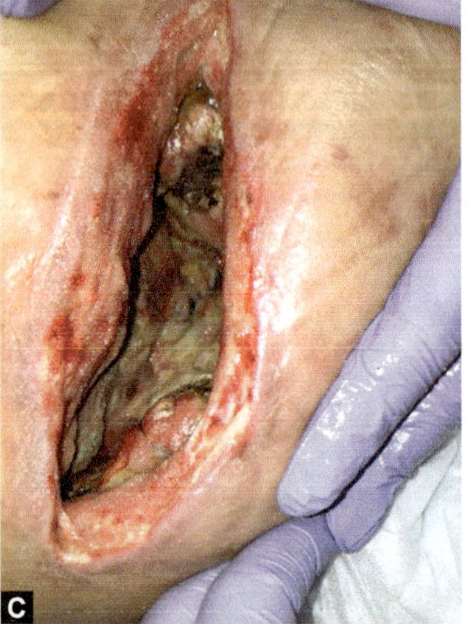

FIGS. 6A TO C: Chest X-ray, CT chest, and chest wall examination revealing right Clagett's window. Note iatrogenic absence of the right posterolateral chest wall.

At times, these aspergillomas can invade the surrounding structures causing destruction of the parenchymal tissue and erosion of blood vessels leading to hemoptysis. Resection of the affected area by either a wedge resection, segmentectomy, or even lobectomy may be indicated to obtain control of the bleeding.[15] In patients who are not good surgical candidates, bronchial artery embolization or a cavernostomy is considered. A cavernostomy involves creating an opening into the fungal cavity to allow it to evacuate.[16]

Mucormycosis is an invasive necrotic fungal infection affecting immunocompromised individuals. There is often a poor response to antifungal treatment due to limited blood supply secondary to tissue necrosis and thrombosis. Surgical resection is recommended in patients with limited disease not responding to the antifungals. Tedder et al. reported that patients with mucormycosis treated with medical therapy alone had a 68% mortality as compared to 11% in the combined medical and surgical therapy group **(Figs. 8A and B)**.[17]

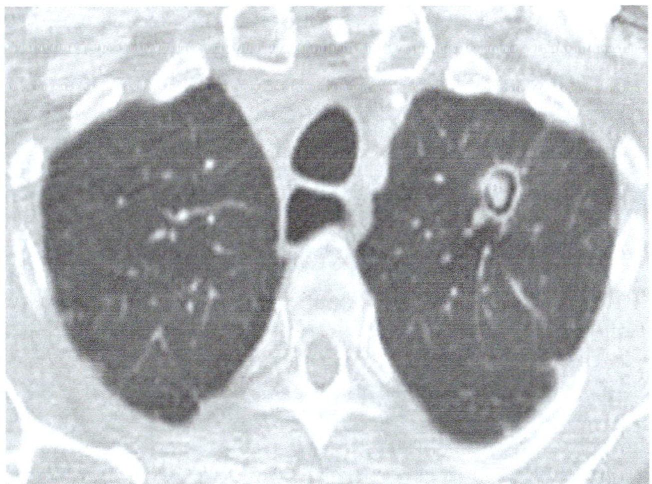

FIG. 7: Left upper lobe shows Monod's sign of aspergilloma. Patient required lobectomy for hemoptysis following failed bronchial artery embolization. The patient was on anticoagulation therapy for paroxysmal atrial fibrillation.

Histoplasma is an endemic fungal infection that often causes asymptomatic pulmonary lymphadenopathy and calcifications. However, sometimes, these calcified nodes can erode into the airway causing compression and inflammation in the airway. They can present as persistent cough, recurrent pneumonias, or, in severe cases, massive hemoptysis. If asymptomatic, conservation management is indicated. If the broncholith is freely mobile in the airway, bronchoscopic removal can be performed. With significant destruction or a fistula formation, surgical resection is indicated.[18] Histoplasmosis can be complicated by fibrosing mediastinitis which causes an invasive fibrosing process in the mediastinum leading to vascular and airway obstruction and destruction. These complications often require surgery to prevent further consequences. Airway involvement causes constrictions and resultant hyperemia that can lead to hemoptysis. Bronchoscopic localization and control of bleed by laser or argon plasma coagulation are indicated in these cases.[19] Stenosis of airways and great vessels may require placement of stents or even bypass grafts in order to maintain patency.[20-22]

Mycobacterial Pneumonia

The late 19th century saw many advances made in the field of thoracoscopic surgery to facilitate the treatment of TB. After the introduction of antitubercular medications, there has been a significant reduction in the use of surgical methods; however, surgery remains an important adjunctive therapy in patients with multidrug-resistant (MDR) and extensively drug-resistant (XDR) TB **(Fig. 9)**. The indications for surgery for TB can be classified as emergent, urgent, and elective **(Box 1)**.

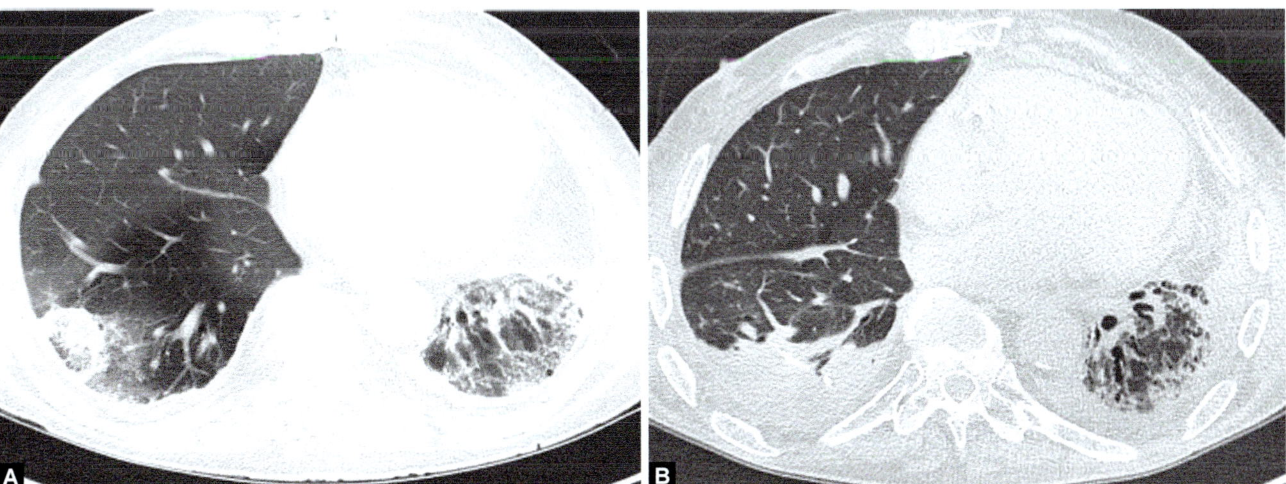

FIGS. 8A AND B: Right lower lobe angioinvasive mucor infection in a patient with single (right) lung transplant for idiopathic pulmonary fibrosis. This was treated surgically with a wedge resection.

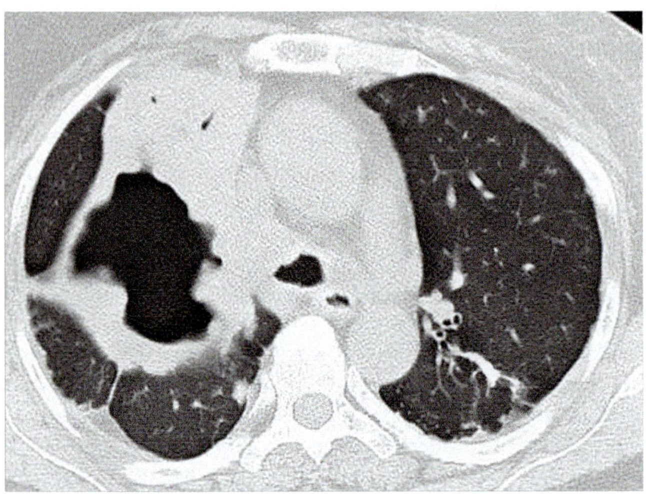

FIG. 9: Multidrug-resistant mycobacterial infection necessitating pneumonectomy to reduce the organism load.

BOX 1 Indications for surgery in pulmonary tuberculosis.

Emergent
- Profuse hemorrhage
- Tension pneumothorax

Urgent
- Irreversible progression (despite anti-TB medications)
- Recurrent hemoptysis, not controlled by other methods

Elective
- Localized cavity with persistent bacillary shedding despite 6 months of therapy
- XDR TB with failure to treat
- Complications of TB:
  - Pneumothorax
  - Empyema
  - Bronchopleural fistula
  - Broncholith
  - Superimposed fungal infection (aspergilloma)
  - Post-TB tracheal or bronchial stenosis
  - Post-TB bronchiectasis

(TB: tuberculosis; XDR: extensively drug-resistant)

For patients with MDR and XDR TB, surgical intervention is associated with successful treatment outcomes. In their meta-analysis of 24 studies, Marrone et al.[23] reported favorable surgical outcomes in subgroups with increased drug-resistant organisms.

Historically, plombage and thoracoplasty were commonly performed surgeries for cavitary TB. Plombage, also known as extraperiosteal or extrapleural pneumonolysis, refers to a surgically created cavity under the upper ribs that is filled with inert material like ping-pong balls, oils, rubber sheets, or gauze **(Figs. 10A and B)**. The theory was that this would cause collapse of the upper lobe resulting in faster healing of the cavitary lesion. In the modern area, hemostatic absorbable oxidized cellulose sheets are used to create a plombage effect, particularly in the management of persistent air leaks **(Fig. 11)**. Thoracoplasty is the resection of ribs from the chest wall resulting in permanent collapse of the cavity. While this procedure resulted in high rates of cavity collapse, it caused some degree of chest wall and shoulder deformity often causing scoliosis and respiratory failure and was associated with a significant operative mortality.

Special Circumstances

Postobstructive Pneumonia

Endobronchial obstruction can lead to infection of the distal lung parenchyma. This obstruction is most commonly caused by a neoplasm; however, retained foreign bodies can also frequently cause postobstructive pneumonia. Neoplasms like squamous cell or small cell lung carcinoma can commonly lead to airway obstruction and pneumonia due to their central location. Carcinoid tumors can also present as an endobronchial mass leading to pneumonia. Antibiotics and relief from obstruction remain the first line of treatment for postobstructive pneumonia.[24]

A computed tomography (CT) scan should be performed in the cases suspected of having postobstructive pneumonia, followed by a bronchoscopy. If a foreign body is identified, retrieval can lead to the resolution of pneumonia. For earlystage cancers, surgical resection for curative intent can be considered. If, however, the tumor is unresectable or has metastasized, debulking of the tumor to relieve obstruction can be performed through either a rigid or a flexible bronchoscope. Debulking can be performed mechanically or by using argon plasma coagulation electrocautery, laser photoresection, or cryoablation.[24] An endobronchial stent may be required to maintain patency of the airway following the debulking if the residual obstruction is >50%. This is a palliative maneuver to reduce the frequency of postobstructive pneumonia and to improve the quality of life.

Lady Windermere Syndrome

Lady Windermere syndrome, first described in 1992,[25] refers to an isolated right middle lobe postobstructive bronchiectasis caused due to voluntary suppression of the cough reflex seen in a middle-aged woman **(Fig. 12)**. This leads to a predisposition for recurrent infections, particularly colonization and infection with nontubercular mycobacteria (NTM) like *Mycobacterium avium complex*. Treatment consists of a combination regimen of macrolide antibiotics (azithromycin or clarithromycin), ethambutol, and rifamycin. Anatomic destruction seen in this disease contributes to the failure of antibiotics, and surgical resection of the area may be required to control recurrent infections. Thoracoscopic lung resection has shown

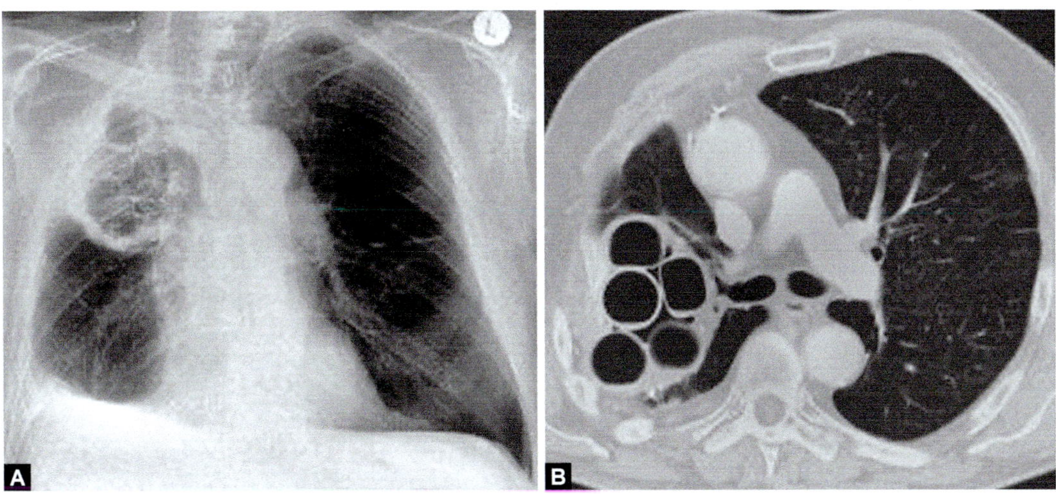

FIGS. 10A AND B: Right upper lobe apical tenting and plombage using ping-pong balls to treat a cavity caused by multidrug-resistant *Mycobacterium tuberculosis* (1989). The procedure had to be reversed in 2005 due to recurrent cellulitis.

Courtesy: Dr S Bal, Sir Gangaram Hospital, New Delhi

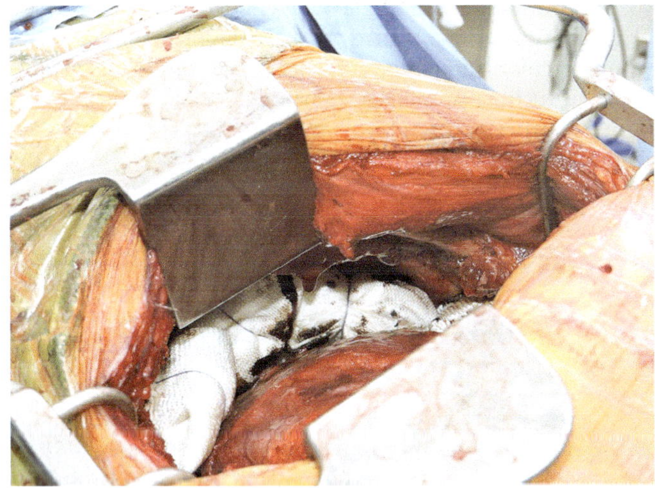

FIG. 11: Extrapleural plombage with hemostatic absorbable oxidized cellulose sheets in a patient with persistent air leak after decortication. These sheets help in parietal and visceral pleural apposition and are eventually reabsorbed by the body.

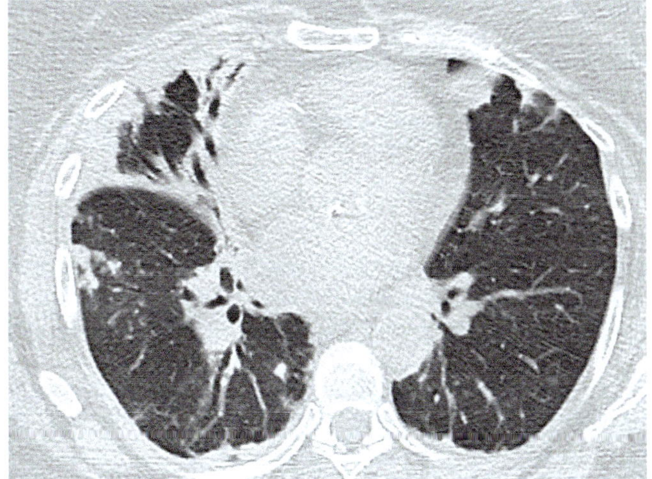

FIG. 12. Right middle lobe bronchiectasis in a middle aged white woman suggestive of Lady Windermere syndrome requiring a lobectomy.

good outcomes[26] and is comparable to lung resection by thoracotomy in appropriate patients with Lady Windermere syndrome.

Right Middle Lobe Syndrome

The right middle lobe bronchus is the longest and the narrowest among all the lobar bronchi. It is also surrounded by multiple lymph nodes. Right middle lobe syndrome refers to the atelectasis of the middle lobe (occasionally lingula as well) due to either obstructive or nonobstructive causes.[27] The obstruction can be intraluminal but commonly caused by enlarged peribronchial lymph nodes causing extrinsic compression. The prevalence is higher in the endemic areas for fungal infections such as histoplasmosis. Nonobstructive middle lobe syndrome has been attributed to poor drainage due to anatomic take of the right middle lobe bronchus or the lack of collateral ventilation preventing re-expansion once atelectasis has taken place. Treatment modalities focus on airway clearance with bronchodilators, mucolytics, and chest physiotherapy with the addition of antibiotics if infection is suspected. Recurrent infections often necessitate surgical intervention, either for the relief of the obstruction or for resection of the affected lobe.[28,29]

Congenital Anomalies

Congenital anomalies leading to developmental issues in the lung can present as bronchopulmonary or vascular abnormalities. Anomalies such as bronchopulmonary sequestration, tracheal bronchus, and bronchial atresia can present as recurrent pneumonias. This occurs due to inadequate clearance of secretions or the blood flow to the affected areas of the lung.

Bronchopulmonary sequestration occurs when a dysplastic segment or lobe of the lung does not communicate with the rest of the tracheobronchial tree and receives an anomalous blood supply. This segment can get repeated infections due to a lack of appropriate ventilation. Surgical excision is the treatment of choice;[30] however embolization is now gaining importance, especially in patients who are poor surgical candidates.[31]

Tracheal bronchus, or bronchus suis, is the aberrant takeoff of an upper lobe bronchus from the trachea. The angle of this takeoff often causes inadequate drainage of secretions leading to recurrent infections. Symptomatic treatment is the first line; however, in patients with recurrent infections, a segmentectomy or lobectomy can be considered.

Congenital bronchial atresia occurs due to interruption and cul-de-sac termination of bronchi at the lobar or segmental levels causing obstruction, mucus impaction and recurrent infections of the parenchyma distal to the affected airway. Surgical resection, either a segmentectomy or a lobectomy, is required to prevent recurrent infections.[32]

Bronchiectasis

Cystic Fibrosis

Cystic fibrosis (CF) is an autosomal recessive disease that has various manifestations involving the respiratory, pancreatic, gastrointestinal, and reproductive systems. In the lungs, CF is characterized by thick viscous secretions leading to recurrent infections that cause bronchiectasis and parenchymal destruction. The basic premise of the treatment of lung disease is airway clearance by bronchodilators, mucolytics, and antibiotics as well as in selected patients, cystic fibrosis transmembrane conductance regulator (CFTR) modulators to improve the function of the defective protein. However, in patients with localized bronchiectasis leading to recurrent infections, resection may be needed, though this is known to have a high rate of complications.[33] Patients with CF often present with hemoptysis. Bronchial artery embolization is an established treatment option in these patients;[34] however, in the setting of uncontrolled bleeding despite embolization, surgical resection of the affected lobe may be indicated.[33] In the last four decades, lung transplantation has been frequently considered in patients with advanced lung disease due to CF; however, the widespread use of CFTR modulators in slowing down the progression of lung disease and thus the frequency of lung transplants due to CF has declined.[35]

Noncystic Fibrosis-related Bronchiectasis

Non-CF bronchiectasis occurs due to various reasons including immunodeficiencies like common variable immunodeficiency (CVID), as a sequela of prior infections like recurrent pneumonias, TB, ciliary clearance defects, and autoimmune diseases. Bronchiectasis airways are prone to colonization and infection which leads to a vicious cycle of further propagating bronchiectasis.[36] In patients with a localized structural change that causes downstream bronchiectasis, surgery may be considered to eliminate the reservoir of infection and provide symptomatic control.[37] Resection can be performed by either segmentectomy, lobectomy, or even pneumonectomy **(Figs. 13A to C)**.

PREOPERATIVE ASSESSMENT AND OPTIMIZATION

Unless it is an emergent procedure, patients should be thoroughly evaluated preoperatively to improve their surgical outcomes. Management of comorbidities like

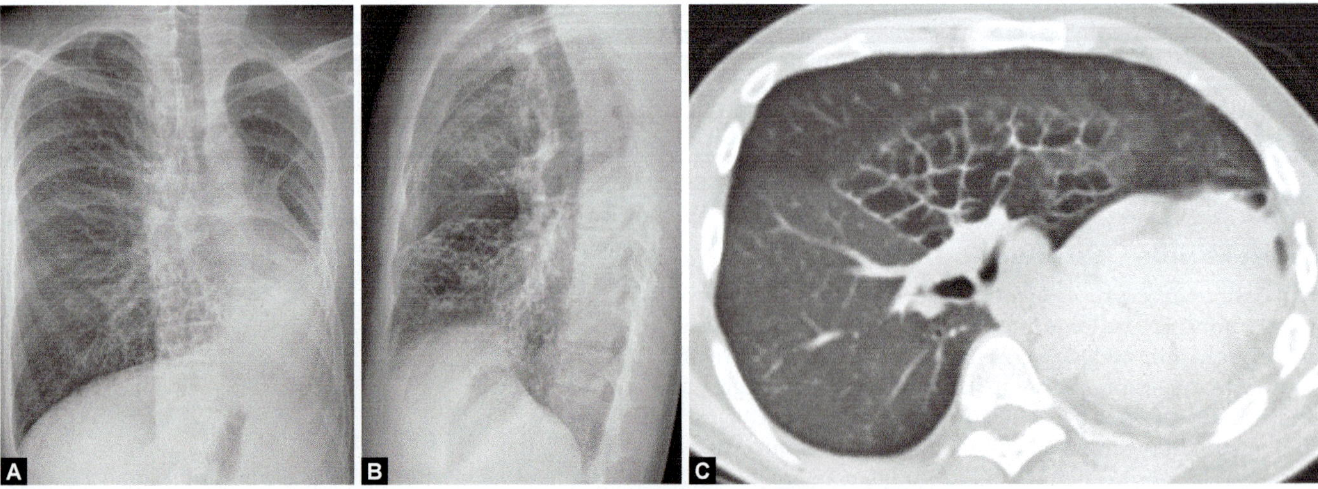

FIGS. 13A TO C: Noncystic fibrosis bronchiectasis requiring left pneumonectomy. Note hyperexpansion and herniation of the right lung into the left hemithorax. There is persistent localized bronchiectasis in the right lung.

diabetes, hypertension, chronic obstructive pulmonary disease, or obstructive sleep apnea should be optimized. All patients should get a computed tomography (CT) scan to aid in surgical or bronchoscopic planning. If feasible, pulmonary function tests should be performed to assess baseline lung function. In select patients, a ventilation/perfusion scan or a cardiopulmonary exercise test may be indicated.

TYPES OF PROCEDURES

The type of procedure depends on the location of lesions as well as the extent of involvement of the lung parenchyma. **Box 2** lists some of the common procedures that can be done for pneumonias. Transthoracic procedures are indicated for peripheral lesions or for those who are poor candidates for surgery. Open debridement of necrotized tissue or cavities is indicated for peripheral lesions.[38] Resection can be nonanatomic or anatomic, and the decision is largely guided by how much lung is involved as well as the overall condition of the patient and the remaining lung **(Figs. 14A and B)**.

BOX 2 Surgical procedures for Pneumonias.

Transthoracic procedures
- Transthoracic needle aspiration
- Thoracostomy tube

Bronchoscopic procedures
- Abscess drainage
- Endobronchial blocker placement for bleeding or bronchopleural fistula
- Bronchoscopic control of bleeding by cold saline, cauterization, tranexamic acid
- Foreign body removal

Surgical procedures
- Debridement
- Wedge resection
- Segmentectomy—single or multiple
- Lobectomy or bilobectomy
- Pneumonectomy
- Decortication of empyema
- Fenestration procedures—Clagette window or Eloesser's flap

POSTOPERATIVE MANAGEMENT AND COMPLICATIONS

Surgical management for pneumonia is generally well tolerated. The less invasive the procedure, the lower the risk of postoperative complications. Routine postsurgical management includes wound care, chest physiotherapy, early mobilizations, and adequate pain control to prevent splinting. Prophylaxis against deep vein thrombosis and pulmonary embolism should be considered in all patients unless absolute contraindications exist. The most common surgical complications specifically related to lung resection include the formation of a bronchopleural fistula which leads to a persistent air leak.[39] Other complications include postoperative atelectasis, pneumonia, or respiratory failure.

SUMMARY

The primary treatment for pneumonias continues to be broad-spectrum antibiotics. Surgical management is reserved for patients not responding to antibiotics or those who have complications or structural abnormalities leading to recurrent pneumonias as detailed above. With the right patient selection, surgery is generally well tolerated

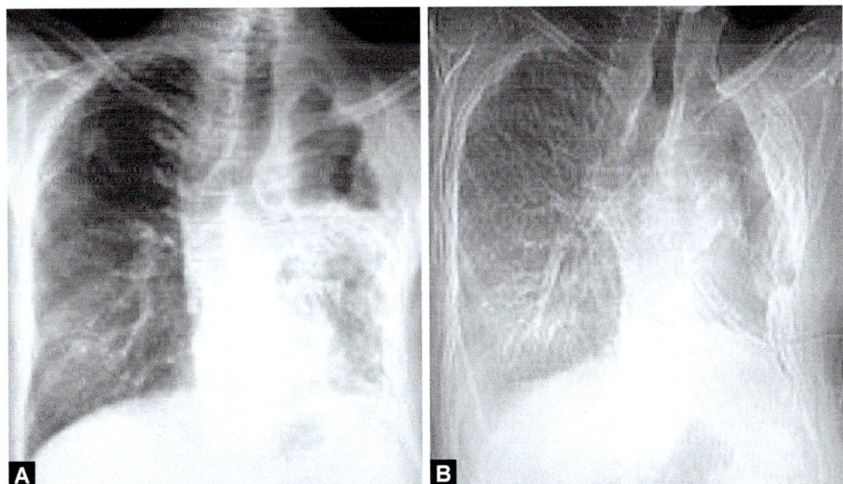

FIGS. 14A AND B: (A) Left bronchopleural fistula. Note hydropneumothorax. (B) Chest X-ray, postpneumonectomy for life-threatening hemoptysis. Note herniation of the right lung into the left chest.

REFERENCES

1. CDC. Underlying cause of death, 2018-2021, Single Race Results Form. [online] Available from https://wonder.cdc.gov/controller/datarequest/D158;jsessionid=0EB57912BC0C6B7FBEC7361DFA05#Citation [Last accessed October, 2024].
2. World Health Organization. (2022). Pneumonia in children. [online] Available from https://www.who.int/news-room/fact-sheets/detail/pneumonia [Last accessed October, 2024].
3. Elsner HL. Pneumonia with Empyemia: Radical Operation-Recovery. Buffalo Med Surg J. 1887;26(12):542-6.
4. NEJM. Certain aspects of pulmonary abscess, from an analysis of 227 cases. [online] Available from https://www-nejm-org.ccmain.ohionet.org/doi/full/10.1056/NEJM192504231921701 [Last accessed October, 2024].
5. Neuhof H, Hurwitt E. Acute putrid abscess of the lung: Relationship of the technic of the one-stage operation to results. Ann Surg. 1943;118(4):656-64.
6. Menendez R, Torres A. Treatment failure in community-acquired pneumonia. Chest. 2007;132(4):1348-55.
7. Wali SO. An update on the drainage of pyogenic lung abscesses. Ann Thorac Med. 2012;7(1):3-7.
8. Pagès PB, Bernard A. [Lung abscess and necrotizing pneumonia: chest tube insertion or surgery?]. Rev Pneumol Clin. 2012;68(2):84-90.
9. Kuhajda I, Zarogoulidis K, Tsirgogianni K, et al. Lung abscess-etiology, diagnostic and treatment options. Ann Transl Med. 2015;3(13):183.
10. Kundu S, Mitra S, Mukherjee S, et al. Adult thoracic empyema: A comparative analysis of tuberculous and nontuberculous etiology in 75 patients. Lung India Off Organ Indian Chest Soc. 2010;27(4):196-201.
11. ScienceDirect. The American Association for Thoracic Surgery consensus guidelines for the management of empyema. [online] Available from https://www-sciencedirect-com.ccmain.ohionet.org/science/article/pii/S0022522317301526?via%3Dihub [Last accessed October, 2024].
12. Benjamin SR, Panakkada RK, Andugala SS, et al. Surgical management of empyema thoracis – experience of a decade in a tertiary care centre in India. Indian J Thorac Cardiovasc Surg. 2021;37(3):274-84.
13. Denlinger CE. Eloesser Flap Thoracostomy Window. Oper Tech Thorac Cardiovasc Surg. 2010;15(1):61-9.
14. Salik I, Vashisht R, Abramowicz AE. Bronchopleural Fistula. In: StatPearls. Treasure Island: StatPearls Publishing; 2023. [online] Available from http://www.ncbi.nlm.nih.gov/books/NBK534765/ [Last accessed October, 2024].
15. Kasprzyk M, Pieczyński K, Mania K, et al. Surgical treatment for pulmonary aspergilloma – early and long-term results. Kardiochirurgia Torakochirurgia Pol Pol J Cardio-Thorac Surg. 2017;14(2):99-103.
16. Beamer S. Surgical management of non-mycobacterial fungal infections. J Thorac Dis. 2018;10(Suppl 28):S3398-407.
17. Tedder M, Spratt JA, Anstadt MP, et al. Pulmonary mucormycosis: results of medical and surgical therapy. Ann Thorac Surg. 1994;57(4):1044-50.
18. Krishnan S, Kniese CM, Mankins M, Heitkamp DE, Sheski FD, Kesler KA. Management of broncholithiasis. J Thorac Dis. 2018; 10(Suppl 28):S3419-27.
19. Scheubel R. Therapie der chronischen Mediastinitis. Chir. 2016; 87(6):486-8.
20. Cimenoglu B, Ozkan B, Basaran M, et al. Pulmonary Arterial Bypass Surgery for Fibrosing Mediastinitis Causing Severe Pulmonary Hypertension. Ann Thorac Surg. 2019;107(6):e411-3.
21. Duan J, Wang S, Liu P, et al. Early prediction of noninvasive ventilation failure in COPD patients: derivation, internal validation, and external validation of a simple risk score. Ann Intensive Care. 2019;9(1):108.
22. Deshwal H, Ghosh S, Magruder K, et al. A review of endovascular stenting for superior vena cava syndrome in fibrosing mediastinitis. Vasc Med Lond Engl. 2020;25(2):174-83.
23. Marrone MT, Venkataramanan V, Goodman M, et al. Surgical interventions for drug-resistant tuberculosis: a systematic review and meta-analysis. Int J Tuberc Lung Dis Off J Int Union Tuberc Lung Dis. 2013;17(1):6-16.
24. Rolston KVI, Nesher L. Post-Obstructive Pneumonia in Patients with Cancer: A Review. Infect Dis Ther. 2018;7(1):29-38.
25. Reich JM, Johnson RE. Mycobacterium avium complex pulmonary disease presenting as an isolated lingular or middle lobe pattern. The Lady Windermere syndrome. Chest. 1992;101(6):1605-9.
26. Yu JA, Pomerantz M, Bishop A, et al. Lady Windermere revisited: treatment with thoracoscopic lobectomy/segmentectomy for right middle lobe and lingular bronchiectasis associated with non-tuberculous mycobacterial disease. Eur J Cardiothorac Surg. 2011;40(3):671-5.
27. Graham EA, Burford TH, Mayer JH. Middle lobe syndrome. Postgrad Med. 1948;4(1):29-34.
28. Sehitogullari A, Sayir F, Cobanoglu U, Bilici S. Surgical treatment of right middle lobe syndrome in children. Ann Thorac Med. 2012;7(1):8-11.
29. Pejhan S, Salehi F, Niusha S, Farzanegan B, Sheikhy K. Ten Years' Experience in Surgical Treatment of Right Middle Lobe Syndrome. Ann Thorac Cardiovasc Surg. 2015;21(4):354-8.
30. Alsumrain M, Ryu JH. Pulmonary sequestration in adults: a retrospective review of resected and unresected cases. BMC Pulm Med. 2018;18(1):97.
31. Thompson TS, Lazarowicz M, Mahmoud A, et al. Endovascular embolization for pulmonary sequestration in adults: An adjunctive technique to delay surgical intervention. Am J Interv Radiol. 2022;6.
32. Macias L, Ojanguren A, Dahdah J. Thoracoscopic anatomical resection of congenital lung malformations in adults. J Thorac Dis. 2015;7(3).
33. Sheikh SI, McCoy K, Ryan-Wenger NA, et al. Lobectomy in patients with cystic fibrosis. Can Respir J J Can Thorac Soc. 2014;21(4):e63-6.
34. Brinson GM, Noone PG, Mauro MA, et al. Bronchial artery embolization for the treatment of hemoptysis in patients with cystic fibrosis. Am J Respir Crit Care Med. 1998;157(6 Pt 1):1951-8.
35. Martin C, Reynaud-Gaubert M, Hamidfar R, et al. Sustained effectiveness of elexacaftor-tezacaftor-ivacaftor in lung transplant candidates with cystic fibrosis. J Cyst Fibros Off J Eur Cyst Fibros Soc. 2022;21(3):489-96.
36. Cole PJ. Inflammation: a two-edged sword--the model of bronchiectasis. Eur J Respir Dis Suppl. 1986;147:6-15.
37. Hiramatsu M, Shiraishi Y. Surgical management of non-cystic fibrosis bronchiectasis. J Thorac Dis. 2018;10(Suppl 28):S3436-45.
38. Sancho LM, Paschoalini MS, Fernandez A, et al. [Surgical treatment of lung abscesses]. Rev Hosp Clin. 1997;52(5):254-7.
39. Clark JM, Cooke DT, Browne LM. Management of Complications After Lung Resection. Thoracic Surg Clin. 2020;30(3):347-58.

Preoperative Evaluation

CHAPTER 178

Mahesh PA, Greeshma MV, Jayaraj BS

INTRODUCTION

Preoperative evaluation is a critical process that involves assessing the patient's overall health status before surgery. This evaluation is particularly important for patients with complex medical conditions as it helps to estimate the risks associated with surgery and anesthesia and formulate a plan to mitigate these risks.[1] One of the key aspects of the preoperative evaluation is assessment of pulmonary risk. This involves evaluating any potential issues that could lead to postoperative pulmonary complications (PPCs), which can lead to increased morbidity, prolonged hospital stays, and increased perioperative mortality.

A thorough preoperative evaluation is critical to identify and manage the risks effectively.[2] In addition to assessing pulmonary risk, the preoperative evaluation also involves estimating cardiac risk and the risk of perioperative venous thromboembolism[2,3] based on a combination of patient-related and procedure-related risk factors. The evaluation may also involve diagnostic testing to further refine the risk estimate. Another important aspect of the preoperative evaluation is the consideration of sleep-disordered breathing, particularly obstructive sleep apnea (OSA). Patients with OSA may be at increased risk of PPCs and special considerations may be needed for airway management in these patients.[4] Finally, the preoperative evaluation also involves shared decision-making and communication of treatment goals and expectations. This ensures that the patient is fully informed about the risks and benefits of surgery and that their preferences and values are taken into account in the decision-making process. The preoperative pulmonary evaluation plays a crucial role in ensuring the safety and success of surgical procedures. The preoperative evaluation is critical, particularly for patients with complex medical conditions. It involves a comprehensive assessment of the patient's overall health status before surgery, with a focus on estimating pulmonary risk, cardiac risk, and the risk of perioperative venous thromboembolism.[5]

This chapter aims to present a preoperative assessment grounded in evidence for patients scheduled for either thoracic or nonthoracic surgery. Following the initial evaluation applicable to all patients, the subsequent focus is on the pulmonary-specific assessment. The primary goal of the preoperative evaluation is to pinpoint individuals with an elevated likelihood of encountering perioperative complications and enduring long-term disability as a result of surgical removal of lung tissue, utilizing the least intrusive diagnostic tests available.

IMPORTANCE OF PREOPERATIVE ASSESSMENT

Preoperative assessment is important to identify patient-related and procedure-related risk factors, determine the need for diagnostic testing, and propose interventions to minimize risk and improve perioperative outcomes. PPCs are a significant concern in the surgical setting. They include conditions such as pneumonia, respiratory failure, atelectasis, chronic obstructive pulmonary disease (COPD) exacerbation, bronchospasm, respiratory arrest due to sleep-disordered breathing, and perioperative pulmonary mortality. These complications can have severe consequences, including the need for mechanical ventilation for >48 hours after surgery or unplanned reintubation.[6] Studies have shown that PPCs are common and can significantly impact patient outcomes. For example, one study found that 14% of patients with severe systemic disease had at least one PPC, leading to increased length of stay and a threefold increase in the need for intensive care unit stays. Therefore, a thorough preoperative evaluation is essential in identifying and managing these risks effectively, ultimately improving patient outcomes in the surgical setting.[7]

PERIOPERATIVE RISK ASSESSMENT

Patient-associated Risk Factors

The pulmonary assessment for surgical risk serves the dual purpose of evaluating risks and devising strategies to mitigate PPCs. The assessment involves analyzing patient related, surgery-related, and anesthesia-related risk factors.

Notably, the preoperative risk assessment places a significant emphasis on surgery-related factors, distinguishing it from preoperative cardiac evaluations where patient-related factors hold more relevance than the intrinsic factors associated with the surgery. A thorough examination of a patient's medical history and physical condition is crucial for assessing overall fitness and identifying comorbid conditions. Several risk factors contribute to the likelihood of PPCs, including age, smoking history, critical illness, and comorbidities such as COPD.[7,8]

Advancing age, especially beyond 50 years, independently increases the risk of surgery, with a fivefold rise in the odds of PPCs observed in individuals aged 80 years or older. Cigarette smoking increases the risk of PPCs, and recent studies have alleviated concerns about heightened complications associated with discontinuing smoking within 8 weeks before surgery. The risk of PPCs and mortality is higher in current smokers compared to ex-smokers and nonsmokers, particularly in those with a history of smoking 10 pack-years or greater. The benefits of preoperative smoking cessation in reducing PPC risk are more pronounced with cessation periods exceeding 8 weeks.[9]

Chronic obstructive pulmonary disease is associated with a doubled risk of PPCs. Physical examinations can reveal specific signs, such as worsening shortness of breath, changes in cough and sputum, oxygen saturation lower than baseline, systemic signs of infection, and active wheezing, and the presence of these signs is linked to a sixfold increase in the risk of PPCs. Well-controlled asthma, regardless of its severity, has a minimal impact on PPC risk. Patients with interstitial lung disease, particularly those with a low diffusing capacity of the lung for carbon monoxide (DLCO) and forced expiratory volume in 1 second (FEV1) or forced vital capacity (FVC) ≤ 60% predicted, are considered less suitable candidates for surgery due to heightened PPC risk. Pulmonary hypertension and preoperative anemia, even in mild forms, are additional factors contributing to an increased risk of PPCs. The presence of anemia, coupled with allogeneic blood transfusions, independently contributes to both PPCs and surgical site infections in surgical patients. The extent of the risk is notable, underscoring the importance of considering these factors in preoperative assessments and decision-making processes.[10,11]

Functional and general health statuses play a significant role in predicting PPCs. Pooled analyses indicate that partial and total physical dependence are associated with a higher risk of postoperative respiratory failure and pneumonia. The American Society of Anesthesiologists (ASA) classification, which considers chronic illness and comorbid conditions, reveals that an ASA class ≥ 2 is linked to a nearly fivefold increase in the odds of PPCs. Congestive heart failure stands out as a strong predictor of postoperative respiratory failure, while neuromuscular weakness and obesity may also increase PPC risk. Obesity, in particular, may be associated with OSA, further elevating perioperative complications. Conditions affecting pulmonary parenchyma function, respiratory muscle function, lung compliance, resistance, or gas exchange elevate the risk of PPCs.[3]

Procedure-related Risk Factors

While certain procedure- and surgery-related factors pose inherent risks for PPCs, it is crucial to acknowledge that the site of surgery, especially its proximity to the respiratory system, significantly influences the likelihood of PPC development. Studies on postoperative pneumonia and respiratory failure highlight that aortic and thoracic surgeries carry the highest risk, followed by upper abdominal and neurosurgical procedures. The urgency level of surgery is another critical determinant, with urgent or emergent procedures increasing the risk of complications. Assessing the urgency level is recommended in preoperative guidelines as it correlates with a higher risk of PPCs. Additionally, the duration of surgery independently contributes to PPC risk, with procedures lasting ≥4 hours, doubling the likelihood of complications. In summary, factors such as increased surgical urgency, proximity to the diaphragm, and prolonged procedure duration are predisposing elements for a higher incidence of PPCs.

Intraoperative volume administration is linked to the development of pulmonary edema. Although certain interventions are necessary during emergent surgeries, caution should be exercised to avoid administering fluids that lack therapeutic benefits and may only increase salt and chloride levels. While blood and crystalloid infusions are often unavoidable in emergent situations, patients receiving more than 4 units of blood appear to face an elevated risk of pneumonia. This emphasizes the importance of judicious fluid management to mitigate the potential for pulmonary complications.[12,13]

Anesthesia-related Risk Factors

Thoughtful planning of anesthesia management during surgery is crucial due to the observed causal relationship between the type of anesthesia and the development of PPCs. General anesthesia, when compared to neuraxial anesthesia, is associated with higher rates of respiratory failure and postoperative pneumonia. The use of inhaled anesthesia can impact surfactant function and alter the oxygen to nitric oxide ratio, potentially increasing gas reabsorption and the development of atelectasis. The utilization of general anesthesia elevates the risk of PPCs, emphasizing the preference for alternatives such as neuraxial or regional anesthesia whenever feasible. This preference is underscored by research, indicating that patients with COPD undergoing surgery with general anesthesia face a higher risk of PPCs, ventilator dependence, and unplanned postoperative intubations compared to those receiving regional anesthesia.

Neuromuscular blockers, commonly used during anesthesia, have lasting effects on respiratory muscle strength that can extend for several days. The use of intermediate and long-acting neuromuscular blockers is associated with postoperative complications, such as atelectasis, reintubation, pneumonia, and pulmonary edema. Studies suggest that postoperative pneumonia and respiratory failure are more common in patients receiving intermediate and long-acting neuromuscular blockers in a dose-dependent manner. Unfortunately, continuous neuromuscular monitoring during surgery and the use of reversal agents do not appear to provide protection against PPCs based on current evidence.[3]

Respiratory complications manifest immediately upon the initiation of general anesthesia. As consciousness levels decrease and controlled mechanical ventilation begins after sedation-induced apnea, the respiratory system's response to hypercapnia and hypoxia undergoes alterations. Simultaneously, the respiratory muscles' function undergoes immediate changes, including a shift in the diaphragm arch's physical shape toward dependent areas and reduced contact with the chest wall. This alteration results in a modification of muscle tone at the end of exhalation, leading to a 15–20% decrease in functional residual capacity (FRC) compared to the awake and upright state. The diminished FRC, combined with uneven regional ventilation distribution during positive pressure ventilation and a reduction in cardiac output from positive pressure mechanical ventilation, contributes to a ventilation/perfusion (V/Q) ratio mismatch. This mismatch leads to an increase in alveolar dead space, hindering oxygen delivery and carbon dioxide removal. Furthermore, over 75% of patients undergoing general anesthesia with neuromuscular blockers experience atelectasis, particularly in dependent lung areas observable on chest imaging. Factors, such as postoperative pain, diaphragm position changes, and decreased FRC elevate the risk of atelectasis, which, if prolonged, predispose individuals to pneumonia.[14]

RISK FACTORS (FIGS. 1 AND 2)

Preoperative risk prediction models aim to offer objective assessments of risk to guide clinical decision-making during the perioperative period. Various prediction models exist to help stratify patient risk for pulmonary complications before surgery. However, the adoption of risk stratification tools in clinical practice varies due to several barriers, including limited awareness among clinicians, uncertainty about the precision of these tools for specific populations and pulmonary complications, and a lack of data on the impact of using these tools on clinical behavior, patient outcomes, and resource utilization. Key observations highlight the specificity of each model as they were derived in distinct populations, influencing their performance.

The ARISCAT (Assess Respiratory Risk in Surgical Patients in Catalonia) score is a risk prediction tool used to estimate the risk of PPCs in patients undergoing noncardiac surgery. The ARISCAT score takes into account various factors, including patient characteristics, type of surgery, and preoperative health status. It assigns points based on these factors and the total score is used to estimate the risk of PPCs.[14,15] PPCs can include complications such as pneumonia, respiratory failure, and other respiratory issues after surgery. The score is particularly designed to assess the risk of pulmonary complications within the first 7 postoperative days. The specific variables considered in the ARISCAT score include age, preoperative oxygen saturation, respiratory infection in the last month, preoperative anemia, and type of surgery. Patients are classified into low-, intermediate-, or high-risk categories based on their total ARISCAT score. The higher the score, the higher the estimated risk of PPCs. It is important to note that while risk prediction tools such as the ARISCAT score can provide valuable information for clinicians, they are not the sole factors in decision-making. Clinical judgment and individual patient characteristics are also crucial considerations.

However, external validation in a larger, European data registry revealed variations in the tool's performance across different geographic populations. To address some of these limitations, the American College of Surgeons introduced the NSQIP (National Surgical Quality Improvement Program), originally devised in the 1990s for risk-adjusted outcomes reporting within Veterans Affairs hospitals. It has since expanded to encompass private-sector hospitals. The NSQIP risk tool predicts the risk of pneumonia and respiratory failure within 30 days of surgery.

Another challenge lies in the differing definitions of PPCs used by each model. While not necessarily negative, this diversity may prompt clinicians to choose different tools to assess specific risks related to patient populations or procedures. Moreover, interobserver variability among physicians in estimating risk and outcome measures using these tools can be attributed to the reliability of nonobjective patient data and the clinical accuracy of administrative data employed for case-mix adjustments in these models. These models typically score patients on a scale to provide a risk category relative to the original study population but do not offer individualized risk predictions of PPCs. Consequently, a comprehensive approach that combines clinical assessment, patient preferences, risk stratification tools, and anesthesiologist/surgeon assessments of intraoperative risk provides a more holistic strategy.[16]

ROLE OF PREOPERATIVE TESTS

Studies are not universally indispensable in preoperative pulmonary risk assessment; certain situations exist where their inclusion plays a crucial role. In many cases, a comprehensive evaluation of the patient's history and physical condition, incorporating pulse oximetry provides sufficient information for an accurate risk assessment. However, there are specific scenarios outlined further where additional studies become essential to enhance the precision of the assessment and guide clinical decision-making.

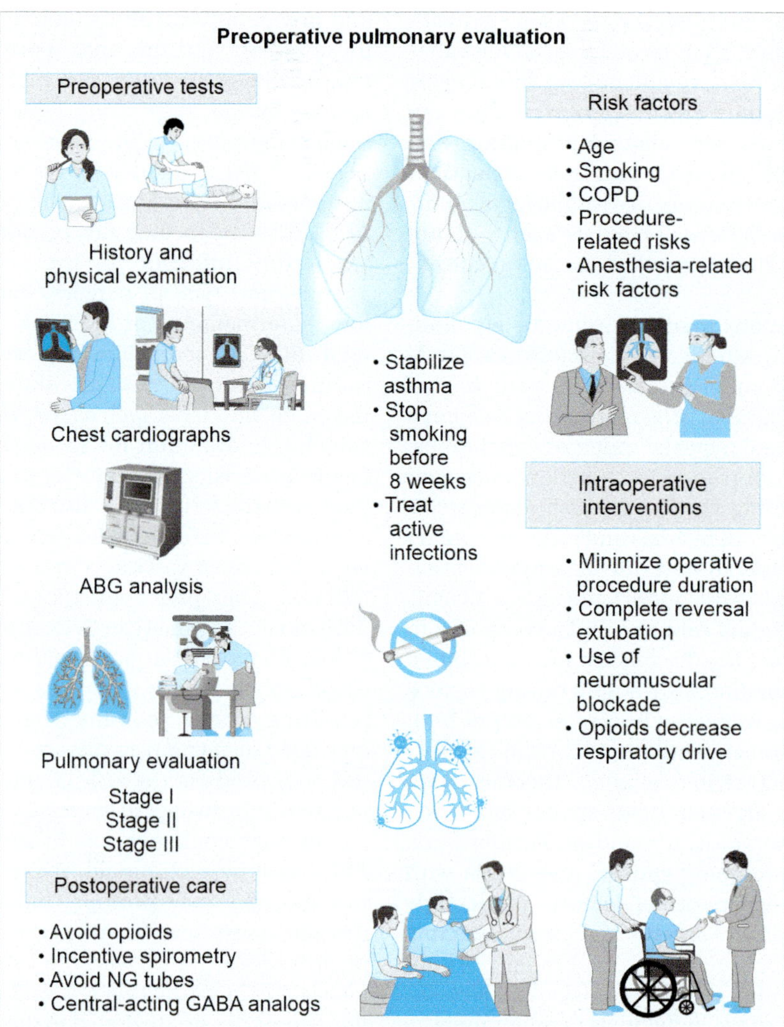

FIG. 1: Risk factors that can impact postoperative pulmonary complications, preoperative evaluation for risk assessment, intraoperative interventions, and postoperative care to reduce postoperative pulmonary complications.

(ABG: arterial blood gas; COPD: chronic obstructive pulmonary disease; GABA: gamma-aminobutyric acid; NG: nasogastric)

History and Physical Examination (Fig. 1)

The cornerstone of preoperative pulmonary risk assessment lies in a meticulous approach to history-taking and physical examination. An exhaustive history should encompass inquiries into respiratory symptoms, such as chronic cough, dyspnea, and chest pain, along with an exploration of potential symptoms related to sleep apnea. The patient's functional capacity and the extent of activity limitation also form crucial components of the history. A detailed examination of the smoking history is essential, and patients should be actively encouraged to embark on smoking cessation. Additionally, it is prudent to delve into any recent history of respiratory tract infections; in cases where such infections are present, it is advisable to consider delaying surgery until the infection is resolved. This comprehensive approach to history and examination serves as a vital foundation for preoperative pulmonary risk assessment. During the physical examination, identifying signs indicative of unrecognized pulmonary disease is crucial. Observations such as decreased breath sounds, dullness to percussion, wheezes, rhonchi, and a prolonged expiratory phase can serve as important indicators of an elevated risk of pulmonary complications. Additionally, the presence of cardiac failure and pulmonary hypertension should be carefully evaluated. This comprehensive physical examination aids in uncovering potential pulmonary issues and contributes to a thorough preoperative risk assessment.[17]

Chest Radiographs

The current evidence suggests that preoperative chest radiographs rarely provide unexpected information that

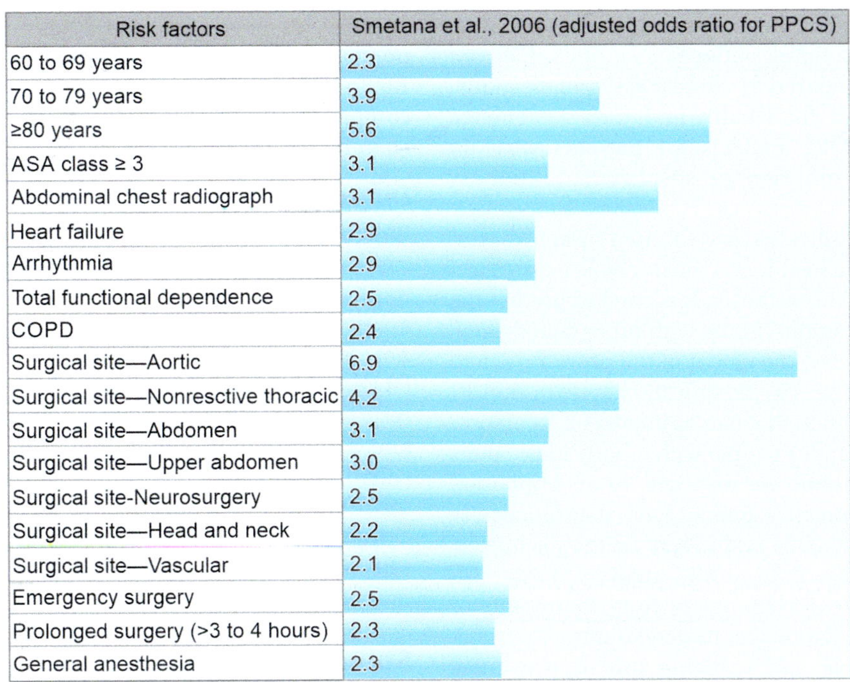

Risk factors	Smetana et al., 2006 (adjusted odds ratio for PPCS)
60 to 69 years	2.3
70 to 79 years	3.9
≥80 years	5.6
ASA class ≥ 3	3.1
Abdominal chest radiograph	3.1
Heart failure	2.9
Arrhythmia	2.9
Total functional dependence	2.5
COPD	2.4
Surgical site—Aortic	6.9
Surgical site—Nonresctive thoracic	4.2
Surgical site—Abdomen	3.1
Surgical site—Upper abdomen	3.0
Surgical site-Neurosurgery	2.5
Surgical site—Head and neck	2.2
Surgical site—Vascular	2.1
Emergency surgery	2.5
Prolonged surgery (>3 to 4 hours)	2.3
General anesthesia	2.3

FIG. 2: Various risk factors and associated odds ratio for postoperative pulmonary complications.
(ASA: American Society of Anesthesiologists; COPD: chronic obstructive pulmonary disease; PPCs: postoperative pulmonary complications)

alters preoperative management. Most abnormal findings on preoperative chest radiographs can be anticipated by thorough history-taking and physical examination. As a result, a preoperative chest radiograph is warranted when there are new or unexplained symptoms, a history of underlying lung disease without recent imaging, or when thoracic surgery is planned. While preoperative chest radiographs do not significantly enhance the predictive value of patient history and physical examination for PPCs, an abnormal chest radiograph, once identified, is associated with an increased risk of PPCs. The Choosing Wisely initiative advises against routine chest radiographs in ambulatory patients without specific indications from history and physical examination. However, obtaining a chest radiograph is deemed reasonable in cases where acute or stable cardiopulmonary disease is suspected, particularly in patients with known cardiovascular or respiratory issues.[8,18]

Spirometry

Spirometry is a widely accessible, cost-effective, standardized diagnostic test for obstructive and restrictive lung diseases. While recommended for candidates undergoing lung resection or coronary artery bypass, its utility before extrathoracic surgery lacks robust evidence, and there is no established prohibitive spirometric threshold for surgery risks. Preoperative spirometry is typically reserved for patients with thoracic surgery plans or those with unexplained chest symptoms, particularly suggestive of COPD or a history of smoking. Initially considered valuable for predicting PPCs, recent studies have shown that physical examination and the ASA class are superior predictors of PPCs compared to spirometry values. While spirometry can aid in identifying unknown obstructive diseases when clinical evaluation is uncertain, specific spirometry values for surgery denial are not established. For lung resection surgery, routine baseline spirometry and estimation of DLCO are recommended. Pneumonectomy, lobectomy, and segmentectomy are associated with varying degrees of decline in FEV1 and DLCO.

To assess predictive postoperative lung function, one can utilize either quantitative V/Q scans or the segment method based on computed tomography scans. This is particularly applicable when the predicted postoperative (PPO) FEV1 or DLCO falls within the range of 30–60%. If the PPO FEV1 or DLCO is <30%, further evaluation with a cardiopulmonary exercise test (CPET) is recommended. Overall, the value of routine spirometry for high-risk procedures beyond lung resection (upper abdominal surgery) or coronary artery bypass remains uncertain.[19]

Arterial Blood Gas Analysis

Partial pressure of arterial carbon dioxide ($PaCO_2$) exceeding 45 mm Hg is recognized as a significant risk factor for pulmonary complications, often indicating chronic respiratory failure. Hypercapnia, reflected by elevated $PaCO_2$, has historically been considered a relative contraindication to lung resection. Therefore, it is recommended to conduct arterial blood gas (ABG) analysis in patients with chronic lung disease, those with a substantial pulmonary condition, and individuals undergoing lung resection. However, routine ABG use is not advised for all patients, as it often does not alter management compared to clinical assessment alone. The National Institute for Health and Care Excellence supports obtaining ABG analysis for patients with an ASA class III with confirmed or suspected pulmonary disease.[20]

The ASA III is a classification system used by anesthesiologists to determine the health of a person before a surgical procedure that requires anesthesia. It is used to predict the risk of surgical complications, along with other factors such as the type of surgery, age, the extent of the procedure, and surgery timeframe. In the ASA classification system, ASA III refers to a serious condition that has an impact on a person's overall health. This includes people with a body mass index (BMI) > 40 kg/m^2, alcohol use disorder, or an implanted pacemaker. In clinical practice, patients with neuromuscular disease, chronic hypercapnia respiratory failure, or obesity hypoventilation may benefit from ABG analysis to establish baseline preoperative gas exchange or to further justify or titrate noninvasive ventilation recommendations.

A widely accessible and valuable tool is the pulse oximeter. In a patient lying supine and breathing room air, low oxygen saturation emerges as an independent risk factor for PPCs. Saturation levels ≤95% double the risk of PPCs, while levels ≤90% increase the risk tenfold. This underscores the utility of pulse oximetry in assessing and identifying patients at risk for pulmonary complications during the preoperative period.[21,22]

Pulmonary-specific Evaluation for Lung Resection Surgeries

Evaluation of pulmonary function is crucial for patients undergoing lung resection surgeries. The goals of pulmonary-specific assessment are twofold: First, to gauge the patient's ability to withstand the surgical procedure, minimizing perioperative mortality and morbidity; and second, to evaluate PPCs, ensuring a reasonable quality of life. Various physiological tests are available for this purpose, although there is not a singular "gold standard" test that perfectly predicts complications. This preoperative evaluation segment is structured into three sequential stages of tests, collectively contributing to the risk stratification of patients before the scheduled surgery.

Stage 1

In the initial stage of pulmonary-specific evaluation, tests focus on assessing the overall functions of both lungs.

Spirometry

Forced expiratory volume in 1 second assessment: Among the indices measured by spirometry, FEV1 is considered the most effective in predicting complications of lung resection and is commonly used in decision-making. There is not a universally agreed-upon cutoff for FEV1; however, suggested preoperative values include 2 liters for pneumonectomy and 1.5 liters for lobectomy. The risk of postoperative respiratory complications significantly rises when the FVC or maximal voluntary ventilation (MVV) is below 50% predicted.

Diffusion Capacity

Reflecting alveolar membrane integrity and pulmonary capillary blood flow, DLCO is a crucial parameter. Studies have identified DLCO as a key predictor of mortality and a key predictor of PPCs. Although absolute cutoffs are not firmly established, individuals with preoperative DLCO < 60% predicted tend to experience more frequent respiratory complications and hospitalizations. PPO DLCO and a combined value known as the PPO product (PPP), calculated by multiplying PPO FEV1 and PPO DLCO, are found to be independent predictors of pulmonary complications, morbidity, and mortality. In one study, a PPP >1,650 was associated with a higher risk of surgical mortality.[23,24]

Stage II

The next stage of pulmonary-specific evaluation tests shift focus to measuring differential lung function and estimating PPO lung function. Three techniques are employed to predict postoperative values: Segment method, radionuclide scanning technique, and quantitative computed tomography.

Segment Method

Predicting postoperative pulmonary function can be achieved through straightforward methods that involve calculating the remaining portion of bronchopulmonary segments after resection. The estimation of postoperative lung function is determined by multiplying the preoperative value by this calculated portion. The conventional approach starts with a baseline of 19 total segments (10 on the right and 9 on the left).[25] The formula for PPO FEV1 is given by:

$$PPO\ FEV1 = Preoperative\ FEV1 \times (19\ segments - x)/19$$

Here, x represents the number of lung segments to be removed. Another method involves using the number of subsegments, adjusted for preoperatively obstructed segments.

For example, let us consider where a patient is scheduled for removal of few segments. The surgeon plans to remove two segments and the patient's preoperative FEV1 is 2.6 liters (2,600 mL).

The formula for PPO FEV1 is given by:

$$\text{PPO FEV1} = \text{Preoperative FEV1} \times (19 \text{ segments} - x)/19$$

Given an example where x = 2 and preoperative FEV1 = 2,600 mL

PPO FEV1 = 2,600 × (19 – 2)/19

PPO FEV1 = 2,600 × 17/19

PPO FEV1 = 2,600 × 0.89
PPO FEV1 = 2,326.32

So, in the given example, $x = 2$ and the preoperative FEV1 is 2,600, the estimated PPO FEV1 is approximately 2,326.32. This is the expected lung function after surgery, taking into account the removal of two lung segments.

Radionuclide Scanning Technique

Quantitative V/Q scans, utilizing inhaled ^{133}Xe for ventilation lung scans and ^{99}Tc macro-aggregates for perfusion lung scans, offer an accurate means of calculating PPO FEV1. While both V/Q scans are effective, perfusion scanning is more commonly employed due to its technical simplicity. The underlying principle of this technique aligns with that of segment methods.[26]

Using the quantitative V/Q scan method, we can calculate the PPO FEV1 postlobectomy using the given formula:

PPO FEV1 postlobectomy = Preoperative FEV1 × [1 – (y/z)]

Assuming the patient's preoperative FEV1 is 2.8 liters (2,800 mL), the surgeon plans to remove two functional lung segments ($y = 2$), and one of the segments is nonfunctional. That leaves a total of 16 functional lung segments ($z = 16$) out of 19 segments.

PPO FEV1 postlobectomy = 2,800 mL × (1 – 2/16)
PPO FEV1 postlobectomy = 2,800 mL × (1 – 0.125)
PPO FEV1 postlobectomy = 2,800 mL × (0.875)
PPO FEV1 postlobectomy = 2,450 mL

In this example, the calculated PPO FEV1 postlobectomy is 2,450 mL.

For PPO FEV1 after pneumonectomy

PPO FEV1 postpneumonectomy = Preoperative FEV1 ×
(1 – a fraction of the total perfusion for the resected lung)

Determination of function (%): The function of the affected lung is often determined based on a lung perfusion scan or other imaging studies. The percentage is derived by comparing the perfusion of the affected lung to the total perfusion of both lungs. Usually, the perfusion of the right lung is 55% and the left lung is 45%. The diseased lung may have lower perfusion.

For example, if the affected lung contributes to 40% of the total lung perfusion, then the function of that lung is considered 40%. The fraction of total perfusion for the resected lung (the function) is represented by a decimal. If the function is 40%, the decimal representation would be 0.40.

The formula for PPO FEV1 after pneumonectomy is:

PPO FEV1 postpneumonectomy = Preoperative FEV1 ×
(1 – a fraction of the total perfusion for the resected lung)

Now, let us consider an example of a pneumonectomy. Assuming the preoperative FEV1 is 3.0 liters (3,000 mL) and the perfusion contributions of the right lung are 60% and the left lung 40%.

Now, using the formula:

PPO FEV1 postpneumonectomy = Preoperative FEV1 ×
(1 – a fraction of the total perfusion for the resected lung)

PPO FEV1 postpneumonectomy = 3,000 × (1 – 0.40)
PPO FEV1 postpneumonectomy = 3,000 × 0.60
PPO FEV1 postpneumonectomy = 1,800 mL

So, in this example, considering the right lung contributes 60% and the left lung contributes 40% to the total perfusion, the PPO FEV1 after a left pneumonectomy would be 1,800 mL.

These examples illustrate the application of the quantitative V/Q scan method in predicting postoperative lung function after lobectomy and pneumonectomy.

Predicting DLCO after lung resection

Typically, the right lung contributes 55% of overall lung function, whereas the left lung contributes 45%. The formulas for PPO and the percentage of PPO DLCO following lung resection adhere to the same underlying principle. The correlation between predicted and actual postoperative FEV1 using this method has been observed with high R-values, reaching up to 0.88. The correlation for DLCO has been noted to be around 0.68.

This anatomical approach is applicable not only to lobectomies but also to segmentectomies, as the loss of function in lobectomy is not significantly greater than that in segmentectomy. This suggests the versatility of the method across different types of lung resections.

Quantitative Computed Tomography

Quantitative computed tomography represents a method where the volume of lung with attenuation between –500 and –910 Hounsfield units serves to estimate functional lung volume. By determining the lung volume in the region slated for resection as a fraction of the total lung volume and applying the aforementioned principles, this technique allows for an estimation of PPO pulmonary function. Despite evidence supporting its superiority over radionuclide quantitative perfusion imaging, this method has not been extensively adopted. Additionally, the PPO FEV1 can be computed without conducting a split lung function test. According to the Juhl and Frost formula:

PPO FEV1 = Preoperative FEV1 × [1 – (s × 5.26/100)]

Where s represents the number of bronchopulmonary segments involved and planned to be resected. Alternative tests assessing differential lung function, such as bronchospirometry (measuring oxygen uptake in each lung individually), lateral position testing, and total unilateral pulmonary artery occlusion, are no longer included in preoperative evaluations due to their invasive nature, reliance on specialized equipment, a high level of technical expertise, and concerns over result reproducibility.

Let us consider an example using the Juhl and Frost formula to calculate the PPO FEV1 for a patient undergoing lung resection. Assume the patient's preoperative FEV1 is 2.6 liters (2,600 mL) and the surgeon plans to remove three bronchopulmonary segments, $s = 3$.

The formula is given by:

$$PPO\ FEV1 = Preoperative\ FEV1 \times [1 - (s \times 5.26/100)]$$

PPO FEV1 = 2,600 mL × [1 - (3 × 5.26)/100)]
PPO FEV1 = 2,600 mL × (1 - 0.1578)
PPO FEV1 = 2,600 mL × 0.8422
PPO FEV1 = 2,189.72 mL

In this example, the calculated PPO FEV1 using the Juhl and Frost formula for a patient with a preoperative FEV1 of 2.6 liters and the removal of three bronchopulmonary segments is approximately 2,189.72 mL. This demonstrates how quantitative computed tomography and the Juhl and Frost formula can be applied to estimate postoperative pulmonary function without the need for a split lung function test providing valuable information for preoperative planning.

Stage III

Stage III involves exercise testing, providing confirmatory evidence of operability. Exercise testing serves as a valuable tool to assess whether individuals with compromised lung function can tolerate surgical resection. Various forms of exercise testing, ranging from formal procedures such as symptom-limited cycle ergometry to simpler assessments such as exercise oximetry, stair climbing, and shuttle walking have been explored. Among these, cycle ergometry with incremental workloads, measuring parameters such as oxygen consumption (VO_2), VO_2 max, minute ventilation, and carbon dioxide output, while monitoring electrocardiogram (ECG), blood pressure (BP), and oximetry stands out as a comprehensive method. Exercise testing can be either a fixed exercise challenge, involving sustained work levels, or incremental exercise testing, where the workload is progressively increased to a desired endpoint.

The measurement of exercise capacity, particularly the VO_2 max during CPET, has demonstrated predictive value for postoperative complications, including both short-term and long-term mortality. A VO_2 max below 15–20 mL/kg/min is associated with an elevated risk of postoperative complications. In situations where a complete CPET is impractical, simpler tests prove useful. In a study, a 4% or greater desaturation during exercise oximetry outperformed FEV1 and DLCO in predicting PPCs, including death and respiratory failure. Simpler tests such as the stair-climbing test and the 6-minute walk test have been employed to estimate the risk of lung resection. In particular, patients incapable of climbing two flights of stairs or completing a 6-minute walk of >500 feet are considered unsuitable candidates for lung resection. The shuttle walk test, an incremental exercise test, where individuals walk back and forth over a defined distance at an increasing rate, has shown correlation with VO_2 max obtained on a treadmill, with walking 25 shuttles (10 meters each) approximating a VO_2 max of 10 mL/kg/min. Estimating the specific number of shuttles one should walk to achieve a VO_2 max of >20 mL/kg/min is challenging without a thorough individual assessment. The shuttle walk test provides a rough estimation, but it is important to understand that the relationship between shuttle walks and VO_2 max can vary among individuals due to factors such as age, fitness level, and health status. Moreover, while a VO_2 max of >20 mL/kg/min is often considered a minimal criterion for safe surgery according to some guidelines, other factors, such as the type of surgery and an individual's overall health condition, are crucial considerations. Therefore, it is not appropriate to rely solely on a specific shuttle walk target without a comprehensive evaluation. Considering the surgery, it may be necessary for a more detailed assessment, such as a CPET, which provides a more accurate measurement of aerobic capacity and overall fitness. This test involves monitoring respiratory gases during exercise and can offer valuable information for surgical risk assessment.[27,28]

STRATEGIES TO MINIMIZE PERIOPERATIVE PULMONARY RISK[26]

Preexisting Pulmonary Conditions

- Optimal control of obstructive lung disorders (COPD and asthma) through guideline-based therapy.
- Maintain inhaled medications until the day of surgery for COPD patients and in the postoperative period.
- Consider short-term systemic corticosteroids for active wheezing in COPD; theophylline should be continued.
- Perioperative use of anxiolytic medications to prevent bronchospasm during induction.
- Treat respiratory infections appropriately and consider postponing elective surgery for 4–6 weeks of postinfection.
- Optimize congestive heart failure through guideline-directed medical therapy.
- CPAP initiation for patients with OSA undergoing elective surgery; encourage preoperative adherence.

Smoking Cessation

- Use the preoperative period as a teachable moment for smoking cessation.
- Encourage smoking cessation, supplementing with behavioral therapy, and nicotine substitution.
- Benefits of smoking cessation increase with the duration of the smoke-free period.

Preoperative Interventions

- Implement preoperative aerobic exercise and inspiratory muscle training for thoracic, cardiac, and upper abdominal surgery patients.

- Optimize anemia preoperatively to maintain hemoglobin levels above transfusion thresholds.

Operative Interventions

- Prefer alternative strategies (neuraxial/regional anesthesia) over general anesthesia, especially in high-risk cases.
- Epidural anesthesia with general anesthesia to reduce postoperative pain and preserve lung function, particularly in COPD patients.
- Cautious use of neuromuscular blockers; reversal does not decrease PPCs.
- Mechanical ventilation with low tidal volume (6–8 mL/kg) and moderate positive end-expiratory pressure (PEEP) reduces postoperative respiratory failure and length of hospital stay.
- Avoid high tidal volumes and excessive PEEP to prevent inflammatory cytokine release.
- Optimal PEEP settings are under research; PEEP ≤5 cmH_2O may predispose to atelectasis and high PEEP (>10 cmH_2O) has potential risks.
- Minimize fluid administration, especially in patients prone to lung injury, consider goal-directed fluid therapy using esophageal Doppler for individualized management.

SUMMARY

Preoperative evaluation is important for patients with complex medical conditions to effectively estimate the risks associated with surgery and anesthesia. The evaluation involves diagnostic testing, shared decision-making and communication of treatment goals and expectations of the patient who should be fully informed about the risks and benefits of surgery. It involves a comprehensive assessment of the patient's overall health status before surgery with a focus on estimating pulmonary risk, cardiac risk, and the risk of perioperative venous thromboembolism. For lung resectional surgery, the primary goal of the preoperative evaluation is to pinpoint individuals with an elevated likelihood of encountering perioperative complications and enduring long-term disability as a result of surgical removal of lung tissue, utilizing the least intrusive diagnostic tests available.

REFERENCES

1. O'Donnell FT. Preoperative Evaluation of the Surgical Patient. Mo Med. 2016;113(3):196-201.
2. Smetana GW. Preoperative Pulmonary Evaluation. N Engl J Med. 1999;340(12):937-44.
3. Eren Tuna M, Akgün M. Preoperative pulmonary evaluation to prevent postoperative pulmonary complications. Anesth Perioperative Sci. 2023;1:34.
4. Bae E. Preoperative risk evaluation and perioperative management of patients with obstructive sleep apnea: a narrative review. J Dent Anesth Pain Med. 2023;23(4):179-92.
5. Zambouri A. Preoperative evaluation and preparation for anesthesia and surgery. Hippokratia. 2007;11(1):13-21.
6. UpToDate. (2024). Evaluation of perioperative pulmonary risk. [online] Available from https://www.uptodate.com/contents/evaluation-of-perioperative-pulmonary-risk [Last accessed September, 2024].
7. Bapoje SR, Whitaker JF, Schulz T, et al. Preoperative evaluation of the patient with pulmonary disease. Chest. 2007;132(5):1637-45.
8. Sameed M, Choi H, Auron M, et al. Preoperative Pulmonary Risk Assessment. Respir Care. 2021;66(7):1150-66.
9. Rodgers JL, Jones J, Bolleddu SI, et al. Cardiovascular Risks Associated with Gender and Aging. J Cardiovasc Dev Dis. 2019;6(2):19.
10. AL Wachami N, Guennouni M, Iderdar Y, et al. Estimating the global prevalence of chronic obstructive pulmonary disease (COPD): a systematic review and meta-analysis. BMC Public Health. 2024;24(1):1-16.
11. Iheanacho I, Zhang S, King D, et al. Economic burden of Chronic Obstructive Pulmonary Disease (COPD): a systematic literature review. Int J Chron Obs Pulmon Dis. 2020;15:439-60.
12. Ladha K, Melo MFV, McLean DJ, et al. Intraoperative protective mechanical ventilation and risk of postoperative respiratory complications: Hospital based registry study. BMJ. 2015;351:h3646.
13. Miskovic A, Lumb AB. Postoperative pulmonary complications. BJA Br J Anaesth. 2017;118(3):317-34.
14. Rezaian S, Asadi Gharabaghi M, Rahimi B, et al. Concordance between ARISCAT risk score and cardiopulmonary exercise test values in risk prediction of postoperative pulmonary complications of major abdominal surgeries in a tertiary cancer hospital: A cross-sectional study. Heal Sci Rep. 2023;6(12):e1740.
15. Ulger G, Sazak H, Baldemir R, et al. The effectiveness of ARISCAT Risk Index, other scoring systems, and parameters in predicting pulmonary complications after thoracic surgery. Medicine (Baltimore). 2022;101(30):E29723.
16. Sherrer M, Simmons JW, Dobyns JB. Preoperative Risk Stratification: Identifying Modifiable Risks for Optimization. Curr Anesthesiol Rep. 2022;12(1):10-25.
17. Mills E, Eyawo O, Lockhart I, et al. Smoking cessation reduces postoperative complications: a systematic review and meta-analysis. Am J Med. 2011;124(2):144-54.e8.
18. Smetana GW, Lawrence VA, Cornell JE. Preoperative pulmonary risk stratification for noncardiothoracic surgery: systematic review for the American College of Physicians. Ann Intern Med. 2006;144(8):581-95.
19. American Lung Association. (2023). Spirometry. [online] Available from https://www.lung.org/lung-health-diseases/lung-procedures-and-tests/spirometry [Last accessed September, 2024].
20. Doyle DJ, Hendrix JM, Garmon EH. American Society of Anesthesiologists Classification. In: StatPearls [Internet]. Treasure Island (FL): StatPearls Publishing; 2024.

21. Wedzicha JA, Miravitlles M, Hurst JR, et al. Management of COPD exacerbations: A European Respiratory Society/ American Thoracic Society guideline. Eur Respir J. 2017;49(3): 1600791.
22. Labarca G, Uribe JP, Pacheco C, et al. Bronchoscopic Lung Volume Reduction with Endobronchial Zephyr Valves for Severe Emphysema: A Systematic Review and Meta-analysis. Respiration. 2019;98(3):268-78.
23. Johnson DC. Interpretation of Diffusing Capacity. Chest. 2021; 159(6):2513-4.
24. Neder JA, Berton DC, O'Donnell DE. The lung function laboratory to assist clinical decision-making in pulmonology: evolving challenges to an old issue. Chest. 2020;158:1629-43.
25. Armstrong P, Congleton J, Fountain SW, et al. Guidelines on the selection of patients with lung cancer for surgery. Thorax. 2001;56(2):89-108.
26. Jiang G, Zhang L, Zhu Y, et al. Clinical consensus on preoperative pulmonary function assessment in patients undergoing pulmonary resection (1st edition). Curr Challenges Thorac Surg. 2019;1(0):7.
27. Wyser C, Stulz P, Solèr M, et al. Prospective evaluation of an algorithm for the functional assessment of lung resection candidates. Am J Respir Crit Care Med. 1999;159(5 Pt 1):1450-6.
28. Bechard D, Wetstein L. Assessment of Exercise Oxygen Consumption as Preoperative Criterion for Lung Resection. Ann Thorac Surg. 1987;44(4):344-9.

CHAPTER 179

Lung Transplantation

KT Prasad, Ritesh Agarwal

INTRODUCTION

Many chronic lung diseases including chronic obstructive pulmonary disease (COPD), interstitial lung disease (ILD), and bronchiectasis are relentlessly progressive and result in irreversible decline in lung function despite optimal treatment. Eventually, they result in end-stage lung disease, which profoundly restricts physical functionality and reduces survival. Lung transplantation is the only definitive treatment for patients with end-stage lung diseases who are symptomatic despite the maximum available therapy. In these patients, lung transplantation is generally the only treatment that offers improved survival and enhanced quality of life.

HISTORY

Success in lung transplantation was demonstrated only after several decades of experimental studies in animals and multiple attempts in humans.[1] The first lung transplantation in a human was performed in 1963 by Dr. James Hardy. It was a single lung transplantation (SLT) performed on a patient with lung cancer. Although the procedure was successful and there was no clinical evidence of rejection, the patient died on the 18th postoperative day due to malnutrition and renal failure. Over the next decade, although about 40 patients underwent lung transplantation worldwide, only 2 patients survived beyond 2 months. The principal reasons behind poor outcomes were organ rejection and infection. Anastomotic dehiscence was also common with the surgical techniques employed at that time and was compounded by the deleterious effect of steroids and azathioprine on the healing anastomosis. Thereafter, interest in lung transplantation remained low until improvement in the anastomotic techniques and the introduction of cyclosporine in the 1980s. The first heart–lung transplantation (HLT) was performed in 1981 by the Stanford group. Subsequently, in 1986, the Toronto group for the first time demonstrated improved long-term outcomes with SLT for ILD. The improved success was attributed to the careful selection of patients, the use of cyclosporine that did not interfere with anastomotic healing, and employing an omental pedicle to promote healing of bronchial anastomosis. However, SLT was not considered the best option for COPD as the hyperinflated native lung may interfere with the functioning of the transplanted lung. Thereafter, the Toronto group performed the first *en bloc* double-lung transplantation (DLT) (transplantation of both the lungs along with the trachea and both main bronchi) for COPD in 1986. However, the *en bloc* DLT technique was associated with certain disadvantages like the need for prolonged cardiopulmonary bypass, higher risk of tracheal anastomotic dehiscence, and cardiac denervation. As a result, by the 1990s, bilateral sequential lung transplantation (BLT) (transplantation of each lung with its bronchus without the trachea) had replaced the *en bloc* DLT technique. After these encouraging experiences, there was an exponential increase in the number of lung transplantations in the 1990s. At present, over 4,000 lung transplantations and about 50 HLTs are performed worldwide, annually.[2]

CANDIDATE SELECTION, EVALUATION, AND MANAGEMENT

Indications and Contraindications

In general, lung transplantation should be considered in patients who have a high (>50%) risk of death from the lung disease within the next 2 years.[3] Disease-specific indications for referral and listing for lung transplantation for some of the most common lung diseases are specified in **Table 1**. Over the past decade, idiopathic pulmonary fibrosis (IPF) was the most common indication for lung transplantation, followed by COPD, and cystic fibrosis (CF).[4] Together, these three indications accounted for over two-thirds of the transplantations performed worldwide.[2,4] Conditions associated with an unacceptably high risk of complications or poor post-transplant survival are considered as contraindications for lung transplantation **(Table 2)**. In particular, advanced dysfunction involving other organs is generally considered a contraindication unless multiorgan transplantation is being considered. Patients on life-support

TABLE 1: Disease-specific indications for referral and listing for lung transplantation for some of the most common chronic lung diseases.

Disease	Indications for referral	Indications for listing
COPD	• BODE score 5–6 with additional factors suggestive of increased risk of mortality: ○ Frequent acute exacerbations ○ Increase in BODE score >1 over past 24 months ○ Pulmonary artery to aorta diameter >1 on CT scan ○ FEV_1 20–25% predicted • Clinical deterioration despite appropriate maximal treatment including medication, pulmonary rehabilitation, oxygen therapy, and nocturnal NIV • Poor quality of life unacceptable to the patient	• BODE score 7–10 • Additional factors that may prompt listing include: ○ FEV_1 <20% predicted ○ Presence of moderate-to-severe PAH ○ History of severe exacerbations ○ Chronic hypercapnia
ILD	• Referral should be made at the time of diagnosis, even if a patient is being initiated on therapy, for histopathological UIP or radiographic evidence of a probable or definite UIP pattern • Any form of pulmonary fibrosis with FVC <80% predicted or DLCO <40% predicted • Any form of pulmonary fibrosis with one of the following in the past 2 years: ○ Relative decline in FVC ≥10% ○ Relative decline in DLCO ≥15% ○ Relative decline in FVC ≥5% in combination with worsening of respiratory symptoms or radiographic progression • Supplemental oxygen requirement either at rest or on exertion. • For inflammatory ILDs, progression of disease (either on imaging or pulmonary function) despite treatment	• Any form of pulmonary fibrosis with one of the following in the past 6 months despite appropriate treatment: ○ Absolute decline in FVC >10% ○ Absolute decline in DLCO >10% ○ Absolute decline in FVC >5% with radiographic progression • Desaturation to <88% on 6MWT or >50 m decline in 6MWT distance in the past 6 months • PAH on right-heart catheterization or 2-dimensional echocardiography (in the absence of diastolic dysfunction) • Hospitalization because of respiratory decline, pneumothorax, or acute exacerbation
CF and non-CF bronchiectasis*	Presence of any of the following criteria despite optimal medical management: • FEV_1 <30% predicted • FEV_1 <40% predicted and any of the following: ○ 6MWT distance <400 m ○ $PaCO_2$ >50 mmHg ○ Hypoxemia at rest or with exertion ○ PAH (PASP >50 mm Hg on echocardiogram or evidence of right ventricular dysfunction) ○ Worsening nutritional status despite supplementation ○ Two exacerbations per year requiring IV antibiotics ○ Massive hemoptysis (>240 mL) requiring bronchial artery embolization ○ Pneumothorax • FEV_1 <50% predicted and rapidly declining based on pulmonary function testing or progressive symptoms • Any exacerbation requiring positive pressure ventilation	At least one of the referral criteria in combination with any of the following: • FEV_1 <25% predicted • Rapid decline in lung function or progressive symptoms (>30% relative decline in FEV_1 over 12 months) • Frequent hospitalization, particularly if hospitalized for >28 days in the preceding year • Any exacerbation requiring mechanical ventilation • Chronic respiratory failure with hypoxemia or hypercapnia, particularly for those with increasing oxygen requirements or needing long-term NIV • PAH (PASP >50 mm Hg on echocardiogram or evidence of right ventricular dysfunction) • Worsening nutritional status particularly with BMI <18 kg/m^2 despite nutritional interventions • Recurrent massive hemoptysis despite bronchial artery embolization • WHO functional class IV

Continued

Continued

Disease	Indications for referral	Indications for listing
PAH	• ESC/ERS intermediate or high risk or REVEAL risk score ≥8 despite appropriate PAH therapy • Significant right ventricular dysfunction despite appropriate PAH therapy • Need for IV or SC prostacyclin therapy • Progressive disease despite appropriate therapy or recent hospitalization for worsening PAH • Known or suspected high-risk variants such as PVOD, PCH, scleroderma, and large and progressive pulmonary artery aneurysms • Signs of secondary liver or kidney dysfunction due to PAH • Potentially life-threatening complications such as recurrent hemoptysis	• ESC/ERS high risk or REVEAL risk score >10 on appropriate PAH therapy, including IV or SC prostacyclin analogs • Progressive hypoxemia, especially in patients with PVOD or PCH • Progressive, but not end-stage liver or kidney dysfunction due to PAH • Life-threatening hemoptysis

*For individuals with noncystic fibrosis bronchiectasis, similar criteria as with cystic fibrosis for referral and listing for lung transplantation is reasonable, though providers should recognize that prognosis is highly variable with many patients experiencing a more stable course.

(6MWT: 6-minute walk test; BMI: body mass index; BODE: body mass index, airflow obstruction, dyspnea, and exercise capacity; COPD: chronic obstructive pulmonary disease; CF: cystic fibrosis; CT: computed tomography; DLCO: diffusing capacity of the lung for carbon monoxide; ESC/ERS: European Society of Cardiology/European Respiratory Society; FEV_1: forced expiratory volume in the first second; FVC: forced vital capacity; IV: intravenous; ILD: interstitial lung disease; NIV: noninvasive ventilation; $PaCO_2$: partial pressure of carbon dioxide in arterial blood; PAH: pulmonary arterial hypertension; PASP: pulmonary artery systolic pressure; PCH: pulmonary capillary hemangiomatosis; PVOD: pulmonary veno-occlusive disease; REVEAL: Registry to Evaluate Early and Long-term Pulmonary Arterial Hypertension Disease Management; SC: subcutaneous; UIP: usual interstitial pneumonia; WHO: World Health Organization)

Source: Adapted from Leard et al. (2021).

TABLE 2: Contraindications for lung transplantation.

	Absolute contraindications	Risk factors with high or substantially increased risk for poor outcomes following lung transplantation	Other risk factors associated with poor outcomes following lung transplantation
Age		>70 years	65–70 years
BMI		>35 kg/m^2 or <16 kg/m^2	30–34.9 kg/m^2 or 16–17 kg/m^2
Cardiac disorders	Acute coronary syndrome or myocardial infarction within 30 days (excluding demand ischemia)	Severe CAD that requires CABG at transplant; reduced LVEF <40%	Mild-to-moderate CAD; severe CAD that can be revascularized via percutaneous coronary intervention prior to transplant; reduced LVEF 40–50%
Renal disorders	Acute renal failure with rising creatinine or on dialysis and low likelihood of recovery; chronic renal failure with GFR <40 mL/min/1.73 m^2 (unless being considered for multiorgan transplant)		Chronic kidney disease with GFR 40–60 mL/min/1.73 m^2
Hepatic disorders	Acute liver failure and liver cirrhosis with portal hypertension or synthetic dysfunction (unless being considered for multiorgan transplant)		
Neurologic disorders	Stroke within 30 days and progressive cognitive impairment	Significant cerebrovascular disease	
Gastrointestinal disorders		Severe esophageal dysmotility	Severe gastroesophageal reflux disease and esophageal dysmotility

Continued

Continued

	Absolute contraindications	Risk factors with high or substantially increased risk for poor outcomes following lung transplantation	Other risk factors associated with poor outcomes following lung transplantation
Hematological disorders		Untreatable hematologic disorders including bleeding diathesis, thrombophilia, or severe bone marrow dysfunction	Thrombocytopenia, leukopenia, or anemia with a high likelihood of persistence after transplant
Infections	Septic shock, active extrapulmonary or disseminated infection; active tuberculosis; HIV infection with detectable viral load	Infection with multidrug-resistant organisms like *Mycobacterium abscessus*, *Lomentospora prolificans*, *Burkholderia cenocepacia*, and *Burkholderia gladioli*; Hepatitis B or C infection with detectable viral load and liver fibrosis	*Scedosporium apiospermum* infection and HIV infection with undetectable viral load
Malignancy	Malignancy with a high risk of recurrence or death related to cancer		
Psychosocial factors	Lack of patient willingness or acceptance of transplant and repeated episodes of nonadherence without evidence of improvement	Psychiatric, psychological, or cognitive conditions with potential to interfere with medical adherence without sufficient support systems; unreliable support system or caregiving plan; and lack of understanding of disease or transplant despite teaching	
Substance abuse	Active substance use or dependence including current tobacco use, vaping, marijuana smoking, or intravenous drug use		Edible marijuana use
Life support requirements		Extracorporeal life support	Mechanical ventilation
Other medical conditions			Peripheral vascular disease; connective tissue diseases (scleroderma, lupus, and inflammatory myopathies); osteoporosis; hypoalbuminemia; and diabetes that is poorly controlled
Surgical considerations		Chest wall or spinal deformity expected to cause restriction after transplant	Previous thoracic surgery including CABG and prior pleurodesis
Retransplant considerations		Retransplant in <1 year following initial lung transplant, retransplant for restrictive CLAD, retransplant for AMR as etiology for CLAD	Retransplant >1 year for obstructive CLAD
Others	Other severe uncontrolled medical conditions expected to limit survival after transplantation and limited functional status (e.g., nonambulatory) with poor potential for post-transplant rehabilitation	Limited functional status with potential for post-transplant rehabilitation	Frailty

(AMR: antibody-mediated rejection, BMI: body mass index, CAD: coronary artery disease, CABG: coronary artery bypass grafting, CLAD: chronic lung allograft dysfunction, GFR: glomerular filtration rate, HIV: human immunodeficiency virus, LVEF: left ventricular ejection fraction)

Source: Adapted from Leard et al. (2021).

equipment like mechanical ventilation or extracorporeal support should be considered for surgery in well-experienced centers as they may have poorer outcomes.

Referral

Suitable candidates for lung transplantation should be referred to a center specialized in lung transplantation for further evaluation and possible listing. The timing for lung transplantation referral is crucial. Patients should be referred during the transplant window during which the disease is sufficiently advanced to seriously affect their survival; however, the disease should not be so advanced as to preclude the surgery. In general, it is better to refer patients earlier during the transplant window to allow sufficient time for further evaluation. It should be remembered that not all patients referred for lung transplantation undergo the procedure. Only a proportion of patients referred for lung transplantation are waitlisted for the surgery after an extensive evaluation. The remaining are periodically re-evaluated.

Evaluation and Preparation of Candidates

All prospective lung transplantation candidates undergo a detailed assessment followed by appropriate preparation **(Box 1)**. At the outset, a comprehensive discussion should

BOX 1 Evaluation and preparation of transplant candidates.

- *Cardiorespiratory assessment*
  - Arterial blood gas analysis
  - Spirometry
  - Chest radiograph
  - High-resolution computed tomography of the thorax
  - 6-minute walk test
  - Serum N-terminal pro-B-type natriuretic peptide
  - Electrocardiogram
  - Echocardiogram
  - Right heart catheterization
  - Coronary arteriography (in patients with clinical suspicion of coronary artery disease)
- *Assessment of established or suspected comorbid conditions*
  - Routine lab investigations including hemogram, coagulogram, liver and kidney function tests, and urinalysis
  - *Anemia:* Serum iron studies, serum B_{12}, and folate
  - *Diabetes:* Glycosylated hemoglobin (HbA1C), fasting and 2-hour postprandial blood sugar
  - *Dyslipidemia:* Fasting lipid profile
  - *Osteoporosis:* Vitamin D levels, and dual-energy X-ray absorptiometry scan
  - *Clinical suspicion of gastroesophageal reflux disease:* 24-hour esophageal pH monitoring, radionuclide gastric reflux scan, upper gastrointestinal endoscopy
  - *Clinical suspicion of esophageal dysmotility:* Barium swallow and esophageal manometry
  - Glucose-6-phosphate dehydrogenase (G6PD) deficiency screening in view of risk of hemolysis when trimethoprim–sulfamethoxazole is used for pneumocystis prophylaxis.
  - *Clinical suspicion of peripheral arterial disease:* Doppler evaluation of carotid artery and arteries of the lower limb
- *Assessment for infections*
  - Details of prior treatment for tuberculosis
  - Tuberculin skin test or interferon-gamma release assays
  - Human immunodeficiency virus serology
  - Venereal disease research laboratory test
  - Hepatitis B surface antigen, antihepatitis B surface and core antibodies, and antihepatitis C antibody
  - Cytomegalovirus immunoglobulin M (IgM) and immunoglobulin G (IgG)
  - Epstein–Barr virus IgM and IgG
  - Toxoplasma IgM and IgG
  - Stool for ova and cysts
  - *Sputum evaluation (in patients with expectoration):* Gram stain and culture, fungal smear and culture, smear for acid-fast bacilli, and mycobacterial culture

Continued

Continued

- *Surgical assessment*
  - Body mass index
  - Details of prior thoracic surgery or pleurodesis
  - Assessment for thoracic and spinal deformities
- *Assessment for matching including transplant immunology*
  - Height
  - History of blood transfusions, pregnancy, and prior transplantation
  - ABO and Rh blood typing
  - Pretransfusion screening for antibodies capable of causing hemolysis
  - Highly sensitive, solid-phase assays for human leukocyte antigen (HLA) I and II antibodies [also called donor-specific antibodies (DSA) testing]
  - Panel reactive antibodies (PRA)
- *Others*
  - Psychosocial assessment
  - *Suspicion of ongoing tobacco or drug abuse:* Serum or urine toxicology screen
- *Preparation of transplant candidates*
  - Optimization of medical therapy
  - *Vaccination:* Influenza and *pneumococcus*
  - Pulmonary rehabilitation
  - Treatment of latent tuberculosis

be held with the patient and their caregivers to assess their understanding of the disease, post-transplant outcomes, willingness for the procedure, and psychosocial support. Subsequently, a detailed evaluation of cardiorespiratory function, other organ function, comorbid conditions, and screening for chronic infections should be performed. All transplant candidates should be listed in a comprehensive pulmonary rehabilitation program. Wherever feasible, appropriate vaccinations (influenza and *pneumococcus*) should be administered prior to transplantation. Some centers may also prefer to treat latent tuberculosis.

WAITING LIST AND ORGAN ALLOCATION

There is a huge mismatch between the organ demand and donor pool for lungs. As a result, generally, there is a significant waiting time before lung transplantation. Traditionally, lung allocation was based on the time accrued on the waitlist. Since this system did not consider medical urgency, it resulted in a high mortality rate for patients with more severe diseases like IPF. In 2005, the *lung allocation score (LAS)* was introduced in the United States to place more emphasis on medical urgency rather than the waiting time.[5] The LAS prioritized patients on the waitlist by estimating the risk of death while on the waiting list (waiting list urgency) and the expected post-transplant survival. The LAS was scored from 0 to 100, with higher scores representing greater priority for lung transplantation (greater risk of death on waiting list and greater post-transplant survival benefit). After the introduction of the LAS, median waiting time was reduced from 2–3 years to <200 days, with a waiting time of <35 days for 25% of patients.[5] Further, after the introduction of the LAS, IPF became the most common indication for lung transplantation, displacing COPD,[6] as IPF had a greater risk of death on the waiting list than COPD. In March 2023, the LAS was replaced by lung *composite allocation score (CAS)*, which is also scored from 0 to 100. In addition to waiting list urgency and expected post-transplant survival, the CAS incorporates other factors such as biological compatibility based on calculated panel reactive antibodies and blood group, patient access (priority for pediatric patients and prior living organ donors), and placement efficacy (distance between donor hospital and transplant center and other logistics). The CAS is expected to further reduce the waitlist mortality.

DONOR SELECTION, EVALUATION, MATCHING, AND HARVESTING

Donor Selection

The characteristics of an "ideal" brain-dead lung donor are: Age <55 years, tobacco history <20 pack-years, no prior cardiopulmonary surgery, no chest trauma, ratio of partial pressure of oxygen in arterial blood to fraction of inspired oxygen (PaO_2:FiO_2) >300 on 100% oxygen and a positive end-expiratory pressure (PEEP) of 5 cmH_2O, clear chest radiograph, no evidence of aspiration or sepsis, absence of organisms on sputum Gram stain, and absence of purulent secretions at bronchoscopy.[7] However, strictly adhering to these "ideal" criteria markedly reduces the lungs available for donation. In a study from India, less than one-third of

TABLE 3: Ideal and extended criteria for deceased lung donors.

	Ideal criteria	Extended criteria
Age	<55 years	<70 years
Tobacco history in pack-years	<20	<40
Prior pulmonary disease	Absent	Absent (except asthma)
Chest trauma	Absent	Not relevant if lung function is good
Chest radiography	No lung opacities	Minor diffuse and moderate focal chest radiograph changes are acceptable if good, stable, or improving function
PaO_2/FiO_2 ratio	>300 on PEEP of 5 cmH_2O	>250 on PEEP of 5 cmH_2O
Aspiration	Absent	Not relevant if lung function is good
Sepsis	Absent	Minor sepsis is not relevant if lung function is good
Purulent secretions on bronchoscopy	Absent	Not relevant if lung function is good
Gram stain of sputum	Absent	Not relevant if lung function is good

(FiO_2: fraction of inspired oxygen, PaO_2: partial pressure of oxygen in arterial blood; PEEP: positive end-expiratory pressure)

the brain-dead donors were eligible for lung donation using the ideal criteria.[8] In actual practice, these "ideal" criteria are often relaxed to accept "marginal" or "extended" lung donors (**Table 3**). In a recent study of nearly 25,000 transplants performed over more than a decade, 80% had at least one extended criterion, and >40% of lung transplantations had two or more extended criteria.[9] In particular, the use of donor lungs with abnormal chest radiograph or purulent bronchoscopy had more than doubled over the decade from 30% to 70% and 12% to 25%, respectively. The use of donor lungs with two or more extended criteria also increased from 28% to 48% over this period. Fortunately, even when donors with two or more extended criteria were accepted for lung transplantation, the 1-year post-transplant survival was not affected.[9] However, bacterial colonization of donor airways was not evaluated in this study. Airway colonization with bacteria is common in lung donors and whether transplantation of colonized lung is associated with poor outcomes is not clear.

Donor Evaluation and Management

All brain-dead potential organ donors should be rapidly evaluated within the limited time available (**Box 2**). Evaluation of lung should include arterial blood gas (ABG) analysis, chest radiograph, and flexible bronchoscopy. Appropriate cultures should be obtained and screening for chronic infections should be made. All potential lung donors should be managed with a stringent fluid protocol and lung protective ventilatory strategy (**Box 2**).

BOX 2 Evaluation and management of brain-dead potential lung donors.

- Evaluation
  - *Assessment of lung*
    - History of smoking and prior tuberculosis
    - Chest radiograph
    - Arterial blood gas analysis
    - Endotracheal aspirate or bronchoalveolar lavage for Gram stain and bacterial culture
    - Bronchoscopic inspection of airways
- *Assessment for sepsis and nonpulmonary infections*
    - Blood culture
    - Human immunodeficiency virus serology
    - Hepatitis B surface antigen, antihepatitis B surface and core antibodies, and antihepatitis C antibody
    - Cytomegalovirus IgM and IgG
    - Epstein–Barr virus IgM and IgG
  - *Matching considerations*
    - Height and sex
    - ABO and Rh blood typing
    - Human leukocyte antigen (HLA) typing (optional)
- Management
  - *Antibiotics*
    - Initiate empiric antibiotics based on local bacterial flora and antibiogram
    - Tailor antibiotic regimen after airway culture results
  - *Lung protective ventilatory strategy*
    - Low tidal volume (6–8 mL/kg of predicted body weight)
    - Positive end-expiratory pressure 8–10 cmH_2O
    - Closed airway suctioning
    - Recruitment maneuvers when necessary
    - Performance of apnea test using continuous positive airway pressure (CPAP) rather than T-piece
  - *Prevention of aspiration*
    - Head end elevation by 30–45°
    - Maintenance of endotracheal cuff pressure at 20–25 mm Hg
  - *Stringent fluid protocol*
    - Aim for net neutral or negative balance
    - Restrict fluid intake
    - Use diuretics when necessary

Matching

The donor and the recipient should have compatible blood groups and have a reasonable size match so that the donor's lungs fit the recipient's thoracic cavity. Most centers perform size matching based on the height and chest radiograph. Some centers prefer to use donors with a specific predicted total lung capacity (TLC) (calculated using standard equations based on height and sex), which lies in between the actual and the predicted TLC of the recipient. Although human leukocyte antigens (HLA) mismatched lung transplantation has shown to be associated with higher mortality, routine pre-transplant HLA crossmatching is not recommended at present.[10]

Harvesting

Donor lungs are usually harvested through a median sternotomy. During harvesting, the lungs are flushed with a special organ preservative solution (e.g., Perfadex®). The harvested lungs are inflated and stapled at the trachea and then placed within an ice cooler (4–8 °C) in sterile bags containing the same organ preservative solution. The ischemic time (time elapsed between application of aortic cross-clamp in the donor till the reperfusion of the transplanted lung in the recipient) should preferably not exceed 8 hours.

SURGERY AND POSTOPERATIVE CARE

Lung transplantation can be performed as SLT, BLT, or HLT. During SLT, one of the diseased native lungs is replaced with a donor lung while the other native lung is left in situ. BLT is generally performed as a bilateral sequential lung transplantation in which both the native lungs are replaced with donor lungs, which are sequentially transplanted during the same surgery. Although an *en-bloc* DLT can be performed in which the donor trachea is anastomosed to the recipient trachea, it is not preferred in view of a higher risk of airway-related complications. SLT is performed via a posterolateral thoracotomy. During SLT, anastomoses are performed at the bronchus, pulmonary artery, and pulmonary vein. BLT is usually performed through a transverse thoracosternotomy (clamshell incision) and the lungs are transplanted in a similar manner, sequentially, necessitating two separate bronchial anastomoses. HLT requires a median sternotomy. During HLT, anastomoses are made at the trachea, aorta, superior vena cava, and inferior vena cava. Cardiopulmonary bypass is optional for SLT and BLT but is mandatory for HLT. The entire procedure takes about 4–8 hours for SLT, 6–12 hours for DLT, and longer for HLT. At present, BLT is the most common type of surgery performed accounting for over three-fourths of the lung transplantations performed worldwide.[4] Living donor BLT is typically performed by replacing the entire right and left lungs of a single recipient with the right and left lower lobes obtained from two healthy donors. However, living donor lung transplantation is infrequently performed in view of the high donor morbidity associated with the procedure.[11]

IMMUNOSUPPRESSION AND PROPHYLACTIC THERAPY

Immunosuppression for lung transplantation involves induction therapy and maintenance therapy **(Table 4)**. Induction therapy involves the administration of a potent immunosuppressive agent during the perioperative or immediate postoperative period to reduce the risk of acute

TABLE 4: Agents used for immunosuppression after lung transplantation.

Agent	Dose and administration	Comments
Induction of immunosuppression		
Basiliximab (anti-IL-2 receptor alpha)	20 mg IV over 2–30 minutes during lung implantation and on postoperative day 4	Most commonly used induction agent
Alemtuzumab (anti- CD52)	30 mg IV over 2 hours intraoperatively	Causes profound lymphopenia, which may last for months to years
Antithymocyte globulin (ATG) of rabbit origin or horse origin	*Rabbit ATG:* 1.5 mg/kg/day IV over 6 hours for 3–4 days post-transplant *Horse ATG:* 7.5–15 mg/kg/day for 3–5 days post-transplant	Requires premedication with glucocorticoids, antihistamines, and antipyretics prior to infusion
Maintenance of immunosuppression		
Calcineurin inhibitors		
Tacrolimus	0.03–0.05 mg/kg/day IV infusion for 24 hours after transplantation; thereafter, 0.05 mg/kg PO twice daily; titrate further doses based on drug levels	*Target trough level:* 8–15 ng/mL
Cyclosporine	2–3 mg/kg/day IV infusion for 24 hours after transplantation; thereafter, 3–5 mg/kg PO twice daily; titrate further doses based on drug levels	*Target trough level:* 250–350 ng/mL; target 2-hour post-dose (C2) level: 900–1200 ng/mL

Continued

Continued

Agent	Dose and administration	Comments
Nucleotide blockers		
Mycophenolate mofetil*	250 mg PO twice daily to be started within 72 hours of transplantation; gradually increase to 1000 mg PO twice daily (with tacrolimus) or 1500 mg PO twice daily (with cyclosporine)	Titrate dose based on leukocyte count
Mycophenolate sodium*	360–720 mg PO twice daily	Better gastrointestinal tolerability than mycophenolate mofetil; titrate dose based on leukocyte count
Azathioprine	1–2 mg/kg/day	Titrate dose based on leukocyte count
Mammalian target of rapamycin (mTOR) inhibitors		Since mTOR inhibitors can interfere with wound healing, they should not be used until the bronchial anastomosis has completely healed (approximately 90 days)
Sirolimus	*Starting dose:* 2 mg PO once daily; titrate further doses based on drug levels	*Target trough level:* 4–8 ng/mL (when used with a calcineurin inhibitor) or 8–12 ng/mL (when used without a calcineurin inhibitor)
Everolimus	*Starting dose:* 1.5 mg PO twice daily; titrate further doses based on drug levels	*Target trough level:* 3–12 ng/mL
Glucocorticoids		
Prednisolone	0.5–1 mg/kg/day initially, tapered to 5–10 mg per day over several months	

*Mycophenolate mofetil and mycophenolate sodium cannot be interchanged indiscriminately as they have different pharmacokinetics of absorption.

(IL: interleukin; IV: intravenous, PO: per oral)

rejection. Over 80% of the centers use induction therapy, with interleukin-2 (IL2) receptor antagonists being the most common agents.[2] Although high-dose methylprednisolone (500–1,000 mg) is given intravenously during lung implantation, its primary purpose is to reduce the reperfusion injury, and hence it is not considered a part of the induction therapy. Regardless of the use of induction therapy, all lung transplant recipients have to receive lifelong maintenance therapy to prevent rejection. Maintenance therapy involves the use of a glucocorticoid, along with one more of the following: Calcineurin inhibitors (cyclosporine or tacrolimus), nucleotide blockers (azathioprine or mycophenolate), or mammalian target of rapamycin (mTOR) inhibitors (sirolimus or everolimus). Worldwide, the combination of prednisolone, tacrolimus, and mycophenolate is the most commonly used regimen for maintenance of immunosuppression.[2] The intensity of immunosuppression is generally reduced after the 1st year of transplantation. As lung transplant recipients are at an increased risk of infectious complications due to the immunosuppression, all patients must receive long-term prophylaxis for fungal infections, pneumocystis, and cytomegalovirus (CMV) **(Table 5)**.

FOLLOW-UP

Patients undergo periodic spirometry and lung imaging. Some centers do periodic transbronchial lung biopsies every 3 months in the initial year after lung transplantation and thereafter, annually for detection of indolent rejection. The immunosuppressive agents used in transplant recipients are associated with several adverse effects. Hence, cell counts, blood glucose, lipid profile, and hepatic and renal function need to be monitored periodically. Drug levels need to be monitored for calcineurin inhibitors and mTOR inhibitors.

COMPLICATIONS

Lung transplantation is associated with several surgical and medical complications **(Table 6)**. In addition, the immunosuppressants used are associated with infection and various drug-related complications. Due to the extensive list of complications, lung transplantation is often referred to as the trading of one illness for another.

Allograft-related Complications

Primary Graft Dysfunction

Primary graft dysfunction (PGD) is a form of reperfusion injury associated with diffuse alveolar damage. PGD presents with diffuse alveolar opacities and hypoxemia within 72 hours of lung transplantation. PGD affects about one-third of all lung transplantation and is the leading cause of early (<30 days) postoperative mortality after lung transplanta-

TABLE 5: Antimicrobial prophylaxis after lung transplantation.

Organism	Indication	Regimen	Duration
Bacterial infections	All patients	As per the local microbial spectrum and antibiogram; typically includes an antipseudomonal agent and an anti-MRSA agent	Typically for 48–72 hours after lung transplantation; further treatment should be based on the clinical assessment including cultures from donor and recipient
Invasive mold and yeast infections	All patients	Nebulized treatment with any one of the following: amphotericin B lipid complex 100 mg (if intubated) or 50 mg (if extubated) once daily for 4 days after transplantation, thereafter once weekly; or liposomal amphotericin B 25 mg thrice weekly; or amphotericin B deoxycholate 5–10 mg twice daily	Until discharge from hospital
	All patients	*No risk factors for mold infection*:* Fluconazole 6 mg/kg IV (or 400 mg PO) once daily *With risk factors for mold infection*:* Voriconazole 6 mg/kg IV (or 400 mg PO) twice daily for two doses, then 4 mg/kg IV (or 200 mg PO) twice daily; or itraconazole 200 mg PO thrice daily for 3 days, then 200 mg PO twice daily; or posaconazole IV or delayed-release tablet 300 mg PO twice daily for 2 doses, then 300 mg PO once daily; or isavuconazole 200 mg PO thrice daily for two days, then 200 mg PO once daily	3–6 months post-transplant
Pneumocystis jirovecii	All patients	Trimethoprim–sulfamethoxazole (TMP–SMZ) one single-strength tablet (TMP 80 mg + SMZ 400 mg) PO daily or one double-strength tablet (TMP 160 mg + SMZ 800 mg) PO three times per week	Continued indefinitely
Cytomegalovirus (CMV)†	CMV D+/R-, D+/R+, D-/R+	Ganciclovir 5 mg/kg IV once daily till the patient can take feeds orally, then tablet valganciclovir 900 mg PO once daily	6–12 months if D+/R+ or D-/R+ 12 months if D+/R-

*Risk factors for mold infection include current or prior airway colonization with mold, airway ischemia, concurrent cytomegalovirus infection, and increased immunosuppression for rejection.
†CMV prophylaxis is not required for CMV D-/R- transplantations.
(IV: intravenous, MRSA: methicillin-resistant *staphylococcus aureus*, PO: per oral)

TABLE 6: Complications associated with lung transplantation.

Allograft-related	• Primary graft dysfunction
	• Acute rejection
	  ○ Acute cellular rejection
	  ○ Antibody-mediated rejection
	  ○ Hyperacute rejection
	• Chronic rejection
	  ○ Bronchiolitis obliterans syndrome
	  ○ Restrictive allograft syndrome

Infections	Bacterial infections, tuberculosis, fungal infections (aspergillosis, mucormycosis, and pneumocystis pneumonia), toxoplasmosis, and cytomegalovirus
Surgical and perioperative	*Airway:* Anastomotic dehiscence, airway stenosis, and bronchopleural fistula *Vascular:* Obstruction of vascular anastomoses at pulmonary artery or pulmonary veins *Pleural:* Pneumothorax, pleural effusion, empyema, chylothorax, and hemothorax *Cardiac:* Atrial arrhythmias, hemodynamic instability, and venous thromboembolism *Other:* Injury to phrenic nerve and recurrent laryngeal nerve

Continued

Continued

Malignancy	Skin cancer, lung cancer, and post-transplant lymphoproliferative disorders
Adverse effects of immunosuppressive agents	*Corticosteroids:* Diabetes mellitus, myopathy, and osteoporosis *Calcineurin inhibitors:* Diabetes mellitus, hyperlipidemia, nephrotoxicity, thrombotic microangiopathy, hypertension, tremors, seizures, and posterior leukoencephalopathy *Mycophenolate:* Diarrhea, anemia, leukopenia, and thrombocytopenia *Azathioprine:* Nausea, vomiting, leukopenia, thrombocytopenia, and transaminitis *Mammalian target of rapamycin (mTOR) inhibitors:* Anemia, leukopenia, thrombocytopenia, diabetes mellitus, hyperlipidemia, nausea, vomiting, diarrhea, constipation, oral ulcers, drug-induced interstitial lung disease, and nephrotoxicity
Others	Gastroparesis and gastroesophageal reflux disease, recurrent primary disease (sarcoidosis, lymphangioleiomyomatosis, pulmonary Langerhans cell histiocytosis, and bronchioloalveolar carcinoma), and hyperammonemia

tion, accounting for 22% of deaths during this period.[2,12] There is no specific treatment for PGD. Management consists of supportive care, including mechanical ventilation when necessary. Pulmonary vasodilators like inhaled nitric oxide and epoprostenol have been tried in severe cases. Retransplantation for PGD is also associated with poor outcomes. PGD is associated with a significant mortality and morbidity. Further, lung transplantation recipients who survive PGD may have a higher risk of chronic rejection over time.

Acute Rejection

Acute allograft rejection can be mediated by T-cells [acute cellular rejection (ACR)] or donor-specific antibodies (DSA) [acute antibody-mediated rejection (AMR)].

- *ACR*: It is the most common form of acute allograft rejection affecting about one-fourth of the lung transplantation recipients in the 1st year after transplantation.[2] ACR is mediated by T-cells directed against the HLA and non-HLA antigens of the donor. Patients with ACR may be asymptomatic or have nonspecific symptoms like fever, cough, and dyspnea. Hence, all lung transplantation recipients must undergo periodic screening with spirometry and transbronchial lung biopsy regardless of the presence of symptoms. ACR is associated with lymphocytic infiltration of the perivascular and peribronchiolar areas. The severity of ACR is graded depending on the intensity of the inflammation in the perivascular, interstitial, and peribronchiolar areas. Treatment of ACR includes high-dose corticosteroids and optimization of the maintenance immunosuppressive regimen. Patients with refractory AMR may require additional treatments like antithymocyte globulin, alemtuzumab, belatacept, mTOR inhibitors, and extracorporeal photopheresis. ACR is responsible for about 5% of deaths that occur in the 1st year after transplantation.[2]
- *Acute AMR:* It is less common than ACR and occurs in <5% of lung transplantations in settings where virtual crossmatching to exclude DSA is performed routinely prior to lung transplantation. Acute AMR generally occurs in the 1st year after transplantation. Acute AMR can be diagnosed in the presence of acute allograft dysfunction associated with circulating DSA and histologic evidence of acute lung injury with subendothelial C4d deposition after excluding alternate etiologies. The treatment of AMR includes therapeutic plasma exchange, intravenous immunoglobulins, and rituximab.
- *Hyperacute rejection (HAR)*: It is a severe form of AMR, which occurs within minutes to hours of lung transplantation due to preexisting DSA in the recipient. In settings where pretransplant virtual crossmatching is performed routinely, HAR is extremely rare. The clinical presentation of HAR is like PGD, with diffuse alveolar opacities and hypoxemia. The treatment of HAR is similar to acute AMR.

Chronic Rejection

Chronic lung allograft dysfunction (CLAD) is diagnosed >3 months after lung transplantation when there is a persistent (lasting for >3 weeks) decline in forced expiratory volume in one second (FEV1) of at least 20% compared to the post-transplant baseline after exclusion of other etiologies.[13] CLAD develops in about half of the lung transplantation recipients by 5 years. CLAD can have obstructive [bronchiolitis obliterans syndrome (BOS)], restrictive [restrictive allograft syndrome (RAS)], mixed, or undefined phenotype.

- *Bronchiolitis obliterans syndrome*: It is the most common type of CLAD. BOS affects about 10% of lung transplantation recipients each year and by 5 years, about half of the lung transplantation recipients would have developed BOS.[2] BOS is the most common cause of death beyond the 1st year of lung transplantation and accounts for about 25% of all deaths during this period.[2] BOS is characterized by obliteration of small airways secondary to granulation tissue, eventually causing fibrous scarring. Risk factors of BOS include

ACR, AMR, PGD, gastroesophageal reflux disease (GERD), CMV pneumonia, and other infections. BOS presents with nonspecific symptoms like cough and dyspnea. The diagnosis of BOS is generally made using serial spirometry showing decline of FEV1 ≥20% along with obstruction [FEV1/ forced vital capacity (FVC) <0.7]. Chest imaging is not very sensitive and may show evidence of hyperinflation. Wherever feasible, a transbronchial lung biopsy should also be performed. There is no proven therapy for BOS and treatment strategies may include intensified immunosuppression, macrolide antibiotics, total lymphoid irradiation, and extracorporeal photopheresis. BOS has a poor prognosis with a median survival of about 3 years after diagnosis.

- *RAS*: It is a type of CLAD characterized by parenchymal and pleural fibrosis. RAS accounts for about 18–30% of patients who develop CLAD.[14] The risk factors for RAS are largely similar to BOS. In patients with a diagnosis of CLAD, RAS can be established in the presence of restriction (FEV1/FVC ≥0.7 and ≥10% reduction of TLC from baseline) along with CT evidence of parenchymal or pleural fibrosis.[14] The most effective treatment strategy for RAS is not clear. Generally, treatment strategies similar to BOS are employed. Antifibrotics have also been tried. Overall, RAS has a significantly worse prognosis compared to BOS.

Infection Complications

Infectious complications are the most common cause of death in the 1st year of lung transplantation, beyond the early (30 days) postoperative period, accounting for 33% of deaths during this period.[2]

Bacterial Infections

Bacterial infections, especially with gram-negative bacilli are the most common infections in the early postoperative period. Candidates with bronchiectasis with prior colonization may be at a higher risk. Donor colonization with gram-negative bacilli could also predispose to postoperative pneumonia.[15] Hence, typically patients receive antibiotic prophylaxis per the local microbial spectrum and antibiogram.

Tuberculosis

Among solid organ transplant (SOT) recipients, lung transplant recipients have the highest risk of tuberculosis (TB).[16] Even in developed countries, the risk is as high as 70 times that of the general population.[17] Although data from India is unavailable, the risk is likely to be even greater. Lung transplant recipients also develop TB much earlier than other solid transplant recipients. The median time to developing TB in lung transplant recipients is 0.2 years compared to 1.2 years for all SOTs combined.[16] Although pulmonary TB is the most common type of post-transplant TB, cavitary disease and smear-positive disease are less common.[16]

Guidelines recommend pretransplant testing of SOT candidates using tuberculin skin test or interferon-gamma release assays and treatment of patients with positive results for latent TB infection (LTBI) after ruling out active TB.[18] However, practices vary across the world and pretransplant screening for LTBI may not be performed in all candidates.[16,19] Even when LTBI screening is performed, a large proportion of transplant recipients can develop TB despite negative results, which could have been due to tuberculin anergy.[16,19]

Fungal Infections

Aspergillus, *Candida*, and non-*Aspergillus* molds are the most common cause of invasive fungal infections after lung transplantation.[20] The majority of fungal infections occur within the 1st year of lung transplantation when the intensity of immunosuppression is the highest. *Aspergillus* infections commonly present as tracheobronchitis and anastomotic-site infections, especially in the early postoperative period, followed by invasive pulmonary aspergillosis. *Aspergillus* colonization is common in lung transplantation recipients, especially, in patients with CF. The most common manifestation of invasive candidiasis in lung transplantation recipients is candidemia.[21] Although invasive pneumonitis due to *Candida* is uncommon, it can cause wound infection, mediastinitis, and empyema. Although *Pneumocystis* infections were common in the preprophylaxis era, they are uncommon now.

Notably, antifungal prophylaxis has not definitively reduced the risk of invasive fungal infections. However, most centers use antifungal prophylaxis for the initial 3–6 months.[22] Typically, a combination of nebulized amphotericin and a systemic azole is used. In patients with prior mold isolation, voriconazole or other azoles with greater activity against *Aspergillus* is preferred over fluconazole. *Pneumocystis* prophylaxis is continued indefinitely.

Viral Infections

Among SOT recipients, lung transplantation recipients have the highest risk of CMV infection,[23] possibly, because of a higher burden of donor CMV infected cells in the lung and the greater degree of immunosuppression. CMV serostatus is the most important risk factor for the development of CMV disease.[23] CMV D+/R- transplants have the highest risk of CMV disease. CMV R+ recipients have an intermediate risk of CMV infection, possibly because of preexisting immunity. The risk is lowest with CMV D-/R- transplants. The intensity of immunosuppression, especially the use of lymphocyte-depleting agent, is another important risk factor for CMV disease. CMV in lung transplantation recipients commonly manifests as CMV pneumonitis or colitis. CMV disease is associated with several complications including a higher risk of other infections and BOS. Hence, all lung transplantation recipients (except CMV D-/R-) should receive universal prophylaxis for CMV. Preemptive treatment for prevention of CMV disease is not recommended in lung transplantation recipients.[23]

Surgical Complications

Airway Complications

Bronchial stenosis is the most common airway complication after lung transplantation.[24] Normally, the bronchi have a dual blood supply from both the bronchial and pulmonary arteries. During anastomosis of the donor and recipient bronchi, the bronchial artery supply is generally not restored. The bronchial artery circulation gets reestablished through collaterals over a period of about 4 weeks. During this period, the bronchi are entirely dependent on the pulmonary artery circulation, which is a low-pressure system with low oxygen content. Hence, bronchial anastomosis is highly susceptible to ischemia and infection. Bronchial necrosis and dehiscence can occur in the early postoperative period (<4 weeks) leading to the development of bronchopleural fistula. Infection of the anastomotic site with bacterial or fungal pathogens (especially *Aspergillus* and *Candida*) can also occur. Some patients may develop exophytic granulation tissue at the site of bronchial anastomoses, which might require bronchoscopic debridement. Bronchial stenosis is generally treated with endobronchial interventions like balloon dilatation, endobronchial ablation, or stenting.

Vascular Complications

Vascular anastomotic complications are less common than airway complications. Obstruction of the vascular anastomoses at pulmonary artery or pulmonary veins can occur due to extrinsic compression, kinking, thrombosis, or stricture.

Pleural Complications

Pleural complications are common after lung transplantation.[25] Pleural effusion is almost universal in the early postoperative period. However, it may not be visible on imaging as patients generally have a chest tube in the immediate postoperative period. The pleural fluid is generally a hemorrhagic, neutrophil-rich exudate. Underlying mechanisms for the pleural effusion include increased production of interstitial fluid due to elevated alveolar permeability, fluid overload, and acute rejection along with decreased clearance of interstitial fluid due to disruption of the lymphatics around the main bronchi. The pleural fluid output reduces rapidly within the first few days after surgery permitting removal of the chest tube within 1–2 weeks in most patients. After removal of the intercostal tube drainage (ICTD), pleural effusion may recur in about one-fourth of the patients.[26] Most of these effusions are still exudative and resolve spontaneously within a few weeks after transplantation when the continuity of the pulmonary lymphatics get restored. About 5% of patients develop pleural infection in the postoperative period which may adversely affect the 1-year survival.[26] Persistent air leaks, lasting for >7 days, maybe secondary to anastomotic dehiscence and will require careful bronchoscopic evaluation.

Other Surgical Complications

Diaphragm dysfunction may occur as a result of phrenic nerve injury. Diaphragm dysfunction is associated with prolonged mechanical ventilation and longer ICU stay. In the perioperative period, patients are at increased risk of venous thromboembolism (VTE). The risk of VTE may be disproportionately high in patients on sirolimus.

Malignancy

In addition to an increased risk of skin cancers, lung transplant recipients have a three-fold higher risk of de novo non-skin cancers compared to the general population.[27] Among subjects who survive beyond the 1st year of transplant, malignancy is the cause of death in 11% of subjects until 5 years, and the proportion increases to 17% for those who survive beyond 5 years.[28] The most common de novo non-skin cancers after lung transplantation are lung cancers, followed by post-transplant lymphoproliferative disorders (PTLD).[27,29] In fact, among the four most common SOTs (kidney, liver, heart, and lungs), lung transplant recipients have the highest risk of lung cancer and PTLD amounting to a 6-fold and 19-fold higher risk, respectively compared to the general population.[30]

Lung Cancer

Common indications for lung transplantation like COPD and IPF are associated with smoking, which is a well-known risk factor for lung cancer. Hence, it is not surprising that lung cancer following lung transplantation occurs predominantly in the native lung of SLT recipients.[31] Although lung cancer in lung transplantation recipients is generally diagnosed in less advanced stages compared to the general population, the outcomes are worse.[31]

Post-transplant Lymphoproliferative Disorders

Post-transplant lymphoproliferative disorders refer to a wide spectrum of benign and malignant proliferations of lymphoid cells that occur in transplant recipients. The pathogenesis of PTLD is closely related to Epstein–Barr virus (EBV) infection and the majority of the PTLDs are EBV-positive. The cumulative incidence of PTLD after lung transplantation is 1%, 2.5%, and 4% at 1, 5, and 10 years.[32]

Advanced age, EBV-seronegative recipient, and use of cytolytic induction immunosuppression therapy (antithymocyte globulin, muromonab-CD3, and alemtuzumab) are some of the risk factors associated with PTLD.[32] Most patients with PTLD respond to a reduction in immunosuppression. Refractory cases may need treatment with rituximab, chemotherapy, or radiotherapy.

Adverse Effects of Immunosuppressive Agents

In addition to increasing the risk of infections, immunosuppressive therapy is associated with several other adverse effects. Bone marrow suppression can occur with the use of mycophenolate, azathioprine, and mTOR inhibitors. Calcineurin inhibitors and mTOR inhibitors are associated with renal dysfunction. By the end of the 1st year of lung transplantation, 6% have severe renal dysfunction (creatinine >2.5 mg/dL or chronic dialysis) and by 5 years, 16% have severe renal dysfunction.[28] Some subjects may even require renal transplantation. Neurologic complications like tremors, confusion, seizures, and reversible posterior leukoencephalopathy syndrome may also be associated with the use of calcineurin inhibitors. Both calcineurin inhibitors and corticosteroids are associated with glucose intolerance, diabetes mellitus, and hyperlipidemia. By the end of the 1st year of lung transplantation, about 20% have diabetes and by 5 years, about one-third have diabetes.[28] Chronic corticosteroid therapy may also be associated with myopathy and osteoporosis.

OUTCOMES

The median survival after lung transplantation is 6.7 years.[2] In comparison with other SOTs, survival rates are much lower with lung transplants. The 5-year survival rate for primary kidney, pancreas, heart, liver, and lung transplants are 87%, 84%, 79%, 76%, and 56%, respectively.[33] Survival benefit with lung transplantation is highest for patients with CF and ILD and lowest for COPD.[34] Post-transplant survival is also highest for CF patients (9.5 years).[28] Advanced recipient age (≥55 years), pretransplant ventilator support, and retransplantation have been associated with higher mortality while BLT has been associated with lower mortality.[28]

Nevertheless, lung transplantation significantly improves the quality of life, especially in the domains related to physical functioning.[35] Most lung transplant recipients report a significant improvement in their physical activity levels in the initial months following the transplantation. About 80% of the lung transplant recipients report no activity limitation at 1 year after transplantation. However, their activity levels and exercise capacity generally do not match that of healthy controls. Nonetheless, about one-third of lung transplant recipients are able to return to work within 1 year after the transplantation.

LUNG TRANSPLANTATION IN INDIA

Chronic respiratory diseases account for over 10% of the total deaths in India.[36] Hence, chronic respiratory diseases could have resulted in approximately 13 lakh deaths in India in 2021.[37] Even with a conservative assumption that 5% of these subjects would have been eligible for lung transplantation, the estimated number of patients who would need lung transplantation annually amounts to over 50,000.[38] However, lung transplantation rates in India are much lower compared to developed countries. In 2021, only 133 lung transplants were performed in India (0.1 per million population) compared to 2,569 (7.7 per million population) in the USA. There are several reasons for this huge gap. Deceased organ donation rate in India is dismal (0.4 per million population) compared to developed countries like the USA (41.6 per million population). The poor deceased organ donation rate, coupled with a low donor conversion rate for lung transplants (the proportion of deceased organ donors from whom lungs could be transplanted) of about 25% in India, produces a drastic reduction in the lungs available for transplantation. Another important reason is the high cost of lung transplantation. Majority of the lung transplantation surgeries in India are performed in the private sector with an estimated cost of about ₹ 20–40 lakh (25,000–50,000 USD).[38] Although this expenditure is much lower than developed countries, it is still out of the reach of most patients in India due to the lack of adequate health insurance. Nevertheless, the number of lung transplantations in India is expected to rise through the continued and coordinated efforts of the National Organ and Tissue Transplant Organization (NOTTO) and the increasing number of institutions offering lung transplantation across India.

SUMMARY

Lung transplantation offers a beacon of hope to individuals grappling with end-stage lung diseases. Over the past several decades, there have been significant advances in surgical techniques including lung preservation strategies, immunosuppressive therapies, and postoperative care. However, challenges persist, ranging from organ scarcity to the intricacies of graft rejection and infection management, and the overall survival is still unsatisfactory. Hopefully, as our understanding of immunology and transplantation biology continues to expand, outcomes of lung transplantation will improve further.

REFERENCES

1. Venuta F, Van Raemdonck D. History of lung transplantation. J Thorac Dis. 2017;9(12):5458-71.
2. Chambers DC, Cherikh WS, Harhay MO, et al. The International Thoracic Organ Transplant Registry of the International Society for Heart and Lung Transplantation: Thirty-sixth adult lung and heart-lung transplantation Report-2019; Focus theme: Donor and recipient size match. J Heart Lung Transplant. 2019;38(10):1042-55.
3. Leard LE, Holm AM, Valapour M, et al. Consensus document for the selection of lung transplant candidates: An update from the International Society for Heart and Lung Transplantation. J Heart Lung Transplant. 2021;40(11):1349-79.
4. Perch M, Hayes D, Jr., Cherikh WS, et al. The International Thoracic Organ Transplant Registry of the International Society for Heart and Lung Transplantation: Thirty-ninth adult lung transplantation report-2022; focus on lung transplant recipients with chronic obstructive pulmonary disease. J Heart Lung Transplant. 2022;41(10):1335-47.
5. Kotloff RM, Thabut G. Lung transplantation. Am J Respir Crit Care Med. 2011;184(2):159-71.
6. Gries CJ, Mulligan MS, Edelman JD, et al. Lung allocation score for lung transplantation: Impact on disease severity and survival. Chest. 2007;132(6):1954-61.
7. Orens JB, Boehler A, de Perrot M, et al. A review of lung transplant donor acceptability criteria. J Heart Lung Transplant. 2003;22(11):1183-200.
8. Prasad KT, Sehgal IS, Dhooria S, et al. Underutilization of potential donors for lung transplantation at a tertiary care center in North India. Lung India. 2019;36(5):399-403.
9. Christie IG, Chan EG, Ryan JP, et al. National trends in extended criteria donor utilization and outcomes for lung transplantation. Ann Thorac Surg. 2021;111(2):421-6.
10. Dick A, Humpe A, Kauke T. Impact, screening, and therapy of HLA antibodies in patients before and after lung transplantation. Transfus Med Hemother. 2019;46(5):337-47.
11. Yusen RD, Hong BA, Messersmith EE, et al. Morbidity and mortality of live lung donation: Results from the RELIVE study. Am J Transplant. 2014;14(8):1846-52.
12. Diamond JM, Arcasoy S, Kennedy CC, et al. Report of the International Society for Heart and Lung Transplantation Working Group on Primary Lung Graft Dysfunction, part II: Epidemiology, risk factors, and outcomes-A 2016 Consensus Group statement of the International Society for Heart and Lung Transplantation. J Heart Lung Transplant. 2017;36(10):1104-13.
13. Verleden GM, Glanville AR, Lease ED, et al. Chronic lung allograft dysfunction: Definition, diagnostic criteria, and approaches to treatment-A consensus report from the Pulmonary Council of the ISHLT. J Heart Lung Transplant. 2019;38(5):493-503.
14. Glanville AR, Verleden GM, Todd JL, et al. Chronic lung allograft dysfunction: Definition and update of restrictive allograft syndrome-A consensus report from the Pulmonary Council of the ISHLT. J Heart Lung Transplant. 2019;38(5):483-92.
15. Prasad KT, Sehgal IS, Dhooria S, et al. Experience of the first lung transplantation performed in public sector in India. Lung India. 2019;36(1):66-9.
16. Katrak S, Han E, Readhead A, et al. Solid organ transplant recipients with tuberculosis disease in California, 2010 to 2020. Am J Transplant. 2023;23(3):401-7.
17. Torre-Cisneros J, Doblas A, Aguado JM, et al. Tuberculosis after solid organ transplant: Incidence, risk factors, and clinical characteristics in the RESITRA (Spanish Network of Infection in Transplantation) cohort. Clin Infect Dis. 2009;48(12):1657-65.
18. Subramanian AK, Theodoropoulos NM. Mycobacterium tuberculosis infections in solid organ transplantation: Guidelines from the infectious diseases community of practice of the American Society of Transplantation. Clin Transplant. 2019;33(9):e13513.
19. Singh N, Paterson DL. Mycobacterium tuberculosis infection in solid-organ transplant recipients: Impact and implications for management. Clin Infect Dis. 1998;27(5):1266-77.
20. Pappas PG, Alexander BD, Andes DR, et al. Invasive fungal infections among organ transplant recipients: Results of the Transplant-Associated Infection Surveillance Network (TRANSNET). Clin Infect Dis. 2010;50(8):1101-11.
21. Andes DR, Safdar N, Baddley JW, et al. The epidemiology and outcomes of invasive Candida infections among organ transplant recipients in the United States: Results of the Transplant-Associated Infection Surveillance Network (TRANSNET). Transpl Infect Dis. 2016;18(6):921-31.
22. Pennington KM, Baqir M, Erwin PJ, et al. Antifungal prophylaxis in lung transplant recipients: A systematic review and meta-analysis. Transpl Infect Dis. 2020;22(4):e13333.
23. Razonable RR, Humar A. Cytomegalovirus in solid organ transplant recipients-Guidelines of the American Society of Transplantation Infectious Diseases Community of Practice. Clin Transplant. 2019;33(9):e13512.
24. Crespo MM, McCarthy DP, Hopkins PM, et al. ISHLT Consensus Statement on adult and pediatric airway complications after lung transplantation: Definitions, grading system, and therapeutics. J Heart Lung Transplant. 2018;37(5):548-63.
25. Tang A, Siddiqui HU, Thuita L, et al. Natural history of pleural complications after lung transplantation. Ann Thorac Surg. 2021;111(2):407-15.
26. Wahidi MM, Willner DA, Snyder LD, et al. Diagnosis and outcome of early pleural space infection following lung transplantation. Chest. 2009;135(2):484-91.
27. Magruder JT, Crawford TC, Grimm JC, et al. Risk factors for de novo malignancy following lung transplantation. Am J Transplant. 2017;17(1):227-38.
28. Chambers DC, Cherikh WS, Goldfarb SB, et al. The International Thoracic Organ Transplant Registry of the International Society for Heart and Lung Transplantation: Thirty-fifth adult lung and heart-lung transplant report-2018; Focus theme: Multiorgan Transplantation. J Heart Lung Transplant. 2018;37(10):1169-83.
29. Sampaio MS, Cho YW, Qazi Y, et al. Posttransplant malignancies in solid organ adult recipients: An analysis of the U.S. National Transplant Database. Transplantation. 2012;94(10):990-8.
30. Engels EA, Pfeiffer RM, Fraumeni JF Jr, et al. Spectrum of cancer risk among US solid organ transplant recipients. JAMA. 2011;306(17):1891-901.

31. Triplette M, Crothers K, Mahale P, et al. Risk of lung cancer in lung transplant recipients in the United States. Am J Transplant. 2019;19(5):1478-90.
32. Zaffiri L, Long A, Neely ML, et al. Incidence and outcome of post-transplant lymphoproliferative disorders in lung transplant patients: Analysis of ISHLT Registry. J Heart Lung Transplant. 2020;39(10):1089-99.
33. Organ Procurement and Transplantation Network: Kaplan-Meier Patient Survival Rates For Transplants Performed between 2008-2015. [online]. Available from https://optn.transplant.hrsa.gov/data/view-data-reports/national-data/#
34. Vock DM, Durheim MT, Tsuang WM, et al. Survival benefit of lung transplantation in the modern era of lung allocation. Ann Am Thorac Soc. 2017;14(2):172-81.
35. Singer JP, Singer LG. Quality of life in lung transplantation. Semin Respir Crit Care Med. 2013;34(3):42.
36. Nations within a nation: Variations in epidemiological transition across the states of India, 1990-2016 in the Global Burden of Disease Study. Lancet. 2017;390(10111):2437-60.
37. United Nations. Data Portal Population Division. (2024). Interactive access to global demographic indicators. [online]. Available from https://population.un.org/dataportal/[Last accessed September, 2024].
38. Divyaveer S, Nagral S, Prasad KT, et al. Health system building blocks and organ transplantation in India. Transplantation. 2021;105(8):1631-4.

SECTION

19

Perspectives of Respiratory Care

SECTION OUTLINE

Ethics in Respiratory Care

CHAPTER 180

Basil Varkey

INTRODUCTION

Ethics is an inseparable part of clinical medicine in all physician-patient interactions and settings. In some interactions, such as a decision to withdraw a ventilator on a patient, the ethical component is obvious, while in others, such as a decision on treatment options for end-stage diseases in an office setting or a long-term care facility, it is less obvious. Patient care decisions involve more than selecting a treatment or intervention on a scientific basis. A physician's ethical obligation is to benefit the patient and to avoid or minimize harm while respectfully considering the values and preferences of the patient and his or her family.

MEANING AND SCOPE OF ETHICS

Ethics is a generic term, covering different ways of examining the moral life. Normative ethics attempts to answer the question "Which general moral norms for the guidance and evaluation of conduct should we accept and why?"[1] Some moral norms about right conduct are common to humankind—transcend cultures, regions, religions, and other group identities and constitute common morality, examples of which include not to kill or harm or cause suffering to others, not to steal, not to punish the innocent, to be truthful, to obey law, to nurture the young and dependent to help the suffering, and rescue those in danger. Particular morality norms bind groups, especially because of their culture, religion, profession, etc., and include responsibilities, ideals, professional standards, etc., and the explication or adjudication in some cases may need experts or religious authorities.

Moral codes and standards of clinical practice are one form of particular morality. Physicians have specialized knowledge and training and a commitment to providing services to patients. The standards and rules of their organizations attempt to keep them competent and trustworthy so that they can fulfill their obligations to their patients. These obligations based on the accepted role of a physician then form on a basic level the ethics of the profession. Physicians' organizations have also codified their standards to reduce the vagueness of professional morality based on "the accepted role of a physician." Codes, although well-intentioned, may simplify moral requirements and may lead physicians to mistakenly consider that they are fulfilling moral norms by complying with the codes. Critics have observed that these codes have inconsistently appealed to general ethical standards or a source of moral authority and "has often appeared to protect the profession's interests more than to offer a broad and impartial moral viewpoint or to address issues of importance to patients and society."[2]

Ethics, specifically bioethics, has evolved rapidly due to several factors that include the deplorable abuses in research on people without informed consent, experimentation in World War II concentration camps, societal changes, and advances in medicine and medical technology. Bioethics has an extensive scope that includes research ethics, public health ethics, organizational ethics, and clinical (medical) ethics. Ethics, because of its familiarity, rather than the more precise term clinical ethics will be used in this chapter.

FUNDAMENTAL PRINCIPLES OF ETHICS

Beneficence, nonmaleficence, autonomy, and justice constitute the four principles of ethics. The first two can be traced back to the time of Hippocrates "to help and do no harm," while the latter two evolved later. Thus, in Percival's book on ethics in the early 1800s, the importance of keeping the patient's best interest as a goal is stressed, while autonomy and justice were not discussed. However, with the passage of time, both autonomy and justice gained acceptance as important principles of ethics. In modern times, Beauchamp and Childress' Book on Principles of Biomedical Ethics is a classic for its exposition of these four principles and their application while also discussing alternative approaches.[1]

Beneficence

The principle of beneficence is the obligation of the physician to act for the benefit of the patient and supports a number of moral rules to protect and defend the rights of others, prevent harm, remove conditions that will cause harm, help persons with disabilities, and rescue persons in danger. It is worth emphasizing that, in distinction to nonmaleficence, the language here is one of the positive requirements. The principle calls for not just avoiding harm but also to benefit patients and to promote their welfare. While physicians' beneficence conforms to moral rules and is altruistic, it should also be recognized that it can be reasonably considered payback for the debt to society for education (often subsidized by governments), to ranks and privileges, and to the patients themselves (learning and research).

Nonmaleficence

Nonmaleficence is the obligation of a physician not to harm the patient. This simply stated principle supports several moral rules—do not kill, do not cause pain or suffering, do not incapacitate, do not cause offense, and do not deprive others of the goods of life. The practical application of nonmaleficence is for the physician to weigh the benefits against the burdens of all interventions and treatments, to eschew those who are inappropriately burdensome, and to choose the best course of action for the patient. This is particularly important and pertinent in difficult end-of-life (EOL) care decisions on withholding and withdrawing life-sustaining treatment, medically administered nutrition and hydration, and pain and other symptom control. A physician's obligation and intention to relieve the suffering (e.g., refractory pain or dyspnea) of a patient by the use of appropriate drugs, including opioids, override the foreseen but unintended harmful effects or outcome [doctrine of double effect (DDE)].[1,3]

Autonomy

The philosophical underpinning for autonomy, as interpreted by philosophers Immanuel Kant (1724–1804) and John Stuart Mill (1806–1873), and accepted as an ethical principle, is that all persons have intrinsic and unconditional worth, and therefore should have power to make rational decisions and moral choices and each should be allowed to exercise his or her capacity for self-determination.[4] This ethical principle was affirmed in a United States (US) court decision by Justice Cardozo in 1914 with the epigrammatic dictum, "Every human being of adult years and sound mind has a right to determine what shall be done with his own body."[5]

Autonomy, as is true for all four principles, needs to be weighed against competing moral principles, and in some instances may be overridden; an obvious example would be if the autonomous action of a patient causes harm to another person(s). The principle of autonomy does not extend to persons who lack the capacity (competence) to act autonomously as in infants and children. Caution must be used in judging incompetence due to developmental, mental, or physical disability as one should not assume that individuals with disabilities are not capable of making decisions.[6] Ableism, a form of discrimination that treats individuals with disabilities as lesser or less valuable than those without disabilities, is pervasive and extends to healthcare.[7,8] The impact of ableism may harm patients with autism and Down syndrome who now increasingly grow into adulthood when they fall seriously ill and need intensive care.[7]

Healthcare institutions and state governments in the US have policies and procedures to assess incompetence. However, a rigid distinction between incapacity to make healthcare decisions (assessed by health professionals) and incompetence (determined by the court of law) is not of practical use, as a clinician's determination of a patient's lack of decision-making capacity based on physical or mental disorder has the same practical consequences as a legal determination of incompetence.[9]

Detractors of the principle of autonomy question the focus on the individual and propose a broader concept of relational autonomy (shaped by social relationships and complex determinants such as gender, ethnicity, and culture)[10] as a person's identity, needs, interests, and autonomous preferences are shaped by their relationships with others. Relational autonomy may then be expressed through group decision-making or even ceding decision-making to another person.

Resistance to the principle of patient autonomy and its derivatives (informed consent and truth-telling) in nonwestern cultures is not unexpected. In countries with ancient civilizations, rooted beliefs and traditions, and the practice of paternalism (parentalism) by physicians emanate mostly from the principle of beneficence. However, culture (a composite of the customary beliefs, social forms, and material traits of a racial, religious, or social group) is not static and autonomous and change with other trends over the passing years. It is presumptuous to assume that the patterns and roles in physician–patient relationships that have been in place for half a century and more still hold true. Therefore, a critical examination of paternalistic medical practice is needed for reasons that include technological and economic progress, improved educational and socioeconomic status of the populace, globalization, and societal movement toward an emphasis on the patient as an individual rather than as a member of a group. This needed examination can be accomplished by research that includes well-structured surveys on demographics, patient preferences on informed consent, truth-telling, and role in decision-making.

Family members, with the good intention of protecting their loved ones, may ask physicians to lie or not disclose to the patient the diagnosis, prognosis, or treatment options. Though it is appropriate to acknowledge the sentiments and cultural, religious, and social norms that underlie such a request, physicians must recognize such a request is co-opting the autonomy of an adult with decision-making capacity.[11-13] Respecting the principle of autonomy obliges the physician to disclose medical information and treatment options that are necessary for the patient to exercise self-determination and this principle further supports informed consent, truth-telling, and confidentiality.

Informed Consent

The requirements of informed consent for a medical or surgical procedure, or for research, are that the patient or subject (1) must be competent to understand and decide, (2) receives a full disclosure, (3) comprehends the disclosure, (4) acts voluntarily, and (5) consents to the proposed action.

The universal applicability of these requirements, rooted and developed in the western culture, has met with some resistance and a suggestion to craft a set of requirements that accommodate the cultural mores of other countries.[14] In response and vigorous defense of the five requirements of informed consent, Angell wrote, "There must be a core of human rights that we would wish to see honored universally, despite variations in their superficial aspects... The forces of local custom or local law cannot justify abuses of certain fundamental rights, and the right of self-determination on which the doctrine of informed consent is based, is one of them."[15]

As competence is the first of the requirements for informed consent, one should know how to detect incompetence. Standards (used singly or in combination) that are generally accepted for determining incompetence are based on the patient's inability to state a preference or choice, inability to understand one's situation and its consequences, and inability to reason through a consequential life decision.[16]

In a previously autonomous but presently incompetent patient, his/her previously expressed preferences (i.e., prior autonomous judgments) are to be respected.[17] Incompetent (nonautonomous) patients and previously competent (autonomous) but presently incompetent patients would need a surrogate decision-maker. In a nonautonomous patient, the surrogate can use either a substituted judgment standard (i.e., what the patient would wish in this circumstance and not what the surrogate would wish), or a best interests standard (i.e., what would bring the highest net benefit to the patient by weighing risks and benefits). Snyder and Sulmasy[18] provide a practical and useful option when the surrogate is uncertain of the patient's preference(s) or when patient's preferences have not been kept abreast of scientific advances. They suggest the surrogate use "substituted interests," i.e., the patient's authentic values and interests to base the decision.

Truth-telling

Truth-telling is a vital component in a physician-patient relationship; without this component, the physician loses the trust of the patient. An autonomous patient has not only the right to know (disclosure) of his/her diagnosis and prognosis but also has the option to forgo this disclosure. However, the physician must know which of these two options the patient prefers.

In the US, full disclosure to the patient, however, grave the disease is, is the norm now but was not so in the past. Significant resistance to full disclosure was highly prevalent in the US, but a marked shift has occurred in physicians' attitudes on this. In 1961, 88% of physicians surveyed indicated their preference to avoid disclosing a diagnosis[19]; in 1979, however, 98% of surveyed physicians favored it.[20] This marked shift is attributable to many factors that include—with no order of importance implied—educational and socioeconomic progress, increased accountability to society, and awareness of previous clinical and research transgressions by the profession.

In contrast to the US, full disclosure to the patient is highly variable in other countries.[21] A continuing pattern in nonwestern societies is for the physician to disclose the information to the family and not to the patient. The likely reasons for the resistance of physicians to convey bad news are concerns that it may cause anxiety and loss of hope, some uncertainty on the outcome, or belief that the patient would not be able to understand the information or may not want to know. However, this does not have to be a binary choice as careful understanding of the principle of autonomy reveals that autonomous choice is a right of a patient, and the patient, in exercising this right, may authorize a family member or members to make decisions for him/her.

Importantly, surveys in the US show that patients with cancer and other diseases wish to be fully informed of their diagnoses and prognoses. Providing full information, with tact and sensitivity, to patients who want to know should be the standard. The sad consequences of not telling the truth regarding cancer include depriving the patient of an opportunity to complete important life tasks: Giving advice to and taking leave of loved ones, putting financial affairs in order, including division of assets, reconciling with estranged family members and friends, attaining spiritual order by reflection, prayer, rituals, and religious sacraments.[22,23]

Confidentiality

Physicians are obligated not to disclose confidential information given by a patient to another party without the patient's authorization. An obvious exception (with implied patient authorization) is the sharing of necessary medical information for care of patient from the primary physician to consultants and other healthcare teams. In the present-day, modern hospitals with multiple points of tests and consultants and the use of electronic medical records, there has been an erosion of confidentiality. However, individual physicians must exercise discipline in not discussing patient specifics with their family members or in social gatherings[24] and social media. There are some noteworthy exceptions to patient confidentiality. These include, among others, legally required reporting of gunshot wounds and sexually transmitted diseases and exceptional situations that may cause major harm to another [e.g., epidemics of infectious diseases, partner notification in human immunodeficiency virus (HIV) disease, relative notification of certain genetic risks].

Justice

Justice is generally interpreted as fair, equitable, and appropriate treatment of persons. Of the several categories of justice, the one that is most pertinent to ethics is distributive justice. Distributive justice refers to the fair, equitable, and appropriate distribution of healthcare resources determined by justified norms that structure the terms of social cooperation.[25] How can this be accomplished? There are different valid principles of distributive justice. These are distribution to each person (1) an equal share, (2) according to need, (3) according to effort, (4) according to contribution, (5) according to merit, and (6) according to free-market exchanges. Each principle is not exclusive and can be often combined in application. It is easy to see the difficulty in choosing, balancing, and refining these principles to form a coherent and workable solution to distribute medical resources.

Although an in-depth review of distributive justice that has multiple stakeholders exceeds the scope of this chapter, a few examples of issues encountered in hospital and office practice need to be mentioned. These include allotment of scarce resources (equipment, tests, medications, organ transplants), care of uninsured patients, and allotment of time for outpatient visits (equal time for every patient? based on need or complexity? based on social and or economic status?). The principle of justice is severely stressed when faced with increased demand over available resources as we faced in the coronavirus disease 2019 (COVID-19) pandemic.[26] Examples are the disparities in the admission policies and the allocation of intensive care unit (ICU) resources to various subgroups of patients, such as older individuals, females, those from diverse racial backgrounds, those with chronic neurological disabilities, and those with developmental disabilities.[6-8]

Difficult as it may be, and despite the many constraining forces, physicians must accept the requirement of fairness contained in this principle.[27] Fairness to the patient is of primary importance when there are conflicts of interest. A flagrant example of violation of this principle would be when a particular option of treatment is chosen over others, or an expensive drug is chosen over an equally effective but less expensive one because it benefits the physician financially or otherwise.

CONFLICTS BETWEEN PRINCIPLES

Each one of the four principles of ethics is to be taken as a prima facie obligation that must be fulfilled, unless it conflicts, in a specific instance, with another principle. When faced with such a conflict, the physician has to determine the actual obligation to the patient by examining the respective weights of the competing prima facie obligations based on both content and context. Consider an example of a conflict that has an easy resolution: A patient in shock treated with urgent fluid resuscitation and the placement of an indwelling intravenous catheter caused pain and swelling. Here, the principle of beneficence overrides that of nonmaleficence. Many of the conflicts that physicians face, however, are much more complex and difficult. Consider a competent patient's refusal of a potentially life-saving intervention (e.g., instituting mechanical ventilation) or request for a potentially life-ending action (e.g., withdrawing mechanical ventilation). Nowhere in the arena of ethical decision-making is conflict as pronounced as when the principles of beneficence and autonomy collide.[28]

Beneficence has enjoyed a historical role in the traditional practice of medicine. However, giving it primacy over patient autonomy is paternalism (parentalism) that makes a physician–patient relationship analogous to that of a father/mother to a child. A father/mother may refuse a child's wishes and influence a child in a variety of ways—nondisclosure, manipulation, deception, coercion, etc., consistent with his/her thinking of what is best for the child. Paternalism can be further divided into soft and hard.

In soft paternalism, the physician acts on grounds of beneficence (and, at times, nonmaleficence) when the patient is nonautonomous or substantially nonautonomous (e.g., cognitive dysfunction due to severe illness, depression, or drug addiction).[29] Soft paternalism is complicated because of the difficulty in determining whether the patient was nonautonomous at the time of decision-making but is ethically defensible as long as the action is in concordance with what the physician believes to be the patient's values. Hard paternalism is action by a physician, intended to benefit a patient but contrary to the voluntary decision of an autonomous patient who is fully informed and competent and is ethically indefensible.

On the other end of the scale of hard paternalism is consumerism, a rare and extreme form of patient autonomy, that holds the view that the physician's role is limited to providing all the medical information and the available choices for interventions and treatments while the fully informed patient selects from the available choices. In this model, the physician's role is constrained and does not permit the full use of his/her knowledge and skills to benefit the patient, and is tantamount to a form of patient abandonment and therefore is ethically indefensible.

Faced with the contrasting paradigms of beneficence and respect for autonomy and the need to reconcile these to find a common ground, Pellegrino and Thomasma[29] argue that beneficence can be inclusive of patient autonomy as "the best interests of the patients are intimately linked with their preferences" from which "are derived our primary duties to them."

One of the basic and not infrequent reasons for disagreement between physician and patient on treatment issues is their divergent views on the goals of treatment. As goals change in the course of the disease (e.g., a chronic neurologic condition worsens to the point of needing ventilator support or a cancer that has become refractory to treatment), it is imperative that the physician communicates with the patient in clear and straightforward language, without the use of medical jargon, and with the aim of defining the goal(s) of treatment under the changed circumstance. In doing so, the physician should be cognizant of patient factors that compromise decisional capacity, such as anxiety, fear, pain, lack of trust, and different beliefs and values that impair effective communication.[30]

The foregoing theoretical discussion on principles of ethics has practical application in clinical practice in all settings. In the resource book for clinicians, Jonsen et al.[31] have elucidated a logical and well-accepted model **(Table 1)** along the lines of the systematic format that practicing physicians have been taught and have practiced for a long time (Chief Complaint, History of Present Illness, Past History, pertinent Family and Social History, Review of Systems, Physical Examination, and Laboratory and Imaging studies). This practical approach to problem-solving in ethics involves:

- Clinical assessment (identifying medical problems, treatment options, goals of care)
- Patient (finding and clarifying patient preferences on treatment options and goals of care)
- Quality of life (QOL) (effects of medical problems, interventions, and treatments on patient's QOL with awareness of individual biases on what constitutes an acceptable QOL)
- Context (many factors that include family, cultural, spiritual, religious, economic, and legal)

TABLE 1: Application of principles of ethics in patient care.

Beneficence, nonmaleficence	*Clinical assessment:* • Nature of illness (acute, chronic, reversible, terminal) • Goals of treatment • Treatment options and probability of success for each option • Adverse effects of treatment and does the benefit outweigh harm • Effects of no medical/surgical treatment • If treated, plans for limiting treatment? Stopping treatment?
Respect for autonomy	*Patient rights and preferences:* • Information given to patient on benefits and risks of treatment • Patient understood the information and gave consent? • Patent mentally competent? If competent, what are his/her preferences? • If patient is mentally incompetent, are patient's prior preferences known? • If preferences are unknown, who is the appropriate surrogate?
Beneficence, nonmaleficence, respect for autonomy	*Quality of life (QOL):* • Expected QOL with and without treatment • Deficits—physical, mental, social—may have after treatment? • Judging QOL of patient who cannot express himself/herself? Who is the judge? • Recognition of possible physician bias in judging QOL? • Rationale to forgo life-sustaining treatment(s)?
Distributive justice	*External forces and context:* • Conflicts of interests—does physician benefit financially, professionally by ordering tests, prescribing medications, and seeking consultations? • Research or educational considerations that affect clinical decisions, physician orders? • Conflicts of interests based on religious beliefs? Legal issues? • Conflicts of interests between organizations (clinics, hospitals), third-party payers? • Public health and safety issues? • Problems in allocation of scarce resources?

Ethics in End-of-life Care

"Over and over, we in medicine inflict deep gouges at the end of people's lives and then stand oblivious to the harm done."

—**Atul Gawande**[32]

Though EOL care is covered in another chapter, a few focused comments on ethical issues in EOL care are of particular importance to pulmonary and critical care physicians as they care for seriously ill patients with advanced disease in ICUs and other settings. A substantial number of patients die with unrelieved symptoms that are poorly recognized and poorly treated; physicians are often unaware of patients' wishes regarding EOL care and interventions are often done that are not consistent with patients' preferences,[33,34] while a significant number of patients end their lives in the hospital, hooked up to machines and surrounded by strangers and not by their family.

End-of-life care demands a diverse set of physician skills,[35] professionalism, and ethics.[36,37] Besides cognitive skills, the physician needs to have affective skills to provide emotional support to the patient while respecting the patient's values, skills to communicate with patient and family, and the ability to coordinate and communicate with the care team. Dealing with EOL issues, more than any other patient/family and physician interactions, has the potential to compromise decision-making that is influenced by the physician's personal and cultural values and religious and spiritual beliefs.[38,39]

Pulmonary and critical care physicians provide care in various milieus (outpatient, inpatient hospital, ICU) for patients with cancer and chronic life-limiting diseases such as chronic obstructive pulmonary disease (COPD) and pulmonary fibrotic diseases. In the latter group, prognostication is difficult and therefore, it is hard to decide when to initiate advanced care planning and EOL care. The quality of EOL care in chronic lung disease is poor[40,41] and patients with COPD are more likely to die in the ICU than patients with cancer while on mechanical ventilation and with dyspnea.[37] In the US, approximately 20% of all deaths occur in the ICU and a substantial number of them involve a decision to withhold or withdraw life-supporting therapy.[42]

Communication and Decision-making in End-of-life Care

The initial communication step for a physician is to inquire about the patient's preference regarding decision-making—self or a designated family member or members. The patient or designated family member(s) may also defer some of the responsibility, especially for a difficult decision (e.g., do not resuscitate order) to the physician.[43] In such a case, the physician is obligated to provide periodic updates and affirm that there has been no change in the delegated responsibility. As many critically ill patients in the ICU are not able to fully participate in discussions on their own EOL care, their family members often play a key role in EOL decisions. Hence, the physician should be sensitive to the stresses and burdens of the family, help them understand the clinical status and prognosis, elicit from them the patient's values, and in partnership with them develop goals of care and treatment plan that is based on the patient's prognosis, values, and preferences.[44]

Sorrily, in one European study, only one half of the ICU's involved patients and families in decision-making and wide variations in practice were noted between countries.[45] Even when guidelines are in place, the practice patterns may vary greatly.[46] There is a dearth of information on EOL decision-making process in the ICUs from the most populous countries—India and China.

Seriously ill patients and their families identify communication skills as one of the most important skills for physicians[47] and communication successes and failures generate more gratitude and complaints than any other aspect of EOL care.[48] Several components of communication are shown to improve the quality of EOL and one useful mnemonic for family conferences is VALUE; *v*alue the statements family members make, *a*cknowledge emotions, *l*isten to family members, *u*nderstand the patient as a person (values, characteristics, preferences), and *e*licit questions from the family.[49]

Medical Futility and Conflicts

The concept of medical futility is controversial and the term is fraught with ambiguity. Futility can be used to cover various situations of predicted improbable outcomes, improbable success, and unacceptable benefit-burden ratios. Typically, the term is used in a situation in which dying patients have reached a point at which further treatment provides no physiologic benefit or is hopeless and becomes optional. "Clinically nonbeneficial interventions" have been proposed as a better alternative term for futility.[1]

Invoking medical futility as the reason to withhold or withdraw life-sustaining treatments against the wishes of a patient or surrogate decision-maker is ethically very problematic. Such conflicts can be substantially reduced with timely and structured communications that build trust between the physician and the patient and family. To incorporate the provision to avoid interventions of no benefit (medical futility) into a framework of EOL decision-making is essential, provided "benefit" is defined with reference to the patient's preferences and values.[50] The American Medical Association recommends that when a patient or surrogate decision-maker insists on a therapy that the physician believes is futile, a communication and negotiation process should be started to reconcile these differences and the treatment should be provided until the differences are reconciled.[51]

Withholding or Withdrawing Life-sustaining Measures

Most of the deaths in the ICU and acute care wards occur after a decision to withdraw life-sustaining treatments.[44,52,53] Some physicians are uncomfortable in withdrawing treatment that is already in place but feel justified in withholding (not started) treatment. This distinction from an ethical standpoint is unclear, irrelevant, and morally untenable.[1] Assigning a preference and priority to withholding over withdrawal can lead to undertreatment (not using it to avoid the decision to withdraw later) of some patients who may possibly benefit from it and overtreatment (continuation of treatment that is no longer beneficial) in others.

Pulmonologists, critical care physicians, and others practicing in ICUs should understand the goal of withdrawing life-sustaining treatments is to remove all treatments no longer desired or indicated while ensuring patient comfort. Discussion with families should include an explanation of the process, assurance that a palliative approach to alleviate all symptoms and to provide comfort will be provided, the expected length of survival (range and if uncertain state so), and learning of specific patient and family preferences (especially religious and cultural) prior to death.[54,55] Documentation should include the rationale for withdrawal of life-sustaining treatments, plans on how the procedure will be done, and how complications, if any, will be handled.

Modalities such as vasopressors, antibiotics, and nutrition can be discontinued without a taper. As abrupt mechanical ventilation withdrawal may cause discomfort from dyspnea and secretions, a protocol for ventilator withdrawal[56] and a protocol for analgesia and sedation[57] should be followed. There is no set upper limit for the sedative and analgesic drugs used in this setting as symptom control is the overriding objective (see the following section under DDE). Moreover, higher doses of opioids and benzodiazepines used in the context of withdrawal from ventilator do not consistently decrease the time from withdrawal to death.[58]

The reasons for the use of increased sedation and analgesia and monitoring of symptoms and treatments used from withdrawal of life-sustaining treatment until death should be documented. Prior to the withdrawal, the family should be given time with the patient and also after withdrawal and control of symptoms.

Doctrine of Double Effect

The DDE makes a distinction between the intended effect and unintended but foreseen effect of a single act that has double effects—one good and one harmful. Under the DDE, if the action satisfies four elements, it is morally permissible.[1] The four elements are (1) the nature of the act, (2) the intention of the doer, (3) the distinction between means and effects, and (4) the proportionality between the good effect and the bad effect (the bad effect is permissible only if the intended good effect is proportionally more than the bad effect). The classic clinical situation in which DDE comes into play is in severe symptom (e.g., pain, dyspnea) management in EOL.[3] In this context, the physician's obligation and intention to relieve the suffering of the patient by appropriate drugs, such as opioids, overrides the foreseen but unintended harmful effects or outcomes.

Meeting the Needs of the Family

In acute care settings, especially in ICUs, the needs of family members of the patient are largely unmet. The modern ICU is not designed to be family friendly. Family members are often excluded from the bedside.[59,60] Supportive and compassionate care to the family from physicians and other healthcare providers falls short due to factors that include a lack of role models, deficiencies in attitude and skills, competing demands for time, and constraints placed by the hospital and physical layout of the ICU.

To meet the basic and minimum requirements of the family, any ICU anywhere in the world should provide a designated place/room (with chairs and toilet facility) for family members to rest, periodic updates on the patient's condition, and access to the patient. Policies regarding visitation restrictions that are generally more stringent in ICUs in the developing world should be reexamined. Issues that need to be addressed include: Are some of the restrictive policies more for the convenience of the healthcare providers than for patient benefit? Are risks of infections (not influenza, coryza, and other viral infections) transmitted from the family to the patient proven and quantitated? Are simple protocols such as hand washing and disposable face masks for visitors in place? Do these risks outweigh the positive benefits to the patient of having a loving family member at the bedside?

Culturally Sensitive Care

Culture is commonly defined as the customary beliefs, social forms, and material traits of a racial, religious, or social group and has a clear influence on the group's values, perspectives, and decision-making. Recognition of culture-based differences that may exist between physician and patient is a critical step in providing culturally sensitive care[61] and skillfully managing these differences improves patient and family satisfaction and may also lead to better outcomes.[62]

However, this critical step of recognition of culture-based differences should be based on communication and the expressed opinions of the patient and not on assumptions based on religion, caste, race, socioeconomic status, gender, or age as differences may exist within each group. Cultural differences are also present, as expected, between countries and as a consequence, some practices of medical ethics of the western world are either not accepted or resisted in other parts of the world; examples are the moral and legal equivalence of withholding and withdrawing life-sustaining treatment (previously discussed) and the definition of brain death.[63,64]

One major component of culturally sensitive care is respecting and accommodating religious beliefs of the patient and family.[65-67] This is particularly important in EOL care when death is imminent. Some religious scholars have offered their views to guide their believers.[68] Prayers and rituals provide solace to the patient and family. Policies in ICUs and wards should be flexible within reason to honor rituals and prayers specific to the dying person's religion. At times, a simple provision for a ritual (e.g., sipping Ganges water) may be all that is needed to fulfill the last wish of a dying patient.[69]

EDUCATION AND CHALLENGES WITH TECHNOLOGICAL ADVANCES

Knowledge, skills, and attitudes of ethics among practicing physicians and resident physicians are variable and often less than satisfactory. Although the obligation to respect patient preferences on care at the end of life is accepted in the US, a seminal nationwide study found significant deficiencies in physician performance.[33] Another study found that physicians often failed to disclose medical errors although disclosure is an ethical duty.[70] Other studies have documented deficiencies in knowledge and skills in resident physicians.[71,72] These and similar studies along with an increased recognition of the importance of ethics in medical practice have spurred educational efforts at all levels in the US.

Ethics is a formally required part of the curriculum for medical students in the US and is incorporated into the core competencies in internal medicine residency. Resident physicians are graded on their professionalism, interpersonal and communication skills, and patient care. Continuing education programs in ethics are offered or required by several states. The goals of ethics education are (1) to appreciate the ethical dimensions of patient care, (2) to understand ethical principles (principlism) of the medical profession, (3) to have competence in core ethical behavioral skills—obtaining informed consent, assessing decision-making capacity, discussing resuscitation status and use of life-sustaining treatments, advanced care planning, breaking bad news, and effective communication, (4) to know the commonly encountered ethical issues in general and in one's specialty, (5) to have competence in analyzing and resolving ethical problems, (6) to appreciate cultural diversity and how it impacts ethics, and (7) to share one's knowledge in ethics with colleagues, trainees, and students.[73]

Ethics education has been shown to improve learner awareness, attitudes, confidence, knowledge, and moral reasoning[73,74] and to improve the quality of care in certain areas.[70,74-76] It is hoped that physician leaders in academia and practice in all countries of the world with support from their organizations and private and governmental grants develop and promote ethics education at all levels—students, trainees, and practitioners.

The advent of electronic medical records posed an ethical challenge to patient confidentiality. In response to this challenge, educational interventions and protective laws were put in place in the US. A much greater challenge awaits us as the nascent artificial intelligence (AI) technology matures. AI is a term used to describe a computer program's capacity to execute tasks associated with human intelligence, such as reasoning and learning. It also includes processes such as adaptation, sensory understanding, and interaction. AI learns the functions from data input and through learning from these data has the potential to change healthcare. Harnessed effectively AI can have an immense positive impact on many areas of healthcare delivery.[77] These include providing evidence-based management and decision-making to the physician and helping in clinical and imaging diagnosis, drug discovery, personalized medicine, and operational efficiency. However, a sound governance framework is required to protect humans from harm, including harm resulting from unethical behavior.[77,78] Many ethical issues may arise with wide-ranging effects on individuals, groups, institutions, sectors, and society due to factors that include misguided, inconclusive, or inscrutable evidence, related to unfair outcomes, traceability, and others.[78-80]

A NEW COVENANT FOR PHYSICIANS

The Hippocratic oath, attributed (authorship is questionable) to Hippocrates (460–370 BC), expressed physicians' obligations to patients of beneficence (to help the sick) and non-maleficence (never to use it to injure or harm them) and was the standard for ethical medical practice. However, the Hippocratic oath, which had run for many centuries, has become outdated (elements of sexism, self-aggrandizement, sorcery) and inadequate (autonomy and justice not included). Consequently, many academic medical centers and physician leaders have proposed new oaths appropriate to our times. I have selected seven elements from one among them[81] and paraphrased them (listed further) as they are consonant with the theme of this chapter and together they form an appropriate new covenant for physicians.

1. I will remain a student all my professional life, attempting to learn not only from formal medical sources but from my patients as well.
2. I will attempt to function as a teacher for my patients so that I can care for them more effectively and apply the lessons they provide to the care of other patients.
3. Knowing my own inadequacies and those of medicine generally, I will strive to cure when possible but to comfort always.
4. I will do unto patients and their families only what I would want done unto me or my family. I will not experiment on patients unless the patients give truly informed consent. I will strive to instruct patients fully so their informed consent is possible.
5. I will be honest with my patients in all medical matters. When this honesty reveals bad news, I will deliver it with understanding, sympathy, and tact.
6. I will provide my patients with acceptable alternatives for various forms of diagnosis and medical and surgical treatment, explaining the risks and benefits as best I know them.
7. I will allow my patients to make the ultimate decision about their own care within the options I have explained to them. In circumstances where my patients are incapable of making decisions, I will accept the decision of family members or loved ones, encouraging them to decide as they believe the patient would have decided.

A CONCEPTUAL MODEL FOR PATIENT CARE

In this concluding segment, I define professionalism and its alignment with ethics, elucidate the virtues desired of a physician, and present an integrated model for patient care. Professionalism "demands placing the interest of patients above those of the physician, setting and maintaining standards of competence and integrity, and providing expert advice to society on matters of health."[27,82] The core of professionalism is a therapeutic relationship built on competent and compassionate care by a physician that meets the expectations and benefits a patient. In this relationship, rooted in the ethical principles of beneficence and nonmaleficence, physicians can fulfill their obligations **(Box 1)** to patients.

Drawing on a lifetime of experience as a physician, teacher, and mentor, I envisage physicians with qualities of both "heart" and "head." Ethical and humanistic values shape the former, while knowledge (e.g., by study, research, and practice) and technical skills (e.g., medical and surgical procedures) form the latter. **Flowchart 1** is a representation of this model. Morality that forms the base of the model and the ethical principles that rest on it were previously explained. Virtues are linked, some more tightly than others, to the principles of ethics. Compassion, a prelude to caring, presupposes sympathy, and is expressed in beneficence. Discernment is especially valuable in decision-making when principles of ethics collide. Trustworthiness leads to trust and is a needed virtue when patients, at their most vulnerable time, place themselves in the hands of physicians. Integrity involves the coherent integration of emotions, knowledge, and aspirations while maintaining moral values. Physicians need both professional integrity and personal integrity, as the former may not cover all scenarios (e.g., prescribing ineffective drugs or expensive drugs when effective inexpensive drugs are available, performing invasive treatments or experimental research modalities without fully informed consent, any situation where personal monetary gain is placed over patient's welfare). Conscientiousness is required to determine what is right by critical reflection on good versus bad, better versus good, logical versus emotional, and right versus wrong.

BOX 1 Physician's obligations.

- Cure of disease when possible
- Maintenance or improvement of functional and quality of life (relief of symptoms and suffering)
- Prevention of untimely death
- Avoidance of harm to the patient in the course of care
- Education and counseling of patients (condition and prognosis)
- Providing palliative care throughout the course of illness and especially near the time of death
- Communicating with and supporting families of patients
- Promotion of health and prevention of disease

SUMMARY

As shown in my model, medical knowledge, technical skills, practice based learning, and communication skills are partnered with ethical principles and professional virtues. The virtues of compassion, discernment, trustworthiness, integrity, and conscientiousness are the necessary building blocks for the virtue of caring. Caring is the defining virtue of all healthcare professions. In all interactions with patients, besides the technical expertise of a physician, the human element of caring (one human to another) is needed. In different situations, caring can be expressed verbally and nonverbally (e.g., the manner of communication with both physician and patient closely seated, and with unhurried, softly spoken words); a gentle touch, especially when conveying "bad news;" a firmer touch or grip to convey reassurance to a patient facing a difficult treatment choice; to hold the hand of a patient dying alone). Thus, "caring" is at the center of the depicted integrated model, and as Peabody succinctly expressed it nearly 100 years ago, "The secret of the care of the patient is caring for the patient."[83]

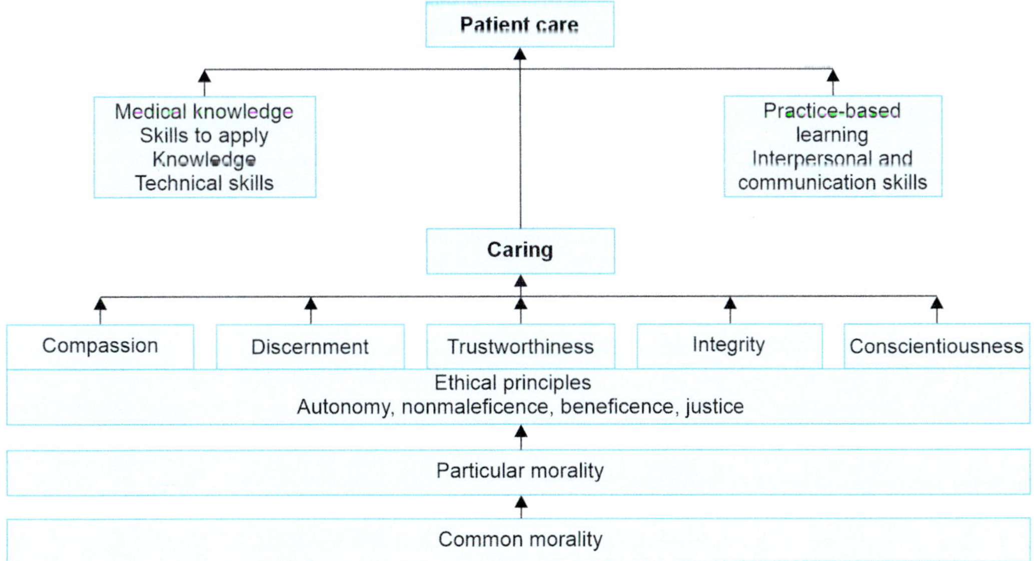

FLOWCHART 1: A conceptual model of patient care by a physician who integrates morality, ethical principles, virtues, and competencies.

REFERENCES

1. Beauchamp TL, Childress JF. Principles of biomedical ethics, 9th edition. New York, NY: Oxford University Press; 2019.
2. Berkman ND, Wynia MK, Churchill LR. Gaps, Conflicts and Consensus in the Ethics Statements of Professional Associations, Medical Groups and Health Plans. J Med Ethics. 2004;30: 395-401.
3. Mularski RA, Puntillo K, Varkey B, et al. Pain management within the palliative and end-of-life care experience in the ICU. Chest. 2009;135(5):1360-9.
4. Guyer P. Kant on the theory and practice of autonomy. Soc Philos Policy. 2003;20(2):70-98.
5. Cardozo B. Basic right to consent to medical care – Schlendorff v. the Society of the New York Hosp., 105 N.E. 92, 93 (N.Y. 1914). [online] Available from https://biotech.law.lsu.edu/cases/consent/schoendorff.htm [Last accessed September, 2024].
6. Morris MA. Death by ableism. N Engl J Med. 2023;388(1):5-7.
7. Taccone FS. Ableism in the intensive care unit. Intensive Care Med. 2023;49:898-99.
8. Baksh RA, Pape SE, Smith J, et al. Understanding inequalities in COVID-19 outcomes following hospital admission for people with intellectual disability compared to the general population: a matched cohort study in the UK. BMJ Open. 2021;11:e052482.
9. Grisso T, Appelbaum PS. Assessing competence to consent to treatment: A guide to physicians and other health professionals. New York: Oxford University Press; 1998. p. 11.
10. Mackenzie CM, Stoljar N. Relational autonomy: Feminist perspectives on autonomy, agency, and the social self. New York: Oxford University Press; 2000.
11. McCabe MS, Wood WA, Goldberg RM. When the family requests withholding the diagnosis: who owns the truth? J Oncol Pract. 2010;6(2):94-6.
12. Hallenbeck J, Arnold R. A request for nondisclosure: don't tell mother. J Clin Oncol. 2007;25(31):5030-4.
13. Jotkowitz A, Glick S, Gezundheit B. Truth-telling in a culturally diverse world. Cancer Invest. 2006;24(8):786-9.
14. Levine RJ. Informed consent: Some challenges to the universal validity of the western model. In: Vaughn L (Ed). Bioethics: Principles, Issues and Cases. New York (NY): Oxford University Press; 2010. pp. 183-8.
15. Angell M. Ethical imperialism? Ethics in international collaborative clinical research. N Engl J Med. 1988;319(16):1081-3.
16. Appelbaum PS, Grisso T. Assessing patients' capacities to consent to treatment. N Engl J Med. 1988;319:1635-8.
17. Davis JK. The concept of precedent autonomy. Bioethics. 2002; 16(2):114-33.
18. Sulmasy DP, Snyder L. Substituted interests and best judgments: an integrated model of surrogate decision making. JAMA. 2010; 304(17):1946-7.
19. Oken D. What to tell cancer patients. A study of medical attitudes. JAMA. 1961;175(13):1120-8.
20. Novack DH, Plumer R, Smith RL, et al. Changes in physicians' attitudes toward telling the cancer patient. JAMA. 1979;241(9): 897-900.
21. Surbone A. Truth telling to the patient. JAMA. 1992;268(13): 1661-2.
22. Rayson D. A piece of my mind. Lisa's stories. JAMA. 1999; 282(17):1605-6.
23. Fallowfield LJ, Jenkins VA, Beveridge HA. Truth may hurt but deceit hurts more: communication in palliative care. Palliat Med. 2002;16(4):297-303.
24. Weiss BD. Confidentiality expectations of patients, physicians, and medical students. JAMA. 1982;247(19):2695-7.
25. Fleishacker S. A short history of distributive justice. Cambridge (MA): Harvard University Press; 2005.
26. Varkey B. Palliative care considerations and ethical issues in the care of Covid-19 patients. Curr Opin Pulm Med. 2021;27:64-5.
27. ABIM Foundation; ACP-ASIM Foundation; European Federation of Internal Medicine. Medical professionalism in the new millennium: a physician charter. Ann Intern Med. 2002;136(3): 243-6.
28. Tonelli MR, Misak CJ. Compromised autonomy and the seriously ill patient. Chest. 2010;137(4):926-31.
29. Pellegrino E, Thomasma D. For the patient's good: The restoration of beneficence in health care. New York: Oxford University Press; 1988. p. 29.
30. Dubler NN, Liebman CB. Bioethics Mediation: A Guide to Shaping Shared Solutions. New York, NY: United Hospital Fund of New York; 2004.
31. Jonsen AR, Siegler M, Winslade WJ. Ethics: A practical approach to ethical decisions in clinical medicine, 8th edition. United States: McGraw Hill; 2015.
32. Gawande A. Being Mortal: Medicine and What Matters in the End. India: Penguin Books; 2014.
33. The SUPPORT Principal Investigators. A controlled trial to improve care for seriously ill hospitalized patients: the study to understand prognoses and preferences for outcomes and risks of treatments (SUPPORT). JAMA. 1995;274:1591-8.
34. Hofmann JC, Wenger NS, Davis RB, et al. Patients' preferences for communication with physicians about end-of-life decisions. Ann Intern Med. 1997;127:1-12.
35. Curtis, JR, Wenrich MD, Carline JD, et al. Understanding physicians' skills at providing end-of-life-care: perspectives of patients, families, and health care workers. J Gen Intern Med. 2001;16:41-9.
36. Curtis JR, Vincent J-L. Ethics and end-of-life care for adults in the intensive care unit. Lancet. 2010;376:1347-53.
37. Thorns A. Ethical and legal issues in end-of-life care. Clin Med. 2010;10:282-5.
38. Goold SD, Stern DT. Ethics and professionalism: what does a resident need to learn? Am J Bioeth. 2006;6:9-17.
39. Weissmann DE. Decision making at a crisis near the end of life. JAMA. 2004;292:1738-43.
40. Lynn J, Ely EW, Zhong Z, et al. Living and dying with chronic obstructive lung disease. J Am Geriatr Soc. 2000;48:S91-100.
41. Varkey B. Unfulfilled palliative care needs of chronic obstructive pulmonary disease patients. Curr Opin Pulm Med. 2006;12: 103-5.
42. Angus DC, Barnato AE, Linde-Zwirble WT, et al. Use of intensive care at the end of life in the United States: an epidemiologic study. Crit Care Med. 2004;32:638-43.
43. Curtis RA, Burt RA. Point: the ethics of unilateral "do not resuscitate orders: the role of the "informed assent". Chest. 2007;132:748-51.
44. Torke AM, Alexander GC, Lantos J, et al. The physician-surrogate relationship. Arch Intern Med. 2007;167:1117-21.

45. Vincent J-L. Forgoing life support in western European intensive care units. Crit Care Med. 1999;27:1626-33.
46. Ravenscroft AJ, Bell MDD. End-of-life decision making within intensive care: objective, consistent, defensible? J Med Ethics. 2000;26:435-40.
47. Hickey M. What are the needs of families of critically ill patients? A review of the literature since 1976. Heart Lung. 1990;19:401-5.
48. Abbott KH, Sago JG, Breen CM, et al. Families looking back: one year after discussion of withdrawal or withholding of life-sustaining support. Crit Care Med. 2001;29:197-201.
49. Shanawani H, Wenrich MD, Tonelli MR, et al. Meeting physicians. responsibilities in providing end-of-life-care. Chest. 2008;133:775-86.
50. Curtis JR. Communicating about end-of-life care with patients and families in the intensive care unit. Crit Care Clin. 2004; 20:363-80.
51. Council on Ethical and Judicial Affairs AMA. Medical futility in end-of-life care. JAMA. 1999;281:937-41.
52. Smedira NG, Evans BH, Grais LS, et al. Withholding and withdrawing of life support from the critically ill. N Engl J Med. 1990;322:309-15.
53. Keenan SP, Busche KD, Chen LM, et al. A retrospective review of a large cohort of patients undergoing the process of with-holding or withdrawal of life support. Crit Care Med. 1997;22: 1020-5.
54. Brody H, Campbell ML, Faber-Langendoen K, et al. Withdrawing intensive life-sustaining treatment; recommendations for com-passionate clinical management. N Engl J Med. 1997;336:652-7.
55. Rubenfeld GD, Crawford S. Principles and practice of with-drawing life-sustaining treatments in the ICU. In Curtis JR, Rubenfeld GD, eds. Managing death in the intensive care unit: transition from cure to comfort. New York, NY: Oxford University Press; 2001. pp. 127-48.
56. Treece PD, Engelberg RA, Crowley L, et al. Evaluation of a standardized order form for withdrawal of life support in the intensive care unit. Crit Care Med. 2004;32:1141-8.
57. Curtis JR, Rubenfeld GD. Improving palliative care for patients in the intensive care unit. J Palliat Med. 2005;8:840-54.
58. Chan JD, Treece PD, Engelberg RA, et al. Association between narcotic and benzodiazepine use after withdrawal of life support and time of death. Chest. 2004;126:286-93.
59. Shannon SE. Helping families prepare for and cope with a death in the ICU. In: Curtis JR, Rubenfeld GD (Eds). Managing Death in the ICU: The Transition From Cure to Comfort. New York, NY: Oxford University Press; 2001. pp. 165-82.
60. Levy MM. A view from the other side. Crit Care Med. 2007;35: 603-4.
61. Pachter LM. Culture and clinical care: folk illness beliefs and behaviors and their implications for health care delivery. JAMA. 1994;271:690-4.
62. Carrese JA, Perkins HS. Ethics consultation in an culturally diverse society. Public Aff Q. 2003;17:97-120.
63. Blackhall LJ, Frank G, Murphy ST, et al. Ethnicity and attitudes towards life sustaining technology. Soc Sci Med. 1999;48:1779-89.
64. Byrne PA, O'Reilly S, Quay PM. Brain death: an opposing viewpoint. JAMA. 1979;242:1985-90.
65. Crawley LM, Marshall PA, Lo B, et al. Strategies for culturally effective end-of-life-care. Ann Intern Med. 2002;136:673-9.
66. Kagawa-Singer M, Blackhall LJ. Negotiating cross-cultural issues at the end of life: "You got to go where he lives". JAMA. 2001;286:2993-3001.
67. Lo B, Ruston D, Kates LW, et al. Discussing religious and spiritual issues at the end of life: a practical guide for physicians. JAMA. 2002;287:749-54.
68. Mobasher M, Aramesh K, Zahedi F, et al. End-of-life care ethical decision making: Shiite scholars view. J Med Ethics Hist Med. 2014;7:2.
69. Jindal SK. Holy water- the last wish. Stories at the End of Life: Final Days. Northbrook, Illinois: American College of Chest Physicians; 2003. pp. 20-3.
70. Manser T, Staender S. Aftermath of an adverse event: supporting health care professionals to meet patient care expectations through open disclosure. Acta Anaesthesiol Scand. 2005;49: 728-34.
71. Gisondi MA, Smith Coggins R, Harter PM, et al. Assessment of resident professionalism using high-fidelity simulation of ethical dilemmas. Acad Emerg Med. 2004;11:931-7.
72. Wayne DB, Muir JC, DaRosa DA. Developing an ethics curriculum for an internal medicine residency program: use of a needs assessment. Teach Learn Med. 2004;16:197-201.
73. Carrese JA, Sugarman J. The inescapable relevance of bioethics for the practicing clinician. Chest. 2006;130:1864-72.
74. Sulmasy DP, Geller G, Levine DM, et al. A randomized trial of ethics education for medical house officers. J Med Ethics. 1993;19:157-63.
75. Self DJ, Olivarez M, Baldwin DC. Clarifying the relationship of medical education and moral development. Acad Med. 1998;73:517-20.
76. Clarke EB, Curtis JT, Luce JM, et al. Quality indicators for end-of-life care in the intensive care unit. Crit Care Med. 2003;31: 2255-62.
77. Naik N, Hameed BMZ, Shetty DK, et al. Legal and Ethical Consideration in Artificial Intelligence in Healthcare: Who Takes Responsibility? Front Surg. 2022;9:862322.
78. Stephenson J. Who offers guidance on use of Artificial Intelligence in medicine. JAMA Health Forum. 2021;2:e212467.
79. Gerke S, Minssen T, Cohen G. Ethical and legal challenges of artificial intelligence-driven healthcare. Artif Intell Healthcare. 2020;295-336.
80. Rodrigues R. Legal and human rights issues of AI: gaps, challenges and vulnerabilities. J Respons Technol. 2020;4:100005.
81. Robin ED, McCauley RF. Cultural lag and the Hippocratic Oath. Lancet. 1995;345:1422-4.
82. Dugdale LS, Siegler M, Rubin DT. Medical professionalism and the doctor-patient relationship. Perspect Biol Med. 2008;51(4):547-53.
83. Peabody FW. The care of the patient. JAMA. 1927:877-82.

Psychosocial Aspects of Respiratory Diseases

CHAPTER 181

Kranti Garg, Nitin Gupta

INTRODUCTION

Diagnosis of a respiratory illness affects the patient's ability to carry on his work and day-to-day activities and could lead to loss of livelihood. Besides physical disability due to respiratory illness, chronicity of the disease burdens the patients with pain, suffering, helplessness, lowered self-esteem, social stigma, and isolation. The added problems of fear of spreading the disease to others, dependency, financial costs, familial and emotional trauma, frequent hospital visits/ admissions, poor health-related quality of life (HRQoL), and premature mortality contribute to psychological distress and development of psychiatric disease. It has been observed that the seriousness of somatic disease is directly proportional to the risk of the patient suffering from mental illness. Failure to identify and manage psychiatric comorbidities increases the patient's probability of suffering from complications and may even turn lethal over a period of time.

The perceptions of the people within the society are of paramount importance in determining the self-perception of the patients with respect to his illness. Diseases known to be associated with societal negativity have a significant negative impact on the psychological makeup of the patient and further add to psychological distress and psychiatric illnesses.

There can also be a coincidental co-occurrence of psychiatric and respiratory illness without any direct etiological cause-and-effect relationship. In such situations, it may become extremely difficult to identify whether the psychological symptoms are because of a coexistent psychiatric disorder, or as a result of the underlying respiratory disease, or both. However, their coexistence complicates the diagnosis and management of an underlying illness and can even alter their course. Patients with poor mental health do not approach specialized healthcare services, increasing the severity and unprecedented burden of the underlying respiratory disease over a period of time. The relationship between respiratory disease and psychiatric illness is thus bidirectional, with one directly impacting the other and vice versa. In a similar vein, substance abuse (harmful use/dependence on nicotine, alcohol, cannabis, etc.) can also have a cause-and-effect relationship with respiratory disease and psychiatric illness.

Psychiatric consultations, in general, are only sought in rare circumstances. Assessment of mental health and HRQoL, and diagnosis of psychiatric comorbidities are not routinely practiced, with majority remaining underestimated, unrecognized, untreated, and grossly neglected.

COMMON LUNG DISEASES

Tuberculosis (TB) is known to be associated with social stigma since decades.[1] Extremes of psychological distress and stressful situations are the known reasons for exacerbations in asthmatic patients.[2] The myths about inhaler use have always clouded the appropriate management of bronchial asthma (BA) and chronic obstructive pulmonary disease (COPD).[2,3] The impact of the diagnosis of a terminal illness like lung cancer on mental health, particularly in relation to physical suffering and end of life decisions, has remained almost always forgotten in evaluation of the patient.[4,5] The physicians have, in one way or the other, accepted them to be a part and parcel of the underlying lung disease. Hardly anything is done about their formal assessment, diagnosis, and specific treatment.

Time and again, the recommendations pertaining to various respiratory diseases have proposed for early identification and treatment of mental illnesses. The Global Initiative for Obstructive Lung Diseases (GOLD) recommends the need to investigate COPD patients for anxiety and depression as a part of multimorbidity care plan. It has been repeatedly stressed that underdiagnosis of psychiatric comorbidities is associated with poor health status and prognosis.[6] Similarly, the Global Initiative for Asthma (GINA) has observed that anxiety and depression are more prevalent in asthmatics and are associated with poor symptom control, increased exacerbations, poor treatment adherence, and poor HRQoL.[2]

Hence, it is important to identify psychosocial issues/ psychological distress and psychiatric comorbidities. It is even more important to differentiate psychosocial issues/psychological distress from a psychiatric illness, as

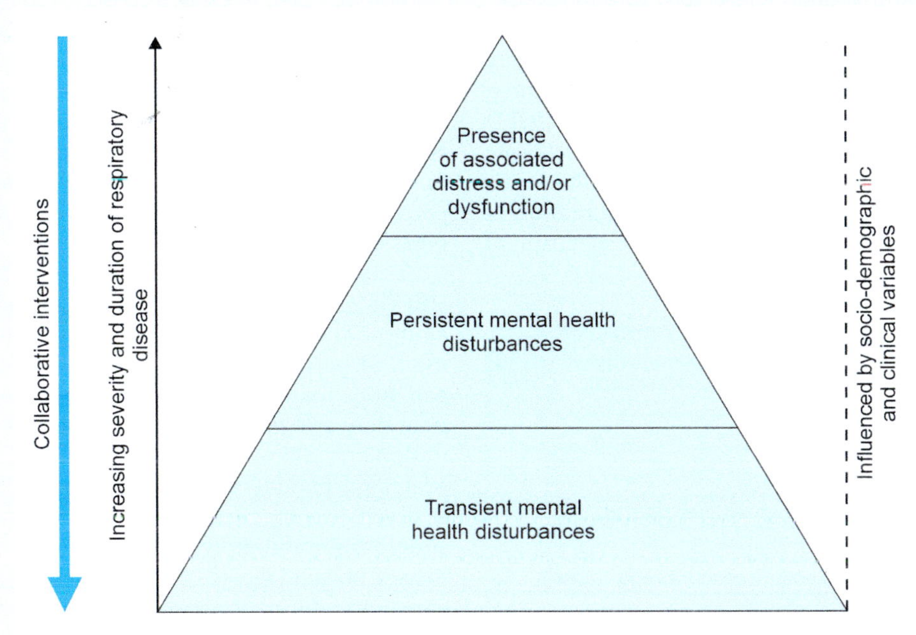

FIG. 1: Pyramid model of psychological suffering in patients with respiratory diseases.

different interventions are required for managing the two different entities. Early management of psychosocial issues/ psychological distress can prevent the development of psychiatric illnesses in majority of the sufferers over a period of time **(Fig. 1)**.

ASSESSMENT OF BASELINE MENTAL HEALTH BY THE PULMONOLOGIST

As a pulmonologist/physician, it may not be possible to reach at a diagnosis of psychiatric disorder or to treat it appropriately. However, being the doctor of first contact, it is necessary to screen the patients for any psychological distress at the initial workup and at regular intervals during follow-ups. Those who screen positive at any point of time should undergo a detailed formal assessment by psychiatrists. The World Health Organization (WHO) defines health as a state of complete physical, mental, and social well-being and not merely the absence of disease or infirmity.[7] It is important to maintain a record of psychological status/comorbidity along with underlying disease and other systemic illnesses.

Procedure for Screening

The casual assessment of the patient for mental well-being should be started from the point of first contact itself. It may provide a baseline of the extent and severity of the psychological distress in relation to the extent and severity of the underlying illness. It is not necessary that the patients suffer mental trauma only after the diagnosis of a respiratory illness is delivered, and its repercussions discussed. Years of physical suffering, compounded by a variety of fears in the minds of the patient and his family, may have affected the mental health already. Breaking the diagnosis may have an additive/multiplicative effect in such a mentally compromised patient.

After the diagnosis of the illness to the patient, a period of 2 weeks should preferably elapse before a formal mental health assessment is carried out. This period will help curtail his immediate responses to the diagnosis, as his mind accepts his disease. However, in patients with signs and symptoms of impending mental catastrophe on casual assessment, immediate screening and psychiatric referral should be practiced.

The various reasons for nonassessment of psychological distress and HRQoL on a routine basis diminish the probability of identification and/ or treatment of psychological comorbidities **(Box 1)**. Most of the times, the clinicians are also not well versed with the screening tools, lack confidence in using them on a routine basis, and prefer referrals, rather than honing their skills. Despite knowing the fact that management of almost all respiratory diseases includes the component of mental health and well-being and that variable illness perception and lower self-efficacy of symptom management can have an impact on treatment adherence in general and use of inhalational therapy and antitubercular treatment (ATT) in particular, they still fail to screen their patients for psychological distress.

The patient should be convinced for a formal psychological screening/workup in the pulmonology clinic itself, and the impact of the same should be discussed in relation to his lung condition and also in totality. The clinician should use various handy and simple-to-use screening questionnaires. General Health Questionnaire-12 (GHQ-12) is one such general questionnaire which can be used in a variety of patients. As of date, certain disease-specific screening tools such as COPD Assessment Test (CAT), Clinical COPD Questionnaire (CCQ), COPD and Asthma Sleep Impact Scale (CASIS), and COPD and Asthma Fatigue Scale (CAFS) can also be used as per individual needs.[6,8,9] A combination of different questionnaires can provide a broader spectrum of the mental afflictions and HRQoL.

BOX 1 Reasons for nonassessment of psychological distress and quality of life on a routine basis.

Patient:
- Variable psychological responses to disease
- Stigma of psychological comorbidity
- Lack of awareness of psychiatric comorbidity and its management
- Lack of time to undergo detailed assessments and comply with follow-ups
- Lack of knowledge of impact of treatment of psychiatric comorbidity on respiratory disease course and outcomes
- Multimorbidities
- Sociodemographic and cultural differences

Clinician:
- Variable perceptions regarding importance of mental health issues
- Lack of time: Huge patient load
- Lack of knowledge of availability of screening tools
- Lack of confidence to administer different tools
- Lack of coordination with the psychiatrist for a multidisciplinary team approach

If screen positive, the need of psychiatric referrals should be highlighted, and every effort made to obtain an expert psychiatric consult. It will complement the recovery of the patient. Patients who screen positive for psychological distress but not diagnosed with any psychiatric disease should be star marked as vulnerable population; considered for psychological counseling and also followed up over a period of time for development of any possible psychiatric illness.

This process of evaluation of mental well-being and HRQoL should be carried out at regular intervals and/or along with routine follow-ups of the patients. The reassessment of psychological distress and HRQoL at follow-ups can help identify treatment responses early and guide treatment strategies. Natural course and progression of the underlying disease should be carefully considered while evaluating patients at follow-ups. The compliance of patients to psychiatric medications/therapy is equally important and should be noted at every visit. Formal reminders, patient diaries, hospital records, online chartings, and the integration of various information, education, and communication (IEC) tools can help simplify this seemingly cumbersome task.

A BRIEF OVERVIEW OF MENTAL HEALTH IN RESPIRATORY DISEASES

The spectrum of respiratory illnesses with psychiatric comorbidities include both acute and chronic diseases **(Table 1)**.

Acute illnesses, if not associated with some long-term sequelae, are usually accompanied by transient changes in mental health and HRQoL. On the other hand, long-term complications/sequelae of acute illnesses, chronic

TABLE 1: Commonly reported psychiatric comorbidities in respiratory diseases and their impact on the disease outcomes.

Respiratory disease	Psychiatric comorbidity	Impact on the disease outcomes
Chronic obstructive pulmonary disease (COPD)	Anxiety, depression, dysthymia, panic disorders, phobia, somatoform disorders, suicidal tendencies	Poor medication adherence, poor HRQoL, poor response to nonpharmacological therapy, increased exacerbations and emergency visits, poor prognosis, higher mortality rates
Bronchial asthma (BA)	Affective disorders, anxiety, depression, panic attacks, phobia, somatoform disorders, suicidal ideation	Worse symptom control, poor medication adherence, poor HRQoL, increased exacerbations and emergency visits, worse asthma outcomes
Tuberculosis (TB)	Adjustment disorder, anxiety, delirium, depression, mood disorders, neurocognitive disorders, obsessive–compulsive disorder, paranoid disorders, personality changes, psychosis, somatoform disorders	Poor medication adherence, increased drug interactions, development of drug resistance, poor prognosis, poor treatment outcomes, higher mortality rates
Diffuse parenchymal lung disease (DPLD)	Anxiety, depression	Poor medication adherence, early dropout from rehabilitation, impaired HRQoL, increased exacerbations, increased hospital admissions and length of hospital stays, premature death
Malignancy	Anxiety, depression	Poor treatment compliance, poor HRQoL, prolonged hospital stay, reduced survival

(HRQoL: health-related quality of life)

respiratory diseases (CRDs), and terminal illnesses exert long-term effects on mental health and, consequently, HRQoL. COVID-19 pandemic has re-taught us the importance of mental well-being. Home isolation, infectiousness of the disease, risk of infection to the close contacts, fear of hospitalization, unpredictable unfavorable outcomes, and death caused mental agony in one and all.[10]

Tuberculosis

Stigma due to TB is a major determinant of poor mental health.[1] Psychiatric illness may develop subsequent to TB infection. Conversely, recipients of psychiatric services are at a higher risk of developing and transmitting TB.[2,4,6,11] Commonly shared risk factors for the development of psychiatric illness and TB (poor socioeconomic status, smoking, substance abuse, HIV, diabetes mellitus, etc.) are the possible reasons.[12,13]

Antitubercular drugs can have significant adverse psychiatric effects. Isoniazid is known to be associated with psychosis. Cycloserine used in drug-resistant TB (DRTB) is known to cause psychiatric illness, and patients usually need drug modification/dose reduction. Ethambutol, ethionamide, and fluoroquinolones have also been reported to cause psychiatric symptoms. Psychopathology is a major barrier to compliance to ATT, leading to multidrug resistance and therapeutic failure. Enzyme inducers like rifampicin may reduce the effective doses of antipsychotics; and enzyme inhibitors like isoniazid may increase the same. The emergence of DRTB complicates the psychological suffering and HRQoL further, due to greater extent of the disease, and enhanced social isolation, longer recovery time, and poor outcomes.[14]

Chronic Respiratory Diseases

Bronchial asthma and inhalational therapy have also remained associated with stigma and lowered self esteem.[2] Patients with CRDs like BA, COPD, diffuse parenchymal lung disease (DPLD), and others have a variable course with frequent exacerbations. The exacerbations cause transient fluctuations in mood and require aggressive management/hospitalizations.[2,6,11] The resultant disabilities, progression of the disease, and fear of an untimely death may be devastating. The "additional" psychological burden and poorer HRQoL during the period of exacerbations make the "daily" psychological distress and HRQoL worse, as there is a downhill course with each and every exacerbation.

Rapid deterioration within a short time frame in terminal illnesses like lung cancer multiplies the psychological distress with every passing day. Concerns regarding end-of-life issues attain priority and need to be addressed meticulously to ease the life of a dying patient.

A variety of other lung conditions like occupational and environmental lung diseases and sleep disorders are also not free of mental afflictions but have almost never received sufficient attention for their psychological comorbidities, neither clinically nor in research settings.

Mental health is an integral part of pulmonary rehabilitation (PR) programs. Evidence for benefit of PR in almost every CRD is generating, and there is an urgent need to emphasize it as a "standard of care" in PR programs. In addition, its routine applicability is also important to prevent compromise of various nonpharmacological therapies like smoking cessation, weight reduction, sleep hygiene, and occupational rehabilitation.

MULTIMORBIDITIES

A variety of other comorbidities and systemic manifestations related/unrelated to the primary illness add to the physical suffering, morbidity, and mortality, thus complicating the mental health issues and HRQoL.

VARIABLE PATIENT RESPONSES AND COPING MECHANISMS

The consequences of any illness on mental health in different individuals are never identical. A variety of responses are generated, with some adapting to the illness in a short period of time while others feeling completely devastated. Social stigma associated with the underlying disease, impaired physical functioning, fear of morbidity and mortality with debilitating and progressive diseases, social blunting, variety of responses generated by the family and society, age, gender, sociodemographics, educational, financial and cultural differences, addictions and substance abuse, etc., may all complicate the behavioral reactions of an individual in a given situation **(Box 2)**.

PSYCHOLOGICAL DISTRESS AND CAREGIVERS

Illness of the patients affects the psychosocial status and HRQoL of their otherwise healthy caregivers too.[15-17] The burden has all the more remained undiagnosed and ever neglected. Coexistence of psychological dysfunction in both the patient and his/her caregiver significantly worsens the functioning of both of them in terms of their personal relationships, social roles, and professional living and has a negative impact on the recovery of the patient. It becomes

BOX 2 **Factors affecting the presence and severity of psychiatric comorbidity.**

- Personality of the patient and general well-being
- Sociodemographics: Age, gender, residence, socioeconomic status, education, employment, family size, available social support mechanisms, presence/absence of disease in the family members
- Respiratory disease related: Duration, severity, cost and type of treatment, impairment and disability due to disease, natural course of the illness, expected outcomes
- Other comorbidities: Number and type
- Addiction and/or substance abuse

demanding in terms of healthcare utilization as continuous psychological care is additionally required for caregivers as well.

SCREENING TOOLS FOR STIGMA AND SELF-ESTEEM, PSYCHOLOGICAL DISTRESS, AND HRQoL

A variety of simple and easy-to-administer screening tools are available for the use of the treating physician or ancillary staff **(Box 3)**.

Screening Tools for Stigma and Self-esteem

- *28-item stigma related scale:* It is a brief scale which assesses patients on three domains: Disclosure, discrimination, and positive aspects. Each response is recorded on a Likert scale.[18]
- *Rosenberg's self-esteem scale:* It is a self-report instrument and consists of 10 questions regarding self-esteem. Response is marked on a Likert scale.[19]
- *Stigma-related social problem scale (SSPS):* It includes items on a broad range of social activities. The responses are aggregated into two domains: Distress (10 items) and avoidance (10 items). Item responses are finally aggregated into summated scale scores.[20]

BOX 3 **Tools for stigma and self-esteem, psychological distress, and health-related quality of life (HRQoL).***

- *Screening tools for stigma and self-esteem*:
  - 28-item stigma-related scale
  - Rosenberg self-esteem scale
  - Stigma-related social problem scale (SSPS)
- *Screening tools for psychological distress*:
  - General Health questionnaire (GHQ)
  - Patient Distress Thermometer (PDT)
  - Thakur's Death Anxiety scale
  - Depression, Anxiety and Stress Scale-21 items (DASS-21)
  - Rotterdam Symptom Check-List (RSCL)
  - Coping Strategy Check-List (CSCL)
  - The 4-item Perceived Stress Scale (PSS-4)
- *Screening tools for HRQoL*:
  - COPD Assessment Tool (CAT)
  - Clinical COPD Questionnaire (CCQ)
  - St. George's Respiratory Questionnaire (SGRQ)
  - COPD and Asthma Sleep Impact Scale (CASIS)
  - Functional Performance Inventory-Short Form (FPI-SF)
  - COPD and Asthma Fatigue Scale (CAFS)
  - World Health Organization Quality of Life Instrument (WHO-QOL)

*These are some of the commonly used tools. For a more comprehensive list, the reader is advised to refer to scholarly review articles on this subject.

Screening Tools for Psychological Distress

- *GHQ:* This is a measure of the current mental health. It was originally developed as a 60-item instrument. Presently, shortened versions of the questionnaire like GHQ-30, GHQ-28, GHQ-20, and GHQ-12 are available. The scale evaluates whether the respondent has experienced a particular symptom or behavior recently. GHQ-12 Hindi version is a 12-item scale, translated in Hindi, with each item rated on a four-point scale (less than usual, no more than usual, rather more than usual, or much more than usual). Bimodal (0-0-1-1) and Likert scoring styles (0-1-2-3) are the most common scoring methods. GHQ-12 is brief, simple, and easy to complete, and its application in research settings as a screening tool is well documented in patients of COPD, BA, DPLD, lung cancer, COVID-19, and general population.[8,17,21,22] It has been translated into other different local languages also.
- *Patient Distress Thermometer (PDT):* This is a modified visual analog scale that resembles a thermometer with a range from 0 (no distress) to 10 (extreme distress). It also contains an accompanying list of 34 problems grouped into five categories (practical, family, emotional, spiritual/religious, and physical) and has been used in patients of COPD, DPLD, lung cancer, and COVID-19.[8,17,22]
- *Thakur's Death Anxiety Scale:* This scale was developed in India, as a self-administered scale to assess death-related fear. The scale consists of 16 items: 11 positively worded and 5 negatively worded. The positive worded items are to be rated on a five-point scale: Quite true (5), True (4), Undecided (3), False (2), and Quite False (1). For the negative worded items, a reverse scoring pattern is followed. The higher the score, the greater the death anxiety. This scale has been used in patients of lung cancer and TB.[17,23]
- *Depression, Anxiety and Stress Scale-21 items (DASS-21):* This scale consists of three groups of seven questions. Each of the three groups measures the degree of depression, anxiety, and stress. For depression, the values 0–9 are normal, 10–13 indicative of mild forms, 14–20 low forms, and ≥21 serious forms of depression. For anxiety, the values 0–7 are normal, 8–9 indicative of mild forms, 10–14 low forms, and ≥15 serious forms of anxiety. Similarly, 0–14 is scored as normal, 15–18 mild, 19–25 low, and ≥26 as serious forms of stress. For convenience, mild and low forms of mental disorders are considered as one entity. This scale has found use in patients of COPD, DPLD, and lung cancer.[17,22]
- *Rotterdam Symptom Checklist (RSCL):* The RSCL was originally developed to measure symptoms reported by cancer patients participating in clinical research. Later,

it proved applicable in monitoring the levels of patients' anxiety and depression and reflects the presence of psychological illness. Two highly reliable subscales of RSCL assess psychological and physical distress. A higher score indicates higher distress. The scale finds application in patients of lung cancer.[17]

- *Coping Strategy Check-List (CSCL):* It is a self-administered checklist, comprising 36 coping strategies used to deal with stressful situations. Scores range from 0 to 36, with higher scores indicating greater use of coping strategies. A factor analysis of these strategies results in five factors: Denial, internalization, externalization, emotional outlet, and anger coping. The scale has been applied in patients of COPD, DPLD, lung cancer, and COVID-19.[17,22]
- *The 4-item Perceived Stress Scale (PSS-4):* This scale is a validated measure of the degree to which situations in a person's life are perceived as stressful. It is scored from 0 to 16. Higher scores are indicative of higher degrees of stress. It has been used in caregivers of asthmatic children in the past.[24]

Screening Tools for HRQoL

- *CAT:* This consists of eight items that reflect most bothersome health-related symptoms and activity limitations in patients of COPD: Cough, phlegm, chest tightness, breathlessness on walking uphill or one flight of stairs, any activity limitation at home, confidence leaving home, sleep, and energy. The scale of each item ranges from 0 to 5 points and in total ranges from 0 to 40 with higher scores indicating poor health status. It has been recommended by GOLD for evaluation of COPD patients and to guide further management.[6]
- *CCQ:* This is composed of 10 items distributed in 3 domains (symptom, functional, and mental states) assessed by a seven-point scale from 0 to 6, directing the best and worst conditions. The total score is calculated by summing the scores of questions applied and dividing it by a number of questions. It has also found mention for use in COPD patients in GOLD recommendations.[6]
- *St George's Respiratory Questionnaire (SGRQ):* This has 50 items distributed into 3 categories: Symptoms, activity, and impact, with 76 weighted responses. The highest possible weight is 100, the lowest being 0. Empirically derived weight of each item is noted, and a total score is calculated. The scale has been used for a variety of respiratory illnesses like COPD, BA, and DPLD.[6,8,22,25]
- *CASIS:* This is a seven-item score to evaluate sleep impairment. Response ranges from 1 = Never to 5 = very often. The item scores are summed together to arrive at a total raw score which is then transformed linearly to a 0–100 total scale score. The scale finds use in patients of COPD and BA.[8,9,26]
- *Functional Performance Inventory-Short Form (FPI-SF):* It is a 32-item self-administered questionnaire to assess the level of difficulty respondents have with physical activities across 6 domains: Body care (5 items), maintaining household (8 items), physical exercise (5 items), recreation (5 items), spiritual activities (4 items), and social interaction (5 items). For each item, respondents are asked to rate how difficult the activity is for them to perform on a three-point scale as no difficulty (Score 3), some difficulty (Score 2), and much difficulty (Score 1). Total score is mean across six domains. It has been used in the past in COPD patients.[8,27]
- *CAFS:* Items on fatigue, associated with respiratory disease and breathing problems, are included in 12-item CAFS. Responses range from 1 = never to 5 = very often. CAFS raw scores are then linearly transformed to 0–100 total scale score with higher scores indicating greater fatigue. The recall time period for the measure is taken as previous week. The scale is used in patients of COPD and BA.[8,28]
- *World Health Organization Quality of Life Instrument (WHO-QOL):* WHO-QOL-100 quality of life assessment was developed by the WHO-QOL Group, who aimed to devise a tool with wider applicability. 100 items were included in the WHO-QOL-100 Field Trial Version. These included four domains: Physical health, psychological health, social relationships, and environment health. WHO-QOL-BREF contains a total of 26 questions. Two items are from overall quality of life and general health facet. One item from each of the 24 facets of the WHO-QOL-100 is included along with. WHO-QOL-BREF has been used in the patients of COPD, BA, DPLD, and lung cancer.[17,22,29]

Other lesser used screening tools in respiratory practice for assessment of psychological distress and HRQoL include Hopkins Symptom Checklist, Modified Distress Thermometer, Chronic Respiratory Disease Questionnaire, King's Brief Interstitial Lung Disease Questionnaire, Living with Asthma Questionnaire, Wisconsin Quality of Life Index, etc.

In addition to the above standardized tools, self-structured questionnaires can also be used to evaluate a particular domain/disease under consideration; however, validity and reliability need to be established before administration.

Use of Multiple Tools in Combinations

The questionnaires for assessment of psychological distress and HRQoL can be used individually, or in different combinations, depending on the issues under consideration. A particular domain of mental well-being and HRQoL can also be evaluated individually or in combination, on a case-to-case basis. Combined use of two or more tools may be more representative of the wider spectrum of mental health and HRQoL.[8,17,22]

It has also been seen in the past that a questionnaire, developed for a particular illness, when tried and used for another disease, found a wider applicability. This potential of each tool should be thoroughly studied and exploited to the fullest for a variety of respiratory illnesses and for the evaluation of a multimorbid patient.

Administration of Screening Tools

The tools can be self-administered and/or physician-administered. Online questionnaires can be shared with the patients in certain conditions where physical contact with the patient is not possible; however, they may be lesser effective than in-person interviews.

It is also assumed that the physician-administered scales are better than self-administered tools for screening purposes. However, it needs to be kept in mind that the information gathered by physician-administered scales may not always be better than self-administered tools because of inherent differences in subjective and objective reporting, as has been proven through the emic versus etic anthropological approach.

Patient-reported Outcome Measures (PROMs)

These have been extensively used for COPD and BA patients and include Asthma Quality of Life Questionnaire (AQLQ), Mini-AQLQ, Rhinasthma, SF-36 questionnaire, MacGill COPD Quality of Life questionnaire, Capacity of Daily Living during the Morning Questionnaire, Living with COPD questionnaire, etc.[30,31] However, scores are less dependable in individuals with low literacy skills, learning disabilities, etc. They can also be administered under supervision, or directly by an interviewer, and can yield reliable scores.

Screening Tools for Caregivers

Majority of the tools used for the assessment of patients can be administered to evaluate caregivers too. In the past, caregiver assessment has received attention for COPD, BA, lung cancer, and COVID-19, with the use of different questionnaires, individually and in combinations. Apparently, healthy caregivers of patients with CRDs and COVID-19 have reported significant psychological distress when measured with discrete tools.[16,17,24] This completely unknown burden of mental ill health needs attention to ensure the well-being of patients, their families, and the society.

PULMONOLOGIST VERSUS PSYCHIATRIST

It is pertinent to mention that various tools listed above are for screening purposes only. If screen positive, referral to a psychiatrist for detailed evaluation and treatment is important after baseline counseling by the clinician himself. The clinician may find it difficult to convince the patients for an expert opinion because of poor understanding of mental well-being. Hence, short but dedicated counseling sessions as a part of every routine visit to the clinician, focusing on mental health, may be imparted to patients/caregivers awaiting/declining psychiatrist intervention. This will address their worries about the disease and infuse a feeling of well-being.

Respiratory physicians should always understand that they cannot replace a psychiatrist. Detailed evaluation, diagnosis, and definitive treatment are essential for management of comorbid psychiatric illnesses and hence should be routinely practiced.

Role of Ancillary Staff

Services of ancillary staff, under supervision of respiratory and mental health specialists, can be taken for dedicated screening and counseling sessions. They can help in structured need assessment and clinical reviews, psychoeducation, health promotion, treatment adherence, and individualized rehabilitation strategies. They can also help in establishing networks with self-help groups and community agencies to address psychosocial issues and bring stigma and discrimination to an end.[32] Their sympathetic attitude can help maintain the continuity of psychosocial support mechanisms at every routine visit even in busy OPDs in patients awaiting/declining expert psychiatrist intervention. Combined and collaborative community-based care plus facility-based care has been shown to yield promising results when implemented as an initial service in resource-poor settings and is sustainable in the long term.

Role of Family, Society, and Healthcare Professionals

Sustained family and social support networking is required at every point in the management cascade. Those screening negative and having sound mental health may also need continuous care and concern for their mental health as they are vulnerable and can deteriorate at any point of time. The empathy of the clinician, staff, and the social circle around is particularly important, in view of the increased risk of development of psychological comorbidities.

Role of Tele-health Interventions

Tele-health interventions can help in managing the physical and mental illness. Tele-monitoring and tele-rehabilitation have been found to improve the patient's underlying respiratory illness, his health status, and HRQoL.[33] They seem more beneficial when compared with physical doctor–patient communication, as they are cost-effective, with services being delivered at the patient's doorstep, in much lesser time. However, the important component of physical contact with the physician is missing, and its importance cannot be set aside. Head-to-head studies are required to establish the superiority/inferiority over physical consultations.

INDIAN SCENARIO

Psychiatric consultations have always remained a taboo in the Indian population. Despite increasing awareness regarding mental health issues in the recent past, there is a

BOX 4 Multidisciplinary approach.

- Policies to screen and treat anxiety, depression, and other psychiatric illnesses
- Integration of mental health services with lung health
- Psychiatrist as a team member for management of patients with chronic respiratory illnesses
- Client-oriented comprehensive efforts to improve patient's HRQoL
- Development of simple, quick, and easy-to-use patient-centered discrete screening tools
- Additional research on risk factors leading to psychiatric distress/illnesses
- Longitudinal studies for determining the interplay of psychological parameters with disease-related variables
- Inclusion of chronic respiratory illnesses in National Mental Health Program

huge gap between the actual disease burden, its identification, and treatment. Mental health awareness programs should be encouraged at the grassroots level to enhance public knowledge and improve day-to-day practices. The physicians at primary contact should be sensitized and taught to screen patients for psychological distress.[34] Strong family and social support system existent in India should be tapped fully to provide the required psychological support.

There is an urgent need for the development of simple, quick, and easy-to-use patient-centered discrete screening tools, which can be applied in routine OPDs by the physicians and ancillary staff. In addition, on a case-to-case basis, a multidisciplinary approach, with the psychiatrist being an integral part of the team, is required for prevention, early detection, and effective treatment of the psychological illnesses in the long run (**Box 4**).

SUMMARY

Psychological sufferings are associated with significant public health implications in terms of poor HRQoL and direct/indirect cost of care. Knowledge and education regarding mental health is a must, for the patient, his care-giver, and the treating physician. Healthcare professionals should be vigilant to identify psychological comorbidities. Simple, quick, and easy-to-use screening tools should be used at every visit as a routine and simultaneous psychiatric consultations sought whenever required. To ease the huge unforeseen burden of psychological comorbidities, task sharing with ancillary staff, community health workers, self-help groups, ex-service users, and their family members should be performed.[32] Holistic management plans with clear-cut recommendations for mental health should be formulated, upscaled, and integrated with public health programs related to respiratory health and delivered to one and all.

REFERENCES

1. Strategy to End Stigma and Discrimination Associated with Tuberculosis: Ministry of Health and Family Welfare [Internet]. [cited 2023 Jul 19]. Available from: https://tbcindia.gov.in/showfile.php?lid=3588
2. 2024 GINA Main Report - Global Initiative for Asthma - GINA [Internet]. [cited 2024 Nov 4]. Available from: https://ginasthma.org/wp-content/uploads/2024/05/GINA-2024-Strategy-Report-24_05_22_WMS.pdf
3. Monteiro C, Maricoto T, Prazeres F, et al. Determining factors associated with inhaled therapy adherence on asthma and COPD: A systematic review and meta-analysis of the global literature. Respir Med. 2022;191:106724.
4. Chambers SK, Dunn J, Occhipinti S, et al. A systematic review of the impact of stigma and nihilism on lung cancer outcomes. BMC Cancer. 2012;12.
5. Ettinger DS, Wood DE, Aisner DL, et al. NCCN Guidelines® Insights: Non-Small Cell Lung Cancer, Version 2.2023. J Natl Compr Canc Netw. 2023;21(4):340-50.
6. 2024 GOLD Report - Global Initiative for Chronic Obstructive Lung Disease - GOLD [Internet]. [cited 2024 Nov 4]. Available from: https://goldcopd.org/2024-gold-report/
7. Constitution of the World Health Organization [Internet]. [cited 2024 Nov 4]. Available from: https://www.who.int/about/governance/constitution
8. Gupta A, Garg K, Chopra V, et al. Assessment of health status and its correlation with lung function in patients with chronic obstructive pulmonary disease: a study from a tertiary care center in north India. Monaldi Arch Chest Dis. 2023;7;94(1).
9. Garrow AP, Yorke J, Khan N, et al. Systematic literature review of patient-reported outcome measures used in assessment and measurement of sleep disorders in chronic obstructive pulmonary disease. Int J Chron Obstruct Pulmon Dis. 2015;9;10:293-307.
10. Krishnamoorthy Y, Nagarajan R, Saya GK, et al. Prevalence of psychological morbidities among general population, healthcare workers and COVID-19 patients amidst the COVID-19 pandemic: A systematic review and meta-analysis. Psychiatry Res. 2020;293:113382.
11. Singh S, Sharma B, Bairwa M, et al. Management of interstitial lung diseases: A consensus statement of the Indian Chest Society (ICS) and National College of Chest Physicians (NCCP). Lung India. 2020;37(4):359-78.
12. National framework for joint TB diabetes: Central TB Division [Internet]. [cited 2024 Nov 4]. Available from: https://mohfw.gov.in/sites/default/files/National%20Framework%20for%20Joint%20TB-Diabetes%20Collaborative%20Activities_1.pdf
13. Lara-Espinosa JV, Hernández-Pando R, Lara-Espinosa JV, et al. Psychiatric Problems in Pulmonary Tuberculosis: Depression and Anxiety. J Tuberc Res [Internet]. 2021;9(1):31-50.
14. Chapter 47. Antimycobacterial Drugs | Katzung & Trevor's Pharmacology: Examination & Board Review, 10e | AccessPharmacy | McGraw Hill Medical [Internet]. [cited 2023

Jul 25]. Available from: https://accesspharmacy.mhmedical.com/Content.aspx?bookId=514§ionId=41817566

15. Fana TE, Sotana L, Tong KW. Exploring the experiences of family caregivers with people with drug-resistant tuberculosis. Cogent Social Sciences. 2021;7(1).
16. Garg RK, Garg K, Chopra V, et al. Psychosocial Impact of Pandemic and State Imposed Lockdown on Caregivers of Patients Presenting with Respiratory Complaints Mimicking COVID-19: A Short-term Follow-up Study. J Clin of Diagn Res. 2022;16(10):LC34-LC39.
17. Dutta K, Saini V, Gupta N, et al. Psychological impact of lung cancer: A cross-sectional study. Indian J Soc Psychiatry [Internet]. 2022;38(3):257-63.
18. King M, Dinos S, Shaw J, et al. The Stigma Scale: development of a standardised measure of the stigma of mental illness. Br J Psychiatry. 2007;190:248-54.
19. Valero-Moreno S, Montoya-Castilla I, Pérez-Marín M. Family styles and quality of life in adolescents with bronchial asthma: The important role of self-esteem and perceived threat of the disease. Pediatr Pulmonol. 2023;14;58(1):178-86.
20. Ohlsson-Nevo E, Karlsson J. Impact of health-related stigma on psychosocial functioning in the general population: Construct validity and Swedish reference data for the Stigma-related Social Problems scale (SSP). Res Nurs Health. 2019;42(1):72–81.
21. Garg RK, Garg K, Gupta N, et al. COVID-19 Vaccine Behaviour among People Attending a Tertiary Care Centre, Punjab, India J Clin of Diagn Res. 2022;16(3):LC26-LC32.
22. Rajpoot A, Garg K, Saini V, et al. Psychological morbidity in interstitial lung disease: a study from India. Monaldi Arch Chest Dis. 2020;90(4).
23. Singh A, Singh UP. Death Anxiety among TB Patients and Normal Persons. Indian Journal of Human Relations. 2019;53(1):132-6.
24. Kopel LS, Petty CR, Gaffin JM, et al. Caregiver stress among inner-city school children with asthma. J Allergy Clin Immunol Pract. 2017;5(4):1132-1134.e3.
25. Apfelbacher C, Paudyal P, Bülbül A, et al. Measurement properties of asthma-specific quality-of-life measures: protocol for a systematic review. Syst Rev. 2014;3:83.
26. Pokrzywinski RF, Meads DM, McKenna SP, et al. Development and psychometric assessment of the COPD and Asthma Sleep Impact Scale (CASIS). Health Qual Life Outcomes. 2009;7.
27. Leidy NK, Hamilton A, Becker K. Assessing patient report of function: content validity of the Functional Performance Inventory-Short Form (FPI-SF) in patients with chronic obstructive pulmonary disease (COPD). Int J Chron Obstruct Pulmon Dis. 2012;7:543-54.
28. Revicki DA, Meads DM, McKenna SP, et al. COPD and Asthma Fatigue Scale (CAFS): Development and Psychometric Assessment. Health Outcomes Res Med. 2010;1;1(1):e5-16.
29. Ozoh OB, Aderibigbe SA, Ayuk AC, et al. Health-related quality of life in asthma measured by the World Health Organization brief questionnaire (WHO-BREF) and the effect of concomitant allergic rhinitis-A population-based study. Clin Respir J. 2023.
30. Worth A, Hammersley V, Knibb R, et al. Patient-reported outcome measures for asthma: a systematic review. NPJ Prim Care Respir Med. 2014;24:14020.
31. Jahagirdar D, Kroll T, Ritchie K, et al. Patient-reported outcome measures for chronic obstructive pulmonary disease: the exclusion of people with low literacy skills and learning disabilities. Patient. 2013;6(1):11-21.
32. Lancet Global Mental Health Group; Chisholm D, Flisher AJ, Lund C, Patel V, Saxena S, Thornicroft G, Tomlinson M. Scale up services for mental disorders: a call for action. Lancet. 2007;370(9594):1241-52.
33. Honkoop P, Usmani O, Bonini M. The Current and Future Role of Technology in Respiratory Care. Pulm Ther. 2022;8(2):167-79.
34. Gaiha SM, Salisbury TT, Koschorke M, et al. Stigma associated with mental health problems among young people in India: a systematic review of magnitude, manifestations and recommendations. BMC Psychiatry. 2020;20(1):538.

End-of-Life Care

CHAPTER 182

Jenifer Jeba S, Jyothsna Kuriakose

INTRODUCTION

The National Institute for Health and Care Excellence (NICE) defines "adults approaching end of life"[1] as those in the final weeks and months of life, although for people with some conditions, this could be months or years. This includes people with:

- Advanced, progressive, incurable conditions
- General frailty and coexisting conditions that mean they are at an increased risk of dying within the next 12 months
- Existing conditions if they are at risk of dying from a sudden acute crisis in their condition
- Life-threatening acute conditions caused by sudden catastrophic events

End-of-life (EoL) care is both an art and science of caring for people with progressive incurable illnesses, to help them live as well as possible until they die, by reducing suffering and distress. The process of care extends beyond the dying person to include the family members or caregivers. It upholds the right of every individual for a dignified death. EoL care is not synonymous with palliative care.

In an era where the healthcare system has medicalized life, dying well has become a challenge. A metasystematic review exploring the components of a good death articulated 11 themes: (1) Relief from pain and other physical symptoms; (2) effective communication and relationship with healthcare providers, (3) performance of cultural, religious, or other spiritual rituals; (4) relief from emotional distress; (5) autonomy with regard to treatment-related decision-making; (6) dying in the preferred place; (7) life not being prolonged unnecessarily; (8) awareness of the deep significance of what is happening; (9) emotional support from family and friends; (10) not being a burden on anyone; and (11) the right to terminate one's life.[2] However, social and cultural norms exert undue influence over the conceptions of good or bad death and any attempt to draft a universal definition for good death would be challenging.[2,3] Good-quality palliative and EoL care should become an integral part of cardiopulmonary medicine.[4]

CHALLENGES WITH PROGNOSTICATION

Identifying EoL is a challenge and requires the clinical skill of prognostication. Transition into this phase may be very acute or subtle, depending on the disease, and varies for malignant and nonmalignant diseases **(Fig. 1)**. The illness trajectory in cancer is often a predictable decline until death, whereas in chronic respiratory diseases, such as chronic obstructive pulmonary disease (COPD), the clinical course is usually a slow deterioration, punctuated by dramatic exacerbations, that often ends in unexpected death. Moreover, in cancer, there is maintenance of good functional status until a short period, with a predictable decline in the last weeks or months of life.[5] The important barrier that precludes provision of good EoL care is the difficulty involved with prognosticating and recognizing dying.

Prognostication tools added with clinical experience can help with better prognostication. The holistic needs of patients with chronic lung diseases should be considered

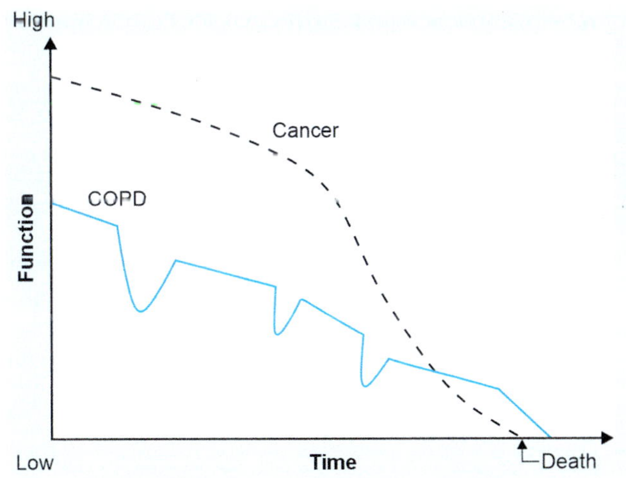

FIG. 1: Difference in illness trajectory in malignancy and COPD.
(COPD: chronic obstructive pulmonary disease)

throughout the disease trajectory. Specific triggers such as unexpected or repeated hospital admissions and visits to the emergency department should be used as points to initiate conversations with the patient and relatives to better understand their values, goals, extent of medical care, and wishes around the place of care and death in case of deterioration. Even when recovery or prognosis is uncertain, it is better to discuss the uncertainty rather than give false hope. Often, the family is able to understand this, develop trust, and perceive it as strength in the doctor–patient relationship. Despite the existing barriers and difficulties, it is crucial for the healthcare team to identify the EoL phase and adopt a sensitive and structured approach of care.

PRINCIPLES OF BEST CARE FOR THE DYING PERSON

The International Collaborative for Best Care for the Dying Person has formulated 10 key evidence-based principles for the care of the dying person that transcend international and cultural boundaries and apply regardless of the place of care.[6,7]

1. Recognition that the person is in the last few days and hours of life should be made by the multidisciplinary team (ideally a doctor and a nurse) and documented by a senior healthcare professional responsible for the person's care.
2. Communication of the recognition of dying should be shared with the person where possible and deemed appropriate and with those important to them.
3. The dying person and those important to them (relative, carer, or advocate) should have the opportunity to discuss their wishes, concerns, feelings, faith, beliefs, and values.
4. Anticipatory prescribing should be available for symptoms that can be expected.
5. All clinical interventions are reviewed in the best interests of the individual person.
6. There should be a review of hydration needs, including the commencement, continuation, or cessation of clinically assisted (artificial) hydration.
7. There should be a review of nutrition needs, including the commencement, continuation, or cessation of clinically assisted (artificial) nutrition.
8. There should be a full discussion of the plan of care with the dying person, where possible and deemed appropriate, and with those important to them.
9. There should be regular reassessments of the dying person at least every 4 hours and review by the multidisciplinary team at least every 48 hours.
10. Care for the dying person and those important to them immediately after death is dignified and respectful.

These principles underpinned by a robust quality improvement process can be used as a framework for setting up local, institutional, and national policies for EoL care.

STEPS OF END-OF-LIFE CARE PROCESS

In the integrated care plan for the dying brought out jointly by the Indian Society of Critical Care Medicine and the Indian Association of Palliative Care,[8] a six-step process has been described for guiding clinicians in providing quality EoL care:

1. *Identify*: "When to initiate", "whom to initiate"
2. *Assess*: Assessment of physical symptoms and distress, nonphysical issues, and communication needs
3. *Plan*: Site of care, review existing care protocol/medication chart and stop unnecessary interventions/medications/investigations, write anticipatory prescription, communication, consensus, and consent
4. *Provide*: Access to essential medication for EoL symptom control, provision of dedicated space and staff for round-the-clock care, attend to the special care needs of the patient and the family, afterdeath care, and bereavement support
5. *Reassess*: Thorough ongoing review and reassessment, ensure adequate symptom control, and initiate prompt action as per variance of symptoms
6. Reflect the care process and identify the gaps.

RECOGNITION OF THE DYING PROCESS

Identifying those who are at the EoL is the first and foremost step for initiation of the care process. An easy and quick way to prognosticate is using clinical prediction of survival which includes a temporal approach (How long will the patient live?), a probabilistic approach (What is the approximate probability that this patient will be alive for six months?), and the surprise question ("Would I be surprised if this patient died in 12 months?").

Diagnosing an actively dying patient is a clinical skill. Various signs have been identified as predictors of the last hours or days of life encompassing changes related to breathing, general condition, skin, intake of food/fluids, and consciousness/cognition **(Table 1)**. Vital signs should not be overly relied upon for predicting impending death and can be only supplemental to the other signs. It has also been demonstrated that laboratory variables including hypoalbuminemia and C-reactive protein are indicators of poor survival. The phase angle, a marker of cellular membrane integrity and hydration, is one of the objective and physiological measurements having prognostic significance. It can range from 4 to 9 in healthy individuals and is known to be lower in patients with shorter survival times. It is assessed by bioelectric impedance measurement. Despite these signs and scores, it is imperative for clinicians to bear in mind that around 1 in 10 might experience sudden or unexpected deterioration and death.[9]

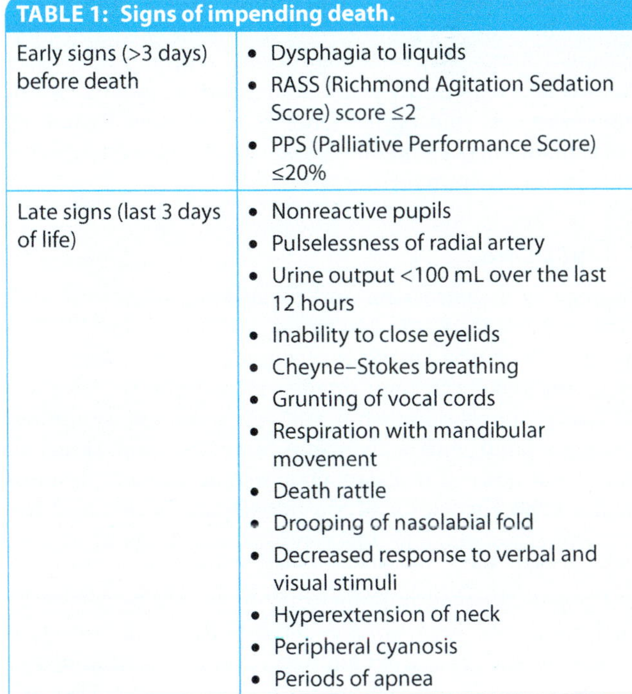

TABLE 1: Signs of impending death.

Early signs (>3 days) before death	• Dysphagia to liquids • RASS (Richmond Agitation Sedation Score) score ≤2 • PPS (Palliative Performance Score) ≤20%
Late signs (last 3 days of life)	• Nonreactive pupils • Pulselessness of radial artery • Urine output <100 mL over the last 12 hours • Inability to close eyelids • Cheyne–Stokes breathing • Grunting of vocal cords • Respiration with mandibular movement • Death rattle • Drooping of nasolabial fold • Decreased response to verbal and visual stimuli • Hyperextension of neck • Peripheral cyanosis • Periods of apnea

COMMON SYMPTOMS AT END-OF-LIFE

One of the essential components in EoL care is achieving maximal symptom control. The most common physical symptoms at the EoL include pain, breathlessness, agitation, nausea and vomiting, constipation, and noisy breathing. Pain, breathlessness, and fatigue are present in more than 50% of patients with end-stage respiratory disease.[10] Anxiety and depression are more common among COPD patients than among patients with lung cancer, 90% versus 52%, respectively.[11] Coexisting depression may play a significant role in EoL decisions and treatment preferences for life-sustaining therapies.[12]

Pain

The prevalence of pain among lung cancer patients attending the outpatient services and those using palliative care services is 27% and 76%, respectively. The pain may relate to cancer (73%) or to treatment (11%); nociceptive in the majority, although 30%, can have neuropathic pain.[13] Pain is often ignored and remains an uncontrolled symptom, as many physicians focus on ordering an array of investigations and making diagnosis and fail to prescribe analgesics at the appropriate dose and frequency. Various aspects relating to pain should be addressed, to ensure "total pain" relief **(Fig. 2)**. Comprehensive pain evaluation, routine assessment, appropriate analgesic prescription, and titration until adequate pain relief are requisites for optimal pain management.[14] Patients who are unconscious should be actively screened for pain. Presence of changes in facial expressions (fully tightened, grimacing), vocalization (sighing, moaning, crying out), tachycardia, and changes in breathing patterns can indicate pain.

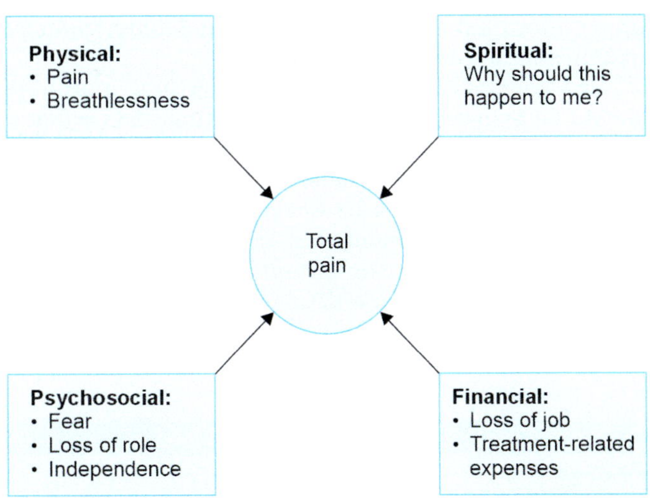

FIG. 2: Concept of total pain.

BOX 1 WHO analgesic ladder with sample prescriptions.

Step 1 (mild pain: nonopioid ± adjuvant)
- Tab Diclofenac sodium 50 mg tid
- Tab Ranitidine 150 mg bd
- (OR Tab Paracetamol 1 gm qid)

Step 2 (moderate pain: weak opioid ± nonopioid ± adjuvant)
- Cap Tramadol 50–100 mg Q6–8H and prn
- Tab Domperidone 10 mg tid
- Tab Bisacodyl 5 mg HSOD

Step 3 (severe pain: strong opioid ± nonopioid ± adjuvant)
- Tab Morphine IR 5–10 mg Q4H and prn (or Tab Morphine SR 10 mg bd)
- Titrate dose upward as needed based on the pain relief)
- Tab Domperidone 10 mg tid
- Tab Bisacodyl 10 mg HSOD

The World Health Organization (WHO) cancer unit has developed simple analgesic prescribing guidelines,[15] which constitute the gold standard in cancer pain management and an effective method to ensure rational titration of analgesia and effective pain relief in nearly 90%.[16] Patients and families can be assured that pain can be relieved safely and effectively in the majority. The WHO analgesic ladder recommends use of analgesics at the right dose, at the right time (round the clock), at the right frequency, and by the right route (oral) background pain. The oral route should be preferred as it is convenient, noninvasive, and cost-effective. The choice of analgesia should be based on the mechanism of pain, severity in a step wise fashion and not on the stage of disease **(Box 1)**. To prevent side effects of opioids, prophylactic antiemetics and laxatives should be prescribed. Nonsteroidal anti-inflammatory drugs (NSAIDs) should be avoided in patients with significant upper intestinal tract bleeding, renal failure, platelet dysfunction, and on anticoagulants.[17]

The general guidelines for starting oral morphine should be followed **(Box 2)**. Opioids should be used at a reduced dose in the elderly and at a reduced frequency in those with renal/hepatic failure. Adjuvants are drugs which are not primarily analgesics but produce analgesic effect in some painful conditions (e.g., corticosteroids, tricyclic antidepressants, anticonvulsants, bisphosphonates). These can be combined with any of the steps, especially in neuropathic pain, spinal cord compression, and bone metastasis. Palliative radiotherapy can also provide pain relief in painful bone metastasis. In difficult pain, appropriate referral for expert opinion should be obtained. An audit on pain assessment and analgesics prescription for cancer patients in a respiratory ward at a tertiary hospital in South India revealed that educational interventions (teaching, provision of pocket guidelines, and use of posters) improved analgesic prescription patterns.[18]

BOX 2 Oral morphine prescribing guidelines.

If opioid naive:
- Start with Tab Morphine IR 5 mg q4h or Tab Morphine SR 10 mg bd
- For breakthrough pain, give an extra dose (same as the 4 hourly dose) one dose up to 1–2 hourly
- Do not omit the next regular dose, if a prn dose has been given

When a patient is already on opioids: If a patient is already on regular tramadol, the starting dose would be at least morphine IR 10 mg q4h.

Increasing morphine dose:
- If pain is not controlled or ≥2 prn doses are needed per day, increase by approximately 50% of the starting dose OR recalculate q4h dose based on the total used in the previous 24 hours
- If the oral route is no longer practical → Give *half* the dose by subcutaneous (SC) injection (10 mg oral = 5 mg SC)

If pain is nonresponsive:
- Check compliance
- Is the patient taking drugs prn only?
- Have you got the cause right?
- Does the opioid dose need to be increased?
- Is there a neuropathic element?
- Are psychosocial aspects being neglected?
- Will an alternate route of administration help?

Adverse effects:
- Sedation can be common at the start of treatment, but resolves within few days
- When starting the patient on opioids, use Tab Domperidone 10 mg q8h × 3 days
- If the patient is constipated on opioids even with Tab Bisacodyl 10 mg HSOD:
  - Consider Bisacodyl 10 mg tid, along with a softener (e.g., Syr Cremaffin 15–30 mL tid)
  - If problem persists, intervene early with rectal measures
  - Rectal examination to rule out impaction and digital rectal evacuation in case of hard impacted stools
  - Bisacodyl suppository
  - High glycerine enema

Dyspnea

Dyspnea is a distressing and frightening symptom with incidence of up to 70% during the last 6 weeks of life.[19] It significantly affects the physical, emotional, and social well-being and results in poor quality of life (QOL).[20] Dyspnea is a bad prognostic indicator and as a refractory symptom, it is associated with a five-time increased probability of sedation at EoL.[21] The approach to management of dyspnea includes the correction of the underlying factors and use of nonpharmacological interventions and drugs to palliate dyspnea **(Fig. 3)**.

Dyspnea is often multifactorial and could be related to the disease, treatment, or other comorbidities. It is important to identify and treat the common reversible conditions in malignant and nonmalignant respiratory diseases **(Box 3)**. Symptomatic treatment is indicated when there is no clear correctable cause or the disease-specific treatment is ineffective, difficult to tolerate, or not consistent with patient preference. Several nonpharmacological measures **(Box 4)** can also help. A respiratory physiotherapist can help with education on nonpharmacological treatments; however, these measures may be difficult toward the EoL.

In advanced respiratory disease due to interstitial lung disease (ILD) or COPD, palliative drugs are indicated when standard treatments have failed to relieve dyspnea or are not feasible on a long-term basis. Opioids in lower doses, than used for pain, have been shown to improve the sensation of breathlessness **(Box 5)**. Opioid titration reduces the respiratory rate without producing significant changes in

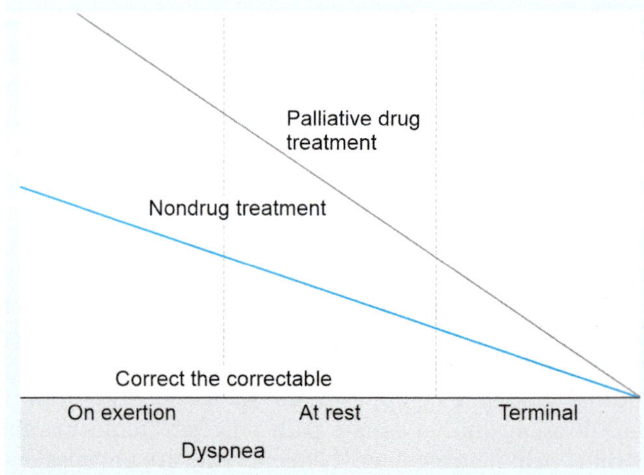

FIG. 3: Approach to management of dyspnea.

SECTION 19: PERSPECTIVES OF RESPIRATORY CARE

BOX 3 Common correctable causes of dyspnea.

Typically in advanced cancer

- Pleural/pericardial effusion
- Superior vena cava obstruction
- Pneumonia
- Pulmonary embolism
- Anemia
- Cardiac failure

Typically in advanced respiratory disease

- Pneumothorax
- Pneumonia
- Pulmonary embolism
- Anemia
- Cardiac failure

BOX 4 Nonpharmacological treatment for palliation of dyspnea.

- Explanation—acknowledge symptom and address anxiety
- Education—handling a sudden episode of dyspnea/panic, activity pacing
- General measures—keep window open, use fan, loose clothing around neck
- Breathing techniques
- Chest physiotherapy
- Relaxation therapy
- Pulmonary rehabilitation

BOX 5 Guideline on the use of morphine for palliation of dyspnea.

In patients who are opioid naive:

- For mild dyspnea, prn doses of immediate-release oral morphine 2.5 mg will suffice
- In others, start with Tab Morphine IR 2.5 mg q4h and as required
- After 24 hours, if little or no improvement, increase to 5 mg q4h and as required
- Assess further response and titrate with 30–50% dose increments
- Relatively small doses should suffice 2.5–10 mg q4h

For patients already on round-the-clock regular morphine:

- Increase morphine dose based on the severity of dyspnea
- Moderate dyspnea: Give morphine at a dose equivalent to 50– 100% of the q4h analgesic dose
- Severe dyspnea: Give morphine at a dose ≥ 100% of the q4h analgesic dose
- Reassess and titrate with 30–50% dose increments

Extreme dyspnea and distress

Give morphine 2.5 mg SC followed by midazolam 2.5 mg SC

(If the patient is not improving, seek advice from specialist palliative care physician)

BOX 6 Management guidelines for severe terminal dyspnea.

- Convert oral to SC morphine (use half the oral dose)
- Increase the dose by 30–50% if the dyspnea was previously uncontrolled (round to the nearest 5 or 10 mg)
- Consider adding midazolam 10 mg as a continuous SC infusion over 24 hours
- In addition, give haloperidol 2.5 mg at night OR along with the morphine and midazolam continuous SC infusion over 24 hours
- Extra prn doses of midazolam 2.5 mg SC with morphine 5 mg SC may be needed
- When reviewing after 24 hours, the dose of morphine and midazolam may need to be revised in the light of the extra doses given
- Patients who are very old, debilitated, or have severe renal or hepatic failure need dose reduction
- Other medications should be reviewed on a daily basis and simplified
- Explain to family that the intent is to reduce distress associated with breathlessness

PaO_2 and $PaCO_2$.[22-24] Morphine when used judiciously with careful titration does not produce respiratory depression.[25,26] During the terminal phase of life, dyspnea and anxiety can worsen, with an increasing chance of delirium which can be managed with appropriate medications **(Box 6)**. The European Respiratory Society task force recommended against the use of opioids for dyspnea in view of very low certainty of evidence. However, it also highlighted the reporting and selection bias, more studies on COPD, lack of sufficient washout periods and small sample sizes and lack of studies at the very EoL when people are more symptomatic. It states that opioids can be tried at the lowest dose to achieve clinical improvement with clear communication and shared decision making and stopped if not beneficial.[27]

Anxiety often coexists with and significantly affects the intensity of dyspnea, resulting in a vicious cycle.[28] Benzodiazepines are considered useful where there is significant anxiety or panic attacks that worsen dyspnea.[29] Combination of benzodiazepine with opioid is often found better than using either of them alone, but needs to be used with caution.[30] Benzodiazepines probably help through anxiolytic and sedative effect and possibly muscle relaxation. Care should be taken with diazepam, as it can accumulate due to its long half-life. Lorazepam (1–2 mg) is shorter acting and when given sublingually, provides immediate relief, hence especially useful during panic attacks. A Cochrane review recommends the use of benzodiazepines as a second- or third-line treatment within an individual therapeutic trial, when opioids and nonpharmacological measures have failed to control dyspnea.[31]

Most COPD patients receive regular bronchodilators. In cancer patients, bronchodilators are useful if there is bronchospasm. Bronchospasm is found in more than half of dyspneic cancer patients.[32,33] A combination of inhaled short-acting beta-2 agonists and anticholinergics is helpful. Use of oxygen is not routinely indicated in advanced cancer. It is not beneficial in those with dyspnea without hypoxia. Oxygen therapy with 2–4 L/min via nasal cannula can be tried along with opioids in those who are dyspneic with persistent hypoxia. The patient should be reassessed after 24 hours, and oxygen should be stopped if symptomatic response is not satisfactory.[24,34] Blowing cool air over the face with a fan is useful. Benefits of long-term oxygen therapy (LTOT) involving continuous oxygen use for more than 15 h/day are well established in COPD patients with hypoxia.[35] There is lack of evidence of benefit in patients without hypoxia, but most breathless patients approaching EoL are commenced on oxygen. Before initiation of oxygen, the pros and cons should be tightly weighed on an individual basis. Patients can become psychologically dependent and may become anxious whenever oxygen is stopped. Oxygen causes dryness of nasal mucosa and limits mobility and the mask impairs communication. There is a risk of combustibility and added cost with oxygen use. So, if oxygen is used outside the indications for LTOT in COPD patients or on a trial basis in cancer patients, it should be used on an N-of-1 randomized controlled trial.[36,37] Nebulized furosemide has also been tried to alleviate dyspnea in cancer and has not been proved beneficial.[38]

Cough

A phase 2, multicentre, randomized, double-blind, placebo-controlled, two-way crossover trial (PACIFY COUGH) showed that low dose controlled-release morphine significantly reduced cough related to idiopathic pulmonary fibrosis over 14 days compared with placebo.[39]

Cough is a normal but complex physiological mechanism that protects the airways and lungs by removing mucus and foreign matter from the larynx, trachea, and bronchi. Pathological cough is common in those with cardiothoracic disorders and can be quite distressing. It is present in more than half the patients with chronic lung disease or lung cancer. Cough can be classified as productive, with or without the patient being able to cough effectively, and nonproductive.

Management of cough depends on the type and cause of cough, the patient's performance status, and prognosis. The first step should be to address and reverse the cause of cough, whenever possible. Nonpharmacological measures like physiotherapy, teaching the patient to cough effectively, and steam inhalation may be helpful. Simultaneously, appropriate drugs to produce symptom relief should be prescribed. The choice of drugs would primarily depend on whether it is productive or nonproductive cough, to aid or suppress expectoration respectively. Protussive agents include nebulized saline, compound benzoin tincture, menthol, guaifenesin, and carbocysteine. Antitussives include simple linctus (demulcent) and opioids (codeine/morphine) and opioid derivatives like dextromethorphan.[40]

Hemoptysis

Massive hemoptysis in advanced lung cancer and chronic lung disease is rare but can be very frightening and visually traumatic. Management depends on the cause and prognosis. If this occurs in a patient who is otherwise terminally ill, with palliative goals, the treatment aims to reduce awareness and fear. Use dark towels (green or red) to cover blood. Being physically present with the patient continually is very supportive. Benzodiazepines (diazepam or midazolam) can be given parenteral to reduce panic and awareness; the intravenous route is preferred if there is peripheral vascular shutdown.[41]

Stridor

Stridor is a harsh inspiratory wheezing sound heard due to the obstruction of the larynx or of major airways. Corticosteroids can be beneficial in the initial stages. Dexamethasone can be given in high doses (8–24 mg/day). However, the symptom will progress and worsen if the primary cause is not reversible. Explanation to the patient and the carers is crucial. In the terminal phase, palliative sedation can be used after discussion with the relatives to reduce the distress.

Terminal Respiratory Secretions

During the last hours of life, reduced ability to swallow and impaired clearance of oropharyngeal secretions result in accumulation of tracheobronchial secretions. This manifests as gurgling or rattling sounds with each breath and is termed "death rattle" or "terminal respiratory secretions". It is present in 12–80% of patients at EoL and signals impending death. Death rattle is of two types. Type 1 death rattle, also known as true death rattle, is caused by accumulation of saliva and secretions in the upper airways. Type 2 death rattle is caused by accumulation of bronchial secretions as a result of tumor-related bronchorrhea, aspiration pneumonitis, and pulmonary edema.

It is important to reassure the family members that it is unlikely to be bothersome for the patient although the noise might feel distressing. Positioning the patient semiprone could help in drainage of secretions. Current evidence does not support the use of oropharyngeal suction.[42] Medications with anticholinergic effects, preferably hyoscine butylbromide or glycopyrrolate, are commonly used to treat secretions. Prophylactic administration of subcutaneous scopolamine butylbromide has been shown to produce significant reduction in death rattle.[43] These drugs can cause dry mouth; hence, extra attention should be given for mouth care.

Delirium

Around 90% of the patients experience delirium at the EoL. Delirium could be hyperactive or hypoactive or mixed. Nonpharmacological measures such as reorientation measures play a pivotal role in preventing delirium. Causes amenable to interventions such as fecal impaction or urinary retention should be addressed depending on the patient's proximity to death and goals of care. When there is no identifiable etiology, this could be "terminal delirium or terminal restlessness". Antipsychotics such as haloperidol can be initiated at the lowest effective dose to treat agitation. Benzodiazepines might be required to attain rapid control of anxiety and agitation; they could occasionally lead to paradoxical worsening of delirium if used alone. In refractory situations, palliative sedation might be required.[44,45]

Nausea and Vomiting

Nausea and vomiting of multifactorial etiology (bowel obstruction, constipation, hypercalcemia, uremia, brain metastasis, drugs) are common in many advanced diseases. The appropriate antiemetic should be chosen based on the understanding of the likely cause.[42]

Constipation

Most patients can be constipated at EoL, because of immobility, poor diet, dehydration, and drugs such as opioids. It is important to assess constipation. Treatment should consist of a combination of stimulant laxative (bisacodyl, senna) and stool softener (milk of magnesia, macrogols). If patients are unable to take orally, use of rectal suppositories can be considered.[42]

Table 2 provides the medications used for common symptoms during EoL.

Nursing Care

Nursing care interventions for morbid patients include care of the pressure areas, bowel and bladder care, especially as patients may be bed-bound, oral care, measures to reduce secretions, dry mouth, and odor. In a patient who is actively dying, routine measurement and recording of vital parameters are not generally recommended.[46]

Psychosocial and Existential Issues

End-of-life can be associated with a mixture of emotions: Fear, remorse, guilt, love, meaning of life, and need to forgive or be forgiven. An awareness of nearing the end can facilitate the time and space for final conversations between patients and their loved ones. Dignity therapy, meaning centered therapy, and professional spiritual care by chaplains are some beneficial interventions in this regard. Use of antidepressants is generally not advisable as there might not be sufficient time for the effect to manifest. Instead, low dose of benzodiazepines is recommended for anxiety, stress-related disorders, and insomnia at EoL.[47]

PALLIATIVE SEDATION

Palliative sedation is defined as the "monitored use of medications intended to induce a state of unconsciousness in order to relieve the burden of otherwise intractable suffering in a way that is ethically acceptable to the patient, family and health care providers." The common symptoms for which palliative sedation is initiated when they become

TABLE 2: Common symptoms at the end of life and medications used.

Symptom	Drug	Dose	Route
• Pain • Neuropathic pain	• Morphine or opioid equivalent • Lidocaine/ketamine/ methadone	• Convert regular dose of oral medication to parenteral or transdermal equivalent • Continue as previously or initiate if required for neuropathic pain	• SC/IV/transdermal • SC/IV
• Dyspnea • With anxiety	• Morphine or opioid equivalent • Lorazepam	• 1–2.5 mg morphine IR q4h in the opioid naïve • 0.25–2 mg HSOD	SC/IV
Cough	Morphine or opioid equivalent	1–2.5 mg morphine q4h in the opioid naïve	SC/IV
Respiratory secretions	• Hyoscine butylbromide • Glycopyrrolate	• 20 mg q8h • 0.2–0.4 mg q4h	• SC • SC
• Nausea and vomiting If prokinetic required • Primarily central	• Metoclopramide • Haloperidol	• 10–20 mg tid–qid • 0.5–1.5 mg bd–tid	• SC/IV • SC/IV
Constipation	Stimulant laxative (e.g., Bisacodyl) plus stool softener (e.g., lactulose)	10 mg HSOD 15 mL HSOD	PO or rectal suppositories PO
Delirium	Haloperidol	1.5–5 mg tid	SC

refractory include pain, dyspnea, and delirium. A symptom is said to be refractory when there are no further therapeutic choices or when those that are accessible lead to unbearable side effects. It differs from medically assisted dying in that treatment is proportionate, intent is reduced consciousness, and medication doses are titrated only until the required sedation is achieved. Medications used for sedation include continuous infusions of benzodiazepines (midazolam), antipsychotics (haloperidol), barbiturates (phenobarbitone), and less commonly anesthetic agents (propofol). Ongoing medications for symptom management such as opioids for analgesia are continued if they have proven beneficial to the patient. Proper communication and documentation are essential considering the emotional impact imposed on families and staff during the process. Clinicians should facilitate final conversations and fulfilling of the last wishes prior to initiation of sedation.[48]

REVIEWING MEDICATIONS AT END-OF-LIFE

Clinicians should review the medication chart so as to identify and deprescribe any potentially inappropriate medications after prudently weighing the benefits versus burdens of continuing the medications.[1] This reduces the burden of polypharmacy, cost, and any potential adverse effects. Examples of such medications include antihypertensives, dyslipidemia medications, multivitamins and minerals, peptic ulcer prophylaxis measures, and complementary and alternative medications.

ANTICIPATORY PRESCRIBING AT THE END-OF-LIFE

Anticipatory prescribing is a clinician-led pragmatic solution wherein medications are prescribed anticipating a symptom in advance and are administered by trained individuals when the need arises. Injectable medications are typically preferred at EoL as the patient may not be able to take orally. Medications are given through the subcutaneous route. The four common symptoms that need anticipatory prescribing include pain, nausea/vomiting, agitation, and respiratory secretions **(Table 3)**. When choosing anticipatory medications, it is vital to consider the likelihood of specific symptoms occurring, the benefits and harms of prescribing versus not prescribing, the potential risk of a person suddenly deteriorating, the location of care, and the time it would take to obtain medicines. It is advisable to use a tailored strategy.[49]

TABLE 3: Common medications used in anticipatory prescribing at end-of-life.

Medication	Symptom	Route and common dose
Morphine	Pain, breathlessness, cough	SC prn (dose depends on regular dose)
Haloperidol	Nausea, vomiting, delirium	1–5 mg SC prn
Midazolam	Anxiety, breathlessness Seizures	2.5–5 mg SC prn 5–10 mg SC prn
Hyoscine butylbromide	Bowel colic, death rattle	20 mg SC prn

ARTIFICIAL NUTRITION AND HYDRATION AT THE END-OF-LIFE

Clinically assisted hydration (CAH) consists of administration of fluids, either enterally (via a tube into the gut) or parenterally (intravenous or subcutaneous). A routine assessment of the hydration status of the patient should be done. It is desirable to follow a personalized approach taking into consideration the level of consciousness, swallowing difficulties, risk of pulmonary edema, level of thirst, and any cultural or spiritual beliefs that may influence the patient/family preferences. If oral hydration is inadequate and the patient develops distressing symptoms attributable to dehydration, a therapeutic trial of hydration can be considered with at least 12 hourly monitoring for benefits and risks.[50]

Near the EoL, cognitive deterioration, fatigue, and risk of aspiration significantly undermine the ability to take orally. Disease-related factors such as anorexia, dysphagia, and bowel obstruction could further impact nutritional status. Often, this causes significant distress to the family members and lead to requests for artificial nutrition. Currently, there is no evidence of benefit for artificial nutrition in prolonging survival or improving QOL of patients. Validating the family members' distress and empathetically explaining to them about the burdens versus benefits are critical for arriving at a plan based on the patient's best interests.[51]

APPLICATION OF ETHICAL PRINCIPLES IN END-OF-LIFE CARE

The fundamental ethical principles of autonomy, beneficence, nonmaleficence, and justice have to be carefully applied when making decisions. A complete and open disclosure of the necessary information is crucial in enabling the patient to make an informed choice and exercise autonomy around decisions. In instances where a patient has lost the capacity to make decisions, decisions are made based on an advance directive if available. If such a directive does not exist, a surrogate decision maker takes the decisions based on previously expressed patient preferences and also by keeping in mind the best interests of the patient. Any intervention that is not in the best interest of the patient or is going to be inappropriate should not be initiated or continued. Patients who may not benefit

3. Sallnow L, Smith R, Ahmedzai SH, et al. Lancet Commission on the Value of Death. Report of the Lancet Commission on the Value of Death: Bringing death back into life. Lancet. 2022;399: 837-84.
4. Selecky PA, Eliasson CA, Hall RI, et al. American College of Chest Physicians. Palliative and end-of-life care for patients with cardiopulmonary diseases: American College of Chest Physicians position statement. Chest. 2005;128:3599-610.
5. Murray SA, Kendall M, Boyd K, et al. Illness trajectories and palliative care. BMJ. 2005;330:1007-11.
6. The 10/40 model of care. [online] Available from https://www.bestcareforthedying.org/10-40-model [Last accessed October, 2024].
7. Ellershaw J E, Lakhani M. Best care for the dying patient. BMJ. 2013;347:f4428.
8. Myatra SN, Salins N, Iyer S. End-of-life care policy: An integrated care plan for the dying: A Joint Position Statement of the Indian Society of Critical Care Medicine (ISCCM) and the Indian Association of Palliative Care (IAPC). Indian J Crit Care Med. 2014;18:615-35.
9. Mori M, Morita T, Bruera E, et al. Prognostication of the Last Days of Life. Cancer Res Treat. 2022;54:631-43.
10. Solano JP, Gomes B, Higginson IJ. A comparison of symptom prevalence in far advanced cancer, AIDS, heart disease, chronic obstructive pulmonary disease and renal disease. J Pain Symptom Manage. 2006;31:58-69.
11. Gore JM, Brophy CJ, Greenstone MA. How well do we care for patients with end stage chronic obstructive pulmonary disease (COPD)? A comparison of palliative care and quality of life in COPD and lung cancer. Thorax. 2000;55:1000-6.
12. Stapleton RD, Nielsen EL, Engelberg RA, et al. Association of depression and life sustaining treatment preferences in patients with COPD. Chest. 2005;127:328-34.
13. Potter J, Higginson IJ. Pain experienced by lung cancer patients a review of prevalence, causes and pathophysiology. Lung Cancer. 2004;43:247-57.
14. Gonzales GR, Elliot KJ, Portenoy RK, et al. The impact of a comprehensive evaluation in the management of cancer pain. Pain. 1991;47:141-4.
15. Report of a WHO Expert Committee. Cancer Pain Relief and Palliative Care. WHO Technical Report Series 804. Geneva: World Health Organization; 1990.
16. Zech DF, Grond S, Lynch J, et al. Validation of World Health Organization Guidelines for cancer pain relief: a 10-year prospective study. Pain. 1995;63:65-76.
17. Risser A, Donovan D, Heintzman J, et al. NSAID prescribing precautions. Am Fam Physician. 2009;80:1371-8.
18. Jeba J, George R, Thangakunam B, et al. Pain assessment and analgesic prescription for cancer patients in a medical ward: The influence of an educational intervention. Natl Med J India. 2009;22:177-80.
19. Reuben DB, Mor V. Dyspnea in terminally ill cancer patients. Chest. 1986;89:234-6.
20. Booth, S, Silvester, S, Todd, C. Breathlessness in cancer and chronic obstructive pulmonary disease: Using a qualitative approach to describe the experience of patients and carers. Palliat Support Care. 2003;1:337-44.
21. Cuervo Pinna MA, Mota Vargas R, Redondo Moralo MJ, et al. Dyspnea—A Bad Prognosis Symptom at the End of Life. Am J Hosp Palliat Care. 2009;26:89-97.
22. Abernethy AP, Currow DC, Frith P, et al. Randomised, double blind, placebo controlled crossover trial of sustained release morphine for the management of refractory dyspnoea. BMJ. 2003;327:523-8.
23. Jennings A, Davies A, Higgins J, et al. A systematic review of the use of opioids in the management of dyspnoea. Thorax. 2002;57:939-44.
24. Kamal AH, Maguire JM, Wheeler JL, et al. Dyspnea review for the palliative care professional: treatment goals and therapeutic options. J Palliat Med. 2012;15:106-14.
25. Estfan B, Mahmoud F, Shaheen P, et al. Respiratory function during parenteral opioid titration for cancer pain. Palliat Med. 2007;21:81-6.
26. Clemens KE, Klaschik E. Symptomatic Therapy of Dyspnea with Strong Opioids and Its Effect on Ventilation in Palliative Care Patients. J Pain Symptom Manage. 2007;33:473-81.
27. Holland AE, Spathis A, Marsaa K, et al. European Respiratory Society clinical practice guideline on symptom management for adults with serious respiratory illness. Eur Respir J. 2024;63: 2400335.
28. Bruera E, Schmitz B, Pither J, et al. The Frequency and Correlates of Dyspnea in Patients with Advanced Cancer. J Pain Symptom Manage. 2000;19:357-62.
29. Cachia E, Ahmedzai SH. Breathlessness in cancer patients. Eur J Cancer. 2008;44:1116-23.
30. Navigante AH, Cerchietti LC, Castro MA, et al. Midazolam as adjunct therapy to morphine in the alleviation of severe dyspnea perception in patients with advanced cancer. J Pain Symptom Manage. 2006;31:38-47.
31. Simon ST, Higginson IJ, Booth S, et al. Benzodiazepines for the relief of breathlessness in advanced malignant and non-malignant diseases in adults. Cochrane Database Syst Rev. 2016;10(10):CD007354.
32. Dudgeon DJ, Lertzman M. Dyspnoea in the advanced cancer patient. J Pain Symptom Manage. 1998;16:212-9.
33. Congleton J, Muers MF. The incidence of airflow obstruction in bronchial carcinoma, its relation to breathlessness, and response to bronchodilator therapy. Respir Med. 1995;89:291-6.
34. Bruera E, de Stoutz N, Velasco Leiva A, et al. Effects of oxygen on dyspnoea in hypoxaemic terminal-cancer patients. Lancet 1993;342:13-4.
35. Eaton T, Lewis C, Young P, et al. Long-term oxygen therapy improves health-related quality of life. Respir Med. 2004;98: 285-93.
36. Uronis HE, Currow DC, Abernethy AP. Palliative management of refractory dyspnoea in COPD. Int J COPD. 2006;1:289-304.
37. Bruera E, Schoeller T, MacEachern T. Symptomatic benefit of supplemental oxygen in hypoxemic patients with terminal cancer: the use of the N of 1 randomized controlled trial. J Pain Symptom Manage. 1992;7:365-8.
38. Jeba J, George R, Pease N. Nebulised furosemide in the palliation of dyspnoea in cancer: a systematic review. BMJ Support Palliat Care. 2014;4:132-9.
39. Wu Z, Spencer LG, Banya W, et al. Morphine for treatment of cough in idiopathic pulmonary fibrosis (PACIFY COUGH): a prospective, multicentre, randomised, double-blind, placebo-controlled, two-way crossover trial. Lancet Respir Med. 2024; 12:273-80.
40. Davis CL. ABC of palliative care: Breathlessness, cough and other respiratory problems. BMJ. 1997;315:931-4.

41. Bennett M, Lucas V, Brennan M, et al. Using antimuscarinic drugs in the management of death rattle: evidence-based guidelines for palliative care. Palliat Med. 2002;16:369-74.
42. Sleeman KE, Collis E. Caring for a dying patient in hospital. BMJ. 2013;346:f2174.
43. Van Esch HJ, van Zuylen L, Geijteman ECT, et al. Effect of prophylactic subcutaneous scopolamine butylbromide on death rattle in patients at the end of life: The SILENCE randomized controlled trial. JAMA. 2021;326:1268-76.
44. Breitbart W, Alici Y. Agitation and delirium at the end of life: "We couldn't manage him". JAMA. 2008;300:2898-910.
45. Hui D, Frisbee-Hume S, Wilson A, et al. Effect of lorazepam with haloperidol vs haloperidol alone on agitated delirium in patients with advanced cancer receiving palliative care: a randomized controlled trial. JAMA. 2017;318:1047-56.
46. Cherny NI, Coyle N, Foley KM. Guidelines in the care of the dying cancer patient. Hematol Oncol Clin North Am. 1996;10: 261-86.
47. Chochinov HM, Hassard T, McClement S, et al. The patient dignity inventory: a novel way of measuring dignity-related distress in palliative care. J Pain Symptom Manage. 2008;36: 559-71.
48. Cherny NI, Radbruch L. European Association for Palliative Care (EAPC) recommended framework for the use of sedation in palliative care. Palliat Med. 2009;23:581-93.
49. Bowers B, Ryan R, Kuhn I, et al. Anticipatory prescribing of injectable medications for adults at the end of life in the community: A systematic literature review and narrative synthesis. Palliat Med. 2019;33:160-77.
50. Kingdon A, Spathis A, Brodrick R, et al. What is the impact of clinically assisted hydration in the last days of life? A systematic literature review and narrative synthesis BMJ Support Palliat Care. 2021;11:68-74.
51. McClement SE, Degner LF, Harlos M. Family beliefs regarding the nutritional care of a terminally ill relative: a qualitative study. J Palliat Med. 2003;6:737-48.
52. Breen CM, Abernethy AP, Abbott KH, et al. Conflict associated with decisions to limit life-sustaining treatment in intensive care units. J Gen Intern Med. 2001;16:283-9.
53. van Doorslaer E, O'Donnell O, Rannan-Eliya RP, et al. Effect of payments for health care on poverty estimates in 11 countries in Asia: an analysis of household survey data. Lancet. 2006;368: 1357-64.
54. Puchalski CM, Zhong Z, Jacobs MM, et al. Patients who want their family and physician to make resuscitation decisions for them: Observations from SUPPORT and HELP. Study to Understand Prognoses and Preferences for Outcomes and Risks of Treatment. Hospitalized Elderly Longitudinal Project. J Am Geriatr Soc. 2000;48:S84-90.
55. Mani RK, Simha S, Gursahani R. Simplified Legal Procedure for End-of-life Decisions in India: A New Dawn in the Care of the Dying? Indian J Crit Care Med. 2023;27:374-6.
56. Curtis JR, Engelberg RA, Nielsen EL, et al. Patient-physician communication about end-of-life care for patients with severe COPD. Eur Respir J. 2004;24:200-5.
57. Knauft E, Nielsen EL, Engelberg RA, et al. Barriers and facilitators to end-of-life care communication for patients with COPD. Chest. 2005;127:2188-96.
58. Maguire P, Pitceathly C. Managing the difficult consultation. Clin Med. 2003;3:532-7.
59. Parker SM, Clayton JM, Hancock K, et al. A systematic review of prognostic/end-of-life communication with adults in the advanced stages of a life-limiting illness: patient/caregiver preferences for the content, style, and timing of information. J Pain Symptom Manage. 2007;34:81-93.
60. Ramirez A, Addington-Hall J, Richards M. ABC of palliative care. The carers. BMJ. 1998;316:208-11.

Health Economics of Pulmonary Care

CHAPTER 183

Sudheendra Ghosh C, Sayujya S Ghosh

INTRODUCTION

Health economics focuses on how the economic behavior of providers and recipients affects the quality and cost of clinical care. During the last decade, the phenomenon of rising healthcare costs has been observed globally due to an aging society that has increased demand for healthcare services. Medical care expenditures brought on by improvements in medical technology and changes in the severity of diseases lead us to analyze the financial burden. Medical science and economics are major topics in health economics. The primary objective in health economics is evaluating the healthcare system operations and clinical phenomena using economic approaches such as econometrics, value evaluation, decision analysis, and behavioral science. Health economics is broadly classified into two types: Those analyzed from the macro and those from the micro perspective **(Table 1)**.

HEALTHCARE MARKET AND PUBLIC HEALTH

Traded commodities have both a use value and an exchange value. The healthcare market has different characteristics **(Table 2)**.[1] The decision of clinicians significantly impacts both the supply and demand in healthcare market. Even though equal distribution of healthcare resource is desired, it is frequently so expensive that everyone cannot afford advanced medical care. So, there is emphasis on the theme that the public medical marketplace requires a system of "exchange value" and "use value" to operate and develop as a component of the social system. The knowledge in health economics is concerned with assessing the efficacy of medical care, the perspective for valuing alternative therapies is that of the society.

TABLE 1: Broad classification of topics.

Topics	Areas
Macroeconomics	• Social security schemes • Healthcare policy
Microeconomics	• Hospital management • Health technology • Clinical care

TABLE 2: Characteristics of healthcare market.

Deals with health and life	Both are precious and cannot be replaced by anything else
Characterized by Information asymmetry	A high degree of specialized knowledge and skills are required in the medical field
Healthcare is essential	So equal distribution is desired

APPRAISAL OF THE EVIDENCE

Many distinct genes can undergo modest alterations impacting the functioning of cells and organisms. Clinical medicine is constantly accompanied by uncertainty regarding the diagnosis, treatment response, and prognosis. Probabilities and other quantitative methods like meta analysis, decision analysis, and cost-effectiveness analysis (CEA) are necessary in clinical decision-making where uncertainty exists as in pandemic. Information thus generated facilitates the practice of evidence-based medicine (EBM). EBM stands for the integration of the best available scientific evidence with clinical expertise and judgment in patient care.[2,3] We are currently applying precision medicine and individualized medicine in pulmonology practice due to the availability of advanced technology as well as biomarkers. The combination of data analytics, deep learning, and translational medicine has made it possible to effectively manage the current pandemic.

Deductive reasoning and economic analysis form the basis for answering many clinical management challenges. When resources are scarce, CEA is a method of choosing among competing desires.[4] In the middle of the 1960s, CEA was initially used in healthcare when it was enthusiastically introduced to clinicians. These strategies have gained widespread understanding and acceptance among the major players in the healthcare industry, including doctors.[5,6] As COVID-19 progressed through its many phases, we have come to understand the importance of applying the criteria of safety, efficacy, effectiveness, efficiency, and equity to generate evidence.[7]

Safety is the most important issue in the evaluation of an intervention. The next critical step is assessing its efficacy. Here, one attempts to respond to the question, "Can the treatment work?". We can find proof of this in random clinical trials and meta-analyses. If it is efficacious, then we want to know how well it performs in real-world clinical settings. Literature-based comparative assessment research investigations will provide a response to our criteria of effectiveness by answering the question, "Does it work?". If so, then we must evaluate the efficiency criterion. The issue of efficiency concerns the clinical outcome in relation to the financial input. We will be able to resolve this problem with the help of CEA. The subject of resource allocation among the people is addressed by equity. The pandemic vaccine program is implemented strictly to comply with the aforementioned standards.

What is the Relevance of Economic Evaluation?

Economic evaluation generates evidence-based information to decision makers for efficient use of available resources for maximizing health benefits. In the economic analysis of healthcare, there are three dimensions that need to be discussed: (1) The perspective of the analysis, (2) the type of costs involved, (3) the type of analysis considered.

PERSPECTIVE OF THE ANALYSIS (WHO PAYS AND WHO GAINS?)

The society, the patient, the hospital administration, and the insurance companies can all have different perspectives on the expenses, results, and benefits. For instance, the fees that are permitted by that payer are equal to the cost to the insurance company of managing a critically ill patient in an intensive care unit (ICU). Regardless of the fee, the hospital bears the full burden of delivering critical care. Only by performing a cost-finding exercise can the exact economic cost of the hospital be revealed. The price to the patient includes both the service fee and the time away from work. The whole net cost of every single aspect of society, including the patient's productivity and the costs associated with providing and receiving intensive care, is what is known as the cost to society.

TYPES OF COSTS INVOLVED

The consumption of a resource that could have been used for another reason is how economists define the cost of critical care management. Since the resource is now being used for managing critical care, there is no longer a chance to use it for something else. Its worth in the alternative usage, which is no longer feasible, is hence known as the "opportunity cost". The investment needed to set up the critical care unit is a fixed expense. The expense needed for the ongoing care of the patient in the ICU is known as a variable cost. Depending on the level of service, this will change. Direct and indirect costs have typically been used to categorize costs associated with resources utilized. The term "direct" is used in economics to refer to productivity gains or losses related to illness or death. It typically refers to costs in resource use attributable to intensive care treatment.

- *Direct cost*: The value of all the products, services, and other resources used to provide intensive care treatment is included in the category of direct expenses. These expenses are frequently considered to involve a monetary data related to resource use. Doctor time, nurse time, support staff time, equipment cost, procedure cost, laboratory cost, medicine cost, and costs for other consumables are all included in direct costs.
- *Indirect cost*: This includes (1) the cost of lost or diminished capacity for work or leisure activities as a result of sickness and (2) lost economic productivity as a result of mortality.

Type of economic analysis: Economic evaluation of clinical management strategies will assist us in selecting the most effective treatment or diagnostic approaches for effective resource utilization. Cost-effectiveness, cost utility, and cost-benefit analyses are thought to be complete economic evaluations that take into account both costs and effects, whereas cost minimization analysis assesses only the cost component and is merely a partial study **(Table 3)**.

Cost-effectiveness analysis is a technique for comparing the relative value of various therapeutic strategies. In its most simple form, a new treatment is compared with the current practice (the "low-cost alternative") in the calculation of the cost-effectiveness ratio. It is also worthwhile to recognize that CEA is only relevant to certain decisions. There are various ways to how a new therapeutic strategy might compare with an existing approach **(Table 4)**. Note that a CEA is relevant only if a new strategy is both more effective and more costly (or both less effective and less costly).

CE ratio = (Cost of new strategy – Cost of current practice)/(Effectiveness of new strategy – Effectiveness of current practice)

MEASURES FOR EVALUATING OUTCOMES AND QUALITY OF LIFE

The World Health Organization has defined quality of life (QoL) as a person's view of his or her place in life in relation to his or her objectives, expectations, standards, and worries, as well as the culture and value systems in which they live.

TABLE 3: Common types of economic analysis.

Type of analysis	Advantages	Disadvantages
Cost-minimization analysis (CMA)	By comparing the cost of two or more alternatives that have identical outcomes, result identifies the least-expensive alternative	It is difficult to compare different diseases due to differences in the measure of primary effectiveness. The definition of cost components should be discussed clearly
Cost-effectiveness analysis (CEA)	• Outcomes are measured in natural units, such as years of life saved and number of cases averted • Its outcomes are commonly used in clinical practice, so they are acceptable for physicians and payers	It is difficult to establish comparisons between different diseases due to differences in the measure of primary outcome
Cost-utility analysis (CUA)	Outcomes are measured in quality-adjusted life-years (QALY), which combines the benefits of the survival and quality of life as a measure of effects. It can simultaneously compare results among different diseases as the outcome is measured in the same unit	In some situations, the sensitivity can be due to the measurement method. The value of QALY is more likely to be lower with the elderly than with younger subjects
Cost–benefit analysis (CBA)	• Outcomes are measured in monetary units resulting in calculation of net benefit • It permits a direct comparison between the incremental cost and its incremental benefits	Converting clinical benefit into monetary benefit is not easy as this analysis is for resource allocation

TABLE 4: Conditions under which cost-effectiveness analysis (CEA) is relevant.

Effectiveness	Cost of new strategy high	Cost of new low
New strategy more effective	CEA relevant	Adopt new strategy
New strategy less effective	New strategy is dominated	CEA relevant

TABLE 5: Common instruments to measure quality of life (QoL) in pulmonary medicine.

Instrument	Measure
St George's Respiratory Questionnaire (SGRQ)	3 aspects (activity, symptoms, impact)
Medical Outcome Study Short Form 36 (SF-36)	8 dimensions
WHOQOL-BREF	6 dimensions, 25 aspects of QoL
EuroQOL 5 D (EQ 5D)	5 dimensions

It is a wide-ranging notion that takes into account a person's relationship to important elements of their environment as well as their physical and psychological well-being, amount of independence, social connections, and personal views **(Tables 5 and 6)**.

The term "disability-adjusted life-years" (DALYs) refers to a measurement that includes both years spent disabled and years lost owing to early mortality (from the disability). Years of life lost (YLL) and years lived with disability (YLD) are two mathematical equations that are used to calculate DALYs. YLL stands for years of life lost as a result of premature death. YLD is the number of healthy years lost until remission or death due to the condition's handicap. Years spent with a disability are calculated by adding these.

MEASURE OF HEALTH-RELATED QUALITY OF LIFE

Health status or health-related QoL measures how disease affects a person's ability to function physically, emotionally, and socially.[8,9] The individual's perspective of their life constitutes the essence of QoL. An individual patient's goals, values, and beliefs are represented by many domains that make up the subjective, dynamic, and multidimensional concept of health-related QoL. Utility is considered a component of health-related quality of life (HRQoL) in the healthcare industry, and assessments are based on preferences, which typically include patient satisfaction. This is multiplied by the number of years in life to get the measurement "quality-adjusted life-years" (QALY).

INCREMENTAL COST-EFFECTIVENESS RATIO

The cost-effectiveness ratio is calculated by contrasting a new treatment with the standard of care (the "low-cost alternative") in its most basic form. It is also important to understand that CEA only applies to particular decisions. Incremental cost-effectiveness ratio (ICER) is a concept that contrasts rising costs with rising benefits incrementally. The "incremental increase in cost/incremental increase in benefit" formula is how ICER is typically expressed. The idea is that even if the cost goes up, the so-called performance

TABLE 6: World Health Organization (WHO) quality of life (QoL) instrument.

Domains	• Items incorporated
Physical health (HRQoL)	• Energy and fatigue • Pain and discomfort • Sleep and rest
Psychological health (HRQoL)	• Body image and appearance • Negative feelings • Positive feelings • Self-esteem • Thinking, learning, memory, and concentration
Level of independence (HRQoL)	• Mobility • Activities of daily living • Dependence on medicines and medical aids • Work capacity
Social relationships (HRQoL)	• Personal relationships • Social support • Sexual activity
Environment	• Financial resources • Freedom, physical safety, and security • *Health and social care*: Accessibility and quality • Opportunities for acquiring new information and skills • Participation in and opportunities for recreation and leisure • Physical environment (pollution, noise, traffic, climate) • Transport • Home environment
Personal values and beliefs	• Religion • Spirituality • Personal beliefs

Source: Adapted from World Health Organization (WHOQOL-100).[9]

of health interventions will increase if there is a bigger improvement in effectiveness.

If new strategy A costs more than the existing strategy B but has a smaller impact, it will be "inferior" to B; however, if A costs less than B but has a greater impact, it would be "superior". Different comparisons between a novel therapeutic technique and an established one are possible. You should be aware that a cost effectiveness analysis (CEA)/cost utility analysis (CUA) is only applicable if a new technique is both more expensive and more effective (or vice versa). If the ICER value is superior, the intervention in question is recognized as having a higher health economy than the comparison intervention, and this becomes a basis for promoting patient access **(Table 7)**.[10-12]

ECONOMICS OF CHRONIC OBSTRUCTIVE PULMONARY DISEASE AND INTERSTITIAL LUNG DISEASES

The cost of managing a condition like chronic obstructive pulmonary disease (COPD) is influenced by a number of variables, most significantly the frequency of acute exacerbations.[13] For COPD, various cost-effectiveness approaches have been applied. The cost-effectiveness of triple-drug therapy for COPD in UK was £4104 (£1646–£19 201) per QALY.[14] The cost and efficacy of ICU treatment are shown differently as daily expenditures for ventilated and nonventilated patients.[15] An Indian study reported INR 44,390 as the median cost per severe COPD admission.[16]

Patients with advanced ideopathic pulmonary fibrosis (IPF) along with interstitial lung diseases (ILD) tend to have similar HRQoL deficits to those with COPD. In addition to the evident impact on physical health, HRQoL in individuals with IPF suggests that overall health, energy level, respiratory symptoms, and level of independence are also harmed. Assessments of dyspnea or pulmonary function do not entirely account for the variation in HRQoL among patients, indicating that HRQoL assessments offer specific information. Significant correlations were seen between the Short Form-36 (SF-36), Quality of Wellbeing Scale (QWB), and Saint George's Respiratory Questionnaire (SGRQ) scores and forced vital capacity (FVC), forced expiratory volume in 1 second (FEV1), and diffusing capacity, especially when antifibrotics are not cost-effective.[17]

INCREMENTAL COST-EFFECTIVENESS RATIO IN COVID-19 (REMDESIVIR AND DEXAMATHAZONE)

Using dexamethasone for all patients was the most cost-effective treatment option; all remdesivir regimens were more expensive and less successful. Remdesivir was unlikely to be a COVID-19 treatment that is cost-effective, according to available data.[18,19]

COST-EFFECTIVENESS OF INTERVENTIONAL PULMONARY PROCEDURES

The major challenges for interventional pulmonary (IP) procedures as we go toward value-based healthcare are validating new technology, demonstrating its cost-effectiveness, and determining the impact on patient outcomes.[20] The majority of IP studies only evaluate the technical success of the procedure, not the patient's QoL .[21] An emphasis on CEA in high-quality technology assessment is crucial for IP since it must transform its practice into patient-centered, evidence-based care **(Table 8)**.

TABLE 7: Estimation of ICER in MDR/XDR, LTB, biologicals, and COVID-19.

Author	Analysis design	Intervention	Comparator	Outcome
Sweeney et al. (2022)	Markov prediction model	Bedaquiline, Pretomanid, and Linezolid (BPaL) with and without Moxifloxacin (BPaLM)	Standard current treatment	BPaL was the most cost-saving regimen, saving $112–$1,173 per person
Shedrawy (2021)	Markov prediction model	LTBI-screening program and retreatment	No screening and treatment	Age group 13–19 years had the lowest ICER, 300,082 Swedish Kronor (SEK)/QALY
Giorgio Walter Canonica PROXIMA Study (2020)	Observational data	1 year post-omalizumab cost-effectiveness	Pre-omalizumab period	0.132 QALYs gained €3729 per patient reduction in direct healthcare cost the ICER €56,847/QALY
Jo and Jamieson (2021)	COVID-19 Clinical outcome Prediction Model	Dexamethasone alone for nonventilated and ventilated patients	Standard care	Scenario of resulting in $231 per death averted

(ICER: incremental cost-effectiveness ratio; LTB: latent tuberculosis; MDR: multidrug resistant; XDR: extensively drug-resistant; QALY: quality-adjusted life-years)

TABLE 8: How to evaluate interventional pulmonary procedures?

Technology	Clinical purpose	Outcome	Type of technology assessment/ economic evaluation
Advanced bronchoscopic imaging techniques—ENB, EBUS (radial and convex) and novel uses of real-time fluoroscopy and CBCT	• Approach to lung nodules • Evaluation of mediastinal/hilar adenopathy	• Procedural safety • Efficacy • Meaningful patient outcomes	• Accuracy of diagnosis • Survival following therapy: CMA, CEA, CUA
Robotic bronchoscopy and real-time imaging	• Early diagnosis and treatment of difficult-to-access peripheral lung lesions • Treatment of early-stage peripheral lung cancer	For intralesional chemotherapy, gene therapy, and immunotherapy outcome	RCT incorporating patient-reported outcome in CEA and CUA leading to measurement of ICER
Promising advances in therapeutic bronchoscopic/ thoracoscopic modalities	Bronchoscopy/thoracoscopy approaches to management of airway diseases and pleural diseases	Optimal treatment of asthma, COPD, bronchiectasis, and patients with pleural diseases	RCTs incorporating CEA to provide new insights

(CBCT: cone-beam computed tomography; CEA: cost-effectiveness analysis; CMA: cost-minimization analysis; COPD: chronic obstructive pulmonary disease; CUA: cost-utility analysis; EBUS: endobronchial ultrasound; ENB: electromagnetic navigation bronchoscopy; ICER: incremental cost-effectiveness ratio; RCT: randomized clinica trial)

SUMMARY

Health economics is an applied topic of study that enables a methodical and thorough analysis of the challenges associated with attaining universal health. Health economics seeks to comprehend how people, healthcare professionals, public and private organizations, and governments behave when making decisions by applying economic theories of consumer, producer, and social choice. Through evidence production, evidence synthesis, and value to support the allocation of healthcare resources and reimbursement decision-making within a healthcare system, health economic approaches have been created to address specific concerns related to the value of new diagnoses and treatments. The capability of modern pulmonology has significantly increased in recent years, thanks to the exponential expansion in technology and its expanding availability. Numerous distributive, ethical, and economic questions are also raised by it. Neither medical necessity nor anticipated medical benefit provides us with a method of decision-making for dealing with these distributive issues. However, economic analysis provides more thorough information that is important to our choices.

REFERENCES

1. Tomoyuki Takura, An Evaluation of Clinical Economics and Cases of Cost-effectiveness. Intern Med. 2018;57(9):1191-200.
2. Timmerman S, Angell A. Evidence Based Medicine, Clinical uncertainty, and learning to doctor. J Health Soc Behav. 2001; 42:342-59.
3. Drummond MF, Richardson WS, O'Brien BJ, et al. Users' guides to the medical literature. XIII. How to use an article on economic analysis of clinical practice. A. Are the results of the study valid? Evidence-Based Medicine Working Group. JAMA. 1997;277:1552-7.
4. Russell LB, Gold MR, Siegel JE, et al. The role of cost-effectiveness analysis in health and medicine. Panel on Cost-Effectiveness in Health and Medicine. JAMA. 1996;276(14):1172-7.
5. Chapman RH, Berger M, Weinstein MC, et al. When does quality-adjusting life years matter in cost-effective analysis? Health Econ. 2004;13:429-36.
6. Weinstein MC, Stason WB. Foundations of cost-effectiveness analysis for health and medical practices. N Engl J Med. 1977; 296(13):716-21.
7. Appleby J. Tackling COVID-19: are the costs worth the benefits? BMJ. 2020;369:m1496.
8. Kaplan RM, Hays RD. Health-related quality of life measurement in public health. Annu Rev Public Health. 2022;43:355-73.
9. World Health Organization. *WHOQOL: Measuring* Quality of Life: The structure of the WHOQOL-100. [online] Available from https://web.archive.org/web/20200814200819/https://www.who.int/healthinfo/survey/whoqol-qualityoflife/en/index4.html [Last accessed October, 2024].
10. Sweeney S, Berry C, Kazounis E, et al. Cost-effectiveness of short, oral treatment regimens for rifampicin resistant tuberculosis. PLoS Glob Public Health. 2022;2(12):e0001337.
11. Shedrawy J, Deogan C, Öhd JN, et al. Cost-effectiveness of the latent tuberculosis screening program for migrants in Stockholm Region. Eur J Health Econ. 2021;22:445-54.
12. Canonica GW, Colombo GL, Rogliani P, et al. Omalizumab for Severe Allergic Asthma Treatment in Italy: A Cost-Effectiveness Analysis from PROXIMA Study. Risk Manag Healthc Policy. 2020;13:43-53.
13. Martin A, Shah D, Ndirangu K, et al. Is single-inhaler triple therapy for COPD cost-effective in the UK? The IMPACT trial. ERJ Open Res. 2022;8(1):00333-2021.
14. Kaier K, Heister T, Wolff J, et al. Mechanical ventilation and the daily cost of ICU care. BMC Health Serv Res. 2020;20:267.
15. Koul PA, Nowshehri AA, Khan UH, et al. Cost of Severe Chronic Obstructive Pulmonary Disease Exacerbations in a High Burden Region in North India. Ann Glob Health. 2019;85(1):13.
16. Dempsey TM, Thao V, Moriarty JP, et al. Cost-effectiveness of the anti-fibrotics for the treatment of idiopathic pulmonary fibrosis in the United States. BMC Pulm Med. 2022;22:18.
17. 17. Glass DS, Grossfeld D, Renna HA, et al. Idiopathic pulmonary fibrosis: Current and future treatment. Clin Respir J. 2022;16: 84-96.
18. Jo Y, Chhatwal J, Basu A. Cost-effectiveness of remdesivir for COVID-19 treatment: what are we missing? Value Health. 2022; 25(5):697-8.
19. Jamieson L, Edoka I, Long L, et al. Cost-effectiveness of Remdesivir and Dexamethasone for COVID-19 Treatment in South Africa. Open Forum Infect Dis. 2021;8(3):ofab040.
20. Shafiq M, Lee H, Yarmus L, et al. Recent Advances in Interventional Pulmonology. Ann Am Thorac Soc. 201916(7):786-96.
21. Wahidi MM, Herth FJF, Chen A, et al. State of the Art: Interventional Pulmonology. Chest. 2020; 157:724-36.

SECTION 20

Appendices

Note: All algorithm figures have been reproduced (with kind permission) from various issues of Chest (References cited with figures).
Explanatory comments for all algorithms by: Anup Singh, Suhail Raoof

SECTION OUTLINE

Appendix A: Algorithmic Approach to Respiratory Diseases

Appendix A.1: Bronchiolar Disorders Algorithm

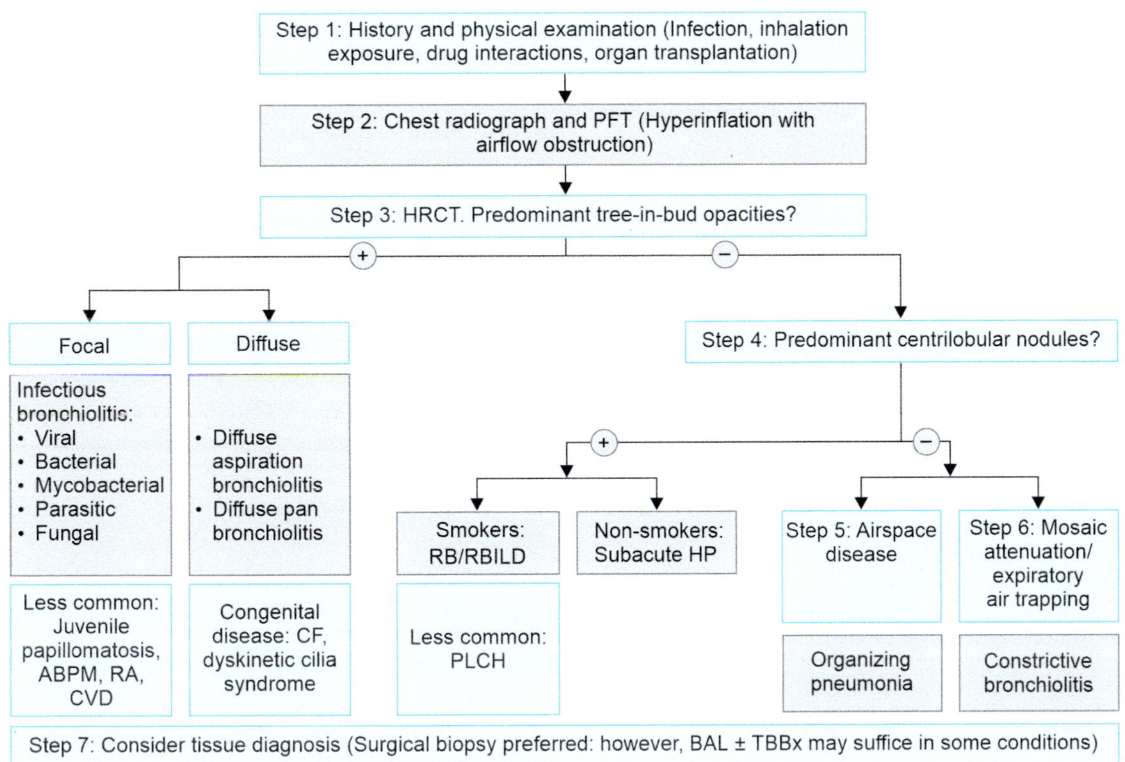

FLOWCHART 1: Algorithmic approach to bronchiolar disease.

Source: Flowchart reproduced with kind permission from Devakonda A, Raoof S, Sung A, et al. Bronchiolar disorders: a clinical-radiological diagnostic algorithm. Chest. 2010;137(4):938-51.

(ABPM: allergic bronchopulmonary mycosis; BAL: bronchoalveolar lavage; CF: cystic fibrosis; CVD: cardiovascular disease; HP: hypersensitivity pneumonitis; ILD: interstitial lung disease; PFT: pulmonary function test; PLCH: pulmonary Langerhans cell histiocytosis; RA: rheumatoid arthritis; RB: respiratory bronchiolitis; TBBx: transbronchial biopsy)

Explanatory Comments

Anup Singh, Suhail Raoof

Bronchioles are small airways with an internal diameter of 2 mm or less. The process of gas exchange takes place in the respiratory bronchioles which are 0.5 mm or less in diameter.

Bronchiolar disease should be suspected in an individual whose symptoms are out of proportion to their physical findings, pulmonary function test (PFT) abnormalities, and chest X-ray (CXR) findings. Patients will complain of dyspnea on exertion, demonstrate significant reduction in diffusing capacity for carbon monoxide (DLCO), and 6-minute walk distance. This is because the disease predominantly affects the very small airways that constitute the silent zones of the lungs where gas exchange takes place.

For the diagnosis of bronchiolar disorders, the following steps are recommended:

Step 1: Pertinent history is important—onset of symptoms (acute: infections; subacute: organizing pneumonia; chronic: atypical mycobacterial disease)

Pertinent history of respiratory infections, inhalational exposure, drug use, collagen vascular disease, and organ transplant

Physical examination (evidence of hyperinflation, fine crackles, expiratory wheezing)

Step 2: CXR which may show some hyperinflation and nonspecific nodules and PFT. PFT findings may vary but may demonstrate a mild predominantly obstructive or restrictive picture. The DLCO may be reduced out of proportion to the degree of obstruction or restriction. Of note, the 6-minute walk distance may be significantly reduced, and the patient may show significant desaturation with exercise.

Step 3: It involves ordering a high-resolution CT chest and observing for the following patterns:

- Is there evidence of tree-in-bud opacities? If so, the etiology may be further categorized as focal (more likely to be infectious from tuberculosis, nontubercular mycobacteria, aspergillus/fungal, parasitic) or diffuse (aspiration or panbronchiolitis).

Step 4: It is considered if the pattern on high-resolution CT (HRCT) scan is that of ground-glass centrilobular nodules. In the case of smokers, the diagnosis is likely to be respiratory bronchiolitis (RB)-interstitial lung disease (ILD). In a nonsmoker, the diagnosis is likely to be nonfibrotic hypersensitivity pneumonitis. Usually, the nodules are more profuse in hypersensitivity pneumonitis.

Step 5: This is to be considered when the HRCT picture indicates air space disease or consolidation. This may be suggestive of organizing pneumonia in the correct clinical settings.

Step 6: This is considered when there is evidence of mosaic attenuation on HRCT scan, suggestive of air trapping. This may be accentuation on expiratory images. Depending on the clinical history, constrictive or obliterative bronchiolitis may be considered.

Step 7: Finally, if the HRCT pattern does not demonstrate any of the four above-mentioned patterns and the patient is significantly symptomatic, a consideration to obtain tissue diagnosis (surgical biopsy or transbronchial lung biopsy) or bronchoalveolar lavage (BAL) may be considered. The procedure chosen for diagnosis would be predicated upon the clinical suspicions for a particular entity. For example, if the working diagnosis is hypersensitivity pneumonitis, a BAL and bronchoscopic biopsy may be considered.

Appendix A.2: Cavitary Lung Disease Algorithm

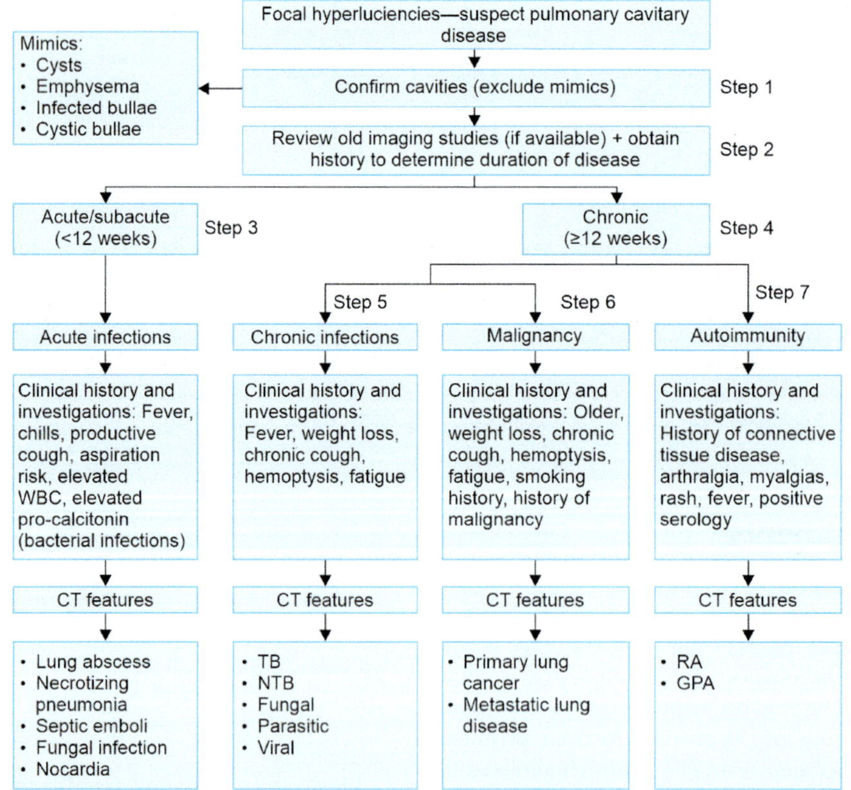

FLOWCHART 2: Algorithmic approach to cavitary lung disease.

(GPA: granulomatosis with polyangiitis; NTM: nontuberculous mycobacteria; RA: rheumatoid arthritis; TB: tuberculosis)

Source: Flowchart reproduced with kind permission of Gafoor K, Patel S, Girvin F, et al. Cavitary Lung Diseases: A Clinical-Radiologic Algorithmic Approach. Chest. 2018;153(6):1443-65.

Cavity is defined as a thick-walled (>4 mm), gas-containing lucent area located within lung consolidation, mass, or a nodule.

For the diagnosis of cystic lung disease, the following steps are recommended:

Step 1: This is to ensure that it is a true cavity. Cystic disease, centrilobular emphysema, infected bullae, and cystic bronchiectasis are common mimickers of a true cavity.

Step 2: Clinical history and chest X-ray review for estimation of duration of the disease. The plan is to follow steps 3 and 4 if the duration of the cavity is <12 weeks (acute) and >12 weeks (chronic), respectively.

Step 3: The infections are the most common cause of acute cavities. Differentials include bacterial infections (lung abscesses, necrotizing pneumonia, septic emboli, pulmonary nocardiosis), fungal infections (coccidioidomycosis, aspergillosis, mucormycosis), and *Mycobacterium tuberculosis which in a few instances may develop an acute cavity*.

Step 4: It includes the identification of chronic cavity and then follow step 5 (chronic infection), step 6 (malignancy), and step 7 (autoimmune disorders).

Step 5: The differentials for chronic cavities due to chronic infection includes *Mycobacterium* (tubercular and non-tubercular mycobacteria), fungal (chronic, necrotizing aspergillosis, histoplasmosis, blastomycosis), parasitic (paragonimiasis, echinococcosis), and viral (human papillomavirus).

Step 6: The differentials for chronic cavities due to malignancy include pulmonary malignancies (squamous cell lung cancer and pulmonary lymphoma) and metastasis from extrapulmonary sources (head and neck, skin or cervical squamous cell carcinoma, sarcoma, or gastrointestinal malignancies).

Step 7: The differentials for chronic cavities due to autoimmune disorders include rheumatoid arthritis and granulomatosis with polyangiitis.

Appendix A.3: Cystic Lung Disease

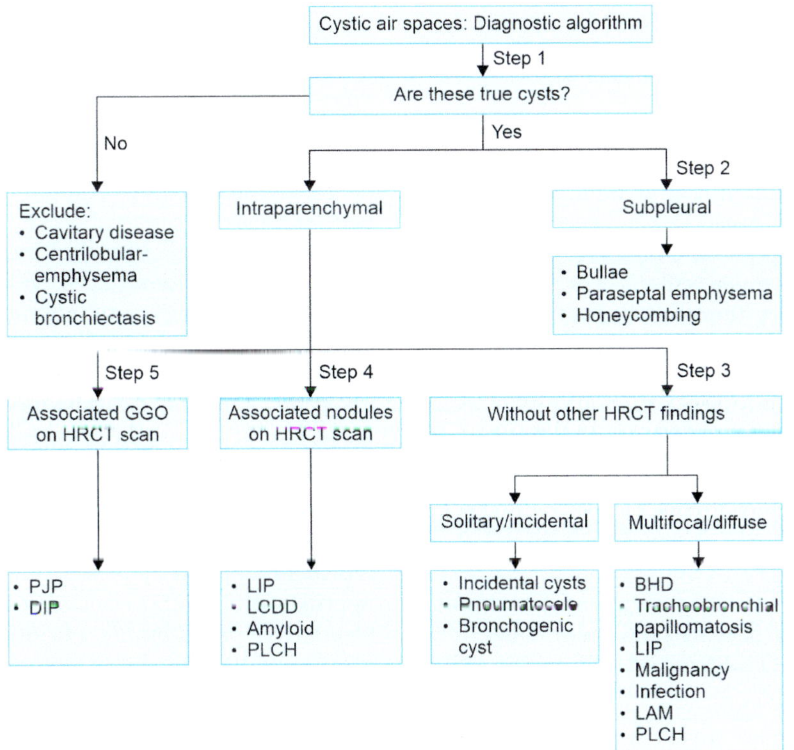

FLOWCHART 3: Detailed algorithmic approach to cystic lung disease.

(BHD: Birt–Hogg–Dubé syndrome; DIP: desquamative interstitial pneumonia; GGO: ground-glass opacity; HRCT: high-resolution CT; LAM: lymphangioleiomyomatosis; LCDD: light-chain deposition disease; LIP: lymphoid interstitial pneumonia; PLCH: pulmonary Langerhans cell histiocytosis; PJP: *Pneumocystis jirovecii* pneumonia)

Source: **Flowchart** reproduced with kind permission from Raoof S, Bondalapati P, Vydyula R, et al. Cystic Lung Diseases: Algorithmic Approach. Chest. 2016;150(4):945-65.

Cysts are round parenchymal lucencies or low attenuation areas on HRCT scans with the well-defined wall that is <2 mm in thickness and with normal adjacent lung parenchyma. They are usually air-filled but may rarely contain fluid or solid material. Cysts may be present in normal individuals, but they may be associated with many different diseases. In contrast to cavities (which have a thicker wall and demonstrate a reaction in the adjacent lung parenchyma and denote a necrotizing infectious or inflammatory or neoplastic process), cysts may be seen as remnants of a prior infection, congenital diseases, or miscellaneous conditions.

To identify the etiology of cystic lung disease, the following steps are recommended:

Step 1: Ensure that we are dealing with a true cyst. Cavities, centrilobular emphysema, and cystic bronchiectasis are common mimickers of cysts.

- Cavity: Thick-walled (>4 mm), gas-containing lucent area located within lung consolidation, mass, or a nodule.
- Centrilobular emphysema: Centrilobular lucent area, around 1 cm in size, without a distinct wall, located predominantly in the upper lobe with a dot (branch of the pulmonary artery in the secondary lobule) in the center.
- Cystic bronchiectasis: Bronchial dilatation without tapering, adjacent to a bronchial artery (signet ring sign), associated with the presence of bronchi within 1 cm of pleural surface.

Step 2: After ensuring that we are dealing with a true cyst, the next step is to determine if cysts are subpleural in location. Bullae, paraseptal emphysema, and honeycombing are differentials for subpleural cysts.

- *Bullae*: Round focal area with a diameter > 1 cm with a thin or almost imperceptible wall.
- *Paraseptal emphysema*: Thin-walled, multiple, separate hyperlucent area bordered by pleural surface or interlobular septa. It is present mainly in the upper lobes in emphysema and rarely in uncommon conditions like Ehlers–Danlos or Marfan syndrome. They vary in size from a few millimeters to several centimeters
- *Honeycombing*: Subpleural, uniform-sized (3–10 mm), thick-walled (1–3 mm), multiple, adjoining cysts. Present in advance fibrotic lung disease.

Step 3: As the next step, cysts are categorized into simple if there is no accompanying parenchymal abnormality. These are further described as (1) solitary and (2) focal (multifocal or diffuse).

- *Solitary*: Single cysts, randomly distributed. Differential includes incidental cysts (seen usually in patients > 55 years of age with or without a smoking history), pneumatocele(s) (usually remnants of acute pneumonia, trauma, or aspiration of hydrocarbon fluids), and bronchogenic cyst(s) (usually in the lower lobes commonly filled with fluid).
- *Multifocal (>1 cyst per lobe) and diffuse (cyst in > 1 lobe)*: Differential includes Birt–Hogg–Dube syndrome (skin lesions, spontaneous pneumothoraces, renal cancer), lymphoid interstitial pneumonia (LIP) (may also be associated with centrilobular nodules and ground-glass opacities, sometimes associated with autoimmune diseases, immune deficiency states like HIV and common variable immunodeficiency, infections, drugs and allogenic hematopoietic stem cell transplants), tracheobronchial papillomatosis (history of tracheostomies and visible nodularity in tracheal and bronchial walls), malignancy, infection, lymphangioleiomyomatosis [diffuse involvement, chylous effusions, spontaneous pneumothoraces with positive HMB-45 and vascular endothelial growth factor-D (VEGF-D) elevation], and pulmonary Langerhans cell histiocytosis (PLCH) (bizarre-shaped cysts in upper and middle lobes sparing costophrenic angles, sometimes associated with nodules).

Step 4: This is to identify complex cysts, i.e., those associated with parenchymal abnormalities. In this step, cysts are associated with lung nodules. The differential diagnosis includes LIP (middle-aged women, associated with collagen vascular disease, HIV, combined variable immunodeficiency disease, Castleman syndrome), PLCH (smoker, age commonly 20–40 years), light-chain deposition disease (middle age, multiple myeloma and other plasma cell dyscrasia), and amyloidosis [Sjögren syndrome, lymphoproliferative diseases including MALTOMA (mucosa-associated lymphoid tissue lymphoma)]

Step 5: This is also the identification of complex cysts, i.e., those associated with parenchymal abnormalities in the form of ground-glass opacities. The differential diagnosis includes *Pneumocystis jirovecii* pneumonia (multiple, upper lobe, thick-walled cysts with diffuse central ground-glass opacities, commonly associated with HIV) and desquamative interstitial pneumonitis (40–60 years of age, smokers, predominantly men, lower zone ground-glass opacities with very thin wall discrete cysts).

Appendix A.4: Lung Hyperlucency: Algorithmic Approach for Interpretation

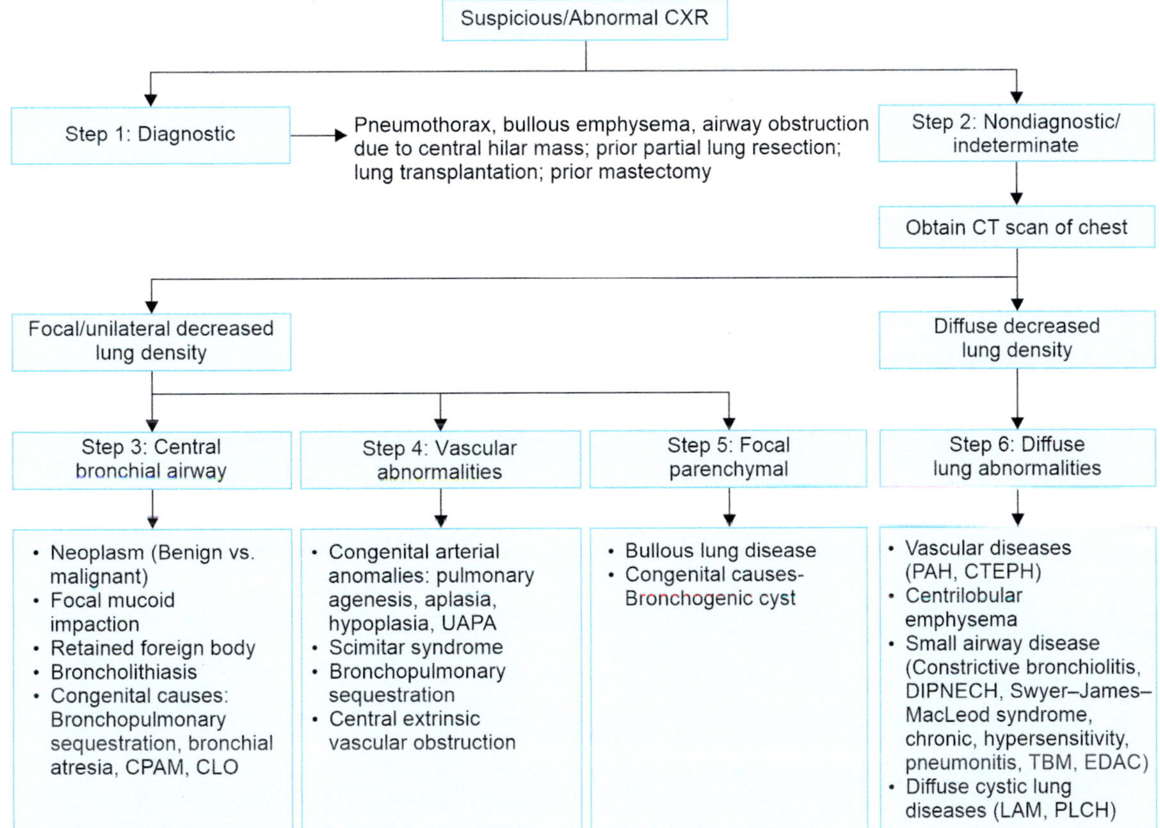

FLOWCHART 4: Lung hyperlucency: Algorithmic approach for interpretation.

(CLO: congenital lobar overinflation; CPAM: congenital pulmonary airway malformation; CTEPH: chronic thromboembolic pulmonary hypertension; CXR: chest radiograph; DIPNECH: diffuse idiopathic pulmonary neuroendocrine cell hyperplasia; EDAC: excessive dynamic collapse of airways; LAM: lymphangioleiomyomatosis; PAH: pulmonary arterial hypertension; PLCH: pulmonary Langerhans cell histiocytosis; TBM: tracheobronchomalacia; UAPA: unilateral absence of the pulmonary artery)

Source: Flowchart reproduced with kind permission from Cherian SV, Girvin F, Naidich DP, et al. Hyperlucent lung. A clinical radiologic algorithmic approach to diagnosis. Chest. 2020;157:119-41. (Figure 1)

The areas of abnormal decreased lung density on chest radiograph (CXR) and CT chest are frequently termed hyperlucent. The algorithmic approach is helpful in identifying the multiple etiologies for hyperlucent areas on the CXR/CT chest.

Step 1: Routine diagnostic radiographic interpretation: Hyperlucent areas are usually first identified on plain CXR. A rotated image or axillary folds are common causes of false hyperlucent areas on CXR. Pneumothorax, bullous emphysema, airway obstruction due to central airway mass, partial lung resection, lung transplant, and prior mastectomy are common causes of hyperlucent lung, which can be diagnosed on CXR without requiring a CT chest.

Step 2: Indeterminate and/or nondiagnostic radiographic findings: A noncontrast high-resolution CT chest should be considered when the diagnosis is not evident on CXR. Intravenous contrast or dynamic CT chest may be considered in select cases. This step includes categorizing the hyperlucent lung on the CT chest as focal/unilateral or diffuse.

Step 3: The next series of steps is pertinent to unilateral or focal lung hyperlucent lesions. It is important to evaluate for possible central airway and/or bronchial obstruction. The etiologies include neoplastic (endobronchial or central lung mass), non-neoplastic (mucus plug, retained aspirated foreign body or a broncholith), and congenital (bronchial atresia, bronchopulmonary sequestration, congenital lobar overinflation, congenital pulmonary airway malformation).

Step 4: Evaluate for possible vascular etiologies: The next step is identifying the vascular etiologies that may lead to unilateral or focal hyperlucent lung on the CT chest. Pulmonary arterial anomalies (pulmonary agenesis, atresia, hypoplasia), bronchopulmonary sequestration, Scimitar syndrome, chronic pulmonary thromboembolism, and acute pulmonary embolism are common differential diagnoses for vascular etiologies.

Step 5: Evaluate for focal parenchymal etiologies: The next step is identifying the lung parenchymal abnormalities leading to focal or unilateral hyperlucent lung. Bullous lung disease [chronic obstructive pulmonary disease (COPD), Marfan syndrome, and Ehler-Danlos syndrome], compensatory emphysema (post lobectomy), and emphysema due to alpha-1 antitrypsin deficiency are common parenchymal etiologies for hyperlucent lungs.

Step 6: In the event of diffuse hyperlucent lung disease, the next step involves identifying various etiologies for diffuse, bilateral hyperlucent lung on CT chest. The differential diagnosis includes centrilobular emphysema, vascular disease (chronic thromboembolism and pulmonary hypertension), small airway disease (constrictive bronchiolitis, diffuse idiopathic pulmonary neuroendocrine cell hyperplasia, Swyer-James-MacLeod syndrome, chronic hypersensitivity pneumonitis, tracheobronchomalacia, and excessive dynamic airway collapse), and diffuse cystic lung disease (lymphangioleiomyomatosis and pulmonary Langerhans cell histiocytosis).

Appendix A.5: Pictorial Essay: Multinodular Disease

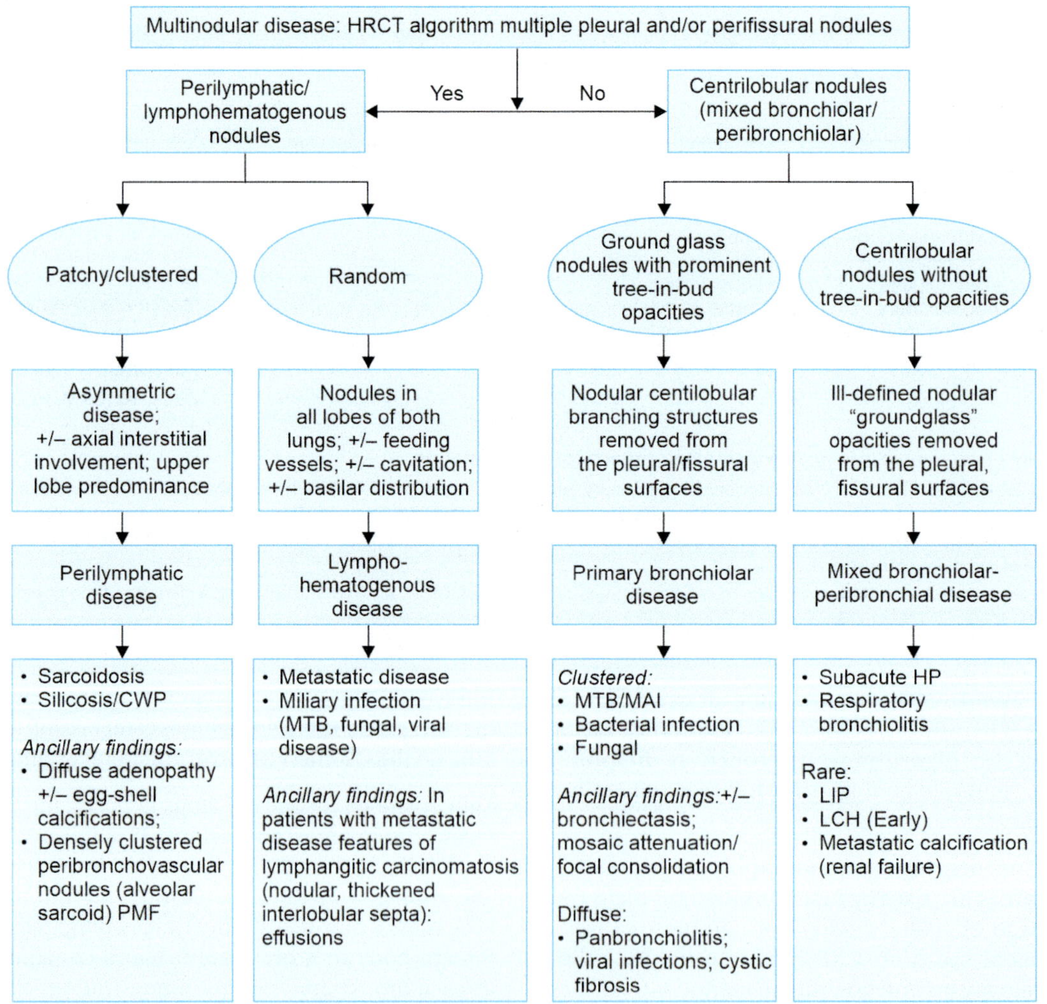

FLOWCHART 5: High-resolution CT (HRCT) diagnostic algorithm.

Note: The nomenclature for subacute HP has been changed to nonfibrotic HP.

(CWP: coal workers pneumoconiosis; LCH: Langerhans cell histiocytosis; LIP: lymphoid interstitial pneumonia; MAI: *Mycobacterium avium* intracellulare; MTB: *Mycobacterium tuberculosis*; PMF: progressive massive fibrosis)

Source: Flowchart reproduced with kind permission from Raoof S, Amchentsev A, Vlahos I et al. Pictorial essay: multinodular disease: a high-resolution CT scan diagnostic algorithm. Chest. 2006;129:805-15. (Table 1)

Multinodular disease is characterized by multiple nodules (<1 cm in average diameter) in all lobes of the lungs which are too numerous to count on the HRCT chest. An important point that needs to be borne in mind is that in contrast to the morphology of the nodules, the single most important determination of the etiology of the nodules is its proximity to the secondary pulmonary lobule structures.

Step 1: The identification of nodules adjacent to pleural or perifissural structures indicates that these nodules are either coming to the secondary pulmonary lobule via lymphatic channels or blood vessels. The origin of these nodules can be ascribed to perilymphatic or lympho-hematogenous channels.

Step 2: This is to further differentiate the patchy/clustered nodules into either lymphatic or hematogenous in origin. The common etiology for a patchy/clustered nodular pattern is sarcoidosis. These nodules are poorly defined, measure only a few millimeters in size, and involve upper to mid-lung fields. The other differential diagnoses for clustered nodules are silicosis and coal worker's disease.

Step 3: The random distribution of nodules throughout the lung including pleural/perifissural distribution and in the center of the secondary pulmonary lobule (adjacent to alveolar units where blood vessels are present in profusion) is due to hematogenous disease. The most common differential diagnosis for random nodules on the CT chest is hematogenous metastasis. These nodules are smooth with well-defined margins, size > 1 cm, with a feeding vessel, and are predominantly present in basal lung fields. The random nodules with a miliary pattern are likely secondary to infectious etiology (miliary tuberculosis fungal or bacterial infections) or malignancy (metastasis from thyroid cancer, renal cancer, and melanoma). The cavitating random nodules could be secondary to septic emboli, invasive fungal infection, and pulmonary vasculitides.

Step 4: This is to identify nodules that have a centrilobular distribution, which is defined by nodules involving centrilobular bronchioles and/or accompanying pulmonary arteries. These nodules have no or occasional pleural/perifissural distribution and stop 5–10 mm short of the pleural surface. These are nodules that are reaching the secondary pulmonary lobule via the small airways and alveolar sacs and alveolar ducts.

Step 5: The next step is to classify these nodules as tree-in-bud or nodules without a branching/tree-in-bud configuration (ground-glass nodules). The tree-in-bud nodules are defined as centrilobular nodules with a micronodular branching pattern that ends several millimeters away from the pleural surface. The tree-in-bud pattern is a result of secretions getting lodged in centrilobular bronchioles. The most common etiology for the tree-in-bud pattern is infective bronchiolitis (*Mycobacterium tuberculosis*, *Mycobacterium avium* complex, bacterial, viral or fungal disease). Other, less common differentials for tree-in-bud opacities include follicular bronchiolitis, diffuse panbronchiolitis, and cystic fibrosis.

Step 6: The last step of the algorithm is to identify the nodules without tree-in-bud opacities. These nodules are localized to the centrilobular portion of the secondary lobule. The disease in this group has peribronchial distribution, resulting in diffuse, poorly defined ground-glass opacities. The differential diagnosis for this group includes subacute hypersensitivity pneumonitis, respiratory bronchiolitis, lymphocytic interstitial pneumonitis, Langerhans cell histiocytosis, respiratory bronchiolitis, and interstitial lung disease.

Appendix A.6: Organizing Pneumonia: Algorithmic Approach

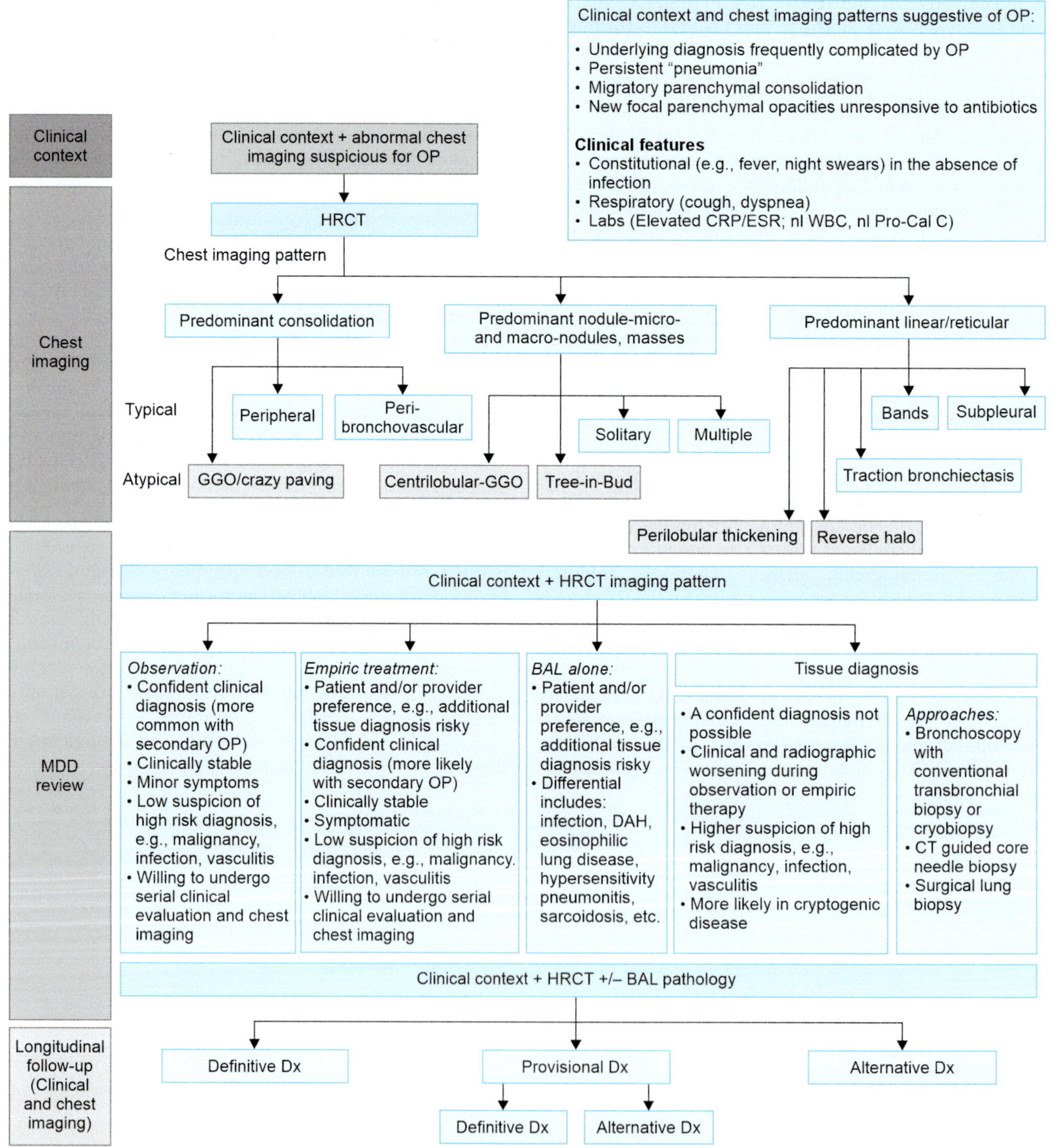

FLOWCHART 6: Organizing pneumonia: Algorithmic approach.

(BAL: bronchoalveolar lavage; CRP: C-reactive protein; DAH: diffuse alveolar hemorrhage; Dx: diagnosis; ESR: erythrocyte sedimentation rate; GGO: ground-glass opacification; HRCT: high-resolution CT; MDD: multidisciplinary discussion; nl Pro-Cal: normal procalcitonin; nl WBC: normal WBC; OP: organizing pneumonia)

Source: Flowchart reproduced with kind permission from Cherian SV, Patel D, Machnicki S, et al. Algorithmic approach to the Diagnosis of Organizing Pneumonia: A Correlation of Clinical, Radiologic, and Pathologic Features. Chest. 2022;162:156-78.

Organizing pneumonia (OP) has multiple etiologies and is histologically defined as the patchy filling of alveoli and bronchioles by loose connective tissue plugs. The management of organizing pneumonia includes a stepwise approach.

Step 1: The first step is to suspect OP based on clinical data. OP does not have a diagnostic clinical symptom or examination findings. The symptoms are nonspecific and present commonly among nonsmokers. Clinicians should suspect OP in patients with nonresolving pneumonia or the occurrence of new lung opacities despite being on antibiotics. The diagnosis is usually delayed by 6–8 weeks because OP is a diagnosis of exclusion.

Step 2: The next step is identifying the radiological pattern associated with OP. There are multiple radiological patterns associated with OP. OP may have a predominant *consolidation pattern* (typically peripheral and/or peri-bronchovascular), *predominant lung nodules (solitary or multiple)*, or predominantly *reticular pattern* (subpleural, associated with traction bronchiectasis and bands).

Step 3: Once the HRCT pattern is identified, a decision to observe closely or treat OP empirically is based on clinical features and radiology patterns. Stable patients with minor symptoms and low suspicion of alternative diagnosis (malignancy, infection, or vasculitis) may be observed with symptom monitoring and serial chest imaging. The symptomatic patient with low suspicion of alternative diagnosis can be treated empirically based on clinical and radiology patterns, especially if the patient is at high risk for procedure-related complications or is averse to undergo invasive testing.

Step 4: This step includes scenarios where clinical features and radiology patterns are not sufficient for diagnosis of OP or suspicion of alternative diagnosis is high. Bronchoscopy with bronchoalveolar lavage may be considered if diffuse alveolar hemorrhage, eosinophilic lung disease, hypersensitivity pneumonitis, or sarcoidosis is suspected. The tissue diagnosis (bronchoscopy with biopsy or CT-guided biopsy) should only be considered in patients suspected of malignancy, chronic infection, or vasculitis.

Step 5: The last step is to continue clinical and radiology follow-up of the patient after starting treatment with a corticosteroid or immunosuppressive agent (cyclophosphamide, azathioprine, mycophenolate, or rituximab) or macrolide.

Appendix B: From our Archives of 1970s–1980s

It is always good to learn from the past. We reproduce a few of the selected images to see how fast the practice of pulmonary medicine has changed in this period.

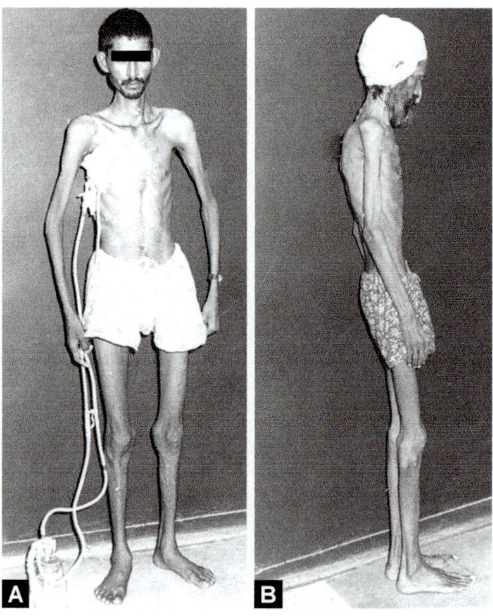

FIGS. 1A AND B: Extreme wasting from tuberculosis (TB) (justifying the older terminology of "consumption") was common to be seen in the TB ward. This degree of severity has become rare with the advent of effective chemotherapy and TB control programs.

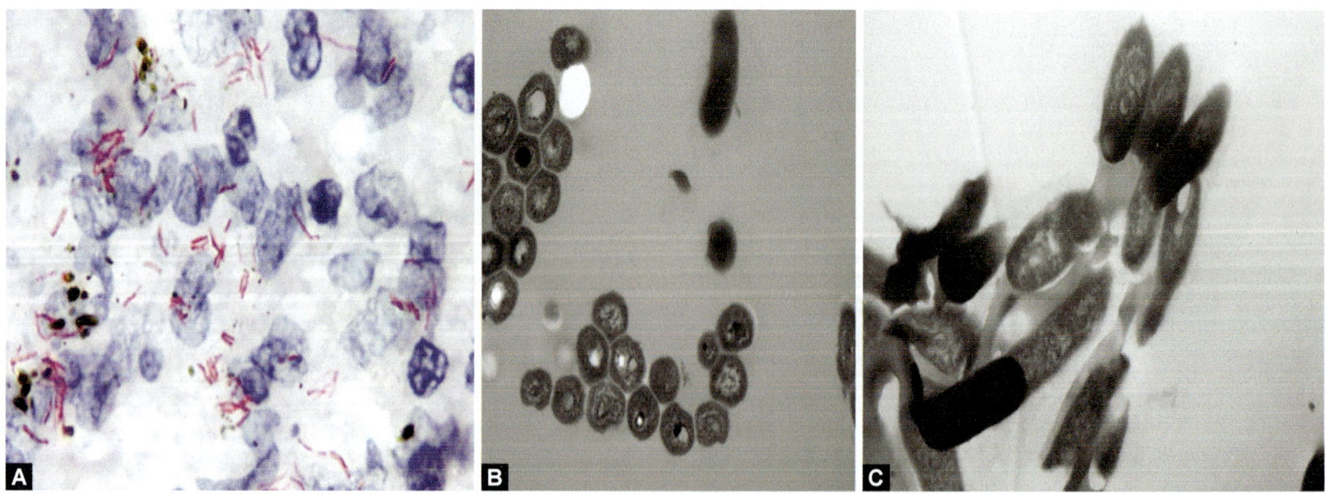

FIGS. 2A TO C: Mycobacteria in the granuloma, engulfed by macrophages and its ultramicroscopic structure.

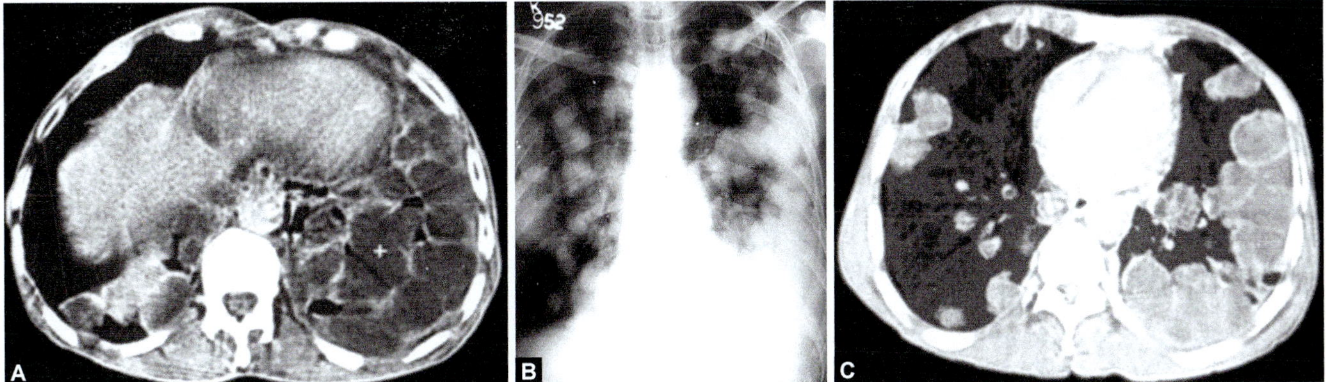

FIGS. 3A TO C: Multiple hydatid cysts in the lung.

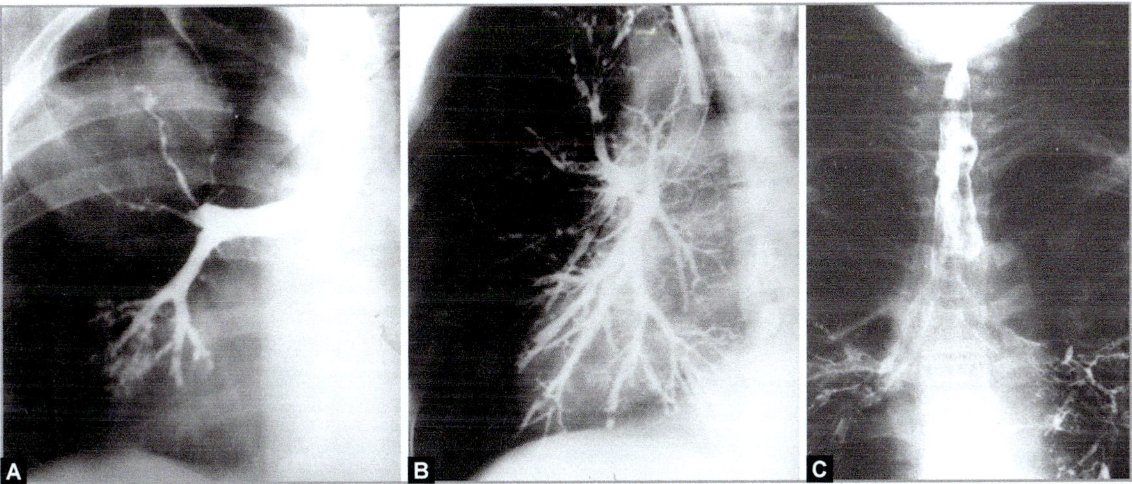

FIGS. 4A TO C: Bronchography with instillation of a radio-opaque marker with the help of a catheter was a common procedure to delineate the bronchial tree and diagnose lesions such as bronchial masses, bronchiectasis, fistulae, and pouches. Endoscopic and scanning procedures have replaced the old, gold standard.

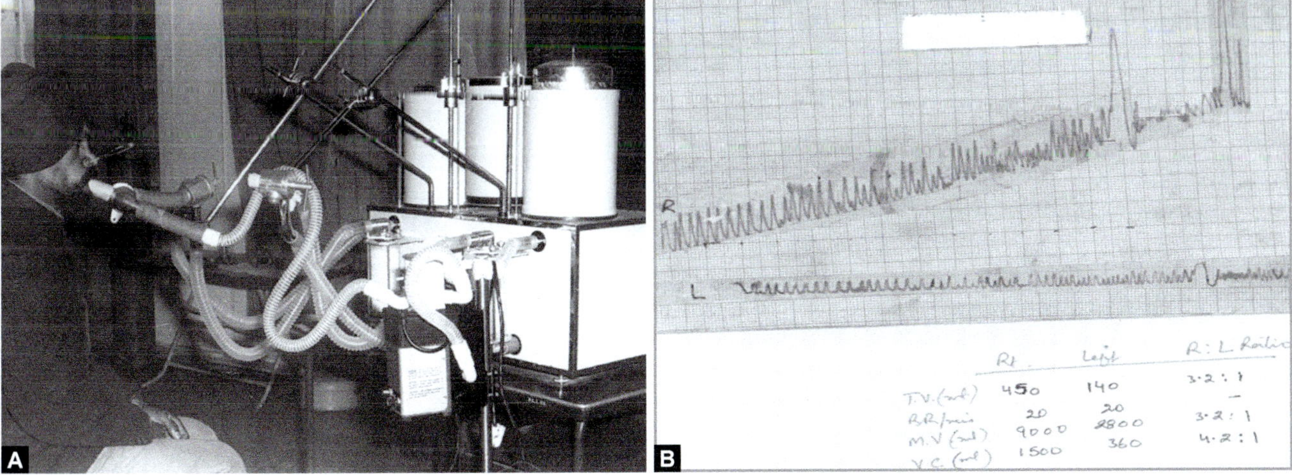

FIGS. 5A AND B: (A) Spirometry with the help of a double barrel, volume displacement spirometer (B) on a graph followed by manual calculations: Differential spirometry showing nonfunctional left lung.

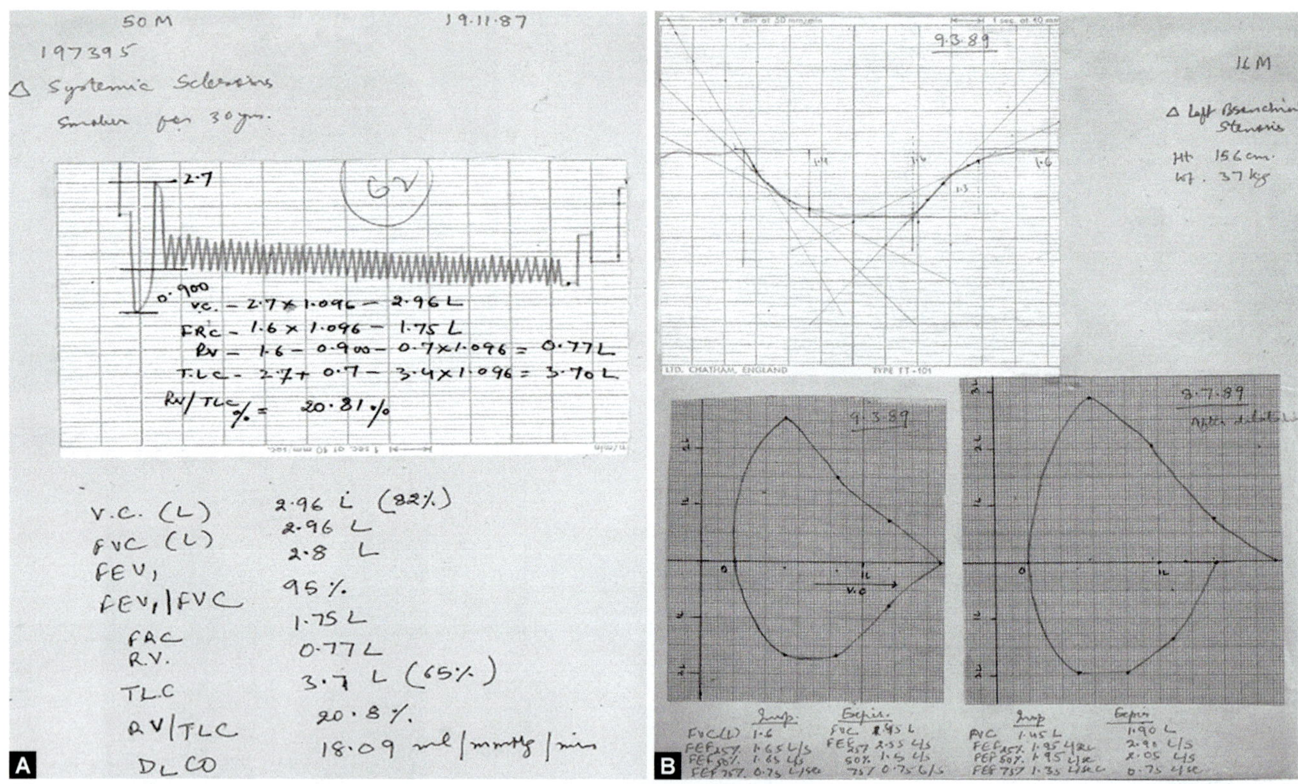

FIGS. 6A AND B: Spirometry in (A) systemic sclerosis and (B) left bronchial stenosis.

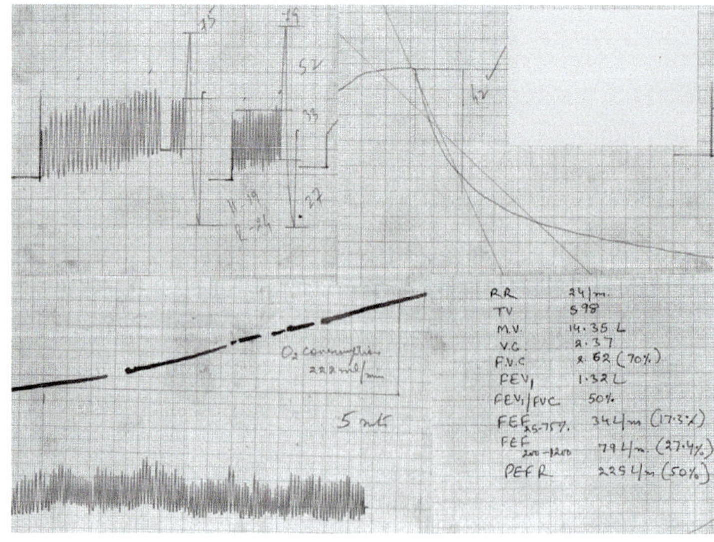

FIG. 7: Oxygen consumption with the help of a spirometer by measuring the amount of oxygen required to replace the consumed volume, after absorption of CO_2 from the exhaled air using the formula: O_2 consumption = VC × FiO_2 – FeO_2.

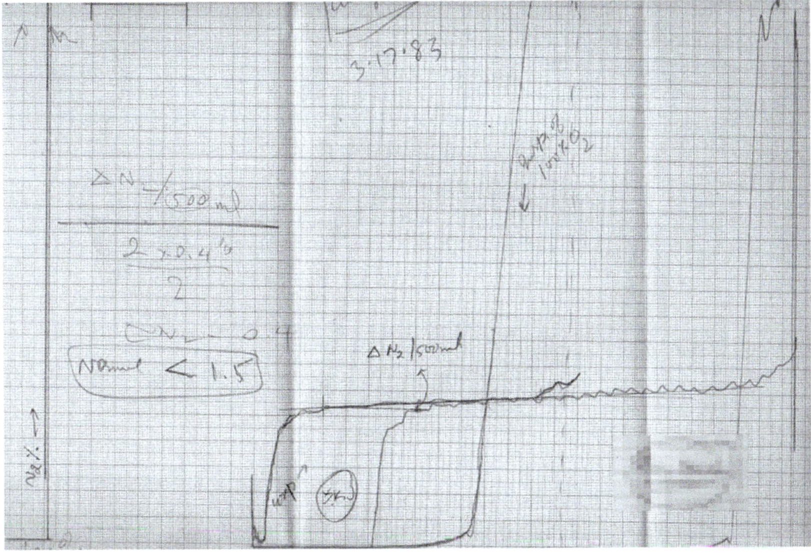

FIG. 8: Single breath nitrogen-washout test to measure closing volume and closing capacity as measures of small airway disease.

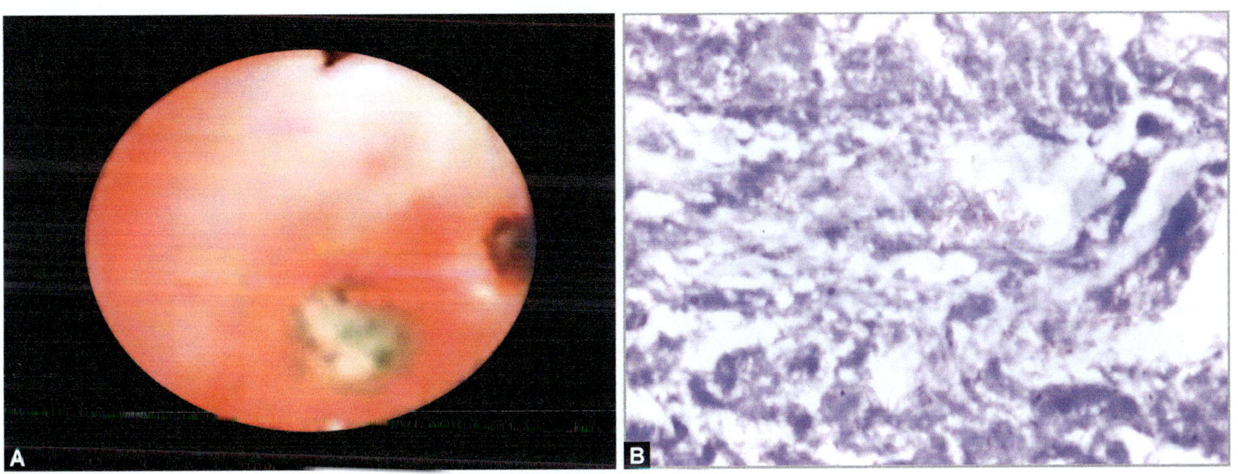

FIGS. 9A AND B: Bronchoscopic biopsy: Endobronchial tuberculosis.

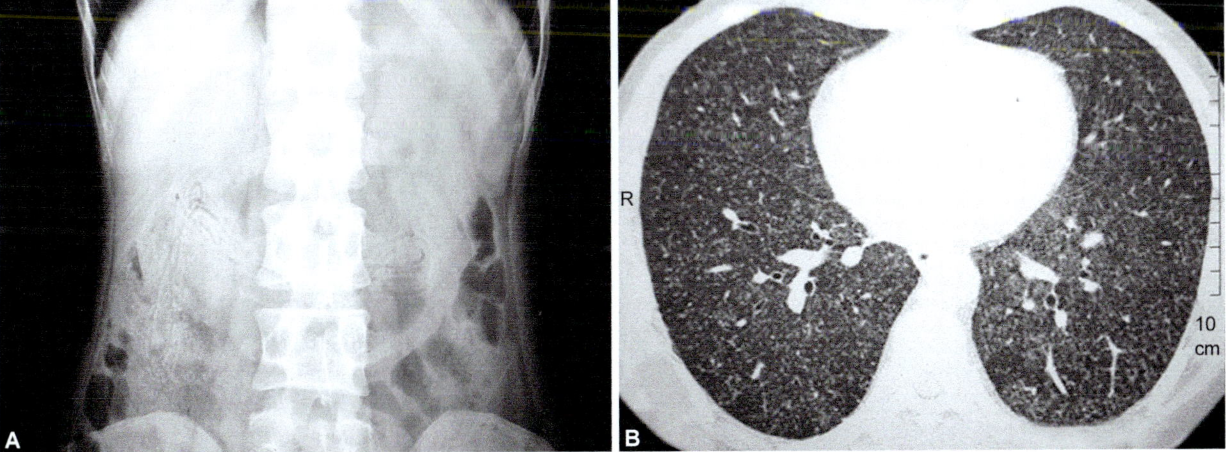

FIGS. 10A AND B: A case of Loeffler's syndrome caused by intestinal roundworms. (A) Abdominal X-ray shows the presence of intra-abdominal worms; (B) High-resolution CT of the chest demonstrates ground-glass opacities and centrilobular nodules secondary to eosinophilic pneumonia.

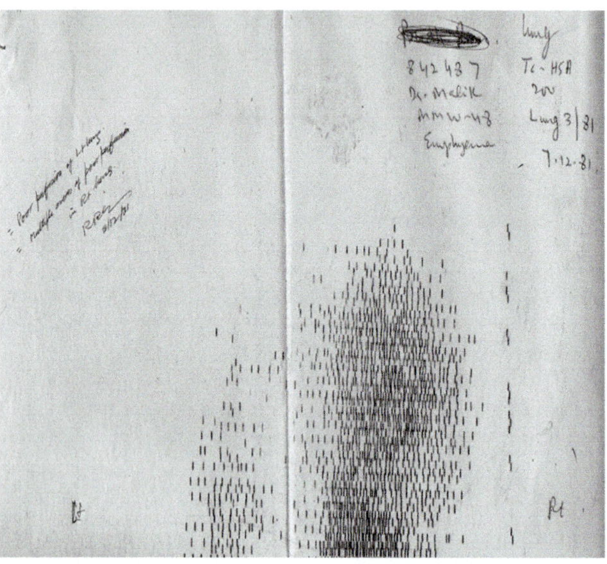

FIG. 11: Lung perfusion scan with TcHSA in a case of emphysema—poor perfusion of the whole of left lung and multiple areas of right lung indicating the presence of extensive bullae formation.

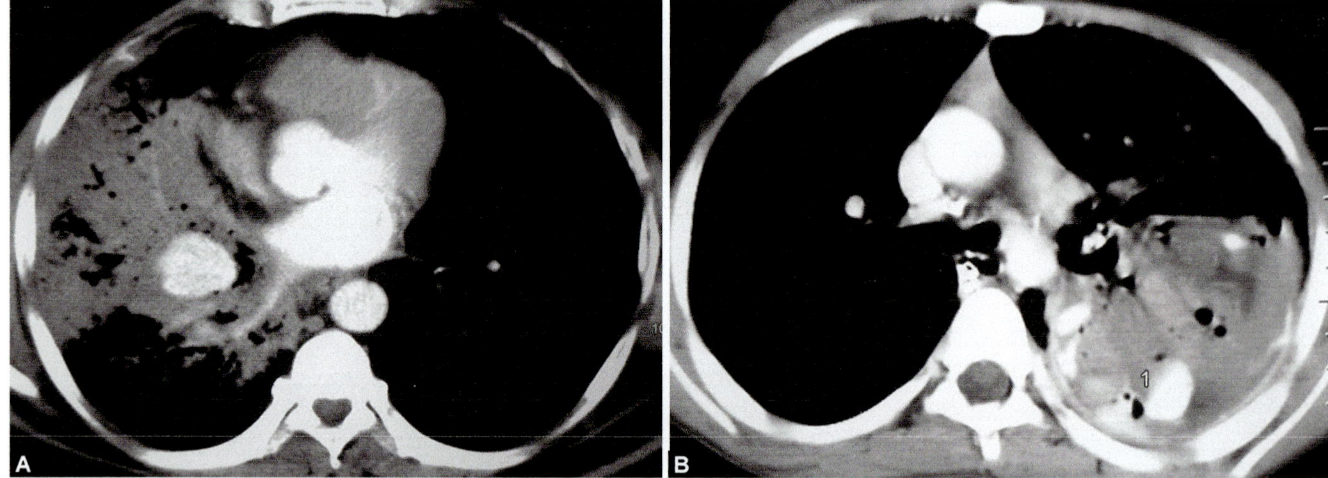

FIGS. 12A AND B: Contrast-enhanced CTs of two different patients with community-acquired necrotizing pneumonia demonstrating an uncommon but potentially life-threatening complication of infective pulmonary aneurysm. The CT films show the presence of contrast-enhanced densities within the areas of consolidation consistent with the presence of vascular aneurysm.

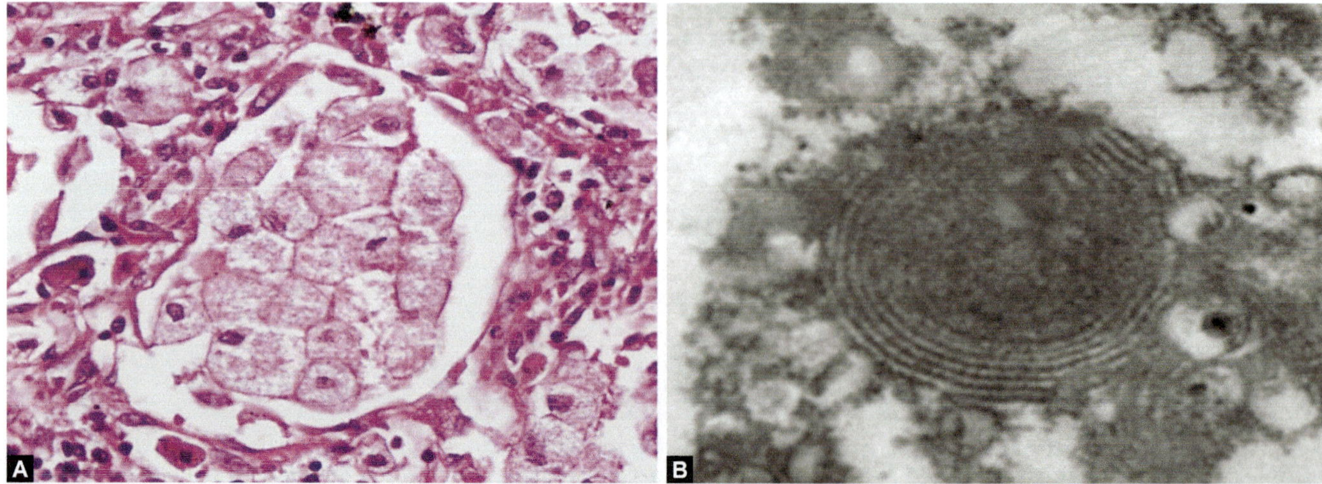

FIGS. 13A AND B: Foamy macrophage with intracytoplasmic granular material in a case of pulmonary alveolar proteinosis (hematoxylin and eosin, ×200). Electron microscopic image of the same patient showing whorled lamellated surfactant bodies (×6450).

Index

Page numbers followed by *b* refer to box, *f* refer to figure, *fc* refer to flowchart, and *t* refer to table.

A

B

C

D

E

F

H

M

N

O

P

Q

R

S

T

U

V